Postgraduate Dermatology

The photographs on the cover of the textbook depict images as under:

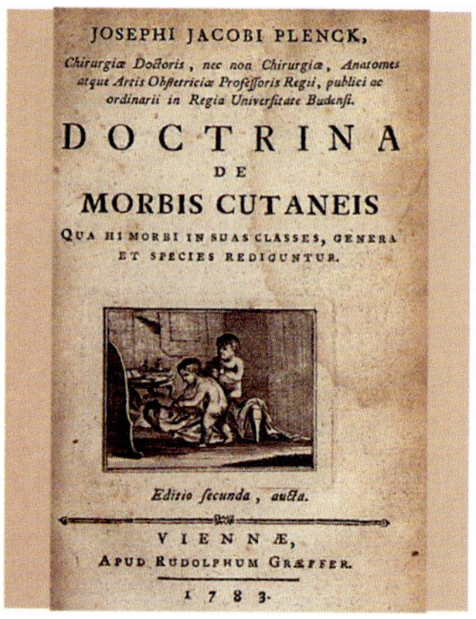

This image from the second edition of (1783) of *Doctrina De Morbis Cutaneis* of Joseph Jacob Plenck (1735–1807), a Viennese Military Surgeon and polymath. Plenck was the first to introduce a method of classifying skin diseases in 1776. This profoundly influenced Robert Willan (1757–1812), the Father of English Dermatology to introduce the modern classification. The first four orders namely Papulae, Squamae, Exanthemata and Bullae published as a book entitled *On Cutaneous Diseases* Vol. I in 1808.

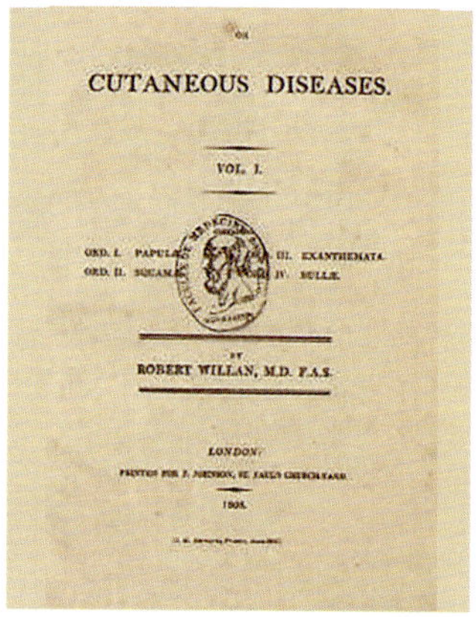

A water color from Willan's book depicting the various orders. Willan was also the first physician to give clear clinical description of psoriasis, another milestone in the history of psoriasis.

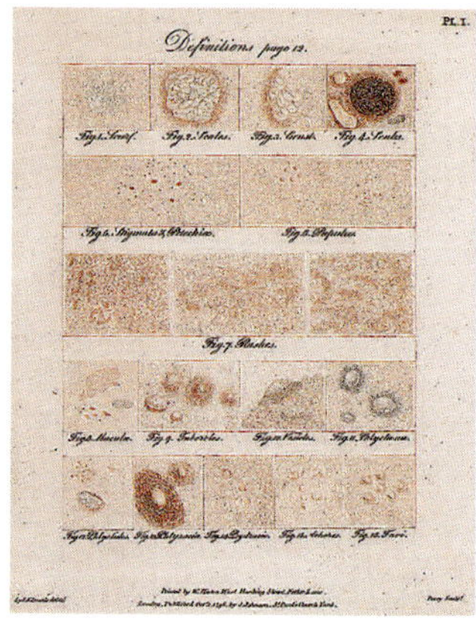

A collage of four landmark images which formed the most important milestones in the history of modern dermatology.

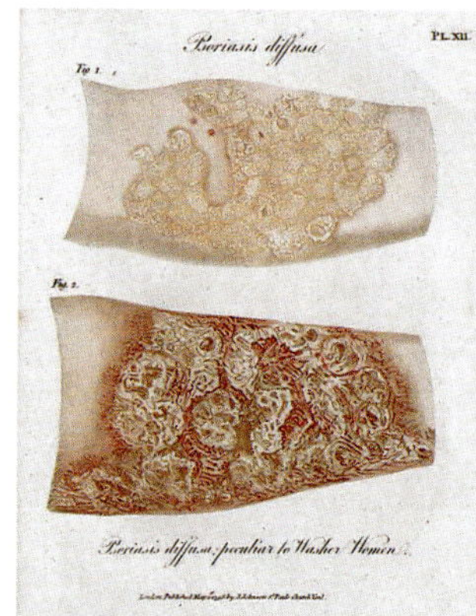

A water color entitled *Psoriasis diffusa*, taken from Willan's aforesaid treatise.

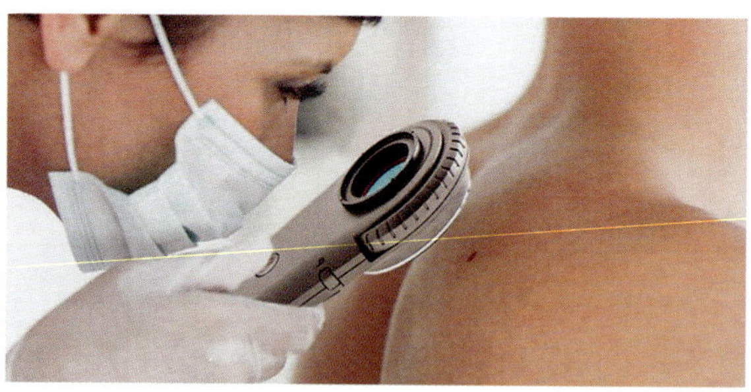

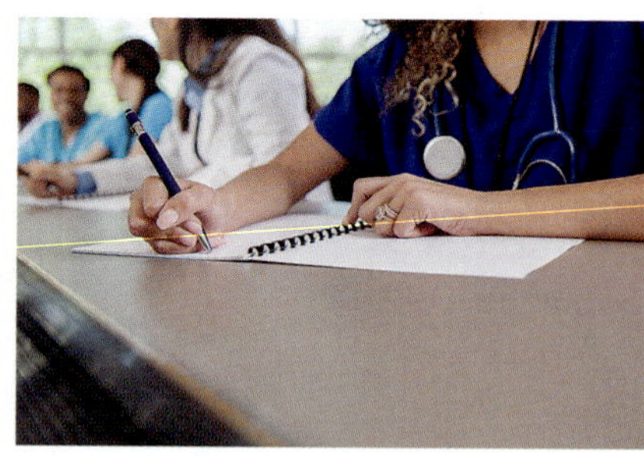

Postgraduate Dermatology

Volume 1

Editors

Koushik Lahiri
MBBS DVD (CAL) FIAD FFAADV FRCP (Glasgow) FRCP (Edin) FRCP (London)
Professor and Distinguished Academician (AHERF)
Senior Consultant Dermatologist
Apollo Multispecialty Hospitals Limited
Honorary Medical Director
Wizderm Speciality Skin and Hair Clinic
Kolkata, West Bengal, India
Vice President, International Society of Dermatology (2017–2021)
President, Association of Cutaneous Surgeons (I) (2013–2015)
Chairperson, ACSI Academy of Dermatosurgery (2017–2019)
Editor, Indian Journal of Dermatology (2012–2017)

Abhishek De
MD FAGE MRCP-SCE (Dermatology)
Associate Professor
Calcutta National Medical College
Kolkata, West Bengal, India
Associate Editor, Indian Journal of Dermatology
Associate Editor, Indian Journal of Skin Allergy
Honorary Secretary, Skin Allergy Research Society of India
Assistant Editor, Journal of Cutaneous and Aesthetic Surgery (JCAS)

Assistant Editors

Aarti Sarda
MD FAGE MRCP-SCE (Dermatology)
Consultant Dermatologist
Department of Dermatology
Wizderm Speciality Skin and Hair Clinic
Kolkata, West Bengal, India

Anupam Das MD
Assistant Professor
Department of Dermatology
KPC Medical College and Hospital
Kolkata, West Bengal, India

Abhijit Saha MD
Consultant Dermatologist
Institute of Child Health
Kolkata, West Bengal, India

Surajit Gorai
MD (Gold Medalist) DNB MNAMS (Dermatology)
Associate Professor (AHERF)
Consultant Dermatologist
Apollo Gleneagles Hospital
Kolkata, West Bengal, India

Barnali Chowdhury MD
Consultant Dermatologist
Rabindranath Tagore International
Institute of Cardiac Sciences
Kolkata, West Bengal, India

Foreword

S Premalatha

JAYPEE

JAYPEE BROTHERS MEDICAL PUBLISHERS
The Health Sciences Publisher
New Delhi | London

Jaypee Brothers Medical Publishers (P) Ltd

Headquarters
EMCA House, 23/23-B
Ansari Road, Daryaganj
New Delhi 110 002, India
Landline: +91-11-23272143, +91-11-23272703
+91-11-23282021, +91-11-23245672
e-mail: jaypee@jaypeebrothers.com

Corporate Office
4838/24, Ansari Road, Daryaganj
New Delhi 110 002, India
Phone: +91-11-43574357
Fax: +91-11-43574314
e-mail: jaypee@jaypeebrothers.com

Overseas Office
JP Medical Ltd.
83, Victoria Street, London
SW1H 0HW (UK)
Phone: +44-20 3170 8910
e-mail: info@jpmedpub.com

EU GPSR Authorised Representative
Logos Europe, 9 rue Nicolas Poussin
17000, La Rochelle, France
Phone: +33 (0) 6 67 93 73 78
e-mail: contact@logoseurope.eu

Website: www.jaypeebrothers.com
Website: www.jaypeedigital.com

Inquiries for bulk sales may be solicited at: jaypee@jaypeebrothers.com

Postgraduate Dermatology (Volumes 1 and 2)

First Edition: **2022**
Reprint: **2026**
ISBN: 978-93-5270-463-7

Printed at: Samrat Offset Pvt. Ltd.

Dedicated to

Our
Parents
Professors
Partners
Progenies
Peers
Patients
And everyone else from whom we have learned something.

Contributors

Aarti Sarda
MD FAGE MRCP-SCE (Dermatology)
Consultant Dermatologist
Department of Dermatology
Wizderm Speciality Skin and Hair Clinic
Kolkata, West Bengal, India

Aayushi Mohan MD
Consultant Dermatologist
Dr Janki Prasad Sevashram Clinic
Gorakhpur, Uttar Pradesh, India

Abhijit Saha MD
Consultant Dermatologist
Institute of Child Health
Kolkata, West Bengal, India

Abhishek De
MD FAGE MRCP-SCE (Dermatology)
Associate Professor
Calcutta National Medical College
Kolkata, West Bengal, India

Adhyatm Bhandari MD (DVL)
Senior Resident
Department of Dermatology, Venereology and Leprosy
Postgraduate Institute of Medical Education and Research
Chandigarh, India

Aditi Chakrabarti MD (DVL)
Associate Professor
Department of Dermatology
KPC Medical College and Hospital
Kolkata, West Bengal, India

Adrija Datta MD (DVL)
RMO cum Clinical Tutor
Department of Dermatology
Institute of Postgraduate Medical Education and Research
Kolkata, West Bengal, India

Ajit B Janagond MD
Assistant Professor
Department of Dermatology, Venereology and Leprosy
Shri BM Patil Medical College and Research Center
BLDE (Deemed to be University)
Vijaypura, Karnataka, India

(Late) AK Bajaj MD
Chief Consultant Dermatologist
Bajaj Skin Clinic
Prayagraj, Uttar Pradesh, India

Akansha Bhargava MD (DVL)
Consultant Dermatolo1gist
Dr Akansha Bhargava's Skin Clinic
Sagar, Madhya Pradesh, India

Akash Agarwal MBBS
Junior Resident
Department of DVL
IMS and SUM Hospitals
Bhubaneswar, Odisha, India

Akhilesh Shukla MD DNB Dip Derm
Consultant Dermatologist
Shri Balaji Super Speciality Hospital
Raipur, Chhattisgarh, India

Amiya Kumar Mukhopadhyay
MD PhD DNB (Derm) DNB (Derm & Vener) MNAMS
Consultant Dermatologist
Sri Durga Medical Mart
Asansol, West Bengal, India

Amrita Sil MD (Pharmacology)
Associate Professor
Department of Pharmacology
Government Medical College
Rampurhat, West Bengal, India

Anil Ganjoo MD
Founder Director
Skinnovation Clinics
(Dermatology and VD)
New Delhi, India

Anita Kulhari MD
Senior Resident
Department of Dermatology and STD
University College of Medical Sciences and Associated Guru Teg Bahadur Hospital
New Delhi, India

Ankur Talwar MD
Consultant Dermatologist
Talwar Skin Institute
Lucknow, Uttar Pradesh, India

Anoosha P MD
Consultant Dermatologist
Amara Hospital
Tirupati, Andhra Pradesh, India

Anup Kumar Tiwary MD (DVL)
Consultant Dermatologist
Yashoda Hospital and Research Centre
Ghaziabad, Uttar Pradesh, India

Anupam Das MD
Assistant Professor
Department of Dermatology
KPC Medical College and Hospital
Kolkata, West Bengal, India

Anuradha Bishnoi
MD (Dermatology, Venereology and Leprology) DNB
Assistant Professor
Department of Dermatology, Venereology and Leprology
Postgraduate Institute of Medical Education and Research
Chandigarh, India

Arghyaprasun Ghosh MD
Professor and Head
Department of Dermatology
Bankura Sammilani Medical College
Bankura, West Bengal, India

Arijit Coondoo DVD MD
Professor Emeritus
Department of Dermatology
KPC Medical College and Hospital
Kolkata, West Bengal, India

Arnab Dutta MD DVL
Senior Resident
Department of Dermatology
Calcutta National Medical College
Kolkata, West Bengal, India

Arun C Inamadar MD FRCP (Edinburgh)
Professor and Head
Department of Dermatology, Venereology and Leprosy
Shri BM Patil Medical College and Research Center
BLDE (Deemed to be University)
Vijaypura, Karnataka, India

Ashish Amrani
MD DNB MNAMS MRCP-SCE
Assistant Professor
NC Medical College
Panipat, Haryana, India

Astha Sharma MD (Dermatology and VD)
Consultant Dermatologist
Lok Clinic and Hospital
New Delhi, India

Balachandra S Ankad MD
Professor and Head
Department of Dermatology
S Nijalingappa Medical College
Bagalkot, Karnataka, India

Balachandran C MD
Professor and Head
Department of Dermatology, Venereology and Leprosy
Sree Narayana Institute of Medical Sciences
Ernakulum, Kerala, India

Banashree Majumdar MD
Consultant
Department of Dermatology
Medica Multispecialty Hospital
Jamshedpur, Jharkhand, India

Barnali Chowdhury MD
Consultant Dermatologist
Rabindranath Tagore International
Institute of Cardiac Sciences
Kolkata, West Bengal, India

Barunesh Gautam MD (DVL)
Senior Resident
Department of Dermatology
MGM Medical College and LSK Hospital
Kishanganj, Bihar, India

BC Sharath Kumar MD DVD DNB
Professor and Head
Department of Dermatology
Kempegowda Institute of Medical Sciences
Bengaluru, Karnataka, India

Bela J Shah MD
Professor and Head
Department of Dermatology,
Venereology and Leprology
BJ Medical College and Civil Hospital
Ahmedabad, Gujarat, India

Belliappa P Raju MBBS DVD DNB MNAMS
Professor
Department of Dermatology,
Venereology and Leprosy
Rajarajeshwari Medical College
and Hospital
Bengaluru, Karnataka, India

Bhabani STP Singh MD
Associate Professor (Dermatology)
IMS and SUM Hospital
Bhubaneswar, Odisha, India

Bhushan Madke MD
Professor and Head
Department of Dermatology,
Venereology and Leprosy
Jawaharlal Nehru Medical College
Datta Meghe Institute of Medical Sciences
Wardha, Maharashtra, India

Binod Kumar Thakur MD
Consultant Dermatologist
Cosmic Dermatology and Hair
Transplant Clinic
Shillong, Meghalaya, India

CR Srinivas MD
Professor
Department of Dermatology
Kalinga Institute of Medical Sciences
Bhubaneswar, Odisha, India

Chander Grover MD DNB MNAMS
Professor
Department of Dermatology and STD
University College of Medical Sciences and
Associated Guru Teg Bahadur Hospital
New Delhi, India

Chethana S Gurumurthy MD (DVL)
Senior Resident
Department of Dermatology
JSS Medical College and Hospital
Mysuru, Karnataka, India

Chinmay Kar MD (DVL)
Assistant Professor
Calcutta National Medical College
Kolkata, West Bengal, India

D Dinesh Kumar MD FIAMS FRCP (Glasgow)
Consultant Dermatologist and Head
Dr Dinesh's Skin and Hair Clinic
Chennai, Tamil Nadu, India

Debatri Datta MD (DVL)
Consultant Dermatologist
Oliva Skin and Hair Clinic
Kolkata, West Bengal, India

Deblina Bhunia MD (DVL)
Assistant Professor
Department of Dermatology
MGM Medical College and LSK Hospital
Kishanganj, Bihar, India

Deep Joshipura MD
Dermatologist and Assistant Professor
Warren Alpert Medical School of
Brown University
Providence, Rhode Island, USA

Deepika Halder MD
Senior Resident
Calcutta National Medical
College and Hospital
Kolkata, West Bengal, India

Deepika Pandhi MD MNAMS
Professor
Department of Dermatology and STD
University College of Medical Sciences and
Associated Guru Teg Bahadur Hospital
New Delhi, India

Devinder Mohan Thappa
MD DHA FRCP (Edin) FRCP (Glasg) FAMS FIMSA
Professor Senior Scale
Department of Dermatology and STD
Jawaharlal Institute of Postgraduate
Medical Education and Research
Puducherry, India

Dinesh Jayaram
MD (DVL) FRGUS (Dermatosurgery)
Junior Consultant
CUTIS Academy of Cutaneous Sciences
Bengaluru, Karnataka, India

Dipankar De MD
Additional Professor
Department of Dermatology
Postgraduate Institute of Medical
Education and Research
Chandigarh, India

Dipayan Sengupta MD (Dermatology)
Consultant
Euro Skin, Hair and Wellness Clinic
Kolkata, West Bengal, India

Falguni Nag MD
Assistant Professor
Department of Dermatology
Government Medical College
Purulia, West Bengal, India

Fenil Patel MBBS DDVL
Consultant Dermatologist,
Venereologist and Leprologist
Shaleen Hospital and Sanjeevani
Heart and Medical Hospital
Ahmedabad, Gujarat, India

Feroze Kaliyadan
MD DNB MNAMS FIMSA SCE-RCP Euro Board
Dermato-venereology FRCP (Lon)
Faculty of Dermatology
College of Medicine
King Faisal University, Saudi Arabia

Fibin Thanveer DVD MD
Senior Consultant Dermatologist
Starcare Hospital
Kozhikode, Kerala, India

Gagan Jot Kaur MD
Medical Officer (Specialist)
and District Leprosy Officer
District Hospital
Faridkot, Punjab, India

Gillian Roga MD DNB Dermatology
Consultant Dermatology, Cosmetologist
and Hair Transplant Surgeon
Dr Gillian's Skin, Hair, Laser and
Cosmetology Clinic
Chikmagalur, Karnataka, India

Gobinda Chatterjee MD
Head
Department of Dermatology
Institute of Postgraduate Medical
Education and Research
Kolkata, West Bengal, India

Gulhima Arora DNB MNAMS
Consultant Dermatologist
Mehektagul Dermaclinic
New Delhi, India

Harsh Tahiliani MD
Consultant Dermatologist
Dr Tahiliani's Clinic
Mumbai, Maharashtra, India

Harsha Siddappa
MD (DVL) FRGUS (Dermatosurgery)
Consultant Dermatologist
Ananthapuri Hospital and
Research Institute
Thiruvananthapuram, Kerala, India

Hemanta Kumar Nath MD (DVL)
Consultant Dermatologist
Pratiksha Hospital
Guwahati, Assam, India

Himanshu Gupta
MD Dermatology FACSI (Dermatosurgery)
FIADVL (LASER & Aesthetics)
Consultant Dermatologist
Skinkonnect Clinic
New Delhi and Ghaziabad,
Uttar Pradesh, India

Imran Majid MD
Consultant Dermatologist
Cutis Institute of Dermatology
Srinagar, Jammu and Kashmir, India

Indrashis Podder
MD (Dermatology) DNB (Dermatology)
Assistant Professor
Department of Dermatology
College of Medicine and Sagore
Dutta Hospital
Kolkata, West Bengal, India

Ishad Aggarwal MD
Consultant Dermatologist
Wizderm Speciality Skin And Hair Clinic
Kolkata, West Bengal, India

Ivoreen Darung MD
Senior Resident
TomoRiba Institute of Health and
Medical Sciences
Naharlagun, Arunachal Pradesh, India

Janaki Chellam MD (Dermatology) DD MAMS
Consultant Dermatologist
Billroth Hospitals
Chennai, Tamil Nadu, India

Janani Adityan MD DVL
Department of Dermatology
PSG Institute of Medical Sciences
and Research
Coimbatore, Tamil Nadu, India

Jayadev Betkarur MD (DVL)
Professor
Department of Dermatology
JSS Medical College and Hospital
Mysuru, Karnataka, India

Jyothi Jayaraman MBBS DVD DNB
Senior Resident
Department of Dermatology
Father Muller Medical College
Mangaluru, Karnataka, India

Kaleem Khan MD
Consultant
Wockhardt Hospitals
Mumbai, Maharashtra, India

Kananbala Sahu MD
Senior Resident
Department of Dermatology
All India Institute of Medical Sciences
Bhubaneswar, Odisha, India

Kapisha Shah MBBS DDV
Consultant Dermatologist
Body Shrine Clinic
Mumbai, Maharashtra, India

Karalikkattil T Ashique
MBBS DDVL PGDHS FRCP (London)
Medical Director and Senior
Consultant Dermatologist
Amanza Skin Clinic
Perinthalmanna, Kerala, India

Kavish Chouhan MD
Consultant Dermatologist and Hair
Transplant Surgeon
Director, DermaClinix—the Complete
Skin and Hair Solution Center
All India Institute of Medical Sciences
New Delhi, India

Kingshuk Chatterjee
MBBS DNB MNAMS FAAD MRCPS (Glasgow)
Assistant Professor
Department of Dermatology
Calcutta School of Tropical Medicine
Kolkata, West Bengal, India

Kinnor Das MD (DVL)
Senior Resident
Department of DVL
Silchar Medical College and Hospital
Silchar, Assam, India

Kiran V Godse MD PhD FRCP (Glasgow)
Professor
Department of Dermatology
Dr DY Patil University School of Medicine
Navi Mumbai, Maharashtra, India

KN Sarveswari MD DD DNB
Consultant Dermatologist
Sundaram Medical Foundation and
Dr Rangarajan Memorial Hospital
Chennai, Tamil Nadu, India

Komal Agarwal
MD (DVL) MRCP-SCE (Dermatology)
Senior Resident
Department of Dermatology
Calcutta National Medical College
Kolkata, West Bengal, India

Koushik Lahiri
MBBS DVD (CAL) FIAD FFAADV FRCP (Glasgow)
FRCP (Edin) FRCP (London)
Professor and Distinguished
Academician (AHERF)
Senior Consultant Dermatologist
Apollo Multispecialty Hospitals Limited
Honorary Medical Director
Wizderm Speciality Skin and Hair Clinic
Kolkata, West Bengal, India

Kshama Talwar MD
Consultant Dermatologist
Talwar Skin Institute
Lucknow, Uttar Pradesh, India

Kumar Abhishek MD DNB MNAMS
Assistant Professor
Department of Dermatology
HiTech Medical College
Bhubaneswar, Odisha, India

Kumar Satyaprakash MD (DVL)
Senior Resident
Department of Dermatology
MGM Medical College and LSK Hospital
Kishanganj, Bihar, India

Kusuma MR
MD(DVL) FRGUS (Dermatosurgery)
Junior Consultant
CUTIS Academy of Cutaneous Sciences
Bengaluru, Karnataka, India

Laila Achampat MD (DVL)
Consultant and Dermatologist
Cutis Institute of Advanced Dermatology,
Aesthetic Medicine and Surgery
Kozhikode, Kerala, India

Loknath Ghosal MD (Derm & Ven)
Assistant Professor
Department of Dermatology
Nil Ratan Sircar Medical College
and Hospital
Kolkata, West Bengal, India

M Ramam MD
Professor
Department of Dermatology
and Venereology
All India Institute of Medical Sciences
New Delhi, India

Madhu Rengasamy
MD (Dermatology) DCH MAMS
Associate Professor
Department of Dermatology,
Venereology and Leprosy
Madras Medical College
Chennai, Tamil Nadu, India

Madhuri Agarwal MD DDV
Founder and Medical Director
Yavana Aesthetics Clinic
Mumbai, Maharashtra, India

Mahajabeen S Madarkar MD
Assistant Professor
Department of Dermatology
S Nijalingappa Medical College
Bagalkot, Karnataka, India

Maitreyee Panda MD (DVL)
Professor
Department of DVL
IMS and SUM Hospitals
Bhubaneswar, Odisha, India

Maitreyee Sengupta MD
Senior Resident
RG Kar Medical College and Hospital
Kolkata, West Bengal, India

Mamatha George MD
Professor
Department of Dermatology
Malabar Medical College Hospital and Research Center
Kozhikode, Kerala, India

Manas Chatterjee MD DNB (Dermatology)
Senior Adviser
Professor and Head
Department of Dermatology
Institute of Naval Medicine, INHS Asvini
Mumbai, Maharashtra, India

Manasa Narayan Kayarkatte MD DNB
Assistant Professor
Department of Dermatology
Kasturba Medical College
Mangaluru, Karnataka, India

Manjyot Gautam MD (DVL)
Professor
Department of Dermatology
Dr DY Patil University School of Medicine
Navi Mumbai, Maharashtra, India

Marisa Pongprutthipan MD
Assistance Professor
Division of Dermatology
Department of Medicine
Faculty of Medicine
Chulalongkorn University
King Chulalongkorn Memorial Hospital
Bangkok, Thailand

Mary Zothanpuii Chhangte MD
Senior Resident Doctor
Department of Dermatology and STD
North Eastern Indira Gandhi Regional Institute of Health and Medical Sciences (NEIGRIHMS)
Shillong, Meghalaya, India

Monali Pattnaik MD DNB
Associate Consultant (Dermatology)
Aditya Ashwini Hospital
Bhubaneswar, Odisha, India

Munisamy Malathi MD DNB
Associate Professor
Department of Dermatology and STD
Jawaharlal Institute of Postgraduate Medical Education and Research
Puducherry, India

Namratha C Manjunath
MD (DVL) FRGUS (Dermatosurgery)
Assistant Professor
Department of Dermatology
Kempegowda Institute of Medical Sciences
Bengaluru, Karnataka, India

Neha Bhardwaj DDVL MRCP-SCE
Consultant Dermatologist
SkinLab
New Delhi, India

Neha Dubey MD
Consultant Medical and Cosmetic Dermatologist
Medical Director
Meraki Skin Clinic
Gurugram, Haryana, India

Nidhi Choudhary MD (DVL)
Senior Resident
Department of Dermatology
All India Institute of Medical Sciences
Bhopal, Madhya Pradesh, India

Nilay Kanti Das MD
Professor
Department of Dermatology
Bankura Sammilani Medical College and Hospital
Bankura, West Bengal, India

Nina Madnani MD FAAD FISSVD
Consultant
PD Hinduja National Hospital
Mumbai, Maharashtra, India

Nisha Chaturvedi DVD MD DNB
Consultant
Surya Mother and Child Hospital
Mumbai, Maharashtra, India

Nishant Choudhary MD
Assistant Professor
LN Medical College and JK Hospital
Bhopal, Madhya Pradesh, India

Niteen Dhepe MD
Medical Director
Skin City India
Postgraduate Institute of Dermatology
Pune, Maharashtra, India

Niti Khunger MD DNB DDV
Consultant Dermatologist
Professor and Head
Department of Dermatology and STD
Vardhman Mahavir Medical College and Safdarjung Hospital
New Delhi, India

PK Srivastava DCD (Cardiff UK)
Dermatologist
Mansi Skin and Allergy Clinic
Prayagraj, Uttar Pradesh, India

Piyush Kumar MD (DVL)
Consultant Dermatologist
Derma Corner
Katihar, Bihar, India

Pragya A Nair MD (DVL)
Professor and Head
Department of Dermatology, Venereology and Leprosy
Pramukh Swami Medical College
Karamsad, Gujarat, India

Preethi B Nayak MD DNB FRGUHS
Consultant Dermatologist and Dermatosurgeon
CUTIS Academy of Cutaneous Sciences
Bengaluru, Karnataka, India

Prerna Raj MD
Senior Resident
BN Bose Subdivisional Hospital
Barrackpore, West Bengal, India

Priyankar Misra MD
Senior Resident
Department of Dermatology, Venereology and Leprology
Jagannath Gupta Institute of Medical Sciences
Kolkata, West Bengal, India

R Raghunatha Reddy
MD DNB FRGUHS (Dermatosurgery)
Professor
Consultant Dermatologist and Dermatosurgeon
Dr Raghu's Mathapitha Polyclinic
Bengaluru, Karnataka, India

Raghavendra Rao MD DNB
Professor and Head
Department of Dermatology
Kasturba Medical College
Manipal Academy of Higher Education
Manipal, Karnataka, India

Rajat Kandhari MD MSc
Consultant Dermatologist
Dr Kandhari's Skin and Dental Clinic
Veya Aesthetics
New Delhi, India

Rajesh K Mondal MD DVL
Associate Professor
Department of Dermatology
North Bengal Medical College
Darjeeling, West Bengal, India

Rajetha Damisetty MD
Additional Medical Director
Oliva Hair and Skin Clinics
Hyderabad, Telangana, India

Rajsmita Bhattacharjee MD
Senior Resident
Department of Dermatology, Venereology and Leprology
Postgraduate Institute of Medical Education and Research
Chandigarh, India

Ramesh Bhat M MD DVD DNB MNAMS
Professor
Department of Dermatology
Father Muller Medical College
Mangaluru, Karnataka, India

Rashmi Sarkar MD MNAMS
Professor
Department of Dermatology
Maulana Azad Medical College and Associated Lok Nayak Jai Prakash Narayan Hospital
New Delhi, India

Rasya K Dixit MD
Dr Dixit Cosmetic Dermatology Clinic
Bengaluru, Karnataka, India

Ravi Ranjan MD (DVL)
Senior Resident
Department of Dermatology
MGM Medical College and LSK Hospital
Kishanganj, Bihar, India

Reema R Baxi MD (DVL)
Resident
Department of Dermatology and Venereology
Government Medical College
Vadodara, Gujarat, India

Reena Rai MD DVL
Head and Professor
Department of Dermatology
PSG Institute of Medical Sciences and Research
Coimbatore, Tamil Nadu, India

Remya Raj R MD (DVL)
Assistant Professor
Department of Dermatology
Jawaharlal Institute of Postgraduate Medical Education and Research
Puducherry, India

Resham Vasani MD DNB FCPS DDV
Consultant Dermatologist
Bhojani Clinic
Mumbai, Maharashtra, India

Riti Bhatia MD
Assistant Professor
Department of Dermatology, Venereology and Leprosy
All India Institute of Medical Sciences
Rishikesh, Uttarakhand, India

Rochit Singhal MD
Assistant Professor
Chirayu Medical College
Bhopal, Madhya Pradesh, India

Roma Dhande MBBS
Resident Doctor
Department of Dermatology, Venereology and Leprosy
Jawaharlal Nehru Medical College
Datta Meghe Institute of Medical Sciences
Wardha, Maharashtra, India

Ruchi Shah MD
Resident
Department of Dermatology and Venereology
Government Medical College
Vadodara, Gujarat, India

Rupika Singh MD
Consultant Dermatologist
Akiya Aesthetics
Ghaziabad, Uttar Pradesh, India

S Sacchidanand
MD DVD DHA FRCP (Glasgow)
Former Head and Professor
Department of Dermatology
Bangalore Medical College and Research Institute, Bengaluru, India
Vice Chancellor, Rajiv Gandhi University of Health Sciences, Bengaluru
Former Director of Medical Education
Government of Karnataka, Bengaluru
Former Registrar (Evaluation)
RGUHS, Bengaluru
Former Dean–Director
Bangalore Medical College and Research Institute
Bengaluru, Karnataka, India

Sabha Mushtaq MD
Resident Dermatologist
Department of Dermatology
Government Senior Medical College
Jammu, Jammu and Kashmir, India

Sachi Gupta MBBS DDVL DNB FAGE
Locum Consultant Dermatologist
Department of Dermatology
Hertford County Hospital
Hertfordshire, UK

Sahana M Srinivas
DNB DVD FRGUHS (Pediatric Dermatology)
Consultant
Department of Pediatric Dermatology
Indira Gandhi Institute of Child Health
Bengaluru, Karnataka, India

Sameena Batool Dip Derm
Resident Dermatology
Cutis Institute of Dermatology
Srinagar, Jammu and Kashmir, India

Samiksha Chavhan MBBS
Resident Doctor
Department of Dermatology, Venereology and Leprosy
Jawaharlal Nehru Medical College
Datta Meghe Institute of Medical Sciences
Wardha, Maharashtra, India

Sandeep Arora MD
Professor
Senior Advisor and Head
Department of Dermatology
Command Hospital Air Force
Bengaluru, Karnataka, India

Sandipan Dhar MD DNB FRCP (Edin)
Professor and Head
Department of Pediatric Dermatology
Institute of Child Health
Kolkata, West Bengal, India

Sanjay Ghosh MD
Professor and Head
Department of Dermatology
MGM Medical College and LSK Hospital
Kishanganj, Bihar, India

Sanjay K Rathi MD
Consultant Dermatologist
Siliguri, West Bengal, India

Sanjeev Handa MD FAMS FAAD FRCP (Edin)
Professor and Head
Postgraduate Institute of Medical Education and Research
Chandigarh, India

Satarupa Mondal MBBS
Resident
Department of Dermatology
RG Kar Medical College
Kolkata, West Bengal, India

Sathish Pai B MD DVD
Professor
Department of Dermatology, Venereology and Leprosy
Kasturba Medical College
Manipal Academy of Higher Education
Manipal, Karnataka, India

Satyaki Ganguly MD (DVL) DNB (DV)
Associate Professor
Department of Dermatology
All India Institute of Medical Sciences
Raipur, Chhattisgarh, India

Saumya Panda MD
Professor and Head
Department of Dermatology
KPC Medical College and Hospital
Kolkata, West Bengal, India

Saurav Kundu MD
Associate Professor
Department of Dermatology
MGM Medical College and LSK Hospital
Kishanganj, Bihar, India

Savitha AS
MD (DVL) DNB FRGUHS (Dermatosurgery)
Associate Professor
Department of Dermatology
Sapthagiri Institute of Medical
Science and Research Center
Bengaluru, Karnataka, India

R Raghunatha Reddy
MD (DVL) DNB FRGUHS (Dermatosurgery)
Professor and Head
Department of Dermatology
Akash Institute of Medical
Sciences and Research
Bengaluru, Karnataka, India

Sejal Chandak MBBS
Resident Doctor
Department of Dermatology,
Venereology and Leprosy
Jawaharlal Nehru Medical College
Datta Meghe Institute of Medical Sciences
Wardha, Maharashtra, India

Sentamilselvi Ganapathi
MD DD PhD FAMS
Former Professor and Head
Department of Dermatology
Madras Medical College, Chennai
Consultant Dermatologist
Chennai, Tamil Nadu, India

Shailvi Banka Biyani
MD (Dermatology)
Consultant Dermatologist
ILS Hospitals
Kolkata, West Bengal, India

Shashank Bhargava MD
Assistant Professor
Department of Dermatology
RD Gardi Medical College
Ujjain, Madhya Pradesh, India

Shashi Kumar BM
MD (DVL) FIADVL (Dermatopath)
Associate Professor
Department of Dermatology
Mandya Institute of Medical Sciences
Mandya, Karnataka, India

Shekhar Neema MD
Associate Professor
Department of Dermatology
Armed Forces Medical College
Pune, Maharashtra, India

Shikha Bansal MD DNB MNAMS
Professor
Department of Dermatology
Vardhman Mahavir Medical College and
Safdarjung Hospital
New Delhi, India

Shouvik Ghosh MD
Senior Resident
Department of Dermatology
KPC Medical College and Hospital
Kolkata, West Bengal, India

Shravya R MBBS
Resident Doctor
Department of Dermatology,
Venereology and Leprosy
Jawaharlal Nehru Medical College
Datta Meghe Institute of Medical Sciences
Wardha, Maharashtra, India

Shrenik Balger MD
Consultant Dermatologist
Skin City India
Postgraduate Institute of Dermatology
Pune, Maharashtra, India

Shrikant Kumavat MBBS DDVL
Senior Resident
Department of Dermatology
Dr Vasantrao Pawar Medical College
Nashik, Maharashtra, India

SK Shahriar Ahmed MD DNB
Senior Resident
Calcutta National Medical College
Kolkata, West Bengal, India

Smitha Prabhu S MD DVD
Associate Professor
Department of Dermatology and
Venereology
Kasturba Medical College
Manipal Academy of Higher Education
Udupi, Karnataka, India

Snehal Siddhesh Kalantri MD DVL
Consultant Dermatologist
Skincare Solutions
Nashik, Maharashtra, India

Somenath Sarkar MD
Associate Professor
Department of Dermatology
Bankura Sammilani Medical College
Bankura, West Bengal, India

Somodyuti Chandra
MD DVL (Gold Medalist) DNB DVL
SCE-Dermatology (UK) FRGUHS Fellowship
in Aesthetic Medicine and Laser
Consultant Dermatologist
Medica Superspeciality Hospital, Kolkata
Wizderm Speciality Skin and Hair Clinic
Kolkata, West Bengal, India

Sonal Singh MD
Consultant Dermatologist
Skinvita Clinic
Kolkata, West Bengal, India

Souvik Sardar MD (DVL)
Consultant Dermatologist
Eleganz Skin and Hair Clinic
Kolkata, West Bengal, India

Subhamoy Neogi MD (DVL)
Tutor
Institute of Postgraduate Medical
Education and Research and
SSKM Hospital
Kolkata, West Bengal, India

Subhra Sankar Sahoo MBBS
Junior Resident
Department of Dermatology
Calcutta National Medical College
Kolkata, West Bengal, India

Sudhir Nayak UK MD DDVL
Associate Professor
Department of Dermatology,
Venereology and Leprosy
Kasturba Medical College
Manipal Academy of Higher Education
Manipal, Karnataka, India

Sudip Das
MD (Derm & Ven) FRCP (EDIN)
Professor and Head
Department of Dermatology
Calcutta National Medical College
Kolkata, West Bengal, India

Sudip Kumar Ghosh
MD DNB MNAMS
Professor of Dermatology
RG Kar Medical College
Kolkata, West Bengal, India

Sudip Sarkar MBBS
Postgraduate Trainee in Dermatology
Calcutta National Medical College
and Hospital
Kolkata, West Bengal, India

Sujala Sacchidanand Aradhya
MD (DVL) FRGUHS (Dermatosurgery)
FIADVL (Trichology) FACSI (Dermatosurgery)
Consultant Dermatologist and
Dermatosurgeon
Sujala Polyclinic and Laboratory
Bengaluru, Karnataka, India

Sujata Sengupta
DCH MD (Derm & Ven)
Professor and Head
Department of Dermatology
KPC Medical College and Hospital
Kolkata, West Bengal, India

Sumit Sen MBBS DTM&H MD
Professor
Department of Dermatology
Institute of Postgraduate Medical
Education and Research and
SSKM Hospital
Kolkata, West Bengal, India

Suneil Gandhi MD (DVL) DNB (Dermatology)
Consultant Dermatologist
Reviva Skin Clinic
Surat, Gujarat, India

Surajit Gorai
MD (Gold Medalist) DNB MNAMS (Dermatology)
Associate Professor (AHERF)
Consultant Dermatologist
Apollo Gleneagles Hospital
Kolkata, West Bengal, India

Surbhi Rajput MD
Dermatologist
Department of Dermatology
Military Hospital
Amritsar, Punjab, India

Suresh Joshipura
MD PhD DVD FRCP (London)
Senior Consultant Dermatologist
Skin Center
Rajkot, Gujarat, India

Sushil Tahiliani MD DVD
Consultant Dermatologist
Dr Tahiliani's Clinic and Hinduja Hospital
and Medical Research Centre
Mumbai, Maharashtra, India

Suyomi Shah MD (DVL)
Junior Resident
Dr DY Patil Medical College
Navi Mumbai, Maharashtra, India

Swetalina Pradhan MD
Assistant Professor
Department of Dermatology
All India Institute of Medical Sciences
Patna, Bihar, India

Thurakkal Salim MD DNB MNAMS
Medical Director
Cutis Institute of Advanced Dermatology,
Aesthetic Medicine and Surgery
Kozhikode, Kerala, India

Umashankar Nagaraju MD
Professor
Department of Dermatology,
Venereology and Leprosy
Rajarajeshwari Medical College
and Hospital
Bengaluru, Karnataka, India

Vandana Mehta MD DNB
Consultant Dermatologist
Dr Hassan Al Abdulla Medical Centre
Doha, Qatar

Vandini Kabra MD
Consultant Dermatologist
Dr Dixit Clinic
Bengaluru, Karnataka, India

Varsha M Shetty MD DNB
Associate Professor
Department of Dermatology
Kasturba Medical College
Manipal, Karnataka, India

Varsha Vaidyanathan MD DNB
Senior Resident
North DMC Medical College and
Hindu Rao Hospital
New Delhi, India

Vasundhara Singh MD
Resident
Dr DY Patil Medical College and Hospital
Navi Mumbai, Maharashtra, India

Vijay P Zawar MD DNB DVD FRCP (Edin)
Professor
Department of Dermatology
Dr Vasantrao Pawar Medical College
Nashik, Maharashtra, India

Vinutha Rangappa MD (DVL)
Assistant Professor
Department of Dermatology
JSS Medical College and Hospital
Mysuru, Karnataka, India

Vishal Chugh MD
Fellow in Dermatosurgery
Bangalore Medical College and
Research Institute
Bengaluru, Karnataka, India

Vivek M Pai MD DNB FRGUHS
Consultant Dermatologist and
Dermatosurgeon
Hairline International Clinic
Bengaluru, Karnataka, India

Vivek V Pai MBBS DVD FCGP FAMSc
Director
Bombay Leprosy Project
Mumbai, Maharashtra, India

Vrushali Lonikar MD
Specialist Dermatologist
Department of Dermatology
NMC Specialty Hospital
Abu Dhabi, UAE

Yashpal Manchanda
MD DNB MNAMS
Senior Consultant Dermatologist
Ministry of Health
Department of Dermatology
Al Farwaniya Hospital, Kuwait

Yogesh S Marfatia MD
Professor and Head
Department of Skin and VD
SSG Hospital
Vadodara, Gujarat, India

Foreword

'There is no end to learning, but there are many beginnings'

– Tim Johnson

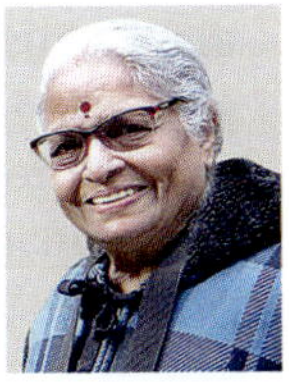

I am very much pleased to go through the ramifying network of various chapters in this wonderful book, *Postgraduate Dermatology* pertaining to various sections of dermatology, leprosy and sexually transmitted diseases.

I would like to congratulate the prime Authors/Editors Dr Koushik Lahiri and Dr Abhishek De, as I consider this book as their 'Brain Child'. I appreciate their endless and sincere efforts to bring out this book exclusively for the benefits of postgraduate students in dermatology.

I also congratulate all the credential authors of this book for their contribution to impart knowledge in-depth to the postgraduate students.

The knowledge has been spread from the 'Overview of Basics in Dermatology' to the 'Procedural Dermatology' at the end... Nothing has been overlooked in the middle.

To put it in a nutshell, the book, *Postgraduate Dermatology* is an inspiring, complete, comprehensive and a crispy recipe book on dermatology for the postgraduate students—easy to digest, recall or ruminate to remember the subject.

This spectacular book is a tell-tale evidence to reveal that a positive attitude with sincere efforts always results in beneficial effects and happiness.

I am sure that the postgraduate students will enjoy reading this book.

S Premalatha
DD MD PhD FAMS FIMSA
Retired Professor and Head
Department of Dermatology and Leprosy
Government Stanley Medical College and Hospital
Former Professor
Department of Dermatology
Sri Ramachandra Medical College and Deemed University
Chennai, Tamil Nadu, India

Preface

"History with its flickering lamp stumbles along the trail of the past, trying to reconstruct its scenes, to revive its echoes, and kindle with pale gleams the passion of former days. What is the worth of all this? The only guide to a man is his conscience; the only shield to his memory is the rectitude and sincerity of his actions. It is very imprudent to walk through life without this shield, because we are so often mocked by the failure of our hopes and the upsetting of our calculations; but with this shield, however the fates may play, we march always in the ranks of honor."

– Winston S Churchill

Rome was not built in a day, and so is this book.

Just as we finished our project *Lasers in Dermatology*, the proposal to start working for the next project reached us immediately and right from the top.

The boss was not only persuasive, but he was also extremely confident and took very little time to convince us about the exigency of such a book for the postgraduates in training.

We realized though we have enough exhaustive, elaborate, outstanding and voluminous textbooks for our students, we do not have a concise, crisp, handy, user friendly yet authentic book for them.

We started working and immediately understood the enormity of the project we were assigned to.

Inspite of the astonishingly rich pool of authors, clinical material and experience in dealing with these disorders, no compendium of this magnitude in dermatology was ever conceived before from this part of the globe.

We tried to keep it simple.

Discussed the concept with teachers across generations and scanned the question papers of last one decade of different universities and most importantly tried to understand what a postgraduate student wants and needs to read. We have never for a moment tried to create yet another exhaustive textbook. Our instruction to the prospective authors was to contribute short and crisp chapters unlike conventional textbooks as the book is focused on the needs of a postgraduate student as well as the clinician as the ready reference. It was our policy position to stay away from compiling elaborate and exhaustive textbook chapters.

We divided the 180 chapters into 15 sections. Worked closely with more than 300 authors involved. Each of the chapters received were thoroughly peer-reviewed and rigorously cross-checked to avoid any smell of plagiarism. We have tried to collect and add as many questions as possible from all over the country. Innumerable tables, flowcharts, bulleted texts, figures, line drawings, graphs have been used keeping the examination orientation intact.

But, the journey, unlike our past projects, was not smooth all along.

It was not a sprint, not even a marathon, rather a life-changing cross-country race. The project got delayed for reasons beyond our control. But thanks to the indulgence of a supportive chief, and an amazingly efficient team of M/s Jaypee Brothers Medical Publishers (P) Ltd, New Delhi, India, we could manage to sail through.

A never before pandemic struck the planet and we utilized the interruption in a most positive way. As Confucius uttered, *"Our greatest glory is not in never falling, but in rising every time we fall."*

We were blessed with a set of young, energetic and amazingly erudite Assistant Editors in Aarti Sarda, Anupam Das, Abhijit Saha, Surajit Gorai, and Barnali Chowdhury. Their help in assigning the authors of the book is special. We also acknowledge Dr Arnab Dutta who has helped us to compile the recent questions at the end of each chapters.

The final result is this magnum opus. A never before compilation on the subject, which we believe suits the taste and requirement of the target readership, just perfectly.

This is just not an examination purpose notebook, but a collective wisdom of key academic opinion leaders bejeweled with the extensive and priceless clinical arsenal of the authors. We hope this cute compendium will be of value to all dermatologists whether postgraduate students, senior practitioners or academicians in India, Asia and the globe.

We sincerely look forward to your feedback.

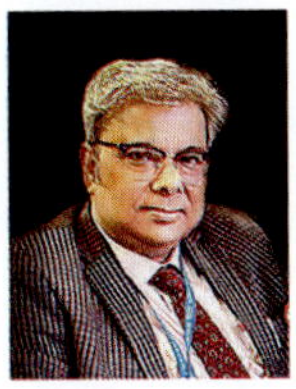

Koushik Lahiri

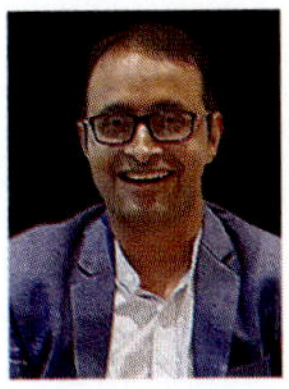

Abhishek De

"Successful and unsuccessful people do not vary greatly in their capabilities.
They vary in their desire to reach their potential."

– John Maxwell

Acknowledgments

We must thank M/s Jaypee Brothers Medical Publishers (P) Ltd, New Delhi, India, one of the most reputed, respected and largest medical publishing houses in the world, to suggest us the title and for giving us the opportunity.

This book comprises of 180 chapters and we had to work closely with more than 300 amazing authors for last few years. They are virtually the topmost key opinion leaders in these topics. We would like to personally thank each of these brilliant authors who came forward to contribute high quality chapters for this project.

We are thankful for huge compilation of DNB questions contributed by our fellow colleagues Dr Arnab Dutta, Dr Ramesh Bhat M, Dr Kiran Godse, Dr Rashmi Sarkar, Dr Shyamanta Barua and Dr Abhishek De.

If only one person is to be credited for the realization of this magnum opus, he is none other than Shri Jitendar P Vij (Group Chairman) himself. From inception to final execution, he took personal care of this project. His patience and trust, almost to the degree of indulgence was the real guiding force.

Ms Chetna Malhotra (Associate Director–Content Strategy) from the publisher side played the role of a seasoned and experienced facilitator.

The delegation of Dr Rajul Jain (Development Editor) was the game changer. She is a thorough professional and a pure perfectionist.

Renowned dermatologist/historian/archivist Dr Amiya Mukhopadhyay has selected and introduced the historically significant images used as the background of the cover. He deserves a bow.

The jewel in the crown is the foreword from the legendary polymath Professor (Dr) S Premalatha. We sincerely appreciate her invaluable contribution. This would certainly augment the credibility and recognition to our humble effort.

Contents

VOLUME 1

SECTION 1 OVERVIEW OF BASICS IN DERMATOLOGY

SECTION 2 PRURITUS, URTICARIA, ALLERGY, AND ECZEMAS

SECTION 6 PAPULOSQUAMOUS DISEASES

SECTION 7 SKIN AND SYSTEMIC DISEASE

SECTION 8 HAIR, NAIL, MUCOSA, ADNEXA AND CONNECTIVE TISSUE

VOLUME 2

SECTION 9 VASCULAR DISEASES

SECTION 10 NEOPLASTIC SKIN DISEASES

SECTION 13 SEXUALLY TRANSMITTED DISEASE

1 SECTION

Overview of Basics in Dermatology

1. History of Dermatology
2. Embryology of Skin
3. Anatomy of Skin and Appendages
4. Functions of the Skin
5. Basic Immunology in Relation to Skin
6. Basics of Genetics in Relation to Skin
7. Basics in Dermatopathology
8. Clinical Signs in Dermatology and Approach to Diagnosis
9. Bedside Tests in Dermatology
10. Laboratory Investigations Specific to Dermatology Disorders
11. Skin through Ages
12. Diet in Dermatology
13. Environment and Skin
14. Evidence-based Dermatology
15. Medical Statistics

1 CHAPTER

History of Dermatology

Amiya Kumar Mukhopadhyay

INTRODUCTION

"... non illa pro simplici habenda est involucro, sed organum constitutit..."

It was 1777. The French physician Charles-Anne Lorry (1726–1783) wrote the above sentence: skin is not merely a cover but an organ.... These few words not only gave his view regarding *skin* but also heralded a new vision that gave birth to the specialty of *Dermatology* within the next 100 years.

If we navigate in the history of medicine, the early medical men like Shamans, faith healers, priest healers and every other whoever dealt with the human disorders never missed to note their observation on the skin in health and diseases. We can find the mortal evidence of skin disease in the Egyptian mummy about 5,000 years old. The Ebers, the Hearst, the Edwin Smith, and other papyri written about 3,500 years back mentioned about skin diseases and various prescriptions, whatever peculiar they may be.

India, one of the cradles of human civilization, developed a methodical thinking about diseases in the form of *Ayurveda* at least 3,000 years back. Ayurvedic tomes such as *Charaka Samhita, Sushruta Samhita, Bhela Samhita*, and many others mentioned about various skin diseases including ring worms, eczema, ichthyosis, skin tags, cellulites, and *leprosy*. It is mandatory here to state that skin diseases were mentioned much earlier in the oldest religious texts of the Indo-Iranian Aryans—the Vedas.[1]

Gradually, the subject of healing metamorphosed from purely magical to a rational form. Hippocrates of Cos (460–377 BC) was the first in the Western world to proclaim that disease is not a wrath of the God but a disorder with reasons behind and prescribed the concept of disturbed *humors* as their etiology. Galen (129–199 AD) was the next towering historical personality whose influence lived actively in the Western world almost till the 16th century and even after. But these are all about more on the history of medicine than of dermatology, though both are integral parts of a single story. As, by *dermatology* we mean Western dermatology by default, so our further discussion will remain limited within this specified space only.

"SKIN DISEASE" OR "*DERMATOLOGY*": WHY AND WHEN?

There is a controversy. Should we use the term dermatology if we write or discuss about diseases of the skin during 300 years or before? Semantically speaking: No! The term *dermatology* came into vogue only during the mid-19th century. Before that period, terms such as *dermology, dermiatry* and *dermatophily* were used.[2] As far as history goes, Antoni Rosner (1831–1896) was appointed as a lecturer of skin diseases under the term *Dermatology* in the year 1858 in Cracow, though Hebra was the first to be appointed as the first ever professor of *only* skin diseases in 1849. So, practically speaking the history of modern *Dermatology* began only little more than one and a half century back, though history of modern skin diseases started another three centuries back when Girolamo Mercuriale (1530–1606) **(Fig. 1)** published the first ever book on skin diseases *"De Morbis Cutaneis..."* in 1572. The first hospital dedicated for the treatment of skin diseases was Hôpital Saint Louis of Paris started as early as November 27, 1801.

EVOLUTION OF MODERN DERMATOLOGY

The sojourn began much earlier with the endeavor of Mercuriale, Paulus Aegineta, Riolan, Haffenreffer, and others. The period between AD 1500 and 1900 witnessed a tremendous development in the field of dermatology. Though syphilis proved its first presence in Europe in 1493 in Spain, it got its

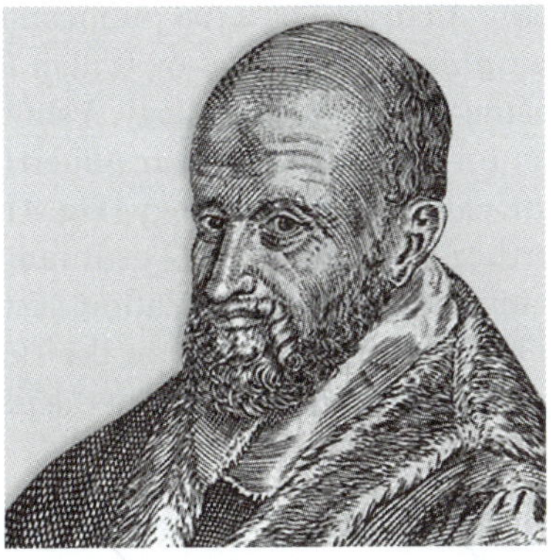

Fig. 1: Portrait of Girolamo Mercuriale.

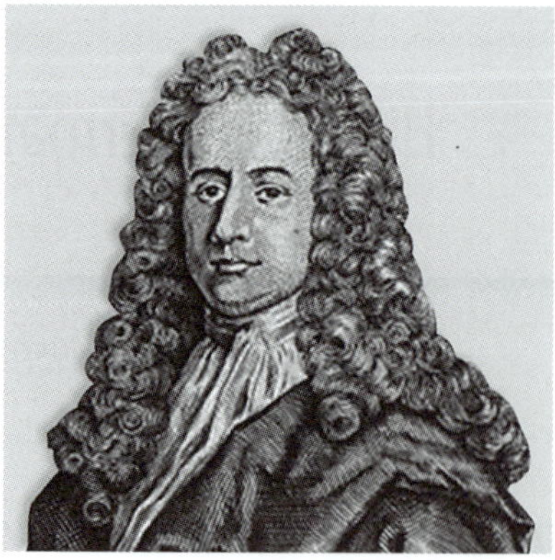

Fig. 2: Daniel Turner.

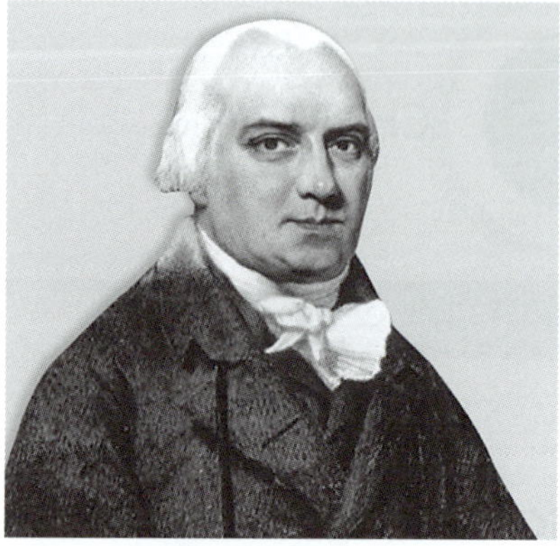

Fig. 3: Robert Willan.

name from Girolamo Fracastoro's poem "Syphilis Sive Morbus Gallicus." Ambroise Paré (1510–1590) described itch mite, and Bonomo in 1687 gave a clinical description and cause of scabies. Bernardino Ramazzini (1633–1714) told about the temporal relation between trades and occupation and various skin problems. Herman Boerhaave (1668–1738) described "cryptae sebacae," the structure of sebaceous glands. Jean Austrac (1684–1766) tried to explain the cutaneous lesion on the basis of anatomical structure. Daniel Turner (1667–1741) **(Fig. 2)**, who authored *de Morbis Cutaneis: A Treatise of Diseases Incident to the Skin*, the first book in English language on skin diseases (1736), described about herpes. Thus, an era of great development and observation began.

The 18th and early-to-mid 19th century became busy with classification of skin diseases. Though the effort started since Hippocrates, it was de Sauvages (1706–1767) who tried to classify skin diseases on the basis of external symptoms. Charles-Anne Lorry found his way of classifying skin diseases in the line of botanical classification of Carl Linnaeus. Joseph Jacob Ritter von Plenck (1735–1807), a man of diverse talent, first gave a relatively more logical classification in 1776 which formed the very basis of Willan's epoch-making classification of skin diseases. Robert Willan (1757–1812) **(Fig. 3)**, rightly considered as the father of modern dermatology, was the man who gave a classification system that changed the way of thinking and interpretation of dermatological diseases on both sides of the Atlantic. The 1798 publication of the first section of *On Cutaneous Diseases* by Willan is considered the birthday of the modern dermatology. A similar but short-lasted effort came from Jean-Louis-Marc Alibert (1768–1837)), the father figure of French dermatology **(Fig. 4)**. The process witnessed further progress when Ferdinand von Hebra (1816–1880) advocated his classification system that was based on the pathological anatomy of the skin in 1845. It rendered all previous systems a record of the past.[3]

INVESTIGATIVE DERMATOLOGY: A LOOK BACK

The discovery of a microscope in 1590 had a direct impact on dermatology. A microscopic view of the skin opened the door of a different world. Nicolaus Steno, a Danish physician, gave an early description of sweat gland. Marcello Malpighi discovered sebaceous gland and told the scientific world about the pigmentation of the Negro skin in the 17th century. The French physician Jean Austrac studied the structure of the skin. The whole phenomena of microscopy and histological approach witnessed a havoc change with the publication of the *Cellular pathology*... the *Magnum opus* by Rudolph Virchow (1821–1902). The process received a further thrust with the publication of Gustav Simon's *Die Hautkrankheiten Durch Anatomische Untersuchungen Erläutert*, the first ever dermatopathology textbook in 1848. The further work of Rokitansky and his ardent follower Hebra consolidated the position of pathological basis of dermatological diseases. The whole story came to its maturity with the publication of *The Histopathology of the Diseases of the Skin* by Paul Gerson Unna.

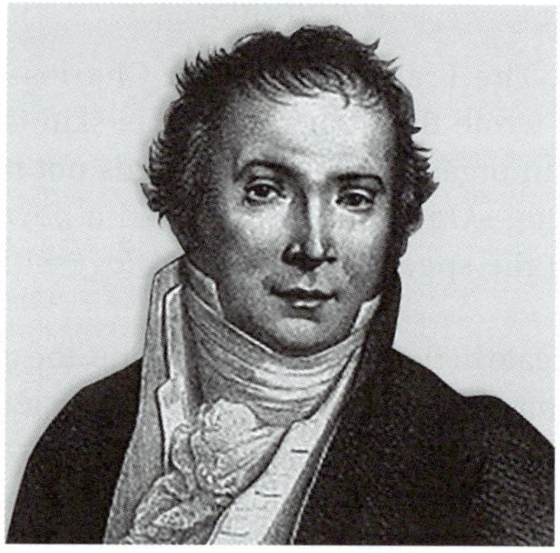

Fig. 4: Jean Louis Alibert.

Another most important landmark in the investigative dermatology is the contribution of the legendary figure of Breslau Clinic Josef Jadassohn (1863–1936) whose "patch test" began a new chapter. It was further enriched by the work of Marion Sulzberger (1895–1984).

EMERGENCE OF NEWER MANAGEMENTS

As skin is easily approachable, almost any and everything has been tried since antiquity. This trial and error, sometimes even the fruit of rich imagination, ultimately led to the development of modern dermatological therapeutics. In the past "medicine" comprised of fat of lion, hippopotamus (in Mesopotamia), milk of ass, herbs and metals and nonmetals were used save the story of leech application.[4,5]

The modern-day treatment started since the last 300 years or so when Paracelsus (1492–1541) first used Mercury in 1529 for the treatment of syphilis. The use of antimonials and arsenics in the various skin diseases is of historical interest. The innovation of "606" (Salvarsan) by Paul Ehrlich became the treatment of choice for many diseases. The discovery of Penicillin in 1928 by Alexander Fleming in London ushered in a new era in the antimicrobial therapy.[6]

It was a work entitled "investigations of the hormones of the adrenal cortex" that brought the Nobel prize to Philip Hench, Edward Kendall, and Tadeus Reichstein in 1950 and began a new age in the field of medicine in general and dermatology in particular. The discovery of corticosteroid not only saved the life of millions but also led us unearthing the etiology of many diseases that were clueless.[7]The journey of heliotherapy that started since antiquity gave birth to the phototherapy and photodynamic therapy of today. Niels Ryberg Finsen (1860–1904) in 1896 cured his friend's lupus vulgaris with his "chemical rays" lamp. He was awarded Nobel Prize in 1903 for his work on treatment of skin diseases with light.[8] In 1904, Bernhard first employed heliotherapy for the treatment of skin ulcer. In 1962, Allyn was a pioneer in using 8-methoxypsoralen (MOP) along with UV radiation in the treatment of psoriasis and in 1969 Fulton used topical 8-MOP in vitiligo. William Pusey first used radiation treatment for skin diseases and Sabouraud along with Noiré used radiation therapy for the management of scalp ringworm.

The story of LASER started in 1917. Gordon Gould coined the term LASER. In 1962, Leon Goldman first tried to destroy melanin in hair follicles with ruby laser. The use of cryotherapy was first used by Arnott to destroy tumors in the mid-19th century. Worth, in 1907, used cryotherapy in the management of warts, naevi, etc.

Dermatologic surgery has a long history. Thermocautery and chemical cautery have been mentioned in ancient Indian Ayurvedic texts such as *Sushruta Samhita*. Today, there are various surgical procedures such as excision, grafting, and repairing of various dermatologic defects and diseases. The availability of dermabrasion, fillers, and botulinum toxins made management of skin diseases most sophisticated now. In 1941, Frederic Mohs published his chemosurgical approach for the removal of skin tumor and this established the very basic of Mohs' surgery widely practiced at present.[6]

BOOKS AND PERIODICALS OF EARLY ERA

Since Mercuriale's publication in 1572, many treatises were published which regularly incorporated the growing knowledge on the subject. In terms of modern dermatology, Willan's *On Cutaneous Diseases* (1798) **(Fig. 5)** marked the beginning. This other remarkable work was by Alibert's *Description des Maladies de la Peau* in 1806 and *Nosology* **(Fig. 6)**. This was followed by various other famous treatises and atlases by Bateman, Cazenave, Worcester, Dowling, Duhring, Fox, and Neligan, to name a few. The foremost dermatology journals were *Syphilidologie* (1839–1845) and *Annales Des Maladies de la Peau* (1844–1851). The *Journal*

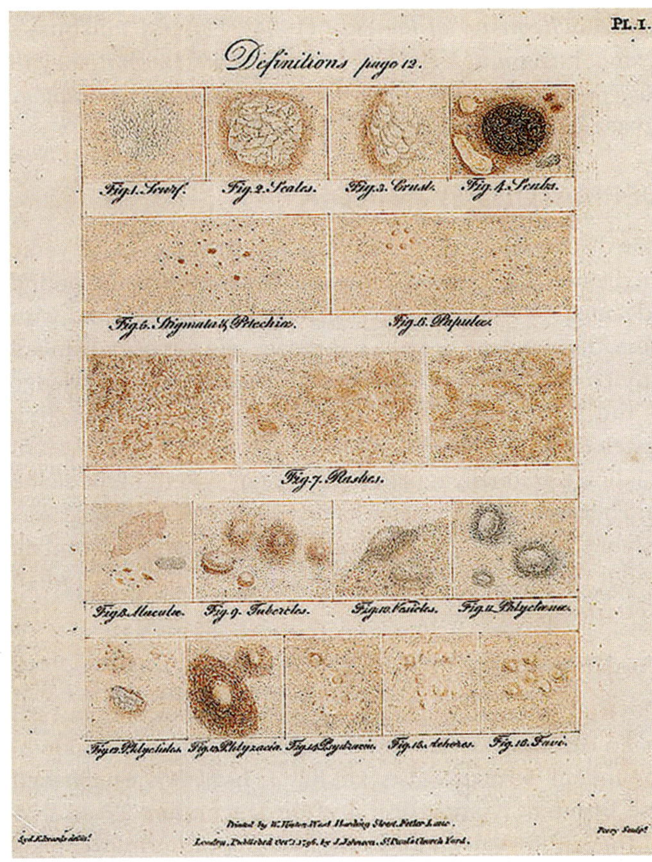

Fig. 5: On cutaneous diseases (1808) by Robert Willan.

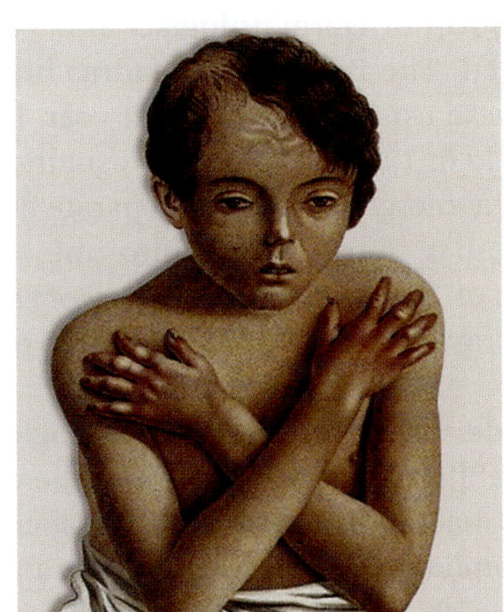

Fig. 6: "Scrophulemomie" by Alibert (1817).

of Investigative Dermatology is another milestone, dedicated to the investigative dermatology. In India, Dr U B Narayan Rao published the "*Indian Journal of Venereal Diseases and Dermatology*" in 1935 which subsequently changed its name to "*Indian Journal of Dermatology and Venereology*" in 1955 to be rechristened as "*Indian Journal of Dermatology, Venereology and Leprology*" in 1973. In 1955, "*Indian Journal of Dermatology*" started its journey and remained the only Indian dermatology journal indexed in Index Medicus from 1962 till 1990. The few "Bibles" of modern-day dermatology need mention. Stephen Rothman's *Physiology and Biochemistry of the Skin* (1954), Donald Pillsbury's textbook *Dermatology* (1956), Fitzpatrick's *Dermatology in General Medicine* (1965), and Rook's *Textbook of Dermatology* (1968) are some of them.[3,9]

DERMATOLOGY IN INDIA

Skin diseases were described since the early days of the Vedic medicine. The Ayurvedic treatises of the later Vedic period advanced to the level of classifying skin diseases and with time, dermatology in India has grown into a most advanced branch of medicine **(Table 1)**.[10] The addition of knowledge of the Siddha and Unani medicine enriched the existing system. With the establishment of the British rule, the Western medicine gradually replaced the Indian system of medicine and became the mainstay. The first chair of dermatology was established in 1875 at the Grant Medical College, Mumbai, under care of Major C Fernandez—the "founder of Indian Dermatology".

Evolution of IADVL

The true Indian dermatology began its journey only in 1935 when UB Narayan Rao first thought about an association of the Indian dermatologists. On July 1, 1947, Rao established the Bombay Association and on December 27 and 28 of the same year an all-India meeting of dermatologists was convened at the JJ Hospital, Mumbai. Dr RV Rajam was the first president. On December 28, 1947, the All-India Association of Dermatologists and Venereologists was established. The Bengal and Madras branches of the association were established the next year. In the second conference held in 1951 at Calcutta, a resolution was passed which led to the merger of all three separate bodies, namely Calcutta, Bombay, and Madras, into one singular body under the title of "The Indian Association of Dermatologists and Venereologists (IADV)." The founder president was Dr AC Rebello.

In a new development, the Dermatological Society of India was established in Calcutta under the chairmanship of Major AM Chakraborty in 1960. This association and the IADV took an initiative to form a single body and accordingly met on August 20, 1972, to formulate the future course of action; this resulted into the development of present-day

TABLE 1: Timeline of major events of dermatology in India.[10]

Time period	*Events*
1500–800 BC	*Vedas* including *Atharvaveda* mentioned many skin diseases
600 BC to AD 800	Evolution of *Ayurveda*. Beginning of systemic approach
600 ? BC	*Sushruta Samhita*
200 BC to AD 100 ?	*Charaka Samhita*
AD 800–1300	Muslim invasion and introduction of Unani system
AD 1757	Establishment of the British Empire in India
AD 1835	Medical colleges established in Calcutta and Madras
AD 1869	Dr Bhau Daji Lad claimed effective treatment of leprosy with Hydnocarpus oil
AD 1871	First leprosy survey
AD 1872	Tilbury Fox and T Farquhar surveyed the prevalence and pattern of skin diseases in India
AD 1881	Donovanosis first recognized by Kenneth Mcleod in Madras
AD 1895	First chair of dermatology (Grant Medical College, Bombay)
AD 1898	"Indian Lepers Act" promulgated
AD 1905	Col. Charles identified causative organism of donovanosis (Madras)
AD 1923	Dermatology department established at the School of Tropical Medicine, Calcutta
AD 1926	First inpatient department of dermatology (Seth GS Medical College and KEM Hospital)
AD 1935	Bombay Association of Dermatology established. Dr UB Narayan Rao first started publication of the "India Journal of Venereal Diseases and Dermatology"
AD 1940	Sulfone became available for leprosy
AD 1942	Dharmendra developed "Lepromin"
AD 1947	The first all-India conference of the association (IADVL): December 27 and 28
AD 1955	Indian Journal of Venereal Diseases and Dermatology changed to Indian Journal of Dermatology and Venereology Indian Journal of Dermatology was first published
AD 1973	"Indian Association of Dermatologists, Venereologists and Leprologists" established on January 28
AD 1981–82	Multidrug Therapy (MDT) for leprosy started in India
AD 1984	International Leprosy Congress held in New Delhi
AD 1987	National AIDS control program launched
AD 1994	"IADVL Textbook and Atlas of Dermatology" published
AD 1996	Indian Society for Pediatric Dermatology established
AD 2000	Goal to eradicate leprosy from the country declared

Contd...

Contd...

Time period	*Events*
AD 2005	Elimination of leprosy at the national level
AD 2006	Website of the IADVL (www.iadvl.org) launched (August 6)
AD 2007	IADVL awarded full member status by ILDS
AD 2010	Indian Dermatology Online Journal (IDOJ) published
AD 2013	IADVL hosted the XI International Congress of Dermatology at New Delhi
AD 2018	The print issue of IDOJ rolled out

Days to remember	
January 28	IADVL Day
January 30	Leprosy Day
May 19	Vitiligo Day
December 1	HIV Day
Second day of DERMACON	IADVL Felicitation Day

Indian Association for Dermatologists, Venereologists and Leprologists (IADVL) on January 28, 1973. The first president of IADVL was Dr BN Banerjee and Hony. General Secretary was Dr LK Bhutani. The association was registered at Lucknow on May 8, 1975. The logo which we see today was designed by Dr SB Mondal. The IADVL website www.iadvl.com that was formed in 2001 initially was subsequently updated to www.iadvl.org under the able guidance of Drs Koushik Lahiri and Suresh Joshipura. IADVL has played an important role in the arena of international dermatology. It is an active member of SARAD (South Asian Regional Association for Dermatologists, Venereologists and Leprologists) and International League for Dermatological Societies (ILDS).[11-13] The seed that was sown had now grown into a big tree with a mammoth strength of more than 13,000 (August, 2020) members with a significant presence in the international fora.[14]

CONCLUSION

It may be summarized that one should know the history of his subject to grasp the underlying philosophy. We should know the deeds of our forerunners to realize the way they strove to deliver us the most developed knowledge with which we thrive and boast today. It can be concluded with words of Rokitansky: *Those about to study Medicine, and the younger Physicians should light their torches at the fire of the Ancients.*

KEY POINTS

- Diseases of the skin were known since antiquity.
- Many ancient texts such as Vedas, Zend Avesta, various papyri and scrolls, Torah, Talmud, and Old Testament mention skin diseases.
- Robert Willan first gave the modern classification of skin diseases.
- Indian dermatology took shape with the effort of Dr UB Narayan Rao who started publishing the first-ever Indian journal in 1935.
- Dermatology has now many subspecialties and is growing further.

REFERENCES

1. Mukhoadhyay AK. Skin diseases ('Dermatology') in India: History and evolution. Calcutta: Allied Book Agency; 2011.
2. Holubar K, Wallach D. History of dermatology: a bicentennial perspective. In: Freedberg IM, Eisen AZ, Wolff K, Austen KF, Goldsmith LA, Katz SI (Eds). Fitzpatrick's Dermatology in General Medicine, 5th edition. New York: McGraw-Hill; 1999. pp. 5-7.
3. Mukhopadhyay AK. On the history of classification in dermatology. Indian J Dermatol. 2016;61(6):588-92.
4. Hunter JA. Turning points in dermatology during the 20th century. Br J Dermatol. 2000;143(1):30-40.
5. Radbill SX. Pediatric dermatology in antiquity. Int J Dermatol. 1975;14(5):363-68.
6. Tan SY, Tatsumura Y. Alexander Fleming (1881-1955): Discoverer of penicillin. Singapore Med J. 2015;56(7):366-7.
7. Burns CM. The history of cortisone discovery and development. Rheum Dis Clin North Am. 2016;42(1):1-14.
8. Al Aboud KM, Al Aboud AM, Hawasawai KA, Ramesh V. Awards in medicine and dermatology. J Ayub Med Col Abbottabad. 2006;18(1):78-80.
9. Potter BS. Bibliographic landmarks in the history of Dermatology. J Am Acad Dermatol. 2000;48(6):919-32.
10. Mukhopadhyay AK. Dermatology in India and Indian dermatology: A medico-historical perspective (editorial). Indian Dermatol Online J. 2016;7(4):235-43.
11. IADVL. The Constitution: Rules and Byelaws, 5th edition. Kolkata: Indian Association of Dermatologists, Venereologists and Leprologists; 2006.
12. Khopkar U, Thappa DM. History of the IADVL (Indian Association of Dermatologists, Venereologists and Leprologists. Mumbai: Medknow Publications; 2010.
13. Thappa DM, Kumari R. Establishment of IADVL and its present day status. Indian J Dermatol Venereol Leprol. 2009; 75:204-10.
14. Feroz K. Honorary Secretary General speaks. In: Feroz K (Ed). IADVL News. 2020;16(2):7-9.

EXAMINATION QUESTIONS

Write short notes on the following:

1. Evolution of dermatology as a separate branch of medicine.
2. Evolution of investigative dermatology.

CHAPTER 2

Embryology of Skin

Deepika Pandhi, Anita Kulhari

INTRODUCTION

The epidermis, the outermost component of the skin, is the primary barrier that protects the body from dehydration, mechanical trauma, and microbial insults. The epidermis is separated from the underlying dermis by the basement membrane, which consists of proteins secreted by epidermal keratinocytes and by dermal fibroblasts.

The two compartments of the skin, the dermis and the epidermis, function cooperatively and together are responsible for the development of epidermal appendages, including hair follicles and mammary glands.

The skin is composed of cell types of both ectodermal and mesodermal origin.

Flowchart 1: Gastrulation.

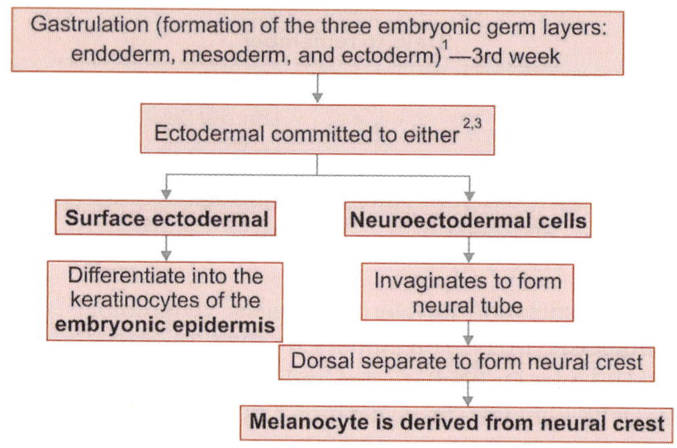

ECTODERMAL

- Epithelial structures, i.e., epidermis (surface and infundibular)
- Apocrine units
- Eccrine units
- Sebaceous units
- Hair follicles
- Nail units

Neuroectoderm

- Melanocytes
- Nerves
- Specialized sensory receptors

Mesodermal

- Langerhans cells (LCs)
- Macrophages
- Mast cells
- Fibrocytes
- Blood vessels
- Lymph vessels
- Muscles
- Adipocytes

EMBRYONIC ORIGIN OF THE SKIN

During the third week, the embryo undergoes gastrulation, a complex process resulting in the formation of the three embryonic germ layers: (1) Endoderm, (2) mesoderm, and (3) ectoderm. During the next stage of embryogenesis, ectodermal cells commit to either a surface ectodermal or neuroectodermal fate **(Flowchart 1)**. The surface ectodermal cells eventually differentiate into the keratinocytes of the embryonic epidermis, whereas the neuroectodermal cells invaginate to create the neural tube in a process called neurulation.

SIGNALING[3]

As development progresses, the single-layered embryonic epidermis expresses Wnts. Some cells fail to respond to Wnts, and these become fated to become epidermal cells through bone morphogenetic protein (BMP), epidermal growth factor (EGF), and Notch signaling. The cells that do respond to Wnt signaling also receive underlying fibroblast growth factor (FGF) and BMP inhibitory signals from the mesenchyme and, together, these signals instruct the cells to make an appendage. Collectively, the inhibition of BMP inhibitory signals and Wnt activating signals produce the hair placode **(Flowchart 2 and Fig. 1)**. Additional dermal messages from below further instruct the placodes to make the follicle.[3]

EPIDERMAL DEVELOPMENT

Surface ectoderm forms the embryonic epidermis **(Fig. 1)**.[3-7]

- *4th week*:
  - Epidermis begins to form from surface ectoderm.

- It is composed solely of a basal layer of cuboidal cells above mesenchyme or future dermis.
- *5th week*:
  - Periderm is formed.
  - It is a single cell layer that covers the developing epidermis until the cornified cell layer is formed above the basal layer.
  - *Function of periderm*: Exchange substances across fetal skin and protect the developing epidermis.
- *8th week*:
  - Intermediate cell layer is formed between the basal layer and the periderm.
  - Beginning of embryonic epidermal stratification
- *8–12 weeks*:
  - Epidermal stratification begins.
  - Appearance of melanocytes, Merkel cells, and LCs
- *20 weeks*: Additional layers of intermediate cells are formed to form four more superficial strata of epidermis.
- *22–24 weeks*:
  - Cells in the intermediate layer withdraw from the cell cycle permanently and differentiate into spinous and granular cells.
  - Cornification begins, occurring first in the skin on the head, palms, and soles [early cornification can be observed within the hair canal at approximately 15 weeks' estimated gestational age (EGA)]

Flowchart 2: Signaling steps in specification of embryonic skin.

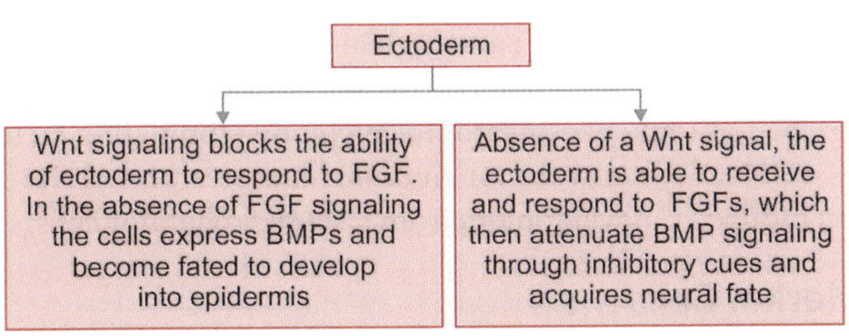

(BMP: bone morphogenetic protein; FGF: fibroblast growth factor)

- *24–26 weeks*: Cornified cell layer composed of dead keratinocyte is formed.
- *24 weeks*: The periderm detaches from the underlying epidermis and is sloughed off into the amniotic fluid, with remnants forming vernix caseosa that coats the newborn.
- During the third trimester, the number of keratohyalin and lamellar granules as well as stratum corneum layers increases.
- By the mid third trimester, the epidermis is morphologically similar to adult skin although it does not acquire full barrier function until a few weeks after birth.

Clinical Significance

Mosaic Skin Conditions

- Follow the lines of Blaschko.
- Represent the migration pathways of epidermal cells during embryonic development.
- Examples include epidermal nevi and sebaceous nevi.

Abnormal Epidermal Barrier Function

Lamellar ichthyosis or congenital ichthyosiform erythroderma results from mutations in the same set of genes that encode proteins essential for formation of the epidermal barrier, including transglutaminase-1 (an enzyme that cross-links lipids to the cornified cell envelope; TGM1), lipid processing enzymes (*ALOXE3, ALOX12B*), and lipid transporters (*ABCA12*). There may be development of collodion membrane.

Premature Infants

Stratum corneum matures rapidly till the end of the first week of life but achieving full maturation may take >4 weeks. The process of maturation differs with gestational age; with <25 weeks of gestational age, it takes 8–10 weeks for stratum corneum to mature, while in those of >27–28 weeks of gestational age it reaches full maturity in about 10 days. Hence, in premature infants, especially those born before 28 weeks, the immaturity of the stratum corneum results in impaired

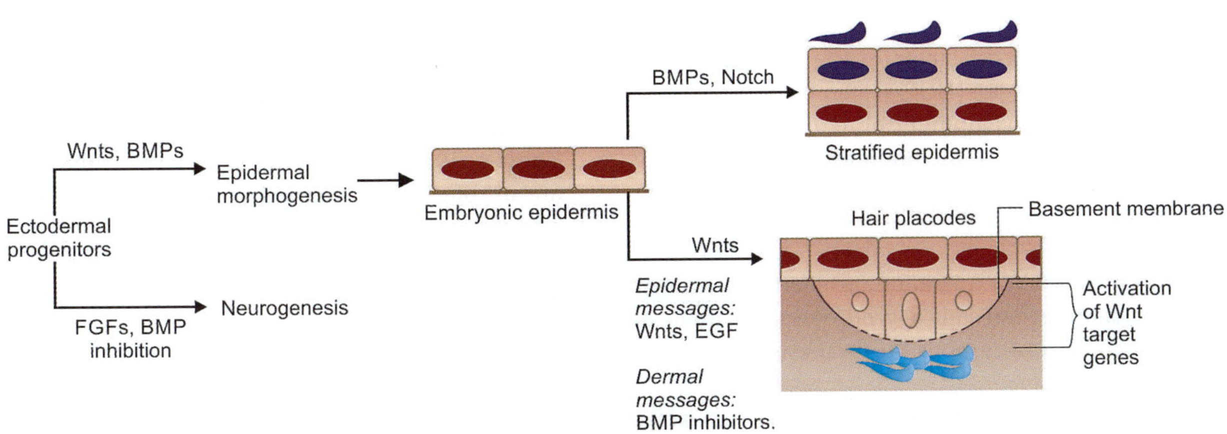

Fig. 1: Early signaling steps in specification of embryonic skin.[3]
(BMP: bone morphogenetic protein; EGF: epidermal growth factor; FGF: fibroblast growth factor)

barrier function, an increased risk of infection, dehydration, and excessive absorption of topical medications or chemicals.[8]

The epidermis is derived from the embryonic surface ectoderm. After epidermal commitment, the surface ectoderm becomes the embryonic epidermal basal layer, which subsequently gives rise to the intermediate layer, spinous layer, granular layer, and cornified layer.[9]

DEVELOPMENT OF SPECIALIZED CELLS WITHIN THE EPIDERMIS

There are three nonkeratinocytic cells in epidermis:

1. Melanocytes
2. LCs
3. Merkel cells

They migrate to the epidermis during early embryonic development.

Melanocytes

- Derived from the neural crest that forms along the dorsal neural tube.
- Melanocyte precursors migrate following a characteristic trajectory, moving dorsolaterally and then ventrally around the trunk to the ventral midline, anteriorly over the scalp and face, and distally along the extremities.
- *50 days*:
  - Melanocytes can be identified within the epidermis.
  - The number initially is approximately 1,000 cells/mm^2.

  At 80–90 days, it is approximately 3,000 cells/mm^2.

  Later, in gestation, it becomes similar to that of adults (800–1,500 cells/mm^2).
- *3–4 months*: Melanin production begins.
- *5 months*: Melanosome transfer to keratinocytes begins.

Signaling Molecules: Significance?

Various signaling pathways are required for the development of melanocytes from their precursors in the embryonic neural crest which are:

- Wnt
- Endothelin (ET)-3
- BMPs
- Steel factor (SF) [stem cell factor (SCF), c-kit ligand]
- Hepatocyte growth factor (HGF/scatter factor)

Wnt promote the development of neural crest cells to melanocytes and signals to melanoblasts to increase the number of melanocytes.

Clinical Significance

- Defects in melanoblast migration, proliferation, and/or survival occur in several clinical syndromes, and many of the genetic mutations responsible for these defects have been identified.
- Failure of an adequate number of melanoblasts to completely supply distal points on their embryonic migration path occurs in the different types of Waardenburg syndrome, as well as in piebaldism, resulting in depigmented patches on the central forehead, central abdomen, and extremities. These defects are associated with mutations in several different genes, including genes encoding transcription factors, as well as membrane receptors and their ligands, such as endothelin 3, endothelin-receptor B, and c-kit.
- In albinism, melanocyte development is normal, but production of pigment or melanin is inadequate. This results from null mutations in the gene encoding tyrosinase, the rate-limiting enzyme in the production of melanin, and mutations in other genes encoding proteins important in melanin assembly in melanosomes or their transportation.
- *Dermal melanocytoses and blue nevi*: Represent melanocytes that have not migrated completely from the neural crest to the epidermis during the embryonic stage

Langerhans Cells[10]

- Langerhans cells reside in the epidermis as a dense network of immune system sentinels. These cells determine the appropriate adaptive immune response.
- They are detectable as early as 40 days' EGA.
- These cells originate from hemopoietic progenitor cells in the yolk sac or fetal liver, the primary sites of hemopoiesis during the embryonic period.
- Until week 14 of EGA, these cells acquire the full phenotypic profile of LC, i.e., the CD1a, Langerin, and Birbeck granules.
- Characteristic dendritic morphology; expression of CD45, HLA-DR, and CD1c; and high levels of ATPase activity
- The density of human LCs decreases with age.
- SCF, granulocyte-macrophage colony-stimulating factor (GM-CSF), and tumor necrosis factor alpha (TNF-α) induce LC development from CD34+ progenitor cells.

Merkel Cells

- They are detected as early as 8–12 weeks' EGA in palmoplantar epidermis and slightly later in interfollicular skin.
- Merkel cells are identified by the presence of cytoplasmic dense core granules and the expression of cytokeratin 20 and neuropeptides.
- These cells are found in the basal layer of the epidermis and are often associated with appendages and nerve fibers and are particularly dense on volar skin.

DEVELOPMENT OF THE DERMIS AND SUBCUTIS

- The origin of the dermis varies depending on the body site.
- The dermal mesenchyme of the face and anterior scalp as well as the underlying muscle and bone is derived from neural crest ectoderm.

- The dermal mesenchyme of the back originates from the dermomyotome of the embryonic somite.
- The dermal mesenchyme of the extremities and ventral trunk arise from the lateral plate mesoderm.
- *6–8 weeks' EGA*: Presumptive dermal fibroblasts are situated under the developing epidermis.
- *9 weeks' EGA*: The demarcation between the dermis and the underlying skeletal condensations becomes distinct.
- *By 12–15 weeks' EGA*: Distinction can be made between fine weave of the papillary and thicker, deeper reticular dermis.
- *22–24 weeks' EGA*: First definitive elastic fibers detected.
- By the end of the second trimester, the dermis shifts from a nonscarring to a scarring form of wound repair.

VASCULAR

- Blood vessels develop according to two fundamental processes. Vasculogenesis refers to embryonic formation of vessels, which arise in situ from primordial endothelial cells and angiogenesis, to the growth of new vessels from the vasculature during development and remodeling in adults.
- By 45–50 days, horizontal vascular plexuses are formed within the subpapillary and deep reticular dermis, which are interconnected by groups of vertical vessels.
- By 3 months, the distinct horizontal and vertical networks are formed.
- By 5 months, vasculogenesis has largely ceased and the formation of the complex vascular plexus is initiated by angiogenesis, the budding and migration of endothelium from pre-existing vessels.
- By approximately 3 months of age, the vascular patterns more closely resemble those of the adult.
- Molecular controls involved in the regulation of angiogenesis are vascular endothelial growth factor (VEGF) family as well as the tyrosine kinase receptors Tie-1 and Tie-2 and their stimulatory (Ang-1) and inhibitory (Ang-2) angiopoietin ligands.

Clinical Significance

Errors in neurovascular morphogenesis likely lead to several relatively common syndromes such as Klippel–Trénaunay, Sturge–Weber, and PHACES syndromes.

NERVES

- The nerves of the skin consist of somatic sensory and sympathetic autonomic fibers that are predominantly small and unmyelinated.
- 7.5-week fetus-free nerve endings can be visualized beneath the epithelium.
- *Mid-to-late first trimester*: Nerve networks are formed but also undergo significant remodeling during later development and early postnatal life.

DEVELOPMENT OF THE HYPODERMIS AND ADIPOSE TISSUE

- The hypodermis can be delineated by 50–60 days' EGA.
- It is a distinct region that is separated from the overlying cellular dermis by a plane of thin-walled vessels.
- Toward the end of the first trimester, the sparse matrix of the hypodermis can be distinguished morphologically from the slightly denser, more fibrous matrix of the dermis.
- In the second trimester, mesenchymally derived pre-adipocytes begin to differentiate and accumulate lipids.
- By the third trimester, the more mature adipocytes are aggregated into large lobules of fat divided by fibrous septa.

Clinical Relevance

- Mutations in genes that encode dermal structural proteins (e.g., collagens, elastic fibers) and their processing enzymes are seen in Ehlers–Danlos syndrome and cutis laxa
- Abnormal dermal development is seen in Goltz syndrome (focal dermal hypoplasia), caused by mutations in *PORCN*, an effector of the Wnt signaling pathway.
- Adipose tissue plays an active endocrine role with effects on vascular and immune function. An example is the gene that encodes leptin, whose abnormal regulation has been implicated in the pathogenesis of obesity.

DERMOEPIDERMAL JUNCTION

- The dermoepidermal junction (DEJ) is the region where the epidermis and dermis abut.
- Both dermal and epidermal compartments contribute to the molecular synthesis, assembly, and integration of this region.
- A simple basement membrane, separating the dermis and epidermis, can be discerned as early as 8 weeks' EGA.
- The basic protein constituents common to all basement membranes can be detected immunohistochemically at this stage which include collagen IV, laminin, heparin sulfate, and proteoglycans.
- Specialized components of the DEJ do not appear until after the embryonic–fetal transition, around the time of initial epidermal stratification.
- All basement membrane antigens are in place by the end of the first trimester.

Clinical Applications

Epidermolysis bullosa (EB) can result from mutations in genes that encode several different components of the DEJ.

NAIL[11,12]

The nail apparatus develops and matures from the primitive epidermis primarily between the 9th and 20th week of intrauterine life **(Fig. 2)**.

Nail development can be divided into two components: (1) Morphogenesis and (2) tissue differentiation.

Morphogenesis

- *8 weeks*: Individual digits are identified. The epithelium that will become a future nail unit at first is indistinguishable from the adjacent epidermis.
- *9 weeks*:
  - The dorsal tip of digit is covered by epidermis, and an invagination of this primitive skin gives rise to the nail analge.
  - Nail analge is the first embryonic element of nail unit.
- *10 weeks*:
  - Primary nail field with proximal, distal, and lateral grooves seen.
  - The primary nail field grows downward and proximally by a wedge of germinative matrix cells extending back from the tip of the digit.
  - These germinative matrix cells forming the nail matrix primordium are presented proximal to both distal groove and ridge.
  - These structures give rise to vestigial distal groove and hyponychium.
- *13–14 weeks*:
  - Differential growth of the slowly developing primary nail field and surrounding tissue results in the emergence of overhanging proximal and lateral nail folds.
  - Nail field is well demarcated, with the matrix primordium underlying a proximal nail fold and four components of the epithelium of a developing nail unit are visualized histologically, namely, the basal, spinous, granular, and cornified layers.
- *By 14 weeks*:
  - The proximal part of a nail bed comes to be covered by a firm plate of cornified cells that is derived from the matrix and represents the developing nail plate that can be visualized underneath the proximal nail fold.
  - By week 16, the morphogenesis is almost complete and a fetal nail is discernible.
- *At 17 weeks*: The nail plate covers most of the nail bed and the distal ridge has flattened.
- *From 20 weeks:*
  - The matrix cells show a postnatal type cell division, differentiation, and keratinization.
  - The nail unit and finger grow in tandem, with the nail plate abutting the distal ridge.
- *By 36 weeks*: The nail plate reaches the tip of digit by growing and extending to the distal groove, and there is well-formed cuticle and lateral nail folds.

Tissue Differentiation

- Keratin synthesis starts early and it can be identified from early stages of differentiation.
- At 12–13th week the nail matrix analge, which is a thin epithelial wedge, is considered to represent the ventral matrix primordium.
- Keratin represents 80% of the intracellular structural protein of epithelial cells.
- At 15 weeks, hard keratin is present throughout nail bed and matrix.

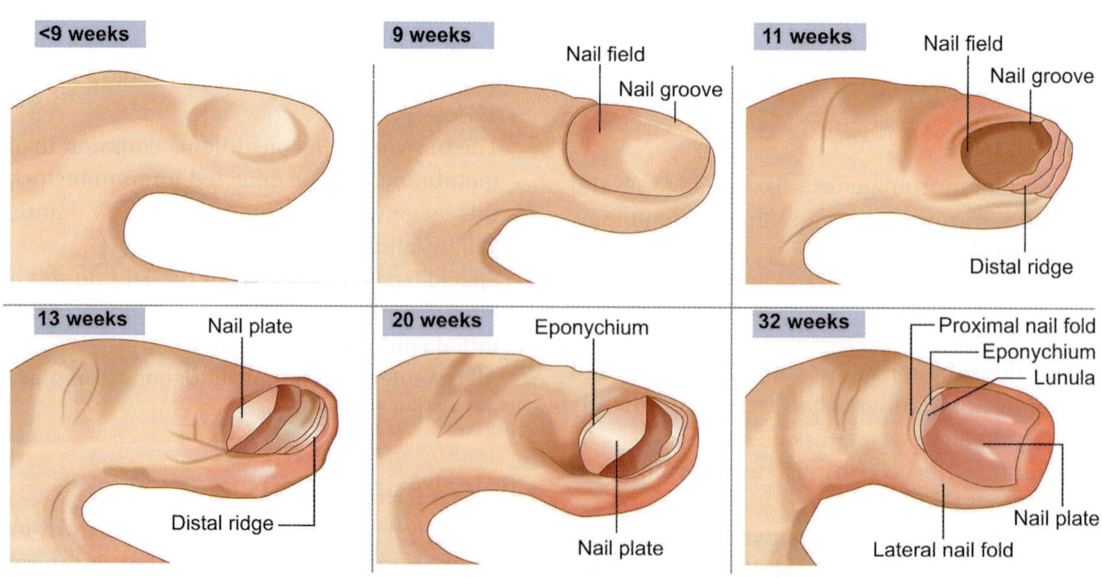

Fig. 2: Fetal development of the nail apparatus.[13]

- At 22 weeks, the proportion of keratinocytes having hard keratin in nail bed is low while it is significantly higher in the matrix.
- Nail differentiation is mostly complete by the 25th week although some chemical alterations in nail constituents may continue till birth.

HAIR[14-20]

Hair follicle formation is the result of complex sequential signaling events between the dermal mesenchyme and the overlying epithelium.

Hair follicle formation events are divided into eight distinct developmental stages.

The development of human hair follicles first starts between the 8th and 12th weeks of gestation:

- *Stage 1*: The first stage is detailed in **Table 1**.
- *Stage 2—Early peg:* The hair placode elongates toward the dermis while the underlying "cap" of dermal fibroblast condensate becomes more evident.
- *Stage 3—Hair peg:* The epidermal cells form a multilayered and elongated column called the hair peg and dermal condensate becomes a spherical dermal papilla (DP) in adjacent to the hair peg.
- *Stage 4—Bulbous hair peg stage:* By 12–14 weeks' gestation, the epithelial base of the hair pegs on the scalp invaginates to envelop the dermal cell condensates and form DP.

  A corn-shaped inner root sheath (IRS) forms above the DP.
- *Stage 5*:
  - *13–16 weeks' gestation*: The superficial portions of the hair follicles subsequently develop two distinct, asymmetrical bulges of cells on the "posterior" side of the follicle, which is at an obtuse angle to the skin surface.
  - The upper bulge closest to the skin surface eventually forms the sebaceous gland.
  - The lower bulge forms the location of the presumptive follicular stem cells and will later anchor the developing arrector pili muscle to the hair follicle.
  - Some hair follicles will develop a third superficial bulge of cells above the cells destined to become the sebaceous gland, which indicates the formation of an apocrine gland, for example, over the face and scalp.
  - In the second trimester, the hair follicles differentiate to eventually form the seven layers of cells in concentric cylinders seen in mature hair follicles.
  - Beginning near the bulb at the end of stage 4 or at the beginning of stage 5, a core of epithelial cells separates from the peripheral epithelial cells which later become the outer root sheath, continuous with the nonfollicular epithelium.
  - The epithelial cell core, resting on the top of the DP, further differentiates into the IRS Henle, Huxley, and cuticle layers, and the central core of matrix cells that proliferate and give rise to the hair fiber cuticle, cortex and, later in terminal hairs, the medulla.
- *Stage 6*: Defined by the visible development and growth of the hair fiber
- *Stage 7*: By 19–21 weeks, hair canals form.
- *Stage 8*:
  - The hair follicles are fully formed and the first hair fibers erupt from the skin.
  - The initial lanugo hair of the first anagen hair growth phase grows until 24–28 weeks of gestation.

TABLE 1: Hair germ or hair placode.

Signals	*Hair follicle morphogenesis*
1st signal	• At 10 weeks • *Epithelial placode:* Collection of primitive epithelium cells to form placodes in response to dermal signaling element • The very first hair follicle placodes are seen in the eyebrow, upper lip, and chin regions • Placode formation subsequently expands in a wave caudally and ventrally over the skin of the fetus
2nd signal	Arise from epithelial placode and induce the aggregation of underlying dermal cells to form mesenchymal condensates—the first visible stage in hair follicle development
3rd signal	• The dermal condensates send signal to initial proliferation and differentiation of placode cells and initiate penetration of the dermis • The hair follicles grow into the dermis at an angle to the skin surface, with the degree of angle determined by the location of the hair follicle

Molecular Mediation of Hair Follicle Morphogenesis[17,18]

Hair follicle morphogenesis is induced by a complex network of sequential activation and inactivation of autocrine, paracrine, and endocrine signaling pathways **(Fig. 3)**.[9]

Various signaling pathways which induce follicle morphogenesis are as follows:

- *β-catenin*: The β-catenin-dependent Wnt pathway signals through cytoplasmic stabilization and accumulation of β-catenin. As it accumulates, it translocates to the cell nucleus where it forms complexes with members of the lymphoid enhancer-binding factor/T cell factor (LEF/TCF) family of DNA-binding factors to activate gene transcription. With the initiation of the first signaling and placode formation, a plethora of extracellular and intracellular mediators is expressed.
- EDA and EDAR
- Noggin
- Transforming growth factor β2 (TGFβ2), TGFβR-II, β1 integrin, and neural cell adhesion molecule.
- Fibroblast growth factors FGF1, FGF2, FGF4, and receptor FGFr2
- Shh important for hair germ and DP formation

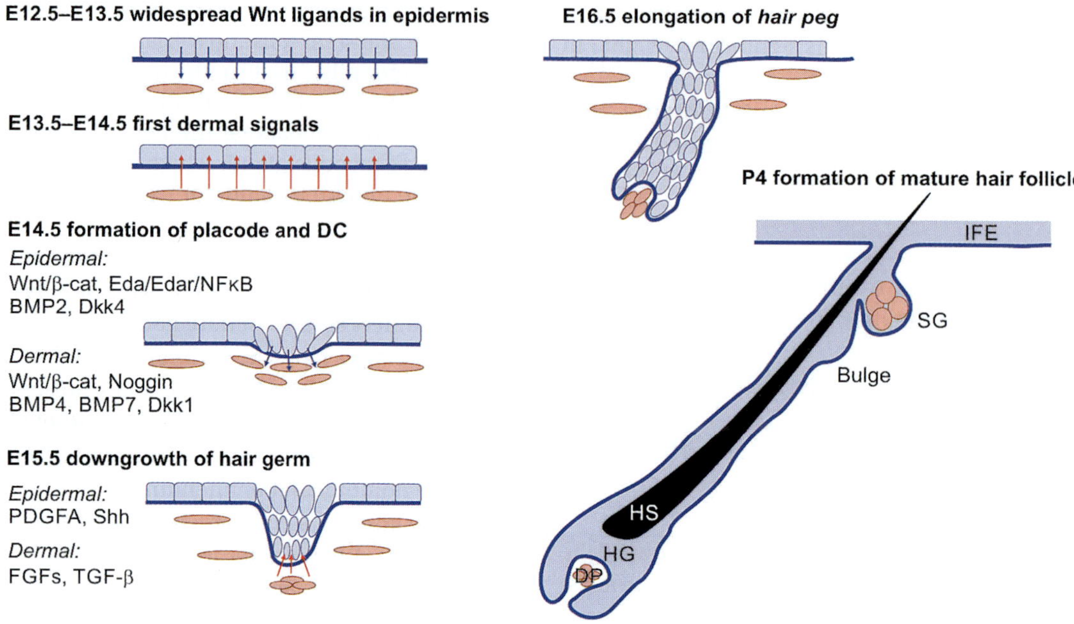

Fig. 3: Events and key regulators during hair follicle morphogenesis.[9]
(DC: dermal condensate; DP: dermal papilla; HG: hair germ; HS: hair shaft; SG: sebaceous gland; IFE: interfollicular epidermis; β-cat: β-catenin)

Various inhibitors of hair follicle placode formation are as follows:

- BMP-2, BMP-4
- p75NTR
- Activin βa-placode inhibitor

SEBACEOUS GLAND[21]

- It develops in the 13th to 16th week of gestation from bulges (epithelial placodes) on the developing hair follicles.
- Wnt/wingless (Wnt) and Sonic Hedgehog (Shh) signaling pathways are involved in embryonic patterning and cell fate decisions.

Signals

- Increased Shh and Myc signaling and decreased Wnt signaling—sebocyte fate
- Intact Wnt signaling promotes hair follicle differentiation **(Fig. 4)**.

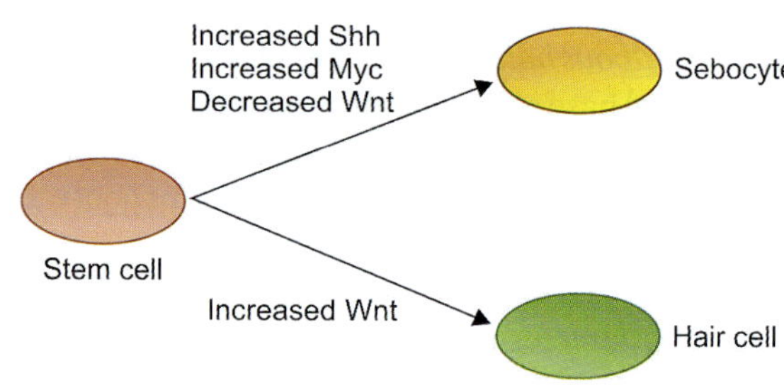

Fig. 4: Signaling pathway and transcription factors in cell lineage determination.

ECCRINE GLAND[22,23]

- The first morphologic indicators of palmoplantar eccrine gland development are the formation of large mesenchymal bulges or pads on the volar surfaces of the hands and feet between 55 and 65 days' EGA, and the induction of parallel ectodermal ridges overlying these bulges between 12 and 14 weeks.
- 5th fetal month—develops in the axillary skin
- 6th fetal month—develops over the entire body
- By 16 weeks, the glandular regions at the terminal portion of this downgrowth are formed, and the secretory and myoepithelial components become discernible. Canalization of the dermal components of the glands occurs by loss of desmosome adhesion along the innermost ectodermal.
- This process is complete by 16 weeks, whereas the opening of the epidermal portion of the duct by vesicular fusion and autolysis and keratinization of the wall are not complete until 22 weeks' EGA.
- By the 8th fetal month, eccrine secretory cells resemble those of the adult.
- By the 9th fetal month, myoepithelial cells form.

APOCRINE GLAND[22]

- 4th month of gestation—develops from the upper bulge of the hair follicle with continued development as long as hair follicles develop.
- Over the next several weeks, the glandular cords of cells elongate.

TABLE 2: Embryological development of cutaneous structure.

Gestational age	*Epidermal development*	*Dermal/subcutaneous development*	*Hair, nail, and gland development*	*Cell development*
~3–4 weeks	Epidermis from surface ectoderm			
~6 weeks	Outer flattened periderm above cuboidal germinal (basal) layer	Germinal layer in contact with underlying mesenchyme		Langerhans cells can be seen
~7 weeks	Fetal basement membrane		Primordial tooth	
~8–12 weeks	Epidermal stratification begins (~8 weeks) *Appearance of:* • Melanocytes • Langerhans cells • Merkel cells	Formation of distinct boundary of dermis and hypodermis		Merkel cells detected
~9–12 weeks	Formation of anchoring filaments/hemidesmosomes		Primordial hair follicle and nail formed	Melanocytes migrate (12 weeks)
~12 weeks	Formation of dermoepidermal junction	Appearance of type III collagen	Nail bed starts to keratinize, proximal nail fold forms	
~12–14 weeks	Parallel ectodermal ridges (fingerprints)	Fibroblasts start synthesizing collagen and elastin	Primordial eccrine and sebaceous gland formed	
~12–24 weeks	• Melanin production (12–16 weeks) • Melanosome transfer (20 weeks)		Hair follicles differentiate in seven concentric layers	
~15–20 weeks		• Formation of distinct boundary of papillary/reticular • Appearance of dermal ridges	• Follicular keratinization begins • Nail plate completely covers nail bed	
~22 weeks		Elastic fiber seen		
~22–24 weeks	• Cornification begins • Periderm detached from epidermis (24 weeks)	Appearance of adipocyte under dermis		

- By 7 months' EGA, the clear cells and mucin-secreting dark cells characteristic of apocrine glands are distinguishable.
- At birth, the secretory portions of nonvolar sweat glands remain high in the dermis but postnatally extend progressively down to the subcutis.
- The apocrine gland functions transiently in the third trimester and then becomes quiescent in the neonate, whereas the eccrine gland does not appear to function in utero but progressively reaches functional maturity postnatally.

Table 2 summarizes the chronological changes in the embryogenesis of skin.

Knowledge about embryology of skin will greatly help in management of preterm neonates and in understanding of several inherited dermatoses. It will also aid in the understanding of physiologic growth processes of skin and its appendages. This could help in identification of appropriate therapeutic targets.

KEY POINTS

- Skin is composed of cells that have origin from both ectoderm and mesoderm.
- Ectoderm is committed to either surface ectoderm or neuroectoderm which forms the epidermis, its appendages, nail unit, and melanocytes.
- Epidermis develops from surface ectoderm at 4 weeks with stratification beginning at 8 weeks.
- By 12–15 weeks, a distinction can be made between the fine weave of the papillary and thicker, deeper reticular dermis.
- By the 12th week, lanugo (fine, soft, unpigmented hair) is visible on the eyebrows, upper lip, and chin.
- Nails begin development in 10 weeks.
- Various cells such as Langerhans cells, macrophages, mast cells, fibroblasts, and adipocytes are derived from mesoderm.
- The development process is under various activating and inhibitory signals such as Wnt, BMP, and FGF.
- Any abnormality in the development of the structures has varied clinical manifestations such as development of nevi and ichthyosis depending on the structure or the process affected during embryogenesis.

REFERENCES

1. Koster MI, Roop DR. Mechanisms regulating epithelial stratification. Annu Rev Cell Dev Biol. 2007;23:93-113.
2. Stern CD. Neural induction: Old problem, new findings, yet more questions. Development. 2005;132:2007-21.
3. Fuchs E. Scratching the surface of skin development. Nature. 2007;445:834-42.
4. Lane AT. Human fetal skin development. Pediatr Dermatol. 1986;3:487.

5. Holbrook KA, Odland GF. The fine structure of developing human epidermis: light, scanning, and transmission electron microscopy of the periderm. J Invest Dermatol. 1975; 65:16-38.
6. Koster MI, Roop DR. Mechanisms regulating epithelial stratification. Annu Rev Cell Dev Biol. 2007;23:93-113.
7. M'Boneko V, Merker HJ. Development and morphology of the periderm of mouse embryos (days 9-12 of gestation). Acta Anat (Basel). 1988;133:325-36.
8. Hoeger PH, Enzmann CC. Skin physiology of the neonate and young infant: a prospective study of functional skin parameters during early infancy. Pediatr Dermatol. 2002;19:256-62.
9. Liu S, Zhang H, Duan E. Epidermal development in mammals: key regulators, signals from beneath, and stem cells. Int J Mol Sci. 2013;14(6):10869-95.
10. Foster CA, Holbrook KA, Farr AG. Ontogeny of Langerhans cells in human embryonic and fetal skin: expression of HLA-DR and OKT-6 determinants. J Invest Dermatol 1986; 86(3):240-3.
11. Lewis BL. Microscopic studies of fetal and mature nail and surrounding soft tissue. AMA Arch Derm Syphilol. 1954;70: 733-47.
12. Warwick R, Williams PL (Eds). Gray's Anatomy, 35th edition. Harlow: Longman; 1973.
13. Jiaravuthisan MM, Sasseville D, Vender RB, Murphy F, Muhn CY. Psoriasis of the nail: anatomy, pathology, clinical presentation, and a review of the literature on therapy. J Am Acad Dermatol. 2007;57(1):1-27.
14. Baran R, de Berker DAR, Holzberg M, Thomas L (Eds). Baran and Dawber's Diseases of the Nails and Their Management, 4th edition. New York: Wiley-Blackwell; 2012;
15. Ebling FJ. The physiology of hair growth. In: Breuer MM (Ed). Cosmetic Science, Vol. 2. London: Academic Press; 1980. pp 181-232.
16. Hardy MH. The secret life of the hair follicle. Trends Genet. 1992;8:55-61.
17. Holbrook KA, Minami SI. Hair follicle embryogenesis in the human. Characterization of events in vivo and in vitro. Ann N Y Acad Sci. 1991;642:167-96.
18. Millar SE. Molecular mechanisms regulating hair follicle development. J Invest Dermatol. 2002;118:216-25.
19. Olivera-Martinez I, Thelu J, Dhouailly D. Molecular mechanisms controlling dorsal dermis generation from the somitic dermomyotome. Int J Dev Biol. 2004;48:93-101.
20. Mou C, Jackson B, Schneider P, Overbeek PA, Headon DJ. Generation of the primary hair follicle pattern. Proc Natl Acad Sci USA. 2006;103:9075-80.
21. Niemann C, Horsley V. Development and homeostasis of the sebaceous gland. Semin Cell Dev Biol. 2012;23:928-36.
22. Fu X, Li J, Sun X, Sun T, Sheng Z. Regeneration science: epidermal stem cells are the source of sweat glands in human fetal skin: Evidence of synergetic development of stem cells, sweat glands, growth factors, and matrix metalloproteinases. Wound Repair Regen. 2005;13:102-8.
23. Solomon LM, Esterly NB. Neonatal dermatology. I. The newborn skin. J Pediatr. 1970;77(5):888-94.

EXAMINATION QUESTIONS

1. Outline the events and key regulators during hair follicle morphogenesis.
2. Outline the steps in the development of nail unit.
3. Enumerate the various signals during hair development.
4. Enumerate disorders of skin development.
5. Write a short note on embryological development of skin and its appendages.

3 CHAPTER

Anatomy of Skin and Appendages

Abhishek De, Arnab Dutta, Aarti Sarda

EMBRYOLOGY

- Human development occurs through 40 weeks of gestation. During the first trimester (weeks 0–12), organogenesis occurs. However, the development continues through the second (weeks 13–26) and the third (weeks 27–40) trimester. Interestingly, full-barrier formation of skin occurs after birth **(Table 1)**.
- The three germ layers that form during gastrulation include the ectoderm, the mesoderm, and the endoderm. The ectoderm forms the epidermis, the melanocytes, and the nervous system. The mesoderm forms fibroblasts, blood vessels, and muscles. The endoderm does not contribute to skin development.
- *Neural crest development:* The ectoderm forms the neural plate in the third week of fetal life. Then, at the junction

TABLE 1: Important developmental stages of skin structures.

	Gestational age	*Epidermal development*	*Appendageal development*	*Dermal and subcutaneous development*
First trimester	2 weeks	• Gastrulation begins and an ectoderm is formed • Single-layer germinativum		
	3 weeks	Periderm forms		
	6 weeks	Outer flattened periderm and inner, cuboidal germinal (basal) layer		Germinal layer in contact with underlying mesenchyme
	7 weeks	Fetal basement membrane appears	Tooth primordia appear	
	8 weeks	• Epidermal stratification begins • Melanocytes appear	Hair follicle and nail primordia are seen	• Dermal-subcutaneous • Boundary becomes distinct • Distinct boundary between epidermis and dermis
	9 weeks		Nail placode appears	
	10 weeks	Langerhans cells appear		
	10–12 weeks	Anchoring filaments/hemidesmosomes appears	Hair follicle primordia are seen	
	12 weeks	Merkel cells appear	• Nail bed starts to keratinize, proximal nail fold forms • Sweat gland placode forms on volar sites	• Formation of dermo-epidermal junction • Type III collagen appears
Second trimester	13–14 weeks	Parallel ectodermal ridges (fingerprints) appear	Sebaceous gland primordia are seen	• Papillary dermis becomes distinct from reticular dermis • Fibroblasts start synthesizing collagen and elastin in dermis
	12–16 weeks	Melanin production starts		
	20 weeks	• Melanosome • Transfer starts • Periderm start shedding (periderm is part of vernix caseosa)	Follicular keratinization	
	22 weeks		• Trunk eccrine gland • Primordia appear	Elastic fiber is seen
	24 weeks	Maturation epidermis is complete with interfollicular keratinization		Adipocytes appear

between the neural plate and the ectoderm, a distinct group of cells, known as the neural crest forms. Neural crest cells lead to the development of the Merkel cells and melanocytes.[1]

EPIDERMIS

Introduction

- Epidermis is the outermost layer of the skin. It performs many important function including:
  - Acts as a mechanical barrier
  - Acts as an antimicrobial barrier
  - It protects against water loss
  - It provides immunological protection
  - It helps in thermoregulation
- Thickness of the epidermis varies from 0.04 (eyelid skin) to 1.5 mm (palmoplantar skin).
- Epidermis is mainly divided into four layers; each layer has a characteristic cell shape, intracellular structure, and proteins. From inside to outside the layers of epidermis are:
  1. Stratum basale (germinativum)
  2. Stratum spinosum
  3. Stratum granulosum
  4. Stratum corneum
- Stratum lucidum is an additional layer in palmoplantar skin. Located between the stratum granulosum and stratum corneum layers, it is composed of three to five layers of dead, flattened keratinocytes.[2]
- Epidermis consists of the following cells:
  - *Keratinocytes:* Consists of 80–85% of total epidermal cell population
  - *Melanocytes:* Located in the basal layer
  - *Langerhans cells (LCs):* Located in the suprabasal layer, consists of 2–8% of total epidermal cell population
  - *Merkel cells:* Located in the basal layer

Keratinocyte

- Keratinocytes are the primary type of cell found in the epidermis. Keratinocytes comprise approximately 80–85% of epidermal cells.
- Keratinocytes originate in the basal layer, produce keratin, and are responsible for the formation of the epidermal water barrier by making and secreting lipids.
- They are derived from ectoderm during the first few weeks of embryonic development.
- The normal transit time for a cell from basal layer to stratum corneum is around 14 days and the transit time through the stratum corneum to desquamation requires 14 days, leading to a total of 28 days.
- Epidermal self-renewal is maintained by the stem cells in the basal layer of interfollicular epithelium and the bulge region of hair follicles. The stem cells in the bulge region of hair follicles are only activated in the event of an epidermal injury.
- Within the epidermis, keratinocytes are associated with other cell types such as melanocytes and Langerhans cells.
- Keratinocytes are able to release, respond to, and produce tumour necrosis factor α (TNFα) which causes increased differentiation.
- Keratinization is part of the physical barrier formation (cornification), in which the keratinocytes produce more and more keratin and undergo terminal differentiation.
- Keratinocytes produce keratin intermediate filaments, which form the cell's cytoskeletal network.
- Microfilaments like actin, myosin, and α-actinin assist in the upward movement of the keratinocytes as they differentiate.
- Integrins regulate adhesion and initiation of differentiation.
- *Functions:*
  - The primary function of keratinocytes is the formation of a barrier against environmental damage by injury, ultraviolet (UV) radiation, water loss, infection, and immunologic challenges.
  - A number of structural proteins (filaggrin, keratin), enzymes (proteases), lipids, and antimicrobial peptides (defensins) contribute to maintaining the important barrier function of the skin.
  - Keratinocytes also regulate calcium absorption by the activation of cholesterol precursors by UVB light to form vitamin D.[3]

Layers of Epidermis

The layers of the epidermis include the stratum basale, stratum spinosum, stratum granulosum, stratum lucidum, and stratum corneum from the deepest to superficial portion.

Stratum Basale

- It is also known as stratum germinativum.
- It is the deepest layer consisting of a single layer of columnar or cuboidal basal cells.
- Stratum basale is separated from the dermis by the basement membrane (basal lamina) and attached to the basement membrane by hemidesmosomes. These cells are attached to each other and to the cells of the overlying stratum spinosum cells by desmosomes.
- About 10% of the basal layer keratinocytes are mitotically active stem cells that give rise to transit-amplifying cells, which allow for maintenance of tissue.
- Structurally, the basal layer of keratinocytes is vertically-oriented columnar or cuboidal cells with large oval nucleus and more basophilic cytoplasm than other keratinocytes.
- This layer also contains melanocytes, Merkel cells, and Langerhans cells (latter mainly in stratum spinosum).
- Basal cells express ornithine decarboxylase which is a marker of proliferative activity. Ornithine decarboxylase is stimulated by trauma, UV, epidermal growth factor (EGF),

estrogens, β-agonists, tumor promoters and inhibited by retinoids, corticosteroid, and vitamin D_3.
- De novo expression of K5 and K14 occurs in the basal layers forming keratin tonofilaments, which insert into both desmosomes and hemidesmosomes and form keratinocyte cytoskeleton.
- K19 found in basal cells at transitional boundaries between different types of epithelia.
- Microfilaments like actin, myosin, and α-actinin assist in upward movement of cells as they differentiate. Integrins regulate adhesion and initiation of differentiation.

Stratum Spinosum

- It is also known as the prickle cell layer or spinous layer. This layer contains keratinocytes and Langerhans cells.
- This layer is composed of 8–10 layers of irregular, polyhedral keratinocytes joined together with desmosomes. These cells have a rounder nucleus, more flattened appearance.
- Keratinocytes in this layer have cytoplasmic processes that extend outward and contact neighboring cells by desmosomes. Their spiny appearance is due to shrinking of the microfilaments between desmosomes that occurs when stained with H&E.
- In stratum spinosum K5/K14 is still present, but not made de novo in this layer.
- There is a new synthesis of K1/K10. These are keratinization-specific keratins, characteristic of epidermis, and markers of terminal differentiation.
- Cells in the upper spinous layer contain lamellar granules (syn: lamellated bodies or Odland bodies) that are intracellular lipid-carrying granules formed within Golgi **(Box 1)**
- *Applied aspects:*
  - In psoriasis, actinic keratoses and wound healing, suprabasilar keratinocytes downregulate K1/K10 and make K6/K16. The mRNAs for K6/K16 are always present but only translated during proliferation.
  - Hyperproliferative state markers are K6, K16, and Ki-67.[2]

Stratum Granulosum

- Stratum granulosum consists of 3–5 cell layers with more flattened diamond-shaped keratinocytes with keratohyalin granules and lamellar granules.
- It is a thin layer of cells in the epidermis lying above the stratum spinosum and below the stratum corneum (stratum lucidum on the soles and palms)
- Granular cells start to lose their nuclei but retain dense keratin filaments.
- Keratohyalin granules are composed of keratins, profilaggrin and loricrin, and other proteins that make up the bulk of the cornified envelopes. The main function of keratohyalin granules is to bind intermediate keratin filaments together (**Box 2**)

BOX 1: Lamellated bodies.

- They are also known as "Odland bodies" or lamellar granules
- These are membrane-bound intracellular structures, 0.2–0.3 µm in diameter; lamellated bodies found intracellularly in upper-level keratinocytes
- These are modified lysosomes with secretory function. Lamellar granules originate in Golgi
- They first appear in upper stratum spinosum, but their primary activity is in stratum corneum
- Odland bodies discharge their contents into the extracellular space at the junction of the granular and horny layers, thus establishing a barrier to water loss, and along with filaggrin, mediate stratum corneum adhesion
- Odland bodies release lipid precursors into intercellular space; including glycoproteins, glycolipids, phospholipids, free sterols, and glucosylceramides. Ceramides are the major lipid for barrier function of the skin
- The glycoproteins and lipid precursors which are discharged into intercellular space between granular and cornified layer; form lamellar sheets (ceramide) or "mortar" which acts as intracellular cement for corneocytes ("bricks"), thus contributing to formation of cutaneous lipid barrier **(Fig. 1)**
- *Applied aspects:*
  - In Flegel's disease there are decreased lamellar granules.
  - In Harlequin ichthyosis, the lamellar granules are uniformly abnormal or absent
  - In X-linked ichthyosis, the enzyme steroid sulfatase is missing in lamellar granules. This leads to an increased level of the β fraction of cholesterol sulfate that can be identified by serum lipoprotein electrophoresis. Prenatal diagnosis of X-linked ichthyosis can be done by measurement of decreased estrogen levels and the presence of nonhydrolyzed sulfated steroids in maternal urine[4]

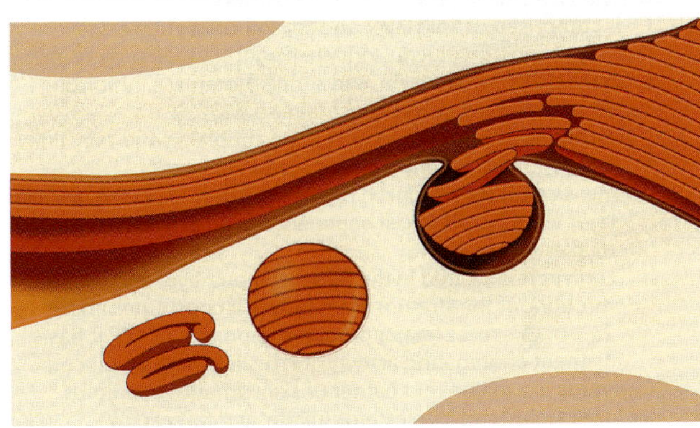

Fig. 1: The epidermal lamellar bodies are also called as Odland bodies, lamellar bodies, and lamellar granules. Epidermal lamellar bodies are vesicles present in keratinocytes of the stratum spinosum and, in larger numbers, in the keratinocytes of the stratum granulosum of the epidermis. They contain lipids and enzymes. After exocytosis in the intercellular space, the lipids are metabolized by the enzymes to give the free ceramides and the fatty acids present in the stratum corneum of the epidermis, thus forming a protective barrier.

- K1 modified to K2 and K10 to K11 by proteolysis and phosphorylation
- There is programmed destruction of the granular cell:
  - Loss of nucleus, yet retention of keratin filaments and filaggrin matrix
  - Destruction involves apoptosis, called transition cells ("T" cells)

BOX 2: Keratohyalin granules.

- Keratohyalin granules of epidermis are dense stellate globules which contain profilaggrin (F granules) and loricrin (L granules contain loricrin at periphery and help form cornified cell envelope) + keratin intermediate filament (KIF)
- Keratohyalin granules can be divided in three classes:
  1. Globular keratohyalin granules (KHG) (found in quickly dividing epithelia, such as the oral mucosa)
  2. Stellate KHG (found in the slowly dividing normal epidermis)
  3. KHG of Hassall's corpuscles or type VI epithelioreticular cells of the thymus gland. The exact purpose of the keratinization of Hassall's corpuscles remains unknown
- *Filaggrin:*
  - These are histidine-rich keratin filament aggregating proteins in KHG; they bind intermediate filaments and organize into fibrils
  - Filaggrin is initially cleaved from profilaggrin (when granular layer transformed into cornified layer) and this is a calcium-dependent process
  - They promote aggregation and disulfide bonding of keratin filaments in cornified cell (like glue)
  - Filaggrin is degraded into urocanic acid (UCA) and pyrrolidone carboxylic acid; both hydrate stratum corneum and block UV radiation
  - *UCA:* Filaggrin degradation product found naturally in the cornified layer; absorbs/blocks UV radiation and forms natural moisturizing factor (NMF) with other filaggrin degradation products (amino acids, pyrrolidone carboxylic acid); NMF allows stratum corneum to remain hydrated even in drying conditions[5]
- *Cornified cell envelope (CE)* ***(Fig. 2):***
  - Cornified envelopes are the products of terminal differentiation in the epidermis. They are acellular and a nuclear structures
  - CE is a highly cross-linked lipid-rich flexible structure enveloping corneocytes serving as insoluble exoskeleton and rigid scaffold for internal keratin filaments. It provides both mechanical and water permeability barriers
  - CE is comprised of lipid layer and several covalently cross-linked proteins: Involucrin, loricrin, filaggrin, small proline-rich proteins (SPRs), envoplakin, and serine proteinase inhibitor called skin-derived antileukoproteinase (SKALP)
    - *Envoplakin:* It is homologous to desmoplakin and may link the CE to desmosomes and to keratin filaments
    - *Involucrin:* It is cross-linked by transglutaminase in the granular layer to an insoluble cell boundary. It is an early differentiation marker
    - *Loricrin:* It is located in the upper spinous layer and throughout the stratum granulosum. It constitutes about 75% of CE's mass (major protein component of CE). It has filament aggregating activity; it crosslinks with involucrin
  - Ceramide is a major lipid barrier of skin; other barrier lipids include cholesterol, cholesterol sulfate, and fatty acids
- *Transglutaminase (TG):*
  - Three versions of TG are present that function in cross-linking the CE (calcium-dependent process)
  - These form γ-glutamyl-lysine isodipeptide bonds in the CE, most prominently with involucrin
  - *TG-1 (type K):* Keratinocyte transglutaminase, membrane associated.
  - *TG-2 (type C):* Fetal epidermis and basal layer of adult epidermis, soluble
  - *TG-3:* Can be present in hair follicles, sublamina densa and differentiated epidermal cells, soluble
- *Applied aspects:*
  - Vohwinkel syndrome variant is associated with a defect in loricrin.
  - Filaggrin defect causes ichthyosis vulgaris
  - TG-1 (type K) defect causes lamellar ichthyosis type I (*TGM1* gene) and nonbullous congenital ichthyosiform erythroderma (T9M1 + ALOX12B + ALOXE3)
  - TG-3, when present in sublamina densa, can be the antigen for dermatitis herpetiformis
  - Involucrin is upregulated in psoriasis

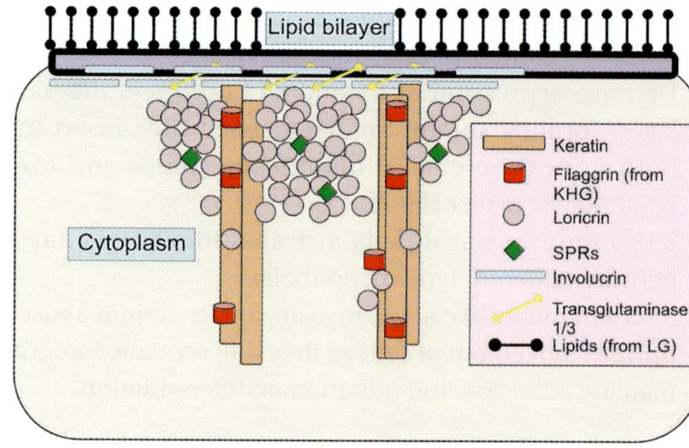

Fig. 2: Cornified cell envelope (CE).
(KHG: keratohyalin granules; SPRs: small proline-rich proteins)

  - Terminal differentiation is initiated by increase in calcium gradient in suprabasal epidermis
- At the transition between this layer and the stratum corneum, cells secrete lamellar bodies containing lipids and proteins into the extracellular space. This results in the formation of the hydrophobic lipid envelope responsible for the skin's barrier properties.

Stratum Lucidum

- This layer is 2–3 cell layers thick, and present in thicker skin found in the palms and soles.
- This is a thin clear layer consisting of eleidin which is a transformation product of keratohyalin.

Stratum Corneum

- The stratum corneum (Latin for "horny layer") is the outermost layer of the epidermis.
- This layer is composed of 15–20 layers of flattened cells with no nuclei and cell organelles.
- This is the layer which varies most in thickness, and is especially thick in callused skin.
- Transition from stratum granulosum is accompanied by loss of 45–86% in dry weight.
- This layer provides mechanical protection, barrier to water loss, and barrier preventing permeation of environmental soluble substances.
- Corneocytes are composed of high-weight keratins embedded in a filaggrin-rich matrix.
- Normal stratum corneum cells have no nuclei; nuclei may persist in incompletely keratinized cells (parakeratosis).
- *Brick and mortar model:* Lipid-depleted, protein-rich corneocytes ("bricks") surrounded by extracellular lipid-rich matrix ("mortar").
- Within this layer, the dead keratinocytes secrete defensins, which are part of our first immune defense.
- *Applied aspects:* A failure to modulate the activity of kallikreins via the disruption of the protease inhibitor LEKTI causes the debilitating disorder Netherton syndrome.

KERATIN

- Keratins (also described as cytokeratins) are polymers of type I and type II intermediate filaments which form the cell's cytoskeletal network **(Tables 2 and 3)**.
- This cytoskeletal network provides resilience, structural integrity, along with serving as a marker for differentiation. The second cytoskeletal network formed by actin filaments.
- The human genome encodes 54 functional keratin genes, located in two clusters on chromosomes 12 and 17.
- Among the total 54 functional keratins 37 are epithelial and 17 are hair keratins.
- Molecular weight of keratins intermediate filaments varies between 40 and 70 kDa.
- Keratins bind to each other in the rod region. Keratins are expressed as either type I (acidic) or type II (basic), and acidic and basic keratins are coexpressed in order to form a filamentous structure: "Obligate heteropolymers."
  - Examples of acidic keratins are Keratin 9 (K9)-K20, their genes are located in the chromosome 17.

TABLE 2: Intermediate filaments.

Type I	*Type II*	*Type III*	*Type IV*	*Type V*	*Type VI*	*Unclassified*
Keratin 9–20 (acidic keratin)	Keratin 1–8 (basic keratin)	• Vimentin • Desmin • Glial fibrillary acidic protein (GFAP) • Peripherin	• Neurofilament light, heavy, and medium polypeptides (NF-L, NF-H, NF-M) • α-Internexin • Syncoilin • Synemin	• Lamin A/C • Lamin B1 • Lamin B2	Nestin	• Filensin • Phakinin

TABLE 3: Keratin filament expression pattern.

Type II (basic keratin)	*Type I (acidic keratin)*	*Location of expression*	*Associated diseases*
K1	K10	Suprabasal keratinocytes	Bullous congenital ichthyosiform erythroderma (epidermolytic hyperkeratosis)
K1		Suprabasal keratinocytes	• Diffuse nonepidermolytic palmoplantar keratoderma (aka Unna- Thost) • Ichthyosis hystrix of Curth-Macklin • Greither syndrome (transgrediens form of PPK)
K1	K9	Palmoplantar suprabasilar keratinocytes	Vorner palmoplantar keratoderma (epidermolytic palmoplantar keratoderma)
K2e	K10	Granular and upper spinous layer	Ichthyosis bullosa of Siemens
K3	K12	Cornea	Meesmann corneal dystrophy
K5	K14	Basal keratinocytes	• *Epidermolysis bullosa simplex:* – Dowling-Meara (head or tail of central rod domain) – Koebner (segment 1A or 2B of rod domain) – Weber-Cockayne (nonhelical parts) • Dowling-Degos disease
K4	K13	Mucosal epithelium	White sponge nevus
K6a	K16	Outer root sheath	• Pachyonychia congenita (Jadassohn-Lewandowsky) • Focal nonepidermolytic PPK
K6b	K17	Nail bed	Pachyonychia congenita II (Jackson-Lawler)
	K17	Nails, hair follicles, palms and soles and sebaceous glands	Steatocystoma multiplex
K8	K18	Simple epithelium	Cryptogenic cirrhosis
K81, K83, K86		Hair follicle	Monilethrix
	K19	Bulge cells and simple epithelium	Paget's disease (Other markers of Paget's disease are CK7 and CK20)
	K20	Basal layers of epidermis	Merkel cell carcinoma
K5		Basal keratinocytes	Epidermolysis bullosa simplex, with Mottled pigmentation (Non-helical V1 domain)
	K14	Basal keratinocytes	• Naegeli-Franceschetti-Jadassohn syndrome • Dermatopathia pigmentosa reticularis • Epidermolysis bullosa simplex, autosomal recessive variant

- Examples of basic keratins are K1-K8; their genes are located in the chromosome 12.
- *Keratins can also be classified as:*
  - *Based on distribution:* Soft keratin (found in the epidermis) and hard keratin (found in nail, hair cortex, and hair cuticle)
  - *Based on X-ray diffraction pattern:* Alpha, beta, feather, and amorphous keratins.
- In the basal layer K5 and K14 expressed; keratin filaments in basal cells insert into desmosomes and hemidesmosomes.
- K19 found in basal cells at transitional boundaries between different types of epithelia.[6,7]
- *Functions of keratins:*
  - Keratins influence the architecture and mitotic activity of the epithelial cell.
  - Keratins and associated filaments provide a scaffold for epithelial cells and tissues to sustain mechanical stress, maintain their structural integrity, ensure mechanical resilience, to protect against variations in hydrostatic pressure and establish cell polarity.
  - Keratins and its filaments are involved in cell signaling, cell transport, cell compartmentalization, and cell differentiation.
  - Keratin filaments also influence cell metabolic processes by regulating protein synthesis and cell growth.
  - Keratins may also be involved in the transport of membrane-bound vesicles in the cytoplasm of the epithelial cells.

INTRAEPIDERMAL ADHESION MOLECULES

- Four types of intercellular junction are present in between keratinocytes especially in the stratum spinosum and stratum corneum: Desmosomes, adherens junctions, tight junctions, and gap junctions.
- All are essential for the development of the embryonic layers and organs as well as adult tissue homeostasis.
- While each junction type is defined as a distinct entity, it is now clear that they cooperate physically and functionally to create a robust and functionally diverse system.

Desmosomes

- Desmosomes are calcium-dependent cell-cell adhesion molecules between keratinocytes.
- Desmosomes emerged from adherens junctions with structural similarities but distinct functions.
- They serve as attachment sites for cytoskeleton (intermediate filaments).
- *Several features set desmosomes apart from adherens junctions:*
  - Their association with intermediate filaments
  - There are two subclasses of desmosomal cadherins, desmogleins (Dsgs) and desmocollins (Dscs), both of which are required for DSM structure and function.
  - DSMs are capable of undergoing a transition from calcium-dependent to calcium-independent status, also known as the "hyperadhesive" state.
- *Each desmosome made up of several proteins:*
  - *Transmembrane proteins:* Desmoglein 1/3, desmocollin 1/2 (desmosomal cadherins)
  - *Desmosomal plaque proteins:* Plakoglobin (γ-catenin), desmoplakin 1/2, keratocalmin, desmoyokin, band 6 protein, and envoplakin
- *Desmosomal cadherins:*
  - Cadherins are a family of calcium-dependent cell–cell adhesion molecules that play an important role in the formation and maintenance of complex tissue integrity.
  - Based on sequence similarity, cadherins have two major subgroups, classic cadherins (e.g., E-, P-, N-cadherins) and desmosomal cadherins (desmogleins and desmocollins).
  - Cadherins associate with the plaque proteins, α-catenin, β-catenin, and plakoglobin, which mediate and regulate binding to the cytoskeleton network.
  - Cadherin molecules form dimers as their functional unit, with the distal extracellular domain of the cadherin from one cell binding to the same region of a second cadherin from an opposing cell.
  - Desmogleins have four isoforms (Dsg1–4). Expression of Dsg1 and Dsg3 is basically restricted to stratified squamous epithelia, while Dsg2 is expressed in simple epithelia and myocardium. Dsg4 plays an important adhesive role primarily in hair follicles.
  - Desmocollins are another group of transmembrane glycoproteins within desmosomes and they have three isoforms (Dsc1–3).
  - Desmosomes always have desmoglein and desmocollin as a pair.
- *Desmosomal plaque proteins:*
  - Plakoglobin and plakophilin, together with β-catenin, are members of the armadillo family of nuclear and junctional proteins, which are not only simple anchoring molecules but also dynamic regulators of cellular adhesion and proliferation.
  - Desmoplakin is a dumbbell-shaped molecule flanked by globular carboxyl- and amino-terminal domains that interact with intermediate filaments and armadillo family members, respectively. They are members of plakin family, and play an important role in the anchorage of the cytoskeleton to filament attachment sites on desmosomes. Desmoplakins are of two types: Desmoplakin I (250 kDa) and II (210 kDa) **(Fig. 3)**.[8]

Adherens Junctions (Zonula Adherens)

- Transmembrane classical cadherins (namely E and P) linked to actin cytoskeleton via cytoplasmic plaque proteins (α, β, γ-catenin).

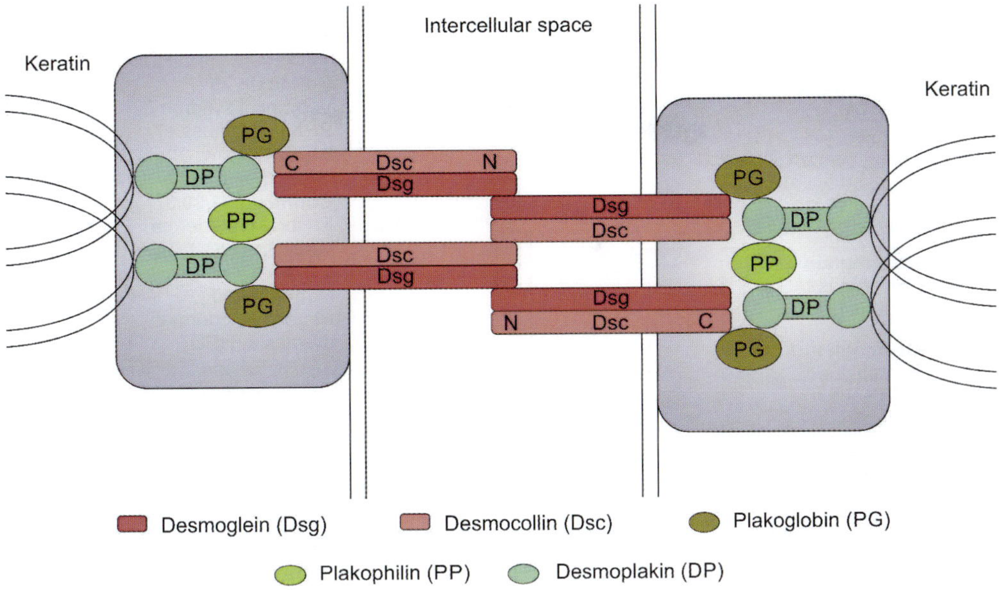

Fig. 3: The desmosome complex: It includes desmogleins and desmocollins as transmembrane constituents, and plakoglobin, plakophilin, and desmoplakin as cytoplasmic constituents. Desmogleins and desmocollins associate with plakoglobin, which in turn binds to desmoplakin, which links keratin to the membrane.

- The adherens junction anchors bundles of actin microfilaments and contains classic cadherins (e.g., E-, P-, N-cadherins) as its transmembrane components and α, β, γ-catenin and plakoglobin as its cytoplasmic components. (In contrast, the desmosome anchors intermediate filaments like keratins and contains desmosomal cadherins as its transmembrane components and plakoglobin, plakophilin, and desmoplakin as its cytoplasmic components.)
- Plakoglobin is the only common protein between adherens junction and desmosome.
- In general, adherens junctions mediate quick but weak cellular adhesion, whereas desmosomes mediate slow but strong cellular adhesion.[9]

Tight Junctions (Zonula Occludens)

- Tight junctions, also known as occluding junctions or zonula occludens are multiprotein junctional complexes whose general function is to seal intercellular space and to prevent diffusion of solutes between cells and maintain cell polarity.
- Tight junctions may also serve as leaky pathways by forming selective channels for small cations, anions, or water.
- Major constituents of tight junctions are claudins and occludins. Other constituents are junction adhesion molecules and angulin.[9]

Gap Junctions

- Gap junctions are a specialized intercellular connection between multitudes of animal cell-types.
- These are also called nexus or macula communicans.
- These are transmembrane channels formed by six connexin monomers.
- They directly connect the cytoplasm of two cells, which allow various molecules, ions and electrical impulses to directly pass through a regulated gate between cells.
- Gap junctions are more abundant in stratum spinosum compared with stratum basale.[10]

Applied Aspects

- *Diseases related to gap junction proteins:*
  - *Connexin 26:* Vohwinkel's syndrome, keratitis-ichthyosis-deafness (KID) syndrome, palmoplantar keratoderma (PPK) with deafness.
  - *Connexin 30.3 and 31:* Erythrokeratoderma variabilis
  - *Connexin 30:* Hidrotic ectodermal dysplasia
- *Diseases related to desmosomal proteins* ***(Fig. 4)****:*
  - *Desmoglein 1:* Pemphigus foliaceus and autosomal dominant strait palmoplantar keratoderma
  - *Desmoglein 3:* Pemphigus vulgaris, paraneoplastic pemphigus
  - *Desmoglein 4:* Monilethrix (autosomal recessive)
  - *Desmocollin 1:* Subcorneal pustular dermatosis
  - *Plakoglobin:* Naxos syndrome
  - *Desmoplakin 1 and 2:* Carvajal syndrome, striate PPK, skin fragility/woolly hair syndrome, paraneoplastic pemphigus
  - *Plakophilin:* Ectodermal dysplasia/skin fragility syndrome
  - *Envoplakin:* Paraneoplastic pemphigus

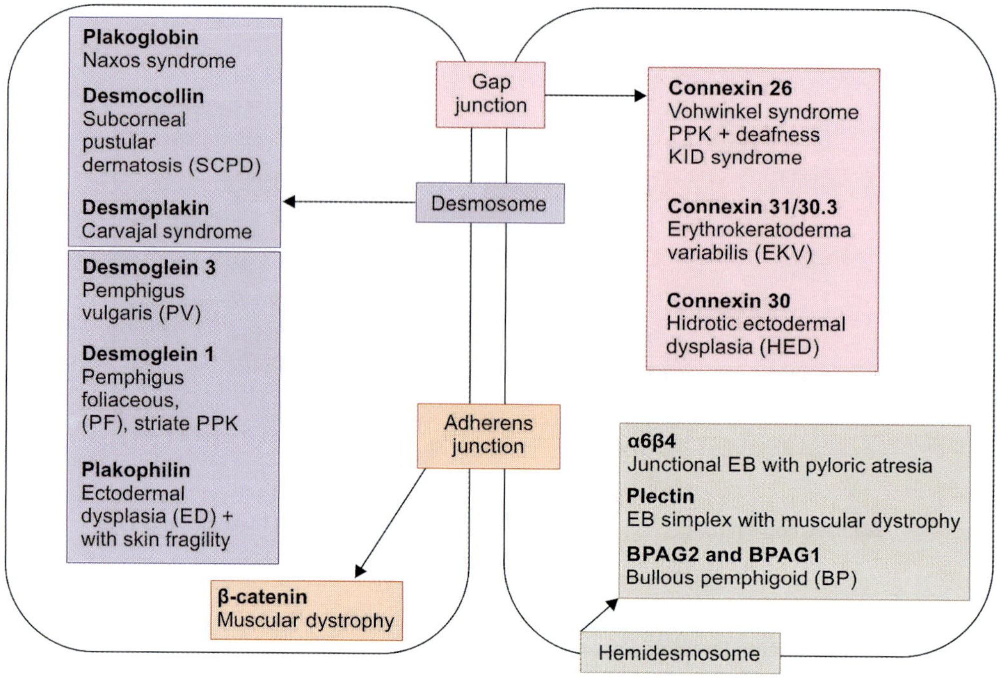

Fig 4: Skin diseases associated with cell junction.

KERATINIZATION

Introduction

- The epidermal thickness and the number and size of epidermal cells remain constant, with the rate of cell production matching the rate of cell loss.
- The keratinocyte stem cells give rise to all the layers of the epidermis, with the majority of these cells committed to terminal differentiation.

Definition

- Keratinization, also termed as cornification, is a process of cytodifferentiation which the keratinocytes undergo when proceeding from their postgerminative state (stratum basale) to finally differentiated, hardened cell filled with protein, constituting a structurally and functionally distinct keratin containing surface layer such as stratum corneum.
- At the cellular level, cornification is characterized by:
  - Production of keratin
  - Production of small proline-rich (SPRR) proteins and transglutaminase which eventually form a cornified cell envelope beneath the plasma membrane
  - Terminal differentiation
  - Loss of nuclei and organelles, in the final stages of cornification.[11]

Epidermal Cell Production (Epidermopoiesis)

- Normally, most epidermal cells are produced in the basal layer of the epidermis, but some (about 30% of the total) are also produced in the first suprabasal layer.
- The proliferative cells go through a cell cycle, which is defined as the time interval between two successive mitoses (intermitotic time).
- *The multiplying cells pass through four phases:* The mitosis phase (M) is followed by the interphase or postmitotic growth phase (G1), a phase of active DNA synthesis (S), and a short resting or premitotic phase (G2).
- Some basal cells may remain quiescent in the so-called G0 phase, which permits them to reenter the cell cycle under appropriate stimuli.
- The duration of the cell cycle for normal epidermis varies from 50 to 457 hours; the time taken in each phase of cell cycle is also variable.
- Mitotic divisions occur in the keratinocytes every 18–19 days.[12]

Total Epidermal Turnover Time

It takes on average 45–60 days (30–50 days from stratum basale to stratum corneum and approximately 14 days from stratum corneum to desquamation).

Steps of Keratinization

- During the process of epithelial differentiation, cells become cornified as keratin protein is incorporated into longer keratin intermediate filaments **(Fig. 5)**.
- Eventually the nucleus and cytoplasmic organelles disappear, metabolism ceases and cells undergo a programmed death as they become fully keratinized.
- Keratinization results in the formation of cornified cell envelope by the following steps:
  - Cross-linking of envoplakin, periplakin, along cell membrane

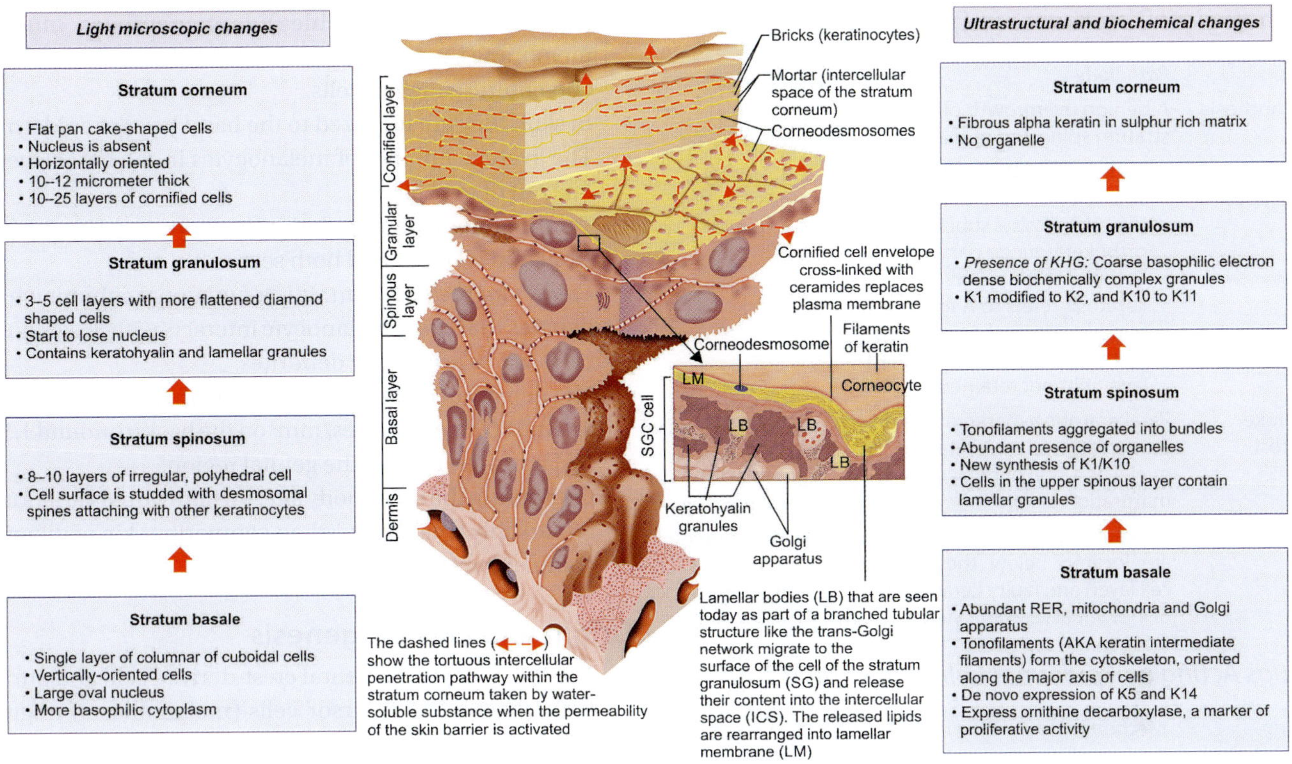

Fig. 5: Keratinization process.

- Lamellar granule extrusion into extracellular space
- Loricrin cross-links envelope
- Keratin and filaggrin cross-link

Regulation of Epidermopoiesis[13]

Stimulatory signals	• Growth factors— EGF, TGF-alpha, amphiregulin, basic FGF, KGF. • Cytokines—interleukin-1, interleukin-6 and GM-CSF • Platelet-derived growth factor (PDGF), TGF-α, IL-1β, and tumor necrosis factor (TNF) induce the keratinocyte growth factor (*KGF*) gene • Arachidonic acid metabolite—LT and HETE • Hormones—androgens • Polyamines—spermine/spermidine
Inhibitory signals	• TGFβ, present in epidermal cells, inhibits the growth of keratinocytes • Interferon (IFN)-α and -γ • TNFα • Vitamin D_3 • Cyclic AMP • PGD2, E2 • Drugs—adrenaline, glucocorticoids
Apoptosis	Programmed cell death is a major cellular homeostatic mechanism in the skin. Terminal differentiation of epidermal keratinocytes occurs by modified apoptotic programs
Signal transduction pathways	Growth factors, cAMP, protein kinase C, inositol phosphate, and protein tyrosine kinase
Integrins	Serve a physical link between matrix molecules (collagen, laminin, fibronectin) and the cytoskeleton of keratinocytes, and act as the route for bidirectional communication that can result in a change in gene expression, pH, and calcium fluxes
Others	• A low calcium level inhibits differentiation of keratinocytes; proliferation is inhibited by high calcium concentrations in vitro • Vitamin A and retinoic acids are required for normal morphogenesis and differentiation

Contd...

Contd...

Applied Aspects

Diseases Caused by Alteration of Important Keratinization Molecule

Filaggrin	• Atopic dermatitis • Ichthyosis vulgaris • Granular porokeratosis
Loricrin	• Progressive symmetric erythrokeratoderma • Mutilating keratoderma with ichthyosis • Vohwinkel (variant)
Keratin	Discussed earlier
Absent steroid sulfatase in lamellar granules	X-linked ichthyosis
Transglutaminase	TG3 → dermatitis herpetiformis, TG1 → lamellar ichthyosis
β-catenin	Pilomatricoma (multiple may be associated with myotonic dystrophy)
Connexin	Discussed earlier

Pathological Disturbance in Epidermal Kinetics

Term	*Pathology*	*Examples*
Acanthosis	A benign overgrowth of the stratum spinosum of the skin	Psoriasis, chronic eczema
Hyper-keratosis	• An increased thickness of the stratum corneum • Hyperkeratosis is subclassified as orthokeratotic or parakeratotic • Orthokeratotic hyper-keratosis refers to A form of hyperkeratosis characterized by thickening of the cornified layer without retained nuclei	• Autosomal recessive congenital ichthyosis • Lichen planus
Parake-ratosis	Parakeratotic hyperkeratosis or parakeratosis shows retained nuclei as a sign of delayed maturation of keratinocytes	• Psoriasis • Axillary granular parakeratosis
Dyskeratosis	A premature (keratinocytes that are located below the granular cell layer) and faulty keratinization of individual keratinocytes	• Darier's disease • Dyskeratosis congenita

Drugs Acting on Epidermal Cells and Keratinization

Drug	*Mechanism*
Retinoids	• Act on retinoic acid receptors RAR and RXR • Modulate epidermal differentiation • Tazarotene causes upregulation of K10
Vitamin D analogs	Regulate keratinocyte proliferation
Coal tar	Atrophogenic effect
Salicylic acid	Dissolve the intercellular substance of the corneocytes

MELANOCYTES

Introduction

Melanocytes are pigment-producing cell derived from neural crest, projects cellular processes that interact with other cells.

Sites

- *Melanocytes are found in multiple tissues:* Epidermis, hair matrix, retinal pigment epithelium, inner ear (stria vascularis of cochlea), leptomeninges, mucous membranes, uveal tract of eye (choroid, iris, ciliary body), and enteric ganglion cells.
- In skin, they are localized to the basal layer of epidermis.
- The average number of melanocytes in the basal layer is one out of ten cells.
- Total melanocyte population is about 2×10^9 which is similar in all races and both sexes.
- *Epidermal melanin unit:* It is a functional subunit which denotes that every melanocyte interacts with 36 keratinocytes via its arborizing dendrites.
- The density of melanocytes varies with the body site from around 900 melanocytes/mm^2 on the back to around 1,500 melanocytes/mm^2 in the genital region.
- Comparing the same body site, the individual variation is remarkably small, even when comparing skin of differing complexion **(Fig. 6)**.

Origin and Embryogenesis

- The melanocyte is a neural crest-derived cell, and during embryogenesis precursor cells (melanoblasts) migrate along a dorsolateral pathway via the mesenchyme to reach the epidermis and hair follicles.
- Melanocytes appear in the eighth week of fetal skin. Melanosomes appear between 4th and 6th months in fetal life.
- Cutaneous melanocytes can also arise from Schwann cell precursors located along nerves in the skin, which also originate from the neural crest.
- Survival and migration of melanocytes during embryogenesis depends on specific interactions such as c-kit activation contributing to migration and development of melanocytes and melanoblasts.
- Melanin production starts postnatally except in nipples and genitalia.
- Parenthetically, choroidal melanocytes may continue to produce melanin and cause darkening of the iris until early adulthood.[14]

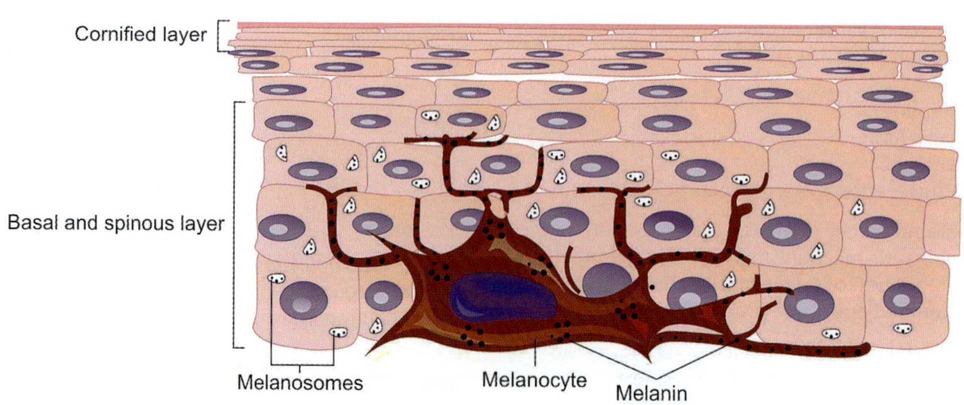

Fig. 6: Association of keratinocytes and melanocytes. The dendritic melanocyte is located in the basal layer of skin and produces melanin. Melanin pigments in melanosomes are transferred to keratinocytes.

Structure of Melanocytes

Light Microscopy

- Melanocytes show artifactual halo on H&E as they do not form junctions with keratinocytes.
- Melanocytes can be differentiated from keratinocytes by:
  - Smaller nucleus
  - Presence of dendritic processes
  - Absence of tonofilaments and desmosomes

Special Stains

- The commonly used Fontana-Masson ("melanin stain") stain relies upon the melanin granules to reduce ammoniacal silver nitrate (but argentaffin, chromaffin, and some lipochrome pigments also will stain black as well).
- Schmorl's method uses the reducing properties of melanin to stain granules blue-green.
- The most specific method of all is an enzyme histochemical method called DOPA-oxidase. It requires frozen sections for best results.
- Bleaching techniques remove melanin in order to get a good look at cellular morphology. They make use of a strong oxidizing agent such as potassium permanganate or hydrogen peroxide. Ocular melanin takes hours to bleach, while that from skin takes minutes.

Immunohistochemistry

- The S100 antigen is expressed in melanocytes.
- Melan-A (and its closely-related antigen MART-1) is a commonly used alternative to S100 because of its perceived high sensitivity and specificity for melanocytes.
- Microphthalmia-associated transcription factor (MITF) is a newer melanocytic marker that may allow for more accurate estimation of the number of melanocytes within the epidermis.

Electron Microscopy and Ultrastructure of Melanocytes

- Melanocytes contain numerous mitochondria, well-developed RER, Golgi apparatus, and cytoplasmic filaments.
- However, they do not have tonofilaments and desmosomes.
- Melanosomes:
  - Melanosomes are tissue-specific "lysosome-related" organelles of pigment cells in which melanins are synthesized and stored.
  - Melanosomes are relatively large organelles, measuring up to 500 nm in diameter.
  - Melanosomes, via dendritic-like processes, contact keratinocytes and transfer melanosomes to keratinocytes
  - *There are two types of melanosomes:* Eumelanosomes (make eumelanin) and pheomelanosomes (make pheomelanin). In humans most melanosomes switch from making one melanin to another.

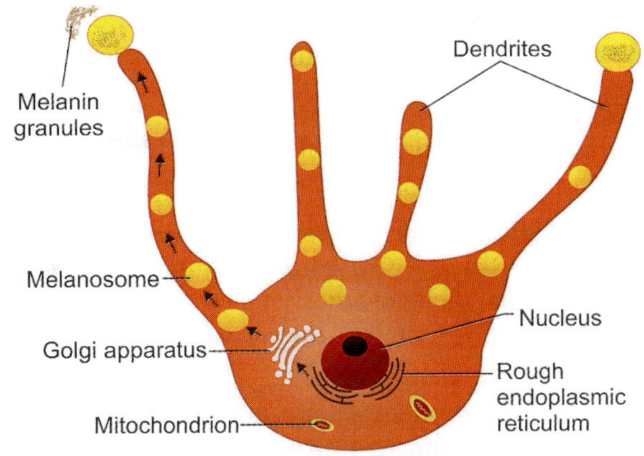

Fig. 7: Ultrastructure of melanocytes.

  - They are bound by a bilipid membrane and contain structural proteins and enzymes like tyrosinase, acid peptidases, and ATPase.
  - Critical enzymes include tyrosinase-related protein 1 (TYRP1) and TYRP2 [also called dopachrome tautomerase (DCT)]. Hormones that drive pigmentation such as MSH induce gene expression of TYR, TYRP1, and TYRP2
  - *Stages of melanosomes:*
    - *Stage 1:* Spherical. Presence of concentric lamellae. No melanin deposition.
    - *Stage 2:* Ellipsoid. Presence of numerous lamellae, some showing crosslinking. Minimal deposition of melanin; high tyrosinase activity.
    - *Stage 3:* Moderate deposition of melanin, partially obscuring lamellar structure. High tyrosinase activity.
    - *Stage 4:* Heavy deposition of melanin, making it electron opaque. Presence of vesiculo-globular bodies. Minimum tyrosinase activity.
  - During the progression from stage 1 to stage 4 of melanosomes the amount of tyrosinase decreases and acid phosphatase increases.
  - Chronic sun exposure results in melanocytes creating larger melanosomes.
- *Racial differences:* Not due to differences in the number of melanocytes, but rather the size, distribution, and number of melanosomes (all races have *same* melanocyte density). Individuals with darker skin tone have a greater production of melanosomes in the melanocytes, individual melanosomes with a higher degree of melanization, larger melanosomes, a higher degree of dispersion of melanosomes in the keratinocytes, and a slower rate of melanosome degradation **(Fig. 7)**.[15]

Stages of Melanogenesis

- Synthesis of melanosomes
- Melanin synthesis

- Intracellular transport
- Melanin transfer to keratinocyte

Melanin:

- Melanin is a high-molecular weight biochrome that results from the oxidation of tyrosine by tyrosinase within melanosomes. There are two varieties:
  1. Eumelanin, a brownish-black melanin present in ellipsoidal melanosomes.
  2. Pheomelanin, a brownish-yellow melanin present in spherical melanosomes.
- Eumelanin and pheomelanin initially have a common biosynthetic pathway; under appropriate physiologic conditions dopaquinone reacts with cysteine to produce intermediate metabolites that form pheomelanin.
- Pheomelanin is found only in red or blond hair.

Melanin synthesis:

- Melanin is formed from the phenolic amino acid precursor L-tyrosine through a series of enzymatic and spontaneous chemical reactions termed as the Raper–Mason pathway.
- Melanin is synthesized through a series of interactions catalyzed by enzyme complexes that are highly similar metalloproteins.
- L-tyrosine serves as the starting material for biosynthesis of melanin. The immediate product, dopa, upregulates melanin synthesis.
- Hydroxylation of L-tyrosine to L-DOPA is the rate-limiting step in melanin synthesis and is catalyzed by tyrosinase, which is a copper-containing membrane-bound located in melanosomes.

Melanin transfer:

- The melanocyte and its associated keratocytes seem to function symbiotically, the melanocyte synthesizing melanosomes and transferring them to the keratocytes.
- This process is known as apocopation (the tip of the dendrite is snipped off and engulfed by the keratocytes).
- Melanosome translocation in these cells involves bidirectional transport along microtubules, facilitated by both dynein and kinesin motors, and peripheral capture on actin filaments.
- In the keratinocytes, the melanosomes arrange themselves in an umbrella-like array in the sunny side of the nuclei.
- Melanin is distributed preferentially to more basally located keratinocytes **(Fig. 8)**.[15,16]

Factors Affecting Melanization

- Race
- UVR exposure
- Age
- *Hormonal changes:* Hormones such as MSH, ACTH, androgens, estrogens, progesterone, and thyroxin have a role in melanin production. The increase in estrogen levels during pregnancy can cause hyperpigmentation.
- *Other physiological stimuli:* PGE2, PGD2, arachidonic acid, and oleic acid.
- *Transcription factors involved in melanogenesis:* MITF plays a key role in the regulation of melanogenic proteins expression; other transcription factors of importance are paired box (PAX) 3, SRY-Box (SOX)9/10, and T-cell factor/lymphoid enhancer factor (TCF/LEF-1).
- *Proteins with supportive roles in the melanin biosynthesis pathway:* Ocular albinism (OA)1 protein, P protein,

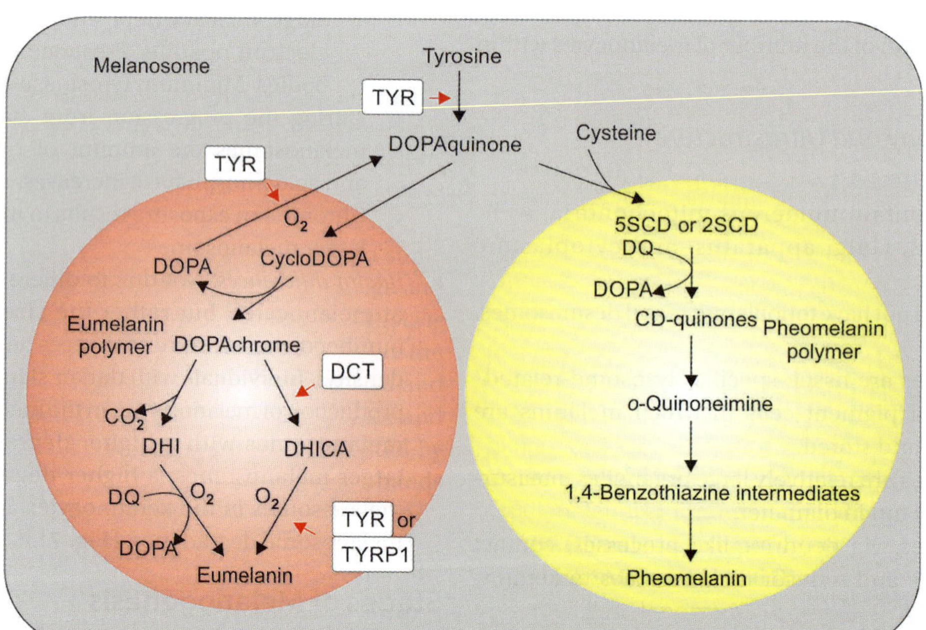

Fig. 8: Melanogenic pathway that occurs within melanosomes, leading to the production of eumelanin and/or pheomelanin.

membrane-associated transporter protein (MATP), copper-transporting P-type ATPase (ATP7A or Menkes protein), and biogenesis of lysosome-related organelles complex 1 (BLOC-1).

- Keratinocytes can produce both growth and inhibitor factors for melanocytes:
  - *Growth:* Basic fibroblast growth factor (bFGF) and transforming growth factor (TGF)-α
  - *Inhibitory:* Interleukin (IL)-1, IL-6, TGF-β.
- *Extrinsic factors affecting melanogenesis:* Magnesium-l-ascorbyl-2-phosphate (MAP), hydroxyanisole, N-acetyl-4-S-cysteaminylphenol, arbutin, and hydroquinone are the most widely prescribed skin whitening products
- *Inflammation:* Melanocytes respond to inflammatory events in the epidermis by producing either more or less melanin (hyperpigmentation or hypopigmentation, respectively).[17]

Hair Melanocytes

- Melanin unit exists in proximal anagen bulb: One melanocyte is paired with five keratinocytes
- Follicular melanogenesis is coupled to hair growth cycle: Melanocyte proliferation occurs during early period of anagen
- Hair follicle contains melanocyte precursors that can repopulate the interfollicular epidermis
- Graying caused by gradual decline in the number of follicular melanocytes; influenced by both age and genes

Functions of Melanocytes

- Production of melanin pigment with subsequent transfer to keratinocytes
- Absorption of UV radiation and protection from UV-induced mutations.
- Biochemically neutralize toxic free radical oxygen derivatives
- Imparts hair color.

Applied Aspects

- *MC1R* gene mutations associated with red hair, increased risk of melanoma and skin cancer.
- Oculocutaneous albinism (OCA) is caused by the defect in melanin synthesis due to loss of:
  - Tyrosinase (OCA1) (melanosomes arrest in stage I or II)
  - *P*-gene (OCA2)
  - *TYRP1* gene (OCA3)
- Giant melanosomes are found in:
  - Chédiak–Higashi syndrome
  - Ocular albinism
  - Café-au-lait spots
- *Hermansky–Pudlak syndrome:* Defective trafficking of organelle-specific proteins to melanosomes, lysosomes, and cytoplasmic granules
- *Griscelli syndrome:* In all three forms, melanosomes are retained in the body of the melanocyte rather than trafficking to the tips of dendrites for transfer to keratinocytes.

LANGERHANS CELL

Introduction

- Langerhans cells are tissue-resident, nonphagocytic, mononuclear dendritic cells which are critical in recognizing and presenting foreign antigens to specific T-lymphocytes.
- Paul Langerhans, while still a medical student, described these cells first in 1868.
- About 120 years later, these cells were ultimately determined to belong to the subset of leukocytes called dendritic cells (DCs) thanks to the work of Nobel Prize Laureate Ralph Steinman and Gerold Schuler.

Origin and Distributions

- LCs make their appearance by 10th to 14th week of fetal life.
- They are bone marrow-derived dendritic cells with monocyte-macrophage lineage originating from the "mesenchymal precursor" in the bone marrow.
- They migrate from bone marrow in embryonic development and continue to repopulate epidermis during their lifetime. Cell cycle of LCs is approximately 16 days.
- They are present in all layers of the epidermis but most prominent in the stratum spinosum.
- LCs reside in the epidermis as a dense network of immune system sentinels. It constitutes 3–5% of cells of epidermis. Concentration of LCs in epidermis varies from 460 nm/mm^2 and 1000/mm^2.
- They also occur in the papillary dermis, particularly around blood vessels, as well as in the mucosa of the mouth, foreskin, and vaginal epithelium.
- Oral mucosa contains about 37 times as many T-lymphocytes as the epidermis of normal skin.
- They can be found in other tissues, such as lymph nodes, particularly in association with the condition Langerhans cell histiocytosis (LCH).

Structure

Light Microscopy

- With hematoxylin and eosin stains in conventional microscopy, they appear as clear spaces due to artifact caused by the cell shrinkage.
- The LCs can be visualized as cells with their bodies generally in the middle portion of stratum spinosum. Delicate dendritic processes can often be observed extending to the level of stratum corneum. Their cytoplasmic processes are found in the stratum corneum and usually directed toward the epithelial surface.

- According to morphology, LCs have been classified into two types, i.e., type 1 LCs, which are pyramidal in shape, located in the suprabasal layer, and type 2 LCs, which are spherical in shape, located in the basal layer. Type 1 contains numerous Birbeck granules, electron lucent cytoplasm, and long-branched dendritic processes whereas type 2 cells, with fewer Birbeck granules, electron dense cytoplasm and shorter dendritic processes.

Special Stains

- One of the first techniques employed to demonstrate LCs was the metal impregnation staining technique using heavy metals such as gold chloride, osmium iodide or zinc osmium iodide, and uranyl acetate-lead staining.
- Zinc osmium iodide, although gives good staining, also stains keratinocytes and melanocytes.

Enzyme Histochemistry

- The actual sites of cellular enzymatic activity can be demonstrated by enzyme histochemical techniques like ATPase, which is an excellent method for the identification of human LCs.
- ATPase is the 1st marker to develop.
- Other enzymes used are adenosine diphosphatase (ADPase), 5 nucleotidases, and amino-peptidases.

Immunohistochemistry

- CD1a immunolabeling is considered to be the most reliable method to identify the human LCs.
- Positive for CD207 (langerin) which induces the formation of Birbeck granules.
- Also positive for S100 and CD34.
- Positive for CD45, Fc receptor, C3, actin, and vimentin.

Electron Microscopy and Ultrastructure

- LCs exhibit a cleaved or folded kidney-shaped nucleus.
- There are no tonofilaments or desmosomes. Adhere to cells by E-cadherin.
- Located in all layers of epidermis, but mostly in the suprabasal layer of stratum spinosum.
- *Birbeck granules:*
    - The Birbeck granules are characteristically present in their cytoplasm, which have a three-dimensional profile of a disk.
    - Their size varies from 100 nm to 1 μm.
    - These granules seem to be the most specific marker for LCs.
    - Birbeck granules show a vesicle at one end and sometimes at both ends.
    - In cross sections, the granule with vesicle at one end shows a characteristic appearance, which is termed as "tennis racket" appearance.
    - Presence of transverse striations has also been observed within the Birbeck granule. It is believed that they are formed due to invagination of the cell membrane.
- Grune and Stratton, 1983, have used six electron microscopic criteria of specificity for LCs:
    1. Indented or lobulated nucleus
    2. Birbeck granules
    3. Absence of tonofilaments
    4. Well-developed Golgi apparatus with a clear cytoplasm
    5. Absence of desmosomes
    6. Absence of melanosomes and premelanosomes.[18,19]

Functions

- They are the most important cells for recognition, uptake, and processing of antigens in the skin and presenting these antigens to naïve T-cells.
- There are two stages in the Langerhans life cycle:
    1. In epidermis, they ingest and process antigens; are weak stimulators of T-cells
    2. Activated LCs that have contacted antigen and can strongly stimulate naïve T-cells
- Once a Langerhans cell encounters and processes a given antigen, it "matures" and migrates to a local lymph node, where it then presents the antigen to a naïve (or resting) T cell, which activates that T-cell.
- They produce IL-1.
- Exposure to UV radiation causes depletion of LCs and decreases ability to present antigen.

Applied Aspects

- LCs are central to the pathogenic processes of atopic dermatitis, psoriasis, allergic contact dermatitis, and infections such as leishmaniasis.
- LC can be infected with HIV.
- *Langerhans cell histiocytosis:*
    - Letterer-Siwe—acute disseminated
    - Eosinophilic granuloma—involves bone (cranium)
    - Hand-Schüller-Christian—triad of diabetes insipidus, exophthalmos, and bone lesions.
    - Hashimoto-Pritzker—self-healing variant **(Fig. 9)**.

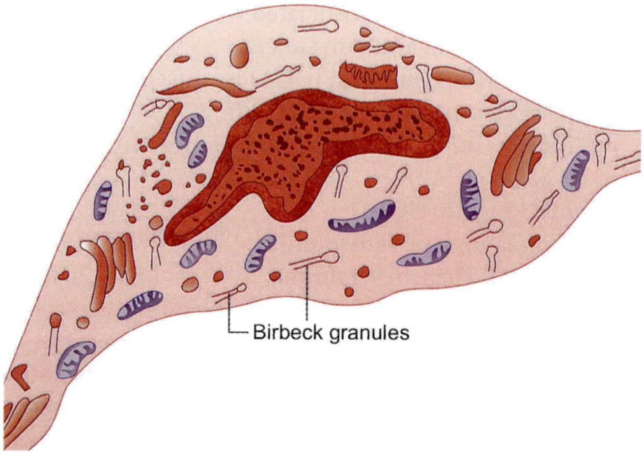

Fig. 9: Langerhans cell with cleaved nucleus and numerous Birbeck granules within the cytoplasm.

MERKEL CELL

Introduction

- It is an oval-shaped cell found in the basal layer of epidermis which acts as a slowly adapting touch receptor.
- Synonyms: Merkel-Ranvier cells, "Tastzellen" (touch cells), "Haarscheibe" (Hair disk), tactile epithelial cells.
- In 1875 Friedrich Sigmund Merkel, using a light microscope, discovered Merkel cells.

Embryology

- The origin of MCs has been debated for over 20 years.
- It is first seen at 12 weeks of gestation.
- There are two prevailing hypotheses concerning the developmental origin of MCs: (1) the neural crest origin hypothesis and (2) the epidermal origin hypothesis (Tachibana, 1995).
- Evidence from skin graft experiments in birds implies that they are neural crest derived, but experiments in mammals now demonstrate an epidermal origin.

Distribution

- Merkel cells are found in the skin and some parts of the mucosa.
- They are commonly seen in masticatory mucosa, but are usually absent in lining mucosa.
- MCs are concentrated near the eccrine glands of glabrous skin, near the hair follicles of hairy skin, and in certain areas of mucosal tissues.
- MCs are found in high numbers in the palms and soles, lips, anterior hard palate, and gingiva.

Structure

Light Microscopy

- Using routine light microscopy of hematoxylin and eosin stained human skin the MCs are clear cells found in the stratum basale of the epidermis approximately 10 μm in diameter.
- It has nerve tissue immediately subjacent and is presumed to be a specialized neural pressure sensitive receptor cell.
- MCs are oval-shaped cells and differ from other nonkeratinocytes in that they are not dendritic.

Immunohistochemistry

- Anticytokeratin 20 (CK20) is a specific and reliable marker of Merkel cells and presents as perinuclear dots. MCs also contain CK8, 18, and 19.
- The dense-core granules stain positively for the neuro-endocrine markers chromogranin A, neuron-specific enolase, and synaptophysin; these markers may be useful as diagnostic adjuncts.
- Vasoactive intestinal polypeptide, serotonin, and substance P show variable positivity.

Fluorescent Microscopy

Other methods of their identification with light microscopy are based on incorporation of fluorescent dyes into the MCs. Live MCs are known to incorporate quinacrine, which fluoresces a light under ultraviolet (UV) illumination.

Electron Microscopy and Ultrastructure

- MCs can be distinguished from other cells of epidermis by electron microscopy.
- By electron microscopy, the uranaffin reaction has been applied to identify MCs. Uranaffin reaction was introduced as an ultrastructural stain for the localization of adenine nucleotide in organelles storing biogenic amines.
- The surface of MCs appears to be attached to the basement membrane.
- MCs show lobulations or spine-like protrusions called microvilli at the cell surface. The spine-like protrusions of highly variable length attached to the neighboring keratinocytes by relatively few, small desmosomes.
- Cytoplasm has low microscopic density and contains loosely arranged intermediate filaments assuming whorled arrangement near the nucleus (dot-like pattern).
- MC possesses a lobulated nucleus, with a characteristic intranuclear rodlet.
- *Dense-core secretory granules:*
  - These are ultrastructural characteristics of MCs.
  - They accumulate near the nerve fiber junction.
  - They have an electron-dense core, surrounded by a clear halo, and a simple membrane.
  - MCs' granules measure about 80–120 nm.
- Most often, but not always, they are associated with sensory nerve endings, when they are known as a Merkel cell-neurite complex.
- *MC contains a battery of neuropeptides and neuro-transmitter-like substances:* Neuron-specific enolase (NSE), vasoactive intestinal peptide (VIP), calcitonin gene-related peptide (CGRP), chromogranin A, synaptophysin, and met-enkephalin

Possible Functions

- *Somatosensation:* MCs are possibly sensory cells that transduce mechanical stimuli and then communicate with sensory afferents via neurotransmission. They are associated with slowly adapting somatosensory nerve fibers. They react to low vibrations (5–15 Hz) and deep static touch such as shapes and edges.
- *Endocrine function:* Merkel cells are sometimes considered APUD cells because they contain dense core granules, and thus may also have a neuroendocrine function.
- *Chemosensation:* MCs may have a possible chemosensitive function, in particular nociceptive function, which are mediated by free nerve endings.[20]

Applied Aspects

- Merkel cell carcinoma:
  - MCC is an uncommon and often aggressive malignancy that has a poor prognosis.
  - It is also known as cutaneous APUDoma, primary neuroendocrine carcinoma of the skin
  - MCC in most cases is caused by a virus MC polyomavirus (MCV). Other factors involved are immunosuppression and ultraviolet exposure.
  - It is more common in people over 60-year-old, Caucasian people, and males.
  - It occurs most frequently on the head, neck, and extremities, as well as in the perianal region and on the eyelids and has a predilection for the periocular region.
  - It most commonly presents as a blue or red, firm, solitary, nontender, dome-shaped nodule and may have a plaque or a subcutaneous mass-like appearance.
  - The overlying skin may be ulcerated but more frequently intact.
  - On light microscopy, MCC shows basaloid tumor nests with neuroendocrine features ("salt and pepper" chromatin, scarce cytoplasm, and brisk mitotic activity).
  - Histologically, MCC has been classified into three distinct subtypes: Trabecular type, Intermediate type, Small cell type.
  - MCC is often positive for CK20. Other markers are PAX5 and neuroendocrine molecular markers such as synaptophysin or chromogranin A.
  - Wide surgical (1-cm to 2-cm margins) excision is the primary mode of treatment for nonmetastatic disease. Sentinel lymph node biopsy may aid in the staging.
  - Adjuvant radiation to the primary site and involved lymph nodes can prevent local recurrences and may improve survival.
  - The mortality rate is approximately 25% **(Fig. 10)**.[21]

STEM CELLS OF EPIDERMIS

- Stem cells are lineage-specific cells that can multiply and differentiate to mediate epidermal renewal/turnover.
  - Keratinocyte stem cells express markers such as Delta 1, MCSP, α6- and β1-integrins, LRIG1; and have low levels of CD71
  - Melanocyte stem cells express markers such as ax3, TYRP1, TYRP2; and are negative for KIT, tyrosinase.
  - Hair follicle stem cells express markers such as SOX9, keratin 15, α6- and β1-integrins, CD200, PHLDA1, follistatin, frizzled homolog 1, LGR5; and have low levels of CD24, CD34, CD71, and CD146.
  - Merkel cell stem cells express markers such as α6-integrin, keratin 17, ATOH1, CD200, GLI1, SOX2.[22]

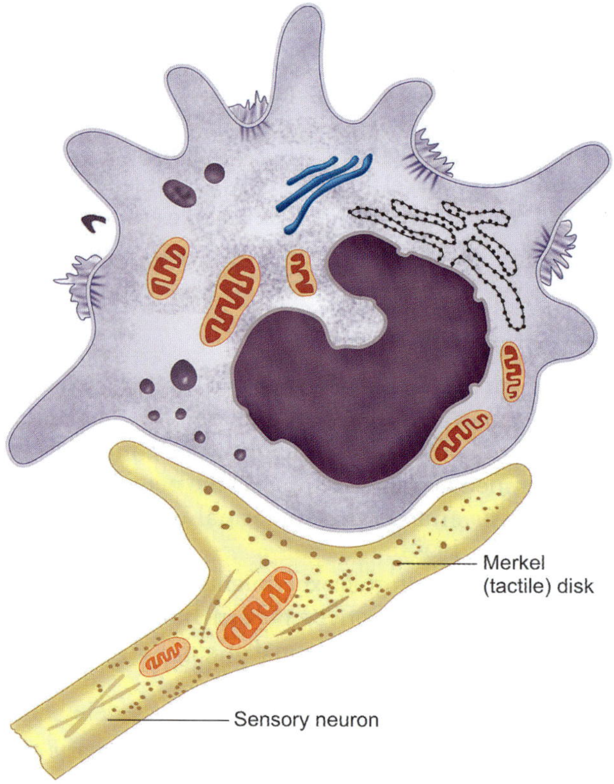

Fig. 10: Merkel cells.

BASEMENT MEMBRANE ZONE

Introduction

- Basement membranes are specialized structures for attachment and interaction between the epidermis and the dermis.
- It is a selective barrier between the epidermis and dermis; allows for interaction between the two areas and provides anchoring of epidermis to dermis.
- This area is also known as the dermal-epidermal junction (DEJ).
- It is matured in fetal skin at the 12th week of gestation.
- The zone is composed of proteins derived from keratinocytes of ectodermal origin as well as dermal fibroblasts of mesodermal origin.
- In the "laminated" model of the basement membrane zone (BMZ), the keratin cytoskeleton in the basal keratinocytes attach to hemidesmosomes. In turn, anchoring filaments connect hemidesmosomes to the lamina densa. The lamina densa is attached to the superficial dermis by anchoring fibrils.

Light Microscopy

- In conventional microscopy BMZ are best visualized after staining with PAS stains where it appears as a thin magenta colored linear band immediately beneath the basal keratinocytes.

- Silver nitrate stains reveal a zone of argyrophilic fibers-oriented perpendicular to and just below the PAS positive region.

Ultrastructure

- The cutaneous BM itself is about 80 nm thick.
- There are four distinct subregions of the epidermal basement membrane. These subregions, from superior to inferior distribution, are:
  - *Inferior portion of basal keratinocyte:* This includes the cytoskeleton, hemidesmosomal plaques, and plasma membranes of the basal keratinocytes
  - *The lamina lucida*: This is an electron-lucent region that contains delicate filaments connecting hemidesmosomes (HDs) in basal keratinocytes to the underlying lamina densa
  - *The lamina densa or basement membrane proper*
  - *The sublamina densa region*: This contains anchoring fibrils, anchoring plaques, and filamentous proteins of the papillary dermis.[23]

Inferior Portion of Basal Keratinocyte

- *Keratin intermediate filaments:*
  - The basal keratinocyte cytoskeleton comprises the intermediate filament cytokeratins 5 and 14
  - Keratin intermediate filaments form part of a continuous network that is indirectly attached to adjacent keratinocytes by desmosomes and to the underlying BMZ and dermis by hemidesmosomes.
- *Hemidesmosome (HD):*
  - Hemidesmosomes are small (i.e., <0.5 μ), electron-dense stud-like units on the basal plasma membranes of the basal keratinocytes.
  - It provides attachment between basal keratinocyte and extracellular matrix (ECM).
  - Their concentration in the skin is constant, without regional variation or differences between sexes or age.
  - *Hemidesmosomes have five main elements:* Integrin α6β4, plectin, tetraspanin protein CD151, BPAG1, or and BPAG2.
  - Tonofilaments (or keratin filaments) insert into hemidesmosomes.
- *Plectin:*
  - Plectin is a 500 kDa intracellular protein, belonging to the plakin family and associated with the cytoplasmic plaque domain of hemidesmosomes.
  - The carboxy terminus of plectin binds intermediate filaments (specifically, keratins or vimentin) and the amino terminus contains domains that bind the cytoplasmic tail of integrin subunit β4, BPAG2, and actin.
  - Therefore, it attaches intermediate filaments to HDs and plasma membranes of basal keratinocytes and cross-links HD proteins.
- *Bullous pemphigoid antigen 1 (BPAG1):*
  - BPAG1, a 230 kD noncollagenous glycoprotein of plakin family, is localized to the cytoplasmic plaque of HD.
  - They promote adhesion of intermediate filaments with plasma membranes.
  - BPAG1 binds to integrin α6β4, BPAG2 and keratin 5 and 14. The main role of BPAG1 is hemidesmosome stability and cytoskeletal organization.
  - It also serves as a potential link between HD biology and Erb-B2 signaling.
- *Bullous pemphigoid antigen 2 (BPAG2):*
  - BPAG2 is a transmembrane (mainly extracellular) protein, belonging to the collagen family (specifically, type XVII collagen) that exists adjacent to integrins.
  - BPAG2 has domains that bind to plectin, integrin β4 subunit in the cytoplasm and integrin α6 and laminin-332 in the extracellular space.
  - It has two forms: Full-length transmembrane and soluble 120-kDa ectodomain that is shed from cell surface
  - It may play a role in the structure or stability of anchoring filaments.
  - Disease associated with BP antigens[24]

Site of involvement of BP antigens	*Disease associated*
BPAg1/BPAg2-NC16A	Bullous pemphigoid
BPAg2	Lichen planus pemphigoides
Portion of BPAg2	Linear IgA disease
BPAg2-NC16A	Pemphigoid gestationis
BPAg2, C-terminal domain	Cicatricial pemphigoid

- *Integrins:*
  - The α6β4 type is the hemidesmosome-associated integrin.
  - They are found at sites where keratin intermediate filaments attach.
  - Expression of α6β4 integrin is limited to basal layer of epidermis.
  - They coordinate linkage between intermediate filaments and ECM of the basement membrane.
  - The α6β4 integrin binds intermediate filaments intracellularly, laminin-332 in lamina lucida, and HD proteins like plectin, BPAG2.
  - *Plasma membrane-associated integrins:* Nonhemidesmosomal integrins expressed in basal keratinocytes are integrins α2β1 and α3β1. Among these α3β1 is seen in the basal aspect plasma membranes. Though integrin α3β1 does not play a role in HD assembly, it is thought to provide key signals regulating cytoskeletal assembly and maintenance of basement membrane integrity.
- *Tetraspan CD151:*
  - Tetraspan proteins with four membrane-spanning domains, form "web-like" networks with other membrane proteins.

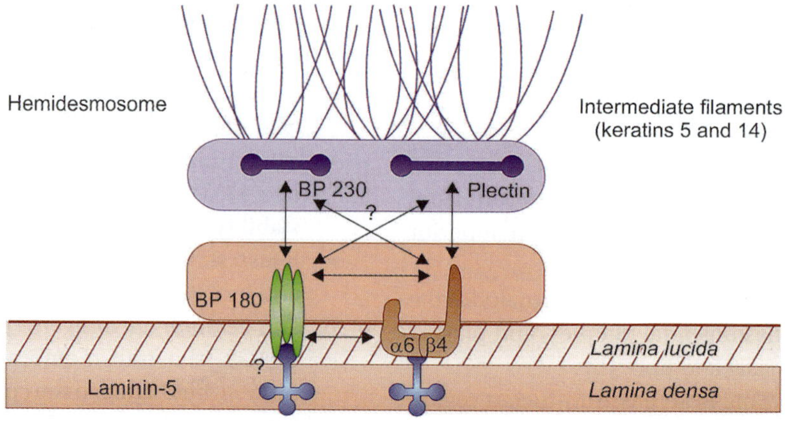

Fig. 11: Hemidesmosome.

- CD151 is the tetraspan concentrated in HD and is associated with integrins α6β4.
- CD151 is thought to provide a framework for the spatial organization of different HD components **(Fig. 11)**.

Lamina Lucida

- This is the electron-lucent zone under the hemidesmosome seen on electron microscopy of BMZ. Lamina lucida is the weakest link of BMZ. Lamina lucida is composed of anchoring filaments (laminin-332), laminin-1, fibronectin, nidogen (entactin), uncein, and a portion of BPAG2.
- It is roughly 40 nm wide.
- *Anchoring filaments:*
  - The major components of anchoring filaments are laminin 5 (also called laminin 332) and BP180.
  - These are proteins composed of three classes of polypeptides. These polypeptides intersect to form a cross-like structure that spans from the plasma membrane of basal keratinocytes to lamina densa.
  - *Anchoring filaments have two major roles:* Structural network in basement membrane and signaling.
- *Laminins:*
  - Laminins are a family of heterotrimeric glycoproteins consisting of three subunits (α, β, and γ)
  - Epidermal basement membranes have three types of laminin like laminin 332 (or laminin 5), laminin 311 (or laminin 6), and laminin 511 (or laminin 10).
  - Laminin 332 or laminin 5 is a major component of anchoring filaments; it is also called epiligrin. Laminin 332 provides the major attachment factor for keratinocytes and binds α6β4 integrin at hemidesmosome
  - Laminin 6 isoforms are found in the dermoepidermal junction (DEJ) of human skin and mucous membranes.

Lamina Densa

- It is the electron-dense zone below lamina lucida appearing as a dense line with closely stippled dots on electron microscopy. Major component of lamina densa is type IV collagen. Other components are laminins, entactin (nidogen-1), and heparan sulfate.
- *Type IV collagen:*
  - Unlike classic fibrillar collagens, type IV collagen is not helical through its entire length which provides increased flexibility. They are highly cross-linked and form a lattice.
  - Functionally, type IV collagen gives structural support and confers flexibility to basement membrane.
  - The collagen IV network is linked to the laminins 5/6/10 complex by the small adhesion molecule, nidogen.
  - Fragments of type IV collagen α-chain subunits like canstatin and tumstatin have important biologic functions like antiangiogenic activity.
- *Nidogen:*
  - Nidogen (entactin) is a 150 kDa glycoprotein localized to the lamina densa of basement membranes.
  - It links type IV collagen networks and various laminin isoforms like laminins 5/6/10.
- *Heparan sulfate proteoglycan:* Heparan sulfate proteoglycans are a diverse group of macromolecules that are negatively charged, and thus function as a permeability barrier.

Sublamina Densa

- Also known as lamina fibroreticularis. This zone contains anchoring fibrils, anchoring plaques, elastic microfibrils (without elastin), and linkin.
- *Anchoring fibril:*
  - Primary constituent of anchoring fibril is type VII collagen. They are larger than anchoring filaments and emanates perpendicularly down from lamina densa into papillary dermis

- Anchoring fibrils begin in the lamina densa and are incorporated into the papillary dermis inserting into amorphous areas of electron-dense material called anchoring plaques.
- Some of the anchoring fibrils curve back up to the lamina densa and reinsert there rather than attaching to the plaques. The attachment of anchoring fibril to the dermis provides adhesion of the BMZ to the underlying dermis.

- *Anchoring plaques:*
  - These are electron-dense oval structures seen under lamina densa on EM
  - They are composed of type IV collagen.
  - Anchoring fibrils attach in these structures from above and fibrillar collagen (type I and III) attach from below.
- *Type VII collagen:*
  - It is the major component of anchoring fibrils. It is a homotrimeric protein consisting of three identical α-chains, each with a molecular weight of approximately 290 kDa.
  - The globular NC1 domains of type VII collagen molecules bind the lamina densa at one end and either loop back into the lamina densa or connect to electron-dense elements in the sublamina densa region termed anchoring plaques
  - Type VII collagen also interacts with laminin 332.
- *Microfibrils:*
  - In the papillary dermis, microfibrillar elements of elastic fibers (also known as oxytalan fibers) insert vertically into the lamina densa and at their inferior aspect, merge with microfibrillar elements-oriented parallel to the skin's surface **(Table 4)**.[23,24]

Functions

- *Attachment:* The primary function of the BMZ is to anchor the epidermis to dermis
- Support
- Regulation of permeability
- The BMZ may act as a mechanical barrier, preventing malignant cells from invading the deeper tissues.
- Role in embryonic differentiation
- The BMZ may also be essential for angiogenesis. The BMZ proteins have been found to accelerate differentiation of endothelial cells **(Fig. 12)**.

Applied Aspects

TABLE 4: Diseases associated with BMZ proteins.[25]

Proteins	*Associated disease*
Plectin	EBS with muscular dystrophy, paraneoplastic pemphigus (PNP)
α6β4 integrin	JEB with pyloric atresia, cicatricial pemphigoid (CP)—ocular
BPAG1	Bullous pemphigoid (BP), PNP
BPAG2	• *NC16A domain (1st extracellular segment):* Typically targeted by bullous pemphigoid (BP), pemphigoid gestationis, linear IgA bullous dermatosis (LABD) • *Carboxy terminus (C-terminal):* Cicatricial pemphigoid (CP) tends to target this portion
Laminin-332 (5)	Junctional EB cicatricial pemphigoid with increased risk of cancer
Type VII collagen	Dystrophic EB, EBA, bullous SLE

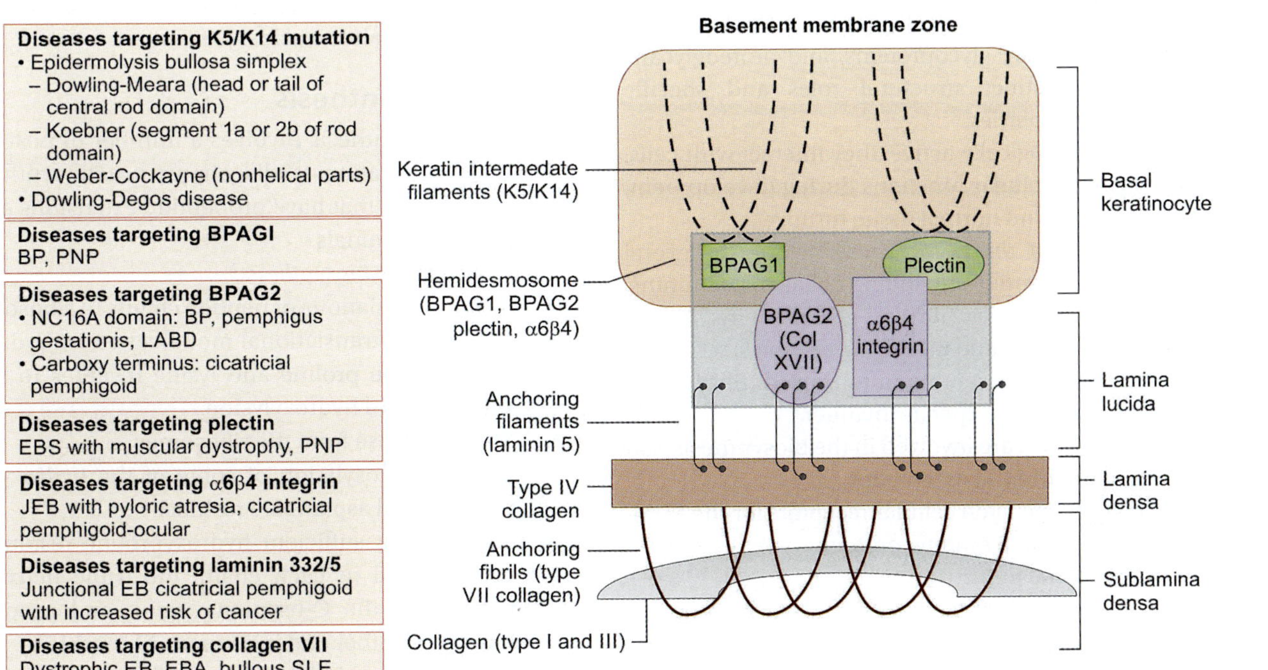

Fig. 12: Anatomy of skin.

DERMIS

- Beneath the epidermis there is a vascularized dermis that provides structural and nutritional support.
- Dermis is composed of mesoderm-derived components. It contains collagen, elastic fibers, matrix (ECM and ground substance made up of proteoglycans and gelatin), dermal cells (fibroblasts, monocytes, phagocytes, mast cells, dermal dendrocytes, glomus cells).
- It can be divided into superficial papillary dermis and deep reticular dermis.
- Reticular dermis has larger collagen bundles and mature branching elastic fibers.
- In pathologic conditions the functions and types of dermal cells change substantially, with a variety of infiltrating cells arriving via vascular routes. The composition of dermal infiltrates provides useful diagnostic clues about the pathological conditions.
- *Papillary dermis:*
  - In young or healthy skin, it consists of small-diameter collagen fibrils and oxytalan elastic fibers
  - In aging or actinically damaged skin, there are more mature elastic fibers that are large and dense
  - Papillary dermis have high density of fibroblast cells that proliferate rapidly
  - Solar elastosis represents degenerated collagen in the upper dermis.
- *Reticular dermis:*
  - It is composed of large-diameter collagen fibers with mature, branching elastic fibers
  - The elastic and collagen bundles progressively increase in size as they move toward the hypodermis
- *ECMs:*
  - ECM represents specifically organized networks of collagens, elastin, glycoproteins, and proteoglycans that have distinct structural roles and specific functional properties.
  - ECMs are biologically active; they interact with cells, and regulate cellular functions during development, regeneration, and normal tissue turnover.
  - *Components of the ECM:* These belong to several protein superfamilies including collagens, laminins, elastin proteoglycans, fibrilins, glycoproteins, LTBPs, integrins, fibulins, and modifying enzymes.
  - The molecules assemble into mixed fibrils and networks in a tissue-specific manner.
  - Several enzymes are involved in the biosynthesis and modification of ECM assemblies.
  - Integrins are the main cellular receptors for the ECM. LTBP, latent TGF-β binding protein.
  - *Functions of the ECM:*
    - ECM provides a structural scaffold that gives organs their shape and consistency.
    - ECMs macromolecules are potent regulators of cellular functions during development, regeneration, wound healing, inflammation, and tumorigenesis.[26]

COLLAGEN

Introduction

- The word collagen is derived from a Greek word κόλλα (kólla), meaning "glue", and suffix -γέν, -gen, denoting "producing"
- It is the most abundant protein of the body making up from 25 to 35% of the whole-body protein content.
- This is a family of fibrous proteins with 28 genetically distinct types. They provide structural stability, tensile strength, and elasticity of dermis and also play an important role in the wound healing process.
- It becomes evident by 13–14 weeks of intrauterine life.

Structure

- A single collagen molecule, tropocollagen, is used to make up larger collagen aggregates, such as fibrils. All collagens consist of three polypeptide chains, known as left handed α-helix, which are folded into a triple helix, a quaternary structure stabilized by many hydrogen bonds.
- Composition of these three chains varies according to collagen type. However, all of them have regular arrangement of amino acids in a Gly-X-Y amino acid motif that repeats, where X and Y are proline and hydroxyproline.
- The prototype collagen (type I) has an uninterrupted Gly-X-Y repeat sequence that is almost 1000 amino acid residues in length. This forms a rigid, rod-like structure of approximately 300 nm in length and 1.5 nm in diameter. In some collagens, the (Gly- X-Y)n repeats are interrupted by one or more amino acids.

Collagen Biosynthesis

- Collagen biosynthesis involves a number of post-translational modifications. Collagens are usually synthesized as procollagens that have propeptide extensions at their one or both terminals.
- *Steps of collagen biosynthesis:*
  - *Step 1:* Translations of peptide chains in ribosomes
  - *Step 2:* Post-translational modification by hydroxylation of some proline and lysine residues to hydroxyproline and hydroxylysine.
  - *Step 3:* Release from the ribosomes
  - *Step 4:* Glycosylation of some of the hydroxylysine residues and asparagine residues
  - *Step 5:* After sufficient hydroxyproline residues are incorporated in each chain, the triple helix starts forming in the C-terminal region and propagates toward the other end in a zipper-like fashion.
  - *Step 6:* The procollagen molecules thus formed are then transported from the endoplasmic reticulum

across the Golgi apparatus. The newly formed triple helical procollagen is then secreted into the extracellular space.
- *Step 7:* In the extracellular space the N- and C-terminal propeptides are cleaved by specific proteases.
- *Step 8:* These tropocollagen molecules then cross-linked to form collagen fibrils

- Lysyl hydroxylase and proline hydroxylase cross-link collagen (desmosine residues); vitamin C is a required cofactor along with copper and vitamin B_6 for the function of the enzymes. Collagen VII-containing anchoring fibrils is transaminated, and collagen VII serves as a substrate for tissue transglutaminase-2.
- Collagen is degraded by interstitial collagenases (metalloproteinases or MMPs).
- Collagen synthesis is stimulated by retinoic acids.
- Collagen synthesis inhibited by IL-1 (↑ MMP expression), glucocorticoids, IFNγ, TNFα, D-penicillamine, and UV irradiation **(Fig. 13)**.

Formations of Collagen

- Most collagens in the skin are products of dermal fibroblasts.
- *Exceptions are:*
  - Collagen XVII produced by epidermal keratinocytes
  - Collagen VII, synthesized by both keratinocytes and fibroblasts
  - Collagens VIII and XVIII, produced by endothelial cells.

Collagens of the Skin

- Collagens are the primary dermal component and it constitutes about 75% of the dry weight of the dermis.
- Different collagens polymerize into distinct suprastructures and have specific functions in the dermis. Most commonly involved in the regularly crossbanded collagen fibrils with periodicity of 64 nm results in the dermis are collagens I, III, V, XII, and XIV.
- Collagen I is the major component of the dermal fibrils but the content of collagen III increases during embryonic development and wound repair.
- Collagen VI, a highly glycosylated and disulfide-bonded collagen, is a component of many tissues, including the skin.
- The collagen IV constitutes the basement membranes.
- *Two collagens are highly important in dermoepidermal junctions:* Collagen VII is the major component of the anchoring fibrils and collagen XVII (also known as bullous pemphigoid antigen 2) is a component of the anchoring filaments.
- Cutaneous vascular basement membranes contain collagens VIII and XVIII.

Demonstration of Collagen

- Histologic special stains for collagen:

Special stain	*Color of collagen*
Masson trichrome	Blue or green
Verhoeff-van Gieson	Red
Aldehyde fuchsin (Gomori)	Red

Contd...

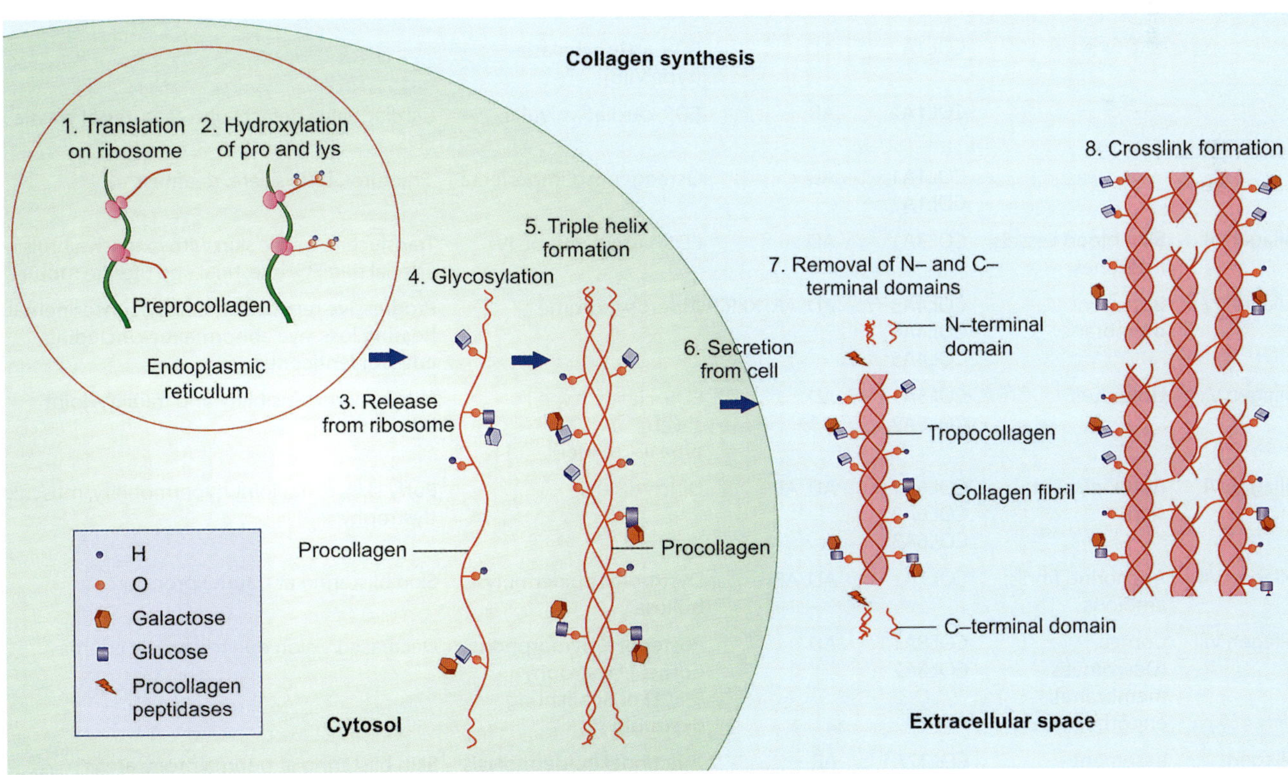

Fig. 13: Steps of collagen biosynthesis.

Contd...

Special stain	*Color of collagen*
Mallory triple stain or trichrome stain (aniline blue)	Blue
PTAH (phosphotungstic acid hematoxylin)	Red
Movat's pentachrome	Yellow

- *Electron microscope:* Collagen fibrils have a characteristic 64 nm banded appearance under the EM, and the fibers are not branched.[27,28]

Applied Aspects

- *Uses of collagen:*
  - Topically used in wound dressing, in cosmeceuticals.
  - Oral collagen supplements increase skin elasticity, hydration, and dermal collagen density.
- Scurvy as a clinical manifestation of severe vitamin C deficiency is caused by the role of ascorbic acids in collagen synthesis. Vitamin C allows hydroxylation and crosslinking of procollagen catalyzed by lysyl hydroxylase. Lack of vitamin C decreases transcription of procollagen. Additionally, a lack of ascorbic acid leads to epigenetic DNA hypermethylation and inhibits the transcription of various types of collagen found in skin, blood vessels, and tissue.
- Homocystinuria is caused by abnormal cross-linking of collagen because of mutated cystathionine synthase.
- Genetic diseases associated with collagen are discussed in **Table 5.**
- Acquired diseases associated with collagen discussed in **Table 6.**

ELASTIC FIBERS

Introduction

- Elastic fibers constitute 4% of the dry weight of the skin.
- They form complex meshwork extending from lamina densa of the DEJ through the dermis and into the hypodermis.
- The elasticity of the skin depends upon the structure of elastic fibers; they make skin return to normal configuration after being stretched.

Structure

- The main components of elastic fibers are: Elastin (amorphous protein at the core) and fibrillin microfibrils (protein filaments at the surroundings).
- *Elastin:*
  - Elastin forms an amorphous core of the elastic fibers and it is surrounded by microfibrils.

TABLE 5: Genetic diseases associated with collagen.

Collagen type	*Distribution*	*Mutation*	*Inheritance*	*Disease associated*	*Key features*
Collagen I	Skin, bone, tendon	COL1A1	AD	EDS, arthrochalasia (type IIA)	Skin hyperextensibility and fragility, joint hypermobility, congenital hip dislocation
		COL1A2	AD	EDS, arthrochalasia (type VIIB)	
		COL1A2	AR	EDS, cardiac valvular	Cardiac valve defects plus features of classic EDS
		COL1A1 COL1A2	AD	Osteogenesis imperfecta	Fractures, blue sclera, deafness
Collagen III	Skin blood vessels, intestines	COL3A1	AD	EDS, vascular (type IV)	Translucent, fragile skin with extensive bruising; arterial fragility, intestinal and uterine rupture
Collagen IV	Basement membrane	COL4A3 COL4A4 COL4A5	AD, AR, XLR	Alport syndrome	Progressive renal insufficiency, sensorineural hearing loss, eye abnormalities including anterior lenticonus
Collagen V	Ubiquitus	COL5A1 COL5A2	AD	EDS, classic (type I – severe; type II – milder)	Skin hyperextensibility and fragility, joint hypermobility
Collagen VI	Aorta, placenta, skin	COL6A1 COL6A2 COL6A3	AD, AR	Ulrich disease	Puffy skin, distal joint hypermobility, muscular dystrophy
Collagen VII	Anchoring fibrils, amnions	COL7A1	AD, AR	Dystrophic epidermolysis bullosa	Skin blistering at trauma prone areas
Collagen VIII	Cornea (Descemet's membrane), endothelial cells	COL8A1, COL8A2	AD	Posterior Polymorphous Corneal Dystrophy (PPCD or Schlichting dystrophy)	Decreased vision due to corneal edema
Collagen XVII	Basement membrane zone	COL17A1	AR	Junctional epidermolysis bullosa (Rarer cause)	Skin blistering at trauma prone areas

TABLE 6: Acquired diseases associated with collagen.

Collagen type	*Disease associated*	*Key features*
Collagen IV	Goodpasture disease	Glomerulonephritis, pneumonitis with hemoptysis
Collagen II	Relapsing polychondritis	Chondritis of ear, larynx, and trachea; arthritis
Collagen XVII	Bullous pemphigoid, cicatricial pemphigoid, and pemphigoid gestationis	Skin blistering
Collagen VII	Epidermolysis bullosa acquisita and bullous systemic lupus erythematosus (SLE)	Skin blistering

- Elastin is a highly cross-linked protein constituting about 90% of the total elastic tissue.
- They are fibrous proteins with a molecular weight of 72,000 kDa.
- The elastin precursor molecule is tropoelastin, which is encoded by a single-copy gene *ELN* in humans located in the chromosomal locus 7q11.2.
- Elastin has a high concentration of alanine and valine, but less hydroxyproline than is present in collagen fibers.
- Desmosine and isodesmosine unique to elastic fibers.
- Lysyl oxidase (copper-dependent enzyme) necessary for formation of elastic-specific amino acids and cross-linking.

- *Microfibrils:*
  - The main component of microfibrils is a glycoprotein called fibrillin.
  - Fibrillin represents the predominant core of the microfibrils in elastic as well as nonelastic extracellular matrices, and interacts closely with tropoelastin and integrins.
  - Fibrillin is important for the assembly of elastin into elastic fibers.
  - The fibrillin-1 and 2 genes (*FBN1* and *FBN2*) are located in chromosome 15 (*FBN1*) and in chromosome 5 (*FBN2*).
- *Fibulin:*
  - A new family of ECM proteins, the fibulins, is being characterized progressively.
  - Fibulins 1, 2, 3, 4, and 5 have been identified.
  - Fibulins are tightly connected with basement membranes, elastic fibers, and other components of ECM, and participate in formation of elastic fibers.
  - Fibulin-5 is essential for dermal elastic fiber assembly.
  - The various fibulins are localized in different parts of the elastic fiber, with fibulin-1 in the amorphous core and fibulin-2 in the fibrillin-containing elastin-associated microfibrils.
- There are two types of elastic fibers forming continuous network spanning from lamina densa of DEJ throughout dermis
  1. *Oxytalan fibers:* These are thin fibers running perpendicular to the skin surface in papillary dermis; contain no elastin. They lack the elastin core. Oxytalan fibers connect the basal lamina to the underlying dermal elastic tissue.
  2. *Eulanin fibers:* These are thicker fibers parallel to the skin surface in reticular dermis. They have less elastin and more fibrillin.

These two types of fibers probably correspond to consecutive stages of normal elastogenesis. These fibers appear to be continuous with the elastic fibers within the reticular dermis, which contains more abundant elastin.

Formation of Elastic Fibers

- Elastic matrix assembly occurs primarily during development and it completes by adolescence.
- Elastic fibers are synthesized by fibroblasts. Elastin is secreted in the form of a precursor, tropoelastin.
- This is ultimately cross-linked with desmosine to form stable elastin by lysyl oxidase.
- Additional elastin is added to the aggregates, which are then transferred onto pre-existing fibrillin-1-containing microfibrils that bind to the cell surface via integrins.
- Fibulin-4 and fibulin-5 interact with the elastin aggregates, enhance cross-linking, and bind to fibrillin-1, thus increasing the transfer of elastin aggregates to the microfibrils.
- Furthermore, fibulin-5 plays an important role as an adaptor molecule between elastin and the matrix scaffold.
- The elastin aggregates and the microfibrils develop into larger structures and are further cross-linked by lysyl oxidase to form a functional elastic fiber **(Fig. 14)**.

Histologic Special Stains for Collagen

- *Verhoeff-van Gieson:* Black
- *Orcein–Giemsa (Pinkus acid orcein):* Black
- *Aldehyde fuchsin (Gomori):* Blue or purple
- *Movat's pentachrome:* Black

Degrading of Elastic Tissue

- Elastin is metabolized by proteolytic enzymes (elastases). Elastases are found in neutrophils, macrophages, platelets, and human fibroblasts.
- Elastase activity is also present in other enzymes, such as cathepsin G, proteinase 3, matrix metalloproteinases 2 and 9, and metalloelastase (MMP12).[29,30]

Applied Aspects

- *Anomalies with increased elastic tissue:*
  - Elastoma (nevus elasticus)
  - Dermatosis lenticularis disseminata

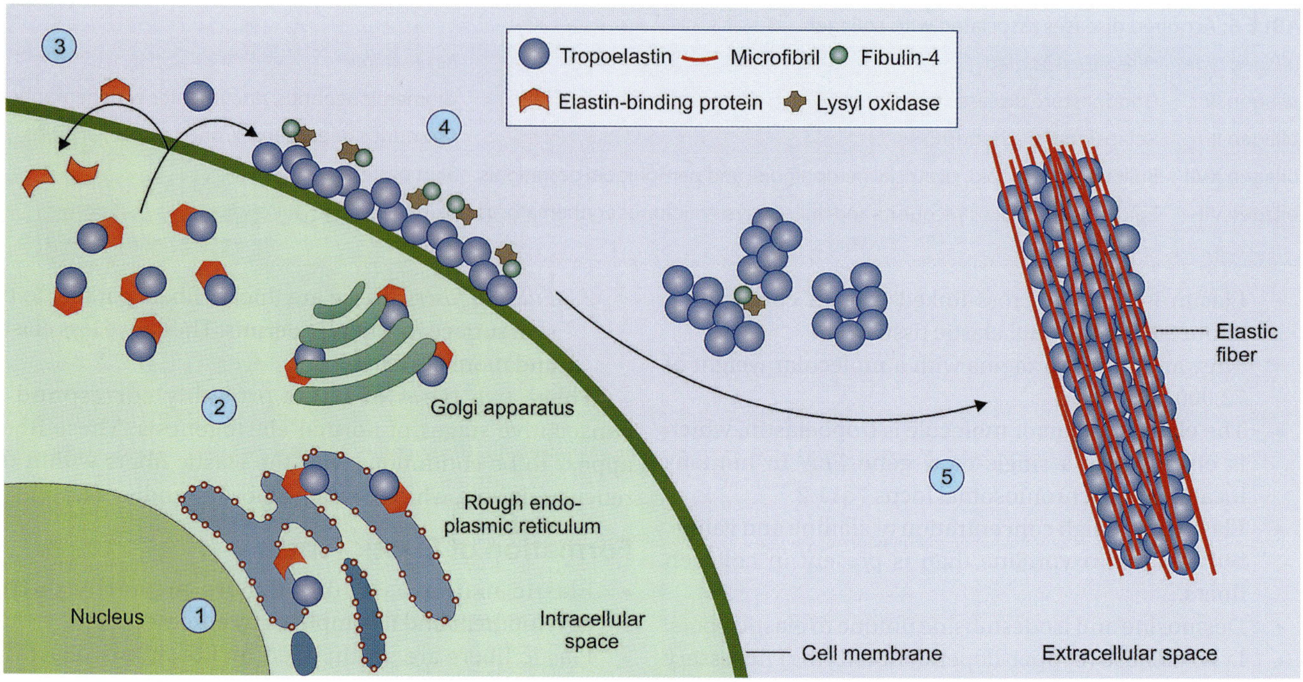

Fig. 14: Schematic representation of the major stages of the elastic fiber assembly: (1) Tropoelastin (TE) is synthesized on the rough endoplasmic reticulum where it binds to the chaperone protein elastin-binding protein (EBP). (2) The EBP-TE complex is transported through the Golgi apparatus and secreted to the cell membrane. (3) TE is released from the chaperone and forms globules at the cell surface, while EBP dissociates as a result of interaction with glycosaminoglycans and is recycled back into the cell. (4) Fibulin-4 is important for the chain alignment of TE mediating the interplay with lysyl oxidase or lysyl oxidase-like enzymes. The oxidation of lysine residues initiates a series of condensation reactions forming covalent intra- and intermolecular cross-links. (5) After clusters of tropoelastin molecules reach a critical size, they are moved from the plasma membrane through the ECM and aggregate onto the microfibril scaffold to eventually form the elastic fiber.

  - Pseudoxanthoma elasticum
  - Late-onset focal dermal elastosis
  - Linear focal elastosis
  - Elastoderma
  - Elastofibroma dorsi
  - Elastosis perforans serpiginosa
- *Anomalies with decreased elastic tissue:*
  - Nevus anelasticus
  - Papular elastorrhexis
  - Perifollicular elastolysis
  - Anetoderma
  - Cutis laxa
  - Postinflammatory elastolysis and cutis laxa
  - White fibrous papulosis of the neck
  - PXE-like papillary dermal elastolysis
  - Mid-dermal elastolysis
- *Cutis laxa (CL):*
  - CL can be caused by *Fibulin 5* gene defect among other causes
  - There are decreased desmosine and lysyl oxidase
  - CL is characterized by fragmentation and loss of elastic fibers
- *Marfan's syndrome:*
  - It is caused by decreased fibrillin 1.
  - Marfan's syndrome shows fragmentation of elastic fibers, especially aortic tissue.
- *Congenital contractural arachnodactyly:* There is mutation in fibrillin 2.
- *Pseudoxanthoma elasticum:*
  - It is also known as Gronblad–Strandberg syndrome.
  - PXE is an autosomal recessive disorder due to mutations in the *ABCC6* (adenosine triphosphate binding cassette subfamily C member 6) gene on the short arm of chromosome 16.
  - This disrupts the function of the ABC cassette transporter MDRP6 (multidrug resistance-associated protein 6) expressed in the liver, kidney, and intestine.
- *Buschke–Ollendorff syndrome:*
  - It is caused by *LEMD3* (also called MAN1) gene defect
  - There is increased desmosine and an increased amount of thickened elastic fibers
- *Anetoderma:* There is decreased desmosine; and loss and fragmentation of elastic fibers.[30]

THE EXTRAFIBRILLAR MATRIX

- Amorphous gel-like material in which connective tissue fibers are embedded is called extrafibrillar matrix (or previously ground substance).
- This constitutes about 0.2% of the dry weight of the dermis.
- It is primarily composed of proteoglycans. Proteoglycans consist of a "core protein" complexed with glycosaminoglycan such as hyaluronic acid binding to the core protein.

Other glycosaminoglycans include dermatan sulfate, heparan sulfate, and chondroitin sulfate.

- Glycosaminoglycans are polysaccharides composed of sulfated and acetylated sugars with negative charges that can bind large amounts of ions and water. The most prominent and ubiquitous protein-free GAG is hyaluronic acid.
- Proteoglycans differ remarkably in their protein content and the number, type and length of their GAG side chains. Proteoglycans can bind up to 1,000 times their volume and regulate the water-binding capability of the dermis.
- Four different proteoglycan-bound GAGs are seen in dermis; those are chondroitin sulfate, dermatan sulfate, keratan sulfate, and heparan sulfate.
- Versican, perlecan, decorin, biglycan, and syndecans are the most important proteoglycans in the dermis.
- Besides water absorption other functions of extrafibrillar matrix include shock-absorbing properties, and lubrication between collagen and elastic fibers.[31]
- *Applied aspects:*
    - Aging results in an increase in dermatan sulfate and decrease in chondroitin sulfate.
    - Mucopolysaccharidoses represent genetic storage diseases resulting from abnormal lysosomal function and subsequent accumulation of these substances. *Examples:*
        - Hurler's (deficiency of the enzyme known as α-L-iduronidase)
        - Hunter's (deficiency of the enzyme known as iduronate sulfatase).

CELLS OF DERMIS

Fibroblasts are the primary cells within the dermis, but histiocytes, mast cells, and adipocytes also play important roles in maintaining the normal structure and function of the dermis.

Dermal Fibroblasts

- Dermal fibroblasts are responsible for generating connective tissue and allowing the skin to recover from injury.
- Dermal fibroblasts are derived from mesenchyme.
- Dermal fibroblast proliferation can be stimulated by the presence of fibroblast growth factor (FGF).
- Upon injury, dermal fibroblasts can give rise to myofibroblasts; these are fibroblast cells with smooth muscle characteristics. Their contraction plays a critical role in wound healing and fibrosis.
- These cells also produce an ECM framework.
- They synthesize soluble mediators that regulate signaling between the dermis and epidermis.
- During wound healing they produce fibroplasia and control wound contraction.[32]

Mononuclear Phagocytic Cells

- Monocytes, macrophages, and dermal dendrocytes are derived from bone marrow.
- All phagocytic skin macrophages expressing CD11c and CD6.
- CR4 (CD11c) = α2-integrin are abundantly expressed in monocytes and macrophages. These bind C3b, leading to stimulation of phagocytosis.
- *Functions of macrophages in dermis:*
    - They have phagocytic and tumoricidal action.
    - They help in the processing and presenting of antigens to naïve T-cells.
    - They are also microbicidal through production and release of lysozyme, peroxide, and superoxide.
    - They have secretory functions as they release cytokines, growth factors, etc.
    - Macrophages are involved in coagulation, atherogenesis, wound healing, and tissue remodeling.
    - They express CD11a or LFA 1 which binds to ICAM.
    - They also express CD11b or Mac-1 on which binds to LCAM.

Dermal Dendrocytes

- Dermal dendrocytes are subset of antigen-presenting cells that function in the afferent limb of the immune response.
- They are derived from the bone marrow.
- Dermal dendrocytes are found in papillary dermis and upper reticular dermis.
- Dermal dendritic cells comprise two distinct populations: CD1+ dendritic cells and CD209+ macrophages
- Dermal dendritic cells comprise a novel part of the innate immune response in the resident skin immune system. They are highly phagocytic, similar to the melanophages in the dermis that contain ingested pigment
- They are likely the cell of origin in benign proliferative tumors such as dermatofibromas or fibroxanthoma.[33]

Mast Cells

- *Introduction:* Mast cells are immune cells derived from the myeloid lineage. Mature mast cells are present only in tissue and are not found in circulation. They are derived from bone marrow CD34+ stem cells
- *Location:* Mast cells are found in mucosal and epithelial tissues throughout the body. In skin mast cells are found in the greatest density in the papillary dermis, in sheaths of the appendages, and around blood vessels and nerves of the subpapillary plexus.
- *Structure:* Mast cells are mononuclear cells containing round or oval nuclei and 50–200 large dark-staining granules that store inflammatory mediators, including histamine, heparin, a variety of cytokines, chondroitin sulfate, and neutral proteases. IgE receptors are found in the plasma membrane.

- *Types:* Two major types of mast cell have been identified: (1) MC (T) cells are found in gastrointestinal or respiratory mucosa and contain granules with mostly tryptase. They predominantly act in the immune response. (2) MC (TC) cells contain tryptase as well as chymase and carboxypeptidase in the secretory granules and are found in the submucosa and connective tissue adjacent to the conjunctiva and skin. MC (TC) cells play a pivotal role in tissue repair.
- *Secretion:*
  - *Preformed mediators:* Many inflammatory mediators, such as histamine, heparin, tryptase, chymase, carboxypeptidase, neutrophil chemotactic factor, and eosinophilic chemotactic factor of anaphylaxis, are produced and stored in preformed secretory granules.
  - *Cells release without storing:* Growth factors (platelet-activating factor), cytokines, and leukotrienes including prostaglandin D2
  - Secretory granule release induced by a variety of stimuli. The release or degranulation process is identical regardless of stimulus **(Fig. 15)**.
- *Functions:*
  - *Angiogenesis:* Mast cells secrete proangiogenic factors, such as VEGF, bFGF, TGF-beta, TNF-alpha, and IL-8.
  - *Homeostasis in the immune system:* The mast cell functions as part of the body's innate immune system.
  - *Innate and adaptive immunity:* Mast cell releases lipid-based prostaglandins and leukotrienes, which have proinflammatory effects. Cytokines released also have direct effects on local tissue, such as increased mucus production or increased gut peristalsis to reduce pathogen invasion.
  - Mast cells also play a role in tissue repair.
  - Mast cells have been implicated in the wound contraction and the regeneration of nerve fibers.
- *Demonstration:*
  - *Light microscopy:* Mast cells are mononuclear oval or irregularly shaped cells with a centrally located nucleus. Under light microscopy, a dense granular cytoplasm is seen, often obscuring the nucleus and other organelles. There are three morphologies noted:
    1. *Intact cells:* Spindle-shaped cells with closely packed granules.
    2. *Spreading cells:* Fewer granules than in the intact cell type.
    3. *Degranulated cells:* Nonmetachromatic, pale staining, appearing light pink with a blue nucleus.
  - *Histochemistry and cytochemistry:* Metachromasia is unique to mast cells and basophils. Stain cells for CD34, c-Kit, SCF or with Giemsa, Teledyne, and Leder stain (naphthol chloroacetate esterase). Mast cells can usually be distinguished from basophils due to their mononuclear morphology, and with special stains such as tryptase or monoclonal antibodies to the mast cell kit (CD117) receptor.
  - *Electron microscopy:* Under scanning electron microscopy, mast cells are characterized by the cytoplasmic granules and finger-like pseudopods projecting out of the cell membrane.[34]
- *Clinical significance:*
  - Mast cell degranulation leads to vascular smooth muscle contraction, increased vascular permeability, tissue edema, and the recruitment of inflammatory cells.

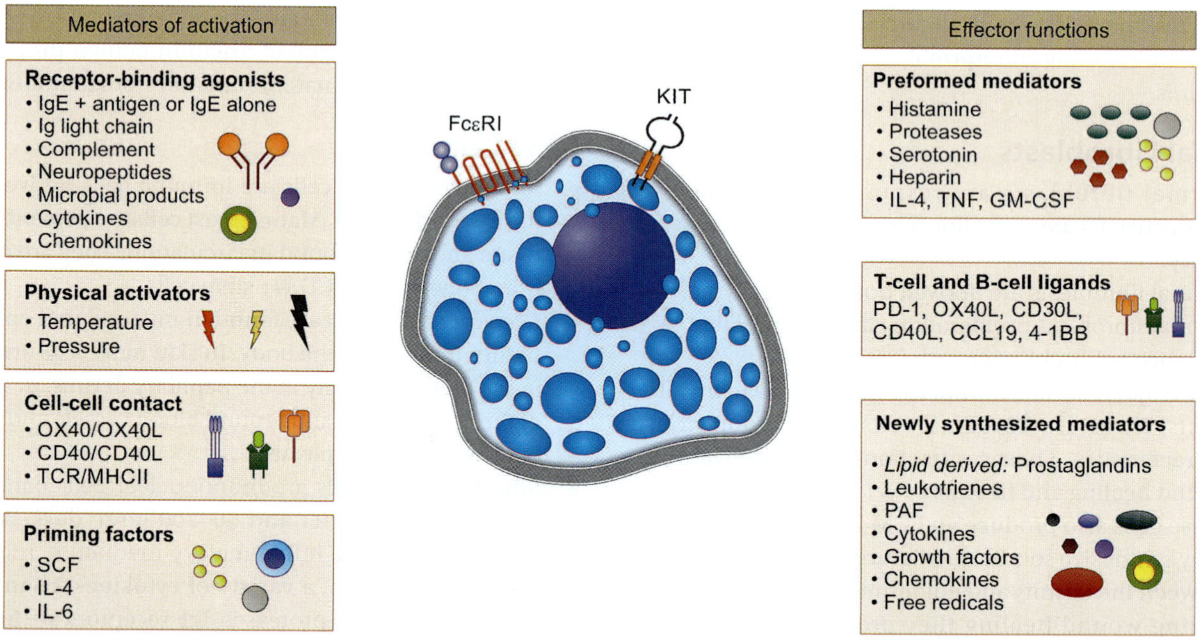

Fig. 15: Mast cell.

- Mast cells are responsible for immediate-type hypersensitivity reactions and participate in chronic inflammatory conditions.
- Mutations in c-Kit (CD117) may result in mastocytosis or piebaldism.
- Mast cells and their mediators are common pharmacological targets. Antihistamines block histamine from interacting with its receptor and are widely used to treat type I hypersensitivity reactions. Cromolyn sodium is a mast cell stabilizer that is thought to act on both chloride channels and signaling proteins in the cell membrane to inhibit degranulation.

Glomus Cells

- These are modified smooth muscle cells found in dermis and involved in body temperature regulation.
- Glomus bodies are specialized arteriovenous shunts consisting of afferent arteriole, Sucquet-Hoyer canal, efferent arteriole, and nerve fibers. Glomus bodies are most numerous in the fingers and toes. The glomus body has a high sympathetic tone and potentiation leads to near complete vasoconstriction.
- Glomus cells are derived from Sucquet-Hoyer canals, and allow shunting of blood from arterioles to venules without going through capillaries.
- *Applied aspects:* Disease processes of glomus cells include glomus tumor and glomangioma.[35]

ECCRINE GLAND

Introduction

- Eccrine glands are the major sweat glands in humans. Other two types of sweat glands are apocrine glands and apoeccrine glands (controversial).
- Most important function of eccrine glands is to regulate body temperature through evaporative heat loss.
- There are approximately 1.5–4 million eccrine sweat glands.

Distribution

- Eccrine glands are present over the entire cutaneous surface except the vermillion border of the lips, nail beds, labia minora, glans penis, clitoris, external auditory canal.
- The highest density of eccrine sweat glands is found on the palms and soles.

Structure

- Eccrine glands are composed of three sections:
  1. *Acrosyringium:* This is the intraepidermal spiral portion of the duct opening to the surface of skin.
  2. *Straight duct:* Straight portion of the duct, runs within the dermis and consists of double layer cuboidal epithelium lined by eosinophilic cuticle on luminal side.
  3. *Secretory eccrine coil:* Secretary coil exists either in the lower portion of the dermis or at the border of the dermis and the subcutaneous fat and contain two cell types interspersed within a single cell layer: (1) large clear cells responsible for the gland's secretion of electrolytes and water; and (2) dark cells, of unknown function, with basophilic granules that are thought to produce sialomucin. Both cell types are surrounded by myoepithelial cells, which probably function to enhance the delivery of sweat to the skin surface.
- Eccrine glands are supplied by postganglionic cholinergic sympathetic fibers.
- Presence of eosinophilic cuticle helps to distinguish eccrine duct from coil histologically.
- Eccrine glands are positive for S100, carcinoembryonic antigen (CEA), and keratin.

Development

- Functional eccrine glands are present at birth.
- Eccrine glands develop first on palms and soles in the 4th month, on the body in the 5th month.
- Eccrine gland stem cells express markers such as keratins 15, 18, and 19.[36]

Functions

- Eccrine sweat is a sterile, dilute electrolyte solution that is formed in two steps: Secretion of primary fluid, isotonic NaCl; and then reabsorption of NaCl by the duct.
- The quantity and quality of eccrine sweat secretion varies greatly, depending on emotional and environmental stimuli.
- Sweating rate is the most important determinant of NaCl concentration in final sweat fluid.
- Other components of sweat include antimicrobial peptides (e.g., dermcidin), lactate, urea, ammonia, amino acids, proteins, and proteases.
- Sweating provides a mechanism for thermoregulation by evaporative heat loss. It also plays a role in maintenance of electrolyte balance. Sweat keeps the stratum corneum moist to insure fine tactile skills and pliability of the palms and soles.

Applied Aspects

- The excretory function of the sweat gland is used in the drug delivery to the stratum corneum (e.g., ketoconazole and griseofulvin).
- It is also responsible for the cutaneous side effects of certain chemotherapeutic drugs.
- Botulinum toxin by blocking the release of acetylcholine at the neuroglandular junction, is effective in the palmoplantar and axillary hyperhidrosis **(Fig. 16)**.

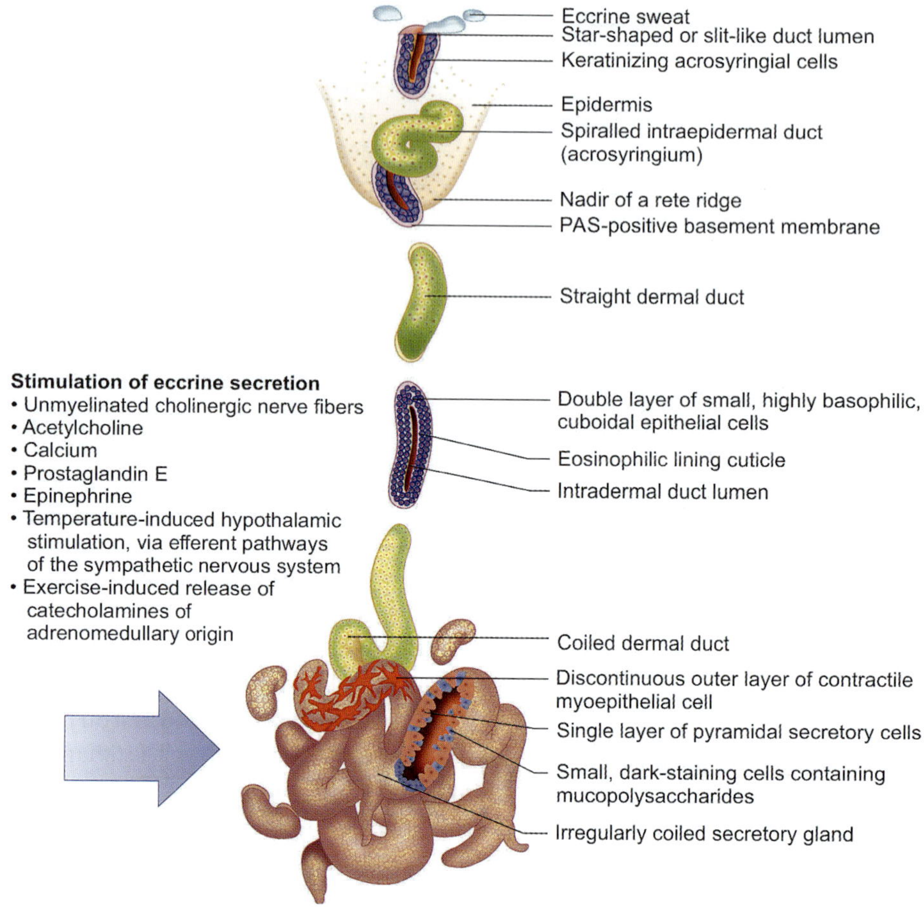

Fig. 16: Eccrine sweat glands.

APOCRINE GLAND

Introduction

- An apocrine sweat gland (from Greek apo "away" and krinein "to separate") is composed of a coiled secretory portion located at the junction of the dermis and subcutaneous fat, from which a straight portion inserts and secretes into the infundibular portion of the hair follicle
- They are larger than eccrine glands.

Distribution

- In humans, apocrine sweat glands are found only in certain locations of the body; mostly confined to axillae, breast (mammary gland), anogenital region, external auditory canal (ceruminous gland), and eyelids (Moll's gland).
- However, in most nonprimate mammals, apocrine sweat glands are distributed over the majority portion of their body.

Structure

- *Like eccrine glands, apocrine glands are also composed of three segments:* Intraepidermal duct, intradermal duct, and secretory portion.
- Duct of apocrine gland usually leads to a pilosebaceous follicle above the entrance of the sebaceous duct.
- The secretory portion is a convoluted tubular structure with a single layer of columnar epithelial cells surrounded by myoepithelial cells.
- The ductal portion consists of a double layer of cuboidal cells and a layer of myoepithelial cells.
- Apocrine glands respond mainly to sympathetic adrenergic stimuli.
- *Immunohistochemistry:*
  - Glands stain positive for keratin, S100, CEA, lysozyme.
  - CD15 staining differentiates between the two types of sweat glands as CD15 stains apocrine but not eccrine secretory cells. Other relatively nonspecific markers include human milk fat globule-1 (HMFG-1), gross cystic disease fluid protein-15 (GCDFP-15)

Development

- Apocrine glands are derived from the primary epithelial germ layer, which also gives rise to the sebaceous gland and hair follicle.
- First seen week 24 on scalp.
- In fetal life, apocrine sweat glands are present all over the skin, but most of them subsequently disappear, giving the characteristic distribution.

- The function of the glands begins at puberty due to hormonal stimulation (primarily by androgens).[37]

Functions

- Apocrine secretion in humans has an unclear role; possibly it participates in olfactory communication.
- Apocrine secretion via decapitation, i.e., a portion of cell pinched off and enters lumen.
- Sweat secretion in response to emotive stimuli mediated by the limbic system—through action of epinephrine/norepinephrine. Denervation does not abolish this response, though apocrine sweating requires intact nerve supply. During sleep, the glands are inactive, which support the idea of emotional control.
- Apocrine secretion is a very small quantity of an oily fluid which is sterile, odorless and viscous, with a pH between 5.0 and 6.5.
- Though the initial sweat secretion is odorless, it later produces a distinct odor. The odor is derived from C6 to C11 acids; the most abundant is 3-methyl-2-hexenoic acid.

Applied Aspects

- *Fox-Fordyce disease:* It is a chronic skin disease caused by occlusion of apocrine ducts. It is most common in women aged 13–35 years. It is characterized by the development of intense itching in the underarm area, the pubic area, and around the nipple of the breast as a result of perspiration which becomes trapped in the sweat gland and surrounding areas.
- Chromhidrosis is a rare condition characterized by the secretion of colored sweat due to lipofuscin context.
- Bromhidrosis is a chronic condition in which excessive odor, usually an unpleasant one, emanates from the skin. Abnormal body odor apocrine gland secretion.

SEBACEOUS GLANDS

Introduction

- Sebaceous gland, a microscopic exocrine gland in the skin, produces an oily or waxy matter, called sebum via holocrine secretion and has multiple biological functions, including hormonal and immune modulation.
- Sebum, produced by the glands, is released into the infundibular portion of the hair follicle.

Distribution

- Sebaceous glands are found throughout skin except palms, soles, and prepuce.
- Distribution of the glands is variable; however, these are more common on the scalp, face, upper back, and chest.
- These glands are always associated with hair follicles, except for the ectopic or free sebaceous glands in the following locations:
  - *Gland of Zeis:* Found on superficial eyelid margin (near Moll's gland)
  - *Meibomian gland:* Present in tarsal plate of eyelids (behind Moll's gland)
  - *Montgomery tubercle:* Present in nipple and areola.
  - *Tyson's gland:* Found in external fold of prepuce (genitalia)
  - *Fordyce spot:* Present in vermilion border of the lips and buccal mucosa
- Though the glands are found in association with hair structures, there is no relationship between the size of the sebaceous gland and the size of the associated hair.

Structure

- *A sebaceous gland structure consists of two parts:* The cauliflower-like convoluted sebaceous gland, and the sebaceous duct which connects the gland with the infundibulum of the hair follicle.
- Sebaceous follicles harbor a diverse microflora including bacteria like *S. epidermidis* and *Propionibacterium acnes*, fungi like *Malassezia* spp. and mites like Demodex.
- These glands are under androgenic hormonal control, and not under neural control.

Development

- Sebaceous glands are derived from the epidermis as buds from developing hair follicle root sheaths and grow downward into the dermis.
- Sebaceous glands are present at birth and they enlarge at puberty in response to increased androgens, especially 5α-dihydrotestosterone (DHT).
- Blimp-1 (B-lymphocyte-induced maturation protein-1) was found to be a marker for sebaceous gland stem cells in mice, and terminally differentiating cells of the sebaceous gland, hair follicle, and interfollicular epidermis in human.

Functions

- Sebum is a light yellow viscous fluid. Lipid composition of sebum is 57% triglycerides, 25% wax esters, 15% squalene, <3% cholesterol, and cholesterol esters.
- Secretion of sebum is holocrine, that is, the sebocytes disintegrate and thereby release their sebum as they migrate toward the central gland and sebaceous duct
- The rate of sebum production is 0.5 mg/10 cm^2 every 3 hours.
- Human sebum differs from other lipids by the presence of wax esters.
- Sebum lubricates the skin to protect against friction and makes it more impervious to moisture. Furthermore, the sebaceous gland transports antioxidants and exhibits a natural light protective activity. It possesses an innate antibacterial activity and has a pro- and anti-inflammatory function. It can regulate the activity of xenobiotics and is actively involved in the wound healing process.[38]

Applied Aspects

- Sebaceous glands play key roles in the pathogenesis of acne vulgaris and rosacea.
- Increased sebum excretion, alteration of lipid composition, and the oxidant/antioxidant ratio characteristic of the skin surface lipids are major concurrent events associated with the development of acne.
- Sebaceous skin tumors are classified into sebaceous adenoma, sebaceoma, and sebaceous carcinoma. An additional group of cystic sebaceous tumors indicates the Muir-Torre syndrome.
- *Muir-Torre syndrome:*
    - MTS is autosomal dominant nonpolyposis colon cancer syndrome.
    - There are mutations in the DNA mismatch repair genes (*MSH2* gene on chromosome 2p), *MSH6*, *MLH1*.
    - The skin signs include sebaceous gland tumors (sebaceous adenoma, sebaceous carcinoma) and keratoacanthomas with sebaceous differentiation.
    - It is associated with colonic carcinoma.

CUTANEOUS NEURAL SYSTEM

Introduction

- The cutaneous neural network consists of somatic sensory fibers and sympathetic autonomic fibers.
- Somatic sensory fibers are myelinated till their terminal ramifications and autonomic fibers are unmyelinated.
- Sensory nerve fibers may exist alone (free nerve endings) or in conjunction with specialized receptors of touch, pain, temperature, itch, and mechanical stimuli.
- The sympathetic motor fibers are distributed along with sensory fibers in the dermis until they branch to innervate the hair follicles, sweat glands, arrector pili muscles, and smooth muscles of the blood vessels.

Neuroanatomy and Neurophysiology of Cutaneous Nerves

- *Sensory nerves are divided into four groups:*
    1. Aα fibers (12–22 mm) are highly myelinated show a fast conduction velocity (70–120 m/s), and are associated with muscular spindles and tendon organs.
    2. Aβ fibers are moderately myelinated (6–12 μm) and capture touch receptors.
    3. Aδ fibers constitute a thin myelin sheath (1–5 μm), an intermediate conduction velocity (4–30 m/s), and are generally polymodal.
    4. The slow-conducting C fibers (0.5–2 m/s) are unmyelinated and small (0.2–1.5 μm).
- Aδ fibers constitute ~80% of primary sensory nerves sprouting from dorsal root ganglia, whereas C fibers make up ~20% of the primary afferents.
- Moreover, the activation threshold of Aδ fibers is higher than that of C fibers.[39]

Sensory Receptors of the Skin

- *Nonencapsulated endings:*
    - *Free nerve endings:* Free nerve endings are the most important and widespread sensory receptors particularly in the papillary dermis. They usually have a Schwann cell sheath and a basal lamina. These are rapidly adapting receptors. Majority of these consist of nonmyelinated C-type fibers and some have myelinated Aδ-type fibers. Terminal endings are within epidermis and papillary dermis and mainly detect touch, pressure, and pain.
    - *Merkel cells:* These cells are found in the basal layer and make close contact with the sensory nerve terminal (Merkel disk), detecting touch.
- *Encapsulated endings:*
    - *Vater-Pacini (Pacinian) corpuscle:* These are up to 1 mm long, ovoid structures present in deep dermis/subcutis. These are rapidly adapting mechanoreceptors with a distinctive capsule and lamellar wrappings resembling an onion. The capsule (perineurium) has 30 or more concentric layers of cells and fibrous connective tissue. These corpuscles detect deep pressure and vibration. They have increased concentration in palms/soles, nipples, and anogenital regions.
    - *Meissner's corpuscle:* These are elongated mechanoreceptors resembling a pine cone which detect light touch. They are located just below DEJ (dermal papillae) and have the highest density in palmoplantar skin.
    - *Ruffini corpuscle:* These are the nerve terminals present in human digits, in which several expanded endings branch from a single, myelinated afferent fiber. The endings are directly related to collagen fibrils. They are thin, encapsulated, fluid-filled slow adapting receptors which are found in deep dermis and detect continuous pressure.
    - *Krause end bulbs:* This is an encapsulated swelling of myelinated fibers situated in the superficial layers of the dermis. These are mucocutaneous receptors found on the vermilion lip, perianal region, glans penis, clitoris, and labia minora.
    - *Golgi-Mazzoni corpuscle:* This is found in the subcutaneous tissue of the human finger and is similarly laminated but of much simpler organization **(Fig. 17)**.[40]

CUTANEOUS BLOOD VESSELS

Introduction

- The skin has a rich vascular network with distributing and collecting channels.

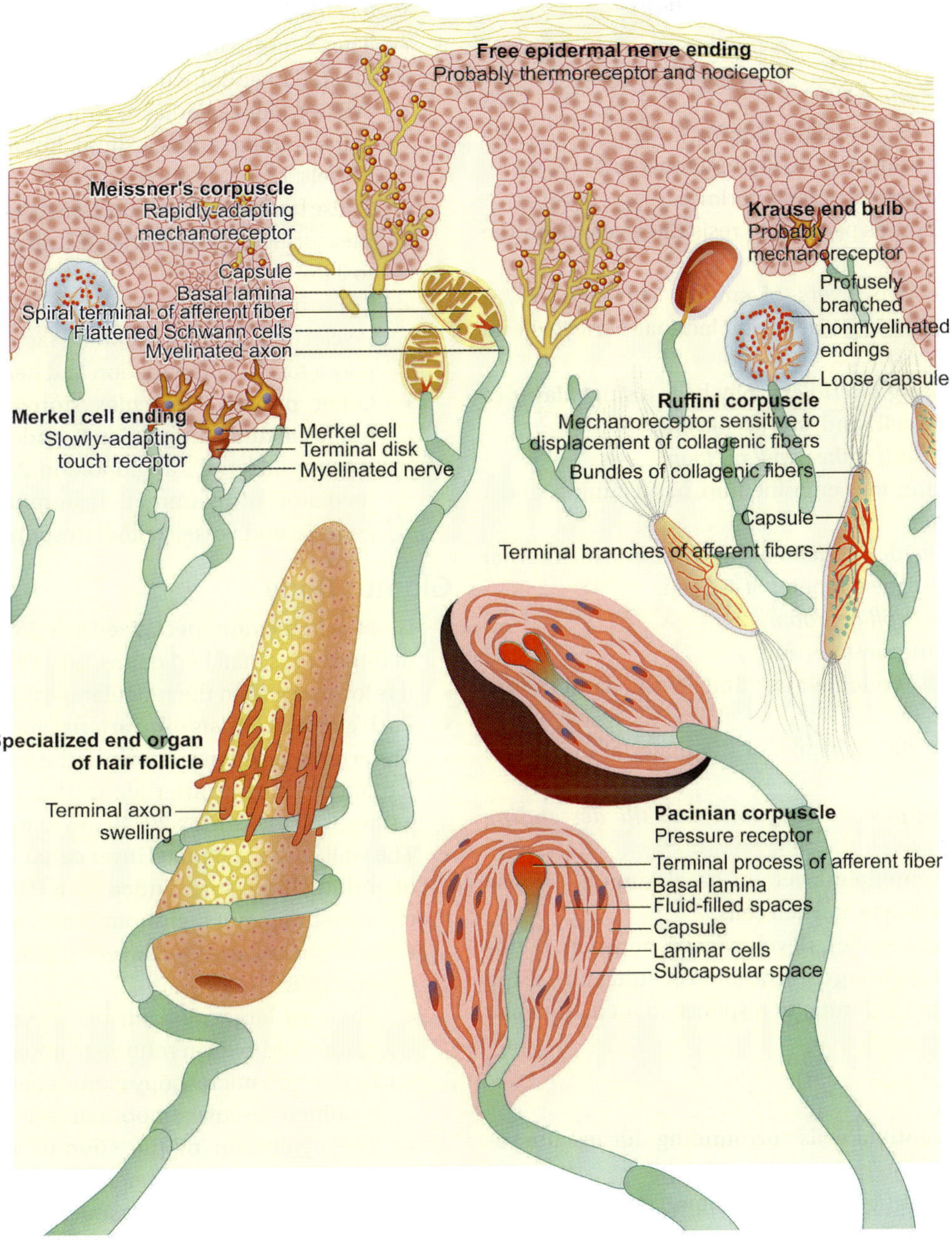

Fig. 17: Cutaneous sensory endings.

- The dermal microcirculation includes arterioles, terminal arterioles, precapillary sphincters, arterial and venous capillaries, postcapillary venules, and collecting venules.

Structure of Cutaneous Vasculature

- The arterioles and venules of the cutaneous microcirculation form two important plexuses in the dermis:
  1. An upper horizontal network in the papillary dermis from which the nutritive capillary loops of the dermal papillae arise. This is situated 1–1.5 mm below the skin surface.
  2. A lower horizontal plexus at the dermal-subcutaneous interface.
- Ascending arterioles and descending venules are paired as they connect the two plexuses.
- From the upper layer, arterial capillaries rise to form the dermal papillary loops that represent the nutritive component of the skin circulation.
- There are sphincter-like smooth muscle cells at the point where the ascending arterioles divide to form the arteriolar component of the upper horizontal plexus.
- At the dermal-subcutaneous junction, there are collecting veins with two cusped valves that are oriented to prevent the retrograde flow of blood.

Ultrastructure

Microvascular Segments

- The ascending arterioles:
  - These are in the papillary dermis.
  - These vary from 17 to 26 μm in diameter.
  - They represent terminal arterioles.
  - They function as part of the resistance vessels in the skin.
  - They have two layers of smooth muscle cells, a discontinuous internal elastic lamina, pericytes and Veil cell.
- *The anastomosing arterioles:* They have a single layer of smooth muscle cells and lack elastic fibers.
- *The ascending limb of the capillary loop:*
  - It has a continuous endothelium, basal lamina, and a few pericytes.
  - It has an outside diameter of 10–12 μm and an internal endothelial tube diameter of 4–6 μm.
- *The apex of the capillary loop:*
  - This is the thinnest portion.
  - Here, both endothelium and basal lamina are attenuated.
  - This allows the transport of the material out of the capillary.
- *The descending postcapillary limb and the descending venule:*
  - They have multiple layers of basal lamina, a loose sheath of pericyte and veil cells.
  - Descending venules develop gaps between endothelial cells allowing extravasation of fluid and escape of cells from the lumen in response to mediators like histamine.[41]

Veil Cells

- These are adventitial cells surrounding dermal microvessels.
- They are long thin cells, with an attenuated cytoplasm, and ultrastructurally resemble fibroblasts.
- The exact nature and function of veil cells are not clear.
- They do not have cell markers for T, B, or Langerhans cells, nor do they stain for HLA-DR.
- Unlike pericyte, which are an integral component of the vascular wall, veil cells are totally external to the wall, demarcating the vessel from the surrounding dermis.

Endothelial Cells

- Endothelial cells are rich in cytoplasmic organelles like Golgi apparatus, rough and smooth endoplasmic reticulum, mitochondria, and lysosomes.
- These cells actively participate in transmural shuttling of macromolecules and trafficking of immune cells.
- Endothelial cells are a rich source of enzymes like angiotensin converting enzymes and cytokines.
- *Weibel–Palade bodies:*
  - These are small characteristic storage granules located in endothelial cells.
  - Weibel–Palade bodies are found in arteries, capillaries, veins, and the endocardium, but not in the lymphatic vessels.
  - These bodies are electron dense rod-shaped structures measuring approximately 0.1 μm in diameter and up to 3 μm in length.
  - These bodies function to store two principal molecules, P-selectin and von Willebrand factor. These two agents play a role in inflammation and hemostasis.
  - Other protein molecules stored in Weibel-Palade bodies include interleukin 8, endothelin 1, eotaxin-3, osteoprotegerin, angiopoietin-2, etc. These are mediators of inflammation, immune response, angiogenesis, and vessel caliber/response to stressors.

Glomus Body

- Glomus bodies are specialized arteriovenous shunts seen in finger pads, nail bed palms, and soles.
- It is located within the reticular dermis.
- Each glomus consists of an arterial and a venous segment.
- The arterial segment is known as the Sucquet–Hoyer canal. It branches from an arteriole and has a narrow lumen and a thick wall measuring 20–40 μm in diameter.
- The wall of the Sucquet–Hoyer canal shows a single layer of endothelium, surrounded by a PAS-positive, diastase resistant basement membrane zone, and a media that are densely packed with 4–6 layers of glomus cells.
- *Glomus cells:*
  - These are large cells with a clear cytoplasm resembling epithelioid cells in routine histopathology.
  - In electron microscopy glomus cells are confirmed as modified vascular smooth muscles.
  - The cytoplasm of the Glomus cells is filled with filaments with a diameter of about 5 nm.
  - Also, there are cytoplasmic and peripheral dense bodies, which are 300–400 nm in diameter. These bodies are present in the glomus cells as a result of condensation of the myofilaments.
  - Numerous unmyelinated nerves ensheathed by Schwann cells are present peripheral to the glomus cells.
  - Glomus bodies are concerned with temperature regulation.

Functions of Skin Vasculature

- *Nutritional function:* Vasculatures of skin are important for delivering nutrients and removing unwanted metabolic waste.
- *Immunological function:* Vasculature of the skin plays a vital role in the immune-surveillance of the skin, serving as a conduit for elements of the immune system.

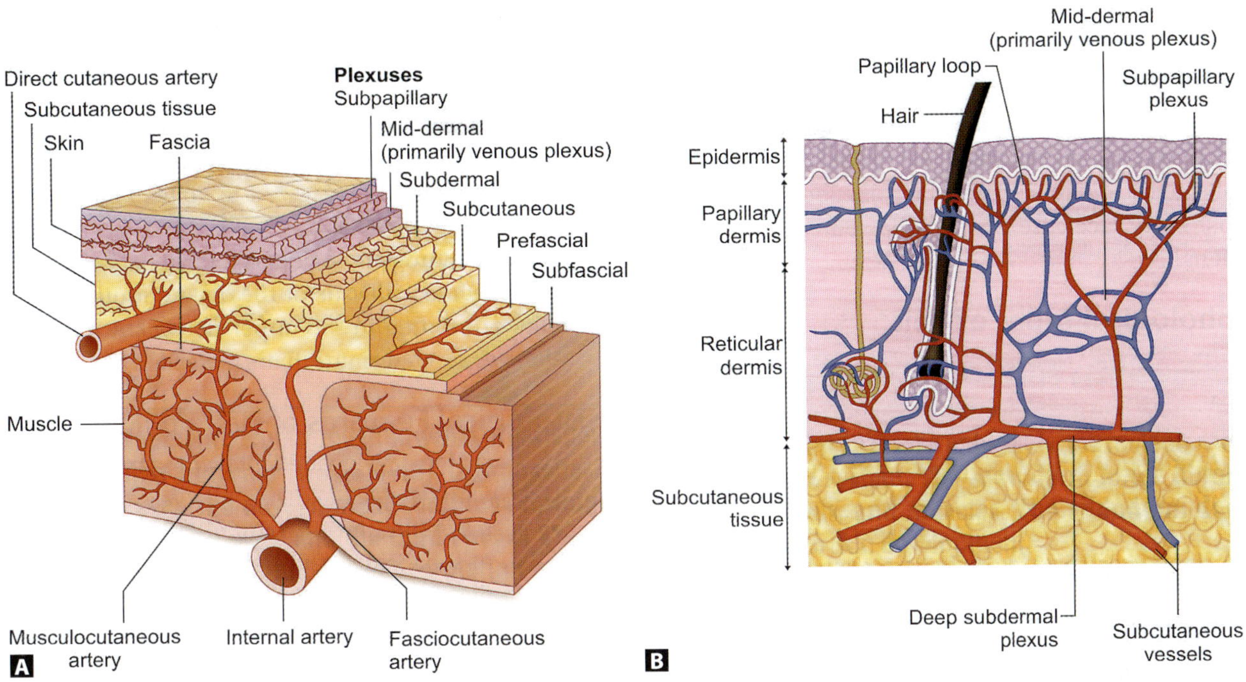

Figs. 18A and B: Cutaneous vasculature.

- *Thermoregulation:* Skin also plays a vital role in thermoregulation, being able to dissipate heat by dilation of superficial vessels and increasing blood flow.

Applied Aspects

- Defects in vascular development can lead to Klippel–Trenaunay and Sturge–Weber syndrome.
- Hereditary hemorrhagic telangiectasia or Osler–Weber–Rendu syndrome is an inherited disorder characterized by vascular dysplasia, hemorrhage, and shunting of blood. Mutations of the *ENG* gene and abnormalities of the protein it produces (endoglin) result in HHT-1. Mutations of the activin receptor-like kinase 1 (*ACVRL1*) gene and abnormalities of the protein in encode (ALK1) result in HHT-2 **(Figs. 18A and B)**.

CUTANEOUS LYMPHATICS

- Lymphatic vessels in skin form two horizontally running networks:
  - *Superficial lymphatic network:* A narrow-meshed network lying subepidermally.
  - *Deeper lymphatic network:* A wide-meshed network.
- These two networks are connected to each other through obliquely running lymphatic vessels.
- *Lymphatics are of two types:*
  1. Smaller, noncontractile, initial lymphatics which initiate the drainage process
  2. Larger, contractile, lymphatic collectors
- *Arrangements of lymphatics:*
  - The blind-ending, interconnecting lymphatic capillaries start in the papillary dermis and then drain into the subpapillary plexus below the venous plexus.
  - From there lymphatics drain into a deeper plexus at the reticular dermis.
  - From deeper plexus lymphatics drain into subcutaneous lymphatic vessels.
  - These vessels drain into the lymph nodes.
- There are bicuspid valves inside the lymphatic vessels that prevent backflow of lymph.
- *Structure:*
  - Lymphatic vessels have a larger lumen and a thinner vessel wall in comparison to blood vessels
  - In the thin walls of lymph vessels there are flattened endothelial cells, discontinuous basal lamina, and elastic fibers.
  - The endothelium lacks Weibel–Palade bodies and fenestrations.
- *Ultrastructure:* Lymphatic endothelial cells contain cytoplasmic filaments that represent vimentin filaments.[42]
- *Functions:*
  - Regulation of the interstitial fluid by resorption of leaked fluid.
  - Clearance of unwanted proteins, lipids, organisms, cells, and degraded material
- *Applied aspects:* Hereditary lymphedema is a genetic developmental disorder affecting the lymphatic system. It is characterized by swelling (edema) of certain parts of the body. Swelling frequently occurs in one or both legs, but may also be present in the trunk, face, genitalia, and arms. Hereditary lymphedema type IA or Milroy's disease occurs because of mutation in the *FLT4* gene which encodes the vascular endothelial growth factor receptor 3 (*VEGFR-3*) gene located on the long arm on chromosome 5.

HAIR FOLLICLES

Introduction

- The entire cutaneous surface is populated by hair follicles (HFs) except for palms, soles, dorsa of terminal phalanges, glans penis, and mucocutaneous junctions.
- Most hairy races are whites followed by Africans and Asians.

Morphological Types of Hair

Types	*Race*
Straight	Asian > white
Spiral	Black
Helical	White
Wavy	White

Development of Hair

- Hair structure development starts after 8 weeks of fetal life.
- It begins with the appearance of placodes in the epidermal basal layer.
- Specialized mesenchymal cells organize in a small condensate directly beneath the basement membrane, stimulating the overlying epithelial stem cells to invaginate and penetrate into the dermis forming an epidermal peg.
- The epidermal peg continues to grow downward enclosing the dermal condensate forming the dermal papilla.
- The tip of the epidermal peg becomes the matrix portion of the hair bulb.
- Cells of the follicular matrix terminally differentiate into inner root sheath and the hair shaft that exits from the surface of the skin. Initial hair population is completed by 22 weeks.
- Fine lanugo hair develops in an advancing wave from the frontal to occipital scalp and it is shed by 36 weeks. A second coat of lanugo hair appears and it is shed in a synchronized wave pattern at 3–4 months of life.[43]

Developmental Types of Hair

- Lanugo—fetus is covered by soft, fine, lightly pigmented hair. It is shed by 8–9 months of gestation or at birth. It is longer than vellus hair.
- Vellus—small with a diameter less than 0.03 mm, are often less than 1 cm in length, and lack melanin and medulla. True vellus hairs have thin, external root sheaths, and short stelae in the upper dermis. Vellus-like miniaturized hairs have thicker external root sheaths and long stelae extending into the lower dermis or subcutaneous fat. Follicular stelae, in the upper dermis only, indicate vellus hairs. Follicular stelae in the lower dermis indicate terminal, catagen, or telogen hairs or miniaturized vellus-like hairs.
- Intermediate—diameter = 0.03–0.06 mm, little thicker than vellus hair. Hair bulbs are situated in the reticular dermis.
- Terminal—long coarse pigmented hairs with larger diameters exceeding 0.03 mm and 1 cm in length are often pigmented and medullated. They can be graded by hair shaft diameter as small (0.031–0.06 mm), medium (0.061–0.09 mm), or large (greater than 0.091 mm). Terminal hairs miniaturized to vellus hair proportions are described as vellus-like hairs such as seen in alopecia areata or androgenetic alopecia. Terminal hairs are rooted in subcutaneous tissue or the deep dermis, while vellus hairs are rooted in the upper dermis. A normal scalp averages seven terminal hairs per vellus hair.[44]

Histological Features of Hair Follicle

- HF is histologically divided into two segments:
  1. *Upper segment:*
     - Infundibulum—ostium of HF above to entrance of sebaceous duct below. An infundibulum has the shape of a funnel, the upper two-thirds of the infundibulum has the shape of a funnel and the lower one-third, referred to as the infrainfundibulum, consists of the narrow tube of the funnel.
     - Isthmus—from entry of sebaceous duct above to site of attachment of erector pili.
  2. *Lower segment:*
     - Stem—from site of attachment of erector pili above to Adamson's fringe where the keratogenous zone ends below
     - Bulb—from Adamson's fringe to the base of HF.
- Upper segment of HF is constant while the lower segment undergoes a process of regression and regeneration as hair passes through its phases of evolution **(Figs. 19A and B)**.[45]

Characteristics of the Segments of HF

Vide **Table 7**.

Ultrastructure

- Hair is formed of hard keratin with high sulfur content that is responsible for its extraordinary tensile strength as against the soft keratin of the skin and the nails that have lower sulfur content.
- The hair cortex is made up of a low sulfur fibrillar component tightly packed in a sulfur-rich matrix.
- The fibrillar component consists of microfibrils, 7 nm thick, arranged in a longitudinal lamellated form, which on cross-section under the electron microscope give a thumbprint appearance.

Nerve Supply and HF Innervation

- Around infundibulum—C and sympathetic fibers
- Around isthmus—C and A delta fibers
- Free nerve endings
- Ruffini end organs
- Merkel nerve endings

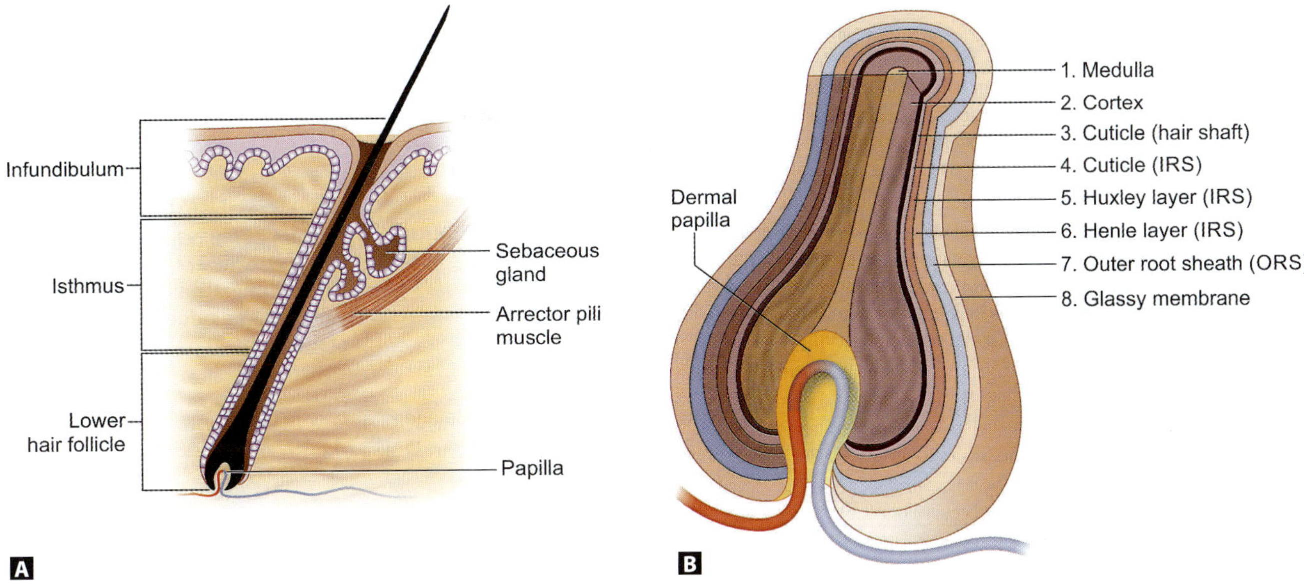

Figs. 19A and B: (A) Longitudinal section of hair follicle; (B) Cross-section of hair follicle.

TABLE 7: Characteristics of the segments of hair follicles (HFs).

Segment	*Description*	*Applied aspects*
Infundibulum	Funnel-shaped infundibulum passes through the epidermis where it is known as acrotrichum and the intraepidermal portion of the eccrine duct is known as acrosyringium. Infundibular epithelium is thinner and lacks rete ridges. Granular layer and stratum corneum (SC) present	Infundibular cyst—occurs on the face and trunk
Isthmus	• This is the narrow part of the follicle between the bulge (attachment of arrector pili) and the opening of the sebaceous duct • Hair follicle stem cells reside at the base of isthmus • Zone of trichilemmal keratinization—outer root sheath (ORS) becomes cornified without presence of granular layer	Isthmus-catagen cyst—situated on the scalp
Stem	The longest section of terminal hair in anagen. Extends from base of isthmus to summit of bulb marked by Adamson's fringe	
Bulb	• The lowermost portion of HF • Present in subcutaneous fat • Base invaginated by dermal papillae • Melanocytes are present spreading dendrites between germinative cells and keratinocytes • Line across widest part of bulb called line of Auber: – Lower region—mitotically active matrical cells – Upper region—lower and lateral cells give rise to inner root sheath (IRS) while the upper and central cells give rise to hair shaft • From outside inward the seven components of hair bulb are: • Outer root sheath—filled with glycogen and composed of pale and clear cells: – Inner root sheath—controls shape of hair shaft. IRS is composed of three layers: 1. Henle's layer—one cell thick and composed of trichohyalin granules and first to cornify 2. Huxle's layer—two cells thick and composed of numerous brightly eosinophilic trichohyalin granules 3. Cuticle of inner sheath—one cell thick • *Cuticle of hair:* It has mainly protective functions. It also maintains the integrity of hair shaft. In cosmetic procedure there is degradation of cuticle which leads to the fracture of the hair shaft • *Cortex of hair:* – It forms the bulk of the hair – Fusiform shape – It is fully hyalinized in suprabulbar region – The major component is alpha hard keratin IFs, these are keratin proteins with high glycine tyrosine proteins, sulfur-rich proteins • Medulla of hair is the last layer to cornify and it is present only in terminal hair	• Pilar sheath acanthoma, trichilemmoma, proliferating trichilemmal cyst, trichilemmal carcinoma- due to abnormality of outer root sheath • Loose anagen hair syndrome – due to absence of IRS

Contd...

Contd...

Segment	*Description*	*Applied aspects*
Adamson's fringe	• Demarcates upper limit of bulb/lower limit of stem • End of the keratogenous zone • The site where Huxley's layer loses trichohyalin granules and begins cornification • Cells of the outer sheath become pink	Site of dermatophyte infection
Dermal papilla	• Flask-shaped • Specialized fibroblast like cells embedded in extracellular matrix • Vascular supply present • Size of hair shaft is proportional to size of dermal papilla • Play a major role in maintenance of hair cycle • Androgen and GF receptors	The thicker the hair, the greater is the number of cells in a papilla and hence papillary cells become sparse when terminal hair transforms into a vellus hair as it does in androgenetic alopecia (AGA)

- Lamellated nerve endings in sinus hair follicle—vibrissae follicles

HAIR CYCLE

Definition

- Hair follicle cycle is defined as autonomous, rhythmic transformation of fully developed HFs through phases of growth, regression, and resting; controlled by the follicle itself by "hair cycle clock," with modulation by numerous systemic/extrafollicular factors.
- The growth of hair is cyclical as a consequence of established cycles of hair follicle **(Fig. 20)**.

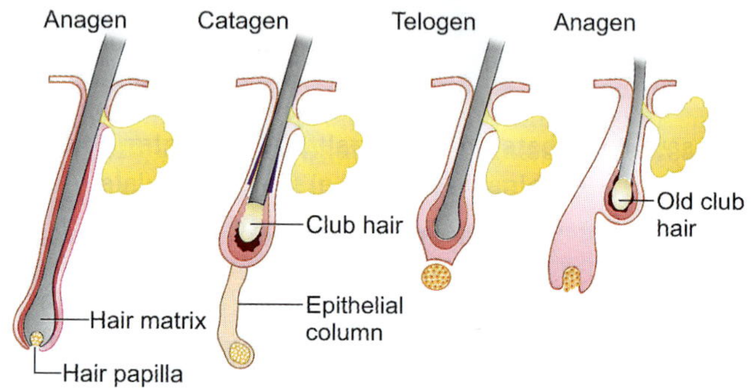

Fig. 20: Hair cycle.

Phases of Hair Cycle

- Growth phase (anagen I–VI)
- Regression phase (catagen)
- Resting phase (telogen)
- Shedding phase (exogen)
- Lag phase (kenogen)[46]

The phases in the cycle of a hair follicle are tabulated in **Table 8**.

Control of Hair Cycle

- Hair cycle control is primarily by individual hair follicles (intrinsic).
- In newborns the hair cycle is coordinated in a wave-like fashion (moult wave).
- In temperate climates the moult wave continues in seasonal fashion in adulthood.
- Synchronicity of hair cycle is lost with increasing age.
- *Regulation of hair cycle can be divided in three major categories:* (1) Intrinsic control, (2) Molecular control, and (3) Hormonal control.[47]

Intrinsic Control of the Hair Cycle

Vide **Table 9**.

Molecular Control of the Hair Cycle

It is described in **Figure 21**.[49]

Hormonal Control of the Hair Cycle

Vide **Table 10.**

NAIL

Introduction

- *The nail unit is made of several components:* The proximal and lateral nail folds, the nail matrix, the nail bed, the hyponychium, and the nail plate itself.
- Nails grow continuously throughout life. Growth rates of fingernails are 2–3 mm/month; and toenails are 1 mm/month.
- Complete replacement of nail requires 6 months for fingernail and 18 months for toenail.

Development

- Nail placode appears in the ninth week of embryonic life from the epidermis of the dorsal tip of the digit as a rectangular area.
- Nail matrix development completes by the 15th week and then it starts producing the nail plate, which will continue to grow until death.

Nail Structure

Nail Plate

- Nail plate consists of fully cornified structure made up of closely packed, adherent, interdigitating cells that lack nuclei or organelles, known as onychocytes.
- Nail plate created by the nail matrix epithelium.
- Pink color of nail plate due to longitudinally situated subungual capillaries.

TABLE 8: The phases in the cycle of a hair follicle (HF).

Growth phase	*Description*	*Applied*
Anagen	• Growth stage of the HF cycle • Duration—2–6 years • Out of 1,00,000 hair in human scalp, 90% in anagen • Stages of development: – Stage 1—cells of dermal papilla increase in size + increased RNA synthesis + increased mitosis of germ cells at base of bulb – Stage 2—lower part of HF grows down into the dermis and partially encloses dermal papilla – Stage 3—differentiation of cells is distinct – Stage 4—melanocytes form dendrites and develop melanin – Stage 5—new hair pushes out original clubbed hair – Stage 6—new hair comes out to the surface • Growth factors (GFs) acting— PDGF-A, TNF	Anagen effluvium—any event or insult that causes abrupt cessation of mitotic activity leads to weakening of the partially keratinized, proximal portion of the hair shaft, resulting in narrowing and subsequent breakage within the hair canal and even complete failure of hair formation. The hair bulb itself may be damaged and the hairs may separate at the bulb and fall out. Causes are chemotherapy and radiation to the head and neck, severe protein energy malnutrition, pemphigus vulgaris, alopecia areata (AA), and exposure to toxic agents like mercury, boron, thallium, etc. Other medications that can rarely cause anagen effluvium include bismuth, levodopa, colchicine, and cyclosporine
Catagen	• Involution of the lower two-thirds of the HF by massive keratinocyte apoptosis • Duration—2–3 weeks • 1% of hair • At the end of anagen, the follicle enters the regressive catagen phase, which is divided into eight substages (catagen I–VIII). The initiation of catagen is characterized by a nearly 50% reduction in the volume of the dermal papilla due to loss of extracellular matrix (ECM) and migration of cells into the surrounding dermal sheath • GFs acting—FGF-5	
Telogen	• Resting phase of the HF cycle • Duration—3 months • 10–15% of hair • Begins when the dermal papilla reaches the base of the permanent portion of the HF • GFs acting—FGF-18, BMP-6	Telogen effluvium (TE)—TE is a nonscarring, diffuse, hair loss from the scalp that occurs around 3 months after a triggering event and is usually self-limiting, lasting for about 6 month
Exogen/ Teloptosis	This refers to the phenomenon of hair shedding that happens as an activity parallel to the hair cycle. It is independent of either the anagen or the telogen phase	Trichostasis spinulosa—defective exogen
Kenogen/Lag phase	It is a phase in the hair cycle where the hair follicle is empty after hair shedding and persists in this stage for a variable duration	The severity of AGA is directly proportional to the total number of hairs in kenogen and the duration of kenogen

TABLE 9: Intrinsic control of the hair cycle.

Chalone hypothesis	At the end of anagen, a local active inhibitor accumulates and causes entry to telogen
Bulge activation hypothesis[6]	The "bulge activation hypothesis" proposes that the stem cells of the follicle reside not in the bulb matrix but in the bulge region at the insertion of the arrector pili muscle, this being the lowermost permanent part of the follicle. These cells divide at the end of telogen to give rise to the "transient amplifying cells" that multiply to form the matrix cells with a fixed life span. After this, the bulb disappears and the follicle returns to telogen only to restart the cycle. The dermal papilla, which moves upward during telogen, may interact with the bulge cells to start their activation. The keratinocytes of the bulge area differ from the surrounding keratinocytes by expressing a different set of keratins, namely, keratin 19, high expression of $\alpha3\beta1$ integrin, and slow cycling nature. This signifies their special role in hair development[48]

- Nail plate has a firm attachment to the underlying nail bed.
- The free edge of the nail plate extends beyond the distal end of the digits.
- It is made up of three horizontal layers: A thin dorsal lamina, the thicker intermediate lamina, and a ventral layer from the nail bed.
- The nail plate is rich in phospholipids and calcium, found as the phosphate in hydroxyapatite crystals.
- Nail keratins comprise about 80% of the dry weight of the nail plate, and they are divided between "soft" and "hard" (sulfur rich, cross-linked).

Nail Matrix

- Wedge-shaped area of specialized epithelium, divided into proximal and distal portions.
- Proximal nail matrix synthesizes the dorsal aspect of the nail plate and the distal nail matrix creates the ventral surface of the nail plate.
- The proximal part of finger nails shows a whitish, opaque, half-moon-shaped area, known as the lunula. This is the visible distal portion of the nail matrix.
- Melanocytes, Merkel cells, and LCs are found in the distal part of the nail matrix.

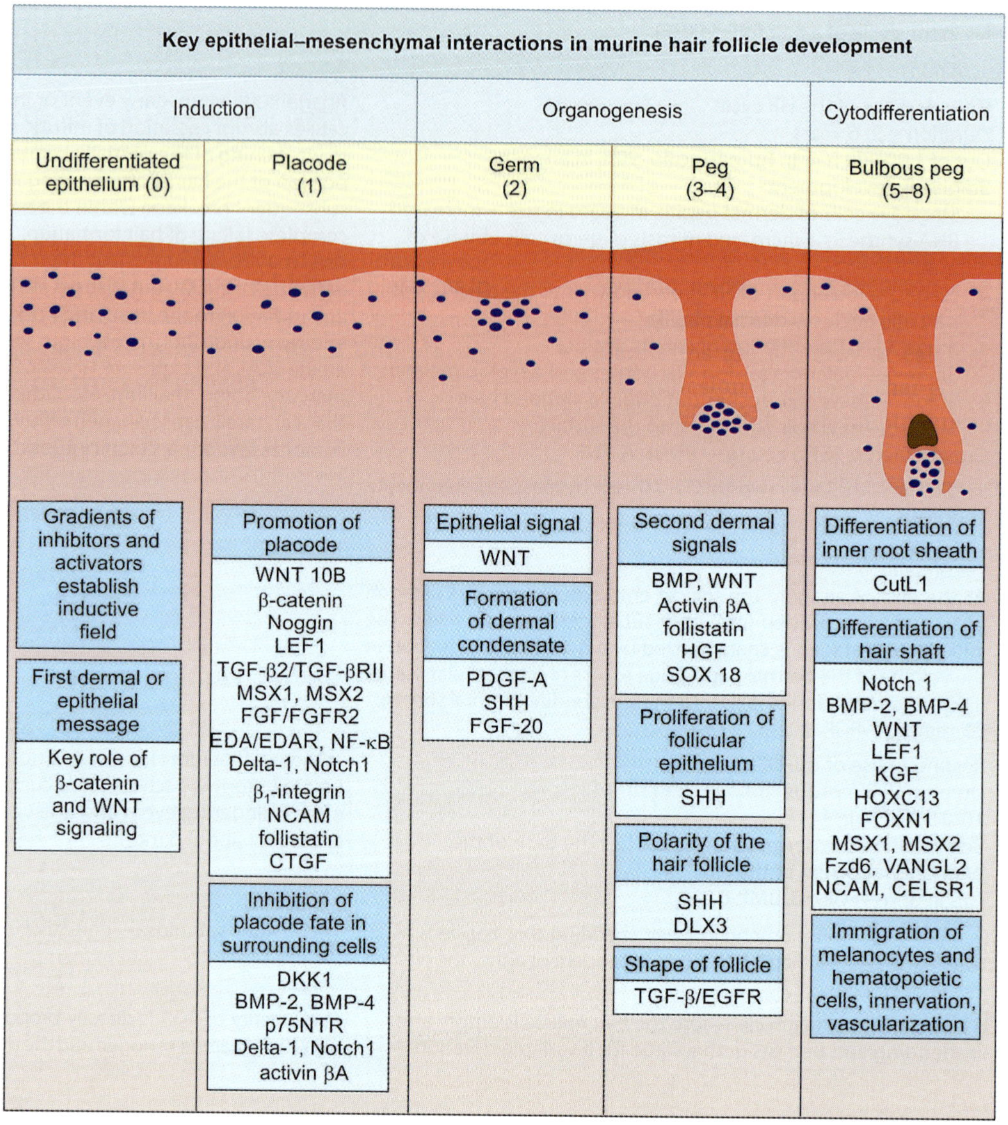

Fig. 21: Molecular control of the hair cycle.

TABLE 10: Hormonal control of the hair cycle.

Androgens	Increases the duration of anagen and hence the thickness of hair shaft; increases the size of the hair follicle
Estrogens	Prolongs anagen and delays transition to telogen
Prolactin	Has androgen-like activity on hairs
Insulin	Acts through IGF-1 and promotes hair growth
Growth hormone	Induces sebocyte differentiation
Thyroid hormones	Both hypo- and hypersecretion can cause alopecia; enhance the onset of the follicular cycle of activity but retard the rate of hair growth and retain the club hair in the follicle

Cuticle or Eponychium

- It is the narrow band of epidermis that extends and adheres to the proximal part of the nail plate.
- Cuticle prevents separation of nail plate and proximal nail fold.

Nail Bed

- Nail bed is present underneath the nail plate and along with the nail matrix contributes to nail plate formation.
- The epithelium of the nail bed is thin and consists of two to five cell layers.

- Nail bed keratinization does not involve formation of a granular layer.

Nail Groove

- It is the indentation between the edges of the nail plate and the nail folds.
- Here the anchoring ligaments are present between the nail matrix and the underlying bone.

Nail Folds

- The nail fold is the tissue that encloses the nail matrix at the root of the nail.
- This is similar in structure to the adjacent skin but is devoid of dermatoglyphic markings and pilosebaceous glands.[50]

Blood Supply of the Nail

- The blood supply of the nail is provided by the lateral digital arteries.
- The nail bed is rich in vascular supply and is supplied by encapsulated neurovascular structures containing one to four arteriovenous anastomoses and nerve endings.

Nerve Supply

The cutaneous sensory nerves, originated from the dorsal branches of the paired digital nerves, supply the nail apparatus.

Applied Aspects

Inherited diseases of the nails:

- *Pachyonychia congenita:*
  - *Type I (Jadassohn-Lewandowsky syndrome):* Autosomal dominant condition with mutations in the *KRT6A/KRT16* genes. This condition is characterized by focal palmoplantar keratoderma, benign oral leukokeratosis, and nail dystrophy with significant subungual hyperkeratosis.
  - *Type II (Jackson-Lawler syndrome):* Autosomal dominant condition with mutations in the *KRT6b, KRT17* genes. This condition is characterized by nail dystrophy, steatocystomas, eruptive vellus hair cysts, natal teeth, and pili torti
  - *Type III (Schafer–Brunauer) syndrome:* Features all the findings of the type I disease associated with leukokeratosis of the corneas, involves mutations in *KRT6A*
  - *Type IV, pachyonychia congenita tarda:* Late onset of the disease during the second or third decade of life and involves mutations in *KRT6B*.
- *Nail-patella syndrome:*
  - Also known as (Hereditary Osteo-Onychodysplasia)
  - Autosomal dominant condition caused by mutation in *LMX1B* gene
  - The condition is characterized by triangular lunulae, hypoplastic nails, absent patella, scapular thickening, Lester iris, radial head abnormalities, and iliac crest exostoses.
- *Dermatopathia pigmentosa reticularis:*
  - It is a rare ectodermal disorder with the diagnostic triad of generalized reticulate hyperpigmentation, noncicatricial alopecia, and onychodystrophy.
  - Autosomal dominant condition with *KRT14* mutation.
  - *Differential diagnosis:* It shares a similar *KRT14* mutation with Naegeli-Franceschetti-Jadassohn syndrome. The shared clinical features in both conditions are adermatoglyphia, palmoplantar keratoderma, and hypohidrosis. However, alopecia is only seen in dermatopathia pigmentosa reticularis and dental abnormalities are seen in only in Naegeli-Franceschetti-Jadassohn syndrome **(Figs. 22A and B)**.

WOUND HEALING

Introduction

- Wound healing is a physiological reaction of tissue injury and involves a complex interplay between numerous cell types, cytokines, mediators, and the vascular system.

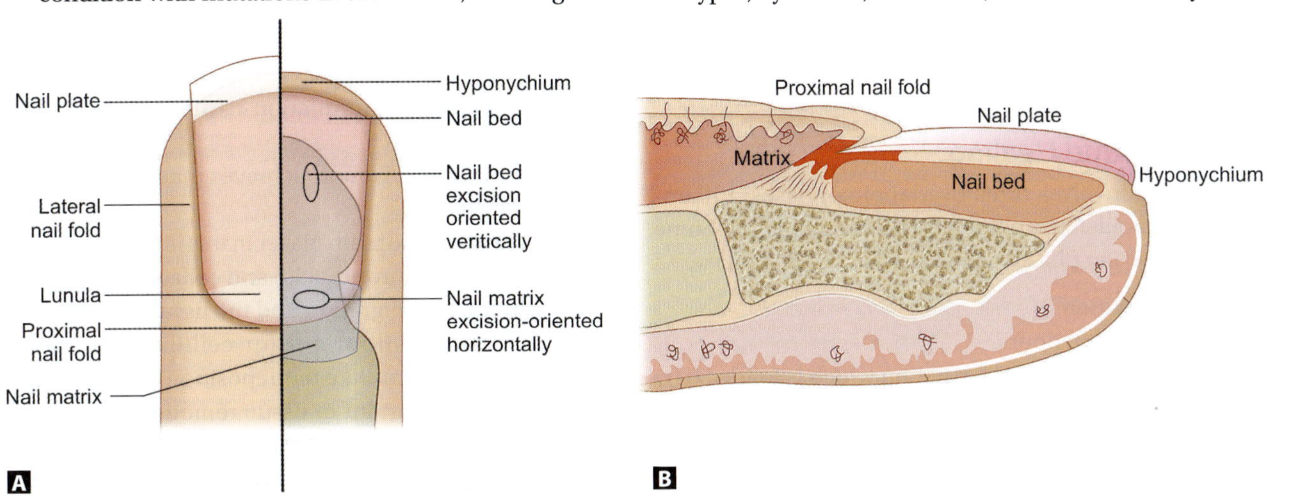

Figs. 22A and B: (A) Nail anatomy; (B) Nail apparatus in transverse section, showing the four structures that contribute to nail plate formation: Proximal nail fold, nail matrix, nail bed, and hyponychium.

- The scar strength is 5% at 1 week, 20% at 3 weeks, and about 70–80% at 1 year.

Cutaneous Stem Cells

- Stem cells are involved in wound healing, and each subtype of stem cells contributes to regeneration of various components of skin and adnexal structures.
- *Keratinocyte stem cells:* Interfollicular epidermis self-renewing stem cells reside within the basal layer, which adheres through $\alpha3\beta1$- and $\alpha6\beta4$-integrins to an underlying basement membrane of laminin-5-rich ECM that separates the epidermis from the underlying dermis. Secreted factors such as FGF-7, FGF-10, insulin-like growth factor (IGF), EGF ligands, and TGF-α from dermal fibroblasts promote the proliferation of basal epidermal cells. Transition from the basal to the spinous layer requires Notch signaling, a highly conserved pathway involved in a wide variety of developmental processes.
- *Hair follicle stem cells:* Hair follicle and melanocyte stem cells reside in the bulge and the hair germ. In anagen, hair follicle stem cells regenerate the lower segment of the follicle. Melanocyte stem cells generate mature melanocytes, which transfer their pigment to differentiating hair cells. Hair follicle stem cells can be subdivided into two populations: A quiescent one located in the bulge and a primed population within the hair germ just below the bulge, which is more prone to proliferation. *Wnt signaling is also critical for hair germ activation:* The downstream Wnt effector, nuclear β-catenin, accumulates in the activated hair germ and leads to target gene activation.
- *Sebaceous gland stem cells:* These are found at or near the bud of the sebaceous gland, and regenerate sebaceous glands during wound repair.
- *Eccrine gland stem cells:* These can form acral epidermis in wound repair.
- *Merkel cell stem cells:* These are located in hairy skin.
- *Melanocyte stem cells:* These are located in the lower bulge region and regenerate hair matrix and epidermal melanocytes.[51]

Stages of Wound Healing

Wound healing involves three overlapping phases: Inflammatory phase, proliferative phase, and tissue remodeling. Some also suggest vascular phase (hemostasis) as the first phase.

Phase 1: Inflammation

- This is the first 6–8 hours.
- In this phase, there is clot formation which is followed by wound debridement by neutrophils and macrophages.
- The inflammatory phase is characterized by hemostasis, chemotaxis, and increased vascular permeability, limiting further damage, closing the wound, removing cellular debris and bacteria, and fostering cellular migration.
- Platelets are the main player in this phase. They release chemotactic factors like fibrinogen, fibronectin, thrombospondin, vWF, ADP, attracting other platelets, WBCs, and fibroblasts. It produces fibronectin which acts as a provisional matrix for fibroblast migration; also releases PDGF, TGFα, and TGFβ.
- Neutrophils appear first and in greater numbers than macrophages. They are attracted by fibrinogen, fibrin split products, leukotrienes, and C5a. This plays an important role in the tissue debridement and bacterial killing.
- Next, macrophages become predominant WBC as the process continues. They aid in tissue debridement and play a critical role in wound healing by helping the transition from inflammation to repair. Macrophages are attracted by fibrin degradation products, fibronectin, fragments of collagen, TGF-β. They release growth factors which stimulate fibroblasts and ECM production.

Phase 2: Proliferative phase

- This phase takes 5–7 days but may take longer.
- The proliferative phase is characterized by the formation of granulation tissue, re-epithelialization, and neovascularization.
- Keratinocytes are the main player in this phase. Re-epithelialization begins several hours after injury; keratinocytes leapfrog over each other from wound edges and adnexal structures. Collagenase which is produced in the wound area, aids in migration of the keratinocytes.
- Fibroblasts are another major player in this stage. They migrate to wound 48 hours after injury, moving along the fibronectin matrix from initial clot. Type III collagen is found in early wounds. Wound contraction by myofibroblasts starts typically the second week of healing.
- Stimulation of new vessel growth occurs in this phase via VEGF, TGF-β, thrombospondin, angiotropin, angiogenin, and secreted protein acidic and rich in cysteine (SPARC).

Phase 3: Tissue remodeling or tissue maturation phase

- It starts after 3rd week
- In this phase the granulation tissue becomes a mature scar tissue.
- In this phase the wound achieves maximum strength as it matures
- Fibroblasts are the main player in this phase. They produce fibronectin, hyaluronic acid, and collagen which play key roles in the cell migration and the tissue support.
- Fibronectin is important for cellular migration and formation of a template for deposition of collagen,
- Collagen is important in tissue remodeling. Granulation tissue is initially composed of type III collagen. As the type III collagen is gradually replaced by the type I collagen and scar's tensile strength increases. Final strength attained is about 70–80% of the preinjured skin (**Fig. 23**).[52]

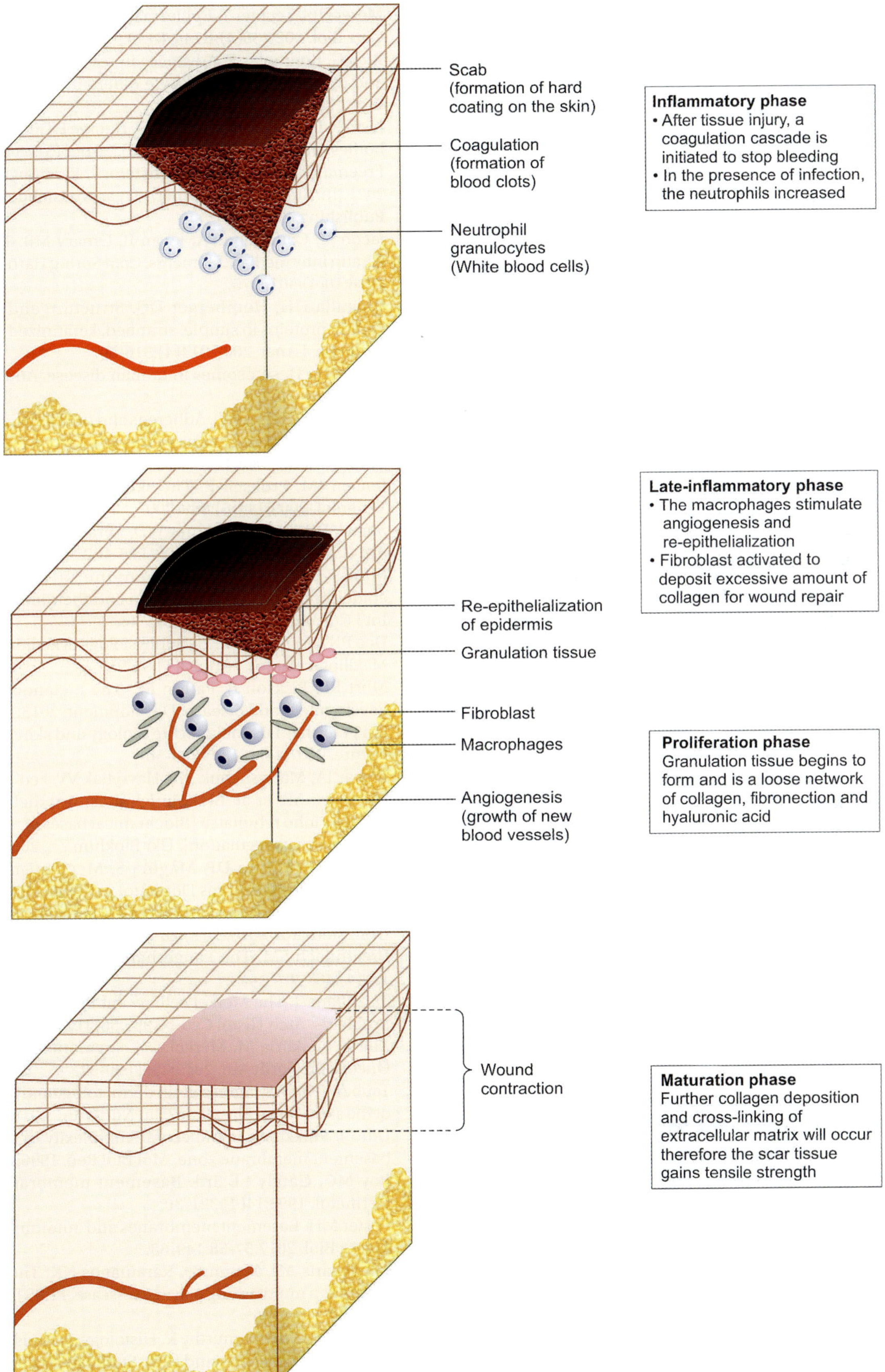

Fig. 23: Stages of wound healing.

KEY POINTS

- The ectoderm forms the epidermis, the melanocytes, and the nervous system. The mesoderm forms fibroblasts, blood vessels, and muscles. The endoderm does not contribute to skin development.
- The layers of the epidermis include the stratum basale, stratum spinosum, stratum granulosum, stratum lucidum, and stratum corneum from the deepest to superficial portion.
- Desmosomes are calcium-dependent cell-cell adhesion molecules between keratinocytes.
- Keratinization, also termed as cornification, is a process of cytodifferentiation which the keratinocytes undergo when proceeding from their postgerminative state (stratum basale) to finally differentiated, hardened cell filled with protein, constituting a structurally and functionally distinct keratin containing surface layer such as stratum corneum.
- Melanocytes are pigment-producing cell derived from neural crest. Epidermal melanin unit is a functional subunit which denotes that every melanocyte interacts with 36 keratinocytes via its arborizing dendrite.
- LCs are tissue-resident, nonphagocytic, mononuclear dendritic cells which are critical in recognizing and presenting foreign antigens to specific T-lymphocytes.
- Basement membranes or dermal-epidermal junction are specialized structures for attachment and interaction between the epidermis and the dermis.
- Collagens are the primary dermal component and it constitutes about 75% of the dry weight of the dermis. Elastic fibers constitute 4% of the dry weight of the skin.
- Eccrine glands are the major sweat glands in humans. Eccrine glands are present over the entire cutaneous surface except the vermillion border of the lips, nail beds, labia minora, glans penis, clitoris, external auditory canal.
- Sebum is a light yellow viscous fluid. Lipid composition of sebum is 57% triglycerides, 25% wax esters, 15% squalene, <3% cholesterol, and cholesterol esters.
- Merkel cells are found in the basal layer and act as the slowly adapting touch receptors.
- Glomus bodies are specialized arteriovenous shunts seen in finger pads, nail bed palms, and soles.
- Phases of hair cycle includes the growth phase (anagen I–VI), the regression phase (catagen), the resting phase (telogen), the shedding phase (exogen), the lag phase (kenogen).
- The scar strength is 5% at 1 week, 20% at 3 weeks, and about 70–80% at 1 year after wounding.

REFERENCES

1. Hu MS, Borrelli MR, Hong WX, Malhotra S, Cheung ATM, Ransom RC, et al. Embryonic skin development and repair. Organogenesis. 2018;14(1):46-63.
2. Moreci RS, Lechler T. Epidermal structure and differentiation. Curr Biol. 2020;30(4):R144-R149.
3. Rice G, Rompolas P. Advances in resolving the heterogeneity and dynamics of keratinocyte differentiation. Curr Opin Cell Biol. 2020;67:92-8.
4. Joshi R. Learning from eponyms: George F. Odland and Odland bodies. Indian Dermatol Online J. 2014;5(3):334-8.
5. Freeman SC, Sonthalia S. Histology, keratohyalin granules. 2021. In: StatPearls [Internet]. Treasure Island, FL: StatPearls Publishing; 2021.
6. Jacob JT, Coulombe PA, Kwan R, Omary MB. Types I and II keratin intermediate filaments. Cold Spring Harb Perspect Biol. 2018;10(4):a018275.
7. Bragulla HH, Homberger DG. Structure and functions of keratin proteins in simple, stratified, keratinized and cornified epithelia. J Anat. 2009;214(4):516-59.
8. Najor NA. Desmosomes in human disease. Annu Rev Pathol. 2018;13:51-70.
9. Hartsock A, Nelson WJ. Adherens and tight junctions: structure, function and connections to the actin cytoskeleton. Biochim Biophys Acta. 2008;1778(3):660-9.
10. Jensen JM, Proksch E. The skin's barrier. G Ital Dermatol Venereol. 2009;144(6):689-700.
11. Smack DP, Korge BP, James WD. Keratin and keratinization. J Am Acad Dermatol. 1994;30(1):85-102.
12. Marks R. The epidermal engine: a commentary on epidermopoiesis, desquamation and their interrelationships. Int J Cosmet Sci. 1986;8(3):135-44.
13. Deo PN, Deshmukh R. Pathophysiology of keratinization. J Oral Maxillofac Pathol. 2018;22(1):86-91.
14. Mort RL, Jackson IJ, Patton EE. The melanocyte lineage in development and disease. Development. 2015;142(4):620-32.
15. Lin JY, Fisher DE. Melanocyte biology and skin pigmentation. Nature. 2007;445(7130):843-50.
16. Makar IA, Martyshchuk MV, Havryliak VV, Fed'kiv OO, Stapaĭ PV, Syvyk AE, et al. Biokhimichni osnovy melanohenezu ta shliakhy ïoho rehuliatsiï [Biochemical bases of melanogenesis and ways of its regulation]. Ukr Biokhim Zh. 2004;76(3):16-24.
17. Videira IF, Moura DF, Magina S. Mechanisms regulating melanogenesis. An Bras Dermatol. 2013;88(1):76-83.
18. Collin M, Milne P. Langerhans cell origin and regulation. Curr Opin Hematol. 2016;23(1):28-35.
19. Breathnach SM. The Langerhans cell. Br J Dermatol. 1988; 119(4):463-9.
20. Tachibana T. The Merkel cell: recent findings and unresolved problems. Arch Histol Cytol. 1995;58(4):379-96.
21. Xue Y, Thakuria M. Merkel cell carcinoma review. Hematol Oncol Clin North Am. 2019;33(1):39-52.
22. Taub AF, Pham K. Stem cells in dermatology and anti-aging care of the skin. Facial Plast Surg Clin North Am. 2018;26(4):425-37.
23. Uitto J, Pulkkinen L. Molecular complexity of the cutaneous basement membrane zone. Mol Biol Rep. 1996;23(1):35-46.
24. Ray MC, Gately LE 3rd. Basement membrane zone. Clin Dermatol. 1996;14(4):321-30.
25. Foster MH. Basement membranes and autoimmune diseases. Matrix Biol. 2017;57-58:149-68.
26. Theocharis AD, Manou D, Karamanos NK. The extracellular matrix as a multitasking player in disease. FEBS J. 2019;286(15): 2830-69.
27. Brown TM, Krishnamurthy K. Histology, Dermis. In: StatPearls [Internet]. Treasure Island (FL): StatPearls Publishing; 2021.
28. Yousef H, Alhajj M, Sharma S. Anatomy, Skin (Integument), Epidermis. In: StatPearls [Internet]. Treasure Island (FL): StatPearls Publishing; 2021.

29. Green EM, Mansfield JC, Bell JS, Winlove CP. The structure and micromechanics of elastic tissue. Interface Focus. 2014;4(2):20130058.
30. Andrés-Ramos I, Alegría-Landa V, Gimeno I, Pérez-Plaza A, Rütten A, Kutzner H, et al. Cutaneous elastic tissue anomalies. Am J Dermatopathol. 2019;41(2):85-117.
31. Theocharis AD, Skandalis SS, Gialeli C, Karamanos NK. Extracellular matrix structure. Adv Drug Deliv Rev. 2016;97:4-27.
32. Thulabandu V, Chen D, Atit RP. Dermal fibroblast in cutaneous development and healing. Wiley Interdiscip Rev Dev Biol. 2018;7(2).
33. Sueki H, Telegan B, Murphy GF. Computer-assisted three-dimensional reconstruction of human dermal dendrocytes. J Invest Dermatol. 1995;105(5):704-8.
34. Fong M, Crane JS. Histology, Mast Cells. In: StatPearls [Internet]. Treasure Island (FL): StatPearls Publishing; 2021.
35. Lawson W. Glomus bodies and tumors. N Y State J Med. 1980;80(10):1567-75.
36. Cui CY, Schlessinger D. Eccrine sweat gland development and sweat secretion. Exp Dermatol. 2015;24(9):644-50.
37. Farkaš R. Apocrine secretion: new insights into an old phenomenon. Biochim Biophys Acta. 2015;1850(9):1740-50.
38. Thody AJ, Shuster S. Control and function of sebaceous glands. Physiol Rev. 1989;69(2):383-416.
39. McGlone F, Reilly D. The cutaneous sensory system. Neurosci Biobehav Rev. 2010;34(2):148-59.
40. Munger BL, Ide C. The structure and function of cutaneous sensory receptors. Arch Histol Cytol. 1988;51(1):1-34.
41. Ryan TJ. The blood vessels of the skin. J Invest Dermatol. 1976;67(1):110-8.
42. Ryan TJ. Structure and function of lymphatics. J Invest Dermatol. 1989;93(2 Suppl):18S-24S.
43. Reynolds AJ, Lawrence CM, Jahoda CA. Human hair follicle germinative epidermal cell culture. J Invest Dermatol. 1993;101(4):634-8.
44. Dawber RPR. Hair follicle structure. Keratinization and the physical properties of hair. In: Rook A, Dawber R (Eds). Diseases of the Hair and Scalp, 2nd edition. Oxford: Blackwell Scientific Publications; 1991. pp. 18-50.
45. Poblet E, Ortega F, Jiménez F. The arrector pili muscle and the follicular unit of the scalp: a microscopic anatomy study. Dermatol Surg. 2002;28(9):800-3.
46. Hashimoto K, Ito M, Suzuki Y. Innervation and vasculature of the hair follicle. In: Orfanos CE, Happle R (Eds). Hair and Hair Diseases. Berlin: Springer-Verlag; 1990. pp. 117-47.
47. Stenn KS, Paus R. Controls of hair follicle cycling. Physiol Rev. 2001;81:449-94.
48. Sun TT, Cotsarelis G, Lavker RM. Hair follicular stem cells: the bulge activation hypothesis. J Invest Dermatol. 1991;96: 77-8.
49. Peus D, Pittelkow MR. Growth factors in hair organ development and the hair growth cycle. Dermatol Clin. 1996;14:559-72.
50. de Berker D. Nail anatomy. Clin Dermatol. 2013;31(5):509-15.
51. Ojeh N, Pastar I, Tomic-Canic M, Stojadinovic O. Stem cells in skin regeneration, wound healing, and their clinical applications. Int J Mol Sci. 2015;16(10):25476-501.
52. Gantwerker EA, Hom DB. Skin: histology and physiology of wound healing. Facial Plast Surg Clin North Am. 2011;19(3): 441-53.

EXAMINATION QUESTIONS

1. Write a short note on Odland bodies.
2. Write a short note of keratohyalin granules.
3. Draw and describe steps of keratinization.
4. Write a short note of desmosome.
5. Draw and describe a melanocyte.
6. Describe the steps of melanogenesis and discuss its applied aspects.
7. Draw and describe a Langerhans cell.
8. Draw and describe a Merkel cell.
9. Draw and describe a basement membrane zone. Discuss its applied aspects.
10. Write a short note on collagen.
11. Write a short note on elastic tissue.
12. Write a short note on extra-fibrillar matrix.
13. Write a short note on dermal cells with applied importances.
14. Draw and describe a mast cell.
15. Draw and describe an eccrine gland.
16. Write a short note on apocrine gland.
17. Write a short note on sebaceous gland and list the diseases of the sebaceous glands.
18. Write a short note on cutaneous nervous system.
19. Write a short note on cutaneous vasculature.
20. Draw and describe a hair follicle.
21. Discuss hair cycle with its applied importances.
22. Draw and describe structure of a nail.
23. Draw and discuss stages of wound healing.
24. Write a short note on disorders of keratinization in dermatology.
25. Write a note on pilosebaceous unit.
26. Write a note on composition of sebum and its function.
27. Outline principles of wound healing, factors responsible for abnormal wound healing, and novel therapies in wound healing.

4 CHAPTER

Functions of the Skin

Varsha Vaidyanathan, Aarti Sarda, Abhishek De

INTRODUCTION

The skin is the largest organ of the human body, measuring about 2 square meters in the average adult. Aside from the obvious function of providing a barrier between the body and the external environment, there are a host of other functions of the skin. It is a vibrant and dynamic entity that allows the individual to interact with the outside world while at the same time provides protection and support to the internal environment. In this chapter, we will further discuss the functions of the skin.

The functions of skin can be discussed under the following headings:

BARRIER FUNCTION[1-3]

The skin has to withstand many insults whether they be physical, chemical, thermal, electrical, or microbial in origin. Resistance to these hazardous external conditions depends upon the integrity of the skin, its permeability, and on the extent to which it allows these agents to penetrate the skin.

Permeability Barrier

The skin is not a rigid, impermeable barrier. In fact, it is selectively permeable to the flow of water and electrolytes. To a very great extent life depends upon this permeability. The regulation of water and electrolytes is a function of the epidermis and to be more precise, the stratum corneum. It is an effective barrier against most substances yet many chemicals can penetrate in minute quantities after prolonged contact. The thickness of this stratum corneum is a key component of this barrier as is evidenced by the fact that penetration through the thick-skinned palms and soles is significantly lower than that of other thin-skinned areas like the eyelids. Secondary to the thickness, the other key factor governing the permeability of the skin is the total lipid concentration of the stratum corneum. The barrier function is provided through patterned lipid lamella existing in the extracellular space between keratinocytes. These keratinocytes contain proteins such as filaggrin and keratin bound to a peripheral envelope formed by protein cross-linking. Multiple layers of these cells in the stratum corneum provide a resilient scaffolding for the intercellular lipid lamella. This lamella is formed by the Odland bodies. Membrane-coating granules or lamellar granules or Odland bodies are found in the upper stratum spinosum and stratum granulosum next to the cell membranes. They fuse with the plasma membrane and release their contents (glycolipids, phospholipids, and sterols) into the intercellular space. Thus, they have an important role in maintaining the barrier function. Lysosomal enzymes cause lipid remodeling to fine tune the process of barrier formation. Tight junctions may also have a role in epidermal barrier function.

Of the three possible routes of percutaneous absorption, as discussed, the stratum corneum is the most important. The other two—the pilosebaceous unit, and the sweat gland apparatus—have a decidedly less important role to play. They act more as diffusion shunts for easy pathways for certain ions and molecules that are too large to pass comfortably or quickly through the stratum corneum.

There are various factors which influence the permeability and absorption through the skin. Increased water content of the skin and increased skin temperature both increase the absorption. The composition of the substances matters too. Lipids and lipid-soluble substances pass through easily whereas organic compounds containing hydrophilic groups pass through with some difficulty. The vehicle, whether it is an ointment, gel, cream, also matters. Factors such as age, external environment, and continuity of skin also influence permeability. Damaged skin, either by disease, drugs or chemicals, is more permeable than intact skin and allows the entry of harmful agents. There is regional variability in absorption such that palms and soles are less permeable compared to face and genitalia. Occlusion increases absorption. This fact is taken advantage of in the clinical approach toward treatment of conditions such as atopic dermatitis where the steroid-emollient combination is applied to the body and then occluded with bandages so that absorption is increased. Dry skin is less permeable so in order to reduce absorption of irritant drugs such as tretinoin, the skin must be thoroughly dried prior to application.

Toxic epidermal necrolysis (TEN): In this condition, there is a generalized and rapid necrosis of keratinocytes which leads to epidermal detachment. The skin is thus unable to perform the basic barrier function. There is a large amount of fluid and electrolyte loss with accompanying dehydration. There is an inability to block entry of pathogens leading to secondary infection and sepsis. Depending upon the extent of involvement, there is an increased risk of death, thus exemplifying the importance of the skin's barrier function to life and health.

Barrier to Pathogens

An intact stratum corneum prevents the entry of microorganisms into the body through the skin. Sebum acts as a fungistatic agent. Glycerophospholipids and free fatty acids have an inhibitory effect on microorganisms. Antimicrobial peptides (AMP) such as cathelicidin and defensins present on the skin surface have the ability to kill bacteria, fungi, and viruses. Even areas such as hair follicles and sweat glands, where there is a natural break in skin continuity and can potentially allow entry of microorganisms, produce small amounts of AMP to counteract the pathogens.

Barrier to Ultraviolet Radiation

Ultraviolet radiation can induce various deleterious skin changes such as immunosuppression, carcinogenesis and premature aging. Melanin present in the epidermis along with the proteins of the stratum corneum absorbs the atmospheric ultraviolet radiation and mitigate its deleterious effects on DNA. With prolonged exposure, there is increase in the number of melanocytes and melanosomes and also a thickening of the epidermis, all of which enhance the barrier effect to ultraviolet radiation.

Oculocutaneous albinism: In this condition, there is reduced or absent melanin in the skin due to loss of function of tyrosinase enzyme. This skin lacking in melanin is unable to combat the effects of UV radiation and patients suffering from OCA are found to have a greater tendency to develop photosensitive disorders, actinic keratoses and squamous cell carcinoma as compared to the rest of the population.

Mechanical Barrier

The elastic property of skin due to the dermal collagen and elastin, along with the cushioning effect of subcutaneous fat counteracts deforming forces and provides protection from blunt trauma.

THERMOREGULATION[4]

Thermoregulation involves the maintenance of the core body temperature at a constant of 37°C irrespective of the external environmental conditions. Although there are minor fluctuations in temperature due to circadian rhythm, menstrual cycle and aging, by and large the body temperature is maintained within a very narrow and tightly-controlled range as deviating from this can be fatal.

The hypothalamus is the co-ordinating center for temperature control. The preoptic anterior hypothalamus is the key area which receives input from peripheral and central thermoreceptors.

Response to Increase in Body Temperature

Skin

The blood vessels in the skin vasodilate in response to the increased temperature. Arteriovenous anastomoses open and blood flows directly from artery to vein without passing through arterioles and capillaries. When the blood is brought close to the skin surface there is dissipation of heat from the body to the outside environment through convection.

Sweat Glands

Increased ambient temperature and exercise both increase sweating which is mediated by sympathetic cholinergic fibers. Sweat collects on the skin surface and gets evaporated resulting in the transfer of heat to the external environment. This causes a cooling-down of the body.

Behavioral Changes

While the body experiences high temperatures, the individual consciously decides to stay in the shade, decrease activity, turn on the cooler, drink cold water, etc.

Response to Decrease in Body Temperature

Skin

In response to cold temperatures, sympathetic vasoconstrictor nerves along with ATP and neuropeptide Y act to constrict the skin blood vessels and shunt the blood away from the skin surface through the dermal veins. This causes heat to be conserved in the body core.

Brown Fat

This adipose tissue is thermogenic through the process of nonshivering thermogenesis. Here oxidative metabolism is delinked from ATP production and energy is released. This results in an increase in the core body temperature.

Piloerection

Cold temperatures cause an increased sympathetic nerve discharge resulting in contraction of the arrector pili muscles. The hairs stand on end (goosebumps) with air trapped between them which form a layer of insulating air around the body and minimize heat loss.

Shivering

Shivering takes place when the body is unable to conserve heat in spite of vasoconstriction and piloerection. It is initiated by the anterior preoptic hypothalamus and mediated through the motor cortex in response to the peripheral thermoreceptors. This indicates that it is the skin temperature rather than the core temperature which is the stimulus for shivering. It is described as involuntary, oscillating and rapid skeletal muscle contraction. During this process, ATP is used up but no work is done so the energy produced is expended as heat. This is important in adults, but in neonates who have immature skeletal muscles, nonshivering thermogenesis through brown adipose tissue is more relevant.

Behavioral Changes

Drop in ambient temperature leads the individual to wear warm clothing, turn on the heater, increase activity, etc.

Failure of Thermoregulation

Excessive heat: In patients who cannot thermoregulate as discussed above, e.g., hypohidrotic ectodermal dysplasia wherein there is a near complete absence of functional sweat glands, the core temperature increases rapidly with increased environmental heat or internal heat generated during exercise, and this may even lead to death from overheating.

Excessive cold: In extreme cold, humans need an external source of heat to maintain the core body temperature since the intrinsic mechanisms to generate heat are insufficient. Without adequate protection by way of warm clothing or heat sources, hypothermia and frostbite can occur which can lead to death and disability.

IMMUNE DEFENSE

The skin acts as the first port of immune response against various microorganisms. The epidermal dendritic cells (Langerhans cells) and the dermal dendritic cells activate on recognizing the foreign antigens and pathogens. These cells then travel to the regional lymph nodes via the draining lymphatics. Within the lymph nodes, the B-lymphocytes produce antibodies and the T-lymphocytes circulate to and from the skin. A subset of memory T-cells reside within the skin and are critical for the immune defense.

Loss or failure of this immune defense function can lead to infections either bacterial, viral or fungal.

Some examples are as follows:

Warts: Trauma to the skin allows implantation of viral particles within the keratinocytes. Ordinarily, the cytotoxic immune response kicks in causing destruction of the virus and brings about resolution. However, a failure of this process or immunosuppression causes results in chronic and recurrent warts. Nowadays, newer therapies have begun to rely on the body's immune response to bring about a faster cure by use of MMR vaccine, topical imiquimod and oral cimetidine.

Leprosy: The same micro-organism causes the disease to take different forms ranging from the tuberculoid to lepromatous spectrum, based on the immune resistance and response of the affected individual.

Autoimmune disorders: At times, the immune system fails to distinguish between "self" and "foreign" antigens, in effect causing the body to fight against itself. This results in the gamut of disorders falling under the umbrella term of "autoimmune disorders". In some cases, there are antibodies formed against the skin antigens which give rise to characteristic disorders. **Table 1** shows some common skin conditions arising due to autoantibodies.

TABLE 1: Skin conditions and their target autoantigen.

Disorder	*Antigen in skin*
Pemphigus foliaceous	Dsg 1
Pemphigus vulgaris	Dsg 1 and 3
Bullous pemphigoid	BPAg 1 and 2
Dermatitis herpetiformis	Transglutaminase 3
Paraneoplastic pemphigus	Dsg 1, Dsg 3, Plectin, Desmoplakin, Envoplakin
Epidermolysis acquisita	Collagen VII

TABLE 2: Mechanoreceptors in skin

	Hairy skin	*Non-hairy skin*
Main receptor	Hair follicle receptor	
Rapidly-adapting receptor	Pacinian corpuscle	Meissner's corpuscle
Slowly-adapting receptors	Ruffini's corpuscle	Merkel's receptors

SENSATION

Multiple sensory receptors, i.e., mechanoreceptors for touch, pressure, and vibration are distributed all over the skin. The predominant mechanoreceptor in the hairy skin is the hair-follicle receptor. Nonhairy skin contains the rapidly adapting Meissner's corpuscle and the slowly adapting Merkel's receptor. Hairy skin too contains a rapidly adapting receptor, the Pacinian corpuscle and a slowly adapting Ruffini's corpuscle. In addition to these mechanoreceptors, multiple thermoreceptors for hot and cold sensation, nociceptors for pain, and itch and neuropeptides acting as neurotransmitters are present throughout the skin. All of these put together contribute to the various sensations experienced by the individual **(Table 2)**.

Excessive sensitivity: Sometimes, the receptors or the mediating nerve fibres may demonstrate hyper-reactivity without any structural abnormality. This can lead to sensations of extreme pruritus or pain.

Leprosy: Nerve involvement leads to decreased sensations. Patients fail to perceive cutaneous trauma and this leads to the development of multiple wounds and ulcers especially on the hands and feet.

CIRCULATION

There are two circulatory systems which mediate the transport of cells and solutes to and from the skin.

1. *The hematological system:* This is a two-way system in which blood flows both to and from the skin. It contains nutritive vessels (arteries, veins and capillaries) and anastomosing vessels helping in thermoregulation. This system functions to supply nutrients to the skin, deliver leukocytes to the required areas of the skin and also aids in heat regulation.

2. *The lymphatic system:* This is a one-way system which transports leukocytes, macrophages, Langerhans cells and interstitial fluids from the lymphatic capillaries into the central venous system via the lymph nodes and the thoracic duct.

Arterial embolism: A failure of the circulatory mechanism in the arteries results in embolus formation which occludes the arteries. Within a few hours, there is necrosis of skin distal to the occlusion due to the dependence of the skin on the hematological system for its nutrition.

Vasculitis: Inflammation of the blood vessels, most often in the background of autoimmune disorders such as SLE, Sjögren syndrome, systemic sclerosis, leads to various cutaneous changes depending upon the size of the vessels involved.

Venous insufficiency: Valvular incompetence in the venous system of the lower limbs leads to varicosities, stasis changes and finally chronic venous ulcers in the legs.

Failure of lymphatic drainage: Various infections such as staphylococcal, streptococcal and filariasis lead to blockage of lymphatic drainage due to scarring. As a result, there is an inability to drain the interstitial fluid which leads to edema distal to the blockage. Eventually, there is a verrucous thickening of the overlying skin known as elephantiasis nostras verrucosa.

WOUND REPAIR/REGENERATION

In order to maintain the integrity of the skin, there are repair mechanisms in place which attempt to re-establish a functional skin barrier in response to wounds, trauma, burns, etc. In an ideal situation, this wound-healing response would lead to complete regeneration with both skin structure and function fully. When this is not possible there is repair instead of regeneration and the quality of the newly-formed skin varies. The process of repair and regeneration is complex and involves inflammation, tissue formation, and tissue remodeling. There is interaction of epidermal and dermal cells and immune responses to form a scaffolding for the new tissue.

Keloids and hypertrophic scars: These occur when the skin responds to an injury by an exuberant overgrowth of dermal tissue due to increased TGF-beta activity. The resultant scar tissue does not lie flat with the surrounding skin and is instead raised.

Delayed wound healing: When the skin fails to effectively repair injuries due to factors such as diabetes mellitus, peripheral arterial disease, etc., there is delay in wound healing leading to chronic ulcers especially on the lower limbs.

APPEARANCE

The appearance of the skin, hair, and nails has a major role to play in the social and sexual attraction between humans. They have an impact on interpersonal relations and psychological well-being. Enhancement of these natural endowments via use of cosmetics is now a huge industry. Aside from the visual appearance, secretions from the apocrine glands called pheromones are theorized to influence social interactions, although evidence demonstrating this in humans is lacking.[5,6]

Aging skin: Wrinkles and sagging skin are a natural part of aging. However not many consider them to be attractive. Lasers, fillers, botox are some of the ways by which these can be dealt with.

Pigmentary disorders: Vitiligo can be mistaken for leprosy in many parts of the world and patients have to deal with the resulting stigma. An uneven skin tone as in the case of melasma can be the source of great distress to the affected individual.

Hair loss: Patterned hair loss especially in males can make the affected individual look prematurely aged.

VITAMIN D SYNTHESIS

Vitamin D is an essential vitamin crucial for bone formation and maintenance. Increasingly, there is evidence that vitamin D also plays a role in inflammation and immune defense.[7] 7-dehydrocholestrol is synthesized in the skin and is converted to cholecalciferol on exposure to sunlight. This cholecalciferol is taken by liver and kidneys and is hydroxylated into calciferol, which is the active form of vitamin D.

VITAMIN E SECRETION

Vitamin E is a fat-soluble vitamin which is secreted by the sebaceous glands of the face onto the skin surface. This protects the surface lipids from oxidation.

MISCELLANEOUS

- Aside from cushioning trauma, subcutaneous fat provides insulation and acts as a calorie reserve. The hormone leptin is released from fat tissue and acts on the hypothalamus to control hunger and satiety.[8]
- Nails protect the tips of fingers and toes. They also help in scratching, pinching, and picking up objects.
- Dermatoglyphics of the fingertips (fingerprints) provide a unique identity to each individual.
- Sweat glands cause lubrication of the palms which help to provide a better grip.
- Scalp hair may have a slight role in providing insulation. Other hair like eyelashes have a protective effect by preventing foreign objects from entering the eyes.

Table 3 briefly summarizes the chief functions of the skin and a few examples of what a functional failing entails.

TABLE 3: The chief functions of the skin and a few examples of what a functional failing entails.

Function	*Disorder due to loss of function*
Barrier function	TEN, dehydration, infection, SCC
Thermoregulation	Heat stroke, hypothermia, frostbite
Immune defense	Fungal, bacterial and viral infections, autoimmune disorders
Sensations	Pruritus, leprosy
Circulation	Venous insufficiency, vasculitis, elephantiasis nostras verrucosa, arterial embolism and cutaneous necrosis
Wound repair/ regeneration	Keloids, hypertrophic scars
Appearance	Aging, vitiligo, melasma, patterned hair loss
Vitamin synthesis	Vitamin deficiency

KEY POINTS

- The skin is a dynamic entity that has multiple functions essential for maintenance of health and homeostasis.
- Any failure or loss of integrity of the skin can have devastating consequences.

REFERENCES

1. Thappa DM. Structure and functions of the skin. In: Valia RG, Valia AR (Eds). IADVL Textbook of Dermatology, 3rd edition. New Delhi: Bhalani Publishing House; 2008. pp. 7-36.
2. McGrath JA, Uitto J. Structure and function of the skin. In: Griffiths C, Barker J, Blelker T, Chalmers R, Creamer D (Eds). Rook's Textbook of Dermatology, 9th edition. New Jersey, USA: Wiley-Blackwell Publication; 2016. pp. 2.1-48.
3. Madison KC. Barrier function of the skin: "la raison d'etre" of the epidermis. J Invest Dermatol. 2003;121(2): 231-41.
4. Tansey EA, Johnson CD. Recent advances in thermoregulation. Adv Physiol Educ. 2015;39(3):139-48.
5. Doty RL. Human pheromones: do they exist? In: Mucignat-Caretta C (Ed). Neurobiology of Chemical Communication. Boca Raton (FL): CRC Press/Taylor & Francis; 2014.
6. Grammer K, Fink B, Neave N. Human pheromones and sexual attraction. Eur J Obstet Gynecol Reprod Biol. 2005;118(2): 135-42.
7. Bartley J. Vitamin D: emerging roles in infection and immunity. Expert Rev Anti Infect Ther. 2010;8(12):1359-69.
8. Triantafyllou GA, Paschou SA, Mantzoros CS. Leptin and hormones: energy homeostasis. Endocrinol Metab Clin North Am. 2016;45(3):633-45.

EXAMINATION QUESTION

1. Describe in detail the functions of skin and its applied importance.

5 CHAPTER Basic Immunology in Relation to Skin

Surajit Gorai, Shailvi Banka Biyani, Kinnor Das

INTRODUCTION

The skin is a highly composite organ, which provides not only a mechanical barrier, but also an immune system for protection. The ability of the skin to generate an immune response is given the term "skin-associated lymphoid tissues" (SALT).[1]

SKIN-ASSOCIATED LYMPHOID TISSUES

The subset of the lymphoid system is associated with the dermis and epidermis. It includes Langerhans cells (LCs) and resident phagocytes **(Fig. 1)**.

Immune system is divided into innate and adaptive immunity based on specificity of response and immunologic memory **(Flowchart 1)**.[2]

The term immunity has traditionally referred to the resistance exhibited by host toward injury caused by microorganisms and their products.

Factors Affecting Immunity

- Age
- Nutrition
- Hormonal influences
- Infections

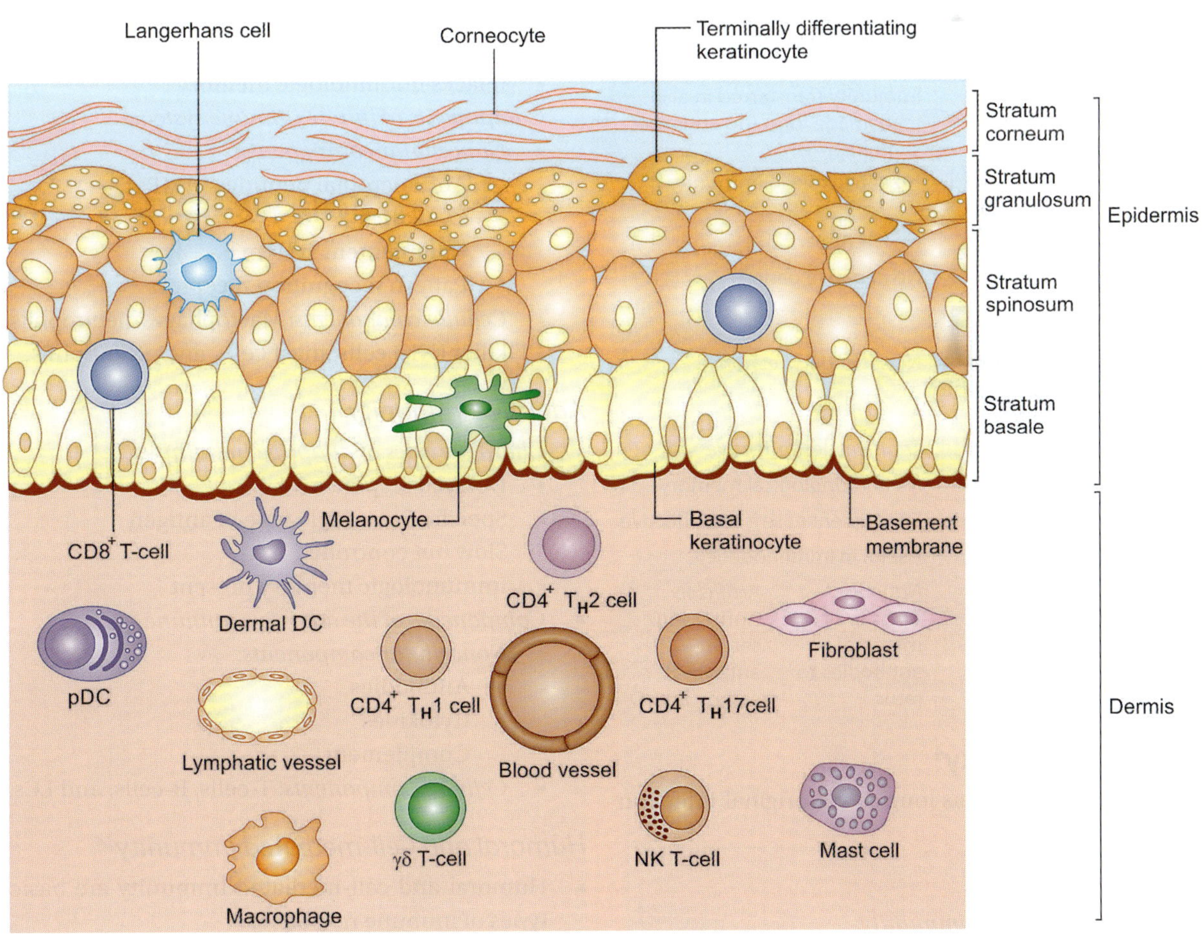

Fig. 1: Skin immunity and cellular effectors.
(NK: natural killer)

Flowchart 1: Components of immune system.[6]

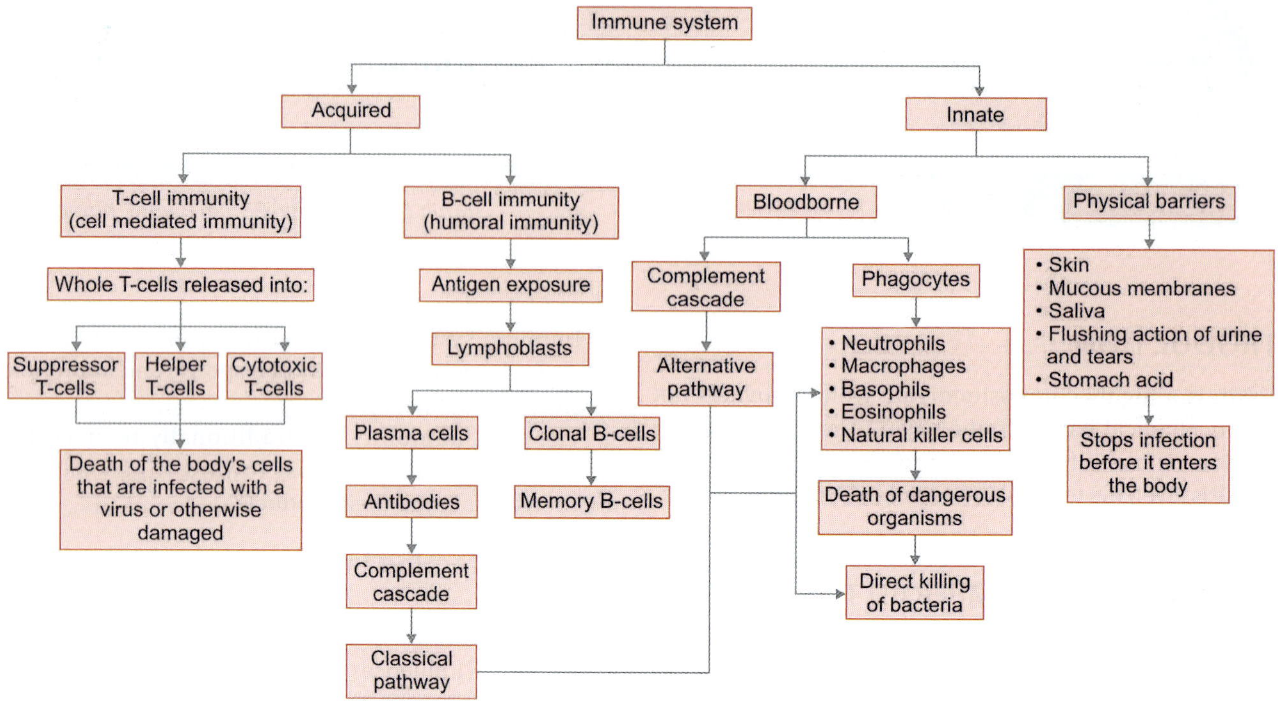

TABLE 1: Differences between adaptive and innate immunity.

Adaptive	*Innate*
Immunity develops after antigenic stimulus	Immunity transferred in a readymade form (no antigenic stimulus)
Involves host immune system leading to production of antibodies	No active role in immunity
After a *latent period*	No latent period
Negative phase (level of immunity decrease after stimulation for a short period)	No negative period
Secondary response (subsequent infection by same antigen cause quick and rapid response)	No secondary response
Durable *effective* response	*Transient*, less effective
Immunological memory present	*No* immunological memory
Booster effect on subsequent dose	Subsequent dose is less effective
No use in immunodeficit	Useful in immunodeficit
Natural: Immunity after varicella; *Artificial*: By vaccination	*Natural*: Transfer of maternal antibodies to fetus; *Artificial*: Antitetanus serum, antirabies serum, anti-D,

Premunition Immunity[4]

Immunity to infection lasts as long as the original infection remains active, e.g., syphilis

Innate Immunity[3,5]

- *Characteristics of innate immunity*:
  - It forms the first-line defense
  - It is primitive
  - It is nonspecific for any type of antigen
  - Fast acting
  - It lacks immunologic memory
- *Components of innate immune system*:
  - *Noncellular components:*
    - Antimicrobial peptides (AMPs)
    - Cytokines
    - Complement system
    - Pattern recognition receptors
  - *Cellular components*: Macrophages, neutrophils, natural killer (NK) cells, mast cells, and eosinophils.

Adaptive Immunity[3,5]

- *Characteristics of adaptive immunity:*
  - Delayed response
  - Specific for a single type of antigen
  - Slow but controlled
  - Immunologic memory present
- *Components of the adaptive immune system:*
  - *Noncellular components*:
    - Antibodies
    - Cytokines
    - Complement
  - *Cellular components*: T-cells, B-cells, and LCs.

Humoral and Cell-mediated Immunity[3,4]

- Humoral and cell-mediated immunity are basically the types of immune response.
- As the name implies cell mediated means immune response is from cells.

- Humoral immunity is mediated by macromolecules found in extracellular fluids such as secreted antibodies, complement proteins, and certain AMPs.
- Humoral immunity is so named because it involves substances found in the humors, or body fluids (ancient Greek and Roman physicians).
- It should be kept in mind that complement activation and functioning, which is a part of innate immunity, is also an humoral response.
- Its aspects involving antibodies are often called antibody-mediated immunity.

Antigen[3,5]

Any substance foreign to the body that evokes an immune response either alone or after forming a complex with a larger molecule (such as a protein) and that is capable of binding with a product (such as an antibody or T-cell) of the immune response.

- *Complete antigen*:
  - *Immunogenicity*: Induction of immune response
  - *Immunological reactivity*: Specific reaction with antibody
- *Hapten*:
  - Incapable of inducing antibody response but react with antibody
  - *Nonimmunogenic*: But has immunological reactivity
- *Epitope*: Antigenic determinant:
  - Smallest unit of antigenicity
  - *T-cell*: Linear or sequential epitope
  - *B-cell*: Conformational epitope
- *Paratope*:
  - Combining area of an antibody corresponding to epitope
  - Specific antigen determinants on paratopes are called idiotypes.

Superantigen (Table 2)[7]

- Antigen which does not require antigenic processing and not specific for a T-cell receptor (TCR)
- Attaches itself outside the antigen-binding groove directly to the lateral aspect of TCR-β chain [conventional antigens bind to the αβ heterodimer groove of the major histocompatibility complex (MHC) molecules through the V regions of the T-cell antigen receptor (TCR) α and chains]
- Resistant to proteases and denaturation by CD4+ T-cells
- Activates up to 20% of T-cells and massive release of cytokines [tumor necrosis factor-α (TNF-α), interleukin-1 (IL-1)] (conventional antigens activate only 0.001%).

INNATE IMMUNE RESPONSE[3,5]

Antimicrobial peptides: The first AMP to be found in human skin was human β-defensin-2 (hBD-2). The up- and downregulation of these peptides in psoriasis and atopic dermatitis explain why superinfections are so rare in the former and common in the latte. Increased expression of these peptides is seen atopic skin. The AMP LL-37 helps in dendritic cell activation in psoriasis by stimulating toll-like receptor 9 (TLR9) and hence induce interferon (IFN) production **(Table 3)**.[8]

TABLE 2: Superantigen.

Organism	*Superantigen*	*Disease*
Staphylococcus aureus	Enterotoxin or toxic shock syndrome (TSS) toxin	• TSS • Multiple sclerosis
Group A streptococci	Pyrogenic exotoxin	• Shock • Guttate psoriasis
HIV	Nef (negative regulatory factor)	AIDS
EBV	Not identified	B-cell lymphoma

(AIDS: acquired immunodeficiency syndrome; EBV: Epstein-Barr virus; HIV: human immunodeficiency virus)

Cytokines (Table 4)

- Low-molecular-weight protein
- Play major role in intercellular communication, proliferation, differentiation, activation of cells, and intercellular communication
- They can be soluble or membrane bound
- Act in autocrine, paracrine, or endocrine manner
- *Types*: Interleukins, lymphokines, or chemokines

Complement (Fig. 2)[3]

- System of small proteins which destroy microorganism either by opsonization or direct membrane damage[7]
- Also help in chemotaxis, anaphylaxis, immune complex stabilization, and B-cell activation
- Three pathways—(1) classical, (2) alternative, and (3) mannose-binding lectin pathway
- End-product is membrane attack complex or MAC (C5b–C9) which results in osmotic lysis of cell
- Human cells are resistant to complement killing, since they express the complement receptor type 1 (CR1, CD35), decay-accelerating factor (DAF, CD55), and membrane cofactor protein (MCP, CD46) which inhibits C3 convertase.
- *Complement synthesis*:
  - C1: Intestinal epithelium
  - C2, C4: Macrophages
  - C5, C8: Spleen
  - C3, C6, C9: Liver
- Complement is activated by three pathways given in **Table 5**.
- *Complement inhibitor*:
  - C1 esterase inhibitor
  - S protein
- *Complement inactivator*:
  - Factor I (by human keratinocytes)
  - Factor H (by human keratinocytes)

TABLE 3: The names of the antimicrobial peptide found in human skin.

Name	Origin	Target		Inducibility
		Bacteria	Fungi	
Human β-defensin-1 (hBD-1)	Keratinocytes	++	+	• Constitutive expression • Direct chemoattractant for immature dendritic cell and memory T-cells
Human β-defensin-2 (hBD-2)	• Keratinocytes • Airway epithelium • Intestinal tract	+	++	Inducible
Human β-defensin-3 (hBD-3)	• Keratinocytes • Airway epithelium	+++	+++	Inducible
Human β-defensin-4 (hBD-4)	• Keratinocytes • Airway epithelia (mRNA)	++	+	Inducible
Canthelicidin (LL-37)	• Keratinocytes • Airway epithelia • Urogenital tract • Granulocytes	++	++	Inducible
Psoriasin	• Keratinocytes Sebocytes	+	+	Inducible
Antileukoprotease (ALP)	• Keratinocytes • Airway epithelia	++	++	Noninducible
Lysozyme	• Keratinocytes • Airway epithelia	++	–	Noninducible
Demcidin	Sweat glands	+++	++	Noninducible

Source: Bolognia J, Schaffer J, Cerroni L. Dermatology, 4th Edition. Gurugram: Elsevier India; 2017.

TABLE 4: Types of cytokines.

Type	Origin	Function
IL-1	Monocytes, macrophages, keratinocyte	Proinflammatory, innate immunity
IL-2	Activated T-cells	T-cell stimulator, adaptive immunity
IL-3	T-cells	Growth of mast cells and increased basophil production
IL-4	TH 2 cells	Increased TH2 response, adaptive immunity
IL-5	TH 2 cells, mast cells	Eosinophil stimulator
IL-6	Lymphoid cells, endothelial cells	Proinflammatory, innate immunity
IL-8	Keratinocyte, endothelial cells	Neutrophil chemotaxis
IL-10	TH 2 cells, keratinocytes	Anti-inflammatory
IL-12	Mononuclear phagocytes, dendritic cells	Increased TH1 response, adaptive immunity
TNF-α	T-cell, mononuclear phagocyte, mast cell, keratinocytes	Proinflammatory, innate immunity
IFN-α,β	Leukocytes, fibroblasts	Antiproliferative, innate immunity
IFN-γ	T-cells, NK cells	Increased TH1 response
TGF-β	Activated platelets, keratinocyte	Anti-inflammatory

(IL: interleukin; INF-α: interferon-α; NK: natural killer; TGF-β: transforming growth factor-β; TNF-α: tumor necrosis factor-α)
Source: Sima J. Dermatology, 2nd edition. Berlin/Heidelberg: Springer; 2017.

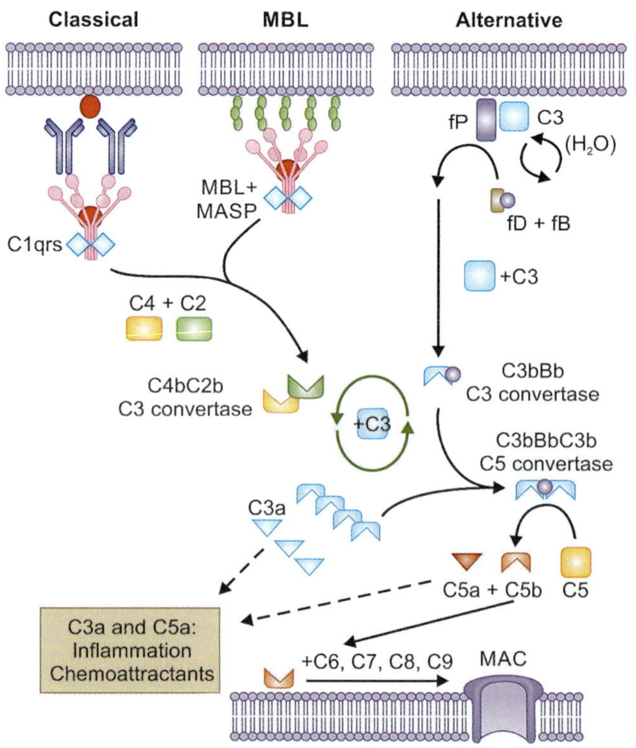

Fig. 2: Overview of complement system.
(MAC: membrane-attack complex; MBL: mannose-binding lectin; MASP: mannose-binding lectin-associated serine protease)
Source: Mathern DR, Heeger PS. Molecules great and small: the complement system. Clin J Am Soc Nephrol. 2015;10(9):1636-50.

TABLE 5: Three pathways of complement activation.

Classical pathway	*Alternative pathway*	*Lectin pathway*
• Ag-Ab complex • IgM > IgG • DNA • C-reactive protein • Trypsin	• Bacterial endotoxin • IgA > IgD • Cobra venom • Nephritic factor	Binding of mannose-binding lectin to mannose residues on the surfaces of microorganisms such as *Salmonella, Neisseria, Listeria, Cryptococcus, Candida*

(Ag-Ab: antigen-antibody; IgM: immunoglobulin M)

TABLE 6: Complement deficiency.

Deficit complement	*Disease*
C1 esterase inhibitor	Hereditary angioneurotic edema
C2 deficiency	*Most common*, little or no increase in susceptibility to infection
C1, C2, C4	*SLE* and collagen vascular disease
C3 and its regulatory protein C3b inactivator	Severe recurrent pyogenic infections (immune complex-mediated glomerulonephritis)
C5-C8	*Bacteremia (mainly gram-negative diplococci)*, toxoplasmosis
C9	No particular diseases

(SLE: systemic lupus erythematosus)
Source: Sima J. Dermatology, 2nd edition. Berlin/Heidelberg: Springer; 2017.

- Anaphylatoxin inctivator C4-binding protein
  - Major serum opsonin: 3b
  - Membrane-attack complex: C5 to C9
  - Anaphylatoxin (potency): C5a > C3a.

The deficiencies of complement are given in **Table 6**.

Pattern Recognition Receptors (Fig. 3)

- Germline-encoded host sensors, which detect molecules typical for the pathogens.
- They are proteins expressed, mainly, by *sentinel cells* of the innate immune system, such as dendritic cells, macrophages, monocytes, neutrophils, and epithelial cells, to identify two classes of molecules: pathogen-associated molecular patterns (PAMPs), which are associated with microbial pathogens, and (DAMPs), which are associated with components of host's cells that are released during cell damage or death.

Types of pattern recognition receptors:

- Toll-like receptors
- C-type lectin receptors
- Retinoic acid-inducible gene (RIG)-like receptors
- Nucleotide-binding oligomerization domain (NOD)-like receptors.

Toll-like Receptors

- These are single membrane spanning noncatalytic receptors usually expressed in sentinel cells (macrophages, dendritic cells)

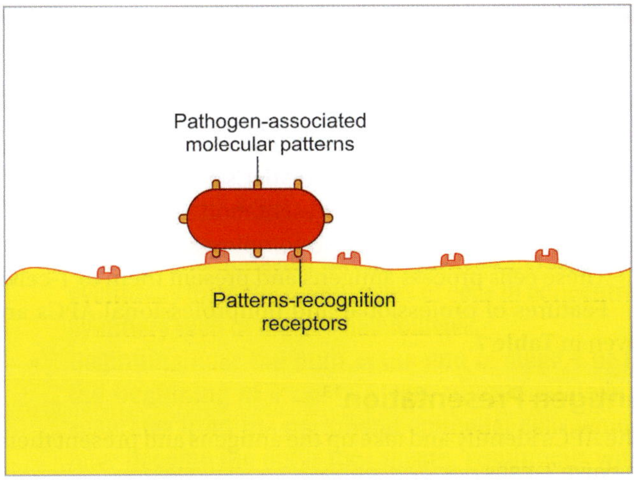

Fig. 3: Pattern recognition receptors.

- Form a bridge between innate and adaptive immunity[8]
- Help in nuclear factor kappa B (NF-κB) activation
- Recognizes PAMP on surface of microorganisms, activation causes release of inflammatory mediators
- Dendritic cells express several types of TLRs
- Dendritic cells stimulated by the innate immune system instruct T-cells to respond how and where.

Different TLRs can recognize different antigens as listed below:

- *TLR 1:* Bacterial lipoprotein and peptidoglycans
- *TLR 2:* Bacterial peptidoglycans
- *TLR 3:* Double-stranded RNA
- *TLR 4:* Lipopolysaccharides (LPSs)
- *TLR 5:* Bacterial flagella
- *TLR 6:* Bacterial lipoprotein
- *TLR 7:* Single-stranded RNA, bacterial and viral
- *TLR 8:* Single-stranded RNA, bacterial and viral, phagocytized bacterial RNA
- *TLR 9:* CpG DNA
- *TLR 10:* Triacylated lipopeptides.

Clinical correlate of TLR:

- Imiquimod signals to the innate arm of the immune system through the toll-like receptor 7 (TLR7)
- *In pathogenesis of systemic lupus erythematosus (SLE)*:
  - There is abnormal TLR-7 signaling in response to RNA
  - TLR-9 signaling in response to DNA
  - Increased expression of TLR-9 on peripheral blood B-cells, plasma cells, and dendritic cells
- TLR2 is required for recognition of bacterial LPS and is associated with inflammatory acne
- Anti-inflammatory effect of retinoids is via TLR2.

ADAPTIVE IMMUNE RESPONSE[5,10]

Adaptive immunity requires the production of specific T-lymphocytes to identify an antigen with precision and

B-cells to produce specific antibodies that bind to the microbe in a "lock-and-key" fashion.

Antigen Presenting Cells[11,12]

An antigen-presenting cell (APC) or accessory cell is a cell that displays antigen complexed with MHCs on their surfaces; this process is known as antigen presentation.

- T-cells may recognize these complexes using their TCRs.
- These cells process antigens and present them to T-cells.

Features of professional and nonprofessional APCs are given in **Table 7**.

Antigen Presentation[13]

The APCs identify and take up the antigens and present them to naive T-cells.

The process of antigen presentation occurs in the following way:

APC bind pathogens to their TLRs

↓

Internalization and processing of the pathogen

↓

Display of a short peptide on the surface on a major histocompatibility complex (MHC) molecule.

The human leukocyte antigen (HLA) system or complex is a gene complex encoding the MHC proteins in humans **(Fig. 4** and **Table 8)**.

TABLE 7: Features of professional and nonprofessional APCs.

Professional APC	*Nonprofessional APC*
• Dendritic cell • Macrophage • Langerhans cells	• Astrocyte • Oligodendrocytes • Ependymal cells • Endothelial cells • Some epithelial cells
Present foreign antigens to helper T-cells express MHC class II molecules	• Display endogenous peptides on the cell membrane • All nucleated cell types in the body • Nonprofessional APCs express MHC class I molecule

(APC: antigen-presenting cell; MHC: major histocompatibility complex)

Human Leukocyte Antigen Association and Skin Disease[14]

Human leukocyte antigen association and skin disease are described in **Table 9**.

T-cells

The skin contains resident T-cells and recruits circulating T-cells. Antigen presentation leads to maturation of naïve T-cells → effector T-cells, → differentiation into two varieties **(Table 10)**:

1. Cytotoxic CD8+ T-cells
2. CD4+ T helper (Th) cells.

B-cells

B-cells are responsible for creating a memory of prior antigen exposure to ensure a faster immune response and a lasting immunity. B-cells produce antibodies [immunoglobulins (Igs)] that can bind to specific antigens **(Fig. 5)**.

To produce antibodies, B-cells require cytokine signaling and stimulatory signals from Th cells. This takes place in secondary lymphoid organs such as lymph nodes.

- The B-cells and T-cells must bind via the B-cell receptor (BCR) and the TCR, respectively. This is mediated by costimulatory signals on Th cells.
- The proliferation of B-cells leads to the production of a specific antibody, either IgG, IgA or IgE, depending on the antigen.

Upon re-exposure to the same antigen and follicular dendritic cells, B-cells are activated to produce specific antibodies. This process allows for the generation of memory B-cells and long-lived plasma cells for long-lasting immunity from infection.

Types of Antibodies[3]

Types of antibodies are given in **Table 11**.

Antigen-antibody (Ag-Ab) binding would cause five different protective mechanism:

1. *Agglutination*: Reduces number of infectious units to be dealt with

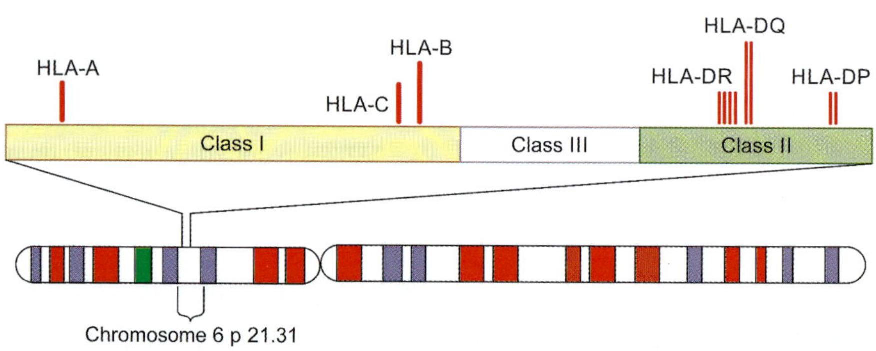

Fig. 4: Human leukocyte antigen (HLA) complex on chromosome 6 in humans.

TABLE 8: HLA system encoding MHC in human.

HLA I → MHC I			*HLA II → MHC II*			*HLA III → MHC III*
A	*B*	*C*	*DP*	*DQ*	*DR*	• Encode components of the complement system • C2, C4 • TNF • Heat shock protein
• Against intra-cellular infection • All nucleated cell and platelets			Extracellular defense			
Presents to CD8			Presents to CD4			• No role in restriction • Have physiologic role unlike MHC I/II
Prevent autoimmune system to be activated						

(HLA: human leukocyte antigen; MHC: major histocompatibility complex; TNF: tumor necrosis factor)

TABLE 9: Human leukocyte antigen (HLA) association and skin disease.

Disease	*HLA*
Psoriasis vulgaris	HLA CW-06-02
Psoriatic arthritis	HLAB27
Atopic dermatitis	HLA DR4
Behcet's disease	HLA B5
Vitiligo	HLA A24
Pemphigus vulgaris	HLA DR4, HLA DQ1
DLE	HLA B8, HLA DR3
SCLE	HLA B8, DR3
SLE	HLA DR2, HLA DR3
Dermatitis herpetiformis	HLA DR3
Reiter's syndrome	HLA B27
Bullous pemphigoid	HLA DQ7
Tuberculoid leprosy	HLA DR2, DR3
Lepromatous leprosy	HLA DQ1
Cutaneous leishmaniasis	HLA DQw3 (risk marker) HLA DR2 (protective)
Scabies	HLA A11 (increased susceptibility: resistant to treatment, multiple nodular lesions)

(DLE: discoid lupus erythematosus; SCLE: subacute cutaneous lupus erythematosus; SLE: systemic lupus erythematosus)

TABLE 10: Antigen presentation.

Cytotoxic CD8+ T-cells	*CD4+ Th cells*
• They bind to MHC-I molecules • They bind to the Fas receptor → initiates the perforin–granzyme pathway and cytokine-mediated apoptosis → which directly kills virally infected cells or tumor cells	• They bind to MHC-II molecules • They activate B-cells to produce specific antibodies • Upon re-exposure to the same antigen, memory T-cells responds immediately via division and clonal expansion • Th cells include the Th1, Th2, Th17

(MHC: major histocompatibility complex)

2. *Activation of complement*: Causes inflammation and cell lysis
3. *Opsonization*: Coating antigen with antibody enhances phagocytosis
4. *Antibody-dependent cell-mediate cytotoxicity*: Antibodies attached to target cell cause destruction by macrophages, eosinophils, and NK cells
5. *Neutralization:* Blocks adhesion of bacteria and viruses to mucosa.

Antigen-Antibody Reaction Used in Immunodiagnostics[16]

Bonds between Ag-Ab are weak non-covalent bonds like:

1. Van der Waals forces,
2. Hydrogen bonds,
3. Ionic bonds, etc.

Affinity: Intensity of attraction between antigen and antibody.

Avidity: Strength of bond after the formation of the Ag-Ab complex.

CELLS OF IMMUNE SYSTEM[3,5]

- *Lymphocytes*: Natural killer (NK) cells, B-cells, and T-cells
- *Monocytes*: Macrophages and dendritic (Langerhans) cells
- *Granulocytes*: Neutrophils, eosinophils, and mast cells

NK Cells

- Form 2% circulating lymphocytes
- Derived from bone marrow
- Target tumor or virally infected cells
- Express CD2, CD56, and CD16, produce IFN-γ, IL-4 and IL-10
- Destroy cells via granzyme and perforins
- Involved in UV-induced immunosuppression, down-regulate immune responses to UV-induced tumors.[9]

Langerhans Cells

- Dendritic shape, act as antigen presenting cell, derived from bone marrow
- Identified by Birbeck granules (racket-shaped granules) on electron microscopy
- Markers—CD1a, S100, vimentin, langerin, express CD80, or CD86 after activation
- CD1a is a useful marker and is exclusively expressed on LCs
- Found in epidermis (mainly stratum spinosum), lymph nodes, and spleen
- Intricated with nerve fibers, through the release of neuropeptides such as calcitonin gene-related peptide (CGRP)
- Numbers is reduced on the palms and soles, genitalia, and buccal mucosa
- The density decreases with age and is reduced in chronically UV-exposed skin
- Langerhans cells are responsible for inciting immune reaction in Langerhans cell histiocytosis, HIV, and HPV infection.

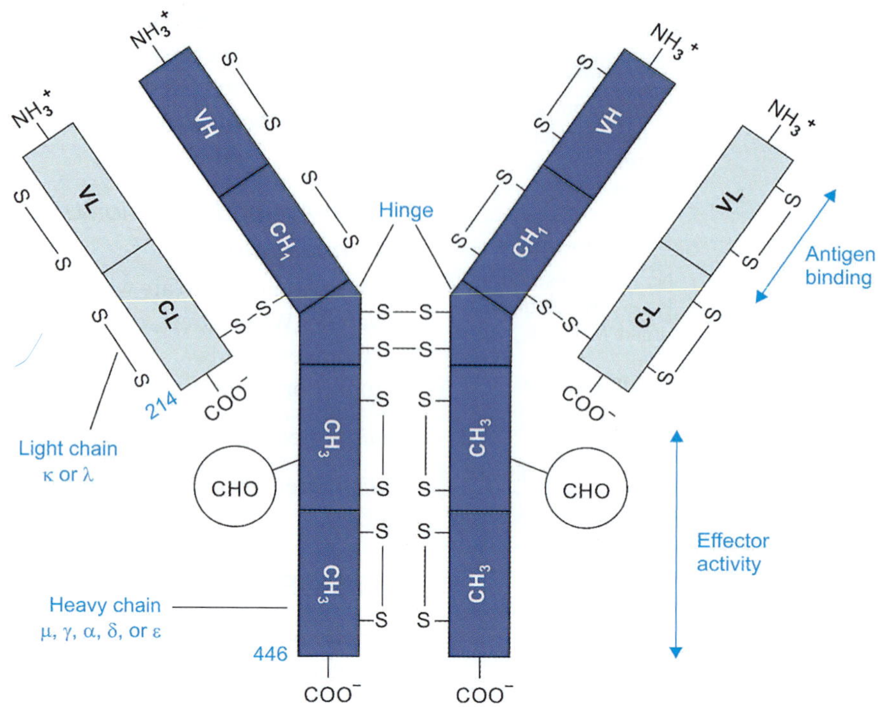

Fig. 5: Schematic diagram of the structure of immunoglobulins derived from amino acid sequence analysis.[3]
Source: Owen J, Punt J, Stranford S. Kubys Immunology, 7th edition. New York: WH Freeman and Company; 2013.

TABLE 11: Types of antibodies.

	The antibody/immunoglobulin types				
	IgM pentamer	*IgG monomer*	*IgA dimer*	*IgE monomer*	*IgD monomer*
Number of antigen-binding sites	10	2	4	2	2
Heavy chains	μ	γ	α	ε	δ
Molecular weight (Daltons)	900,000	150,000	385,000	200,000	180,000
Percentage of total antibody in serum	6%	80%	13%	0.002%	1%
Cross placenta	No	Yes	No		
Fixes complement	Yes		No		
Function	Best antibody of primary responses, best at fixing complement; the IgM monomer act as B-cell receptor	Main blood antibody of secondary responses, neutralizes toxins, causes opsonization	Found in secretions such as mucus, tears, saliva, colostrum	Allergic and antiparasitic activity	B-cell receptor

Mast Cells

- Derived from bone marrow (CD34+ cells), often present in perivascular spaces
- Similar in both appearance and function to basophil
- High affinity receptors for IgE, on activation release new and preformed mediators
- Preformed mediators are serine proteases, histamine, serotonin, proteoglycans, ATP, lysosomal enzymes
- Newly formed lipid mediators (2), cytokine, reactive oxygen species
- Express high-affinity receptor for IgE (FceRI) on their surface; cross-linking of receptor-bound IgE and results in release of mast cell granule contents (preformed or newly formed)
- Has receptor for c-kit which is involved in mastocytosis
- Involved in wound healing, allergy, anaphylaxis, urticaria, and angioedema
- Mastocytomas, mast cell sarcoma, and mast cell leukemia are mast cell tumors
- IL-3, stem cell factor (SCF), C3a, C4a, C5a (anaphylatoxin), nonsteroidal anti-inflammatory drugs (NSAIDs), opiates, aspirin, vancomycin, polymyxin B, curare, radiocontrast media, neuropeptides like substance P are triggers for mast cells.

Flowchart 2: Different types of T-cell response.

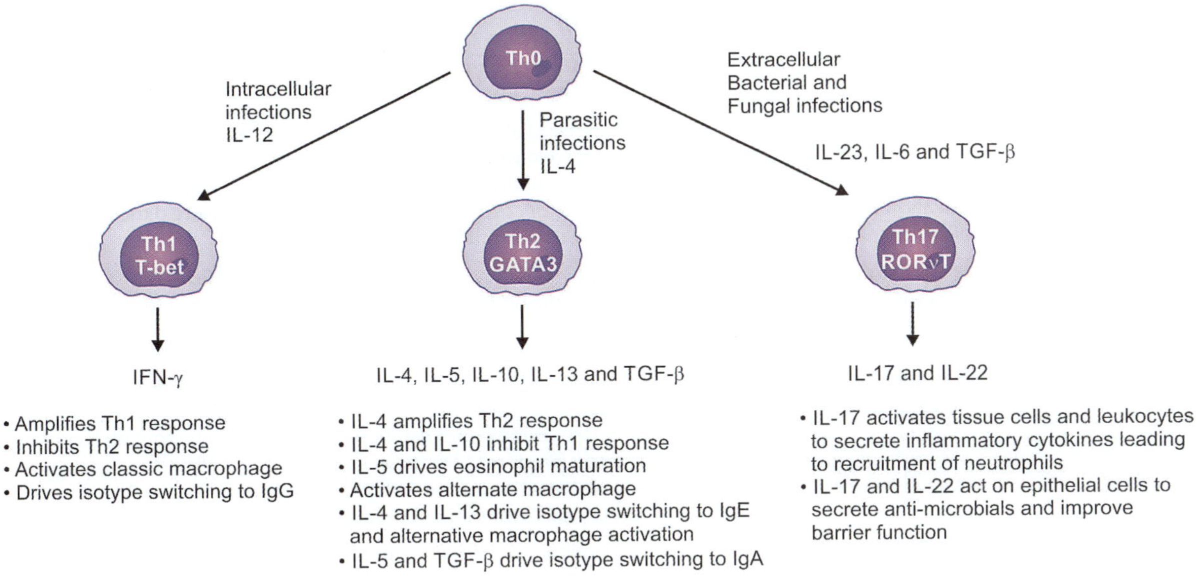

(IgG: immunoglobulin G; IL: interleukin; RORγ: retinoic acid-related orphan receptor γ; TGF-β: transforming growth factor-β)
Source: USMLE Step 1 Lecture Notes 2017: Immunology and Microbiology, 1st edition. New York: Kaplan Publishing; 2017. p. 512.[15]

B-cells

- Form 5–10% of circulating lymphocyte
- *Function*: Antibody production
- Naïve B-cells → recognizes Ag → differentiate into memory cells or plasma cells → produce antibody[13]
- Possess both primary and secondary immune response
- Isotype switching helps in keeping long-term memory.

T-cells

- About 70–75% of circulating lymphocyte
- Formed from bone marrow mature in thymus
- It is of two types—(1) helper T-cells (CD4) and (2) cytotoxic T-cells (CD8) **(Flowchart 2)**
- In their early stage of development, T-cells express both CD4 and CD8
- Helper T-cells are of Th1 and Th2 type.

Th1

- Involved in delayed-type contact hypersensitivity reactions, active against viruses and intracellular bacteria and antitumor response
- *Diseases associated*: Allergic contact dermatitis, tuberculoid leprosy, cutaneous leishmaniasis, psoriasis.

Th2

- Upregulate humoral immunity, active against viruses, extracellular bacteria, and parasites
- *Diseases associated*: Atopic dermatitis, lepromatous leprosy, disseminated leishmaniasis, Sezary syndrome, and parasitic infections. Th17–IL-17 secreated that activates inflammatory cells. Important for psoriasis pathogenesis.

Cytotoxic (CD8) Cells

- Result in lysis of cells
- CD8 cell releases perforin, granzymes, and granulysin → apoptosis of target cell[17]
- CD8+ T-cell-mediated cytolysis appears to be involved in lichen planus, fixed drug eruptions, cutaneous graft-versus-host disease (GVHD), and herpes simplex virus infections.

T-cell anergy: It is a tolerance mechanism in which the lymphocyte is intrinsically functionally inactivated following an antigen encounter, but remains alive for an extended period of time in a hyporesponsive state.[17]

Tolerance[18]

- Only non-self-reacting B- and T-cells are automatured
- Self-reactive B- and T-cells are killed by apoptosis
- Tolerance (unresponsiveness) to self-antigens is a fundamental property of the immune system and breakdown of tolerance is the basis of autoimmune diseases.

Central tolerance: Immature lymphocytes that recognize self-antigens in the central (generative) lymphoid organs are killed by apoptosis; in the B-cell lineage, some of the self-reactive lymphocytes switch to new antigen receptors that are not self-reactive.

Peripheral tolerance: Mature lymphocytes that recognize self-antigens in peripheral tissues become functionally inactive

TABLE 12: Hypersensitivity reactions and its types.

Type 1	*Type 2*	*Type 3*	*Type 4*
IgE-mediated hypersensitivity	IgG-medicated cytotoxic hypersensitivity	Immune complex-mediated hypersensitivity	Cell-medicated delayed type of hypersensitivity
Antigen induces crosslinking of IgE bound to mast cells and basophils with release of vasoactive mediators	Antibody directed against cell surface antigens mediates cell destruction via complement activation or antigen-dependent cell killing	Antigen and antibody complexes get deposited in various tissues and induce complement activation and an ensuing inflammatory response mediated by massive PMNL infiltration	Specialized Th1 cells release cytokines that activate macrophages to Tc cells which mediate direct cellular damage
• Anaphylaxis • Angioedema • Urticaria (hives) • Penicillin and cephalosporin allergy • Food allergy	• Autoimmune hemolytic anemia • Autoimmune thrombocytopenic purpura • Pemphigus vulgaris • Bullous pemphigoid • Vasculitis caused by ANCA • Myasthenia gravis • Graves' disease	• SLE • Erythema nodosum • ENL • HSP • Pan • FDE • Jarisch–Herxheimer reaction • *Insect bite*: It may first have a rapid type I reaction. Some 4–8 hours later a typical Arthus reaction develops	• ACD • Type 1 lepra reaction • Mantoux test • DRESS • SJS/TEN • EM • Lichenoid drug eruption • GVHD

(ACD: anemia of chronic disease; ANCA: antineutrophil cytoplasmic autoantibody; DRESS: drug reaction with eosinophilia and systemic symptoms; EM: erythema multiforme; ENL: erythema nodosum leprosum; FDE; fixed drug eruption; GVHD: graft-versus-host disease; HSP: Henoch-Schonlein purpura; PMNL: polymorphonuclear leukocyte; SJS/TEN: Stevens-Johnson syndrome/toxic epidermal necrolysis; SLE: systemic lupus erythematosus)

(anergic), or are suppressed by regulatory T lymphocytes, or die by apoptosis.

The variables that lead to a failure of self-tolerance and the development of autoimmunity include inheritance of susceptibility genes that may disrupt different tolerance pathways, and infections and tissue alterations that may expose self-antigens and activate APCs and lymphocytes in the tissues.

HYPERSENSITIVITY REACTIONS[3,5]

Hypersensitivity reactions and its types are given in **Table 12**.

IMMUNODEFICIENCY DISEASES[3]

Inherited Immunodeficiency

- *Cellular immunodeficiency*:
  - DiGeorge syndrome (thymic hypoplasia)
  - Purine nucleotide phosphorylase deficiency
  - Chronic mucocutaneous candidiasis
  - Nude syndrome
- *Humoral immunodeficiency*:
  - X-linked (Brutons) agammaglobulinemia
  - Common variable immunodeficiency
  - Selective Ig deficiency or dysgammaglobulinemia
- *Combined immunodeficiency*:
  - Wiskott–Aldrich syndrome
  - Severe combined immunodeficiency (X-linked and autosomal recessive type)
  - Ataxia telangiectasia
  - X-linked lymphoproliferative syndrome
  - Cellular immunodeficiency with abnormal Ig synthesis (Nezelof syndrome)
  - Hyper-IgM syndrome
- *Disorders of phagocytosis*:
  - Chronic granulomatous disease of childhood
  - Job syndrome (hyper IgE—recurrent infection syndrome)
  - Chediak–Higashi syndrome
  - Leukocyte adhesion deficiency
  - Myeloperoxidase deficiency
  - Leukocyte glucose-6-phosphate dehydrogenase (G6PD) deficiency
  - Tuftsin deficiency
  - Actin-binding protein deficiency
  - Shwachman's disease

Acquired Immunodeficiency

- Human immunodeficiency virus infection
- Irradiation and chemotherapy for cancer
- Involvement of bone marrow due to cancers
- Protein-calorie malnutrition
- Post-splenectomy

IMMUNE PREVILAGE[19,20]

Certain sites of the human body have immune privilege, meaning they are able to tolerate the introduction of antigens without eliciting an inflammatory immune response. In immune privileged sites, tissue grafts can survive for extended periods of time without rejection occurring.

Immunologically privileged sites were thought to include:

- The brain, but this is now known to be incorrect and indeed immune cells of the central nervous system (CNS) contribute to the maintenance of neurogenesis and spatial learning abilities in adulthood

- The eyes
- The placenta and the fetus
- The testicles
- Bulge area of hair
- Nail epithelium—proximal nail matrix.

NEW DISCOVERY[21,22]

- Keratinocytes are important contributors in cutaneous immune response.
- Keratinocytes provide signals to APC via the release of mediators, particularly cytokines, eicosanoids, and neurohormones.
- IL-1, IL-6, TNF-α, and IL-8 are cytokines released.
- Keratinocytes also produce prostaglandins and leukotrienes.
- Keratinocytes do not express MHC class II molecules under normal conditions; they can be induced to do so in inflammatory settings.

KEY POINTS

- Adaptive immunity acquired by antigenic challenge whereas innate is readymade, transferred from mother.
- Superantigen, released from *Staphylococcus* or *Streptococcus* may cause severe immune damage like TSS that may be fatal.
- TLR, different pattern recognition receptors are now found to be associated with many immune disorders. They are also act as drug targets.
- Antigen presentation and different MHCs determines type of lymphocytic cells to be involved in further immune reaction down the line thus it decides pathomechanism of many immune disorders.
- Four types of hypersensitivity reactions are involved in multiple immune-mediated disorders such as anaphylaxis, serum sickness like reaction, etc.
- Keratinocytes and melanocytes are found to play many important roles in cutaneous immunity.

REFERENCES

1. Streilein JW. Skin-associated lymphoid tissues (SALT): origins and functions. J Invest Dermatol. 1983;80 Suppl:12s-16s.
2. Parkin J, Cohen B. An overview of the immune system. Lancet. 2001;357(9270):1777-89.
3. Owen JA, Punt J, Stranford SA, Jones PP. Kuby Immunology, 7th edition. New York: W H Freeman & Co; 2013.
4. Ray CG, Ryan KJ. Sherris Medical Microbiology, 6th edition. New York: McGraw-Hill Education/Medical; 2014.
5. Steinhoff M. Inflammation, immunology and allergy. In: Griffiths C, Barker J, Bleiker TO, Chalmers R, Creamer D (Eds). Rook's Textbook of Dermatology, 9th edition. Oxford: Wiley-Blackwell; 2016.
6. Paul S, Hmar EB, Sharma HK. Strengthening immunity with immunostimulants: a review. Curr Trends Pharm Res. 2020;7(1):35-64.
7. Fleischer B. Superantigens. APMIS. 1994;102:3-12.
8. Lei J, Sun L, Huang S, Zhu C, Li P, He J, et al. The antimicrobial peptides and their potential clinical applications. Am J Transl Res. 2019;11(7):3919-31.
9. Mathern DR, Heeger PS. Molecules great and small: the complement system. Clin J Am Soc Nephrol. 2015;10(9):1636-50.
10. Medzhitov R, Janeway CA. Innate immune induction of the adaptive immune response. Cold Spring Harb Symp Quant Biol. 1999;64:429-36.
11. Hughes CE, Benson RA, Bedaj M, Maffia P. Antigen-presenting cells and antigen presentation in tertiary lymphoid organs. Front Immunol. 2016;7:481.
12. den Haan JMM, Arens R, van Zelm MC. The activation of the adaptive immune system: cross-talk between antigen-presenting cells, T-cells and B-cells. Immunol Lett. 2014;162(2 Pt B):103-12.
13. Guermonprez P, Valladeau J, Zitvogel L, Théry C, Amigorena S. Antigen presentation and T-cell stimulation by dendritic cells. Annu Rev Immunol. 2002;20(1):621-67.
14. Alves C, Vieira N, Meyer I, Alves CO, Toralles MBP, Oliveira M de FSP. Human histocompatibility antigens and dermatology: from research to clinical practice. An Bras Dermatol. 2006;81(1):65-73.
15. USMLE Step 1 Lecture Notes 2017: Immunology and Microbiology, 1st edition. New York: Kaplan Publishing; 2017. p. 512.
16. Edwards R (Ed). Immunodiagnostics: A Practical Approach. Oxford: OUP Oxford; 1999. p. 300.
17. Schwartz RH. T-cell anergy. Annu Rev Immunol. 2003;21(1):305-34.
18. Sakaguchi S, Yamaguchi T, Nomura T, Ono M. Regulatory T-cells and immune tolerance. Cell. 2008;133(5):775-87.
19. Streilein JW. Unraveling immune privilege. Science. 1995;270(5239):1158-9.
20. Ito T, Meyer KC, Ito N, Paus R. Immune privilege and the skin. Curr Dir Autoimmun. 2008;10:27-52.
21. Luger TA, Schwarz T. The role of cytokines and neuroendocrine hormones in cutaneous immunity and inflammation. Allergy. 1995;50(4):292-302.
22. Volc-Platzer B, Majdic O, Knapp W, Wolff K, Hinterberger W, Lechner K, et al. Evidence of HLA-DR antigen biosynthesis by human keratinocytes in disease. J Exp Med. 1984;159(6):1784-9.

EXAMINATION QUESTIONS

1. Explain antimicrobial peptide.
2. Explain complement and skin.
3. Describe interleukins in dermatology.
4. Write a short note on different types of cells.
5. Write a short note on superantigens.
6. Write a short note on haptens.
7. Describe neutrophil and its applied importance.
8. Describe eosinophil and its applied importance.

6 CHAPTER Basics of Genetics in Relation to Skin

Surajit Gorai, Kinnor Das

Genetics etymology is derived from Greek word *genesis*. The term was coined by William Bateson in 1905.[1]

DEOXYRIBONUCLEIC ACID (DNA), RIBONUCLEIC ACID (RNA), CHROMOSOME, GENE, ALLELE, AND RELATED TERMS[2]

DNA and RNA

They are polymer of nucleotides. DNA is made up of two strands, arranged in a double helix *(model given by James Watson and Francis Crick in 1953)*[3] whereas RNA contains of one strand only **(Fig. 1)**.

The length of DNA is usually denoted by the number of paired nucleotides (called base pairs) present in it **(Fig. 2)**.

> Haploid content of human DNA is 3.3×10^9 base pairs[4]

Nucleotide vs. *nucleoside*: Nucleosides is composed of a nitrogenous base, (purine or pyrimidine), and a five-carbon carbohydrate (ribose in case of RNA, and deoxyribose for DNA). A nucleotide is a nucleoside with a phosphate group.

Nitrogenous bases: There are two types of nitrogenous bases.

1. Purines (Adenine and Guanine)
2. Pyrimidines (Cytosine, Uracil and Thymine)

Cytosine is common for both DNA and RNA and thymine is present in DNA. Uracil is present in RNA at the place of thymine.

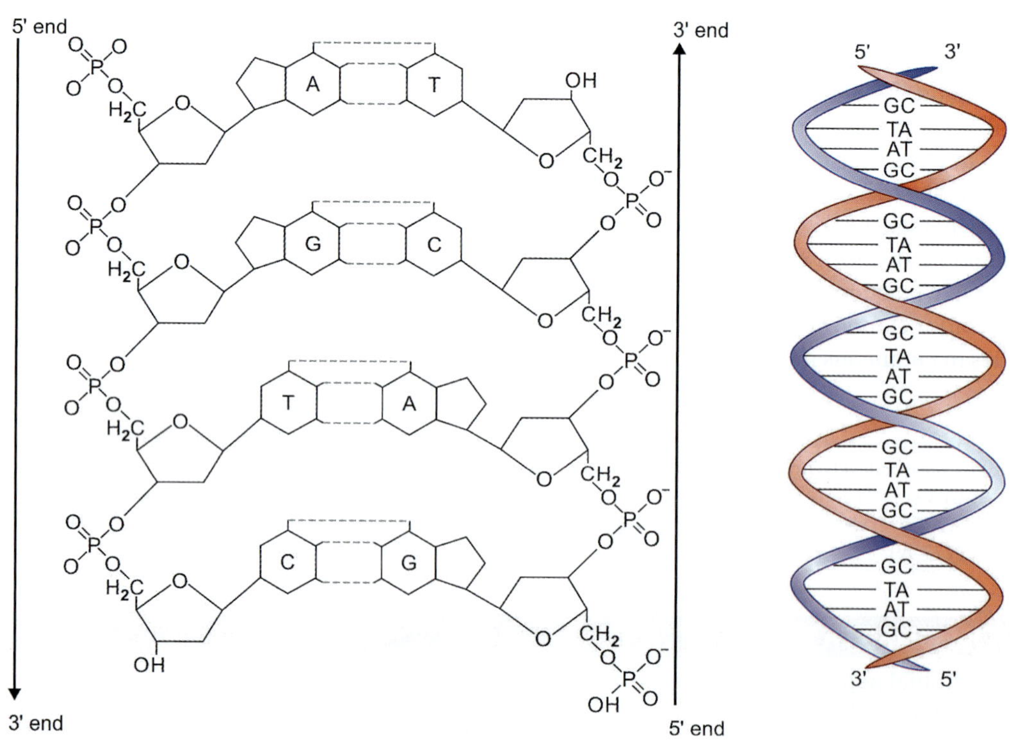

Fig. 1: Diagram of DNA. It contains two polynucleotide chains and forms a double-stranded helix. The two chains are "antiparallel," one in 5′-3′ and another in 3′-5′ direction. The nitrogenous bases attached to deoxyribose projects into the center of the helix. Purine form bond with pyrimidine and vice versa.
Source: Adapted from Molecular Genetic Pathology by Cheng, Liang, Zhang, David Y.[2]

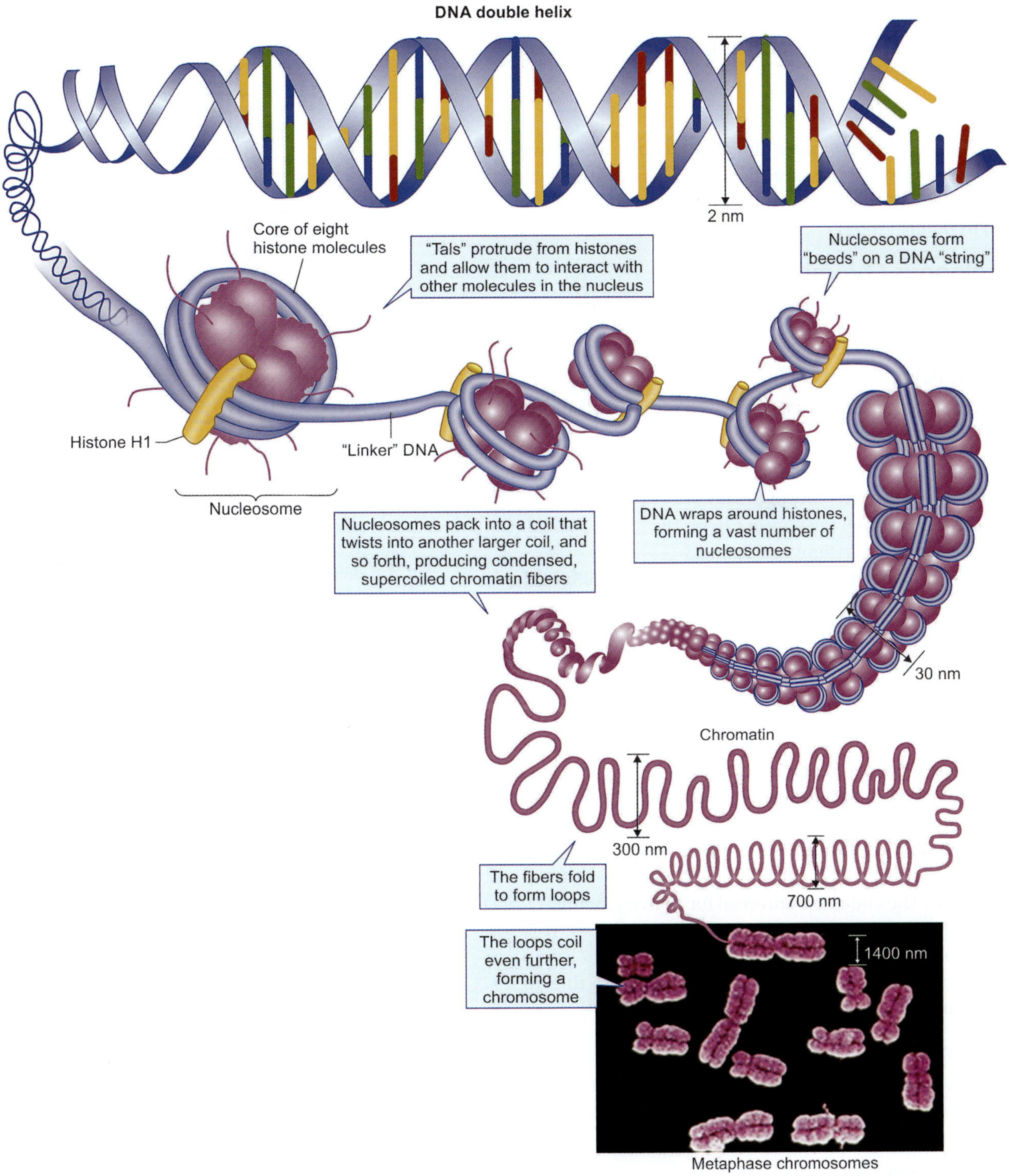

Fig. 2: DNA and its packaging inside the nucleus.[5]

Chromosome

A strand of convoluted and tightly wrapped DNA **(Fig. 2)**. Humans have 46 chromosomes = 23 pairs.

- 22 pairs called autosomes (they are numbered from 1 to 22)
- 1 pair of sex chromosomes (X and Y)
- "Ploidy": Number of sets of chromosomes that are found within the nucleus.
  - *Haploid cells* contain only one set of chromosomes (n).
  - *Diploid,* contains two sets of chromosomes (2n).

Gene

A part of DNA that holds information for encoding or making certain type of protein.

Allele

They are the different variety of a gene (Those who carry two different alleles at the same genetic locus are known as *heterozygotes* and those who carry same pairs of alleles are known as *homozygotes*).

Homologous Chromosome

A chromosomes containing same genes but not necessarily the same alleles.

Aneuploidy

It refers to abnormal number of chromosomes (Ch.) in the nucleus.

Diseases owing to aneuploidy:

- *Down syndrome:* Trisomy of Ch. no 21
- *Edwards syndrome:* Trisomy of Ch. no 18
- *Patau syndrome:* Trisomy of Ch. no 13
- *Klinefelter syndrome:* Disomy of X Ch. (genotype 45,XXY)
- *Turner syndrome:* Monosomy of the sex Ch. (genotype 45,X)

Genetic Code[7]

In the genetic code, three consecutive nucleotides (called triplet/codon) code for an amino acid **(Fig. 3)**.

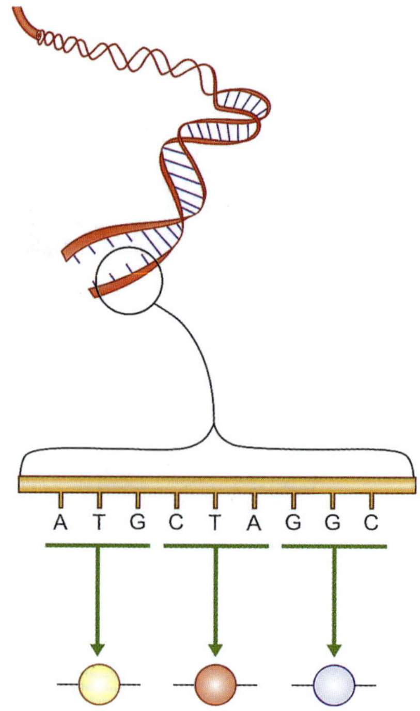

Fig. 3: Genetic code: Three consecutive nucleotides code for an amino acid.

Characteristic of genetic code include:

- *Degenerate*: Most amino acids are encoded by more than one codon.
- *Unambiguous and specific*: One codon encodes for only one amino acid.
- *Universal*: The codes are universal for all living being.
- *Genotype*: Genetic composition of an individual. It is determined by the set of alleles that are present.
- *Phenotype*: Observable/visual physical traits due to genotype (genetic composition).

Mutation[2]

Mutation is a phenomenon which results in alteration of DNA sequences and in consequence changes the genotype and the phenotype of an individual.

Types of mutation:

1. *Substitutions*: Substitution of a single base (also called point mutations). They can be:
   - *Silent*: Substitution which leads to synonymous codon generation, consequently same protein is translated.
   - *Missense*: Substitution which leads to different codon generation.
   - *Nonsense*: Substitution which leads to formation of a stop codon (UAG, UAA, and UGA) consequently terminates the translation process.
2. *Deletions*: As the name suggests it occurs when one or more base pairs are lost. It results in a frameshift.
3. *Insertions*: It occurs due to insertion of base pairs. It can also cause frameshifts.

Causes of mutation:

- Faulty DNA replication
- Faulty DNA recombination
- Any damage to DNA due to chemicals
- Any damage to DNA due to radiations.

DNA repair mechanisms:

- Mismatch repair
- Nucleotide excision repair (NER)
- Direct DNA repair by virtue of specialized enzymes
- Recombination repair.

DNA repair is regulated in mammalian cells by protein *p53*.

- *p53 is encoded by TP53 gene*
- p53 is also called as "Guardian of the Genome."[8]

Penetrance

It is the proportion of individuals carrying mutated gene and exhibit the clinical phenotype of the underlying mutated genotype. Some individuals may not exhibit the phenotype although they carry the mutated gene; this condition is termed as reduced penetrance or incomplete penetrance.

Linkage and Recombination[9]

Genetic linkage is the probability of recombination between two loci of a chromosome resulting from crossing-over of sister chromatids.

Genetic recombination is a programmed feature of cell machinery which involves rearrangement of DNA sequences due to breaking and rejoining of chromosomes its segments.

Polymorphism

A gene is said to be polymorphic if more than one allele of that particular gene occupies that gene's locus in a certain population. Additionally, each allele must occur in at least 1% of the population for being considered as polymorphic.[1]

Mosaicism and Chimerism (Figs. 4A and B)[10]

- *Mosaicism*: Occurrence of two or more cell populations with different genotypes in a single individual who has developed from one fertilized egg.
  - Pigmentary mosaicism (like hypomelanosis of Ito)
  - Verrucous epidermal nevus syndrome
  - Nevus comedonicus syndrome
  - McCune-Albright syndrome
  - Multiple syringomas
  - Buschke-Ollendorff syndrome.
- *Chimerism*: It is said to occur when a one organism composed of multiple cells with distinct genotype. Chimerism occur in:
  - Twins
  - Organ transplantation.

Modes of Inheritance[11]

Autosomal means that the gene containing a trait is located on one of the autosomes (nonsex, chromosomes). *X linked* or *Y linked* means that the gene containing a trait is located in either of the sex chromosome (X or Y).

Dominant vs. recessive: Dominant signifies that a single copy of the gene in question enough to exhibit the phenotype or trait. Whereas, two copies of the gene in question are needed to exhibit the phenotype or trait.

Autosomal dominant (AD)	• Both male and female equally affected • There is a 50% chance the offspring will inherit the disease from one affected parent • They are seen in every generation
Autosomal recessive (AR)	• Both parents of an affected person are carriers • They are not seen in every generation • Common in offsprings of consanguineous parents
X-linked dominant (XLD)	• Males and females can be affected • Males are more severely affected. Even some XLD disorders are lethal in males • There is a 50% chance the offspring will inherit the disease from one affected mother • From an affected male, all his daughters are affected, whereas all sons are normal
X-linked recessive (XLR)	• Affected males transmit the mutated allele to all of their daughters (the daughters become carriers), but to none of their sons • Women are affected when they are homozygous. From an affected mother all the sons are affected, whereas their daughters are unaffected carriers

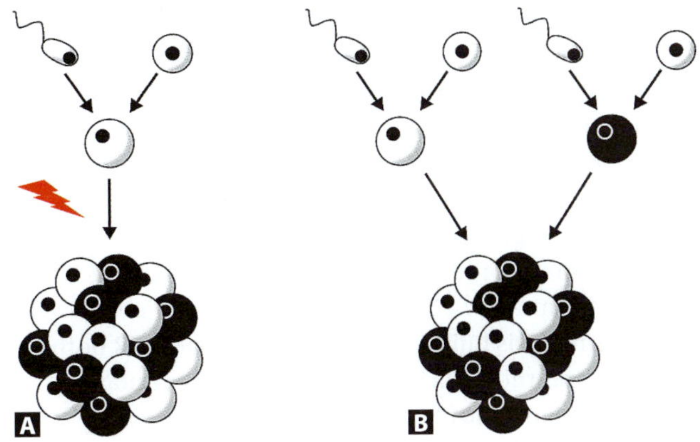

Figs. 4A and B: Diagram illustrating: (A) Mosaicism; (B) Chimerism.[10]

Autosomal Dominant Diseases[12]

- Neurofibromatosis type 1 (*NF1* gene mutation Ch. segment 17q11.2)
- Tuberous sclerosis (*TSC1* and *TSC2* gene mutation)
- Dariers disease (*ATP2A2* gene mutation)
- Acrokeratosis verruciformis of Hopf (distinct clinical entity of Dariers disease)
- Porphyria (AIP, VP, HCP, PCT)
- Clouston syndrome (hidrotic ectodermal dysplasia) (connexin gene, GJB6 or connexin-30 mutation)
- Ectrodactyly ectodermal dysplasia-cleft (EEC) syndrome (*p63* gene missense mutation)
- Rapp–Hodgkin syndrome (RHS) (distinct clinical entity of EEC syndrome)
- Epidermolysis bullosa simplex (*KRT5*, *KRT14* gene mutation)
- Nail-patella syndrome (gene located on Ch. 9q34 mutated)
- Noonan syndrome (*PTPN11*, *SOS1*, *RAF1*, and *KRAS* gene mutation)
- Peutz–Jeghers syndrome [*STK11* (*LKB1*) gene mutation on Ch. 19]
- White sponge nevus (*KRT4* or *KRT13* gene mutation)
- Nevoid basal cell carcinoma syndrome (*PTCH1* gene mutation, occasionally *SUFU* and *PTCH2* genes mutated)
- Gardner syndrome (*APC* gene mutation)
- Cowden syndrome (*PTEN* gene mutation)
- Carney complex (mutations in the *PRKAR1A* gene) which includes:
  - LAMB syndrome (lentigines, atrial myxomas, and blue nevi)
  - NAME syndrome (nevi, atrial myxoma, myxoid neurofibromas, and ephelides)

Autosomal Recessive Diseases[12]

- Netherton syndrome (*SPINK5* gene mutation on Ch. 5q32)
- Oculocutaneous albinism (OCA) group of diseases (*OCA1* to *OCA7* gene mutated depending upon subset of OCA)

- Xeroderma pigmentosum [nucleotide excision repair (NER) defect]
- Cockayne syndrome (aka Neill-Dingwall syndrome) (defective DNA repair mechanism)
- Trichothiodystrophy (defective DNA repair mechanism, *C7orf11* gene mutation)
- Ataxia telangiectasia (*ATM* gene mutation)
- Junctional epidermolysis bullosa (*LAMA3, LAMB3, LAMC2*, and *COL17A1* gene mutation)
- Epidermolysis bullosa dystrophica (AD and AR both)
- Pseudoxanthoma elasticum (*ABCC6* gene mutation)
- Bloom syndrome (*BLM* gene mutation)
- Omenn syndrome (*RAG* gene mutation)
- Lamellar ichthyosis (nonbullous congenital ichthyosis) (*ABCA12* gene mutation)
- Harlequin ichthyosis (loss-of-function mutation in the *ABCA12* gene)
- Erythrodysplasia verruciformis (*EVER1* or *EVER2* gene mutation on chromosome 17q25)
- Papillon-Lefevre syndrome [Cathepsin C (*CTSC*) gene mutation]
- Werner syndrome (*WRN* gene mutation)
- Leukocyte adhesion deficiency (LAD) (LAD 1, 2 and 3 caused by mutation in *ITGB2, SLC35C1*, and *FERMT3* gene respectively)
- Wilsons syndrome (*ATP7B* gene mutation)
- Schopf-Schulz-Passarge syndrome (*WNT10A* gene mutation on Ch. 2)
- Rothmund-Thomson syndrome (DNA repair mechanism affected due to mutations in the DNA helicase *RECQL4* gene)
- Kindler syndrome (mutation in *KIND1* gene).

X-linked Dominant Diseases[12]

- Incontinentia pigmenti [*IKBKG* gene (formerly known as *NEMO* or *NF-kappaB* gene) on Ch. Xq28)
- XLD porphyria (*ALAS2* gene mutation on Ch. X)
- Bazex syndrome [Unknown (gene linked to Xq24–q27 is mutated)]

X-linked Recessive Diseases[12]

- X-linked ichthyosis (*STS* gene mutation on Ch. Xp22.3)
- Hypohydrotic ectodermal dysplasia (*EDA, EDAR*, or *EDARADD* genes mutation)
- Lesch-Nyhan syndrome (*HPRT1* gene mutation)
- Ocular albinism (*GPR143* gene mutation)
- Wiskott-Aldrich syndrome (*WAS* gene mutation on Ch. Xp11.23)
- X-linked severe combined immunodeficiency (SCID) (*IL2RG* gene mutation)
- Menkes disease (*ATP7A* gene mutation)
- Androgen insensitivity syndrome (*AR* gene mutation)
- Fabrys disease (*GLA* gene mutation)
- X-linked dyskeratosis congenita (DKC) also known as Zinsser-Engman-Cole syndrome (DKC is mostly XLR but it may be polygenic as well) (*DKC1* gene mutation).

Y-linked Diseases

- Hairy pinna (HEY genetic locus on Ch. Yq)[13]
- Azoospermia (AZF microdeletions)[14]

Mitochondrial Inheritance

Mitochondrial inheritance means the gene in question is located in mitochondrial DNA (mtDNA). They are inherited solely from mother as after fertilization only maternal mitochondria is transmitted. Father with mtDNA mutations have no chance of transmitting the disease to their offspring, e.g., Leber's hereditary optic neuropathy, Kearns-Sayre syndrome.

> mtDNA are small circular DNA inside mitochondria. They contain around 16k base pairs. They are haploid and do not have any repair mechanism.

Codominant Inheritance

In codominant inheritance, each parent contributes a different version of a particular gene, and both versions influence the resulting genetic trait.[15]

Polygenic Inheritance

A polygenic trait is one whose phenotype is determined by multiple genes. Example of such trains in human include height and skin color. They do not follow Mendelian inheritance rules. Some polygenic traits are also affected by the environmental factors and are called multifactorial. Example of cutaneous diseases with polygenic inheritance are psoriasis vulgaris and melanoma.[1,15]

GENETIC COUNSELING[16,17]

It is a process of communication and imparting education to address the concerns related to development and/or transmission of a genetic disorder.

The steps involved in genetic counseling include:

1. Diagnosis of disorder
2. Risk assessment
3. Communication (with the parents)
4. Discussion (of options)
5. Long term contact and support.

Medical knowledge should be imparted by a specialist having in-depth understanding of the disease.

Parents should be explained regarding the:

- Inheritance mode
- Probability of having an affected child
- Risk of transmission to next generation (through carriers)
- Grades of severity (in subsequent generations)
- Prognosis of the disorder if parents are already having an affected child.

TABLE 1: Methods of prenatal diagnosis of skin diseases.

Method(s)	*Skin disorders tested for*	*Timing*	*Technique*
Preimplantation genetic diagnosis	• Harlequin ichthyosis • Severe ectodermal dysplasia syndromes	3 days after in-vitro fertilization	• Genetic testing of embryos after fertilization • Embryos confirmed to be free of the disorder are implanted in the uterus
Chorionic villus sampling	• Epidermolysis bullosa • Oculocutaneous albinism	• Weeks 10–13 of pregnancy • Not before 10 weeks	• Cells from placental villi are collected using a needle inserted either through the cervix or transabdominally under ultrasound guidance • Fetal DNA is extracted and analyzed for a known genetic mutation
Amniocentesis	• Epidermolysis bullosa • Oculocutaneous albinism	From week 14 of pregnancy	• Fetal cells are collected from the amniotic fluid by a needle inserted transabdominally under ultrasound guidance • Fetal DNA is investigated for a known genetic mutation
Fetal skin biopsy	Skin conditions with unknown genetic mutation	From week 19 of pregnancy (once fetal skin adequately formed)	• Biopsy of fetal skin is performed under ultrasound guidance • The biopsy is examined by immunohisto-chemistry and electron microscopy
Maternal serum screening	X-linked ichthyosis (identified by low levels of estriol)	During second trimester of pregnancy (weeks 14–26)	Maternal serum levels of specific hormones and proteins are measured by a blood test to assess the risk of different conditions
Ultrasound	Harlequin ichthyosis (suggested by echogenic amniotic fluid, joint and digital contractions plus facial dysmorphism)	From 12 weeks of pregnancy onwards	• Trans-abdominal ultrasound performed to assist with diagnosis • Useful in identifying conditions with no known family history

PRENATAL DIAGNOSIS

Prenatal diagnosis is the identification of a disorder before birth. This may be done either during pregnancy, prior to implantation or while in-vitro fertilization.[18]

Methods of prenatal diagnosis of skin diseases have been described in **Table 1**.[18]

KEY POINTS

- Mosaicism can explain many dermatology disorders such as hypomelanosis of Ito that involves a few clones of cells in the disease process.
- AR diseases are usually more severe than AD diseases. Concept of inheritance is important in many pediatric dermatosis.
- Mitochondrial inheritance is found to be important in many genetic disorders and its transmission is purely maternal.
- Genetic counseling plays an important role in prevention of genetic diseases.

REFERENCES

1. Kumaran MS, De D. Basic genetics for dermatologists. Indian J Dermatol Venereol Leprol. 2013;79(4):457.
2. Zhang S, Davidson DD, Zhang DY, Parks JA, Cheng L. Principles of clinical molecular biology. In: Cheng L, Zhang DY (Eds). Molecular Genetic Pathology. Totowa, NJ: Humana Press; 2008. pp. 3-32.
3. Watson JD, Crick FHC. Molecular structure of nucleic acids: a structure for deoxyribose nucleic acid. Nature. 1953;171(4356):737-8.
4. Vasicek TJ, McDevitt BE, Freeman MW, Fennick BJ, Hendy GN, Potts JT, et al. Nucleotide sequence of the human parathyroid hormone gene. Proc Natl Acad Sci. 1983;80(8):2127-31.
5. Sadava D. DNA is Packed into a Mitotic Chromosome. Learn Science at Scitable [Internet]. [online] Available from: https://www.nature.com/scitable/content/DNA-is-Packed-into-a-Mitotic-Chromosome-3497/ [Last accessed January, 2021].
6. Crick F. Central dogma of molecular biology. Nature. 1970;227(5258):561-3.
7. Crick FHC. The origin of the genetic code. J Mol Biol. 1968;38(3):367-79.
8. Efeyan A, Serrano M. p53: guardian of the genome and policeman of the oncogenes. Cell Cycle. 2007;6(9):1006-10.
9. Bodmer WF, Parsons PA. Linkage and recombination in evolution. In: Caspari EW, Thoday JM (Eds). Advances in Genetics. Cambridge, Massachusetts: Academic Press; 1963. pp. 1-100.
10. Castori M, Tadini G. Discoveries and controversies in cutaneous mosaicism. G Ital Dermatol E Venereol Organo Uff Soc Ital Dermatol E Sifilogr. 2016;151(3):251-65.
11. Genetic Alliance, New York-Mid-Atlantic Consortium for Genetic and Newborn Screening Services. Understanding Genetics: A New York, Mid-Atlantic Guide for Patients and Health Professionals Washington (DC): Genetic Alliance; 2009. p. 104.
12. Jain S. Dermatology: Illustrated Study Guide and Comprehensive Board Review. New York: Springer Science & Business Media; 2012. p. 375.
13. Baryah N, Krishan K, Puri S, Kanchan T. Inheritance of hypertrichosis pinnae auris-a review of literature. J Clin Diagn Res. 2018;12.

14. Fernando L, Gromoll J, Weerasooriya TR, Nieschlag E, Simoni M. Y-chromosomal microdeletions and partial deletions of the Azoospermia Factor c (AZFc) region in normozoospermic, severe oligozoospermic and azoospermic men in Sri Lanka. Asian J Androl. 2006;8(1):39-44.
15. Wakim S, Grewal. Non-Mendelian Inheritance. Biology LibreTexts. 2018. [online] Available from: https://bio.libretexts.org/Bookshelves/Human_Biology/Book%3A_Human_Biology_(Wakim_and_Grewal)/08%3A_Inheritance/8.5%3A_Non-Mendelian_Inheritance [Last accessed January, 2021].
16. Durmaz A, Durmaz B. Chapter 12 - The role of next generation sequencing in genetic counseling. In: Demkow U, Płoski R (Eds). Clinical Applications for Next-Generation Sequencing. Boston: Academic Press; 2016. pp. 241-58.
17. Delatycki M. Genetic counseling. In: Maloy S, Hughes K (Eds). Brenner's Encyclopedia of Genetics, (2nd edition). San Diego: Academic Press; 2013. pp. 240-1.
18. Georgina H. Prenatal diagnosis of inherited skin conditions. DermNet NZ. 2015. [online] Available from: https://dermnetnz.org/topics/prenatal-diagnosis-of-inherited-skin-conditions/ [Last accessed January, 2021].

EXAMINATION QUESTIONS

1. Explain mosaicism and chimerism with examples.
2. Write the definition and types of pigmentary demarcation lines.
3. Discuss genetic counseling.
4. Explain the procedure of prenatal diagnosis of skin diseases.

7 CHAPTER

Basics in Dermatopathology

Riti Bhatia, M Ramam

INTRODUCTION

Dermatopathology involves learning the process manifesting on the skin through microscopy. The vastness of the field makes it look like a herculean task to master. Like any other skill, strong basics form a good foundation in learning the subject.

This chapter is an overview of basics in dermatopathology. The initial part will focus on findings in a normal biopsy while the later part broadly covers features of major histopathological reaction patterns in various skin disorders.

NORMAL SKIN BIOPSY

Broadly, normal skin biopsy has three parts:

1. *Epidermis*: The thickness varies from 0.05 to 1.5 mm depending on the site. Eyelids and scrotum have thin epidermis and acral areas and back are thickest. There are four layers in a normal epidermis, except in palms and soles.[1] As we go down the layers are:
   a. Stratum corneum consisting of flattened keratinocytes without nuclei. The normal stratum corneum shows a basket-weave orthokeratosis due to the crisscross pattern of arrangement of keratinocytes. The exception is palms and soles where stratum corneum is compact.
   b. Stratum lucidum is a thick translucent layer seen only in skin of the palms and soles, it is absent elsewhere.
   c. Stratum granulosum consists of 1–3 layers of polygonal cells with basophilic granules.
   d. Stratum spinosum consists of 3–10 layers of keratinocytes interconnected through desmosomes that can be appreciated in certain disorders noted as thin, hair-like strands between keratinocytes.
   e. Stratum basale consists of single layer of cuboidal keratinocytes intermingled with melanocytes in a ratio of 1:10.
2. *Dermis*: The thickest layer of skin is dermis, varying from 1.5 to 4 mm. It consists of vessels, adnexal structures (hair follicles, glands), and the stroma.
3. *Subcutis*: The part of skin below the dermis consisting of adipocytes is the subcutis. Adipocytes are arranged in clusters/lobules that are separated by delicate fibrous septae.

The various cells that are normally seen in a skin biopsy are described below.

- *Keratinocytes form the epidermis*: These are cuboidal to polygonal cells with eosinophilic cytoplasm and vesicular nuclei that are connected to each other with desmosomes. The cells in the basal layer are more basophilic and become pinker as keratin accumulates in the upper layers. Certain stains are helpful in distinguishing basal from suprabasal keratinocytes, and can be used in the diagnosis of epidermal neoplasms. High molecular weight cytokeratins 5 and 6 are expressed in all the layers. While basaloid proliferations stain with BerEP4, the squamoid/suprabasal proliferations stain with epithelial membrane antigen (EMA).[2]
- *Melanocytes are found in the basal layer*: They have a dark nucleus surrounded by condensed cytoplasm that is retracted from the surrounding keratinocytes giving the appearance of a vacuolated cell. Various immunohistochemical markers useful for staining melanocytes are S-100, HMB45 for melanosomes, and Melan-A, microphthalmia transcription factor for membrane antigens.
- Langerhans cells are dendritic cells found in the epidermis and are increased in number in certain disorders. The nucleus is characteristically kidney-shaped or reniform. These stain positively with S100 and CD1a. The latter is taken up by Birbeck granules, otherwise seen only with electron microscopy.
- Lymphocytes are seen normally in a skin biopsy in small numbers especially around vessels. These are roughly of the size of a red blood cell (7–10 µm). The nucleus is round and basophilic and there is hardly any discernible cytoplasm.
- Histiocytes are cells that usually accompany lymphocytes in small numbers. These have abundant cytoplasm and a vesicular nucleus.
- Mast cells are about twice the size of a red blood cell. The nucleus is round, central, and basophilic like that of a lymphocyte and there is abundant cytoplasm as in a histiocyte giving the cell a "fried-egg appearance." Occasional mast cells can be seen in a normal skin biopsy, usually around vessels. Mast cell granules stain with toluidine blue, Giemsa, Leder's stain (chloroacetate esterase), and alcian blue. CD117 stains the membrane antigen.
- Plasma cells are normally seen in the mucosa and in biopsies from the head and neck. These large cells have

an eccentric nucleus with a cart wheel appearance due to focally condensed chromatin, a perinuclear halo and abundant amphophilic cytoplasm.

The various special stains and immunohistochemical stains are enlisted in **Tables 1 and 2**.

Some commonly used dermatopathological terms and their definitions include:[3]

- *Acantholysis:* Separation of keratinocytes due to loss of adhesion between the keratinocytes.
- *Acanthosis:* Thickening of the epidermis, seen as increase in the number of layers of stratum spinosum to more than 10.
- *Atrophy:* Reduction in number of layers of epidermis or thinning of the dermis, usually attributed to loss of collagen or elastin.
- *Dermal edema:* Accumulation of fluid within the dermis, leading to loosening of collagen fibers. It is often accompanied with dilated capillaries or lymphatic channels.
- *Exocytosis:* Migration of inflammatory cells, such as lymphocytes, eosinophils, into the epidermis.
- *Hypergranulosis:* Increase in the number of layers of stratum granulosum to more than 3.
- *Hyperkeratosis:* Thickening of stratum corneum, leading to a compact or laminated appearance, in contrast to the basket-weave pattern of normal stratum corneum.
- *Necrobiosis:* Indistinct basophilic appearance of collagen fibers, due to accumulation of mucopolysaccharides.
- *Necrotic keratinocytes:* Pyknotic eosinophilic keratinocytes, lying singly in the papillary dermis, due to the pathological degeneration of basal keratinocytes

TABLE 1: Special stains in dermatopathology.

Name	*Target tissue*	*Color*
Verhoeff-Van Gieson	Collagen	Red
	Elastic fibers	Black
Masson trichrome	Collagen	Blue-green
Gomori's aldehyde fuchsin	Collagen	Red
	Elastic fibers	Blue
	Acid MPS	Blue
Oil-red-O	Fat	Red
Sudan black B		Black
Scarlet red		Red
Fontana-Masson	Melanin	Black
Silver nitrate		Black
Orcein-Giemsa	Melanin	Brown
	Elastic fibers	Black
	Amyloid	Light blue
Congo red	Amyloid	Green birefringence with polarization
Crystal violet		Purple
Thioflavin T		Yellow fluorescence
Perls	Hemosiderin	Blue
Prussian blue		Blue
Alizarin red S	Calcium	Orange
Von Kossa		Black
Toluidine blue	Acid mucopoly-saccharides	Purple
Alcian blue		Blue
Crystal violet		Purple
Giemsa		Purple
Periodic acid Schiff	Neutral mucopoly-saccharides	Pink
	Fungal wall	Red
Leder (chloro-acetate esterase)	Mast cells	Red
Brown-Brenn (modified Gram stain)	Bacteria	Blue/Red
Fite Faraco	Leprosy	Red
Warthin-Starry	Leishmania, Histo-plasma, Rickettsia	Purple
Grocott	Fungal wall	Black
Gomori		Black
Bodian	Nerve	Black

(MPS: mucopolysaccharides)

TABLE 2: Immunohistochemical stains.

Cells	*Stain*
Macrophage/histiocyte	CD68
Natural killer cell	CD56
Langerhans cells	CD1a, S100
Melanocytes/Melanoma	S-100, Melan-A, HMB45
B-cell	CD20, 79a
T-cell	CD2-8
Plasma cell	CD138
Merkel cell	CK20
Paget cell	CK7, CAM5.2
Endothelial cell/Blood vessel	CD31, CD34
Angiosarcoma	CD31
Lymphatic channels	D2-40
Dermatofibrosarcoma protuberans	CD34
Dermatofibroma	Factor XIII a
Mast cell	CD117, c-kit
Eccrine gland	CEA
Sebaceous gland	EMA, keratin
Apocrine	GCDFP-15
SCC	EMA
BCC	BerEP4
Lymphomatous papulosis and anaplastic large cell CA	CD30
Follicular center lymphoma	BCL 2
Lymphoma	CD45
Glomus cells	Vimentin, smooth muscle actin

(CEA: carcinoembryonic antigen; EMA: epithelial membrane antigen)

- *Papillomatosis:* Undulating appearance of the epidermis, seen in disorders such as verruca vulgaris.
- *Parakeratosis:* Retention of nuclei of keratinocytes within stratum corneum.
- *Pigment incontinence:* Presence of melanin laden macrophages in the papillary dermis, as a result of damage to the melanocytes in the basal layer in interface dermatitis.
- *Spongiosis:* Edema within the epidermis leading to swollen keratinocytes and prominent desmosomes/intercellular junctions.

REACTION PATTERNS

Correlating the histopathological findings with the clinical diagnosis is a key component of the diagnostic process. However, an important initial step in the assessment of a skin biopsy is the recognition of a set of findings that are suggestive of broad groups of disorders.[4] These findings are collectively referred to as a reaction pattern. Recognizing the reaction pattern is an essential skill for dermatopathology and leads logically to the next step of recognizing further clues that help differentiate the various disorders that produce the same pattern and to the final step of clinicopathological correlation. Some of the important reaction patterns are described in the following sections.

Lichenoid or Interface Dermatitis

The characteristic feature is basal cell degeneration leading to a loss of continuity of basal layer. Basal keratinocytes may show vacuolization or necrosis/apoptosis and in advanced disease, complete loss of the basal layer. Necrotic/apoptotic keratinocytes are visualized as round eosinophilic bodies with a pyknotic or absent nucleus which drop down into the upper dermis as colloid bodies. These changes are accompanied by an upper dermal infiltrate of lymphocytes impinging on the overlying epidermis **(Fig. 1)**. The infiltrate is milder and accompanied by edema in acute lichenoid disorders while it is dense and band-like in chronic disorders such as lichen planus, which also show acanthosis of the epidermis. Melanophages are a prominent component of the lichenoid tissue reaction and lead to the bluish color of skin lesions. The presence or absence of additional features such as parakeratosis, acanthosis, basement membrane thickening, eosinophils in the infiltrate, localization of the infiltrate to the papillary dermis, or around hair follicles helps to identify the various disorders that share this reaction pattern.[5]

Lichen planus is a prototype disorder. Apart from basal cell damage, it shows hypergranulosis, an intense band-like infiltrate of lymphocytes along the basal layer and pigment incontinence. Parakeratosis is absent, except in mucosal lichen planus, hypertrophic variant of lichen planus, and lichenoid drug eruptions. Vacuolization of basal cells is a feature of connective tissue disorders such as lupus erythematosus and dermatomyositis. Important disorders in this group are shown in **Table 3**.

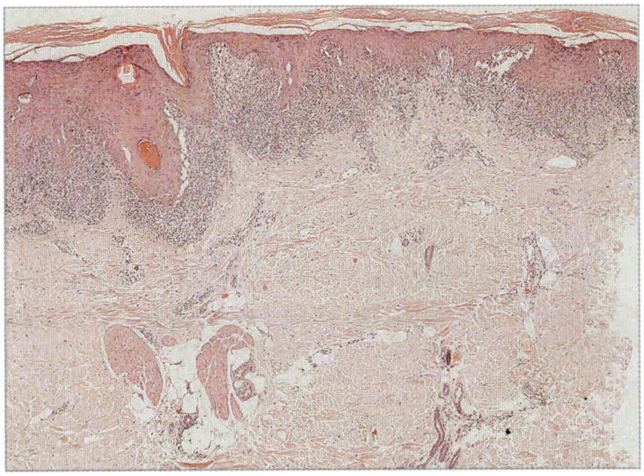

Fig. 1: Lichenoid tissue reaction. Dense band-like infiltrate of lymphocytes in upper dermis impinging on overlying epidermis with basal layer degeneration in lichen planus (H&E, ×200).

Psoriasiform Reaction Pattern

This reaction pattern is characterized by acanthosis or epidermal hyperplasia as the prominent change accompanied by varying degrees of infiltrates in the epidermis and underlying dermis. Hyperkeratosis may be accompanied by parakeratosis and infiltrates of neutrophils within the stratum corneum (Munro's microabscess). The granular layer is usually deficient or absent below zones of parakeratosis (hypogranulosis). Neutrophils may be seen in the spinous layers, singly or in collections that extend between keratinocytes separated by edema (spongiform pustule of Kogoj). The papillary dermis is edematous and shows changes in the capillaries. There may be thinning of the epidermal plates overlying the dermal papillae (suprapapillary thinning). The diseases that show this reaction pattern can be differentiated by the type of parakeratosis: confluent, patchy, or alternating, the uniformity of the acanthosis, the presence or absence of neutrophils in the stratum corneum and stratum spinosum, dilatation and tortuosity of dermal capillaries, and suprapapillary thinning.[6]

Psoriasis is the prototype disorder in this group which shows regular acanthosis with parakeratosis, Munro's microabscesses and spongiform pustules of Kogoj, hypogranulosis, suprapapillary thinning, upper dermal edema, and dilated capillaries **(Fig. 2)**. However, diagnostic histopathological findings are seen in only a minority of biopsies of psoriasis. Other disorders in this group include pityriasis rubra pilaris, reactive arthritis, and secondary syphilis **(Table 4)**.

Spongiotic Reaction Pattern

Spongiotic reaction pattern is characterized by edema between keratinocytes in the epidermis which stretches the

TABLE 3: Disorders with lichenoid reaction pattern.

Lichen planus—Classic variant	• *Basal layer degeneration*: Damage of basal layer with presence of necrotic keratinocytes, eosinophilic round keratinocytes without nuclei, along the basal layer. Rete ridges appear "saw toothed" • *Band-like infiltrate* of lymphocytes in upper dermis • Wedge-shaped hypergranulosis • Pigment incontinence
Lichen planus hypertrophicus	• Basal layer degeneration less extensive and usually confined to tips of rete ridges of acanthotic epidermis • Parakeratosis and eosinophils in upper dermis • *Differential diagnosis*: Lichen simplex chronicus/prurigo nodularis
Lichen planus pigmentosus	• Minimal basal degeneration, usually not seen • Prominent pigment incontinence • *Differential diagnosis*: Postinflammatory pigmentation
Lichen planopilaris	• Basal degeneration centered around hair follicles • Few follicles with preserved sebaceous glands, in established cases • *Differential diagnosis*: Discoid lupus erythematosus
Lichen nitidus	• Localized basal layer degeneration • Localized infiltrate of epithelioid cells, lymphocytes and histiocytes, clutched by "claw-like" acanthotic epidermis, present beneath areas of basal damage
Lichen striatus	• Localized basal degeneration • Superficial and deep infiltrate of lymphocytes and histiocytes around follicles and eccrine glands
Lupus erythematosus	*Acute* • Basal layer vacuolization • *Differential diagnosis*: dermatomyositis *Subacute* • Basal layer vacuolization, less than acute LE • Interstitial mucin • Perifollicular and perivascular infiltrate of lymphocytes and histiocytes in upper dermis *Discoid* • Follicular plugging • Atrophic epidermis • Perifollicular and perivascular infiltrate of lymphocytes and histiocytes in upper and deep dermis, more than SCLE • Interstitial mucin, less than SCLE • *Differential diagnosis*: Other diseases with superficial and deep infiltrates, memorized easily with mnemonic 8Ls plus drugs (**l**ight reactions, **l**eprosy, **l**ichen striatus, **l**epidoptera/insect bite hypersensitivity, **l**ues/syphilis, **l**upus erythematosus, pseudo**l**ymphomas, necrobiotic **l**ipoidica, and drug reactions)[4]
Lichenoid drug reaction	• Parakeratosis • Necrotic keratinocytes higher up in the epidermis • Eosinophils in upper dermis

(SCLE: subacute cutaneous lupus erythematosus)

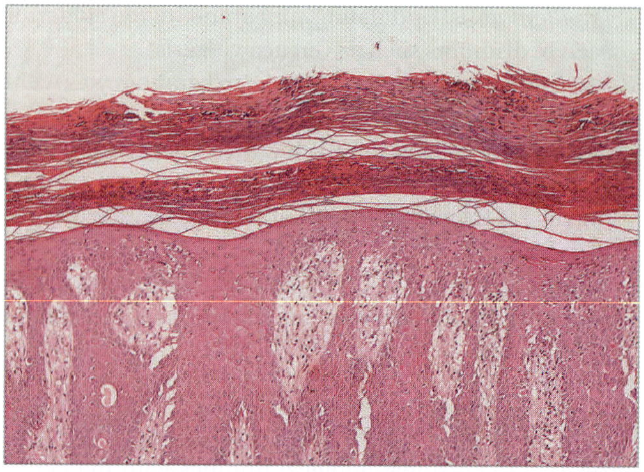

Fig. 2: Psoriasiform tissue reaction. Regular acanthosis with hyperkeratosis, parakeratosis, collections of neutrophils within stratum corneum (Munro's microabscess), suprapapillary thinning, and dilated capillaries in upper dermis in psoriasis (H&E, ×200).

TABLE 4: Disorders with psoriasiform reaction pattern.

Psoriasis vulgaris	• Dilatation and congestion of vessels in papillary dermis and a mild, perivascular, lymphocytic infiltrate—*earliest change*, in lesions of less than 24 hours' duration • Parakeratosis • Hypogranulosis • Suprapapillary thinning • Dilated vessels in upper dermis
Pustular psoriasis	• Intraepidermal pustules • Clusters of neutrophils in stratum corneum and stratum spinosum, Munro's microabscesses and spongiform pustules of Kogoj, respectively • Acanthosis develops in late stage • Perivascular infiltrate of lymphocytes, and sometimes neutrophils, seen in upper dermis • *Differential diagnosis*: Cutaneous lesions of reactive arthritis
Reactive arthritis	*Similar to pustular psoriasis, except:* • Thicker massive stratum corneum • Regular acanthosis
Pityriasis rubra pilaris	• Changes seen best in erythematous nonfollicular lesions • Alternating orthokeratosis and parakeratosis in both vertical and horizontal directions (checkerboard pattern), not seen in all cases • Regular acanthosis • Suprapapillary thickening • Focal/confluent hypergranulosis
Inflammatory linear verrucous epidermal nevus	• Alternating zones of orthokeratosis and parakeratosis horizontally • Hypogranulosis underlying the zones of parakeratosis • Regular acanthosis • Focal mild spongiosis

intercellular bridges and makes them more prominent, an appearance that has been awkwardly likened to a sponge **(Fig. 3)**. Spongiosis is often accompanied by the infiltration of inflammatory cells such as lymphocytes into the epidermis,

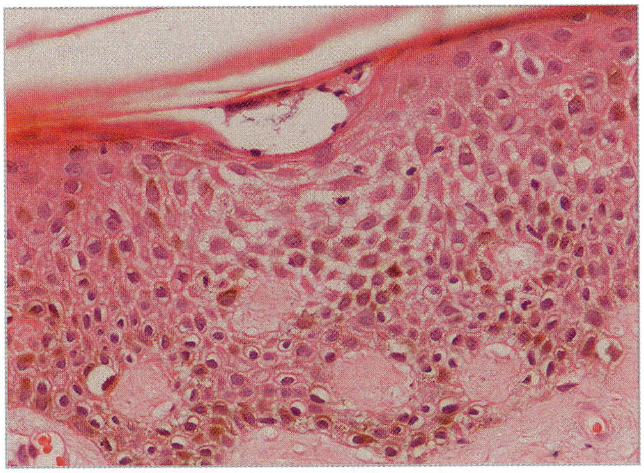

Fig. 3: Spongiotic tissue reaction. Edema in epidermis with stretching of keratinocytes, exocytosis of lymphocytes and cup-shaped collection of Langerhans cells in epidermis (H&E, ×400).

a process known as exocytosis.[5] Small cup-shaped collections of Langerhans cells in the upper epidermis are frequently seen. When edema is marked, the collection of fluid in the epidermis leads to the formation of spongiotic vesicles. Additional features include scale crust consisting of formed by the admixture of parakeratosis and fibrin/plasma with neutrophils and red blood cells and dilated superficial dermal vessels with a superficial perivascular infiltrate of lymphocytes, histiocytes, and occasional neutrophils or eosinophils.

Depending on the age of the lesion biopsied, there is a variation in the histopathological pattern. An acute irritant dermatitis shows necrosis of keratinocytes, which may be accompanied by exocytosis of neutrophils. Acute dermatitic lesions show prominent spongiosis, spongiotic vesicles, and a scale-crust. Subacute lesions show epidermal hyperplasia with milder spongiosis and exocytosis. Chronic rubbing in lichen simplex chronicus and prurigo nodularis leads to pronounced psoriasiform hyperplasia, parakeratosis, little or no spongiosis, and fibrosis of the dermal papillae with vertically oriented collagen fibers.

Important disorders in this group are allergic and irritant contact dermatitis, atopic dermatitis, nummular dermatitis, pityriasis rosea, and seborrheic dermatitis **(Table 5)**. There is considerable overlap in the histopathological features and it is often a lot easier to tell these conditions apart on clinical grounds than on biopsy. Spongiosis of the infundibulum of follicle is seen in follicular lesions of atopic dermatitis, disseminate infundibulo-folliculitis and seborrheic dermatitis. Parakeratosis surrounding the follicles is seen in seborrheic dermatitis. In miliaria, spongiosis is centerd around the acrosyringium, the portion of the sweat duct in the epidermis. Eosinophilic spongiosis is seen in precursor lesions of pemphigus, urticarial phase of bullous pemphigoid, arthropod bite reactions, allergic contact dermatitis, and incontinentia pigmenti.

TABLE 5: Disorders with spongiotic reaction pattern.

Atopic dermatitis	• Parakeratosis • Fibrin globules in stratum corneum • Spongiosis or intercellular edema in the epidermis with prominent intercellular bridges • Spongiotic vesicles containing Langerhans cells and lymphocytes • Presence of cells like neutrophils or eosinophils in the epidermis, also known as "exocytosis" • *Differential diagnosis*: Pityriasis rosea, allergic contact dermatitis
Seborrheic dermatitis	• Scale crust in stratum corneum centered on hair follicle • Spongiosis • Exocytosis of lymphocytes • Dilated capillaries and edema in papillary dermis • Perivascular infiltrate of lymphocytes, histiocytes and sometimes, neutrophils in papillary dermis
Irritant dermatitis	• Variable necrosis of epidermis • Spongiosis • Exocytosis of lymphocytes, neutrophils or eosinophils • Ballooning degeneration of keratinocytes • Edema in papillary dermis • Perivascular infiltrate of lymphocytes, neutrophils and histiocytes in upper dermis
Dermatophytic and candida infections	• Collections of neutrophils in epidermis and stratum corneum • Spongiosis • Periodic-acid Schiff staining reveals hyphae and spores

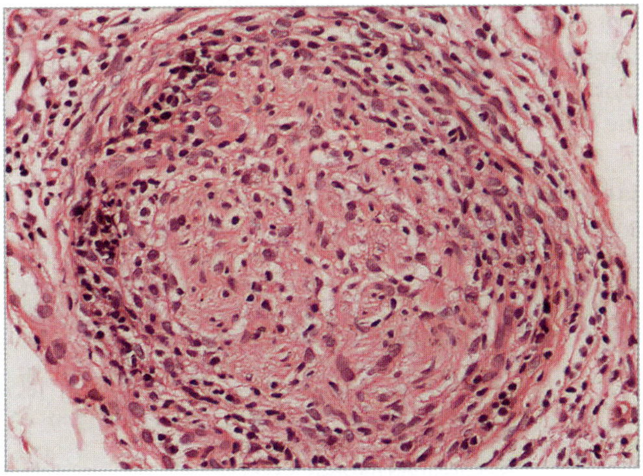

Fig. 4: Granulomatous tissue reaction. Well defined granuloma composed of collection of epithelioid cells in the center surrounded by collar of lymphocytes and histiocytes (H&E, ×400).

Granulomatous Reaction Pattern

The unifying feature of this group is a focal aggregation of epithelioid cells, usually surrounded by a collar of lymphocytes and histiocytes **(Fig. 4)**.[7] Epithelioid cells are large cells, about 20–40 microns in diameter, with an elongated vesicular nucleus that has a prominent nucleolus and abundant eosinophilic cytoplasm. They have indistinct cell borders. Epithelioid cells may fuse to form multinucleate giant cells of different types. *Langhans* giant cells have a neatly arranged rim of nuclei at the periphery while *foreign body* giant cells have nuclei arranged haphazardly through the cytoplasm. Other cells seen that may be seen in a granuloma include plasma cells, eosinophils and neutrophils, depending on the disorder and chronicity of lesion. Necrosis may be seen at the center of the granuloma and may be prominent in some diseases. Dermal fibrosis accompanies some granulomas. The overlying epidermis may be normal, atrophic, or thickened in different disorders. The diseases that show this reaction pattern can be differentiated by the arrangement of the granulomatous infiltrate, the tendency of granulomas to coalesce or stay discrete, the nature of the accompanying infiltrate, the presence and type of giant cells and any inclusions within them, type and extent of necrosis, alterations in the dermal collagen, and presence of foreign materials or organisms.

Granulomas have been classified into tuberculoid granuloma, which shows a mantle of lymphocytes around a core of epithelioid cells; sarcoidal granuloma which shows small, noncoalescing aggregates of epithelioid cells with a paucity of lymphocytes; suppurative or mixed cell granuloma which shows a mixture of acute inflammatory cells such as neutrophils and eosinophils accompanying the granuloma often with edema, congestion of blood vessels and many plasma cells; necrobiotic granulomas which show an alteration in collagen at the center of the granuloma; and foreign body granulomas usually have a disproportionately high number of giant cells of the foreign body type accompanied by a foreign body that may be seen in sections examined with ordinary or polarized light **(Table 6)**. Some biopsies show more than one type of granuloma and some cannot be easily categorized.

TABLE 6: Disorders with granulomatous reaction pattern.

Cutaneous tuberculosis	*Lupus vulgaris* • Distinctive pattern with a confluent granulomatous infiltrate in upper dermis with lichenoid damage of the overlying epidermis (lichenoid-granulomatous pattern). Accompanied by more discrete, epithelioid cell granulomas in the deep dermis. Fibrosis may be seen • Overlying epidermis usually hyperplastic with parakeratotic follicular plugs • Caseation necrosis is rare • Acid-fast bacilli (AFB) hardly ever seen *Tuberculosis verrucosa cutis* • Similar to lupus vulgaris but hyperplastic epidermal changes are more prominent *Scrofuloderma* • Epidermis may be ulcerated or acanthotic if biopsied at sinus edge • Diffuse dense mixed infiltrate of neutrophils and eosinophils along with epithelioid cells, lymphocytes and histiocytes, with many plasma cells accompanied by edema, congested vessels and fibrosis (suppurative granuloma)
Leprosy	*Leprosy pattern (across the entire spectrum)* • Superficial and deep, well circumscribed, perivascular, and periappendageal, oval, oblong, curvilinear infiltrates with minimal interstitial spill. The overlying epidermis is normal *TT/BT leprosy* • Well-defined compact granulomas in the leprosy pattern, focally encroaching on epidermis • AFB almost always absent *BB/BL lesions* • Epithelioid cell granulomas in the leprosy pattern are accompanied by foamy histiocytes. Foamy histiocytes and lymphocytes predominate in borderline lepromatous (BL) leprosy. In mid-borderline (BB) leprosy, two patterns may be seen: in one, epithelioid cells predominate while in the other, they are accompanied by a roughly equal proportion of foamy histiocytes • Edema is frequent in BB leprosy as Type 1 reaction is commonly associated • AFB is seen on biopsy, in larger numbers in BL leprosy
Sarcoidosis	• Round to oval, small, compact, collections of epithelioid cells; usually lymphocyte-poor but numbers are variable • Typically, granulomas are closely aggregated but discrete and do not coalesce • Asteroid and Schaumann bodies may be seen in giant cells • *Differential diagnoses:* Foreign body granulomas
Deep fungal infections	• Suppurative granulomatous reaction pattern • Diffuse dermal infiltrates of lymphocytes and histiocytes admixed with neutrophils, eosinophils along with focal aggregates of epithelioid cells • Periodic-acid Schiff and Grocott (or Gomori) methenamine silver stains may reveal fungal organisms • *Differential diagnosis*: Scrofuloderma, atypical mycobacterial infections, hidradenitis suppurativa
Granuloma annulare	• Necrobiosis of collagen is a feature and recognized as altered dermal collagen showing blurring of margins, separation of fibers, decrease in nuclei, altered staining • Histiocytes, giant cells, and some epithelioid cells arranged in a palisading manner around areas of necrobiosis • Mucin within the granuloma
Foreign body granuloma	• Granuloma shows many giant cells, including large foreign body type • Foreign body may be seen in H&E stain or as birefringent bodies in polarized light

In granulomatous diseases, the biopsy should always be screened carefully for infective organisms, though several noninfective conditions can also lead to granulomas. Special stains, including acid-fast bacilli (AFB) and periodic-acid Schiff (PAS) should be done to look for organisms especially in suppurative granulomas.

Vesiculobullous Reaction Pattern

This pattern is identified by a split in the epidermis or at the dermoepidermal junction that occurs due to a defect in adhesion within the epidermis or between epidermis and dermis. The split usually contains some plasma/fibrin and varying amounts of infiltrate. The mechanism leading to the formation of an intraepidermal vesicle can be *acantholysis* **(Fig. 5)**, characterized by rounded keratinocytes detached from adjacent cells; *spongiosis*, in which intracellular edema leads to separation of keratinocytes; *ballooning degeneration*, which occurs due to swelling and rupture of keratinocytes; *necrosis*, in which there is cell death, confluent enough leading to formation of blisters.

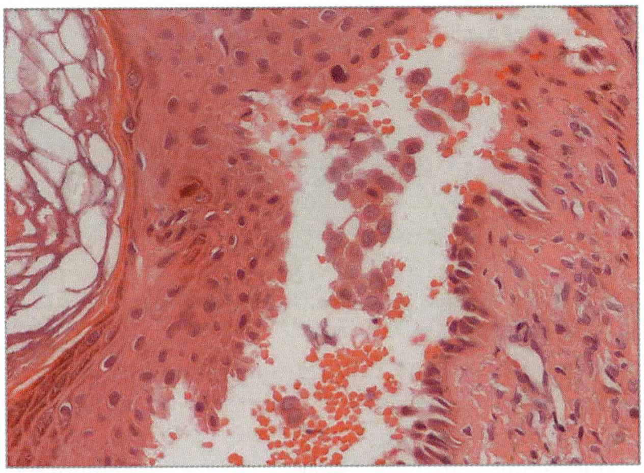

Fig. 5: Vesicobullous tissue reaction. Suprabasal split containing acantholytic cells, RBCs, and fibrin. Separation of basal keratinocytes from each other while being attached to basement membrane, forming 'row of tombstones' in pemphigus vulgaris (H&E, ×400).

The disorders in this group can be differentiated on the basis of level of split, type of cells in the split, and mechanism of formation of blisters. According to the level of split, these disorders can be classified as subcorneal, intraepidermal, suprabasal, and subepidermal **(Table 7)**. A paucicellular split is seen in inherited disorders like epidermolysis bullosa while immune-bullous disorders usually show numerous cells.

Histopathological findings vary according to the age of the lesion biopsied. Early stage may show only edema and an infiltrate without a split. On the other hand, one may see features of regeneration and epidermal hyperplasia at late stages. Hence, well developed lesions should be biopsied.

Important disorders showing this reaction pattern are pemphigus, pemphigoid, dermatitis herpetiformis, linear IgA disease, and epidermolysis bullosa.

Vasculitic Reaction Pattern

This reaction pattern is characterized by inflammation directed at blood vessels manifesting as fibrin deposition in the walls of vessels and around them, extravasation of RBCs and a tight perivascular and interstitial infiltrate usually of neutrophils and eosinophils **(Fig. 6)**. Degeneration of

TABLE 7: Disorders with vesicobullous reaction pattern.

Subcorneal blistering disorders	*Pemphigus foliaceus* • Split in subcorneal region with acantholytic cells in the split. Dyskeratotic keratinocytes are commonly seen, in addition • *Differential diagnosis*: Pemphigus herpetiformis, IgA pemphigus (subcorneal type), pemphigus erythematosus
Suprabasal blistering disorders	*Pemphigus vulgaris* • Suprabasal split containing acantholytic keratinocytes • *Differential diagnosis*: IgA pemphigus (intraepidermal type) • DIF shows a intercellular, fish-net pattern of IgG deposition *Pemphigus vegetans* • Pseudoepitheliomatous hyperplasia, downward prolongation of rete ridges • Eosinophilic microabscesses in epidermis • Upper dermal edema with heavy infiltrate of lymphocytes and eosinophils • Acantholytic cells may be seen *Paraneoplastic pemphigus* • Variable features owing to the polymorphous clinical features • Combination of suprabasal acantholysis and lichenoid tissue reaction with lymphocyte exocytosis, dyskeratotic keratinocytes • Upper dermal band-like infiltrate of lymphocytes and histiocytes • DIF shows deposits of C3 and IgG both in a fish-net pattern and also at the basement membrane *Darier's disease* • Suprabasal cleft with acantholysis and dyskeratotic cells • Dyskeratotic cells in the form of corps ronds and grains in stratum corneum and spinosum, respectively • Overlying keratin plug with parakeratosis • *Differential diagnosis*: Pemphigus vulgaris (no hyper- and parakeratosis, fewer dyskeratotic keratinocytes), Hailey-Hailey disease (more acantholysis) *Hailey-Hailey disease* • Suprabasal cleft with acantholytic cells lining and within the cleft • "Dilapidated brick wall" appearance due to widespread acantholysis at different levels of the epidermis • Negative direct immunofluorescence

Contd...

Contd...

Subepidermal blistering disorders	*Bullous pemphigoid* • Subepidermal split containing inflammatory cells, predominantly eosinophils. Clinically noninflammed blister are paucicellular on biopsy • Eosinophilic spongiosis with upper and deep perivascular infiltrates of eosinophils and lymphocytes, is the only finding in early urticarial stage • DIF shows homogeneous linear deposits of C3 and IgG at basement membrane zone
	Linear IgA bullous dermatosis/chronic bullous disease of childhood • Subepidermal split containing predominantly neutrophils with occasional eosinophils • DIF shows linear homogeneous IgA deposits at basement membrane
	Dermatitis herpetiformis • Collections of neutrophils in papillary dermis, also known as, papillary dermal microabscesses • Granular IgA deposits at basement membrane seen in DIF
	Epidermolysis bullosa acquisita • Subepidermal split, paucicellular or with neutrophils and eosinophils in the split • DIF shows linear deposits of C3 and IgG (similar to bullous pemphigoid). Salt split skin studies are required for differentiation

(DIF: direct immunofluorescence)

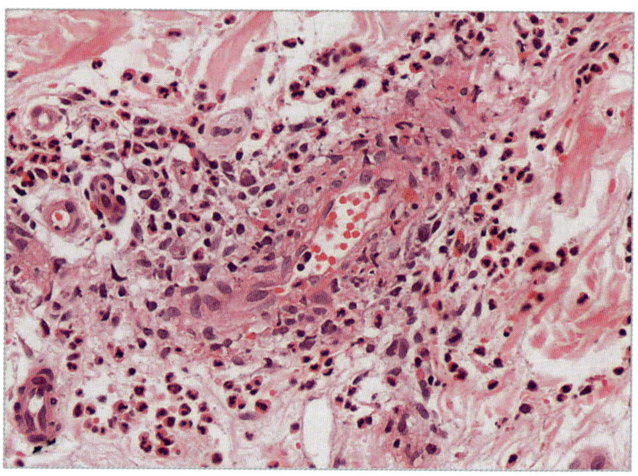

Fig. 6: Vasculitic tissue reaction. Fibrin deposition in vessel wall, multiple neutrophils, RBCs and fragmented neutrophils (leukocytoclasia) within and surrounding a small caliber vessel in vasculitis (H&E, ×400).

TABLE 8: Disorders with vasculitic/vasculopathic pattern.

Vasculitis	• Neutrophils in the vessel walls • Leukocytoclasia or fragmented nuclear dust of neutrophils surrounding vessel walls • Extravasation of red blood cells • Fibrinoid necrosis of vessel walls, seen as eosinophilic thickened walls • Depth and type of vessel involved (small, medium or large) depends on the type of vasculitis
Vasculopathy	• Thickening of vessel walls with deposition of fibrinoid material • Thrombi in vessels • Absent inflammation

neutrophils with fragmentation of their nuclei, referred to as leukocytoclasia, is a feature **(Table 8)**. Endothelial swelling is noted. Henoch-Schönlein purpura is the prototypical disorder but all these findings may not be present in every case and finding 2–3 features, in the appropriate clinical context, is diagnostic.

In some cases, the infiltrates around vessels may be lymphocytes (lymphocytic vasculitis) or epithelioid cells (granulomatous vasculitis).

The finding of an infiltrate within the wall of medium sized vessels is evidence for vasculitis but does not have the same significance in small vessels which may show diapedesis as a normal finding. When fibrin deposits within lumina and in the walls of vessels dominate the picture without significant inflammatory infiltrates, the term vasculopathy is used. Some vasculitic disorders may show this picture but the differential diagnosis primarily includes prothrombotic states.

The various disorders in this group can be differentiated on the basis of the caliber of vessel affected, the composition of the infiltrate, and additional findings including direct immunofluorescence (DIF).

Panniculitis

This reaction pattern is characterized by inflammation by of the subcutaneous tissue, exclusively or predominantly. The process may involve lobules of adipocytes or the fibrous septae separating them, or both. Lobular panniculitis is characterized by an infiltrate that extends between individual adipocytes and pushes them apart. In septal panniculitis, infiltrate, and edema pushes fat lobules apart. Septal infiltrates may spill into the adjacent lobule but the center of the lobule is typically spared. Similarly, lobular infiltrates may extend into the septae but the bulk is within the lobule. In some condition, both septum and lobule are affected **(Fig. 7)**. Adipocyte damage manifests as fatty microcysts and macrocysts and lipophages, which may persist as markers of lobular inflammation even after the infiltrate has subsided. Long standing septal inflammation results in thickening and fibrosis of the septae. Early stages of most panniculitides have infiltrates of neutrophils while chronic

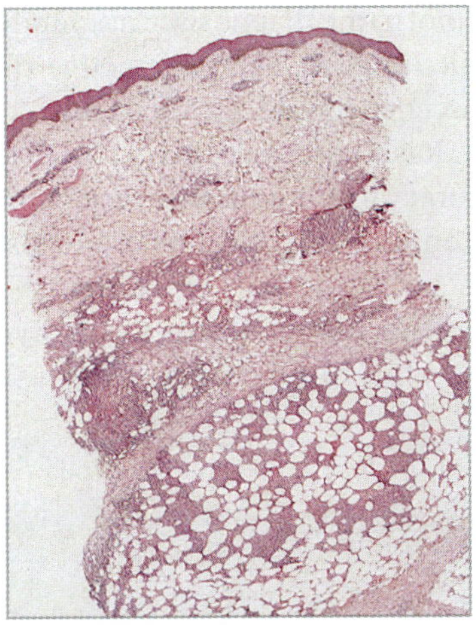

Fig. 7: Panniculitis. Inflammatory infiltrate in fat lobules extending between individual adipocytes and in the septae between adjacent lobules (H&E, ×100).

lesions show admixture of lymphocytes, histiocytes, and giant cells. This is followed by fibrosis.

The part of the subcutis affected the composition of the infiltrate, the presence or absence of associated vasculitis, and other additional findings are useful to differentiate the different panniculitides.

Erythema nodosum is the prototype septal panniculitis. Histopathological findings vary with the age of lesion. Early lesions show predominance of neutrophils. This is followed by an infiltrate of lymphocytes, histiocytes, epithelioid cells variably forming giant cells in the septae. Histiocytes arranged radially around minute slits constitute Miescher's radial granulomas. However, these are not specific to erythema nodosum and may be seen in a number of other panniculitides. Septal fibrosis is noted in later stages.

Lobular panniculitis is seen in erythema induratum. There is an infiltrate of neutrophils, lymphocytes, histiocytes, plasma cells within the lobule accompanied by small, focal aggregates of epithelioid cells, and giant cells. Vasculitis of small and/or medium vessels is noted.

Other disorders showing this reaction pattern include lupus panniculitis, panniculitic lymphoma, morphea, subcutaneous fat necrosis of newborn, and lipodermatosclerosis **(Table 9)**.

TUMORS AND PROLIFERATIONS

The skin shows both benign and malignant neoplasms which may arise from the many cells types that are seen in the skin including keratinocytes, melanocytes, adnexal structures, and soft tissues. Benign neoplasms are usually well circumscribed, symmetrical, show smooth borders and bland looking cells. Malignant neoplasms are poorly circumscribed with an infiltrative margin, asymmetrical, and show cytological atypia, mitotic figures, and necrosis.[8] The number of different neoplasms in the skin is too large to cover each separately

TABLE 9: Disorders with panniculitic reaction pattern.

Septal panniculitis	*Erythema nodosum* • Inflammation centered in the septae of fat lobules • Acute stages show infiltrate of neutrophils, lymphocytes, histiocytes, and epithelioid cells in the septae • Fibrosis of septae and paucity of cells in chronic lesions • Miescher radial granulomas, although considered pathognomonic, are nonspecific, also found in Behcet's syndrome, Sweet's syndrome, erythema induratum *Morphea* • Septal thickening with presence of plasma cells, lymphocytes and histiocytes • Squaring-off of edges of biopsy due to thick collagen bundles • Homogenized collagen bundles in lower dermis • Obliteration of spaces around appendages
Lobular panniculitis	*Erythema induratum* • Infiltrate of lymphocytes, histiocytes, and epithelioid cells in lobules • Spilling of infiltrate can occur in adjacent septae • Fibrosis in later stages • Vasculitis of small/medium vessels, seen occasionally *Lupus panniculitis* • Lobular panniculitis with prominent lymphoplasmacytic infiltrate • In up to half the cases there are epidermal and dermal changes of lupus erythematosus (particularly in those complicating discoid lupus erythematosus) • Lymphoid follicles adjacent to fibrous septa, seen in about 20–50% • Lipophages and lipomembranous changes may be seen • *Differential diagnosis*: Subcutaneous panniculitis-like T-cell lymphoma (SPTCL) shows overlapping features and can be histopathologically impossible to distinguish. Epidermal involvement, lymphoid follicles, prominent plasma cells point toward lupus panniculitis while atypical lymphocytes with bean bag cells indicate SPTCL *Subcutaneous fat necrosis of newborn* • Infiltrate of lymphocytes, histiocytes, foreign-body type giant cells and occasional plasma cells in lobules • Focal fat necrosis with cyst formation • Fine, needle-like crystals representing triglycerides, seen in narrow clefts radiating from a point near the periphery of the cell • Calcification foci in older lesions • *Differential diagnosis*: Needle-shaped crystals are also seen in sclerema neonatorum and steroid panniculitis. Inflammation is absent in former and of mixed type in latter *Lipodermatosclerosis* • Septal lymphocytic infiltrate rims the fat lobules • Associated capillary congestion and thrombosis, hemorrhage with hemosiderin deposition • Later stages show septal thickening, hyaline sclerosis with lipophage formation • Advanced lesions show marked septal sclerosis and lipomembranous change with reduced inflammation

but the **Table 10** describes the prominent histopathological findings in some important and/or commonly encountered tumors.

IMMUNOFLUORESCENCE

Immunofluorescence is an immunohistochemical technique to detect antibodies to the tissue bound antigens in DIF or circulating antibodies in indirect immunofluorescence. It is a valuable tool in the diagnosis of autoimmune disorders, especially vesicobullous and connective tissue diseases. Immunofluorescence should not be considered as a substitute for skin biopsy. It is a complementary tool that enhances the diagnostic accuracy in autoimmune vesicobullous disorders, when used in conjunction with clinical and histopathological findings.

It involves the use of fluorescent dye-conjugated antibodies that bind to the target antigen. The dyes used

TABLE 10: Histopathological findings in commonly seen tumors.

Basal cell carcinoma (Fig. 8)	• Islands of basaloid proliferation in dermis, an attachment to epidermis is usually seen • Peripheral palisading of cells • Retraction clefts between cells and stroma • Mitotic figures common, may be atypical • Necrotic keratinocytes seen commonly • Surrounding newly formed stroma may show variable amount of mucin • Amyloid may be seen in stroma in about 50% cases • Lymphocytic infiltrate in dermis seen in actively regressing tumors • Diffusely express BerEP4, CD10 • Histopathological types include superficial, pigmented, nodular (solid), micronodular, cystic, infiltrating, infundibulocystic, adenoid, sclerosing, keratotic, metatypical, basosquamous, and fibroepitheliomatous • *Differential diagnosis*: Trichoepithelioma (cribriform/racemose pattern, absent peripheral palisading and retraction clefts, negative for BerEP4 immunostaining)
Squamous cell carcinoma (Fig. 9)	• Nests of proliferating keratinocytes extending beyond basement membrane upto variable depths • Full thickness epidermal atypia • Keratinocytes show abundant cytoplasm and large hyperchromatic nuclei • Depending on degree of keratinization and nuclear atypia, can be graded into: well, moderately and poorly differentiated • Keratin pearls form in well differentiated tumors • Mitotic figures frequently seen • Perineural and vascular invasion seen in aggressive tumors • Immunostaining for epithelial membrane antigen, cytokeratins 5/6 positive • Histopathological types include verrucous, spindle cell or sarcomatoid, acantholytic, desmoplastic, follicular, keratoacanthoma-like, clear cell, signet-ring, adenosquamous, metaplastic, inflammatory, basaloid, pseudohyperplastic, basaloid, infiltrated, pigmented
Melanoma	• Asymmetrical and poorly circumscribed proliferation of melanocytes in dermis • Cells show hyperchromatic nuclei with clear cytoplasm containing melanin pigment • Atypical melanocytes often extend into epidermis (pagetoid spread) and often leading to consumption of epidermis with cleft formation • Lymphocytic infiltrate may be seen surrounding tumor aggregates in dermis • Extension into follicular epithelium may be seen • Atypical mitosis are seen but are not frequent • Lack of maturation of melanocytes at the base of tumor • Dermal fibrosis may be seen • Immunostaining for HMB45, Melan A, and S-100 is usually positive • Histopathological variants include *Lentigo maligna melanoma* shows atypical melanocytes irregularly distributed in basal layer of epidermis and dermal invasion; *superficial spreading melanoma* has scattered atypical melanocytes in epidermis (*buckshot scatter*); *nodular melanoma* shows bundles and nests of atypical melanocytes; *acral lentiginous melanoma* shows elongated rete ridges and scattered atypical melanocytes close to basal layer, *desmoplastic melanoma* with predominant spindle shaped atypical melanocytes in a fibrotic stroma in dermis often with lymphoplasmacytic infiltrate
Melanocytic nevus	• Nests of cuboidal and oval pigmented cells with clear cytoplasm in dermis • Aggregates show symmetrical architecture, vertically, and horizontally • Smaller, nonpigmented nests and sheets of cells that diminish in size deeper in the lesion, also called maturation, differentiates it from melanoma • Classified into: *Junctional nevi* that are limited to dermoepidermal junction, *compound* with both junctional and dermal component and *intradermal* with only dermal component
Dermato-fibroma	• Reactive proliferation of histiocytes, also known as benign fibrous histiocytoma • Acanthotic epidermis with elongated rete ridges and increased basal layer pigmentation • Grenz zone seen beneath epidermis

Contd...

Contd...

	• Poorly demarcated proliferation of histiocytes and fibrocytes in dermis, often arranged with the long axis parallel to the epidermis • Entrapment of collagen fibers, often at the periphery of lesion • No extension into subcutis • Histopathological variants include *cellular, atypical, aneurysmal, hemosiderotic, lipidized, palisading,* and *clear cell dermatofibroma* • Immunostaining positive for factor XIIIa and CD68 • *Differential diagnosis*: Other spindle cell proliferations including neurofibroma, vascular tumors, dermatofibrosarcoma protuberans- storiform arrangement of spindle cells, extension into subcutis and, stains positively for CD34 and negatively for factor XIIIa, CD68, unlike dermatofibroma
Neurofibroma	• Noncapsulated, proliferation of pale spindle cells in dermis • Proliferation of all elements of peripheral nerves • Cells have wavy slender nuclei with pointed ends • Stroma may show increased mucin • Mast cells often increased in number • Proliferation of nerve bundles in plexiform neurofibroma
Syringoma	• Dermal tumors composed of multiple small ducts lined by two layers of cuboidal epithelium • Multiple islands of cuboidal cells arranged in nests, cords and tubules limited to upper dermis • "Comma" or "tadpole" shaped epithelial islands appearing as *paisley tie pattern* • Sclerosis of surrounding stroma • No extension in subcutis • Stain positively for carcinoembryonic antigen (CEA) • *Differential diagnosis: Desmoplastic trichoepithelioma* consisting of multiple keratinous cysts, with a peripheral basaloid layer and several layers of stratified squamous epithelium with central loosely laminated horn, stain positive for CK20 and involucrin and negative for CEA, *desmoplastic basal cell carcinoma, microcystic adnexal carcinoma* which usually extends into subcutis and shows aggressive growth with perineural invasion
Mycosis fungoides	• Multiple biopsies recommended as diagnosis may be missed with single biopsy • Epidermotropism, seen as lymphocytes in the epidermis in the absence of significant spongiosis; lymphocytes may be aligned along the basal layer of epidermis, have haloes around them and are larger than lymphocytes in the dermis; most pronounced in plaque stage and absent in tumors and erythrodermic stages • Atypical lymphocytes show enlarged hyperchromatic nuclei and convoluted or cerebriform nuclear contours; intraepidermal collections are known as Pautrier's microabscesses • Wiry collagen bundles in papillary dermis • Tumor stage shows a diffuse infiltrate of atypical lymphocytes with pleomorphic and hyperchromatic nuclei and prominent nucleoli throughout the dermis which may extend into subcutis, epidermotropism is absent • Erythrodermic mycosis fungoides often shows nonspecific spongiotic reaction pattern, with parakeratosis, spongiosis, absent epidermotropism. Atypical lymphocytes may be seen in dermis • Immunostaining usually positive for CD3 and CD4 and negative for CD7 • Histopathological variants include *folliculotropic, hypopigmented, granulomatous slack skin, pagetoid reticulosis* and *syringotropic mycosis fungoides*

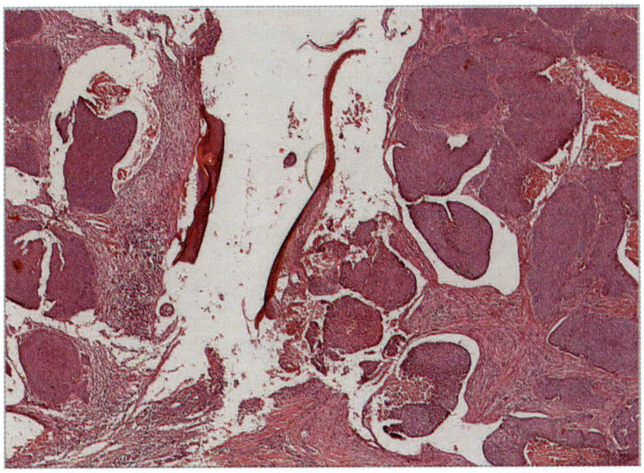

Fig. 8: Basal cell carcinoma. Multiple islands of basaloid cells with prominent retraction clefts between the cells and stroma in dermis (H&E, × 400).

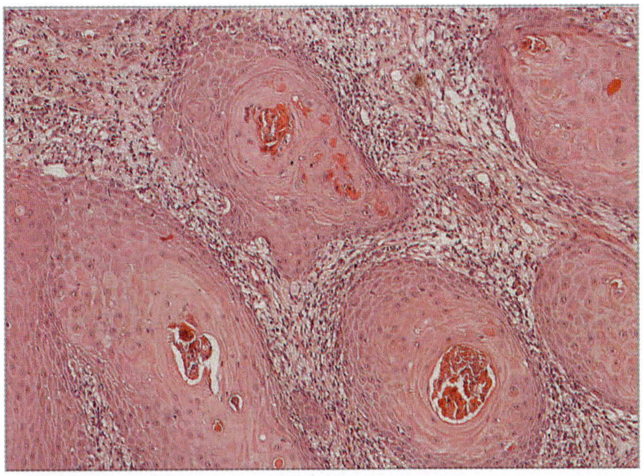

Fig. 9: Squamous cell carcinoma. Nests of proliferating keratinocytes in dermis with differentiation into keratin along with dyskeratotic keratinocytes in the center of nests. Mixed infiltrates of lymphocytes, histiocytes, and neutrophils seen surrounding the neoplastic cells (H&E, × 400).

include fluorescein isothiocyanate (FITC) and tetramethyl rhodamine isothiocyanate (TRITC). The resulting immune complexes are visualized under an ultraviolet microscope. Collection of skin biopsy from appropriate site is of utmost importance. Biopsy in vesicobullous diseases should be obtained from the uninvolved perilesional area, within 1 cm and 3–5 mm of the lesion, in the skin and mucosa, respectively. Lesional biopsy from a lesion not more than 24 hours old, is preferred in vasculitides.[9] Skin biopsy in lupus erythematosus is best taken from sun-protected sites, as the staining in these sites correlates with a diagnosis of systemic lupus erythematosus and renal involvement. Ideally, a fresh lesion, not more than 48 hours old, should be taken. The biopsy is transported to a laboratory in Michel's or Zeus medium. In case the laboratory is nearby, normal saline may be used.[10] The salient direct immunofluorescence findings seen in autoimmune disorders are mentioned in **Table 11**.

A general approach to diagnosis of skin biopsy is depicted in **Flowchart 1**. *Certain "named" histological findings and diagnostic histological findings in dermatological disorders are mentioned in **Tables 12 and 13**.*

Flowchart 1: Approach to diagnosis of skin biopsy.

Examine slide under low power to identify the broad reaction pattern

↓

Examine under medium and high power to confirm findings of the reaction pattern

↓

Look for additional findings that characterize individual conditions

↓

- Reach a specific diagnosis
- If a specific diagnosis cannot be made, describe the reaction pattern and any additional findings

TABLE 11: Direct immunofluorescence findings in autoimmune disorders.

Disorder	*Direct immunofluorescence findings*
Pemphigus vulgaris	• Intraepidermal deposits of IgG and C3, in a fish-net pattern • The staining is more intense in the basal layers of epidermis
Pemphigus foliaceus	Similar to pemphigus vulgaris, except that the staining may be more intense in the superficial layers of epidermis
Bullous pemphigoid	• Linear homogeneous deposition of IgG and C3 at the dermoepidermal junction • The deposits are seen at the roof of blister in a salt-split skin
Pemphigoid gestationis	Linear homogeneous deposition of C3, and rarely IgG, at the dermoepidermal junction
Epidermolysis bullosa acquisita	• Linear homogeneous deposits of IgG and C3 at the dermoepidermal junction • Deposits are seen at the floor in a salt-split skin
Dermatitis herpetiformis	Granular deposition of IgA at the tips of dermal papillae
Linear IgA bullous disease/chronic bullous disease of childhood	Linear homogeneous deposition of IgA at dermoepidermal junction
Mucous membrane pemphigoid	Linear homogeneous deposition of IgG and C3 at the dermoepidermal junction
Bullous systemic lupus erythematosus	Linear deposits of C3, fibrin and multiple immunoglobulins at the dermoepidermal junction
Lupus erythematosus	• Linear deposition of C3 and immunoglobulins in a speckled pattern at the basement membrane • Deposition of immunoglobulins other than IgM at non-sun exposed sites correlates with a diagnosis of systemic lupus erythematosus and renal involvement
Vasculitides	Immunoglobulins, chiefly IgA, and complement in the vessel walls

TABLE 12: Histologic bodies and entities in dermatology.

Name	*Description*	*Found in*
Arao-Perkins bodies	Small fibrous bodies at the base of dermal papilla in hair follicle	Normal hair follicle
Asteroid bodies	Eosinophilic star-shaped bodies	Sporotrichosis, sarcoidosis, other granulomatous disorders
Banana bodies	Exogenous yellow to brown material, with curvilinear/ banana shape, in papillary dermis	Ochronosis
Bean bag cells	Phagocytosis of lymphocytes, RBCs or neutrophils in histiocytes	Cytophagic histiocytic panniculitis
Caterpillar bodies	Elongated , segmented eosinophilic PAS positive globules arranged linearly in papillary dermis	Porphyria cutanea tarda,

Contd...

Contd...

Name	*Description*	*Found in*
Cholesterol clefts	Small empty spaces filled with cholesterol/fat	Sclerema neonatorum, subcutaneous fat necrosis of newborn, necrobiotic xanthogranuloma, erythema elevatum diutinum, necrobiosis lipoidica diabeticorum
Civatte bodies/colloid bodies	Round eosinophilic pyknotic nuclei in the epidermis (civatte bodies) or papillary dermis (colloid bodies/ necrotic keratinocytes)	Lichen planus, systemic lupus erythematosus
Cowdry Type A inclusion bodies	Eosinophilic nuclear inclusion bodies	Herpes virus infection
Cowdry Type B inclusion bodies	Basophilic nuclear inclusion bodies	Polio virus
Donovan bodies	Rod-shaped organisms inside macrophages, basophilic with Giemsa stain	Granuloma inguinale
Flame figures	Degranulation of eosinophils around collagen fibers	Eosinophilic cellulitis
Gargoyle cells	Large oval cell, around 20 µm diameter, with a pale central nucleus and cytoplasm appearing clear (H&E) or granular (toluidine blue)	Hurler disease
Grains and Corp ronds	Two types of dyskeratotic cells are seen in Darier's disease-grains are oval cells with elongated nuclei and abundant keratohyaline granules, located in stratum corneum; corps ronds consist of irregular eccentric pyknotic nucleus with perinuclear halo and eosinophilic cytoplasm, seen in stratum spinosum and stratum granulosum	Darier's disease
Gamma-Favre body	Large, intracytoplasmic basophilic inclusion bodies in endothelial cells	Lymphogranuloma venereum
Henderson-Patterson bodies	Eosinophilic intracytoplasmic inclusion bodies	Molluscum contagiosum
Kamino bodies	Dull-pink globules at the tips of dermal papilla	Spitz nevi
Copper penny bodies/ sclerotic/muriform/medlar bodies	Brown colored oval bodies, representing fungal spores, seen in the dermis	Chromomycosis
Miescher's radial Granuloma	Histiocytes arranged radially around a central cleft	Erythema nodosum, Behçet's disease, Sweet's syndrome, nodular vasculitis
Miescher's granuloma/ O'Brien's granuloma	Annular plaques on face/sun-exposed areas, that show granulomatous tissue reaction with elastophagocytosis in skin biopsy	Annular elastolytic giant cell granuloma
Michaelis-Gutmann bodies	Concentric basophilic inclusions measuring 2–10 µm	Malakoplakia
Mikulicz cell	Large foamy macrophages containing gram negative bacilli	Rhinoscleroma
Munro microabscess	Collection of neutrophils in stratum corneum due to squirting from papillary dermis	Psoriasis
Negri bodies	Round or oval cytoplasmic inclusions within nerve cells	Rabies
Pautrier microabscesses	Collection of atypical lymphocytes within the epidermis	Cutaneous T-cell lymphoma
Russell bodies	Large eosinophilic homogeneous inclusions composed of immunoglobulins in a plasma cell	Plasma cell diseases
Verocay body, Antoni A and B	Architectural patterns seen in Schwannomas: Type A is highly cellular and demonstrates nuclear palisading; type B shows loose stroma, fewer cells, and myxoid change	Schwannoma
Schaumann bodies	Basophilic inclusion bodies composed of calcium and protein	Sarcoidosis
Koilocytes	Vacuolated keratinocytes with pyknotic nucleus and perinuclear halo	Verruca

TABLE 13: Characteristic histologic findings in certain disorders.

Characteristic histologic findings	*Found in*
Follicular plugging	Pityriasis rubra pilaris, lupus erythematosus (LE), lichen planopilaris (LPP), lichen sclerosus
Cornoid lamella	Porokeratosis
Alternating parakeratosis	Actinic keratosis (AK)
"Checkerboard" and "shoulder" parakeratosis	Pityriasis rubra pilaris
"Church spire" papillomatosis	Acrokeratosis verruciformis
Max Joseph space	Lichen planus
"Claw" clutching a "ball" appearance	Lichen nitidus
Windblown appearance	Bowen's disease
Eosinophilic spongiosis	Arthropod bite, pemphigoid, pemphigus, incontinentia pigmenti (IP), drug eruption, contact dermatitis
Pagetoid cells	Bowen's disease, melanoma, recurrent nevus, Paget's disease, CTCL, lymphomatoid papulomatosis (LyP), Langerhans cell histiocytosis (LCH)
Dilapidated brick wall	Hailey-Hailey disease
Row of tombstone appearance	Pemphigus vulgaris
Squamous eddies	Irritated seborrheic keratosis (SK), inverted follicular keratosis (IFK), SCC, trichoblastoma
Horn pseudocysts	Seborrheic keratosis (SK), IFK, trichoepithelioma,
Grenz zone	Lepromatous leprosy, granuloma faciale, lymphocytoma cutis, leukemia cutis
Thickening of basement membrane	Discoid lupus erythematosus, porphyria cutanea tarda
Extravasated red blood cells	Pityriasis rosea, pityriasis lichenoides et varioliformis acuta (PLEVA)
Vertically oriented collagen	Acquired digital fibrokeratoma
Necrobiosis	Granuloma annulare (GA), necrobiosis lipoidica diabeticorum (NLD), rheumatoid nodule, necrobiotic xanthogranuloma (NXG)
Tadpole-shaped structures	Syringoma
Jigsaw puzzle and hyalinized droplets	Cylindroma
Cannon balls in dermis	Eccrine spiradenoma
Coat-sleeving or perivascular cuffing of lymphocytes	Erythema annulare centrifugum (EAC)
"Naked" granulomas	Sarcoidosis
Touton giant cell	Xanthelasma, atypical fibroxanthoma (AFX), necrobiotic xanthogranuloma (NXG)
Ground glass giant cell	Multicentric reticulohistiocytosis
Ghost cells	Pilomatricoma, Pancreatic panniculitis
Swarm of bees	Alopecia areata
Needle-shaped clefts	Subcutaneous fat necrosis, sclerema neonatorum
Clear multivacuolated cells in fat	Hibernoma
Promontory sign, slit-like spaces	Kaposi sarcoma
Hob nailing (endothelial cells protrude into vessel)	Angiolymphoid hyperplasia with eosinophilia
Staghorn appearance	Hemangiopericytoma
"Indian" filing of cells	GA, congenital melanocytic nevus, lymphoma, leukemia
Painful tumors of skin	Blue rubber bleb, eccrine spiradenoma, neurilemmoma, glomus tumor, angiolipoma, leiomyoma
Chunks of coal appearance	Lymphomatoid papulosis
Promontory sign	Kaposi's sarcoma

KEY POINTS

- Epidermis is about 0.05–1 mm in thickness and consists of four layers: (1) Stratum corneum, (2) stratum granulosum, (3) stratum spinosum, and (4) stratum basale.
- Dermis measures around 1.5–4 mm in thickness and consists of connective tissue, blood vessels, and adnexal structures including hair follicles and glands, muscle, and nerves.
- Reaction pattern refers to a set of findings that are suggestive of broad groups of disorders. Recognition of reaction patterns in a biopsy is an important initial step in the assessment.
- Major reaction patterns and their prototype disorders are: Lichenoid tissue reaction—lichen planus, psoriasiform—psoriasis, spongiotic—dermatitis, granulomatous—tuberculosis, vesicobullous—pemphigus, panniculitis—septal in erythema nodosum and lobular in erythema induratum, and vasculitis—Henoch-Schönlein purpura.
- Benign and malignant neoplasms may arise from the many cell types that are seen in the skin including keratinocytes, melanocytes, adnexal structures, and soft tissues. Immunohistochemistry is a helpful complementary tool in making diagnosis in neoplasms.
- Immunofluorescence is a valuable adjunct to clinical and histopathological findings in autoimmune disorders.

REFERENCES

1. McGrath JA, Uitto J. Structure and function of the skin. In: Griffiths C, Barker J, Bleiker T, Chalmers R, Creamer D (Eds). Rook's Textbook of Dermatology, 9th edition. New York: John Wiley & Sons Ltd.; 2016. pp. 2.1-2.48.
2. Schach CP, Smoller BR, Hudson AR, Horn TD. Immunohistochemical stains in dermatopathology. J Am Acad Dermatol. 2000;43:1094-100.
3. Calonje E, Brenn T, Lazar A, McKee P. McKee's Pathology of the Skin with Clinical Correlations, 4th edition. New York: Elsevier Mosby; 2011.
4. Ackerman AB, Boer A, Bennin B, Gottlieb GG. Histologic Diagnosis of Inflammatory Skin Diseases, 3rd edition. New York: Ardor Scribendi; 2004.
5. Panth A, Ramam M. Epidermal reaction patterns. Indian J Dermatopathol Diagn Dermatol. 2015;2:1-7.
6. Tirumalae R. Psoriasiform dermatoses: microscopic approach. Indian J Dermatol. 2013;58(4):290-3.
7. Yadav D, Ramam M. Epithelioid cell granuloma. Indian J Dermatopathol Diagn Dermatol. 2018;5:7-18.
8. Khandpur S, Ramam M. Skin tumours. J Cutan Aesthet Surg. 2012;5:159-62.
9. Elston DM, Stratman EJ, Miller SJ. Skin biopsy: biopsy issues in specific diseases. J Am Acad Dermatol. 2016;74:1-24.
10. Patel AN, Simpson RC, Cohen SN. In a patient with an immunobullous disorder, is transportation of the skin biopsy in normal saline adequate for direct immunofluorescence analysis? A critically appraised topic. Br J Dermatol. 2013;169:6-10.

EXAMINATION QUESTIONS

1. Enlist the major reaction patterns and prototype disorder for each pattern.
2. Classify panniculitis according to histopathological features.
3. Describe the histopathological features of epidermal neoplasms—basal cell carcinoma and squamous cell carcinoma.
4. Write a short note on HPE of erythema multiforme.
5. Write a short note on acantholysis and dyskeratosis.
6. Write a short note on interface dermatitis. Discuss dermatologic disease having interface dermatitis, with their characteristic histological features.
7. Define and classify granulomas in dermatology.
8. What are the major reaction patterns in dermatology? Briefly describe any three reaction patterns.
9. Discuss noninfective granuloma in dermatology.
10. Define necrobiosis. Write a short note on necrobiotic granuloma.
11. Write a short note on giant cell.

8 CHAPTER

Clinical Signs in Dermatology and Approach to Diagnosis

Monali Pattnaik

INTRODUCTION

All students of dermatology need a basic foundation and framework upon which to accumulate knowledge. The secret for learning dermatology is to adapt the same skill sets that enable you to recognize primary and secondary skin lesions clinically and relate them to the history or findings. In contrast to other fields, patient should be examined before a detailed history is taken because patients can see their lesion and thus often present with a history that is flawed with their own interpretation. History can be more focused following the objective findings. Thus, a proper physical examination and analysis are essential.

TAKING A DERMATOLOGICAL HISTORY

Using the standard structure of history taking, following are the important points to consider when taking a history from a patient with a skin problem.

- *Presenting complaint*: Nature, site, and duration of problem
- *History of presenting complaint*:
  - Initial appearance and evolution of lesion
  - Symptoms (particularly itch and pain)
  - Aggravating and relieving factors
  - Previous and current treatments (effective or not)
  - Recent contact, stressful events, illness, and travel
  - History of sunburn and use of tanning machines
  - Skin type **(Table 1)**
- *Past medical history*:
  - History of atopy, i.e., asthma, allergic rhinitis, eczema, and tuberculosis
  - History of skin cancer and suspicious skin lesions

TABLE 1: Skin types.

Skin type	*Color*	*Feature*
I	Pale white skin, blue/green eyes, blond/red hair	Always burns, does not tan
II	Fair skin, blue eyes	Burns easily, tans poorly
III	Darker white skin	Tans after initial burn
IV	Light brown	Burns minimally, tans easily
V	Brown skin	Rarely burns, tans easily
VI	Dark brown	Never burns, always tans

- *Family history*: Family history of skin disease
- *Social history:*
  - Occupation (including skin contacts at work)
  - Improvement of lesions when away from work
- *Medication and allergies*: Regular, recent, and over-the-counter medications
- *Impact on quality of life*: Impact of skin condition and concerns

Physical examination: General examination of all systems

Vital signs: Pulse, respiration, and temperature

Whether uncomfortable, well, sick

EXAMINING THE SKIN

- *Inspect in general*:
  - General observation
  - Site and number of lesions
  - If multiple, pattern of distribution and configuration
- *Describe the individual lesion*: **SCAMM S**ize (the widest diameter), **S**hape, **C**olor, **A**ssociated secondary change, **M**orphology, **M**argin (border)
- *Palpate the individual lesion surface*: Consistency, mobility, tenderness, temperature
- *Systemic check*: Examine the nails, scalp, hair, and mucous membranes

The entire skin should be examined including all mucous membranes, hairs, and nails

Classically skin lesions are classified into:

- *Primary lesion* representing the initial basic lesion **(Table 2)**
- *Secondary lesion* which may result from evolution of primary lesion or may be created by scratching or infection **(Table 3)**

The *prerequisite* of dermatologic diagnosis includes:

- Type of lesion
- Color **(Table 4)**
- Margination
- Shape
- Arrangement
- Distribution of lesions **(Figs. 1 to 10)**
- Palpatory findings of lesions **(Box 1)**.

TABLE 2: Types of primary lesion.

Term	*Clinical feature*	*Clinical disorder*
Macule	Flat (nonpalpable), circumscribed, differs in color from surrounding skin, neither elevated nor suppressed • <1 cm in diameter	Ephelides (freckles) • Lentigo • Idiopathic guttate hypomelanosis • Petechiae • Flat component of viral exanthems
Patch	Flat (nonpalpable), circumscribed, differs in color from surrounding skin • >1 cm in diameter	Vitiligo • Melasma • Dermal melanocytosis (Mongolian spot) • Café-au-lait macule • Nevus depigmentosus • Solar purpura
Papule (Fig. 10)	Elevated (palpable), circumscribed • <1 cm in diameter May have secondary changes (e.g., scale, crust) • The profile can be flat-topped (lichenoid), dome-shaped	Seborrheic keratosis Compound melanocytic nevus, verruca, molluscum contagiosum • Lichen nitidus • Small-vessel vasculitis
Plaque	Elevated (palpable) circumscribed • >1 cm in diameter • May have secondary changes (e.g., scale, crust)	Psoriasis • Lichen simplex chronicus • Nummular dermatitis • Hypertrophic scar **(Fig. 4)**, keloid, morphea
Nodule	Palpable, circumscribed • Larger volume than papule, usually >1 cm in diameter • Involves the dermis and/or the subcutis	Lipomas, neurofibromas, panniculitis, e.g., erythema nodosum • Lymphoma
Wheal	Transient elevation of the skin due to dermal edema, often pale centrally with an erythematous rim	Urticaria
Vesicle	Elevated, circumscribed • <1 cm in diameter, filled with fluid—clear, serous, or hemorrhagic	Herpes simplex, varicella or zoster • Dyshidrotic eczema
Bulla	Elevated, circumscribed • >1 cm in diameter • Filled with fluid	Bullous pemphigoid • Bullous fixed drug eruption
Pustule	Elevated, circumscribed • Usually <1 cm in diameter • From its onset, filled with purulent fluid	*Follicularly centered* • Folliculitis • Acne vulgaris *Non-follicularly centered* • Pustular psoriasis • Acute generalized exanthematous

TABLE 3: Secondary feature.

Term	*Description*	*Example*
Crust (Fig. 2)	• Dried serum, blood or pus on the surface of the skin • May include bacteria (usually *Staphylococcus*)	Secondarily infected hand dermatitis • Eczema/dermatitis (multiple types) • Impetigo • Later phase of herpes simplex, varicella or zoster • Erythema multiforme
Scale	• Hyperkeratosis • Accumulation of stratum corneum due to increased proliferation and/or delayed desquamation	• Psoriasis [silvery (micaceous) scale] • Tinea (leading scale) • Erythema annulare centrifugum (trailing scale) • Pityriasis (tinea) versicolor [powdery (furfuraceous)] scale
Excoriation	Exogenous injury to all or part of the epidermis (epithelium) • May be linear or punctate	Pruritic conditions like atopy, acne excoriee
Fissure	Linear cleft in skin • Often painful • Results from marked drying, skin thickening, and loss of elasticity	Angular cheilitis • Hand dermatitis • Sebopsoriasis (intergluteal fold) • Irritant cheilitis
Erosion	Partial loss of the epidermis (epithelium)	Pemphigus vulgaris, trauma

Contd...

Contd...

Term	*Description*	*Example*
Ulcer	Full-thickness loss of the epidermis (epithelium) • May have loss of the dermis or even subcutis • The size, shape, and depth should be described as well as the characteristics of the border, base, and surrounding tissue	Ecthyma, pyoderma gangrenosum
Infarct	Ischemia of tissue • Color can vary from gray–white to purple to black	Can be due to vascular compromise (e.g., atherosclerosis, calciphylaxis), thrombosis, vasculitis, emboli (infectious or noninfectious), or vasospasm
Atrophy	Looks shiny and wrinkled (if thinning of the epidermis) or Depressed (if loss of dermal collagen)	Striae anetoderma
Lichenification	Accentuation of natural skin lines, reflecting thickening (acanthosis). Often due to rubbing	Lichen simplex chronicus

TABLE 4: Diagnosis of dermatologic disorders based on color of the lesions.

Color	*Example*	*Color*	*Example*
Erythema (pink to red-brown, depending upon the skin phototype)	Dermatitis • Psoriasis • Morbilliform drug eruption • Viral exanthems • Any insult that causes vasodilation	**Purple**	Purpura, nonpalpable (e.g., solar purpura) • Purpura, palpable (e.g., small vessel vasculitis) • Vascular neoplasms (e.g., angiokeratoma, angiosarcoma) • Lichen planus • Lymphoma cutis • Pyoderma gangrenosum—border • Morphea—border
Black	• Vasculitis (granulomatosis with polyangiitis) • Thrombosis (e.g., DIC, monoclonal cryoglobulinemia) • Emboli (e.g., ecthyma gangrenosum) • Vasospasm (e.g., severe Raynaud's phenomenon) • Vascular compromise (e.g., atherosclerosis, calciphylaxis) – Eschar (e.g., anthrax) – Cutaneous melanoma – Traumatic tattoos	**White**	Absence of melanocytes or melanin production (e.g., vitiligo, piebaldism, OCA1A) • Scarring (e.g., scarring in discoid lupus erythematosus) • Vasospasm (e.g., Raynaud's phenomenon, nevus anemicus) • Deposits (e.g., calcinosis cutis, gouty tophi) • Macerated stratum corneum—mucosal surfaces (e.g., leukoplakia)
Blue	Dermal melanocytosis (e.g., Mongolian spot, nevus of Ota) • Dermal melanocytomas (e.g., blue nevi) • Cyanosis • Ecchymoses • Venous congestion (e.g., venous malformations) • Drugs/deposits (e.g., minocycline, traumatic tattoos)	**Green**	*Pseudomonas* infection • Tattoo • Chloroma • Green hair due to copper deposits
Brown	Pigmented lesions • Lentigines • Seborrheic keratoses melanocytic nevi • Café-au-lait macules • Dermatofibromas • Melanoma • Pigmented AKs, Bowen disease	**Orange red**	Pityriasis rubra pilaris, xanthogranulomas • Mycosis fungoides
Yellow	Carotenoderma • Xanthomas (e.g., xanthelasma, eruptive) • Necrobiosis lipoidica	**Gray**	Dermal pigmentation (e.g., erythema dyschromicum perstans) • Drugs/deposits (e.g., argyria, chrysiasis) • Combined melanocytic nevus • Traumatic tattoo

(AKs: actinic keratoses; DIC: disseminated intravascular coagulation; OCA1: oculocutaneous albinism type 1)

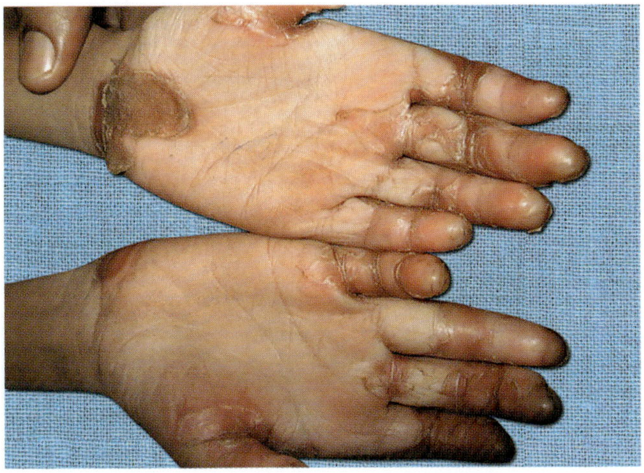

Fig. 1: Acral distribution in acrodermatitis enteropathica.

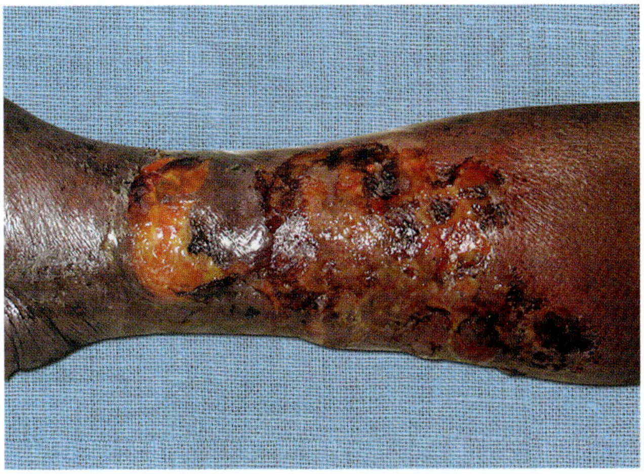

Fig. 2: Secondary lesions in form of crust, erosion over an ulcer.

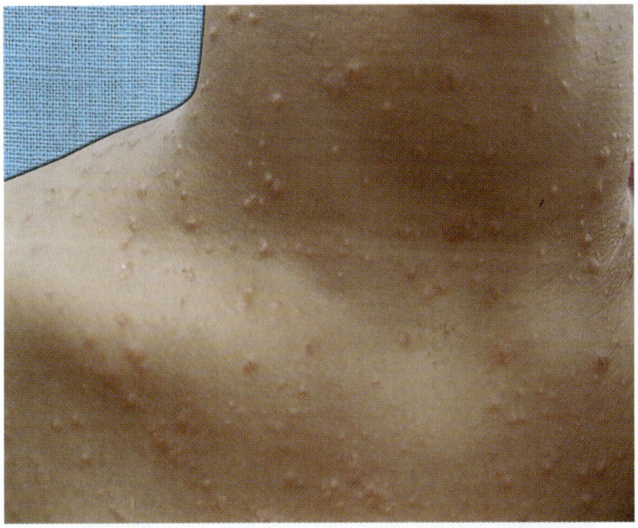

Fig. 3: Vesicles in generalized distribution (varicella).

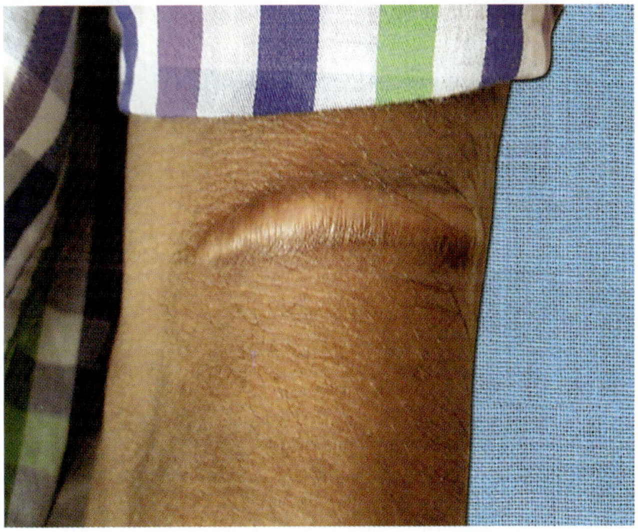

Fig. 4: Hypertrophic scar in site of previous cut.

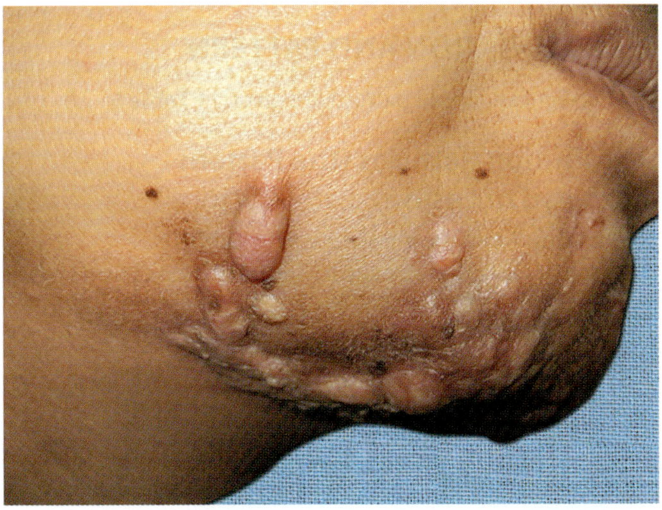

Fig. 5: Cystic lesions over face.

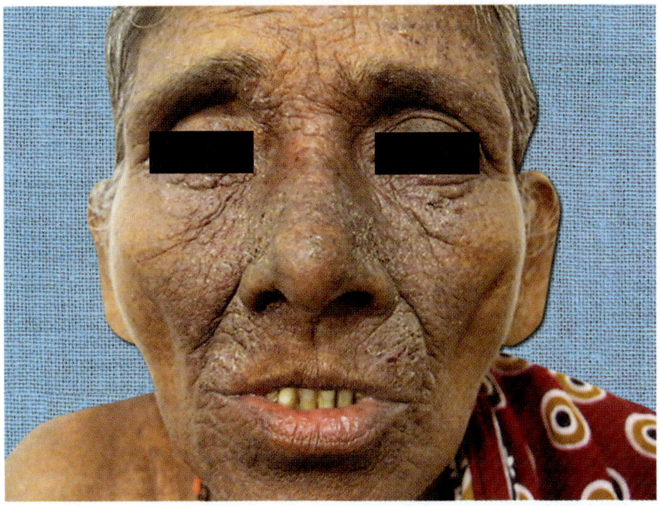

Fig. 6: Involvement of eyebrow, nasolabial fold, face in photoaggravated seborrheic dermatitis.

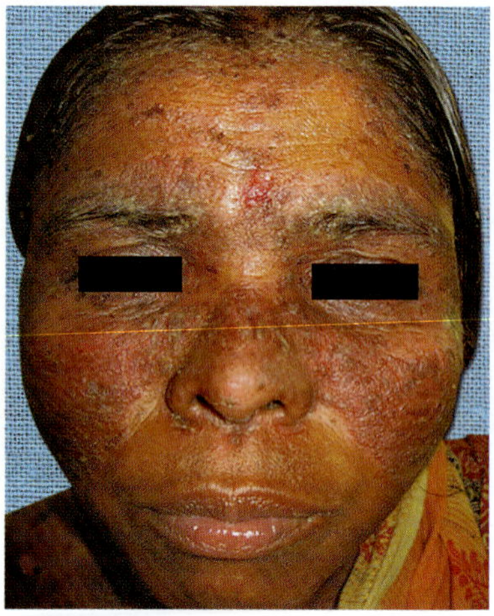

Fig. 7: Sparing of folds (nasolabial), involvement of malar area in photosensitive dermatoses: Pemphigus foliaceus here.

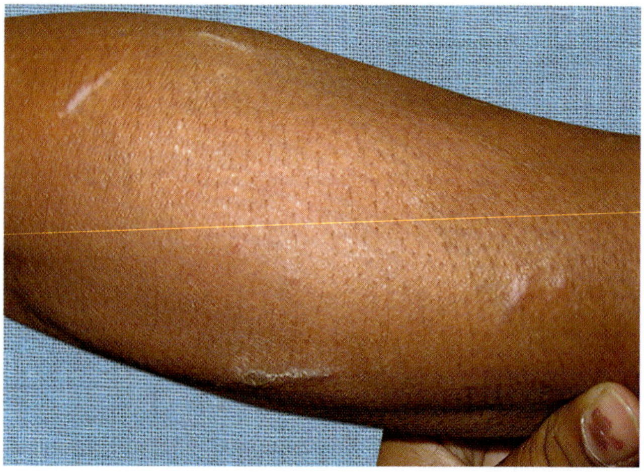

Fig. 8: Linear lesions in lichen planus due to koebnerization.

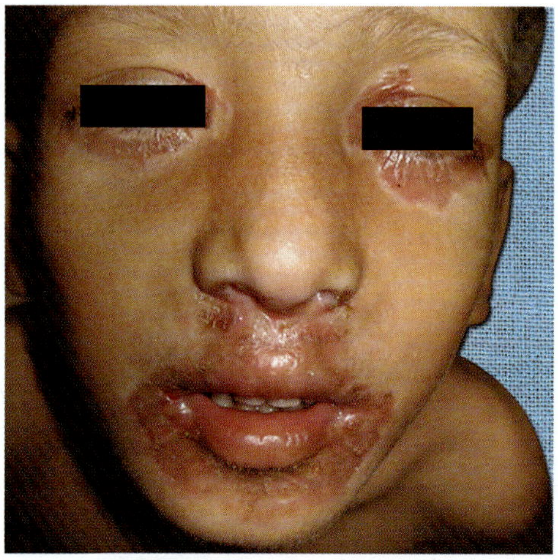

Fig. 9: Periorificial distribution in zinc deficiency.

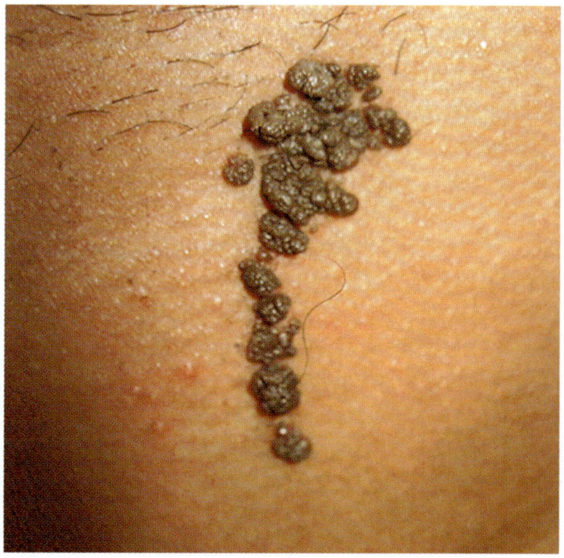

Fig. 10: Verrucous papules in linear distribution in epidermal verrucous nevus.

BOX 1: Palpation of cutaneous lesions.

- Soft (e.g., intradermal nevus) versus firm (e.g., dermatofibroma) versus hard (e.g., calcinosis cutis, osteoma cutis)
- Compressible (e.g., venous lake) versus noncompressible (e.g., fibrous papule)
- Tender (e.g., inflamed epidermoid inclusion cyst, angiolipoma, leiomyoma) versus nontender
- Blanchable (e.g., erythema due to vasodilation) versus nonblanchable (e.g., purpura)
- Rough versus smooth
- Mobile versus fixed to underlying structures
- Dermal versus subcutaneous
- Temperature—normal versus warmer versus cooler
- Others, e.g., thrill, pulsatile

CONFIGURATION AND PATTERN

The configuration and pattern are given in **Table 5**.

Distribution Patterns (the Pattern of Spread of Lesion)

The distribution patterns are given in **Table 6**.

Different clinical signs and method to description are described in **Table 7**.

TABLE 5: Configuration and pattern.

Pattern type	*Example*
Annular	Tinea corporis, granuloma annulare
Serpiginous	Cutaneous larva migrans
Clustered/grouped	Piloleiomyomas, herpetiform vesicles

Contd...

Contd...

Pattern type	*Example*
Reticulated	Erythema ab igne
Retiform	Purpura fulminans, purpura due to calciphylaxis
***Linear* (Fig. 8)**	Excoriations due to scratching, Koebner phenomenon
***Linear* and following the lines of Blaschko**	Epidermal nevus
Sporotrichoid pattern	Atypical mycobacterial infection
Dermatomal	Herpes zoster: Segmental
Target	*Erythema multiforme:* Concentric rings (like a dartboard)
Confluent	*Pityriasis versicolor* (lesions merging together)

TABLE 6: Distribution patterns.

Pattern	*Description*	*Examples*
Generalized (Fig. 3)	All over the body	Viral exanthem, drug rash, erythroderma
Widespread	Extensive	Toxic epidermal necrolysis
Localized	Restricted to one area of skin only	Irritant contact dermatitis
Solitary	Single lesion	Basal cell carcinoma, skin tumors
Discrete	Individual lesions separated from each other	Excoriations in scabies, Prurigo simplex
Flexural	Body folds, i.e., groin, neck, behind ears, popliteal, and antecubital fossa	Atopic dermatitis in adults
Extensor	Knees, elbows, shins	Psoriasis
Seborrheic (Figs. 5 and 6)	Scalp, body folds (postauricular, nasolabial), sterna, intrascapular, neck	Seborrheic dermatitis, acne vulgaris, and pityriasis versicolor
Pressure areas	Sacrum, buttocks, ankles, heels	Bed sore
Dermatome	An area of skin supplied by a single spinal nerve	Herpes zoster
Photosensitive (Fig. 7)	Affects sun-exposed areas such as face, neck, and back of hands	Polymorphic light eruption, phototoxic drug reactions (e.g., to doxycycline, SLE)
Symmetry	Bilateral involvement in similar distribution	Epidermal nevus syndrome
Acral (Fig. 1)	Fingers, toes, nose tip, ears	Vitiligo
Periorificial (Fig. 9)	Around orifices such as mouth, anus, nose	Zinc deficiency
Palmoplantar	On palm, sole	Eczema, psoriasis

(SLE: systemic lupus erythematosus)

Of note, sometimes a disorder will display a combination of distribution patterns; e.g., in dermatomyositis, lesions can be both photodistributed and involve extensor surfaces.

TABLE 7: Different clinical signs and method to description.

Name of clinical sign	*Classically seen in*	*Also seen in*	*Method to elicit/description*
Albright's dimple sign	Albright's hereditary osteodystrophy		Presence of a dimple over the knuckle of the typically affected fourth metacarpal and can be enhanced by clenching of the fist
Antenna sign	Keratosis pilaris		When examined in tangentially incident light individual follicles show a long strand of keratin glinting
Asboe–Hansen sign (blister spread sign) first described by Gustav Asboe–Hansen	Pemphigus vulgaris	Bullous pemphigoid	A small, intact, tense bulla is selected and pressure is applied at the center in perpendicular fashion after marking its boundary causing enlargement of bulla
Auspitz sign (named after Heinrich Auspitz)	Classical plaque psoriasis	Darier's disease Actinic keratosis	On doing a grattage test, there occurs pinpoint bleeding on removal of scales from the lesions
Barnett's sign/scleroderma neck sign	Scleroderma		On asking to extending the head a palpable tight band is visible over platysma along with ridging and tightening of skin of neck

Contd...

Contd...

Name of clinical sign	*Classically seen in*	*Also seen in*	*Method to elicit/description*
Berliner sign (first described by Benjamin C Berliner)	Roseola infantum (exanthem subitum or sixth disease)		Eyelid edema in a child giving clinical look of "heavy eyelids," or a "droopy" or "sleepy" appearance and disappears after appearance of rash
Breakfast, lunch, and dinner sign	Bed bugs bite *(Cimex lectularius)*		The bites in a linear pathway in a group of three to five caused due to blood meals of the bugs
Buerger's sign	Lower limb ischemia due to arterial disease		Elevation of the lower limb causes pallor, most evident on the soles while dependency leads to a delayed but exaggerated hyperemia of the limb, most pronounced on the dorsa of feet
Buschke–Ollendorff sign	Secondary syphilis (papular type)	Cutaneous vasculitis	Occurrence of deep dermal tenderness on pressing the lesion with a pinhead
Butterfly sign	Prurigo nodularis	Neurodermatitis	Mid scapular area is spared as they are unable to reach the region for scratching
Carpet tack sign (tin-tack sign, cat tongue sign)	Discoid lupus erythematosus (DLE)	Seborrheic dermatitis	On removing an adherent scale from the lesions the undersurface of the scale shows horny plugs that have occupied patulous hair follicles
Chagas–Mazza–Romaña's sign/Romaña's sign	Chagas' disease (American trypanosomiasis, *Trypanosoma cruzi)*		Occurrence of unilateral swelling of eyelids and orbit when conjunctiva is the portal of entry
Coral bead sign	Multicentric reticulohistiocytosis		Papules seen around the nail fold
Coudability sign (first described by *Shuster* in 1984)	Alopecia areata		Select normal-looking hairs tapered at the proximal end in the perilesional area and push inward or bend it. Look for kink on it
Crowe's sign	Type I neurofibromatosis		Presence of axillary freckling
Cullen's sign	Acute hemorrhagic pancreatitis	Ruptured ectopic pregnancy	Periumbilical ecchymosis Similar changes in the flank is called as *Grey-Turner sign*
Deck-chair sign	Papuloerythroderma of Ofuji		Flat-topped red papules which may become generalized erythrodermic plaques without the involvement of abdominal skin folds
Darier's sign	Mastocytoma	Leukemia cutis, Juvenile xanthogranuloma, and Langerhans cell histiocytosis	Occurrence of urtication, flare, swelling, and sometimes blister formation on rubbing due to release of histamine In contrast, *pseudo-Darier's sign* is seen in smooth muscle hamartoma where there is increase in induration and piloerection after firm stroking
Dimple sign (Fitzpatrick sign, pinch sign)	Dermatofibroma		Squeezing the skin adjacent to lesion causes a dimpled appearance on its surface
Dory-flop sign	Syphilitic chancre		Upon retracting the foreskin the entire ulcer on coronal border flips out all at once because it is too hard to bend due to underlying button-like induration. Demonstratable in an uncircumscribed male
Doughnut sign	Scleromyxedema		Induration of skin with central depression over proximal interphalangeal joint
Dubois sign	Congenital syphilis		Presence of a very short little finger
Flag sign	Kwashiorkor- or Marasmus-type malnutrition		Look for presence of sharply demarcated alternating band of normally pigmented and hypopigmented zone of hair (indicating episodes of normal nutrition and intermittent malnutrition respectively)
Forscheimer's sign	Rubella	Infectious mononucleosis	Enanthem consisting of dull-red macules or petechiae confined to the soft palate. Occur during the prodromal period or on the first day of the rash
Frank's sign	Predictor of atherosclerotic heart disease		Diagonal crease in the earlobes of adult

Contd...

Contd...

Name of clinical sign	*Classically seen in*	*Also seen in*	*Method to elicit/description*
Friar Tuck sign	Trichotillomania		Alopecia of the vertex with sparing of occipital region
Gorlin's sign	Ehlers–Danlos		Ability to touch the tip of the nose with the tip of their tongue
Gottron's sign	Dermatomyositis		Presence of scaly erythematous eruption seen on the dorsa of hands, metacarpophalangeal joints, and proximal interphalangeal joints
Groove sign	Eosinophilic fasciitis (Shulman's syndrome)		Linear groove or indentation along the superficial veins of the medial aspect of the upper extremity
Groove sign of Greenblatt	Lymphogranuloma venereum (LGV)		Enlargement of both inguinal and femoral group of lymph nodes separated by Poupart's ligament which produces a groove
Hair collar sign	Cranial dysraphism, (encephalocele, meningocele)		Presence of a collar of hypertrichosis around smooth dome-shaped hairless nodules (representing heterotopic neural tissue)
Hanging curtain sign	Pityriasis rosea		When the skin is stretched across the long axis of the herald patch, the fine and light scales tend to fold across the line of stretch
Head light sign	Atopic eczema		Perinasal and periorbital pallor
Hertoghe's sign (Queen Anne's sign)	Leprosy, myxedema, atopic dermatitis, and hypothyroidism	Follicular mucinosis, trichotillomania, ectodermal dysplasia, DLE, alopecia areata, syphilis, ulerythema ophryogenes, systemic sclerosis, HIV infection	Loss of lateral one-third of eye-brows (superciliary madarosis)
Higoumenaki's sign	Late congenital syphilis		Enlargement of the sternal end of the (right) clavicle
Holster sign	Dermatomyositis		Confluent macular violaceous erythema present on the lateral side of hip and thighs is called as "Holster sign" corresponding to the site of hanging a holster
Hutchinson's sign (named after *Sir Jonathan Hutchinson*)	(i) Subungual melanoma (ii) Affection nasociliary nerve, a branch of trigeminal nerve in herpes zoster		(i) Melanonychia with pigmentation of proximal nail fold (ii) Presence of papulovesicular lesions on the tip of nose
Hypopyon sign	Linear immunoglobulin A (IgA) dermatosis	Pyodermas, secondarily infected vesiculobullous disorders	There is a transverse fluid level comprising purulent material at the bottom when the patient is in a standing position
Name of clinical sign	*Classically seen in*		*Method to elicit/description*
Ingram's sign	Progressive systemic sclerosis		Inability to retract the lower eye-lid by using finger
Jellinek's sign (Rasin's sign)	Hyperthyroidism		Pigmentation of the eyelids seen in hyperthyroidism
Kaposi–Stemmer sign	Chronic lymphedema		Inability to pinch or pick up a fold of skin at the base of the second toe because of its thickness
Leser–Trelat sign (*Edmund Leser and Ulysse Trelat*)	Marker of internal malignancy [gastrointestinal (GI) tract or lungs]		Sudden appearance of numerous seborrheic keratosis Usually associated with pruritus
Love's sign	Glomus tumor		Locating point of tenderness with the help of pin head
Matchbox sign	Delusion of parasitosis (acarophobia, entomophobia)		Patient collects skin debris with mistaken belief that such collected material contains alleged parasite in a matchbox, tissue paper, or small container
Meffert's sign	Fordyce's disease sign		Leaving a lipstick like mark on the rim of a glass mug after consuming a hot beverage due presence of ectopically located sebaceous glands

Contd...

Contd...

Name of clinical sign	*Classically seen in*	*Method to elicit/description*
Milian's ear sign		Sign used to distinguish between erysipelas and cellulitis of the facial region, where there is involvement of ear in erysipelas and sparing in cellulitis, as there is no deeper dermal tissue and subcutaneous fat
Mizutani's sign (Round finger pad sign)	Raynaud's phenomenon associated with systemic sclerosis	Fingertip contour looks hemisphere-like especially on ring fingers instead of peak like
Nazzaro's sign	Multiple myeloma	Presence of horny follicular spicules commonly on the face which shows compact follicular hyperkeratosis
Nikolskiy's sign named (*Piotr Vasiliyevich Nikolskiy*, 1894)	Pemphigus	Tangential pressure over a bony prominence causing easy peeling of skin. Elicited in the oral cavity with the help of cotton tipped applicator
Nose sign (Pavithran's nose sign)	Exfoliative dermatitis	Sparing of nose while other areas extensively involved. Possible cause may greater sun-exposure of nose or mechanism of island of normal skin
Oil drop sign	Nail psoriasis	Circular areas of discoloration of nail bed and hyponychium occur as a result of involvement of these resembling oil drops
Osler's sign	Alkaptonuria (endogenous ochronosis)	Blue black pigmentation in the sclera near insertion of rectus muscle
Pastia's sign	Streptococcal scarlet fever	Linear petechial eruption in the skin folds especially on the antecubital fossa and axillary folds
Patrick Yesudian sign	Type 1 neurofibromatosis	Palmar melanotic macules (palmar freckling)
Pitaluga's sign	Kala-azar	Acquired hypertrichosis of eyelashes
Prayer sign	Diabetic cheiroarthropathy	When asked to bring both the palmar surface of the hands together at the time of prayer if unable to do so completely due to limited joint mobility, it is called positive
Punshi's sign	Vitiligo	The original white color of vitiligo macules turns to red-pink during menstruation and returns to original color soon after Seen in young women and girls
Pup-tent sign	Nail lichen planus	Nail splits and elevates longitudinally with downward angle of lateral nail edge
Raccoon sign/panda sign/owl eye	Systemic amyloidosis	Eruption on the face and periorbital skin due to laxity of blood vessels. Often seen after proctoscopic examination (postproctoscopic periorbital purpura)
Reverse Namaskar sign	Ehlers–Danlos syndrome	Ability to fold forearms at the back and oppose their palms to say "Namaskar," due to the hyperextensible joints
Rope sign	Ackerman's syndrome with arthritis	Thick indurated inflammatory cord-like structure that extends from the lateral trunk to the axillae
Russell's sign	Bulimia	Crusted callosity on the knuckles of dominant hand due to repeated self-induced vomiting
Scratch sign (*coup d'ongle sign, Besnier's sign, stroke of the nail*)	Pityriasis versicolor	The barely perceptible scales are made to stand out by scratching the lesion with fingernail
Shawl sign	Dermatomyositis	Confluent macular violaceous erythema on the posterior neck and shoulders
Samitz's sign	Dermatomyositis	Dystrophic and ragged cuticle
Shuster's sign	DLE	Scarring of the concha
Stafne's sign	Progressive systemic sclerosis	An increase in the width of the periodontal ligament space due to increased collagen synthesis which gets accommodated at the expense of alveolar bone
Thumb sign (Steinberg sign)	Marfan syndrome	Thumbs protrude from the clenched fist beyond the ulnar border of hand

Contd...

Contd...

Name of clinical sign	*Classically seen in*	*Method to elicit/description*
Tongue sign of uremia (by M Thomas Mathew)	Uremia	Large pale tongue with prominent impression of teeth all around the edges
Ugly duckling sign (by Grob and Bonerandi, 1988)	Melanoma	Nevi in the same individual tend to resemble one another while an atypical mole often deviates from the individual's nevus pattern. Hence, a nevus that does not resemble other nevi is more likely to be suspicious
Umbilical sign	Marfan syndrome	Ability to touch the umbilicus with the right hand, crossing the back, and approaching from the left side (indicates increased length of upper extremity)
V-sign	Dermatomyositis	Confluent macular violaceous erythema on the anterior neck and chest
Volcano sign	Old World cutaneous leishmaniasis	Presence of an erythematous rim along border of a crusted ulcer. The initial lesion may be a papule which enlarges and ulcerates centrally
Wartenberg's sign	Ulnar nerve paralysis in leprosy	The little finger assumes the position of constant abduction secondary to paralysis of adductor digiti minimi (*earliest sign of ulnar nerve affection*)
Wimberger's sign	Congenital syphilis	Presence of bilateral, symmetrical, and well-defined metaphyseal defects on the medial surface of upper tibia, can result in pseudoparalysis
Winterbottom's sign	African trypanosomiasis caused by *Trypanosoma brucei rhodesiense* and *Trypanosoma brucei gambiense* known as sleeping sickness	Enlargement of lymph nodes in the posterior cervical chain. It is seen in early stages
Wrist sign (Walker's sign)	Marfan syndrome	The distal phalange of the first and fifth fingers of the hand overlaps when wrapped around the opposite wrist

CONCLUSION

Proper history taking and correct approach to assessment of lesions are essential for proper diagnosis. This visibility of skin lesions often enables the physician to make an instant or spot diagnosis. A proper history recording, clinical signs and clues go a long way in establishing a diagnosis and judge the severity of disease in an individual.

These signs reflect close observatory quality and can help a postgraduate student in making a clinical diagnosis more easily. In the coming years, more and more such clinical signs are likely to improve our clinical diagnostic skills.

FURTHER READING

1. Al Aboud K, Al Hawsawi K, Ramesh V, Al Aboud D, Al Githami A. Cutaneous signs. Skinmed. 2003;2:104-7.
2. Freiman A, Kalia S, O'Brien EA. Dermatologic signs. J Cutan Med Surg. 2006;10:175-82.
3. High WA, Tomasini AF, Argenziano G, Zalaudek I. Basic principles of dermatology. In: Bolognia J, Schaffer J, Cerroni L (Eds). Dermatology: 2-Volume Set, 4th edition. Gurugram: Elsevier India; 2017. pp. 10-34.
4. Kangle S, Amladi S, Sawant S. Scaly signs in dermatology. Indian J Dermatol Venereol Leprol. 2006;72:161-4.
5. Madke B, Nayak C. Eponymous signs in dermatology. Indian Dermatol Online J. 2012;3:159-65.
6. Nast A, Griffiths CE, Hay R, Sterry W, Bolognia JL. The 2016 International League of Dermatological Societies' revised glossary for the description of cutaneous lesions. Br J Dermatol. 2016;174:1351-8.
7. Taylor SC, Cook-Bolden F. Defining skin of color. Cutis. 2002;69:435-7.
8. Teh CL, Wong JS, Soo HH. Polymyositis and dermatomyositis in Sarawak: a profile of patients treated in the Sarawak General Hospital. Rheumatol Int. 2012;32:265-8.
9. Tran H, Chen K, Lim AC, Jabbour J, Shumack S. Assessing diagnostic skill in dermatology: a comparison between general practitioners and dermatologists. Australas J Dermatol. 2005; 46:230-4.

EXAMINATION QUESTIONS

1. Demonstrate Auspitz sign.
2. Write a short note on Koebner phenomenon.

9 CHAPTER Bedside Tests in Dermatology*

Shashi Kumar BM, Savitha AS, R Raghunatha Reddy

DIASCOPY

Diascopy is a common bedside test performed in dermatology with a glass slide. It is a modification of method for assessing superficial erythema by pressing fingertip against the skin and withdrawing suddenly to check for blanching. In diascopy, a glass slide is pressed against the skin and the lesion is observed directly under pressure. This test helps to identify if redness is due to intravascular blood or extravasated blood into the skin like in purpura or petechiae. On pressure, the lesions due to blood in lumen will blanch, unlike the lesions due to extravasation. The glass slides should be pressed carefully as the slide may break under pressure and the sharp edge damage the skin. Two glass slides may be used simultaneously to minimize this risk **(Figs. 1 to 3)**.[1]

Clinical Significance

- To differentiate erythema from extravasation (petechiae and purpura)
- Telangiectasia (in which the central "feeder" vessel may be distinguished)
- Granulomatous nodules, such as sarcoidosis, granuloma annulare, and lupus vulgaris, reveal a brownish-yellow "apple jelly" translucent quality upon diascopy
- To differentiate between nevus anemicus and nevus depigmentosus: Nevus anemicus becomes indistinguishable from surrounding skin.

Auspitz Sign

Auspitz sign is elicited in psoriasis. It is attributed to parakeratosis, suprapapillary thinning of the stratum malpighii, elongation of dermal papillae, and dilatation and tortuosity of the papillary capillaries.[2]

Method: Choose a new scaly papule/plaque, gently scrape the surface of the lesion tangentially with the blunt surface of a glass slide till scales are removed. This test is called Grattage test. Loosely adherent, silvery white powdery scales are suggestive of psoriasis.

- *Positive:* Once the scales are removed, a glistening membrane called Bulkeley membrane appears and once that is removed, dilated capillaries are seen in the form of multiple tiny bleeding points – implying that the Auspitz sign is positive **(Fig. 4)**.
- *Significance*: Seen in psoriasis, Darier's disease, and actinic keratosis. It is not seen in inverse psoriasis, pustular psoriasis, erythrodermic psoriasis, and guttate psoriasis.

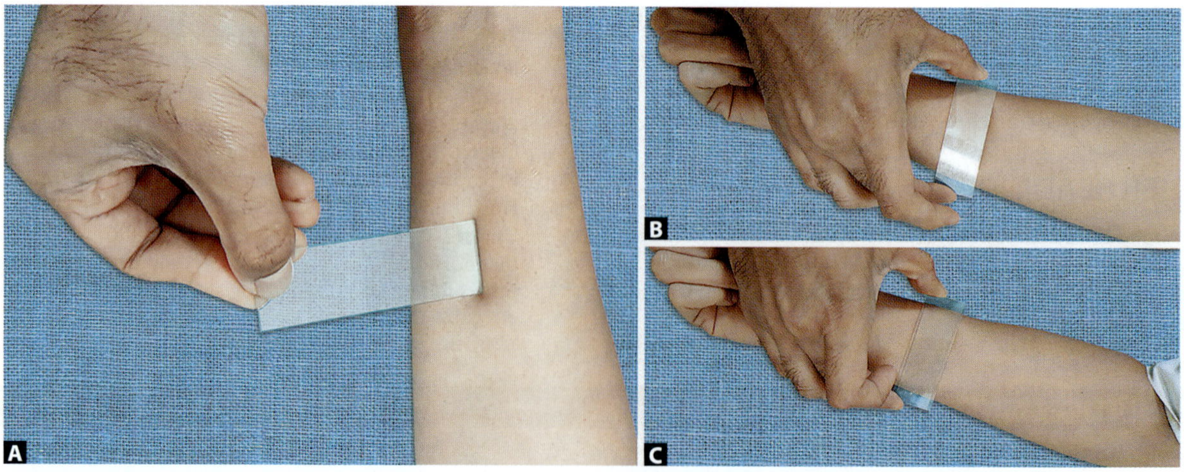

Figs. 1A to C: (A) Wrong method of using glass slide, there is risk of slide breakage and injury to the skin from the edges of the slide; (B) The glass slide is held on both the ends and then placed on the lesion; (C) Using two slides reduces the chances of slide breakage.

* In this chapter, bedside investigations and commonly elicited signs are enumerated.

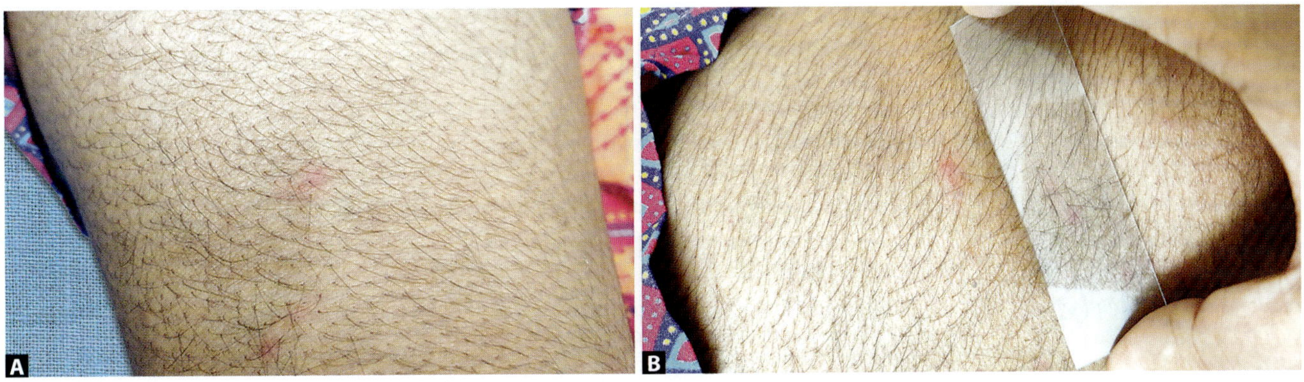

Figs. 2A and B: Blanching of lesions on diascopy.

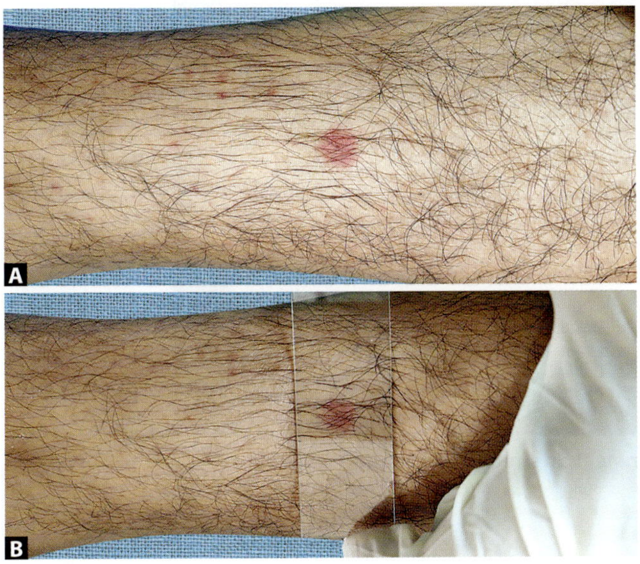

Fig. 3A and B: Purpura over the leg, no blanching seen on diascopy.

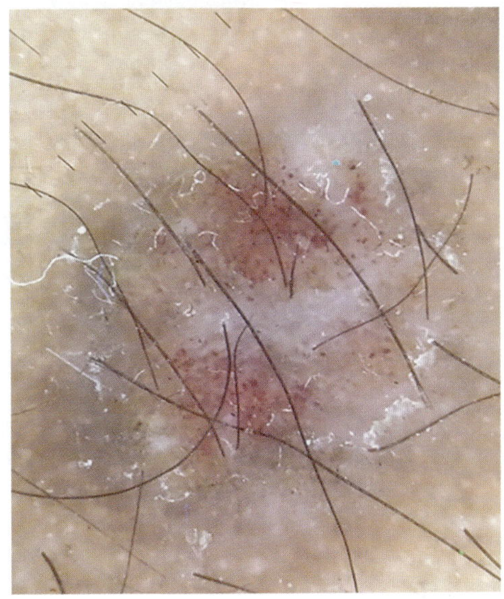

Fig. 4: Multiple bleeding points seen on removal of scales.

Nikolsky Sign[3]

Nikolsky sign is elicited in vesiculobullous disorders.

Method: The sign is elicited by applying lateral pressure with finger pad on normal appearing skin over a bony prominence in a patient with vesiculobullous disease. Shearing of skin is noticed indicating intraepidermal cleavage **(Figs. 5A and B)**, e.g., (pemphigus vulgaris, staphylococcal scalded skin syndrome). Positive test indicates activity of the disease, and helps to monitor treatment.

Variants of Nikolsky sign is enumerated in **Table 1**.

Bulla Spread Sign

This sign is also elicited in vesiculobullous diseases.

Method: Mark the margins of an intact blister with pen, then apply unidirectional pressure with a finger. There will be peripheral extension of bulla beyond margins. If extension has irregular angular borders it is pemphigus vulgaris, if borders are rounded, it is bullous pemphigoid or a subepidermal bullous disorder.

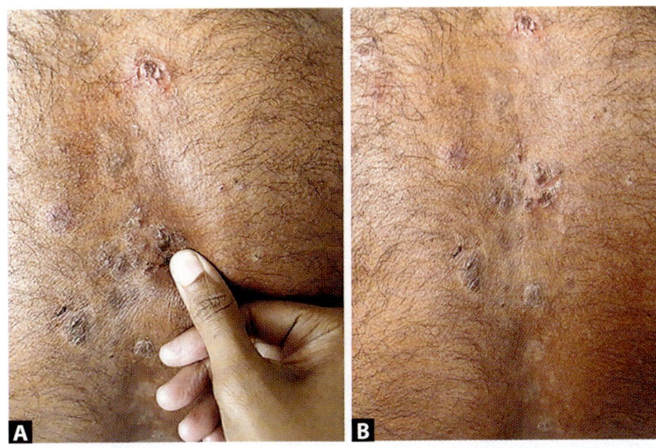

Figs. 5A and B: (A) Application of tangential pressure at the edge of an erosion; (B) Peeling of skin noticed at the edge of the lesion, indicating positive Nikolsky sign.

Variant: Asboe-Hansen sign—pressure is applied over the center of the blister, rather than the edges.

TABLE 1: Variants of Nikolsky sign.

Marginal Nikolsky sign	Elicited on normal appearing skin close to the bulla
Direct Nikolsky sign	Elicited on normal appearing skin away from the bulla
Nikolsky phenomenon	Superficial layer is felt to move over deep layer, but no erosion occurs immediately. Bulla develops after some time
Modified Nikolsky sign	Peripheral extension of blisters on applying pressure to their surface
Sheklakov sign/False Nikolsky sign	Extension of blister when the remnant roof of a ruptured blister is pulled, positive in subepidermal disorders
Pseudo-Nikolsky sign/Epidermal peeling sign	Positive Nikolsky sign due to necrosis of epidermal cells and not acantholysis, e.g., Stevens–Johnson syndrome, toxic epidermal necrolysis

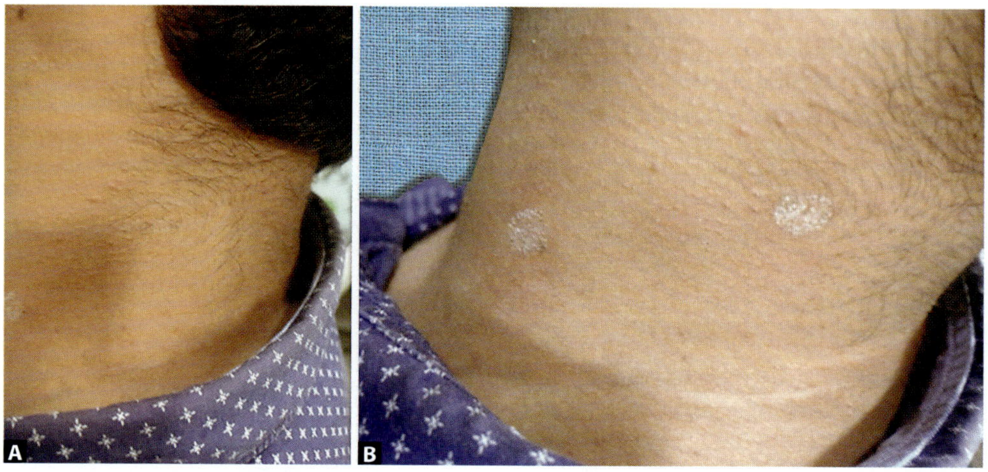

Figs. 6A and B: Lesion is more prominent on stretching the skin.

Scratch Sign (Coup d'ongle Sign, Besnier's Sign, Stroke of the Nail)

Pityriasis versicolor has hypo- or hyperpigmented macules with fine furfuraceous scales. Often the scales are not visible and can be made prominent by stretching or scratching with a finger nail.

Method: Stretching a lesion or gently scratching the lesion loosens the scale and makes it more prominent **(Figs. 6A and B)**. It may be negative if patient has had bath just before eliciting the sign.

Darier's Sign

Darier's sign is elicited in cutaneous mastocytosis.

Method: Rubbing or stroking the lesion gently with a soft blunt object results in itching, erythema, wheal or rarely vesiculation in 2–5 minutes, the symptoms might persist up to 30 minutes. This is also seen in leukemia cutis, juvenile xanthogranuloma, and histiocytosis X.

Pseudo-Darier's sign is transient piloerection and elevation or increased induration of a lesion induced by rubbing and is observed in congenital smooth muscle hamartomas.[4]

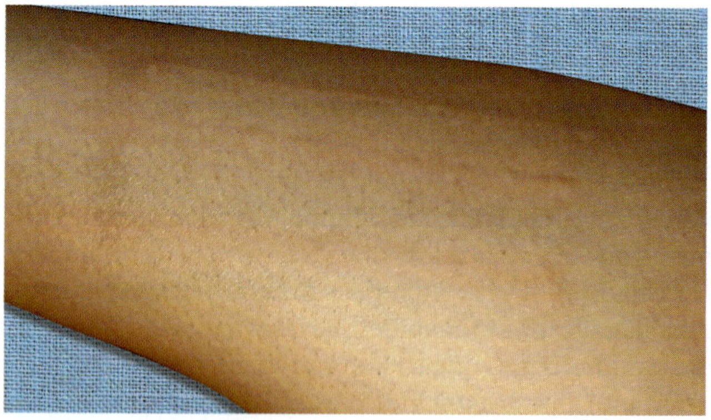

Fig. 7: *Dermatographism:* Erythema and edema along the lines of stroking the skin.

Dermatographism[5]

- *Indications:* Urticaria
- *Method*: Stroking or scratching normal skin with moderate pressure with a blunt object. A calibrated instrument dermatographometer can be used to elicit the sign.
- *Positive:* Itching, erythema, wheal occur at the site in a few minutes **(Fig. 7)**

Table 2 enumerates the types of dermatographism.

TABLE 2: Types of dermatographism.

1	Immediate symptomatic dermatographism	Exaggerated triple response with severe itching
2	Delayed dermatographism	Develops 3–6 hours later
3	Red dermatographism	On repeated rubbing small punctuate wheals are seen
4	Follicular dermatographism	Transient follicular urticarial papules on a red background
5	Cholinergic dermatographism	Grouped urticarial papules
6	Cold-precipitated dermatographism	Dermatographism on chilled skin

Hair Pull Test[6]

This is also known as the "traction test" or "Sabouraud's sign" or the "pull-out sign."

Method

- Approximately 20–60 hairs are grasped between the thumb, index and middle fingers from the base of the hairs near the scalp and firmly, but not forcefully, tugged away from the scalp.
- If more than 10% hairs are pulled away from the scalp, this constitutes a positive pull test and implies active hair shedding.
- The patient must not shampoo for at least a day prior to the pull test.
- The test is positive in cases of telogen effluvium, anagen effluvium, loose anagen syndrome, early cases of patterned alopecia and at the advancing edge of alopecia areata.

Wood's Lamp Examination[7]

Wood's lamp has a filter made of barium silicate with 9% nickel oxide with a wavelength of peak at 365 nm.

Method

The procedure is best performed in a dark room. Allow the Wood's lamp to warm up (about 1 minute), and give your eyes time to adapt to the dark. The light source should be 4–5 inches from the lesion. Shine the light directly above the lesion or sample in question. Carefully inspect the area, paying close attention to zones in fluorescence and their borders. Watch out for lint, topical medications, and soap residue. They all fluoresce, creating false positives, usually red-pink. Washing the area before subjecting it for Wood's lamp examination should be avoided since it may yield false negative results due to dilution of the pigment **(Table 3)**.

TABLE 3: Wood's lamp examination.

Condition	*Pigment*	*Color*
Tinea capitis	Pteridine	Bluish green
Pityriasis versicolor		Yellowish white
Pseudomonas infections	"Pyoverdin" or "fluorescein"	Green
Erythrasma	Coproporphyrin III	Coral red
Acne vulgaris	Coproporphyrin	Orange red

KOH Mount

Specimen collection

Before collecting specimen clear the site of any remnants of medications or debris by cleaning with alcohol or washing.

- *Skin*: Scales are scraped with blunt end of scalpel onto a glass slide or with another glass slide from the active border of a suspected dermatophytic infection.
- *Hair*: Plucked hair from the areas of suspected tinea capitis along with scraping.
- *Nail*: Nail scrapings from affected site for considerable depth, nail clippings, and subungual debris. Specimen is taken from the deeper discolored portion of the nail.

Procedure

- Cover the specimen with a coverslip.
- Apply two drops of KOH on opposite corners of the coverslip allowing it to spread by capillary action throughout.
- A folded paper towel is used to gently press down the coverslip. This absorbs excess KOH and also the pressure helps the KOH solution to digest keratin. Brief heating with care not to overheat or dry the KOH also helps to digest keratin faster. Pressing of the cover slip is better avoided in hair sample, as it might distort the hair.
- View the slide after 5 minutes or longer (30 minutes to 2 hours) if the specimen is thick.

Modifications

- *Cellophane tape method:* A cellophane tape is applied over the site and then stuck on glass slide. In the lab, the tape is lifted, KOH added and then replaced. The slide is viewed after warming the under surface of slide. This method helps in easier transportation and avoids use of fragile coverslip.
- *Parker's ink method:* Adding Parker's ink to KOH stains, the fungal wall blue.
- *Eosin 1% method:* Eosin 1% stains the background pink while the fungal elements remain unstained.
- *Modified Parker's ink and 1% eosin method:* 1% eosin and Parker's ink in 2:1 proportion by volume is prepared and painted over the site. Once it dried collect specimen by cellophane tape technique. No heating is required. The background stains pink due to eosin, while the fungal elements stain blue due to ink.
- *Calcofluor white:* This is a colorless dye, a fluorochrome stain, for rapid detection of fungi in wet mounts, smears and tissue sections, especially in scrapings from skin and mucous membrane. Viewed under ultraviolet light, fungal structures display a brilliant apple-green or a ghostly blue-white color.
- *1% Chicago sky blue stain:* Chicago sky blue (CSB) stain is a new contrast stain used together with KOH as the clearing agent **(Fig. 8)**.

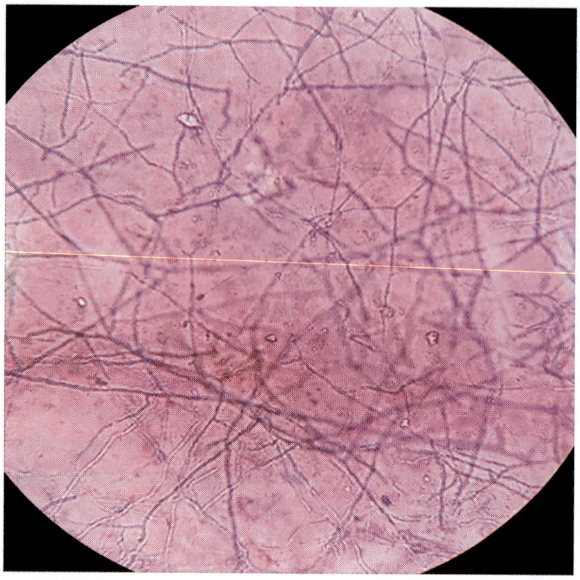

Fig. 8: Hyphae easily visualized with Chicago sky blue stain.

Tzanck Smear[8]

- This is an important cytopathological test for herpetic lesions and vesiculobullous diseases, infections, and malignancies.
- Sample is collected by de roofing and by scraping the base of a fresh blister with No. 15 blade and smeared onto a clean glass slide.
- For tumors or solid nonbullous lesions tissue smear is prepared. After removing crusts if any, sample is obtained with a small curette and specimen is crushed between two slides before staining.
- After it is air dried, Giemsa stain is applied and washed after 15 minutes. Air dry the slide and examine.

Pemphigus vulgaris, Hailey-Hailey disease	Acantholytic cells
Toxic epidermal necrolysis	Necrotic basal cells
Staphylococcal scalded skin	Dyskeratotic acantholytic cells
Leishmaniasis	Leishman-Donovan bodies
Herpes simplex	Ballooning multinucleated giant cells
Molluscum contagiosum	Henderson-Patterson bodies
Darier's disease	Corps ronds, grains

Mineral Oil Preparation[9]

For parasitic infestations

Method

- Place few drops of mineral oil on a glass slide.
- Dip No. 15 blade on to the oil and scrape the burrow repeatedly; the debris is transferred onto the slide. Place a coverslip and examine it for mites, egg casings, and scybala. For Demodex, a facial pustule can be expressed and suspended in mineral oil.

Gram Stain

- Collect the sample onto a glass slide and heat fix the specimen.
- Add crystal violet on to the slide and wash after 30 seconds.
- Add Gram's iodine and rinse in 30 seconds.
- Add the decolorizer solution till the run off is clear and rinse in water.
- Flood the stain with safranin counter stain for 30 seconds and rinse.
- Air dry the slide and view under a microscope.

Urethral Smear

Specimen collection

- In men, urethral discharge is collected directly onto a glass slide after retracting the prepuce and cleaning the meatus. If there is no visible discharge, milk or strip the urethra from the root of the penis to the glans to collect discharge. Collecting the specimen 2 hours after micturition is advisable, as voiding reduces the amount of specimen.
- In women, swab is taken from the endocervical canal using a sterile swab. The swab is inserted 2–3 cm into endocervical canal, rotated from side to side for 5 seconds and withdrawn.

Wet Mount

Wet mount is done to diagnose organisms of trichomoniasis and bacterial vaginosis.

Method: The specimen is collected from the posterior fornix under speculum examination using sterile swab or loop. In men, sample is obtained from urethra.

1 mL normal saline is added to the specimen on the slide, cover slip is placed and examined.

Whiff Test

This test is performed in bacterial vaginosis.

Method

- Specimen collected from the vagina as described above.
- On adding a drop of KOH, a characteristic fishy odor indicates positive test.

CONCLUSION

These simple bedside tests are easy to perform and master, they should be practiced regularly by residents.

KEY POINTS

- Diascopy helps to differentiate erythema from extravasation.
- Wood's lamp is an important bedside test to diagnose infections like erythrasma.
- KOH mount is a rapid bedside test for diagnosis of dermatophytosis.

REFERENCES

1. McKay M. Office techniques for dermatologic diagnosis. In: Walker HK, Hall WD, Hurst JW (Eds). Clinical Methods: The History, Physical, and Laboratory Examinations, 3rd edition. Boston: Butterworth Publishers; 1990.
2. Kangle S, Amladi S, Sawant S. Scaly signs in dermatology. Indian J Dermatol Venereol Leprol. 2006;72:161-4.
3. Sachdev D. Nikolsky and related signs. Indian J Dermatol Venereol Leprol. 2007:5-8.
4. Surjushe A, Jindal S, Gote P, Saple DG. Darier's sign. Indian J Dermatol Venereol Leprol. 2007;73:363-4.
5. Bhute D, Doshi B, Pande S, Mahajan S, Kharkar V. Dermatographism. Indian J Dermatol Venereol Leprol. 2008; 74(2):177.
6. Dhurat R, Saraogi P. Hair evaluation methods: merits and demerits. Int J Trichol. 2009;1(2):108.
7. Ponka D, Baddar F. Wood lamp examination. Can Fam Phys. 2012;58(9):976.
8. Gupta LK, Singhi MK. Tzanck smear: a useful diagnostic tool. Indian J Dermatol Venereol Leprol. 2005;71(4):295.
9. Bronfenbrener R. Stains and smears: resident guide to bedside diagnostic testing. Cutis. 2014;94(6):E29-30.

EXAMINATION QUESTION

1. Explain bedside tests in dermatology.

10 CHAPTER

Laboratory Investigations Specific to Dermatology Disorders

Vijay P Zawar, Shrikant Kumavat

INTRODUCTION

Laboratory tests are frequently used for arriving at the diagnosis, follow-up during treatment, and to judge the prognosis of given patients in the area of dermatology. A thorough clinical examination is must before advising any sort of investigation in dermatology patients. Inadvertent deletion of an important investigation or unnecessary investigations may be avoided by doing careful systematic clinical examination.

TZANCK SMEAR[1]

- Tzanck smear is one of the methods of cytodiagnosis in which the characteristics of cell are studied.
- It was used initially by Tzanck in 1947 for the diagnosis of herpes simplex.
- This technique is simple, rapid, and cheap. In few diseases, the findings of Tzanck smear are diagnostic while in some they are only suggestive of a disease.

Technique

- In case of viral infections, a fresh vesicle is ruptured and the base of the vesicle is gently scraped by the blunt side of the scalpel and smeared over the clean glass slide.
- For blistering disorders, intact bulla is chosen. The roof of the blister is opened along one side, folded back, and the floor is gently scraped by the blunt side of the scalpel. It is then smeared over the clean glass slide and allowed to air dry.
- A suspected tumor is incised with a sharp scalpel and a sample is collected by a blunt scalpel or curette. If the tumor is ulcerated, the sample is collected from the floor of the ulcer. This sample is pressed between two slides.
- Fixative fluid prevents denaturization and cross linking of proteins and autolysis so that cellular morphology is preserved.
- Fixative fluids contain formalin, glutaraldehyde, methanol, ethanol, other alcohols, acetone, acetic acid, chromates, and picric acid depending on purpose.
- After air drying, it is immediately fixed by fixation fluid such as formol-Zenker solution.
- Tzanck smear can be stained by a variety of methods such as Giemsa stain, hematoxylin and eosin, Wright, methylene blue, Papanicolaou, and toluidine blue.
- The most commonly used stain is Giemsa stain. A diluted (1:10) solution of the Giemsa stain is kept for 15 minutes over a slide. After washing the slide with water, it is examined under a microscope. It stains nuclei from reddish blue to purple to pink and cytoplasm stains bluish. **Table 1** states diseases and their findings on Tzanck smear.

POTASSIUM HYDROXIDE MOUNT[2]

Potassium hydroxide (KOH) mount is a simple and outpatient departmental procedure to detect fungal infection in skin, hairs, and nails.

TABLE 1: Diseases and their findings on Tzanck smear.

Disease	*Findings*
Pemphigus vulgaris	Acantholytic cells or Tzanck cells (large, round keratinocytes with a hypertrophic nucleus with condensation of basophilic cytoplasm at the periphery giving appearance of a perinuclear halo)
Bullous pemphigoid	No acantholytic cells, plenty of leukocytes
Toxic epidermal necrolysis	Necrotic basal cells, leukocytes, fibroblasts
Staphylococcal-scalded syndrome	Dyskeratotic acantholytic cells, very few inflammatory cells
Leishmaniasis	Multiple, light blue, ellipsoid, Leishman-Donovan bodies within the macrophage in a "swarm of bees" fashion
Herpes simplex, varicella, zoster	Multinucleated giant cells with ballooning degeneration. Giant cells have a tadpole, bipolar, or irregular teardrop shape with a smooth external contour. Multiple nuclei (eight or more) of giant cell fit together in a jigsaw puzzle-like fashion **(Fig. 1)**
Molluscum contagiosum	Deeply basophilic, ovoid, hyaline, homogeneous intracytoplasmic inclusion bodies called Henderson-Patterson bodies or molluscum bodies

Contd...

Contd...

Disease	*Findings*
Vaccinia, Orf, milker's nodules, and variola	Variable number of acantholytic cells or detached, squamous keratinocytes. They may contain an eosinophilic cytoplasmic inclusion body called "Guarnieri body"
Hailey-Hailey disease	Acantholytic cells
Darier's disease	Corps ronds (isolated keratinocytes with a round shape with peripherally dense acidophilic cytoplasm) Grains (small, hyaline, acidophilic ovoid bodies resembling pomegranate seeds)
Basal cell epithelioma	Clusters of basaloid cells (little larger and more deeply basophilic than normal basal cells with a central oval, intensely basophilic nucleus)
Squamous cell carcinoma (nodular, soft or non-ulcerated, nonketotic variant)	Absence of clusters, pleomorphism, and nuclear alterations (hypertrophic, hyperchromatic, lobated or multiple nuclei, and abnormal mitoses)
Histiocytosis-X	Atypical Langerhans cells (multinucleate cells with wide, pale, weakly eosinophilic or amphophilic, micro-vacuolates or granular cytoplasm and a large, lobulated, convoluted, reniform, or centrally grooved nucleus)
Paget's disease	Paget's cells (round-to-oval cells with vacuolated cytoplasm and hypertrophic nucleus)
Erythroplasia of Queyrat	Polyhedral, spindle shaped, and round cells with poikilokaryosis
Mastocytoma	Plenty of mast cells (irregular-shaped cells with metachromatic staining of granules)

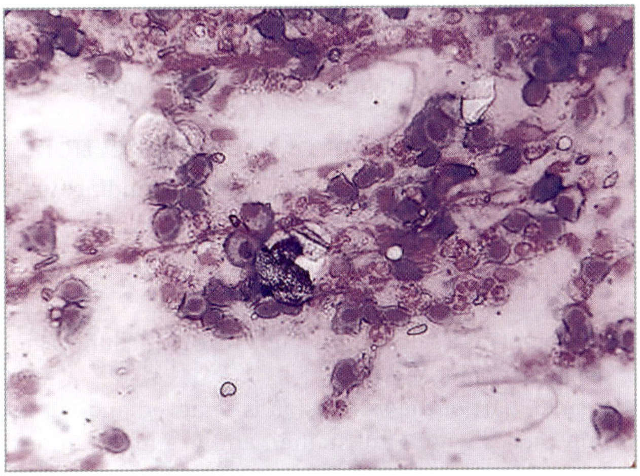

Fig. 1: Multinucleate giant cell in herpes zoster (H&E, ×100).

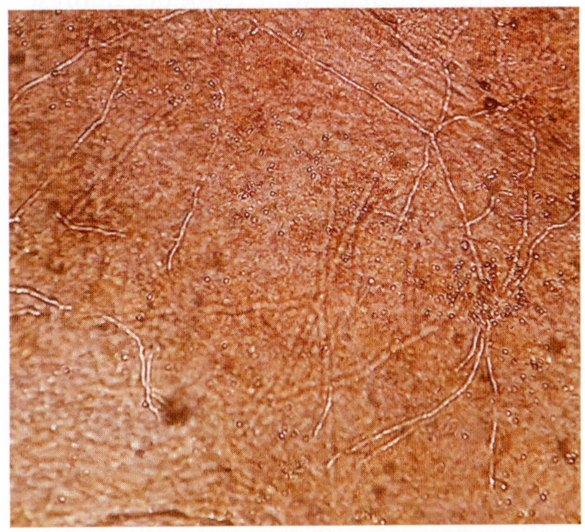

Fig. 2: Branching and septate hyphae of dermatophyte (KOH, ×40).
Courtesy: Dr Shwetal Rathi, Dr Vasantrao Pawar Medical College Hospital and Research Centre, Nashik.

Method

1. Select a high yielding site such as the outer edge of an annular lesion or a pustule.
2. Wipe the target area with alcohol.
3. Take no. 15 scalpel and scrape the scale or pustule perpendicular to the skin.
4. Collect scales over a clean glass slide.
5. Add a drop of 10% KOH over the slide and keep for 10 minutes. KOH dissolves keratinocytes and enhances visualization of hyphae or yeast forms.
6. Cover it by cover slip.
7. Reduce the light by lowering the condenser of the microscope until epithelial cells are visible. This improves contrast under a microscope and makes visualization easy as no stain is used in this method.
8. Do direct microscopic examination of the slide initially under low magnification and then on higher magnification for details of fungus morphology.
9. In case of onychomycosis, scrape the undersurface of nail and mount with 20% KOH.
10. Identify hair specimens with the help of Wood's lamp. Collect scales by a scalpel, toothbrush, or cotton tip.

TABLE 2: Diseases and their findings on KOH mount.

Disease	*Finding*
Dermatophyte infection	Branching and septate hyphae **(Fig. 2)**
Endothrix	Fungal spores packed inside the hair cortex
Ectothrix	Fungal spores grouped and attached outside the hair cortex
Candidiasis	Budding yeast cells
Pityriasis versicolor	Spaghetti and meatball appearance

Table 2 mentions diseases and their findings on KOH mount.

FUNGAL CULTURE

- Culture of fungus can identify the species of fungus which may not be possible on KOH mount.
- A new culture medium, named dermatophyte testing medium (DTM), has been devised for the simplified diagnosis of dermatophytosis.

- DTM inhibits bacteria and saprophytic contaminants while allowing dermatophytes to grow and produce alkaline metabolites which change the phenol red indicator from yellow to red.[3]
- DTM enables unskilled personnel to determine the presence of dermatophytic fungi from skin and hair.

Method

1. Clean the suspected lesion with 70% ethyl alcohol. This will remove any dirt and contaminating bacteria.
2. Collect the sample from the erythematous, peripheral, actively growing margins of the lesions.
3. Scrape across the inflamed margin of the lesion using the blunt edge of a sterile surgical blade onto a clean glass slide.
4. For suspected hair infections, pluck hair by epilating forceps. Scrape the surface near the hair root using the blunt edge of a sterile surgical blade. Wood's lamp can help to find out infected hairs which produce fluorescence.
5. Apply the collected material gently to Sabouraud dextrose agar or dermatophyte test medium.
6. Observe the rate of growth, colony morphology, and pigment on obverse and reverse daily for 2–3 weeks.

Appearance of Fungal Culture Colonies

Table 3 states species and the appearance of fungal culture colonies.

TABLE 3: Species and the appearance of colony after fungal culture.

Name of species	*Appearance of colony after culture*
Microsporum canis	White and fluffy center with a golden yellow border
Epidermophyton floccosum	Olive green to yellow-mustard color
Trichophyton mentagrophytes	Buff and powdery or white and downy **(Fig. 3)**
Trichophyton rubrum	White to buff, fluffy and downy

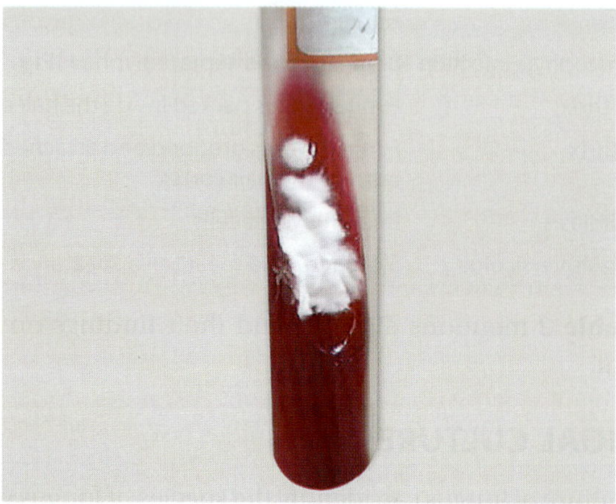

Fig. 3: White fluffy colonies of *Trichophyton rubrum* on dermatophyte testing medium.
Courtesy: Dr Shwetal Rathi, Dr Vasantrao Pawar Medical College Hospital and Research Centre, Nashik.

WET MOUNT

- Wet mounts are used to study water-bound organisms or body fluids such as saliva, blood, urine, and vaginal discharge.
- In dermatology, wet mount is commonly used for study of vaginal discharge.

Method

1. Take a sample with a cotton-tipped applicator. Use a speculum to obtain a sample of vaginal discharge.
2. Place the sample on a clean glass slide.
3. Put a drop of clean water or saline over the slide.
4. Place the edge of the cover slip over the sample and lower the cover slip slowly into place using a toothpick.
5. This will prevent air bubble formation under cover slip.
6. Examine the glass slide immediately under a microscope with a phase-contrast objective.
7. Normal findings include mature epithelial cells, parabasal cells, and lactobacilli.
8. Leukocytes in a 1:1 ratio to epithelial cells are also seen.

Findings in Wet Mount of Vaginal Infections[4]

Table 4 mentions vaginal infections and their findings in wet mount.

SKIN BIOPSY

- Skin biopsy is a safe, simple, and office procedure of great diagnostic value.
- A small part of the skin lesion is removed and cut into thin pieces which are stained and examined under a microscope.
- Skin biopsy ensures that the documentary evidence of diagnosis has been made and the basis for treatment started.

Based on the technique, skin biopsy is classified into the following:

- *Punch biopsy*: It is a simple and office procedure. Local anesthesia of 1% lignocaine is injected 15 minutes before. A punch made up of steel is used to obtain 2–5 mm diameter of lesional tissue. For example, punch biopsy of the lichen planus lesion.

TABLE 4: Findings in wet mount of vaginal infections.

Name of the disease	*Findings on wet mount*
Candidiasis	Pseudohyphae, budding yeast cells
Bacterial vaginosis	Clue cells (epithelial cells with bacteria adherent to the cell wall so that they appear ragged), lack of lactobacilli
Trichomoniasis	A pear-shaped morphology and whip-like processes of motile *Trichomonas vaginalis* organisms, increase in leukocytes

- *Incisional biopsy*: A part of the lesion is removed by a scalpel if the lesion is large in size.
- *Excisional biopsy*: The whole lesion and its surrounding normal skin is removed. This technique has a therapeutic role also. For example, melanoma biopsy.
- *Shave biopsy*: The superficial part of the protuberant lesion is shaved off by a sharp blade. For example, seborrheic keratosis.

Fixation

- After taking biopsy, the specimen is transferred into 10% formalin or buffered 10% formalin. For immunofluorescence studies, the sample is kept in Michel's medium as it preserves immune-reactants for several weeks. Alternatively, the specimen can be frozen in liquid nitrogen for immunofluorescence.
- The tissue specimen is then dehydrated by 50–100% alcohol. It is defatted by xylene or chloroform. Finally, it is passed through paraffin at 60°C.
- The tissue block is then mounted on a microtome machine to take cut sections of 5-μm thickness.
- These sections are mounted on a slide and stained by hematoxylin and eosin staining.

IMMUNOFLUORESCENCE

In this technique, antigen or antibodies are identified from the specimen by binding of fluorescent agents.

Direct Immunofluorescence Test[5]

- This test demonstrates antibodies in tissue.
- Biopsy specimen is carried in Michel's medium.
- It is stained by fluorescein-labeled conjugates which bind tissue-bound autoantibodies, C3 and fibrin. This produces a typical pattern which is characteristic to disease.

Table 5 mentions diseases and their patterns of immunofluorescence.

Indirect Immunofluorescence Test

This test demonstrates and quantify the amount of circulating antibody.

TABLE 5: Diseases and their patterns of immunofluorescence.

Disease	*Pattern of immunofluorescence*
Pemphigus vulgaris	Fishnet pattern
Bullous pemphigoid	Linear, homogeneous deposits of IgG at the dermoepidermal junction
Linear IgA	Linear homogeneous deposits of IgA at the dermoepidermal junction
Dermatitis herpetiformis	Focal granular deposits of IgA at the papillary tips
Systemic lupus erythematosus	Granular deposits along the basement membrane zone

(IgG: immunoglobulin G)

- Antibodies specific to disease are identified and by serial dilutions titer is calculated.
- It is useful for diagnosis and for monitoring of disease process as titer indicates change in the activity of disease.

Salt-split Immunofluorescence

- Few subepidermal blistering disorders show similar findings on immunofluorescence.
- To differentiate between them, normal human skin is incubated in 1 mol/L sodium chloride for 48–72 hours.
- This results in split at the level of lamina lucida. In bullous pemphigoid, fluorescent antibodies bind to the epidermal side (roof) and floor of the blister.
- Epidermolysis bullosa acquisita shows fluorescence on the dermal side (floor) only.

PATCH TEST[6]

- Patch testing is useful to find out the cause of allergic contact dermatitis (ACD).
- It is a gold standard for diagnosing ACD.
- It is a simple procedure to perform and can be done in the outpatient department.
- In 1895, the German physician Joseph Jadassohn used patch testing for the first time as a diagnostic tool.
- Bruno Blotch graded the intensity of the reaction to patch tests and suggested a standardized battery of tests.
- Jadassohn and Blotch initially used a small patch of linen cloth or blotting paper dipped in antigen which was covered by cellophane or other impermeable film, hence the name patch test.
- Later on, aluminum chambers, called Finn chambers, were developed and the term "chamber test" was coined.

Indications

- It is indicated in patients of acute or chronic, pruritic, eczematous or lichenified dermatitis where underling or secondary ACD is suspected.
- It is done in patients of atopic dermatitis with suspected ACD in whom there is no response to treatment and with a change of pattern of dermatitis.
- It is done in those patients in whom history and physical examination alone are not adequate to find out the allergen.

Patch Test Kits (Fig. 4)

- The Indian Standard Series (ISS) consists of 28 allergens approved by the Contact and Occupational Dermatoses Forum of India (CODFI).
- The allergens in the ISS are similar to those of the European standard series, with the exception of primin and the sesquiterpene lactone (SL) mix.

- The American Academy patch test kit and the European Standard Series (ESS) have already been well established for patch testing.

Common Antigens used in Patch Testing

Common antigens used in patch testing and their sources are given in **Table 6**.

Instructions to Patient

- Oral immunosuppressants should be stopped before applying patch test.
- Topical corticosteroids, topical calcineurin inhibitors, or ultraviolet light should be stopped at least 5–7 days before application of the patch test.
- Do not expose back to sun or use sunbed before patch test application.
- Do not swim, rub, or exercise after the patch test is applied.

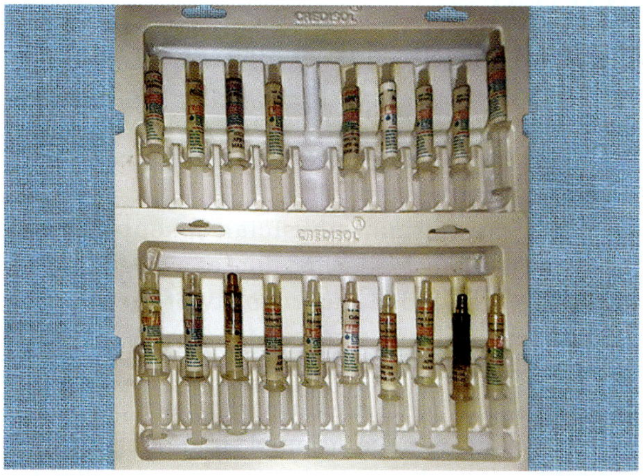

Fig. 4: Patch test kit showing syringes filled with antigens.

TABLE 6: Common antigens used in patch testing and their sources.

Antigens	*Source*
Balsam of Peru	Cement, topical medications, cosmetics
Benzocaine	Topical anesthetic
Cetrimide	Antiseptic, shampoo
Cobalt chloride	Tattoos, pottery, clays, cement
Colophony	Adhesive tape, polish
Epoxy resins	Adhesives, surface coatings
Fragrance mix	Perfumes, deodorants, toothpastes
Mercapto mix	Rubber, fungicides
Monobenzyl ether of hydroquinone	Shoes, chappals
Neomycin	Topical medications
Nickel sulfate	Earrings, bangles, buttons, coins
Paraben mix	Pharmaceuticals, cosmetics
Paraphenylenediamine free base	Hair dyes
Parthenium	Parthenium hysterophorus
Potassium dichromate	Leather, cement, bleaches

Method

1. The preferred site for patch testing is back as it is the biggest flat surface area available for testing.
2. Shave the back by an electric razor a day before, if there are hairs. Do not use chemical hair-removal products.
3. Do not apply oil or any moisturizer over the back before patch testing.
4. Clean the back with water and pat dry. Do not use alcohol.
5. Tell the patient to sit erect with shoulders dorsiflexed.
6. Small aluminum chambers, called Finn chambers, mounted on an adhesive tape are filled with allergens to be tested.
7. The strips are applied over the patient's upper back from below upward. Avoid development of air pouches by giving firm pressure over the adhesive tape.
8. For liquid antigens, soak a filter paper disk into the antigens and then apply over the back with an adhesive tape.
9. Mark the top and bottom of each strip with a marking pen.
10. Keep patches in place and dry for 48 hours.
11. Take the first reading after the 48 hours of application of patch.
12. Remove the patch and take reading after 20 minutes. This allows erythema to settle down caused by occluding pressure or stripping of the tape.
13. If contact urticaria is considered, then reading can be taken after 20–30 minutes after the patch application.
14. Take the second reading between 3 and 7 days. The 5th day (96 hours) after patch application is optimal for second reading.

Interpretation of Patch Testing

If the patient is allergic to the allergen applied, the area shows reaction ranging from mild erythema to blister formation. Various kits containing allergens are available in the market.

Grading of Patch Test Reactions

Grading of patch test reactions is given in **Table 7**.

False-positive Reaction

It can result from causes such as:

- Irritant substances
- Allergic substances applied in large quantity
- Pressure reaction from fin chamber
- Angry back or excited skin—Patients with more than five reactions in close proximity to each other

TABLE 7: Grading of patch test reactions.

Grade	*Clinical observation*
–	Negative
±	Doubtful (faint erythema)
+	Weak (definite erythema)
++	Strong (edema/vesicles) **(Fig. 5)**
+++	Extreme (bullous/erosion)
Ionizing radiation	Irritant reaction (pustules and sharp edge)

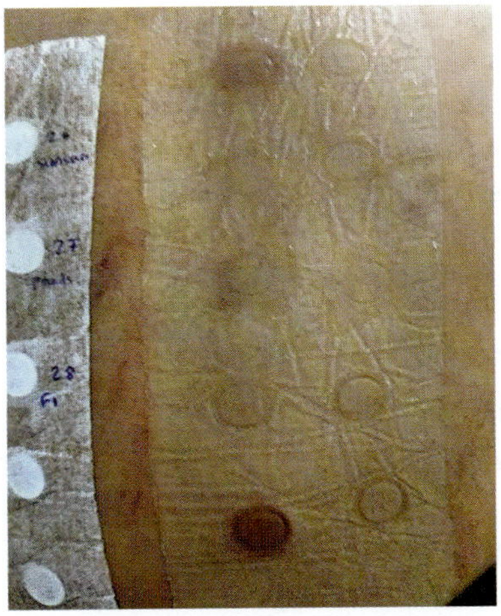

Fig. 5: Patch test response after 48 hours showing erythema and edema for two antigens.

- Pustular patch reaction to metals such as nickel, copper, arsenic, and mercuric chloride in atopic dermatitis

False-negative Reaction

It can result from following reasons:

- Too low concentration of antigen
- Wrong carrier vehicle
- Prior ultraviolet light exposure, topical corticosteroids, topical calcineurin inhibitors, or immunosuppressive therapies.
- Errors in performing patch test such as insufficient occlusion

Complications of Patch Testing

- Exacerbation of the patient's eczema
- Reaction to occlusive strapping or sticking
- Positive reaction may persist for a longer period
- Rare anaphylactic reaction to formaldehyde antigen
- Activation of the patient's eczema leading to flare-up of a positive patch test reaction
- Depigmentation, scars, and keloids

Patch Testing in Atopy[7]

- Patients with atopic dermatitis appear to have an increased risk of developing ACD.
- ACD remains an important comorbidity and potential exacerbant of atopic dermatitis in clinical practice.
- Patients with atopic dermatitis have increased penetration of allergens, immune dysregulation including shared cytokine pathways, frequent use of emollients and topical medications, all of which may predispose toward developing ACD.
- Patch testing should be considered in adolescent- or adult-onset atopic dermatitis, worsening or more generalized dermatitis, localized or atypical lesional distribution, refractory disease, prior to systemic immunosuppressive treatment, or when atopic dermatitis worsens with topical therapy.
- Common relevant allergens include lanolin, neomycin, formaldehyde, SL mix, compositae mix, and fragrances that are commonly found in atopic dermatitis patients' personal care products.
- The patch test antigen series should be at least a Thin-layer Rapid Use Epicutaneous (TRUE) test or preferably expanded patch testing series, e.g., American Contact Dermatitis Society (ACDS).
- Patients with atopic dermatitis have a lower irritancy threshold, which may lead to higher rates of irritant or false-positive reactions.
- Use of systemic immunosuppressive medications, ultraviolet therapy, or excessive solar radiation can decrease the sensitivity threshold of patch testing and lead to false negatives.

TRUE Test[8]

- The TRUE test is a new patch test.
- It is a ready-to-apply test with good stability.
- The allergens are dissolved, emulsified, or micronized into a gel, which is printed on an adhesive layer on a plastic, paper-plastic, or aluminum foil backing.
- After application of the adhesive layer to the human skin, the salts liquefy and become rapidly accessible to the skin surface at a high concentration.
- The TRUE test produces an exact dosage, even surface spread, and high bioavailability for the allergens.

PHOTOPATCH TESTING[9]

- It is the primary investigation for the detection of photodermatitis.
- Though European or Scandinavian photopatch test trays are available, those might not be relevant in Indian patients.
- The Indian standard kit can be used for the photopatch testing.
- Other than Parthenium, photosensitizing agents include chemicals present in sunscreens, antiseptic agents, fragrances, and nonsteroidal anti-inflammatory drugs.
- Photodermatitis due to parthenium is prevalent in India.

Method

1. Apply antigens filled in Finn chambers over the back on one side of the spine.
2. Apply similar antigens on the other side of the spine.
3. Patches are removed after 24 hours.
4. Interpret as done in patch testing.
5. Cover the back with an opaque sheet or material.
6. Irradiate the other side of the back by UVA (14 J/cm^2).
7. If an allergic reaction develops after 48 hours only on the irradiated side, it is called a positive photopatch test.

8. If both sides show a positive reaction with the irradiated side showing >1+ positivity, it is termed contact dermatitis with photoaggravation.
9. If both sides show an equal reaction after irradiation, it is because of contact allergy.

INTRADERMAL TESTS

- Intradermal tests in dermatology help in the diagnosis of infectious and noninfectious diseases.
- These tests detect immediate (type I) hypersensitivity and delayed (type IV) hypersensitivity to the exogenous as well as endogenous antigens.
- Although the whole-skin surface is capable of producing response to injected antigen, regional variations are still observed. Hence, a symmetric area for the control is selected for the testing.
- Conventionally, the proximal part of the flexor aspect of the forearm is used.
- Antigen is injected into the superficial layer of dermis through a fine bore (26 or 27-G) needle with its bevel pointing upward. Universally, 0.1-mL antigen is injected.
- A control solution (normal saline) is always injected at the symmetric site at the same time.
- The significant difference between the antigen and control site is taken as a positive test.
- For type 1 hypersensitivity reaction testing, reading is taken after 20–30 minutes after intradermal injection.
- Reading is taken at 48 hours after injection in the delayed type of hypersensitivity reaction.

Intradermal Tests for Infectious Diseases[10]

- This test detects delayed (type IV) hypersensitivity to the bacterial, fungal, and parasitic antigens.
- A positive test means that the person was exposed to antigens previously and does not necessarily mean that person has infection currently.
- *Tuberculin test*:
  - The antigen, known as tuberculin, is a purified protein extract of bacilli grown on 5% glycerol broth.
  - The quantity injected is 0.1 mL intradermally and reading is taken after 48 hours.
- *Interpretation of test*: The interpretation of the tuberculin test is given in **Table 8**.
- *Lepromin test*:
  - It is a prognostic test.
  - Earlier, this test was used for classification of leprosy.
  - Mitsuda lepromin antigen is prepared from autoclaved tissue of experimentally infected armadillos.
  - After intradermal injection of antigen, it shows two types of reaction.
  - The first type of reaction is called Fernandez reaction which develops within 48–72 hours after injection.
  - The second type of reaction, known as Mitsuda reaction, develops at 3–4 weeks.
  - This test measures cell-mediated immunity toward antigen.
  - It is positive in majority of healthy individuals of non-endemic area and negative in lepromatous pole of leprosy.
- *Interpretation of lepromin test*: The interpretation of the lepromin test is given in **Table 9**.

Other Intradermal Tests for Bacterial Infections

Other intradermal tests for bacterial infections are given in **Table 10**.

- *Trichophytin test:*
  - This test detects hypersensitivity toward dermatophytes.

TABLE 8: Interpretation of the tuberculin test.

Size of induration	*Result*	*Inference*
>10 mm	Positive	Past or present infection with *M. tuberculosis* or vaccination with BCG or active infection in children <2 years of age
<5 mm	Negative	Nonexposure to *M. tuberculosis* or absent/decreased DTH as in AIDS, disseminated tuberculosis, lymphoreticular malignancies, and sarcoidosis
Between 6 and 9 mm	Doubtful	Atypical mycobacterial infection

(AIDS: acquired immunodeficiency syndrome; BCG: Bacillus Calmette-Guérin; DTH: delayed-type hypersensitivity)

TABLE 9: Interpretation of the lepromin test.

Response	*Reading*	*Inference*
Fernandez reaction	Erythema or induration <5 mm	Negative
	Erythema and induration 5–10 mm	Weakly positive (*)
	Erythema and induration 11–15 mm	Moderately positive (**)
	Erythema and induration >16 mm	Strongly positive (***)
Mitsuda reaction	No reaction	Negative
	Papule < 3 mm	Doubtful
	Erythematous papule 4–7 mm	One plus positive (*)
	Erythematous papule 7–10 mm	Two plus positive (**)
	Erythematous papule >10 mm or any-size papule with ulceration	Three plus positive (***)

TABLE 10: Intradermal tests for bacterial infections.

Intradermal test	*Disease*
Frei's test	Lymphogranuloma venereum
Ito–Reenstierna test (Ducrey test)	Chancroid
Foshay test	Cat-scratch disease
Dick's test	Scarlet fever

- The trichophyton antigen is extracted from the spores and mycelia of *Trichophyton mentagrophytes*.
- After injection of antigen, an immediate reaction is seen after 20 minutes and delayed response after 24–72 hours.
- A wheal >10 mm in diameter at 20 minutes and induration >5 mm at 72 hours is a positive response.

- *Candidin test*:
  - This is not a diagnostic test.
  - It demonstrates cellular immune response in patients of reduced cell-mediated immunity.
  - Antigen is derived from two strains of *Candida albicans*.
  - Induration of >5 mm at 48 hours of injection indicates a good immune response in an immunocompetent person.
  - The response to test is significantly reduced in patients with AIDS, Hodgkin's disease, and sarcoidosis.
- *Coccidioidin test*: This test differentiates chronic pulmonary disease caused by fungus *Coccidioides immitis* from other chronic cavitary, nodular, and fibrotic diseases such as tuberculosis and malignancies.
- *Histoplasmin test*: This test is useful in epidemiological studies.
- *Leishmanin test*:
  - It is also called Montenegro test as it was initially done by Montenegro in 1926 in Brazil.
  - It is useful for epidemiological, immunological, and diagnostic studies.
  - A palpable nodule >5 mm in diameter developing in 48–72 hours is a positive test.
  - It detects early cutaneous and mucocutaneous leishmaniasis.
- *Onchocerca skin test*: It is a sensitive test which detects active onchocerciasis.

Intradermal Tests for Noninfectious Diseases[11]

- These tests detect immediate (type I) hypersensitivity to antigen.
- *Autologous serum skin test (ASST)*:
  - This test is done in patients of chronic idiopathic urticaria to find out autoantibodies against IgE antibody.
  - Around 25–45% of patients of chronic idiopathic urticaria have autoantibodies against IgE receptor FcεRI or IgE.
  - The positive test confirms the diagnosis of autoimmune urticaria.
  - A patient's 5-mL venous blood is collected and kept for 45 minutes for separation to obtain serum.
  - A patient's own serum (0.05 mL) is injected intradermally on the left forearm.
  - Saline control is injected into the right forearm.
  - A red wheal of diameter of >1.5 mm than control is interpreted as a positive test.
- *Kveim–Siltzbach test*:
  - It is done for the diagnosis of sarcoidosis. Around 0.1 mL of antigen is injected intradermally. A nodule develops at the site of injection after 4–6 weeks.
  - Sarcoid granuloma in histopathological examination of biopsied nodule confirms the diagnosis of sarcoidosis.
  - This test is of historical importance now.
- *Pathergy test*:
  - A prick by a sterile 20–22G needle is done over the proximal part of the forearm.
  - A sterile substance such as normal saline can be injected by the needle.
  - After 48 hours of prick, the development of an erythematous papule >2 mm at the site of injection shows a positive pathergy test.
  - This test is one of the diagnostic criteria for Behçet's disease.
  - It is also positive in pyoderma gangrenosum, hairy cell leukemia, and Hodgkin's lymphoma and in chronic myeloid leukemia treated with interferon alpha.
- *Histamine test*:
  - It is done to test the integrity of dermal nerves in cases of tuberculoid leprosy.
  - One drop of histamine acid diphosphate 1 in 1,000 (1 mg/mL) is placed on the skin surface.
  - A superficial prick is made through the drop.
  - Development of bright flare within 1 minute confirms intact axon reflex within dermal nerves.
  - Histamine flare is absent if sympathetic nerves are damaged in and around the lesions of leprosy.
- *Pilocarpine test*:
  - This test detects the integrity of dermal nerves in cases of tuberculoid leprosy.
  - Impairment of sweat function is seen early in the skin lesions of leprosy.
  - It is helpful when demonstration of loss of sensory function is difficult as in children.
  - Around 0.2 mL of 1 in 1,000 solution of pilocarpine nitrate is injected intradermally into the lesion. Around 0.05 mL of 0.1% acetylcholine or 0.02 mg of prostigmin can also be used instead of pilocarpine.
  - The injection site is painted with tincture of iodine and then dusted with starch powder.
  - If sweating is present, iodine and starch mix together producing a blue color after 2 minutes.

PRICK TEST

- This test measures the immediate type of hypersensitivity.
- A small amount of test solution is put on the skin and superficial prick is made to the epidermis at 45° with a sharp needle.

- A very small amount of test solution goes into the epidermis producing wheal and flare which are measured after 15 minutes.
- One positive control of histamine 10 mg/mL and glycerol 50% as a negative control are compared with test.
- House dust mite, pollen, dairy products, nuts, fish, and wheat can be tasted for skin allergy.

SCRATCH TEST

- A drop of solution containing antigen is placed on the skin.
- A linear scratch, around 1 cm long, is made through drop up to the level of epidermis.
- Development of wheal within 30 minutes is a positive test.
- Allergy to penicillin can be tested by this technique.

SERUM IMMUNOGLOBULIN E TEST

- Immunoglobulin E (IgE) has the lowest concentration in blood as compared to five isotypes of human immunoglobulins (IgG, IgA, IgM, IgD, and IgE).
- It has the shortest half-life among them.
- It primarily provides protective immunity against helminth parasites but can also respond to foreign substances.
- Serum IgE levels are increased in atopic diseases (asthma, allergic rhinitis, atopic dermatitis, and urticaria), parasitic diseases, cutaneous diseases, neoplastic diseases, and immune deficiencies.
- Patients of autoimmune urticaria have shown elevated levels of total IgE.
- It is also well reported that the level of serum IgE corresponds to the severity of urticaria except in atopics.
- The serum IgE level in serum >100 IU indicates atopy.

RADIOALLERGOSORBENT TEST

- Radioallergosorbent test (RAST) measures antigen-specific IgE.
- Allergens are linked to paper disks or polyurethane caps and reacted with the individual's serum.
- Specific IgE antibody and allergen form a complex which is detected by the use of an enzyme-linked antihuman IgE antibody in a colorimetric reaction.
- Kits having various antigens are available which can detect specific antibody, e.g., house dust mite allergy, pollen, and food allergens.
- RAST has a much higher reproducibility and is not influenced by ongoing symptoms or treatment, e.g., antihistamines or anti-inflammatory therapy.

SLIT-SKIN SMEAR EXAMINATION[12]

- In 1874, G A Hansen stated that leprosy is an infectious disease and is caused by *Mycobacterium leprae*.
- Later, in 1884, he used methyl violet to stain bacteria and described morphological characteristics such as rod-like structures, chains of coccoid forms, and clumps of bacilli.
- Patrick Manson in 1884 suggested squeezing the nodule of leprosy before piercing it to obtain exudates for staining.
- Instead of piercing, Alvarez surgically removed a piece of skin, grinded it, and added a drop of saline to make smears.
- The current and widely used technique, known as slit-skin smear technique, was developed by Wade and Rodriguez in 1927.

Objective of Technique

Demonstration of lepra bacilli in skin smear not only confirms the diagnosis of leprosy but also helps to classify and monitor the disease activity.

Morphology of *Mycobacterium leprae*

- It is a straight or slightly curved rod-shaped organism with parallel sides and rounded ends.
- Its length is around 1–8 µm and diameter is 0.3 µm.
- It is gram-positive bacteria.
- It is an acid-fast bacillus.
- It is an intracellular organism and commonly seen in clumps or globi.

Methodology (Slit and Scrape Method of Wade)

A sample is taken from at least four sites:
1. Right ear
2. Right forehead
3. Chin
4. Left buttock in men and left upper thigh in women
5. Active or suspicious lesion

Method

1. Take clean and numbered glass slides.
2. Clean the skin site by cotton swab dipped in methylated alcohol.
3. Pinch the skin between the thumb and the index finger of the left hand.
4. Make a cut by a surgical blade (BP no. 15), 2 mm deep and 5 mm long.
5. Turn the blade by 90° and smear fluid from bottom and side of cut.
6. Transfer the material from blade over the slide.
7. Apply antibiotic cream over skin.
8. Take the remaining smears by separate blades.
9. After air drying of slides, fix the smear by the moving slide over the flame.
10. Stain slides by the Ziehl-Neelsen technique.
11. Examine smears under oil immersion lens **(Fig. 6)**.

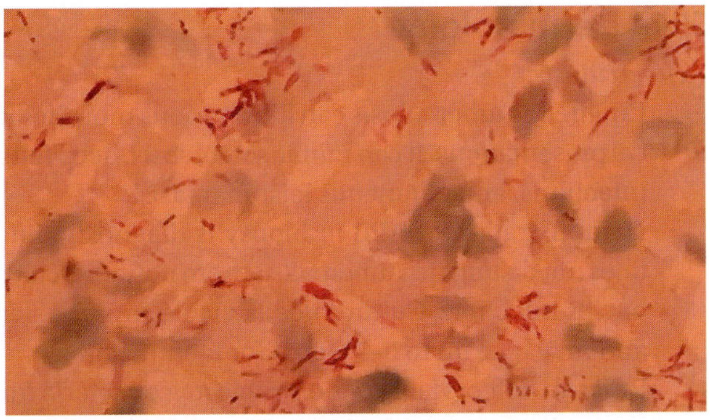

Fig. 6: *Mycobacterium leprae* in slit-skin smear (Z&N, ×100).

ZIEHL-NEELSEN STAINING TECHNIQUE FOR *MYCOBACTERIUM LEPRAE*

Method of Staining

1. Place the slides on staining rods over a sink after fixing by heat.
2. Flood the slides by carbol fuchsin and keep for 20 minutes.
3. Gently heat the slides using a gas flame under the slide, just to produce the steam to rise from all parts of the slide.
4. Wash the slides gently in running water.
5. Pour 5% sulfuric acid over the slides for 10 minutes to de-stain.
6. Again wash the slides gently in running water.
7. Keep counter stain 0.2% methylene blue for 1 minute over the slides.
8. After washing the slides by running water, dry the slides by keeping them inclined.
9. Examine the smears using a light microscope under an oil immersion objective.

Bacterial Index

- When the smear is found positive, bacilli are counted in the field and noted.
- Dharmendra in his bacterial index (BI) scale recommends examination of at least 50 fields for calculation of BI.
- The average BI is calculated by adding the total grades of different sites and dividing by the number of sites examined.
- The universally accepted standard method for assessment of BI as defined by Ridley is based on logarithmic scale (**Table 11**).

TABLE 11: Ridley's logarithmic scale.

Clinical observation	*Grade*
1–10 bacilli in 100 fields	1+
1–10 bacilli in 10 fields	2+
1–10 bacilli per field	3+
10–100 bacilli per field	4+
100–1,000 bacilli per field	5+
>1,000 bacilli, clumps, and globi in every field	6+

Morphological Index

- Morphological index (MI) is the percentage of solid-stained bacilli, calculated after examining 200 bacilli lying singly under the microscope.
- Acid-fast bacilli (AFBs) are considered solid staining if the organisms satisfy the following criteria:
  - The entire organism must be uniformly stained.
  - The longitudinal sides are parallel.
  - Both ends are rounded.
  - The length is five times its width.
- Solid-stained bacteria indicate viability of the organism.
- The World Health Organization does not recommend MI for routine use as it lacks standardization and poor reproducibility.

Ridley's Solid-fragmented-granular Index

- Ridley concluded that fragmentation and granularity are the stages of degenerating bacilli.
- He divided organisms into three categories:
  1. Solid staining-regular staining unbroken rods
  2. Fragmented-acid fast substance is interrupted at one or more points.
  3. Granular-round granules either in line or in clumps.
- Sequential changes in the solid-fragmented-granular (SFG) index can indicate the effect of treatment more precisely.

GRAM'S STAINING TECHNIQUE

Method

1. Fix the smear by gentle heating.
2. Pour Gentian violet stain over the slide and keep for 1 minute.
3. After washing the slide with tap water, pour Gram's iodine over the slide and keep for 1 minute.
4. Iodine is removed by washing and decolorize the slide by acetone.
5. Again after washing, counter stain the slide by safranine for 1 minute.
6. Air dry the slide.
7. Examine the slide under oil immersion.

Mechanism

- Gram-positive cells have more acidic protoplasm so they retain the first basic dye more than gram-positive cells and appear violet.
- Gram-positive cells permit the outflow of dye iodine complex during decolorization and appear red.

GIEMSA STAINING TECHNIQUE

- Giemsa staining is used for staining Tzanck smear.
- The stained nuclei appear as reddish blue to purple and cytoplasm appears as bluish.

TABLE 12: Types of hair and their characteristics.

Type of hair	*Characteristic of hair root observed*
Anagen hair	Preserved inner root sheath and outer root sheath, 20° angle with shaft
Telogen hair	Club-shaped end, smooth shaft, and straight shaft
Catagen hair	Bulb is covered by loose thick outer and inner root sheath
Traumatized anagen hair	No outer root sheath, with angulated end
Dystrophic hair	Pointed root, absent root sheath, e.g., alopecia areata, drug-induced anagen effluvium

Method

1. Fix smear by methanol for 2–3 minutes and air dry.
2. Pour diluted Giemsa stain (1 in 19-mL distilled water) into the dish and cover with a lid.
3. Keep the slide in a dish to stain for 10–15 minutes.
4. Wash the slide with distilled water and air dry.
5. Observe the slide under the oil immersion lens of a microscope.

TRICHOGRAM/HAIR PLUCK TEST[13]

- In this test, hair roots are examined under a microscope for abnormality and predominant type is found.
- At a time, 5–10 hairs are plucked with the help of epilators in the direction of hair growth and by sudden jerk. A total of 60–80 hairs are removed.
- Hair roots are examined under a microscope (**Table 12**).
- The normal values for anagen, telogen, and catagen are 80–88%, 10–20%, and 1–2%, respectively.

POLYMERASE CHAIN REACTION BASED MOLECULAR DIAGNOSTIC ASSAYS[14]

- Polymerase chain reaction (PCR) test is a rapid, sensitive, and specific test for identification of many pathogens.
- In comparison to routine microscopy, PCR requires a very less number of organisms for detection.
- Culture of organisms requires special media and a long period for growth whereas PCR can give result within minutes.
- Depending on the stage of the infection, the serologic test may show variability in sensitivity but PCR can detect small amounts of organisms as long as they are present in body or tissue.
- The PCR assay technique involves exponential multiplications of a desired specific DNA sequence.
- With the help of heat-stable DNA polymerase enzyme and two primers (short DNA strands complimentary to ends of DNA to be amplified), multiple cycles of reaction are carried out.
- Amplified DNA is then put on agarose gel for electrophoresis.

PCR in Dermatology

- *Tuberculosis*:
  - Cutaneous tuberculosis can have various morphological presentations. It can mimic sarcoidosis, deep fungal infections, and cutaneous leishmaniasis.
  - Demonstration of AFB in biopsy is diagnostic but it does not distinguish tuberculosis from nontuberculosis bacilli infection. Culture needs viable mycobacteria and may take up to 6–7 weeks for identification.
  - PCR can detect viable or nonviable mycobacteria from a sample containing <10 organisms in 48 hours. It also allows differentiation of *M. tuberculosis* from atypical mycobacteria.
  - PCR can be performed on formalin-fixed paraffin-embedded tissue.
- *Leprosy*:
  - As *M. leprae* cannot be grown on synthetic culture media, diagnosis of leprosy depends on demonstration of AFB in slit-skin smears and in skin biopsy.
  - Slit-skin smears give positive results in 100% cases of the lepromatous type where bacterial load is high. But in tuberculoid leprosy, it is difficult to demonstrate AFB.
  - Due to gene amplification in the PCR technique, specimens containing as low as 1–10 organisms can be detected.
  - The PCR technique in leprosy targets 16S rRNA, 16S rDNA, and 530bp protein genes.
- *Syphilis*:
  - Diagnosis of syphilis by dark-field microscopy requires 10^5 organisms per milliliter in a sample and is useful only in primary and secondary stages.
  - Serological tests done in secondary and tertiary syphilis cannot differentiate from recent and past infections.
  - The PCR method detects *tpf-1* gene, basic membrane protein gene, and *tmpA* and *tmpB* genes.
  - Newer assays use *polA* gene, are highly sensitive and specific, and do not require confirmatory tests.
- *Rickettsial disease*:
  - Serological tests for diagnosis in rickettsial diseases are useful after 15–26 days when antibodies are developed. Culture may take 60 days for growth.
  - PCR allows early diagnosis and species identification. It can help by starting antimicrobials early and improve treatment outcome.
- *Cutaneous leishmaniasis*:
  - Identification of Leishmania amastigotes, either in tissue smears or in biopsy, is the gold standard of diagnosis.
  - However, an organism cannot be demonstrated in all clinical stages and culture takes lot of time.

- Molecular testing is rapid, specific, and has the advantage that it can identify different species of organism.
- PCR assays target *Leishmania* ribosomal repeats such as ribosomal internal transcribed spacer 1 (ITS1) and small subunit ribosomal RNA.

- *Fungal infections*:
  - PCR testing has been used for diagnosis of systemic fungal infections.
  - The conventional method of diagnosis by culture can take 2–4 weeks.
  - It is useful in systemic fungal infection such as *Aspergillus* spp, Blastomycosis, Candidiasis, coccidiomycosis, cryptococcosis, Histoplasmosis, and Paracoccidioidomycosis.
- *Viral infections*:
  - The PCR technique is used for diagnosis of herpes simplex virus (HSV) infection, varicella zoster virus, and cytomegalovirus.
  - Blister fluid or fresh tissue is used for testing.
  - The test can differentiate between HSV 1, HSV 2, and varicella zoster virus infection.

ULTRASOUND IN DERMATOLOGY[15]

- Alexander and Miller in 1979 used a unidirectional USG device (A-mode) to measure skin thickness.
- Nowadays, in dermatology, high-frequency transducers are used.
- As the frequency increases, the wavelength becomes shorter giving good resolution.
- Devices of 20–25 MHz can reach up to the dermis. Frequencies between 50 and 100 MHz are limited to epidermis.
- The epidermis appears as a hypoechoic line and the dermis as a hyperechoic band.
- Subcutaneous tissue is a hypoechoic layer with hyperechoic longitudinal structures corresponding to fibrous septa.

Applications

- *Skin tumors*:
  - Skin tumors, whether malignant or benign, appear as hypoechoic in contrast to the surrounding normal tissue.
  - Basal cell carcinoma (BCC) presents as a hypoechoic area, well defined, with irregular contour, usually in the dermis.
  - Hyperechoic spots inside tumor represent corneal cysts, microcalcifications, and cluster of apoptotic cells.
  - BCC and squamous cell carcinoma appear similar on ultrasound (USG) except that the latter does not show hyperechoic areas inside the tumor.
  - Melanoma on USG appears as a homogeneous hypoechoic area, oval or spindle shaped. USG is used for measuring tumor thickness, margins, and vascularization. Metastasis of melanoma in the lymph nodes can also be demonstrated.
- *Inflammatory diseases*:
  - The stages of the systemic sclerosis such as edematous, fibrotic, and atrophic can be differentiated. This helps in treatment planning and estimating prognosis.
  - Thickening of epidermis and dermis on USG and increased blood flow in dermis on color Doppler are demonstrated in psoriatic plaques.
  - The size, shape, and depth of acne scars can be studied by USG.
- *Infections*:
  - Hypoechoic lesions affecting epidermis and dermis with interruption of the epidermis are observed in plantar warts.
  - USG can locate the wart and can measure its depth, enabling to choose an appropriate therapeutic choice.
  - It can be used to find out the extent of infection in severe forms of cellulitis.
- *Skin aging*:
  - Thinning of dermis, decrease in collagen, and elastic fiber degeneration show changes in echogenicity on USG.
  - Subepidermal low echogenicity band is seen in photoaging.
  - Dermal fillers can be applied at the correct location and in accurate quantity with the help of USG.

KEY POINTS

- In dermatology, laboratory test are used for arriving at the diagnosis, follow-up during treatment, and to judge the prognosis.
- Tzanck smear is simple, rapid, and cheap technique in which characteristics of cell is studied. It is commonly used as bedside test in vesicobullous disorders and viral infections in dermatology.
- Acantholytic cells or Tzanck cells are diagnostic of pemphigus vulgaris.
- KOH mount is a simple and outpatient departmental procedure to detect fungal infection in skin, hairs, and nails.
- Fungal culture can find out species of fungus which is not possible in KOH mount.
- In dermatology, wet mount is commonly used for study of vaginal discharge.
- Skin biopsy is a safe, simple and office procedure of great diagnostic value. Depending on the size of lesion, location and suspected clinical diagnosis, method of performing biopsy is determined.
- Other than hematoxyline and eosin staining, skin biopsy can be used for special stains and immunofluorescence study.

- Patch test is a gold standard for diagnosing allergic contact dermatitis. Allergen causing contact dermatitis can be found out by patch testing.
- Intradermal tests in dermatology help in the diagnosis of infectious and noninfectious diseases.
- These tests detect immediate (type I) hypersensitivity and delayed (type IV) hypersensitivity to the exogenous as well as endogenous antigens.
- Patients with atopic dermatitis appear to have increased risk of developing allergic contact dermatitis. Hence, it is important to find out allergens and decrease exacerbations in atopic patients.
- The TRUE test is a newer ready-to-apply patch test.
- The photopatch test is used for the detection of photo-dermatitis.
- The PCR test is a rapid, sensitive, and specific for identification of many pathogens. It involves DNA amplification of specific gene or genetic sequence of pathogen which gives typical pattern over gel electrophoresis.
- High-frequency ultrasound is newer investigative modality in dermatology. It can be used for detection of lymphadenopathy, tumor thickness measurement, extent of thickness in scleroderma, and extent of infection in sever cellulitis.

REFERENCES

1. Gupta LK, Singhi MK. Tzanck smear: A useful diagnostic tool. Indian J Dermatol Venereol Leprol. 2005;71:295-9.
2. Kurade SM, Amladi SA, Miskeen AK. Skin scraping and a potassium hydroxide mount. Indian J Dermatol Venereol Leprol. 2006;72:238-41.
3. Taplin D, Zaias N, Rebell G, Blank H. Isolation and recognition of Dermatophytes on a New Medium (DTM). Arch Dermatol. 1969;99(2):203-9.
4. Mylonas I, Bergauer F. Diagnosis of vaginal discharge by wet mount microscopy: a simple and underrated method. Obstet Gynecol Surv. 2011;66(6):359-68.
5. Mohan KH, Pai S, Rao R, Sripathi H, Prabhu S. Techniques of immunofluorescence and their significance. Indian J Dermatol Venereol Leprol. 2008;74:415-9.
6. Fonacier L. A practical guide to patch testing. J Allergy Clin Immunol Pract. 2015;3(5):669-75.
7. Owen JL, Vakharia PP, Silverberg JI. The role and diagnosis of allergic contact dermatitis in patients with atopic dermatitis. Am J Clin Dermatol. 2018;19(3):293-302.
8. Fischer TI, Maibach HI. The thin layer rapid use epicutaneous test (TRUE-test), a new patch test method with high accuracy. Br J Dermatol. 1985;112(1):63-8.
9. Rai R, Thomas M. Photopatch and UV-irradiated patch testing in photosensitive dermatitis. Indian Dermatol Online J. 2016;7(1):12-6.
10. Nagar R, Pande S, Khopkar U. Intradermal tests in dermatology-I: tests for infectious diseases. Indian J Dermatol Venereol Leprol. 2006;72(6):461-5.
11. Pande S, Nagar R, Khopkar U. Intradermal tests in dermatology-II: tests for noninfectious diseases. Indian J Dermatol Venereol Leprol. 2007;73(1):57-9.
12. Sehgal VN, Joginder. Slit-skin smear in leprosy. Int J Dermatol. 1990;29(1):9-16.
13. Dhurat R, Saraogi P. Hair evaluation methods: merits and demerits. Int J Trichol. 2009;1(2):108-19.
14. Swick BL. Polymerase chain reaction-based molecular diagnosis of cutaneous infections in dermatopathology. Semin Cutan Med Surg. 2012;31(4):241-6.
15. Barcaui Ede O, Carvalho AC, Lopes FP, Piñeiro-Maceira J, Barcaui CB. High frequency ultrasound with color Doppler in dermatology. An Bras Dermatol. 2016;91(3):262-73.

EXAMINATION QUESTIONS

1. Define Tzanck smear. Briefly discuss the technique and utility of the test in various vesicobullous diseases.
2. Cytodiagnosis in dermatology.
3. Patch test.
4. Write a note on photopatch testing.
5. Write a short note on lepromin test.
6. Describe briefly autologous serum skin test in urticaria and its significance in the management.
7. Write a note on uses of ultrasonography in dermatology.

11 CHAPTER

Skin through Ages

KN Sarveswari

INTRODUCTION

From birth till death, the skin and its appendages show many structural and functional alterations. Aging modifications in the skin reflect analogous changes that occur in internal organs.

EMBRYOLOGY

In the embryo, signaling pathways including the wingless-related (Wnt) signaling pathway, the bone morphogenic pathway, Sonic Hedgehog pathway, Notch pathway as well as the receptor tyrosinase kinase and fibroblast growth factors are used frequently to develop various structures in the body.[1]

Epidermis

- In 2 weeks, a single layer of cuboidal epithelium is present.
- In 4 weeks, the second outer layer periderm is formed.
- In 8 weeks, stratum intermedium starts to appear.
- In 9 weeks, rudimentary hair begins to develop.
- In 12 weeks, dendritic cells begin to appear.
- Between the 16th and 28th weeks, Merkel cells are seen.
- In 24 weeks, the granular and the horny layers form after the periderm sloughs.

Dermis

- In 4–8 weeks, stellate mesenchymal cells embedded in a matrix of hyaluronic acid and glycogen is seen.
- In 12 weeks, immature elastic fibers are present.
- In 16–20 weeks, papillary and reticular compartments are distinguished.
- During the fourth week, subcutaneous fat cells appear beneath dermis.

SKIN IN PRETERM INFANTS, NEONATES, AND INFANTS

Infants born before 37 weeks of pregnancy are considered "preterm infants". The first month after birth is considered the "neonatal period", while the whole of the first year is considered "infancy".

Skin of Preterm Infants[2]

- Stratum corneum is thin, leading to barrier dysfunction.
- The infants are susceptible to infections, react easily to irritants and are prone to toxicity from topically applied substances.
- Transepidermal water loss (TEWL) is increased.
- They have high blood flow through the skin and more water per kilogram body mass which aggravates TEWL.
- Skin damage such as removal of dressings, tapes, and monitors increases TEWL.[3]
- Application of emollients enhances barrier function.
- Sweat glands are functionally immature and sweating is not an effective mechanism for thermoregulation in preterm infants. Strict care should therefore be taken to avoid overheating.
- Vernix is very minimal.
- Vernix consists of lipids and prevents infections.

Skin of Neonates and Infants

- Thin stratum corneum
- Papillary dermis is thinner than adults
- Collagen fibers are smaller
- Elastic fibers are immature
- TEWL is similar to that of adults
- Infants are more susceptible to percutaneous toxicity
- High surface area to volume ratio, decreased subcutaneous fat stores, and immature drug metabolism system—these factors increase absorption while decreasing the volume of drug or toxin. It is thus important to apply only essential products to the skin during the first year of life.[4]
- In infants, the subcutaneous fat is rich in saturated fats which have higher melting point (unlike unsaturated fats of adults) and can freeze easily. This causes fat necrosis easily in infants manifesting as "subcutaneous fat necrosis of newborn", when they are exposed to lower temperatures. Hence, it is essential to avoid extreme cold exposure.

Disorders in Neonates and Infants

- Certain infantile disorders like infantile acne occur between 3 months and 1 year.
- Comedones and inflammatory papules occur similar to adult skin.

- Infantile acne is thought to be triggered by endogenous androgens.
- Prompt search for signs of hyperandrogenism should be made in an infant with severe acne.[5]
- Neonatal acne lacks comedones and is due to *Malassezia* yeast species. This condition can be treated with topical ketoconazole.
- Staphylococcal scalded skin syndrome caused by "exfoliatin", a toxin from *Staphylococcus,* can occur in infants. Prompt diagnosis and treatment with systemic antibiotics is important.
- Infantile skin is fragile and is susceptible to irritant dermatitis, especially napkin dermatitis.
- Other pustular eruptions in infants include transient neonatal pustulosis, eosinophilic pustular folliculitis, candidiasis, and congenital syphilis.

SKIN DURING CHILDHOOD

There is gradual acquisition of structural and functional features of the adult prior to development of sexual characteristics of puberty.

- Children are likely to be more exposed to infections and pyodermas, warts, molluscum contagiosum, tinea capitis, scabies, and chickenpox.[6]
- Endogenous eczemas such as atopic eczema, seborrheic eczema, and pityriasis alba occur increasingly.
- There is also increased incidence of exogenous eczema due to contact and irritant dermatitis.
- Other causes of eczemas maybe due to genodermatoses such as Leiner's disease, Hartnup syndrome, and phenylketonuria.
- Skin diseases maybe due to nutritional and endocrine disorders.
- Increased stress levels brought on by factors including competitive education, family issues, and peer pressure can lead to psychocutaneous disorders such as "dermatitis artefacta".
- One must also keep in mind symptoms of sexual abuse in children.

SKIN DURING ADOLESCENCE[7]

With the onset of puberty, the childhood skin undergoes several changes to transform into adult skin. These changes are due to a surge in the sex hormones such as estrogen, testosterone, and progesterone which bring about maturation of hair follicles, sebaceous glands, and sweat glands in the skin.

- In adolescent boys, testosterone derived from the Leydig cells of the testis causes secondary sexual changes such as growth of pubic hair, axillary hair, moustache, beard, and enlargement of larynx and penis.
- Testosterone is also responsible for axillary hyperhidrosis and increased sebaceous secretion.
- In girls, development of breasts is the first sign of puberty. It is due to the secretion of estrogen from the ovaries and occurs between 8 and 13 years of age.
- Sex hormones also cause development of apocrine gland which becomes localized in the axillary and pubic region. They produce the thick apocrine sweat, which along with bacteria on the surface of the skin is responsible for body odor.
- Sebaceous gland activity and sex hormones are also responsible for the common teenage problem acne vulgaris.
- In puberty, there is also a risk of sexually transmitted diseases. Teenagers are also exposed to new exogenous hazards.
- Androgenic alopecia occurs in genetically susceptible males and females.
- Certain disorders such as atopic dermatitis tend to improve during puberty.
- Becker's Nevus starts during puberty.
- Other disorders that tend to occur in puberty include seborrheic dermatitis, hidradenitis suppurativa, polymorphic light eruptions, and Fox-Fordyce disease.

SKIN DURING MENSTRUAL CYCLE

Cyclical fluctuations in estrogen and progesterone levels that occur during the menstrual cycle are responsible for many of the cutaneous changes and disorders like autoimmune progesterone dermatoses.

- Many women report premenstrual flare of acne.
- Some report dry skin while others find their skin and hair more greasier.
- Diseases which undergo premenstrual flare include psoriasis, recurrent aphthae, rosacea, herpes simplex, and atopic dermatitis.
- Premenstrual edema involving feet, ankles, and even face and ankles can occur.
- Some women experience premenstrual flushing as part "premenstrual syndrome". This might be due to hormonal influences, nutritional changes like depletion of essential fatty acids, fluid balance abnormalities, neurotransmitters, and psychological factors or a complex of all this into related problems.
- Increased melanocyte-stimulating activity can cause darkening of skin around eyes and nipples premenstrually.
- Autoimmune progesterone dermatitis consists of variable skin manifestations such as pompholyx-like eczema, erythema multiforme, and urticarial dermatitis herpetiformis.[8] These lesions occur premenstrually in some women and are thought to be due to hypersensitivity to progesterone. It is refractory to treatment with topical steroids and antihistamines, but some respond to estrogen or tamoxifen.

SKIN AND MENOPAUSE[9]

Menopause marks the end of reproductive life and is characterized by cessation of menses for 12 months. Average age of onset is around 50 years (45–55 years), and most women will live at least one-third of their lives in the post-menopausal state. Phase of waning ovarian activity 2–3 years before and 2–5 years after menopause is called as "climateric" or "menopause transition (MT)".

Hormones during Menopause[10]

- Ovaries become atrophic, resulting in decreased levels of ovary-derived estrogen.
- Progesterone production by corpus luteum ceases. This results in increased production of follicle-stimulating hormone and luteinizing hormone (LH).
- Relative increase of testosterone due to reduced estrogen.
- Estrogen is now derived from the conversion of androstenedione of the adrenals into estrogen.

Effect of Estrogen on Skin

- Estrogen receptors are found in keratinocytes, sebaceous glands, eccrine and apocrine glands, hair follicles, dermal fibroblasts, and melanocytes.
- Skin thus appears to be the target organ for estrogens and its decrease during menopause may aggravate the deleterious effect of intrinsic and extrinsic aging.
- Estrogens are essential for essential hydration because of their increased water retaining capacity, increased production of glycosaminoglycans, and improved barrier function of stratum corneum.
- They prevent aging by increasing collagen content, skin thickness, and their hydrating capacity.
- Low estrogen levels cause atrophy of the vagina epithelial cells.
- pH of vagina increases and can cause recurrent infections.
- Decreased estrogen levels also cause thin epidermis and dermis, loss of elastic tissue, and reduced vasculature.
- These receptors are found in greater numbers in women than in men.

Disorders Common in Menopause[9]

- Pruritus
- Menopausal flushing (due to pulsatile release of LH)
- Atrophic vaginitis
- Hirsutism
- Androgenic alopecia
- Chronic telegenic effluvium
- Brittle nails
- Frontal fibrosing alopecia
- Impaired wound healing
- Keratoderma climactericum
- Lichen sclerosus et atrophicus
- Hormone replacement therapy (HRT) used to treat menopausal symptoms can cause urticaria or eczematous reactions.
- HRT can also exacerbate chloasma, acanthosis nigricans, and spider angioma.

AGING SKIN

As in other organs, passage of time does not leave the skin unaltered. Both its structure and functions are affected.

Skin aging can be:

- *Intrinsic (chronological)* ***(Flowchart 1):***
  - Genetic background
  - Time bound
  - Inevitable
- *Extrinsic (results in premature aging)*:
  - Photodamage
  - Constant facial movements
  - Poor nutrition
  - Stress
  - Pollution
  - Smoking

Photoaging

Photoaging is premature aging of the skin caused by repeated exposure to ultraviolet (UV) radiation, primarily from the sun but also from artificial UV sources. It is the super imposition on intrinsic aging triggered by chronic sun exposure. Photoaging is different from chronological aging, as the damaging effects of UV rays from the sun (or artificial tanning sources) alter the normal structures of the skin **(Flowchart 2)**.

Features of Photodamaged Skin

- Coarse skin
- Furrows

Flowchart 1: Chronological aging pathogenesis.

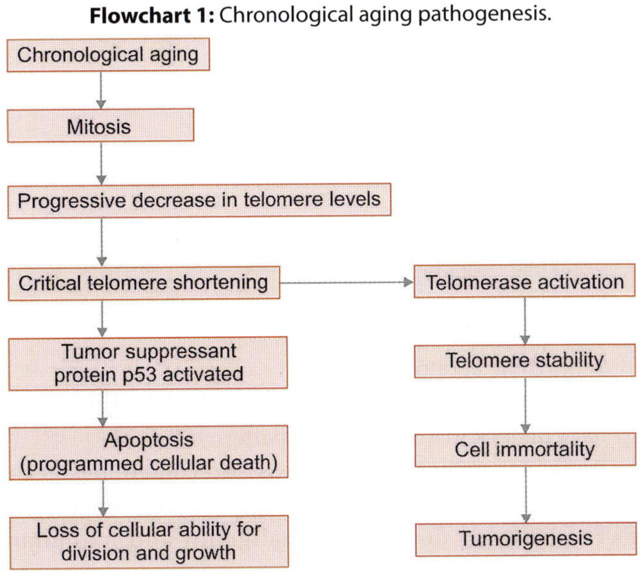

Flowchart 2: Photoaging pathogenesis.

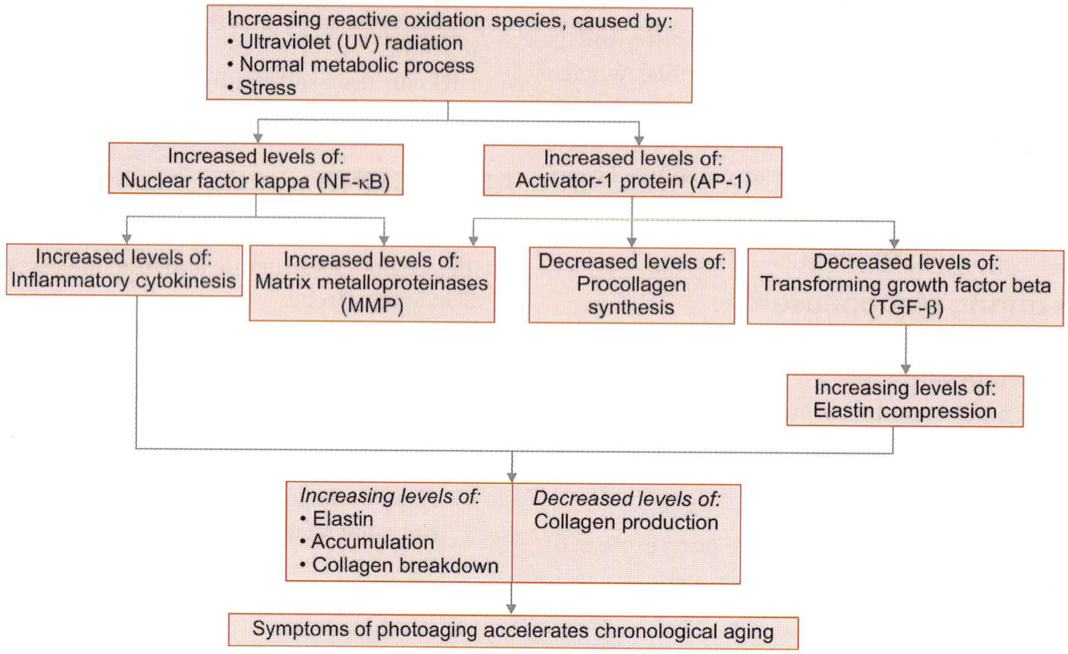

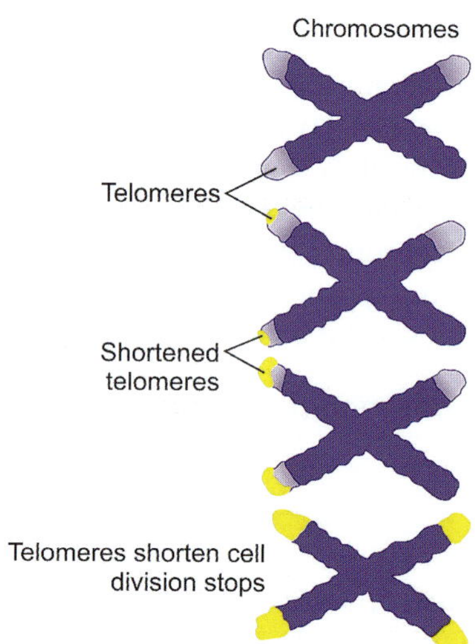

Fig. 1: Telomere shortening.

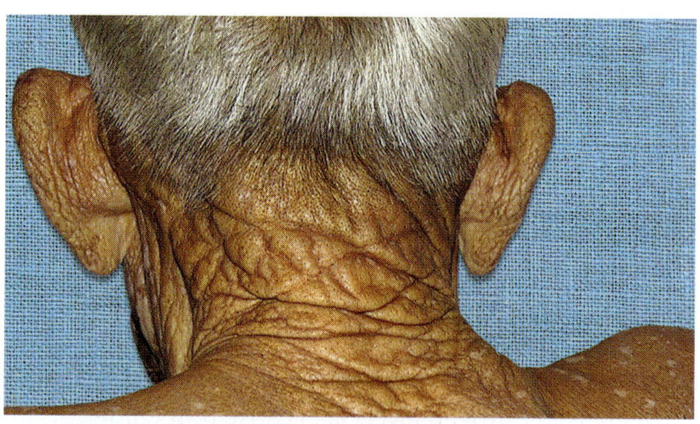

Fig. 2: Cutis rhomboides nuchae.
Courtesy: Dr Koushik Lahiri.

- Deep wrinkles
- Dry
- Lax and sagging
- Freckles
- Solar lentigines
- Telangiectasia (over cheeks)
- Seborrheic keratosis
- Cutis rhomboidalis nuchae (sun-induced wrinkling on back of neck in a rhomboidal pattern) **(Fig. 2)**
- Favre-Racouchot disease (cysts and comedones in the periorbital region due elastic degenerative changes)
- Tendency to develop premalignant and malignant neoplasms

Cutaneous Disorders in Old Age

- Senile pruritus (probably due to increased touch and pain thresholds)
- Senile lentigines (over dorsal of hands and face)
- Graying of hair
- Xerosis (avoid harsh soaps)
- Brittle nails, trachyonychia, onychogryphosis, onycholysis, onychauxis, infections, subungual hematomas, splinter hemorrhages, subungual exostosis, and malignancies
- Asteatotic eczema (rule out internal malignancy, if severe)
- Allergic contact eczema (from products containing perfumes, lanolin, and local anesthetics)
- Stasis eczema (due to insufficient venous drainage)

TABLE 1: Cutaneous problems related to chronological aging.

Chronologic changes	*Problems in skin*
Epidermis	
• Reduced epithelial melanocytes • Reduced adhesion of epithelial corneocytes	• Increased cancer susceptibility • Skin gets dry
Disappearance of rete ridges with reduced adhesion of epidermis and dermis	Wound healing gets delayed and blisters occur easily
Increased skin permeability	Occurrence of allergic contact dermatitis is common
• Reduced photosynthesis of vitamin D • Reduced Langerhans cell	• Bone fractures and osteomalacia • Increased susceptibility of infection
Dermis	
Disappearance of capillary network	Persistence of allergens
Increased matrix metalloproteinases (MMPs)	Loss of collagen
Muffled inflammatory response	Increased sunburns and irritant eczema
Delayed "dermal clearance"	Persistence of topical medications persist ("depot formation")
• Fragmented collagen fibers • Reduced collagen and elastic fibers	• Purpura and wound healing gets delayed • Reduced tensile strength in wounds
Reduced secretion of eccrine gland	Thermoregulatory disorders
Solid state of hyaluronic acid	• Reduced water-binding capacity • Appearance of more wrinkles
Disappearance of Pacinian corpuscles	Lead to more injuries and reduced sensations
Reduced cell-mediated immunity	Increased carcinomas, infections, and allergic contact dermatitis
Reduced subcutaneous fat	Hypersensitivity to cold
Immune dysfunction of B-cell, autoantibodies	Increased autoimmune disease
Disappearance of antibodies to common infections	Increased chance of infections

Source: Sarveswari KN, Premalatha S. Skin at different ages. In: Sacchidanand S (Ed). IADVL Textbook of Dermatology, 4th edition. New Delhi: Bhalani Publishing House; 2015. p. 179.

- Leg ulcers (due to venous hypertension and arterial diseases)
- Decubitus ulcers
- Infections like bacterial cellulitis due to venous stasis, candidal intertrigo in skin folds (unable to reach and dry skin folds, especially toe webspaces)
- Herpes zoster (especially postherpetic neuralgia)
- Ectoparasitic infestations such as scabies and pediculosis
- Bullous disorders such as bullous pemphigoid
- Benign and malignant skin tumors

Cutaneous problems related to chronological aging are given in **Table 1**.

CONCLUSION

The integumentary system typically reflects the process of aging that occurs through all the tissues and organs of the body. While this intrinsic chronological aging is progressive, protection from sun damage and environmental toxins can slowdown the progress of aging.

KEY POINTS

- The skin and its appendages show many structural and functional changes from womb to tomb.
- In the full-term infant, the epidermis, the epidermal appendages, and dermoepidermal junction are fully developed. But the dermis is thinner than that of adults.
- The ratio of skin surface area to volume is high in infants thus making them more susceptible to toxicity from absorption of toxins and drugs.
- During childhood there is a gradual acquisition of structural and functional features of the adult prior to development of sexual characteristics of puberty.
- Low levels of estrogen during menopause accelerate intrinsic aging.
- Both intrinsic (chronological) and extrinsic (environmental) factors contribute to skin aging.

REFERENCES

1. Sarveswari KN, Premalatha S. Skin at different ages. In: Sacchidanand S (Ed). IADVL Textbook of Dermatology, 4th edition. New Delhi: Bhalani Publishing House; 2015. p. 179.
2. Jurica SA, Čolić A, Gverić-Ahmetašević S, Lončarević D, Filipović-Grčić B, Stipanović-Kastelić J, et al. Skin of the very premature newborn: physiology and care. Paediatr Croat. 2016;60:21-6.
3. Dhar S. Newborn skin care revisited. Indian J Dermatol. 2007; 52:1-4.
4. Sarkar R, Basu S, Agarwal RK, Gupta P. Skin care for the newborn. Indian Pediatr. 2010;47(7):593-8.

5. Puttegn B, Cohen BA. Neonatal dermatology. In: Cohen BA (Ed). Pediatric dermatology, 4th edition. Philadelphia: Saunders; 2013. p. 21.
6. Sladeen IN, Johnston GA. Common skin infections in children. BMJ. 2004;329(7457):95-9.
7. Graham Brown RAC. The ages of man and their dermatoses. In: Burns T, Breathnach S, Cox N, Griffiths C (Eds). Rook's Textbook of Dermatology, 7th edition. New Jersey: Wiley-Blackwell; 2008. p. 70.6.
8. Graham Brown RAC. The ages of man and their dermatoses. In: Burns T, Breathnach S, Cox N, Griffiths C (Eds). Rook's Textbook of Dermatology, 7th edition. New Jersey: Wiley-Blackwell; 2008. p. 70.10.
9. Duarte GV, Trigo AC, Oliveria MFDP. Skin disorders during menopause. Cutis. 2016;97:E16-E23.
10. Hall G, Phillips TJ. Estrogen and skin: the effects of estrogen, menopause and hormone replacement therapy on the skin. J Am Acad Dermatol. 2005;53(4):555-68.

EXAMINATION QUESTIONS

1. What are the skin manifestations associated with aging?
2. Discuss the physiological neonatal disorders.

12 CHAPTER Diet in Dermatology

Devinder Mohan Thappa, Munisamy Malathi

Food explains some, but by no means all, skin conditions.

—Burton JL

INTRODUCTION

Diet is derived from the Greek work "dieta" which means "way of life". Nutrients in the diet are essential for various metabolic processes in the body, and any imbalance in the form of nutritional deficiency or specific nutrient deficiency or excess can disturb the equilibrium of the body and with the skin being the largest organ of the body, most of the manifestations are evident on the skin. Moreover, the role of diet in the induction of certain skin disorders and skin disorders per se resulting in nutritional deficiencies is well known. The photoprotective effect of antioxidants and the immunomodulatory effect of micronutrient supplementation and fatty acids have been researched and well documented. Similarly, the role of diet in the management of certain dermatological diseases is proven and in some diseases, it probably plays a role. In conditions such as dermatitis herpetiformis and food allergies, the role of diet is well established; in conditions such as acne and pemphigus, dietary interventions might influence the course of the disease; in conditions such as skin cancer and aging of the skin, dietary change might have a role in the prevention; in conditions such as inborn errors of metabolism, definitive dietary modifications are an essential component in planning the therapeutic strategies; in conditions such as psoriasis and acanthosis nigricans which are linked to systemic diseases, dietary changes might affect health outcomes and finally systemic drugs prescribed for dermatological disease, such as steroids and cyclosporine, are known to raise the risk of other diseases or might be associated with interactions, and dietary change might be beneficial.

This chapter summarizes the possible associations between diet and dermatology which will be useful for the dermatologist to keep some dietary information handy to recommend to patients and to deal with the occasional patient who does not seem to show adequate response despite the best, scientific and evidence-based therapy.

NUTRITIONAL DERMATOSES[1-3]

Nutritional dermatoses are given in **Table 1**.

CUTANEOUS DISORDERS ASSOCIATED WITH EXCESS DIETARY INTAKE[3,4]

Cutaneous disorders associated with excess dietary intake are given in **Table 2**.

CUTANEOUS DISORDERS ASSOCIATED WITH FOOD[1-4]

Cutaneous disorders associated with food are given in **Table 3**.

TABLE 1: Nutritional deficiency and its cutaneous manifestations and source.

Nutritional deficiency	*Cutaneous manifestations*	*Source of nutrients*
Marasmus	Failure to thrive, emaciation, loss of subcutaneous fat and muscle mass, loss of buccal fat (monkey facies); dry, thin, loose, wrinkled skin; loose skin folds; angular cheilitis; fine brittle hair, alopecia; fissuring and impaired growth of nails	Food rich in calorie with balanced diet
Kwashiorkor	Failure to thrive, edema; generalized dermatitis with "flaking enamel paint," "cracked pavement" appearance, xerosis, erosions, brittle, lusterless, reddish brown hair with flag sign (altered bands of light and dark-colored hair), soft and brittle nail, increased pigmentation on arms and legs	Foods containing mainly proteins
Vitamin A deficiency	Xerosis, generalized hyperpigmentation, sparse and fragile hair, phrynoderma	Liver, heart, kidney, milk, cod liver oils, silver oils, butter, eggs, carrots, cabbage, vegetables, green leaves, mangoes, potatoes tomatoes, spinach, papaya

Contd...

Contd...

Nutritional deficiency	*Cutaneous manifestations*	*Source of nutrients*
Niacin deficiency (Pellagra)	Photosensitive dermatitis, angular stomatitis, cheilitis, glossitis (dermatitis, diarrhea, dementia, and death)	Fish, lean meats, whole grains, seeds, legumes, coffee and tea, green vegetables, and milk
Riboflavin deficiency	Angular stomatitis, cheilitis, xerosis, fissuring, glossitis, seborrheic dermatitis-like dermatitis	Eggs, organ meats (kidneys and liver), lean meats, milk, green vegetables
Vitamin B_{12} deficiency	Skin hyperpigmentation, vitiligo, angular stomatitis, and hair changes	Milk, liver, kidney, muscle, butter, chicken, fish, yeast, cheese, raw egg, white grains, green vegetable such as spinach, peanuts, fruits such as apple, orange
Vitamin C deficiency (scurvy)	Bleeding gums, perifollicular purpura, corkscrew hairs, follicular keratotic plugging, ecchymosis, poor wound healing	Guava, amla, green chili, amaranth leaves, citrus fruits, green vegetables, potatoes, tomatoes, cheese, milk
Vitamin D deficiency	Photodamage	Fish liver oils (cod liver oil, halibut liver oil), butter, milk, eggs, liver
Biotin deficiency	Erythematous, crusting, scaly dermatitis around eyes, nose, mouth, and other periorificial areas, alopecia, glossitis	Eggs, almonds, nuts, legumes, whole grains, milk, meat
Zinc deficiency (acrodermatitis enteropathica)	Weeping dermatitis (acute), psoriasiform (chronic) secondary infection, poor wound healing, excessively fragile hair and sparse or no scalp and pubic hair; nail defects	Turmeric, red pepper, cloves, ginger, cumin, anise, fennel, basil, rosemary, garlic, and pomegranate
Selenium deficiency	Hypopigmentation of skin and hair, whitening of the nails	Wheat germ, seafood such as tuna and salmon, garlic, Brazil nuts, eggs, brown rice, and whole wheat bread
Iron deficiency	Spoon-shaped nails (koilonychia), hair loss, glossitis with loss of papillae, angular cheilitis, and pruritus	Liver, eggs, meat, dark and green vegetables, lentils, potatoes, soybeans, chickpeas, black beans, spinach
Fatty acid deficiency	Dry, itchy, scaly skin, phrynoderma	Diet rich in fish and seafood
Anorexia nervosa	Low weight, lanugo hair, xerosis, pruritus, loss of buccal fat pad, yellow tinge, alopecia, Russel's sign	Balanced diet
Bulimia	Normal to overweight, Russell's sign, pharyngitis, caries teeth, dental enamel erosion, bald tongue, purpura, subconjunctival hemorrhage	Balanced diet

TABLE 2: Dermatological manifestations associated with excess dietary intake.

Excess dietary intake	*Dermatological manifestations*
Hypervitaminosis A	Diffuse alopecia, scaling
Hypercarotenemia (excessive consumption of carrots)	Orange discoloration of palms and soles
Lycopenemia (excessive consumption of tomatoes, rosehips, beets, and chili beans)[4]	Yellowish orange pigmentation of the skin and palms
High glycemic food	Acne, acanthosis nigricans

TABLE 3: Cutaneous disorders associated with food and their recommendations.

Cutaneous disorders	*Diets known to precipitate or flare up various skin diseases*	*Recommendations/Comments*
Dermatologic disorders in which diet has a definite role		
Dermatitis herpetiformis (DH)	• *Gluten-containing food:* Wheat, rye, oats, barley trigger • Rash of DH is gluten-dependent • *Iodine-containing food:* Fish, kelp, iodized salt, and vitamin precipitate • DH is worsened by iodides—local chemotaxis and stimulate neutrophil migration	• Gluten-free diet • Rice, corn, and potatoes—safe • Gluten-free diet—protective against the development of lymphoma • Iodides—avoided in patients nonresponsive to gluten-free diet

Contd...

Contd...

Cutaneous disorders	*Diets known to precipitate or flare up various skin diseases*	*Recommendations/Comments*
Dermatologic disorders in which diet has a probable role in etiopathogenesis		
Atopic dermatitis (AD)	• Prevalence of food allergy—30–40% • Prevalence of food allergy-*induced* AD—<30% • *"Western" affluent diet:* High intake of refined grains, cured and red meats, saturated and unsaturated fatty acids—increased risk of AD • Dairy products, beef, eggs, chicken, fish, wheat, soy, citrus and berry fruits, food additives, chocolate and nuts, cheese, caffeine, wheat, tomatoes—implicated as food allergens causing urticarial reactions or flare of dermatitis or nondermatological symptoms	• Benefit from supplementation with vitamin D, evening primrose oil, borage oil, fish oil, zinc sulfate, selenium, vitamin E, pyridoxine, sea buckthorn seed oil, hempseed oil, sunflower oil, and docosahexaenoic acid has insufficient evidence • Prebiotic supplementation in infants and prenatal period followed by postnatal probiotic supplementation decrease the risk of AD • Elimination diets for patients who have a food allergy that is proven by oral food challenge • Exclusive breastfeeding for 4 months or breastfeeding supplemented with hydrolyzed formula is protective against AD in high-risk infants[5]
Acne vulgaris	• Western diet with high glycemic index and higher concentration of omega-6 polyunsaturated fatty acids promotes acne • Frequent milk consumption is associated with higher risk of acne but insufficient evidence for recommendation	• Association of diet with acne—no solid evidence for dietary recommendation • Low glycemic diet comprised mainly of unprocessed fresh fruits, vegetables, lean meats, fish and sea food and low in saturated fats and free of processed food, cereal grains, dairy products, refined sugar, and refined oil has been beneficial • Increased consumption of dietary omega-3 polyunsaturated fatty acids may be therapeutic[5,6]
Psoriasis vulgaris	• Iodides (sea food, iodized salt) can precipitate pustular psoriasis • Deficiency of calcium and zinc can precipitate pustular psoriasis of pregnancy	• Weight loss and decreased alcohol consumption—improve symptoms and increase the efficacy of antipsoriatic medications • Low calorie diets—improve psoriasis • Dietary supplementation with polyunsaturated fatty acids (fish and fish oil rich in eicosapentaenoic acid and docosahexaenoic acid), folic acid, vitamin D, and antioxidants (vitamin C, vitamin E, beta carotene and selenium) and high content of carotenoids and flavonoids (fresh fruits and vegetables, such as carrots and tomatoes)—adjuncts • Gluten-free diet—efficacious in patients with celiac disease-related antibodies • Supplementations of food containing calcium and zinc in pustular psoriasis of pregnancy[7]
Pemphigus	• Thiols, thiocyanates, phenols and tannins containing foods—precipitate pemphigus as they have been found to induce acantholysis in vitro • *Vegetables*: Onion, turnip, broccoli, radish, cabbage, cauliflower, potato, leek, shallots, chives, tomatoes, cassava, eggplant • *Fruits*: Mango, cashew apple, guava, raspberry, cherry, cranberry, blackberry, avocado, banana, apple, peach, grape, pineapple, pear • *Nuts*: Kola nut, walnut, cashew, peanut, pistachio • *Masticatories*: Betel nut leaf, *katha* • *Beverages*: Coffee, tea, beer, cocoa, wine, soft drinks • *Spices*: Ginger, ginseng, garlic, red chilies, asafetida, coriander, cumin, black pepper, *ajwain*, mustard • *Miscellaneous*: Ice cream, candy, baked foods, aspartame, sodium benzoate, tartrazine, coloring agents, nutritional supplements • *Water*: High tannin content in water	Dietary restriction of implicated substances can be beneficial in the management of refractory cases and in the prevention of flares

Contd...

Contd...

Cutaneous disorders	*Diets known to precipitate or flare up various skin diseases*	*Recommendations/Comments*
Urticaria	• Acute urticaria or chronic intermittent urticaria—mostly allergic reactions to food • Chronic urticaria—mostly pseudoallergic reactions to food additives such as salicylates, benzoates, and azo-dyes—tartrazine, amaranth, sunset yellow, carmoisine—and to aromatic volatile ingredients in tomatoes, white wine, and herbs	• Pseudoallergen-free diet and vitamin D supplementation for patients with chronic urticaria • Gluten-free diet in patients with concomitant celiac disease[7]
Pruritus	–	• Restriction of dietary protein reduces the symptoms of uremic pruritus • Supplementation of dietary PUFA is beneficial in cholestatic pruritus
Allergic contact dermatitis	• Latex–fruit syndrome—patients with latex allergy have hypersensitivity to freshly consumed avocado, banana, chestnut, kiwi, peach, tomato, potato, bell pepper, turnip, zucchini, and cassava • *Systemic contact dermatitis—nickel-sensitive individuals—Nickel-rich food:* Whole wheat, whole grain, rye, oat, millet, buckwheat, cocoa, chocolate, tea, gelatin, baking powder, soy products, red kidney beans, legumes such as peas, lentils, peanut, soya beans and chickpeas, dried fruits, canned foods, beverages, strong licorice, beer, red wine, mackerel, tuna, herring and shellfish, sunflower seeds, linseeds, hazelnuts, marzipan, walnuts, tomatoes, onion, raw carrots, spinach, garlic, tea, coffee, vitamin supplements; canned food; food contaminated during processing or by kitchen utensils[8]	Dietary restriction of implicated substances has been found to be beneficial in the management of these specific dermatitis
	• Balsam of Peru dermatitis—aggravation of dermatitis with wine, candy, chocolate, cinnamon, curry, citrus fruit, tomatoes, and flavorings • *Chromium allergy—diet rich in chromium:* Meat, whole grains, legumes, nuts, brewer's yeast, black pepper and other spices, raw sugar, bran cereals, green beans, broccoli, grape juice, orange juice, apple, banana, potato, garlic, red wine, tea, and coffee[9] • *Protein contact dermatitis:* Fruits, vegetables, spices, plants, animal protein, grains, amylase, lactase	
Dermatologic disorders in which specific factors in the diet are directly implicated in the etiopathogenesis of the disorder		
Fish odor syndrome (Trimethylaminuria)	• Foods containing high amounts of choline or of trimethylamine *N*-oxide (TMAO) • *Foods with a high TMAO:* Sea or saltwater fish, especially deep sea fish, cephalopods, and crustaceans • *Foods with high choline content:* Eggs, liver, kidney and other offal, peas, beans, peanuts, soya products, and other legumes	Dietary restriction of foods with a high TMAO or high choline content and use of soaps with a pH value of 5.5–6.5 to remove any traces of free TMA from the skin has been beneficial
Toxic oil syndrome	Consumption of oils containing fatty acid esters of 3-(N-phenylamino)-1,2-propanediol	• Outbreak in Spain in 1981, due to consumption of food grade rapeseed oil containing aniline derivatives • Toxicity symptoms resemble scleroderma and graft versus host disease
Fixed drug eruption	Artificial flavors, colors and preservatives in foods, and dyes in medications	Should be suspected in the absence of definitive drug history
Genetic and metabolic disorders wherein either an elimination diet is mandatory or dietary supplementation of specific factors is beneficial		
Phenylketonuria	*Phenylalanine-containing diet:* Beef, poultry, pork, fish, milk, yogurt, eggs, cheese, soy products (including soy protein isolate, soybean flour, and tofu), and certain nuts and seeds, artificial sweetener aspartame	• Dietary restriction of phenylalanine • Excess intake of milk, egg, meat, and aspartame used as artificial sweetener should be avoided • Natural protein should be restricted to 2 g/kg/day in infants and 1 g/kg/day in childhood

Contd...

Contd...

Cutaneous disorders	*Diets known to precipitate or flare up various skin diseases*	*Recommendations/Comments*
		• A supplement of tyrosine/phenylalanine-free amino acids is usually given even if the allowance of natural protein provides enough substrate for growth • Essential fatty acids, vitamins, and minerals supplementation
Tyrosinemia	*Tyrosine-containing diet:* Chicken, turkey, milk, cheese, yogurt, cottage cheese, peanuts, almonds, avocados, bananas, lima beans, pumpkin seeds, and sesame seeds	• Dietary restriction of tyrosine • Excess intake of milk, egg, meat, and aspartame used as artificial sweetener should be avoided • Daily protein requirement is 3 g/kg for those ≤2 years of age, 2.5 g/kg for those between 3 and 5 years of age, and 2 g/kg for those ≤10 years of age • Natural protein and amino acid supplements should provide 10–12% of the daily intake
Homocystinuria	*Methionine-containing diet:* Milk and milk products, meat and fish, wheat, maize, rice, pulses, legumes, nuts and dried fruits	• Low methionine diet • Fruits and vegetables to be consumed in moderate amounts • Sago, arrowroot, corn flour, custard, sugars, fats, tea and coffee—not restricted
Galactosemia	*Galactose- and lactose-containing diet:* Milk	• Throughout childhood—dietary exclusion of galactose and lactose • Infancy—nutritionally adequate galactose/lactose-free milk • Later childhood—occasional lactose-free milk and calcium and vitamin supplements
Refsum's disease	• Phytanic acid-containing diet • Fish, beef, lamb, and dairy products	• Limit phytanic acid intake to 10–20 mg/day • Phytanic acid in vegetables is in bound form (phytol) which is converted to phytanic acid by ruminants which is present in their meat • Since low phytanic acid-containing diet is unpalatable, poultry, pork, fruit and vegetables are allowed. The diet should contain enough calories to prevent weight loss and subsequent mobilization of phytanic acid from fat • Neurological, cardiac, and dermatological sequelae are reversible, but visual and hearing impairments are less responsive
Glucose-6-phosphate dehydrogenase (G6PD) deficiency	• Fava beans is the most common trigger of hemolytic anemia • Role of other legumes, especially peas, is unknown and reports of symptoms after eating green beans and chickpeas have been reported.	–
Xanthomas	High intake of fats and lipids	Foods containing high concentrations of cholesterol, such as fat, eggs, meat, and dairy products, to be avoided
Gout	*High purine-containing diet:* Organ meat (liver, kidney), fish and shellfish, meat and yeast extract brewer, baker's yeast, pulses, spinach, asparagus, and fermented milk products	Low-fat dairy products, ascorbic acid, and wine consumption is protective
Porphyria	–	• *Dietary supplementation of carotene-containing foods:* Carrots and green leafy vegetables • A 3-week high-fiber diet of natural vegetable/fruit products with a daily caloric content of 1,676 kJ/day—beneficial in porphyria cutanea tarda
Miscellaneous disorders with an uncertain relationship to diet		
Rosacea	Tea, coffee, hot beverages, tobacco, alcohol, and spicy food—precipitate flushing	–
Vitiligo	–	• Supplementation with antioxidants containing alfa-lipoic acid and vitamin B_{12} improves the clinical effectiveness of phototherapy • No scientific data to support or refute the role of elimination diet including citrus fruits, sour yoghurt, sour pickles, and simultaneous consumption of milk and fish

Contd...

Contd...

Cutaneous disorders	*Diets known to precipitate or flare up various skin diseases*	*Recommendations/Comments*
Aphthous ulcers	Allergy or intolerance to figs, cheese, walnuts, tomatoes and various fruits, gluten, cows' milk protein, azo dyes, and preservatives	• Elimination diet in selected cases might result in remission • Recurrent aphthous stomatitis with celiac disease markers respond to gluten-free diet
Cutaneous vasculitis	Food additives such as dyes and preservatives such as tartrazine and ponceau	Elimination diets in selected cases of refractory hypersensitivity vasculitis after ruling out other causes
Telogen effluvium	Iron, zinc, and biotin deficiency	• Minimum intake of at least 0.8 g/kg protein and 1,200 kcal/day • Adequate dietary intake of iron and oral iron supplementation—lean meats, beef, nuts, seeds, legumes, bean products, raisins, dark green leafy vegetables, whole grains, and iron-fortified cereals • No concrete evidence to prove deficiencies of zinc and biotin
Nonmelanoma skin cancer	• Selenium supplementation— increase the risk of nonmelanoma skin cancer, especially squamous cell carcinoma • Meat and fat dietary pattern was found to increase squamous cell carcinoma risk	• No significant association between dietary factors and nonmelanoma skin cancer • Antioxidant supplementation—no role in skin cancer prevention • Dietary consumption of whole foods such as fruits and vegetables rich in antioxidants and phytochemicals decreased the risk of squamous cell carcinoma[5]
Melanoma	–	• Supplementation with polyunsaturated fats, vitamins D and E, selenium, green tea, resveratrol, and lycopene to prevent the development or progression of melanoma in general population—insufficient evidence • Decreased alcohol intake and vitamin D supplementation—lower melanoma risk in high-risk patients[7]
Scleroderma	–	• Avoidance of high-fiber diet • Improvement in the skin of scleroderma on vitamin E supplementation
Herpes	Ingestion of refined sugar or arginine-rich food—recurrence	Mix of nutrients found in fruits and vegetables—vitamins, zinc, and iron supplementation improve immunity and prevent recurrences
Flushing	• Alcohol-related flushing • Food additives—mono sodium glutamate (MSG), sodium nitrite and nitrate, sulfites in processed food, cheese	• Relative deficiency of acetaldehyde dehydrogenase • Tyramine and histamine in fermented alcohol • Alcohol containing industrial solvents • Drugs such as chlorpropamide cause severe alcohol-induced flushing • Cheese and pickles induce flushing in patients on mono amine oxidase inhibitors • Chinese restaurant syndrome (with MSG)

NAMED SIGNS AND SYNDROMES WITH NUTRITIONAL ISSUES

Named signs and syndromes with nutritional issues are given in **Table 4**.

DIET AND NAIL DISORDERS

Visible changes in the nails can be observed in the nail plate or nail matrix or nail bed and can occur in patients with malnutrition or in those with systemic diseases resulting in malnutrition as summarized in **Table 5**, requiring correction of deficiencies and supplementation of vitamins, especially biotin in case of brittle nails.

DIET AND HAIR DISORDERS

Healthy-appearing hair is a sign of good health and changes in hair and hair growth can occur due to general malnutrition **(Table 6)** since vitamins and minerals are required as cofactors for structural proteins in hair.

DIETARY ALLERGENS/PSEUDOALLERGENS

Dietary allergens and pseudoallergens have been implicated in urticaria and atopic dermatitis. In contrast to allergic reactions which are immunoglobulin E (IgE)-mediated reactions, pseudoallergic reactions are non-IgE-mediated reactions resulting in mast cell release. In acute urticaria, while

TABLE 4: Named signs and syndromes with nutritional issues.

Nutritional deficiency/excess	*Named syndromes and signs*
Vitamin A deficiency	Xerophthalmia, Nyctalopia, Bitot's spots, Phrynoderma
Vitamin A excess	• Hypercarotenemia • Hypervitaminosis A
Vitamin D deficiency	Rickets; rachitic rosary
Vitamin K deficiency	Neonatal vitamin K deficiency bleeding
Vitamin B_2 (riboflavin) deficiency	Oro-oculo-genital syndrome
Vitamin B_3 (niacin) deficiency	Pellagra, seborrheic dermatitis-like eruption
Vitamin B_6 (pyridoxine) deficiency	Pellagra-like dermatitis, seborrheic dermatitis-like eruption
Vitamins B_9 (folic acid, folate) and B_{12} deficiency	Hunter glossitis, Addisonian pigmentation
Vitamin C deficiency	• Scurvy, corkscrew hair, swan neck deformity of hair • *X-ray changes:* Pelkan spurs, Wimberger ring, white line of Frankl, scurvy line or Trümmerfeld zone
Biotin deficiency	Acrodermatitis enteropathica-like eruption
Zinc deficiency	Acrodermatitis enteropathica
Protein energy malnutrition	• Marasmus—Monkey facies • Kwashiorkor—"flaky paint," "crazy paving," or "enamel paint" dermatosis; flag sign
Obesity	Horseshoe-shaped plantar hyperkeratosis, adiposis dolorosa (Dercum disease), elephantiasis nostras verrucosa
Eating disorders: Anorexia nervosa and bulimia nervosa	Lanugo-like body hair, carotenoderma, perimylolysis, Russell sign

TABLE 5: Nail changes and their causes.

Nail changes	*Causes*
Involvement of nail matrix, nail bed, and nail plate—chromonychia	• Lunula—bluish discoloration due to copper overload in Wilson's disease; blackish-gray discoloration due to silver overload in argyria • Nail bed—pallor seen in anemia • Nail plate—longitudinal melanonychia seen in malnutrition, vitamins D and B_{12} deficiencies, and hemochromatosis
Involvement of nail bed	• Splinter hemorrhages seen in scurvy and hemochromatosis • Terry nails seen in chronic liver disease • Muehrcke lines seen in hypoalbuminemia, malnutrition, and acrodermatitis enteropathica • Onycholysis seen in iron deficiency anemia, pellagra, and Cronkhite-Canada syndrome
Nail plate changes	• Transverse leukonychia seen in acrodermatitis enteropathica, pellagra, low calcium levels, hemochromatosis, arsenic poisoning (Mee's line) • Clubbing seen in citrullinemia, phosphorus, arsenic, alcohol, mercury or beryllium poisoning, hypervitaminosis A, and cretinism due to iodine deficiency • Koilonychia seen in sideropenic anemia, riboflavin deficiency, pellagra, and vitamin C deficiency • Hapalonychia seen in hypochromic anemia, arsenic poisoning, deficiency of vitamins A, B_6, C, and D, and low serum calcium • Beau's lines seen in protein deficiency, pellagra, hypocalcemia, chronic alcoholism (malnutrition and malabsorption), arsenic toxicity • Onychomadesis seen in arsenic and lead poisoning • Onychorrhexis seen in iron-deficiency anemia, arsenic poisoning, and zinc deficiency • Trachyonychia seen with poor or decreased dietary water and food intake
Brittle nail syndrome	• Onychorrhexis and onychoschizia • Deficient production of intercellular cement substance due to nutritional deficiencies • Treatment options tried include vitamin C, pyridoxine, iron, vitamin D, calcium, amino acids, gelatin, and biotin supplementation

type 1 food allergy is commonly implicated, pseudoallergy to nonsteroidal anti-inflammatory drugs (NSAIDs) is more common than to food. But, in chronic urticaria, pseudoallergy to food has been commonly implicated. The dietary allergens include milk, egg, wheat, soy, peanut, tree nuts, shellfish, fish, cheese, vegetables, fruits, chocolate, alcohol, etc., while dietary pseudoallergens include aromatic compounds found in vegetables (especially tomatoes, herbs), white wine and

TABLE 6: Nutritional disorders and hair changes.

Nutritional disorders	*Hair changes*
Marasmus	• Fine or brittle hair • Alopecia due to telogen effluvium • Increase in lanugo hairs
Kwashiorkor	• Soft and fine hair • Fine and unruly eyelashes—broomstick appearance • Hypochromotrichia—lightening of hair color • Banded pattern of scalp hair—flag sign
Zinc deficiency	Progressive, diffuse, patchy nonscarring alopecia, hair dryness, and brittleness
Essential fatty acid deficiency	Diffuse alopecia of the scalp and eyebrows, and lightening of the remaining hair
Selenium deficiency	Alopecia with hypopigmentation of hair (pseudoalbinism)
Biotin deficiency	• Severe alopecia of scalp, eyebrows, and eyelashes • Lanugo hairs can be absent
Vitamin C deficiency	Corkscrew hairs on the arms, trunk, and legs
Vitamin A deficiency	Follicular hyperkeratosis on extensor surfaces
Anorexia nervosa and bulimia nervosa	• Hypertrichosis lanuginosa—back, abdomen, and forearms • Opaque, dry, and fragile hairs • Diffuse alopecia with a frontal predominance due to telogen effluvium • Pili torti
Iron deficiency	Chronic telogen effluvium
Hypervitaminosis A	Loss of scalp, axillary, and pubic hair

food, and food additives and preservatives (such as salicylates, benzoates and azo-dyes—tartrazine, amaranth, sunset yellow, carmoisine). In atopic dermatitis, food allergy is both IgE- and cell-mediated. Cow's milk, egg, fish, wheat, soy, nuts, and citrus fruits are the proven allergens while pseudoallergens, especially food additives though reported, have a controversial role in aggravation of atopic dermatitis.

Clinical diagnosis of dietary pseudoallergy might be difficult owing to differences in clinical features and diagnostic tests when compared to food allergy. Type 1 allergic reactions can be diagnosed by skin prick test or specific serum IgE or oral food challenge. However, the gold standard test for diagnosis for food allergy is double-blind, placebo-controlled food challenge (DBPCFC). But the diagnosis of pseudoallergy is difficult owing to nonavailability of in vitro tests and skin tests. During provocation tests also, in contrast to type I allergy, symptoms usually occur after a latency of >4 hours and symptoms stop only after an omission of the suspected pseudoallergen for >10 ± 14 days.

The various elimination diets that have been tried in chronic urticaria include low-histamine diet, pseudoallergen-free diet, gluten-free diet, and diet without fish products. In atopic dermatitis, preventive strategies including avoidance measures, diet supplements, and early complementary food introduction have been advocated with a patient-tailored approach.

TABLE 7: Nutricosmetics and their benefits.

Nutricosmetic	*Benefits*
Vitamin D	Prevents skin cancer (melanoma)—cutaneous aging spectrum
Vitamin C	Lightening of skin dyspigmentation
Vitamins E and A	Antiaging benefits
Carotenoids: Astaxanthin (from salmon fish), lutein (green leafy vegetables, such as spinach and kale), lycopene (tomatoes, watermelon, pink grapefruit, papaya, red bell pepper, pink guava)	Antiaging benefits
Pycnogenol (extract of French marine pine bark)	Potent free radical scavenger used as an ideal antiaging additive

DIET IN AESTHETIC DERMATOLOGY AND ANTIAGING PRACTICES

Consumption of high glycemic food can result in production of advanced glycation end products which results in cross linking of collagen, thereby accelerating aging **(Table 7)**. Herbs and spices, such as oregano, cinnamon, cloves, ginger, and garlic, can prevent the production of these advanced glycation end products. Hydration of the skin is essential which can be achieved by drinking adequate quantity of water and consuming food rich in omega-3 essential fatty acids (fish, oats, flaxseeds) and sorbitol (grapes, berries, plums, pears, and seaweeds and algae) which help to retain moisture.[10] This approach to antiaging is known as the "inside-out" approach, wherein oral food supplements and topical agents are combined to improve efficacy. Despite the absence of double-blind placebo-controlled studies to confirm this concept and lack of adequate evidence, this inside-out approach has led to the development of a new product category called "nutricosmetic".

CONCLUSION

The relation between health and food has gained interest in recent years. Dermatologic conditions linked with nutrition can range from nutritional deficiencies, excess nutrients, or metabolic disorders. While the association between skin disorders and nutritional deficiencies and few dermatoses is well established, recent research in this area has uncovered significant evidence that dietary considerations may be important in some dermatological conditions, although a significant lacuna still exists that needs to be addressed. Since patients often link their skin disorders to diet and invariably inquire about dietary modifications, it is quite often challenging to the dermatologists owing to the vast and conflicting evidence that exists on this topic. Hence, dermatologists must take the lead in providing clear, well-substantiated dietary recommendations separating the myths from the facts from a practical point of view.

KEY POINTS

- The role of diet in the induction of certain skin disorders and skin disorders per se resulting in nutritional deficiencies is well known.
- In conditions such as dermatitis herpetiformis and food allergies, the role of diet is well established.
- In conditions such as acne and pemphigus, dietary interventions might influence the course of the disease.
- In conditions such as skin cancer and aging of the skin, dietary change might have a role in the prevention.
- In conditions such as inborn errors of metabolism, definitive dietary modifications are an essential component in planning the therapeutic strategies.
- In conditions such as psoriasis and acanthosis nigricans which are linked to systemic diseases, dietary changes might affect health outcomes.
- Dietary allergens and pseudoallergens have been implicated in urticaria and atopic dermatitis.
- Consumption of high-glycemic food can result in production of advanced glycation end products which results in cross linking of collagen, thereby accelerating aging.
- Herbs and spices, such as oregano, cinnamon, cloves, ginger, and garlic, can prevent the production of these advanced glycation end products.

REFERENCES

1. Basavaraj KH, Seemanthini C, Rashmi R. Diet in dermatology: present perspectives. Indian J Dermatol. 2010;55:205-10.
2. Prabhu SS, Nayak SU, Shenoi SD, Pai SB. Synopsis of Diet in Dermatology: A one day CME conducted by the Department of Dermatology, Kasturba Medical College, Manipal, March 3, 2013. Indian Dermatol Online J. 2013;4:358-64.
3. Katta R, Desai SP. Diet and dermatology: the role of dietary intervention in skin disease. J Clin Aesthet Dermatol. 2014;7:46-51.
4. Kaimal S, Thappa DM. Diet in dermatology: revisited. Indian J Dermatol Venereol Leprol. 2010;76:103-15.
5. Bronsnick T, Murzaku EC, Rao BK. Diet in dermatology: Part I. Atopic dermatitis, acne, and nonmelanoma skin cancer. J Am Acad Dermatol. 2014;71:1039.e1-1039.e12.
6. Melnik BC. Diet in acne: further evidence for the role of nutrient signalling in acne pathogenesis. Acta Derm Venereol. 2012;92:228-31.
7. Murzaku EC, Bronsnick T, Rao BK. Diet in dermatology: Part II. Melanoma, chronic urticaria, and psoriasis. J Am Acad Dermatol. 2014;71:1053.e1-1053.e16.
8. Sharma AD. Low nickel diet in dermatology. Indian J Dermatol. 2013;58:240.
9. Sharma AD. Low chromate diet in dermatology. Indian J Dermatol. 2009; 54:293-5.
10. Nguyen G, Torres A. Systemic antioxidants and skin health. J Drugs Dermatol. 2012;11:e1-4.

EXAMINATION QUESTIONS

1. Discuss nutritional dermatoses in detail.
2. Briefly discuss the role of diet in deramtology.
3. Explain the role of dietary allergens/pseudoallergens in atopic dermatitis and urticaria.

13 CHAPTER

Environment and Skin

Rashmi Sarkar, Neha Dubey, Akansha Bhargava

INTRODUCTION

Skin forms an important interface between humans and environment. With its large surface area it functions as the primary organ of defense and thus provides the first barrier against environmental stresses and becomes the most vulnerable target. Cutaneous responses vary according to different environmental conditions and so does the seasonal and geographical variations of different types of skin ailments. Environmental factors affecting skin include physical [e.g., heat, cold, ultraviolet radiation (UVR), ionizing radiation (IR), and mechanical factors], chemical (e.g., cosmetics, food items, and pharmacological products), biological (virus, bacteria, fungi, and parasites), and psychosocial (e.g., stress, inter human contact components). All of these can manifest as an acute or chronic skin disease. Few studies have also reported gender differences in the biology of skin and its response to various environmental insults. Skin conditions such as atopic dermatitis, psoriasis, carcinomas of skin, and autoimmune diseases involves the interactions between genetic risk factors and environmental triggers **(Table 1)**.[1]

CUTANEOUS REACTIONS TO COLD[3]

Physiology (Flowchart 1)

The body's thermoregulatory mechanism maintains a constant core temperature of approximately 37°C against the external temperature ranging between 15 and 54°C. Persistent exposure to cold causes repeated cycles of vasodilatation followed by vasoconstriction, this is also known as "*hunting reaction of Lewis*". Persistent vasoconstriction jeopardizes the vascular supply causing the arteriovenous (AV) anastomoses in the skin to open up causing transient vasodilatation and hence preventing cutaneous necrosis. Classification of cold injuries is given in **Table 2**.

Frostbite[4]

Definition: It is localized damage to skin and tissues due to freezing by extreme cold environment.

Pathophysiology: It can be divided into four overlapping pathologic phases: (1) prefreeze, (2) freeze thaw, (3) vascular stasis, and (4) a later ischemic phase, which are described in **Table 3**.

Clinical features—mentioned in **Table 4**.

Risk factors:

- *Environmental factors*: Temperature, cold exposure, altitude, and degree of wetness.
- *Host factors*: Neuroleptic and sedative drugs, old age, immobility, diabetes, malnutrition, tobacco addiction,

Flowchart 1: Physiology of cutaneous response to cold.

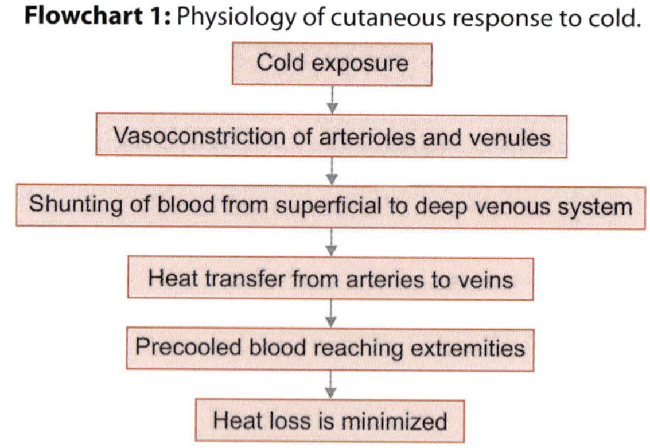

TABLE 1: Cutaneous reaction patterns.[2]

Reaction pattern	*Allergic skin*	*Atopic skin*	*Irritative skin*	*Reactive skin*
Trigger	Exposure to allergens	Abnormal cutaneous barrier	Environmental factors (heat, cold, ultraviolet radiation)	Physical, psychological, and chemical factors
Response	Pruritus, erythema ± vesicles	Excessive dryness, pruritus ± erythema	Dry, cracked, erythematous skin	Inflammation, tingling, pins and needle sensation

TABLE 2: Classification of cold injuries.[2]

Diseases of cold exposure	*Diseases with abnormal cold susceptibility*
Frostbite	Acrocyanosis
Chilblain (pernio)	Cryoglobulinemia
Trench foot	Paroxysmal cold hemoglobinuria
Erythrocyanosis	Livedo reticularis
Raynaud's phenomenon (primary)	Raynaud's phenomenon (secondary)
Cold urticaria	
Cutis marmorata	

TABLE 3: Pathophysiology of frostbite.

Prefreeze	Decrease in blood flow resulting in skin cooling and vasoconstriction
Freeze thaw	Ice crystals form intra- or extracellularly, causing protein and lipid derangement, cellular shifts of electrolytes, dehydration, cell membrane lysis, and death. This may initiate ischemia-reperfusion injury and inflammatory response
Vascular stasis	• Vessels constrict and dilate • Blood may leak from vessels
Ischemic phase	Tissue ischemia and infarction

TABLE 4: Clinical features.

First-degree injury	Characterized by epidermal involvement, seen as erythema, mild edema
Second-degree injury	Full-thickness skin freezing with substantial edema and formation of clear blisters, which contract and dry within 2–3 weeks, forming a dark eschar
Third-degree injury	Formation of hemorrhagic blisters, blue-gray discoloration of the skin, deep burning pain on rewarming, thick gangrenous eschar formation, and the sequelae of trophic ulceration and severe cold sensitivity
Fourth-degree injury	Characterized by involvement of fourth-degree injury

peripheral neuropathy, cardiac disease, constricting clothing, and footwear. Exposed areas such as nose, cheeks, toes, and fingers are frequently affected.

Treatment: Rapid rewarming is done by immersing the affected area in warm water for 15–20 minutes. Tetanus prophylaxis and antibiotics might be required if the wound is contaminated. Other modalities include ibuprofen, thrombolytic therapy, heparin, vasodilators, and hyperbaric oxygen. Surgery should be avoided until the demarcation of viable tissue is clear (6–12 weeks).[4]

Trench Foot

It is a "wet cold" disease which results from exposure to moisture from one to several days at or near the freezing point. It is commonly associated with dependency and immobility. Trench foot on rewarming undergoes a stage of prehyperemia with anesthesia and edema, paresthesia, and anhidrosis. Severe cases show muscular weakness or atrophy and ulceration or gangrene on distal superficial areas. Within few days or week, a posthyperemic stage develops that is characterized by hypersensitivity to cold which may last for years.[5]

Chilblains

It is a nonfreezing tissue injury due to cold in a predisposed individual which leads to vasoconstriction of the deep cutaneous arterioles with simultaneous dilatation of the smaller superficial vessels.

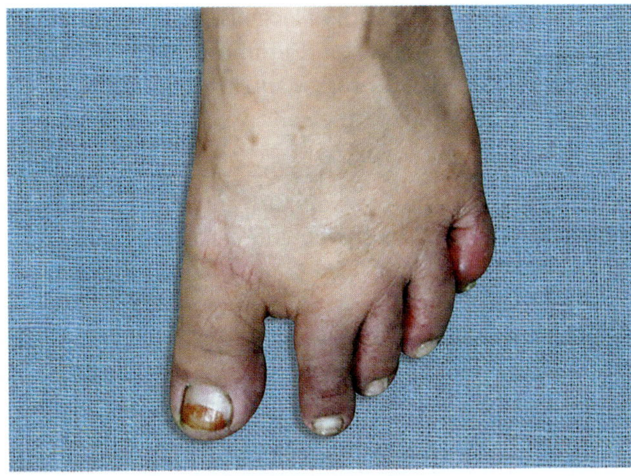

Fig. 1: Chilblains of the foot.
Courtesy: Dr Vivek Kumar Dey.

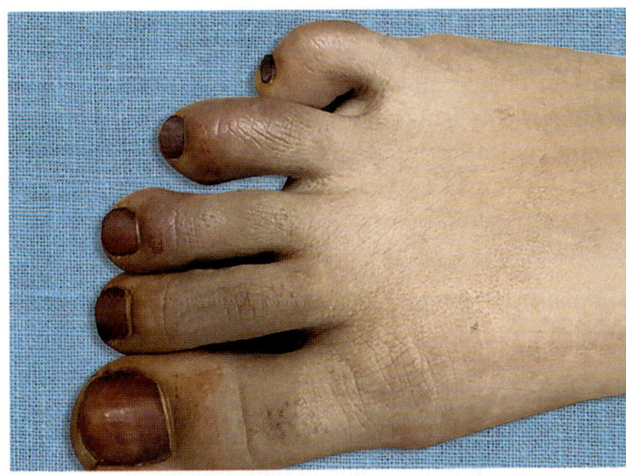

Fig. 2: Chilblains of the foot.
Courtesy: Dr Akansha Bhargava.

Risk factors: Genetic predisposition, dampness, poor nutrition, systemic diseases, alcohol, nicotine.

Clinical features: Presents 12–24 hours after cold exposure as red or violaceous macules, papules, nodule, plaques, or vesicles over acral areas which can ulcerate **(Figs. 1 and 2)**. Also associated with burning and pain.

Treatment: Rest, warmth, and calcium channel blockers in mild cases. Thyrocalcitonin and hemodilution for severe cases.

Acrocyanosis

It is characterized by bluish discoloration of skin and mucous membrane due to chronic vasospasm of small cutaneous arteries with capillary and postcapillary venules dilatation as a compensatory mechanism leading to cyanosis and sweating.

Etiology: Classified into primary and secondary to psychiatric, infective, metabolic, neurologic, autoimmune, or other causes.

Clinical features: Presents with violaceous, dusky discolorations of hands, and sometimes feet. Commonly seen in females. Extremities appear cold, swollen and sweaty. Ear, nose, lips, and nipples might also get affected.

Treatment: No standard treatment is available. Diet and lifestyle changes, counseling about hygiene, and avoidance of cold are the important preventable measures.

Erythrocyanosis

Reddish-blue blanchable discoloration of the skin over thighs, lower legs, and gluteal area in girls and young females. The discoloration is cold to touch.

Treatment: Warm clothing, weight reduction, and calcium channel blockers.

Cold Urticaria

It is a rare form of physical urticaria. It is a localized or generalized eruption of papules on exposure to cold air, liquids, or objects and can be associated with angioedema and anaphylaxis. It may be acquired or autosomal dominant. Acquired cold urticaria often presents in young adulthood with a mean duration of 4–5 years and remission or improvement of symptoms after 5 years in 50% of cases. Familial variant presents in early childhood and persists lifelong.

Treatment: Antihistamines, leukotriene receptor antagonists, biologics, and glucocorticoids.

Cryoglobulinemia

Cryoglobulins are immunoglobulins that precipitate when incubated at low temperature and disappears at 37°C. They are classified into three types:

- *Type I* consists of monoclonal immunoglobulin G (IgG) or IgM antibody that are produced due to underlying lymphoproliferative disease. These precipitates to inflammatory vasculitis and vessel obstruction, clinically seen as erythematous or purpuric papules on lower extremities and at times ulcers.
- *Types II and III* are called mixed cryoglobulins as they contain two immunoglobulins of different isotypes. These are produced due to hyperactivation and/or proliferation of β-cells. Chronic inflammatory states, including collagen diseases and viral infections [hepatitis C virus (HCV)], may initiate β-cell hyperactivation. Skin manifestations are less common. Arthralgia, myalgia, peripheral neuropathy, respiratory manifestations, and membranoproliferative glomerulonephritis are more commonly seen in mixed cryoglobulinemia.

Treatment: Nonsteroidal anti-inflammatory drugs (NSAIDs) to relieve arthralgia, myalgia, and fatigue. Progressive renal failure, necrosis of the distal extremities or uncontrolled neuropathy requires plasmapheresis and/or steroids and cytotoxic drugs. Associated lymphoproliferative disorder requires chemotherapy and radiation. For chronic HCV infection-associated cryoglobulinemias ribavirin, pegylated interferon (IFN) and rituximab are recommended.

Raynaud's Phenomenon[6] (Figs. 3A and B)

It is characterized by episodic vasospasm of the fingers and toes, precipitated by cold exposure which classically manifests as triphasic color changes—pallor, cyanosis, and erythema. It is classified as primary (idiopathic) when there is no underlying illness present and as secondary, when associated with systemic disorders. Difference between primary and secondary Raynaud's phenomenon are given in **Table 5**.

Criteria for primary Raynaud's phenomenon:

- Vasospastic attacks precipitated by cold or emotional stress
- Symmetric manner
- Absence of tissue necrosis or gangrene
- No history or physical finding suggestive of a secondary cause

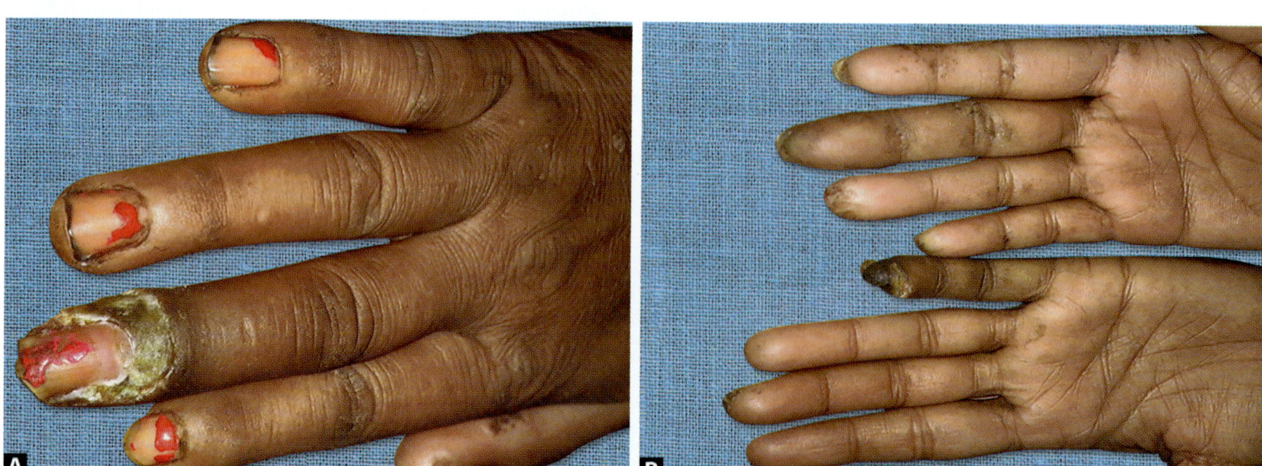

Figs. 3A and B: Raynaud's phenomenon with pits and ulcerations in a patient of systemic sclerosis.
Courtesy: Dr Akansha Bhargava.

TABLE 5: Difference between primary and secondary Raynaud's phenomenon.[6]

Primary Raynaud's	*Secondary Raynaud's*
Cold or stress leading to vasospastic attack, no underlying systemic disease associated	Associated with underlying systemic diseases such as connective tissue disorders, atherosclerosis and others
Symptoms are usually mild	Symptoms are severe
Spontaneous improvement	Progression or resolution depends on causative agent
Symmetric attacks involving both hands	Asymmetric attacks
Normal ESR	ESR increased
Absence of tissue necrosis and gangrene	Can lead to ischemia and gangrene
Normal nailfold capillaries	Abnormal microvasculature
ANA negative	ANA positive
Females are affected more	Gender affliction depends upon cause
Onset occurs in teens or 20s	Onset in third and fourth decade or later
Treatment is symptomatic	Treat the underlying cause

(ANA: antinuclear antibody; ESR: erythrocyte sedimentation rate)

- Normal nail fold capillaries
- Normal erythrocyte sedimentation rate (ESR)
- Negative serologic findings particularly negative test for antinuclear antibody (ANA)

Factors associated with secondary *Raynaud's phenomenon* are given in **Box 1**.

Treatment

- *Pharmacological*: Calcium channel blockers, sympatholytic agent, angiotensin II receptor type I antagonist, selective serotonin reuptake inhibitors, vasodilators, vasoactive drugs such as pentoxifylline and prostaglandins.
- *Nonpharmacological*:
  - Avoidance of cold temperature and keeping the body warm
  - Reducing emotional stress
  - Avoiding agents which lead to vasoconstriction
  - Avoid smoking
  - Surgery—sympathectomy

Paroxysmal Cold Hemoglobinuria

It is an autoimmune intravascular hemolytic anemia that results in a biphasic hemolysin in the blood, usually polyclonal IgG. This antibody binds to glycosphingolipid P antigen on the RBC surface at low temperatures. This interaction leads to complement lysis within vascular circulation.

Etiology: Usually seen in young children within 2–3 weeks of upper respiratory and gastrointestinal infection. Neoplasms could be an underlying pathology.

BOX 1: Factors associated with secondary Raynaud's phenomenon.[6]

Rheumatological disease:
- Scleroderma
- Systemic lupus erythematosus (SLE)
- Dermatomyositis or polymyositis
- Rheumatoid arthritis
- Takayasu arteritis
- Giant cell arteritis
- Primary biliary cirrhosis

Mechanical injury:
- Vibration
- Frostbite

Recurrent trauma or injury to large vessels:
- Crutch pressure
- Thoracic outlet syndrome

Arterial diseases:
- Brachiocephalic atherosclerosis

Vasospastic disorders:
- Migraine or vascular headaches
- Prinzmetal angina

Endocrine disorders:
- Carcinoid syndrome
- Pheochromocytoma
- Hypothyroidism

Malignant diseases:
- Ovarian cancer
- Angiocentric lymphoma

Abnormal blood elements:
- Cryoglobulins
- Cryofibrinogenemia
- Cold agglutinins
- Paraproteinemia
- Polycythemia

Infections:
- Parvovirus B19
- *Helicobacter pylori*

Chemicals or drugs:
- Bleomycin
- Vinblastine
- Polyvinyl chloride
- Beta blockers
- Interferon α and β

Clinical features: Constitutional symptoms with dark red-brown colored urine.

Investigations: Direct antiglobulin, Donath–Landsteiner test, and indirect antiglobulin test.

Treatment: Supportive care and avoidance of cold is the mainstay of treatment. Other modalities includes: RBC transfusion in severe anemia. Infusion of humanized monoclonal anti-C5 antibody eculizumab.

CUTANEOUS REACTIONS TO HEAT[7]

Physiology

Skin plays a crucial role in thermoregulation. A balance between heat creation and heat dissipation regulates our body temperature. Heat dissipation takes place via conduction, convection, radiation, and evaporation **(Flowchart 2 and Table 6)**.

Flowchart 2: Physiology of cutaneous reaction to heat.

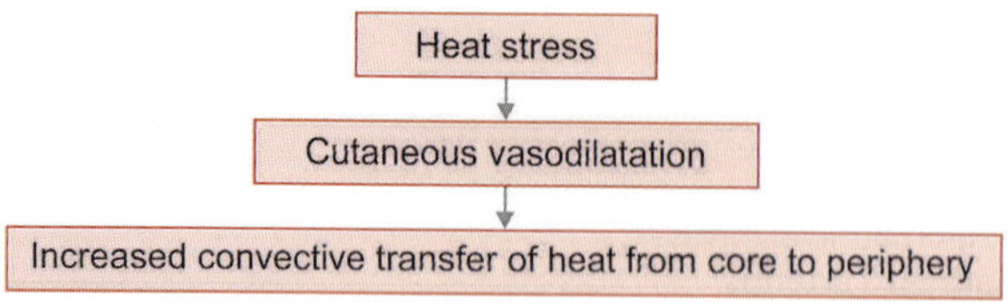

TABLE 6: Cutaneous reaction patterns to heat.

Immediate	*Delayed*	*Long term*
Erythema	Miliaria	Photoaging
Sweating	Acne	Squamous cell carcinoma
Heat contact urticaria	Erythema ab igne	Merkel cell carcinoma
Cholinergic urticaria		Marginal zone lymphoma

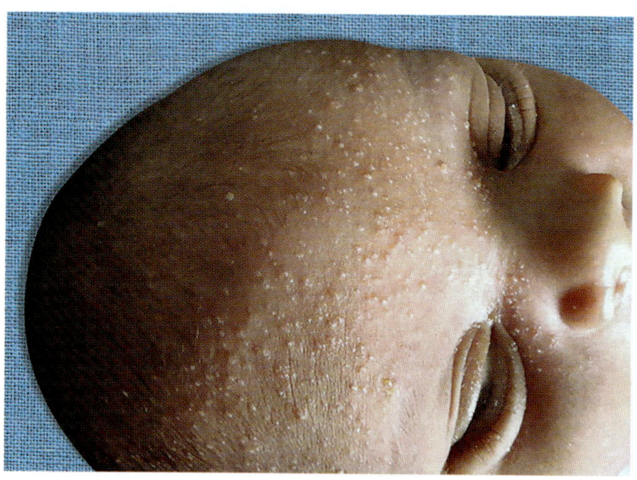

Fig. 4: Miliaria.
Courtesy: Dr Vivek Kumar Dey.

Miliaria

A disorder of sweat glands, this commonly occurs in tropics. It is classified into four subtypes depending upon level of obstruction—(1) *miliaria crystallina, (2) miliaria rubra, (3) miliaria pustulosa, and (4) miliaria profunda* **(Fig. 4)**. Exercise, hot and humid climate, UVR, and normal flora on skin aggravate this condition.

Treatment: Cooling, avoidance of sweating, excessive clothing, calamine lotion, topical or oral antibiotics, and isotretinoin for more severe and resistant to treatment cases.

Cholinergic Urticaria

It is a type of physical urticaria occurring due to increased core body temperature mainly after exercise, exposure to stress or after having spicy meals. It is characterized by multiple 1–5 mm papules or wheals, mainly over trunk and limbs lasting for a few minutes to an hour. Provocation test is performed to differentiate between cholinergic urticaria and exercise-induced urticaria. Exercise-induced urticaria is induced by exercise while cholinergic urticaria is induced by warming.

Heat Contact Urticaria

It is a rare form of physical urticaria. Urticarial lesions typically occur at the site of heat contact. Provocation test is performed by applying hot object at 45°C over the volar aspect of forearm for around 5 minutes. Test is read after 10 minutes, if wheal and flare occurs it is considered as positive.

Tropical Acne

It is a form of acne seen in tropics or hot and humid climate. Presents as multiple large inflammatory nodules over trunk and buttocks.

Treatment: Systemic antibiotics and climatic change.

Erythema Ab Igne

It is a reticular erythematous pigmented dermatoses occurring due to prolonged or repeated exposure to infrared radiation at 43–47°C. Presents as multiple hyperpigmented reticulated patches with telangiectasia.

Treatment: Removal of heat source, topical retinoids, hydroquinone for pigmentation.

Heat-associated Carcinomas

- Kangri cancer is a type of squamous cell carcinoma (SCC) of skin. It is a heat-induced skin carcinoma found mainly in Kashmir because of the use of kangri "a traditional firepot" in winters, which is kept close to thighs or abdomen to maintain continuous warmth.
- Kang cancer in Chinese workers occurs due to hydrocarbon-fuelled heat exposure from sleeping on coal-fire-heated bricks.
- Other cancers include Kairo cancer in Japanese due to carrying metallic benzene-burning flasks. In Ireland peat fire cancer on the legs of rural irish women due to prolonged standing over peat fires, and epithelioma in Australia caused by spectacles focusing infrared radiations on the cheeks.

CUTANEOUS REACTIONS TO ULTRAVIOLET RADIATION[8] (TABLE 7)

Ultraviolet B (UVB) is more erythematogenic than UVA. UVR creates reactive oxygen species and induce DNA damage. This in turn causes the release of autoantigens which can lead to apoptosis or malignant transformation of autoreactive immune processes. UVR induce immunosuppression and inflammation by depletion of Langerhans cell and T-cells and cytokine-mediated immune activation respectively. UVR also have the potential to cause photoallergic and phototoxic reactions.

TABLE 7: Normal responses of skin to ultraviolet radiation.

Acute	*Chronic*
Tanning	Photoaging
Sunburn	Photodermatoses
Vitamin D synthesis	Carcinogenesis
Epidermal hyperplasia	

Types of ultraviolet radiation:

UVC (200–280 nm)
↓
UVB (280–320 nm)
↓
UVA (320–400 nm)

Acute Effects

- *Tanning:*
    - Immediate—transient darkening of exposed skin induced by UVA and other visible radiation. Evident within 5–10 minutes of exposure, it fades within 1–2 hours.
    - Delayed—becomes evident after 1–2 days of exposure and may persist for weeks or months.
- *Sunburn*: An acute injury following excessive exposure to solar radiation characterized by erythema. Longer exposure can cause pain and blistering **(Fig. 5)**.
- *Vitamin D synthesis*: UVB exposure causes vitamin D synthesis in the skin.

Chronic Effects

- *Photoaging:* Also known as *dermatoheliosis*, it is mainly a result of UVB exposure. It is characterized by a heterogeneous response of epidermal cells, connective tissue of dermis and the cutaneous vasculature. Seen as xerosis, deep wrinkles, loss of elasticity, telangiectasia, and mottled pigmentation. Other features include senile comedones, solar lentigines, and seborrheic keratosis.
  Treatment: Use of broad-spectrum sunscreen, restricted UV exposure and topical retinoids.
- *Photodermatoses:* These are a heterogeneous group of dermatoses characterized by polymorphic cutaneous eruptions secondary to UV and/or visible light exposure **(Fig. 6)**.
- *Carcinogenesis:* Most of the nonmelanoma skin cancers (basal cell carcinoma, squamous cell carcinoma) are a result of chronic exposure to UVB and to some extent UVA exposure.

Favre–Racouchot Syndrome (Senile Comedones)

These are characterized by multiple, open and closed comedones superimposed on sun-damaged skin in the periorbital region **(Fig. 7)**.

Treatment: Comedone extraction and regular use of sunscreen and topical retinoids.

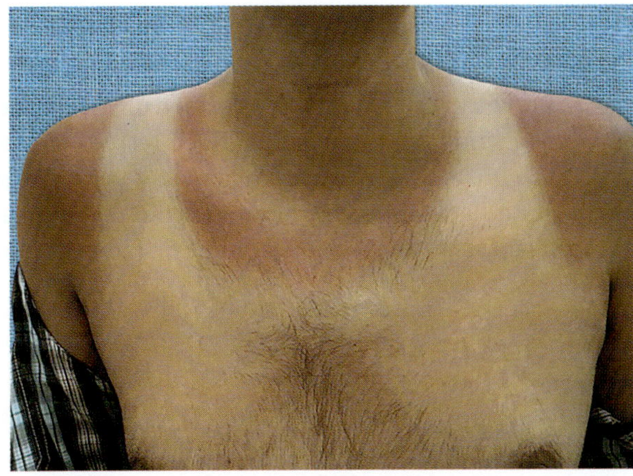

Fig. 5: Acute sunburn reaction in photoexposed parts.
Courtesy: Dr Vivek Kumar Dey.

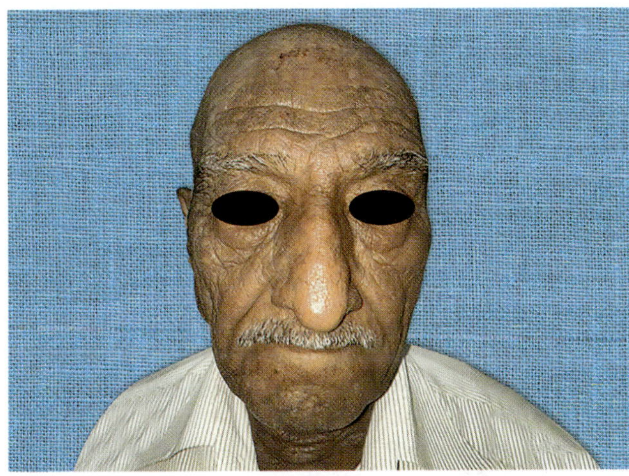

Fig. 6: Chronic actinic dermatitis.

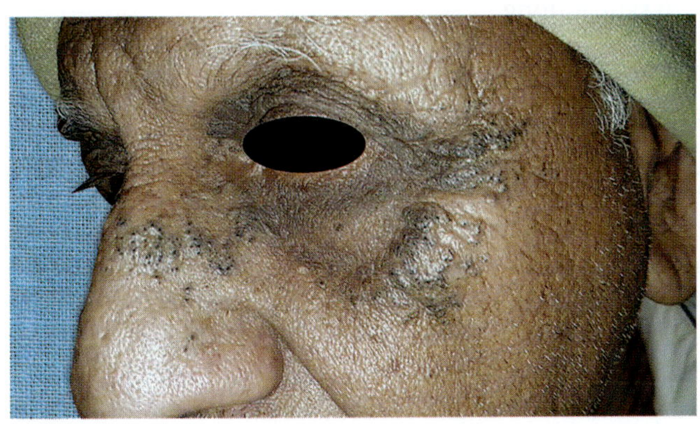

Fig. 7: Senile comedones.
Courtesy: Dr Vivek Kumar Dey.

Solar Urticaria[9]

It is a type of physical urticaria caused by direct exposure to sunlight.

Clinical features: Appearance of wheals within few minutes of UVR exposure associated with erythema, itching, and burning sensation which usually subside within a few hours. Systemic features such as headache, dizziness, and syncope are seen in case larger surface areas are involved.

Diagnosis: Provocative tests can be performed on the buttocks using the solar simulators with filters. UVA is tested at 6 J/cm^2 and UVB at 60 mJ/cm^2. Positive test reaction is characterized by a wheal and flare within 10 minutes at the reaction site. Visible light is tested using a projector at a distance of 10 cm in case of negative reaction.

CUTANEOUS REACTIONS TO IONIZING RADIATION[10]

Ionizing radiation is usually used for the treatment of malignant conditions but can lead to radiation-induced skin changes in many. Radiation-induced cutaneous reactions are graded as acute, consequential-late or chronic changes. Acute changes present within 90 days of exposure as erythema and pain. Severe acute reactions cause blistering, erosions, and ulcerations. Chronic radiation dermatitis is permanent, progressive and irreversible characterized by pigmentary changes, fibrosis, atrophy, and telangiectasia. It can lead to development of cutaneous malignancies.

Acute reactions can be managed by use of moisturizers, low- to mid-potency steroids for pruritus and irritation, and hydrocolloid dressing. And for severe acute reactions surgical excisions, reconstruction, and amputation might be required.

For chronic reactions, appropriate wound care in case of ulcers and erosions and surgical intervention for nonhealing ulcers is required.

Fibrosis is managed by physical therapy, massage and pain management, pentoxifylline, superoxide dismutase, interferon-γ, hyperbaric oxygen therapy, and laser therapy with skin grafting.

CUTANEOUS REACTIONS TO FRICTION AND PRESSURE[11,12]

Corns and Callosities

Chronic exposure of the skin to mechanical shearing and friction results in corns and callosities. If the force is focused at a particular area it results in development of corn and if the area is larger than 1 cm^2 a callus develops. Commonly affecting the feet these can develop due to faulty footwear, deformities, bony prominences, and sometimes autosomal inheritance. They can develop on extrapedal sites as well owing to personal habits for example gnaw warts and prayer nodules.

Management: Keratolytics, paring, cushioning of footwear, and surgical removal.

Pressure Ulcers

Definition: A pressure ulcer is a localized injury to the skin or underlying tissue, usually over a bony prominence, as a result of unrelieved pressure.[12]

Predisposing factors: *Intrinsic*—limited mobility, comorbidities, and poor nutrition. *Extrinsic*—pressure, shear, and friction.

Causative factors: Muscle necrosis due to pressure and friction, microvascular damage, and disuse atrophy due to neural dysfunction. They generally develop over the bony prominences of the lower limbs and pelvic region.

The National Pressure Ulcer Advisory Panel classifies the stages of development of a pressure ulcer as:

- *Stage 1:* Nonblanchable erythema of intact skin
- *Stage 2:* Partial thickness skin loss
- *Stage 3:* Full thickness skin loss
- *Stage 4:* Extensive tissue necrosis

Management: Release of pressure and friction, proper wound care, nutritional support, and corrective surgeries.

CONCLUSION

Our environment affects our body in many ways and our skin being one of the first barriers tends to be very responsive to any external insult by manifesting as various types of dermatoses. Proper knowledge about these skin and environmental factors interactions aid in their proper management.

KEY POINTS

- Skin forms the first barrier against environmental stresses.
- Environmental factors affecting the skin could be *physical, chemical, and biological.*
- It is imperative to have a sound knowledge of various cutaneous reaction patterns.
- Persistent cold exposure causes repeated cycles of vasodilatation followed by vasoconstriction—"hunting reaction of Lewis".
- Raynaud's phenomenon manifests as triphasic color changes, namely, pallor, cyanosis, and erythema.
- Miliaria, tropical acne and cholinergic urticaria are common reaction pattern to heat.
- Ultraviolet B rays are more erythematogenic than UVA rays.
- IR can induce many skin changes, ranging from blisters, erosions to ulceration.

REFERENCES

1. Misery L. How the skin reacts to environmental factors. J Eur Acad Dermatol Venereol. 2007;21 suppl 2:5-8.
2. Pierard-Franchimont C, Henry F, Pierard GE. Cold injuries. In: Wolff K, Goldsmith LA, Katz SI, Gilchrest BA, Paller AS, Leffell DJ (Eds). Fitzpatrick's Dermatology in General Medicine, 7th edition. New York: McGraw Hill; 2008. pp. 844-51.
3. Creamer D. Reactions to cold. In: Burns T, Breathnach S, Cox N, Griffith C (Eds). Rook's Textbook of Dermatology, 8th edition. Oxford: Wiley-Blackwell; 2010. pp. 28.63-28.74.

4. McIntosh SE, Hamonko M, Freer L, Grissom CK, Auerbach PS, Rodway GW, et al. Wilderness medical society practice guidelines for the prevention and treatment of frostbite. Wilderness Environ Med. 2011;22:156-66.
5. Meryman HT. Tissue freezing and local cold injury. Physiol Rev. 1957;37:233-50.
6. Block JA, Sequeira W. Raynaud's phenomenon. Lancet. 2001;357:2042-8.
7. Kellogg DL Jr. In vivo mechanisms of cutaneous vasodilation and vasoconstriction in humans during thermoregulatory challenges. J Appl Physiol (1985). 2006;100(5):1709-18.
8. Maverakis E, Miyamura Y, Bowen MP, Correa G, Ono Y, Goodarzi H. Light, including ultraviolet. J Autoimmun. 2010;34(3):J247-57.
9. Botto NC, Warshaw EM. Solar urticaria. J Am Acad Dermatol. 2008;59(6):909-20.
10. Hymes SR, Strom EA, Fife C. Radiation dermatitis: clinical presentation, pathophysiology, and treatment 2006. J Am Acad Dermatol. 2006;54(1):28-46.
11. Cambiaghi S, Morel P. Hereditary painful callosities with associated features. Dermatology. 1996;193(1):47-9.
12. Bluestein D, Javaheri A. Pressure ulcers: prevention, evaluation, and management. Am Fam Physician. 2008; 78(10):1186-94.

EXAMINATION QUESTIONS

1. What are the effects of UVR on skin?
2. Elaborate the cutaneous reaction patterns to cold.

14 CHAPTER

Evidence-based Dermatology

Saumya Panda

INTRODUCTION

What is evidence-based medicine, evidence-based practice, and evidence-based dermatology?

David Sackett, a clinical epidemiologist, defined evidence-based medicine (EBM) in a landmark article in the British Medical Journal (BMJ) in 1996 as "the conscientious, explicit and judicious use of current best evidence about the care of individual patients."[1] This definition is a comprehensive one, and encapsulates the core concepts of the discipline **(Box 1)**. However, the most important phrase in the definition is the frequently forgotten one that is "the care of individual patients." It means that EBM is not an ivory tower concept, for scoring intellectual brownie points in academia, or ego boosting in journal clubs. Rather, its place is in the clinics, or at the bedside. Its processes start and end with the patient. In short, EBM is a system of learning, with improved outcome of health of patients being its primary aim.

These days, the term "evidence-based practice" is being increasingly used in place of EBM. Evidence-based practice is defined as integrating clinical expertise with best external evidence obtained from systematic research.[2] The concept of evidence-based practice is more appealing to many as it implies *applying knowledge* in contrast to EBM, which focuses on the *process of acquiring knowledge.*

Evidence-based dermatology (EBD) simply denotes the application of the principles of EBM to people with skin diseases.[3]

What is EBD and what it is not?

Despite such comprehensive definitions, there are many misconceptions about EBD that abound in the literature, as also among the general population of practicing dermatologists. EBD, to use RE Clerk's metaphor, stands on a three-legged stool—that of external evidence, clinical expertise, and patients' values and preferences **(Fig. 1)**. Take any one leg away, and the stool falls apart.[4]

Thus the popular concept of EBM having everything to do only with the best external evidence is a woefully inadequate one, and it engenders many of the wrong notions prevalent about the discipline. While systematic search for the best evidence is at the heart of EBD, so too is the clinical expertise of the general dermatologist. The ordinary patient with his/her individual clinical problem, values, and expectations is the best source for generating evidence-based questions, and thus forms the fulcrum of evidence-based practice. Generating an answerable clinical question, or being able to critically appraise a randomized clinical trial (RCT) report or a systematic review about a dermatological treatment should be regarded as basic core competencies for a dermatologist as much as the ability to clinically examine, perform clinicopathological correlation to diagnose, or to perform a skin biopsy, or do an electrosurgery to remove a wart.

It should be clear then, that EBD/EBM is not simply a form of cookbook medicine, and is not a simple assemblage of a recipe of desirable treatments. It must be remembered that, being a young discipline, many of the methods of EBM are of fairly recent vintage, like those used to conduct RCTs or systematic reviews. Many of the lynchpins of dermatologic treatment, such as steroids or methotrexate, have been in use much longer than the RCTs have been in vogue. Lack of RCT evidence of efficacy in such cases should not be interpreted

BOX 1: Key concepts of evidence-based medicine (EBM).

- *Conscientious:* An active process requiring learning, doing, and thinking
- *Explicit:* A process that is transparent in its description and is replicable
- *Judicious:* A process needing clinical judgment in application of evidence
- *Current:* A process that requires being up to date
- *Best:* A process that searches for the most reliable source of evidence to apply in practice

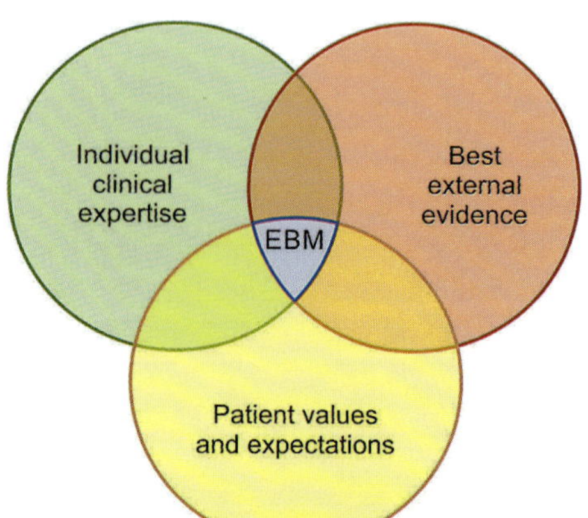

Fig. 1: The triad of evidence-based medicine (EBM).

as evidence of lack of efficacy of such agents. Thus, the relative lack of RCT evidence of efficacy of topical steroids in seborrheic dermatitis should not imply that these should not be used in this condition when there is so much of clinical experience to support its use.

A similar situation obtains regarding guidelines. Guidelines should not be equated with evidence. Like every other source of knowledge, these can either be based on evidence or not. Mere use of the Grading of Recommendations Assessment, Development and Evaluation (GRADE) or the Strength of Recommendation Taxonomy (SORT) system does not make guidelines foolproof. Favoring expensive novel treatments based on placebo-controlled RCTs conducted by the pharmaceutical industry (e.g., biologics in severe psoriasis) over long-established efficacious cheaper agents (e.g., methotrexate), simply because the former pass the "Level A" evidence criteria, is a valid source of criticism against for guideline developers.

EMPIRICAL EVIDENCE BASED ON PATHOMECHANISM

Basing clinical decisions and treatment choice on etiopathogenesis of disease is problematic, because these understandings are dynamic, they change over time, and so must the logically derived treatments. Sometimes, because of our partial understanding of the pathophysiology, these treatments can have unexpected consequences. A classic example is provided by the clinical trial of thalidomide in toxic epidermal necrolysis (TEN). Thalidomide, an inhibitor of tumor necrosis factor-α (TNF-α), was used on the basis of the observation that TEN is associated with high levels of TNF-α. The trial had to be stopped early as 10 out of 12 patients in the thalidomide group died, compared to 3 out of 10 on placebo.[5]

EVIDENCE-BASED VERSUS EXPERIENCE-BASED MEDICINE

Experience is an invaluable ingredient of a competent physician. However, the dangers of depending solely or too much on personal experience is widely documented **(Box 2)**.[4,6]

It is to be understood that experience is also a source of evidence, only evidence at the bottom of the hierarchy of evidence. Thus, in clinical practice, experience should be relied upon only in situations where no other form or source of evidence exists.

BOX 2: Pitfalls of experiential medicine.

- Overemphasis on anecdotes, habitually overlooking statistically strong evidence
- Recall bias in favor of evidence supporting pre-existing knowledge and against evidence rejecting the same
- Ignorance of statistical principles such as sample size, selection bias, regression to the mean, etc. that characterize population data
- Inability to distinguish statistical and causal association
- Persistence of belief in dated knowledge despite contrary evidence

HIERARCHY OF EVIDENCE

An important principle of EBM is the concept of a hierarchy of evidence that is the understanding that there is a hierarchy according to the strength or quality of evidence. It implies a hierarchy of evidence that starts with systematic reviews at the top with anecdotes and case reports at the bottom **(Fig. 2)**.[7]

The hierarchy of evidence is linearly arranged from the top to the bottom in ascending scale of the degree of bias in the source of evidence. However, it is not to be understood as a linear phenomenon, as the relevance of evidence is as important as its quality. Thus, a well-conducted cohort study with adequate sample size may be more reliable as evidence than a shabbily done RCT with a sample size inadequate to answer the research question **(Fig. 3)**.[8] Quality is a multidimensional concept that includes an appropriate design, conduct, data analysis, and clinical relevance.

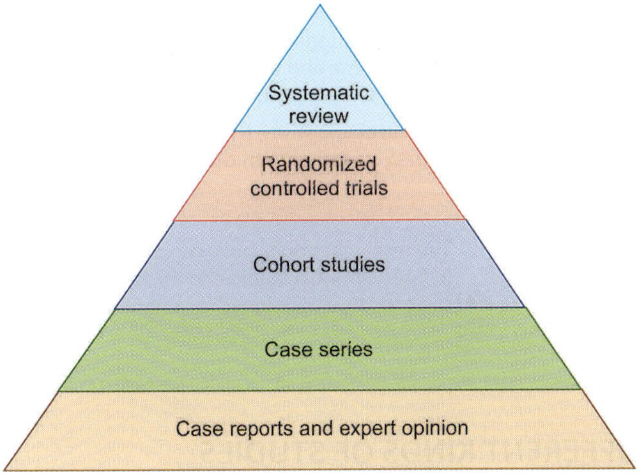

Fig. 2: The hierarchy of evidence.

Source: Adapted from Williams H. Why is the center of evidence-based dermatology relevant to Indian dermatology? Indian J Dermatol. 2009;54:118-23.

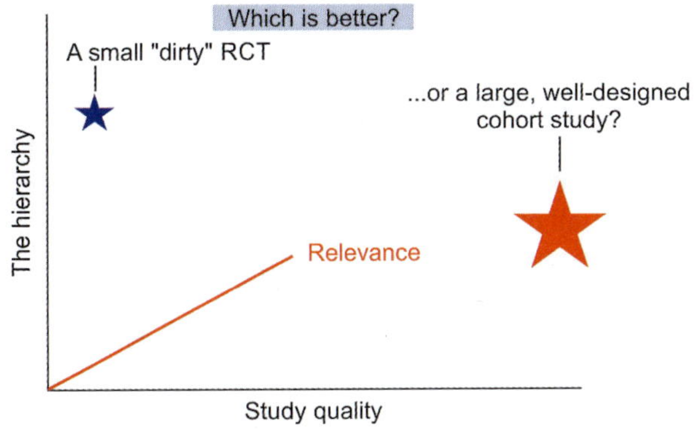

Fig. 3: The dimensions of hierarchy.

Courtesy: Hywel Williams.

TABLE 1: Some common study designs and their application.

Study design	*Definition*	*Application*	*Example*
Systematic review (SR)	An overview that answers a specific clinical question, contains a thorough, unbiased search of the relevant literature, explicit criteria for assessing studies, and structured presentation of the results	• Therapy • Diagnostic tests • Etiology • Mechanisms	An SR of 20 studies to compare 23 different interventions used for melasma[9]
Meta-analysis	An objective and quantitative summary of evidence that is amenable to statistical analysis	Meta-analysis is always conducted within the context of a SR	The role of *Bacillus Calmette–Guérin* (BCG) in prevention of leprosy[10]
Randomized controlled trial	A clinicoepidemiological experiment in which subjects are randomly allocated into groups, usually called the test and control groups, to receive or not a preventive or a therapeutic procedure or an intervention	Effectiveness and safety of treatment	Effectiveness and safety of clofazimine and pentoxifylline in the treatment of type 2 lepra reactions[11]
Cohort study	An observational study in which the participants are selected based on exposure status and they are followed over time to evaluate for the occurrence of the outcome of interest	• Cumulative incidence and incidence rate • Prognosis • Causation and risk factors	Estimate the incidence of cardiovascular events in patients with psoriasis
Case–control study	An observational study in which the participants are selected based on the outcome status, some having the outcome of interest (cases), and others not having the outcome (controls), with the investigator assessing the exposure in both these groups	Causation and risk factors	The association between smoking and lung cancer
Cross-sectional study	An observational study in which the investigator measures the outcome and the exposures in the study participants at the same time	• Diagnosis • Screening • Prevalence	Prevalence of vitiligo in a village
Ecologic study	In an ecologic study, the unit of analysis is a group or aggregate rather than the individual	Hypothesis generation	Correlation between per capita intake of dietary fat and incidence of breast cancer in 21 countries[12]
Natural experiments	The researcher does not assign the exposure (as is the case in interventional studies) to the groups in the study; rather, the exposure is assigned by a natural process	• In situations when it is not ethical to assign exposures • Evaluation of policies and laws	Evaluation of eye injuries in the UK before and after the introduction of seat belt laws[13]

DIFFERENT KINDS OF STUDIES AND THEIR RELEVANCE

Evidence-based medicine places considerable emphasis on the randomized controlled clinical trial as the building block for informing clinical practice and places systematic reviews and meta-analyses at the very acme of the evidence pyramid.[7] It is because a well-conducted RCT is the most efficient mechanism to minimize bias when seeking an answer to the most effective way to treat a disease. *Bias is defined as a systematic error resulting in an incorrect estimation of true effect.* However, it must be stressed that RCTs are not the be-all and end-all of EBD. Different study designs are needed to answer different research questions **(Table 1)**.

STEPS OF PRACTICING EVIDENCE-BASED DERMATOLOGY

The process of practicing EBD may be summed up in five steps **(Box 3)**.[4]

BOX 3: The steps of evidence-based practice.

- Asking an answerable structured question, generated from a patient encounter or a clinical problem
- Searching for the best external evidence
- Critically appraising the evidence for relevance and validity
- Applying the results of appraised evidence back to the patient or the problem
- Recording the data for future

Framing a Structured Research Question

Developing a structured answerable question is a learnable skill. Such a question has four essential components:

1. *P*atient/*P*roblem belonging to the population to which one wishes to generalize
2. *I*ntervention (in experimental studies)/*E*xposure (in observational studies)
3. *C*omparator/*C*ontrol
4. *O*utcome(s) of interest

This structure is thus known by the acronyms PICO (for interventional studies), and PECO (for observational studies).

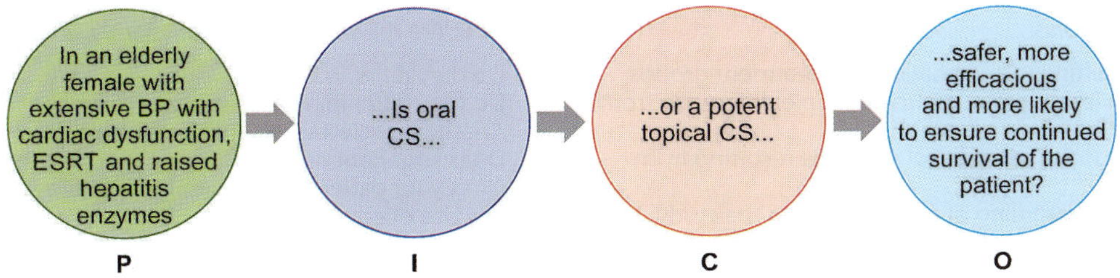

Fig. 4: The four elements of PICO (*p*opulation, *i*ntervention, *c*omparator, *o*utcome).

Example: "What is the best treatment of extensive bullous pemphigoid?" is of no use as there cannot be a specific answer. A real patient, generating a real clinical problem drawn from a real clinical encounter, will, on the other hand, lead to the following question **(Fig. 4)**:

"In an elderly female with extensive bullous pemphigoid with cardiac dysfunction, end-stage renal disease and raised hepatic enzymes, is an oral corticosteroid or a potent topical corticosteroid safer, more efficacious and more likely to ensure continued survival of the patient?"

Searching for the Best External Evidence

This is a crucial step in evidence-based practice and requires resources, access, and necessary skills of performing electronic search. **Table 2** summarizes some of the major resources for carrying out meaningful electronic search necessary for evidence-based practice.

Critical Appraisal of Evidence for Relevance and Validity

The utility of an evidence is the product of its clinical relevance, multiplied by its validity, divided by its accessibility.[14] Relevance simply means looking for the best kind of evidence in properly designed studies. For example, one should not try finding out prevalence from case-control studies, or should not waste time taking a look at case report of topical aloe vera improving oral lichen planus when there are already RCT reports addressing the issue.

Applying the Evidence Back to the Patient

This is one of the most critically important yet least discussed aspects of EBM. There are two aspects of a valid evidence: (1) the results must be true (*internal validity*) and (2) the results must be applicable to real-life patients (*external validity*).

Internal validity is assessed by critically appraising the study design. The moot questions to be asked are:

- What is the role of chance as an alternative explanation of the study results?
- What is the potential for bias?

Answering the first question requires basic knowledge in statistical analysis. Statistically significant difference is generally expressed in statistical shorthand by means of p-values. A statistically significant result means that the result did not happen simply by chance. But one must remember that p-value is not the be-all and end-all in assessing the results of a study. In a word, statistical significance is not the same as clinical significance.

Assessing bias requires skill and expertise in methods of EBM. **Box 4** lists some of the major kinds of bias regularly encountered.

TABLE 2: Useful resources for evidence-based dermatology (EBD).

Sources of previously appraised information	
Collections of systematic reviews, databases, and websites of groups that evaluate health interventions	
Cochrane Library Cochrane access via Cochrane Collaboration Cochrane Skin Group CRD database	www.cochranelibrary.com www.cochrane.org skin.cochrane.org www.crd.york.ac.uk/CRDWeb/
Secondary information sources	
ACP Journal Club Evidence-based Medicine (EBM)	www.acponline.org/clinical-information/journals-publications/acp-journal-club ebm.bmj.com
Books and resources based on the principles of EBM	
Evidence-based Dermatology *BMJ* Clinical Evidence UpToDate	www.evidencebasedseries.com/dermatology www.bmj.com/specialties/clinical-evidence www.uptodate.com/home
Clinical practice guidelines	
US National Guideline Clearinghouse Guidelines International Network British Association of Dermatologists American Academy of Dermatology	www.ahrq.gov/gam/index.html www.g-i-n.net/home www.bad.org.uk/healthcare-professionals/clinical-standards/clinical-guidelines www.aad.org/practicecenter/quality/clinical-guidelines
Critically appraised topics	
BestBETs The CAT Bank	bestbets.org www.minervation.com/
Metasearch engines	
TRIP Database SUMsearch	www.tripdatabase.com sumsearch.org/
Primary information sources	
PubMed Embase LILACS Google Scholar	www.ncbi.nlm.nih.gov/pubmed/ www.embase.com lilacs.bvsalud.org/en/ scholar.google.com

BOX 4: Major kinds of bias.

- *Selection bias:* Resulting in an imbalance in treatment groups
- *Performance bias:* Treating one group of people differently from the other
- *Detection bias:* Biased assessment of outcome resulting from lack of blinding
- *Attrition bias:* Biased handling of deviations from the study protocol and those lost to follow-up
- *Publication bias:* The tendency to conceal or delay publishing negative studies

BOX 5: Applying the evidence.

- Is my patient sufficiently similar to the trial patients?
- Do the outcomes make clinical sense to me?
- Is the magnitude of benefit clinically worthwhile for my patient?
- What are the treatment drawbacks?
- How does the treatment fit in with my patient's beliefs, values, and social station?

BOX 6: Are the trial patients sufficiently similar to mine?

- Do they differ in biological ways, e.g., age, sex, etc.?
- Do they differ in disease subtype?
- Are there social factors that diminish adherence?
- Does your patient suffer from other comorbidities?
- Does your patient have a similar baseline risk of benefit/adverse effects?

BOX 7: Do the outcomes make clinical sense to you?

- If a composite scale has been used, what does a change in score of 10 points mean?
- Has a scale been chosen deliberately to enhance treatment effects?
- Do the outcome measures capture the appropriate time points?
- Does the outcome include simple categorical measures of patients' views?

To give an example, bias assessment of an RCT may be initiated by asking three questions:

1. Is the method of generating the randomization sequence and subsequent concealment of allocation of participants clearly described and appropriate?
2. Were participants and study assessors blind to the intervention?
3. Were all those who originally entered the study accounted for in the results and analysis (i.e., was an intention-to-treat analysis performed)?

In assessing the applicability of an evidence drawn from a clinical trial in an individual patient (external validity), the five key questions to be asked have been summarized in **Box 5.**[15]

Box 6 delineates the questions to be asked to determine whether any individual patient is sufficiently similar to the patients in a trial.[15] **Box 7** summarizes the key points for making clinical sense of the outcome measures.

A profusion of scales make appraisal difficult, because these can be selected or modified in order to amplify statistical changes. Thus, the properties of these scales are to be carefully assessed to see whether these add or multiply by extent and to find out whether twice the score means twice as bad, etc.

The worth of the clinical magnitude of an intervention has to be assessed in addition to its statistical and clinical significance. This is most usefully expressed as the number needed to treat (NNT), which is simply the reciprocal of the difference in effectiveness of the intervention over its comparator. Suppose treatment A produces 30% response and treatment B 20%. The difference being 10%, NNT (number of patients who need to be treated to achieve on additional response) will be 1/0.10 = 10.

Similarly, the spread (or range) of response is always more relevant than mean response **(Fig. 5)**. Thus, confidence interval (CI) is a more useful measure of the true estimate of treatment effect than the p-value, the overemphasis on which has led to the common tendency to divide all clinical trials into those that are significant at the arbitrary 5% level and those that are not.

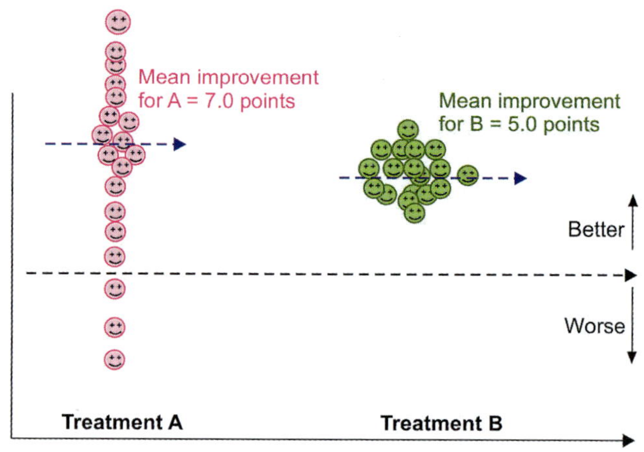

Fig. 5: Would you choose mean response or spread of response?

It is important to correctly interpret the application of aggregate data to individuals and not equate group probabilities with individuals. If the result of a study of treatment A in plaque psoriasis is achieving PASI90 in 75% of patients at the end of 4 months, one cannot tell the patient that "you have 75% chance of 90% reduction of your psoriasis at the end of 4 months." The correct statement would be "75% of patients like you have 90% reduced psoriasis at the end of 4 months with this treatment." Likewise, if an ecologic study finds that districts with a higher proportion of the upper socioeconomic status (SES) individuals have a high prevalence of psoriasis, one should not immediately jump to the conclusion that higher SES is associated with psoriasis. This will be an example of "ecologic fallacy" that is interpreting ecologic level analysis at the individual level.

CONCLUSION

The best way to achieve good clinical practice in the age of EBD is to successfully marry individual clinical expertise with the best available external evidence. Without systematically appraised current best evidence, practice gets rapidly outdated. Without clinical expertise, practice may be nothing but a systematized tyranny of evidence.

KEY POINTS

- Evidence-based medicine is the "conscientious, explicit, and judicious use of current best evidence about the care of individual patients."
- Evidence-based practice is defined as integrating clinical expertise with best external evidence obtained from systematic research.
- EBM/EBD has a triad of equally important domains—external evidence, clinical expertise, and patients' values and preferences.
- The hierarchy of evidence starts with systematic reviews at the top with anecdotes and case reports at the bottom.
- Systematic review is an overview that answers a specific clinical question, contains a thorough, unbiased search of the relevant literature, explicit criteria for assessing studies, and structured presentation of the results.
- RCT is a clinicoepidemiological experiment in which subjects are randomly allocated into groups, usually called the test and control groups, to receive or not a preventive or a therapeutic procedure or an intervention.
- The structured format of a research question for an experimental study is known by the acronym PICO (*p*opulation, *i*ntervention, *c*omparator, *o*utcome).
- Bias is defined as a systematic error resulting in an incorrect estimation of true effect.
- NNT (number of patients who need to be treated to achieve on additional response) is the reciprocal of the difference in effectiveness of the intervention over its comparator.
- Confidence interval is a more useful measure of the true estimate of treatment effect than the p-value.
- Cochrane Library (www.cochranelibrary.com) is the most useful repository of systematic reviews and RCTs.
- The best way to achieve good clinical practice in the age of EBD is to successfully marry individual clinical expertise with the best available external evidence.

REFERENCES

1. Sackett DL, Rosenberg WM, Gray JA, Haynes RB, Richardson WS. Evidence-based medicine: what it is and what it isn't. BMJ. 1996;312:71-2.
2. Sackett DL, Strauss S, Richardson W, Rosenberg W, Haynes R. Evidence-based Medicine: How to Practise and Teach EBM, 2nd edition. London: Churchill Livingstone; 2000.
3. Bigby M. Snake oil for the 21st century. Arch Dermatol. 1998;134:1512-4.
4. Williams HC, Bigby M. The rationale for evidence-based dermatology. In: Williams HC, Bigby M, Herxheimer A, Naldi L, Rzany B, Dellavalle RP, Ran Y, Furue M (Eds). Evidence-based Dermatology, 3rd edition. Chichester: John Wiley; 2014.
5. Wolkenstein P, Latarjet J, Roujeau JC, Duquet C, Boudeau S, Vaillant L, et al. Randomized comparison of thalidomide versus placebo in toxic epidermal necrolysis. Lancet. 1998;352:1586-9.
6. Hines DC, Goldheizer JW. Clinical investigation: a guide to its evaluation. Am J Obstet Gynecol. 1969;105:450-87.
7. Williams H. Why is the center of evidence-based dermatology relevant to Indian dermatology? Indian J Dermatol. 2009; 54:118-23.
8. Bigby M. The hierarchy of evidence. In: Williams HC, Bigby M, Herxheimer A, Naldi L, Rzany B, RP Dellavalle RP, Ran Y, Furue M (Eds). Evidence-based Dermatology, 3rd edition. Chichester: John Wiley; 2014.
9. Rajaratnam R, Halpern J, Salim A, Emmett C. Interventions for melasma. Cochrane Database Syst Rev. 2010;(7): CD003583.
10. Setia MS, Steinmaus C, Ho CS, Rutherford GW. The role of BCG in prevention of leprosy: a meta-analysis. Lancet Infect Dis. 2006;6:162-70.
11. Roy K, Sil A, Das NK, Bandyopadhyay D. Effectiveness and safety of clofazimine and pentoxifylline in type 2 lepra reaction: a double-blind, randomized, controlled study. Int J Dermatol. 2015;54:1325-32.
12. Prentice RL, Kakar F, Hursting S, Sheppard L, Klein R, Kushi LH. Aspects of the rationale for the women's health trial. J Natl Cancer Inst. 1988;80:802-14.
13. Cole MD, Clearkin L, Dabbs T, Smerdon D. The seat belt law and after. Br J Ophthalmol. 1987;71:436-40.
14. Shaughnessy AF, Slawson DC, Bennett JH. Becoming an information master: a guidebook to the medical information jungle. J Fam Pract. 1994;39:489-99.
15. Williams HC. Applying the evidence back to the patient. In: Williams HC, Bigby M, Herxheimer A, Naldi L, Rzany B, Dellavalle RP, Ran Y, Furue M (Eds). Evidence-based Dermatology, 3rd edition. Chichester: John Wiley; 2014.

EXAMINATION QUESTIONS

1. Write a short note on evidence-based dermatology.
2. What are the common study designs? Discuss the merits and demerits of each of them.
3. Define bias. Discuss the different types of bias with relevant examples from dermatology research.
4. Describe the types and merits of controlled trials.

15 CHAPTER Medical Statistics

Amrita Sil

INTRODUCTION

Statistics is the science of collecting, collating, describing, and analyzing data. In this age of evidence-based medicine, statistics play a great role. Understanding statistics makes the medical researcher put forward his data in a presentable fashion and inferences to be drawn more specifically. The practitioner can critically review the literature presented to him and make an informed decision regarding a treatment.

Development of new drugs, new cosmetology products, and equipment depends on statistics to prove their merit. Thus, it is imperative for a medical professional to be updated on the basics of biomedical statistics.

TYPES OF DATA (FLOWCHART 1)

Knowing the type of data one is about to analyze is the first step in biomedical statistics. The type of data determines the further statistical tests one is going to use.

Other types of data:

- *Derived data*:
  - *Percentages*: e.g., percentage of patients improved after treatment
  - *Ratios*: e.g., body mass index (BMI) = weight in kg/ height in meter^2
  - *Rates*: e.g., disease rates = disease events/time period under consideration
  - *Scores*: e.g., quality-of-life score
- *Parametric data*: Data whose distribution in the underlying population can be represented by the normal distribution curve. For such data, only parametric tests should be used while hypothesis testing and calculating *p* value.
- *Nonparametric data*: Data following some distribution other than normal distribution curve or does not follow any distribution or follows some unknown distribution. For such data, only nonparametric tests should be used while hypothesis testing and calculating *p* value.

NORMAL DISTRIBUTION

The bell-shaped (or unimodal) curve is the most important distribution in statistics because it is frequently distributed in nature **(Fig. 1)**. The curve is symmetrical about its mean. The mean, median, and mode all coincide.

The central limit theorem: As the number of observations increase (say sample size > 100), the shape of the sampling distribution will approximate a normal distribution.

How to know which variable is parametric?

Parametric data are usually "numeric" data and are "normally distributed." Statistical software are provided with "goodness of fit" normality tests which test the normality of the distribution. The result of the test is given as a "*p* value." If the *p* value is >0.05, it is assumed that the data is in a normal distribution. These tests are as follows:

- Kolmogorov-Smirnov normality test
- Shapiro-Wilk normality test

Flowchart 1: Types of data.

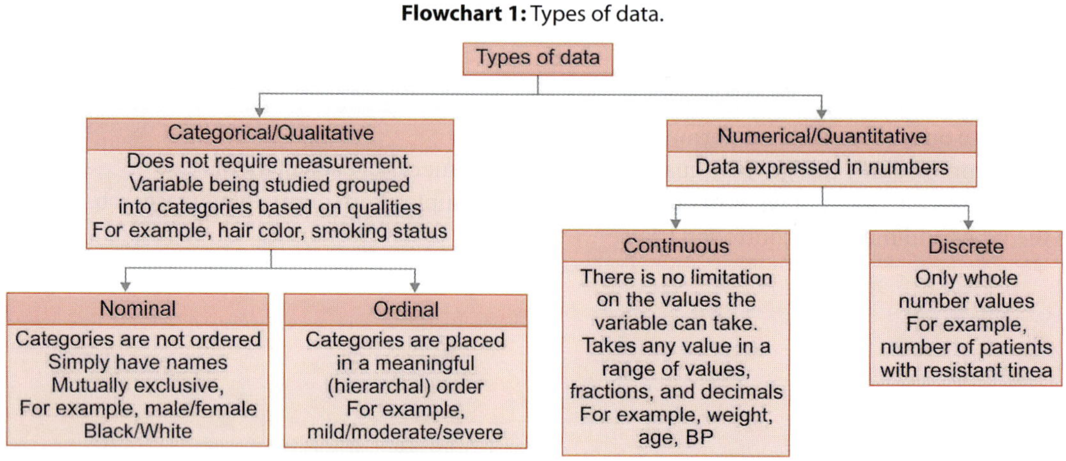

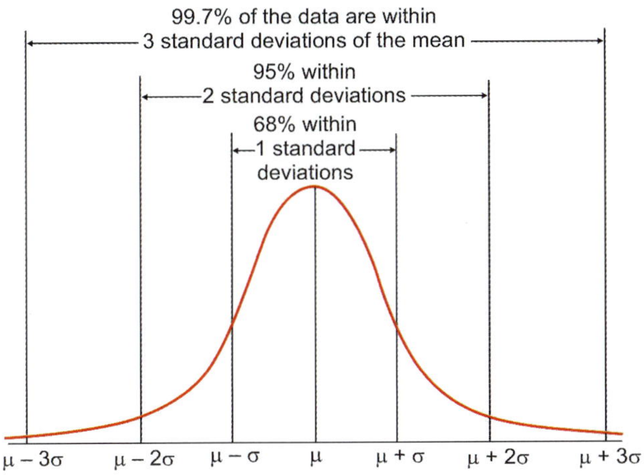

Fig. 1: The normal distribution curve.

DESCRIPTIVE STATISTICS (TABLE 1)

Descriptive statistics summarizes a dataset into evaluable results. Categorical data is summarized using percentages or proportions. While summarizing numerical data, the extent to which observations cluster about a central location is expressed as "measures of central tendency" and the spread can be expressed as "measures of dispersion".

Measures of Central Tendency

- *Mean*: It is the average of the data. The arithmetic mean is severely affected by "outliers" and distorted by "skewed data".
- *Median*: It is the 50th percentile of the sample. The median should be reported when the data has "outliers" or is "skewed".
- *Mode*: It is the expression of the most commonly occurring value. It is most appropriate for categorical and discrete data.

Measures of Dispersion

- *Range*: It is the difference between the highest and the lowest values in a dataset.
- *Interquartile range*: It is the difference between the 3rd quartile (75th percentile) and the 1st quartile (25th percentile). It is robust to outliers and works well for skewed data and should be reported when the data has outliers or is skewed.
- *Variance*: One way of measuring the spread of data is to determine the extent to which each observation deviates from the mean. Variance is the mean square deviation.
- *Standard deviation (SD)*: It is a special form of average deviation from mean. It is the square root of variance. Since SD is expressed in the same units as those of the raw data, it is the most important measure of variation.

CONFIDENCE INTERVAL

The confidence interval or CI is a measure of the precision of the results obtained from the sample. By convention, we usually quote 95% CI. 95% CI is the range of values within which we can be sure with 95% confidence that the true population value lies.

Wide CI → indicates the estimate is imprecise.
Narrow CI → indicates the estimate is precise.

TABLE 1: Example of calculation of measures of central tendency and dispersion of the numerical variable of a dataset. The categorical variables are expressed as a percentage.

Category	*Olopatadine group (n = 54)*	*Levocetirizine group (n = 51)*	*p value (between groups)*
Age (in years)			
Range	19–80	19–80	
Mean ± SD	31.06 ± 13.98	33.02 ± 12.05	0.442
Median (IQR)	26.5 (20.0–38.0)	32 (24.25–39.50)	
Sex			0.162
Male	38 (70.37%)	29 (56.86%)	
Female	16 (29.63%)	22 (43.14%)	
Residence			0.696
Urban	26 (48.15%)	22 (43.14%)	
Rural	28 (51.85%)	29 (56.86%)	

HYPOTHESIS TESTING

Null hypothesis: It is the conservative position of no change or no difference in comparison to baseline or between groups. That is: Group A = Group B; Baseline = Study end. A research study always aims at rejecting the null hypothesis.

P value: It is the maximum probability of getting an observed result by chance. It is accepted that there can be 1 in 20 chance of an accidental result; thus, the cutoff for *p* value is taken as 0.05 or 5%. Thus, the *p* value has to be <0.05 to consider the outcome significant.

Steps of Testing Hypothesis

1. Define the "null" hypothesis and the "alternate hypothesis".
2. Select a research design and sample size appropriate to the hypothesis to be tested.
3. Decide the statistical test that is to be applied.
4. Determine *p* value. If *p* value < 0.05, reject null hypothesis and accept alternate hypothesis.

Tests of Statistical Significance

Tests-to-test the Difference between Study Groups

There can be two types of data groups: (1) Paired and (2) unpaired. Paired data means the result of one set influences the result of the other. For example, test of two topical agents on either the right or the left part of the body in symmetric lesions like psoriasis, test of an antihistamine on chronic urticaria at baseline and study end at 4 weeks **(Flowchart 2)**. Unpaired data means the result of one set does not influence the results of the other set. For example, test of two antihistamines on chronic urticaria at study end **(Flowchart 3)**.

Flowchart 2: Tests of significance for paired data when there is a comparison between groups.

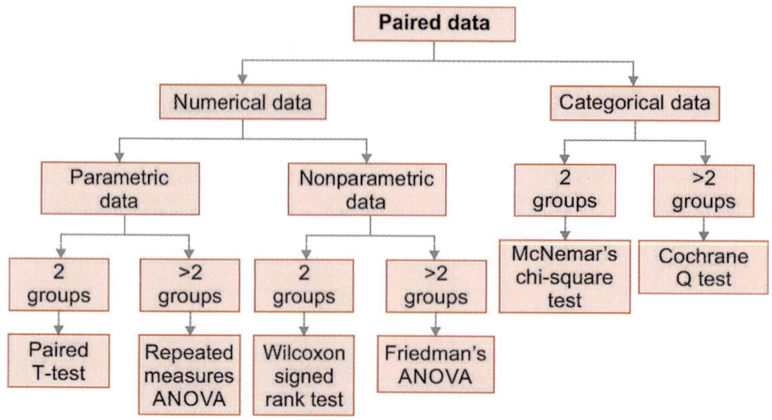

(ANOVA: analysis of variance)

Flowchart 3: Tests of significance for unpaired data when there is a comparison between groups.

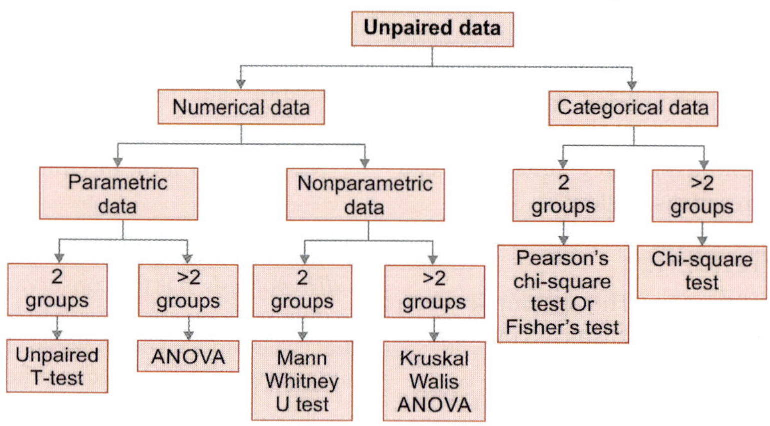

(ANOVA: analysis of variance)

Post hoc tests: If there is a statistical significance in >2 groups, the exact position of difference needs to be identified. Post hoc tests (Dunnett's test and Tukey's test for parametric data and Dunn's test for nonparametric data) determine the position. For example, if there is a significant difference within three visits namely baseline, first follow-up, and second follow-up visit on repeated measures ANOVA, post hoc Dunnett's test finds out whether the significance is from baseline and first follow-up or baseline and second follow-up or between first and second follow-up.

Tests-to-test Association between Two Variables

Correlation: It quantifies the strength of association between two numerical variables which are in a linear relationship between each other. The correlation takes a value between –1 and +1. If both the variables are parametric, Pearson's product moment correlation coefficient (r) is calculated. If the variables are not parametric, Spearman's rank correlation (ρ) or Kendall's rank correlation (τ) coefficient is estimated. A value near +1 indicates a strong positive correlation whereas a value near –1 indicates a strong inverse correlation. A value close to 0 indicates no correlation. However, correlation does not imply causation.

Odds ratio: Certain studies estimate risk. Risk is the association between an observed outcome (e.g., adverse effect) and exposure to certain factors that might contribute to the event. Odds ratio (OR) estimates the risk between two categorical data variables.

$$\text{Odds ratio} = \frac{\text{Odds of outcome in exposed group}}{\text{Odds of outcome in nonexposed group}}$$

When the odds of an outcome in two groups are identical, then OR = 1; if exposure increases risk, OR > 1; if exposure reduces risk, OR < 1.

The 95% confidence interval should be presented along with OR and preferably the interval should not include 1.

SAMPLE SIZE CALCULATION

The sample size should be such that it is enough to draw meaningful inferences. Too large a sample leads to wastage of resources and quality issues. Too small a sample might not be representative of the population or ethically just.

1. *Sample size for comparison of means or proportions between groups:* Calculation of sample size requires:

- *Significance level*: It is taken as 0.05.
- *Power of the study (1 – β)*: β is the probability of making Type II error. β is usually taken as 80 or 90%, i.e., power becomes 0.2 or 0.1 respectively.
- *Effect size*: The magnitude of the effect that is clinically important. For example, difference of 3 units of Urticaria Activity Score (UAS) between chronic urticaria patients receiving two antihistamines. Here, 3 will be the effect size.
- *Standard deviation*: Obtained from previously reported similar studies or pilot studies for the primary outcome variable.

These four values can be inserted in statistical software, and the sample size for each study group can be found out. Adjustment for dropouts is to be done. For example, if 10% dropout is estimated, it should be added to the sample size.

2. *Sample size for surveys:* Calculation of sample size for surveys requires the following:
   - *Population size*: Exact sample size not relevant for large population. Usually taken as 20,000 as sample size does not change much for populations larger than 20,000.
   - *Confidence level*: It is the amount of uncertainty one can allow. It is taken as 95%.
   - *Margin of error*: The error one can tolerate. It is taken as 5%.
   - *Crude estimate of prevalence rate*: It is obtained from published data or pilot surveys.

KEY POINTS

- Data which follows the normal distribution curve is called parametric data. Rest are known as noparametric data.
- Descriptive statistics summarizes a dataset into evaluable results. Categorical data is summarized using percentages or proportions. While summarizing numerical data, the extent to which observations cluster about a central location is expressed as "measures of central tendency" (mean, median, and mode) and the spread can be expressed as "measures of dispersion" (range, interquartile range, variance, standard deviation).
- Null hypothesis is the conservative position of no change or no difference in comparison to baseline or between groups. A research study always aims at rejecting the null hypothesis. *P* value is the maximum probability of getting an observed result by chance. If *p* value < 0.05, the null hypothesis is rejected and alternate hypothesis is accepted. A research study always aims at rejecting the null hypothesis.
- Tests of statistical significance compares groups of data, provide difference between study groups, finds association between datasets.
- For calculating sample size for comparison of means or proportions between groups, power of study, effect size, standard deviation, significance level is taken into account. To calculate sample size for surveys, population size, confidence level, margin of error, and prevalence rate should be considered.

SUGGESTED READING

1. Charan J, Biswas T. How to calculate sample size for different study designs in medical research? Indian J Psychol Med. 2013;35(2):121-6. doi:10.4103/0253-7176.116232.
2. Kaliyadan F, Kulkarni V. Types of variables, descriptive statistics, and sample size. Indian Dermatol Online J. 2019;10:82-6.
3. Parikh MN, Hazra A, Mukherjee J, Gogtay N. Research Methodology Simplified: Every Clinician a Researcher, 1st edition. New Delhi: Jaypee Brothers Medical Publishers; 2010.
4. Sil A, Betkerur J, Das NK. P-value demystified. Indian Dermatol Online J. 2019;10:745-50.
5. Wasserstein RL, Lazar NA. The ASA Statement on p-values: context, process, and purpose. Am Stat. 2016;70:129-33.

EXAMINATION QUESTIONS

1. Name the different types of data by which you can classify your thesis results.
2. Discuss the types of clinical studies.
3. What is p-value? Briefly elaborate on sampling and sample size calculation.
4. Write a short note on meta-analysis in medical research.

2 SECTION

Pruritus, Urticaria, Allergy, and Eczemas

16 CHAPTER Pruritus and Prurigo

Balachandran C, Sudhir Nayak UK

INTRODUCTION

Pruritus can best be defined as an undesirable, but sometimes desirable sensation causing an urge to scratch. Pruritus is a symptom and not a disease. It is perhaps the most common of all dermatological symptoms. Although commonly reported as a cutaneous symptom itch can also be perceived in the conjunctiva, oral and genital mucosa, pharynx, laryngeal, and tracheal mucosa.[1] Just like urticaria, pruritus is classified into acute (when <6 weeks) and chronic (when >6 weeks); chronic pruritus having a poorer prognosis in comparison to acute.

Pruritus causes may be cutaneous, systemic, psychogenic, neurogenic, neuropathic, and sometimes a combination of two or more.

Mediators of itch: Histamine, substance P, opioids, nerve growth factors, neurotrophin 4, proteases/proteinases, interleukins (IL-2, IL-6, and IL-31), prostaglandins (PGE_1 and PGE_2), gastrin-releasing peptides, serotonin, bradykinin, calcitonin gene-related peptide, vasoactive intestinal peptide, and acetylcholine.[1-4]

PATHWAY FOR ITCH

Cutaneous receptors/free nerve endings → C fibers → dorsal root ganglion → synapse with second order neuron in substantia gelatinosa → synapse with neurons in posterior horn cross over to other side → lateral spinothalamic tract → thalamus (ventroposterolateral nucleus) → anterior cingulate cortex and insular cortex → premotor cortex.[3,4]

The C nerve fibers associated with the itch pathway are different from the C fibers that conduct pain. C fibers transmitting itch are unmyelinated histamine sensitive and nonhistamine sensitive. Acute and chronic itch is considered to be mediated by histamine sensitive and nonsensitive C fibers respectively. Inhibition of pruritus by rubbing and scratching of skin is due to stimulation of inhibitory local circuits in the brain and spinal cord.

Receptors for pruritus on sensory-free nerve endings: Transient receptor potential ankyrin 1 A1 (TRPA1), TRPV1, TRPM8, CB1 and 2, mas-related G protein-coupled receptor 3 (Mrgpra3), Mrgpra C11, gastrin-related peptide receptor (GRPR), proteinase-activated receptors 2, opioid receptors, endothelin (ET-A, ET-B).[4]

THEORIES OF PRURITUS[4]

- *Intensity theory*: Weaker stimulation of receptors evokes itch; stronger stimuli evokes pain. Specificity theory: Different afferent fibers for itch and pain.
- *Occlusion theory*: Larger stimuli may occlude itch and produce pain by occluding itch response in the pruritus-specific subset of dorsal root ganglion.

International Forum for the Study of Itch classifies pruritus into two tiers:

1. *Tier I:* When diagnosis is unknown.
2. *Tier II:* When diagnosis is known.[5]

Tier I is subdivided into three:

1. *Group 1:* Pruritus on inflamed/diseased skin
2. *Group 2:* Pruritus on noninflamed/nondiseased skin
3. *Group 3:* Pruritus presenting with severe chronic secondary scratch lesions

Tier II is subclassified into:

- *Cutaneous causes of pruritus*: Scabies, pediculosis, urticaria, dermatophytoses, lichen planus, atopic dermatitis, lichen simplex chronicus, prurigo, bullous pemphigoid, xerosis, keloids, folliculitis, seborrheic dermatitis, psoriasis, mycosis fungoides, eosinophilic folliculitis, autoimmune connective tissue disorder (scleroderma, dermatomyositis, primary Sjögren's syndrome), etc. Very rarely nonpruritic conditions such as acne and pityriasis versicolor may be associated with pruritus.
- *Systemic causes of pruritus*: Endocrine diseases (hypo-/hyperthyroidism, diabetes mellitus), end-stage renal disease, hepatic (cholestatic/cirrhosis), blood dyscrasias (iron deficiency anemia/polycythemia vera/lymphomas, carcinoid tumors). Generalized pruritus in diabetes is due to associated conditions such as dermatophytoses, candidiasis, and neuropathy rather than due to diabetes per se.

Neuropathic itch: Itch occurring in the afferent pathway: Brachioradial pruritus, notalgia paresthetica, meralgia paresthetica, postherpetic neuralgia, etc.

Neurogenic itch: Itch occurring in the central nervous system without any neural pathology. Postcerebrovascular accident, postmorphine administration, multiple sclerosis, etc.

Psychogenic: Delusional parasitosis, anorexia nervosa, anxiety, depression, obsessive-compulsive disorder.

Mixed: When more than one cause is implicated.

Quality/description of itch: Tickle, burning, pricking, crawling, twitching, dysesthesia.

Itch is sometimes very specific of some diseases.

Nocturnal itch, web space itch, itch in family members, itch in genitalia: Scabies

Itch associated with wheals: Urticaria

Itch and/or wheals on exposure to cold: Cold urticaria

Itch after hot water bath followed by cooling: Polycythemia vera.

Cutaneous examination of skin may sometimes show lesions specific to the disease such as wheals (in urticaria/early bullous pemphigoid), burrows (scabies), etc., or nonspecific lesions such as excoriations, postinflammatory de-/hypo-/hyperpigmentation. Lichenified plaques in nape of neck, external genitalia and dorsa of feet may suggest lichen simplex chronicus. *Butterfly sign:* Area in the center of back inaccessible to patient spared from signs of scratching due to chronic itch.

SPECIFIC PRURITUS

Aquagenic pruritus: Itch occurring after contact with water irrespective of the temperature.

Brachioradial pruritus: Itch occurring in the dorsolateral aspect of forearm with symptomatic relief with ice pack application (ice-pack sign).

Scalp pruritus: Causes—seborrheic dermatitis, pediculosis, contact dermatitis to hair dyes, urticarial, psoriasis, folliculitis, psychogenic.

Pruritus ani: Contact dermatitis to toiletries, pinworm infestation, fecal incontinence, poor hygiene, verruca, hemorrhoids.

Pruritus vulvae: Lichen simplex chronicus, lichen sclerosus et atrophicans, candidiasis, trichomoniasis, foreign body (in prepubertal), contact dermatitis to toiletries, condoms, etc.

Scrotal pruritus: Lichen simplex chronicus, dermatophytosis, contact dermatitis.

Winter itch: Synonym for eczema craquele/xerotic eczema.

Mitempfindung (referred pruritus): Stimulus applied on one part of the body perceived in another part.[4]

Contagious pruritus: Those provoked by visual stimuli.[4]

Willan's itch: Synonym for senile pruritus.

Mechanism of renal itch (chronic renal failure): Dry skin, hyperparathyroidism, pruritogenic metabolites, hypercalcemia, abnormal mast cells in skin.

Mechanism of hepatic itch: Bile acid accumulation, increased opioidergic tone, and increased lysophosphatidic acid.

Mechanism of paraneoplastic pruritus: Immunologic reaction to tumor antigens, IL-31, secondary to therapy with molecular targeted therapies and opioids.

Mechanism of pruritus in human immunodeficiency virus (HIV): Eosinophilic folliculitis, seborrheic dermatitis, xerosis, dermatophytosis, etc.

Measurement of pruritus: Visual analog scale, pruritus severity scale, 5D scale, color analog scale (for children), Symtrack computerized continuous pruritus-rating system.[4]

INVESTIGATIONS

The investigations depend upon the etiology of pruritus. The common investigations usually performed in undiagnosed pruritus are complete blood counts including differential counts and erythrocyte sedimentation rate, urine microscopy, liver function test, renal function test, thyroid function test, screening for HIV, serum immunoglobulin E (IgE) levels, histopathology, and immunofluorescence.

TREATMENT

Emollients: Usually, most causes of chronic pruritus tend to be associated with dryness of skin. It is thus imperative to treat skin with emollients, humectants, or moisturizers.

Topical agents: Calamine lotion, menthol (1%), capsaicin, camphor (0.5–2%), pramoxine (1%), polidocanol, steroids, calcineurin antagonists (tacrolimus, pimecrolimus), doxepin (5%), salicylic acid, anesthetics (eutectic mixture of local anesthetic), strontium nitrate.[4]

Systemic: Antihistamines, bepotastine, mirtazapine, doxepin, opioid antagonists (naltrexone, naloxone), opioid agonist-antagonist (butorphanol), gabapentin, thalidomide, selective serotonin reuptake inhibitors, aprepitant.[4]

Phototherapy: Narrowband ultraviolet B therapy (NB-UVB) is the most common type of phototherapy used in generalized pruritus. Other forms of UV-light such as UVA, UVA_1, psoralen and ultraviolet A (PUVA), and UVA/UVB have been used.[1]

Other nonpharmacologic therapies: Pouring of hot/cold water, central field stimulation, biofeedback, behavioral therapy, transcutaneous nerve stimulation, acupuncture.[1,4]

Antihistamines (H_1 antagonists):

- *First generation/classical*: Hydroxyzine, embramine, cyproheptadine
- *Second generation*: Cetirizine, levocetirizine, fexofenadine, loratadine, desloratadine

Treatment of uremic pruritus: Gabapentin, activated charcoal, cromolyn sodium, nalfurafine, naltrexone, correction of calcium and magnesium levels, UVB phototherapy, dialysis, renal transplant.

Treatment for hepatic pruritus: Cholestyramine, colestipol, rifampicin, sertraline, mirtazapine, phenobarbitone, UVB phototherapy, albumin infusion, ondansetron, naloxone, γ-interferon.

Prurigo is a term which has been used to describe a group of diseases characterized by extremely itchy papules or nodules on the skin.[6]

Prurigo papule is an erythematous papule surmounted by a vesicle.

Actinic prurigo: Rare photodermatitis characterized by itchy papules on a photodistributed pattern primarily to UVB.

Besnier's prurigo: Chronic lichenified flexural lesions of atopic dermatitis.[6]

Dermographic prurigo: Symptomatic dermographism occurring at sites of occlusive clothing.

Hebra's prurigo: Old terminology used to describe atopic dermatitis/prurigo simplex.[4,6]

Hutchinson's summer prurigo: Synonym for actinic prurigo.

Hyde's prurigo: Synonym for prurigo nodularis.[6]

Prurigo of pregnancy (prurigo gestationis): Itchy papules seen on the distal extremities of gravid females in midtrimester and subsiding subsequent to delivery.

Prurigo pigmentosa: Itchy papules coalescing to form reticulated pigmentation reported primarily in Japanese females responsive to minocycline.

Prurigo simplex (prurigo ferox, chronic prurigo, prurigo mitis, prurigo agria): Perhaps the most common of all prurigos. It is characterized by excoriated papules usually on the exposed parts of children. More common in atopics than nonatopics. Treated with covering exposed areas, especially at dusk, emollients, topical corticosteroids, and antihistamines.

Prurigo nodularis: Refers to intensely itchy and distressing nodular lesions usually seen on the distal extensor aspect of limbs and characterized by inward elongation of epidermis. Any other part of the body may be involved.

Associated factors: Atopic dermatitis, stress, insect bites

Differential diagnosis: Pemphigoid nodularis

Treatment: Antihistamines (preferably sedative, emollients, topical/intralesional steroids, thalidomide, cyclosporine, azathioprine, NB-UVB).

Prognosis: Chronic protracted course. Often can lead to psychological problems such as depression.

Subacute prurigo: Synonym for chronic papular urticaria or chronic prurigo of adults.

KEY POINTS

- Pruritus is an undesirable, but sometimes desirable sensation causing an urge to scratch.
- The common mediators of itch are histamine, substance P, opioids, nerve growth factors, neurotrophin 4, proteases/proteinases, interleukins, prostaglandins, gastrin-releasing peptides, serotonin, bradykinin, calcitonin gene-related peptide, vasoactive intestinal peptide, and acetylcholine.
- Topical agents used in management of itch are calamine lotion, menthol (1%), capsaicin, camphor (0.5–2%), pramoxine (1%), polidocanol, steroids, calcineurin antagonists (tacrolimus, pimecrolimus), doxepin (5%), salicylic acid, anesthetics (eutectic mixture of local anesthetic), strontium nitrate.
- Antihistamines are preferred systemic agents used for management of itch. Other agents are bepotastine, mirtazapine, doxepin, opioid antagonists (naltrexone, naloxone), opioid agonist-antagonist (butorphanol), gabapentin, thalidomide, selective serotonin reuptake inhibitors, aprepitant.
- Phototherapy and other non-pharmacological therapies are often used in itch management.
- Prurigo is a term which has been used to describe a group of diseases characterized by extremely itchy papules or nodules on the skin.

REFERENCES

1. Weisshar E, Fleischer AB Jr, Bernhard JD, Cropley TG. Pruritus and dysesthesia. In: Bolognia JL, Jorizzo JL, Schaffer JV (Eds). Dermatology, 3rd edition. China: Elsevier Saunders; 2012. pp. 111-26.
2. Yosipovitch G, Patel TS. Pathophysiology and clinical aspects of pruritus. In: Goldsmith LA, Katz SI, Gilcherst BA, Paller AS, Leffell DJ, Wolff K (Eds). Fitzpatrick's Dermatology in General Medicine, 8th edition. New York: McGraw Hill; 2012.
3. Greaves M. Pruritus. In: Burns T, Breathnach S, Cox N, Griffiths C (Eds). Rook's Textbook of Dermatology, 8th edition. Singapore: Wiley-Blackwell; 2010. pp. 21.1-18.
4. Riyaz N, Arakkal FR. Pruritus and prurigo. In: Sachidanand S, Oberoi C, Inamadar A (Eds). IADVL Textbook of Dermatology, 4th edition. Mumbai: Bhalani Publishing House; 2015. pp. 1979-97.
5. Ständer S, Weisshaar E, Mettang T, Szepietowski JC, Carstens E, Ikoma A, et al. Clinical classification of itch: a position paper of the International Forum for the Study of Itch. Acta Derm Venereol. 2007;87:291-4.
6. Berth-Jones J. Eczema, lichenification, prurigo and erythroderma. In: Burns T, Breathnach S, Cox N, Griffiths C (Eds). Rook's Textbook of Dermatology, 8th edition. Singapore: Wiley-Blackwell; 2010. pp. 23.42-6.

EXAMINATION QUESTIONS

1. Describe the itch pathway and mediators of itch.
2. How will you approach to a case of generalized pruritus in dermatology?

17 CHAPTER Psychodermatology

BC Sharath Kumar, Namratha C Manjunath, Barnali Chowdhury

INTRODUCTION

Psychodermatology or psychocutaneous medicine refers to any aspect of dermatology which overlaps with psychiatry.[1] Although this realm of dermatology is old; this domain is gaining popularity in the recent days.[2] It has been estimated that at least 30–40% of patients attending the skin department have an underlying psychological problem.[1] Dermatologists have limitations in understanding mind and psychiatrists lack the skills in diagnosis and intervention of skin lesions. Hence, it is important for both to have a reasonable knowledge of the other, to provide a complete holistic treatment approach to the patient.

PATHOGENESIS

Embryologically, the brain, skin, and nerve are derived from the neural plate in the ectoderm.[1] O'Sullivan et al. proposed, the neuro-immuno-cutaneous-endocrine model.[3] This forms the basis of many inflammatory cutaneous dermatoses that are triggered or aggravated by psychological factors. In response to psychological stress, hypothalamic pituitary axis secretes stress hormones (corticotrophin-releasing hormone, adrenocorticotropin releasing hormone, cortisol, and prolactin), causes sympathetic nervous system activation leading to elevated catecholamine levels, and the release of neuropeptides and neuromediators (substance P and calcitonin gene-related peptide). These stress hormones and mediators targets skin mast cells which suppresses Th1 immune response, upregulates Th2 immune response, and increases skin serotonin levels. This leads to immune dysregulation and various autoimmune and allergic skin diseases.

CLASSIFICATION[4]

- *Primary psychiatric disorders*: They are primarily psychiatric in nature; skin findings are self-induced or secondary.
- *Secondary psychiatric disorders*: Patient develops psychological problems secondary to skin disease.
- *Psychophysiologic disorders*: Emotional factors aggravate or precipitate primary skin disorders **(Box 1)**.

BOX 1: Classification of psychodermatologic disorders.[4]

Primary psychiatric disorders:
- Delusions of parasitosis
- Dermatitis artefacta
- Body-focused repetitive behavior disorder—Trichotillomania
- Obsessive-compulsive disorder (OCD)
- Dysmorphophobia
- Phobic states
- Eating disorders
- Neurotic excoriations
- Psychogenic pruritus

Secondary psychiatric disorders:
- Alopecia areata
- Vitiligo
- Generalized psoriasis
- Chronic eczema
- Ichthyosiform syndromes
- Rhinophyma
- Neurofibroma
- Albinism

Psychophysiologic disorders:
- Psoriasis
- Atopic dermatitis
- Acne excoriee
- Hyperhidrosis
- Urticaria
- Herpes simplex virus infection
- Seborrheic dermatitis
- Aphthosis
- Rosacea
- Pruritus

Miscellaneous:
- Cutaneous sensory syndromes
  - Glossodynia
  - Vulvodynia
  - Chronic itching in scalp
- Psychogenic purpura syndrome
- Pseudopsychodermatologic disease
- Suicide in dermatology patients

PRIMARY PSYCHIATRIC DISORDERS

Delusion of Parasitosis [Ekbom's Syndrome, Delusional Infestation (DI), Pseudoparasitic Dysesthesia, Monosymptomatic Delusional Hypochondriasis]

It is a somatic type of delusional disorder with fixed, false belief that the skin is infested with parasites or has foreign objects extruding from their skin, despite evidence to the contrary.

Incidence: Bimodal in onset, peak prevalence in 20–30 years of age and more than 50 years of age. F:M = 2:1 among patients more than 50 years old. Folie a deux is demonstrated in 8–12% of patients.

Pathogenesis: Excess of extracellular dopamine due to decrease in dopamine transport is found in cerebral striatum.[5]

It can be primary or secondary to psychiatric disorders such as schizophrenia, bipolar depression with psychotic symptoms, borderline personality disorder, anxiety disorder or organic disorders like substance abuse (amphetamine), alcohol, anti-Parkinsonian medication (ropinirole), tuberculosis, HIV, endocrine disorders, thyroid disease, chronic or acute liver disease, renal failure, vitamin B_{12} deficiency, autoimmune disorders, systemic lupus erythematosus, multiple sclerosis, cerebrovascular disease, and Parkinson disease.

Clinical features: Present with cutaneous dysesthesias due to crawling, biting, and stinging ("pins and needles" sensation). Self-imposed erosions, ulcers, prurigo nodules, and lichenification are produced in attempts to remove the organisms with fingernails or tools

They present with the "specimen sign," where they bring specimens (skin particles or hair, fibers from clothing, crusts, and rarely insects) as proof of infestation in small box or container—the "match box sign". The patient pick and dig their skin with nail clipper and tweezers (tweezers sign) and bring debris in small box.

Special forms of DI are:[6]

- *DI as a shared delusion (folie à deux)*: Family members, carers, and friends may believe that they too are infested.
- *DI by proxy*: Despite all evidence to the contrary, patients complain that their child, friend, or pet is infested.

Morgellons disease: It is a form of delusions of parasitosis where patient claims to observe "fibers" exuding from their skin, and it has received widespread media and Internet coverage (folie a'internet); associated with joint, muscle pain, fibromyalgia, fatigue, cognitive dysfunction, poor concentration, and memory.

Differential diagnosis: Schizophrenia, psychotic depression, formication without delusion, vitamin B_{12} deficiency, multiple sclerosis, syphilis, cerebrovascular disease, and drugs like cocaine, alcohol, amphetamines.

Rx: Establish rapport with the patient and counsel regarding the illness. Historically, the treatment of choice has been pimozide (extrapyramidal adverse effects, cardiotoxic), now atypical antipsychotic risperidone (0.5–6 mg/day), olanzapine (2.5–20 mg/day), quetiapine (25–600 mg/day), and aripiprazole (2–30 mg/day) are used.[7]

Dermatitis Artefacta (Factitial Dermatitis)

It is a factitious disorder in which a fully aware patient creates his own skin lesions to satisfy a psychological need of which they are usually not consciously aware.

It is classified in the DSM-5 (*Diagnostic and Statistical Manual of Mental Disorders, 5th edition)* as a factitious disorder imposed on self.

Incidence: F:M is 20:1 to 4:1.Onset is in adolescence and in adults <30 years.

Clinical features: Lesions are polymorphic, bizarre, well-demarcated with sharp borders and geometric shapes and are often result of thermal, chemical, or instrumental injury. Common sites of involvement are face, dorsum of hands, forearm, most frequently of the nondominant limb. Self-inflicted chemical burn may show a "drip sign," corrosive liquids have been uncontrolled and allowed to run over the skin.[6]

The patients show a "belle indifference," where he is indifferent inspite of fearsome nature of lesions.

Variants are:[6]

- Factitious cheilitis
- Factitious nail disease
- Hair artifact
- Witchcraft syndrome
- Dermatitis artefacta with artifact of patch tests
- *Constriction artifact*: Edema of limbs as a result of tied bands (Secretan syndrome)
- Purpura artifact
- Dermal artifact
- Postsurgical artifact

Dermatitis simulata: Patient used external objects like lipstick, printing dyes to simulate a disease and there is no significant damage.

Complications: Pigmentation disturbances, scarring, cutaneous infection, osteomyelitis, fistulae, and severe infection such as cerebral abscess.

Differential diagnosis: Delusions of parasitosis, excoriation disorder, malingering, pyoderma gangrenosum, vasculitis, irritant contact dermatitis, and dermatitis para artefacta (impulse control disorder where patient semiconsciously manipulates pre-existing minimal lesion, e.g., acne excoriee)

Management: Treatment of skin lesion, psychotherapy for restructuring the patient's personality, pharmacologic therapy for the psychiatric condition. Selective serotonin reuptake inhibitor (SSRI), antipsychotic [aripiprazole (2–5 mg/day), pimozide (0.5–1 mg/day), risperidone (0.5–2 mg/day), and olanzapine (2.5–5 mg/day), anxiolytics (Benzodiazepines, buspirone), and relaxation exercises are helpful.

Body-focused Repetitive Behavior Disorder

It is characterized by repetitive behavior that causes physical injury and significant distress. It includes cheek/lip biting, nose/ear picking, and knuckle cracking, onychophagia (nail biting), dermatophagia, and onychotillomania (nail picking)

Clinical features: Recurrent picking, peeling, or scratching of the skin may cause complications. Severe nail biting cause paronychia and gingival injuries. Chronic biting of the skin can cause localized thickened plaques, differential diagnosis includes callosities. In cheek biting changes in the transverse ridges of the oral mucosa is seen, the differential diagnosis includes lichen planus, candidiasis, and white sponge nevus.[7]

Rx: Habit reversal training is used as first-line treatment, mild aversion (applying a bitter substance to the nails) is used for treating chronic nail biting. Clomipramine, SSRIs, and N-acetylcysteine are helpful.

Trichotillomania (Trichotillosis, Hair Pulling Disorder)

It is body-focused repetitive behavior disorder characterized the recurrent pulling out of one's hair, resulting in noticeable hair loss **(Box 2)**.

Incidence: Bimodal age distribution—childhood cases (5–15 years) with a good prognosis and adult cases presenting in later life with a poor prognosis. F:M is 4:1 in adults but equal in children.

Clinical features: Common sites are scalp, eyebrows, eyelashes, and pubic region. The classic finding is hairs of varying lengths distributed within the area of alopecia. The hairs are referred as "irregularly irregular." The hair loss is seen on the side contralateral to the dominant hand.

The pattern of plucking activity is centrifugal from a single starting point or linear, in wave-like activity which removes all hair except that on the occiput referred as "Friar Tuck sign" **(Fig. 1).**

Associated with anxieties, depression, body dysmorphic disorder family dysfunction (common), eating disorders, and substance abuse.

Complications:[5,6]

- Scarring alopecia
- Folliculitis
- Keloid formation
- Trichobezoar

BOX 2: DSM-5 diagnostic criteria for trichotillomania.[7]

- Recurrent pulling out of one's hair, resulting in hair loss
- Repeated attempts to decrease or stop the hair pulling
- Significant distress or impaired functioning related to the hair pulling; no underlying medical condition or other mental disorder that explains the hair loss/pulling

(DSM-5: Diagnostic and Statistical Manual of Mental Disorders, 5th Edition)

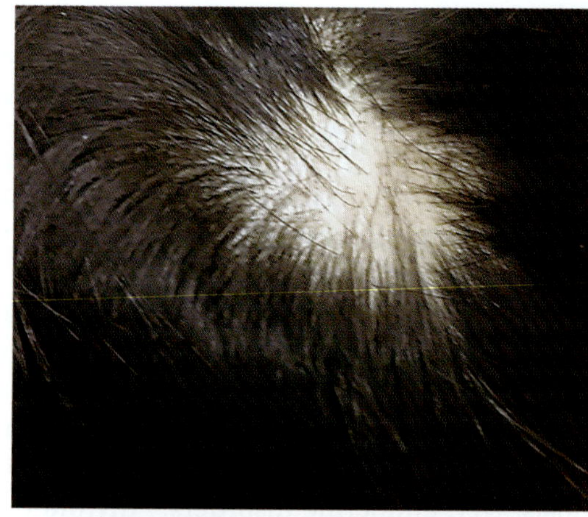

Fig. 1: Alopecia due to hair pulling.

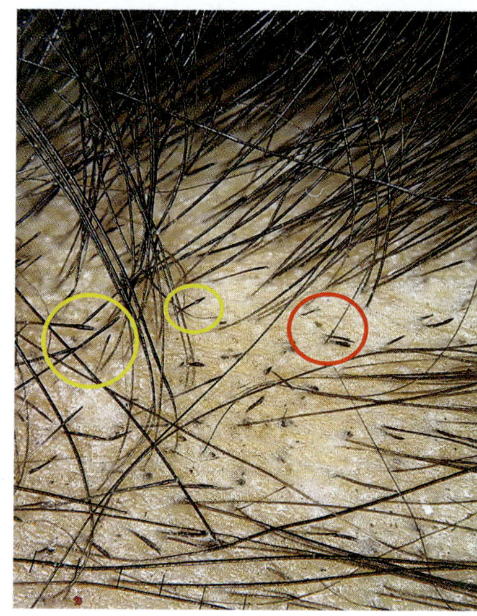

Fig. 2: Trichoscopy showing decreased hair density, hair broken at different length, trichoptilosis (red circle), and tulip hair (yellow circle).

- Changes in color and texture of hair
- Carpel tunnel syndrome, shoulder, and neck pain

HPE: In initial stage empty hair follicles with growing hair, perifollicular hemorrhage is seen, followed by perifollicular fibrosis, pigmented hair casts, follicular plugging with keratin debris, and trichomalacia in late stages.

There is vertically oriented split of hair shafts, within the split proteinaceous material and erythrocytes are present resembling "hamburger within the bun"—Hamburger sign.

Dermoscopy: Irregularly broken hairs, decrease in hair density, short hairs with trichoptilosis, coiled hairs, the "V-sign", flame hairs, tulip hair **(Fig. 2)** and follicular hemorrhages, sprinkled hair residue described as "hair powder."[8]

Differential diagnosis: Nonscarring alopecia (alopecia areata), tinea capitis.

Rx: Behavior modification therapy (e.g., habit reversal training, cognitive behavioral therapy) is the mainstay of treatment. SSRIs and N-acetyl cysteine are used as adjuvant agents

Obsessive-compulsive Disorders

It is a common anxiety disorder characterized by repeated and unwanted thoughts, with behavioral ideas and patterns which drive the patient to act upon it giving them short-term relief.

Incidence: Common in middle aged women. Childhood OCD common in boys.

Associations in OCD:[5]

- Facial tics
- Tourette syndrome
- Depression
- PANDAS (pediatric autoimmune neuropsychiatric disorder associated with streptococcal infection)
- Eating disorders

"*Washing eczema*": Patient obsessed with cleanliness repeatedly wash hands and bathe with soap and also clean the house with detergents which results in irritant contact dermatitis.

Trichotillomania, rhinotillexomania (nose picking), body dysmorphic disorders, dermatophagia, neurotic excoriations and onychophagia will have component of OCD.

Rx: Cognitive behavioral therapy is effective therapy. SSRIs are first line of treatment. Tricyclic antidepressants, low-dose atypical antipsychotics can be used.

Body Dysmorphic Disorder (Dysmorphophobia or Dermatological Nondisease)

It is characterized by a preoccupation with a real or an imagined defect in physical appearance, or an excessive concern over a trivial defect **(Box 3)**.

Incidence: F:M is 2:1.

Clinical features: It is rich in symptoms, poor in sign. Women present with complaints related to face, breast, hair, nose, and stomach, while men related to hair, nose, ear, genitals, and body build.

Symptoms include facial hair, excessive redness, blushing, scarring, large pores, hair loss, red scrotum, urethral discharge, and AIDS phobia. Associated with chronic skin picking, depression, social phobia, substance abuse, anorexia nervosa, and suicidal tendency

BOX 3: DSM-5 diagnostic criteria for body dysmorphic disorder.[7]

- Preoccupation with ≥1 perceived defects in physical appearance that are not observable or appear slight to others Individual has performed repetitive behaviors or mental acts in response to appearance concerns
- Preoccupation causes significant distress in social, occupational, functional aspects of life
- The appearance preoccupation is not better explained by concerns with body fat or weight in an individual whose symptoms meet diagnostic criteria for an eating disorder

Rx: SSRIs, clomipramine, haloperidol, and cognitive-behavioral therapy have been helpful in this condition.

Eating Disorders

It includes anorexia nervosa (AN), bulimia nervosa (BN), binge eating disorder (BED), and eating disorders not elsewhere classified.

Incidence: Women comprise 90% of the patients.

Clinical features: Skin changes occur in AN when BMI is ≤16. The Russell sign (knuckle calluses) is the most characteristic sign of vomiting in purging type AN. The key diagnostic feature in AN is amenorrhea and polycystic ovary syndrome. It has been linked to polycystic ovary syndrome **(Table 1)**.

Rx: It includes psychotherapy combined with attention to medical complications and nutritional needs. Cognitive behavioral therapy is the front-line treatment. Olanzapine may promote weight gain in AN. Fluoxetine, an SSRI, is approved for BN. Lisdexamfetamine, a stimulant, is USFDA-approved for BED.[7]

Neurotic Excoriations (Psychogenic Excoriations, Dermatillomania, Psychogenic Skin Picking)

It is characterized by noticeable tissue damage due to repeated skin picking. Acne excoriee is a variant of neurotic excoriation, where acne lesions are scratched and picked, predominantly on face.

Incidence: F:M is 3:1. Onset during childhood or adolescence and later in life (30–45 years). May have underlying anxiety disorder, OCD, trichotillomania, depression, and body dysmorphic disorders.

Clinical features: The picking targets imaginary flaws or real blemishes. Patients pick at areas until they can pull the material out of the skin, referred as "pulling a thread from

TABLE 1: Skin signs in eating disorders.[7]

Causes	*Skin signs*
Starvation	Lanugo-like hair, asteatosis/xerosis and follicular hyperkeratosis, alopecia, opaque and fragile hair, carotenoderma, acne, hyperpigmentation, seborrheic dermatitis, acrocyanosis, perniosis, and caries
Self-induced vomiting	Perimylolysis, Russell sign (knuckle calluses)
Drug consumption	Adverse reactions to laxatives, diuretics, appetite suppressants, photosensitivity, fixed drug eruption, urticarial eruptions, finger clubbing with laxative containing senna
Psychiatric comorbidity	Self-mutilation, trichotillomania, and dissatisfaction with the appearance of the skin

Lanugo-like hair, perimylolysis, Russell sign, self-mutilation are guiding signs. Occult eating disorder is suspected when there is presence of ≥4 frequent signs and 1 guide sign.

the skin."[1] The scalp, face, dorsal hands and forearms, upper outer arms, upper back, and buttocks are common sites of involvement.

Polymorphic lesions are seen. Newer lesions are angulated excoriated crusted erosions; older lesions have depigmented scarred center and hyperpigmented periphery.

Differential diagnosis: Dermatitis artifacts, trigeminal trophic syndrome, dermatitis herpetiformis, polycythemia, scabies, obscure food allergy, and paraneoplastic pruritus.[5]

Rx: Cognitive-behavioral therapy and habit reversal training are effective. N-acetylcysteine (1200–3000 mg/day) reduces skin picking symptoms. SSRIs, antipsychotics, and antidepressants are helpful.

Psychogenic Pruritus (Somatoform Pruritus, Functional Itch Disorder)

It is intractable or persistent itch in the absence of dermatologic, systemic, and neurologic etiologies (**Box 4**).

Clinical features: Abrupt onset and termination, occurring at the time of relaxation. It can be generalized or localized. The common sites of involvement are face, scalp, legs, arms, and genitals. It is associated with depression, anxiety, and delusion of parasitosis **(Table 2)**.

Differential diagnosis: Neuropathic itch, other causes of generalized itch (lymphoma, hepatic or renal pathology polycythemia).

BOX 4: Diagnostic criteria proposed by Misery et al.[1]

Three compulsive criteria:
1. Localized or generalized pruritus without primary skin lesions
2. Chronic pruritus (>6 weeks)
3. No somatic cause

Three of seven optional criteria:
1. A chronological relationship of pruritus with one or several life events that could have psychological repercussions
2. Variations of intensity associated with stress
3. Nocturnal variation
4. Predominance during rest or inaction
5. Associated psychological disorders
6. Pruritus that is improved by psychogenic drugs
7. Pruritus that is improved by psychotherapy

TABLE 2: Subtypes of psychogenic pruritus.[1]

Compulsive type	*Impulsive type*	*Mixed type*
Skin excoriation performed to avoid anxiety or to prevent a dreaded event elicited by obsession	Skin excoriation liked with arousal, pleasure or reduction of tension	Features of both the types are present
Executed in full awareness	Executed at times with minimal awareness (automatically)	
Associated with some resistance to behavior	Resistance is lesser	

Rx: Sedative antihistamines, SSRI, antidepressants, and atypical antipsychotics are found useful. Patient education, support, and behavior therapies are helpful.

SECONDARY PSYCHIATRIC DISORDERS

Skin disorders are associated with significant morbidity and affects quality of life. Psychiatric symptoms associated with skin diseases refer **Table 3**.

MISCELLANEOUS

Cutaneous Sensory Syndrome (Regional Cutaneous/Mucosal Dysesthesia)

Patients with abnormal skin sensations (e.g., itching, burning, stinging, and biting or crawling) that is unrelated to any known medical condition.

Various subsets are:[5]
- *Orodynia and glossodynia*: Unexplained pain in oral cavity and tongue respectively.
- *Trichodynia*: Unexplained pain of hair associated with scalp dysesthesia.
- *Vulvodynia and phallodynia*: Prolonged pulling type of genital pain. In vulvodynia, the pain is triggered by physical contact (sexual, nonsexual, or both)

Rx: Education, psychological counseling; sexual counseling (vulvodynia), antidepressants, venlafaxine, duloxetine, gabapentin, and pregabalin are helpful.

Psychogenic Purpura Syndrome (Gardner-Diamond Syndrome, Autoerythrocyte Sensitization Syndrome)

Incidence: Common in middle-aged females who are emotionally disturbed.

Etiology: Abnormalities in the neuro-immuno-cutaneous-endocrine network.
- Hypersensitivity reaction to the extravasated red blood cells.
- Autoimmunity
- Increased fibrinolysins in the blood.

Clinical features: Patients manifest with recurring tender purpura and ecchymotic patches on upper limbs and lower

TABLE 3: Psychiatric symptoms associated with skin diseases.[5]

Diseases	*Associated psychiatric symptoms*
Psoriasis	Poor body image, low self-esteem, depression, anxiety, dysthymia, alcohol abuse, suicidal tendency
Vitiligo	Poor body image, low self-esteem, depression, anxiety, adjustment disorder
Alopecia areata	Depression, anxiety, adjustment disorder, phobic state, paranoid disorder
Atopic dermatitis	Anxiety, depression

limbs which is either spontaneously or secondary to minor trauma, surgery, and physical or mental stress.

Diagnosis: By autoerythrocyte sensitization test (0.1 mL of autologous blood or RBCs is intradermally injected into uninvolved skin to see a positive response within few hours.[5]

Rx: It is unsatisfactory. Antihistamines, corticosteroids, antimalarials etc., have been tried.

MANAGEMENT OF PSYCHOCUTANEOUS DISORDERS

It includes treatment of skin disease and underlying psychiatric condition, treatment of latter divided into pharmacotherapy and nonpharmacological intervention.

Pharmacotherapy[5,6,9]

Antidepressants **(Tables 4 to 7)**

Nonpharmacological Interventions (Tables 8 to 10)[1,5]

TABLE 4: Selective serotonin reuptake inhibitors.

Drug	*Indications*	*Side effects*
Escitalopram	Depression, panic disorder, anxiety disorder	Weight gain, sexual dysfunction
Fluoxetine	Depression, OCD, BDD, bulimia nervosa	Anxiety, insomnia, sexual dysfunction
Fluvoxamine	Depression, OCD	DM, weight gain, sexual dysfunction
Paroxetine	Depression, OCD, panic disorder, PTSD, anxiety disorder	DM, weight gain,
Sertraline	Depression, OCD, panic disorder, PTSD (women)	Insomnia, sexual dysfunction

(PTSD: post-traumatic stress disorder DM: diabetes mellitus)

TABLE 5: Serotonin norepinephrine reuptake inhibitors.

Drug	*Indications*	*Side effects*
Venlafaxine	Depression, anxiety	DM, insomnia, nervousness, hypertension, sexual dysfunction
Duloxetine	Depression, anxiety (Also diabetic neuropathy and stress incontinence)	Impairs glycemic control, fatal liver failure

TABLE 6: Tricyclic antidepressants.

Drug	*Indications*	*Side effects*
Amitriptyline	Depression, neuropathic, pain	DM, cardiotoxic, sedation, weight gain, decrease seizure threshold
Nortriptyline		
Doxepin (antipruritic)		

TABLE 7: Antipsychotic drugs.

Drug	*Indications*	*Side effects*
Pimozide	Schizophrenia	Jaundice, dyskinesia, drowsiness, extrapyramidal side effects, prolonged QT interval
Risperidone	Psychoses, mania	Somnolence, insomnia, agitation, rhinitis, metabolic changes (hypoglycemia, dyslipidemia, weight gain, hyperprolactinemia)
Olanzapine	Schizophrenia, mania	
Quetiapine		Somnolence, orthostatic hypotension, anticholinergic
Aripiprazole	Schizophrenia	Headache, somnolence, agitation, dyspepsia

TABLE 8: Nonpharmacological interventions.

Behavior therapy	*Systematic desensitization* • Modeling • Relaxation • Habit reversal • Assertiveness and social skills training • Guided imagery
Cognitive behavior therapy	• Problem solving • Cognitive restructuring • Modeling and guided imagery
Group therapy	• Psychoeducation • Social and assertiveness skills training • Role play
Psychodynamic therapy	• Past regression • Hypnotherapy
Biofeedback	• Electromyography • Blood flow training

TABLE 9: Nonpharmacological interventions for common skin disorders.[4]

Hypnosis	*Biofeedback*	*Cognitive behavior therapy*
Acne excoriee, alopecia areata, atopic dermatitis ichthyosis, erythroderma, dyshidrotic eczema, glossodynia, herpes simplex, hyperhidrosis, lichen planus, nummular eczema, postherpetic neuralgia, pruritus, psoriasis, rosacea, trichotillomania, urticaria, warts, vitiligo	Hyperhidrosis, Raynaud's disease, psoriasis, atopic dermatitis, herpes simplex	Acne excoriee, atopic dermatitis, factitious cheilitis, hyperhidrosis, lichen simplex, onychotillomania, prurigo nodularis, trichotillomania, urticaria, body dysmorphic disorder, neurotic excoriations

TABLE 10: Complementary psychocutaneous therapy.[1]

Therapy	*Indications*
Lavender oil aromatherapy/ magnolia bark	Anxiety
Lemon balm/passion flower	Nervousness, insomnia
St. John's wort	Depression
S-adenosyl-L-methionine	
Melatonin/valerian	Insomnia due to nervousness

KEY POINTS

- Psychodermatology refers to any aspect of dermatology which overlaps with psychiatry.
- It is classified as primary psychiatric disorders, secondary psychiatric disorders, and psychophysiologic disorders.
- Delusion of parasitosis is characterized by fixed, false belief that the skin is infested with parasites or have foreign objects extruding from their skin, despite evidence to the contrary. They present with specimen sign and matchbox sign. Atypical antipsychotics are helpful.
- Dermatitis artefacta is a factitious disorder in which a fully aware patient creates his/her own skin lesions but denies responsibility. Lesions are polymorphic, bizarre, and geometric shapes. Management includes treatment of skin lesions, SSRI, and antipsychotics.
- Trichotillomania is characterized by recurrent pulling out of one's hair, resulting in alopecia. On dermoscopy there is decrease in hair density, trichoptilosis, coiled hairs, V-hairs, flame hairs, tulip hair, follicular hemorrhages, and hair powder. Behavior modification therapy is the mainstay of treatment.
- Dysmorphophobia is rich in symptoms, poor in sign. They present with complaints related to face, breast, hair, genitals, and body build. SSRIs and cognitive-behavioral therapy are helpful.
- Management of psychocutaneous disorders includes treatment of skin disease and underlying psychiatric condition (pharmacological and nonpharmacological intervention).
- Pharmacotherapy includes treatment with antidepressants, antipsychotics, anxiolytics.
- Nonpharmacological interventions are divided into behavior therapy, cognitive behavior therapy, group therapy, psychodynamic therapy, and biofeedback.

REFERENCES

1. Yadav S, Narang T, Kumaran MS. Psychodermatology: a comprehensive review. Indian J Dermatol Venereol Leprol. 2013;79:176-92.
2. França K, Chacon A, Ledon J, Savas J, Nouri K. Pyschodermatology: a trip through history. An Bras Dermatol. 2013; 88(5):842-3.
3. O'Sullivan RL, Lipper G, Lerner EA. The neuro-immuno-cutaneous-endocrine network: relationship of mind and skin. Arch Dermatol. 1998;134:1431-5.
4. Jafferany M. Psychodermatology: a guide to understanding common psychocutaneous disorders. Prim Care Companion J Clin Psychiatry. 2007;9(3):203-13.
5. Shenoi SD, Prabhu S. Psychocutaneous disorders. In: Sacchidanand S, Oberai C, Inamdar AC (Eds). IADVL Textbook of Dermatology, 4th edition. India: Bhalani Publishing House; 2015. pp. 1998-2014.
6. Bewley A, Taylor RE. Psychodermatology and psychocutaneous disease. In: Griffiths CEM, Barker J, Bleiker T, Chalmers R, Creamer D (Eds). Rook's Textbook of Dermatology, 9th edition. West Sussex, UK: Wiley Blackwell; 2016. pp. 86.1-86.40.
7. Kuhn H, Mennella C, Magid M, Stamu-O'Brien C, Kroumpouzos G. Psychocutaneous disease. J Am Acad Dermatol. 2017; 76(5):779-91.
8. Ankad BS, Naidu M V, Beergouder SL, Sujana L. Trichoscopy in trichotillomania: a useful diagnostic tool. Int J Trichol. 2014; 6:160-3.
9. Jerajani H, Jerajani R. Psychocutaneous disorders. Indian J Dermatol. 2006;51:5-7.

EXAMINATION QUESTIONS

Write short notes on the following:

1. Dermatitis artefacta
2. Trichotillomania
3. Body dysmorphic disorder
4. Psychocutaneous disorders in dermatology
5. Culture bound syndromes in dermatology
6. Dhat syndrome

18 CHAPTER

Urticaria and Urticarial Syndrome

Kiran V Godse, Vasundhara Singh

INTRODUCTION

Urticaria is a disease which is characterized by the appearance of wheals and angioedema or both; either inducible or spontaneous in nature and encompassing several subtypes.[1]

NOMENCLATURE

The mention of the term "urticaria" dates to the 18th century. It is derived from the Latin word "urtica" showing its resemblance to stinging sensation caused by nettle weed (*Urtica dioica*).[2]

HISTORY

Earliest description of the disease is found in Chinese literature around 1000 BC, mentioned as "Feng Yin Zheng" meaning concealed rash. Ayurveda mentions urticaria as sheeta pitta. Hippocrates studied the association of wheals and ingestion of certain foods. In 20th century, Gilchrist and Torok proposed the theory of inflammation followed by theory of hypersensitivity by Prausnitz and Küstner.

CLASSIFICATION

Depending upon the duration of the disease urticaria can be acute, i.e., <6 weeks or chronic, i.e., >6 weeks. Recurrent, intermittent, or episodic presentations are also seen. **Table 1** summarizes the subtypes of urticaria.[1]

ETIOPATHOGENESIS OF URTICARIA

Multiple etiologies are proposed for urticaria such as infections, pseudoallergen, autoimmune, vasculitis, physical, and idiopathic.

Mast cell is believed to be involved in most forms of urticaria, along with other cells. Mast cells have high affinity to immunoglobulin E (IgE) receptors (FcεRI); cross-linking of two or more receptors on the mast cells initiates a chain of calcium and energy-dependent steps which cause mast cell degranulation. Degranulation of mast cell causes histamine release which is central to the formation of wheals and developing angioedema.[3] The increase in vascular permeability is due activation of various mediators such as histamine. There are two types of histamine receptors H_1 is responsible for erythema, flare, itching, smooth muscle contraction whereas H_2 receptor is responsible for wheals and erythema of the skin. Few other important mediators are leukotrienes, bradykinin, substance P, vasoactive intestinal polypeptide, etc.[4]

Another entity called mast cell independent urticaria is a hereditary/acquired condition with C1 esterase deficiency. Hereditary angioedema is of two types:

- *Type 1:* Reduced C1 esterase
- *Type 2:* Reduced function of normal levels of C1 esterase

Acquired deficiency may results from formation of autoantibodies against C1 esterases along with low complement C4 levels.[5]

Dermographism (Fig. 1)

First described by Lewis, dermographism is a triple response due to capillary vasodilation, followed by edema and surrounding flare due to reflex-induced dilation of arterioles after stroking the skin. However, <5% of times it can be associated with itching. It is seen mostly in young adults but there is no correlation of dermographism with severity of the disease.

TABLE 1: Subtypes of urticaria.

Physical urticaria	Solar urticaria	Elicited by light (UV/visible)
	Delayed pressure urticaria	Elicited after 2–6 hours after applying vertical pressure 100 g/mm³ for 70s
	Cold contact urticaria	Elicited by cold objects
	Heat contact urticaria	Elicited by heat stimulus 38–44°C for 5 minutes
	Urticaria factitia/ dermographic urticaria	Elicited by mechanical shearing force
	Vibratory urticaria/ angioedema	Elicited by vortex mixer
Spontaneous urticaria	Acute	<6 weeks
	Chronic	>6 weeks
Others	Contact urticaria	Elicited by contact with triggering agent
	Aquagenic urticaria	Elicited by water
	Cholinergic urticaria	Elicited by exercise/hot shower
	Exercise-induced anaphylaxis/urticaria	Elicited by physical exercise

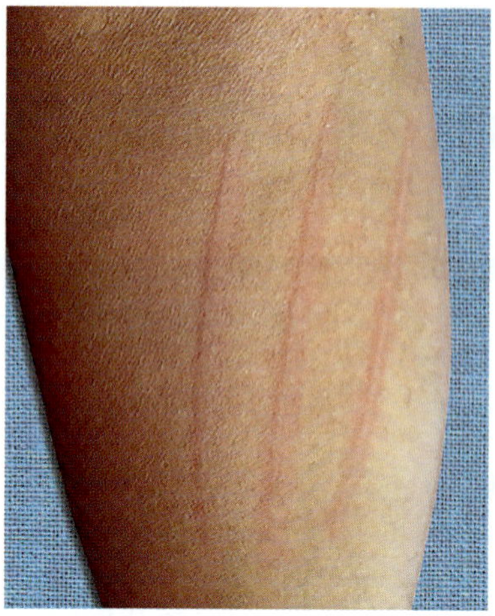

Fig. 1: Dermographism.

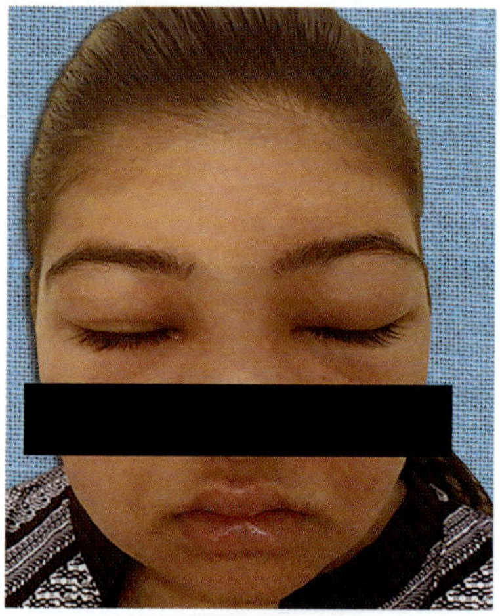

Fig. 2: Perioral and periorbital swelling: Angioedema.

It can be demonstrated with the help of a dermographometer. Stroking the skin at the tip pressure of <36 g/mm^3 induces a linear wheal which is apparent after 10 minutes.

Other forms of dermographism are:

- *Red dermographism*: Due to repeated rubbing forming small punctate wheals
- *Cholinergic dermographism*: Seen in patients of cholinergic urticaria
- *Delayed dermographism*: Wheals return at the previous site of response and persist for 48 hours
- *White dermographism*: Seen in atopic patients due to capillary vasoconstriction
- *Black dermographism*: It is the discoloration seen after pressure from metallic objects.

DIAGNOSIS

There is no need for extensive diagnostic procedures to be performed in case of acute urticaria. The diagnosis of acute urticaria is based on thorough history taking, which should cover the possible trigger.

The following points should be asked in the case of chronic urticaria:[6]

- Frequency, duration, size, and number of wheals
- Stressful life events?
- Angioedema **(Fig. 2)**
- Family history
- Previous allergies
- Psychosomatic and psychiatric illness
- Drug history
- Smoking/alcohol consumption
- Gastric/intestinal problems
- Quality of life impairment
- Previous therapies

Diagnostic procedure for chronic spontaneous urticaria (CSU):[7]

- Urticaria activity score
- Urticaria control test
- Fric test

Extended diagnostic procedures:

- Differential blood count, erythrocyte sedimentation rate (ESR), C-reactive protein (CRP)
- Omission of suspected drug [nonsteroidal anti-inflammatory drugs (NSAIDs)]
- *Ruling out autoreactive CSU*: Autologous serum skin test (ASST); if positive then test for serum IgE where indicated; thyroid and antithyroid hormones, antinuclear antibody (ANA)
- *Ruling out other infections*: *Helicobacter pylori* test, aspartate aminotransferase (AST), liver function test, stool for parasite, urine routine, ENT, and dental examination
- *Ruling out pseudoallergens*: Histamine low diet followed by provocation
- *Ruling out type 1 allergy*: Skin prick test, total and specific IgE
- Tryptase, as indication of severe systemic disease
- If persistence of wheals for >24 hours, then lesional biopsy is advised.

TREATMENT

The main goal should be identifying the underlying cause and treating for symptomatic relief. A step-by-step approach for individual patient should be taken for the management.

General measures: Drugs precipitating urticaria such as NSAIDs and aspirin should be avoided. Although there is no published study on food items causing urticaria, in clinical practice, foods such as tomato, egg, wine, nuts, and herbs may worsen urticaria. Viral infections are one of the common factors precipitating urticaria. Bacterial infections such as sinusitis, dental carries, sepsis, and urinary tract infections are seen in association with the disease. Fungal infections and parasitic infections such as amebiasis, giardiasis, strongyloidiasis, etc., are seen commonly in chronic urticaria patients in developing countries. Treatment of the identifiable cause and avoiding the triggers precipitating attacks should be the initial goal.

Flowchart 1: New GA²LEN/EDF/EAACI/WAO 2016 guidelines.

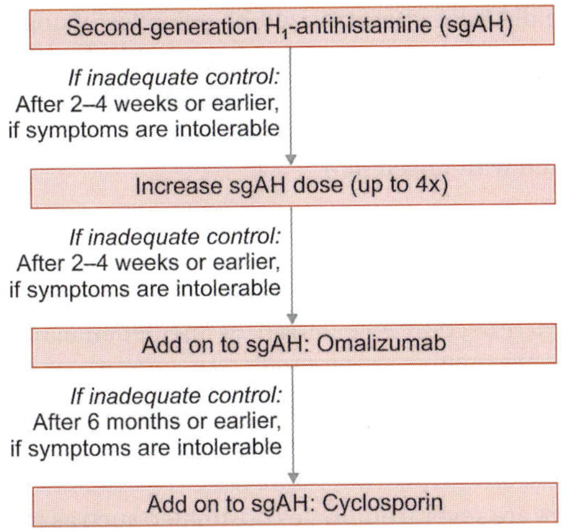

Note: Other treatment options are mentioned below with not remarkably high quality of published data:

- Dapsone
- Methotrexate
- Autoserum therapy
- Azathioprine
- Tranexamic acid
- Colchicine
- H_2 antihistamines
- Phototherapy
- Sulfasalazine
- Intravenous immunoglobulin (IVIg)

Medical measures: Drug of choice is antihistaminics preferably, a nonsedating H_1 class such as levocetirizine, loratadine, desloratadine, ebastine, mizolastine, olopatadine, rupatadine, etc. Classic H_1 antihistamines with sedation include chlorpheniramine, hydroxyzine, diphenhydramine, etc. H_2 antihistamines such as ranitidine and famotidine can be helpful in combination therapy.

New GA²LEN/EDF/EAACI/WAO 2016 guidelines[8] recommend against sedating antihistamines and long-term use of corticosteroids are given in **Flowchart 1**.

In pregnant females' antihistamines should be limited to loratadine with the possible extrapolation to desloratadine; whereas in children first-generation antihistamine use is discouraged.

Omalizumab is a humanized, monoclonal recombinant antibody against IgE. It competitively binds to the FcεRI receptor, thereby preventing IgE—mast cell interaction and inflammatory process. It is given subcutaneously 300 mg monthly for 6–9 months. Severe adverse effects have been noted so far. It was FDA approved for CSU in 2014.

SYNDROMES ASSOCIATED WITH URTICARIA

Cryopyrin-associated Periodic Syndrome

It is a paradigm of interleukin-1 (IL-1)-mediated autoinflammation. The syndrome includes three partially overlapping entities—Muckle-Wells syndrome, familial cold autoinflammatory syndrome (FCAS), CINCA/NOMID (chronic infantile neurological cutaneous and articular/neonatal-onset multisystem inflammatory disease). Within

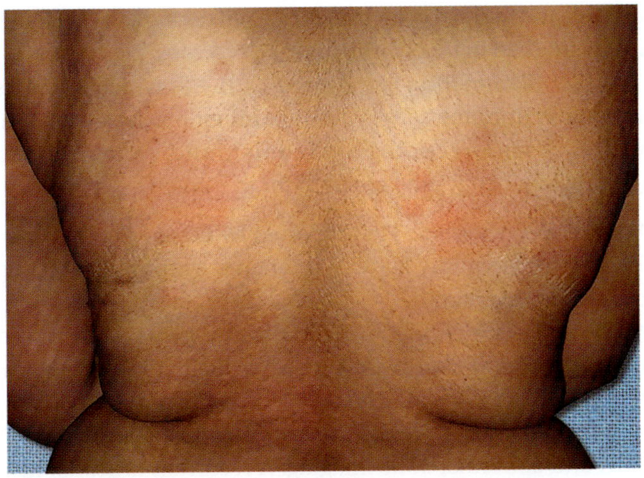

Fig. 3: Erythematous plaques present over the back: Wheals/hives.

the cryopyrin-associated periodic syndrome (CAPS) spectrum CINCA is the most severe entity whereas FCAS is the least. These overlapping entities are related to mutation in the *NLRP3/CIAS1* gene.

These are autosomal dominant disorders and all patients of CAPS have a persistent neutrophilia, chronic anemia, and acute phase reactant proteins with histology showing perivascular and interstitial linear neutrophilic infiltrates.

A newborn presents with flu-like syndrome and rash. Flares are triggered by cold in case of FCAS and partially in Muckle-Wells syndrome, while they are continuous in CINCA. Rash is a nonitchy, symmetrical urticarial rash with angioedema arising from the trunk and involving the limb. It is frequently associated with fever and malaise.

Familial cold autoinflammatory syndrome is characterized by fever, joint pain, conjunctival erythema, rash, fatigue, thirst occurring after 1–2 hours of cold exposure. Symptoms last for a day and patient may experience profuse sweating and intense thirst.

CINCA/NOMID is characterized by continuous flare with mental retardation, sensorineural deafness, neutrophilic aseptic meningitis, and deforming arthropathy. Cutaneous lesions consist of urticarial erythematous papules and plaque often figurate and nonpruritic **(Fig. 3)**. Face shows central bossing, midfacial hypoplasia, and saddle nose. Arthralgia can be severe progressing to large joint polyarthritis with loss of function. There is risk of renal amyloidosis in these patients. Radiological findings show abnormal endochondral ossification, leading to calcified masses in the joint.

Muckle-Wells syndrome: First described in 1962 by Thomas James Muckle, it is an autosomal dominant syndrome associated with acute febrile inflammatory episodes comprising abdominal pain, arthritis, urticaria, sensorineural deafness, and multisystem amyloidosis of AA type.

It is caused by a defect in *CAI1s* gene which forms cryopyrin; therefore, it comes under the CAPS. It is associated with NOMID, i.e., neonatal-onset multisystem inflammatory disease and familial cold urticaria.[9] Cold dependency of flares is less marked in this syndrome.

The inflammation is triggered by IL-1β, which interacts with other immune cells to produce inflammation. Anakinra, which is IL-1 receptor antagonist, and canakinumab (monoclonal antibody) are used for treatment.

Schnitzler's syndrome: First reported by Liliane Schnitzler in 1972, it is a sporadic autoinflammatory syndrome affecting the adults.[10]

It comprises chronic urticaria with a persistently raised monoclonal IgM along with any two of the following features: recurrent fever above 40°C, bone or joint pain, lymphadenopathy, hepatomegaly or splenomegaly, neutrophilia, elevated ESR/CRP, and abnormal bone imaging. A recurrent urticarial rash is usually the first sign with few patients complaining of bone/joint pain. Lesions resolve with hyperpigmentation.

Pathogenesis is similar to other CAPS; symptoms improve with IL inhibitors. An IgG variant has also been reported. Strasbourg diagnostic criteria have been recently proposed for diagnosis.

Profound alteration in quality of life, AA amyloidosis, and refractory inflammatory anemia are severe complications of Schnitzler's syndrome. Possible comorbidities include autoimmune peripheral neuropathy, pseudoxanthoma elasticum, antiphospholipid antibodies, C4 deficiencies, and hearing loss.

Management consists considering the impact of disease on quality of life and levels of inflammatory markers ranging from NSAIDs, colchicine, hydroxychloroquine to anakinra 100 mg/day.

Well's syndrome: Described in 1971, this disease is acute in onset and characterized by plaques resembling cellulitis that may persist for weeks. It can occur in all age groups and is commonly associated with pruritus. With its recurrent nature in the subsequent episodes the duration of symptoms gets prolonged. The lesion in its late phase may show morphea-like residual skin atrophy and hyperpigmentation.

Histopathological features are flame figures due to dermal degradation of eosinophils. Some suggest a type IV hypersensitivity reaction in response to a variety of exogenous and endogenous stimuli as a mode of pathogenesis. Treatment with oral corticosteroids 2 mg/kg/day for a week has been found effective with gradual tapering dose.

Gleich's syndrome: Episodic angioedema with eosinophilia is a rare disorder characterized by episodes of angioedema and eosinophilia that occur at monthly intervals and resolve spontaneously without therapy. There is a female preponderance seen in this disease and few cases are associated with raised IgM.

KEY POINTS

- Urticaria (*Synonym:* Nettle weed) is a cutaneous disorder characterized by wheals and/or angioedema, which may be spontaneous or inducing.
- Based on the duration of symptoms, it can be classified as:
  - Acute urticaria—<6 weeks
  - Chronic urticaria—>6 weeks
- There are several etiologies postulated such as infections, pseudoallergen, autoimmune, vasculitis, physical, and idiopathic.

REFERENCES

1. Zuberbier T, Asero R, Bindslev-Jensen C, Walter Canonica G, Church MK, Giménez-Arnau A, et al. EAACI/GA(2)LEN/EDF/WAO guideline: definition, classification and diagnosis of urticaria. Allergy. 2009;64(10):1417-26.
2. Juhlin L. The History of Urticaria and Angioedema. ESHDV Annual Lecture, Geneva, October 11th 2000.
3. Ferrer M, Nakazawa K, Kaplan AP. Complement dependence of histamine release in chronic urticaria. J Allergy Clin Immunol. 1999;104:169-72.
4. Sachdeva S, Guta V, Amin SS, Tahseen M. Chronic urticaria. Indian J Dermatol. 2011;56:622-8.
5. Grattan C. Aetiopathogenesis of urticaria. In: Maurer M, Zuberbier T, Grattan C (Eds). Urticaria and Angioedema. Berlin Heidelberg: Springer Verlag; 2010.
6. Zuberbier T, Chantraine-Hess S, Hartmann K, Czarnetzki BM. Pseudoallergen-free diet in treatment of chronic urticaria. A prospective study. Acta Derm Venereol. 1995;75:484-7.
7. Maurer M, Grabbe J. Urticaria: its history-based diagnosis and etiologically oriented treatment. Dtsch Arztebl Int. 2008;105:458-65; quiz 465-6.
8. Godse KV. Updosing of antihistamines to improve control of chronic urticaria. Indian J Dermatol Venereol Leprol. 2010;76:61-2.
9. Farasat S, Aksentijevich I, Toro JR. Autoinflammatory disease: clinical and genetic advances. Arch Dermatol. 2008;144(3):392-402.
10. Simon A, Asli B, Braun Falco M, De Koning H, Fermand JP, Grattan C, et al. Schnitzler's syndrome: diagnosis, treatment, and follow-up. Allergy. 2013;68:562-8.

EXAMINATION QUESTIONS

1. Classify urticaria and add a note on dermographism.
2. Elaborate and explain etiopathogenesis of urticaria.
3. Classify antihistamines and write a note on treatment of urticaria.
4. Mention syndromes associated with urticaria and write a short note on Schnitzler's syndrome.
5. Explain recent advances in pathophysiology of urticaria.
6. Explain recent treatment advances in urticaria.
7. Classify angioedema and how will you approach to a case of recurrent angioedema without wheals?

19 CHAPTER

Figurate Erythema

Sudhir Nayak UK, Rupika Singh

INTRODUCTION

Figurate or gyrate erythemas are a heterogeneous group of muti-nomenclatured reactive erythemas which tend to migrate and spread peripherally.[1] Descriptions used to describe this group of diseases include annular, polycyclic, circinate, arcuate, serpiginous, etc.[1]

The common figurate erythemas are:

- Erythema annulare centrifugum (EAC)
- Erythema marginatum rheumaticum (EMR)
- Erythema chronicum migrans
- Erythema gyratum repens (EGR)
- Annular erythemas of infancy (AEI)

ERYTHEMA ANNULARE CENTRIFUGUM

Synonyms: Superficial or deep gyrate erythema, erythema perstans, and palpable migrating erythema.

Probably the most common of all gyrate erythemas. This was first described by Darier in 1916.[2] Occasionally, this term is used to include all annular erythemas which do not fit into the pattern of other gyrate erythemas. This is mostly a chronic delayed hypersensitivity reaction to various stimuli.

Predisposing Causes

Predisposing causes of erythema annulare centrifugum are given in **Table 1**.

TABLE 1: Predisposing causes of erythema annulare centrifugum.

Infection	Dermatophyte, *Candida*, Epstein–Barr virus, molluscum, bacteria, and mycobacteria
Infestation	*Borrelia, Ascaris, and Trypanosoma*
Drugs	Aldactone, amitriptyline, thiacetazone, finasteride, piroxicam, hydroxychloroquine, penicillin, gold, and thiazides
Carcinoma/blood dyscariasis/malignancy	Lymphoma and leukemia
Dysproteinemia	
Autoimmune disease	
Food	
Stress	
Pregnancy	
Idiopathic–most common	

Clinical Features

- Although seen in all age groups, EAC is usually seen in adults, with a female preponderance.[2]
- Clinically it presents as annular, arcuate, serpiginous or polycyclic erythematous or urticarial plaques. Lesions may be single or multiple in number.[3] Polycyclic lesions or serpiginous lesions occur due to the coalescing of annular or arcuate lesions.
- The border of the lesions often depends on whether it is of superficial type or deep type. The superficial forms have an indistinct border and a peripheral trailing scale while the deep forms have a firm, distinct, and nonscaly border.[4]
- Lesions are commonly seen on the trunk or lower limbs. Margins are indurated and of 4-6 mm wide.[5]
- Lesions tend to spread at a rate of 2–3 mm/day and size ranges from 6 to 8 cm.[3] Lesions may last for days to months or even years.[3]
- Lesions become less prominent by the day and appear only erythematous. Mild pruritus and vesicles, hyperpigmentation, and familial forms have been described in EAC.[2]
- EAC has a chronic course which tends to wax and wane and then spontaneously resolve over weeks to months. Investigations for EAC will depend on the predisposing factor.

Histopathology

- Histopathology shows a coat sleeve like distribution of lymphocytic perivascular infiltrate.
- The superficial forms tend to have epidermal changes whereas the deep forms have usually a normal epidermis.[4]
- Vasculitic-like picture has occasionally been reported in the histopathology.[4] But fibrin extravasation is not seen.[5]

Treatment

The treatment of the underlying condition often leads to faster resolution of EAC:

- Topical and/or intralesional corticosteroids are often used.
- Other topical agents tried include tacrolimus and calcipotriol.[2]
- Systemic antihistamines, nonsteroidal anti-inflammatory drugs, antimalarials, oral steroids, etanercept, and phototherapy have been tried.[2,3]

ERYTHEMA MARGINATUM RHEUMATICUM

The term EMR was coined by Cheadle in in 1889 and was in Jones criteria in 1944.[6] EMR is one of the five major diagnostic Jones criteria for rheumatic fever (RF) although it is seen in less than 6% of the cases.[7] The other criteria are carditis and valvulitis, arthritis, central nervous system involvement, and subcutaneous nodules. Although highly specific for RF, EMR is seen only in a minority of patients. More commonly seen in children (5–15 years) than in adults.[2,3]

Clinical Features

- Asymptomatic transient pink to faintly erythematous rash extending peripherally with central clearing and appears with onset of fever. Lesions may become pronounced with a hot bath as well as cold exposure.[2]
- The border which is sharply defined in the outer aspect and diffuse in the inner side; giving an annular appearance and hence the name erythema annulare.
- This is usually seen over the trunk in a bathing suit distribution, especially periumbilical. Facial involvement is not seen although it may occur on the limbs, axillae, and glutei.
- Individual lesions often appear, disappear and reappear over hours to days. Lesions usually spread at a rate of 2–10 mm/12 hours.[3]
- Although transient, it can be persistent and rarely recurrent.
- Usually noticed in acute phase of RF and is associated with acute carditis.
- Rare cases have been seen later in the course of RF and also with chronic carditis.
- Erythema papulatum are rarely occurring papular lesions seen over the elbows and knees, mimicking granuloma annulare, and often disappear after 7 days.[2]
- Subcutaneous nodules are another manifestation of RF.[6]

Associations

Beta-hemolytic streptococcal infection, psittacosis, and angioedema.

Histopathology

Neutrophilic perivascular infiltrate of the superficial dermal vasculature without any vasculitic feature. Occasionally, eosinophils and lymphocytes may be seen.[5]

Treatment

Penicillin is the drug of choice for treatment of RF. Other drugs include erythromycin, aspirin, and nonsteroidal anti-inflammatory drugs (NSAIDs).[3] Treatment of EMR is predominately symptomatic.[2]

ERYTHEMA CHRONICUM MIGRANS

This was first described by the Swedish dermatologist Arvind Afzelius in 1912. This is the figurate erythema which has been described in association with Lyme disease caused by *Borrelia* species and transmitted by *Ixodes* ticks. Lyme disease has been named after the town where it was first noticed—Lyme, Connecticut, USA in 1977. The species of *Borrelia* implicated include *B. burgdorferi* sensu lato, *B. burgdorferi* sensu stricto, *B. afzelii*, and *B. garinii*. The *Ixodes* ticks implicated are *Ixodes scapularis* (*dammini*), *I. ricinus*, and *I. persulcatus*.

Clinical Features

- A red papule is usually seen at the site of the tick bite. Recollection of tick bite is reported retrospectively by 50% of the patients.[8]
- Prior to the onset of rash, patients often exhibit nonspecific symptoms and signs such as fatigue, fever, chills, myalgia, arthralgia, headache, neck stiffness, etc.
- After an interval of few days (1–28 days: mean 9 days) an erythematous macule is seen which then expands to form the characteristic lesion of erythema chronicum migrans.
- The intensity of erythema also varies from patient to patient.[8] The classical lesion is characterized by warm slowly expanding (over days to weeks) of annular erythematous plaque with central clearing often reaching 20 cm located usually over the axilla, popliteal fossa, inguinal or waist. The central clearing is often noticed only after increase in size of the lesion.
- Usually asymptomatic, some patients report itching or burning sensations. Untreated lesions fade over a duration of few weeks (mean—1 day to 14 months).[8]
- Target or bull's eye appearance, vesicular or necrotic center may be seen. Multiple lesions (25%) are common in patients not diagnosed and treated early and are considered to be due to hematogenous spread. Disseminated lesions are smaller, less obvious, and occur days to weeks after primary lesion.[6]

Investigations

Biopsy, enzyme-linked immunosorbent assay (ELISA), Western blot, and indirect immunofluorescence.[8]

Histopathology

The dermis shows interstitial and perivascular lymphocytic infiltrate. Plasma cells, eosinophils, and rarely neutrophils may be seen. In 40–50% of the biopsy, samples stained with Warthin–Starry silver stains show spirochetes in the papillary dermis close the dermoepidermal junction.[8,9]

Treatment

Doxycycline 100 mg BD for 14–21 days is first line of treatment. Amoxicillin 500 mg TID. Other alternatives are cefuroxime 500 mg BD or erythromycin 500 mg QID for 2–3 weeks.[2,8]

ERYTHEMA GYRATUM REPENS

This was first described by Gammel in 1952.[6] EGR, although considered majorly as a paraneoplastic phenomenon (80%), has been described with non-neoplastic conditions too.[2,3] Male:female ratio of 2:1, white races, and age from 16 to 75 years are common.[2,3]

Pathogenesis

Although the exact pathogenesis is unknown, various hypotheses include cross reaction of tumor antigens with cutaneous antigens, modifications of preexisting cutaneous antigens, and immune complex deposition.

Clinical Features

- Characterized by severely pruritic concentric rings of rapidly expanding erythematous plaques with a trailing collarette of scale mainly over the trunk and extremities. The classical description of EGR is described as wood grain or marble- or zebra-like appearance.[2,5,6]
- The rate of spread of EGR is rapid (1 cm/day) and hence tends to involve large parts of the body. Lesions occur within existing lesions as waves, swirls or rings leading to the characteristic description.[3]
- Palmoplantar hyperkeratosis is seen in 10% of the patients irrespective of the underlying condition.[3]
- EGR like other paraneoplastic dermatoses may appear before, during or after diagnosis of underlying malignancy and resolves with treatment of the underlying malignancy, but usually precedes diagnosis of malignancy by 9 months.[2]
- Resolution of EGR occurs 6 weeks after resolution of underlying problem.[2]

Associations

It is usually associated with bronchogenic carcinoma. Other associated malignancies include those of the breast, esophagus, stomach, urinary bladder, prostrate, uterus, and/or cervix. Benign conditions associated with EGR include psoriasis, pityriasis rubra pilaris, pulmonary tuberculosis, lupus erythematosus, CREST (calcinosis, Raynaud's phenomenon, esophageal dysmotility, sclerodactyly, and telangiectasia) syndrome, adverse drug reaction to azathioprine, and other autoimmune conditions.[2]

Histopathology

The epidermal changes seen include focal parakeratosis, spongiosis, and acanthosis while the dermal changes include varying amount of perivascular lymphohistiocytic infiltrate around the superficial vascular plexus. Rarely, extension to the deeper vascular plexus and eosinophils in the infiltrate are seen.[5]

Investigations

Investigation aims mainly to rule out underlying malignancy or other benign conditions.

Treatment

No specific treatment for skin lesions. Intralesional steroid injections have been found to be beneficial in reduction of pruritus. Lesions usually subside on treatment of the primary disease.[2] Treatment of the primary malignancy often results in resolution of EGR and recurrence has been noted with recurrence of malignancy.[5]

ANNULAR ERYTHEMAS OF INFANCY

This refers to a heterogeneous group of erythemas seen in infancy.[5] Controversy exists whether to consider this as a separate entity of whether it is EAC occurring in children. Association with maternal lupus erythematosus is found in many cases.[5] The first case was reported in 1981.

Annular erythemas of infancy include the following earlier described entities, i.e., familial annular erythema, annular erythema of infancy, persistent annular erythema of infancy, erythema gyratum atrophicans transiens neonatale, and infantile epidermodysplastic erythema gyratum.[5] Organisms associated with AEI include *candida albicans*, Epstein–Barr virus (EBV), and *Malassezia* species.

Clinical Features

- Nonpruritic annular or polycyclic erythema or erythematous plaques single/grouped of varying sizes on the face, trunk, and proximal extremities.
- Lesions expand at the rate of 2–3 mm/day and individual lesions last for two to few days.
- No systemic features are seen.
- Lesions occur in cyclical pattern every 5–6 weeks.

Histopathology

Epidermis is usually normal. In the dermis perivascular lymphohistiocytic infiltrate is seen along the superficial and deep vasculature. Eosinophils are also seen.[5] Neutrophilic variant has also been described.

Investigations

Blood eosinophilia is noted. Other required tests include skin biopsy, antibodies to double-stranded deoxyribonucleic acid (dsDNA), Smith antigen (Sm), and Ro and La antigens. Electrocardiogram is also advisable.

Treatment

Treatment is usually not required as it is self-limiting. Topical steroids and tacrolimus have been advocated. Any underlying infection is to be treated.[3]

KEY POINTS

- Erythema occurs usually due to the dilatation of blood vessels, mostly of the papillary and reticular dermis. A heterogeneous group of skin disorders can manifest as erythemas.
- The erythemas discussed in this chapter are figurate erythemas which can be annular, arciform or polycyclic in appearance.
- The four classic types of figurate erythemas are EAC, erythema marginatum, erythema migrans, and EGR.
- The etiology or trigger varies from infections to neoplasms though often the etiology remains idiopathic, especially in the case of EAC.
- Prior to labeling the disorder as idiopathic histological, microbiologic, and serologic evaluation should be done.
- Treatment can either be specific (antibiotics) or nonspecific (topical corticosteroids).

REFERENCES

1. White JW Jr. Hypersensitivity and miscellaneous inflammatory disorders. In: Moschella SL, Hurley HJ (Eds). Dermatology. 2nd edition. New Delhi. Jaypee Brothers Medical Publishers;1985. pp. 473-8.
2. Ghosh S, Haldar S. Cutaneous vascular responses. In: Sacchidanand S, Oberai, C, Inamadar AC (Eds). IADVL Textbook of Dermatology, 4th edition. Mumbai: Bhalani Publishing House; 2015. pp. 1164-72.
3. Rustin M, Cerio R. Reactive inflammatory erythemas. In: Griffiths C, Barker J, Bleiker T, Chalmers R, Creamer D (Eds). Rook's Textbook of Dermatology, 9th edition. Singapore: Wiley Blackwell; 2016. pp. 47.6-47.13.
4. Nayak SU, Shenoi SD, Prabhu SM. Erythema annulare centrifugum: deep variant with vasculitis like histopathology. Indian J Dermatol. 2013;58:329.
5. Patterson JW. The vasculopathic reaction pattern. In: Patterson JW (Ed). Weedon's Skin Pathology, 4th edition. China: Churchill Livingstone Elsevier; 2016. pp. 245-6.
6. Espana A. Figurate erythemas in dermatology. In: Bolognia JL, Jorizzo JL, Rapini RP (Eds), 2nd edition. Spain: Mosby Elsevier; 2008. pp. 277-86.
7. UpTodate (2020). Acute rheumatic fever: Clinical manifestations and diagnosis. [online] Available from: https://www.uptodate.com/contents/acute-rheumatic-fever-clinical-manifestations-and-diagnosis? [Last accessed January, 2021].
8. Rooks Hay RJ, Morris-Jones R. Bacterial infections. In: Griffiths C, Barker J, Bleiker T, Chalmers R, Creamer D (Eds). Rook's Textbook of Dermatology, 9th edition. Singapore: Wiley-Blackwell; 2016. pp. 2669-71.
9. Patterson JW. Spirochetal infections. In: Patterson JW (Ed). Weedon's Skin Pathology, 4th edition. China: Churchill Livingstone Elsevier; 2016. p. 654.

EXAMINATION QUESTION

1. Name and briefly describe the common figurate erythemas.

20 CHAPTER

Eczema: Concept and Classification

Manasa Narayan Kayarkatte, Varsha M Shetty

INTRODUCTION

The word eczema is derived from Greek and translates to "boil over". It is a heterogeneous group of inflammatory disorders which is usually characterized by pruritus, erythema with oozing and vesiculation in early stages, edema and scaling in subacute stage, and later by lichenification in chronic stage.

Eczema is a nonspecific term that describes the morphological appearance of several forms of dermatitis and hence its use to refer to atopic dermatitis alone is now considered imprecise. The disparate nomenclature has deleterious ramifications for research and clinical care, hence the term should be used to denote only morphological appearance and use of a prefix suggestive of the cause such as "atopic" eczema is encouraged for precise understanding.[1]

PREVALENCE

The incidence of each type of eczema varies according to the geographic area, ethnicity, environment and lifestyle. There are numerous studies on the prevalence of atopic dermatitis, but fewer in other types of eczema. Large scale population survey has shown eczema in 11.5% of adults at any given point of time.[2]

Despite an overlap in clinical features and etiopathogenesis, eczema can be classified into two broad groups: (1) exogenous and (2) endogenous based on the causative factors—if they are largely external or internal **(Table 1)**.[3]

ETIOPATHOGENESIS

The pathogenesis of exogenous eczemas, particularly primary irritant and allergic contact dermatitis, is well understood but that of endogenous eczemas is not very clear. Broad outline of difference in allergic and irritant contact dermatitis is given in **Table 2.**[4]

TABLE 1: Classification of eczema based on causative factors.[3]

Exogenous	*Endogenous*
• Irritant contact dermatitis • Allergic contact dermatitis • Photodermatitis • Infective dermatitis • Dermatophytide • Post-traumatic eczema	• Atopic dermatitis • Seborrheic dermatitis • Nummular eczema • Asteatotic eczema • Stasis dermatitis • Pompholyx • Juvenile plantar dermatosis • Eczema associated with systemic disease • Metabolic eczema • Eyelid dermatitis • Hand eczema

TABLE 2: Difference between allergic and irritant contact dermatitis.[3,4]

	Allergic contact dermatitis	*Irritant contact dermatitis*
Definition	Delayed type of hypersensitivity response and skin inflammation mediated by antigen-specific T-cell in a previously sensitized person	Nonspecific inflammatory dermatoses due to toxic chemical on the skin that triggers activation of innate immunity
	Constitutes 20–30% of all contact dermatitis (CD)	Constitutes 70–80% of all CD
Pathogenesis	Involves activation of T-cells	Only innate immunity is activated
Mediators involved	CD8 cell—Th1 mediated; IFN-γ, IL-2, IL-17 with decreased T regulatory cell activity	IL-1, IL-6, IL-8, and TNF-α
Clinical features	Appears 24–48 hours after contact	Appears immediately
	Itching more than burning	Burning more than itching
	Occurs in susceptible individuals	Occurs in most of the population
	Skin lesions can occur at the site of contact as well as at distant sites	Skin lesions tends to occur only at the site of contact
Histology	Spongiosis, exocytosis	Epidermal necrosis may be seen
Patch test, ROAT	Positive	Negative

(IFN-γ: interferon gamma; IL-1: interleukin-1; ROAT: repeated open application test; TNF-α: tumor necrosis factor alpha)

Predisposing Factors

Host factors: Individuals with atopy, and those who are fast acetylators are susceptible to eczema.

Age: Sensitivity to allergens decreases after the age of 70 years.

Sex: As female sex is more commonly exposed to ornamental metal, hence the frequency of eczema is higher.

Hormones: Hormones are known to increase sensitization to allergens and allergic tendencies have been noticed with oral contraceptives

Race: White race is more susceptible than others.

Medication: Patients on immunosuppressive medications are less susceptible to sensitization.

Local factors: Pre-existing local disease causes skin barrier disruption and increase in local mononuclear cells leading to increased risk of sensitization. It is important to maintain skin barrier, so as to prevent the entry of further allergen and thereby disrupting the itch-scratch cycle of eczema. Also, area such as eyelid, where the skin is thinner is easily prone to eczema **(Fig. 1)**.

Environmental Factors

- *Climate*: Ultraviolet (UV) exposure acts as local immunosuppressive, hence decreased risk of sensitization is expected. However, photoactivation of allergens may occur with UV exposure causing increased risk of eczema.
  - *Winters*: Resulting dryness leads to increased sensitization.
  - *Summer*: Sweating and occlusion also leads to easy sensitization
- *Flora*: Certain plants such as Parthenium, Asteraceae family causes sensitization, which may be seasonal.
- *Socioeconomic and cultural*: Cheaper metal jewelry, hair dyes, cosmetics, and tattoo can all cause allergic contact dermatitis.
- *Chemical*: The risk of sensitization depends on the dose of chemical, duration of contact, and area of contact.

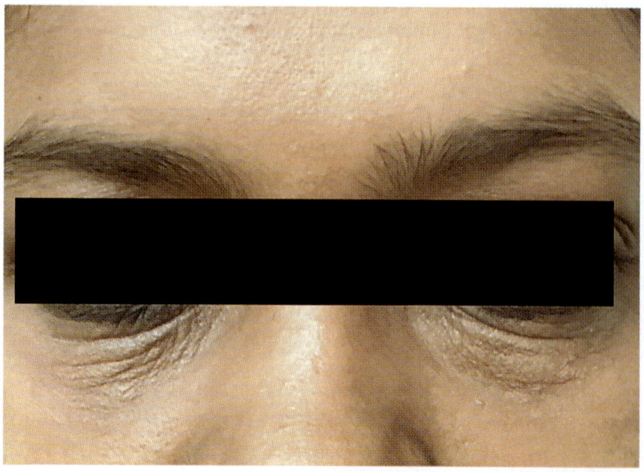

Fig. 1: Eyelid dermatitis.

In a predisposed individual, the interaction of triggering factors with keratinocytes and T-lymphocytes produces an inflammatory cytokine milieu, causing increased intercellular edema, increased keratinocyte turnover, leading to the histological changes and thus the clinical findings[5] **(Fig. 2)**.

- In allergic contact dermatitis, there is an initial phase of sensitization where the allergen is recognized and immunological memory is produced. Then, during elicitation phase, the lesions are produced as the immunological memory gets translated to active T lymphocytes. It is basically a type IV mediated delayed hypersensitivity reaction, and the responsible allergen can be detected by patch test.[5]
- In irritant contact dermatitis, there is a localized, nonimmunologically driven inflammatory reaction with the activation of innate immunity leading to epidermal necrosis.[5,6]

Skin prick test can be employed in the diagnosis wherein a type I hypersensitivity is suspected to inhalants, food, drug, or occupational allergens.[7]

Endogenous eczema is multifactorial similar to atopic eczema wherein genetic factors, diet, environment, infections, stress, allergens all contribute to its pathogenesis **(Fig. 3)**.[5]

CLINICAL FEATURES

The clinical features mainly depend on the stage of the disease—acute, subacute, or chronic **(Figs. 4A and B; Table 3)**.

Autosensitization dermatitis/secondary dissemination refers to a phenomenon in which an acute dermatitis develops at cutaneous sites distant from an inflammatory focus, and where the secondary acute dermatitis is not explained by the inciting cause of the primary inflammation. The classic example quoted is that noted in patients with venous stasis, where nearly one-third develop at least one episode of autosensitization.

Conditioned hyperirritability is a phenomenon where an area of inflamed skin on one part of the body results in a generalized hyperirritability of the skin at distant sites. *Example:* angry back phenomenon during patch testing of a patient suffering from active dermatitis.[3]

HISTOPATHOLOGY

Similar to the clinical features, the histopathology evolves through the different stages of lesions from predominant spongiotic pattern in acute stage to a psoriasiform pattern in chronic stage.[8]

INVESTIGATIONS

- *Clinical examination*: This is usually sufficient to make a diagnosis of eczema. Appropriate laboratory tests to identify secondary bacterial or fungal infection can be advised.

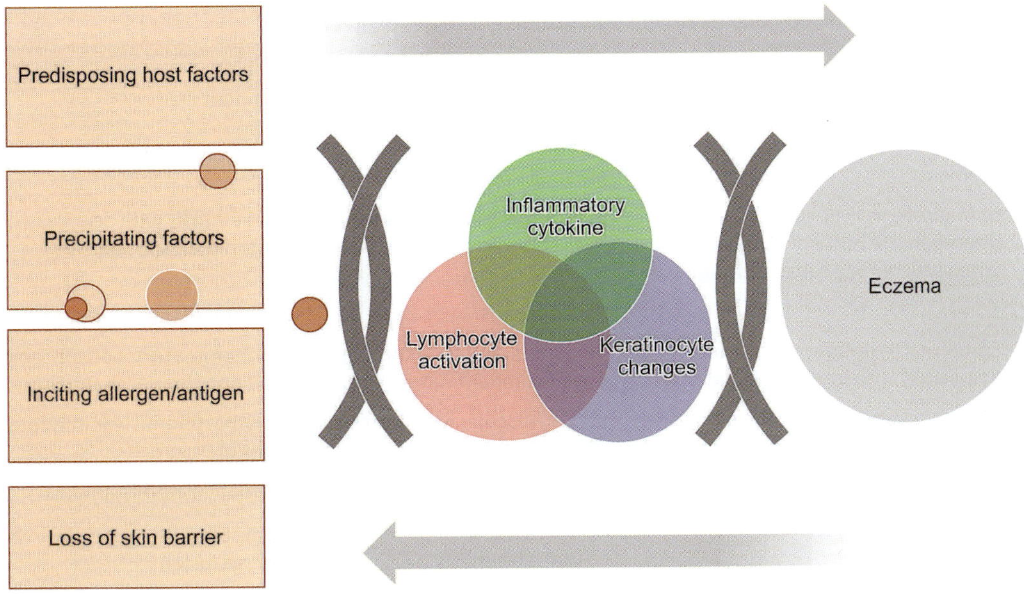

Fig. 2: Pathogenesis of eczema—an outline.

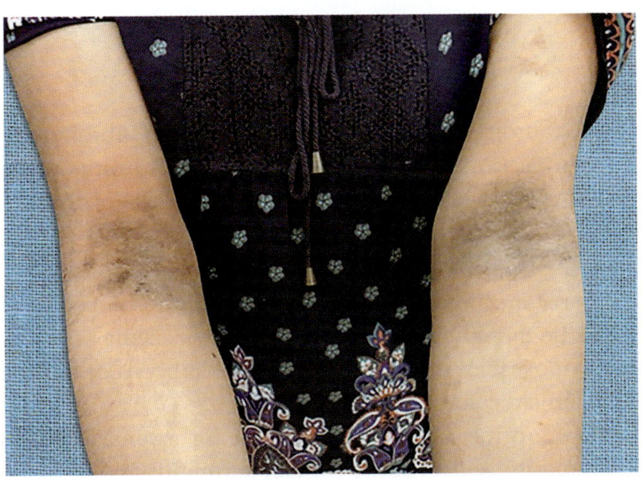

Fig. 3: Atopic eczema showing involvement of cubital fossa.

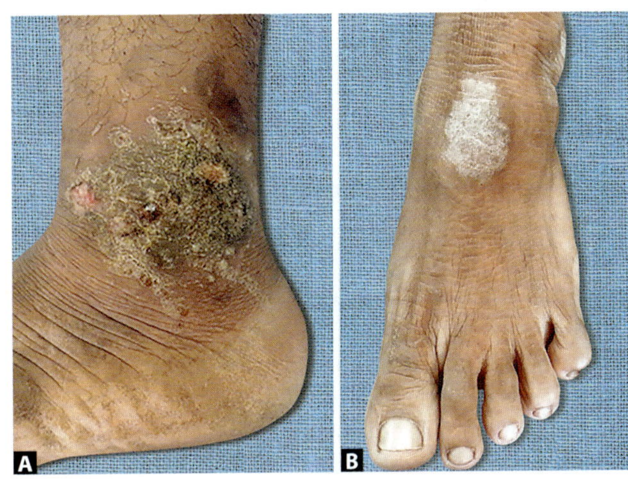

Figs. 4A and B: (A) Subacute eczema with pustules, crusting and ulceration; (B) Chronic eczema showing lichenification.

- *Biopsy*: This is very rarely indicated, as the diagnosis is mainly clinical.
- *Patch testing:* This is based on the principle of delayed hypersensitivity and is primarily employed in the diagnosis of allergic contact dermatitis. Additionally, when the eczema involves the face, hands, and feet or in a case of asymmetrical or atypical dermatitis, patch testing is recommended. The positive patch test does not necessarily mean that the patient has developed the eczema secondary to that antigen. Routine patch testing for atopic or seborrheic dermatitis is not warranted.[9]
- *Skin prick test*: This test is recommended in the setting of a suspected type I hypersensitivity reaction such as protein contact dermatitis.[6,7] This test is utilized in identifying the sensitivity to inhalant, drug, food, or occupational allergens. However, the test results should be carefully interpreted based on the clinical history so that necessary avoidance of the allergen can be appropriately advised.[7]

MONITORING

Multiple scoring systems are available, one of the easy ones being eczema area severity index (EASI) which is similar to psoriasis area severity index (PASI). In EASI, four parameters: (1) erythema, (2) induration, (3) excoriation, and (4) lichenification, are scored from 0 to 3 in individual area of head and neck, upper limbs, trunk, and lower limbs. Each area is scored from 0 to 6 based on the surface area involved and final score is added with a maximum scoring of 72.[10]

Serial photography also helps to monitor the response to therapy.

TABLE 3: Clinical features, histopathology, and treatment during different stages of eczema.[3,8]

	Acute	*Subacute*	*Chronic*
Clinical features	Edema	Erythema	Lichenified plaque
	Vesiculation	Scaling	
	Erythema	Minimal vesicles	
Histopathology	Spongiosis, may be diffuse, but most intense in the mid-epidermal region—when severe may cause clefting	Acanthosis more prominent than spongiosis	Hyperkeratosis with acanthosis, which is more common than spongiosis
		Parakeratosis	Elongation of rete ridges
	Epidermal lymphocytic infiltrate, associated with intercellular edema	Epidermis shows pyknotic nuclei of inflammatory cells	The inflammatory cells in epidermis are less prominent, dermal changes are more marked
	Vascular changes in the form of dilation and perivascular lymphocytic and polymorphonuclear infiltrate and eosinophils in case of drug-induced dermatitis, are appreciated in all the stages of eczema		
Treatment	Sedative antihistamines	Nonsedative antihistamines	Nonsedative antihistamines
	Astringents	• Paste wraps • Topical steroids	Topical steroids—twice-daily regimen, tar under occlusion
	Systemic steroids	Topical tacrolimus	Topical tacrolimus
	Ciclosporin		• Methotrexate • Azathioprine • Alitretinoin • Phototherapy

TREATMENT

Precautions and Supportive Therapy

- Elimination of the underlying etiological factors is essential.
- Patients should be educated to avoid the predisposing and aggravating factors.
- Wet wraps in patients with oozing lesions (acute eczema), emollients in dry lesions is advised.
- Astringents such as potassium permanganate 1:100,000 is useful in edematous lesions.
- Sedative antihistamines in acute eczema and nonsedative ones for chronic lesions is advocated.
- Other adjuvants that can be added with lesser evidence of benefit include omega-3 fatty acid, probiotics, and vitamin D.[9]

Topical Therapy

- Topical steroids are the mainstay in the treatment of eczemas; potency can be based on the morphology of the lesions, clinical picture, and the site of involvement.
- Topical therapy in the form of liberal usage of emollients, which is free from added constituents such as fragrance and preservative, is advised along with topical steroids. Apart from providing hydration, it forms a layer of barrier to the inciting allergen as well.[11]
- Immunomodulators, such as tacrolimus and pimecrolimus, are being used, especially in children >2 years of age.[9]
- Crisaborole, a topical phosphodiesterase 4 inhibitor, has been approved by the Food and Drug Administration (FDA) for atopic dermatitis in children >2 years of age.[11]

Immunosuppressives

- Short tapering course of oral steroids can be used as a rescue therapy in cases of severe acute eczema.
- Low dose methotrexate (5 mg/week) has been used to treat chronic recalcitrant eczema.
- Azathioprine is a common choice for extensive photodermatitis and airborne contact dermatitis.[3]

Other Therapies

- Alitretinoin is FDA approved for chronic hand eczema.
- Phototherapy is used frequently after ruling out photodermatitis.[9]
- Nonlaser 308 nm monochromatic excimer light (MEL) has been tried in chronic localized hand dermatitis.[12]
- Biologics such as dupilumab (IL-13 and IL-4 receptor antagonist) is FDA approved drug for atopic dermatitis.[11]
- The treatment of autoeczematization involves alleviating the original focus of sensitization.[3]

KEY POINTS

- The term eczema denotes morphologic appearance of erythema, vesiculation, edema, progressing to lichenification in later stages.
- It can be classified based on cause—exogenous/endogenous; based on evolution of lesion—acute, subacute,

or chronic; and based on pathogenesis—allergic, irritant, or unclassified.

- Similarly, in acute stage, lesions are edematous with vesiculation and chronic stage shows lichenification.
- Histopathology in acute stages show spongiotic reaction pattern and in chronic stage the psoriasiform pattern predominates.
- Diagnosis is mainly clinical and investigations are directed toward identifying the cause.
- Alleviating the inciting factors, barrier maintenance with emollients, with topical or systemic immunosuppression, based on the severity remains the mainstay of treatment.

REFERENCES

1. Kantor R, Thyssen JP, Paller AS, Silverberg JI. Atopic dermatitis, atopic eczema, or eczema? A systematic review, meta-analysis, and recommendation for uniform use of "atopic dermatitis." Allergy. 2016;71(10):1480-5.
2. Rönmark EP, Ekerljung L, Lötvall J, Wennergren G, Rönmark E, Torén K, et al. Eczema among adults: prevalence, risk factors and relation to airway diseases. Results from a large-scale population survey in Sweden. Br J Dermatol. 2012;166(6):1301-8.
3. Ingram JR. Eczematous disorders. In: Griffiths C, Barker J, Bleiker T, Chalmers R, Creamer D (Eds). Rook's Textbook of Dermatology, 9th edition. United Kingdom: John Wiley & Sons, Ltd.; 2016. pp. 39.1-39.35.
4. Nosbaum A, Vocanson M, Rozieres A, Hennino A, Nicolas JF. Allergic and irritant contact dermatitis. Eur J Dermatol. 2009;19(4):325-32.
5. Mozzanixa N. Pathogenetic aspects of allergic and irritant contact dermatitis. Clin Dermatol. 1992;10(2):115-21.
6. Fonacier L, Noor I. Contact dermatitis and patch testing for the allergist. Ann Allergy Asthma Immunol. 2018;120(6): 592-8.
7. Heinzerling L, Mari A, Bergmann KC, Bresciani M, Burbach G, Darsow U, et al. The skin prick test—European standards. Clin Transl Allergy. 2013;3(1):3.
8. Wu H, Brandling-Bernet HA, Harrist TJ. Noninfectious vesiculobullous and vesiculopustular diseases. In: Elder DE (Ed). Lever's Histopathology of Skin, 10th edition. Philadelphia: Lippincott Williams & Wilkins; 2009. pp. 235-78.
9. Brasch J, Becker D, Aberer W, Bircher A, Kränke B, Jung K, et al. Guideline contact dermatitis: S1-Guidelines of the German Contact Allergy Group (DKG) of the German Dermatology Society (DDG), the Information Network of Dermatological Clinics (IVDK), the German Society for Allergology and Clinical Immunology (DGAKI), the Working Group for Occupational and Environmental Dermatology (ABD) of the DDG, the Medical Association of German Allergologists (AeDA), the Professional Association of German Dermatologists (BVDD) and the DDG. Allergo J Int. 2014;23(4): 126-38.
10. Hanifin JM, Thurston M, Omoto M, Cherill R, Tofte SJ, Graeber M. The eczema area and severity index (EASI): assessment of reliability in atopic dermatitis. EASI Evaluator Group. Exp Dermatol. 2001;10(1):11-8.
11. Lee JH, Son SW, Cho SH. A Comprehensive Review of the Treatment of Atopic Eczema. Allergy Asthma Clin Immunol. 2016;8(3):181-90.
12. Shroff A, Malajian D, Czarnowicki T, Rose S, Bernstein DM, Singer GK, et al. Use of 308 nm excimer laser for the treatment of chronic hand and foot eczema. Int J Dermatol. 2016;55(8):e447-53.

EXAMINATION QUESTIONS

1. Define eczema and discuss classification of eczema based on causative factors.
2. Illustrate the differences between allergic and irritant contact dermatitis.
3. Discuss the pathogenesis of allergic contact dermatitis and add a note on patch test.

21 CHAPTER

Atopic Dermatitis

Sandipan Dhar, Sahana M Srinivas

INTRODUCTION

Atopic dermatitis (AD) is a chronic, relapsing, inherited, inflammatory skin disorder characterized by varying degrees of pruritus, inflammation, and lichenification of skin. It usually manifests in infancy or childhood for the first time and improves with age.[1] AD affects 20% of children and 1–3% of adults in most countries of the world. Majority of the people with AD have a personal or family history of atopic diathesis and is often associated with elevated serum immunoglobulin (IgE) levels. Atopic diathesis refers to presence of allergic rhinitis, bronchial asthma, or AD. AD is often the first step for development of other atopic diseases. It is a constellation of clinical features such as pruritus, facial, and extensor eczema in infants and children and flexural eczema in adults.[2,3]

NOMENCLATURE

The term atopy is derived from the ancient Greek word "atopia" meaning out of place or placelessness. The term atopy was first coined by American allergists "Coca & Cooke" in 1923 to describe an abnormal type of hypersensitivity reactions against environmental allergy. The name "atopic dermatitis" was named by Sulzberger and associates. In 1892, Besnier described the association of hay fever, asthma with AD.

EPIDEMIOLOGY

Atopic dermatitis is a result of complex interplay of several environmental, food, drugs, and behavioral and immunological factors in genetically predisposed individuals. It severely affects the quality of life of an individual not only at the societal level but also at the global level **(Fig. 1)**. There is a worldwide increase in the incidence and prevalence of AD. The lifetime prevalence in different geographical regions varies from as low as 1% to as much as 20%.[4] Most data on the prevalence of AD has come from one of the largest studies, the ISSAC (International study of Asthma and Allergies in childhood), which was a multicentric study using validated questionnaires in school children aged 6–7 years and 13–14 years. It was conducted in 233 centers across 98 countries and the study included large number of centers in developing countries. The prevalence was estimated at 7.9% and 7.3% in 6–7 years and 13–14 years age groups.[5] Among them, the Indian subcontinent had lowest prevalence of 3–4.2%. A recent systematic review of 69 cross-sectional and cohort studies showed a prevalence of over 20% in many affluent countries.[6] Population-based studies on epidemiology of AD in India are very few and most of the data available is from hospital-

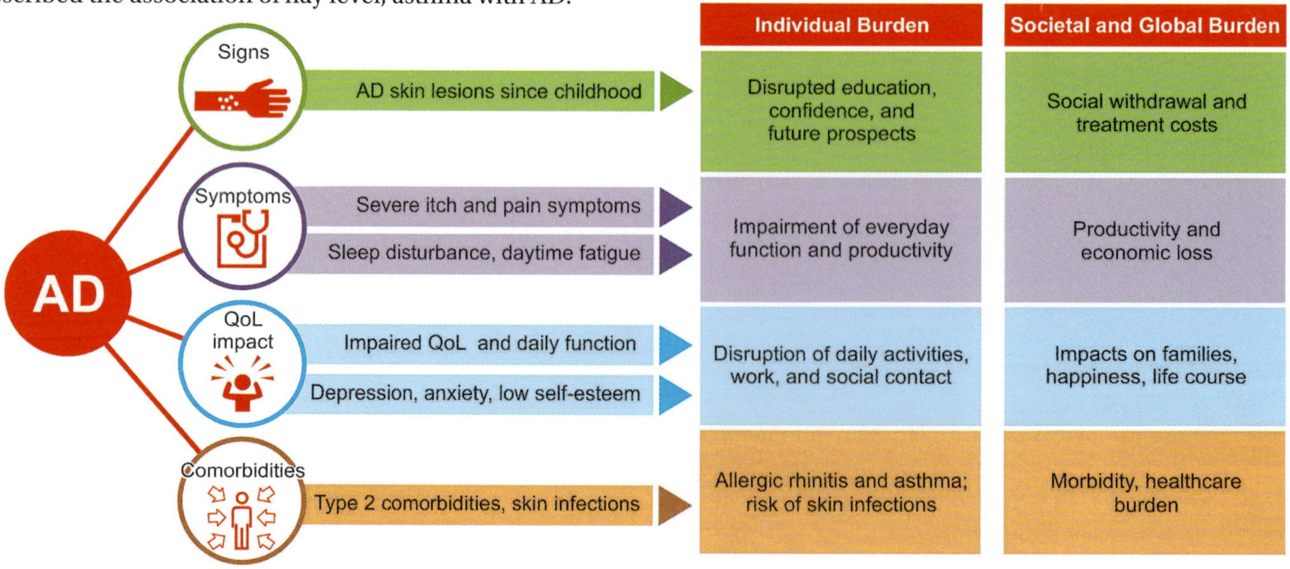

Fig. 1: Burden of atopic dermatitis (AD) on an individual at societal and global levels. (QoL: quality of life)

based studies. A recent study of AD in Eastern India showed a prevalence of 7.21%.[7]

A clinicoepidemiological study, conducted by the first author Dhar S, et al. on North Indian pediatric population, showed that mean age of onset and mean duration of the disease were 4.2 months and 3.3 months in the infantile AD and in the childhood AD group, the figures were 4.1 years and 1.9 years, respectively. Aggravation of AD was seen more in winter in infantile (67.14%) than in childhood AD group (58%). Personal and family history of AD was more associated in childhood AD group than infantile AD group. [8] In another study conducted by Dhar S, et al. among 100 children from East India, the prevalence rate was 0.55%. The mean age of onset was 4.9 years; 54% had personal history of atopy, 65% had family history of atopy, and majority of them had summer exacerbation (40%).[9]

The factors involved in increased prevalence include genetic predisposition, higher socioeconomic status, education, increased urbanization, and increased exposure to environmental pollutants, modernized housing, and exposure to pets, diet, and psychosomatic factors.[4] Recent studies show no association with increased prevalence of AD with higher socioeconomic status or urban areas. There is a significant difference in prevalence not only between but within countries suggesting that environmental factors play a major role in change of disease burden rather than genetic factors.[10]

ETIOPATHOGENESIS

Atopic dermatitis has a complex pathophysiology **(Fig. 2)**. The current understanding of AD is that genetics play an important role in the modulation of disease, but the recent increased prevalence shows that there must be a strong role of exogenous factors. Defect in the physical barrier of skin has been proposed to play a primary role in the pathogenesis of AD rather than immune dysregulation.[11] This defective barrier with altered stratum corneum along with antimicrobial defense results in allergen penetration, leading to immune dysregulation manifesting clinically as pruritus and inflammation in AD. Recent model of AD in the pathogenesis is the complex interplay between genetic predisposition, environmental factors and inflammatory response **(Figs. 2 and 3)**.

Genetics

The role of genetics is complex and not completely understood. There is strong evidence that genetic factors play an important role in predisposition of AD. Atopic disorders runs in the family and this is clearly demonstrated by twin studies, which have shown high concordance rate in monozygotic

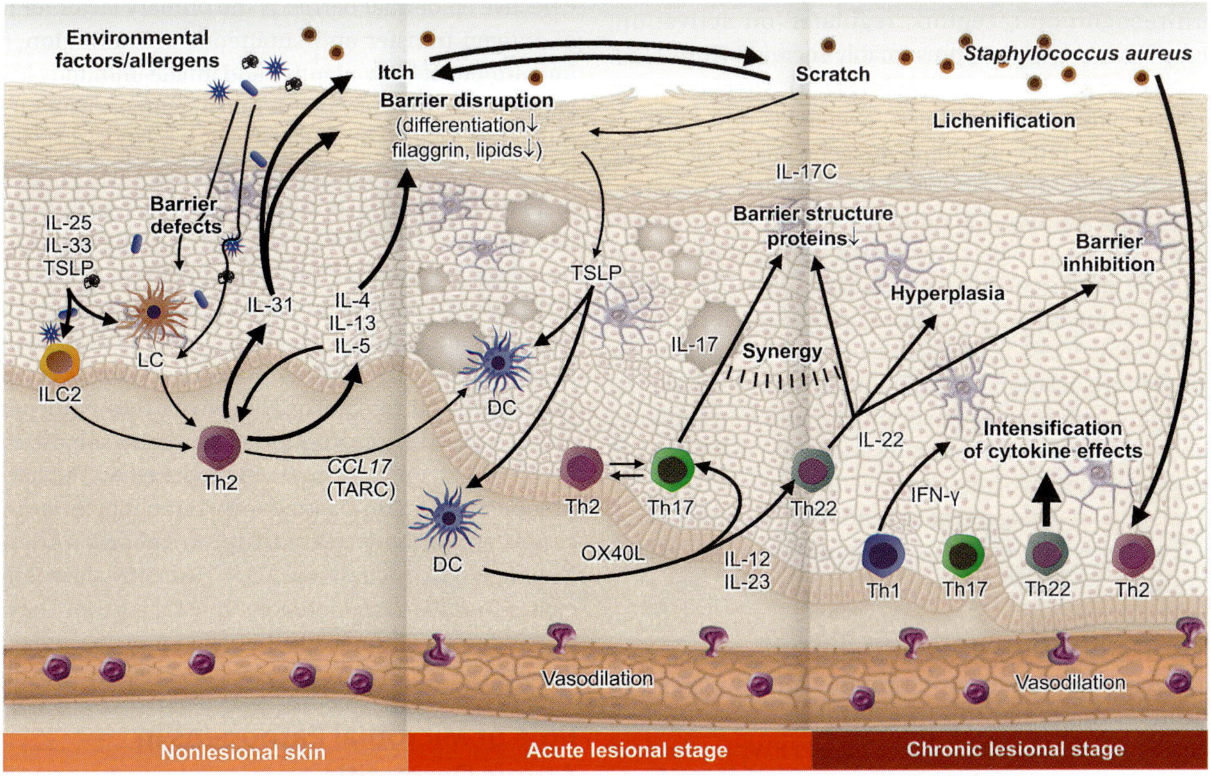

Fig. 2: Complex interplay between environmental factors, barrier disruption, and inflammatory response.
(*CCL17*: CC chemokine ligand 17; DC: dendritic cell; IFN-γ: interferon gamma; IL: interleukin; ILC2: type 2 innate lymphoid cells; OX40L: OX40 ligand; TARC: thymus- and activation-regulated chemokine; Th: T helper cells; TSLP: thymic stromal lymphopoietin)

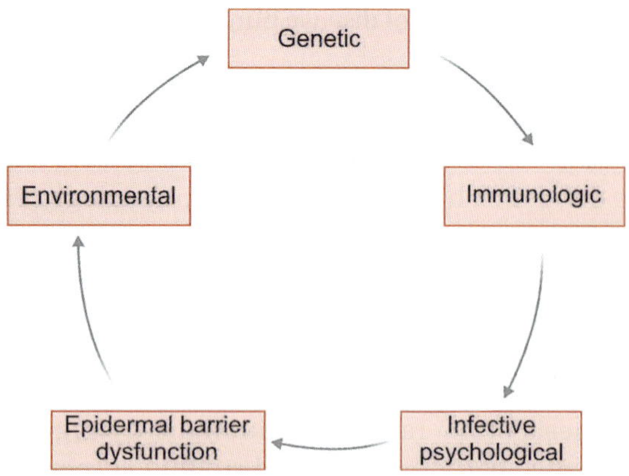

Fig. 3: Etiopathogenesis of atopic dermatitis (AD).

twins (0.77%) as compared to dizygotic twins (0.15%).[12] Atopic disorders are complex poly-or oligo- genetic traits and environmental factors are thought to precipitate the polygenic risk background to disease manifestation.[13] The family history of AD has been demonstrated in 43–73% of cases. There are over 80 candidate genes that have been identified with AD. Until recently whole-genome association studies in eczema have focused on adaptive and innate immune response genes, which have yielded inconsistent results. But in the past few years, a lot of research has been going on the role of barrier dysfunction genes.[14]

Adaptive and innate immune response genes include those encoding for CD14, IL-4, IL-5, IL-13, toll-like receptors, pattern recognition receptors, regulated on activation, normally T-expressed, and presumably secreted (RANTES), a chemotactic factor for eosinophils **(Fig. 2)**. There has been a controversial linkage finding between AD and markers on chromosome 11q3, including the gene encoding for the beta chain of the high-affinity receptor for IgE suggesting that AD has a common genetic basis with other atopic diseases.[15] Genes associated with skin barrier dysfunction reside in the epidermal differentiation complex (EDC) locus on chromosome 1q21. The most widely associated gene with AD at this locus is *filaggrin* gene and is a risk factor with proven association with AD. Interaction between the susceptibility genes, host's environment, and immunologic factors contribute to pathogenesis of AD.[16,17] There are various syndromes involving single-gene defect with AD-like ichthyosis vulgaris (*filaggrin* gene) and Netherton syndrome (*spink5* gene) which explains the complex pathological mechanism.

Filaggrin Mutation and Skin Barrier

Profilaggrin, an important component of the stratum corneum, is degraded into filaggrin that functions in preventing transepidermal water loss (TEWL), prevents intrusion of allergens and microorganisms, and maintains internal fluid and electrolyte homeostasis. Acidic breakdown products of filaggrin has antimicrobial function and maintains the pH of the skin. Filaggrin deficiency leads to reduced natural moisturizing factors (NMF) which probably contributes to xerosis seen in AD.[18] Loss of function mutations in *filaggrin* gene results in decreased or complete absence of epidermal filaggrin which leads to skin barrier dysfunction. Recently filaggrin null mutation has been detected in various populations of the world which has given new dimension in understanding the pathogenesis of AD.

Studies have shown that filaggrin mutations are seen only in 25–50% of children with AD.[19] Presence of mutation predicts early onset and severe disease, worse prognosis and persistence of the disease in adulthood, tendency for eczema herpeticum, allergen sensitization, and development of IgE-mediated food allergies with a positive predictive value of 100%.[20-22] Filaggrin mutation has also been reported as a risk factor for development of atopic march and transition from eczema to asthma.[22] Filaggrin may serve as a prognostic marker for clinical use. Filaggrin null mutation has also been associated with ichthyosis vulgaris, an inherited keratinizing disorder which has close association with AD. Majority of the children may not carry filaggrin, suggesting the possibility of other skin barrier genes of EDC-like genes for loricrin, proteases, and tight junctions for the barrier defects in AD.[23]

Immune Dysregulation in Atopic Dermatitis

In the past few years, the hypothesis of immune dysregulation was the key to pathogenesis of AD, but in the past few years, defective epidermal barrier is the primary factor for initiation of antigen transfer and cutaneous inflammation. There is impairment of both adaptive and innate immunity in children with AD and this may play a role in patients with no filaggrin mutations. There is dysbalance between Th1 and Th2 responses in AD with a predominance of Th2 response in AD. There is increased production of Th2 cytokines such as IL-4, IL-5, IL-13, and deceased Th1 cytokines IL-12, IFN-r. The response in AD is usually biphasic with Th2 predominance in acute lesions and Th1 response in late/chronic lesions.[12] There is increased IgE response and eosinophilia in AD which reflects the increased response of type 2 T-helper cytokines. There is an increased expression of IgE receptor on Langerhans cells and dendritic cells in epidermis which capture the antigen and present it to adaptive immune system. IL-4 and IL-13 produced by Th2 have shown to suppress filaggrin expression by keratinocytes and clinically correlates with the decreased filaggrin expression in lesional AD as compared to nonlesional AD.[24,25] Recently, there is increased expression of IL-22 in AD lesions. IL-22 along with Th2 cytokines may induce epidermal differentiation proteins and epidermal hyperplasia.[26,27]

Role of Microbial Pathogens in Atopic Dermatitis

There is increased susceptibility to bacterial, viral, and fungal infections in AD and they play an important role in triggering and aggravating AD. The colonization of microbes on the skin depends on anatomical sites **(Fig. 4)**. There is downregulation of innate immune responses against microbial pathogens in AD with an increased expression of thymic stromal lymphopoietin (TSLP), a proTh2 IL-2 like cytokine in the keratinocytes of AD lesions.[28] There is decreased expression and secretion of antimicrobial peptides and may contribute to increased susceptibility to skin infections.[29,30] These microbial pathogens induce host production of superantigen or pathogen-specific IgE, leading to basophilic activation and histamine release. Several studies have documented 90% of children with AD showing increased colonization with *Staphylococcus aureus* infection even in uninvolved skin with increased rates of nasal carriage. *S. aureus* secretes toxins which act as superantigen which activate T-cells, inducing IgE production and mast cell degranulation thus contributing to inflammation **(Fig. 5)**.[31] *Malassezia* colonization is commonly seen in variant of AD presenting on the face and neck. *Malassezia* species induces *Malassezia*-specific IgE positivity thus contributing to inflammation.[32] The persistent colonization of *S. aureus* and *Malassezia* species may be influenced by epigenetics and microbiome which are emerging areas of research in AD. The fungus has shown to induce histone acetylation of antimicrobial peptide genes in keratinocytes.[33-35] Bacterial components have been found in the dermis suggesting that the microbiome of skin may extend beyond skin surface.[36] Few patients are prone to develop viral infections such as eczema herpeticum and recently shown to be associated with filaggrin mutation.[37]

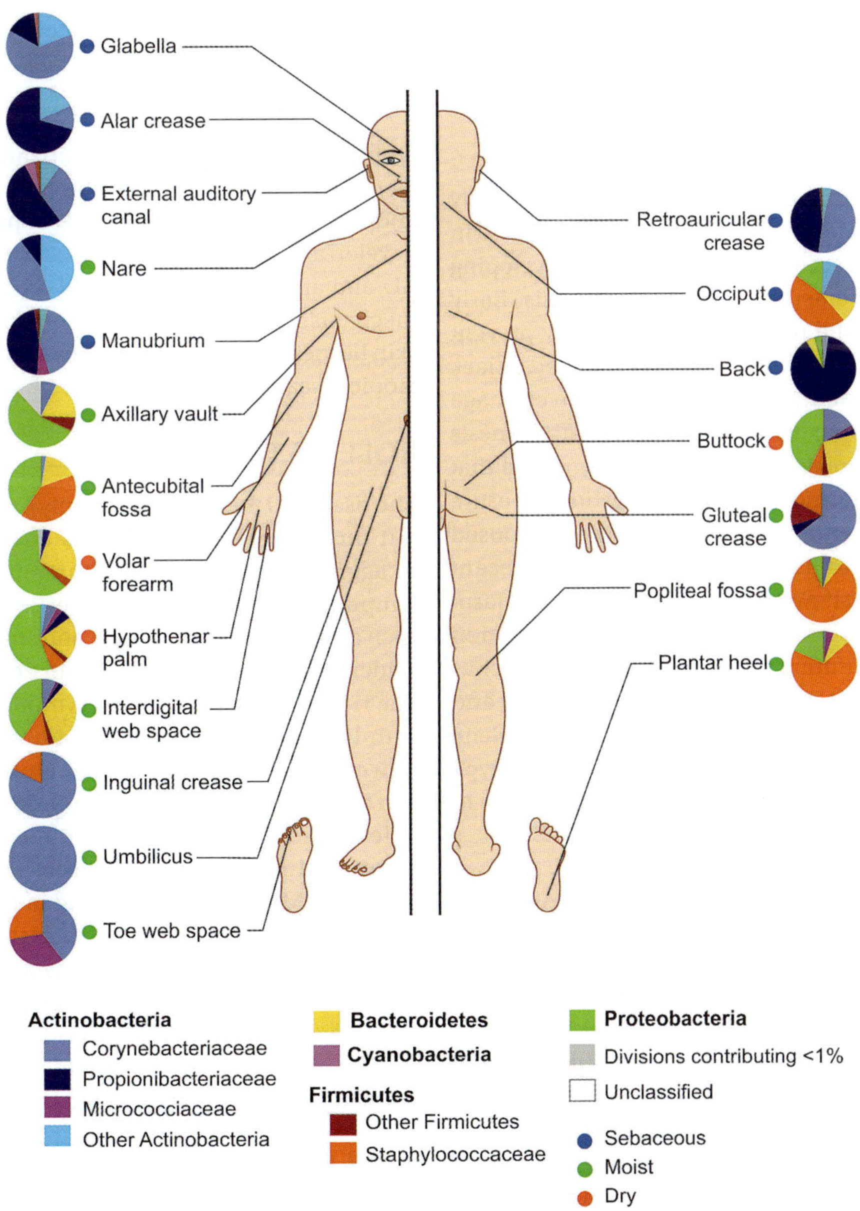

Fig. 4: The colonization of microbes at different anatomical sites.

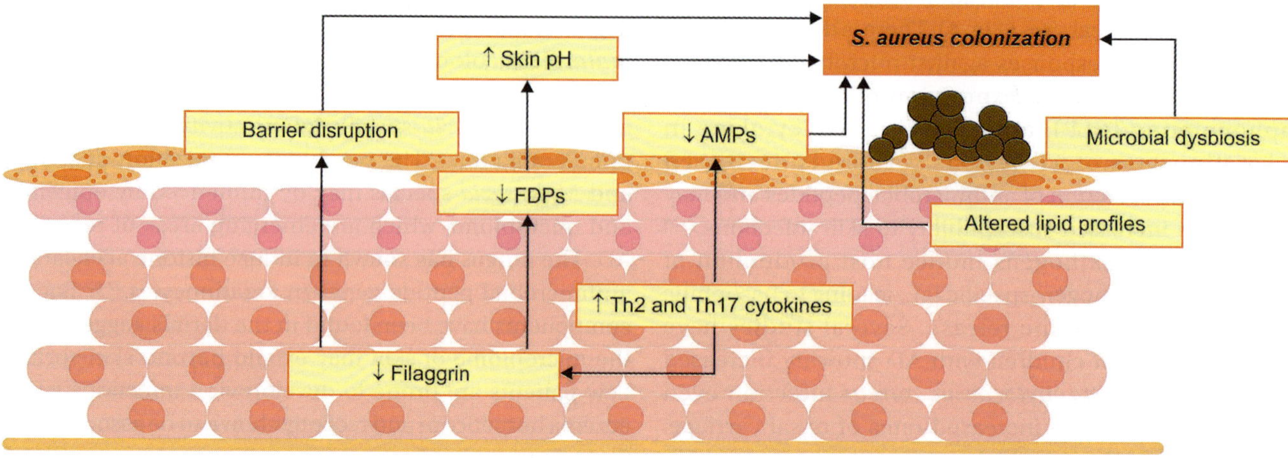

Note: Multiple factors include skin barrier dysfunction, deficiency of AMPs, and decreased levels of filaggrin and FDPs, altered skin pH, overexpressed Th2/Th17 cytokines, microbial dysbiosis and altered lipid profiles.

Fig. 5: *Staphylococcus aureus* colonization on the skin and its interaction causing inflammatory response. (AMPs: antimicrobial peptides; FDPs: filaggrin degradation products; Th: T helper cells)

Hygiene Hypothesis

Hygiene hypothesis was widely accepted theory for many years. The increased incidence of AD in western world and in families with improved socioeconomic status in developing countries may be explained by hygiene hypothesis. Early exposure to microbes and unhygienic contact may prevent development of allergic diseases. This was explained as lack of stimulation of immune system by microbes at an early age and failure of balanced gut flora may act in the pathogenesis of AD.[38] Recent immunological models have suggested that there is evidence of parasitic or helminth infection exposure can prevent development of AD, especially when exposed in pregnancy but not to bacterial infections.[39-41] A recent systematic review has shown exposure to endotoxin, farm animals, and dogs may protect against AD. Consumption of unpasteurized milk during first 2 years of life may act as a protective factor for AD. Early antibiotic exposure and smoking have not shown to effect AD development. Hygiene hypothesis may partially explain some features of AD, as type of infection, timing, and degree of exposure are important to relate to the pathogenesis of AD.

ATOPIC DERMATITIS AND ATOPIC MARCH

Atopic march is the tendency for atopic eczema to precede the development of food allergies, asthma, and allergic rhinitis. Filaggrin mutation has shown to be a risk factor for development of each step of atopic march. AD is the first step in the presentation of atopy and is supported by many cross-sectional and longitudinal studies. Children with eczema with specific IgE antibodies to common environmental triggers, present by the age of 2–4 years and are at high risk of progressing into allergic rhinitis and asthma than those with eczema without IgE sensitization.[42] The risk factors associated with progression are early onset, IgE sensitization, and severity. Approximately 70% of patients with severe AD develop asthma compared with 20–30% of patients with mild AD and approximately 8% in the general population.[43] The mechanism of atopic march is not clearly understood, but skin barrier dysfunction is the key for development of further atopic diseases.

ROLE OF TRIGGERS

The rise in AD is explained not only on genetic predisposition but due to various exogenous factors. Factors involved in aggravating AD are environmental triggers; change in temperature; humidity; aeroallergens; foods; and irritants such as wool, chemicals, soap, and stress. There is increasing evidence for environmental factors causing AD early in life. The ISSAC has shown that AD symptoms correlate positively with latitude, and negatively with outdoor temperatures.[5] Lower outdoor temperatures along with skin irritants can worsen AD in contrary to indoor temperature which is less significant.[44] Aeroallergens are most frequently associated with atopic diathesis. The role of house dust mites (HDM), pets, and smoking in the pathogenesis of AD is controversial. Researchers claim that HDM allergy is just an epiphenomenon, occurring as a result of impaired skin barrier and does not have a direct causative role in AD.[45] Direct contact with farm animals reduces the risk of AD in early life in few instances.[46] A meta-analysis of studies has shown uniform protective effect of dog exposure but not to cats.[47]

Food Allergens

Role of diet in the cause and treatment of atopic dermatitis is controversial and is not well defined. Around 60% of children develop AD by first year of life with food allergies developing early in this group. Clinical studies have documented prevalence of food allergy in atopic dermatitis from 20–80%.[48,49] Common food allergens triggering AD are milk and milk products, peanuts, eggs, soy, wheat, seafood, and shell fish. Exacerbation of AD by food occurs by increased binding of antigen to immature gut microvillus and increased intestinal permeability that initiates immune responses, with primarily altered antigen transfer. The gut bacterial pathogen acts as infectious agent and superantigen thus exacerbating AD by food. Food allergy in AD may result in IgE-mediated immediate and non-IgE-mediated late eczematous reactions. 40–60% constitute IgE-mediated food allergy. Reactions can occur in the skin, oropharynx, gastrointestinal, respiratory, and cardiovascular systems.[50] Immediate IgE-mediated reactions occurs within few minutes to hours after ingestion of food. Cutaneous reactions include urticaria, angioedema, pruritus, erythema, morbilliform eruptions, contact urticaria, and allergic contact dermatitis. In a recent study of soy allergy in patients suffering from AD, early reactions was seen in 2.8% cases. One-third of patients (27.2%) were sensitized to soy without clinical symptoms.[51] Late non IgE-mediated eczematous reactions rarely occur and their pathogenesis is not very clear. Delayed reactions develop after 6–2 days following ingestion of allergen food. Rowlands et al. in their study described that out of the 58 double-blind placebo-controlled food challenges, only one had eczematous food reactions.[52] Dietary elimination is not recommended routinely as there is not much evidence that has demonstrated in improving AD. Few studies have shown good improvement in AD with dietary elimination.[49] A Cochrane systematic review based on randomized controlled trials (RCTs) have shown that eliminating egg or cow's milk did not show any benefit and do not support the concept of dietary elimination.

Alkaline soaps increases the pH of skin, dryness, and increased TEWL. Previous studies have shown that pH of water (hardness) has been associated as a risk factor for aggravating AD, but recent study in Spain has questioned the validity of this association.[53]

Other Risk Factors Associated with Atopic Dermatitis

Personal and family history of atopy was found to increase the severity of AD, but study from the first author on Indian children has found low frequency of personal and family history of atopy thus less severity of AD in this region.[54-56] Dhar S, et al. in their study have shown that there may be an association with growth retardation and severity of the disease and surface area involvement.[57,58] Previously, it was thought that breastfeeding and delayed weaning would prevent AD. Recent data from cross-sectional studies from developed and developing countries including 51,119 children in the ISAAC phase two did not support this data.[59] Meta-analysis of 22 prospective cohort studies did not find any statistically significant results.[60] Type of delivery and dietary modifications in pregnancy and infancy do not help in preventing AD. Exposure to farm animals and pet in pregnancy may reduce the risk of AD and this is due to endotoxins.[61] There is no association with obesity, vitamin D levels, and routine childhood vaccinations in AD.[10] Daycare may influence the risk of development of AD but more studies are required. There is no conclusive evidence that early antibiotic exposure is associated with risk of AD.

OUTGROW OF ATOPIC DERMATITIS: HOW TRUE?

An important aspect of AD is the number of children outgrowing their disease. Many children with AD improve with age. In 60% of the children, the disease clears by age of 10 years.[62] The mechanism of outgrow of AD is unknown and could be attributed to genetic and environmental factors. Although there is improvement of skin, they may develop other atopic diseases. Now AD is thought be a "lifelong disease".

CLINICAL FEATURES

- Onset of AD is most commonly between 3 and 6 months of age, with approximately 60% of patients developing within first year of life.
- Majority of them resolve by adulthood, while 10–30% do not resolve and few of them develop symptoms for the first time as adults.
- Atopic march is the tendency for atopic eczema to precede the development of food allergies, asthma, and allergic rhinitis.
- AD is classified into infantile phase, childhood phase, and adult phase **(Table 1 and Figs. 6 to 10)**.
- *Other variants of AD:* Eyelid dermatitis, hand and foot eczema, cheilitis, vulvar and perianal dermatitis, nipple dermatitis, infra-auricular, retroauricular, and infranasal fissuring and nummular variants **(Figs. 11 to 16)**.

DIAGNOSTIC CRITERIA

Diagnosis of AD is based clinically based on the morphology and distribution as there are no specific laboratory tests. Diagnostic criteria put forward by Hanifin and Rajka in 1980 have been considered as the gold standard for clinical diagnosis of AD **(Box 1)**. The UK working party criteria is simpler and have been extensively used in clinical trials **(Box 2)**.[63]

Significance of minor clinical features was evaluated by conducting many studies by first author. The observations made by first author showed that cheilitis, nipple eczema, perifollicular accentuation, white dermographism, recurrent conjunctivitis, and anterior neck folds was similar to controls.

TABLE 1: Classification of atopic dermatitis.

Classification	*Clinical features*
Infantile phase (Birth to 2 years)	Erythema, scaling, excoriation, edema, exudation, crusting and secondary infection distributed on cheeks, forehead, chin, scalp, sparing the perioral, nasolabial fold and diaper region
Childhood phase (2–12 years)	• Erythema, scaling, oozing, crusting, and lichenification distributed on the flexures, elbows, knees, neck, wrists, and ankles • Reticulate hyperpigmentation of the sides of the neck known as "atopic dirty neck"
Adult phase (12 years to adult)	• Flexures with prominent involvement of wrists and ankles, along with facial and neck eczema • Lichenification, nummular eczema, and prurigo nodularis

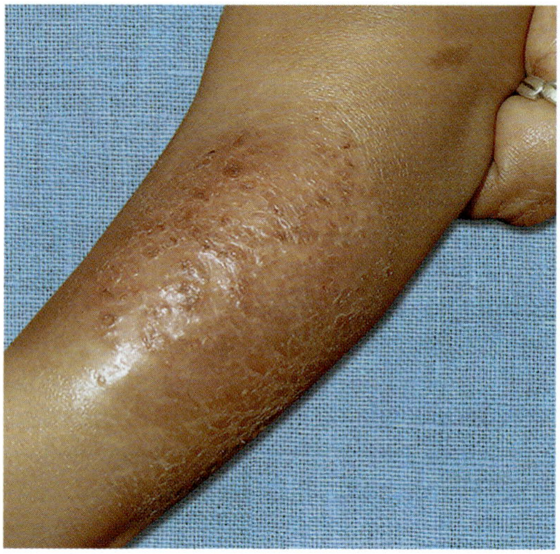

Fig. 8: Erythema, scaling, and excoriation on the extensor aspect of forearms.

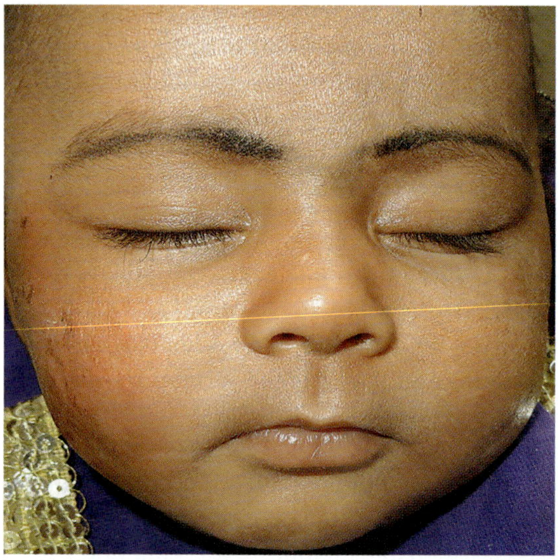

Fig. 6: Erythema with scaling on cheeks in infantile phase of atopic dermatitis.

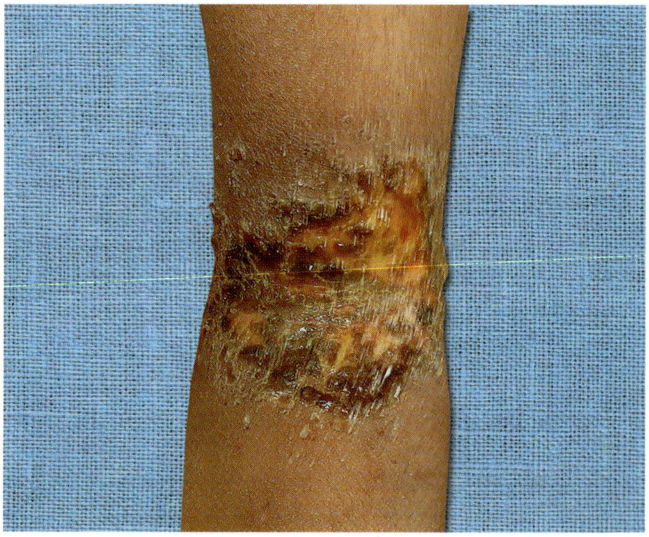

Fig. 9: Atopic dermatitis on cubital fossa with secondary bacterial infection.

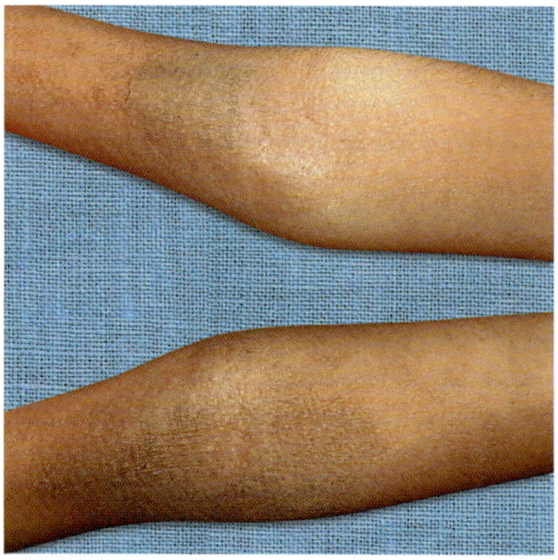

Fig. 7: Mild erythema with lichenification in cubital fossa in childhood phase of atopic dermatitis.

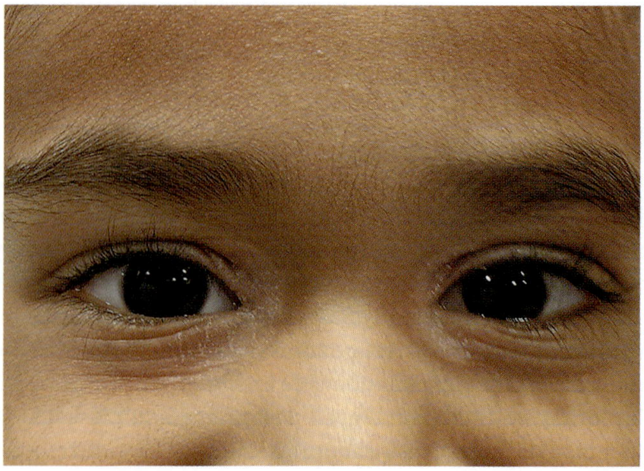

Fig. 10: Eyelid dermatitis with Dennie–Morgan fold.

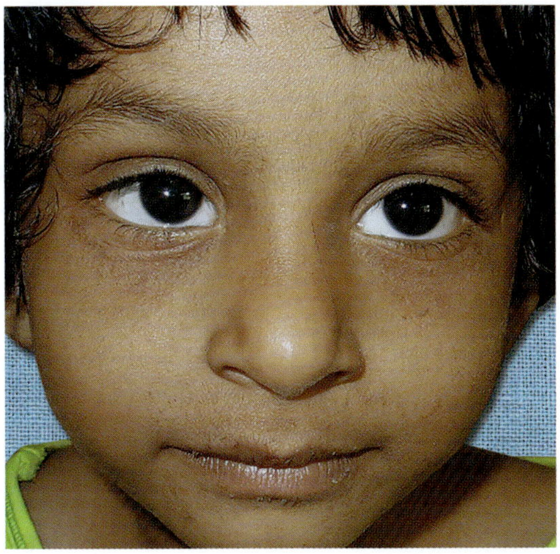

Fig. 11: Eyelid dermatitis with chelitis in atopic dermatitis.

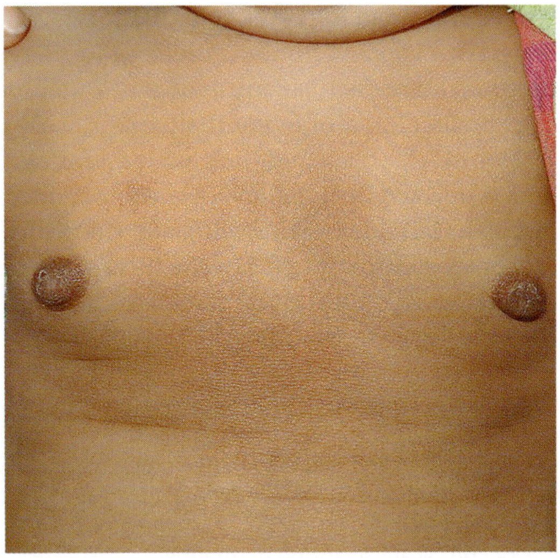

Fig. 12: Nipple eczema with follicular papules on the chest.

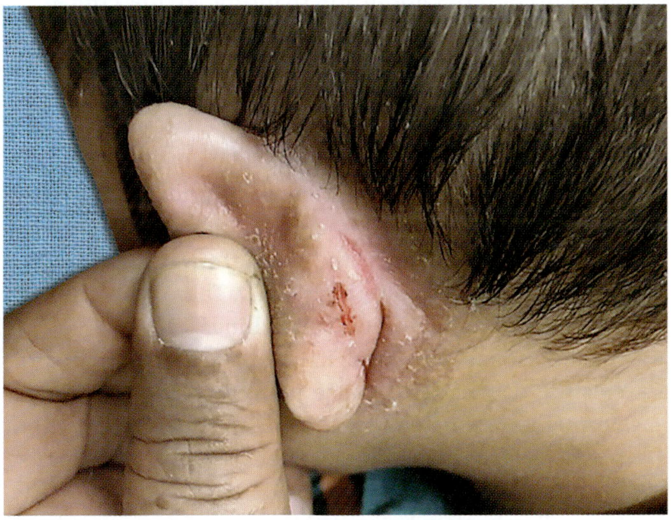

Fig. 13: Retroauricular dermatitis.

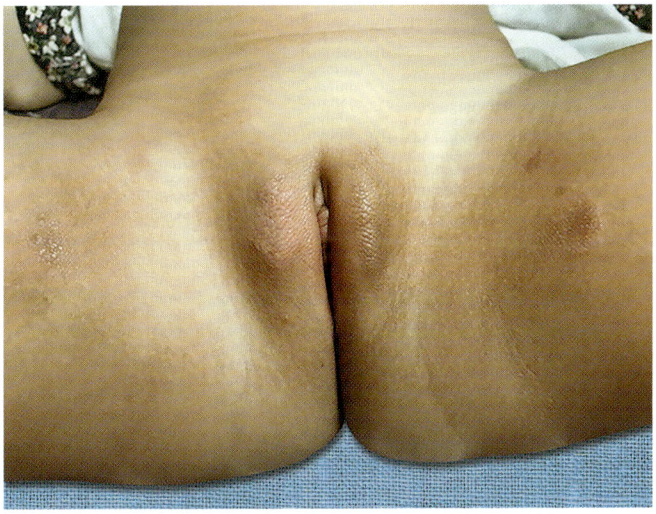

Fig. 14: Atopic dermatitis of the vulval region.

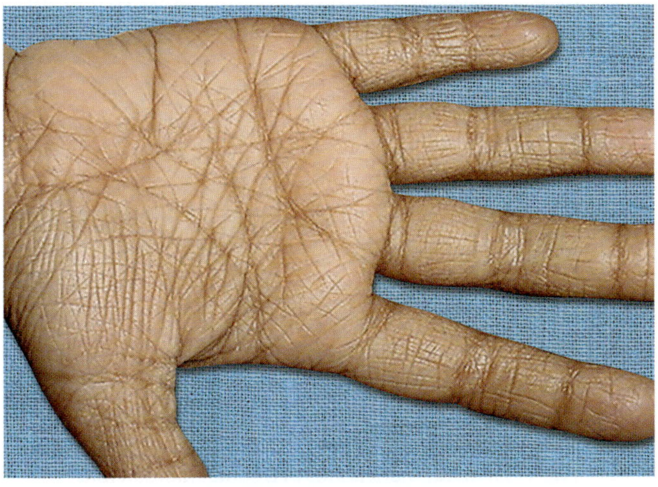

Fig. 15: Palmar hyperlinearity.

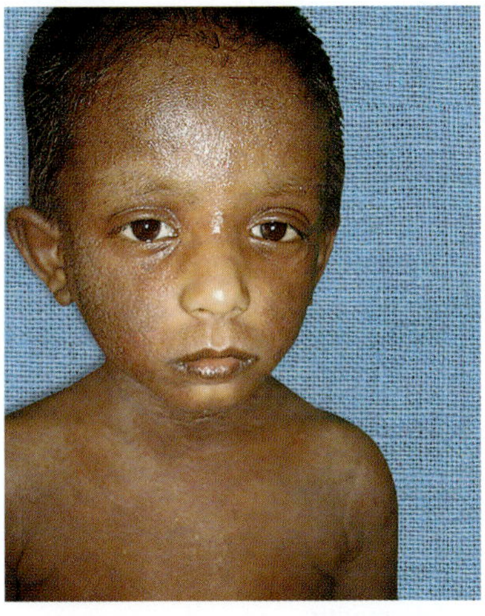

Fig. 16: Severe atopic dermatitis.

Diffuse scalp scaling and infra-auricular fissuring was more significantly associated as minor indicators for diagnosis which could be due to high colony counts of *Pityrosporum* species. The first author also found that xerosis, early onset infection, Dennie–Morgan fold, itch with sweating, wool intolerance, and facial erythema were important minor features, whereas infra-auricular scaling and Hertoghe's sign (thinning of outer eyebrows) were not significant features.[64-70]

BOX 1: Hanifin and Rajka criteria for the diagnosis of atopic dermatitis.

Major or basic features (must have three or more):

1. Pruritus
2. Typical morphology and distribution (flexural lichenification or linearity in adults and facial and extensor involvement in infants and children)
3. Chronic or chronically relapsing dermatitis
4. Personal or family history of atopy (asthma, allergic rhinitis, or atopic dermatitis)

Minor or less characteristic features (must have three or more):

1. Xerosis
2. Ichthyosis, palmar hyperlinearity, or keratosis pilaris
3. Immediate (type 1) skin test reactivity
4. Elevated serum IgE
5. Early age of onset
6. Tendency toward cutaneous infections [especially *Staphylococcus aureus* and herpes simplex virus (HSV) infection]/impaired cell-mediated immunity
7. Tendency toward nonspecific hand or foot dermatitis
8. Nipple eczema
9. Cheilitis
10. Recurrent conjunctivitis
11. Dennie–Morgan infraorbital folds (bilateral symmetrical folds formed by two additional creases beneath the eyelids)
12. Keratoconus (conical cornea resulting from degenerative changes, leading to the cornea being pushed outward due to intraocular pressure)
13. Posterior and anterior subcapsular cataracts (small opacities and translucent globules seen in the lens at the pole in front of the posterior or anterior capsule)
14. Orbital darkening (bluish-to-grayish periorbital pigmentation, possibly following chronic rubbing)
15. White dermographism/delayed blanch (development of a delayed white line on firm stroking of the skin, instead of the usual red line seen normally)
16. Facial pallor/facial erythema
17. Pityriasis alba
18. Anterior neck folds
19. Itch when sweating
20. Intolerance to wool or lipid solvents
21. Perifollicular accentuation
22. Food intolerance

BOX 2: UK working party criteria.

Itchy skin plus (three of the following features):

1. History of flexural dermatitis
2. Onset under the age of two years
3. Personal history of asthma
4. History of dry skin
5. Visible flexural dermatitis

Investigations

Serum IgE is elevated in 80% patients with AD but it does not correlate with the severity of the disease. Tests to confirm food allergy include RAST (radioallergosorbent test), skin prick test, atopy patch test, and double-blind placebo controlled food challenge (DBPCFC) which is considered as a gold standard test.

MANAGEMENT

The main aim of the treatment is not to cure the disease but to control the disease. Treatment is directed to reduce the signs and symptoms, prevent or reduce the recurrences, modify the course of the disease, prevent children from school abstinence, and improve family interactions. Management issues to be dealt in AD are summarized in **Figure 17**. Management of atopic dermatitis is outlined in **Table 2**. Counseling, avoidance of triggers, emollients, and topical steroids form the cornerstone of the management in AD.[71-73] Counseling parents about the disorder, giving education materials, and discussing with them about the avoidance of triggers, and management protocols are necessary.

General Skin Care

Basic skin care regimens include the following: [74,75]

- Bathing helps to remove the crusts and irritants such as sweat allergens and bacterial components. Bathing time should be short with lukewarm water to improve hydration. Avoid bubble bath in AD. There is no standard for frequency and duration of bathing.[59]
- Alkaline soaps may cause irritation and worsen the pre-existing dryness and cause irritant or allergic contact dermatitis.[76] Nonsoap cleansers or syndet soaps with a pH of 5.5 is more preferable. There is no evidence for use of antiseptic soaps.[77]
- Immediately after bath patting dry in cotton towel and applying moisturizing cream are recommended within 3–5 minutes to slightly damp skin.
- Apply moisturizing cream all over the body two to three times per day.

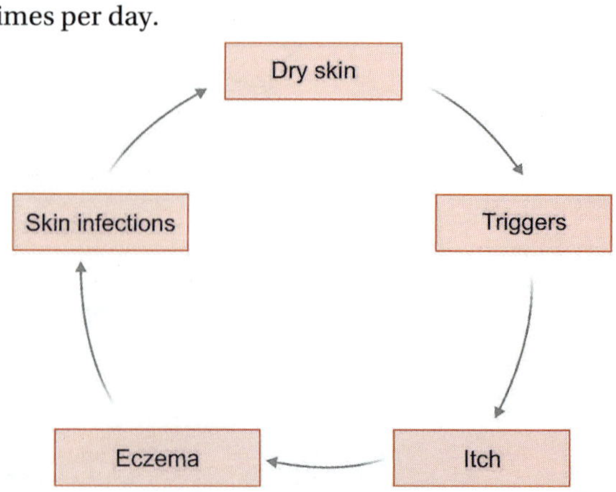

Fig. 17: Management issues in Dennie–Morgan fold atopic dermatitis (AD).

TABLE 2: Management of atopic dermatitis (AD).

Mild AD	• Basic skin care • Avoidance of triggers • Emollients • Counseling
Moderate AD	• Basic skin care • Avoidance of triggers • Emollients • Topical steroids • Topical immunomodulators—calcineurin inhibitors • Oral antihistamines • Counseling
Severe AD	• General skin care • Avoidance of triggers • Emollients • Systemic corticosteroids • Immunosuppressants • Oral antihistamines • Counseling

- Addition of oil or emollient to bath water may help but there is lack of evidence.
- Bleach baths decrease staphylococcal colonization and decreases severity of AD. This involves soaking the body neck down in a tub filled with water (about 150 L) in which half a cup of 6% household bleach has been added. In Indian scenario, one teaspoonful (around 5 mL) of bleach can be added to a bucket of around 15 L of water. A soft cloth soaked into this well-mixed solution can be used for compresses on the skin for around 10 minutes.[78,79]

Avoidance of Triggers

- Extremes of temperature such as very hot, humid, or dry or cold environment should be avoided as they can alter the skin barrier function.[80]
- Woolen and synthetic fabrics can irritate the skin and aggravate pruritus; hence these coarse fabrics much be avoided. Full sleeves, loose, soft cotton clothes must be encouraged. Woolen if worn should not come in contact with the skin.
- Sweating can irritate the skin, hence contact with skin for a long time is not recommended.
- Harsh cloth detergents and disinfectants must be avoided. Clothes after washing should be rinsed thoroughly to take off excess detergents. Fabric softeners can be used.[74]
- Avoid exposure to pets. Early exposure to dog and farm animals may reduce the risk of AD.[46]
- Fur soft toys should be avoided. Washable toys should be preferred in children.
- Avoid swimming in acute flares.
- Airborne allergens such as pollen and HDM should be avoided and this is controversial.[74] Encasing of mattresses and beddings is important to prevent HDM.
- Diet restriction should not be followed unless there is a documented evidence of food allergy as this should not compromise the nutritional status of the child and this will not replace the standard topical or systemic treatment in AD.

Emollients

Emollients form the cornerstone of management in AD. Emollients are occlusive agents that make skin soft, pliable by increasing the hydration of skin. Emollients not only moisturize the skin but have anti-inflammatory, antimicrobial, and steroid-sparing effects thus reducing the flares, improving itch, skin barrier function, and reducing exposure to irritants.[75] Emollients with fragrances, propylene glycol, and urea must be avoided. Emollients should be applied liberally at least two to three times a day to whole body in AD.[81] Emollients should be used in active and maintenance phases. There is strong evidence that regular use of emollients reduces disease severity and also prevents flare in mild form of AD. There is no evidence regarding use of bath emollients.[82] The order of application of emollient and topical corticosteroid (TCS) does not matter in treatment of AD. Emollient application followed by TCS after 15 minutes or reverse order can be tried.[83]

Recent concepts in the pathogenesis of AD have led to the development of modern emollients, called prescription emollient devices (PED). They contain ceramides, cholesterol, and free fatty acids such as palmitoylethanolamide, glycyrrhetinic, and hydrolipid. They act by repairing the defective skin barrier, thus preventing atopic pruritus and inflammation.[84] Recent concept is that use of barrier protection creams form birth may prevent AD.[85]

Topical Corticosteroids

There is sufficient evidence of use of TCS as the first line of management in mild-to-moderate AD. It has anti-inflammatory, antiproliferative, vasoconstrictive, and immunosuppressive properties **(Fig. 18)**. Choosing a TCS depends on the site, age, type of lesion, chronicity, potency, and frequency of application. Several guidelines suggest use of mild TCS on face and flexure while mid potent and potent. TCS can be used on trunk and extremities. TCS should be applied for the shortest possible period to the sites with active percutaneous absorption such as in face and neck.[79] Initially moderately potent steroids can be used for short period followed by mild TCS to avoid tachyphylaxis and side effect of TCS. The finger-tip-unit (FTU) should be used as a guide for application of TCS. Monthly application of TCS should not exceed 15 g in infants and 30 g in children and 60–90 g in adolescents and adults.[86] Long-term usage of TCS may give rise to atrophy, telangiectasia, striae, hypertrichosis, perioral dermatitis, ocular abnormalities, osteopenia, adrenal suppression, and growth retardation. Another important aspect of TCS is "steroid phobia" which should be addressed meticulously with the parents.

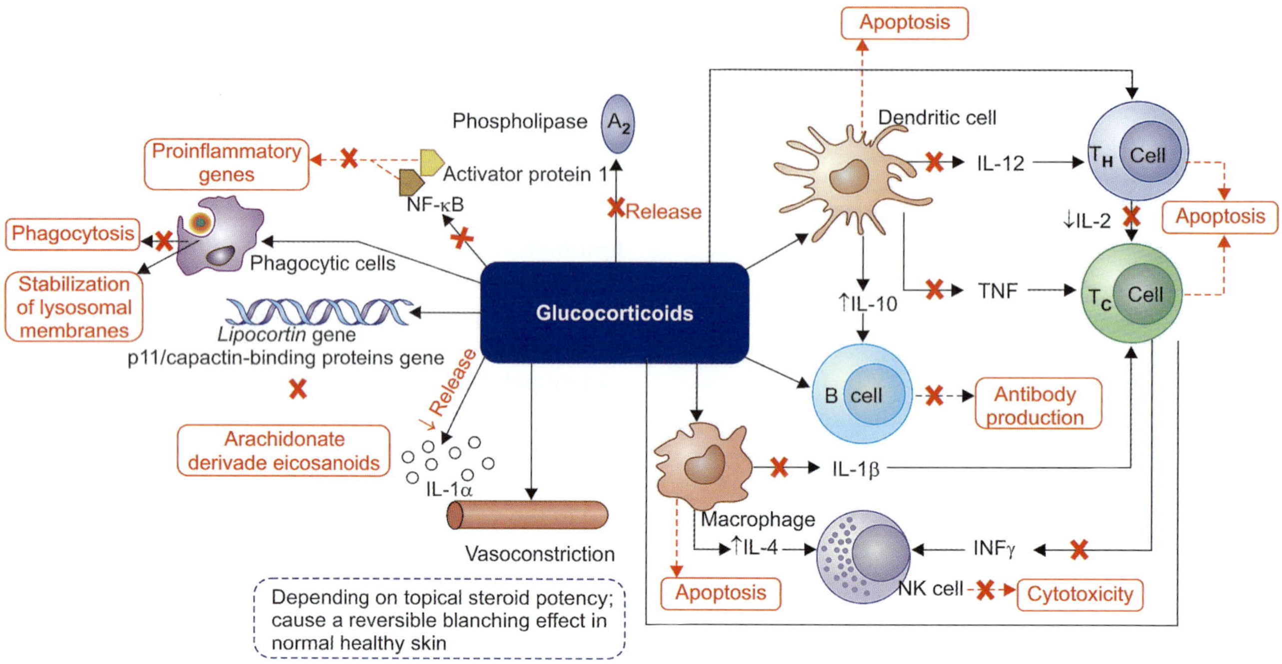

Note: Glucocorticoids possess numerous functions such as anti-inflammatory, antimitotic, apoptotic, vasoconstrictive, and immunomodulatory functions. These properties are closely associated with their efficacy in the skin disease treatment.

Fig. 18: Mechanism of action of topical corticosteroid.

(IL: interleukin; IFN-γ: interferon gamma; NK cells: natural killer cells; Tc cell: cytotoxic T cells; Th cell: T helper cells; TNF: tumor necrosis factor)

TCS should be used once or twice daily. There is no evidence for higher efficacy with application more than twice daily.[87] To prevent the long-term side effects and in patients with recurrent flares at the same time, and for maintenance "proactive therapy" can be tried. Proactive approach consists of predefined, long-term, low-dose, intermittent (twice/week) application of anti-inflammatory agent to previously affected areas of skin along with intensive emollient therapy to the unaffected skin. Proactive, once-to-twice weekly application of mid-potency TCS for up to 40 weeks has not shown any adverse events in clinical trials.[88] This theory was based that normal looking, nonlesional skin of AD is not normal and shows signs of subclinical infection. Studies has shown that proactive therapy reduces flares, delays flares, and increases the duration between flares thus reducing the repeated dosing of steroids.[76,89] Combination therapy with TCS and antibiotics has been tried but the disadvantage is that there will be development of antibiotic resistance. Steroid with topic calcineurin inhibitors is not useful.

Wet Wrap Therapy

Wet wrap therapy may be indicated as an adjuvant therapy in children with severe or refractory AD along with topical anti-inflammatory therapy. In this method, topical emollient or topical steroids are applied, over which two layers of tubular cotton bandages are applied. The first layer is wetted with lukewarm water followed by a second dry layer.[90] If tubular bandages are not available, soft cotton body suits can be used. The first layer can be rewetted every 2–3 hours. This method can be left on for 24 hours. Wet wrap therapy can be done for whole body or whole limbs or localized areas. It is safe but contraindicated in children <6 months.

Topical Calcineurin Inhibitors

Topical calcineurin inhibitor is an immunomodulatory agent which suppresses T-cell activation and reduces production of proinflammatory cytokines. It is a second line of treatment as steroid-sparing agent. Tacrolimus 0.03% or pimecrolimus 1% is used in treatment of acute or chronic AD or in maintenance of AD. Tacrolimus is safe to use in children above 2 years (off-label use <2 years).[91] Pimecrolimus can be used in children of <2 years of age. It can also be used in proactive management once or twice per week on the repeated areas of outbreaks of AD along with emollients. A meta-analysis of 19 RCTs (n = 7,378), 10 of pimecrolimus (n = 2,959) and 9 of tacrolimus (n = 4,419) showed that pimecrolimus 1% was as effective as mild TCS and Tacrolimus 0.1% was more effective than mild TCS and as effective as moderately potent topical steroid.[92] Topical calcineurin inhibitors have shown good safety profile when used up to 1 year. Side effect includes itching, burning, and folliculitis. Studies have not shown an increased risk of bacterial or viral infections on long-term use of topical calcineurin inhibitors. There is insufficient evidence of association with lymphoma though its risk should be counseled with parents before initiation of therapy.[93] Routine blood monitoring is not recommended.

Treatment of Infections in Atopic Dermatitis

The prevalence of colonization of skin and nose by *S. aureus* varies from 60 to 100% in AD, and there is a positive correlation between bacterial colonization and severity of eczema.[94,95] Eczematous skin lesions in AD are prone to staphylococcal and streptococcal infections. Bleach baths and topical antibiotics (fusidic acid/mupirocin) can be used for short term to treat localized bacterial infections. Systemic antibiotics are recommended if there is generalized bacterial infection or bacterial impetiginization. Amoxycillin–clauvalinic acid or cephalosporin (cefadroxil/cefuroxime/cefixime) is usually preferred.[96] For recurrent bacterial infection, decolonization with mupirocin can be effective. Studies have shown that decolonization treatments are followed by prompt recolonization in AD.[97] Recently silver-impregnated textile and antimicrobial silk fabrics have shown to reduce staphylococcal colonization in AD but there is lack of evidence.[98] Many studies have shown that combination treatment of topical antibacterials with topical steroid may be helpful in improving AD.[99] Eczema herpeticum as a complication of AD should be treated as emergency condition and managed with systemic antiviral agents. Oral antifungal therapy may be effective in recalcitrant head and neck variant of AD.[100]

Other Topical Therapies

Some studies have shown topical doxepin 5% cream to improve pruritus in AD. First author in their study has made observations that topical doxepin along with topical steroid may be useful for treatment of itching in AD than alone doxepin or topical steroid.[101]

Oral Antihistamines

There is no evidence regarding general use of oral antihistamines in AD. Sedating antihistamines may be used for short duration where there is sleep disturbance. Nonsedating antihistamines have no role in management of AD.[102]

Systemic Therapy in Atopic Dermatitis

Systemic therapies are given as third line of management. It is indicated in severe, widespread, and recalcitrant AD. Current literature suggests that cyclosporine, methotrexate (MTX), azothioprine (AZT), and mycophenolate mofetil (MMF) are efficacious in treating AD.[103] Oral steroids should be avoided in AD. It is used in acute and severe exacerbation and acts as a bridge therapy to other systemic therapy. Cyclosporine is the only Food and Drug Administration (FDA)-approved treatment of AD in children and is approved as the first line of therapy in Europe for treating severe AD. There are many RCTs regarding efficacy of short-term use of cyclosporine in AD. Cyclosporine is given in the dosage of 3–5 mg/kg/day for a period of 1 year. Initially it is started at 5 mg/kg/day until clinical response and later tapered to 1.5–3 mg/kg in the next few months. Monitoring of blood pressure and serum creatinine is necessary.[104,105]

MTX is given at the dose of 0.2–0.7 mg/kg/week in divided doses. A recent retrospective uncontrolled study showed good improvement in 75% of children with AD.[106] In another study, MTX was effective in clearing refractory discoid eczema in children aged 3–15 years.[107] AZT is a purine analog that blocks the synthesis of DNA and RNA, thus inhibiting the proliferation of T- and B-cells there by reducing the inflammation in AD. Several studies have shown clinical efficacy of AZT between 2 and 4 mg/kg/day from a period of 12 weeks to 12 months. Metabolism of AZT is based on individual TPMT levels (thiopurine methyltransferase). Genetic polymorphisms in TPMT activity are linked to individual susceptibility to AZT toxicity. Adverse effects include gastrointestinal disturbances, hepatotoxicity, leukopenia, and myelosuppression. [108] Pre-evaluation of complete blood count, liver enzymes, HIV, hepatitis B and C, Mantoux test and TPMT levels is necessary.[109] There are no sufficient studies regarding efficacy of MMF in children. MMF blocks purine biosynthesis pathway of T- and B-cells by inhibiting inosine monophosphate dehydrogenase and decreases inflammation. In an uncontrolled retrospective study of 14 children (age above 2 years) treated with MMF for recalcitrant AD, efficacy was present at dosage of 40–50 mg/kg/day in younger children, and 30–40 mg/kg /day in adolescents. Clinical improvement was seen at 8–12 weeks.[110] MMF has a favorable long-term side effect profile than cyclosporine, but cyclosporine has greater efficacy than MMF. Side effects known with MMF are gastrointestinal effects such as nausea, diarrhea, anorexia, abdominal cramps, emesis, and headache and hematological effects such as anemia, leukopenia, and thrombocytopenia.

Phototherapy

Phototherapy should be considered if AD is not responding to conventional treatment and before starting systemic immunosuppressants. Narrow-band UVB (NB UVB) is very safe and effective form of phototherapy in children. NB UVB can be combined with emollients, TCS, and methotrexate. [111]

Role of Prebiotics and Probiotics

Prebiotics are nondigestible food components that benefit the host by stimulating the growth of bacteria in the gut. Probiotics are live organisms when administered in adequate amounts modulate the immune response in the gut-associated lymphoid tissue (GALT). Few studies have shown the benefit of probiotics in prevention of AD if given in pregnancy and infants but on the contrary, many studies have shown to be ineffective.[112]

Recent Therapies in Atopic Dermatitis

Newer topical agents which includes extract of bacteria *Rhodobacter sphaeroides*, UR-1505, with immune modulator properties and thiol derivative N-acetylcysteine (NAC) have been tried in AD but there is no convincing evidence.[113] Newer topical therapies such as MASO63DP have been tried

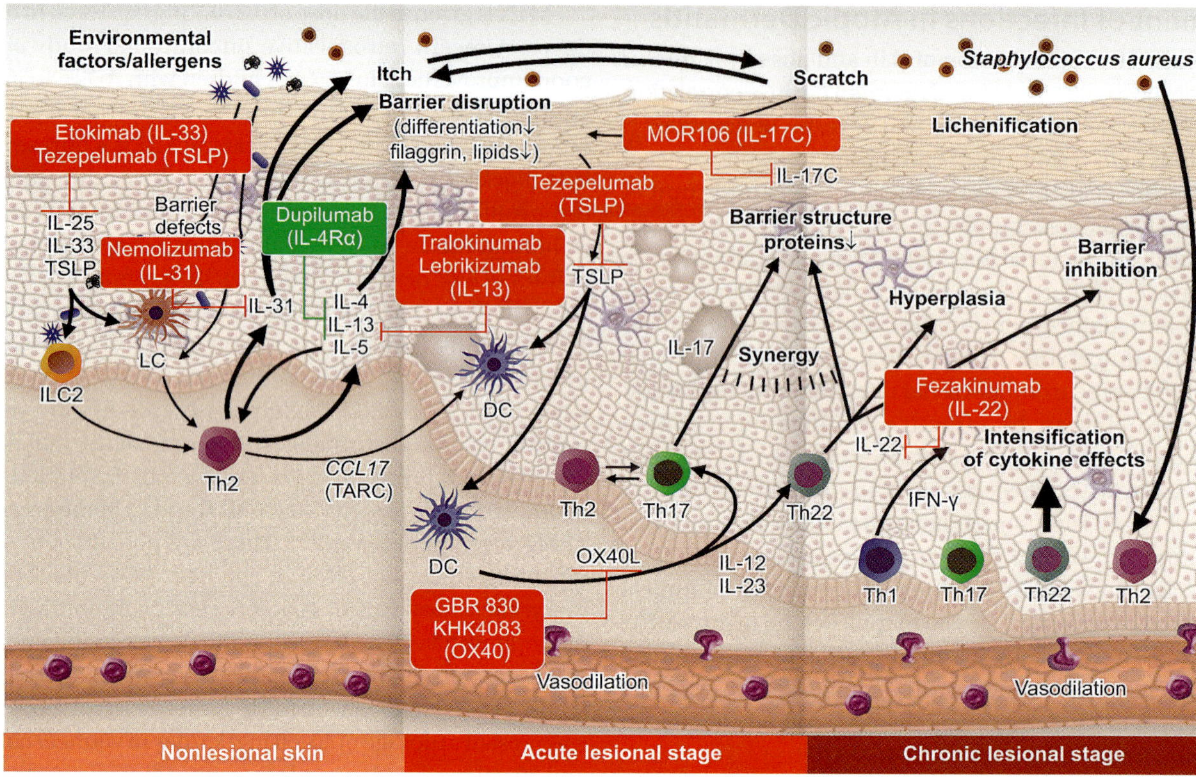

Fig. 19: Biologics in atopic dermatitis (AD).
(*CCL17:* CC chemokine ligand 17; DC: dendritic cell; IFN-γ: interferon gamma; IL: interleukin; ILC2: type 2 innate lymphoid cells; OX40L: OX40 ligand; TARC: thymus- and activation-regulated chemokine; Th: T helper cells; TSLP: thymic stromal lymphopoietin)

in AD which along with other components have antioxidant properties, antiprotease, moisturizing, and anti-inflammatory properties, but recent studies have shown statistically no significant effect.[114] Few trials have been going on topical decoy oligodeoxynucleotides that block transcription factors which act by reducing inflammation. Interferon gamma, intravenous immunoglobulin, and allergen-specific immunotherapy, alitretinoin have been tried in AD but there is lack of data of its usage in children and hence not recommended.[115] Biologicals that have shown promising results and are still in trial are omalizumab, rituximab, alefacept, mepolizumab, dupilumab, efalizumab, infliximab, pitrakinra, etanercept, and apremilast.[116]

Immunomodulators and Cytotoxic Agents

Biologic therapies target specific molecules and therefore theoretically have less harmful effects than other systemic agents used in AD **(Fig. 19)**. Trials done in biologic therapies and their mechanism of action have been summarized in **Table 3**.[114,116]

Though serum IgE is elevated in AD, its exact role in pathogenesis is unclear. Omalizumab is a monoclonal antibody that prevents the proinflammatory effects of IgE by blocking it from binding to its receptors on mast cells. There are many pilot studies regarding beneficial effect of Omalizumab in AD, but a recent double-blind controlled study has not shown statistical significant effects on AD.[117] Though infliximab has shown to inhibit tumor necrosis factor alpha (TNF-α) studies have not shown substantial clinical improvement in AD. Efalizumab and alefacept interfere with T-cell-mediated inflammation. Efalizumab acts as an antibody against CD11a and disrupts the recruitment of T-cells and

TABLE 3: Trials in biologics for atopic dermatitis.

Agent	*Mechanism of action*
Omalizumab	Antibody against IgE, competes with IgE high-affinity receptor
Infliximab	Antibody against tumor necrosis factor alpha
Efalizumab	Antibody against CD11a (anti-T-cell recruitment and activation)
Alefacept	Fusion protein, interferes with LFA-3/CD2 interaction
Mepolizumab	Antibody against IL-5
Rituximab	Antibody against CD20 (anti-B cell)
Pitrakinra	Antibody against IL4-13
Secukinumab	Antibody against IL17
Dupilimab	Antibody against IL-4, IL-17

(CD: cluster of differentiation; IL: interleukin; LFA-3: lymphocyte function-associated antigen 3)

alefacept impairs T-cell activation. There are conflicting results in literature regarding its efficacy in AD. Efalizumab has shown serious side effects and hence not recommended in AD. There are only two studies regarding mepolizumab. It has limited efficacy and large trials are required.[116] There are not many trials regarding rituximab and its efficacy is still being evaluated. Development of pitrakinra has been stopped after phase I and II studies.

Dupilumab New Era in the Treatment of Atopic Dermatitis

Among the recent trials of biologicals in AD, dupilumab has shown promising results in the treatment of AD. Dupilumab is a fully human monoclonal antibody that inhibits the actions of both IL-4 and IL-13. Clinical trials have shown marked improvement in pruritus and clinical symptoms, anxiety, and depression in moderate-to-severe AD with systemic dupilumab. Dupilumab recently received the US FDA breakthrough therapy designation AD, with ongoing trials in both adult and pediatric populations. In a randomized control study of dupilumab in 380 adult patients, 80% reduction was there in the eczema area severity index in 16 weeks.[118] Dupilumab has also shown to improve moderate-to-severe asthma (phase II studies). Long-term trials are required to assess the effectiveness and safety of dupilumab.

Other Recent Therapies

Topical tofacitinib 1% ointment, a potent inhibitor of JAK-3, has been used in adults with mild-to-moderate AD with significant clinical improvement. Crisaborole, a selective low molecular weight topical PDE-4 inhibitor has shown to be effective in mild-to-moderate AD. It is available as 2% ointment and has been approved in US in management of mild-to-moderate AD aged 2 years and above.[119,120]

REFERENCES

1. Dhar S. Banerjee R. Atopic dermatitis in infants and children in India. Indian J Dermatol Venereol Leprol. 2010;76:504-13.
2. Dhar S. Current concepts about the management of atopic dermatitis in infants and children. Ann Inst Child Health. 2004;4:19-28.
3. Dhar S, Kanwar AJ. Atopic diathesis. Ind J Dermatol. 1996;13: 81-2.
4. DaVeiga SP. Epidemiology of atopic dermatitis: a review. Allergy Asthma Proc. 2012;33: 227-34.
5. Mallol J, Crane J, Von Mutius E, Odhiambo J, Keil U, Stewart A. The international study of asthma and allergies in childhood (ISAAC) phase three: a global synthesis. Allergol Immunopathol. 2013;41(2):73-85.
6. Deckers IA, McLean S, Linssen S, Mommers M, van Schayck CP, Sheikh A. Investigating international time trends in the incidence and prevalence of atopic eczema 1990-2010: a systematic review of epidemiological studies. PLoS ONE. 2012;7:e39803.
7. Kumar MK, Singh PK, Ali Tahir MM. The clinic epidemiological profile and the risk factors associated with the severity of atopic dermatitis in Eastern Indian Children. J Clin Diagnostic Research. 2012;6:1162-66.
8. Dhar S, Kanwar AJ. Epidemiology and clinical pattern of atopic dermatitis in a north Indian population. Pediatric Dermatol. 1998;15:347-51.
9. Dhar S, Mandal B, Ghosh A. Epidemiology and clinical pattern of atopic dermatitis in 100 children seen in a city hospital. Indian J Dermatol. 2002;47:202-4.
10. Flohr C, Mann J. New insights into the epidemiology of childhood atopic dermatitis. Allergy. 2014;69:3-16.
11. Elias PM, Hatano Y, Williams ML. Basis for the barrier abnormality in atopic dermatitis: outside-inside-outside pathogenic mechanism. J Allergy Clin Immunol. 2008;121: 1337-43.
12. Boguniewicz M, Leung DY. Atopic dermatitis: a disease of altered skin barrier and immune dysregulation. Immunol Rev. 2011;242:233-46.
13. Novak N, Yu CF, Bussmann C, Maintz L, Peng WM, Hart J, et al. Association of a TLR9 promoter polymorphism with atopic eczema. Allergy. 2007;62:766-72.
14. Barnes KC. An update on the genetics of atopic dermatitis: scratching the surface in 2009. J Allergy Clinical immunology. 2010;125:16-29.
15. Leung DY, Boguniewicz M, Howell MD, Nomura I, Hamid QA. New insights into atopic dermatitis. J Clin Invest. 2004;113: 651-7.
16. Irvine AD, McLean WH, Leung DY. Filaggrin mutations associated with skin and allergic diseases. N Engl J Med. 2011;365:1315-27.
17. Brown SJ, McLean WH. Eczema genetics: current state of knowledge and future goals. J Invest Dermatol. 2009;129: 543-52.
18. Agrawal R, Woodfolk JA. Skin barrier defects in atopic dermatitis. Curr Allergy Asthma Resp. 2014;14:433.
19. Palmer CN, Irvine AD, Terron-Kwiatkowski A, Zhao Y, Liao H, Lee SP, et al. Common loss of function variants of the epidermal barrier protein filaggrin are a major predisposing factor for atopic dermatitis. Nat Genet. 2006;38:441-6
20. Barker JN, Palmer CN, Zhao Y, Liao H, Hull PR, Lee SP, et al. Null mutations in the *filaggrin* gene (FLG) determine major susceptibility to early-onset atopic dermatitis that persists into adulthood. J Invest Dermatol. 2000;127:564-7.
21. Brown SJ, Asai Y, Cordell HJ, Campbell LE, Zhao Y, Liao H, et al. Loss-of-function variants in the *filaggrin* gene are a significant risk factor for peanut allergy. J Allergy Clin Immunol. 2011;127:661-7.
22. Brown SJ, McLean WH. One remarkable molecule: filaggrin. J Invest Dermatol. 2012;132:751-62.
23. Marenholz I, Rivera VA, Esparza-Gordillo I, Bauerfeind A, Lee-Kirsch MA, Ciechanowicz A, et al. Association screening in the epidermal differentiation complex (EDC) identifies an *SPRR3* repeat number variant as a risk factor for eczema. J Invest Dermatol. 2011;131:1644-9.
24. Howell MD, Kim BE, Gao P, Grant AV, Boguiewicz M, DeBenedetto A, et al. Cytokine modulation of atopic dermatitis filaggrin skin expression. J Allergy Clin Immunol. 2009;124:3:R7-12.
25. Pellerin L, Henry J, Hsu CY, Balica S, Jean-Decoster C, Mechin MC, et al. Defects of filaggrin-like proteins in both lesional and non lesional atopic skin. J Allergy Clin Immunol. 2013;131: 1094-102.

26. Nograles KE, Zaba LC, Shemer A, Duculan JF, Cardinale I, Kikuchi T, et al. IL-22-producing “T22” T cells account for upregulated IL-22 in atopic dermatitis despite reduced IL-17-producing TH17 T cells. J Allergy Clin Immunol. 2009;123:1244-52.e2.
27. Gittler JK, Shemer A, Suárez-Fariñas M, Fuentes-Duculan J, Gulewicz KJ, Wang CQF, et al. Progressive activation of T(H)2/T(H)22 cytokines and selective epidermal proteins characterizes acute and chronic atopic dermatitis. J Allergy Clin Immunol. 2012;130:1344-54.
28. Soumelis V, Reche PA, Kanzler H, Yuan W, Edward G, Homey B, et al. Human epithelial cells trigger dendritic cell mediated allergic inflammation by producing TSLP. Nat Immunol. 2002;3:673-80.
29. Kuo IH, Yoshida T, De Benedetto A, Beck LA. The cutaneous innate immune response in patients with atopic dermatitis. J Allergy Clin Immunol. 2013;131:266-78.
30. Zaniboni MC, Samorano LP, Orfali RL, Aoki V. Skin barrier in atopic dermatitis: beyond filaggrin. An Bras Dermatol. 2016;91:472-8.
31. Dhar S, Kanwar AJ, Kaur S, Sharma P, Ganguly NK. Role of bacterial flora in the pathogenesis and management of atopic dermatitis. Ind J Med Res. 1992;95:234-8.
32. Lange L, Alter N, Keller T, Rietschel E. Sensitisation to Malassezia in Infants and children with atopic dermatitis: prevalence and clinical characteristics. Allergy. 2008;63: 486-7
33. Schauber J, Oda Y, Büchau AS, Yun QC, Steinmeyer A, Zugel U, et al. Histone acetylation in keratinocytes enables control of the expression of cathelicidin and CD14 by 1,25-dihydroxyvitamin D3. J Invest Dermatol. 2008;128:816-24.
34. Kong HH, Segre JA. Skin microbiome: Looking back to move forward. J Invest Dermatol. 2012;132:933-9.
35. Angrisano T, Pero R, Paoletti I, Keller S, Lembo L, Baroni A, et al. Epigenetic regulation of IL-8 and β-defensin genes in human keratinocytes in response to Malassezia furfur. J Invest Dermatol. 2013;133:2101-4.
36. Nakatsuji T, Chiang HI, Jiang SB, Nagarajan H, Zengler K, Gallo RL. The microbiome extends to subepidermal compartments of normal skin. Nat Commun. 2013;4:1431.
37. Gao PS, Rafaels NM, Hand T, Murray T, Boguniewicz M, Hata T, et al. FLG null mutations that confer risk of atopic dermatitis confer greater risk for eczema herpeticum. J Allergy Clin Immunol. 2009;124:507-13.
38. Flohr C, Yeo L. Atopic dermatitis and the hygiene hypothesis revisited. Curr Probl Dermatol. 2011;41:1-34.
39. Erb KJ. Can helminths or helminth-derived products be used in humans to prevent or treat allergic diseases? Trends Immunol. 2009;30:75-82.
40. Mpairwe H, Webb EL, Muhangi L, Ndibazza J, Akishule D, Nampijja M, et al Anthelminthic treatment during pregnancy is associated with increased risk of infantile eczema: randomised-controlled trial results. Pediatr Allergy Immunol. 2011;22: 305-12.
41. Flohr C, Tuyen LN, Quinnell RJ, Lewis S, Minh TT, Campbell J, et al Reduced helminth burden increases allergen skin sensitization but not clinical allergy: A randomized, double-blind, placebo-controlled trial in Vietnam. Clin Exp Allergy. 2010;40:131-42
42. Dhar S, Malakar R, Chattopadhyay S, Banerjee R, Ghosh A. Correlation between the severity of atopic dermatitis with absolute counts in peripheral blood and serum IgE. Ind J Dermatol Venereol Leprol. 2005;71:246-9.
43. Alduraywish SA, Lodge CJ, Campbell B, Allen KJ, Erbas B, Lowe AJ, et al. The march from early life food sensitization to allergic disease: A systematic review and meta-analyses of birth cohort studies. Allergy. 2016;71:77-89.
44. Langan SM, Silcocks P, Williams HC. What causes flares of eczema in children? Br J Dermatol. 2009;161:640-6.
45. Van Bever HPS, Llanora G. Features of childhood atopic dermatitis. Asian Pac J Allergy Immunol. 2011;29:15-24.
46. Douwes J, Cheng S, Travier N, Cohet C, Niesink A, McKenzie J, et al. Farm exposure in utero may protect against asthma, hay fever and eczema. Eur Respir J. 2008;32:603-11.
47. Langan SM, Flohr C, Williams HC. The role of furry pets in eczema: A systematic review. Arch Dermatol. 2007;143:1570-77.
48. Katta R, Schlichte M. Diet and dermatitis: Food triggers. J Clin Aesthet Dermatol. 2014;7:30-6.
49. Dhar S, Malakar R, Chakraborty S, Chakraborty J, Mukherjee S. An uncontrolled open pilot study to assess the role of dietary eliminations in reducing the severity of atopic dermatitis in infants and children. Indian J Dermatol. 2009;54:183-5.
50. Celakovska J, Bukac J. Analysis of food allergy in atopic dermatitis patients-association with concomitant allergic diseases. Indian J Dermatol. 2014;59:445-50.
51. Jamila C, Kvetuse E, Karel, Jarostava V, Josef B. Soy allergy in patients suffering from atopic dermatitis. Indian J Dermatol. 2013;58:325.
52. Rowlands D, Tofte SI, Hanifin JM. Does food allergy cause atopic dermatitis? Food challenge testing to dissociate eczematous from immediate reactions. Dermatol Ther. 2006;19:97-103.
53. Font-Ribera L, Gracia-Lavedan E, Esplugues A, Ballester F, Jiménez Zabala A, Santa Marina L, et al. Waterhardness and eczema at 1 and 4 y of age in the INMA birth cohort. Environ Res. 2015;142:579-85.
54. Dhar S, Kanwar AJ, Nagaraja. Personal and family history of ‘atopy’ in children with atopic dermatitis in North India. Ind J Dermatol. 1997;42:9-13.
55. Kanwar AJ, Dhar S. Severity of atopic dermatitis in North India. Br J Dermatol. 1994;131:733-4.
56. Dhar S, Kanwar AJ. Grading of severity of atopic dermatitis in north Indian children. Ind J Dermatol. 1995;40:67-72.
57. Dhar S, Banerjee R, Dutta AK, Gupta AB. Comparison between the severity of atopic dermatitis in Indian children born and brought up in UK and USA and that of Indian children born and brought up in India. Ind J Dermatol. 2003;48:200-2.
58. Dhar S, Mondal B. Malakar R, Ghosh A, Gupta AB . Correlation of the severity of atopic dermatitis and growth retardation in pediatric age group. Ind J Dermatol. 2005;50:129-35.
59. Flohr C, Nagel G, Weinmayr G, Kleiner A, Strachan DP, Williams HC, et al. Lack of evidence for a protective effect of prolonged breastfeeding on childhood eczema: lessons from the international study of Asthma and Allergies in childhood (ISAAC) phase two. Br J Dermatol. 2011;165:1280-9.
60. Kranner MS, Kakuma R. Optimal duration of exclusive breastfeeding. Cochrane Database Syst Rev. 2012;8:CD003517.
61. Okada H, Kuhn C, Feillet H, Bach JF. The ‘hygiene hypothesis’ for autoimmune and allergic disease: an update. Clin Exp Immunol. 2010;160:1-9.
62. Margolis JS, Abuabara K, Bilker W, Hoffstad O, Margolis DJ. Persistence of mild to moderate atopic dermatitis. JAMA Dermatol 2014;150:593-600.
63. William HC, Burney PGJ, Hay RJ, Archer CB, Shipley MJ, Hunter JJ, et al. The UK Working Party’s diagnostic criteria for atopic dermatitis I. Derivation of a minimum set of discriminators for atopic dermatitis. Br J Dermatol. 1994;131:383-96.

64. Dhar S. Diagnostic criteria for atopic dermatitis. Pediatr Dermatol. 1999;16:136.
65. Dhar S, Kanwar AJ, Nagraja. Personal and family history of 'atopy' in children with atopic dermatitis in north India. Ind J Dermatol. 1997;42:9-13.
66. Nagraja, Kanwar AJ, Dhar S, Singh S. Frequency and significance of minor clinical features of atopic dermatitis in various age related subgroups of children. Pediatr Dermatol. 1996;13; 10-13.
67. Kanwar AJ, Dhar S. Frequency and significance of major and minor clinical features of atopic dermatitis. Dermatology 1995;190:317.
68. Dhar S, Kanwar AJ. Atopic dermatitis of the scalp? Ind J Dermatol Venereol Leprol. 1994;59:302-3.
69. Kanwar AJ, Dhar S. How specific are major criteria for the diagnosis of atopic dermatitis? Dermatology. 1993;189:102.
70. Kanwar AJ, Dhar S, Kaur S. Evaluation of minor clinical features of atopic dermatitis. Paediatric Dermatol. 1991;8:114-6.
71. Dhar S. Current concepts about the diagnosis of atopic dermatitis. Ind J Paediatr Dermatol. 1999;2:16-8.
72. Dhar S. Atopic dermatitis: Indian Scenario. Ind J Dermatol Venereol Leprol. 1999;65:253-4.
73. Dhar S. Atopic dermatitis in Indian children. The Child and the New born. 2001;4:47-51.
74. Eichenfield LF, Tom WL, Berger TL, Krol A, Paller AS, Schwarzenberger K, et al. Guidelines of care for the management of atopic dermatitis; section 2. Management and treatment of atopic dermatitis with topical therapies. J Am Acad Dermatol. 2014;71:116-32.
75. Ring J, Alomar A, Bieber T, Deleuran M, Fink-Wagner A, Gelmetti C, et al. Guidelines for the treatment of atopic eczema (atopic dermatitis) part I. J Eur Acad Dermatol Venereol. 2012;26:1045-60.
76. Sidbury R, Tom WL, Bergman JN, Cooper KD, Silverman RA, Berger TG, et al. Guidelines of care for the management of atopic dermatitis: Section 4. Prevention of disease flares and use of adjunctive therapies and approaches. J Am Acad Dermatol. 2014;71:1218-33.
77. Huang JT, Abrams M, Tlougan B, Rademaker A, Paller AS. Treatment of *Staphylococcus aureus* colonization in atopic dermatitis decreases disease severity. Pediatrics. 2009;123: 808-14.
78. Wong SM, Ng TG, Baba R. Efficacy and safety of sodium hypochlorite (bleach) baths in patients with moderate to severe atopic dermatitis in Malaysia. J Dermatol. 2013;40:874-80.
79. Katayama I, Kohno Y, Akiyama K, Aihara M, Kondo N, Saeki H, et al. Japanese Guideline for Atopic Dermatitis 2014. Allergology International. 2014;63:377-98.
80. Engebretsen KA, Johansen JD, Kezic S, Lenneberg A, Thyssen JP. The effect of environmental humidity and temperature on skin barrier and dermatitis. J Eur Acad Dermatol Venereol. 2016; 30:223-49.
81. Rubel D, Thirumoorthy T, Soebaryo RW, Weng SC, Gabriel TM, Villafuerte LL, et al. Consensus guidelines for the management of atopic dermatitis: An Asia-Pacific perspective. J Dermatol. 2013;40:160-71.
82. Shams K, Grindlay DJ, Williams HC. What's new in atopic eczema? An analysis of systematic reviews published in 2009–2010. Clin Exp Dermatol. 2011;36:573-8.
83. NG SY, Begum S, Chong SY. Does order of application of emollient and topical corticosteroids make a difference in the severity of atopic eczema in children? Pediatr Dermatol. 2016;33:160-4.
84. De Belilovsky C, Roo-Rodriguez E, Baudouin C, Menu F, Chadoutaud B, Msika P. Natural peroxisome proliferator-activated receptor-alpha agonist cream demonstrates similar therapeutic response to topical steroids in atopic dermatitis. J Dermatolog Treat. 2011;22:359-65.
85. Eric L, Simpson MD, MCR, Joanne R, Chalmers, Jon M Hanifin. Emollient enhancement of the skin barrier from birth offers effective atopic dermatitis prevention. J Allergy Clin Immunol. 2014;134:818-23.
86. Darsow U, Wollenberg A, Simon D, Taieb A, Werfel T, Orange A, et al. ETFAD/EADV eczema task force 2009 position paper on diagnosis and treatment of atopic dermatitis. J Eur Acad Dermatol Venereol. 2010;24:317-28.
87. Tollefson MM, Bruckner AL. Section On Dermatology. Atopic dermatitis: skin-directed management. Pediatrics. 2014;134:e1735-44.
88. Schmitt J, von Kobyletzki L, Svensson A, Apfelbacher C. Efficacy and tolerability of proactive treatment with topical corticosteroids and calcineurin inhibitors for atopic eczema: systematic review and meta-analysis of randomized controlled trials. Br J Dermatol. 2011;164:415-28.
89. Saraswath A. Topical corticosteroid use in children: Adverse effects and how to minimize them. Indian J Dermatol Venereol Leprol. 2010;76:225-8.
90. Devillers AC, Orange AP. Wet wrap treatment in children with atopic dermatitis: a practical guideline. Pediatr Dermatol. 2012;29:24-7.
91. Dhar S, Banerjee R. Topical tacrolimus in atopic dermatitis: a placebo controlled study with 15 children. Indian J Dermatol. 2004;49:22-4.
92. El-Batawy MM, Bosseila MA, Mashaly HM, Hafez VS. Topical calcinuerin inhibitors in atopic dermatitis: a systematic review and meta-analysis. J Dermatol Sci. 2009;54:76-87.
93. Luger T, De Raeve L, Gelmetti C, Kakourou T, Katsarou A, Lambert J, et al. Recommendations for pimecrolimus 1% cream in the treatment of mild to moderate atopic dermatitis: from medical needs to anew treatment algorithm. Eur J Dermatol. 2013;23:758-66.
94. Park HY, Kim CR, Huh IS, Jung MY, Seo EY, Park JH, et al. Staphylococcus aureus colonization in acute and chronic skin lesions of patients with atopic dermatitis. Ann Dermatol. 2013;25:410-6.
95. Petry V, Liphnarski G, Bessa GR, Silveria VB, Weber MB, Bonamigo RR, et al. Prevalence of community-acquired methicillin-resistant Staphylococcus aureus and antibiotic resistance in patients with atopic dermatitis in Porto Alegre, Brazil. Int J Dermatol. 2014;53:731-5.
96. Sidbury R, Davis DM, Cohen DE, Cordoro KM, Berger TG, Bergman JN, et al. Guidelines of care for the management of atopic dermatitis: section 3. Management and treatment with phototherapy and systemic agents. J Am Acad Dermatol. 2014;71:327.
97. Petry V, Bessa GR, Poziomczyck CS, Oliveria CF, Weber MB, Bonamigo RR, et al. Bacterial skin colonization and infections in patients with atopic dermatitis. Ann Bras Dermatol. 2012;87:729-34.
98. Gauger A, Mempel M, Schekatz A, Schafer T, Ring J, Abeck D. Silver coated textiles reduce Staphylococcus aureus colonization in patients with atopic eczema. Dermatology. 2003;207:15-21.
99. Dhar S. Should topical antibacterials be routinely combined with topical steroids in the treatment of atopic dermatitis. Ind J Dermatol Venereol Leprol. 2005;71:71-2.

100. Darabi K, Hostetler SG, Bechtel MA, Zirwas M. The role of Malassezia in atopic dermatitis affecting the head and neck of adults. J Am Acad Dermatol. 2009;60:125-36.
101. Dhar S, Malakar S. Evaluation of the efficacy of topical doxepin alone or in combination with topical corticosteroid in the management of atopic dermatitis. Ind J Dermatol. 1999;44: 58-60.
102. Ohsawa Y, Hirasawa N. The role of histamine H1 and H4 receptors in atopic dermatitis: from basic research to clinical study. Allergol Int. 2014;63:533-42.
103. Notaro ER, Sidbury R. Systemic agents for severe atopic dermatitis in children. Paediatr Drugs. 2015;17:449-57.
104. Haw S, Shin MK, Haw CR. The efficacy and safety of long-term oral cyclosporine treatment of patients with atopic dermatitis. Ann Dermatol. 2010;1:9-15.
105. Van Der Schaft J, van Zulienz AD, Deinum J, Bruijnzeel-Koomen CA, de Bruin-Weller MS. Serum Creatinine levels during and after long term treatment with cyclosporine A in patients with severe atopic dermatitis. Acta Derm Venereol 2015;95: 963-67.
106. Deo M, Yung A, Hill S, Rademaker M. Methotrexate for treatment of atopic dermatitis in children and adolescents. Int J Dermatol. 2014;53:1037-41.
107. Robert H, Orchard D. Methotrexate is safe and effective treatment for paediatric discoid (nummular) eczema: a case series of 25 children. Australas J Dermatol. 2010;51: 128-30.
108. Caufield M, Tom WL. Oral azathioprine for recalcitrant pediatric atopic dermatitis: clinical response and thiopurine monitoring. J Am Acad Dermatol. 2013;68:29-35.
109. Fuggle NR, Bragoli W, Mahto A, Glover M, Martinez AE, Kinsler VA. The adverse effect profile of oral azathioprine in pediatric atopic dermatitis, and recommendations for monitoring. J Am Acad Dermatol. 2015;72:108-14.
110. Heller M, Shin HT, Orlow SJ, Schaffer JV. Mycophenolate mofetil for severe childhood atopic dermatitis: experience in 14 patients. Br J Dermatol. 2007;157:127-32.
111. Darne S, Leech SN, Taylor AE. Narrowband ultraviolet B phototherapy in children with moderate to severe eczema: a comparative cohort study. Br J Dermatol 2014;170:150-6.
112. Van der Aa LB, Heymans HS, van Aalderen WM, Sprikkelman AB. Probiotics and prebiotics in atopic dermatitis: Review of the theoretical background and clinical evidence. Pediatr Allergy Immunol. 2010;21:e355-67.
113. Nakai K, Yoneda K, Murakami Y, Koura A, Maeda R, Tamai A, et al. Effects of Topical N-Acetylcysteine on Skin Hydration/ Transepidermal Water Loss in Healthy Volunteers and Atopic Dermatitis Patients. Ann Dermatol. 2015;27:450-1.
114. Chase EP, Armstrong AW. Advances in management of atopic dermatitis: new therapies and novel uses of existing treatments. Semin Cut Med Surg. 2012;31:17-24.
115. Jee SJ, Kim JH, Baek HS, Lee HB, Oh JW. Long term efficacy of intravenous immunoglobulin therapy for moderate to severe childhood atopic dermatitis. Allergy Asthma Immunol Res. 2011;3:89-95.
116. Montes-Torres A, Llamas-Velasco M, Perez-Plaza A, Salano-Lopez G, Sanchez-Perez J. Biological treatments in atopic dermatitis. J Clin Med. 2015;4:593-613.
117. Heil PM, Maurer D, Klein B, Hultsch T, Stingl G. Omalizumab therapy in atopic dermatitis: Depletion of IgE does not improve the clinical course - A randomized, placebo-controlled and double blind pilot study. J Dtsch Dermatol Ges. 2010;8:990-8.
118. Simpson EL, Bieber T, Guttman-Yassky E, Beck LA, Blauvelt A, Cork MJ, et al. Two phase 3 trials of dupilumab versus placebo in atopic dermatitis. N Engl J Med. 2016;375(24):2335-48.
119. Ruzicka T, Mihara R. Anti-interleukin-31 receptor A antibody for atopic dermatitis. N Engl J Med. 2017;376:826-35.
120. Hoy SM. Crisaborole ointment 2%: a review in mild to moderate atopic dermatitis. Am J Clin Dermatol. 2017;18:837-43.

EXAMINATION QUESTIONS

1. Explain etiopathogenesis of atopic dermatitis.
2. What are the recent treatment advances in atopic dermatitis?
3. Write a short note on biologicals in atopic dermatitis.
4. Write a short note on dupilumab.

22 CHAPTER

Seborrheic Dermatitis

Debatri Datta, Indrashis Podder

INTRODUCTION

Seborrheic dermatitis is a frequently encountered chronic inflammatory disorder of the sebaceous glands. It clinically presents with erythematous patches and greasy yellowish scales, often associated with itching. The areas rich in sebaceous glands are most affected, such as scalp (where it presents commonly as dandruff), central face, anterior chest, and back. It can affect infants, adolescents, and adults but has a bimodal peak of incidence. It has been associated with a common skin yeast, *Malassezia*. Multiple treatment modalities are available including antifungal shampoos and topical agents, topical steroids, and topical immunomodulators like tacrolimus.

EPIDEMIOLOGY[1]

The first peak of incidence occurs in infancy, while the other peak is observed around third to fourth decade in adults. Almost 70% infants below 3 months of age may be affected with this disorder.

Seborrheic dermatitis is more common in patients with human immunodeficiency virus (HIV) infection and low CD4 T-cell count, Parkinson's disease, and intake of drugs such as haloperidol and lithium. Nutritional deficiencies such as riboflavin and zinc may also trigger seborrheic dermatitis.

PATHOGENESIS[1,2]

Seborrheic dermatitis has a strong association with the commensal skin yeast *Malassezia* species. Studies have demonstrated increased colonization of *Malassezia* on skin of these patients and the disease responds to antifungal therapy targeting the yeast, thus proving a conclusive link. However, the exact pathophysiology of how the fungus causes seborrheic dermatitis is not yet determined. It is hypothesized that fungal metabolites react with triglycerides in sebum, or lipid layer of fungus can incite keratinocytes to generate an inflammatory reaction. A cellular immune response is most likely.

CLINICAL FEATURES AND DIFFERENTIAL DIAGNOSIS[2,3]

In infants, the typical presentation is thick, adherent, and yellowish greasy scales on scalp (cradle cap). This form is usually self-limiting, without any acute inflammation or pruritus. Fine scaling may be observed on face and around ears. If body folds like axilla or inguinal region are involved, it can form exudates and become generalized. However, severe generalized seborrheic dermatitis in infants is usually seen in immunodeficiencies with failure to thrive (Leiner's disease).

In adults, the lesions are chronic and relapsing, initially presenting with mild greasy scaling and erythema on scalp. It often involves the areas rich in sebaceous glands such as nasolabial folds, retroauricular skin, beard area, eyes and eyebrows, chest (especially midline area), and body folds. The lesions appear as pink colored or erythematous macules to thin plaques with scaling ranging from dry, fine, and white to yellowish and greasy. Pruritus may be associated.

Clinical Types

- *Classical*: Already described.
- *Petaloid*: Small, reddish-brown papules, and patches with follicular and perifollicular greasy scales; resembling flower petals, usually occurs on chest.
- *Pityriasiform type*: Generalized macules and patches such as pityriasis rosea. Less common in occurrence.
- *Generalized type*: Severe variety where lesions involve whole body, can progress to erythroderma rarely.

Differential Diagnoses

Some of the common differential diagnoses with their characteristic distinguishing features include:

- *Psoriasis*: Thicker, scaly, and well-defined plaques.
- *Atopic dermatitis*: Diagnostic criteria need to be fulfilled such as Hanifin and Rajka or UK Working Group.
- *Tinea capitis and other dermatophytoses*: Positive potassium hydroxide (KOH) test and/or culture to show fungal elements.
- *Cutaneous lupus erythematosus*: Typical clinical features, raised antinuclear antibody (ANA) titer is indicative, and Systemic Lupus International Collaborating Clinics (SLICC) criteria.
- *Langerhans cell histiocytosis*: More severe disease, hemorrhagic lesions involving the folds, and failure to thrive.
- *Rosacea*: Erythema and flushing on face, aggravated by stress, hot temperature, spices, and cold climate; dermoscopy shows more vascular pattern.

- *Cutaneous lymphoma*: Nodular swellings, skin biopsy is diagnostic.
- *Contact dermatitis*: Short duration, history of contact with irritant chemical.
- *Erythrasma*: Wood's lamp examination is diagnostic.

DIAGNOSIS[2,3]

- *Clinical*: The diagnosis is essentially clinical, based on the appearance of lesions and their characteristic distribution.
- *Dermoscopy/trichoscopy*: Arborizing thin vessels, perifollicular white scales, yellowish scales, structureless areas, honeycomb pigment, comma vessels, and thick hair shafts.
- *Histopathology*: In case of confusion, biopsy can show inflammatory infiltrate with spongiosis, hyperplasia with parakeratosis in the epidermis, and plugged follicular ostia.

TREATMENT[4,5]

Seborrheic dermatitis has no permanent cure. Treatment is aimed at control of symptoms and prevention of relapse. Topical therapies are summarized in **Table 1** and systemic therapies in **Table 2** along with their notable features.

TABLE 1: Topical therapies.

Class	*Drug*	*Remarks*
Keratolytics	Urea	• Keratolytics may help in breaking thick and adherent scales • Used in combination only, not a first-line treatment
	Propylene glycol	
	Lactic acid	
	Salicylic acid	• Shampoo/lotion, may be combined with steroids or antifungals • Used weekly to daily in increased scaling
Topical antifungals	Azoles such as ketoconazole 2% and bifonazole 1%	• First-line treatment, may be combined with steroids/urea • Shampoo, ointment, and lotion available • Two to three times weekly for treatment, less frequently for maintenance and prophylaxis
	Allylamines like butenafine	
	Zinc pyrithione	• Used in combination shampoo • Zinc transport facilitator, antifungal effect by increasing copper in fungal cells which inhibit metabolism
	Ciclopirox olamine 1%	• Broad spectrum antifungal and anti-inflammatory effect • Shampoo/cream/gel form available
	Selenium sulfide	• Shampoo/lotion/cream/foam available • Causes easily reversible orange-brown discoloration in scalp
	Tea tree oil	• Shampoo for regular use in mild cases
Topical steroids	Fluocinolone, desonide, betamethasone, beclomethasone, etc.	• Short-term daily use for symptom control to avoid adverse effects • Shampoo/lotion/cream form, may be used on scalp and body
Topical calcineurin inhibitors	Tacrolimus and pimecrolimus	• Immunomodulatory effect, safer than steroid • Short-term daily use on face and scalp
Topical antibiotic	Metronidazole	• Gel form, shown efficacy with daily use
Miscellaneous	Tar	• Shampoo for regular use, avoided due to local adverse effects such as folliculitis and irritant dermatitis

TABLE 2: Systemic therapies (short-term use for severe cases).

Class		*Use*
Antifungal—azole	Itraconazole	200 mg/day for 7 days with monthly pulse for maintenance
	Fluconazole	Daily or monthly pulse therapy, varying doses from 150 to 300 mg/day
	Ketoconazole	• 200 mg/day for 2–4 weeks • Less used due to adverse effects
Antifungal—allylamine	Terbinafine	250 mg/day continuous or monthly pulse
Systemic steroid	Prednisone/prednisolone	Short-term for very severe unresponsive cases and erythroderma
Miscellaneous	Isotretinoin	For resistant cases, long-term use for 1 year or more

COMPLICATIONS

Complications include blepharitis with meibomian gland occlusion and abscess formation, otitis externa, and other secondary bacterial infection causing discomfort or local lymphadenopathy. Concomitant acne vulgaris may occur due to oily skin common in both disorders.

KEY POINTS

- Seborrheic dermatitis is a common disease seen in infants and adults.
- Characterized by yellowish greasy scales and erythematous patches with occasional itching.
- Lesions seen in scalp, face, anterior chest, and back.
- Can be controlled by antifungals and topical steroids commonly; no permanent cure.

REFERENCES

1. Berk T, Scheinfeld N. Seborrheic dermatitis. Pharm Ther. 2010;35(6):348-52.
2. Clark GW, Pope SM, Jaboori KA. Diagnosis and treatment of seborrheic dermatitis. Am Fam Physician. 2015;91(3):185-90.
3. Widaty S, Pusponegoro EH, Rahmayunita G, Astriningrum R, Akhmad AM, Oktarina C, et al. Applicability of trichoscopy in scalp seborrheic dermatitis. Int J Trichology. 2019;11(2):43.
4. Gupta AK, Richardson M, Paquet M. Systematic review of oral treatments for seborrheic dermatitis. J Eur Acad Dermatol Venereol. 2014;28(1):16-26.
5. Dessinioti C, Katsambas A. Seborrheic dermatitis: Etiology, risk factors, and treatments. Clin Dermatol. 2013;31(4):343-51.

EXAMINATION QUESTION

1. What is seborrheic dermatitis? Mention the common clinical variants.

23 CHAPTER

Contact Dermatitis

AK Bajaj, PK Srivastava

INTRODUCTION

It is an inflammation of the skin with intercellular edema of the epidermis that result from the interaction of the chemical with the skin. Contact dermatitis is of two major types, irritant contact dermatitis (ICD) which accounts for 80% and allergic contact dermatitis (ACD) which constitutes 20%.

Factors affecting the individual cutaneous response are related to the chemical and physical properties, duration and area of exposure, concentration of chemicals, occlusion, individual age, and other skin pathology along with environment where humidity and temperature most of the times plays pivotal role.

IRRITANT CONTACT DERMATITIS (FIG. 1)

Introduction

It is defined as an eczematous reaction to the skin or damage to the keratinocytes caused by the exposure to the external agents/chemicals. The agents are usually acids, alkalies, surfactants, solvents, various oxidants, and enzymes. The concentration of the substance is important factor in determining ICD.

Pathomechanism

Usually, there is genetic predisposition and sensitization but lag phase is not necessary. Irritant reaction causes damage directly to the keratinocytes and this damage induces the activation of various cytokines, phospholipids, and other leukotrienes compounding cellular and vascular damage.

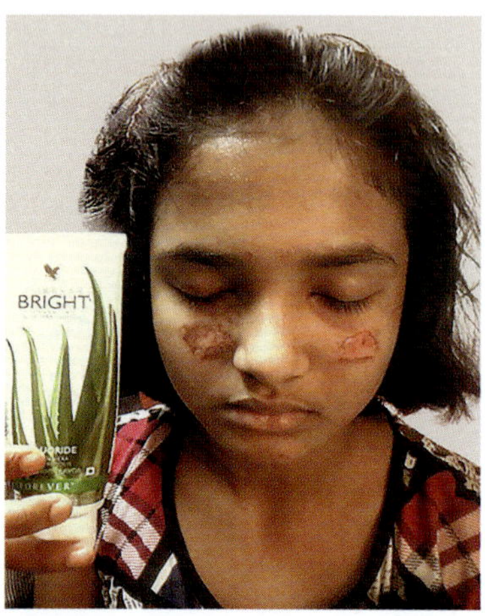

Fig. 1: Irritant contact dermatitis.
Courtesy: Dr Aarti Sarda.

Clinical Spectrum

- Subjective ICD (stinging)
- Acute ICD
- Chronic ICD
- Chemical burn

In acute ICD, the reaction is usually seen after single exposure. The manifestations vary from little dryness, redness to the extreme of vesiculation. Reactions are localized to the site of exposure, which often subside in a few days to weeks.

Chronic ICD also known as cumulative insult or wear and tear dermatitis and as the name suggest is the result of cumulative exposure of the skin to the irritants. Patients complain of dryness, redness, scaling, fissuring more than the vesiculation which may sometimes be seen in chronic ICD. The lesions are located on hands and characteristic feature is the continuing chronicity of the lesions despite of removing the offending agents. The commonly used agents which come into contact with the skin include water, detergents, organic solvents, oils, alkalies, acids, multiple trauma, and frictions.

Other two types of ICD are: (1) stinging (which is also called subjective irritant reaction) and (2) chemical burns. In subjective irritant reaction, there is a lack of clinical manifestation and the only complaints of patients is stinging or burning feeling after contact with chemical within seconds to minutes after exposure, for example, application of chloroform and menthol to the skin, though there are interindividual variations in elicitation.

As far as chemical burn are concerned, reaction seen after skin interaction with highly alkaline or acidic compounds, which causes severe damage to the skin. Clinical picture is like appearance of painful erythema, vesiculation, and formation of necrotic scar, for example, cement ulcer also known as chrome ulcers.

ALLERGIC CONTACT DERMATITIS (FIG. 2)

It is a classical type IV immunological reaction which by definition is mediated by the immune cells (T-cells). Reaction usually occurs in two phases, initially a sensitization phase and later an elicitation phase.

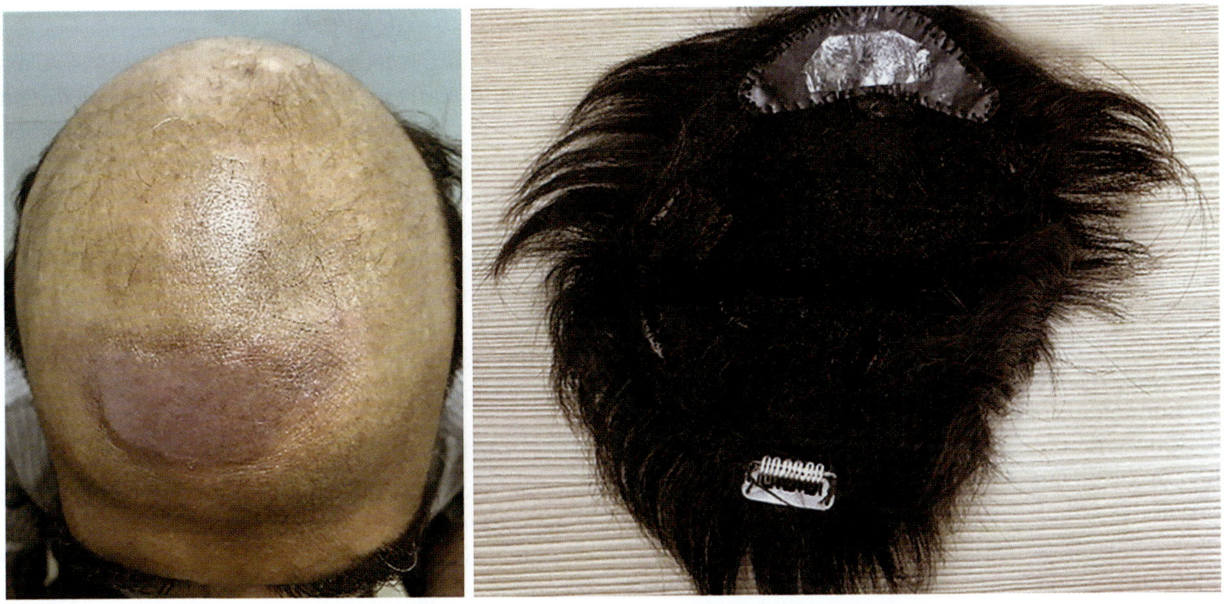

Fig. 2: Allergic contact dermatitis to adhesive on hair piece.
Courtesy: Dr Aarti Sarda.

Sensitization or Induction Phase

The sensitization or induction phase starts when an allergen binds to the skin and finishes when the individual is sensitized enough to produce positive ACD or reaction.

The entire process of induction phase takes at least 3 days to a few weeks. On the other hand, elicitation phase or effector phase occurs on re-exposure and results in the clinical picture of ACD. This phase develops within 1–2 days. Elicitation phase even may be shorter up to a few hours in case of strong sensitizer such as paraphenylene diamine (PPD), *Parthenium*.

During the sensitization phase, allergens penetrate the skin and present themselves to the Langerhans cells [also known as antigen-presenting cells (APCs)]. Now this complex, i.e., Allergen–Langerhans cell complex reaches to the regional lymph nodes via afferent lymphatics and settles down in the paracortical T-cells area. Usually in nonsensitized individuals, the population of T-cells with certain specificities is very low. This increases when APC helps in binding of an allergen and activation of allergen specific T cells. Under the influence of interleukin-1 (IL-1) which is released from the antigen APC complex and IL-1 (which is secreted from the Langerhans cell) activates T-cells which in-turn releases IL-2 which helps in proliferation of T-cell clones.[1] This expanded generation of specific T-cells reaches to the blood via the efferent lymphatics and migrates to the peripheral tissue.

Elicitation Phase

Upon re-exposure, the APC and specific T-cells meet within the skin and release various cytokines and proinflammatory mediators and arrival of more specific T-cells to the skin which in turn further release local mediators leading to an eczematous reaction within 48 hours.

TABLE 1: Clinical and histological differences between allergic and irritant contact dermatitis.

Feature	*Allergic*	*Irritant*
Itch	++++ (Early)	+++ (Late)
Pain/burning	++	++++ (Early)
Erythema	++++	++++
Vesicles	++++	+
Pustules	+	+++
Hyperkeratosis	++	++++
Fissuring	++	++++
Sharp demarcation	Yes	Yes
Reaction delay after contact	Days	Minutes to hours
Spongiosis	++++	++++
Dermal edema	++++	++++
Necrotic keratinocytes	+	+++
Ballooning degeneration	+	+++
Lymphocyte infiltrate	++++	++++
Neutrophilic infiltrate	+	+++

Source: Adapted from Marks JG Jr, Anderson BE, DeLeo VA. Contact and Occupational Dermatology. New Delhi: Jaypee Brothers Medical Publishers; 2016.

Allergic versus Irritant Contact Dermatitis: Clinical and Histological Differences

Clinical and histological differences between allergic and irritant contact dermatitis are given in **Table 1**.[1]

Evaluation of Patient of Allergic Contact Dermatitis

Who is to be patch tested?

Any patients who present with the eczema or dermatitis needs to be patch tested. ACD may also be considered in patient with erythroderma, photosensitivity, and symptoms of burning and itching. The distribution of dermatitis most of the time is strongly suggestive of ACD, for example, eyelid dermatitis to nail cosmetics or deodorant allergy in the axillae. Sometimes patients need to be patch tested while having different cutaneous diseases, for example, atopic eczema, dyshidrotic eczema, or pompholyx, stasis dermatitis, seborrheic dermatitis outside the hairy area or chronic fungal infections of the hands and feet.

Detailed history and complete clinical examination is mandatory if one is suspecting ACD. *Do not test the patients if the dermatitis is acute or severe.* It is always preferable to test after discontinuation of systemic or topical steroids for at least 1 week prior. When the physical examination is completed and there is suspicion of contact allergy patch testing with standard series which varies from country to country and suggestive occupational series should be done.

Indian standard series of 25 antigens shown in **Table 2** needs to be updated. Final diagnosis in ACD always depends upon the results of the patch test and establishing their relevance.

TABLE 2: The Indian Standard Battery of patch test allergens suggested by CODFI.

Test substance	*Vehicle*	*Concentration (%)*
Potassium dichromate	P	0.5
Neomycin sulfate	P	20
Cobalt chloride	P	1.0
Benzocaine	P	5.0
p-phenylenediamine	P	1.0
Paraben mix	P	15.0
Nickel sulfate	P	5.0
Colophony	P	20.0
Gentamicin sulfate	P	20.0
Mercapto mix	P	2.0
Epoxy resin	P	1.0
Fragrance mix 1	P	8.0
Mercaptobenzothiazole	P	2.0
Nitrofurazone	P	1.0
p-chlorocresol	P	1.0
Lanolin alcohol	P	30.0
Balsam Peru	P	5.0
Thiuram mix	P	1.0
Clioquinol	P	5.0
Black rubber mix	P	0.6
p-tertiary butylphenol formaldehyde resin	P	1.0
Formaldehyde	A	1.0
PEG 400	–	100.0
Parthenolide/parthenium extract	P	0.1

(CODFI: Contact and Occupational Dermatoses Forum of India; P: petrolatum; PEG 400: polyethylene glycol 400)

Technique of Patch Testing

Education in the technique of patch testing is as essential to the clinicians as the learning of most of the surgical procedures (Fisher 1986). For doing patch test antigens are applied on the disks which are supplied in strip of tens on the Micropore adhesive tape and are pasted on the upper back. For liquid antigens place a filter paper on the disk and then put a drop of antigen in that chamber. Apply additional tape to secure patches if needed. After 48 hours (D-2), patches are removed and sites are marked. First reading should be taken 30 minutes after the removal of disk as pressure might obscure positive response.

Interpretation of Patch Test

Interpretation of patch test done according to the International Contact Dermatitis Research Group (ICDRG) grading system shown in the **Table 3**, and should be made after second reading, i.e., after 96 hours (D-4) and (seventh day for corticosteroids and neomycin). Exposure list should be used both for determining the clinical relevance of a positive reaction and for assisting patient in allergen/s avoidance.

Causes of false-negative reactions

Negative patch test result means either no allergy exists or there was improper patch test done which means testing with very low concentration, improper technique, or failure to test for a culprit allergen.

Causes of false-positive reactions

Too high concentration of tested allergen, too much test substance applied, current or recent dermatitis at the patch test site, and adhesive tape reactions are the main causes of false-positive reactions.

Test with unknown substance

Ideally, one should avoid patch testing with nonstandard antigens or to unknown substances but if there is strong suspicion then the cosmetic products which are leave on should be tested as it is and wash-off products should be diluted in the ratio of 1:10 dilution. Household products such

TABLE 3: Evaluation of patch test result based on the guidelines of ICDRG.

Symbol	*Morphology*	*Interpretation*
–	No reaction	Negative
? (+)	Erythema, no infiltrate	Questionable
+	Erythema, infiltrate, may be small papules	1+
++	Erythema, infiltrate, papules, vesicles	2+
+++	Erythema, infiltrate, confluent vesicles	3+
Ir	Sharply defined erythema, blisters, necrosis	Irritant

(ICDRG: International Contact Dermatitis Research Group)

as detergents, bleach, solvents, and cleansers should be tested with the dilution of 1:10–1:100. Topical medications such as antibacterials, eye, and ear preparations should be tested as it is. Wart, industrial products, anthralin, benzoyl peroxide, and tretinoin should be tested in the dilution of 1:100–1:1,000. Clothing and shoes should be soaked with saline or water for 10–20 minutes. Leave in place for 96 hours. If one sees positive reactions with unknown substance, test 5–10 normal controls to rule out irritancy of the substance.

Other Patch Test Variants

TRUE test

All necessary material is prepared in advance and the dermatologist, nurse, or technician only has to remove the covering material, apply the test strips, and mark. The allergens are incorporated in hydrophilic gels and the patches are 9 mm by 9 mm. At present, this system is commercially available for the standard series **(Fig. 3)**.[2]

Photopatch test

Allergic contact dermatitis may be accentuated by UV light or rarely visible light when patients skin exposed sufficiently to ultraviolet light present as a dermatitis which predominantly affects sunlight exposed areas such as the face, V of the neck, the back of the hands, and the dorsal forearms.

Photopatch is diagnostic of choice and testing should be conducted on skin that has been clinically normal for the preceding 2 weeks. Two identical sets of allergens are applied as parallel series on either side of the back using conventional patch test techniques. Two days later, both are discarded and the sites are examined for reactions, which are recorded using the standard scoring system.

One set of sites is shielded while the other is irradiated with ultraviolet A (UVA). A reading immediately after irradiation (up to 20 minutes later) is sometimes performed, and detects immediate phototoxic urticarial reactions. Photoallergic reactions may be more obvious and more easily distinguished from phototoxic reactions by the “crescendo” pattern. A later reading after 1 week has also been proposed.

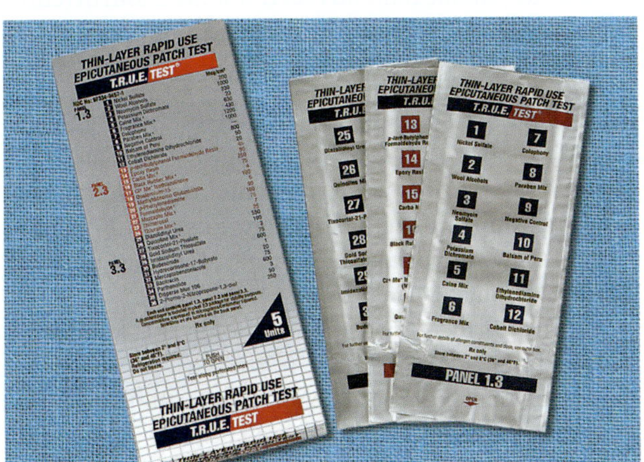

Fig. 3: TRUE test kit.[2]

Semi-open test

This method was introduced by An Goossens. Mainly used for products—brought by the patients—with suspected irritant properties due to solvents or emulsifiers, e.g., detergents, shampoos, paints, resins, varnishes, glues, waxes, cooling fluids, pharmaceuticals, and cosmetics. The product (solution or suspension) is applied with a cotton swab as is in a small amount (about 15 μL) to an area of 2 cm × 2 cm. After complete drying it is covered with acrylate tape for 2 days. The site is checked for contact urticaria and at days 2 and 4 for signs of contact eczema, respectively.

Repeated open application test

The repeated open application test (ROAT) in a standardized form was introduced by Hannuksela and Salo. Test substances, either commercial products or special test substances, are applied twice daily for 7 days to the outer aspect of the upper arm, ante cubital fossa or back skin (scapular area).

If the product is a cleanser or shampoo, wash it off in a minute or so. If the treated skin continues to look normal by the end of the week of testing, the person is unlikely to have a significant allergy to the substance tested. If the individual develops, a patch of red skin, dry skin, itching, or frank dermatitis at the site of application, there may be an allergy to the substance or to one of its ingredients. Immediate signs of skin irritation are usually due to an ICD, rather than an allergic contact dermatitis. An allergic reaction is often only evident several days after applying the substance. A positive reaction to open application testing may indicate formal patch tests should be undertaken to identify a specific contact allergen. The amount of test substance should be approximately 0.1 mL to 5 cm × 5 cm area and 0.5 mL to a 10 cm × 10 cm area.

SYSTEMIC CONTACT DERMATITIS

Systemic contact dermatitis (SCD), better termed systemically reactivated allergic contact dermatitis, is a type of contact hypersensitivity reaction in which ingestion or other systemic exposure to a contact allergen occurs in an already sensitized person. Although the initial sensitizing exposure is usually by topical application, re-exposure by the oral, intravenous or inhalation routes can cause SCD. Sensitized individuals may develop skin eruptions within hours of systemic allergen exposure. This suggests that mechanisms other than type IV delayed-type hypersensitivity are involved. There is evidence that systemic reactions to ingested haptens can be mediated by a type III immunologic reaction.[3] Urticaria and anaphylaxis-type reactions, e.g., those occurring in latex-sensitive patients upon eating bananas, tomatoes, etc., involve immunoglobulin E (IgE)-mediated type I reactions.[4,5]

Clinical patterns of systemic contact dermatitis are given in **Box 1**, and some topical sensitizers with corresponding systemic agents are given in **Table 4**.[6]

BOX 1: Clinical patterns of systemic contact dermatitis.

- Pompholyx, vesicular hand eczema
- Cheilitis, perioral eczema, stomatitis
- Flare-ups of earlier patch test reactions
- Generalized maculopapular-vesicular rash ("baboon syndrome" is a subtype)
- Erythema multiforme
- Vasculitis and purpuric lesions
- Urticaria and anaphylaxis

Source: Adapted from Bajaj AK, Saraswat A. Systemic contact dermatitis. Indian J Dermatol Venereol. 2006;72(2):99-102.

TABLE 4: Some topical sensitizers with corresponding systemic agents that may cross-react with them.

Sensitizing agent	*Possible systemic cross-reactants*
Neomycin	Streptomycin, kanamycin, gentamicin, paromomycin, ambutyrosin
Sulfonamides, para amino benzoic acid, benzocaine, paraphenylenediamine	Thiazide diuretics and antihypertensives; Oral hypoglycemics, e.g., chlorpropamide, tolbutamide, glibenclamide; Sulfonamides; Artificial sweeteners, e.g., saccharin, cyclamates
Phenothiazine antihistamines, e.g., promethazine, methdilazine	Phenothiazine antipsychotics, e.g., chlorpromazine, prochlorperazine, trifluoperazine
Ethylenediamine	Aminophylline, meclizine, hydroxyzine
Dexpanthenol (pro-vitamine B5)	Pantothenic acid, calcium pantothenate
Thiuram	Disulfiram, monosulfiram
Cobalt	Cyanocobalamin (vitamin B_{12})
Balsam of Peru, perfume ingredients	Cinnamon, vanilla, cloves, cola drinks, throat tablets

Source: Adapted from Bajaj AK, Saraswat A. Systemic contact dermatitis. Indian J Dermatol Venereol. 2006;72(2):99-102.

Baboon Syndrome

A clinically distinct type of SCD is termed "baboon syndrome." This refers to the erythema of buttocks and upper inner thighs, reminiscent of the red rump of a baboon. In addition to these sites, the eyelids and other body folds may also be involved and severe cases may show pustules on a background of bright erythema.

Systemic contact dermatitis is an important entity to remember when faced with such diverse conditions as widespread "nonspecific" or "allergic" rashes, extensive eczematous eruptions, vesicular hand eczema, "idiopathic" urticaria, vasculitis, or even erythroderma. The cornerstones of its diagnosis remain the same as in other cases of contact dermatitis: meticulous history taking, thorough examination, and judicious patch testing. Oral provocation may be done in some cases, but only in an inpatient environment and with the understanding that severe reactions may result from this procedure.

Noneczematous Contact Dermatitis

As the name suggests, contact dermatitis develops without eczema. It can be of various types.

Different Types of Noneczematous Contact Dermatitis

- Erythema multiforme-like contact dermatitis
- Purpuric contact dermatitis
- Lichenoid contact dermatitis
- Bullous eruption
- Papular and nodular eruption
- Granulomatous eruption
- Scleroderma-like eruption
- Vascular occlusive contact dermatitis
- Lymphomatoid contact dermatitis
- Pigmented contact dermatitis
- Pustular contact dermatitis
- Dyshidrosiform contact dermatitis

Suspected allergens can be identified by performing patch test and by other patch test variants.

TREATMENT

Avoidance of allergens is a pertinent step when identified. Patient should be given list of common objects containing those allergens and training in avoidance measures. Topical corticosteroids of appropriate potency should be given to provide symptomatic relief. Topical calcineurin inhibitors have also been used. In severe cases, systemic corticosteroids and systemic immunosuppressives may need to be given.

Immunosuppressive Drugs

Methotrexate, azathioprine, cyclosporine, mycophenolate mofetil, and systemic retinoids such as alitretinoin in (chronic hand eczema) can be used depending upon the severity of the dermatitis.

KEY POINTS

- Contact dermatitis is an inflammatory skin condition caused by the interaction of chemicals with the skin.
- Almost 80% of contact dermatitis is irritant and rest is allergic contact dermatitis.
- Patch test is the only scientific tool in the evaluation of allergic contact dermatitis.
- Eczemas which are not responding to the conventional treatment should always be patch tested.
- Testing with patients own material or with unknown substances should be tested as per guidelines.

REFERENCES

1. Marks JG Jr, Anderson BE, DeLeo VA. Contact and Occupational Dermatology. New Delhi: Jaypee Brothers Medical Publishers; 2016.
2. Frosch PJ, Menne T, Lepoittevin JP (Eds). Contact Dermatitis, 4th edition. Heidelberg: Springer; 2006.
3. Veien NK, Svejgaard E, Menne T. In vitro lymphocyte transformation to nickel: a study of nickel sensitive patients before and after epicutaneous and oral challenge with nickel. Acta Derm Venereol (Stockh). 1979;59:447-52.
4. Rodriguez M, Vega F, Garcia MT, Panizo C, Laffond E, Montalvo A, et al. Hypersensitivity to latex, chestnut and banana. Ann Allergy. 1993;70:31-4.
5. Bonamonte D, Foti C, Vestita M, Angelini G. Noneczematous contact dermatitis. ISRN Allergy. 2013;2013:361746.
6. Bajaj AK, Saraswat A. Systemic contact dermatitis. Indian J Dermatol Venereol Leprol. 2006;72:99-102.

EXAMINATION QUESTION

1. What are the differences between irritant and allergic contact dermatitis?

24 CHAPTER Occupational Dermatoses

Sanjay Ghosh, Deblina Bhunia, Kumar Satyaprakash, Barunesh Gautam

INTRODUCTION

Occupational dermatosis denotes any alteration in the skin, mucosa, and annexes, which is direct or indirectly caused, conditioned, maintained, or aggravated by agents present in the occupational activity or work environment.[1]

The types of hazardous exposure may be categorized as:[2]

- *Chemicals*: Organic, inorganic, or protein compounds
- *Mechanical*: Frictions, pressure, and vibration
- *Physical*: Heat, cold, ionizing, and nonionizing radiations
- *Biological*: Bacteria, fungus, virus, and parasites

EPIDEMIOLOGY

Occupational dermatosis is one of the major health problems worldwide. In the Western countries, notification systems exist for occupational dermatoses. Asian countries do not have an established system of reporting these diseases; hence, there is paucity of data. The incidence of various occupational dermatoses depends on the degree of socioeconomic and industrial development in an area, resulting in a lot of geographical variation.[3] The most common occupational dermatosis is contact dermatitis (90–95%).[4]

CLINICAL CLASSIFICATION

- Contact dermatitis
- Chemical burn
- Contact urticaria
- Mechanical injury-related disorders
- Follicular diseases
- Connective tissue disorders
- Foreign body reactions
- Pigmentary disorders
- Hair and nail disorders
- Malignancies
- Infections

Occupational Contact Dermatitis

Occupational contact dermatitis is the most common occupational dermatosis and it predominantly affects the hands. Direct contact with the offending agent is the most common mode of incitation of the dermatitis, but other mechanisms may also be involved. Particulate matter such as dust or smoke, or vapors from volatile substances, may give rise to airborne contact dermatitis, whereas a photocontact dermatitis is induced when a contactant becomes activated by exposure to ultraviolet light **(Table 1)**.[5,6] In the cases of solvents, inhalation may result in widespread dermatitis, sometimes associated with systemic involvements.[2]

Predisposing Factors[5]

- *Age*: Younger workers are more prone due to their less experience and careless attitude toward safety measures.
- *Race*: Skin of most Caucasians are less resistant to the effects of irritants than oriental and black skin.
- *Pre-existing disease*: Atopic individuals.
- *Temperature and humidity*: Under conditions of extreme heat, workers neglect to wear gloves or protective gear. High humidity reduces the effectiveness of the epidermal barrier, while low humidity and cold cause chapping and desiccation of the epidermis.
- *Working condition*: Worksites which are dirty, contaminated with toxic or allergenic chemicals, have obsolete equipment, or lack protective measures. Some workers are at higher risk because they are exposed to strong irritants or allergens (e.g., agricultural workers, construction workers, bakers, hairdressers, cooks, florists, healthcare workers, dental technicians, etc.).

Irritant Contact Dermatitis

Irritant contact dermatitis is a type of inflammatory reaction due to direct cell damage by chemical irritants. Acid and alkalis, soaps and detergents, solvents, petroleum products, and water are common irritants. Most occupational dermatitis results from repeated subthreshold exposure to mild irritants which cause cumulative damage of skin (cumulative irritant contact dermatitis). On the other hand, exposure to potent irritants can elicit acute eczematous dermatitis which may overlap with chemical burns.[6]

Allergic Contact Dermatitis

Occupational allergic contact dermatitis is less common than irritant contact dermatitis. Common allergens are metals (nickel, chrome, cobalt, mercury), rubber additives

TABLE 1: Examples of skin irritants and sensitizers with occupations where contact can occur.[5,6]

Occupation	*Irritants*	*Sensitizers*
Construction workers	Turpentine, thinner, fiberglass, glues, acid, solvents	Chromates, epoxy and phenolic resins, colophony, turpentine, woods, nickel
Farmers, florists, gardeners	Fertilizers, disinfectants, soaps and detergents, pesticides, plants, dust, oils	Plants, woods, fungicides, insecticides
Food handlers, cooks, bakers	Soaps and detergents, vinegar, fruits, vegetables, raw meat and fish, spices, sugar, and flour	Vegetables, spices, garlic, rubber, benzoyl peroxide, sodium metabisulfite (antioxidants for vegetables), formaldehyde
Hairdressers, beauticians	Shampoos, bleach, peroxide, permanent wave, acetone	Paraphenylene diamine in hair dye, ammonium persulfate in bleach, glyceryl monothioglycolate in permanent wave, surfactants in shampoos, nickel, perfume, essential oils, preservatives in cosmetics
Metal workers, machinists and mechanics	Soaps and detergents, oils, petroleum distillates, acids, degreaser, abrasives	Nickel, cobalt, chrome, biocides in cutting oils, hydrazine and colophony in welding flux, epoxy resins and amine catalysts, rubber
Medical personnel	Disinfectants, alcohol, soaps and detergents, medications	Rubber, colophony, formaldehyde, glutaraldehyde, disinfectants, antibiotics, local anesthetics, phenothiazines, benzodiazepines
Dental technicians	Detergents, disinfectants, adhesives, essential oils, orthodontic plasters, amalgam mixtures, solvents	Rubber, epoxy and acrylic monomer, amine catalysts, local anesthetics, mercury, gold, nickel, eugenol, formaldehyde, glutaraldehyde
Printers and photographers	Solvents, acetic acid, ink, acrylic monomer	Nickel, cobalt, chrome, rubber, colophony, formaldehyde, paraphenylene diamine and azo dyes, hydroquinone, epoxy and acrylic monomer, amine catalysts, color developers
Textile workers	Solvents, bleaches, natural and synthetic fibers	Formaldehyde resins, azo- and anthraquinone dyes, rubber, biocides
Painters	Paints, solvents, adhesives, paint removers, paintbrush cleaners, soaps and detergents	Turpentine, thinners, chromium, formaldehyde, epoxy products, polyester resins

(mercaptobenzothiazole, thiurams, carbamates, thioureas), dyes (paraphenylenediamine, photographic color developers, disperse textile dyes), plants (urushiol, sesquiterpene lactones, primin, tulipalin A), plastics (epoxy monomer, acrylic monomer, phenolic resins), biocides (formaldehyde, kathon CG, thimerosal).[5] After initial sensitization, very small amount of allergen is required to induce the dermatitis.

Photocontact Dermatitis

Chemical photosensitivity can occur when a chemical is activated through interaction with light. These photoactivated chemicals can cause direct tissue damage (phototoxic dermatitis) or may induce immunological response (photoallergic dermatitis). Most common occupational photosensitivity is phototoxic in nature and often occurs after exposure to naturally derived psoralens from plants.[2]

Chemical Burn

Chemical burn is irreversible damage of skin with cell death due to contact with acid, alkali, or other chemicals. Common chemicals are acids (sulfuric, nitric, hydrochloric, chromic), alkalis (sodium, potassium, calcium hydroxides; wet concrete, etc.), organic and inorganic chemicals (dichromate, arsenate, phenolic compound), solvents and gases (acrylonitrile, ethylene oxide, carbon disulfide, mustine). Onset is usually acute, but in some chemicals (phenol, weak hydrofluoric acid), reaction may be delayed. Initially, there is pain and burning sensation with progressive development of erythema, blister, erosion, and ulceration.[2]

Contact Urticaria

Contact urticaria is commonly seen among food handlers, agricultural workers, animal laboratory and veterinary workers due to plant or animal-derived proteins. It may be classified as irritant/nonimmune mediated, or allergic/ immune mediated. In some cases, (ammonium persulfate in hairdressers) the mechanism is uncertain. Clinically, it may present with nonspecific symptoms such as pruritus, tingling and burning sensation, or typical urticaria with wheal and flare. Systemic symptoms such as respiratory and gastrointestinal symptoms or anaphylaxis may be associated with immunologically-mediated contact urticaria.[2]

Mechanical Injury-related Skin Disorders

- The effects of trauma are modified by humidity, sweating, age, gender, nutritional status, infection, genetic, and racial factors.[7]
- Slowly increasing friction, pressure may induce callus and blisters, hyperpigmentation, and lichenification.
- Sudden friction or trauma can cause blistering, erosions, and lacerations.
- Repeated trauma increases susceptibility to effects of irritants and allergens.
- Secondary neoplasms may occur at the site of repeated trauma, burn or scar.
- Abrasions and tissue disruption predispose to secondary infection by bacteria or fungi.
- Psoriasis or lichen planus may be aggravated because of the Koebner phenomenon.

- Vibration white finger is associated with exposure to vibrations between 30 and 300 Hz mostly due to increased activity of sympathetic nervous system. There is development of white fingers due to vasospasm in response to cold associated with transient loss of sensation. Operators of chainsaws and pneumatic tools are susceptible to this condition.

Follicular Diseases

Folliculitis, acne, and chloracne are follicular disorders which are caused or aggravated by exposure to certain chemicals.

Common chemicals inducing folliculitis or acne are asphalt, creosote, different oils (e.g., crude, cutting, or lubricating oils), pitch, tar, etc.[8]

Occupational folliculitis is inflammation of hair follicle due to contact with irritants or infection. It commonly affects hair follicles of face, neck, extremities, lower abdomen, and buttocks in workers with heavy soilage.[8] Oil acne and tar acne occurs due to occupational exposure to different industrial oils, pitch, and tar. These chemicals can induce as well as aggravate acne. They can appear both in the usual site for acne and unusual sites such as arms and abdomen where contacts with chemicals occur.[2]

Acne mechanica is a type of inflammatory acne which is exacerbated by repeated frictional trauma that occludes the follicle and it is localized to site of pressure.[2] Acne cosmetica occurs due to contact with certain cosmetic ingredients (e.g., lanolin, petrolatum) used by models or thespians.[2] Chloracne is mostly induced by halogenated hydrocarbons.[8] The lesions are mostly seen over malar crescents and behind the ears. There is predominance of comedones, which may be accompanied by cystic lesions and hypertrichosis.[2]

Connective Tissue Disorders

Systemic sclerosis or scleroderma-like conditions are common occupational exposure-associated connective tissue disorder.

Chemicals inducing systemic sclerosis are silica, chlorinated or aromatic hydrocarbons. Scleroderma-like condition may be induced by plastics (vinyl chloride, epoxy resins), solvents (chlorinated, aromatic, aliphatic hydrocarbons, pesticides), drugs (e.g., bleomycin, pentazocine), and others (aniline and fatty acid, paraffin, silicon). Persons with enhanced genetic susceptibility are predisposed to these disorders.[7]

Persons working in mining industry or underground workplaces are predisposed to silica exposure.

Silica-induced systemic sclerosis is almost similar to classical disease, characterized by progression and remission. Once silica is incorporated in body, it cannot be removed and its deleterious effects are unavoidable.[7]

Scleroderma-like disorders are differentiated from idiopathic scleroderma by the following features:[7]

- Types of skin manifestations such as acrosclerosis, morpheaform plaques, fibrotic nodules, or joint contracture
- Visceral involvement of liver, kidney, nervous system, and muscles
- Laboratory findings—absent autoantibodies, discrete thrombocytopenia
- Cessation or reversal of the disease process following early discontinuation of exposure
- Female preponderance, which is common in idiopathic scleroderma, is often not observed in occupation-associated disorder.

Silica exposure has also been reported with the development of other connective tissue disorders such as lupus erythematosus, Sjögren's syndrome, dermatomyositis, and rheumatoid arthritis.

Foreign Body Reactions

A number of insoluble, nondegradable, and slowly released substances may give rise to a foreign-body granulomatous reaction when they are penetrated into the skin.

These substances include wood, silk, nylon, paraffin, silicon, talcum powder, starch, oils, animal and vegetable spines or bristles, vaccine, and human hair.[7]

Histologically, two types of granuloma may be seen: the more frequent foreign-body granuloma and another is allergic granuloma. This contact allergic granulomatous reaction has been described in subjects sensitized to zirconium, beryllium, and some tattoo colorants.

A foreign-body granuloma may transform into an allergic skin granuloma when the etiologic agent remains in the lesion for some time and behaves as an allergen.[7]

Pigmentary Disorders

Occupationally-induced hyperpigmentation may result from an antecedent inflammatory dermatosis or infections, physical causes, exposure to excessive sunlight, chemical photosensitivity, and other nonphotosensitive chemical exposures.[7]

Occupational causes of hypopigmentation are physical agents (X-rays, UV rays, ionizing radiations), mechanical trauma, burn, postinflammatory hypopigmentation, specific chemical leukoderma. Chemical leukoderma is caused by various chemicals such as phenol/catechol derivatives (e.g., hydroquinone and its derivatives), metals (arsenic, mercurial), etc.[7]

Hair and Nail Disorders

Occupation-related increased shedding of hair and alopecia may occur due to following causative factors:[9]

- *Physical*: Trauma (by caps or strings worn for longer time), burns, and radiations (radiology technicians)

- *Chemical*: Thallium (glass, firework industries), boric acid (glass, nuclear industries), chloroprene (tyre manufacturing)
- *Biological*: Tuberculosis, tinea capitis (medical professionals)
- *Pharmacological*: Coumarin (rat pesticides), colchicine (lily bulb)

Occupational nail disorders may occur due to physical (trauma, burn, cold, ionizing radiations, foreign bodies, vibrating tools, etc.), chemical (alkali, acid, dyes, metals), or biological (bacteria, fungus) factors. Common nail changes include discoloration of nail units, nail dystrophy, Beau's line, onycholysis, nail shedding, koilonychia, ridging, subungual hemorrhage, paronychia, and pterygium depending upon the nature of insult.[7]

Malignancies

- Common inciting factors for occupational malignancies are arsenic, polycyclic hydrocarbons, ultraviolet and ionizing radiations, burn, repeated trauma.[10]
- Basal cell carcinoma, squamous cell carcinoma, and malignant melanoma are common occupation-related skin malignancies.
- Exposure to sun, ionizing radiations, and chemical carcinogens such as tar are predisposing factors for basal cell carcinoma.[10]
- Squamous cell carcinoma may be related to exposure to sunlight or other sources of irradiation, including localized heat. Scarring from a variety of causes such as burn, trauma, and chemical carcinogens including coal tar products are other predisposing factors.[10]
- Outdoor workers who have sustained repeated episodes of severe sunburn might be at risk of malignant melanoma.[10]
- Premalignant occupational exposure-related disorders are actinic keratosis, arsenical keratosis, tar keratosis, Bowen's disease, keratoacanthoma, lentigo maligna, etc.[10]

Infections

Infections which are acquired at workplaces may be transmitted via direct contact, inhalation, ingestion, inoculation of the organism, or by arthropod bites **(Table 2)**.

TABLE 2: Workers with risk of occupational infection.[2,11]

Worker group	*Occupational infection/infectious agents*
Healthcare worker	HIV, hepatitis B, tuberculosis, SARS
Veterinary and farm workers	Cryptosporidiosis, leptospirosis, *Salmonella* infections, Q fever, rabies, anthrax, schistosomiasis, dermatophytosis
Abattoir worker	Nipah virus, *Streptococcus suis*, trichinosis, Q fever
Rice farmers	Melioidosis, "sawah itch"
Forestry workers, forest rangers	Lyme disease, plague, rabies
Miners, sandblasters, grinders, stone cutters, quarry workers, ceramic and foundry workers	Silicotuberculosis
Construction workers	Histoplasmosis
Military personnel	Biological warfare agents such as smallpox, anthrax, and plague
Sex workers	Sexually transmitted diseases
Sewer workers	Leptospirosis, hantavirus infection, hepatitis A, gastrointestinal pathogens

(HIV: human immunodeficiency virus; SARS: severe acute respiratory syndrome)

DIAGNOSIS

Clinical

Most occupational dermatoses are diagnosed by:

- Typical clinical symptoms of the disorders
- History of occupational exposure, the concurrence between the onset of symptoms and the start of exposure, as well as the localization of lesions in areas exposed to suspected agents
- Improvement with avoidance of the inciting factors or workplaces and aggravation upon return to work.

Laboratory

- Patch test is most important test to determine the causative factor in case of allergic contact dermatitis.
- Microbiological investigations are required to diagnose infective diseases.
- Skin biopsy and histopathological examinations are often required to confirm diagnosis.
- Biochemical analysis of blood, urine, hair, and nails may be required for detection of occupational exposure to certain chemicals.

PREVENTION AND MANAGEMENT

Identification of occupational hazards and taking appropriate protective measures are necessary to prevent occupational disease.

The primary preventive measures are:

- Substitution of hazardous working materials
- Technical measures such as use of encapsulated machines or automated cleaning equipment
- Organizational measures, e.g., divide tasks, longer buffer zones to allow drying of equipment and materials
- Individual protective wear (gloves) and special protective skin care
- Selecting suitable individual for work
- Training regarding safety measures

When symptoms are already manifested, early detection of disease, its treatment, and prompt initiation of preventive measures are necessary.

In clinically severe and/or chronic occupational diseases, where the aforesaid measures are inadequate, discontinuation of the activity may be required.

KEY POINTS

- Contact dermatitis is the most common occupational dermatosis.
- Identification can easily be done by medical inspection during heath surveillance.
- Identification of hazardous agents and taking appropriate protective measures are necessary to prevent occupational dermatosis.
- Occupational dermatoses are mostly diagnosed clinically by their typical presentation and temporal relationship with the exposure to the inciting factors and onset of the disease; sometimes aided with few laboratory tests.
- Early diagnosis and treatment are important objectives in the management of these diseases. Discontinuation of the occupation may be required in severe and chronic cases.
- Patch testing is useful to diagnose the causative agents in occupational allergic contact dermatitis and avoidance of those allergens can prevent it.

REFERENCES

1. Alchorne AO, Alchorne MM, Silva MM. Occupational dermatosis. An Bras Dermatol. 2010;85:137-45.
2. Wilkinson SM. Occupational Dermatoses. In: Bolognia JL, Jorizzo JL, Rapini RP (Eds). Dermatology, 3rd edition. London: Elsevier Saunders; 2012. pp. 261-72.
3. Bhatia R, Sharma VK. Occupational dermatoses: An Asian perspective. Indian J Dermatol Venereol Leprol. 2017;83: 525-35.
4. Diepgen TL. Occupational skin diseases. J Dtsch Dermatol Ges. 2012;10:297-313.
5. ILO (2011). Encyclopaedia on Occupational Health and Safety, 4th edition. Geneva: International Labour Organization; 2011. [online] Available from: http://www.ilocis.org/en/contilo.html [Last accessed January, 2021].
6. Honary G, Tailor JS, Sood A. Occupational skin diseases due to irritants and allergens. In: Goldsmith LA, Katz SI, Gilchrest B, Paller AS, Leffell DJ, Wolff K (Eds). Fitzpatrick's Dermatology in General Medicine, 8th edition. New York: McGraw Hill; 2008. pp. 2611-22.
7. Kanerva L, Elsner P, Wahlberg JE, Maibach HI (Eds). Handbook of Occupational Dermatology. Berlin: Springer; 2000. pp. 135-313.
8. Cohen DE, Moore MM. Occupational skin disease. In: Rom WN, Markowitz SB (Eds). Environmental and Occupational Medicine, 4th edition. Philadelphia, PA: Lippincott-Williams & Wilkins; 2007. pp. 617-39.
9. Frati C, Bevilacqua B, Battisti MG, Pizzutelli G. Occupational alopecia in various workers after exposure to chemical agents. Acta Dermatovenerologica Alpina Pannonica et Adriatica. 1993;2:124-6.
10. Gawkrodger DJ. Occupational skin cancers. Occup Med. 2004;54:458-63.
11. Lim VK. Occupational infections. Malays J Pathol. 2009;31: 1-9.

EXAMINATION QUESTIONS

1. Describe different types of occupational contact dermatitis.
2. Describe preventive measures and management of occupational diseases.

25 CHAPTER Plant Dermatoses

CR Srinivas, Smitha Prabhu S

INTRODUCTION

Plant dermatitis is not uncommon and constitutes upto 6–8% of occupational dermatoses, and 5–10% of all dermatitis cases. The causative plants and pattern of dermatitis may vary depending upon geographic area.

Plant dermatitis can be occupational or nonoccupational.

The different types of dermatitis have been shown in **Table 1**.

People at risk: Agriculturists, gardeners, florists, horticulturists, vegetable vendors, home makers, nature walk enthusiasts, cooks, and salad makers.

Though an estimated 400,000 species of plants exist on earth, most dermatitis-inducing plants belong to a few families such as Alliacae, Anacardiaceae, Cactaceae, Compositae, Cruciferae, Hennadiaceae, Lilliaceae, Orchidaceae, Primulaceae, Urticaceae, and most sensitizers are chemicals related to catechols and lactones.

Plants can cause dermatitis by many mechanisms:

- Trauma induced by their sharp parts like thorns, spines, leaf edges, microtrauma by bristles, barbs or calcium oxalate crystals which penetrate skin and disrupt dermoepidermal junction, thereby also enabling the allergens to penetrate and cause allergic contact dermatitis in addition.

TABLE 1: Types of dermatitis.

Type of reaction	*Mechanism*	*Causative plants*	*Pattern*
Nonimmunological contact urticaria	Direct degranulation of mast cell releasing histamine	Nettle, Balsam of Peru, Capsicum	Urticaria
Immunological contact urticaria	IgE-mediated mast cell degranulation. May also generalize, or involve conjunctiva, nasal mucosa or lungs	Fruits and vegetables, *Birch*, rubber	Urticaria, conjunctivitis, rhinitis, asthma
Protein contact dermatitis	In atopics, food handlers.	Onion, lettuce, potato, carrot	Contact urticaria, along with worsening of previous hand dermatitis
Irritant contact dermatitis: • Macrotrauma (spines, thorns) • Microtrauma (bristles) • Chemical irritation → acute or chronic	• Due to spines, thorns → granulomatous reaction • Trichromes glochids, raphides → dermoepidermal penetration of sap → irritant or allergic contact dermatitis	• Cacti, rose • Agave, tubers • Primula, toxicodendron (Poison ivy), marking nut, onion, garlic, cashew	Dryness, cracking, hyperkeratosis, acute edema, vesicles, oozing; Dermatitis usually limited to site of contact
Allergic contact dermatitis (ACD): • Acute ACD • Chronic ACD • Erythema multiforme-like ACD • Airborne contact dermatitis	Delayed type hypersensitivity reaction mediated by T-lymphocytes and their cytokines • Due to air borne oleoresins	• Tulip, narcissus, garlic • Primula, Toxicodendron, pyrethrum, rosewood • *Parthenium, Chromolaena, Pyrethrum*, other Compositae plants	Initially limited to site of contact, later diffuse Maculopapular or vesicular lesions, rarely full blown erythroderma • Fingertip eczema with painful fissuring • Dermatitis with confluent cockades pattern • Dermatitis involving flexures, creases, and exposed areas
Phytophoto dermatitis: • Phytophototoxicity (dermatosis bullosa striata pratensis; meadow dermatitis) • Phytophotoallergy—very rare	Phytophotoallergy is very rare, It is often sunlight induced worsening of ACD	• Asteracea/Umbillifera family • Furocoumarins/psoralens • Fluoroquinolones • Bergamot • Parthenium, psoralens	Linear, figurate, vesiculobullous lesions on sun exposed areas, often heal with hyperpigmentation

Contd...

Contd...

Type of reaction	*Mechanism*	*Causative plants*	*Pattern*
Chronic actinic dermatitis/ persistent light reaction/ actinic reticuloid	Initial contact sensitization progresses to a generalized photosensitivity that persists throughout the year	• Oleoresins • Sesquiterpene lactones, especially Compositae plants	Extensive dermatitis and lichenification, often erythroderma
Pseudophytodermatitis (due to contaminants and insects on plants)	Allergic or irritant, depending on the cause	• Insecticides • Pesticides • Arthropods (e.g., hay itch mite) • Contaminant fungus • Micuim larvae • Sporotrichosis • Paracoccidioidomycosis	Pruriginic maculopapular rash

This is commonly seen with plants like rose, orange and lemon trees, *Bougainvillea*, and cactus.

- Chemical irritant dermatitis is caused by sesquiterpene lactones (cashew), marking nut, etc.
- Urticaria can be induced by nettle, quince
- IgE-mediated contact urticarial can be evoked by celery, pineapple, mango (or almost any plant)
- Acute allergic contact dermatitis (ACD) as well as chronic ACD are seen in the form of painful fissuring and erythema of fingertips (tulip, daffodil, narcissus, garlic). Parthenium, a Compositae plant, which is rampant in India is notorious to cause airborne-contact dermatitis.

Approach to a Suspected Case of Plant Dermatitis

Thorough history taking pertaining to occupation, activities, hobbies, gardening, evening walks, new furniture, or wood work is essential.

Clinical examination should be performed to ascertain the morphology and pattern of dermatitis, like whether localized to hands, photo-exposed sites, whether generalized, acute or chronic lichenified.

Patch test can be performed with readymade plant series, or with suspected indigenous plants pulverized with acetone, ethanol, or petrolatum. Care should be taken when plants are used, as often these can be irritants at relatively higher concentrations and allergens at very low concentrations. Plant series of patch test allergens are shown in **Table 2**.

Photopatch test may be attempted in suspected cases.

Management consists of avoidance of the causative plant, photoprotection, and use of topical or oral steroids, depending upon the intensity and extent of dermatitis.

TABLE 2: Plant series of patch test allergens.

Chemotechnique diagnostics	*Manipal battery of plant allergens*
Anthemis nobilis extract 1.0% pet	*Parthenium hysterophorus* 1%, 3% pet
Diallyl disulfide 1.0% pet	*Chromolaena odoratum* 5%, 10% pet
Arnica montana extract 0.5% pet	*Holigarna ferruginea* 10% pet
Taraxacum officinale extract 2.5% pet	*Smithia salsuginea* 10% in 95% ethanol base
Achillea millefolium extract 1.0% pet	*Geissaspis cristata* 10% in 95% ethanol base
Propolis 10.0% pet	*Ischaemum indicum* 10% in 95% ethanol base
Chrysanthemum cinerariaefolium extract 1.0% pet	*Hopea ponga* 10% in 95% ethanol base
Sesquiterpene lactone mix 0.1% pet	*Vanilla planifolia* 10% in 95% ethanol base
Alfa-methylene-gamma-butyrolactone 0.01% pet	*Oryza sativa* 10% in 95% ethanol base
Tanacetum vulgare extract 1.0% pet	Sesquiterpene lactone mix (SLM)
Alantolactone 0.033% pet	
Lichen acid mix 0.3% pet	
Parthenolide 0.1% pet	
Chamomilla recutita extract 1.0% pet	
(+) Usnic acid 0.1% pet	
Atranorin 0.1% pet	
Evernic acid 0.1% pet	

PLANT DERMATITIS IN INDIA

Compositae dermatitis is the most common plant dermatitis in India represented by *Parthenium* dermatitis; other plants include *Chrysanthemum, Dahlia, Toxicodendron, Nerium variabilis, Lantana camara, Tradescantia, Calotropis procera, Argemone mexicana, Cynodon dactylon, Azadirachta indica, Acacia nilotica*, Ficus, Hibiscus, *Arborvitae*, Silver Oak, and *Bougainvillea*.

Parthenium Dermatitis

Parthenium hysterophorus (syn: bitterweed/feverfew/congress grass, family Asteraceae of Compositae plants) was introduced to India by the US Congress in the 1950s, and grew rampant, first detected in Pune by Lonikar, but later spread to other parts.

Parthenium dermatitis is mainly a T-cell mediated delayed type hypersensitivity disorder, with an early sensitization, and a later elicitation phase. Pathogenesis is similar to allergic contact dermatitis with antigen presentation by Langerhans cells and dendritic cells which take the plant particles to regional lymph nodes, where it is presented to T-cells with further proliferation and production of effector and memory T-cells, which infiltrate the re-exposed skin resulting in inflammation and visible dermatitis. Additional type I immediate hypersensitivity is also postulated for initiation and perpetuation of parthenium dermatitis, especially in atopics. It also causes allergic rhinitis and asthma in susceptible individuals.

Allergens of parthenium: Sesquiterpene lactones (SQLs), namely, *parthenin, ambrosin,* coronophillin, tetraneurin A, hymenin are implicated which are chiefly present in trichomes, dried leaves, pollen, and stem.

Patient profile: Middle-aged men, agriculturists, and outdoor workers.

Parthenium allergy manifests in diverse clinical forms **(Table 3)**, though initial presentation is invariably intense pruritus with erythema, vesiculation, and crusting, which later becomes lichenified and chronic, and may slowly progress to involve unexposed areas. As the condition progresses, there is a general tendency to evolve from air borne pattern to chronic actinic dermatitis pattern, which may persist lifelong with exacerbations and remissions.

Photosensitivity and parthenium dermatitis: SQLs are not photosensitizers, and do not have phototoxicity or photoallergy, though there is photoaggravation with parthenium. There are reports of reduction in MED to UVB and MPD to UVA in people with parthenium dermatitis. In people with chronic actinic dermatitis due to parthenium, there is reduced sensitivity to UVA and UVB.

Diagnosis:
- *Patch test with parthenium 5–15%:* Any part of the plant to be extracted with acetone
- *Prick test with parthenium:* Immediate reaction at 15–20 minutes as well as late reaction at 24–48 hours to be noted
- RAST (Radio-allergo-sorbent test) is less sensitive, not routinely done.
- Histopathology is nonspecific and shows dermatitis in varying severities.

Management

Management of parthenium dermatitis has been shown in **Table 4**.

TABLE 4: Management of parthenium dermatitis.

General measures	*Specific treatment*
• Removal of plant from vicinity, regular deweeding of garden • Adequate protection by clothes, shawl, mask, cap • Wash exposed area with soap and water at the earliest • Use barrier cream and sunscreens • Drying of clothes indoors • Keep doors and windows closed • Air conditioning of residence	*Topical* (mild-to-moderate cases)—topical steroids, tacrolimus, pimecrolimus, barrier creams, moisturizers *Systemic:* • *Corticosteroids:* Topical in mild-to-moderate cases, systemic in severe and extensive cases (starting with 0.5–1 mg/kg of prednisolone, tapering within 3–4 months) • Azathioprine 1–2 mg/kg/day • Cyclosporine 2–3 mg/kg/day • Methotrexate 15 mg/week • PUVA/NB-UVB • Oral hyposensitization

TABLE 3: Diverse clinical forms of parthenium allergy.

Type	*Morphology*	*Areas involved*
Allergic contact dermatitis	Erythema, edema, papules, papulovesicles, oozing crusting → chronic lichenified dermatitis	Dermatitis over sites of contact
Air borne contact dermatitis (ABCD)	Erythema, scaling, papules, and plaques	Eyelids, face, neck, retroauricular, V area of chest, cubital, and popliteal fossae
Chronic actinic dermatitis (CAD)	Lichenified papules plaques, nodules	Lichenified papules, plaques or nodules on sun-exposed sites, Leonine facies
Erythroderma	Erythema and scaling, lichenification	Generalized, >90% BSA
Hand and feet dermatitis	Erythema, scaling, crusting, vesiculation, lichenification	Mostly confined to dorsae of hands and feet
Mixed pattern dermatitis	Scattered infiltrated papuloplaques on exposed parts along with dermatitis over eyelids, neck and flexures	Combination of ABCD and CAD
Photosensitive lichenoid dermatitis	Discrete, flat, violaceous papules, and plaques	Sun-exposed areas
Other types: Pseudo-phytodermatitis Prurigo like lesions, lichenoid type, seborrheic type, atopic type, vesicular hand eczema, lichen nitidus like perianal dermatitis		Site and morphology specific

Azathioprine in Parthenium Dermatitis

It works well by inhibiting T-lymphocytes. It is immunosuppressive, anti-inflammatory, and is used as steroid-sparing agent. Treatment to be continued for 6–12 months past remission.

Pretreatment tests: Thiopurine methyl transferase (TPMT) level estimation - if levels low, there is increased hematopoietic toxicity with azathioprine as its thioguanine nucleotide metabolites accumulate

Complete blood count (CBC), liver function test(LFT), renal function test (RFT): CBC and LFT to be monitored at monthly intervals.

Various schedules:

- Daily dose of 50–100 mg
- Monthly bolus of 300 mg (along with daily dose)
- Pulse azathioprine (weekly 300 mg)

Major side effects: GI intolerance, hepatic dysfunction, bone marrow suppression

Cyclosporine (2–3 mg/kg/day): Potent anti-inflammatory effect, quicker onset of action, suppresses acute phase reactions as well as delayed hypersensitivity. Side effects include hypertension and renal toxicity.

Oral hyposensitization—proposed mechanism is depletion of T-cells without causing frank dermatitis, but has many drawbacks including inconsistency of results, exacerbation of dermatitis, cheilitis, and gastritis.

Immunotherapy with recombinant hybrid proteins containing epitopes from different allergens in a single molecule is under trial.

Biological control of parthenium: This is as important as treatment of the patient so as to prevent further exposure, and is theoretically possible by use of plant eating beetle, using fungal pathogens such as *Ascomycotina, Sphaerotheca, Alternaria, Fusarium* spp., etc. for biocontrol, antagonistic plants, and bioherbicides such as *Cassia uniflora* (Leguminosae), marigold, and use of herbicides; however, Parthenium is a tough plant to eliminate, and grows tenaciously despite hard attempts at eradication.

Other plants of Compositae family include American ragweed, Arnica, Pyrethrum, tansy, Chrysanthemum, sunflower, marigold, dandelion, lettuce, safflower, liver wort, and magnolia. Parthenium and rag weed are shown to cross react, whereas Xanthium, Helianthus and Chrysanthemum, which are other common Compositae seen in India do not cross react with Parthenium, though a person can be sensitized to all four at the same time.

Cashew and mango: These contain SQLs which cause irritant contact dermatitis, which is seen in perioral area if the fruits are consumed, especially raw, and in the fingertips and hands of workers in cashew industry. Occupational dermatoses in cashew workers is well-documented and consists of cauterization type reaction with thickened pigmented skin on areas of contact, with thickened discolored nails, maceration, pits and loss of dermatoglyphics in those who are exposed to cashew shell oil.

Allergic contact dermatitis in up to 30% of tulip and saffron workers of Kashmir valley, especially finger tips and hands is well documented. The term tulip fingers denote fissured hyperkeratotic dermatitis, sometimes with paronychia, more predominant in the dominant hand of tulip workers.

Other than exposure in the natural media, plant products incorporated in daily use articles and substances can cause dermatitis as exemplified in the **Table 5**.

TABLE 5: Dermatitis caused by plant products incorporated in daily use articles.

Turpentine	Pine trees
Balsam	Balsam of Peru, Canada balsam, Chinese lacquer
Perfumes, creams and cosmetics	Amyris, jasmine, eucalyptus, narcissus, aloe vera, rose, lavender, calendula, arnica, Lawsonia, jojoba, tea tree, geranium, citrus, eugenol, isoeugenol, cinnamaldehyde, colophony
Food additives	Vanilla, lavender, mint, cinnamon
Wooden furniture	Teak, oak
Medicaments	Eucalyptus, lemon grass, Citronella, psoralens, witch hazel bark
Alta	Betel, lac
Clothing	Cotton, hemp, jute
Rubber footwear, gloves	Latex from rubber tree

KEY POINTS

- Though there are more than 400,000 plants on the earth, only a few families of plants such as *Alliacae, Anacardiaceae, Cactaceae, Compositae, Cruciferae, Hennadiaceae, Lilliaceae, Orchidaceae, Primulaceae, Urticaceae* are responsible for dermatitis.
- Catechols and lactones are the responsible chemicals.
- Plants can cause dermatitis by various mechanisms such as micro- and macrotrauma, via chemicals, IgE-mediated urticarial and angioedema, allergic, and irritant dermatitis
- Types of plant dermatitis include urticarial, angioedema, contact urticaria, protein contact dermatitis, allergic and irritant contact dermatitis, airborne contact dermatitis, and photodermatitis.
- Parthenium is the most common plant causing dermatitis in India, others include *Chromolaena, Chrysanthemum, Dahlia, Cashew*.

REFERENCES

1. Sharma VK, Verma P. Parthenium dermatitis in India: Past, present and future. Indian J Dermatol Venereol Leprol. 2012; 78:560-8.

2. Lakshmi C, Srinivas CR. Parthenium the terminator: An update. Indian Dermatol Online J. 2012;3:89-100.
3. Lakshmi C, Srinivas CR. Type I hypersensitivity to Parthenium hysterophorus in patients with parthenium dermatitis. Indian J Dermatol Venereol Leprol. 2007;73:103-5.
4. Jerath VP, Jerath P, Sood M, Nishchal R. Immunotherapy in parthenium dermatitis. Indian J Allergy Asthma Immunol. 2014;28:83-5.
5. Davis SV, Shenoi SD, Prabhu S, Shirwaiker A, Balachandran C. Clinical evaluation of patients patch tested with plant series: A prospective study. Indian J Dermatol. 2011;56:383-8.
6. Sharma SC, Kaur S. Air borne contact dermatitis from Compositae plants in Northern India. Contact Derm. 1989; 21:1-5.
7. Reis Vitor Manoel Silva dos. Dermatosis due to plants (phytodermatosis). An Bras Dermatol. 2010;85(4):479-89.
8. Hassan I, Kamili A, Rasool F, Nehvi F, Rather P, Yasmeen S, et al. Contact dermatitis in saffron workers: Clinical profile and identification of contact sensitizers in a saffron-cultivating area of Kashmir Valley of North India. Dermatitis. 2015;26:136-41.
9. Hassan I, Rasool F, Akhtar S, Kamili A, Rather P, Kanth R, et al. Contact dermatitis caused by tulips: Identification of contact sensitizers in tulip workers of Kashmir valley in North India. Contact Dermatitis. 2017;78:64-9.
10. Lakshmi C, Srinivas CR. Parthenium: A wide angle view. Indian J Dermatol Venereol Leprol. 2007;73:296-306.
11. Srinivas CR, Balachandran C, Shenoi SD, Acharya S. Azathioprine in the treatment of Parthenium dermatitis. Br J Dermatol. 1991;124:394-5.
12. Srinivas CR. Parthenium dermatitis treated with azathioprine weekly pulse doses. Indian J Dermatol Venereol Leprol. 2006;72:234.
13. Verma KK, Sethuraman G, Kalavani M. Weekly azathioprine pulse versus daily azathioprine in the treatment of Parthenium dermatitis: A non-inferiority randomized controlled study. Indian J Dermatol Venereol Leprol. 2015;81:251-6.
14. Lakshmi C, Srinivas CR, Jayaraman A. Ciclosporin in parthenium dermatitis—a report of 2 cases. Contact Dermatitis. 2008;59:245-8.
15. Nandakishore T, Pasricha JS. Pattern of cross-sensitivity between 4 Compositae plants, Parthenium hysterophorus, Xanthium strumarium, Helianthus annuus and Chrysanthemum coronarium, in Indian patients. Contact Dermatitis. 1994;30:162-7.
16. Pasricha JS, Srinivas CR, Krupashanker DS, Shenoy K, Subba Rao PV, Singh KK. Occupational dermatoses among the cashew nut workers in Karnataka. Ind J Dermatol Venereol Leprol. 1988;54:15-20.

EXAMINATION QUESTION

1. Illustrate phytophotodermatosis and its management.

26 CHAPTER

Photodermatitis

Sathish Pai B, Sudhir Nayak UK

INTRODUCTION

Photodermatitis encompasses a group of skin diseases characterized by inflammation of skin due to sun exposure. Photodermatitis is a type of contact dermatitis caused by exposure of ultraviolet (UV) irradiation and is characterized by erythema, edema on the photoexposed areas with relative sparing of the photo-covered areas.

The ultraviolet spectrum comprises UVC (200–290 nm), UVB (290–320 nm), and UVA (320–390 nm). The visible spectrum exists from 390 to 700 nm and is occasionally implicated in photodermatitis.

Photodermatitis is usually subclassified into phototoxic reactions, photoallergic reactions, and phytophotodermatitis.

Phototoxic dermatitis (PTD) are nonimmunologic-mediated reactions on the skin caused by interaction of UV light with photosensitizing substances.

Photoallergic dermatitis (PAD), on the other hand, are immunologically mediated reactions on the skin which are caused by interaction of UV light with photosensitizing substances.

Sometimes, a single compound can cause both PAD and PTD, and clinically also it may be impossible to differentiate between both.

The differences between phototoxic dermatitis and photoallergic dermatitis are given in **Table 1**.

Phytophotodermatitis is a type of PTD caused by exposure to phototoxic substances present in plants, fruits, or vegetables followed by sunlight exposure. Some of the substances implicated in causing this include lime, lemon, celery, parsley, and figs. Usually present as linear streaks of lesions which may be erythema, vesicles or even bullae and subsequently heals with hyperpigmentation. Burning sensation is reported rather than itch. Photochemotherapy with psoralens is an example of therapeutic phytophotodermatitis. Berloque dermatitis is a type of phytophotodermatitis due to 5-methoxypsoralen (Bergapten) present in perfumes. Washing of the exposed area after contact with suspected plants is recommended.

All dermatitis occurring in a photodistribution are not a photodermatitis. For example, allergic contact dermatitis (ACD) to sunscreens which are applied on sunexposed areas may be mistaken for photodermatitis. Concomitant airborne contact dermatitis (ABCD), ACD, and extreme photosensitivity may lead to the involvement of photoprotected regions.

Chronic actinic dermatitis (CAD) is a rare idiopathic and chronic photodermatosis seen in elderly males which is characterized clinically by persistent eczematous eruptions on the photoexposed parts, chronic dermatitis (with or without lymphomatous changes) on histopathology and a reduced minimal erythema dose (MED) to UVB and occasionally to UVA.[2,3] The pathogenesis is not clearly understood. Immunological delayed hypersensitivity mechanism by cytotoxic CD8+ T-cells to photo-induced endogenous antigen or a persistent exogenous photosensitizer **(Table 2)**.

Sites involved: Face, neck, V-area of chest, extensors of forearms, dorsa of hands, and feet

Areas spared on face: Creases, upper eyelid, nasolabial fold, below lower lip, submental region, and retroauricular region. In the forearms, the extensor and lateral sides are more affected with relative sparing of flexor and medial aspects of forearms and cubital fossa. The upper limbs usually show a clear demarcation from the line where the garment stops.

TABLE 1: Differences between phototoxic dermatitis and photoallergic dermatitis.

	Phototoxic dermatitis	*Photoallergic dermatitis*
Type of reaction	Direct tissue injury	Type IV hypersensitivity reaction
Population predisposed	All	
Incidence[1]	7–15%	4–8%
Occurrence on first exposure	Yes	No
Concentration of substance required	High	Low
Irradiation type[1]	Usually UVA	Usually UVA
Clinical picture	Exaggerated sunburn like	Allergic contact dermatitis like
Onset	Short—minutes to hours	1–2 days
Implicated drug	Usually systemic drugs	Usually topical drugs
Histopathology	Necrotic keratinocytes	Dermatitis like
Cross reaction	No	Yes

(UVA: ultraviolet A)

TABLE 2: Clinical variants of CAD.[3]

Type	Characteristic
Actinic reticuloid	• Infiltrated erythematous/reticuloid plaques on erythematous/eczematous/normal skin • *Histopathology*: Resembles cutaneous lymphoma • *Photopatch test*: Usually normal
Persistent light reaction	Eczema on photoexposed areas which persists in spite of removal of causative agent
Photosensitive dermatitis	Eczema with photosensitivity to both UVA and UVB spectra
Photosensitive eczema	Eczema with photosensitivity to UVB spectrum alone

(CAD: chronic actinic dermatitis; UVA: ultraviolet A; UVB: ultraviolet B)

Areas spared on face in photodermatitis and involved in airborne contact dermatitis: upper eyelid, nasolabial folds, facial grooves, submental area, retroauricular region. A small triangular area behind the ear lobe called as Wilkinson's triangle is spared in photodermatitis.

Other areas which can give clue to photodermatitis are:

- Balding scalp usually involved
- *Finger and toe webspaces*: Usually spared

Although photodermatitis is bilateral, it can be unilateral in certain instances such as people sitting in offices with one side of the body next to the window, people driving in cars with windows down with the same side being exposed on both to-and-fro journey like on north to south drive every day, and the passenger side being exposed to sunlight on their left side during morning as well as evening.

Drugs associated with phototoxic contact dermatitis: Diuretics (furosemide, thiazides), antiarrhythmic drugs (amiodarone, quinidine), psoralens, antibiotics (quinolones, demeclocycline, doxycycline, sulfonamides), nonsteroidal anti-inflammatory drugs (NSAIDs), and phenothiazines.[1,3,4]

Drugs associated with photoallergic contact dermatitis: Sunscreens, fragrances, antiseptics (chlorhexidine, hexachlorophene), NSAIDs, phenothiazines, griseofulvin.[1,3]

HISTOPATHOLOGY[5]

Phototoxic reaction: Necrotic keratinocytes, sparse dermal infiltrate. In severe PTD, intraepidermal/subepidermal split may be seen.

Photoallergic: Spongiosis, exocytosis, superficial perivascular lymphohistiocytoses. Deep perivascular eosinophilic infiltrate is seen in systemic PAD. In chronic PAD, spongiosis decreases and acanthosis increases.

INVESTIGATIONS

Patch test: Basically to rule out contact dermatitis mimicking photodermatitis.

TABLE 3: Interpretation of results.

Irradiated side	Nonirradiated side	Interpretation
+	–	Photoallergy
+	+	Contact allergy
++	+	Contact allergy and photoallergy

Photopatch test: Allergens are applied in duplicate on either side of the back. Reading is taken after 48 hours as per the International Contact Dermatitis Research Group (ICDRG) guidelines. Then one side is covered with an opaque material and other side is irradiated with 15 J/cm^2 of UVA irradiation. This is then covered. Both sides are again read after 24 and 48 hours of irradiation.

The interpretation of results is given in **Table 3**.

MED detection: An opaque template with multiple windows is kept on the back and increasing doses of UVB are delivered through the windows and reading taken after 24 hours. Usually, MED is defined as dose of UVB needed to produce just perceptible erythema. MED is usually reduced in CAD in comparison to ABCD.

Biopsy: Rarely biopsy may be needed to rule out malignancy (cutaneous T-cell lymphoma) in long-standing CAD.

MANAGEMENT

Detailed history and clinical examination is a must.

Avoidance of any offending drug: A detailed history on the use of any drug likely to cause photodermatitis must be elicited. Over the counter medication, herbal, and alternative medications need to be asked specifically.

Substitution of offending drug-by-drug without any photosensitizing property can be done. Essential medications such as antihypertensive medications with photosensitizing properties need to be substituted by other nonphotosensitizing drugs.

Patient education on photoprotective measures. Simple day-to-day modifications in lifestyle alterations can significantly reduce the recurrence of photodermatitis. The patient education measures are given in **Box 1**.

UV index (UVI): It is a means of informing general public on the ambient erythemal UV irradiation at a given place. It ranges from 1 to 11+; any score >3 requires photoprotection for fair-skinned individuals.[6]

Sun-protective clothing: In western countries such as Australia, New Zealand, and United States, the concept of sun-protective clothing is widely prevalent. Strict guidelines exist in the manufacture of sun-protective clothing. The protective ability of a cloth is defined by the fabric UV protection factor (UPF).

UPF is the ratio of MED of photoprotected skin/ nonprotected skin.

BOX 1: Patient education measures in photodermatitis.

- Avoid sun exposure as far as possible. Keep outdoor activities after sunset and sunrise.
- Avoid peak sunlight time from 10 AM to 4 PM, especially closer to noon.
- Seek shades of trees and buildings while outdoors.
- Physical protective measures such as umbrellas, goggles, caps and hats, and fully covered clothing.
- Avoid water, snow, and sand as these tend to reflect sunrays more.
- Use tinted and sun-protective glasses/films for windows of home, office, and vehicles.
- Use shades, blinders, and curtains for the windows of buildings.
- Shift the place of work away from the window in offices.
- Use sun-protective lenses for the eyes.
- Avoid outdoor recreational activities, especially during flare.

The factors which influence the UPF include color, shades of colors, weave, number of washes, type of fabric, optical whiteners, UV absorbant molecules, fabric thickness, stretching, laundering, number of layers, and hydration. Among the fabrics, the protective effect is as follows: polyester > wool, silk, nylon > cotton, rayon.[7] Darker shades such as saffron (orange), red, and black have better protective property than lighter shades.

Sunscreens: This is perhaps the most common photoprotective agent used. Sunscreens are basically divided as given in **Table 4**.[7]

Micronized and nanoparticles of physical sunscreens are available which increase the compliance of patients due to avoiding the whitening effect of inorganic sunscreen.

Some of the terms associated with sunscreens are given in **Table 5**.[7]

Topical corticosteroids: Low-potent to mid-potent topical corticosteroids are the first choice. Rarely super-potent corticosteroids for short course may be preferred in CAD.

Calcineurin inhibitors: Tacrolimus and pimecrolimus have also been used. Tacrolimus under occlusion may be preferred in CAD in view of its steroid-sparing effects.

Systemic immunosuppressants: Corticosteroids, azathioprine may be sometimes required. Immunosuppressants used include azathioprine (1–2.5 mg/kg), cyclosporine (3.5–5 mg/kg), mycophenolate mofetil (25–40 mg/kg), and thioguanine (0.5–1.5 mg/kg).[2]

Antihistamines: First and second-generation antihistamines may be required to control the associated itch in photoallergic reactions.

NSAIDs: Rarely NSAIDs such as indomethacin may be needed to reduce phototoxic reaction.

TABLE 4: Classification of sunscreens.

Inorganic (physical) sunscreen		• Zinc oxide • Titanium dioxide • Iron oxide
Organic (chemical) sunscreen	UVA protective	• Benzophenones • Avobenzone • Meradimate
	UVB protective	• Salicylates • Cinnamates • PABA and its derivatives • Others—octocrylene, ensulizole

(PABA: p-aminobenzoic acid; UVA: ultraviolet A; UVB: ultraviolet B)

TABLE 5: Terms associated with sunscreens.

Sun protection factor (SPF)	Defines the UVB protective effect of sunscreen: $SPF = \frac{\text{MED of photoprotected skin}}{\text{MED of unprotected skin}}$
Substantivity	Property of sunscreen to remain on skin even after sweating, washing, etc.
Critical wavelength	Measure of breadth of protection offered by sunscreen where 90% of irradiation is absorbed
Boots star rating	Measure of UVA protection of sunscreen. Rated from 0 to 5
PA system	Measure of UVA protection followed in Japan and other Asian countries
Immune protection factor	Ability of sunscreen to prevent immunosuppression
Persistent pigment darkening	Measure of UVA protection
Water resistant	Ability of sunscreen to retain its SPF after two sequential immersions in water of 20 minutes each
Very water resistant	Ability of sunscreen to retain its SPF after four sequential immersions in water of 20 minutes each
Sun block	Misnomer. Often used synonymously with sunscreen

(MED: minimal erythema dose; UVA: ultraviolet A; UVB: ultraviolet B)

KEY POINTS

- Photodermatitis is usually subclassified into phototoxic reactions, photoallergic reactions, and phytophotodermatitis.
- It is important to examine all photoexposed areas which tends to depend on the dress worn by a patient.
- Clinical types of CAD are actinic reticuloid, persistent light reaction, photosensitive dermatitis, and photosensitive eczema.
- Minimal erythema dose (MED) and photopatch test are very important investigative tools in a case of photodermatitis.
- Photoprotective measure includes lifestyle modifications, physical modalities, and sunscreens.

REFERENCES

1. Lim HW, Hawk JLM. Photodermatologic disorders. In: Bolognia JL, Jorizzo JL, Schaffer JV (Eds). Dermatology, 3rd edition. China: Elsevier Saunders; 2012. pp. 1467-86.

2. Pai S. Photosensitive Disorders. In: Viswanath V (Ed). IADVL's Concise Textbook of Dermatology. New Delhi: Wiley-Blackwell; 2012. pp. 184-93.
3. Krupashankar DS, Sashikala K. Photodermatology and photodermatoses. In: Sachidanand S, Oberoi C, Inamadar A (Eds). IADVL's Textbook of Dermatology, 4th edition. Mumbai: Bhalani Publishing House; 2015. 887-932.
4. Photocontact dermatitis. In: Rietschel RL, Fowler JF (Eds). Fischer's Contact Dermatitis, 6th edition. New Delhi: CBS Publishers and Distributor; 2008. pp. 454-69.
5. Wu H, Brandling-Bennett HA, Harrist TJ. Noninfectious vesiculobullous and vesiculopustular diseases. In: Elder DE (Ed). Lever's Histopathology of the Skin, 10th edition (South Asian). New Delhi: Wolters Kluwer (India); 2009. pp. 235-78.
6. Young AR. Photobiology. In: Burns T, Breathnach S, Cox N, Griffiths C (Eds). Rook's Textbook of Dermatology, 8th edition. Singapore: Wiley-Blackwell; 2010. pp. 9.1-13.
7. Lim HW. Photoprotection. In: Goldsmith LA, Katz SI, Gilcherst BA, Paller AS, Leffell DJ, Wolff K (Eds). Fitzpatrick's Dermatology in General Medicine, 8th edition. New York: McGraw Hill; 2012. pp. 2707-13.

EXAMINATION QUESTIONS

1. Classify suncreens and its use in dermatology.
2. Explain sunscreen as a double-edged sword.
3. How will you approach to a case of photodermatitis?
4. Describe solar spectrum in chronic actinic damage on skin. What are the clinical features, complications, and management of chronic actinic dermatitis?

27 CHAPTER Autosensitization Dermatitis

Sanjay Ghosh, Saurav Kundu

INTRODUCTION

Autosensitization, autoeczematization or "id" reaction is a generalized cutaneous reaction which is acute in nature in response to a variety of stimuli including infectious and inflammatory skin conditions. The id reaction has been referred to as dermatophytid, pediculid,[1] or bacterid depending on the triggering infectious process. These reactions are immunologically mediated. Clinical features vary depending on the etiology of the eruption.

PATHOGENESIS[2,3]

Although the exact cause of autosensitization is not clear, the following factors are thought to be responsible:

- Hematogenous dissemination of allergens from the primary site
- Decreased sensitization threshold in distant skin sites after primary inflammation
- Abnormal immune recognition of autologous skin antigens
- Hematogenous dissemination of activated memory T-cells and cytokines

EPIDEMIOLOGY

Exact prevalence of autosensitization dermatitis not known. It is reported in 4–5% cases of dermatophyte infection and in 37% of patients with stasis dermatitis. More than 60% of patients with contact dermatitis and stasis dermatitis develop id reactions.

It has no age, sex, and racial predilection.

CAUSES[3-5]

- *Infections*:
  - Fungal infection such as dermatophytic infection, histoplasmosis
  - Mycobacterial infections
  - Parasitic infections such as pediculosis
- Contact dermatitis, stasis dermatitis
- Immunization reactions such as bacillus Calmette-Guérin (BCG) vaccinations

CLINICAL FEATURES

Classically, the lesions of id reaction are:

- At a site distant from the primary infection or dermatitis
- Occurs 1–2 weeks after the primary infection or dermatitis
- Distributed symmetrically
- Exacerbation of pre-existing dermatitis induced by secondary infection, scratching, and inappropriate therapy

Clinical patterns are as follows:

- An acute onset of pruritic, maculopapular, popular, or papulovesicular eruption that involves the forearms, thighs, legs, face, and hands which is typically associated with stasis dermatitis.
- Symmetrical eruption of small follicular papules associated with kerion.
- Vesicular eruption on the lateral aspects of fingers similar to pompholyx is associated with inflammatory tinea pedis.
- Erysipelas-like eruption over the legs has been reported in dermatophytosis.
- Erythema multiforme-like cutaneous lesions have also been reported.[6]
- Extracutaneous features include fever, anorexia, splenomegaly, and leukocytosis.

DIFFERENTIAL DIAGNOSIS

- Systemic contact dermatitis
- Maculopapular drug eruption
- Atopic dermatitis
- Scabies
- Dermatitis herpetiformis
- Gianotti–Crosti syndrome
- Pityriasis lichenoides
- Insect bite hypersensitivity
- Eosinophilic pustular folliculitis
- Pityrosporum folliculitis
- Idiopathic vesicular hand eczema

INVESTIGATIONS

- Routine tests such as complete hemogram, blood glucose level, liver function tests, serum creatinine, serum immunoglobulin E (IgE), hepatitis B virus (HBV), HCV, and human immunodeficiency virus (HIV).

- Skin scraping and culture to confirm dermatophyte infection.
- Patch testing to exclude allergic contact dermatitis.
- Biopsy must be done to exclude other morphologically similar diseases.

Histopathology of a papulovesicular lesion shows spongiotic epidermis with superficial perivascular lymphohistiocytic infiltrate admixed with small number of eosinophils.

TREATMENT[7]

- The primary aim is to identify the underlying infection or dermatitis and adequately treat it.
- *Treatment of the rash includes*:
    - Systemic and topical corticosteroids
    - Wet compresses
    - Systemic antihistamines.

SPECIAL TERMINOLOGY[8]

As per International Contact Dermatitis Research Group (ICDRG) guideline, allergic contact dermatitis has been broadly termed as "allergic contact dermatitis syndrome." Allergic contact dermatitis at a primary site with generalized dissemination or id eruption has been categorized as "allergic contact dermatitis stage IIIA."

KEY POINTS

- Secondary eczematous lesions develop at sites distant from the primary exposure site.
- More than 60% of id reactions develop from contact dermatitis or stasis dermatitis. Tinea pedis is also an important cause.
- Disseminated lesions appear days to week after primary lesion.
- Lesions are usually ill-defined and symmetric and occur in anatomical analogous sites.
- *Pathogenesis is uncertain and is possibly related to*:
    - Hematogenous dissemination of allergens
    - Circulating activated memory T-cells
- Treatment options include treatment of underlying cause, topical and systemic steroids, and antihistamines.

REFERENCES

1. Brenner S, Ophir J, Krakowski A. Pediculid. An unusual id reaction to pediculosis capitis. Dermatologica. 1984;168(4): 189-91.
2. Kasteler JS, Peterson MJ, Vance JE, Zone JJ. Circulating activated T lymphocytes in autoeczematization. Arch Dermatol. 1992; 128(6):795-8.
3. Lowther C, Miedler JD, Cockerell CJ. Id-like reaction to BCG therapy for bladder cancer. Cutis. 2013;91(3):145-6, 151.
4. Crum N, Hardaway C, Graham B. Development of an idlike reaction during treatment for acute pulmonary histoplasmosis: a new cutaneous manifestation in histoplasmosis. J Am Acad Dermatol. 2003;48(Suppl 2):S5-6.
5. Choudhri SH, Magro CM, Crowson AN, Nicolle LE. An id reaction to *Mycobacterium leprae*: first documented case. Cutis. 1994;54(4):282-6.
6. Atzori L, Pau M, Aste M. Erythema multiforme ID reaction in atypical dermatophytosis: a case report. J Eur Acad Dermatol Venereol. 2003;17(6):699-701.
7. Fritch P, Reider N. Eczematous Group. Bolognia JL, Lorizzo J, Rapini R (Eds). Dermatology. Mosby: St Louis; 2003. pp. 221-2.
8. Lachapelle JM, Maibach HI. Patch Testing Prick Testing: A Practical Guide. Berlin: Springer; 2003. pp. 7-26.

EXAMINATION QUESTION

1. Write briefly about the triggering factors of autosensitization dermatitis.

28 CHAPTER

Erythroderma

Bhushan Madke, Roma Dhande, Sejal Chandak, Shravya R, Samiksha Chavhan

DEFINITION

Erythroderma is defined as diffuse erythema and scaling of >90% of body skin surface area along with diffuse hair loss.

ETIOPATHOGENESIS

Clinically, erythroderma can be classified as acute and chronic, while etiologically, it can be either primary (no cause identified) or secondary (arising from preexisting skin diseases). Typically, secondary erythroderma has a gradual and insidious onset except in the drug-induced cases, where it tends to be sudden. Erythroderma leads to a constellation of signs and symptoms collectively referred to as "skin failure." Either manifesting as *de novo* or arising from secondary causes, erythroderma patients present as diffuse scaling and redness all over body surface area. There is an overwhelming disruption of barrier function of cornified cell envelope. Loss of barrier function has a cascading effect on various physiologic and homeostasis functions. Stratum corneum (SC) disruption leads to increased rate of transepidermal water and electrolyte loss. Disturbed SC barrier and pH alteration allows easy entry of various pathogenic organisms and sensitizing allergens. Increased cutaneous blood flow due to intense vasodilatation allows more loss of body heat, which is perceived by thermoregulatory centers as fall in core body temperature. This leads to shivering attempt to generate heat and maintain core body temperature. A patient with erythroderma behaves as a poikilothermic organism and cannot maintain the body temperature in accordance to changing ambient temperature.

Keratinocytes possess various important proteins and small molecules (e.g., calcium). Excessive shedding of keratinocytes in the scales leads to increased loss of protein molecules. Initially, this is compensated by blood reservoir pool of plasma proteins; however, eventual exhaustion of this circulating pool leads to hypoalbuminemia, which in turn causes reduction in plasma oncotic pressure. A normal plasma oncotic pressure is necessary to maintain the intravascular volume and any reduction in plasma oncotic pressure leads to extravasation of intravascular fluid into the interstitial space. Increased fluid in the interstitial space causes edema in the dependent body parts (pedal edema). Another factor contributory in pedal edema is increased skin blood flow and leaky dermal capillaries. Some cases of erythroderma (especially psoriasis) may lead to increased serum uric acid levels secondary to high nucleic acid (purine) turnover. Some authors used the term "red man syndrome" to refer to idiopathic erythroderma (which must not be confused with the cutaneous reaction associated to rapid intravenous infusion of vancomycin)

CAUSES OF ERYTHRODERMA

Primary/idiopathic—no cause identified after exhaustive work-up.

Secondary:

- *Disorders of keratinization*:
  - Psoriasis (unstable, generalized pustular psoriasis)
  - Pityriasis rubra pilaris
  - Darier's disease
  - Nonbullous ichthyosiform erythroderma
- *Eczema*:
  - Atopic dermatitis
  - Seborrheic dermatitis
  - Contact dermatitis
  - Stasis eczema
- *Infection*:
  - Crusted scabies
  - Extensive dermatophytosis
  - Pityriasis rosea
- *Drugs*:
  - Drug reaction with eosinophilia and systemic symptoms (DRESS)
  - Drug hypersensitivity syndrome (dapsone, allopurinol, phenytoin)
- *Vesiculobullous*: Pemphigus foliaceus
- *Malignancies*:
  - Mycosis fungoides
  - Sézary syndrome
  - B-cell lymphoma
- *Autoimmune connective tissue disorders (AI-CTD)*: Dermatomyositis

CLINICAL PRESENTATION

A patient in erythroderma may be either wheeled in on a stretcher or chair in the OPD. The patient may be swollen from head to toe which may mimic anasarca of organ dysfunction (cardiac, renal, or hepatic origin). The patient can have shivering with multiple layers of clothing on (swaddling). Acute erythroderma has large loosely adherent scales on body with underlying bright red erythema, while erythroderma of chronic duration (compensated) may have fine branny scales with dull erythema. Increased body temperature in a patient of erythroderma can be either of infectious (disrupted SC barrier allowing organisms to gain entry) or noninfectious origin (increased blood flow through cutaneous vascular bed) or both. It must be kept in mind that fever can be a manifestation of drug-induced erythroderma.

On examination, the patient may appear toxic with increased pulse rate (high cardiac output), symmetrical/bilateral pitting pedal edema (reduced plasma oncotic pressure), collection of scales on bedding and clothing. Other clinical features which can be seen are pruritus, palmoplantar keratoderma, nail changes (Beau's lines, onychodystrophy, pitting, discoloration, subungual hyperkeratosis, onycholysis, and paronychia). A peculiar nail change seen in chronic erythroderma is called as ebonization of nails (appearance similar to ebony wood) giving smooth shiny nails due to chronic scratching of skin. There can be liver or spleen enlargement along with lymphadenopathy. Lymph node enlargement in most cases of nonlymphomatous erythroderma is due to reactive hyperplasia (dermatopathic lymphadenopathy).

One must diligently search for cutaneous signs of dermatoses (plaque of psoriasis, silvery white scales), flexural lichenification (atopic eczema), and nail changes (psoriasis, Darier's disease, pityriasis rubra pilaris), hyperkeratotic follicular papules (pityriasis rubra pilaris) and fissured painful palmoplantar keratoderma (T-cell lymphomas)

History taking must be thorough and detailed to find the cause of erythroderma. History of allergic rhinitis, conjunctivitis, and asthma may point toward atopic eczema while long-standing erythematous plaques with slivery white scales on extensors of knees and elbows can provide a clue of psoriasis. Scaly red patches on eyebrows, nasolabial folds, ears, chest, and back may suggest seborrheic dermatitis. Classical images of dermatoses from an Atlas of Dermatology (preferably country specific) can be shown to a patient to gather more information about preexisting dermatoses. History of epilepsy or postherpetic neuralgia can suggest anticonvulsant-induced erythroderma. A detailed history of contact sensitization must be obtained in a patient with unknown cause of erythroderma (nickel, hair dye, parthenium, and cement). Multiple involvements of close family members with itchy rash may suggest scabies or dermatophytosis. In spite of best efforts, in a case of fully established erythroderma, it is difficult to differentiate between its various causes.

Patients from villages and tribal areas usually take treatment from local quacks who in turn can prescribe irritant topical treatment. Irritant application history must be elicited in all patients with erythroderma. Patients with limited pre-existing dermatoses may self-treat themselves with neem leaves paste (*Azadirachta indica*) or bath which may lead to unstable dermatoses and resultant erythroderma. Various herbal and ayurvedic medicines are known to aggravate stable plaque type psoriasis by provoking uncontrolled koebnerization. Sudden withdrawal of oral corticosteroids can make psoriasis unstable and lead to generalized pustular psoriasis or erythroderma.

INVESTIGATIONS

Following investigations should be obtained in patients with erythroderma:

- Complete blood count with differential count, erythrocyte sedimentation rate (ESR), C-reactive protein (CRP), serum protein levels, serum electrolytes, blood sugar, liver and kidney function tests, urine test, chest radiography, abdominal ultrasound, and electrocardiogram. Skin scrapping with KOH mount and mineral oil preparation should be obtained in suspected cases of dermatophytosis and scabies.
- Skin biopsies (multiple and serial), lymph node biopsies, bone marrow investigation, flow-cytometry, immuno-phenotyping, patch testing, and CT scan can be done based on history and relevant clinical features.

MANAGEMENT

General Measures

All patients of erythroderma must be managed in indoor settings preferably in isolation. Disrupted barrier function puts the patient at risk of acquiring nosocomial infections; hence, nursing staff and health professionals must observe principles of reverse barrier nursing. All vital parameters should be monitored on periodic basis based on severity of skin failure.

Patients of erythroderma have skin failure and staff must be aware of managing such patients. A warm humidified environment of 30–32°C will make patient comfortable and reduce the shivering, eventually decreasing heat and energy loss (A practical tip: humidified environment should make visiting consultant sweat). Hemodynamic monitoring includes pulse rate, urine output, and urine osmolality. A urine output of 50–100 mL/h and an osmolality lower than 1,020 are indicative of adequate tissue perfusion. A wide-bore intravenous access should be secured for fluid and drug administration. Fluid and electrolyte replacement should be done in consultation with intensivist and internist to avoid catastrophic fluid overload leading to cardiac failure and alveolar edema. Empirical antibiotic can be instituted based on local infectious organism profile. Appropriate fluid and tissue samples should be sent as per standard operating protocols for culture studies and rational use of parenteral antibiotic must be instituted.

Topical Treatment

The aim of topical treatment is to repair damaged SC barrier function. Use of emollient will repair the barrier function and reduce shedding of scales. Physiologic lipid (mixture of cholesterol, ceramide, and free fatty acids in a ratio of 3:1:1) will repair the barrier function and prevent water loss and energy loss.

Definitive Treatment

All attempts must be made to identify the cause of erythroderma and further treatment must be carried out as per established guidelines for respective dermatoses (e.g., cyclosporine, methotrexate for psoriasis, oral corticosteroids with appropriate tapering for eczemas, antifungal regimens for seborrheic dermatitis, dermatophytosis). Appropriate referral services should be taken in proven cases of malignancies.

KEY POINTS

- Erythroderma is a reactive condition and one must strive to identify the cause.
- Erythroderma leads to acute and chronic skin failures along with its complication.
- Management is aimed at tailored made investigations and disease-specific therapy.
- Symptomatic treatment plays a crucial role in restoration of disturbed epidermal barrier function.

SUGGESTED READING

1. Cuellar-Barboza A, Ocampo-Candiani J, Herz-Ruelas ME. A practical approach to the diagnosis and treatment of adult erythroderma. Actas Dermosifiliogr. 2018;109(9): 777-90.
2. Fraitag S, Bodemer C. Neonatal erythroderma. Curr Opin Pediatr. 2010;22(4):438-44.
3. Maldonado-García CA, Orozco-Anahuati AP. Diagnostic approach of erythroderma in the adult. Rev Med Inst Mex Seguro Soc. 2017;55(3):353-60.
4. Milavec-Puretić V, Zorić Z, Zidanić M, Drcelić A, Stajminger G. Exfoliative erythroderma. Acta Dermatovenerol Croat. 2007; 15(2):103-7.
5. Sarkar R, Garg VK. Erythroderma in children. Indian J Dermatol Venereol Leprol. 2010;76(4):341-7.

EXAMINATION QUESTIONS

1. What are the causes of erythroderma?
2. What are the causes of erythroderma in neonates and infants?
3. Explain acute skin failure and its management.
4. How will you approach to a case of erythroderma?

29 CHAPTER Eosinophilic Dermatoses

BC Sharath Kumar, Namratha C Manjunath, Barnali Chowdhury

INTRODUCTION

Eosinophils are derived from bone marrow which comprises of upto 6% of circulating leukocytes, with average tissue life span of 2–5 days. The name "eosinophil" was given by Paul Ehrlich, because of staining of its cytoplasmic granules with acidic dye eosin. There are five highly toxic proteins in the granules of eosinophils: The major basic protein-1, major basic protein-2, eosinophil peroxidase, the eosinophil protein X/eosinophil derived neurotoxin, and eosinophil cationic protein that kills microbes, parasites, tumor cells and also plays a role in inflammatory reactions leading to tissue damage and fibrosis.[1] Cytokines, chemokines, lipid mediators, and superoxide are other eosinophil derived inflammatory mediators which play a role in inflammatory processes.

EOSINOPHILIC DERMATOSES

Eosinophilic dermatoses comprises of wide variety of inflammatory dermatoses and malignancy characterized by infiltration of few to many eosinophils and/or evidence of eosinophil degranulation in skin and/or mucosa, with and without increased eosinophils in peripheral blood.

CLASSIFICATION[2]

Classification of eosinophilic dermatoses has been shown in **Box 1**.

GRANULOMA FACIALE

Definition: Benign, chronic inflammatory dermatosis characterized by red-brown papules and plaques primarily on face.

History: Described by Wigley.

Epidemiology: Middle-aged Caucasian men.

Etiology: Remains unknown. Sun exposure maybe a precipitating factor.[3] Other hypotheses propose that it may be an Arthus-like reaction or a localized persistent immune complex disease in the form of vasculitis. Interferon - gamma and IL-5 was found to be increased.

Clinical features: Single, asymptomatic, reddish brown to violaceous, well-demarcated plaque on the face. Trunk, extremities, and/or scalp are occasionally involved.

BOX 1: Classification of eosinophilic dermatoses.

Diseases Characterized by Tissue Eosinophils

- Annular erythema of infancy
- Eosinophilic, polymorphic, and pruritic eruption associated with radiotherapy
- *Eosinophilic pustular folliculitis:*
  - Classical (Ofuji disease)
  - Infantile/neonatal
  - Human immunodeficiency virus associated
- Eosinophilic annular erythema
- Eosinophilic cellulitis (Wells' syndrome)
- Eosinophilic dermatosis of hematologic malignancy
- Erythema toxicum neonatorum
- Eosinophilic ulcer of oral mucosa
- Hypereosinophilic dermatitis of Nir-Westfried
- Hypereosinophilic syndrome
- *IgG4-related cutaneous diseases:*
  - Angiolymphoid hyperplasia with eosinophilia
  - Granuloma faciale
  - Kimura disease
- Juvenile temporal arteritis
- Pachydermatous eosinophilic dermatitis

Diseases Commonly Associated with Tissue Eosinophils

- Arthropod bite and sting reactions
- *Autoimmune blistering diseases:*
  - Pemphigoid
  - Pemphigus
  - Epidermolysis bullosa acquisita
- *Dermatoses of pregnancy:*
  - Pemphigoid gestationis
  - Polymorphic eruption of pregnancy, pruritic urticarial papules, and plaques of pregnancy
- *Drug reactions:*
  - DRESS (drug reaction with eosinophilia and systemic symptoms) also known as drug-induced hypersensitivity syndrome
  - Interstitial granulomatous drug reaction
- *Hereditary syndromes:*
  - Incontinentia pigmenti
  - Hyper-IgE syndromes and other immunodeficiency syndromes
  - Autoimmune lymphoproliferative syndrome
- *Histiocytic diseases:*
  - Langerhans cell histiocytosis
  - Juvenile xanthogranuloma
- Papuloerythroderma of Ofuji
- Oid-Oid disease (exudative discoid and lichenoid chronic dermatosis of Sulzberger and Garbe)

Contd...

Contd...

- *Parasitic diseases/infestations:*
  - Cysticercosis, dirofilariasis, fascioliasis, gnathostomiasis, larva migrans, loiasis, myiasis, onchocerciasis, paragonimiasis, schistosomiasis, strongyloidiasis, tungiasis
  - Scabies, pediculosis, phthiriasis, cimicosis
  - Swimmer's itch (cercarial dermatitis) and Seabather's itch
- Pruritic papular eruption of human immunodeficiency virus disease
- *Sclerosis or fibrosis:*
  - Eosinophilic fasciitis
  - Eosinophilia myalgia and toxic oil syndromes
  - Drugs including statins
  - Iron infusion
  - Lymphoma and leukemia
  - Graft versus host disease after stem cell or bone marrow transplantation
- Urticaria and angioedema
- *Vasculitis:*
  - Eosinophilic granulomatosis with polyangiitis (Churg–Strauss syndrome)
  - Eosinophilic vasculitis

Histologic Patterns Defined by Eosinophils

- *Eosinophilic spongiosis:*
  - *Acute dermatitis:* Allergic contact dermatitis
  - Arthropod bite
  - *Autoimmune bullous diseases:* Pemphigoid, Pemphigus
  - Incontinentia pigmenti
- *Eosinophilic panniculitis:*
  - Arthropod bite
  - Erythema nodosum
  - Gnathostomiasis
  - Injection granuloma
  - Vasculitis
  - Wells' syndrome

Eosinophils of Limited or Unreliable Value in Histopathologic Diagnosis

- Granuloma annulare
- Interstitial granulomatous dermatitis
- *Lymphoproliferative disorders (except HES variants):*
  - Mycosis fungoides
  - Anaplastic large cell lymphoma (except neutrophil-rich and eosinophil-rich variants)
  - Lymphomatoid papulosis
- Mastocytosis
- *Neoplasms:*
  - Keratoacanthoma-type squamous cell carcinoma
  - Invasive squamous cell carcinoma

(HES: hypereosinophilic syndromes)

HPE: Epidermis is unaffected. The dermis is infiltrated by lymphocytes, neutrophils, and plasma cells with numerous eosinophils. Infiltrates spare the upper papillary dermis, by narrow Grenz zone of normal collagen. Vasculitis with fibrinoid material deposition within and around blood vessels.

Dermoscopy: Translucent white gray background intermingled with white streaks and elongated telengectasia and dilated follicular openings.[4]

Differential diagnosis: Differential diagnosis of granuloma faciale has been shown in **Box 2**.

BOX 2: Differential diagnosis of granuloma faciale.

Facial: Tumid lesions of lupus erythematosus, sarcoidosis, lymphoma and pseudolymphoma, fixed drug eruption, leprosy, foreign body granuloma, granulomatous variant of rosacea, benign lymphocytic infiltrate of Jessner, basal cell carcinoma, mastocytoma	*Extrafacial:* Erythema elevatum diutinum, granuloma annulare, benign lymphocytic infiltrate of Jessner, fixed drug eruption.

Rx:

	Topical	*Physical*	*Systemic*
First line therapy	Steroids	Cryotherapy Intralesional steroids Pulsed dye laser	Dapsone 50–100 mg/day
Second line therapy	Tacrolimus	Surgical excision	

WELLS' SYNDROME (EOSINOPHILIC CELLULITIS)

Definition: Inflammatory dermatosis characterized by indurated plaques resembling cellulitis.

History: Described by Wells.

Epidemiology: All ages, Male = Female.

Etiology: Nonspecific hypersensitivity reaction in response to exogenous and (or) endogenous stimuli. Triggering factors include myeloproliferative disorder, arthropod bites, viral (parvovirus B19, herpes simplex virus-2, varicella zoster virus, and mumps virus), bacterial infections, parasite infections (ascariasis and *Toxocara canis*), drugs (anticholinergic agents, thyroid medications, thiazide diuretics, anti-tumor necrosis factor agents), and vaccines (thiomersal containing vaccines).

Dysregulated tissue eosinophilia is implicated in the pathogenic process.

Clinical features: Recurrent episodes of prodromal itching or burning preceded by markedly edematous plaques and nodules in form of annular or arcuate configuration and violaceous borders, mostly involving the extremities. The bright red lesions fade to a pink-brown or slate-gray color, resolving over 4–8 weeks. Malaise is the most common systemic complaint followed by fever in less than 25% of cases. Peripheral blood eosinophilia is common.

HPE: Dermal edema, dermal infiltration with eosinophils, lymphocytes, histiocytes, and "flame figures" where collagen fibers are coated with eosinophil granule proteins (**Box 3**).

Differential diagnosis: Urticaria, erysipelas, acute cellulitis, pemphigoid, morphea.

Rx:

- *Mild cases:* Topical steroids.
- *Moderate-to-severe cases:* Systemic steroids. Other options are minocycline, colchicine, antimalarials, dapsone, griseofulvin, IFN-α, cyclosporine, and antihistamines.

EOSINOPHILIC PUSTULAR FOLLICULITIS

Definition: Inflammatory dermatosis presenting with recurrent crops of pruritic follicular papules and pustules, and histopathologically with folliculotropic infiltration of eosinophils.

Etiology: Remains unknown. In skin lesions, intercellular adhesion molecule 1 is expressed by keratinocytes on follicular epithelium, vascular cell adhesion molecule 1 by vascular endothelium around hair follicles, and lymphocyte function-associated antigen 1 on follicular epithelium.[5] These molecules are implicated in the selective migration of eosinophils and lymphocytes to the hair follicles.

Prostaglandin D2 has been implicated in eosinophil infiltration and activation in the pilosebaceous units of skin lesions **(Table 1)**.

Variants

- Classic (Ofuji disease)
- Infantile/neonatal
- Immunosuppression associated

Differential diagnosis: Differential diagnosis of classic and infantile eosinophilic pustular folliculitis has been shown in **Boxes 4 and 5**.

BOX 3: Conditions associated with flame figures.

- Angiolymphoid hyperplasia with eosinophilia
- Arthropod bite and sting reaction
- Churg–Strauss syndrome
- Dermographism
- Drug reaction
- Eczema
- Eosinophilic fasciitis
- Eosinophilic pustular folliculitis
- Fungal disease including dermatophyte infection
- Herpes simplex infection
- Human immunodeficiency virus infection
- Hypereosinophilic syndromes
- Immunobullous diseases (pemphigoid, pemphigoid gestationis, pemphigus vegetans)
- Incontinentia pigmenti
- Kimura disease
- Malignancies, solid organ (bronchogenic carcinoma, colonic adenocarcinoma)
- Mastocytoma
- Molluscum contagiosum
- Myeloproliferative disorders involving skin
- Parasite infestation (ascariasis, gnathostomiasis, onchocerciasis, toxocariasis)
- Urticaria
- Vaccination site reactions
- Varicella

TABLE 1: Differences among variants of eosinophilic pustular folliculitis (EPF).

Variants	*Associated conditions*	*Age of onset and ethnicity*	*Clinical features*	*Predilection sites*	*Elevated serum IgE*	*Histopathology*	*Treatment*
Classic EPF	Rare	35–40 years Asians (Japanese)	Clusters of follicular papules and pustules in annular or arcuate pattern with central clearing and centrifugal extension	Face, trunk, extremities, scalp	Variable	Eosinophilic infiltration with spongiosis in follicular infundibula, with perifollicular involvement, eosinophilic microabscess in the follicular infundibula. Follicular mucinosis and exocytosis of inflammatory cells in the hair follicles are strongly associated with facial EPF	NSAIDs mostly indomethacin. Topical steroids, tacrolimus, ultraviolet B phototherapy, psoralen plus ultraviolet A, systemic steroids, cyclosporine, cetirizine, dapsone, minocycline, dimethyl diphenyl sulfone, colchicine, retinoids, IFNα-2b, and IFN-γ have been tried
Infantile EPF	Rare	Less than 1 year	Isolated or grouped papulo-pustules	Scalp	Uncommon	Either follicular eosinophilic infiltration or perifollicular, interfollicular and/or periadnexal involvement	Topical steroids or observation
Immuno-suppression-associated EPF	HIV or malignancies	16–73 years Asians	Severely pruritic perifollicular erythematous papules and pustules	Upper trunk, upper limbs, head and neck (males), face (females)	Variable	Perifollicular infiltration of eosinophils and mast cells, with CD8+ lymphocytes in infiltrates	Indomethacin, topical steroids, UVB phototherapy

BOX 4: Differential diagnosis of classic EPF.

Facial	*Nonfacial*
Tinea faciei, Demodex folliculitis, lupus miliaris disseminatus faciei, acne, rosacea, seborrheic dermatitis, granuloma faciale, autoimmune annular erythema, and folliculitis.	Palmoplantar pustulosis, subcorneal pustular dermatosis, scabies, follicular mucinosis

BOX 5: Differential diagnosis of infantile EPF.

- Erythema toxicum neonatorum
- Infantile acropustulosis
- Transient neonatal pustular melanosis, miliaria pustulosa
- Arthropod bites
- Acne neonatorum
- Hyper-IgE syndrome (Langerhans' cell histiocytosis)
- Bacterial/viral/fungal infection
- Scabies

TABLE 2: Difference between ALHE and KD.

	Angiolymphoid hyperplasia with eosinophilia	*Kimura disease*
Ethnicity	All races	Asians
Age and sex	3rd–5th decade F > M	2nd–3rd decade M > F
Symptoms	Pruritis, pain, pulsation	Asymptomatic
Clinical features	Small, superficial erythematous papules, nodules, tumors (2 cm) in head and neck region	Subcutaneous nodules (>2 cm), no skin changes in head and neck region with lymph node and salivary glands involvement
HPE	Vascular proliferation with numerous large epithelioid or histiocytoid endothelial cells	Lymphoid proliferation with germinal center with prominent fibrosis
Serum IgE	Normal	Increased
Nephropathy	Absent	Present in upto 20% cases
Dermoscopy	Dotted and irregular linear vessels regularly distributed pale-reddish to light pink background[6]	
Differential diagnosis	Kimura disease, pyogenic granuloma, epithelioid hemangioendothelioma, epithelioid angiosarcoma, Kaposi sarcoma	ALHE, lymphoma
Rx	Surgical excision, intralesional and systemic steroids, INF-α, laser, cryotherapy	Surgical excision, systemic steroids, cyclosporine, radiation therapy

ANGIOLYMPHOID HYPERPLASIA WITH EOSINOPHILIA (EPITHELIOID HEMANGIOMA) AND KIMURA DISEASE

Etiology of angiolymphoid hyperplasia with eosinophilia (ALHE): It may be due to trauma, hormonal changes, infections (HHV-8). IL-5 and vascular endothelial growth factors are increased.

Difference between ALHE and Kimura disease (KD) has been shown in **Table 2**.

HYPEREOSINOPHILIC SYNDROME

It includes spectrum of diseases that have increased blood eosinophils and tissue damage with common clinical features, including skin disease in more than 50% of patients.

Diagnostic criteria for HES have been shown in **Boxes 6 and 7**.

Classification

Classification of HES has been shown in **Table 3.**

Differences between primary and secondary HES have been shown in **Table 4**.

BOX 6: Original diagnostic criteria of HES.

Original criteria[7]

- Peripheral blood eosinophil counts >1500/mm^3 for at least 6 months, or less than 6 months with evidence of organ damage
- Lack of evidence for parasitic, allergic, or other recognized causes of eosinophilia
- Symptoms and signs of organ system involvement

Clinical features: Cutaneous findings range from pruritic erythematous macules, papules, plaques, or nodules on the trunk and extremities to urticaria and angioedema, erythema annulare centrifugum-like lesions, purpuric papules, retiform purpura, livedo reticularis, superficial thrombophlebitis.

Liver, spleen, central and peripheral nervous systems, lungs are affected.

Eosinophilic endomyocardial disease can develop in patient with prolonged peripheral blood eosinophilia. Splinter hemorrhages and/or nailfold infarcts are clues to thromboembolic disease.

HPE: Nonspecific. Urticarial lesions show perivascular or interstitial infiltrates of lymphocytes and eosinophils. Papules or plaques exhibit dermal infiltrate with few eosinophils.

BOX 7: Revised diagnostic criteria of HES.

Revised criteria[8]

- Peripheral blood hypereosinophilia defined as >1.5 eosinophils × 10^9/L blood on two examinations at an interval of 1 month or greater and/or tissue hypereosinophilia defined by:
  - Percentage of eosinophils in bone marrow section exceeds 20% of all nucleated cells, and/or
  - Pathologist is of the opinion that tissue infiltration by eosinophils is extensive, and/or
  - Marked deposition of eosinophil granule proteins is found in the absence or presence of major tissue infiltration by eosinophils
- Organ damage and/or dysfunction attributable to tissue hypereosinophilia*
- Exclusion of other disorders or conditions as major reason for organ damage

* The HES diagnostic criteria are supplemented by defining eosinophil-related organ damage which consist of eosinophil infiltrates associated with organ dysfunction, which can be associated with 1 or more of the following:
1. Fibrosis (lung, heart, digestive tract, skin)
2. Thrombosis with or without thromboembolism
3. Cutaneous (including mucosal) erythema, edema/angioedema, ulceration, or eczema
4. Peripheral or central neuropathy with chronic or recurrent neurologic deficit
5. Less common organ manifestations (liver, pancreas, kidney)

TABLE 3: Classification of HES.

Primary (neoplastic) HES	*Secondary (reactive) HES*	*Idiopathic HES*
• Underlying neoplasm of stem cells, myeloid cells or eosinophils (WHO classification) • Eosinophils are considered (or shown) to be clonal • Male predominance, endomyocardial disease; mucosal ulcers poor prognostic sign • High serum tryptase and vitamin B_{12} levels, tissue fibrosis, splenomegaly, and bone marrow biopsies with increased numbers of CD25+ atypical spindle-shaped mast cells	• Hypereosinophilia is considered to be cytokine-driven, not due to a clonal proliferation of eosinophils • *Subvariant:* lymphocytic (lymphoid) subtype, where clonal T-cells produce Th2 cytokines	• No identified reactive or neoplastic disorder that induces hypereosinophilia

TABLE 4: Differences between primary and secondary HES.

Primary	*Secondary*
• Deletion on chromosome 4 produces tyrosine kinase fusion gene *FIP1L1-PDGFRA* • *PDGFRA, PDGFRB* (encodes platelet-derived growth factor receptor-β), and *FGFR1* (encodes fibroblast growth factor receptor 1) are other rarer fusion genes or rearrangements that are involved • M>F • Presents with fever, weight loss, fatigue, malaise and skin lesions • Heart is often involved, with thrombus formation resulting in subendocardial fibrosis and restrictive cardiomyopathy. • Mucosal ulcers of the oropharynx or anogenital region represent a poor prognostic sign • High serum tryptase and vitamin B_{12} levels, tissue fibrosis, splenomegaly, and bone marrow biopsies with increased numbers of CD25+ atypical spindle-shaped mast cells	• T-cell clone producing Th2 cytokines (IL-5) • M = F • Presents with severe pruritus, dermatitis, erythroderma and/or urticaria and angioedema, lymphadenopathy. • Risk of developing lymphoma

FIP1L1-PDGFRA: factor interacting with PAPOLA and CPSF1- platelet-derived growth factor receptor alpha.

Differential diagnosis: Parasitic infection, urticaria, hereditary angioedema, atopic dermatitis, contact dermatitis, drug reaction, fungal infection, Wells' syndrome, Churg–Strauss syndrome, mycosis fungoides, and Sezary syndrome.

Rx: The aim is to reduce symptoms and to maintain peripheral blood eosinophil count between 1000–2000/mm^3. Failure of corticosteroid monotherapy has worst prognosis. HES is associated with a 5-year survival rate of 80%, with the leading cause of death being congestive heart failure followed by sepsis **(Flowchart 1).**

EOSINOPHILIC FASCIITIS (SHULMAN'S SYNDROME, DIFFUSE FASCIITIS WITH EOSINOPHILIA)

Definition: It is connective tissue disease presenting with rapid onset of symmetrical painful swelling with a progressive woody induration of skin and soft tissues of the distal extremities, with uncertain etiology.

Epidemiology: Middle-aged, M=F

Flowchart 1: Treatment of HES.

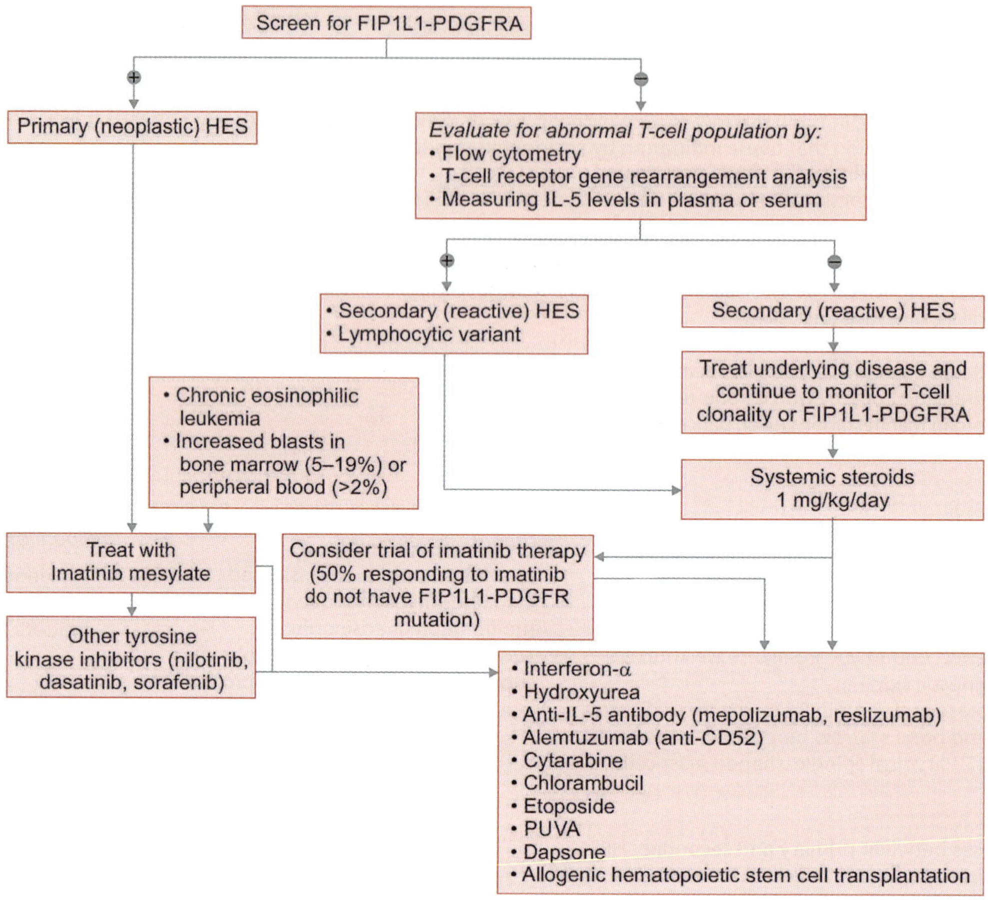

Etiology: Around 30–46% of patients give a history of intense physical exertion or trauma prior to eosinophilic fasciitis onset. Triggering factors are drugs (natalizumab, simvastatin, atorvastatin) and chemical compounds (trichloroethylene), hematological disorders (thrombocytopenia, aplastic anemia, leukemia), infections (borreliosis, *Mycoplasma arginini* infection), arthropod bites, physical factors (radiotherapy, burns), solid tumors, and autoimmune disease.[9]

Clinical features: Abrupt onset of painful, symmetrical, erythematous swelling, and stiffness of the upper and/or lower extremities. Pitting edema progresses resulting in induration of the skin, showing the characteristic "groove sign" (a linear depressions where veins appear to be sunken within indurated skin) and "pseudo-cellulite or peau d'orange" appearance.

Severe skin induration results in joint contracture and tendon retraction. In late stage, extensive skin fibrosis of the trunk may lead hidebound chest.

Diagnosis: Peripheral eosinophilia, elevated serum levels of CRP and ESR, hypergammaglobulinemia, increased serum aldolase, and muscle MRI findings consist of abnormal fascial signal intensity and enhancement.

HPE: The full thickness, or skin-to-muscle, wedge biopsy shows inflammatory and fibrous thickening of fascia, usually 2 to 15 times thicker than normal, with inflammatory infiltrates mainly composed of lymphocytes, plasma cells, and/or eosinophils. The epidermis and dermis are usually unaltered or mildly affected.

Differential diagnosis: Systemic sclerosis, eosinophilia-myalgia syndrome, Churg–Strauss syndrome, hypereosinophilic syndrome.

Rx: Systemic steroids are generally recommended. Methotrexate, azathioprine, cyclophosphamide, cyclosporine, dapsone, rituximab, infliximab, and PUVA can be considered.

EOSINOPHILIA-MYALGIA SYNDROME

It occurs following ingestion of L-tryptophan. TGF-β_1 may play an important role in the development of the connective tissue alterations.

Acute phase presents with severe myalgias, fever, dyspnea, edema, a macular exanthem and peripheral eosinophilia and chronic phase with diffuse, deep sclerodermoid induration of the extremities (with acral sparing), progressive peripheral neuropathy, and myopathy.

Flowchart 2: Approach to diagnosis of a case of eosinophilic dermatoses.

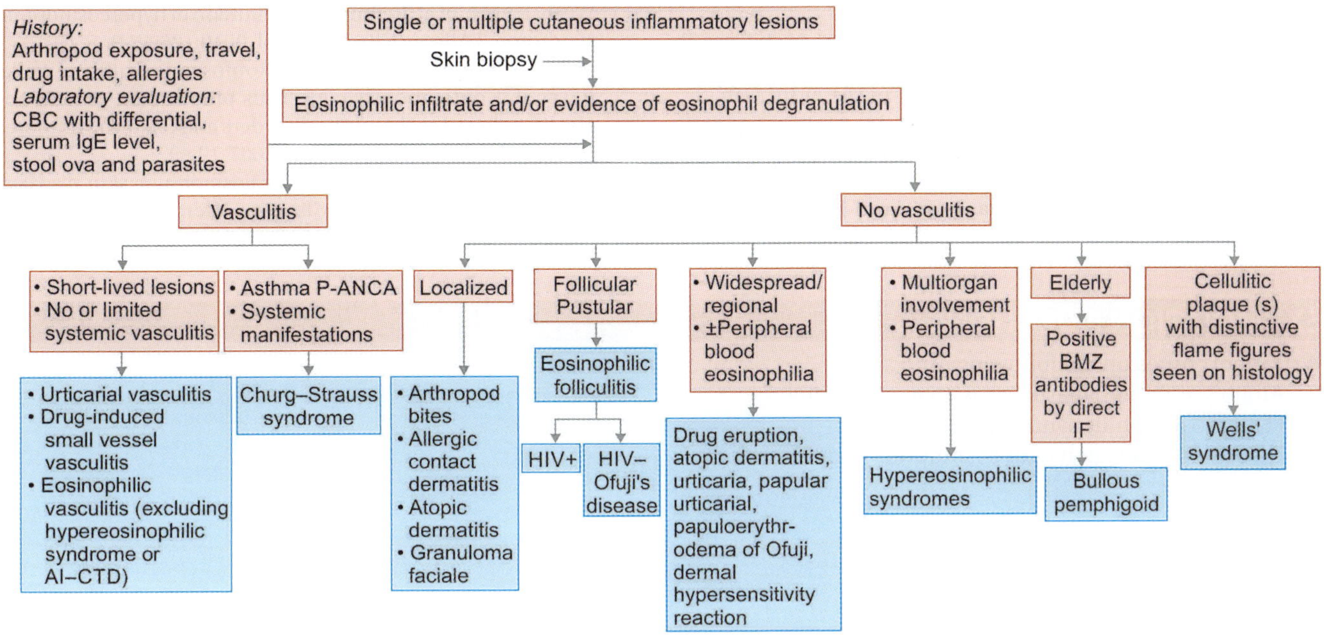

Dermal hypersensitivity reaction includes poorly defined entities (e.g., urticarial dermatitis) in which antigen is unknown.
(AI-CTD: autoimmune connective tissue disease; BMZ: basement membrane zone; IF: immunofluorescence)

There is a prominent inflammatory infiltrate in the perimysium and fascia.

TOXIC OIL SYNDROME

It occurs due to consumption of adulterated rapeseed oil. It starts with nonspecific pruritic erythematous lesions followed by subcutaneous edema of the extremities, accompanied by myalgias, arthralgias, contractures, and peripheral blood eosinophilia. CNS, lungs, and salivary glands are also affected.

APPROACH TO DIAGNOSIS OF A CASE OF EOSINOPHILIC DERMATOSES

Approach to diagnosis of a case of eosinophilic dermatoses has been shown in **Flowchart 2**.

KEY POINTS

- Normal eosinophil count ranges from 50 to 500/mm^3. A count of 500–1500/mm^3 is considered eosinophilia. A count of more than 1500/mm^3 on at least 2 determinations with a minimum time interval of 4 weeks is considered as hypereosinophila.
- Eosinophilic dermatoses include a variety of diseases characterized by eosinophils in inflammatory infiltrates and/or degranulation in skin lesions, with or without blood eosinophilia. Allergy-related dermatoses, drug eruptions, parasitic infestations, and bullous pemphigoid are most common.
- Granuloma faciale characterized by red-brown plaque on face and diffuse, mixed dermal infiltrate, leukocytoclastic vasculitis, grenz zone in histopathology. GF is long-lasting and recalcitrant to treatment. Topical steroids, oral dapsone, and topical tacrolimus are recommended.
- Eosinophilic cellulitis presents with recurrent painful pruritic plaques on extremities or trunk and histologically with diffuse dermal eosinophilic infiltrates and flame figures. It improves dramatically with systemic steroids.
- Eosinophilic pustular folliculitis presents with recurrent crops of pruritic follicular papules and pustules, and folliculotropic infiltration of eosinophils. Variants are classic (Ofuji disease), infantile/neonatal, and immunosuppression associated. Oral indomethacin is effective.
- Primary HES is associated with FIP1L1-PDGFRA fusion gene, responds to Imatinib. In lymphocytic variant of secondary HES there is increase in Th2 cytokines (IL-5) with risk of developing lymphoma.

REFERENCES

1. Bystrom J, Amin K, Bishop-Bailey D. Analysing the eosinophil cationic protein: a clue to the function of the eosinophil granulocyte. Respir Res. 2011;12:10.
2. Leiferman KM, Peters MS. Eosinophil-related disease and the skin. J Allergy Clin Immunol Pract. 2018;6:1462-82.
3. Thiyanaratnam J, Doherty SD, Krishnan B, Hsu S. Granuloma faciale: case report and review. Dermatol Online J. 2009;15:3.
4. Caldarola G, Zalaudek I, Argenziano G, Bisceglia M, Pellicano R. Granuloma faciale: a case report on long-term treatment with

topical tacrolimus and dermatoscopic aspects. Dermatol Ther. 2011;24:508-11.
5. Teraki Y, Konohana I, Shiohara T, Nagashima M, Nishikawa T. Eosinophilic pustular folliculitis (Ofuji's disease). Immunohistochemical analysis. Arch Dermatol. 1993;129:1015-19.
6. Rodriguez-Lomba E, Aviles-Izquidero JA, Molina-Lopez I, Parra-Blanco V, Lazaro-Ochaita P, Suarez-Fernandez R. Dermascopic features in 2 cases of angiolymphoid hyperplasia with eosinophilia. J Am Acad Dermatol. 2016; 75(1):e19-21.
7. Simon HU, Rothenberg ME, Bochner BS, Weller PS, Wardlaw AJ, Wechsler ME, et al. Refining the definition of hypereosinophilic syndrome. J Allergy Clin Immunol. 2010;126:45-9.
8. Valent P, Klion AD, Horny HP, Roufosse F, Gotlib J, Weller PF, et al. Contemporary consensus proposal on criteria and classification of eosinophilic disorders and related syndromes. J Allergy Clin Immunol. 2012;130:607-12.e9.
9. Long H, Zhang G, Wang L, Lu Q. Eosinophilic skin diseases: a comprehensive review. Clin Rev Allergy Immunol. 2016; 50(2):189-213.

EXAMINATION QUESTIONS

Write short notes on the following:
1. Angiolymphoid hyperplasia with eosinophilia
2. Hypereosinophilic syndrome
3. Disorders associated with eosinophils in dermatology

30 CHAPTER Pregnancy Dermatoses

Aarti Sarda, Abhishek De

INTRODUCTION

Skin changes in pregnancy can be either physiological due to the influence of hormones, there may be changes in preexisting skin diseases or development of new pregnancy specific dermatoses. Pregnancy is characterized by many physiological skin changes such as striae gravidarum, linea nigra, chloasma, hair, nail and vascular changes, which are due to hormonal effects. Also the preexisting skin conditions may either improve or exacerbate in pregnancy due to the immunological changes that occur in pregnancy. Due to depressed cell-mediated immunity during normal pregnancy, there is increase in severity and frequency of skin infections such as candidiasis.[1,2]

Physiologic changes during pregnancy and dermatoses influenced by pregnancy are discussed in **Tables 1** and **2** respectively.

Pregnancy-specific dermatoses encompass a heterogeneous group of pruritic skin eruptions, which are seen only in pregnancy.

The dermatoses, which are specific to pregnancy, include:
- Gestational pemphigoid (also known as pemphigoid gestationis)
- Pruritic urticarial papules and plaques of pregnancy (PUPPP, also known as pruritic eruption of pregnancy)
- *Atopic eruption of pregnancy*: Encompasses atopic eczema in pregnancy, prurigo of pregnancy, as well as pruritic folliculitis of pregnancy
- Intrahepatic cholestasis (ICP) of pregnancy

TABLE 1: Physiologic changes during pregnancy.

Pigmentary	• Hyperpigmentation (e.g., areolae, linea nigra) • Chloasma
Hair	• Hirsutism • Postpartum telogen effluvium • Postpartum androgenetic alopecia
Nail	• Subungual hyperkeratosis • Distal onycholysis • Transverse grooving • Brittleness
Glandular	• Increased eccrine function (except palms) • Increased sebaceous function • Decreased apocrine function
Connective tissue	• Striae gravidarum
Vascular	• Spider angiomas • Palmar erythema • Varicosities • Gingival hyperplasia • Pyogenic granuloma • Hemorrhoids

PEMPHIGOID GESTATIONIS (HERPES GESTATIONIS)

Pemphigoid gestationis is an autoimmune subepidermal blistering disease that usually begins in the second or third trimester of pregnancy. It may develop in association with trophoblastic tumors. There is an association with HLA-DR3 and HLA-DR4. The disease could be triggered by a placental antigen that cross-reacts with skin antigens. Immunoglobulin G1 (IgG1) antibodies are directed against bullous pemphigoid (BP 180) in the hemidesmosomal plaque and anchoring filaments.

It presents as itchy urticarial papules, plaques, and vesicles in the umbilical area, which later spreads to other areas forming bullous lesions. Histologically, it is characterized by subepidermal blister formation, and immunopathology shows deposition of C3 and sometimes IgG along the basement membrane zone.[3,4]

The condition may resolve late in pregnancy, but generally flares up at delivery. About 5–10% of newborns may develop

TABLE 2: Dermatoses influenced by pregnancy.

Psoriasis	Improves during pregnancy due to down-regulation of Th1 immune response
• Atopic dermatitis • Systemic lupus erythematosus • Pemphigus vulgaris	Worsens during pregnancy due to shift toward a strong Th2 immune response
Infections (candidiasis, herpes simplex, condyloma acuminata)	Cell-mediated immunity is depressed during normal pregnancy
Acne	Can improve or flare; persistent acne often improves during pregnancy
Rosacea	Often worsens during pregnancy, presumably due to endocrine and vascular changes
Melanocytic nevi	Darken during pregnancy

neonatal pemphigoid. It has been associated with premature birth and small for gestational age babies due to placental failure. Therefore, antenatal surveillance is prudent.

It may recur in subsequent pregnancies and may be triggered by oral contraceptive pills.

POLYMORPHIC ERUPTION OF PREGNANCY

Synonym: Late onset prurigo of pregnancy.

Polymorphic eruption of pregnancy is also known as pruritic urticarial papules and plaques of pregnancy (PUPPP). It is seen in association with multiple gestation pregnancy and increased maternal weight gain. The exact etiology is unknown. It has been postulated that stretching of the skin damages the connective tissue, which in turn leads to an inflammatory process. PUPPP usually occurs in primigravidas in the third trimester although it can first appear in postpartum period. It is characterized by marked pruritus and the onset of itching coincides with the skin lesions, which are seen as erythematous papules, plaques, and sometimes vesicles. The lesions appear over the abdomen, commonly involving the striae gravidarum with sparing of the periumbilical region. The lesions may spread to the breasts, upper thighs, and arms. The face, palms, soles, and mucosal surfaces are usually not involved. Histopathology is nonspecific and immunofluorescence studies are negative. The lesions generally resolve near term or in the early postpartum period. The maternal and fetal prognosis is excellent and recurrence in subsequent pregnancies is unusual.[5,6]

ATOPIC ERUPTION OF PREGNANCY (AEP)

Synonym: Early onset prurigo of pregnancy.

Eczema in Pregnancy

The eruption is seen more commonly in primigravida with singleton pregnancy. Exacerbation of atopic dermatitis may be due to the Th2 shift, which occurs during pregnancy. Patients may have an atopic background with raised total serum IgE levels.

The skin eruption affects all parts of the body including the face, palms, and soles.

Prurigo of Pregnancy

Prurigo of pregnancy is characterized by multiple itchy, excoriated papules over the abdomen and on the extensor surfaces of limbs. It can occur in all trimesters. The etiopathogenesis is not known, although there is sometimes a history of atopy. Histopathology shows parakeratosis and acanthosis, with perivascular lymphocytic infiltrate around upper dermal vessels. Immunofluorescence studies are negative. The lesions generally persist throughout pregnancy and may continue postpartum, although the itching settles shortly after delivery. The mother and fetus are unaffected, but there may be recurrence in successive pregnancies.

Pruritic Folliculitis

Pruritic folliculitis occurs in the second and third trimester of pregnancy. It is characterized by multiple, follicular papules or pustules occurring typically on the shoulders, upper back, arms, chest, and abdomen. Pruritus is not a major feature contrary to its name, and it may be mistaken for acne or folliculitis. The skin lesions usually resolve spontaneously, few weeks following delivery. Histopathology shows nonspecific folliculitis and direct immunofluorescence is negative. There is no association with any maternal or fetal morbidity.[7,8]

PRURITUS GRAVIDARUM (INTRAHEPATIC CHOLESTASIS OF PREGNANCY)

Intrahepatic cholestasis of pregnancy (ICP) is a genetically linked, hormone-dependent, and reversible cholestasis. Patients typically present during the last trimester with severe pruritus. A family history may be present, and there is an association with the HLA-A31 and HLA-B8. There is reduced excretion of bile acids, which leads to increased serum levels. This not only causes severe pruritus in the mother, but may have deleterious effects on the fetus.

It presents with sudden onset of intense, generalized itching, which usually starts on the palms and soles. There are no primary skin lesions, secondary changes due to scratching vary from excoriations to prurigo nodularis in those with pruritus of longer duration. The extensors of extremities, abdomen and buttocks are usually most severely affected.

Jaundice is seen in only 10% of patients, those with the most severe and prolonged episodes of ICP. The itching generally persists till delivery and then it resolves spontaneously within days. Recurrence during subsequent pregnancies occurs in 45–70% of patients, and recurrence with oral contraceptives is routine.[9,10]

Laboratory markers include elevated serum bile acid levels. The condition is associated with a higher risk of premature birth, meconium-stained amniotic fluid, and intrauterine fetal death due to anoxia caused by decreased fetal elimination of toxic bile acids.

Although maternal prognosis is usually good, fetal risk is significant. As a result, ICP is the most important pruritic gestational condition to consider and promptly diagnose and treat in order to prevent fetal impairment **(Table 3)**.[9]

TREATMENT

Polymorphic eruption of pregnancy and atopic eruption of pregnancy respond well to topical emollients and moderately potent steroids along combination with oral antihistamines. For severe cases of PUPPP, systemic steroids may be used. Pruritic folliculitis responds well to topical benzoyl peroxide. Fetal risk is associated with pemphigoid gestationis and ICP

TABLE 3: Dermatosis, risk to fetus, and chances of recurrence.

Dermatosis	*Fetal risk*	*Newborn skin involvement*	*Recurrence*
Pemphigoid gestationis	Increased risk of prematurity and small for gestational age neonates	Mild and transient lesions of pemphigoid gestationis in up to 10%	Commonly recurs recurrences induced by oral contraceptives in 25–50%
Polymorphic eruption of pregnancy	None	None	Usually does not recur
Intrahepatic cholestasis of pregnancy	Increased risk of premature labor (20–60%), intrapartum fetal distress (20–30%), and stillbirths (1–2%)	None	Recurrence in 45–70% of subsequent pregnancies; may be triggered by oral contraceptives
Atopic eruption of pregnancy	None	None	Commonly recurs due to atopic diathesis

and requires specific treatment. Severe cases of pemphigoid gestationis require systemic corticosteroids. PG has also been treated with high-dose intravenous immunoglobulins. For ICP, ursodeoxycholic acid (UDCA) is the most effective treatment.[10]

For ICH, UDCA is considered to be the drug of choice, as it is the only therapy that has been shown to decrease both maternal pruritus and fetal mortality.

REFERENCES

1. Sachdeva S. The dermatoses of pregnancy. Indian J Dermatol. 2008;53(3):103-5.
2. Kroumpouzos G, Cohen LM. Dermatoses of pregnancy. J Am Acad Dermatol. 2001;45:1-19.
3. Vaughan Jones SA, Black MM. Pregnancy dermatoses. J Am Acad Dermatol. 1999;40:233-41.
4. Holmes RC, Black MM. The specific dermatoses of pregnancy. J Am Acad Dermatol. 1983;8:405-12.
5. Shornick JK. Dermatoses of pregnancy. Semin Cutan Med Surg. 1998;17:172-81.
6. Matz H, Orion E, Wolf R. Pruritic urticarial papules and plaques of pregnancy: polymorphic eruption of pregnancy (PUPPP). Clin Dermatol. 2006;24:105-8.
7. Zoberman E, Farmer ER. Pruritic folliculitis of pregnancy. Arch Dermatol. 1981;117:20-2.
8. Fox GN. Pruritic folliculitis of pregnancy. Am Fam Physician. 1989;39:189-93.
9. Lammert F, Marschall HU, Glantz A, Matern S. Intrahepatic cholestasis of pregnancy: molecular pathogenesis, diagnosis and management. J Hepatol. 2000;33:1012-21.
10. Palma J, Reyes H, Ribalta J, Hernandez I, Sandoval L, Almuna R. Ursodeoxycholic acid in the treatment of cholestasis of pregnancy: a randomized, double-blind study controlled with placebo. J Hepatol. 1997;27:1022-8.

EXAMINATION QUESTION

1. Describe pregnancy-specific dermatoses.

31 CHAPTER

Necrobiotic Disorders

Surajit Gorai, Kinnor Das

INTRODUCTION

Necrobiosis means a state of death and life simultaneously.[1]

Necro → Degeneration
Bio → Regenerating

Necrobiotic disorders are those conditions where necrobiotic granulomas, consisting of area of damage (indicated by degenerated collagen) and area of regeneration (indicated by surrounding palisaded granuloma), are seen on histopathology. In this chapter, the commonly encountered necrobiotic disorders have been detailed in a nutshell.

GRANULOMA ANNULARE

Granuloma annulare (GA) is a common inflammatory skin condition typified clinically by annular, smooth, discolored papules and plaques, and necrobiotic granulomas on histology. GA is also known as necrobiotic papulosis.

Etiology:[2]

- *Nonspecific mild trauma:*
  - Bee sting, cat bite, bite of a bug, etc.
  - Tattoo (perforating GA reported)
  - Waxing or threading to remove hairs
- *Occasional disease associations:*
  - EM minor
  - Sarcoidosis
  - Diabetes (type 1 > type 2)
  - Thyroid disorders (thyroiditis, thyroid adenoma)
  - Malignancy
  - *Infections:*
    - Herpes zoster, varicella, EBV
    - Hepatitis B, hepatitis C
    - Tuberculosis
    - *Borrelia burgdorferi*
    - Scabies infestation
  - *Vaccinations:*
    - Tetanus
    - Diphtheria toxoid
    - Hepatitis B immunization
  - Sun exposure and PUVA therapy
  - *Drugs:*
    - Gold
    - Allopurinol
    - Diclofenac
    - Quinidine
    - Intranasal calcitonin
    - Topiramate
    - Amlodipine
    - Thalidomide

Pathogenesis:[2,3]

Exact pathogenesis is yet to be known. Various theories are there:

- Cell-mediated delayed hypersensitivity reaction to an unknown antigen is accepted well. T cell (Th1 to be more precise) mediated reaction that leads to secretion of IFN gamma stimulates macrophages to release matrix metalloproteinase (MMP) leading to damage of dermal collagen.
- Immune complex-mediated vasculitis and post-traumatic primary necrobiosis.
- *Immunological factors*: GA in patients with immunodeficiency and malignancy probably due to release of cytokines by tumor cells might activate fibroblasts and produce an inflammatory cascade leading to granuloma formation.
- Role of TNF-alpha, interferon gamma, and interleukin 2 is also found.
- Primary collagen damage with increased synthesis of collagen that may occur as a reparative process.
- *Perforating GA*: Ischemic epidermal necrosis or transepithelial elimination.

Types of GA and their clinical features ***(Fig. 1)****:*[3,4]

- *Localized*: 75% cases of GA are localized. Most common location → hands. Lesions are annular and skin colored (it may be erythematous or violaceous) Dimensions → usually 1–5 cm in diameter. The margin is firm when palpated.
- *Generalized*: When lesions are seen on trunk as well as on either or both the upper and lower extremities. Associated with HLA BW35. Late onset and poor prognosis. Pruritus is common. May be associated with HIV and diabetes.
- *Subcutaneous*: Occur predominantly in children. Firm to hard, asymptomatic nodules in the deep dermis and subcutaneous tissue and may extend up to underlying muscles. Nodules on scalp and orbit are often adherent to underlying periosteum. Usually 3.5–6 mm in size.

The most common site is anterior leg in pretibial lesion. These are also known as pseudorheumatoid nodule.

- *Perforating variant*: It is characterized by transepidermal elimination of necrobiotic changes.
- *Patch type*: Macular lesions that present as erythematous, reddish brown or violaceous patches without an annular rim are reported in adult women.
- *Disseminated*: Extensive GA lesions, found in extremities. Associated with other disease conditions and drug therapy.
- *Malignancy associated*: Associated with lymphomas, leukemia, solid tumors of prostrate, colon, breast, cervix, testes, lung, and thyroid.
- *Other uncommon variants*:[3]
  - Acute onset painful acral
  - Acute dermal erythema
  - Actinic granuloma
  - Linear
  - Anetodermic
  - Papular
  - Papular umbilicated
  - Plaque like
  - Pustular follicular variant
  - Destructive
  - Giant
  - Targetoid

Investigation: Histopathology is the definite modality for diagnosis of GA.

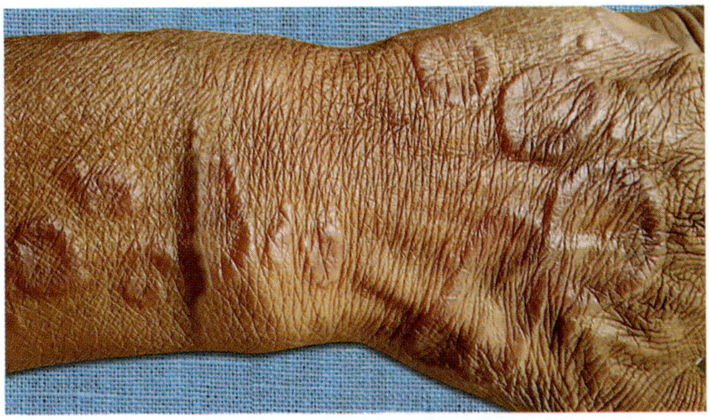

Fig. 1: Granuloma annulare.
Courtesy: Dr Kinnor Das.

Histopathology:[5,6]

Epidermis: Usually normal (perforating type: parakeratosis/areas of perforation) (**Table 1**).

Dermis: Changes usually limited to mid and upper dermis. Ring-shaped necrobiotic areas are found which appear as areas of pale staining, acellular collagen. Blueish strands of mucin can be seen within the granuloma. Palisading histiocytes surround these areas. Eosinophils are often seen large numbers but are insignificant for diagnosis **(Fig. 2)**. Vasculitis may be present occasionally.

Histological variants:[2,3]

- Interstitial type
- Necrobiotic/collagenolytic type
- Tuberculoid type.

Differential diagnosis: Differential diagnosis of granuloma annulare has been shown in **Table 2**.[2]

Treatment:
Overview of therapy of GA: Overview of therapy of granuloma annulare has been shown in **Table 3**.[7]

NECROBIOSIS LIPOIDICA

Necrobiosis lipoidica (NL) is a necrobiotic disorder of unknown etiology which mostly affects the people suffering from diabetes. NL when occurs in association with diabetes is also known as necrobiosis lipoidica diabeticorum (NLD). NL and NLD are used synonymously.

Epidemiology:[3]

- Young-middle aged adults
- Average age of onset: Diabetic patient—34 years[8]
- Overall: Average age of onset 46 years[8]
- Female: Male = 3:1
- Only 0.3–1.2% patient of DM has NL.
- About 22% of patients with NL have or will develop diabetes/glucose intolerance.
- Diabetics + NLD → High risk of complications such as peripheral neuropathy, retinopathy, and immobility of joints.
- *Other associations*: smoking, ulcerative colitis, Crohn's disease, and postjejunal bypass surgery, rheumatoid arthritis, ANCA-positive vasculitis, Hashimoto's thyroiditis, granuloma annulare, and sarcoidosis.

TABLE 1: Histopathological findings of granulomas.[3]

Clinical variant	*Histopathological findings of granulomas*
Perforated GA	Perforator "canal" filled with mucin, collagen, and cellular debris covered by parakeratotic corneal layer or crust
Disseminated GA	Granulomas have minimal necrobiosis and are located in papillary dermis
Subcutaneous GA	Granulomas located in deep dermis and subcutis. Granulomas have larger necrobiotic areas with more mucin and eosinophils than other variants
Juxta-articular GA	Deeper granulomas surrounded by thickened collagen and histiocytes with scanty mucin

Pathophysiology:[3]

- Vascular changes (an explanation for association with diabetes).
- *Contributory factors:* Altered plasma protein profile, elevated factor VIII related antigen, and fibronectin.
- Vascular compromise following immune-deposition in vessel walls or microangiopathic changes due to diabetes → subacute dermal ischemia → dermal collagen degeneration → secondary granulomatous inflammatory response.
- Increased expression of MMP-12, TIMP-1, gelatinase (92 kDa), and urokinase plasminogen activator.
- Elevated anticytoskeleton antibodies (antitroponin, anti-keratin, antidesmin, anti-insulin, and antitrinitrophenol) *[significance unknown]*.

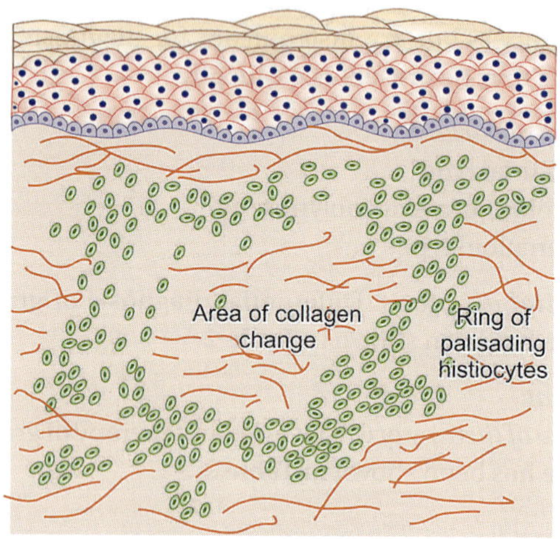

Fig. 2: Granuloma annulare.
Source: Mysore V. Fundamentals of Pathology of Skin, 4th edition. India: Wolters Kluwer India Pvt Ltd; 2015.[5]

Clinical features:[3,7,8]

- Well-defined red-brown indurated plaques with atrophic yellow center.
- Common in legs → pretibial skin, *can occur on other parts of the body, including the trunk and penis, and rarely may diffuse*.
- Originate as a firm, dull-red papule or plaque that progresses to yellowish atrophic plaque with an erythematous edge.
- Surface → glazed in appearance with prominent telangiectatic vessels.
- Hypohidrosis and hypoesthesia or anesthesia may develop and comedo-like plugs can be seen at the periphery of lesions.
- Mostly bilateral
- Persistent and occasionally ulcerate leading to pain.
- Rarely, squamous cell carcinoma may develop.
- Koebnerization at sites of trauma may also occur.

TABLE 2: Differential diagnosis of granuloma annulare.

Annular type	*Generalized type*	*Subcutaneous type*	*Perforating type*	*Patch type*
• Dermatophytosis • SCLE • Annular LP • Acute febrile neutrophilic dermatosis • Erythema chronicum migrans • Actinic granuloma • Necrobiosis lipoidica diabeticorum	• Lichen planus • Lichen nitidus • Molluscum contagiosum	• Erythema nodosum • Dermoid cyst • Rheumatoid Nodules	• Molluscum contagiosum • Insect bites • Pityriasis lichenoides • Perforating collagenosis • Foreign body granuloma • Papulonecrotic tuberculoid • Palisaded neutrophilic and granulomatous dermatitis of immune complex disease	• Morphea • Erythema annulare centrifugum • Parapsoriasis

TABLE 3: Overview of therapy of granuloma annulare.

	Localized	*Generalized*
1st line	• Observation • Cryotherapy • Intralesional corticosteroid • Potent topical corticosteroid	• Narrow band UV-B therapy • PUVA • Dapsone • Ciclosporin • Fumaric acid esters • Methotrexate • Topical antibiotic treatment (Minocycline, ofloxacin, rifampicin)
2nd line	• Topical tacrolimus • Topical pimecrolimus • Topical imiquimod	
3rd line	• Photodynamic therapy • Laser	

HPE:[5,6]

- *Epidermis*: Variable changes (atrophy or hyperkeratosis or ulceration.
- *Dermis*:
    - Horizontal, shelf, or plate-like areas of necrobiosis, vertically alternating with cellular areas.
    - Areas of cellular infiltrate are composed of histiocytes, plasma cells and lymphocytes, and foreign body giant cells. A well-formed granuloma may be seen, referred to as granuloma disciformis of Meissner.
    - Infiltrate extending into lobules of subcutis as panniculitis.
    - Blood vessels often exhibit thickening of their walls with proliferation of their endothelial cells. The process may lead to partial or complete occlusion of the lumen. Vasculitis of the lymphocytic type may be seen sometimes.
    - Foam cells due to lipid deposits.
    - Sclerosis may be present.
    - Dilated blood vessels. Periodic acid-Schiff (PAS)-positive material may be seen in surrounding vessels.

Disease Course and Prognosis

- Slow progression over years is usual, occasionally periods of resolution with variable atrophy and scarring may occur.
- May be complicated by ulceration.

Differential diagnosis:

- Diabetic dermatopathy
- Chronic dermatitis
- Morphea
- Pretibial myxedema
- Lipodermatosclerosis

Management

When NL is associated with diabetes, control of blood sugar forms the first line of management. The treatment is usually unsatisfactory. Prevention of ulcer formation is of utmost importance:

- Topical steroids are mostly used which may halt the progression if used early.
- Intralesional steroids can be given along the borders.
- Topical tacrolimus
- Other immunomodulators can be used with moderate benefit.
- Phototherapy, photodynamic therapy, and pulsed dye laser are the other modalities which has been tried with variable outcome.
- Split skin thickness grafting can be used for ulcerated lesions.

GRANULOMA MULTIFORME[3]

Granuloma multiforme (GM) is a necrobiotic disorder of unknown etiology and is common in the residents of Africa. GM is also known as *Unono Enyl* (meaning elephant ring worm in local Ibo language of Africa) (aged >40 years age).

Clinical features:

- Population affected: >40 years age
- In photoexposed areas
- Pruritic annular papule with mild atrophic changes in center.

Most important differential diagnosis: Tuberculoid leprosy.

HPE:

- Epidermis is usually normal.
- Dermis shows ill-defined, irregular, focal areas of necrobiosis in the upper and mid dermis which are surrounded by a palisading rim of histiocytes.
- Elastoclasia seen in rim as well as center of annular lesion.
- No effective treatment.

NECROBIOTIC XANTHOGRANULOMA[3]

Necrobiotic xanthogranuloma (NXG) is rare non-Langerhans cell histiocytosis.

The associated paraprotein seen in NXG may either be the triggering factor or cofactor in the pathogenesis. This monoclonal protein may resemble a lipoprotein and hence bind to lipoprotein receptors on macrophages.

Clinical features:

- Asymptomatic multiple well-demarcated plaques and nodules with a peripheral erythematous border involving periorbital area.
- Hyperpigmented to violaceous to red-orange or yellow papules and nodules.
- *Around eyes:* Yellowish red color
- *On trunk:* Orange red color
- *Other site:* Trunk and extremities
- Can be associated with ophthalmologic complications.

Histopathology:[5]

- Epidermis and upper dermis are usually normal.
- The necrobiotic areas are seen in the dermis and *subcutis* and are surrounded by histiocytes, foam cells, and multinucleate giant cells, both foreign body and Touton type.
- There is alternation of the necrobiotic areas with areas of xanthogranulomatous infiltration which is considered to be a characteristic feature.
- The granulomas can be band-like (most common), stellate, or nodular.
- Cholesterol cleft and B-cell follicles are common.

- Inclusion bodies such as asteroid bodies, cholesterol clefts, plasma cells, palisade granuloma formation, eosinophils, transepidermal elimination of cholesterol, cellular debris, and blood vessels involvement are rare features.
- The number of foam cells tends to vary and elastic fibers are absent or sparse.
- Histiocytes stain positive for CD68, CD11b, lysozyme, and Mac 387.
- Focus floating microscopes tend to detect the presence of rare spirochetes at periphery of the granuloma.
- Direct immune fluorescence studies show the presence of blood vessel wall deposits of IgM, C3, and fibrin.

It has a chronic and slowly progressive course.

Differential diagnosis:

- Xanthelasma
- Granuloma annulare
- Necrobiosis lipoidica
- Xanthoma disseminatum
- Multicentric reticulohistiocytosis
- Juvenile xanthogranuloma
- Sarcoidosis
- Xanthomas

Recurrence is common after surgical debulking.

RHEUMATOID NODULE[3]

One of the extra-articular manifestation of rheumatoid arthritis (RA).

Clinical features:

- Asymptomatic single or multiple firm, skin colored nodules of size 0.5–4 cm often attached to the underlying periosteum.
- Located mainly on the extensor aspects at sites of pressure commonly on the ulnar side of the forearm and are also seen over the elbows, forearms, finger joints, occiput, Achilles tendon, ischial, and sacral prominences.
- Extracutaneous rheumatoid nodules may also develop in the viscera.
- Histopathology shows homogeneous eosinophilic necrobiotic areas with fibrin deposition at the center.[5]
- Treatment options include intralesional steroid along with management of rheumatoid arthritis.
- Excision leads to recurrence.

RHEUMATIC FEVER NODULES[3,9]

Rheumatic fever nodules are seen in <5% of patients with rheumatic fever (RF).

It is considered as one of the major manifestations of rheumatic fever as per the WHO criteria for diagnosis of rheumatic fever and rheumatic heart disease.

Clinical features: They are 0.5–2 cm, painless, firm subcutaneous nodules often seen over the bony prominences such as elbow, occiput, hands, and feet.

Seen 2–3 weeks after the onset of RF, and usually disappear by 3 weeks.

The development of subcutaneous nodules is often associated with carditis.

Histopathology:

- Rheumatic fever nodules are subcutaneous or deeper.
- These are characterized by few or more foci of *fine fibrinoid necrosis* or fibrinoid change as depicted by separation and swelling of collagen, which are surrounded by histiocytes, which are sometimes arranged in a palisading manner or are multinucleate.
- Mixed inflammatory cell infiltrate is seen perivascular and around the necrobiotic areas. The necrobiotic areas may also contain scattered inflammatory cells or cell debris.
- Lipid deposits are also occasionally seen.
- No definite treatment present.

Histologic Features of Necrobiotic Disorders[10]

Histologic features of necrobiotic disorders are given in **Table 4**.

TABLE 4: Histologic features of necrobiotic disorders.

	Sarcoidosis	*Granuloma annulare*	*Necrobiosis lipoidica*	*Annular elastolytic giant cell granuloma*	*Cutaneous Crohn's disease*	*Interstitial granulomatous dermatitis*	*Palisading neutrophilic and granulomatous dermatitis*	*Rheumatoid nodule*
Typical lesion	Superficial and deep dermis	Superficial and mid dermis	Entire dermis, subcutis	Superficial and mid dermis	Superficial and deep dermis	Mid and deep dermis	Entire dermis	Deep dermis, subcutis

Contd...

Contd...

	Sarcoidosis	*Granuloma annulare*	*Necrobiosis lipoidica*	*Annular elastolytic giant cell granuloma*	*Cutaneous Crohn's disease*	*Interstitial granulomatous dermatitis*	*Palisading neutrophilic and granulomatous dermatitis*	*Rheumatoid nodule*
Granuloma pattern	Tubercle with few peripheral lympho-cytes ("naked")	Palisading or interstitial; patchy with discrete foci	Diffuse palisading and interstitial horizontal "tiers"	Palisading, irregular	Tubercle with surrounding lymphocytes	Interstitial small "rosettes" around single collagen fibers	Palisading and interstitial; prominent neutrophils and leukocytoclasia	Palisading
Necrobiosis (altered collagen)	No	Yes ("blue")	Yes ("red")	No	No	Yes ("blue")	Yes ("blue")	Yes ("red")
Giant cell	Yes	Variable	Yes	Yes	Yes	Variable	Variable	Yes
Elastolysis	No	Variable	Variable	Yes	No	Variable	Variable	No
Elastophago-cytosis	No	Variable	No	Yes	No	No	No	No
Asteroid bodies	Yes	Variable	Variable	Yes	No	Variable	Variable	No
Mucin	No	Yes	Minimal	No	No	Minimal	Variable	Variable
Extracellular lipid	No	Variable	Yes	No	No	No	No	Variable
Vascular changes	No	Variable	Yes	No	No	No	Yes	Yes

Feature	*Granuloma annulare*	*Necrobiosis lipoidica*	*Rheumatoid nodule*
Epidermis	Normal	Thinned (occasionally ulcerated)	Normal
Necrobiosis	Ring-shaped, discrete foci	Plate like, diffuse	Large, sharply defined areas
Location	Superficial or mid dermis	Extensive at all levels	Deep
Infiltration	Single filing	Alternate with necrobiosis	Surrounding the necrobiosis
Types of cells	Palisading histiocytes	Histiocytes, giant cells, tuberculoid granuloma	Histiocytes, giant cells, eosinophils
Appearance of collagen	Pale bluish incomplete degeneration	Pale	Eosinophilic
Vasculitis	Not common	Common	Common
Fibrosis	Rare	Common	Common
Deposited material	Mucin	Lipid	Fibrinoid

Important[5]
Stain for mucin: *Colloidal iron, Alcian blue*
Stain for lipid: *Scarlet red*
Stain for lipid: *Phosphotungstic acid hematoxylin*
Source: Mysore V. Fundamentals of Pathology of Skin, 4th edition. India: Wolters Kluwer India Pvt Ltd; 2015.

Necrobiotic granulomas: Brief overview

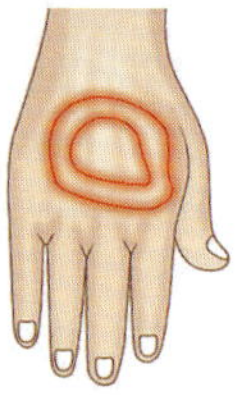

Granuloma Annulare (GA)

Children and young adults, F > M
Sites: Dorsum of hands, feet, ankle, elbow knee (predilection for areas of trauma)
Annular plaques with raised erythematous border and central clearing
Spontaneous regression

Histopathology

Upper and middle dermis involved mainly palisading histiocytes around central mucin (colloidal iron positive) and degenerating collagen

Multinucleate histiocytes may contain intracytoplasmic elastic fibers
Occasional neutrophils in mucinous areas

Subcutaneous variant of GA (as known as *pseudo-rheumatoid nodule*) mainly seen in children

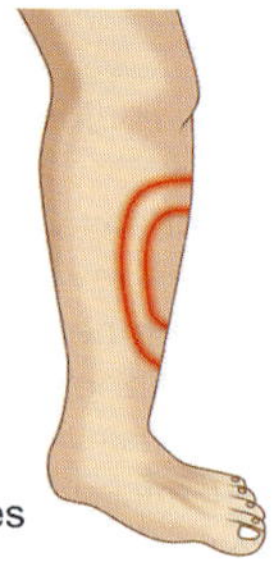

Necrobiosis Lipoidica (NL)

Diabetic patients (5th–6th decades)
Nondiabetic patients (3rd–4th decades)
Female > male (3:1)
Sites: Mostly anterior aspect of tibial surface
Others—Thigh, popliteal fossa, feet and arm

Histopathology

Lower dermis involved mainly
Sandwich sign: Alternating layers of degenerated collagen and granulomatous
Inflammation, comprised of palisading histiocytes predominant *plasma cells* and lymphocytes

Biopsy rectangular in contour

Superficial dermis may show sclerosis and telangiectatic vessels

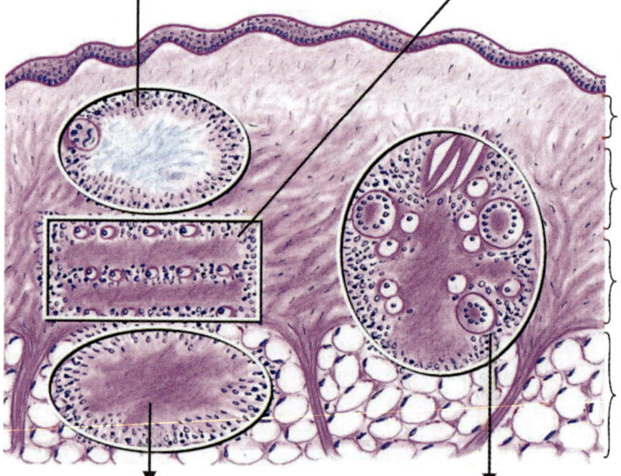

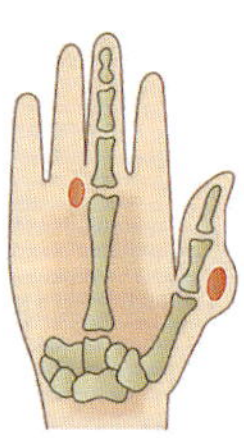

Histopathology

Subcutaneous tissue involved central eosinophilic homogeneous degeneration of collagen

Peripheral palisades of histiocytes and lymphocytes

Chronic deep seated inflammatory nodules 1/3rd cases of rheumatoid arthritis (RA) occasionally a/w SLE
Sites: Single/multiple firm non-tender freely mobile subcutaneous nodules, a/w metacarpophalangeal and proximal interphalangeal joints

Rheumatoid Nodule (RN)

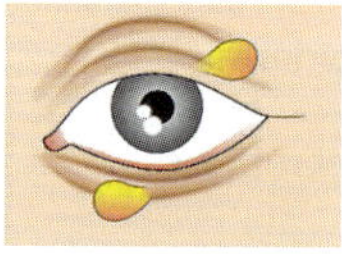

Histopathology

Deep dermis and subcutaneous tissue involved mainly
Granulomatous inflammation composed of foamy histiocytes, Touton gaint cells and lymphoid infiltrate
Interventing broad zone of necrobiosis

Cholesterol clefts present

Middle aged patients
Often associated with paraproteinemia (often IgG monoclonal gammopathy or rare underlying multiple myeloma)

Sites: Mostly periorbital region
Others—Neck, trunk and extremities

Necrobiotic Xanthogranuloma (NX)

Blue necrobiotic granulomas: Granuloma annulare, rheumatoid vasculitis and granulomatosis with polyangiitis (formerly k/a Wegener's granulomatosis)
Red necrobiotic granulomas: Necrobiosis lipoidica, rheumatoid nodule, necrobiotic xanthogranuloma, eosinophilic cellulitis (Well's syndrome) and eosinophilic granulomatosis with polyangiitis (formerly k/a Churg-Strauss syndrome)

Spectrum of granulomatous, neutrophilic and vasculitic dermatoses in patients with rheumatologic disorders

- Erythema elevatum diutinum
- Rheumatoid or other autoimmune connective tissue disease associated vasculitis
- ANCA associated vasculitis

Palisaded neutrophilic and granulomatous dermatitis (PNGD)	Interstitial granulomatous dermatitis (IGD)
• Sweet syndrome • Rheumatoid neutrophilic dermatitis	• Rheumatoid nodule

Source: Rosenbach MA, Wanat KA, Reisenauer A, White KP, Korcheva V, White CR. Non-infectious granulomas. In: Bolognia JL, Schaffer JV, Cerroni L (Eds). Dermatology, 4th edition. Elsevier Limited; 2018. pp. 1644-63.

KEY POINTS

- Necrobiosis indicates degenerative process coupled with regeneration in the surrounding tissue.
- Palisade appearance in histopathology indicates necrobiosis.
- GA is a classical example of necrobiotic disorder.
- Clinically, these disorders usually take annular or arciform in shape.
- Autoimmune process is thought to be involve.

REFERENCES

1. McGuinness M, Padhiar N. Necrobiosis lipoidica diabeticorum. The Foot. 1997;7(1):47-51.
2. Prendiville JS. Granuloma Annulare. In: Kang S, Amagai M, Bruckner AL, Enk AH, Margolis DJ, McMichael AJ, et al., (Eds). Fitzpatrick's Dermatology, 9th edition. New York: McGraw Hill Education; 1990. pp. 564-71.
3. Chandrashekaran B, Kadbet SNU. Necrobiotic disorders. In: Sacchidanand S, Oberai C, Imamdar AC (Eds). IADVL Textbook of Dermatology, 4th edition. Mumbai: Bhalani Publishing House; 2013. pp. 1753-69.
4. Bourke J. Granulomatous disorders of the skin. In: Griffiths C, Barker J, Bleiker T, Chalmers R, Creamer D (Eds). Rooks Textbook of Dermatology, 9th edition. West Sussex: John Wiley & Sons, Ltd; 2016. pp. 97.1-97.13.
5. Mysore V. Fundamentals of Pathology of Skin, 4th edition. India: Wolters Kluwer India Pvt Ltd; 2015. p. 330.
6. Ko CJ, Glusac EJ. Noninfectious granuloma. In: Elder DE (Ed). Lever's Histopathology of the Skin, 11th edition. Philedelphia: Wolters Kluwer; 2015. pp. 427-57.
7. Sardana K, Rani S. Necrobiotic disorders. In: Sardana K, Sinha S, Rani S (Eds). Compendium of Dermatology for Examinations. New Delhi: CBS Publishers & Distributors Pvt. Ltd.; 2020. pp. 390-6.
8. James W, Elston D, Treat J, Rosenbach M, Neuhaus I. Errors in metabolism. In: Andrews' Diseases of the Skin Clinical Dermatology, 11th edition. Philadelphia: Elsevier; pp. 529-30.
9. Hartley M. Rheumatic fever. DermNet NZ. 2010. [online] Available from: https://dermnetnz.org/topics/rheumatic-fever/ [Last accessed January, 2021].
10. Rosenbach MA, Wanat KA, Reisenauer A, White KP, Korcheva V, White CR. Non-infectious granulomas. In: Bolognia JL, Schaffer JV, Cerroni L (Eds). Dermatology, 4th edition. Elsevier Limited; 2018. pp. 1644-63.

EXAMINATION QUESTIONS

1. Define necrobiosis. What are necrobiotic disorders? Discuss in detail any one of them.
2. What is granuloma annulare?

3 SECTION

Pediatric Dermatology

32 CHAPTER

Neonatal Dermatoses

Abhijit Saha, Subhamoy Nyogi

INTRODUCTION

- Most cutaneous lesions in the neonatal period are physiological, benign, transient, and self-limiting conditions that should be differentiated from more serious and potentially life-threatening diseases such as infections and genodermatoses.
- Transient skin disorders are discussed in **Table 1**.

CUTIS MARMORATA

- Benign and generalized cutaneous vasomotor phenomenon induced by hypothermia.
- Due to immaturity of autonomic nervous system in the newborn.
- More common in preterm, although full-term babies may also be affected.
- Transient, blanchable, bluish red, and reticulated areas of mottling that last for minutes. Aggravated by cold and disappear on rewarming.
- Improves spontaneously within first few weeks.[1]
- Has to be differentiated from cutis marmorata telangiectatica congenita, a rare capillary malformation which is fixed and does not disappear with rewarming. It is also associated with extracutaneous findings such as limb growth abnormalities, glaucoma, macrocephaly and other neurological abnormalities.

HARLEQUIN COLOR CHANGE

- Transient and sudden phenomenon characterized by sharply demarcated erythema on one-half of the body with simultaneous blanching on the contralateral half.
- Well-defined line of demarcation in the midline.
- This sudden change of color generally fades within 30 seconds to 20 minutes.
- Appears between the 2nd and 5th day after birth, but may occur up to the 3rd week. Usually a single episode.[2]
- Most commonly observed in lateral decubitus position, the location changes when the baby is rotated.
- Usually observed in healthy newborns, if persists beyond the end of the 4th week, cardiovascular anomalies have to be ruled out.

ERYTHEMA TOXICUM NEONATORUM (FIG. 1) AND TRANSIENT NEONATAL PUSTULAR MELANOSIS (TABLE 2)

Benign and transient self-limited vesicopustular eruptions are seen in term neonates.

DIFFERENTIAL DIAGNOSIS OF PUSTULAR ERUPTIONS IN THE NEONATE

- Miliaria
- Scabies
- Erythema toxicum neonatorum (ETN)
- Transient neonatal pustular melanosis (TNPM)
- Pustular psoriasis
- Congenital or neonatal candidiasis
- Congenital syphilis
- Eosinophilic pustular folliculitis of infancy
- Herpes simplex virus (HSV) infection
- Impetigo
- Benign neonatal cephalic pustulosis
- Infantile acropustulosis
- Neonatal pustulosis of transient myeloproliferative disorder

TABLE 1: Transient skin disorders.

• *Physiological skin disorders:* Vernix caseosa, lanugo, physiological desquamation, milia, miniature puberty, sebaceous hyperplasia, and physiological jaundice • *Transient vascular physiological changes:* Cutis marmorata, salmon patch, harlequin color change, erythema neonatorum, and acrocyanosis • *Transient vesiculopustular eruptions:* Erythema toxicum neonatorum, transient neonatal pustular melanosis, miliaria, benign neonatal cephalic pustulosis, neonatal acne, and infantile acropustulosis	• *Oral lesions:* Epstein pearls, Bohn nodules, dental lamina cysts, natal and neonatal teeth, eruption cyst, and sucking pads of the lips • *Pigmentary skin lesions:* Mongolian spots, pigmentary lines of the newborn, and periungual hyperpigmentation • *Miscellaneous:* Subcutaneous fat necrosis, sucking blisters, adnexal polyps, pedal papules of infancy, and perineal groove

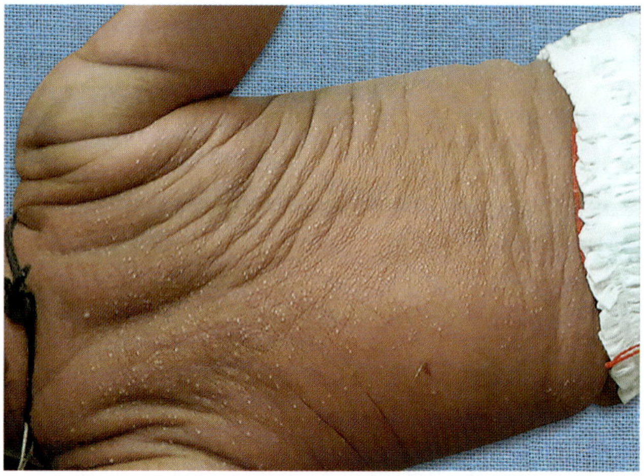

Fig. 1: Erythema toxicum neonatorum.
Courtesy: Dr Abhijit Saha.

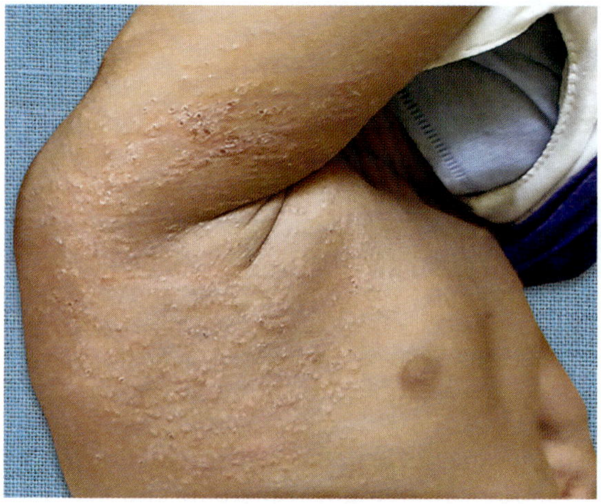

Fig. 2: Flexural accentuation in miliaria rubra.
Courtesy: Dr Abhijit Saha.

TABLE 2: Characteristics of erythema toxicum neonatorum (ETN) and transient neonatal pustular melanosis (TNPM).

Points	*ETN*	*TNPM*
Age of onset	Usually 2–3 days after birth	Almost always present at birth
Ethnicity	In all racial groups	More common in dark-skinned races
Morphology	Erythematous macule 2–3 cm in diameter with central papule or pustule	Fragile pustules or vesicles 1–5 mm in diameter without surrounding erythema
Distribution	Face, trunk, and proximal extremities. Sparing of palms and soles	Forehead, mandibular area, neck, trunk, buttocks, thighs, palms, and soles
Evolution	• Evolve in crops that wax and wane • Spontaneous involution within 1–2 weeks without sequelae[3]	Fragile lesions that break down easily, leaving pigmented macules surrounded by fine, white collarettes of scale Longer time for resolution, few weeks to months[3]
Giemsa or Wright staining	Eosinophils	Predominantly neutrophils with occasional eosinophils
Skin biopsy	Perifollicular dense inflammatory infiltrate composed mostly of eosinophils and subcorneal pustules	Intracorneal or subcorneal collection of neutrophils

Miliaria

- Disorder due to blockage of eccrine sweat ducts
- *Three subtypes according to level of blockage*: Miliaria crystallina (stratum corneum), miliaria rubra (mid epidermal), and miliaria profunda (dermoepidermal junction)
- *Miliaria crystallina*:
  - Superficial, translucent, noninflammatory fragile vesicles 1–3 mm in diameter resembling drops of water.
  - Onset is typically in the first days of life, exacerbated by high humidity, phototherapy, occlusive clothing, and emollients.
  - Most commonly seen in the neck folds, axillae, and on the back.
- *Miliaria rubra **(Fig. 2)***:
  - Crops of nonfollicular papules on an inflammatory base.
  - Flexural areas and neck folds are most prominently affected, also truncal involvement.
  - Type 1 pseudoaldosteronism causes recurrent bouts of miliaria pustulosa.
  - May be mistaken for ETN, however, miliaria has predilection for flexural skin and tends to recur.
- *Miliaria profunda*: Very uncommon in neonates.
- *Differential diagnosis*: Other vesiculopustular eruptions.
- *Treatment*: Cooling measures and removal of predisposing factors such as high heat, humidity, and occlusive clothing.

Milia (Fig. 3)

- Subepidermal keratin containing cysts associated with pilosebaceous apparatus of vellus hair follicles.
- 1–2 mm single or multiple, firm, pinpoint, and pearly white papules located preferentially over nose, cheeks, forehead, chin also scalp, upper trunk, and upper limbs.
- Occur in 40–50% of neonates.
- Primary milia arise spontaneously and secondary milia occur due to medications, diseases, and cutaneous healing after trauma.

- Primary milia in newborn disappear spontaneously without scarring, usually within weeks to months.
- Underlying genodermatoses must be suspected in cases with:[4]
  - Persistent, profuse, and extensive milia
  - With atypical distribution
  - Other associated anomalies
- *Genodermatoses associated with milia*:
  - Orofaciodigital syndrome type 1
  - Gorlin syndrome
  - Brooke-Spiegler syndrome
  - Keratitis-ichthyosis-deafness (KID) syndrome
  - Dystrophic epidermolysis bullosa (EB)
  - Porphyria
  - Bazex syndrome

Neonatal Acne

- Benign, self-limited eruption in neonates, which consists of erythematous papules, pustlules, and less commonly comedones, distributed predominantly on the cheeks, chin, and forehead. No scarring.
- *Age of onset*: Birth to 4–6 weeks, more common in boys.
- Due to hyperactive sebaceous glands stimulated by neonatal and maternal androgens.
- *Differential diagnosis*: Infantile acne, milia, sebaceous hyperplasia, and other neonatal pustular eruptions.
- *Treatment*: Self-limiting. Gentle cleansers, oil-free emollients. If marked pustules, topical azole cream.
- *Neonatal cephalic pustulosis*:
  - Variant of neonatal acne, some consider it to be synonymous
  - Uncertain etiologic role of Malassezia colonization
  - *Age of onset*: Typically 2–3 weeks, but may present as late as 6–8 weeks
  - Spontaneous resolution over 1–2 weeks in majority
  - Asymptomatic, nonfollicular erythematous papules and pustules, and lack of comedonal lesions. Distributed on the forehead, cheeks, and chin, less frequently on neck and upper chest.
  - *Treatment*: No treatment required. Parent counseling. In lesions persisting longer than usual and widespread lesions, topical 2% ketoconazole cream (sometimes in combination with 1% hydrocortisone cream) leads to rapid clearance.

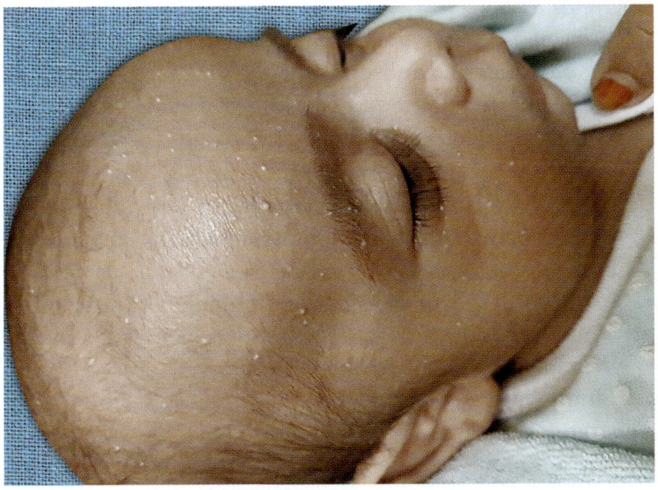

Fig. 3: Multiple milia distributed over nose, cheeks, forehead, and scalp. *Courtesy:* Dr Abhijit Saha.

Caput Succedaneum and Cephalhematoma (Table 3)

Both lesions are due to shearing forces on the scalp skin and skull during labor.

TABLE 3: Characteristics of caput succedaneum and cephalhematoma.

Points	*Caput succedaneum*	*Cephalhematoma*
Anatomy	Subcutaneous edema	Subperiosteal hemorrhage
Onset	At birth, does not increase in size	After birth, increases in size for 2–3 days
Borders	Ill-defined	Well-defined
Suture lines	Crosses suture lines	Does not cross suture lines
Consistency	Soft, pits on pressure	Soft, elastic, but does not pit on pressure
Overlying skin	Ecchymotic	No skin change
Course	Spontaneous resolution, within 7–10 days	Longer time for resolution, usually weeks
Complications	Rare, transient, or permanent alopecia	Underlying skull fracture, hyperbilirubinemia if extensive bleeding
Treatment	No treatment required	No treatment required

SUBCUTANEOUS FAT NECROSIS (FIG. 4) OF THE NEWBORN AND SCLEREMA NEONATORUM (TABLE 4)

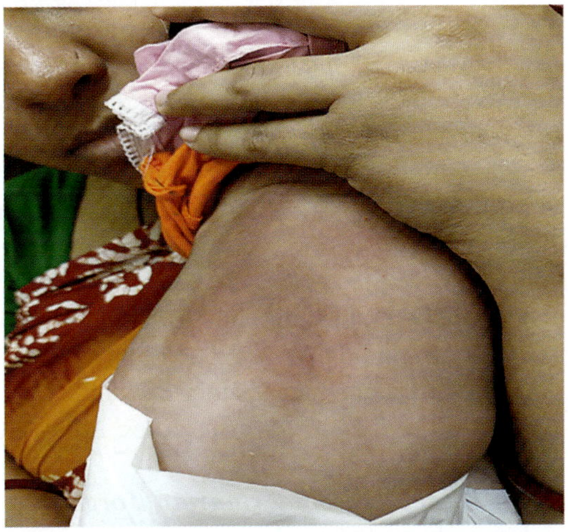

Fig. 4: Erythematous indurated plaque over back in a child with subcutaneous fat necrosis. *Courtesy:* Dr Abhijit Saha.

TABLE 4: Characteristics of subcutaneous fat necrosis of the newborn and sclerema neonatorum.

Points	*Subcutaneous fat necrosis*	*Sclerema*
Incidence	Uncommon	Very rare, usually seen in neonatal ICUs
Age	Usually full-term but also post-term	Premature and small for date babies with severe underlying illness
Predisposing factors	Maternal preeclampsia, gestational diabetes, perinatal asphyxia, hypothermia, maternal drug exposure such as calcium channel blockers (CCBs)	Underlying severe illness such as serious infections, congenital heart disease, and major developmental defects
Onset	1–6 weeks	Almost always during first week
Morphology	Multiple, indurated, nonpitting, painful, subcutaneous nodules, or plaques	Diffuse, yellow-white woody induration
Sites	Back, shoulders, extremities, buttocks, and cheeks	Lower limbs initially, rapidly spread to involve whole body surface except palms, soles, and genitalia
Disease course and prognosis	Spontaneous resolution in several weeks, hypercalcemia can persist for months. Residual subcutaneous atrophy is frequent. Rarely skin ulceration, scarring, and calcification	• Poor prognosis, determined by nature of underlying disease • Mortality >50%
Complications	Hypercalcemia, most common. Others—hypoglycemia, thrombocytopenia, hypertriglyceridemia (rare)[5]	Immobility of extremities, respiratory insufficiency due to restricted chest wall movement
Histology	• Dense inflammatory lobular infiltrate composed of lymphocytes, histiocytes, multinucleated giant cells with fat necrosis • Radially arranged needle-shaped clefts represent crystallized fatty acids dissolved during processing within adipocytes and giant cells	Sparse (if any) inflammatory infiltrate without fat necrosis. Radially arranged needle-shaped clefts within adipocytes
Treatment	• Analgesia • *Monitoring and treatment of hypercalcemia:* Adequate hydration and restriction of calcium and vitamin D_3 intake. Calcium wasting diuretics, glucocorticoids, and bisphosphonates	Treatment of underlying illness

DEVELOPMENTAL ANOMALIES OF THE NEWBORN

Aplasia Cutis Congenita

- Congenital absence of skin or presence of scar.
- Localized and solitary, may be multiple and widespread.
- Around 80% lesions are located on the scalp, most of them in midline in close proximity to the parietal hair whorl.
- 1–3 cm in diameter, round or oval, sharply marginated, hairless atrophic patch with thin parchment-like appearance or can be open with ulceration (larger lesions). Underlying defects in muscle, bone, and even dura may be associated (20%).
- Ring of darker and/or coarser terminal hairs around the defect known as "hair-collar" sign, marker of cranial dysraphism[6] (also seen in encephalocele, meningocele, dermoid cyst, etc.).
- In majority of cases, there are no further abnormalities.
- Most cases are sporadic.
- Anomalies with congenital absence of skin:[7]
    - *With limb reduction abnormalities*: Adams–Oliver syndrome
    - *With associated epidermal and organoid nevi*: Schimmelpenning syndrome
    - Overlying embryological malformations, e.g., meningomyelocele
    - *With EB*: On extremities
    - Aplasia cutis congenita (ACC) caused by specific teratogens, e.g., methimazole
    - *Trisomy 13*: Patau syndrome
- *Differential diagnosis*: Iatrogenic injuries, encephalocele, and meningocele. Other causes of cicatricial alopecia and nevus sebaceous (healed lesions).
- Prognosis for single superficial lesions is excellent, resulting in cosmetic defect only.
- *Treatment*:
    - *Conservative wound management*: With appropriate dressings and antiseptics
    - Deeper lesions require radiological evaluation
    - Early closer of larger defects by skin grafts or local flaps.

Median Raphe Cyst

- Well circumscribed, freely mobile, solitary, or multiple cystic lesions
- *Midline location* along genitoperineal raphe, most commonly on the distal portion of penis.[8] No communication with the urethra
- Lined with pseudostratified columnar, less commonly stratified squamous epithelium
- Asymptomatic, cosmetic concern, and discomfort during sexual intercourse
- *Complication*: Secondary infection
- *Treatment*: Excision with primary closure.

Supernumerary Nipples (Polythelia)

- Most frequent congenital abnormality of the breast.
- Remnants of the embryological milk line.
- *Location*: Chest wall and upper abdomen are the most common location.
- Usually a single lesion, may be multiple and bilateral.
- Brown or pink, small, umbilicated, or elevated papules surrounded by pigmented areola.[9]
- Familial occurrence may be seen.
- Majority of cases, no further anomaly seen.
- *Syndromal association*: Becker nevus syndrome, etc.
- *Differential diagnosis*: Melanocytic nevus.
- *Treatment*: Excision may be done for cosmetic reasons.

Accessory Tragi

- Developmental abnormality of the dorsal portion of first branchial arch.
- Congenital, roundish, solitary or multiple, unilateral or bilateral, soft or cartilaginous, sessile or pedunculated, papules or nodules.
- *Location*: In front of the auricle [medullary carcinoma (MC)], cheek, and anterior to the sternocleidomastoid muscle are less frequent locations.
- Familial occurrence has been reported.
- Usually they are isolated congenital defects.[10]
- Rarely may be associated with other first branchial arch abnormalities such as cleft lip, cleft palate, and branchial fistulae.
- *Rare syndromal associations*:[11]
  - Oculo-auriculo-vertebral syndrome.
  - Treacher–Collins
  - VACTERL (vertebral defects, anal atresia, cardiac defects, tracheoesophageal fistula, renal anomalies, and limb abnormalities).
- *Differential diagnosis*: Macrotragus, hair follicle nevus, and trichofolliculoma.
- *Treatment*: Surgical excision.

Thyroglossal Duct Cysts

- Most common cause of midline neck swellings in childhood (prevalence: 7% of the world population).
- Derived from incompletely obliterated thyroglossal duct (normally involutes by 10th week of gestation).[12]
- *Location*: Most often close to the hyoid bone, in or near the midline but can be located anywhere along the path of thyroid's route of migration from the foramen cecum to the level of thyroid gland.
- *Presentation*: Typically, a painless soft mass of 1–2 cm diameter moves upward on swallowing and tongue protrusion. It can present as an abscess or intermittently draining sinus.
- *Differential diagnosis*: Ectopic thyroid, lipoma, lymphadenopathy, dermoid or epidermoid cysts, second branchial cleft cysts, and carcinoma.
- *Complication*: Recurrent infection, malignant change (most common—papillary CA).
- *Preoperative evaluation*: USG, FNAC, CT, and MRI in some cases.
- *Treatment*: Sistrunk's operation.

Neonatal Erythroderma

- Inflammation of the skin producing fair amount of erythema and scaling involving >90% surface area of the skin.
- Rare, but definitely a life-threatening entity. Needs urgent medical attention and appropriate diagnostic workup to avoid case fatality.
- Causes of neonatal erythroderma are described in **Table 5**.
- Diagnostic clues and management[13] of neonatal erythroderma are given in **Table 6**.
- *Supportive management*:
  - Strict monitoring of temperature, pulse, respiratory rate, blood pressure, and intake-output.
  - Maintaining adequate oral or parenteral fluid intake and mandatory monitoring of serum electrolytes (at risk of hypernatremic dehydration).
  - Bland emollients such as white soft paraffin and wet dressings—for maintaining skin hydration and prevention of fissuring.
  - In case of bullous and erosive lesions—0.01% potassium permanganate soaks (astringent, antibacterial, antifungal action).
  - Maintaining the skin barrier and proper hydration is the cornerstone of management.

Congenital Infections

Newborn baby may acquire infection from pregnant mother. We are trying to throw some light over most important congenital infections of newborn.

Congenital Rubella Syndrome

- Congenital rubella most commonly occurs when mother acquires infection during first 16 weeks of pregnancy.[14]
- Infection in the late pregnancy has a less potential to infect the baby.

TABLE 5: Causes of neonatal erythroderma.

Infections	Staphylococcal scalded skin syndrome (SSSS), toxic shock syndrome, candidiasis
Ichthyoses	Nonbullous ichthyosiform erythroderma, bullous ichthyosiform erythroderma, Conradi–Hunermann syndrome, Netherton's syndrome
Immunodeficiency	Omenn syndrome, graft-versus-host reaction
Metabolic disorders	Disorders of biotin metabolism, essential fatty acid deficiency
Drugs	Ceftriaxone, vancomycin
Cutaneous disorders	Infantile seborrheic dermatitis, psoriasis, atopic dermatitis (AD), pityriasis rubra pilaris, diffuse cutaneous mastocytosis, scabies

TABLE 6: Diagnostic clues and management of neonatal erythroderma.

Disease	*Diagnostic clues*	*Management*
SSSS	• Preceding purulent infection, fever, skin tenderness, superficial blistering, flexural accentuation, irritability, +ve Nikolsky sign • Skin swab—staphylococcal growth • Skin biopsy—subcorneal acantholysis **(Fig. 5)**	IV antibiotics
TSS	• Concomitant maternal infection, scarlatiniform skin rash progressing to erythroderma, fever, hypotension/shock • Skin swab	IV antibiotics, IVIG
Congenital cutaneous candidiasis	• Maternal vaginal Candida infection. Whitish macules on placenta and umbilical cord with neonatal maculopapular exanthem (white dots on the placenta, red dots on the baby) Also in case of listeria infection • Palmoplantar and umbilical regions involved initially • Paronychia, nail dystrophy, sparing of oral cavity, and nappy area (not in case of neonatal candidiasis) • Skin swab, KOH: Pseudohyphae • Urine, blood, and CSF culture to exclude systemic infection	• Topical and oral azoles • IV liposomal amphotericin B
Omenn syndrome	• Generalized eczematous lesions resembling AD, alopecia pachydermia, onychodystrophy • Characteristic triad of erythroderma, hepatosplenomegaly, and lymphadenoptahy along with eosinophilia, raised IgE, hypogammaglobulinemia, decreased B-cells	Cyclosporine, bone marrow transplant curative
GVHR	T-cell immunodeficiency, history of antecedent exchange transfusion, fever, diarrhea	Supportive care and bone marrow transplant
NBIE	Collodion baby, finer scales, ectropion, eclabium, ear canal obstruction, digital autoamputation as sequelae	Emollients, systemic retinoids
Bullous ichthyosiform erythroderma	• Superficial blistering and erosions, ichthyosiform erythroderma, hystrix-like hyperkeratosis, palmoplantar keratoderma, family history • Skin biopsy—epidermolytic hyperkeratosis	Emollients
Netherton's syndrome	• Hypotrichosis, trichorrhexis invaginata, atopy, diarrhea, failure to thrive • Hair microscopy—characteristic, raised IgE, and eosinophilia	Emollients, adequate hydration
Conradi–Hunermann syndrome	• XLD disorder, fatal for male fetuses • Linear and swirled pattern erythroderma, skeletal abnormalities, cataract • Epiphyseal stippling on X-ray	Emollients
Holocarboxylase synthetase deficiency	• Eczematous erythroderma with marked periorificial involvement and alopecia • Lethargy and seizures • *Abnormal ABG:* Ketoacidosis, hyperammonemia, and hypoglycemia. Decreased enzyme activity in fibroblasts	Oral biotin (10 mg/day)
Infantile SD	Cradle cap **(Fig. 6)**, accentuation in the skin folds of axilla, neck, and nappy area	Moisturizer, miconazole-hydrocortisone ointment
AD	Crusting, predominant face **(Fig. 7)** and flexural involvement, sparing of nappy area	• Emollients, weak topical steroid • Short course of oral steroid
Psoriasis	Papulosquamous lesions, can become pustular. Histology—classical	Emollients, cyclosporine, retinoids
PRP	Similar to psoriasis. Follicular keratotic papules, islands of sparing, PPK	Emollients, retinoids
Diffuse cutaneous mastocytosis	• Widespread, yellow-reddish erythema, extensive bulla formation • Darier's sign +ve • Flushing, urticaria, pachydermia • Skin biopsy • Bone marrow biopsy in suspected cases of systemic mastocytosis (hepatosplenomegaly, lymphadenopathy, abnormal blood count, serum tryptase > 100 ng/mL)	• H1 and H2 antagonists. Oral sodium cromoglycate • Avoidance of triggers

(AD: atopic dermatitis; CSF: cerebrospinal fluid; GVHR: graft-versus-host disease; IgE: immunoglobulin; IVIG: intravenous immunoglobulin; NBIE: nonbullous ichthyosiform erythroderma; PPK: palmoplantar keratoderma; PRP: pityriasis rubra pilaris; SD: seborrheic dermatitis; SSSS: staphylococcal scalded skin syndrome; TSS: toxic shock syndrome; XLD: X-linked lymphoproliferative disease)

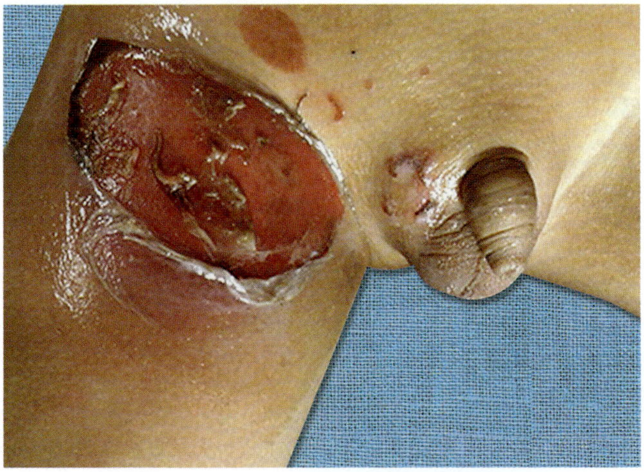

Fig. 5: Staphylococcal-scalded skin syndrome.

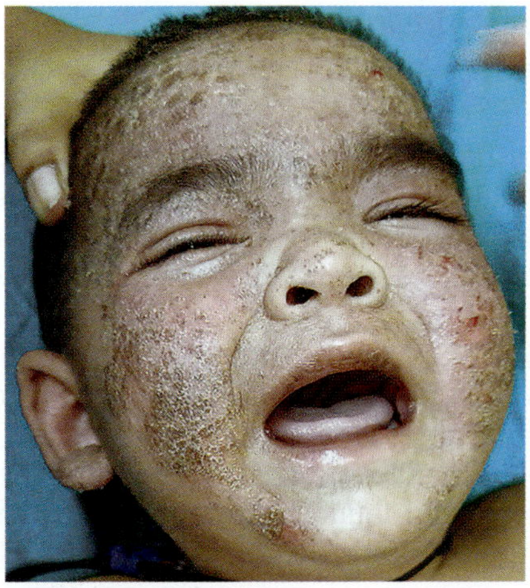

Fig. 7: Severe atopic dermatitis with facial involvement.

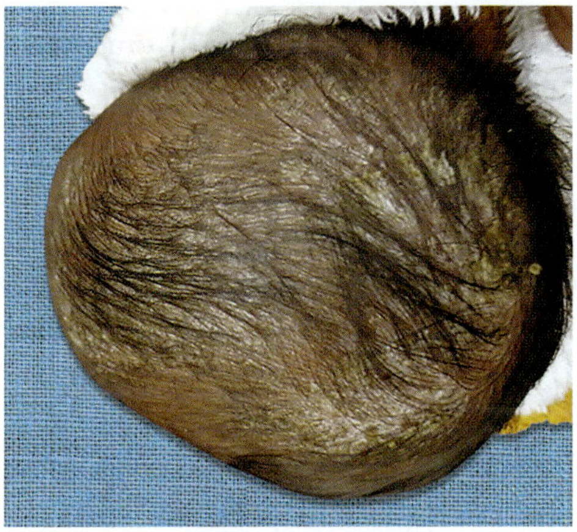

Fig. 6: Cradle cap.
Courtesy: Dr Abhijit Saha.

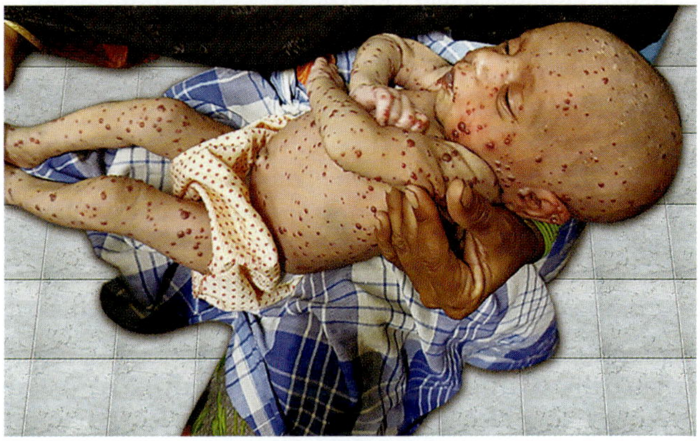

Fig. 8: Blueberry muffin baby.
Courtesy: Dr Abhijit Saha.

- Incidence has declined to a great extent after institution of universal vaccination in 1969.
- Clinical features can be divided into cutaneous and extracutaneous features.
- Most characteristic cutaneous feature is blue berry muffin lesions.[15]
- These lesions represent extramedullary hematopoiesis.
- These lesions present since birth or within first 2 days of life.
- These lesions clinically present as purpuric macules or infiltrative red blue papule and nodule of 2–8 mm in diameter.
- Blueberry muffin lesions **(Fig. 8)** are not specific for rubella, can be seen in other diseases include:
  - Congenital infections such as cytomegalovirus (CMV) infection, toxoplasmosis, enterovirus
  - Erythroblastosis fetalis
  - Twin-twin transfusion syndrome
  - Malignancy such as leukemia, histiocytosis
- Other cutaneous features could be—maculopapular rash, generalized mottling, reticulated erythema of face and extremities, hyperpigmentation, and urticaria.
- *Extracutaneous features*:
  - *Classical traid*: Congenital cataract, deafness, and cardiac defect such as patent ductus arteriosus (PDA)
  - Growth retardation, mental retardation, microcephaly, meningoencephalitis, pigmentary retinopathy
  - Hepatosplenomegaly, jaundice, thrombocytopenia
  - Radiolucent bony lesion
- *Diagnosis*: Confirmed case of congenital rubella syndrome (CRS) is defined as presence of one or more clinical features and presence of laboratory evidences
  - Isolation of virus from cerebrospinal fluid (CSF), urine, or respiratory secretion
  - Rubella-specific IgM antibody
  - IgG antibody which is not due to passive transfer from mother
  - Real-time reverse transcription-polymerase chain reaction (rRT-PCR) from urine, serum or nasopharyngeal secretions.
- *Treatment* is mainly supportive to prevent potential disabilities.
- It only can be prevented by vaccination.
- If mother acquires infection in early pregnancy, abortion is suggested.

Congenital Varicella Syndrome and Neonatal Varicella

- Congenital varicella most commonly occurs when mother acquires infection during first 20 weeks of pregnancy.
- Congenital varicella is extremely rare because primary varicella infection during pregnancy is rare as majority of woman develop immunity during child-bearing age group.
- Newborn of a mother with primary varicella during pregnancy is often normal either due to lack of transmission of infection or self-limiting infection in fetus.
- Cutaneous manifestation is presence of vesicles often in dermatomal distribution with scarring and pigmentation.
- Dermatomal lesions point toward intrauterine herpes zoster.
- Other findings are growth retardation, mental retardation, developmental delay, seizure, microphthalmia, cataract, chorioretinitis, unilateral limb shortening, and flexion contracture.
- Abortion is not usually recommended as risk of fetal malformation is little.
- Neonatal varicella occurs when mother get infected during last few weeks of pregnancy or first few days following delivery.
- In neonatal varicella, timing of onset of infection in neonate and mother is crucial as far as treatment and prognosis is concerned.
- Infection is usually mild if mother get infected 5 days or more before delivery and neonatal varicella starts within 4 days of birth.
- Infection is often severe if mother gets infected within 5 days before delivery and 2 days after delivery or neonatal varicella starts within 5–10 days of birth.
- This severe group should be treated with intravenous acyclovir or intravenous immunoglobulin.

Congenital Syphilis (Fig. 9)

- Caused by transplacental passage of *Treponema pallidum* from infected mother to her fetus.
- Serological evidence of syphilis in mother mandatory to prove congenital syphilis.
- Possible outcomes—spontaneous abortion, stillbirth, live syphilitic child.
- *Classification*:
  - Early congenital syphilis—presenting <2 years of age.
  - Late congenital syphilis—presentation/features appearing >2 years of age.

Early Congenital Syphilis

- May present at birth (severe cases) or within 3–8 weeks of age and in nearly all cases within 3 months. Corresponds to secondary stage of acquired syphilis.
- *Skin lesions*:
  - Vesiculobullous—multiple, discrete, tense bullae, containing serous or seropurulent fluid mainly over palm and soles

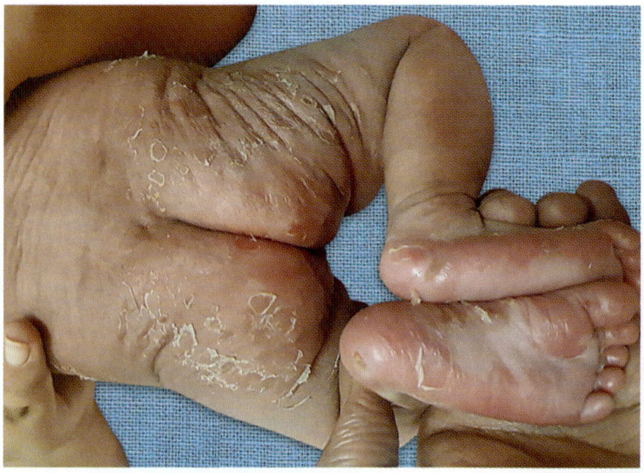

Fig. 9: Congenital syphilis.
Courtesy: Dr Abhijit Saha.

  - Papulosquamous—coppery red, similar to secondary syphilis, distributed over extremities, especially palm and soles
  - Condyloma lata—flat topped, hypertrophic, moist papules at angle of mouth, nose, perianal area
  - Radiating fissures—at the angles of the mouth, on healing leave linear, radiating scars, known as rhagades (late syphilis)
  - Paronychia, patchy alopecia
- *Mucous membrane lesions*:
  - Syphilitic rhinitis/snuffles—profuse, serous, nasal discharge that contains high concentration of treponemes (most important and frequent sign). Inflammatory process may cause nasal cartilage or bone destruction, causing flattening of nasal septum, saddle nose (late manifestation).
  - Mucous patch—smooth, grayish white patches on the palate, tongue, buccal and genital mucosa, pharynx, larynx (may cause hoarse cry).
- *Generalized lymphadenopathy*: Multiple, discrete, firm and nontender. Epitrochlear lymph nodes are considered pathognomonic.
- *Skeletal*:
  - Osteochondritis—common early sign, at the end of long bones, upper end of tibia, distal end of radius and ulna (zone between bone and cartilage becomes involved)
  - Diaphyseal periostitis
  - Wimberger sign—destruction of proximal metaphyses of tibia, X-ray finding
  - Pseudoparalysis of Parrot—pain, tenderness, impairment of movement of extremity due to bone involvement
  - Syphilitic dactylitis—fusiform swelling of the digits, due to osteochondritis of phalanges.
- *Ocular:* Chorioretinitis, uveitis, glaucoma.
- *Central nervous system (CNS)*:
  - Asymptomatic with abnormal CSF findings

- Meningitis and meningoencephalitis—neck stiffness, bulging fontanel, convulsions, hydrocephalus.
- *Gastrointestinal (GI):* Hepatosplenomegaly, sometimes jaundice, ascites.
- *Hematological:* Anemia, thrombocytopenia.

Late Congenital Syphilis

- Correspond to tertiary stage of acquired syphilis
- Stigmata and hypersensitivity/inflammatory reactions
- *Mucocutaneous:*
  - Gummas—nodular/noduloulcerative lesions
  - Nasal/septal perforation
- *Interstitial keratitis*:
  - Onset between 5 and 16 years of age, most common late manifestation, both eyes affected
  - Pain, photophobia, lacrimation, blurred vision, clouding of cornea
  - Circumcorneal vascularization, infiltrating into deeper layers of cornea, slit-lamp diagnostic
  - Not directly influenced by antisyphilitic treatment, good response with corticosteroids
- *Clutton's joint*:
  - Bilateral synovitis of knee joints, presenting as painless hydroarthrosis with no functional impairment
  - Uninfluenced by antisyphilitic treatment
- *Bone involvement*:
  - Thickening and anteroposterior bowing of tibia—sabre tibia
  - Parrot's nodes—round, bony swellings on skull due to localized osteoperiostitis
  - Higoumenakis's sign—thickening of medial part of clavicle
- *Neural deafness*:
  - Due to involvement of cochlear part of eighth nerve
  - Vertigo, tinnitus, loss of hearing
  - Uninfluenced by antisyphilitic treatment
- *CNS*: Juvenile paresis, juvenile tabes
- *Stigmata*: Scars and defects caused by congenital syphilis, diagnostic importance in distinguishing it from acquired syphilis
  - Hutchinson's teeth—deformity of permanent, upper central incisors. Shorter, widely spaced, conical/barrel shaped, notch in the biting edge
  - Hutchinson triad—interstitial keratitis, Hutchinson's teeth and eighth nerve deafness
  - Mulberry molar—first lower molars are commonly affected. Dome-shaped biting edge with ill-developed cusps
  - Frontal and parietal bossing, saddle nose, prominent mandible with short maxillae (bull dog jaw)
  - Corneal opacity, salt and pepper fundus
  - Rhagades

Diagnostic Criteria and Management[16]

Diagnostic criteria and management of congenital syphilis are given in **Table 7**.

TABLE 7: Diagnostic criteria and management of congenital syphilis.

Diagnostic scenarios	*Treatment*
Proven or highly probable congenital syphilis: Any neonate with: • Abnormal physical examination • Serum VDRL/RPR titer >4 times maternal titer (not always true) • Positive dark field test or PCR of lesions/body fluids	Aqueous crystalline penicillin G 1–1.5 lac units/kg/day administered as 50,000 units/kg/dose IV every 12 hours during first 7 days of life, every 8 hours thereafter for a total of 10 days Or Procaine penicillin G 50,000 units/kg/dose IM in a single dose for 10 days
Possible congenital syphilis: Any neonate with normal physical examination and serum VDRL/RPR titer ≤4 times maternal titer and one of the following: • Mother not treated/inadequately treated/no documentation of treatment • Treatment with erythromycin and other non-penicillin G regimen • Mother received recommended treatment <4 weeks before delivery	Aqueous crystalline penicillin G 1–1.5 lac units/kg/day administered as 50,000 units/kg/dose IV every 12 hours during first 7 days of life, every 8 hours thereafter for a total of 10 days Or Procaine penicillin G 50,000 units/kg/dose IM in a single dose for 10 days Or Benzathine penicillin 50,000 units/kg/dose IM single dose
Congenital syphilis less likely: Any neonate with normal physical examination and serum VDRL/RPR titer ≤4 times maternal titer and both of the following are true: • Mother was adequately treated, for the stage of infection and >4 weeks before delivery • No evidence of reinfection/relapse in mother	Benzathine penicillin 50,000 units/kg/dose IM single dose Or No treatment of the infant, rather close serological follow-up in those whose mother's VDRL/RPR titers decreased fourfold after appropriate treatment for early syphilis or remained low or stable for late syphilis
Congenital syphilis unlikely: Any neonate with normal physical examination and serum VDRL/RPR titer ≤4 times maternal titer and both of the following are true: • Mother was adequately treated before pregnancy • Mother's VDRL/RPR titer remained low and stable before and during pregnancy and at delivery (VDRL < 1:2/RPR < 1:4)	No treatment required Or Benzathine penicillin G 50,000 units/kg/dose IM, single dose where follow-up is uncertain

(PCR: polymerase chain reaction; RPR: rapid plasma regain; VDRL: venereal disease research laboratory)

Treatment in Older Infants and Children

Aqueous crystalline penicillin G 2–3 lac units/kg/day administered as 50,000 units/kg/dose every 4–6 hours for 10 days

Second-line treatment: No proven alternative to penicillin. Ceftriaxone IV/IM may be given where penicillin is not available or in penicillin allergic people.

Follow-up:
- All seroreactive infants should have repeat VDRL/RPR titer every 2–3 months, until it becomes nonreactive or there is four-fold decrease (titer should decline by the age of 3 months and should be nonreactive by 6 months, if there is passive transfer of antibody and if the infant was adequately treated)
- If titers are stable or increase after age 6–12 months, the child should be evaluated and treated with 10-day course of parenteral penicillin G.

Recommended Evaluation in Infants with Proven/Highly Probable Disease

- Direct dark-field examination/FTA/PCR from mucocutaneous lesions, lymphnodes, or body fluids
- Serum quantitative nontreponemal and treponemal serological titer (IgM serology highly recommended)
- Complete blood count (CBC) and differential count
- CSF analysis for cell count, protein, VDRL (diagnostic)
- Other tests as clinically indicated (long bone X-ray, chest X-ray (CXR), cranial ultrasound, liver function test (LFT), ophthalmological examination, etc.).

NEONATAL HERPES (FIG. 10)

- Potentially life-threatening disease caused by HSV type 2 (80%) and HSV type 1 (20%).
- *Mode of transmission*: Perinatal (85%), during passage through birth canal and rarely (5%) transplacental intrauterine transmission. Also postnatal, by contact with nongenital sites.

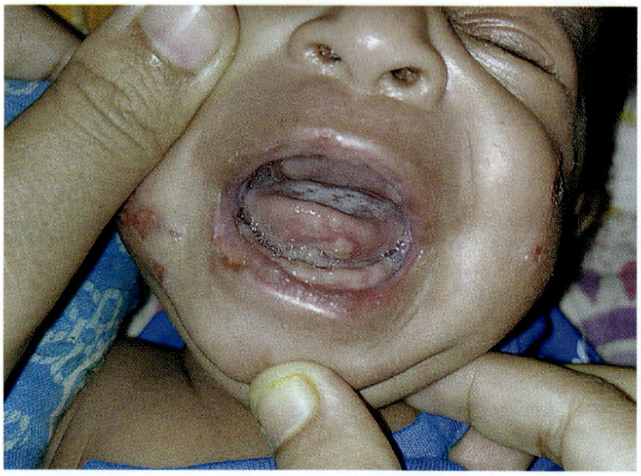

Fig. 10: Neonatal herpes.
Courtesy: Dr Abhijit Saha.

- *Risk factors for transmission*:
  - Primary genital herpes at delivery [>50% risk as compared to recurrent herpes (2%)][17]
  - Vaginal delivery
  - Involvement of cervix
  - Premature infant

However, most neonatal infections occur in mothers who have no previous history of genital HSV and exhibit no overt clinical signs at delivery.

- *Clinical presentation*:
  - Skin, eye, mouth involvement (45% of cases)
  - Encephalitis
  - Disseminated disease affecting multiple organs.

The last two forms account for >50% cases and in 20% of them skin lesions may be absent.

- Isolated or grouped vesicles are most common type of lesion. Others—pustules, petechiae, widespread erosions (may occur without obvious vesiculobullous lesions).
- Scalp and face are most common sites, can occur anywhere, and may become generalized. Oral erosions on the tongue, palate, gingivae, and buccal mucosa.
- *Onset*—first week to 10 days life (more common, suggests perinatal transmission). Onset during first 24 hours denotes intrauterine transmission.
- *Disseminated disease*—lethargy, seizures, hypotension, respiratory distress, thrombocytopenia, hepatosplenomegaly, deranged LFT.
- *Course and prognosis*: In untreated cases, mortality is 60–80%. Even when treated mortality can be 25–30%.
- *Investigations*: Tzanck smear, DFA, PCR of samples (skin lesions, CSF, eyes, nasopharynx).
- *Management*:[18,19]
  - Primary herpes infection in the mother at delivery—CS and prophylactic acyclovir for neonate
  - Primary genital herpes during third trimester—treatment with oral acyclovir (although unclear if it reduces risk of neonatal herpes)
  - Active recurrent herpes—suppressive treatment starting from 36 weeks and delivery by CS.
  - Mothers with previous history of genital herpes but no active lesions during pregnancy/at delivery—asymptomatic shedding needs to considered and strict monitoring of the neonate for presence of HSV.
- Prompt recognition and earliest therapeutic intervention, essential to reduce the risk of progressive infection.
- *Treatment* with IV acyclovir, 20 mg/kg, every 8 hours for 2–3 weeks followed by oral acyclovir for 6 months.

Congenital Candidiasis

- Congenital infection of the child as a result of maternal chorioamnionitis caused by *Candida* (usually ascending infection acquired from genital tract).

- *Risk factors*: Foreign bodies in uterus/cervix, especially intrauterine contraceptive devices (IUCDs), cervical encirclage, invasive procedures, extensive instrumentation, gestational age of child <27 weeks, birth weight <1,000 g.
- *Onset*: At birth or within 6–7 days of life.
- *Clinical presentation*:
  - Extensive maculopapular eruption, progressing to vesicles and pustules on erythematous base in 1–3 days. Rarely—bullae, burn-like exfoliative dermatitis (indicative of onset of systemic involvement).
  - Site—head and neck, back, umbilicus, skin folds, palmoplantar involvement (considered as hallmark). Oral mucosa and napkin area spared (involved in neonatal candidiasis).
  - Onychia, paronychia, nail dystrophy.
  - Systemic involvement—premature and very low birth weight (LBW) neonates at risk. Bronchopneumonia, meningitis, arthritis, endocarditis, microabscess in liver, spleen, kidney, brain.
  - Features suggesting systemic involvement—burn-like skin lesions, respiratory distress, leukocytosis, persistent hyperglycemia, glycosuria, positive cultures from blood, urine, and CSF.
  - *Differential diagnosis*: Neonatal candidiasis and other neonatal vesiculopustular eruptions.
  - *Investigations*: Skin swabs for KOH, routine blood biochemistry, blood/urine/CSF culture (to rule out systemic involvement).
  - *Treatment*: Topical and oral antifungals in skin limited disease, IV liposomal amphotericin B (0.5–1 mg/kg/day), first-line for 3–4 weeks, if systemic involvement. Also fluconazole (6–12 mg/kg/day).

Neonatal Candidiasis

- Relatively common, neonatal *Candida* infection, manifesting usually after 6 days of life
- Mode of transmission—perinatal
- It is of two types: (1) Superficial and (2) disseminated infections.
- Superficial candidiasis—oral thrush with or without perianal napkin dermatitis
  - Moist, erythematous, beefy red napkin dermatitis in perianal location with pustules at the periphery which is often scalloped in outline. Just beyond the margin, in unaffected skin, there may be punctuate and erythematous lesions (satellite lesions).
  - Rash may extend to involve inner thighs and perineum.
- Disseminated candidiasis—premature and very LBW infants at risk. May present as vesiculobullous, pustular or burn-like exfoliative dermatitis.
- *Differential diagnosis*: Other causes of napkin dermatitis such as CD, AD, SD, and psoriasis.
- *Diagnosis*: Clinical. KOH mount.
- *Treatment*: Topical azoles. IV antifungal treatment in disseminated disease.

KEY POINTS

- Most cutaneous lesions in neonatal period are physiological and self-limiting.
- Cutis marmorata has to be differentiated from cutis marmorata telangiectatica congenita, a rare capillary malformation.
- Harlequin color change is usually seen in healthy newborns.
- Transient neonatal pustular melanosis lesions take longer time to resolve when compared to ETN and both of them have to be differentiated from other neonatal vesiculopustular eruptions.
- Primary milia in newborn disappear spontaneously without scarring.
- Neonatal cephalic pustulosis is considered a variant of neonatal acne.
- Both caput succedaneum and cephalhematoma are self-resolving conditions and usually no treatment is required.
- Calcium levels have to be monitored in subcutaneous fat necrosis even after improvement of skin lesions.
- Deeper lesions of aplasia cutis require radiological evaluation.
- Maintaining the skin barrier and proper hydration is the key to managing most of the cases of neonatal erythroderma.
- Blueberry muffin lesions are not specific for rubella, can be seen in other diseases.
- Serological evidence of syphilis in mother mandatory to prove congenital syphilis and penicillin is the only approved treatment.
- Neonatal herpes is a fatal disease, prompt and timely treatment is required to halt systemic progression.
- Premature and very LBW neonates are at risk of systemic involvement in cases of congenital cutaneous candidiasis.

REFERENCES

1. Eichenfield L, Lee P. Transient physiologic changes and cutaneous lesions in the newborn. In: Schachner L, Hansen R (Eds). Pediatric Dermatology, 4th edition. Philadelphia: Mosby Elsevier; 2011. pp. 301-8.
2. Afsar FS. Physiological skin conditions of preterm and term neonates. Clin Exp Dermatol. 2010;35:346-50.
3. Larralde M, Luna PC. Vesicopustular, bullous and erosive diseases of the newborn. In: Schachner L, Hansen R (Eds). Pediatric Dermatology, 4th edition. Philadelphia: Mosby Elsevier; 2011. pp. 328-42.
4. Berk DR, Bayliss SJ. Milia: a review and classification. J Am Acad Dermatol. 2008;59:1050-63.
5. Tran JT, Sheth AP. Complications of subcutaneous fat necrosis of the newborn: a case report and review of the literature. Pediatr Dermatol. 2003;20:257-61.
6. Drolet B, Prendiville J, Golden J, Enjolras O, Esterly NB. 'Membranous aplasia cutis' with hair collars. Congenital

absence of skin or neuroectodermal defect? Arch Dermatol. 1995;131:1427-31.
7. Frieden IJ. Aplasia cutis congenita: a clinical review and proposal for classification. J Am Acad Dermatol. 1986;14:646-60.
8. Krauel L, Tarrado X, Garcia-Aparicio L, Lerena J, Suñol M, Rodó J, et al. Median raphe cysts of the perineum in children. Urology 2008;71:830-1.
9. Brown J, Schwartz RA. Supernumerary nipples: an overview. Cutis. 2003;71:344-6.
10. Solak SS, Altunay IK, Demirci GT, Can B. Prevalence of congenital cutaneous anomalies in 1000 newborns and a review of the literature. Am J Perinatol. 2016;33:79-83.
11. Bahrani B, Khachemoune A. Review of accessory tragus with highlights of its associated syndromes. Int J Dermatol. 2014;53:1442-6.
12. Kepertis C, Anastasiadis K, Lambropoulos V, Mouravas V, Spyridakis I. Diagnostic and surgical approach of thyroglossal duct cyst in children: ten years data review. J Clin Diagn Res. 2015;9:PC13-5.
13. Hoeger PH, Harper JI. Neonatal erythroderma: differential diagnosis and management of the "red baby". Arch Dis Child. 1998;79:186-91.
14. Miller E, Cradock-Watson JE, Pollock TM. Consequences of confirmed maternal rubella at successive stages of pregnancy. Lancet. 1982;2:781-4.
15. Duszak RS. Congenital rubella syndrome—major review. Optometry. 2009;80:36-43.
16. Centers for Disease Control and Prevention. (2015). 2015 sexually transmitted diseases treatment guidelines. [online] Available from: www.cdc.gov/std/tg2015/ [Last accessed February, 2021].
17. Brown ZA, Wald A, Morrow RA, Selke S, Zeh J, Corey L. Effect of serologic status and cesarean delivery on transmission rates of herpes simplex virus from mother to infant. JAMA. 2003;289:203-9.
18. ACOG Committee on Practice Bulletins. ACOG Practice Bulletin. Clinical management guidelines for obstetrician-gynecologists. No. 82 June 2007. Management of herpes in pregnancy. Obstet Gynecol. 2007;109:1489-98.
19. Pinninti SG, Angara R, Feja KN, Kimberlin DW, Leach CT, Conrad DA, et al. Neonatal herpes disease following maternal antenatal antiviral suppressive therapy: a multicenter case series. J Pediatr. 2012;161:134-8.e1-3.

EXAMINATION QUESTIONS

1. Name and describe some transient skin disorders of neonates.
2. Describe mucocutaneous changes of early congenital syphilis.

33 CHAPTER

Nevi

Ajit B Janagond, Arun C Inamadar

INTRODUCTION

The term nevus (plural nevi) originates from Latin word *nævus* meaning birthmark and refers to a circumscribed abnormality of the skin or mucosa presenting at or shortly after birth or in the early adulthood. Very commonly, the phrase nevus is used for a benign tumor of melanocytes also known as mole.

Proposed definition of nevus by Happle: Nevi are visible, circumscribed, long-lasting lesions of the skin or the neighboring mucosa, reflecting genetic mosaicism. With the exception of melanocytic nevi, they do not show neoplastic growth. They never show malignant neoplasia.[1]

CLASSIFICATION

Nevi are classified on the basis of cells of origin:

- Nevomelanocytic nevi
- Dermal and subcutaneous nevi
- Epidermal nevi (EN)
- Vascular nevi
- Epidermal nevus syndrome

Nevomelanocytic Nevi

These are composed of nevocytes or nevus cells which are altered melanocytes.

Nevus cells are located in the lower epidermis and/or upper dermis and form clusters or nests.

They are classified into two types depending upon the time of onset:

1. Congenital melanocytic nevi (CMN)
2. Acquired melanocytic nevi (AMN)

Congenital Melanocytic Nevi

These lesions are usually present at birth and occasionally observed during the first year **(Fig. 1)**.

Consensus classification is based on greatest diameter in projected adult size **(Table 1)**.[2] This classification also includes other factors such as number of satellite nevi, anatomic localization, color heterogeneity, surface rugosity, hypertrichosis, and presence of dermal, or subcutaneous nodules.

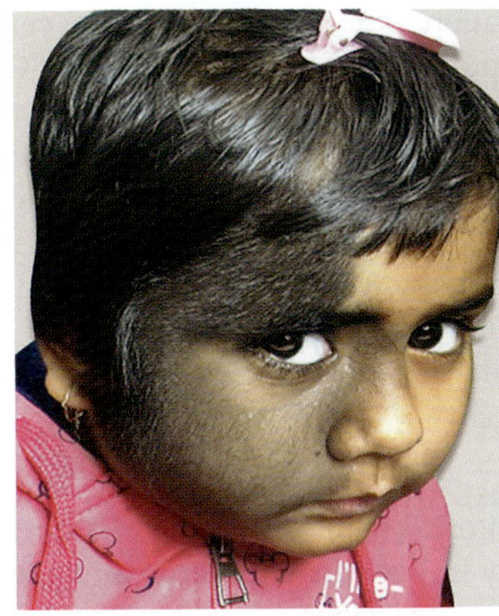

Fig. 1: Congenital melanocytic nevus. *Courtesy:* Dr Koushik Lahiri.

TABLE 1: Consensus classification of congenital melanocytic nevi.

Type of nevus	*Projected adult diameter (cm)*
Small	<1.5
Medium	
M1	1.5–10
M2	10–20
Large	
L1	>20–30
L2	>30–40
Giant	
G1	>40–60
G2	>60

Clinical features

Small and medium CMN present as brown-to-black macules, papules or well-circumscribed patches or plaques. Pigment variation and hypertrichosis may be present.

Large and giant CMN present as dark brown-to-black plaques with varying degrees of overlying surface changes such as verrucosity, nodularity, hypertrichosis, erosions, and ulcerations. Satellite nevi, which are brown-to-black macules and papules with varying degrees of hypertrichosis, may be seen in association with these lesions.

Complications

- *Malignancy*: Malignant melanoma (MM) is the most feared complication of CMN. Melanoma may occur within the skin or in extracutaneous sites such as central nervous system. The risk of developing MM in small and medium-sized lesions is low whereas it is between 2–10% with large and giant CMN.[3] Atypical clinical features, abnormal nevus phenotype, and strong family history of MM are associated with increased risk of MM development.

Incidence of other malignancies such as rhabdomyosarcoma, liposarcoma, malignant peripheral nerve sheath tumor, and other sarcomas is increased in individuals with CMN.[4]

- *Neurocutaneous melanosis (NCM)*: It is characterized by proliferation of nevocytes within the central nervous system (leptomeningeal melanocytosis). Children with large and giant CMN, especially located over head, neck and back are at risk. Patients with greater number of satellite lesions are also prone for developing NCM. About 4.5–11% patients may be symptomatic and manifest with seizures and symptoms related to raised intracranial tension and spinal cord compression.[5] Prognosis in symptomatic patients is poor with mortality rate of almost 90%.[6]

Management

- Close monitoring of the lesions for any surface change—particularly in patients with large and giant CMN and multiple satellite lesions.
- Surgical excision

Acquired Melanocytic Nevi

They commonly appear in early childhood, increase in size and number until the third decade of life, and later regress gradually.

Based on the microscopic location of nevus cells, AMN are classified into three types:

1. Junctional nevi (nevocyte nests within the dermoepidermal junction)
2. Compound nevi (nevocyte nests in both dermoepidermal junction and superficial dermis)
3. Dermal nevi (nevocyte nests in deep dermis)

Histologic descriptions of some AMN correlate with clinical progression. Morphologically, this corresponds with the evolution of lesions from brown-to-black macules in children (junctional) to raised skin colored to brown papules in older children and adults (compound), and lastly to dome-shaped, skin-colored fleshy papules and nodules seen in adults (dermal).

Complications

Lifetime risk of developing malignancy is very low for AMN.[7]

Management

Longitudinal observation of the lesions.

Speckled and Lentiginous Nevus

It is also called as nevus spilus. Generally, it presents at birth but may first become noticed during infancy, childhood, or even later. It is considered as a variant of CMN.[8]

Clinical features

It has two components: Dark brown-to-light black pigmentary background superimposed with darker melanocytic macules or papules. Occasionally, it may be associated with hypertrichosis. The macular spots are usually uniformly distributed and resemble polka dot whereas papular lesions are unevenly distributed.

Histopathology

Background pigmentation shows lentiginous pigmentation. Overlying macules demonstrate nests of nevus cells at dermoepidermal junction and papules show features of compound and dermal nevus.

Associations

- *Speckled and lentiginous nevus (SLN) syndrome:* SLN ipsilateral sensory and/or motor neuropathy, spinal muscular atrophy/hypertrophy and no organoid or capillary nevi.
- *Phakomatosis pigmentovascularis type III*: SLN, nevus flammeus ± nevus anemicus.
- *Phakomatosis pigmentokeratotica*: SLN, organoid nevus with sebaceous differentiation.

Treatment

Q-switched ruby laser, Nd:YAG laser and alexandrite laser

Phakomatosis Pigmentovascularis

It is characterized by combination of different vascular and melanocytic nevi.

Types

Types of phakomatosis pigmentovascularis and their components are given in **Table 2**.

Each type may either have only cutaneous involvement (subtype a) or both cutaneous and systemic manifestations (subtype b).

Spitz Nevus

It is a rare variant of melanocytic nevus usually seen in children over the face.

Clinical features

It presents as a solitary dome-shaped, reddish-brown papule or nodule. It may show initial rapid growth till it reaches a size

TABLE 2: Types of phakomatosis pigmentovascularis and their components.

Type	*Components*
I	Nevus flammeus, nevus depigmentosus, and verrucous epidermal nevus
II	Nevus flammeus, dermal melanocytosis, and nevus anemicus
III	Nevus flammeus, SLN, and nevus anemicus
IV	Nevus flammeus, dermal melanocytosis, SLN, and nevus anemicus
V	Cutis marmorata telangiectatica congenita and dermal melanocytosis

(SLN: speckled and lentiginous nevus)

of 1–2 cm in diameter, and then it remains inactive for years. Lesion morphology may mimic pyogenic granuloma, juvenile xanthogranuloma, and melanoma.

Histopathology

Kamino bodies—amorphous pink bodies formed by degenerated keratinocytes are seen at dermoepidermal junction.

Treatment

Surgical excision

Halo Nevus

It is characterized by a centrally placed pigmented nevus encircled by a 1- to 5-mm halo of hypopigmentation or depigmentation. Halo nevi are frequently seen in children and young adults. Back is the most commonly involved site, though any part of the body can be affected. The loss of pigmentation occurs spontaneously. The precise reason for this loss is still not known.

On histopathology, a marked decline or complete absence of melanin and a dense inflammatory infiltrate around the central nevus is seen which indicates a possible immune-mediated destruction of melanocytes and nevus cells.[9]

Halo nevi are commonly seen in association with compound or dermal nevi but may also be observed along with Spitz nevi, neurofibromas, and melanomas. Halo nevi may finally result in complete disappearance of the original melanocytic lesion and complete repigmentation of the halo occurs gradually over a period of months to years.

Dermal Melanocytic Lesions

During fetal life, melanocytes migrate from neural crest to dermoepidermal junction. Sometimes, the migrating melanocytes remain within the dermis and lead to dermal melanocytic lesions. Skin absorbs blue light less readily than the rest of the visible spectrum and these lesions appear blue because of the optical effects of blue light reflecting from melanin located deep in the dermis (Tyndall effect).

Common dermal melanocytic lesions include:

- Mongolian spots
- Nevus of Ota
- Nevus of Ito

Mongolian Spots

These are the most common dermal melanocytic lesions and present at birth as macular areas of blue-gray pigmentation on the lumbosacral area.

Clinical features

Lesions present as diffuse blue-gray macules of varying sizes and shapes over the lumbosacral area. They are usually solitary but multiple lesions may also occur. If multiple, lesions may involve buttocks, flanks, shoulders, and legs. During infancy, the lesions become more darker and then fade gradually by the age of 4 years. Rarely, they may persist into adulthood.

Histopathology

Presence of increased numbers of elongated dendritic melanocytes deep in the dermis and scattered between collagen bundles in a ribbon-like pattern is characteristic.

Associations

Down syndrome, Hurler syndrome, GM1 gangliosidosis type 1, and mucolipidosis.[10,11]

Treatment

Reassurance

Nevus of Ota (Fig. 2)

It is also known as nevus fuscoceruleus ophthalmomaxillaris and more commonly seen in females at birth or in infancy. It is more common in Japanese population.

Clinical features

They manifest as blue-brown speckled macules or patches distributed along the first and the second branches (ophthalmic and maxillary) of the trigeminal nerve. The blue and brown components may not always coincide, and hence sclera appears blue and conjunctiva brown. Lesions usually affect periorbital region, bulbar, and palpebral conjunctiva and the sclera. They may also extend to involve temple, forehead, scalp, nose, ears, palate, and malar area. Lesions are usually unilateral but bilateral involvement may also be present. Lesions tend to increase in size with age and cause cosmetic concern.

Histopathology

Elongated dendritic melanocytes are seen scattered mainly among collagen bundles of the superficial dermis.

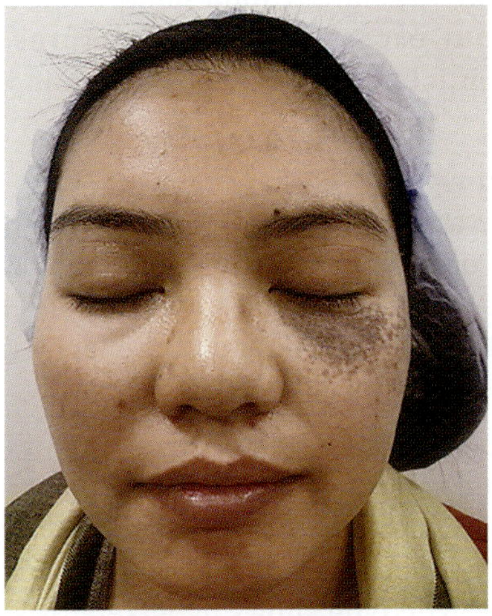

Fig. 2: Nevus of Ota.
Courtesy: Dr Aarti Sarda.

Associations

Nevus of Ito, Mongolian spots, Sturge-Weber, and Klippel-Trenaunay syndromes.

Complications

Melanoma of meninges, choroid, iris, orbit, and very rarely skin.[12,13]

Treatment

Q-switched laser

Nevus of Ito

It is also known as nevus fusoceruleus acromiodeltoideus and commonly seen in Chinese and Japanese population.

Clinical features

It presents as unilateral, blue-grayish macule or patch over acromioclavicular area and chest along the distribution of posterior supraclavicular and lateral cutaneous brachial nerves. As with nevus of Ota, lesions increase in size with age.

Histopathology

It is similar to nevus of Ota.

Treatment

Q-switched laser

Epidermal Nevi

These are benign hamartomatous lesions characterized by hyperplasia of epidermal components caused by underlying cutaneous mosaicism. They are classified into two types based on the principal cell type of differentiation:

1. *Nonorganoid EN*: Differentiation toward keratinocytes [e.g., verrucous epidermal nevus (VEN), inflammatory linear verrucous epidermal nevus (ILVEN)].
2. *Organoid EN*: Differentiation toward adnexal structures such as sebaceous glands, hair follicle, apocrine, or eccrine glands (e.g., nevus sebaceous, follicular nevi, apocrine nevi, and eccrine nevi).

Verrucous Epidermal Nevus **(Fig. 3)**

It is a cutaneous hamartoma composed of keratinocytes without excess adnexal structures. It usually presents at birth but may also appear later in infancy or in adolescence.

Clinical features

Lesions begin as skin colored to pink papule or plaque which gradually become hyperpigmented and attain a warty surface. Based on the histopathologic features they are classified into two types: (1) Epidermolytic and (2) Nonepidermolytic. The two variants cannot be differentiated clinically.

Histopathology

Epidermolytic variant shows perinuclear vacuolization of the keratinocytes with excessive keratohyaline granule formation which are features of epidermolytic hyperkeratosis. Nonepidermolytic type shows hyperkeratosis, acanthosis, papillomatosis, and focal hypergranulosis.

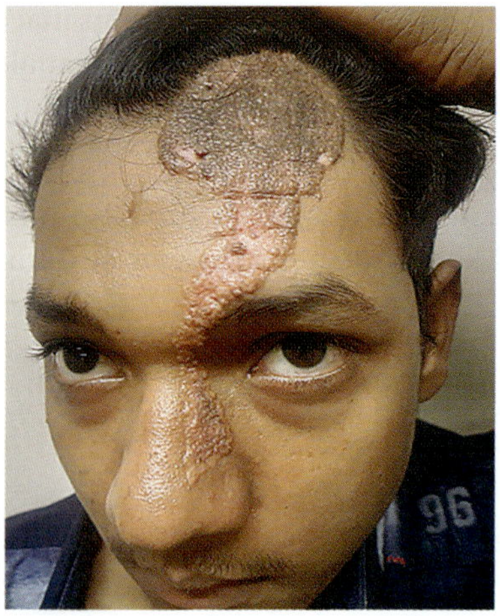

Fig. 3: Verrucous epidermal nevus.
Courtesy: Dr Abhijit Saha.

Treatment

- Topical salicylic acid, lactic acid, retinoic acid, and calcipotriol—may help to reduce the thickness of the lesion.
- Destructive therapies—CO_2 laser, Er:YAG laser, cryotherapy, and cauterization
- Deep surgical excision

Inflammatory Linear Verrucous Epidermal Nevus

It is a distinctive variant of epidermal nevus characterized by inflammation. Lesions are usually present at birth or may develop during early childhood.

Clinical features

It clinically manifests as erythematous, itchy, scaly, verrucous papules which coalesce to form a linear plaque often over an extremity. Lesions show psoriasiform or eczematous morphology.

Histopathology

Columns of hypergranulosis with orthokeratotic hyperkeratosis alternating with columns of agranulosis and parakeratotic hyperkeratosis are observed.

Treatment

- The condition is difficult to treat.
- Potent topical steroids and vitamin D analogs may provide symptomatic relief.
- Destructive therapies—CO_2 laser, pulsed dye laser, and cryotherapy
- Deep surgical excision

CHILD Nevus and CHILD Syndrome

The acronym CHILD stands for congenital hemidysplasia with ichthyosiform nevus and limb defects. CHILD syndrome is characterized by presence of various extracutaneous manifestations in association with CHILD nevus. It is an X-linked dominant condition affecting only females and is lethal for males.

Clinical features

It presents as an asymptomatic well-circumscribed area of erythema with verrucous surface. Lesions have a tendency to involve flexures. Linear lesions may be difficult to distinguish from ILVEN. Extracutaneous manifestations include bone abnormalities, brain hypoplasia, mental retardation, and sensory defects.

Nevus Sebaceous

Nevus sebaceous of Jadassohn is a common epidermal hamartoma predominantly composed of sebaceous glands. It is typically present at birth but may occasionally be noted during early childhood and uncommonly in adults.

Clinical features

It classically presents as a hairless, flat to slightly raised yellow to pink plaque with a waxy surface on scalp or face. The growth of sebaceous nevus occurs in three phases: initial slightly raised lesion at birth under the influence of maternally derived androgens followed by flattening of the lesion during the first year of life and at puberty it becomes verrucous and may also develop oozing and crusting.

Histopathology

Large mature sebaceous glands are noted unusually high in the dermis almost replacing the hair follicles.

Complications

A number of benign and malignant tumors are known to develop within the sebaceous nevus. Syringocystadenoma papilliferum and trichoblastoma are the most common benign tumors whereas basal cell carcinoma is the most common malignant tumor arising from these lesions.[14] The risk of secondary tumor increases with age and majority of them are seen after the third decade.

Associated syndromes

Sebaceous nevus is associated with two syndromes:

1. *Linear nevus sebaceous syndrome (Schimmelpenning syndrome)*: Linear nevus sebaceous associated with neurological, ophthalmic, skeletal, cardiac, and genitourinary abnormalities.
2. *Muir–Torre syndrome*: Sebaceous nevus, keratoacanthoma, and internal malignancy.

Treatment

Surgical excision

Follicular Nevus

It is also known as nevus comedonicus or comedo nevus. It is usually present at birth or may develop during childhood or adolescence.

Clinical features

The lesions present as a plaque composed of grouped or linear dilated follicles or comedones, often filled with keratinaceous plugs. Face, neck, trunk, and upper limbs are commonly affected sites.

Treatment

- Topical retinoids and ammonium lactate may be effective.
- Surgical excision

Syringocystadenoma Papilliferum

It is a rare adnexal hamartoma with apocrine or apoeccrine differentiation. It is usually present at birth but may also appear during infancy or childhood.

Clinical features

It presents either as a solitary plaque, linear group of papules or nodules or a single nodule. The plaque and linear types usually present at birth or develop during infancy whereas the solitary nodular variant develops at puberty. The plaque variant typically presents as a patch of hairless area on the scalp and the linear variant is often seen over neck or face. Solitary forms are seen mostly as domed or umbilicated nodules with a friable or crusted surface over the shoulders. About 30–40% of syringocystadenoma papilliferum lesions develop within a sebaceous nevus.

Histopathology

Duct-like invaginations lined by a two layered epithelium and cyst-like cavities are seen extending from the epidermal surface into the body of the lesion.

Complications

Malignant transformation into basal cell carcinoma and rarely adenocarcinoma.

Treatment

Surgical excision

Eccrine Nevi

Eccrine nevi are classified into three types: (1) Pure eccrine nevus, (2) eccrine angiomatous nevus, and (3) porokeratotic eccrine ostial and dermal duct nevus (PEODDN). The first two types are very rare.

Porokeratotic Eccrine Ostial and Dermal Duct Nevus

These present at birth or in the early childhood as asymptomatic area of plugged pores. On palms and soles, the lesions manifest as linearly arranged small keratotic papules with a central plug and appear like comedo nevus. At other places, they are more verrucous and resemble VEN. Localized anhidrosis or hyperhidrosis may also be present.[15]

Histopathology

Dilated comedo-like epidermal invaginations filled with parakeratotic plugs and columns of parakeratosis extending above the rest of stratum corneum from the adjoining epidermis. Eccrine ducts are usually present in the lower portion of epidermal invaginations.

Treatment

Surgical excision

Becker's Nevus

This is characterized by an area of irregular, well-circumscribed macular hyperpigmentation often associated with hypertrichosis.

Clinical features

Becker's nevi are more common in males and are noted during adolescence. Upper trunk is the most common site but can occur elsewhere. They often have a number of satellite lesions nearby, which eventually combine with the main lesion. Developmental anomalies such as breast hypoplasia, aplasia of underlying pectoralis major, limb hypoplasia, scoliosis, supernumerary nipples, short limbs, and segmental odontomaxillary dysplasia may also be present.[16,17]

Histopathology

Acanthosis, hyperkeratosis, and elongation of rete ridges. Hyperplasia of pilosebaceous structures may be present. Hyperpigmentation of basal layer is seen. Thick bundles of smooth muscle fibers may be present in the dermis. Nests of nevus cells are not seen in the dermis or epidermis.

Associations

Becker nevus syndrome: Becker nevus and associated ipsilateral cutaneous or extracutaneous abnormalities.

Treatment

- Q-switched ruby laser, Er:YAG laser
- Diode or alexandrite lasers for hypertrichosis

Vascular Nevi

Vascular abnormalities have been broadly classified into two types: (1) Vascular malformations and (2) vascular tumors. Vascular malformations are localized defects of development of vasculature without endothelial cell proliferation presenting at birth and persist through the life without regressing. They are further divided into various subtypes depending upon the type of vessel involved (e.g., capillary, vein, artery, lymphatics, and combined) and also on flow characteristics through the lesion (low flow and high flow). The common vascular malformations are discussed in the following text.

Salmon Patch

It is also called nuchal stain or stork bite. These are the most common vascular malformations with their prevalence ranging from 30 to 40%. They manifest as irregular, red-to-pink macular lesions with or without fine telangiectasia. Nape of the neck, forehead and upper eyelids are most often involved sites. Facial lesions almost always fade spontaneously within 1–2 years whereas neck and truncal lesions are more persistent. Sacral lesions may be associated with spinal dysraphism.

Nevus Flammeus (Port-wine Stain)

Port-wine stains (PWSs) are malformations involving capillaries and postcapillary venules which are present at birth and remain throughout life. They may occur either as isolated localized or extensive lesions affecting a whole extremity or as a part of various syndromes.

Clinical features

They present as macular telangiectatic pale pink-to-red patches. With advancing age, they may become dark, remain static or turn lighter and may develop papulonodular changes over the surface. The lesions may involve any part of the body but most commonly seen over face along the distribution of trigeminal nerve followed by limbs. Facial lesions may extend to involve the adjacent mucosal surfaces such as lips and gingiva. Soft tissue hypertrophy in the form of bone overgrowth and early dentition may occur with facial lesions. Limb lesions may cause unilateral limb hypertrophy and lymphatic abnormalities.

Port-wine stains may be seen as a component of various syndromes **(Table 3)**.

Treatment

- Pulsed tunable dye laser
- Nd:YAG (1064 nm) laser

Sturge–Weber Syndrome

Sturge–Weber syndrome (SWS) is a neuroectodermal syndrome characterized by facial PWS distributed along the ophthalmic branch of trigeminal nerve (V1) in association with leptomeningeal angiomatosis and ocular abnormalities.

Clinical features

Patients with SWS have PWS always involving the V1 distribution but may also be multidermatomal and extensive. Typically, the upper eyelid is involved but may also extend to lower lid. In half the patients, PWS can extend beyond the midline and is bilateral. Leptomeningeal involvement affects the normal development of the brain leading to seizures, neurological deficits, delayed developmental milestones and hemiparesis or hemiplegia. Ocular involvement can lead to glaucoma, ipsilateral choroidal vascularity, retinal detachment, and blindness.[18]

Investigations

- Plain X-ray shows sinuous tramline opacification characteristic of intracranial cortical calcification.

TABLE 3: Syndromes associated with port-wine stains.

Sturge–Weber syndrome (SWS)	Cobb syndrome
Klippel–Trenaunay syndrome (KTS)	Bannayan–Riley–Ruvalcaba syndrome
Parkes–Weber syndrome	Beckwith–Wiedemann syndrome
Phakomatosis pigmentovascularis	Von Hippel–Lindau disease
Proteus syndrome	Coat's disease
Macrocephaly-capillary malformation (M-CM) syndrome	Roberts syndrome
Rubinstein–Taybi syndrome	Wyburn–Mason syndrome

- Contrast-enhanced magnetic resonance imaging (MRI) helps in early detection of cerebral and ocular defects

Treatment

Control of convulsions, treatment of glaucoma, and PWS treatment by vascular lasers.

Klippel–Trenaunay Syndrome

It is a slow-flow, complex combined capillary–venous malformation (CVM) or capillary-venous-lymphatic malformation (CVLM) associated with progressive limb overgrowth.

Clinical features

Capillary malformations in Klippel–Trenaunay syndrome (KTS) are generally present at birth or become apparent during early infancy. Lower limb involvement is more common than upper limb. Superficial veins may become prominent and varicose veins develop in late childhood or adolescence. The varicosities are associated with increased risk of thrombophlebitis, deep venous thrombosis, and pulmonary embolism. Hypertrophy of the affected body part presents as increased limb girth and length which may be present at birth or develop rapidly until the end of puberty. Digital anomalies such as macrodactyly, syndactyly, ectrodactyly, clinodactyly, and camptodactyly may also be present.[19]

Investigations

- X-ray of the limbs to assess the limb growth
- Doppler scan to evaluate vascular abnormalities
- MRI scan to detect the extent of soft tissue and bone hypertrophy and lymphatic abnormalities

Treatment

- Multidisciplinary approach involving surgeons and orthopedicians for vascular and bony abnormalities
- Lasers for capillary malformations

Epidermal Nevus Syndrome

Epidermal nevus syndrome (ENS) is a heterogeneous group of mosaic conditions characterized by coexistence of organoid or nonorganoid epidermal with other cutaneous and extracutaneous lesions. The following conditions are included under ENS:[20,21]

Condition	Group
1. Schimmelpenning syndrome.	Organoid nevus syndromes
2. Phakomatosis pigmentokeratotica	
3. Nevus comedonicus syndrome	
4. Angora hair nevus syndrome	
5. Becker's nevus syndrome	
6. Proteus syndrome	Keratinocytic nevus syndromes
7. Type 2 segmental Cowden disease	
8. Fibroblast growth factor receptor 3 (FGFR3) ENS	
9. CHILD syndrome	

Dermatologists come across nevi very frequently. Majority of them are only of cosmetic concern but progression to malignancy is associated with a few, and hence require close monitoring. Nevi may also occur as a part of various syndromes and compel for more detailed examination.

KEY POINTS

- Consensus classification of CMN
- Complications of CMN
- Phakomatosis pigmentovascularis types and components
- Nevus sebaceous, associated complications and syndromes
- Port-wine stain and associated syndromes

REFERENCES

1. Happle R. What is a nevus? A proposed definition of a common medical term. Dermatology. 1995;191:1-5.
2. Krengel S, Scope A, Dusza SW, Vonthein R, Marghoob AA. New recommendations for the categorization of cutaneous features of congenital melanocytic nevi. J Am Acad Dermatol. 2013;68:441-51.
3. Vourc'h-Jourdain M, Martin L, Barbarot S, aRED. Large congenital melanocytic nevi: therapeutic management and melanoma risk. J Am Acad Dermatol. 2013;68: 493-8.e1.
4. Karvonen SL, Vaajalahti P, Marenk M, Janas M, Kuokkanen K. Birthmarks in 4346 Finnish newborns. Acta Derm Venereol. 1992;72:55-7.
5. Hale EK, Stein J, Ben-Porat L, Eichenbaum MS, Marghoob AA, Osman I, et al. Association of melanoma and neurocutaneous melanocytosis with large congenital melanocytic naevi: results from the NYU-LCMN registry. Br J Dermatol. 2005;152:512-7.
6. Kadanaga JN, Frieden IJ. Neurocutaneous melanosis: definition and review of the literature. J Am Acad Dermatol. 1991;24: 747-55.
7. Bauer J, Garbe C. Acquired melanocytic nevi as risk factor for melanoma development: a comprehensive review of epidemiological data. Pigment Cell Res. 2003;16: 297-306.
8. Schaffer JV, Orlow SJ, Lazova R, Bolognia JL. Speckled lentiginous nevus: within the spectrum of congenital melanocytic nevi. Arch Dermatol. 2001;137:172-8.
9. Zeff RA, Freitag A, Grin CM, Grant-Kels JM. The immune response in halo nevi. J Am Acad Dermatol. 1997;37:620-4.
10. Tang TT, Esterly NB, Lubinsky MS, Oechler HW, Harb JM, Franciosi RA. GM1-gangliosidosis type 1 involving the cutaneous vascular endothelial cells in a black infant with multiple ectopic Mongolian spots. Acta Derm Venereol. 1993;73:412-5.
11. Ochiai T, Ito K, Okada T, Chin M, Shichino H, Mugishima H. Significance of extensive Mongolian spots in Hunter's syndrome. Br J Dermatol. 2003;148:1173-8.
12. Theunissen P, Spincemaille G, Pannebakker M, Lambers J. Meningeal melanoma associated with nevus of Ota: case report and review. Clin Neuropathol. 1993;12:125-9.
13. Gerami P, Pouryazdanparast P, Vemula S, Bastian BC. Molecular analysis of a case of nevus of ota showing progressive evolution to melanoma with intermediate stages resembling cellular blue nevus. Am J Dermatopathol. 2010;32:301-5.
14. Kaddu S, Schaeppi H, Kerl H, Soyer HP. Basaloid neoplasms in nevus sebaceus. J Cutan Pathol. 2000;27:327-37.

15. Jamora MJ, Celis MA. Generalized porokeratotic eccrine ostial and dermal duct nevus associated with deafness. J Am Acad Dermatol. 2008;59:43-5.
16. Happle R, Koopman RJ. Becker nevus syndrome. Am J Med Genet. 1997;68:357-61.
17. Sharma R, Mishra A. Becker's naevus with ipsilateral areolar hypoplasia in three males. Br J Dermatol. 1997;136:471-2.
18. Celebi S, Alagoz G, Aykan U. Ocular findings in Sturge-Weber syndrome. Eur J Ophthalmol. 2000;10:239-43.
19. Redondo P, Aguado L, Martinez-Cuesta A. Diagnosis and management of extensive vascular malformations of the lower limb. Part I. Clinical diagnosis. J Am Acad Dermatol. 2011;65:893-906.
20. Happle R. Epidermal nevus syndromes. Semin Dermatol. 1995;14:111-21.
21. Sugarman JL. Epidermal nevus syndromes. Semin Cutan Med Surg. 2007;26:221-30.

EXAMINATION QUESTIONS

1. Classify nevi. Discuss in detail about the nevomelanocytic nevi.
2. Enumerate dermal melanocytic lesions. Write in detail about nevus fuscoceruleus ophthalmomaxillaris.
3. Explain the clinical features, types, and management of verrucous epidermal nevus.
4. Explain the clinical features, complications, associated syndromes, and management of nevus sebaceous.
5. List the syndromes associated with port-wine stain. Explain in detail about Sturge-Weber syndrome.
6. Write a short note on congenital melanocytic nevi.
7. Write a short note on dysplastic nevi.

34 CHAPTER Genodermatosis

Kshama Tawar, Ankur Talwar

INTRODUCTION

The genodermatoses are a large group of inherited disorders with skin manifestations. Many of these disorders are rare. However, the recognition of their skin findings is important not only for the initiation of appropriate therapy but also for the detection of other associated abnormalities, including malignancy, in these frequently multisystem disorders.

CLASSIFICATION OF GENODERMATOSIS

Classification of genodermatosis is given in **Table 1**.

Xeroderma Pigmentosum

- Autosomal recessive trait
- Defects in the excision repair and/or postreplication repair mechanism of DNA
- Inability of the epithelial cells to repair ultraviolet (UV) light-induced damage
- Photosensitivity, tendency to sunburn
- Atrophy, freckled pigmentation, and patchy depigmentation
- Actinic keratoses may develop early. These lesions quickly progress to squamous cell carcinoma

TABLE 1: Classification of genodermatosis.

Type of genodermatosis	*Prototype conditions*
Photosensitive genodermatoses	• Xeroderma pigmentosum • Cockayne's syndrome • Bloom's syndrome • Rothmund–Thomson syndrome
Neurocutaneous genodermatosis	• Neurofibromatosis • Tuberous sclerosis • Sturge–Weber syndrome
Ectodermal dysplasias	• Anhidrotic ectodermal dysplasia • Hidrotic ectodermal dysplasia (Clouston syndrome) • Ectrodactyly-ectodermal defects-cleft lip/palate (EEC) syndrome • Ankyloblepharon-ectodermal defects-cleft lip/palate (AEC or Hay–Wells) syndrome
Disorders with malignant potential	• Basal cell nevus syndrome • Gardner syndrome • Peutz–Jeghers syndrome
Others	• Incontinentia pigmenti • Pachyonychia congenita

- Basal cell carcinoma, melanoma, and nonmelanoma skin cancer may develop at an early age
- Ocular manifestations—photophobia, corneal ulceration, and blindness
- Median age for development of the first nonmelanoma skin cancer is about 9 years while median age for first malignant melanoma is about 22.[1]

Cockayne's Syndrome

- In about two-thirds of cases, it is due to the mutation of the *ERCC6* gene, which plays a vital role in the repair and "decoding" of DNA.[2]
- It is an autosomal recessive inherited disorder whose diagnosis depends on the presence of three signs:
  1. *Growth retardation*: Leading to very short stature, and delayed development
  2. *Photosensitivity*: Even a small amount of sun exposure can cause a sunburn or blistering of the skin
  3. *Prematurely aged appearance (progeria)*: Skin appears wrinkled and aged. Loss of subcutaneous adipose tissue, microcephaly, and prognathism
- Neurological signs and symptoms may be present including seizures, spasticity, ataxia, incontinence, mental deficiency, etc.
- *Eye and vision issues*: Hollow eyes (enophthalmos), pigmentary retinopathy (60–100%), cataracts (15–36%), optic atrophy.

Bloom's Syndrome

- Autosomal recessive genetic trait
- *Photosensitivity*: Skin is erythematous, telangiectatic, infiltrated, and scaly. The rash typically appears in a "butterfly" pattern on the cheeks and across the nose
- Distinctive facial features including a long, narrow face, small lower jaw, large nose, and prominent ears. However, they have normal body proportions
- *Immune deficiency*: Increased number of middle ear infections (otitis media) and/or pneumonia
- *Malignancy*: 50% of people with this disorder eventually develop any one of a variety of malignancies, especially leukemia and cancers of the gastrointestinal tract such as the colon
- Male sterility is common because, for reasons that are not well understood

Rothmund–Thomson Syndrome

- *Photosensitivity*: Erythema, edema and telangiectasia which start over the exposed area and spreads to other areas. Later atrophy and poikiloderma
- *Bilateral juvenile cataracts*: Between the ages of approximately 2 and 7 years.
- Radial ray defect, which is manifest as small, malformed or missing thumbs or shortened forearms. Other skeletal abnormalities including absent or malformed bones, fused bones, and low bone mineral density (osteopenia or osteoporosis)
- Increased risk of developing cancer, particularly osteosarcoma

Neurofibromatosis

Neurofibromatosis Type 1

- As known as Von Recklinghausen's disease. Neurofibromatosis type 1 (NF1) is inherited as autosomal dominant inheritance pattern.
- Mutations in neurofibromin (neurofibromin 1 located on chromosome 17). This gene is believed to function as a tumor suppressor.
- *Diagnostic criteria*:
  - Family history of NF1
  - Six or more café-au-lait spots on the skin—more than six café-au-lait spots is a strong indication of NF1
  - Freckling under the arms or in the groin area
  - Presence of neurofibromas on/just under the skin
  - Plexiform neurofibromas
  - Lisch nodules—on the eye's iris—cannot easily be seen and does not affect vision
  - Skeletal abnormalities such as bowing of the legs (tibial dysplasia), thinning of the shin bone, and scoliosis
  - Tumor on the optic nerve that may interfere with vision—these tumors usually appear by age 3 years, rarely in late childhood and adolescence

Neurofibromatosis Type 2

- Bilateral vestibular schwannomas (VS), also called acoustic neuromas, are definitive signs of neurofibromatosis type 2 (NF2)
- Probable signs of NF2 include family history of NF2, unilateral VS or any two of the following: (1) Meningioma, glioma, schwannoma, juvenile posterior subcapsular lenticular opacity, and (2) juvenile cortical cataracts

Treatment for NF1 and 2 is clinical monitoring and medical intervention when appropriate[3]

Tuberous Sclerosis

- Autosomal dominant inheritance. Arises from mutations in the genes *TSC1* and *TSC2*, encoding hamartin and tuberin, respectively.[4]
- *Skin abnormalities*:
  - *Facial angiofibromas*: Noted first in childhood and exhibit progression during puberty and adolescence
  - *Ash-leaf macule*: Few mm to as much as 5 cm in length. Sometimes "confetti" like depigmented skin lesions may be seen
  - *Shagreen patch*: Present in the lumbar region
  - *Fibrous plaques:* Seen over forehead or face
  - *Koenen's tumor*: Nontraumatic ungual or periungual fibroma
- *Seizures*: In small children, infantile spasm shows up as repetitive spasms of the head and legs
- Cognitive disabilities. Tuberous sclerosis can be associated with developmental delays and sometimes intellectual disability or learning disabilities
- *Renal involvement:* Polycystic kidney disease (presents as hypertension and renal failure) and angiomyolipomas (flank pain, hematuria/retroperitoneal hemorrhage, or abdominal masses)
- Cortical tuber, subependymal nodule, and subependymal giant cell astrocytoma
- Cardiac rhabdomyoma

Sturge–Weber Syndrome

- *Port-wine stain*: Typically in the ophthalmic (V1) and maxillary (V2) distributions of the trigeminal nerve
- *Ocular changes*: Buphthalmos, glaucoma, tomato-catsup color of the fundus, conjunctival, and episcleral hemangiomas
- *Progressive neurological injury*: Seizures, cortical atrophy, hemiparesis, focal seizures, and calcification

Anhidrotic Ectodermal Dysplasia

- As known as Christ–Siemens–Touraine syndrome
- X-linked inheritance, males are affected, while the affected females show partial forms
- *Reduced or absent sweating*: May lead to hyperthermia and seizures. Female carriers may display a blaschkoid distribution of hypohidrosis
- *Typical facies*: Frontal bossing; sunken cheeks; saddle nose; thick, everted lips; wrinkled, hyperpigmented, periorbital skin; and large, low-set ears
- Dental manifestations include conical or pegged teeth, hypodontia or complete anodontia, and delayed eruption of permanent teeth
- Most patients have fine, sparse, lusterless, and fair hair
- Onychodystrophy may occur but is not common

Hidrotic Ectodermal Dysplasia (Clouston Syndrome)

- Inherited in an autosomal dominant manner
- Scalp hair is very sparse, fine, and brittle and alopecia is common. Eyebrows are thinned or absent

- Nail dystrophy is common. Persistent paronychial infections are frequent
- Polydactyly, syndactyly, and bulbous fingertips may be present
- Patients have normal facies, no specific dental defects, and normal sweating
- Other reported findings include reticulate hyperpigmentation of the knees, elbows, and fingers; palmoplantar keratoderma; and eccrine poromatosis

Ectrodactyly-ectodermal Defects—Cleft Lip/palate Syndrome

- Autosomal dominant trait of low penetrance
- Ectrodactyly with tetramelic 3–4 syndactyly results in the characteristic lobster-claw deformity of the hands and feet
- Cleft lip and palate create a characteristic nasal contour
- Other ectodermal anomalies include mild hypohidrosis; coarse, dry hair with hypotrichosis; xerostomia

Ankyloblepharon-ectodermal Defects—Cleft Lip/palate (AEC or Hay–Wells) Syndrome

- The characteristic facies is due to ankyloblepharon (congenital adhesion of the upper and lower eyelid margins by fibrous bands)
- Cleft palate is common; cleft lip is rare
- Nails are absent or dystrophic; pegged teeth are common. Mild hypohidrosis is common. Hair may be sparse and coarse
- Recalcitrant, crusted, and inflammatory scalp dermatitis may cause scarring alopecia

Basal Cell Nevus Syndrome

- As known as Gorlin syndrome or Gorlin–Goltz syndrome or nevoid basal cell carcinoma syndrome (NBCCS)
- Mutations in the patched (*PTCH*) gene on chromosome 9q
- Basal cell carcinomas during adolescence or early adulthood. These cancers occur most often on the face, chest, and back
- Noncancerous (benign) tumors of the jaw called keratocystic odontogenic tumors. First appear during adolescence. May cause painful facial swelling and tooth displacement
- Asymmetric palmar and/or plantar pits are seen in 65–87% of all people with NBCCS
- *Characteristic facies*: Increased head circumference; a broadened nasal root; frontal and biparietal bossing
- Other cancers early in a person's life, including: Medulloblastoma, breast cancer, non-Hodgkin's lymphoma (NHL), and ovarian cancer

Gardner Syndrome

- Mutation in the adenomatous polyposis coli (*APC*) gene which mediates the production of APC protein
- *Epidermoid cysts*: Occur at an earlier age (around puberty), multiple and tend to occur in less common locations such as the face, the scalp, and the extremities
- Colonic adenomatous polyps have a 100% risk of transformation to colonic adenocarcinoma
- Dental abnormalities in this syndrome include multiple impacted or unerupted teeth, supernumerary teeth, hypodontia, and compound odontomes
- *Osteomas*: Mandible is the most common location. They may be widespread in the jaw. It may occur in the skull and the long bones

Peutz–Jeghers Syndrome

- *Lentigines*: Characteristic dark blue to dark brown macules around the mouth, eyes, buccal mucosa, and nostrils. These spots may also occur on the hands and feet. They commonly appear during childhood and often fade as the person gets older
- *Hamartomatous polyps*: Most commonly seen in the small intestine. They are associated with many health problems including anemia, chronic bleeding, bowel obstruction, and intussusception
- High lifetime risk of developing cancer. Cancers of the gastrointestinal tract, breast, pancreas, cervix, ovary, and uterus

Incontinentia Pigmenti

- X-linked dominant trait—lethal in males. Only females present full spectrum of disease
- Disorder of chromosomal instability. Primarily affecting the skin, eyes, and central nervous system (CNS). There are four stages:
  1. *Stage 1*: Vesicular stage—first few weeks of infancy. Vesiculobullous lesions appear on the skin of the trunk and limbs. Spontaneous resolution occurs within 4 months
  2. *Stage 2*: Verrucous stage—verrucous cutaneous plaques develop, affecting the limbs. These clear by 6 months of age
  3. *Stage 3*: Hyperpigmentation stage—macular, brown skin lesions appear, characterized by a strange swirling pattern
  4. *Stage 4*: Atrophy and depigmentation stage—atrophy and depigmentation of the skin ultimately occur
- Neurologic complications occur in 30% patients and are a major cause of morbidity and mortality.[5] CNS abnormalities mental retardation, seizure disorders, and motor difficulties
- *Ocular problems*: Strabismus, cataracts, retinal vascular abnormalities, and optic nerve atrophy

Pachyonychia Congenita

- Inherited as an autosomal dominant trait
- *Type 1*: Jadassohn–Lewandowsky type. Mutations in the *keratin 6A* or *keratin 16* gene

- *Type 2*: Jackson–Lawler form. Mutations of the *keratin 6B* or *keratin 17* gene

Jadassohn–Lewandowsky Type

- *Oral lesions*: Whitish plaques (leukokeratosis) on the mucosa of the cheeks, tongue
- *Nail lesions*: Subungual hyperkeratosis, onycholysis, nail dystrophy, and painful paronychia
- *Keratoderma*: Marked hyperkeratosis of the palmar and plantar surfaces, producing thick, and callous-like lesions.
- *Plantar pain*: Mostly involving weight-bearing areas such as the plantar surfaces
- Keratosis pilaris

Jackson–Lawler Type

- Development of natal teeth
- Widespread steatocystomas

KEY POINTS

- Xeroderma pigmentosum is a photosensitive genodermatosis that presents with atrophy, freckled pigmentation, and patchy depigmentation with risk of early development of basal cell carcinoma and other skin cancers.
- Cockayne's syndrome presents with a triad of severe photosensitivity, prematurely aged appearance (progeria) and severe growth retardation. Neurological abnormalities (such as seizures and mental retardation) and vision anomalies are common.
- Bloom's syndrome presents with facial photosensitive lupus-like skin lesions, type 2 diabetes mellitus and hypogonadism. Up to 50% of patients develop malignancy (leukemia and cancers of the gastrointestinal tract) leading to shortened life expectancy.
- Rothmund-Thomson syndrome is characterized by facial erythema and poikiloderma associated with short stature, sparse scalp hair, sparse eyelashes and eyebrows, and juvenile cataracts.
- Cutaneous manifestations of NF1 include café-au-lait macules, neurofibromas, freckling over the axilla or groin, and plexiform neurofibroma. Other features include Lisch nodules, skeletal abnormalities and tumors on the optic nerve.
- Cutaneous manifestations of tuberous sclerosis include facial angiofibromas, ash-leaf macule, shagreen patch, fibrous plaques, Koenen's tumor (periungual fibroma).
- Sturge–Weber syndrome is characterized by "port-wine stain" or "nevus flammeus" in the territory of the trigeminal nerve along with ocular changes (buphthalmos, glaucoma) and progressive neurological injury.
- Hypohidrotic ectodermal dysplasia presents with a constellation of hair (scalp hair is sparse or absent) and tooth anomalies (teeth are usually peg-shaped with a reduced number) along with an inability to sweat. Facial dysmorphism is a diagnostic feature.
- Hydrotic ectodermal dysplasia primarily affects the hair and nails with sparing of teeth and eccrine glands. Palmoplantar keratoderma is a prominent feature.
- Basal cell nevus syndrome presents with multiple basal cell carcinoma syndrome (BCCS) and superficial pits on the palms and soles. Epidermal inclusion cysts and milia are common.

REFERENCES

1. Black JO. Xeroderma Pigmentosum. Head Neck Pathol. 2016;10(2):139-44.
2. Pascucci B, Fragale A, Marabitti V, Leuzzi G, Calcagnile AS, Parlanti E, et al. CSA and CSB play a role in the response to DNA breaks. Oncotarget. 2018;9(14):11581-91.
3. Boyd KP, Korf BR, Theos A. Neurofibromatosis type 1. J Am Acad Dermatol. 2009;61(1):1-14; quiz 15-6.
4. De Waele L, Lagae L, Mekahli D. Tuberous sclerosis complex: the past and the future. Pediatr Nephrol. 2015;30(10):1771-80.
5. Minić S, Trpinac D, Obradović M. Systematic review of central nervous system anomalies in incontinentia pigmenti. Orphanet J Rare Dis. 2013;8:25.

EXAMINATION QUESTIONS

1. What are the diagnostic criteria for neurofibromatosis type 1?
2. What are the cutaneous changes associated with tuberous sclerosis?
3. Classify the various photosensitive genodermatosis.
4. Write a short note on incontinentia pigmenti.
5. Write a short note on ectodermal dysplasia.

35 CHAPTER Epidermolysis Bullosa

Komal Agarwal, Abhishek De, Aarti Sarda

INTRODUCTION

Epidermolysis bullosa (EB) is an inherited, heterogeneous group of rare disorder characterized by mucocutaneous fragility due to minimal trauma, which clinically presents as vesicles/bullae. It adversely affects the quality of life of the child as well as the parents and contributes to significant morbidity and mortality.[1]

The estimated prevalence and incidence of EB in the US are 8.2 per 1 million population and 19.6 per 1 million live births, respectively.[1]

HISTORY

- von Hebra was the first to distinguish pemphigus from inherited blistering (1870).
- The name, "epidermolysis bullosa hereditaria," was coined by Koebner in 1886.
- Hallopeau recognized the simplex and dystrophic forms of EB.
- Junctional EB was first described by Herlitz and named "EB letalis".
- A comprehensive classification of EB based on a combination of ultrastructural and clinical findings was done by Gedde-Dahl.[2]

CLASSIFICATION

Epidermolysis bullosa is classified by the level of blister cleavage, to the pattern of genetic inheritance, morphology of the lesions and genetic mutations involved. It is classified into four major forms as seen in **Table 1 (Fig. 1)**.[3]

CLINICAL FEATURES

Epidermolysis Bullosa Simplex[4-6]

General Features

- Epidermolysis bullosa simplex (EBS) is characterized by a disorder of keratinocytes and intraepidermal blistering
- There are mutations in the *K5* and *K14* genes, which encode the production of keratin and type I and II intermediate filament proteins.[1,3]
- EBS is subdivided into 3 main clinical types: EBS Generalized severe (previously known as Dowling-Meara type), EBS generalized intermediate (previously known as Koebner type), and EBS localized (previously known as Weber-Cockayne type) **(Table 2)**
- There is usually negligible systemic involvement.
- Nail dystrophy, alopecia and mucosal lesions may occur in more severe forms of the disease.
- Blistering improves with age and there is usually minimal scarring[4] **(Table 1) (Figs. 2 and 3)**.

Generalized Severe Epidermolysis Bullosa Simplex

- It is also known as the Dowling Meara, herpetiformis variant of EBS
- It is regarded as the most severe of the EBS subtypes
- Presents at birth
- Either presents as crops of herpetiform blisters or presents as extensive blisters in a generalized distribution
- Herpetiform blisters occur on the trunk and proximal extremities and heal without scarring
- Oral mucosa is commonly involved, occasionally shows extensive erosions. Rarely other mucosal involvement including esophageal or laryngeal mucosal involvement are seen
- Milia formation may occur in infancy
- Often nails get shed and regrow with dystrophy
- Hyperkeratosis of the palms and soles
- Most patients with EBS-gen/sev live a normal lifespan, with a minority of the most severely affected dying during early infancy from overwhelming sepsis or failure to thrive

Generalized Intermediate Epidermolysis Bullosa Simplex

- It is also known as the Koebner EBS
- It shows an onset of generalized blistering at birth or at latest during early infancy
- Most commonly involved areas are hands, feet, and extremities
- Lesions heal with post-inflammatory hyper- or hypo-pigmentation, and occasional atrophy, and milia.
- Palmar-plantar hyperkeratosis
- Oral mucosa may show mild erosive activity.

TABLE 1: Classification of epidermolysis bullosa (EB).

Types	*Subtypes*	*Level of blister*	*Inheritance*	*Affected gene*	*Affected pattern*
EB simplex	EBS generalized severe (previously known as Dowling-Meara type)	Basal	AD	*KRT5/KRT14*	Keratin 5/Keratin 14
	EBS generalized intermediate (previously known as Koebner type)	Basal	AD	*KRT5/ KRT14*	Keratin 5/Keratin 14
	EBS localized (previously known as Weber-Cockayne type)	Basal	AD	*KRT5/KRT14*	Keratin 5/Keratin 14
	EBS with mottled pigmentation	Basal	AD	*KRT5*	Keratin 5
	EB with muscular dystrophy	Basal	AR	*PLEC1*	Plectin
	EBS superficialis	Subcorneal	AD	Unknown	Unknown
	Lethal acantholytic EBS	Subcorneal	AR	*DSP, JUP*	Desmoplakin, plakoglobin
	EBS with plakophilin deficiency	Suprabasal	AR	*PKP1*	Plakophilin 1
	EBS Ogna	Basal	AD	*PLEC*	Plectin
	EBS with BP230 deficiency	Basal	AR	*DST-e*	BP230/BPAG1
	EBS with exophillin-5 deficiency	Intraepidermal	AR	*EXPH5*	Exophillin 5
	Acral peeling skin syndrome	Subcorneal	AD	*TGM5*	Transglutaminase 5
EB junctional	JEB with pyloric atresia	Intralamina lucida	AR	*ITG4/ITG6/PLEC1*	Integrin 6, integrin 4, plectin
	JEB, generalized severe (Herlitz-type)	Intralamina lucida	AR	*LAM3/LAM3/ LAMC2*	Laminin-332
	JEB generalized Intermediate (non-Herlitz-type)	Intralamina lucida	AR	*LAM3/LAM3/ LAMC2/COL17A1*	Laminin-332, collagen XVII
	JEB Localized	Intralamina lucida	AR	*LAM3/LAM3/ LAMC2/COL17A1*	Laminin-332, collagen XVII
	JEB inversa	Intralamina lucida	AR	*LAM3/LAM3/ LAMC2*	Laminin-332
	JEB laryngo-onychocutaneous JEB	Intralamina lucida	AR	*LAMA3A*	Laminin 3
	Junctional / Mixed EB with Respiratory and Renal involvement	Intralamina lucida	AR	*ITGA3*	Integrin 3
EB dystrophic	DEB, generalized dominant	Sublamina densa	AD	*COL7A1*	Collagen VII
	DEB, localized dominant	Sublamina densa	AD	*COL7A1*	Collagen VII
	DEB, generalized severe Recessive (formerly known as Hallopeau-Siemens)	Sublamina densa	AR	*COL7A1*	Collagen VII
	DEB, generalized intermediate recessive	Sublamina densa	AR	*COL7A1*	Collagen VII
	DEB, localized recessive	Sublamina densa	AR	*COL7A1*	Collagen VII
	DEB, inversa recessive	Sublamina densa	AR	*COL7A1*	Collagen VII
	Bullous dermolysis of the newborn	Sublamina densa	AD/AR	*COL7A1*	Collagen VII
Kindler syndrome		Variable	AR	*KIND1*	Kindlin-1

(AD: autosomal dominant; AR: autosomal recessive; DEB: dystrophic epidermolysis bullosa; EBS: epidermolysis bullosa simplex; JEB: junctional epidermolysis bullosa)

Localized Epidermolysis Bullosa Simplex

- Previously known as the Weber-Cockayne subtype of EBS
- A mild form of EB
- It is the most common form of EB
- Usually presents during infancy or childhood
- Occasionally, first noted in early adulthood, typically after marching during military service.
- Associated with hyperhidrosis of the palms and soles
- Postinflammatory pigmentary abnormalities occur after healing of blisters but milia and scarring are absent.
- Mild oral erosions can rarely be present.

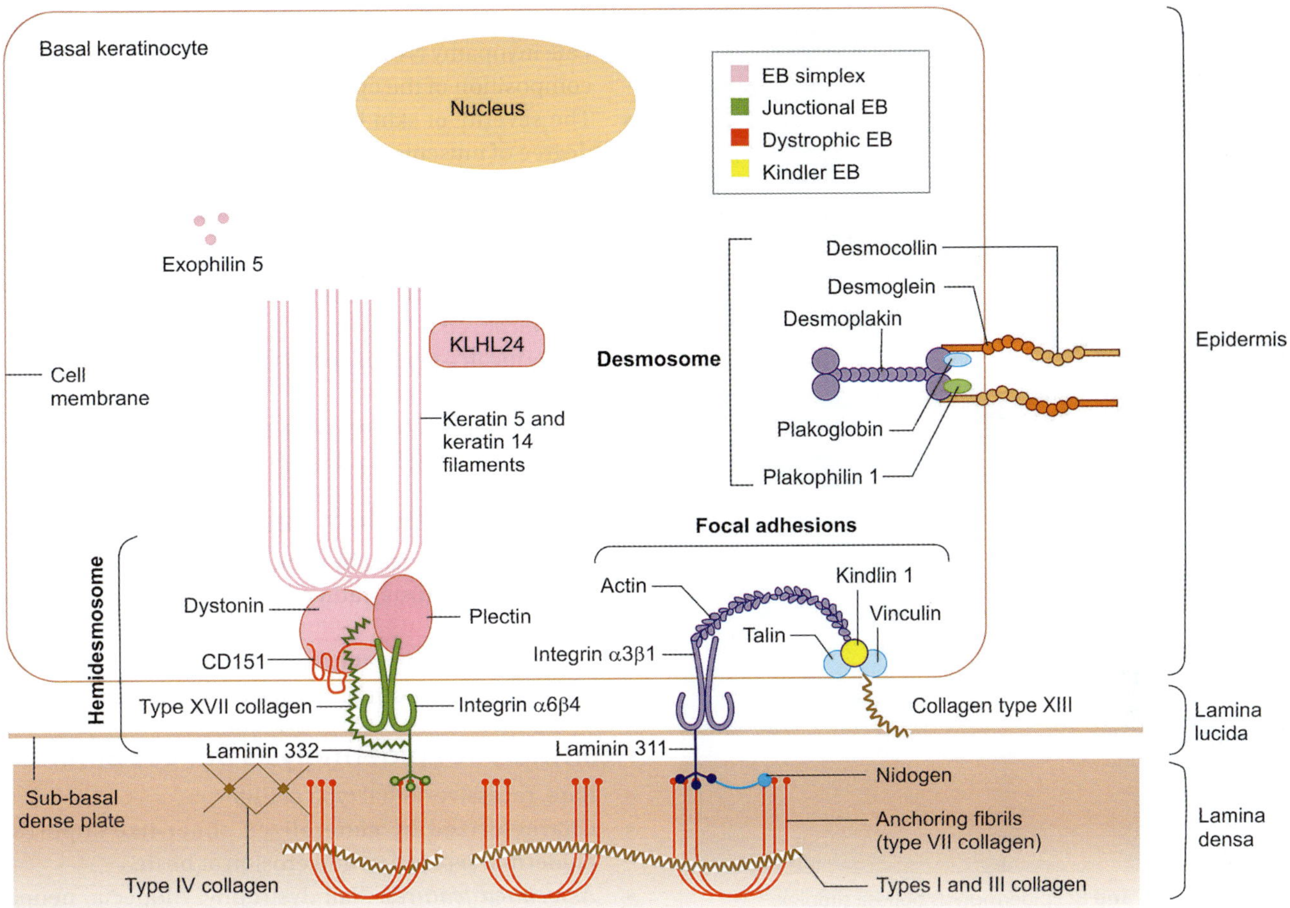

Fig. 1: Schematic representation of the complexes and proteins associated with the different subtypes of epidermolysis bullosa.

TABLE 2: Features of major subtypes of EBS.

Features	*Localized EBS (Earlier, Weber-Cockayne variety)*	*Generalized severe EBS (Earlier, Dowling Meara variety)*	*Generalized intermediate EBS (Earlier, Koebner variety)*
Onset	Infancy or early childhood	Birth	Birth to early infancy
Distribution	Palms and soles	Generalized, herpetiform blisters in an arcuate pattern	Generalized, but more commonly involves hands, feet, and extremities
Scarring	No	Minimal	No
Oral involvement	Rarely, mild oral erosions	Common, occasionally extensive	May show mild erosive activity
Nail dystrophy	No	May be present	No
Mortality	Normal life-expectancy	Most has normal lifespan, some death occurs in infancy	Normal lifespan
Palms and soles	Focal PPK	Diffuse PPK	Focal PPK
Others	Localized congenital absence of skin on legs	Hoarseness of voice, gastroesophageal reflux	Localized congenital absence of skin on legs
Prognosis with age	Persistent	Reduces	Improves

Epidermolysis Bullosa Simplex of Ogna

- Originally reported from Norway
- Onset is in infancy
- Seasonal blistering (summer) on the acral areas (hands and feet)
- Hemorrhagic bullae.
- Healing occurs without scarring
- Generalized bruising tendency
- Shows typical onychogryphosis of the great toenails.

Epidermolysis Bullosa Simplex with Muscular Dystrophy

- Generalized blistering of the skin at birth or infancy

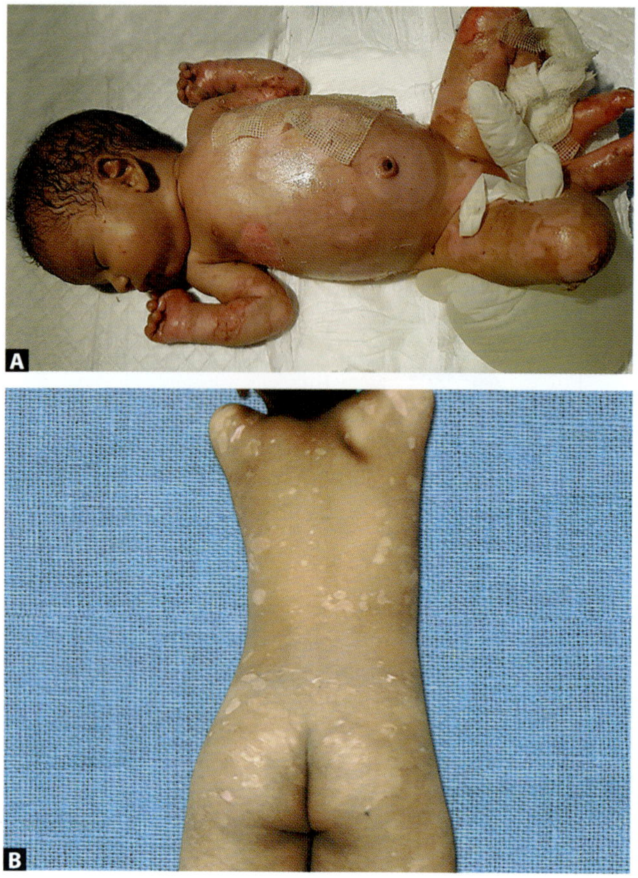

Figs. 2A and B: Epidermolysis bullosa simplex.
Courtesy: For Figure (A) Dr Abhijit Saha.

- Progressive muscular dystrophy in adulthood
- Late myopathy is due to the fact that there is plectin in the composition of the cytoskeleton of skeletal muscles
- The severity of skin lesions does not correlate with the degree of muscular dystrophy

Epidermolysis Bullosa Simplex with Mottled Pigmentation

- Reticulate pigmentation of trunk and proximal extremities with localized blistering
- Blistering in a generalized distribution beginning at birth or early infancy
- Pigmentation improves with age
- Mild oral mucosal involvement may be present

Epidermolysis Bullosa Simplex Superficialis

- Blisters are produced by subcorneal separation
- Erosions and crusts, rather than intact bullae, are usually seen
- Lesions heal with postinflammatory pigmentary changes
- Nail involvement, atrophic scarring, and milia may be seen

Acantholytic Epidermolysis Bullosa Simplex

- Rare, recessive, lethal type of EBS
- Characterized by generalized sheet-like superficial epidermal separation and erosion at birth.
- *Associated features:* Nail dystrophy. Alopecia, neonatal teeth, oral erosions, and respiratory involvement.

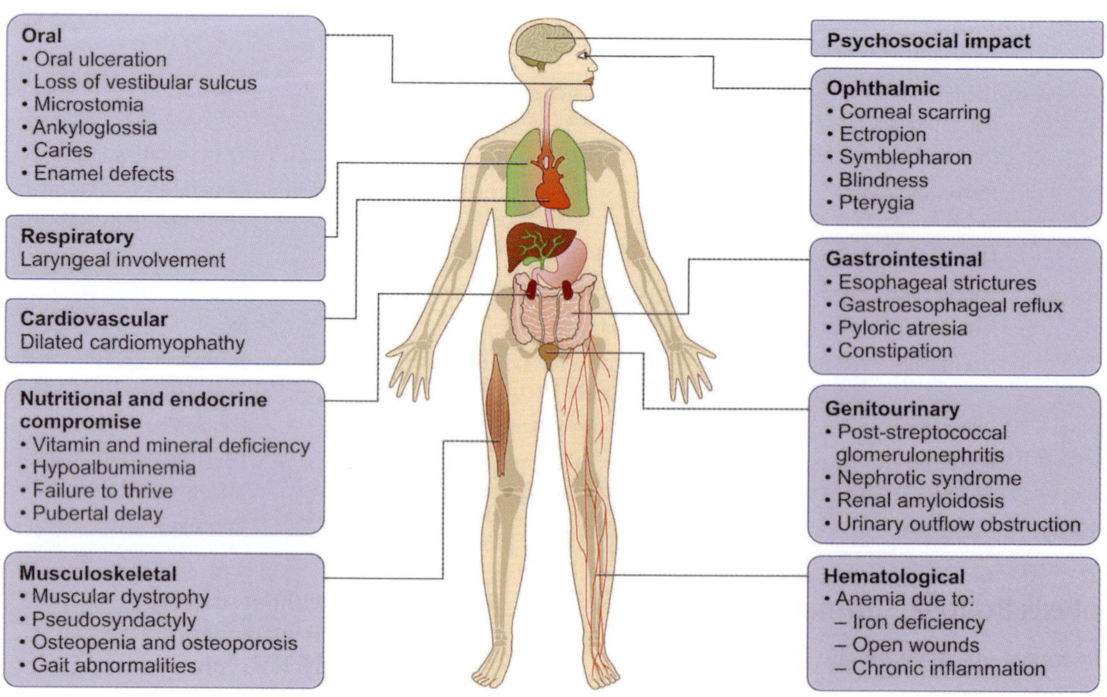

Fig. 3: Extracutaneous manifestations in EB. Extracutaneous manifestations are more frequent in severe forms of epidermolysis bullosa (EB) than in milder forms. However, some specific subtypes may present with specific disease complications. For example, junctional EB can present with interstitial lung disease and nephrotic syndrome and EB simplex can occur with pyloric atresia. Microstomia, ankyloglossia and pseudosyndactyly are common in severe recessive dystrophic EB.

Plakophilin Deficiency

- *Synonym:* Ectodermal dysplasia skin fragility syndrome.
- Characterized by generalized erosions and sometimes superficial blisters at birth.
- *Common association:* Alopecia, dystrophic nails, palmoplantar keratoderma, painful fissures, and nail dystrophy.
- *Rarer association:* Failure to thrive, cheilitis, hypohidrosis, and pruritus.

BP230 Deficiency EBS

- Extremely rare form, seen in Middle East
- Mutations found in the DST-e gene
- Characterized by localized blisters, mainly affecting the feet
- Blisters heal with post-inflammatory pigmentation without scarring.

Exophillin-5 Deficiency

- Very rare autosomal recessive EBS variant
- Caused by mutations of the *EXPH5* gene
- Mild disease with no extracutaneous involvement

Junctional Epidermolysis Bullosa[5-8]

General Features

- Two principal forms of junctional epidermolysis bullosa (JEB) are: severe generalized JEB (JEB Herlitz) and JEB generalized intermediate (non-Herlitz-type) **(Table 3)**.
- Patients with severe generalized JEB (previously termed JEB Herlitz, JEB gravis, or lethal JEB) present with the most severe and the most common disease phenotype. JEB Herlitz is due to premature termination codon in both alleles of any one of the three genes (*LAMA3, LAMB3, LAMC2*).
- JEB non-Herlitz is due to premature termination codon in one alleles and a less disruptive mutation in the paired allele.[1,6]
- Most JEB begins at birth and is characterized by generalized blisters, milia, atrophy/scarring, and nail dystrophy.
- Mucosa, teeth (dental pitting, caries), and systemic organs are often involved.[6]
- There is corneal, conjunctival, tracheobronchial, oral, pharyngeal, esophageal, rectal, and genitourinary mucosal involvement. Hoarseness, coughing, and other respiratory symptoms are frequent.
- Patients with Herlitz JEB are at high risk of death from sepsis during early childhood.

Generalized Severe Junctional Epidermolysis Bullosa

- Also known as junctional epidermolysis bullosa, Herlitz-type (JEB Herlitz), JEB gravis, or lethal JEB
- Most severe and most common EB subtypes
- *Inheritance:* Autosomal recessive
- *Prevalence:* 1–9/1,000,000
- *Age of onset:* Infancy, neonatal
- *Caused by mutations in one of the three laminin-332 coding genes: LAMA3* (18q11.2), *LAMB3* (1q32), and *LAMC2* (1q25-q31). In most cases, null mutations are found on both alleles of the causative gene.
- Characterized by generalized and often extensive blistering at birth.
- Distinctive periorificial granulation tissue around the mouth, eyes, and nares develops later in infancy.
- Associated with severe nail dystrophy and nails are often lost during infancy.
- Erosions of nasal, conjunctival, esophageal, tracheal, laryngeal, rectal, and urethral mucosa.
- *Associated features:* Significant hoarseness, tracheolaryngeal stenosis or obstruction, failure to thrive and growth retardation and sepsis.

Generalized Intermediate Junctional Epidermolysis Bullosa

- Also known as generalized junctional epidermolysis bullosa, non-Herlitz type (JEB non-Herlitz)
- *Inheritance:* Autosomal recessive
- Generalized non-Herlitz junctional epidermolysis bullosa is caused by mutations in the *COL17A1* (10q24.3) and *LAMA3* (18q11.2), *LAMB3* (1q32), and *LAMC2* (1q25-q31) genes.
- Patients initially present with phenotype like that of a generalized severe variety. However they survive infancy and eventually have a less severe pattern of blistering and mucosal erosions.
- Associated with nail dystrophy, scalp involvement, periorificial nonhealing erosions.
- Absence of significant hoarseness is a differentiating feature from JEB Herlitz.
- May be associated with severe epithelial adhesion abnormalities, and tracheostomies or gastrostomy tubes may help in patient survival.
- *Generalized atrophic benign epidermolysis bullosa (GABEB):* A subtype with generalized cutaneous involvement but minimal mucosal disease. Blisters heals with a characteristic atrophic debilitating widespread scarring. Patients usually have enamel pitting, dental caries, nail dystrophy, progressive alopecia of the scalp and terminal hairs elsewhere in the body. Extracutaneous features are otherwise not present.

Localized Junctional Epidermolysis Bullosa

- Also known as minimus JEB
- Rare and milder subtype
- Localized blisters, most commonly affecting the hands, feet, and pretibial regions.

- Occasional nail dystrophy and enamel pitting
- Mild oral or nasal erosions
- Usually a favorable prognosis and a normal lifespan is seen.

Junctional Epidermolysis Bullosa with Pyloric Atresia (JEB-PA)

- Also known as Carmi syndrome
- Severe subtype of JEB characterized by generalized blistering at birth and congenital atresia/stenosis of the pylorus and rarely of other portions of the gastrointestinal tract
- *Inheritance:* Autosomal recessive
- It is caused by mutations in either of the genes encoding the two subunits of alpha6-beta4 integrin, *ITGA6* (2q31.1) and *ITGB4* (17q11-qter).
- *Age of onset:* Infancy, neonatal
- Genitourinary malformations and acquired genitourinary abnormalities (polypoid bladder wall lesions, hemorrhagic cystitis, urethral strictures) are relatively frequent and characteristic.
- Associated with atrophic scarring, nail dystrophy, oral cavity involvement, enamel hypoplasia, aplasia cutis congenita (in approximately 20% of cases), and ear anomalies.
- JEB with pyloric atresia presents at birth and has a poor prognosis.
- It is often associated with hydronephrosis.

Junctional Epidermolysis Bullosa with Respiratory and Renal Involvement

- Also known as interstitial lung disease, nephrotic syndrome, and epidermolysis bullosa, congenital
- Caused by homozygous mutation in the *ITGA3* gene on chromosome 17q21.
- *Inheritance:* Autosomal recessive
- Blistering, usually mild, starts early in life and may be associated with a diffuse alopecia and nail dystrophy.
- Interstitial lung disease, results in respiratory distress and lung infections.
- Kidney involvement includes renal failure, nephrotic syndrome, renal hypoplasia, and hydronephrosis.

Laryngo-Onycho-Cutaneous Syndrome

- Laryngo-onycho-cutaneous (LOC) syndrome presents in infancy with erosions around the mouth and face.
- Hoarseness is always present and teeth may be notched.
- Exuberant granulation tissue leads to delayed wound healing, laryngeal obstruction, and blindness.

JEB Inversa

JEB inversa affects mainly the flexures due to warmth and it heals with small atrophic white streaks.

TABLE 3: Features of major subtypes of JEB.

Features	*Generalized severe junctional epidermolysis bullosa (JEB Herlitz)*	*Generalized intermediate junctional epidermolysis bullosa (JEB non-Herlitz)*
Onset	Birth	Birth
Distribution	Generalized	Generalized
Granulation tissue	Perioral, axilla, neck	Minimal/Absent
Hair	Normal	Scarring alopecia
Palms and soles	PPK absent	Focal PPK
Anemia	++++	++
Growth retardation	++++	++
Soft tissue abnormality	++++	++
GIT, respiratory, ocular	Frequently affected	Less common
Mortality	Common	Uncommon, improves with age

Dystrophic Epidermolysis Bullosa[5,6,8-10]

General Features

- Dystrophic epidermolysis bullosa (DEB) is due to mutations in the gene encoding type VII collagen, resulting in defective anchoring fibrils.[1,7]
- In DEB, milia is very commonly seen due to destruction of hair follicles.[1]
- DEB may be associated with autosomal recessive or dominant inheritance.
- In the dominant subtype (DDEB) clinical manifestations usually occur at birth or during childhood with generalized blistering which become more localized with increasing age. Nail dystrophy and anonychia are common features **(Fig. 4)**.

Generalized Autosomal Dominant Dystrophic Epidermolysis Bullosa

- Also known as DDEB, Pasini type
- It is a subtype of DEB, characterized by generalized blistering, milia formation, atrophic scarring, and dystrophic nails.
- *Inheritance:* Autosomal dominant
- *Age of onset:* Infancy, neonatal
- It is caused by mutations within the type VII collagen gene (*COL7A1*) that lead to an alteration of function or a reduction in the amount of collagen VII. This impairs collagen VII assembly into anchoring fibrils which anchor the basement membrane to the underlying dermis.
- Severe and widespread blisters which heal with scarring plaques and milia.
- Multiple distinctive ivory-white colored scar-like papules and plaques, known as albopapuloid lesions, may occur more frequently on the trunk. These albopapuloid lesions are not pathognomonic because these lesions can also be seen in other EB subtypes.

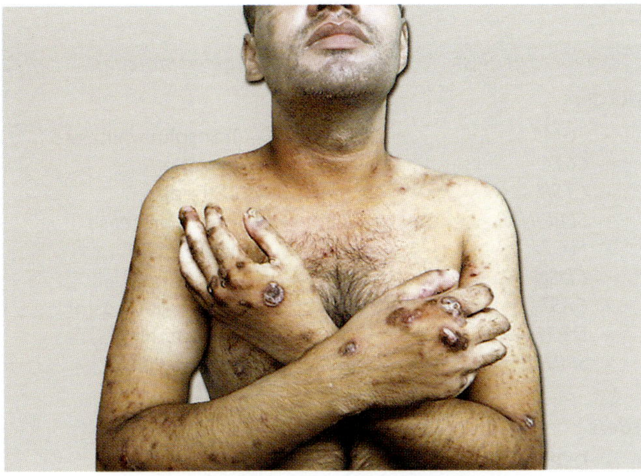

Fig. 4: Dystrophic epidermolysis bullosa.

- Blisters develop in the mucosa, mainly in the oral cavity and, less commonly, the esophagus, where they can cause strictures.
- *Associated features:* Aplasia cutis congenita, nail dystrophy and nail loss, dental caries
- *Uncommon associations:* Corneal and genitourinary tract involvement, anemia, and growth delay.
- *Bullous dermolysis of the newborn:* A rare variant of self-remitting generalized DDEB, termed, consists of generalized blistering that gradually recedes after infancy.

Localized Autosomal Dominant Dystrophic Epidermolysis Bullosa

- Also known as Cockayne-Touraine type of DDEB
- *Onset:* At birth or early childhood
- It is characterized by localized blistering to trauma-prone areas such as the knees, sacrum, and acral surfaces.
- However, generalized blistering can sometimes take place, especially early in life
- *Associated features:* Hypertrophic scar, nail dystrophy/loss, milia, atrophic scarring of the distal digits.
- Oral lesions are uncommon, and teeth are unaffected.
- Patients have a good prognosis and a normal lifespan.

Recessive Dystrophic Epidermolysis Bullosa

- *Two subtypes:* (1) Autosomal recessive generalized dystrophic epidermolysis bullosa, severe form, and (2) Autosomal recessive generalized dystrophic epidermolysis bullosa, intermediate form.
- Severe generalized recessive dystrophic epidermolysis bullosa (RDEB-sev gen) is the most severe subtype of dystrophic epidermolysis bullosa, formerly known as the Hallopeau-Siemens type, and is characterized by generalized cutaneous and mucosal blistering and scarring associated with severe deformities and major extracutaneous involvement. Denudation of an entire region of skin at birth, often involving one of the limbs, sometimes seen with RDEB-sev gen.
- RDEB-sev gen is caused by null mutations within the type VII collagen gene (*COL7A1*) that usually lead to a lack of functional collagen VII, the main constituent of anchoring fibrils.
- *Associated features of RDEB-sev gen:* Congenital absence of skin (Bart syndrome), progressive scarring, pseudo-syndactyly, "mitten" hands and flexion contracture of the hand, teeth shows enamel pitting, and caries, esophageal strictures, malnutrition, and growth retardation.
- A localized form of RDEB that can occasionally be seen that has been previously termed RDEB mitis. Localized RDEB is usually confined to repetitively traumatized skin surfaces, most often in an acral distribution. Blisters heal with scarring and milia formation. Mucosal involvement in localized RDEB is usually mild.

Kindler Syndrome[11,12]

- Kindler syndrome is a rare genodermatosis with onset early in life and traumatic acral blistering, progressive poikiloderma, skin atrophy, and photosensitivity.
- Also known as "bullous acrokeratotic poikiloderma of Kindler and Weary"
- Kindler syndrome was named after Theresa Kindler who considered the disease to be a simultaneous occurrence of two rare diseases—hereditary epidermolysis bullosa and poikiloderma congenitale. Later Weary et al. described the disease as hereditary acrokeratotic poikiloderma and the disease was also known as Weary-Kindler syndrome.
- Inheritance is an autosomal recessive.
- Kindler syndrome is caused by the *KIND1* gene mutation, which codes for the protein kindlin-1.
- It is characterized by trauma-induced blistering at birth and during infancy, with atrophic changes during healing.
- In late childhood, the blistering is replaced by progressive poikiloderma, in sun-exposed areas. Skin changes include atrophy and hyperkeratosis, hypopigmentation, hyperpigmentation, and telangiectasias. The cutaneous manifestations usually improve with age, but systemic complication may arise.
- *Associated features:* Photosensitivity, nail changes, webbing of the toes and fingers, and squamous cell carcinoma
- *Systemic complications:* Mucosal ulcerations and stenosis leading to esophageal strictures, anal stenosis, urogenital strictures, ocular complications such as ectropion, etc.

Other disorders with skin fragility have been shown in **Table 4**.[3]

DIAGNOSIS

Clinical Diagnosis[13]

- Diagnosis of EB is mainly clinical, but investigations are required to confirm the subtype of EB.
- A precise diagnosis and the correct subclassification of EB allow a prognosis of the severity of the disease, genetic

TABLE 4: Other disorders with skin fragility.

Level of skin cleavage	*Disorder name*	*Inheritance*	*Mutated gene(s)*	*Targeted protein(s)*
		Peeling skin disorders		
Intraepidermal	Peeling skin disorders	Autosomal recessive	• *TGM5* • *CSTA* • *CTSB* • *SERPINB8* • *FLG2* • *CDSN* • *CAST* • *DSG1* • *SPINK5*	• Transglutaminase 5 • Cystatin A • Cathepsin B • Serpin protease inhibitor 8 • Filaggrin 2 • Corneodesmosin • Calpastatin • Desmoglein 1 • LEKTI
		Erosive disorders		
Intraepidermal	Erosive skin fragility disorders	Autosomal recessive	• *DSP* • *JUP* • *PK1* • *DSC3* • *DSG3*	• Desmoplakin • Plakoglobin • Plakophilin 1 • Desmocollin 3 • Desmoglein 3
		Hyperkeratotic disorders with skin fragility		
Intraepidermal	Keratinopathic ichthyoses	Autosomal dominant	*KRTI1, KRT10, KRT2*	Keratin 1, 10, 2
		Autosomal recessive	*KRT10*	Keratin 10
Intraepidermal	Pachyonychia congenita	Autosomal dominant	*KRT6A, KRT6B, KRT6C, KRT16, RT17*	Keratin 6A, 6B, 6C, 16, 17
		Connective tissue disorder with skin fragility		
Dermal	Syndromic conncective tissue disorder with skin fragility	Autosomal recessive	*PLOD3*	Lysyl hydroxylase 3

counseling for the patient and family, prenatal or preimplantation genetic diagnosis, inclusion in clinical trials, and precision medicine.

- Thorough history should include the age of onset of blistering and the presence of blistering in other family members. Evaluation systemic involvements such as gastrointestinal, respiratory, ocular, dental, and genitourinary systems along with evaluation of general growth and development are of prime importance.
- Physical examination should include not only a complete skin examination but also a thorough evaluation of mucosa, hair, nails, and teeth.
- Routine laboratory measurements for anemia and such as serum albumin should also be included.

Skin Biopsy[14]

- It is ideal to take a biopsy from an artificially induced blister. A blister may be induced by gently rubbing the skin to produce mild erythema. Rubbing is performed by applying firm downward pressure with an eraser or finger and then rotating it laterally (at least 180° each way). This should be continued for at least 20 times or till the area turns red. One should ideally wait for 5 minutes for a blister to develop microscopically before taking the biopsy.
- A 3-mm punch or shave biopsy should be taken after proper antiseptic precautions and anaesthetization. Shave biopsy is the preferred method as the rate of cleavage has been found to be unacceptably high with punch biopsy.
- It is important to stress that routine histological examination of skin is not recommended in EB, since it may be difficult or impossible to distinguish at the light microscopy level between even lower intra-epidermal and subepidermal cleavage; but it can be done to exclude other blistering disorders.

Immunofluorescence Antigen Mapping[15-17]

- In 1981, Hintner et al. described the technique of immunofluorescence antigen mapping (IFM); using antibodies against BMZ components, they described different staining patterns in the major types of EB.
- IFM could be considered as a modified indirect immunofluorescence technique.
- It is a cheap and simple procedure.
- The biopsy specimen is usually placed in Michel's medium and transported to the laboratory.
- The primary antibodies are mostly monoclonal belonging to IgG class and are raised in mice against human proteins. Then, a secondary antibody tagged with fluorochrome is used to reveal this immune-complex. The secondary antibodies are usually anti-IgG mouse-specific antibodies.
- Most commonly four types of monoclonal antibodies, e.g., Type XVII collagen (BP antigen), collagen VII, collagen IV, and laminin 332 are used. Additional EBS-specific

antibodies (keratin 5 and 14, plectin and α6β4 integrin) may be employed.

Interpretation:

- *Epidermolysis bullosa simplex:* In cases of EBS, all antibodies are found at the base of the blister. In general, expressions of proteins are normal, except in autosomal recessive EBS, when patients may have absent keratin 14 staining. In patients with EBS-muscular dystrophy (EBS-MD), plectin is mostly absent, and in the rare case of EBS Ogna, it is markedly reduced. In EB subtypes with pyloric atresia (either EBS or JEB), plectin or α6β4 integrin are reduced or absent. Collagen IV staining, which highlights the lamina densa, is along the base of the blister.
- *Junctional epidermolysis bullosa:* Collagen XVII is expressed on the roof of split skin whereas other antibodies are seen on the floor of the blister. In the severe Herlitz form of JEB (JEB-H), expression of laminin 332 is absent or markedly reduced. In cases of non-Herlitz JEB (JEB-nH), there is reduced staining of laminin 332. In JEB with pyloric atresia, staining to α6 and β4 integrin is reduced or absent. Type IV collagen staining in all forms of JEB localizes to the blister floor.
- *Dystrophic epidermolysis bullosa:* The level of cleavage occurs in the sublamina densa with collagen XVII and laminin 332 staining seen in the roof of the blister. In patients with severe generalized RDEB, IFM shows absent or barely detectable type VII collagen. Other generalized or localized subtypes of DEB may show a reduced or normal expression of type VII collagen. Type IV collagen staining in all forms of DEB localizes to the blister roof.
- *Kindler's syndrome:* IFM using a standard panel of BMZ antibodies does not show any reduction or major alteration in staining intensity. Labeling of normal skin with a novel, polyclonal antibody against kindlin-1 shows a bright staining in the basal keratinocytes without any dermal alterations. In contrast, in Kindler syndrome skin there is a marked reduction and, in some cases, a complete absence of staining in the epidermis.

Transmission Electron Microscopy[18]

- Transmission electron microscopy (TEM) enables visualization of the structural organization of the cutaneous basement membrane zone to a resolution not possible with light microscopy.
- TEM is considered the gold standard laboratory test for differentiation between the various forms of EB.
- It helps to directly visualize ultra-structural abnormalities and provide a semi-quantitative assessment of specific BMZ structural deficits.
- *Disadvantages:* Expensive, labor intensive, time-consuming, requires specialized equipment which is unavailable in most places, and needs highly skilled technical work.
- Primary fixative for TEM contains 2.5% glutaraldehyde and 2% formaldehyde in 0.1M phosphate buffer at pH 7.4. Once the TEM sample has been immersed in fixative, it can be dispatched to the laboratory at ambient temperature.
- Semi thin (0.5–1.0 μm thick) resin embedded sections are used instead of paraffin embedded tissue **(Table 5)**.

Genetic Confirmation[6,13]

- Molecular fingerprinting confirms diagnosis, underpins genetic counselling and prenatal diagnosis; and ultimately guides optimal management.
- *Sanger sequencing:* DNA sequencing using polymerase chain reaction is done by DNA obtained from saliva or peripheral blood of the patient. In the case of mosaicism, a sample has to be collected from affected and unaffected skin as well.
- *Next generation sequencing:* The whole genome is sequenced at one go (all coding regions of 22000 genes), that is, whole exon. The disease causing mutations are thus identified. Whole-exome sequencing and whole-genome sequencing have accelerated expansion of the EB mutational database. This is a tedious process and takes 1 week or longer.
- Advances in sequencing technology have resulted in faster, less expensive tests with improved mutational detection rates, such that genetic screens using EB-specific panels are now being introduced as a primary investigation
- Molecular testing in EB is quite expensive and is used in special circumstances like:
  - Prenatal or pre-implantation diagnosis
  - When mode of transmission cannot be determined by pedigree analysis
  - Gene replacement therapy
  - To confirm the diagnosis of EB variants.

Diagnostic Algorithm for Epidermolysis Bullosa[6,13]

The approach to EB diagnosis has evolved with advances in sequencing technology and the development of EB-specific gene panels. However, electron microscopy and immunofluorescence antigen mapping retain a place as fundamental tools in the diagnostic armamentarium for EB—for instance, in cases in which sequencing does not yield a diagnostic result or for exploring mosaicism **(Flowchart 1)**.

Prenatal Diagnosis[6,13]

- Fetal skin biopsy (FSB) obtained endoscopically or under ultrasound guidance can be used for subsequent TEM and IAM.
- However, prenatal diagnosis is perhaps the best benefit of molecular diagnostics. As the molecular biology of EB has progressed, FSB has largely been superseded by extraction and examination of fetal DNA derived via chorionic villus sampling or, amniocentesis. Amniocentesis,

TABLE 5: Transmission electron microscopy (TEM) features in EB.

EB subtype	*Level of split*	*Other features*
Generalized severe epidermolysis bullosa simplex EBS Dowling-Meara	Lower epidermis	Tonofilament clumps
Generalized intermediate epidermolysis bullosa simplex EBS Koebner	Lower epidermis	Basal cell lysis
Localized epidermolysis bullosa simplex EBS Weber-Cockayne	Lower epidermis	Basal cell lysis
EBS-muscular dystrophy (plectin deficiency)	Lower epidermis	Small hemidesmosome plaques
EBS mottled pigmentation	Lower epidermis	Abnormal clustering of melanosomes
EBS pyloric atresia	Lower epidermis, just above hemidesmosomes	Diminutive hemidesmosomes lacking normal sub-basal dense plates
EBS superficialis	Upper epidermis	Cleavage present usually at interface between stratum granulosum and stratum corneum
JEB Herlitz	Lamina lucida	Diminutive hemidesmosomes; absent or attenuated sub-basal dense plates; reduced anchoring filaments
JEB non-Herlitz	Lamina lucida	Hemidesmosomes diminutive or normal size. Sub-basal dense plates normal or attenuated.
JEB pyloric atresia	Lamina lucida	Diminutive hemidesmosomes; absent or attenuated sub-basal dense plat
Generalized autosomal dominant dystrophic epidermolysis bullosa	Sublamina densa	Intracytoplasmic inclusions in basal cells; reduced anchoring fibrils
Recessive dystrophic epidermolysis bullosa	Sublamina densa	Absence of normal anchoring fibrils

Flowchart 1: Diagnostic algorithm for epidermolysis bullosa.

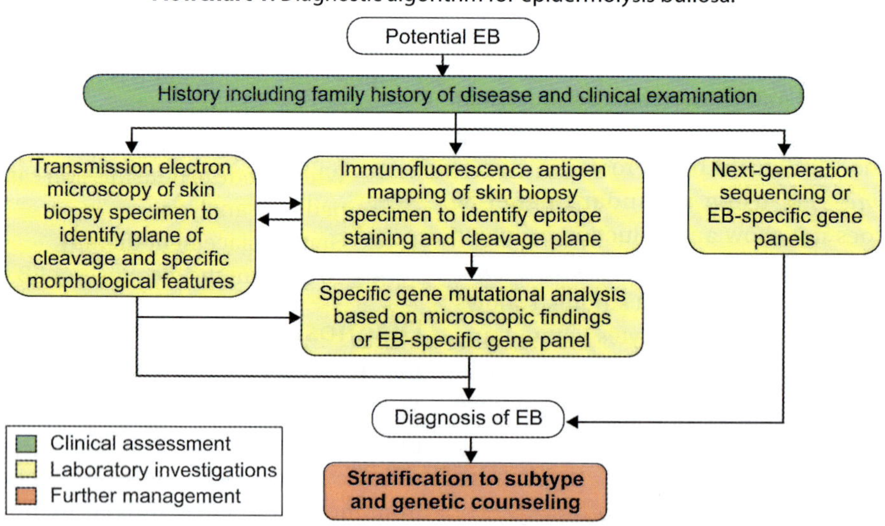

undertaken at around 16 weeks of gestation, is also an option.

- Various modalities of noninvasive prenatal diagnosis have been explored (for instance, ultrasonography and maternal blood tests for fetal DNA) but none has been developed successfully for routine practice.

Preimplantation Genetic Diagnosis[6,13]

Preimplantation genetic diagnosis (PGD) entails genetic screening of cells from oocytes or early embryos before pregnancy. PGD is a highly specialized technique undertaken in few centers globally.

MANAGEMENT[3,6,19,20]

General Management

- In the absence of any curative treatment for EB, current management strategies focus on amelioration of symptoms and prevention of complications.
- The goal of management of EB is:
  - Prevention of new blisters
  - Wound healing
  - Nutritional support
  - Management of extracutaneous complications
  - Psychological support to patient and family members

- *Prevention of new blisters:*
  - Babies should be nursed on thick foam pads covered with silk sheet to minimize trauma.
  - Limit handling of the baby
  - Babies should be rolled and lifted.
  - Clothing should be soft with seams cut inside-out
  - Cotton mittens to reduce self-inflicted trauma
  - Palms and soles should be kept cool and dry during summers.
  - Well-fitting footwear with lining
  - Corn flour should be sprinkled in the shoes to minimize friction.
  - Serial digital photographs and a modified MEASURE method (measure size, exudate, appearance, undermining, re-evaluate, and edge) are helpful for monitoring response to intervention over time.
- *Wound healing:*
  - Erosions should be cleaned with normal saline and covered with nonadherent dressing.
  - Secondary foam dressing provides protection from movement in neonates and infants.
  - Antibiotic usage should depend on culture and sensitivity report.
  - Common infections are *Staphylococcus aureus*, *S. epidermidis*, and *Pseudomonas aeruginosa*.
  - Purulent exudate, pain, malodor and beefy red color of wound are suggestive of wound infection.
  - Topical agents such as hydrogen peroxide and chlorhexidine are preferred over mupirocin due to risk of resistance with the latter.
  - If needed, mupirocin may be used upto 7 days
  - Silver sulfadiazine cream should not be used due to risk of systemic absorption.
  - Nonadherent foams, modified absorbent pads, lipidocolloid dressings, and contact layers can be used for protection and open nonexudative wounds. Hydrogels such as duoderm, are recommended for minimally exudative wounds that may assist with symptomatic relief of pain, itch, or discomfort through wound hydration.
  - Common dressings that may be used in EB include—hydrocolloid, silicon mesh, Vaseline gauze dressing, dermal allograft, collagen based dressings, amniotic membrane, bioengineered skin products such as fibroblast-derived skin substitute from neonatal skin, etc.
- *Nutritional support:*
  - A high fiber diet should be encouraged.
  - Fecal softeners, glycerol suppositories may be used in special cases.
  - Gastrostomy tube may help those who are unable to take oral feeds.
  - Calcium, vitamin D, and iron supplements may be added.
- *Management of extracutaneous complications:*
  - Dental—use of pediatric electric toothbrush, chlorhexidine mouthwash, and daily fluoride supplementation
  - Gastrointestinal—calcium-channel blockers for esophageal spasm, proton-pump inhibitors for gastroesophageal reflux, laxatives for constipation.
  - Eyes—artificial tear substitutes and eye pads may be needed to prevent corneal ulcer.
  - Bone—calcium supplements, vitamin D and bisphosphonates on the basis of DEXA scan
  - Musculoskeletal—surgical release of contractures
  - Anemia—intravenous sucrose iron or packed red cell transfusion if hemoglobin below 7g/dL
  - Pain—topical opiates (not systemic, since systemic opiates aggravate constipation), amitriptyline.
  - Squamous cell carcinoma—serial photographs should be taken every 6 months starting from the age of 5 years. All doubtful lesions should be biopsied. EGFR antagonists help to decrease the carcinoma progression in early stages.

NEWER TREATMENT MODALITIES

Curative

- *Gene therapy:* Keratinocytes from affected patients are propagated and transduced with cDNA containing vector in culture. These corrected keratinocytes are allowed to grow to epithelial sheets and grafted to the donor skin at a prepared affected area. The major limitation is the risk of carcinogenesis.
- *Protein replacement therapy:* A protein therapy approach using intravenous or intradermal recombinant collagen VII injections for treatment of DEB seemed promising at preclinical level.
- *Cell therapy:* It involves the use of human fibroblast and bone marrow stem cells. The cells are directly injected to the skin of affected patients.
- *Antisense oligonucleotides:* The rationale here is that antisense oligonucleotide treatment of cells can lead to skipping of the mutated exons at the RNA level, and thus restore the synthesis of a nearly normal protein that lacks a small fragment encoded by the deleted exon. Diseases caused by collagen gene mutations are especially suitable candidates for this strategy.
- *Premature termination codon read-through:* This approach is based on the fact that approximately 10% of genetic diseases are caused by mutations that generate premature termination codons (PTC) and lead to nonsense-mediated mRNA decay. Gentamicins have demonstrated some efficacy for *COL7A1* and *LAMB3* mutations in vitro. Also, Amlexanox, an anti-inflammatory drug approved in some countries can induce PTC read-through and was shown to enhance collagen VII protein synthesis in vitro in DEB cells carrying nonsense mutations.

Symptomatic

Topical

- Diacerein, an anti-inflammatory compound isolated from rhubarb root has been shown to increase skin stability in EBS.
- Betulin-based oleogel derived from birch bark promotes re-epithelialization and enhances wound healing.
- Topical 2% sirolimus, an mTOR inhibitor, as treatment of plantar blistering in patients with EBS.
- Subcutaneous injections of granulocyte colony stimulating factor (GCSF)

Systemic

- Apremilast
- Oral Epigallocatechin 3 gallate (Polyphenon E), a proteinase inhibitor
- AT-1 receptor antagonist losartan counteracts TGF-β signaling and helps to decrease fibrosis and contractures
- High mobility group box 1 (HMGB1) derived peptide—in EB it increases a specific bone marrow-derived mesenchymal stem cell population that migrates to the circulation, homes to damaged skin, and suppresses inflammation. At preclinical level, in the DEB mouse model, the HMGB1-derived peptide was effective against both skin fibrosis and gastrointestinal strictures.

KEY POINTS

- Epidermolysis bullosa is a condition characterized by inherited skin fragility.
- Children born with epidermolysis bullosa may have lifelong, complex medical needs.
- Comprehensive care of epidermolysis bullosa patients requires the integration of multidisciplinary management
- Recent developments in this complex rare disease aim to restore the skin integrity, by targeting aberrations through molecular interventions.
- Protein, cell, and gene therapies may improve current standard of care in patients with epidermolysis bullosa, from newborns into the decades.

REFERENCES

1. Fine JD. Epidemiology of Inherited Epidermolysis Bullosa based on incidence and Prevalence Estimates from the National Epidermolysis Bullosa Registry. JAMA Dermatol. 2016;152(11):1231-8.
2. Fine JD. Inherited epidermolysis bullosa: past, present, and future. Ann NY Acad Sci. 2010;1194:213-22.
3. Has C, Bauer JW, Bodemer C, Bolling MC, Bruckner-Tuderman L, Diem A, et al. Consensus reclassification of inherited epidermolysis bullosa and other disorders with skin fragility. Br J Dermatol. 2020;183(4):614-27.
4. Pfendner EG, Bruckner AL. Epidermolysis bullosa simplex. 1998. In: Adam MP, Ardinger HH, Pagon RA, Wallace SE, Bean LJH, Stephens K, Amemiya A (Eds). GeneReviews® [Internet]. Seattle, WA: University of Washington; 1993–2020.
5. Sarkar R, Bansal S, Garg VK. Epidermolysis bullosa: where do we stand? Indian J Dermatol Venereol Leprol. 2011;77:431-8.
6. Bardhan A, Bruckner-Tuderman L, Chapple ILC, Fine JD, Harper N, Has C, et al. Epidermolysis bullosa. Nat Rev Dis Primers. 2020;6(1):78.
7. Pfendner EG, Lucky AW. Junctional epidermolysis bullosa. 2008. In: Adam MP, Ardinger HH, Pagon RA, Wallace SE, Bean LJH, Stephens K, Amemiya A (Eds). GeneReviews® [Internet]. Seattle, WA: University of Washington; 1993–2020.
8. Mariath LM, Santin JT, Schuler-Faccini L, Kiszewski AE. Inherited epidermolysis bullosa: update on the clinical and genetic aspects. An Bras Dermatol. 2020;95(5):551-69.
9. Pfendner EG, Lucky AW. Dystrophic epidermolysis bullosa. 2006. In: Adam MP, Ardinger HH, Pagon RA, Wallace SE, Bean LJH, Mirzaa G, Amemiya A (Eds). GeneReviews® [Internet]. Seattle, WA: University of Washington; 1993–2021.
10. Rashidghamat E, McGrath JA. Novel and emerging therapies in the treatment of recessive dystrophic epidermolysis bullosa. Intractable Rare Dis Res. 2017;6(1):6-20.
11. Youssefian L, Vahidnezhad H, Uitto J. Kindler syndrome. 2016. In: Adam MP, Ardinger HH, Pagon RA, Wallace SE, Bean LJH, Mirzaa G, Amemiya A (Eds). GeneReviews® [Internet]. Seattle, WA: University of Washington; 1993–2021.
12. Saleva M, Has C, He Y, Vassileva S, Balabanova M, Miteva L. Natural history of Kindler syndrome and propensity for skin cancer: case report and literature review. J Dtsch Dermatol Ges. 2018;16(3):338-41.
13. Has C, Fischer J. Inherited epidermolysis bullosa: new diagnostics and new clinical phenotypes. Exp Dermatol. 2019;28(10):1146-52.
14. Intong LR, Murrell DF. How to take skin biopsies for epidermolysis bullosa? Dermatol Clin. 2010;28(2):197-200.
15. Rao R, Mellerio J, Bhogal BS, Groves R. Immunofluorescence antigen mapping for hereditary epidermolysis bullosa. Indian J Dermatol Venereol Leprol. 2012;78(6):692-7.
16. Basu K, De A, Karmakar S, Chatterjee G, Rao R, Bandopadhyay M. Role of immunofluorescence antigen mapping in the diagnosis of epidermolysis bullosa: a rare genetic blistering disorder. Int J Clin Diagn Pathol. 2020;3(1):461-8.
17. De A, Gharami RC, Datta PK, Rao R. Does there exist a steroid responsive inflammatory variant of dystrophic epidermolysis bullosa? A case report. J Pakistan Assoc Dermatol. 2010;20:115-9.
18. Eady RA, Dopping-Hepenstal PJ. Transmission electron microscopy for the diagnosis of epidermolysis bullosa. Dermatol Clin. 2010;28(2):211-22.
19. Cohn HI, Teng JM. Advancement in management of epidermolysis bullosa. Curr Opin Pediatr. 2016;28(4):507-16.
20. Prodinger C, Reichelt J, Bauer JW, Laimer M. Epidermolysis bullosa: advances in research and treatment. Exp Dermatol. 2019;28(10):1176-89.

EXAMINATION QUESTIONS

1. Classify epidermolysis bullosa. Write a short note on junctional epidermolysis bullosa.
2. Write a short note on antigen mapping.
3. Write briefly about the pathogenesis of epidermolysis bullosa.

36 CHAPTER Genetic Acantholytic Disorders of Skin

Pragya A Nair, Rochit Singhal

INTRODUCTION

Acantholytic diseases are a heterogeneous group of disorders with overlapping clinical and histological features. Acantholysis can result from a genetically determined defect resulting in desmosomal instability. Important genetic acantholytic disorders include:

- Hailey–Hailey disease (HHD)
- Darier's disease (DD)
- Grover's disease (GD)

Among these, DD and HHD have similar molecular pathogenesis with mutation in intracellular calcium pump of endoplasmic reticulum (SERCA2) and Golgi apparatus (SPCA1).

HAILEY–HAILEY DISEASE (FIGS. 1 AND 2)

Synonym: Familial benign chronic pemphigus

Hailey–Hailey disease was described by the Hailey brothers in 1939. It is a rare genodermatosis with autosomal dominant mode of inheritance. It affects both sexes equally and usually manifests in the late teenage or at 30–40 years of age.[1]

Etiology

Hailey–Hailey disease occurs due to defect in Ca^{2+}/Mn^{2+}-ATPase (adenosine triphosphatase) protein 1 (hSPCA1) due to mutation in ATP2C1 located on chromosome 3. It results in lack of Ca^{2+} signaling, irregular sorting and glycosylation of desmosomal proteins in keratinocytes which leads to epidermal defects, thus the cells do not adhere together properly due to malformation of intercellular desmosomes causing acantholysis, and blisters.

Clinical Features

Hailey–Hailey disease has tendency of remission and exacerbations. It gets aggravated by trauma, heat, sweating, ultraviolet (UV) light, and infections caused by scabies, bacteria, herpes virus, and yeasts. Initially flaccid vesicles and papules develop on erythematous base which turn into macerated or crusted erosions.[2] Lesions have tendency to spread peripherally and form chronic, moist, painful, malodorous vegetations with fissures. Common sites are intertriginous areas such as neck, axillae, inframammary areas, and groin. They leave behind postinflammatory hyperpigmentation without scarring. Mucosal involvement is not common but oral, esophageal, vulvar, and conjunctival involvement can occur. Nail changes are seen in the form of longitudinal white lines and fine palmer pits. Variants of HHD are hyperkeratotic, verrucous, lichenified, papular, papulovesicular, generalized, and vesiculopustular forms.

Differential Diagnosis

Hailey–Hailey disease needs to be differentiated from fungal infection, intertrigo, candidiasis, contact or friction dermatitis,

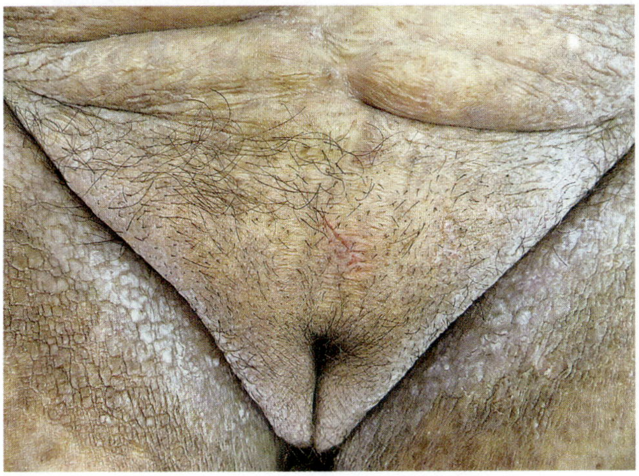

Fig. 1: Multiple hyperkeratotic papules forming plaques with maceration over groins.

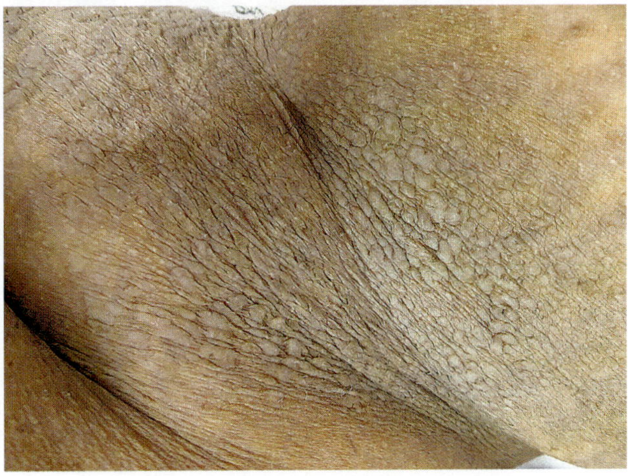

Fig. 2: Multiple papules involving axillae.

inverse psoriasis, extramammary Paget's disease, acanthosis nigricans, pemphigus vegetans, and DD.

Diagnosis

Histopathology is diagnostic. Lacunae formed by suprabasilar clefting with acantholytic cells either singly or in clumps lining the clefts, progress to broad, acantholytic vesicles and bullae. Intercellular edema leads to partial acantholysis and gives rise to areas with characteristic dilapidated brick wall appearance. Dermal papillae lined by single layer of basal cells protrude into blister cavity called as villi.

Complications

Secondary bacterial, fungal, or viral (Kaposi's varicelliform eruption) infection, cellulitis, abscess formation, and scarring are the complications. Depression can occur due to chronic and refractory nature of the disease. Long-term complications include squamous cell carcinoma and adverse effects due to use of steroids in the form of osteoporosis, cataracts, striae, and ulcers.

Severity of the disease decreases with age.

Treatment

General measures include weight reduction, wearing lightweight clothes, and avoiding activities that result in sweating or friction. This will reduce the frequency of exacerbations.

Topical modalities include tacrolimus, antibiotics, steroids (moderate and ultrapotent), tacalcitol or calcitriol, and cyclosporine.[3]

Systemic treatment includes antibiotics, steroids (prednisolone—20–30 mg/day to be gradually reduced), cyclosporine (2.5 mg/kg), dapsone (100 mg daily), methotrexate (10–15 mg/week), and thalidomide.[1]

Dermabrasion or laser abrasion with CO_2 or erbium: yttrium-aluminum-garnet (Er:YAG) laser is effective with long postoperative care. Wide excision and grafting, photodynamic therapy with 5-aminolevulinic acid has been used for recalcitrant cases.

Botulinum toxin is used to reduce sweating in recalcitrant flexural involvement.

DARIER'S DISEASE (FIGS. 3A AND B)

Synonyms: Darier–White disease, keratosis follicularis, dyskeratosis follicularis

Darier's disease was first reported by Darier and White in 1889. It is a rare autosomal dominantly inherited acantholytic disorder characterized by greasy hyperkeratotic papules in seborrheic areas, nail abnormalities, and mucous membrane changes.

Epidemiology

Darier's disease occurs worldwide. Males and females are equally affected. The onset of the disease is often insidious and slowly progressive, it begins during childhood but can manifests at any time.

Etiopathogenesis

Mutations in the gene *ATP2A2* located on 12q23-24.1, encode the sarcoplasmic/endoplasmic reticulum Ca^{2+}-ATP isoform 2 protein (SERCA2), which is a calcium pump.[4] This pump maintains a low cytoplasmic Ca^{2+} level by actively transporting calcium ions from the cytosol into the lumen of the endoplasmic reticulum. Thus mutation leads to defects in protein expression and transport function leading to severe disruption of Ca^{2+} homeostasis, thus causing DD.

Clinical Features

Most patients with DD have a family history of the disease. It is a pruritic disease with chronic, unremitting course.

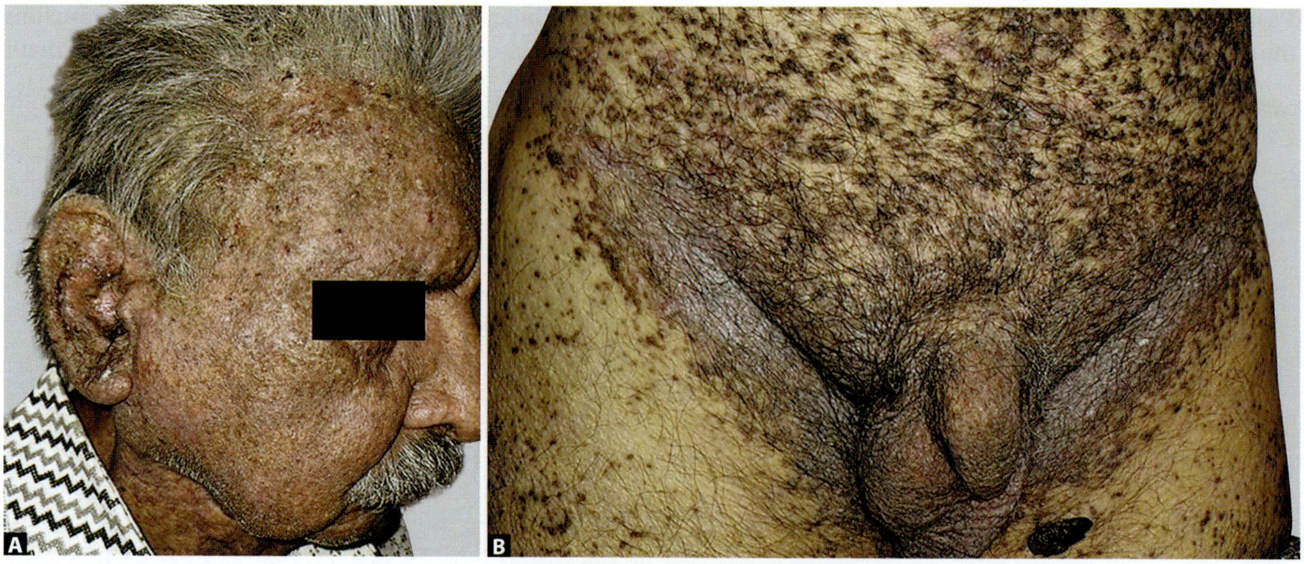

Figs. 3A and B: Greasy, dirty and warty hyperpigmented papules affecting: (A) Forehead, cheeks and ears over face; (B) Lower abdomen and groins.

Aggravating factors include heat, sweat, humidity, sunlight, UVB exposure,[5] lithium, oral corticosteroids, mechanical trauma, and menstruation in females. Initially lesions appear as skin-colored or yellow-brown papules with a greasy, warty texture commonly in seborrheic areas such as the forehead, scalp, margin of the scalp, nasolabial folds, ears, chest, and back.

Flexural areas such as axillae, groin, or perineum have large, warty, and vegetative plaques which are malodorous.

Lesions on the palms present as punctate keratoses, palmar pits, and hemorrhagic macules.

Acrokeratosis verruciformis-like lesions in the form of flat skin colored to brownish papules which resembles flat warts are also present over dorsum of hands and feet. Acrokeratosis verruciformis of Hopf is also due to mutations in ATP2A2, which suggests that it may be a localized form of DD.

Nail changes seen are white and red longitudinal bands, longitudinal nail ridges, longitudinal splitting, triangular nicking of free edges, and subungual hyperkeratosis.

White papules with a central depression called as cobblestoning are commonly found in buccal mucosa, but can involve anogenital mucosa also.

Clinical variants include hypertrophic, vesiculobullous, and linear or segmental types.

Complications

- Infections include secondary bacterial infection, fungi, Kaposi varicelliform eruption due to herpes simplex virus (HSV)
- Oral salivary gland obstruction due to swelling[6]
- Ocular complications such as corneal ulceration, staphylococci endophthalmitis

Differential Diagnosis

Clinical differentials of DD include HHD, seborrheic dermatitis, acrokeratosis of Hopf, and GD. Transient acantholytic dermatosis, pyoderma vegetans, and pemphigus vegetans also need to be differentiated by histopathology.

Histopathology

Acantholysis (loss of epidermal adhesions) and dyskeratosis (abnormal premature keratinization) are the two main features of DD. Acantholysis frequently results in the formation of characteristic suprabasal clefts (lacuna). The underlying dermal papillae, covered by a single layer of epithelium (stratum basale), project into these clefts and form villus-like structures.

Two types of dyskeratotic cells present are corps ronds and grains. Corps ronds are predominantly located in the stratum spinosum and the stratum granulosum. Corps ronds are characterized by an irregular eccentric and pyknotic nucleus, a clear perinuclear halo, and a brightly eosinophilic cytoplasm. Grains are mostly located in the stratum corneum, and they consist of oval cells with elongated cigar-shaped nuclei and abundant keratohyaline granules. Dermis shows mild lymphoid infiltrate.

Nonspecific features include hyperkeratosis, acanthosis, and papillomatosis.

Dermoscopy

Several polygonal, star-like or roundish-oval-shaped yellowish/brownish areas of various sizes are present surrounded by a thin whitish halo.[7]

Treatment

General Measures

General measures such as sunscreen, cool cotton clothing, and avoidance of hot environments can help prevent flares, especially during summer.

Oral or topical antibiotics are often necessary for secondary bacterial infection.

Topical Agents

- Keratolytic agents such as topical retinoids (tazarotene, tretinoin, and adapalene (0.1%), salicylic acid, or sulfur are effective in hyperkeratotic lesions.
- Topical 5-fluorouracil (5-FU)[8] and tacrolimus are also used in localized lesions.

Systemic

- Oral retinoids such as isotretinoin (0.5–4 mg/kg/day) for a period of 16 weeks, acitretin (0.6 mg/kg/day)and etretinate has been reported useful if isotretinoin fails.[9]
- Cyclosporin 2.5 mg/kg/day is also effective in resistant cases.

Surgery and Lasers

Dermabrasion, electrosurgery, and Mohs micrographic surgery have been used to treat localized areas with good results. Laser ablation (Er:YAG or CO_2) and surgery are indicated in recalcitrant plaques over flexural and gluteal region.

GROVER'S DISEASE

Synonym: Transient acantholytic disorder

Transient acantholytic disorder (TAD) was first described by Grover in 1970.[10] It is a rare acquired acantholytic disorder of unknown cause. It is characterized clinically by polymorphic pruritic papules and papulovesicles distributed mainly on the trunk and histologically by acantholysis with or without dyskeratosis.

Epidemiology

Transient acantholytic disorder is mainly seen in males over the age of 40 years. It affects mainly white adults in the fifth decade or later and is less common in darker-skinned individuals. TAD is 1.6–2.1 times more common in men than in women.[10]

Etiology

The etiology of TAD is unknown. It is seen to be associated with heat or sweating, obstruction of sweat ducts due to mechanical irritation or prolonged bed rest, and exposure to sunlight. Medications such as sulfadoxine-pyrimethamine, ribavirin, cetuximab, interleukin-4, ionizing radiation, as well as melanoma therapy with CTLA-4 inhibition have also been associated with the disease. It seems to occur more frequently in patients with atopic dermatitis and asteatotic dermatitis. Association with lymphoma, end-stage renal disease/hemodialysis, xerosis, pyoderma gangrenosum, bacterial and viral infections, and malignancies is also seen.

Clinical Features

Transient acantholytic disorder is a self-limited disorder that resolves over weeks to months, but it can persist and may repeatedly recur for years. One of the hallmarks of TAD is pruritus.

Individual lesions are erythematous to red brown keratotic papules that remain discrete or rarely may have zosteriform or unilateral distribution. Lesions may be acneiform, vesicular, pustular, or even bullous. Common sites of involvement are anterior part of the chest, upper part of the back, and lower part of the rib cage but can affect neck, shoulders, arms, and legs. The scalp is usually not affected, and the palms and the soles are almost always spared.

No systemic symptoms are present, but occasionally, oral lesions can develop resembling aphthae, which are painful.

Complication

Postinflammatory pigmentation and scarring

Differential Diagnosis

Clinical differential diagnoses include dermatitis herpetiformis, folliculitis, insect bite, miliaria rubra, drug eruption, disseminated herpes simplex or herpes zoster, scabies, papular pityriasis rosea, secondary syphilis, acne, acute febrile neutrophilic dermatosis, bullous impetigo, candidiasis, and seborrheic dermatitis.

Histopathology

Two characteristic histopathological features of TAD are focal acantholysis and dyskeratosis. Spongiosis is also commonly seen, and the presence of spongiosis and acantholysis in the same specimen should raise the possibility of transient acantholytic dermatosis. Acrosyringeal acantholysis and multinucleated cells may suggest herpetic infection. Five distinct histologic patterns of TAD have been described: (1) a pattern that simulates HHD; (2) a pattern that simulates DD; (3) a pattern characterized mainly by spongiotic dermatitis; (4) a pattern that simulates pemphigus vulgaris; and (5) a pattern that simulates pemphigus foliaceus. Although one pattern may predominate, each pattern may be seen in different lesions from the same patient or, in some cases, within a single specimen.

Dermoscopy

Two different dermoscopic patterns are found. Early lesions have pinkish-white background with polymorphous vessels, which could be linear, glomerular, or hairpin; whereas late stage lesions have a pinkish-yellow background, a yellowish central keratotic plug (described as a plug with a central, yellowish to brown, star-like pattern), and a white radiating pattern with linear and hairpin vessels.[11]

Treatment

General Measures

Patients should avoid activities that cause excessive sweating such as exercise and prolonged sun exposure.

Topical treatment includes potent topical corticosteroids (fluocinonide gel 0.05%) which are effective in diminishing inflammation and controlling itching. Menthol, zinc oxide, and glycerol-containing lotions are helpful in itching.

Systemic

Retinoids: Isotretinoin 40 mg/day for 2–12 weeks may be effective.[12] It decreases the cohesiveness of abnormal hyperproliferative keratinocytes and reduces the potential for malignant degeneration, and also affects keratinocyte differentiation.

Vitamin A: It is a cofactor in many biochemical processes, given in dose of 50,000 U three times a day for 2 weeks then daily for up to 12 weeks.

Oral corticosteroids, UVB exposure, psoralen plus ultraviolet-A light (PUVA), grenz radiation, and methotrexate have been reported to be effective in severely resistant cases.

KEY POINTS

- Genetic acantholytic disorders include HHD, DD, and GD.
- Hailey-Hailey disease presents as vesicles and papules which form chronic, moist, painful, malodorous vegetations with fissures over intertriginous areas such as neck, axillae, inframammary areas, and groin.
- Histopathology shows partial acantholysis giving rise to areas with characteristic dilapidated brick wall appearance.
- Treatment involves taking care of aggravating factors. Topical modalities such as tacrolimus, steroids, and systemic drugs like steroids, cyclosporine, dapsone, and methotrexate help in controlling the flares. Dermabrasion, laser abrasion, wide excision, and grafting are used for recalcitrant cases.

- Darier's disease is a rare autosomal dominantly inherited acantholytic disorder characterized by greasy hyperkeratotic papules in seborrheic areas, nail abnormalities, and mucous membrane changes.
- Acantholysis and dyskeratosis are the two main histological features of DD.
- Keratolytic agents are effective in hyperkeratotic lesions. Topical 5-FU and tacrolimus are also used in localized lesions. Oral retinoids, surgery, and laser are indicated in recalcitrant lesions.
- Transient acantholytic disorder is a rare acquired acantholytic disorder characterized clinically by polymorphic pruritic papules and papulovesicles distributed mainly on the trunk and histologically by acantholysis with or without dyskeratosis.
- Retinoids, oral corticosteroids, UVB, PUVA, and methotrexate are effective in severely resistant cases.

REFERENCES

1. Valia AR, Ramesh V, Jerajani HR, Fernandez RJ. Blistering disorder. In: Valia RG, Valia AR (Eds). IADVL Textbook of Dermatology, 3rd edition, Volume 1. Bhalani Publishers; 2008. pp. 1127-8.
2. Warycha M, Patel R, Meehan S, Merola JF. Familial benign chronic pemphigus (Hailey-Hailey disease). Dermatol Online J. 2009;15:15.
3. Persić-Vojinović S, Milavec-Puretić V, Dobrić I, Rados J, Spoljar S. Disseminated Hailey-Hailey disease treated with topical tacrolimus and oral erythromycin: case report and review of the literature. Acta Dermatovenerol Croat. 2006;14:253-7.
4. Sakuntabhai A, Ruiz-Perez V, Carter S, Jacobsen N, Burge S, Monk S, et al. Mutations in ATP2A2, encoding a Ca^{2+} pump, cause Darier disease. Nat Genet. 1999;21(3):271-7.
5. Otley CC, Momtaz K. Induction of Darier-White disease with UVB radiation in a clinically photo-insensitive patient. J Am Acad Dermatol. 1996;34(5 Pt 2):931-4.
6. Bernabé DG, Kawata LT, Beneti IM, Crivelini MM, Biasoli ER. Multiple white papules in the palate: oral manifestation of Darier's disease. Clin Exp Dermatol. 2009;34(7):e270-1.
7. Lacarrubba F, Verz AE, Errichetti E, Stinco G, Micali G. Darier disease: dermoscopy, confocal microscopy, and histologic correlations. J Am Acad Dermatol. 2015;73:e97-9.
8. Schmidt H, Ochsendorf FR, Wolter M, Geisslinger G, Ludwig RJ, Kaufmann R. Topical 5-fluorouracil in Darier disease. Br J Dermatol. 2008;158(6):1393-6.
9. Suzuki K, Aoki M, Kawana S. Localized Darier's disease of the scalp: successful treatment with oral etretinate. Dermatology. 2004;208(1):83-4.
10. Grover RW. Transient acantholytic dermatosis. Arch Dermatol. 1970;101(4):426-34.
11. Abreu LD, Cordeiro NGG, Bucard AM, Quintella DC, Argenziano G. Dermoscopy of Grover disease. J Am Acad Dermatol. 2017;76:S60-3.
12. Helfman RJ. Grover's disease treated with isotretinoin. Report of four cases. J Am Acad Dermatol. 1985;12(6):981-4.

EXAMINATION QUESTIONS

1. Write a short note on Darier–White disease.
2. Write a short note on Hailey–Hailey disease.
3. Write a short note on Grover's disease.
4. Write a short note on acantholysis and dyskeratosis.
5. Explain the histopathological features of genetic acantholytic diseases.

37 CHAPTER Porphyrias

Sandeep Arora, Gulhima Arora

INTRODUCTION

Porphyrias are a group of metabolic disorders resulting from disorders of the heme biosynthetic pathway. Inherited or acquired alterations in this pathway's enzymes manifest with neurovisceral, cutaneous, or as a mixed picture. This chapter aims to provide the postgraduate student with salient features of porphyrias with an ability to recognize the prototype porphyria phenotypes and outlines their management.

EPIDEMIOLOGY

Porphyrias are rare with the reported European incidence of 1 in 10,000 of porphyria cutanea tarda (PCT); 1 in 20,000 of acute intermittent porphyria (AIP); and 1 in 50,000 of erythropoietic protoporphyria (EPP). Still rarer forms such as congenital erythropoietic porphyria (CEP) are reported as 1 in 1,000,000, and only six cases of aminolevulinic acid dehydratase porphyria (ADP)[1] have been mentioned in the literature. Variegate porphyria (VP) is reported most frequently in South Africa (1 in 300) due to founder effect while other areas have a much lower incidence.[2] Literature search of porphyria in India reveals AIP as the most common reported porphyria. The authors too have encountered AIP more commonly followed by PCT and CEP in their practice.[3]

PATHOPHYSIOLOGY

Heme Cycle (Flowchart 1)

Heme biosynthesis involves eight enzymes. Mutation in these enzymes results in their reduced function, accumulation of heme cycle intermediates, and the resultant phenotype.

Certain facts must be remembered along with this heme biosynthetic pathway:

- Majority of heme production occurs in the bone marrow which is utilized for hemoglobin production.
- Smaller amounts are synthesized in the liver. These are utilized for cytochrome P450 system enzymes.
- 5-aminolevulinic acid (5-ALA) synthase is the key enzyme in this process. It regulates the rate-limiting step of the formation of delta-ALA in the liver. ALA synthase 1 is found in liver and other tissues while ALA synthase 2 is exclusive to the bone marrow erythroblasts.
- Upregulation of heme synthesis in the bone marrow occurs when heme and iron are available, while in the liver, it is downregulated in presence of adequate heme concentration.
- After formation of heme, a small part of protoporphyrin remains chelated to zinc.
- Rarer causes of heme synthesis disruption include lead poisoning, hereditary tyrosinemia with accumulation of succinylacetone, drugs, nutritional disorders, and hormonal influences. Total erythrocyte protoporphyrin and zinc protoporphyrin may be elevated in lead poisoning, iron deficiency, hemolytic anemias, and certain bone marrow disorders. It is hence essential to differentiate the levels of metal free and zinc protoporphyrin to establish the exact cause.

Basis of Disease

Porphyrin is a special type of tetrapyrolle with four cyclic ring structures with methine bridges. Insertion of a central ferrous iron into the porphyrin (protoporphyrin IX) forms heme. As the double bonds alternate with single bonds the porphyrin structure lets the iron moiety to be utilized for electron transfer, reversible binding of oxygen as well as its participation in oxidation and reduction reactions.

The free electrons in this structure are excited by wavelengths of light peaking at 400–410 nm, known as the Soret band. These electrons may return to the basal state resulting in the characteristic fluorescence created by emission wavelengths of 620–640 nm. Alternatively, they may form triplet states and thereafter transfer excess energy to the surrounding structures resulting in phototoxic biological effects via formation of free radicals and reactive oxygen species with complement activation and release of histamine, kinins, and other factors. Deficiency of any enzyme in the heme metabolism results in accumulation of a porphyrin precursor.

These porphyrins exhibit differential water solubility which affects their localization in tissue and transport in blood.[4] In blood, transport depends upon their binding to albumin and lipoproteins; hence, they exist as free or bound form. Albumin-bound hydrophobic protoporphyrin shall accumulate in cells such as erythrocytes while hydrophilic uroporphyrin and coproporphyrin pass freely through

Flowchart 1: Heme cycle.

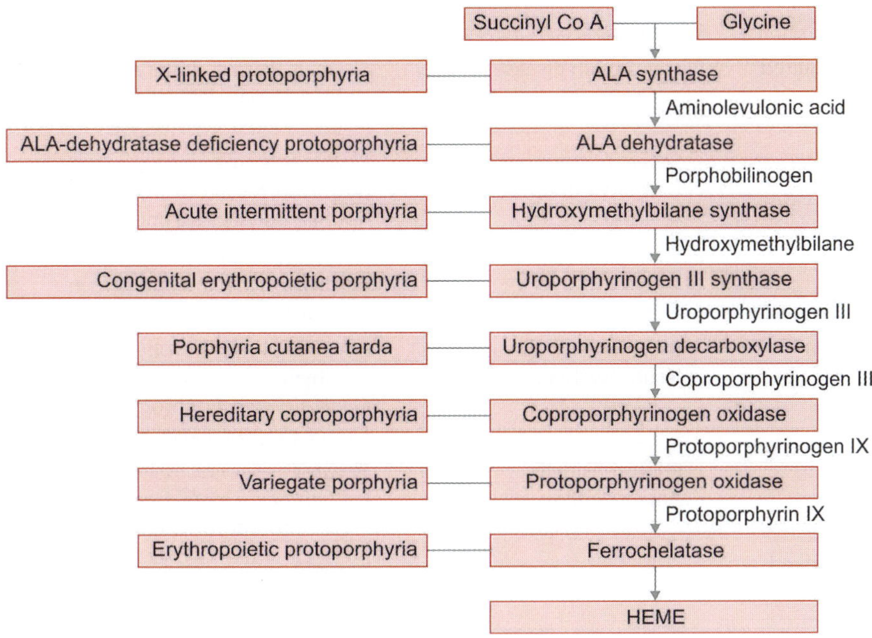

interstitium. The vessel-bound porphyrin in dermal capillaries, upper dermis, or neural localization results in immediate burning sensation on exposure to the offending wavelengths with erythema, edema, or neurological effects.

The pathology of the above process results in repeated insults to vessel walls, resulting in excess basement membrane repair, and their consequent leakiness leads to laying down of amorphous hyaline material in the surrounding tissues.[5-7]

However, the pathogenesis of skin fragility and blistering is not fully explained. Diffusion of porphyrins, their lysosomal uptake, and their breakdown on irradiation with resultant cytolysis in the subepidermal zone also has been proposed.[6,8] Friction of rigid exposed skin subsequently worsens the process. Variable split levels are reported, but the subepidermal split is characteristic.[5]

CLINICAL MANIFESTATIONS

Skin manifestations in porphyrias are predominantly photosensitivity with either acute nonblistering or chronic blistering cutaneous involvement.

It is easier to remember the skin manifestations if a few prototype cutaneous phenotypes are kept in mind **(Table 1)**.

Cutaneous Porphyrias

Type A Phenotype

Type A phenotype is typically characterized by PCT with CEP, hepatoerythropoietic porphyria (HEP), and hereditary coproporphyria sharing its cutaneous features with some variations.

- Chronic photosensitivity often with a delayed reaction to sun exposure
- Face, ears, neck, extensor upper extremities, and feet manifest the disease more.
- Increased skin fragility with recurrent blistering often from trivial trauma, leading to pigmentary changes and scarring. Bullae typically appear on noninflamed skin. Persistent inflammation may be considered a sign of secondary infection in these cases **(Fig. 1)**.
- Repeated scarring may lead to milia and secondary sclerodermatous changes with contractures in severely affected and otherwise a generally atrophic skin.[9]
- Hirsutism on the exposed areas—face and arms—is common **(Fig. 2)**. Temporal hirsutism and exuberant eyebrows have been described commonly.
- Itching may be particularly distressing in females which is reported more at night and cause greatly reduced quality of life and depression.[10]
- Alopecia has been reported.[9]

The above manifestations typify PCT. This is the most common porphyria worldwide manifesting in the 4th to 5th decade. Type I is the more common, sporadic or the acquired variant wherein the hepatic uroporphyrinogen decarboxylase enzyme is defective while type II expresses enzyme defect in all tissues. The rare type III (familial) expresses normal enzyme activity with features of this porphyria.[11] Aggravating factors include iron overload, alcohol, smoking, estrogens, ascorbates and carotenoids, hepatitis C and HIV infection, and end-stage renal disease.

Specific management includes reduction of iron stores by serial phlebotomy (450 mL once a fortnight) to reduce the serum ferritin to 15–25 ng/mL and plasma porphyrin

TABLE 1: Principal features of porphyrias.

Phenotype	*Porphyria*	*Inheritance*	*Principal clinical manifestation*	*Diagnostic investigations*
Type A	PCT I	Acquired	Blistering skin disease	*Elevated*: Plasma, urinary porphyrin, fecal total porphyrin *Normal*: Urinary PBG and ALA *Mildly elevated*: Erythrocyte total porphyrin (Zn)
	PCT II	AD	Blistering skin disease	
	CEP	AR	• Severe blistering skin disease • Hemolytic anemia	*Elevated*: Plasma, urinary porphyrin, erythrocyte total porphyrin, fecal total porphyrin *Normal*: Urinary PBG and ALA
	HEP	AR	Blistering skin disease	*Elevated*: Plasma, urinary porphyrin, erythrocyte total porphyrin, fecal total porphyrin *Normal*: Urinary PBG and ALA
	HC	AD	• Blistering skin disease • Neuropsychiatric features	*Elevated*: Urinary porphyrin, urinary PBG and ALA, fecal total porphyrin *Mildly elevated*: Erythrocyte total porphyrin (Zn) *May be elevated*: Plasma porphyrin
Type B	EPP	AR	• Photosensitivity • Anemia (mild)	*Elevated*: • Erythrocyte metal free protoporphyrin • Zinc protoporphyrin (0–15%)
	XLP	X-linked		*Elevated*: • Erythrocyte metal free protoporphyrin • Zinc protoporphyrin (15–50%)
Type C	AIP	AD	• Abdominal pain • Motor neuropathy • Gastrointestinal symptoms	*Elevated*: • ALA, PBG • Urinary porphyrins
	ALA	AR	Abdominal pain	*Elevated*: ALA *Normal*: Plasma and fecal porphyrin *Reduced*: Erythrocyte ALAD activity
	VP	AD	• Blistering skin disease • Neuropsychiatric features	*Elevated*: Plasma, urinary porphyrin, urinary PBG and ALA, fecal total porphyrin *Mildly elevated*: Erythrocyte total porphyrin (Zn)
	HC	AD		*Elevated*: Urinary porphyrin, urinary PBG and ALA, fecal total porphyrin *Mildly elevated*: Erythrocyte total porphyrin (Zn) *May be elevated*: Plasma porphyrin

(AD: autosomal dominant; AIP: acute intermittent protoporphyria; ALA: aminolevulinic acid; ALAD: aminolevulinic acid dehydrase; AR: autosomal recessive; CEP: congenital erythropoietic porphyria; EPP: erythropoietic protoporphyria; HC: hereditary coproporphyria; HEP: hepatoerythropoietic porphyria; PCT: porphyria cutanea tarda; XLP: X-linked porphyria; VP: variegate porphyria)

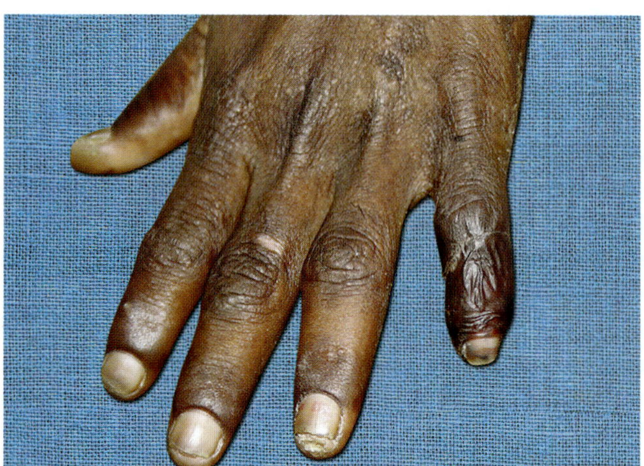

Fig. 1: Bullae on the dorsa of fingers in a boy of congenital erythropoietic porphyria.

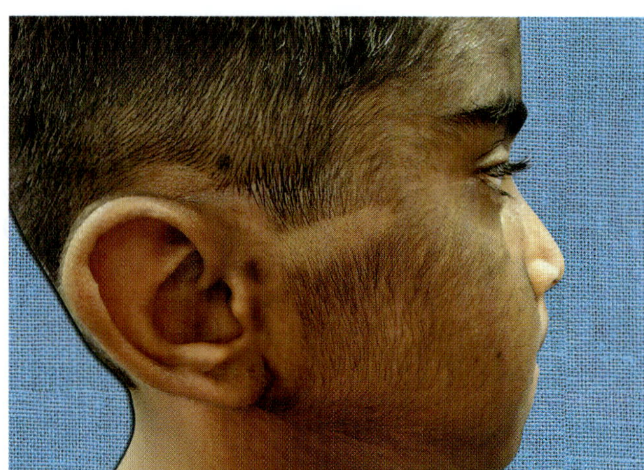

Fig. 2: Hirsutism in a 7-year-old boy of congenital erythropoietic porphyria.

level to approximately 1 μg/dL, iron chelators such as desferrioxamine,[12] diet low in iron-rich red meat, and having tea with meals which reduces iron absorption. Avoidance of the above aggravating factors is a must.[13] Hydroxychloroquine in doses of 100 mg twice daily may achieve the desired plasma porphyrin level as quickly as phlebotomy.[14]

Hepatoerythropoietic porphyria, the homozygous variant of CEP, presents similarly when it appears early in life. Sun protection is probably the only intervention needed in them.

Congenital erythropoietic porphyria presents in infancy with severe manifestations with type A symptoms.[15] Also, known as Gunther's disease, it is an extremely rare autosomal recessive disorder with reported cases numbering <200. Staining of diapers in infancy itself may serve as an early marker of the disease. Higher porphyrin levels in erythrocytes lead to hemolysis, compensatory ineffective erythropoiesis, and subsequent splenomegaly which may be marked. Porphyrin deposition in teeth leads to their discoloration and erythrodontia **(Figs. 3 and 4)** and in urine leads to its characteristic port-wine color **(Fig. 5)**, both fluorescence under Wood's lamp. Photo-mutilation is not uncommon, and corneal involvement may lead to blindness. This marked photosensitivity, red urine, erythrodontia, and the longer duration of symptomatic disease leading to mutilating deformities characterize the rare disorder. These infants are often treated for secondary infections unless they are reviewed at a dermatology or pediatric center.[3] General measures of sun avoidance, prevention of infections, and their prompt treatment are advised. However, as these cases do not exhibit the very acute photosensitivity on sun exposure, they tend to overexpose themselves to sunlight. School-going children must be advised accordingly with intimation to school authorities. Other interventions include hypertransfusion, hemin administration, splenectomy, and cord and bone marrow transplantation. Intracellular uroporphyrinogen III synthase (UROS) enzyme rescue has been tried.[16,17]

Variegate porphyria manifests with the above cutaneous features, usually after puberty or early adulthood, with some presenting still later in life while others may remain asymptomatic throughout life.[18] Severity has been correlated with the longer duration of intense sunlight exposure and some manifesting only cutaneous features in absence of neurovisceral symptoms. Photosensitivity is not as marked as in others.[19] Neurovisceral symptoms are discussed below with AIP.

Hereditary coproporphyria phenotype presents like VP, but skin manifestations are reported in only 20% of those experiencing neurovisceral symptoms.

Type B Phenotype

Type B phenotype presents with acute non-blistering photosensitivity in absence of neurovisceral manifestations unless complicated by hepatic failure. EPP and X-linked protoporphyria present with:

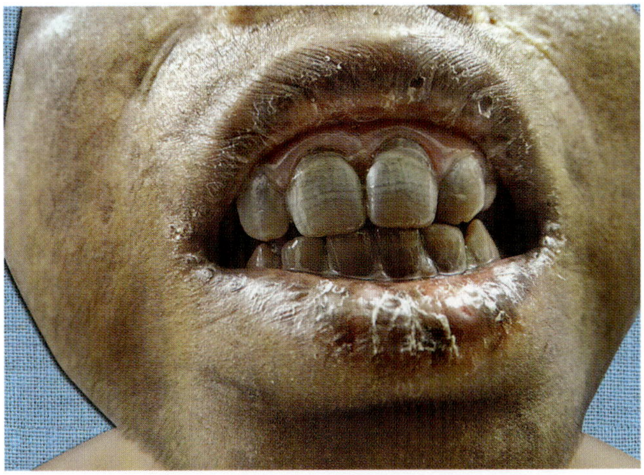

Fig. 3: Discoloration of teeth in congenital erythropoietic porphyria.

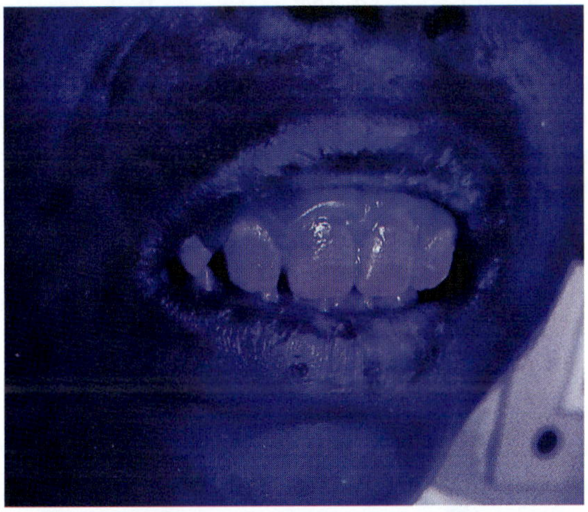

Fig. 4: Erythrodontia in congenital erythropoietic porphyria.

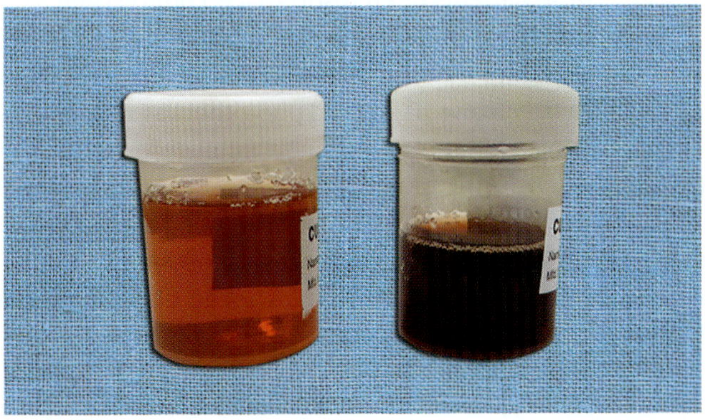

Fig. 5: Port-wine discoloration of urine in two cases of congenital erythropoietic porphyria.

- Onset in early childhood with exacerbations during summer months.
- Acute painful photosensitivity characterized by intense pain, burning, and/or itching occurring almost immediately on exposure to sunlight, and fluorescent light sources, persisting for minutes to days in the severely

affected leading to erythema, edema, and hemorrhagic crusting.

- Skin recovers after the acute episode with no residual changes.
- Longer duration exposures may lead to small papulovesiculation, and such recurrent episodes give rise to an aged look to the dorsa of the hands, particularly the knuckles and the face with a leathery/wax-like appearance. Fissuring of lips and perioral pseudo-rhagades are characteristic. These may be the only tell-tale signs in an otherwise asymptomatic or undiagnosed patient.[20,21]
- Persistent pain following photoexposure reduces the quality of life.
- Seasonal palmoplantar keratoderma has been described as an indicator of autosomal inheritance.[22]

X-linked protoporphyria is an extremely rare disorder with a reported incidence of 2–10% of the type B phenotype.[23,24]

Erythropoietic protoporphyria, an inherited deficiency of ferrochelatase, which inserts iron/metals such as zinc in the protoporphyrin IX ring, manifests in early life as the most common porphyria of childhood.[23] Late-onset EPP is extremely rare and usually associated with a myeloproliferative disorder.[25] Delta-ALA synthase defects (ALAS2 expressed in bone marrow erythroblasts) with a gain of function mutation leads to a similar biochemical defect; however, the zinc protoporphyrin is higher as compared to EPP. Metal-free potoporphyria predominates here too.

Bullae seen in PCT are rarer here. Photosensitivity is elicited with not only sunlight but also incandescent light sources. Iron deficiency with anemia, gallstones, cholestatic protoporphyrin hepatopathy, and peripheral neuropathy may be seen. These patients often resort to ice-cooling their skin.

Apart from general measures, afamelanotide as 16 mg subcutaneous implants administered every alternate month has been tried. Narrow-band UVB phototherapy may help by skin hardening.[26] Childhood cholecystectomy for gallstones, intravenous hemin, plasmapheresis, ursodeoxycholic acid (5 mg/kg twice daily), cholestyramine 4 g up to twice daily, cimetidine, and vitamin E have all been described as beneficial.[26,27] Liver transplant in advanced disease may be necessary.

Type C Phenotype: Neurovisceral Porphyrias

Acute intermittent porphyria typifies this phenotype with the neurovisceral component manifesting in ALA dehydratase porphyria, VP, and hereditary coproporphyria.

- Usually present in the 3rd to 4th decade
- No cutaneous manifestation unless renal failure results in elevated porphyrins resulting in blistering
- Episodes are usually precipitated by one of the exacerbating factors—infections, drugs, smoking, ethanol, starvation, and stress
- Acute episodes may present commonly with a generalized neuropathic colicky, usually lower abdominal pain, in the absence of localizing signs lasting hours to days, preceded sometimes with acute sensory motor, autonomic neuropathy, cerebellar or central nervous involvement, neuropathic bladder, and reddish discoloration of urine. Tachycardia is a useful clinical marker in acute episodes.
- Chronic pain, hypertension, neuropsychiatric manifestations, and hepatic and renal involvement characterize chronic disease.

Variegate porphyria and hereditary coproporphyria manifest with the above symptoms in only 10–20% cases with milder episodes than AIP. ALA dehydratase is an extremely rare disorder reported in only six confirmed cases.[28,29]

Neurovisceral porphyria diagnosis is mainly on clinical suspicion, and an elevated porphobilinogen based on a spot test is preferable before initiating therapy.

Treatment of acute attack is aimed at arresting the episode and provision of symptomatic care.

Hospitalization is a must as the episode is likely to last a few days. Hemin in the dose of 3–4 mg/kg/day as an intravenous infusion for 4 days is recommended; it can be extended further if complete recovery is not observed. Glucose loading of 300–400 g daily as a 10% IV infusion is better tolerated than oral glucose administration. Milder attacks may benefit from only glucose; severe cases need hemin. Hemodialysis may help if hemin is not available.[30,31] It is essential to provide systemic care of respiratory, neurological, alimentary, and renal systems by involving the respective specialists in the team. Chronic disease needs pain management.

Avoidance of precipitating causes such as drugs, smoking, alcohol, early and prophylactic management of infections, avoiding hypoglycemia along with annual screening for hepatocellular carcinoma, and renal disease are essential for long-term management.[32] Cyclic episodes may need prophylactic hemin therapy. RNA interference-mediated hepatic *ALAS1* suppression has recently been described to help abate acute attacks.[33]

LABORATORY DIAGNOSIS OF PORPHYRIAS (FLOWCHARTS 2 TO 4)

The principle of laboratory diagnosis in porphyria is to detect porphyrins or their precursors. Clinical suspicion must be followed up with either bed-side spot tests which detect porphyrins >6 mg/L and confirmed with thin-layer chromatography or high-performance liquid chromatography, quantification of individual porphyrin precursors or porphyrins in urine and feces, and rarely enzyme tests for latent disease in asymptomatic family members.

Specimens collected include urine, feces, and blood. Gross examination of urine may reveal a reddish port wine color **(Flowchart 2)** in case of uroporphyrins or brownish in case

Flowchart 2: Porphyrin assessment in type A phenotype.

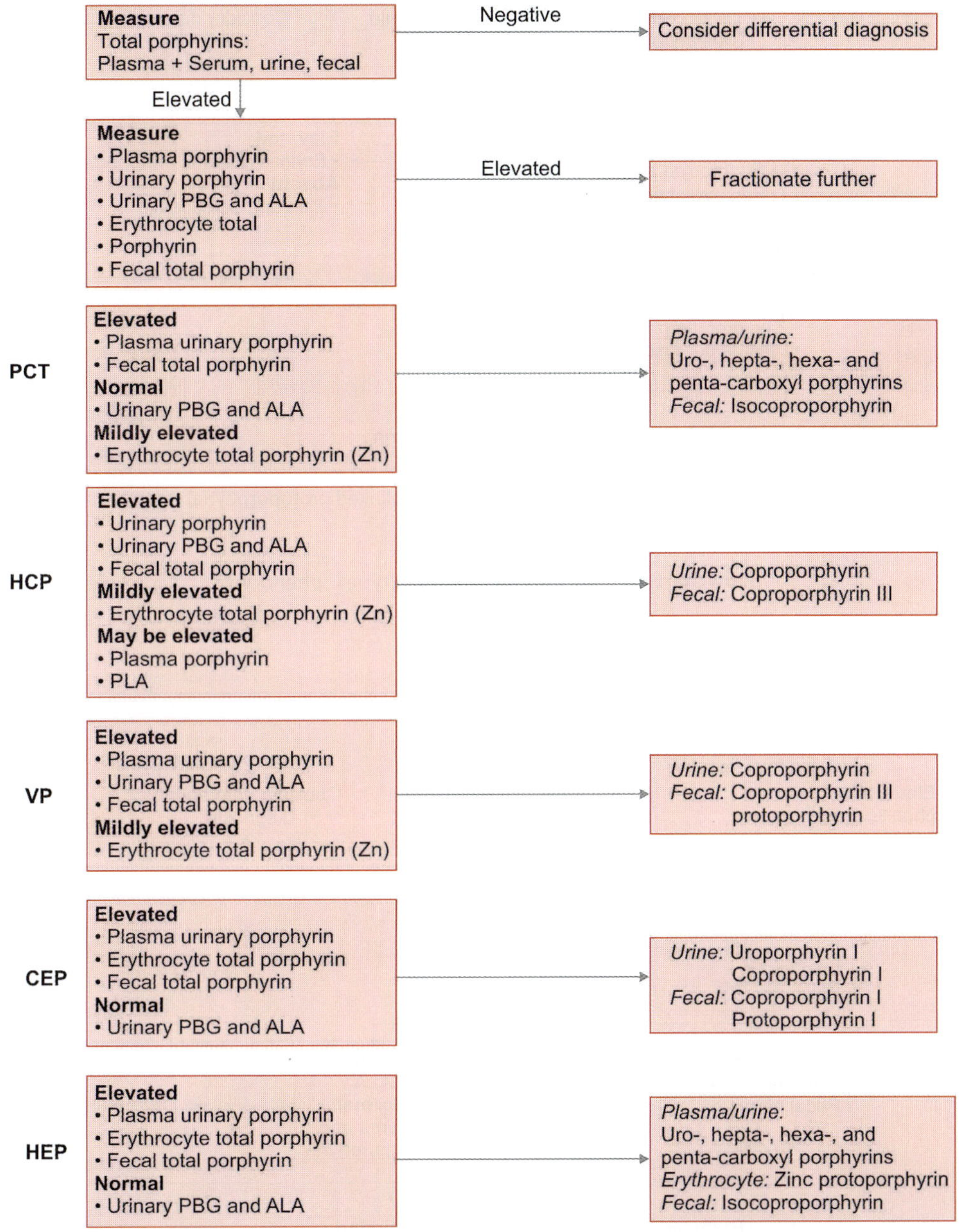

(ALA: aminolevulinic acid; CEP: congenital erythropoietic porphyria; HCP: hereditary coproporphyria; VP: variegate porphyria; PBG: porphobilinogen; PCT: porphyria cutanea tarda)

of porphobilinogen. Porphyrins need to be protected from light with dark paper or aluminum foils and are otherwise reasonable stable. Porphobilinogen may, however, polymerize to uroporphyrin and porphobilin (brownish-red), particularly in the presence of acid.

Urine porphyrins stay stable for 36 hours if preserved protected from light at 4°C, at neutral pH. Longer storage must be at 20°C with pH between 7 and 7.5. Urine creatinine concentration is measured along with samples with levels <4 mmol/L must be discarded. Fecal samples must be analyzed within 36 hours. Wet feces 5 g kept at room temperature may be used within 36 hours and for months at 20°C. Blood samples protected from light, with ethylenediaminetetraacetic acid (EDTA), preserve protoporphyrin levels at room temperature up to 8 days and 8 weeks below 8°C.[34]

Early detection of porphobilinogen in fresh random 25-mL urine samples must be used for cases with unexplained acute abdominal pain. Quantification and other tests can follow. Acute photosensitivity not explained otherwise in absence of blistering may need total porphyrin estimation in blood and followed up further with other tests. Blistering porphyrias must have their urine, feces, and blood samples checked as half of VP may have just skin involvement in absence of any other evidence of acute porphyria symptoms.[35]

Flowchart 3: Porphyrin assessment in type B phenotype.

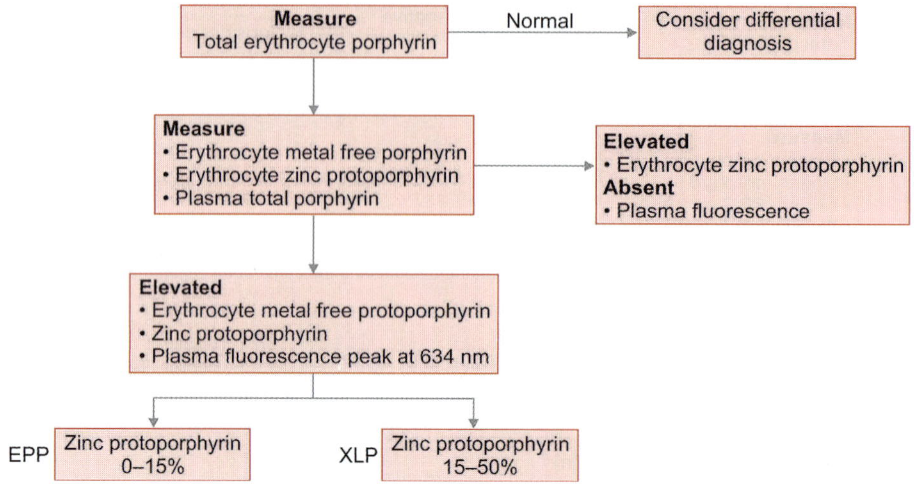

(EPP: erythropoietic protoporphyria; XLP: X-linked protoporphyria)

Flowchart 4: Porphyrin assessment in type C phenotype.

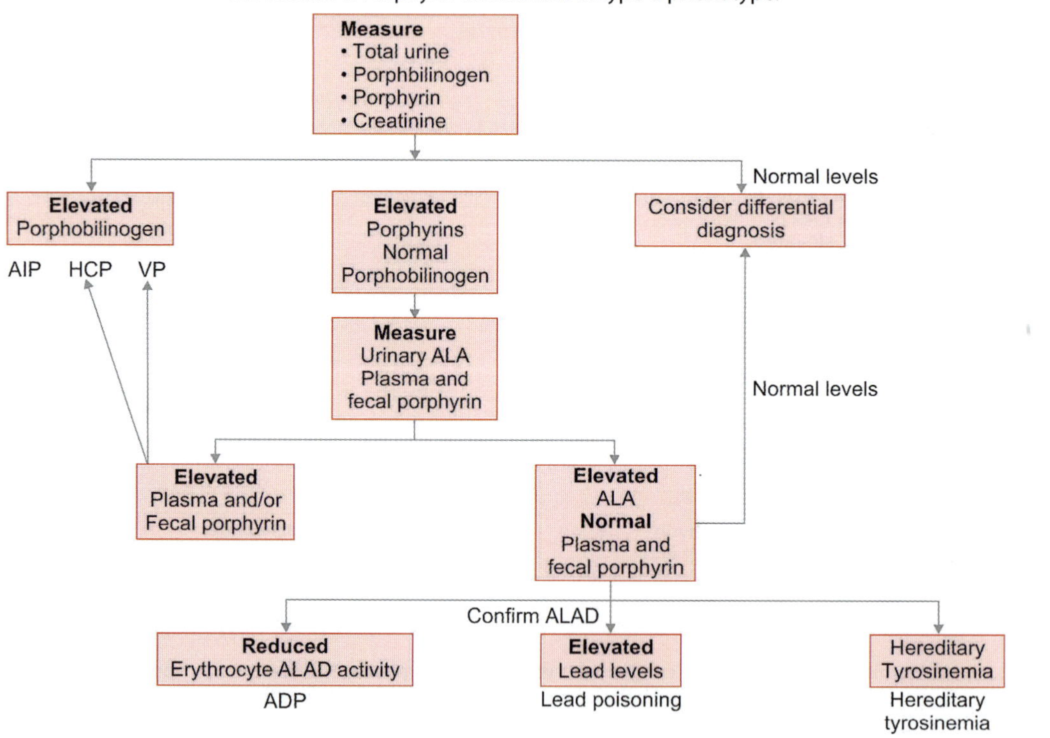

(ADP: aminolevulunic acid dehydratase porphyria; AIP: acute intermittent porphyria; ALAD: aminolevulinic acid deficiency; HCP: hereditary coproporphyria; VP: variegate porphyria)

Thus, in those presenting with acute episodes (hours to weeks) screen for urine porphobilinogen, chronic duration of weeks to months' urine porphobilinogen and delta ALA, feces for porphyrins. Typing of porphyria shall need a run of all tests mentioned above in urine, feces, and blood.

Specific enzyme analysis along with the above may be needed in carriers for specific diagnosis.

Histopathology reveals homogeneous pale eosinophilic material which is periodic acid–Schiff stain positive and diastase negative around thickened blood vessel basement membrane and eccrine glands.

Blister biopsy is rarely needed for confirmation, but if done it reveals subepidermal split with scant inflammation. In some cases, blisters may form in the lamina lucida. Festooning of dermal papillae into the blister is characteristic. Blister roof often has eosinophilic caterpillar bodies which are elongated and sometimes segmented, periodic acid–Schiff stain positive, and diastase negative. Direct immunofluorescence shows immunoglobulin G (IgG) deposits along the vessels in the papillary dermis. Complement deposition is observed only in the active phase.[36]

Wood's Lamp Examination

A useful bedside test to detect fluorescence of porphobilinogen and delta ALA in urine and deposition in teeth is Wood's lamp examination. A coral red fluorescence is characteristic **(Fig. 5)**. Teeth fluoresce similarly **(Fig. 4)**.

SUN PROTECTION IN PORPHYRIAS

Cutaneous porphyrias, i.e., type A and B phenotypes, need adequate sun protection. Physical sunscreens containing titanium oxide or zinc oxide are needed as the conventional sunscreens are ineffective. Sun-protective clothing with use of hats or umbrellas is necessary. Vehicle glasses need tinting or adequate films to cut-off visible light after permission from local authorities.

Beta-carotene in doses of 60–180 mg/day in adults and 30–90 mg/day in children reduces photosensitivity up to 80%,[16,37] usually observed after 12 weeks of administration.[38] Narrow-band UVB phototherapy may be attempted as mentioned above. Dihydroxyacetone alone or as sun- tanning lotion may be a useful adjunct.[39]

Sun avoidance leads to vitamin D deficiency and this must be addressed.

DIFFERENTIAL DIAGNOSIS

Pseudoporphyria

Bullous photodermatosis similar clinically and histologically to PCT with no abnormalities of porphyrin metabolism. It is often induced as a phototoxic drug reaction caused by nonsteroidal anti-inflammatory drugs, antibiotics, retinoids, and neoplastic agents. Other precipitating factors include prolonged hemodialysis or peritoneal dialysis and use of tanning beds.[40]

Autoimmune Bullous Disorders

Bullous pemphigoid and pemphigus group of disorders may present with tense blisters; however, their histopathology is typical and porphyrin levels are normal.

Other Bullous Dermatoses

Hydroa vacciniforme presents in children with blistering on the face and other sun-exposed sites, healing with atrophic scars.[41] Porphyrins are not detectable. Bullous lupus erythematosus too has tense bullae with characteristic histopathology and normal porphyrin levels. Epidermolysis bullosa acquisita present with tense blisters over sites of friction healing with scarring, milia, pigmentary changes, and normal porphyrin levels.

Plumboporphyria

Lead inhibits ALA dehydratase as well as ferrochelatase resulting in accumulation of ALA and protoporphyrin. These present clinically with features of acute porphyria with positive urinary porphyrins. Native medicines consumed over a long period are a cause of lead and other heavy metal ingestion and subsequent toxicity.[42]

KEY POINTS

- Porphyrias are inherited or acquired disorders of heme synthesis characterized by increased excretion porphyrins or porphyrin precursors.
- Porphyrins exhibit differential water solubility which affects their localization in tissue and transport in blood.
- Albumin-bound hydrophobic protoporphyrin shall accumulate in cells such as erythrocytes while hydrophilic uroporphyrin and coproporphyrin pass freely through interstitium.
- Skin manifestations in porphyrias are predominantly photosensitivity with either acute nonblistering or chronic blistering cutaneous involvement.
- Cutaneous porphyrias must be considered when an individual presents with photosensitive blistering on the exposed areas, particularly the hands.
- Immediate photosensitivity with intense pain, discomfort, itching, and edema must be considered as nonblistering cutaneous porphyrias. Total erythrocyte protoporphyrin must be done to diagnose followed by demonstration of elevated metal-free protoporphyrin.
- Severe systemic symptoms in neurovisceral porphyrias need urine spot tests to show elevated porphobilinogen.
- Total porphyrin levels are a useful screening test, followed by measurement of porphyrin fractions in urine, blood, and feces.
- Sun protection is the cornerstone of treatment of cutaneous porphyrias.
- PCT responds to serial phlebotomy or hydroxychloroquine. Neurovisceral porphyrias need urgent hemin infusions. Intravenous glucose is not as effective.

REFERENCES

1. Ramanujam V-MS, Anderson KE. Porphyria diagnostics-part 1: A brief overview of the porphyrias. Curr Protoc Hum Genet. 2015;86:17.20.1-26.
2. Meissner PN, Dailey TA, Hift RJ, Ziman M, Corrigall AV, Roberts AG, et al. A R59W mutation in human protoporphyrinogen oxidase results in decreased enzyme activity and is prevalent in South Africans with variegate porphyria. Nat Genet. 1996;13:95-7.
3. Arora S, Harith A, Sodhi N. Congenital erythropoietic porphyria with undescended testis. Indian J Dermatol. 2016;61:467.
4. Epstein JH, Tuffanelli DL, Epstein WL. Cutaneous changes in the porphyrias: a microscopic study. Arch Dermatol. 1973;107:689-98.

5. Wolff K, Hönigsmann H, Rauschmeier W, Schuler G, Pechlaner R. Microscopic and fine structural aspects of porphyrias. Acta Derm Venereol Suppl (Stockh). 1982;100:17-28.
6. Ryan EA. Histochemistry of the skin in erythropoietic protoporphyria. Br J Dermatol. 1966;78:501-18.
7. Wick G, Hönigsmann H, Timpl R. Immunofluorescence demonstration of type IV collagen and a non-collagenous glycoprotein in thickened vascular basal membranes in protoporphyria. J Invest Dermatol. 1979;73:335-8.
8. Caputo R, Berti E, Gasparini G, Monti M. The morphologic events of blister formation in porphyria cutanea tarda. Int J Dermatol. 1983;22:467-72.
9. Khayat R, Dupuy A, Pansé I, Bagot M, Cordoliani F. Sclerodermatous changes in porphyria cutanea tarda: six cases. Ann Dermatol Venereol. 2013;140:589-97.
10. Muñoz-Santos C, Guilabert A, Moreno N, To-Figueras J, Badenas C, Darwich E, et al. Familial and sporadic porphyria cutanea tarda: Clinical and biochemical features and risk factors in 152 patients. Medicine (Baltimore). 2010;89:69-74.
11. Bissell DM, Anderson KE, Bonkovsky HL. Porphyria. N Engl J Med. 2017;377:862-72.
12. Pandya AG, Nezafati KA, Ashe-Randolph M, Yalamanchili R. Deferasirox for porphyria cutanea tarda: a pilot study. Arch Dermatol. 2012;148:898-901.
13. Ryan Caballes F, Sendi H, Bonkovsky HL. Hepatitis C, porphyria cutanea tarda and liver iron: an update. Liver Int. 2012;32:880-93.
14. Singal AK, Kormos-Hallberg C, Lee C, Sadagoparamanujam VM, Grady JJ, Freeman DH, et al. Low-dose hydroxychloroquine is as effective as phlebotomy in treatment of patients with porphyria cutanea tarda. Clin Gastroenterol Hepatol. 2012;10:1402-9.
15. Harith A, Arora S, Kapoor S, Mukherjee B. Congenital erythropoietic porphyria: insight into the molecular basis of the disease. Indian J Paediatr Dermatol. 2016;17(1):1.
16. Balwani M, Desnick RJ. The porphyrias: advances in diagnosis and treatment. Blood. 2012;120:4496-504.
17. Fortian A, González E, Castaño D, Falcon-Perez JM, Millet O. Intracellular rescue of the uroporphyrinogen III synthase activity in enzymes carrying the hotspot mutation C73R. J Biol Chem. 2011;286:13127-33.
18. Bales L, Day RS, Blekkenhorst GH. The clinical and biochemical features of variegate porphyria: an analysis of 300 cases studied at Groote Schuur Hospital, Cape Town. Int J Biochem. 1980;12:837-53.
19. Kirsch R, Meissner P, Hift R. Variegate porphyria. Semin Liver Dis. 1998;18:33-41.
20. Lecha M, Puy H, Deybach J-C. Erythropoietic protoporphyria. Orphanet J Rare Dis. 2009;4:19.
21. Todd DJ. Erythropoietic protoporphyria. Br J Dermatol. 1994;131:751-66.
22. Alexander Holme S, Whatley SD, Roberts AG, Anstey AV, Elder GH, Ead RD, et al. Seasonal palmar keratoderma in erythropoietic protoporphyria indicates autosomal recessive inheritance. J Invest Dermatol. 2009;129:599-605.
23. Balwani M, Doheny D, Bishop DF, Nazarenko I, Yasuda M, Dailey HA, et al. Loss-of-function ferrochelatase and gain-of-function erythroid-specific 5-aminolevulinate synthase mutations causing erythropoietic protoporphyria and X-linked protoporphyria in North American patients reveal novel mutations and a high prevalence of X-linked protoporphyria. Mol Med Camb Mass. 2013;19:26-35.
24. Whatley SD, Mason NG, Holme SA, Anstey AV, Elder GH, Badminton MN. Molecular epidemiology of erythropoietic protoporphyria in the UK. Br J Dermatol. 2010;162:642-6.
25. Frank J, Poblete-Gutiérrez P, Neumann NJ. Photosensitivity in the elderly—think of late-onset protoporphyria. J Invest Dermatol. 2013;133:1467-71.
26. Dawe R. An overview of the cutaneous porphyrias. F1000Res. 2017;6:1906.
27. Thapar M, Bonkovsky HL. The diagnosis and management of erythropoietic protoporphyria. Gastroenterol Hepatol. 2008;4:561-6.
28. Doss MO, Stauch T, Gross U, Renz M, Akagi R, Doss-Frank M, et al. The third case of Doss porphyria (delta-amino-levulinic acid dehydratase deficiency) in Germany. J Inherit Metab Dis. 2004;27:529-36.
29. Besur S, Schmeltzer P, Bonkovsky HL. Acute porphyrias. J Emerg Med. 2015;49:305-12.
30. Prabahar MR, Manorajan R, Sathiyakumar D, Soundararajan P, Jayakumar M. Hemodialysis: a therapeutic option for severe attacks of acute intermittent porphyria in developing countries. Hemodial Int. 2008;12:34-8.
31. Attarian S, Yu C, Anderson KE, Friedman EW. Effects of hemin and hemodialysis in a patient with acute intermittent porphyria and renal failure. Blood Adv. 2017;1:915-7.
32. Stewart MF. Review of hepatocellular cancer, hypertension and renal impairment as late complications of acute porphyria and recommendations for patient follow-up. J Clin Pathol. 2012;65:976-80.
33. Yasuda M, Gan L, Chen B, Kadirvel S, Yu C, Phillips JD, et al. RNAi-mediated silencing of hepatic Alas1 effectively prevents and treats the induced acute attacks in acute intermittent porphyria mice. Proc Natl Acad Sci. 2014;111:7777-82.
34. Chisolm JJ, Brown DH. Micro-Scale photofluorometric determination of "free erythrocyte porphyrin" (protoporphyrin IX). Clin Chem. 1975;21:1669.
35. Elder GH, Smith SG, Smyth SJ. Laboratory investigation of the porphyrias. Ann Clin Biochem Int J Biochem Lab Med. 1990;27:395-412.
36. Vieira FMJ, Aoki V, de Oliveira ZNP, Martins JEC. Study of direct immunofluorescence, immunofluorescence mapping and light microscopy in porphyria cutanea tarda. An Bras Dermatol. 2010;85:827-37.
37. Mathews-Roth MM, Pathak MA, Parrish J, Fitzpatrick TB, Kass EH, Toda K, et al. A clinical trial of the effects of oral beta-carotene on the responses of human skin to solar radiation. J Invest Dermatol. 1972;59:349-53.
38. Lee J, Jiang S, Levine N, Watson RR. Carotenoid supplementation reduces erythema in human skin after simulated solar radiation exposure. Proc Soc Exp Biol Med. 2000;223:170-4.
39. Asawanonda P, Oberlender S, Taylor C. The use of dihydroxyacetone for photoprotection in variegate porphyria. Int J Dermatol. 1999;38:916-8.
40. Masmoudi A, Hajjaji Darouiche M, Ben Salah H, Ben Hmida M, Turki H. Cutaneous abnormalities in patients with end stage renal failure on chronic hemodialysis. A study of 458 patients. J Dermatol Case Rep. 2014;8:86-94.
41. Lecluse ALY, Kuck-Koot VCM, van Weelden H, Sigurdsson V, Russel IM, Frank J, et al. Erythropoietic protoporphyria without skin symptoms: you do not always see what they feel. Eur J Pediatr. 2008;167:703-6.
42. Akshatha LN, Rukmini MS, Mamatha TS, Sadashiva RP, Prashanth B. Lead poisoning mimicking acute porphyria! J Clin Diagn Res. 2014;8:CD01-2.

EXAMINATION QUESTIONS

Write short notes on the following:

1. Heme cycle
2. Porphyrin metabolism
3. Assessment of a suspected case of porphyria
4. Approach to a case of acute photosensitivity
5. Congenital erythropoietic porphyria/Gunther's disease
6. Variegate porphyria
7. Cutaneous porphyrias
8. Porphyria cutanea tarda

38 CHAPTER

Genetic Disorders of Connective Tissue

Ramesh Bhat M, Jyothi Jayaraman

INTRODUCTION

Inherited disorders of connective tissue comprise a clinically and genetically diverse group of conditions of collagen, elastin, and dermal matrix affecting skin, joints, and internal organs.

CLASSIFICATION[1]

Classification of inherited disorders of connective tissue are given in **Table 1**.

EHLERS–DANLOS SYNDROME (CUTIS HYPERELASTICA)

Introduction

It is a group of inherited disorder of the connective tissues that arise from altered collagen tissue in skin, blood vessels and bones.

Epidemiology

Incidence of various types of Ehlers–Danlos syndrome (EDS) is 1/5,000–560,000 cases and hypermobility type is most common.[2] Most cases present with characteristic features in childhood and sex predilection in females is seen in hypermobility type. Association with osteogenesis imperfecta (OI), pseudoxanthoma elasticum (PXE), and Marfan syndrome (MFS) has been observed.[1]

Pathophysiology

Ultrastructural defects in fibrillar collagen, fibronectin, tenascin-X, and other extracellular molecules leading to disordered collagen framework in dermis, blood vessels, and bones.

Genetic Factors

Autosomal dominant inheritance in 30–50% cases and less commonly autosomal recessive (AR), sporadic X-linked pattern have been observed. Common genetic factors are listed in **Table 2**.[1]

Other subtypes of genetic factors are given in **Table 3**.

In 2017, the International EDS consortium has proposed a revised international classification of EDS with 13 distinct subtypes. A set of clinical criteria was also proposed for each subtype. The definite diagnosis of all EDS subtypes, except for the hypermobile type mandates molecular confirmation with identification.[4]

Management

Investigations and Clinical Assessment Tools

- *Gorlin's sign*: Ability to touch the nose with the tip of the tongue
- Beighton score to test for joint hypermobility. Score 4 or more is diagnostic **(Table 4)**.

TABLE 1: Classification of inherited disorders of connective tissue.

Disorders of collagen	*Disorders of elastin*	*Premature aging syndromes*	*Disorders of abnormal mineralization*	*Infantile stiff skin syndrome*	*Miscellaneous*
Ehlers–Danlos syndrome	Inherited generalized cutis laxa*	Progeria	Pseudoxanthoma elasticum	Hyaline fibromatosis syndrome	Adermatoglyphia
Prolidase deficiency	Michelin tire baby*	Werner syndrome	Fibrodysplasia ossificans progressiva	Stiff skin syndrome	Lipoid proteinosis
Osteogenesis imperfecta	Williams–Beuren syndrome*	Acrogeria	Primary hypertrophic osteoarthropathy	Winchester syndrome	Pterygium syndrome
	Marfan syndrome$^{\infty}$	Familial mandibuloacral dysplasia		Restrictive dermopathy	
		Mulvihill–Smith syndrome			
		Neonatal progeroid syndrome			

*Elastinopathy; $^{\infty}$Fibrillinopathy

TABLE 2: Villefranche classification of molecular and clinical subtypes.

Type	*Inheritance*	*Defect*	*Molecular defect*	*Prominent clinical features*	*Prognosis*
Classical (type I—Gravis, type II—Mitis)	AD	Altered type V collagen	COL5A1 and COL5A2 mutations in up to 90% cases	• Soft velvety hyperextensible skin **(Fig. 1)**, easy bruising, gaping wounds; atrophic (cigarette paper or fish mouth) scars[2] **(Fig. 2)**, blepharochalasis, hypermobile joints, genu recurvatum, kyphoscoliosis and molluscoid pseudotumors (hematomas with calcification and fibrosis), subcutaneous fat herniation (piezogenic pedal papules) • Milder form—Mitis[2]	• High mortality in pregnancy, premature delivery • Cardiac involvement (mitral valve, tricuspid valve prolapse) warrants regular echocardiography
Hypermobile (type III)	AD	Cauliflower fibrils	Haploinsufficiency of tenascin-X (TNXB) in some cases	Increased joint mobility, dislocation and joint pains (complex regional pain syndrome) are common. Extra-articular manifestations such as syncope, palpitations, and fatigue	Normal life expectancy
Vascular or Acrogeric or ecchymotic (type IV)	AD	Small variable fibrils	Point mutations and null mutations in collagen III gene (*COL3A1*)	Prematurity, acrogeric features, thin translucent skin with a prominent venous pattern, easy bruising, rupture of arteries and viscera, keloidal scars	The major complications arise following spontaneous rupture of large arteries, colon, and gravid uterus (12–25% mortality in pregnancy)[2]
Other type or X-linked (type V)	XLR	Unknown (reduced lysyl oxidase)	Unknown	Similar to classical type. Increased bruising seen	Normal life expectancy
Kyphoscoliosis or Oculoscoliotic (type VIA)	AR	Small collagen (type 1 and 3) fibrils	Lysyl hydroxylase (PLOD1) mutations in type A. Normal lysyl pyridinoline/hydroxylysyl pyridinoline (LP/HP) ratios and/or absence of mutations in PLOD1 in type B which was discovered after original classification	Soft hyperextensible skin, hypermobile joints, scoliosis, ocular fragility, keratoconus, marfanoid habitus	Delayed motor development, bleeding from wounds may impair quality of life
Arthrochalasis multiplex congenita (type VIIA, B)	AD	Angular fibrils reduced cross-link formation in collagen 1	A-COL1A1 and B-COL1A2 mutations, result in loss of exon 6 (procollagen N-proteinase/ ADAMTS2 cleavage site)	Hypermobility, recurrent joint dislocations, typically bilateral congenital hip dislocation, criss-cross pattern on palms and soles	Normal life expectancy
Dermatosparaxis (type VIIC)	AR	Hieroglyphic fibrils	Procollagen N-proteinase (ADAMTS2) mutations result in inability to cleave N-propeptide of type I and II procollagens	Markedly hypermobile joints; extremely soft and fragile skin **(Fig. 1)**, premature rupture of the membranes, blue sclera, puffy eyelids, epicanthic folds, micrognathia with gingival hyperplasia and dental anomalies	Serious complications noticed are spontaneous rupture of the bladder or diaphragm
Other form periodontal (type VIII)	AD	Small fibrils	Occasionally collagen III deficient	Severe periodontitis; pigmented pretibial plaques and scarring	Normal life expectancy
Other form Fibronectin (type X)	AR	Large, irregular fibrils	Fibronectin deficiency abnormality	Similar to mild classical type with prominent easy bruising	Normal life expectancy except for easy bruising
Other form Progeroid	AR		XGPT1/B4GALT7 mutations leading to reduced galactosyltransferase I and glycosaminoglycans synthesis	Atrophic scars **(Fig. 2)**, lax skin and joints, aged appearance, short stature, osteopenia, mental retardation	Normal life expectancy

(AD: autosomal dominant; AR: autosomal recessive; XLR: X-linked recessive)

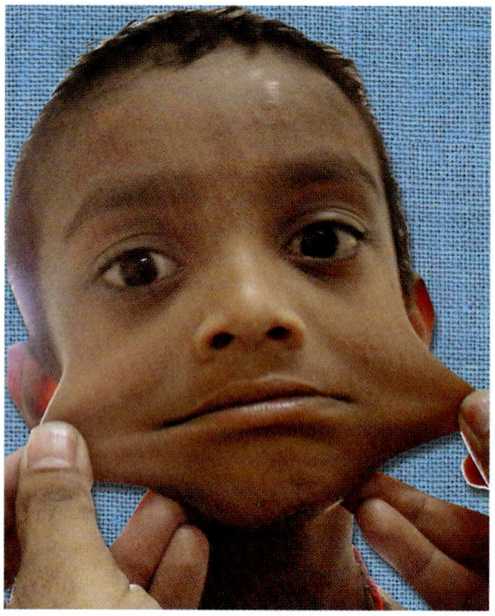

Fig. 1: Hyperelastic skin in Ehlers–Danlos syndrome.
Courtesy: Dr Sahana Srinivas, Bengaluru, Karnataka, India

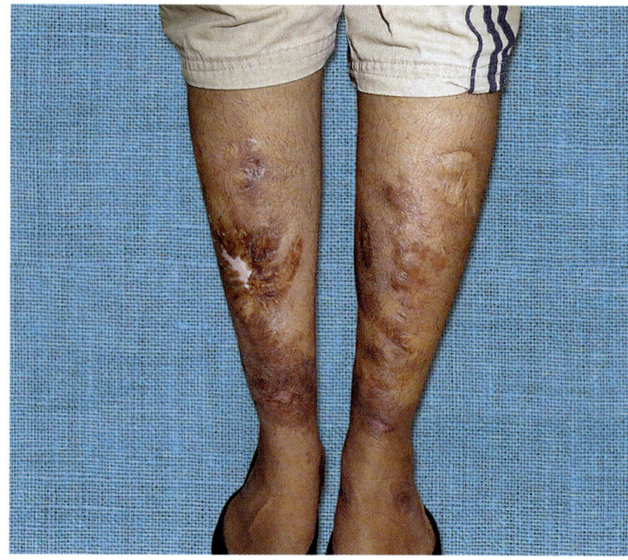

Fig. 2: Atrophic scars in Ehlers–Danlos syndrome.
Courtesy: Dr Sahana Srinivas, Bengaluru, Karnataka, India

TABLE 3: Other subtypes of genetic factors.

Type	*Inheritance*	*Molecular defect*	*Clinical features*
Tenascin-X	AR	Normal fibrils but reduced density due to TNXB mutations	Similar to mild classical type except scarring
Spondylocheirodysplastic	AR	SLC39A13 mutations and reduced activity of transmembrane zinc transporter	Thin skin, easy bruising and wrinkling of palms. Small joint hypermobility with late onset contractures. Tapered fingers, platyspondyly with moderate short stature, osteopenia and widened metaphyses
Musculocontractural (VIB)	AR	CHST14 mutations leading to reduced flexibility of the glycosaminoglycan and abnormal collagen bundle formation	Typical EDS features with distinctive craniofacial appearance, congenital multiple contractures, kyphoscoliosis and variable congenital defects in various systems such as cardiovascular, gastrointestinal, renal, ocular, and CNS. Phenotypic overlap with adducted thumb–clubfoot syndrome
Kyphoscoliosis with myopathy and deafness	AR	• FKBP14 mutations leading to enlarged fibroblast endoplasmic cisterns • Disorganized myofibrils	Typical skin changes of EDS, severe muscle hypotonia at birth, progressive scoliosis, joint hypermobility, myopathy and sensorineural hearing impairment
β3GalT6 deficiency	AR	B3GALT6 mutations leading to glycosaminoglycans production	Skeletal dysplasia and deformities, kyphoscoliosis, intellectual impairment, hypotonia and progeroid features
EDS with periventricular nodular heterotopia	Sporadic and X-linked	FLNA mutations and focal distorted arrangement of fibrils	Periventricular nodular heterotopia with hypermobility
EDS (type IX) occipital horn syndrome[3]	XLR	Defective efflux of copper bound to copper-dependent enzymes such as lysyl oxidase leading to decreased oxidation of collagen and elastin Reclassified as a disorder of copper transport[1]	Soft, lax skin at birth, bladder diverticulae during childhood, bony occipital horns during adolescence

(AD: autosomal dominant; AR: autosomal recessive; CNS: central nervous system; EDS: Ehlers-Danlos syndrome; XLR: X-linked recessive)

TABLE 4: Beighton score to test joint hypermobility.

Movement	*Score*
• Dorsiflex L and R 5th finger >90°	2
• Apposition L and R thumb to forearm	2
• Hyperextend L and R elbow >10°	2
• Hyperextend L and R knee >10°	2
• Palms to floor	1
Total	9

(L: left; R: right)

- Molecular studies if facilities are available, baseline echocardiogram to assess valvular prolapse, and dual energy X-ray absorptiometry to determine bone mineral density loss.

Treatment

Triad of anticipatory guidance, pain management, and physiotherapy (nonweight bearing exercises to strengthen muscles, protective braces to stabilize joints). Steps to prevent injury, gentle skin care encouraged—mild soaps, nonadherent bandages.[2] Sun protection critical to prevent UV rays induced damage, scar revision, use of buttressed sutures, and sutured left for longer duration (double the usual time) to strengthen the scar.

Nonsteroidal anti-inflammatory drugs (NSAIDs) and tricyclic antidepressants for pain relief, closed reduction for joint dislocations. Pregnant women with EDS should be referred to high-risk obstetric practices assessed with increased pregnancy risks.

Celiprolol, a long-acting β1 antagonist with partial β2 agonist properties may be used to reduce the incidence of arterial dissection rupture.[1]

Supportive therapy: Vitamin D and calcium supplements, vitamin C (to improve bruising of skin) may be beneficial.[2]

CUTIS LAXA

(*Synonyms*: Generalized elastorrhexis, generalized elastolysis, generalized dermatochalasis)

Introduction

Generalized cutis laxa is rare heterogenous group of connective tissue disorders. It is clinically characterized by lax pendulous skin which recoils slowly on being pulled.[1]

Pathophysiology

Cutis laxa is caused by disruption of normal elastic tissue function. There are three noted types of genetic transmission:

1. *Autosomal dominant type*: Mutation in the Elastin gene, which encodes for main structural component of elastic fibers.[5]
2. *Autosomal recessive type*: Type 1 is associated with mutation in *Fibulin-5* genes which encode for a family of extracellular matrix proteins with six known members that interact with other extracellular matrix proteins basement membrane components and elastic fibers. Patients often present with severe clinical manifestations. Type 2 is associated with mutations in lysyl oxidase gene.[6]
3. *X-linked cutis laxa (occipital horn syndrome)*: Mutation in the *ATP7A* Cu^{+} transporter gene allelic to Menkes syndrome. Cu^{+} is an essential cofactor of lysyl oxidase which facilitates cross linking fibrillar collagen and elastins.[5]

Syndromes Associated with Cutis Laxa

Geroderma osteodysplastica, SCARF (skeletal abnormalities, cutis laxa, craniostenosis, ambiguous genitalia, retardation, facial abnormalities) syndrome, anterior tortuosity syndrome, Costello syndrome, transaldolase deficiency, and Lenz-Majewski syndrome.

Clinical Features

Prevalence at birth is 1/1,000,000. Autosomal recessive form is the most common.[1] Presentation is usually at birth or early infancy and autosomal dominant forms may present later in life.

Autosomal Dominant Cutis Laxa

Primarily affects the skin and has a later onset than AR form. Distinctive facies (aged appearance), inguinal hernias, bronchiectasis, and soft and hyperextensible skin that fails to resume its normal shape after stretching. Skin fragility, easy bruisability, poor wound healing are not seen.[5]

Autosomal Recessive Cutis Laxa

Autosomal Recessive Cutis Laxa Type I

Facial dysmorphism, broad flat nose, large ears, anti-mongoloid slant of palpebral fissures and sagging cheeks. Associated features such as diaphragmatic and other hernias, diverticula of the gastrointestinal tract (GIT), cardiomegaly, cor pulmonale, and aortic aneurysms. Mortality is high and usually in the first year of life.

Autosomal Recessive Cutis Laxa Type II

Prenatal and postnatal growth deficiency. Large fontanel with delayed closure and congenital hip dislocation and lax joints.

Autosomal Recessive Type III (De Barsy Syndrome)

Corneal opacities, mental retardation, pseudoathetoid movements.

X-linked Recessive Cutis Laxa (Occipital Horn Syndrome)

Bladder diverticula, inguinal hernias, slight skin laxity and hyperextensibility, joint laxity and coarse hair, and skeletal abnormalities such as persistent open anterior fontanel and occipital exostosis.

Management

Investigations

Histopathological examination of skin biopsy granular degeneration and sparse, fragmented elastin fibers in upper dermis.[1] Elastic fibers may separate from an amorphous matrix, and show a "wood grain" pattern.[5] Staining for calcium with Von Kossa stain and abnormal elastin with orcein or Verhoeff stain may be useful in diagnosis. Most significant change on electron microscopy is electron dense amorphous or granular aggregates in and around elastin fibers.[7]

Other investigations required are echocardiography, chest X-ray, lung function testing, and neurological examination and imaging are mandatory in AR cutis laxa type 2. Molecular testing for congenital or inherited cutis laxa.[1]

Treatment

Cutis laxa is a progressive disorder that worsens as age progresses. Although, surgery may be a temporary cure but there are high intraoperative risks. Hernia repairs may be needed frequently. Pulmonary emphysema and other cardiopulmonary complications may necessitate ventilator support.

PSEUDOXANTHOMA ELASTICUM

(*Synonyms*: Systematized elastorrhexis, Grönblad–Strandberg syndrome)

Introduction

Pseudoxanthoma elasticum is a multisystem disorder with significant morbidity characterized by abnormal fragmentation and progressive calcification of the elastic tissues. The cause of progressive calcification is poorly understood despite identification of underlying molecular defect.[1]

Pathophysiology

Pseudoxanthoma elasticum is caused by mutation in the *ABCC6* gene located on chromosome 16p13.1 and inheritance pattern is AR. This gene encodes an adenosine triphosphate (ATP)-binding cassette subfamily C member 6 which is a transmembrane transporter of anionic peptides. This leads to deficiency circulating factors which usually prevent mineralization of elastic fibers.[1,5]

Clinical Features

Precise prevalence rate is unknown but thought to occur 1/50,000. Skin manifestations may appear in adolescence or in childhood, slightly more in women than in men (<2:1).[1]

Skin Lesions

Soft, wrinkled skin hanging in folds over neck axillae, and groin. Yellow colored confluent papules arranged in a reticular pattern giving it a pebbly or cobblestone appearance. It is likened to Moroccan leather or chicken neck. Similar lesions may occur in soft palate, mucosa of lips, stomach, rectum, and vagina.[1] Spontaneous perforating lesions with transepidermal elimination of fragmented elastic fibers (akin to elastosis perforans serpiginous) may be seen.[5]

Ocular Lesions

A "peau-de orange" fundus due to yellowish lesions of the retinal pigment epithelium may be the earliest sign.[1] Angioid streaks of retina or reddish brown curvilinear bands radiating from optic disk, resulting from gaps in the lamina elasticum of the retina due calcified elastic fibers of the Bruch's membrane. They are bilaterally symmetrical and are first visible in early adulthood, seen in 85% of all PXE patients. Fibrovascular ingrowth causes retinal hemorrhage, retinal detachment, and visual loss. Peripheral vision often spared.[5] There may be speckled yellowish mottling (Leopard spotting) and pearly white drusen on Bruch's membrane.[1]

Cardiovascular Changes

Vascular involvement is generalized, predominantly involving large arteries, mesenteric, and visceral arteries or those of the extremities. Calcification of the elastic media and intimal proliferation of blood vessels producing intermittent claudication are the most common manifestation. Hypertension is also common because of renal artery involvement. Mitral valve prolapse has higher prevalence in PXE than in general population. Other features are diminished peripheral pulses, angina pectoris, myocardial infarction, seizures, subarachnoid hemorrhage.[5]

Gastrointestinal Changes

Fragility of calcified mucosal vessels of mainly gastric mucosa leading to GI hemorrhages may be the earliest presenting sign occurring without warning in second to fourth decades of life.[5]

Obstetric Risk

There is an increased risk of abortion in the first trimester, possibly because of failure of placental development.[5]

Associated Abnormalities

Pseudoxanthoma elasticum has been reported in association with osteoectasia, osteitis deformans (Paget's disease), sickle cell anemia, thalassemia, and tumoral calcinosis.

Diagnostic Criteria[5]

- *Major criteria*:
  - Flexural yellow cobble stone lesions
  - Characteristic histological features in lesional skin, using elastic tissue and calcium stains (e.g., Van Gieson and Von Kossa)
  - Angioid streaks in the retina

TABLE 5: Other inherited disorders of connective tissue.

Disorder	*Epidemiology*	*Molecular defect and pathophysiology*	*Clinical features*	*Management*
Osteogenesis imperfecta	Mild forms manifest in adulthood, lethal in perinatal period	• AD inheritance • *COL1A1* and *COL1A2* gene mutation leading to defective collagen 1	Blue sclera, dentinogenesis imperfecta, mitral valve prolapse deafness, skeletal deformity Type 1—classic form Type 2— lethal perinatal form Type 3—progressively deforming form Type 4—mild with normal sclerae Types 5–15—heterogeneous	Multidisciplinary-medical, orthopedic care, physiotherapy, bisphosphonates, allogenic bone marrow, and mesenchymal stromal cell transplantation
Prolidase deficiency	Manifests in infants and young adults. Association with systemic lupus erythematosus	• Decreased prolidase activity in fibroblasts leading to impaired collagen synthesis and wound healing • Abnormal fibroblasts on electron microscopy, imidopeptide secretion in urine	Abnormal facies (high forehead, saddle nose, micrognathia, hypertelorism), skin scarring, photosensitivity, recurrent leg ulcers, recurrent chest infections	Leg ulcers—topical (proline 5% + glycine 5%) ointment, dapsone, topical and systemic growth hormone, pulse corticosteroids, transfusion of prolidase-containing RBCs.
Williams–Beuren syndrome	Manifests in early adulthood	Deletion of genes in a particular region (1.5–1.8 Mb) on chromosome 7	Elfin-like facies, supravalvular aortic stenosis, canities, inguinal hernia, abnormal skin laxity, hypercalcemia	Regular monitoring of calcium monitoring, echocardiography for detecting stenosis
Michelin tire baby (circumferential skin folds syndrome)	Heterogeneous group	Sporadic, inherited—AD or AR	Circumferential skin fold, abnormal elastin fibers, and adipose tissue hyperplasia	
Marfan syndrome	Can manifest at any age	AD inheritance abnormality in fibrillin-1 and transforming growth factor-β signaling	Dolichocephalic skull, high arched palate, ectopia lentis, iridodonesis, pectus excavatum, kyphoscoliosis, increased upper to lower segment ratio, positive thumb sign or Steinberg sign (extension of thumb beyond ulnar border in an opposed clenched hand (Fig. 3) and wrist signs (overlapping of thumb and little finger on wrapping completely around opposite wrist), aneurysmal dilatation of ascending aorta and mitral valve prolapse	Beta blockers, angiotensin-converting enzyme inhibitors to reduce cardiac morbidity, aortic root surgical intervention
Hyaline fibromatosis syndrome (systemic hyalinosis)	Presents in infancy or childhood	Defect in anthrax toxin receptor 2 leading to defective transmembrane protein, deposition of hyaline material in dermis and defective collagen 3	Skin papules, nodules, contractures, and chronic pain	Symptomatic, physiotherapy
Stiff skin syndrome	Presents in infancy or childhood	AD inheritance and mutations in *FBN1* gene encoding for fibrillin-1	Diffuse thickening of skin, short stature, lipodystrophy, joint contractures	Slow progression of skin tightening regular physiotherapy to limit disability
Winchester syndrome	Manifests in infancy with female preponderance	• AR inheritance • Mutations in matrix metalloproteinase14 leading to abnormal collagen 1	Dwarfism, corneal opacity, osteolysis, joint contractures, thick, leathery skin	Radiographs to determine osteolysis, symptomatic relief
Restrictive dermopathy	Presents at birth	• AR inheritance • Mutations in ZMPSTE24 and LMNA leading to accumulation of prelamin A which affects DNA repair	• Abnormal facies with low set ears, micrognathia, choanal atresia, enlarged fontanels, shares features to progeria • Severe joint flexion deformity and restricted respiratory movements	Radiographs, molecular analysis may aid diagnosis, no specific treatment
Progeria (Hutchinson–Gilford syndrome)	• Presents in early childhood (2–3 years) • M : F = 1.5:1.2	Mutations in LMNA which produces progerin that leads to genomic instability and early cell death	Bird-like facies with premature aged appearance wrinkled, mottled skin with scleroderma-like changes, subcutaneous fat loss, coxa valga, angina, strokes	• Care to maintain nutrition, reduce risk of atherosclerosis, physiotherapy • Farnesyltransferase inhibitor (lonafarnib) may be useful

Contd...

Contd...

Disorder	*Epidemiology*	*Molecular defect and pathophysiology*	*Clinical features*	*Management*
Progeria (Werner syndrome)	Manifests at 20–30 year (after puberty)	• AR trait • *RECQL2* gene mutation (codes for DNA helicase) leading to genomic instability	Small stature, beaked nose, canities (earliest at temple area), bilateral juvenile cataracts, glaucoma, atrophic skin with mottled hyperpigmentation and telangiectasias, sclerodactyly and leg ulcers	• Low life expectancy due to myocardial infarction and malignancy • Symptomatic treatment, cataract surgery, care of ulcers
Acrogeria (Gottron syndrome, metageria, acrometageria)	Presents at birth, female preponderance	Thin clumped collagen bundles in dermis	Short stature, pinched face with owl eye appearance, atrophic skin with telangiectasia predominantly over extremities	No specific treatment. Normal life expectancy
Familial mandibuloacral dysplasia	Progressive illness	• AR inheritance • Mutations in LMNA (type A), ZMPSTE24 (type B), and leading to changes in lamin A that affects DNA repair	Progeroid features, mandibular hypoplasia, club-shaped terminal phalanges (tree frog appearance), insulin resistance lipodystrophy in type A and loss of subcutaneous fat in type B	Monitoring for risk of developing metabolic syndrome, cardiovascular damage
Mulvihill–Smith syndrome	Presents in childhood	• AR inheritance • Abnormal fibroblasts	Progeroid features, mental disability, sensory neural hearing loss, cataract, abnormal dentition, IgG immunodeficiency	Symptomatic with clinical watch for development of GIT, skin cancers
Neonatal progeroid syndrome (Wiedemann–Rautenstrauch syndrome)	Early onset (prenatal)	• AR inheritance • DNA repair defect	Intrauterine growth retardation, small face, mouth with beaked nose, sparse hair, and subcutaneous fat, thin limbs with large hands, and mental disability	• Lethal in infancy due to respiratory infections • Symptomatic treatment
Fibrodysplasia ossificans progressiva	Manifests as age progresses	• AD inheritance • Mutations in *ACVR1* gene encoding for type 1 Bone morphogenetic protein (BMP) that leads to progressive ossification on minor trauma or trigger by infection	Malformed big toes, progressive ossification particularly in trunk and proximal limb muscles, functional limb restriction	Severe disability by early adulthood
Primary hypertrophic osteoarthropathy (Touraine–Solente–Gole syndrome, Pachydermo-periostosis)	• Type 1 presents in infancy • Type 2 in pubertal age • Male preponderance	• AR inheritance • Type 1–mutation in *HPGD* gene coding for enzyme involved in prostaglandin degradation • Type 2—*SLCO2A1* gene involved in cellular prostaglandin transport	• Type 1—Pachyderma and furrowing of face and scalp, oily skin, hyperhidrosis, osteoarthropathy • Type 2—myelofibrosis and severe cutis verticis gyrata	Nonsteroidal anti-inflammatory drugs, corticosteroids, colchicine, retinoids
Adermatoglyphia (immigration delay disease)	Congenital	• AD inheritance • Mutation in *SMARCAD1* gene coding for helicase protein superfamily	Congenital absence of epidermal ridges, abnormal palmoplantar sweating, milia on face, fissures	No specific treatment
Lipoid proteinosis (Urbach-Wiethe disease, hyalinosis cutis et mucosae)	Manifests in early infancy	Mutations in extracellular matrix protein 1 (ECM1) that leads to deposition of extracellular hyaline material in dermis	Earliest symptom is hoarseness of voice. Nodular thickening of vocal cords and epiglottis, blisters on skin healing with pock like scars and warty plaques, beading of eyelids (moniliform blepharosis), intracranial calcification leading to epilepsy and psychiatric disorders	Blepharoplasty for blepharosis, retinoids, penicillamine, microdermabrasion, chemical peels, carbon dioxide laser therapy for skin scars, microlaryngoscopy and dissection of vocal cord nodules
Pterygium syndromes	Presents at birth	Type (Inheritance) – Gene mutation 1 (AD) – IRF6 2 (AR) – RIPK4 3 (AR) – CHRNG 4 (AR) – CHRNA1, CHRND or CHRNG	Webbing (pterygium) at neck, antecubital and popliteal fossae, joint contractures due to muscle weakness (arthrogryposis), syndactyly, cleft lip	• Type 2 and 4 are lethal and death in intrauterine or in early infancy is noted • Milder forms surgical treatment to limit disability and physiotherapy

(AD: autosomal dominant; AR: autosomal recessive; DNA: deoxyribonucleic acid; GIT: gastrointestinal tract; IgG: immunoglobulin G; RBCs: red blood cells)

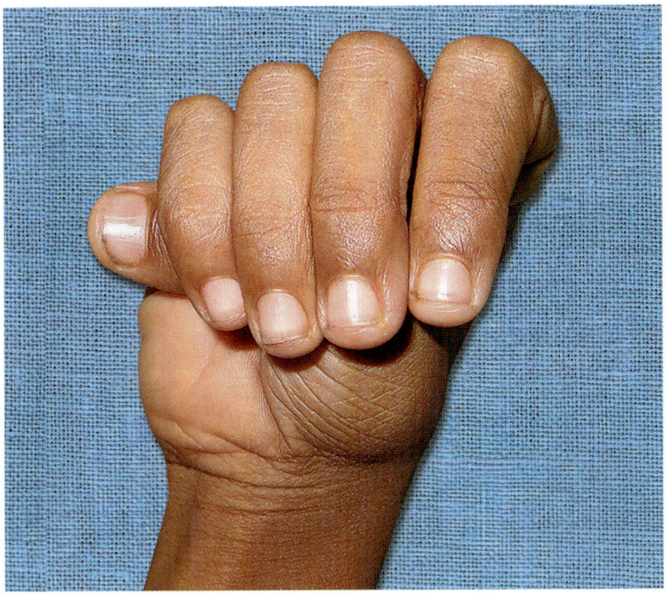

Fig. 3: Thumb sign in Marfan syndrome.
Courtesy: Dr Sahana Srinivas, Bengaluru, Karnataka, India

- *Minor criteria*:
  - Characteristic histologic changes in nonlesional skin
  - Family history of PXE in first-degree relative

Management

Investigations

Histopathologic examination of skin lesions shows clumped, fragmented and calcified elastic fibers, particularly in middle and lower dermis.[8] The normal elastic fibers may also appear blue because of calcium deposition. Staining for calcium with Von Kossa stain and abnormal elastin with orcein or Verhoeff stain may be useful in diagnosis. Serum calcium and phosphate levels should be tested and vitamin K clotting factor levels if *GGCX* gene deficiency is suspected.[1] Radiological investigations such as echocardiogram to evaluate cardiac involvement, radiograph to detect soft tissue calcification.[1] Definitive diagnosis by molecular analysis of the *ABCC6* gene.[5]

Treatment

Dietary restriction of calcium to 600–1 200 mg/dL.[5] Laser photocoagulation, verteporfin photodynamic therapy for retinal hemorrhage. Intravitreal injection of bevacizumab is a newer therapy to reduce choroidal neovascularization. Amsler grid helps in early detection of visual loss. Low lipid diets, avoidance of smoking, control of blood pressure, and safe aerobic exercises may be beneficial. Balloon embolization or surgery GI bleeding may be needed and use of anticoagulants should be minimized.[5]

Other inherited disorders of connective tissue are summarized in **Table 5**.

KEY POINTS

- Inherited connective tissue disorders are clinically and genetically diverse conditions affecting the skin and other extracutaneous tissues.
- The nature and severity of the disorders is based on the type of mutation and role of the affected dermal structural protein.
- Ehlers–Danlos syndrome is characterized by hyper-extensible skin, hypermobile joints, and abnormalities in cardiovascular system such as aneurysms produced by defects in genes coding for collagen fibrils.
- Molecular diagnostic techniques may be useful in diagnosis of various types of EDS.
- High risk of organ rupture, aortic dissection, and uterine rupture in pregnancy is associated with vascular type.
- Generalized cutis laxa is clinically characterized by lax pendulous skin which recoils slowly on being pulled due to abnormality in elastic tissue and has four known genetic subtypes.
- Autosomal recessive is the most common type of cutis laxa characterized by facial dysmorphism. AD type has a late onset presentation and associated with bronchiectasis, inguinal hernias.
- Pseudoxanthoma elasticum is a multisystem disorder with significant morbidity characterized by abnormal fragmentation and progressive calcification of the elastic tissues with AR inheritance.
- Genetic abnormality in ABCC6 leads to abnormal mineralization of elastic fibers in skin, GIT, Bruch's membrane, cardiovascular system (CVS).
- Yellow cobblestoned appearances of flexural skin, angioid streaks in retina, GIT bleeding, hypertension, and renal artery stenosis are common manifestations of PXE.

REFERENCES

1. Burrows N. Genetic disorders of collagen, elastin and dermal matrix. In: Griffiths C, Barker J, Bleiker T, Chalmers R, Creamer D (Eds). Rook's Textbook of Dermatology, 9th edition. West Sussex: Wiley Blackwell; 2016. pp. 72.1-72.8.
2. Dyer JA. Lipoid Proteinosis and Heritable Disorders of Connective Tissue. In: Goldsmith Lowell A, Katz SI, Gilchrest BA, Paller A, Leffell DJ, Wolff K (Eds). Fitzpatrick's Dermatology in General Medicine, 8th edition. USA: McGraw Hill; 2012. pp. 1624-48.
3. Byers PH. Ehlers-Danlos syndrome: recent advances and current understanding of the clinical and genetic heterogeneity. J Invest Dermatol. 1994;103(5):47-52.
4. Malfait F, Francomano C, Byers P, Belmont J, Berglund B, Black J, et al. The 2017 international classification of the Ehlers-Danlos syndromes. Am J Med Genet C Semin Med Genet. 2017;175(1):8-26.
5. Pai GS, Kamath NK, Kuruvila M. Disorders of connective tissue. In: Sacchidanand S, Oberai C, Inamdar AC (Eds). IADVL Textbook of Dermatology, 4th edition. Mumbai: Bhalani Publishing House; 2015. pp. 1666-70.

6. Loeys B, Van Maldergem L, Mortier G, Coucke P, Gerniers S, Naeyaert JM, et al. Homozygosity for a missense mutation in fibulin-5 (FBLN5) results in a severe form of cutis laxa. Hum Mol Genet. 2002;11(18):2113-8.
7. Arkin L, Lee LW, Rubin AI, Yan AC. Congenital diseases (Genodermatoses). In: Elder DE (Ed). Lever's Histopathology of the Skin, 11th edition. Philadelphia: Wolters Kluwer; 2015. pp. 182-3.
8. Arkin L, Lee LW, Rubin AI, Yan AC. Congenital diseases (Genodermatoses). In: Elder DE (Ed). Lever's Histopathology of the Skin, 11th edition. Philadelphia: Wolters Kluwer; 2015. pp. 178-9.

EXAMINATION QUESTIONS

Write short notes on the following:
1. Ehlers-Danlos syndrome
2. Cutis laxa
3. Pseudoxanthoma elasticum

4 SECTION | Infections and Infestations

39 CHAPTER

Normal Skin Flora and its Implication

Priyankar Misra, Anupam Das

INTRODUCTION

The human body is home to trillions of microbes and multicellular organisms which are far greater than the number of human cells. These organisms live upon the host which provides the necessary nutrients, favorable habitat, and shelter.[1] In return, the organisms play an important role in the developing innate immunity in the host, thus forming a symbiotic relationship. This alliance might breakdown when factors such as diet or the use of antibiotics changes the microbial population that result in the development of various chronic inflammatory disorders.[2]

The bulk of microorganisms that are associated with the human body are found in the gut, while the rest inhabit the epithelial surfaces such as the vagina, upper and lower airways, mouth, and skin. The skin has a large surface area (approximately 2 m^2) and is inhabited by 106 bacteria per square centimeter, mounting up to a total of 1,012 skin microbes. The relative paucity of microbes on the skin is a result of the highly unsuitable environment that includes temperature variations, a slightly acidic pH and lack of nutrients, high levels of salt and antimicrobial molecules, and constant exposure to sun, wind, and other external factors.[3] Before delving further into the apparently invisible yet so lively community of living beings on our body, let us go through some terminologies.

BASIC TERMINOLOGIES[4-6]

- *Microbiome*: It is defined as the whole range of microorganisms, including bacteria, fungi, viruses and parasites, their genes and metabolites, and the environmental conditions within which they survive.
- *Microbiota*: It a more limited term which is defined as a collection of microorganisms in a defined micro-environment. This term is now preferred instead of microflora, which refers to microscopic plants.
- *Operational taxonomic units (OTUs)*: It refers to clusters of organisms grouped by deoxyribonucleic acid (DNA) sequence and characteristic of a specific taxonomic marker gene.
- *Alpha diversity*: Measures used to calculate number (richness) and distribution (evenness) of species of microorganisms within a sample.
- *Beta diversity*: Measures used to estimate shared OTUs (microbial species) between different samples and/or subjects.
- *Cutaneous dysbiosis*: It is defined as imbalance in the composition of microbial populations, leading to human and animal inflammatory skin disorders.

COMPOSITION OF SKIN MICROBIOME

Various studies have been conducted to elucidate the nature, diversity, and characteristics of the microbes inhabiting human skin and salient points are as follows:[7,8]

- The microbiota present on the skin can be transient or resident; the latter are considered being members of the "normal" commensal skin microbiota that is in homeostasis with the host, whereas the former are microbes from the environment that temporarily live on the skin.
- Most of the resident skin bacteria are categorized into four different phyla: Actinobacteria, Firmicutes, Proteobacteria, and Bacteroidetes.
- In the sebaceous areas (glabella, alar crease, external auditory canal, occiput, manubrium, and back) the predominant species are *Propionibacterium* and *Staphylococci.*[7]
- In moist sites, such as nares, axillary vault, antecubital fossa, interdigital web space, inguinal crease, gluteal crease, popliteal fossa and plantar heel, and *Corynebacteria and Staphylococcal* species predominate.
- In dry sites, such as the volar forearm, hypothenar palm, and buttock, a mixed population of bacteria are found.
- The drier areas show a higher diversity, but a lower absolute number of organisms.
- There is considerable variation when comparing different sites in a same individual, but the symmetrical sites showed less variation.
- The superficial layers of stratum corneum show higher colonization than the deeper layers.
- Although fetal skin is sterile in utero, colonization begins following the birth process. Vaginally delivered neonates get their skin coated with organisms present in the birth canal such as *Lactobacillus, Prevotella* or *Sneathia* species whereas skin of cesarean section neonates get colonized by microbes predominant over maternal skin such as *Staphylococcus, Corynebacterium*, and *Propionibacterium* species.[9]

ROLE OF COMMENSALS IN PROVIDING INNATE IMMUNITY

The role of gastrointestinal microbiome and chronic inflammatory bowel disorders have been extensively studied and substantially proven. *Bacteroides fragilis* in the gut produces polysaccharide A (PSA) that provides protection from inflammatory bowel disorders. In case of skin microbiome, it is still unclear whether microbial dysbiosis is the cause or the result of inflammatory skin conditions in humans:

- *Lipoteichoic acid (LTA)*: *Staphylococcus epidermidis* plays an important role through the release of LTA which is recognized by the toll-like receptors 2 (TLR2) on the keratinocytes followed by inhibition of TLR3. Ribonucleic acid (RNA) from damaged host cell activates TLR3 that leads to the inflammatory response.
- *Ribosomally synthesized and post-translationally modified peptides (RiPPs)*: These are small molecules and have a narrow spectrum of activity and mediate interactions among closely related species. They are toxic for a limited set of species closely related to the producer and likely determine niche colonization. RiPPs include numerous subclasses, including lantibiotics, bacteriocins, microcins, thiaxole/oxazole-modified microcins and thiopeptides. Lantibiotics are short peptides of less than 40 amino acids that contain thioether bonds, which are redox-stable and the modified amino acids form ring structures that are important for bactericidal activities such as pore formation in bacterial cell membranes. Predominantly, Firmicutes produce lantibiotics, for instance *S. epidermidis* produces the structurally unique lantibiotic epidermin, Pep5, and epilancin K7 and *Staphylococcus aureus* produces Au-26 (also known as Bsa) which inhibits the growth of lactobacilli.[10]
- Serine protease produced by *S. epidermidis* prevents the nasal colonization of *S. aureus* by breaking the biofilm and inhibiting the biofilm formation.

ROLE OF SKIN MICROBIOTA IN VARIOUS DERMATOLOGICAL CONDITIONS[9]

- *Atopic dermatitis (AD)*:
  - In a longitudinal study, it was shown that affected skin of children during flare of AD has lower microbiota diversity, but a significant increase in relative proportions of *S. aureus*. It was also found that the relative proportion of *S. aureus* increased before eruption of skin lesion and the proportion decreased following subsidence of lesion. Those children receiving intermittent therapy showed reduced levels of *S. aureus* almost similar to healthy children.
  - It has been reported that AD individuals have higher abundances of *Malassezia sympodialis* than observed in healthy individuals.
  - It is also seen that the diversity of opportunistic fungi such as *Candida albicans, Cryptococcus diffluens, Cryptococcus liquefaciens, Cladosporium* spp., and *Toxicocladosporium irritans* increase in patients with active lesions of AD.
- *Psoriasis*:
  - The strong clinical correlation of streptococcal beta-hemolytic group A throat infection and guttate psoriasis was reported in 1955, but later it was found that antistreptococcal treatment or removing *Streptococcus* infected tissue did not improve psoriasis.
  - Recent studies to find out association of skin microbes with psoriasis were conducted and it was found that skin of patients with psoriasis was dominated by *Proteobacteria, Firmicutes, and Actinobacteria.*
  - It was also seen in other studies that the microbial diversity is less in patients of psoriasis in comparison to healthy subjects.
  - Stressed keratinocytes release antimicrobial peptides like LL-37 which combine with self-DNA released from damaged keratinocytes to activate the plasmacytoid dendritic cells (pDCs). These pDCs then release interferon-gamma (IFN-gamma). Tumor necrosis factor (TNF), interleukin-1 (IL-1) beta, and IL-6 released from keratinocytes along with IFN-gamma from pDCs activate the dermal dendritic cells which then move to the regional lymph node to activate the naive T-cells.[11]
- *Acne vulgaris*:
  - *Propionibacterium acne* has an important role in the pathogenesis of acne vulgaris though the release of lipase, protease, and hyaluronidase that injure the wall of pilosebaceous unit and activate the complement-mediated inflammatory response. *P. acne* is also found as commensal flora. It was later found that *P. acne* causing acne is of six different strains whereas the commensal group consists of a single strain.
  - The pilosebaceous units involved in acne vulgaris also contain other commensals like *S. epidermis* which are absent in uninvolved hair follicles.
- *Chronic wound*:
  - Wounds that take more than 6 months to heal are considered chronic. In a study of chronic diabetic and venous ulcer wounds, it was found there was a decreased bacterial diversity, along with presence of anaerobic bacteria, including *Serratia* and *Clostridium* species indicating that a drastic microenvironmental alteration allows for the opportunistic colonization of these microbes.
  - Along with the bacteria, there is a wide variety of fungus and viral particles. The bacteria respond to the antibiotic but the others do not, leading to the chronicity of the wounds.

DETERMINATION OF SKIN MICROBIOME[7]

- Before the advent of molecular methods, culture was the only technique to determine the microorganisms of skin but the organisms that do not readily grow were easily missed.
- *16S ribosomal RNA (rRNA)*: This gene is conserved in all bacteria. The transcribed protein has a constant area followed by a hypervariable region sequencing of which gives us an idea of the species.
- *18S rRNA, 28S rRNA, and internal transcribed spacer (ITS)*: These areas are highly conserved in the genomes; and sequencing helps in identifying fungal communities.
- *Whole genome shotgun sequencing*: In this method, bits and pieces of DNA fragments from whole genomes in a sample are sequenced and then they are assembled into longer and almost complete sequences. In microbiome studies, this method is used to characterize any genes that are sequenced in a nontargeted manner from host and microorganisms, allowing phylogenetic characterization and identification of microbial gene.
- *Next-generation sequencing (NGS)*: Here multiple samples are sequenced simultaneous from both targeted DNA clones and randomly acquired DNA fragment from shotgun technique.
- *Virome*: These are used to assemble all types of viral particles such as bacteriophages, single-stranded and double-stranded DNA and RNA viruses from the sample, but it is challenging due to variability of the viral genome and continuous process of evolution.

KEY POINTS

- There are 106 bacteria per square centimeter of skin, mounting up to a total of 1,012 skin microbes which maintains a symbiotic relationship by providing protection against some diseases.
- Most of the resident skin bacteria are categorized into four different phyla: *Actinobacteria*, *Firmicutes*, *Proteobacteria*, and *Bacteroidetes*.
- They also provide important role in maintaing the innate immunity.
- Advent of molecular methods and genetic studies have made determining skin flora easily.

REFERENCES

1. Brestoff JR, Artis D. Commensal bacteria at the interface of host metabolism and the immune system. Nat Immunol. 2013;14:676-84.
2. Belkaid Y, Segre JA. Good and recent review about host-microbe. Science. 2014;346:954-9.
3. Grice EA, Segre JA. The skin microbiome: Up-to date article about new methods exploring the skin microbiome and future perspectives. Nat Rev Microbiol. 2011;9:244-53.
4. Marchesi JR, Ravel J. The vocabulary of microbiome research: a proposal. Microbiome. 2015;3:31.
5. Lozupone CA, Knight R. Species divergence and the measurement of microbial diversity. FEMS Microbiol Rev. 2008;32:557-78.
6. Morgan XC, Huttenhower C. Human microbiome analysis. PLoS Comput Biol. 2012;8:e1002808.
7. Hoffman AR. The cutaneous ecosystem: the roles of the skin microbiome in health and its association with inflammatory skin conditions in humans and animals. Vet Dermatol. 2017; 28:60-e15.
8. Zeeuwen PLJM, Kleerebazem M, Timmerman HM, Schalkwijk J. Microbiome and skin. Curr Opin Allergy Clin Immunol. 2013;13:514-20.
9. Weyrich LS, Dixit S, Farrer AG, Cooper AJ. The skin microbiome: Associations between altered microbial communities and disease. Australas J Dermatol. 2015;56:268-74.
10. Fyhrquist N, Salava A, Auvinen P, Lauerma A. Skin Biomes. Curr Allergy Asthma Rep. 2016;16:40.
11. Morizane S, Gallo RL. Antimicrobial peptides in the pathogenesis of psoriasis. J Dermatol. 2012;39:225-30.

EXAMINATION QUESTIONS

1. Write a short note on the role of skin flora in psoriasis.
2. Write a short note on the role of skin flora in atopic dermatitis.
3. Describe the normal skin flora and its implication in various dermatological disorders.

40 CHAPTER

Bacterial Skin Disease

Shouvik Ghosh, Anupam Das

INTRODUCTION

In dermatology outpatient department, patients presenting with bacterial skin infections are very common. In immunocompetent patients, streptococci and staphylococci are the major causative organisms. Antibiotics with good gram-positive coverage are available for most of the cutaneous bacterial infections. But an increase in community-associated and healthcare-associated strains of methicillin-resistant *Staphylococcus aureus* (MRSA) is an emerging problem nowadays. Due to systemic diseases and immunodeficiency state there may be an increased risk for some specific bacterial skin diseases.[1]

STAPHYLOCOCCAL SKIN INFECTIONS

- *Direct infection of skin and adjacent tissue*:
  - Folliculitis
  - Furuncles
  - Carbuncle
  - Impetigo (both bullous and nonbullous)
- *Cutaneous disease due to bacterial toxins*:
  - Staphylococcal scalded skin syndrome (SSSS)
  - Toxic shock syndrome (TSS)

STREPTOCOCCAL SKIN INFECTIONS

- Impetigo (nonbullous)
- Ecthyma
- Erysipelas
- Cellulitis
- Necrotizing fasciitis
- Blistering distal dactylitis
- Perianal dermatitis
- Streptococcal intertrigo
- Scarlet fever

CLASSIFICATION OF SKIN INFECTIONS ACCORDING TO DEPTH OF INVOLVEMENT

- *Superficial*:
  - *Follicular*:
    - Superficial pustular folliculitis (Bockhart's impetigo)
    - Chronic folliculitis of leg
  - *Nonfollicular*:
    - Impetigo
- *Deep*:
  - *Follicular*:
    - Sycosis barbae
    - Furuncle
    - Carbuncle (with perifollicular involvement)
  - *Nonfollicular*:
    - Ecthyma
    - Erysipelas
    - Cellulitis
    - Necrotizing fasciitis

Acute Superficial Folliculitis (Bockhart's Impetigo)

Bockhart's impetigo is superficial folliculitis where pustules are seen in the follicular orifices. Common locations are the extremities and scalp, although facial lesions are also seen. These small, fragile, yellowish white, pustules with a rim of erythema develop in crops and heal without scarring within few days. *S. aureus* is the most frequent cause.

Treatment: Antibacterial ointments such as fusidic acid, mupirocin, or clindamycin can be used for 7–10 days for localized lesions. When staphylococcal folliculitis is widespread or recurrent, appropriate β-lactam antibiotics (e.g., a β-lactamase-resistant penicillin or first-generation cephalosporin), tetracyclines or (depending on local resistance patterns) macrolides and can be prescribed. Chronic *S. aureus* carriage can be treated with mupirocin 2% ointment applied twice daily to the nares, axillae/groin and/or submammary area for 5 days.

Chronic Folliculitis of the Legs

It is a chronic and recurrent form of folliculitis caused by *S. aureus.* Clinically, it presents as symmetrical follicular pustules on the anterior surface of the legs and may extend to thighs also. This condition is recurrent, recalcitrant and heals with atrophic scarring.

Sycosis Vulgaris (Sycosis Barbae)

Sycosis vulgaris, also known as "barber's itch" or sycosis barbae, is a type of deep folliculitis caused by staphylococcal infection and presents as perifollicular, chronic, erythematous papules, and pustular lesions of the bearded region. Sometimes they coalesce to form plaques studded with pustules and crusts. It has a tendency to recur.

Pseudofolliculitis barbae: A common chronic disorder occurring most often in the beard area of men who shave. The etiology is tightly curved hairs curving back into the skin when shaved. Lesions range from inflammatory papules and pustules to firm papules and keloidal scars.

FURUNCLE AND CARBUNCLE

Furuncle (boil) is a deep follicular infection with perifollicular abscess formation at the level of dermis and subcutaneous tissue and, as such, occur only in hair-bearing area of the skin where sweating and friction is also more. The most common locations are the neck, face, axillae, groin, buttocks, and thighs. Furuncles usually begin as a hard, tender, red nodules that enlarge to become tender and fluctuant with central suppuration. Rupture results in decreased pain. Recurrent furuncles can be associated with chronic *S. aureus* carriage. Conditions such as malnutrition, diabetes mellitus, HIV infection, and systemic steroid also cause increased frequency and severity.

Carbuncle is a deep infection of a group of contiguous hair follicles associated with intense inflammatory collections that extend deep into the subcutaneous tissue. On inspection, the surface shows multiple draining sinus tracts. They usually occur in areas with thicker skin, e.g., nape of neck, back, and thigh. Systemic symptoms are usually present. Carbuncles are slow to heal and scar formation is inevitable.

Treatment: For simple ones, treatment may not be needed. Hot compresses may promote maturation, followed by rupture, drainage and resolution of pain. Fluctuant lesions require incision and drainage. Systemic antibiotics should be used (in conjunction with incision and drainage if possible) in some instances such as furuncles around the nose, within the nares or in the external auditory canal; large and recurrent lesions; lesions with surrounding cellulitis; and lesions not responding to local supportive care. Given the high proportion of infection that are caused by MRSA, empiric coverage with antibiotics such as doxycycline, trimethoprim-sulfamethoxazole or clindamycin (depending on the local resistance patterns) should be considered. Patient with recurrent furunculosis may benefit from eradication of *S. aureus* from the nares, axilla, and perineum. Chronic *S. aureus* carriage can be treated with mupirocin 2% ointment applied twice daily to the nares, axillae/groin and/or submammary area for 5 days.

IMPETIGO

Impetigo is a common, highly contagious, superficial skin infection that primarily affects children. The condition presents in both nonbullous and bullous forms. The primary pathogens in nonbullous and bullous impetigo are *S. aureus* and, less commonly, group A β-hemolytic *Streptococcus* (*Streptococcus pyogenes*).[2]

Nonbullous impetigo presents as single erythematous macule that rapidly evolves into a short-lived vesicle or pustule followed by superficial erosion with a typical "honey-colored" crust and rapid direct extension of infection to surrounding skin. It may arise as a primary infection or a secondary infection of preexisting dermatoses, e.g., pediculosis, scabies, and eczemas.

Bullous impetigo: At early stage, small vesicles are seen which enlarge into superficial bullae. Later flaccid and transparent bullae are seen measuring up to 5 cm in diameter, which persists for 2–3 days and ruptureless rapidly. There is no thick crust and usually no surrounding erythema.

Treatment: Local wound care, cleansing, removal of crusts, and proper dressings. For healthy cases with a few lesions and no systemic symptoms, either mupirocin ointment or fusidic acid cream or ointment can be given. For patients with limited disease, these topical medications are at least equally (if not more) effective than oral antibiotics.

BOTRYOMYCOSIS

It is a suppurative infective condition caused by *S. aureus* presenting on the lower extremities as nodular, crusted purulent lesion. Sinus tracts draining purulent material are seen. These heal with atrophic scars.

STAPHYLOCOCCAL SCALDED SKIN SYNDROME (RITTER'S DISEASE)

Staphylococcal scalded skin syndrome is a widespread desquamative infectious disease in which the skin exfoliates in sheets and occurs most often in neonates and young children <6 years of age. Skin does not separate at the dermoepidermal junction, as in toxic epidermal necrolysis (TEN), but within the granular layer. This superficial loss of skin happens far beyond areas of actual staphylococcal infection, by action of the exfoliative exotoxins types A and B, produced by the bacteria. Clinical manifestations of SSSS begin with sudden onset of diffuse erythema, skin tenderness, and fever. Classically, flexural areas are first to exfoliate. There is sparing of the palms, soles, and mucous membranes. Nikolsky's sign is positive usually after 12 hours. Generalized exfoliation takes place within the next few hours to days, with sheets of epidermis separation. Phage group 2 strains (e.g., types 55, 71) of *S. aureus* are the causative agent in most cases. Cultures should be taken from the mucous membranes because the skin erythema and exfoliation are caused by the distant effects of the exfoliative toxins. Rapid diagnosis of SSSS can be made by biopsy with frozen sections from a blister roof and observing superficial epidermal split not full thickness of the epidermal necrosis as in TEN. Exfoliative toxins blind and cleave desmoglein 1 (Dsg1), which is also targeted by autoantibodies in pemphigus foliaceus.[3]

Treatment: Patients with extensive, generalized forms of SSSS require hospitalization and parental antibiotics. Oral treatment with a β-lactamase-resistant antibiotic (e.g., dicloxacillin and cephalexin) for a minimum of 1 week is usually sufficient for milder disease. Moist and erosive areas should be lubricated with a bland emollient.

TOXIC SHOCK SYNDROME

Toxic shock syndrome is an acute multisystem illness caused by an exotoxin produced by *S. aureus*. TSS is due to infection or colonization with certain strains of *S. aureus* that are able to produce a particular protein, toxic shock syndrome toxin-1 (TSST-1). TSST-1 is thought to cause deleterious effects by acting as a "superantigen". Clinical features of TSS is characterized by a sudden onset of high fever with myalgias, vomiting, diarrhea, headache, and pharyngitis. Rapid progression to shock can occur. Clinically, the illness can vary from relatively mild disease to being rapidly fatal. Patients usually develop a diffuse erythema that starts on the trunk and spreads to peripheral extremities. There is erythematous eruption and desquamation of palms and soles; palmar edema, erythema of the mucous membranes, a strawberry tongue, conjunctival redness, and a generalized nonpitting edema are also present. Desquamation of the hands and feet occurs 1–3 weeks after the onset of symptoms. After recovery, Beau's lines and nail shedding can be seen. In severe cases, telogen effluvium may occur.[4]

Treatment: Severe cases of TSS require intensive supportive therapy. Patient should be treated with intravenous fluids and vasopressor agents. Drainage of *S. aureus*-infected site is done. Any nidus of infection (e.g., nasal packing and tampon) should be removed. Beta-lactamase-resistant antibiotics are used to eradicate any foci of toxin-producing staphylococci.

ECTHYMA

Ecthyma is considered an ulcerated deeper variant of nonbullous impetigo in which the early lesion extends into the dermis to produce a shallow ulcer. It is thought to be due to either a primary infection with *S. pyogenes* or streptococcal superinfection of a preexisting ulceration. Clinically, it is characterized by thick chocolate-colored crust with indurated base and surrounding erythema. The crust is adherent and on removal reveals shallow ulcers, which often heals with scarring. Lower limbs are the most preferred site **(Fig. 1)**.

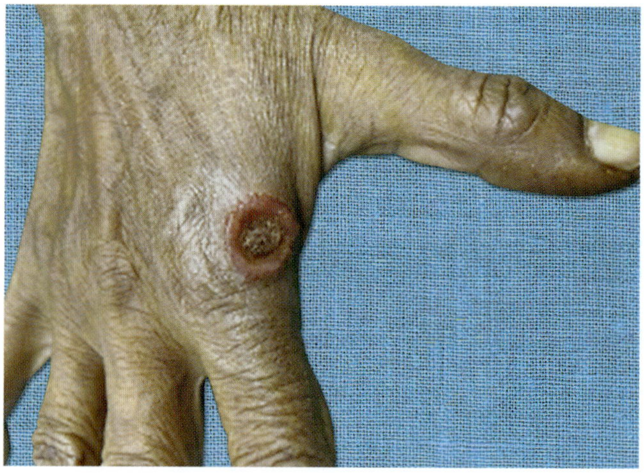

Fig. 1: Ecthyma.
Courtesy: Subhra Sankar Sahoo.

CELLULITIS

Cellulitis is an acute suppurative infection of the skin involving deep dermis and subcutaneous tissue caused most commonly by *S. pyogenes* and *S. aureus*. Cellulitis is often preceded by systemic symptoms such as fever, chills, and malaise. It starts a mild local erythema and tenderness and then rapidly intensifies and spreads. The area is warm on touch and becomes infiltrated and pits on pressure. The lesion usually has ill-defined, nonpalpable borders. In severe infections, vesicles, bullae, pustules, or necrotic tissue may be present. Ascending lymphangitis and regional lymph node involvement may occur. Cellulitis is more common in the lower legs. On the leg, tinea pedis or interdigital candidiasis is the most common portal of entry.

Treatment: Mild cases require a 10-day course of an oral antibiotic with good gram-positive coverage. Hospitalization should be done only to patients who are seriously ill and those with facial involvement. And, parenteral antibiotics should be given to them. Diabetic or decubitus ulcers associated with cellulitis require broad-spectrum coverage (e.g., piperacillin/tazobactam or, in penicillin-allergic patients, metronidazole plus ciprofloxacin). Immobilization and elevation should be recommended.

ERYSIPELAS

Erysipelas is a superficial form of cellulitis caused most commonly by group A β-hemolytic *Streptococcus*. This is manifested as erythematous-edematous infiltrated plaque with a characteristic raised and sharply demarcated advancing edge involving the face; nowadays, however, the lower extremity is the most common location. After an incubation period of 2–5 days, there is an abrupt onset of fever, chills, malaise, and nausea. A few hours to a day later, a small plaque of erythema develops that progressively spreads. The area is clearly demarcated from uninvolved tissue, hot, tense, and indurated. The affected area is painful to palpation. Regional lymphadenopathy is normally present.

Treatment: Systemic penicillin is rapidly effective and 10–14-day course should be given. Although macrolides such as erythromycin may be used in penicillin-allergic cases, there has been an increase in macrolide resistance among certain strains of *S. pyogenes*. Hospitalization and parenteral antibiotics should be reserved for children and debilitated patients.

BLISTERING DISTAL DACTYLITIS

Blistering distal dactylitis classically presents as a localized infection of the volar fat pad of the phalanx of a finger or thumb or, less often, a toe. There is tense superficial blister formation on an erythematous base. Darkening of the surrounding skin is commonly observed for several days to a week before blister formation. The infection most commonly occurs in children aged 2–16 years. Group A β-hemolytic *Streptococcus* and *S. aureus* are the responsible organisms.

STREPTOCOCCAL PERIANAL DISEASE

Streptococcal perianal disease due to *S. pyogenes* presents as superficial, well demarcated, and perianal rim of erythema extending around the anal verge. Patients may complain of painful defecation, blood-streaked stools, prolonged perianal irritation or pruritus, anal leakage and soiling of undergarments. It may also penile and vulval tissues. Systemic symptoms are absent. Children, especially those under the age of 4 years streptococcal perianal disease can be diagnosed with skin culture and treated with approximately 14-day course of systemic penicillin or erythromycin combined with a topical antibiotic.

STREPTOCOCCAL INTERTRIGO

Group A β-hemolytic streptococcal intertrigo affects infants and young children and is easily amenable to treatment. Infants are particularly vulnerable due to irritation and frictional forces in moist deep skin folds of the neck, axillae, and inguinal folds. Sharply demarcated, fiery red erythematous patches and maceration are observed in an intertriginous zone, and a distinct foul smell is suggestive. Penicillin-sensitive group A streptococci are usually isolated, although there are reports of *S. aureus* and *Proteus mirabilis*. The differential diagnosis includes primarily cutaneous candidiasis, seborrheic dermatitis, and irritant contact dermatitis. Simple intertrigo responds to general measures to minimize friction and moisture, and a bacterial cause should be suspected when patients fail to respond to initial conservative treatment. A 10-day course of oral penicillin is effective in most instances.

NECROTIZING FASCIITIS

Necrotizing fasciitis is an acute infection characterized by a rapidly progressing necrosis involving subcutaneous fat and the fascia. It occurs after surgery, or may follow penetrating or blunt traumatic injury, but can develop in the absence of preceding noticeable injury. The sequence of infection begins with an exquisitely tender, erythematous, hot, and swollen area of extensive cellulitis. The disease progresses at an alarming rate, with the skin changing from red to a pathognomonic dusky gray-blue ill-defined patches within 36 hours after onset. Necrosis of the superficial fascia and fat produces a thin, watery, malodorous fluid. By the fourth or fifth day, the areas become gangrenous. The area later become characteristically anesthetic, as cutaneous nerves are destroyed. Many forms of virulent bacteria have been cultured from necrotizing fasciitis, including microaerophilic β-hemolytic streptococci, hemolytic *Staphylococcus*, coliforms, enterococci, *Pseudomonas*, and *Bacteroides*. Both aerobic and anaerobic cultures should always be taken. The most definitive confirmatory test is MRI, which can often aid in delineating the depth of tissue involvement. If done, a biopsy should be obtained from normal-appearing tissue near the necrotic zone. Early and extensive surgical debridement is the mainstay of treatment along with appropriate IV antibiotics, and supportive care. On occasion, amputation is necessary. Antimicrobial therapy is directed toward the results of the initial Gram stain. Initial therapy with a β-lactam/β-lactamase inhibitor with broad-spectrum coverage against gram-negative bacilli, staphylococci, streptococci and anaerobes (e.g., piperacillin/tazobactam) is effective.[5]

SCARLET FEVER

Scarlet fever is a diffuse, erythematous exanthem that occurs shortly after an episode of streptococcal pharyngitis. It affects primarily children. The tonsils are red, edematous, and covered with exudate. The tongue has a white coating through which reddened, hypertrophied papillae project, giving the so-called white strawberry tongue appearance. By the fourth or fifth day the coating disappears, the tongue is bright red, and the red strawberry tongue remains. The cutaneous eruption is characterized by papular erythematous "sandpaper rash" on the trunk and extremities. A linear petechial eruption, called Pastia lines, is often present in the antecubital and axillary folds. There is facial flushing and circumoral pallor. A branny desquamation occurs as the eruption fades, with peeling of the palms and soles. The eruption is produced by erythrogenic exotoxin producing group A streptococci. Cultures of the pharynx will recover these organisms. An elevated antistreptolysin O (ASO) titer may provide evidence of recent infection if cultures are not taken early. Penicillin, erythromycin, or dicloxacillin treatment is curative for scarlet fever, and the prognosis is excellent.[6]

MISCELLANEOUS GRAM-POSITIVE SKIN INFECTIONS

- Cutaneous diphtheria
- Erythrasma (caused by *Corynebacterium minutissimum*)

- Pitted keratolysis (caused by *Kytococcus sedentarius*)
- Trichomycosis axillaris (caused by *Corynebacterium tenuis*)
- Erysipeloid of Rosenbach (caused by *Erysipelothrix rhusiopathiae*)
- Pneumococcal cellulitis
- Anthrax
- Listeriosis
- Clostridial skin infections (anaerobic cellulitis, myonecrosis/gas gangrene)

PSEUDOMONAL SKIN INFECTIONS

- *Ecthyma gangrenosum* is a well-defined but uncommon cutaneous manifestation of pseudomonal septicemia, which occurs primarily in patients who are debilitated and immunocompromised. This begins as an erythematous macule, located in the anogenital area or on an extremity, which turns into a hemorrhagic bulla that ruptures and becomes a gangrenous ulcer with a central gray–black eschar. The surrounding tissue is inflamed and tender. There is often fever, hypotension, tachycardia, and other systemic symptoms
- *Green nail syndrome*
- *Pseudomonal pyoderma and blastomycosis-like pyoderma*
- *Otitis externa and malignant otitis externa*
- *Pseudomonal folliculitis (hot-tub folliculitis)*
- *Pseudomonas hot-foot syndrome*

OTHER GRAM-NEGATIVE SKIN INFECTIONS

- *Gram-negative folliculitis* (seen in acne vulgaris patients treated with long courses of oral antibiotics)
- *Cutaneous malakoplakia* (malakoplakia) a rare granulomatous disease occurs primarily in immunocompromised hosts, e.g., solid organ transfer recipients. The etiology is a chronic bacterial infection due to *Escherichia coli*, although *Pseudomonas, Proteus, Klebsiella, Staphylococcus* also been implicated. The disease is thought to result from defective phagocytic killing by mononuclear cells. Cutaneous lesions usually involve the perianal region and are clinically nonspecific. On histologic examination of involved tissue characteristic findings are Michaelis–Gutmann bodies (intracytoplasmic accumulations of calcified, iron-containing, non-exocytosed phagolysosomes) and von Hansemann cells (large histiocytes that contain Michaelis–Gutmann bodies and immunohistochemically stain positively for CD68, lysozyme and α1-antitrypsin)[7]
- *Cat scratch disease* (*Bartonella henselae*)
- *Trench fever* (*Bartonella quintana*)
- *Bartonellosis* (*Bartonella bacilliformis*)
- *Bacillary angiomatosis* (*B. henselae or B. quintana*)
- *Brucellosis* (*Brucella*, a genus of gram-negative coccobacilli)
- *Glanders* (*Burkholderia mallei*, strictly aerobic, nonpigment-producing, gram-negative bacillus)
- *Melioidosis* (*Burkholderia pseudomallei*)

KEY POINTS

- Common skin infections include cellulitis, erysipelas, impetigo, folliculitis, and furuncles, and carbuncles.
- Bacterial skin infections are fairly common and can range in severity from mild to life-threatening.
- The most common organisms include *Staphylococcus, Streptococcus, Pseudomonas,* and a few others.

REFERENCES

1. Ki V, Rotstein C. Bacterial skin and soft tissue infections in adults: a review of their epidemiology, pathogenesis, diagnosis, treatment and site of care. Can J Infect Dis Med Microbiol. 2008;19(2):173-84.
2. Cole C, Gazewood J. Diagnosis and treatment of impetigo. Am Fam Physician. 2007;75(6):859-64.
3. Patel GK, Finlay AY. Staphylococcal scalded skin syndrome: diagnosis and management. Am J Clin Dermatol. 2003;4(3): 165-75.
4. Ross A, Shoff HW. Toxic Shock Syndrome. In: StatPearls [Internet]. Treasure Island (FL): StatPearls Publishing; 2020. [online] Available from: https://www.ncbi.nlm.nih.gov/books/NBK459345/ [Last accessed February, 2021].
5. Hakkarainen TW, Kopari NM, Pham TN, Evans HL. Necrotizing soft tissue infections: review and current concepts in treatment, systems of care, and outcomes. Curr Probl Surg. 2014;(8): 344-62.
6. Centers for Disease Control and Prevention. (2018). Scarlet Fever. [online] Available from: https://www.cdc.gov/groupastrep/diseases-hcp/scarlet-fever.html [Last accessed February, 2021].
7. Gliddon T, Proudmore K. Cutaneous malakoplakia. N Engl J Med. 2019;380(6):580.

EXAMINATION QUESTIONS

1. Enumerate the skin infections caused by *Pseudomonas aeruginosa*.
2. Enumerate the superantigens in dermatology and its applied importance.
3. Describe the clinical features, pathophysiology and management of SSSS.
4. Write a short note on toxic shock syndrome.
5. Write a short note on bacillary angiomatosis.
6. Write a short note on necrotizing fasciitis.

41 CHAPTER

Mycobacterial Skin Diseases

Sanjeev Handa, Rajsmita Bhattacharjee

INTRODUCTION

Closely following HIV, tuberculosis (TB) is the second largest cause of infectious disease-related deaths; causing a huge drain on global resources.[1] Approximately one-third of the world's population is estimated to be infected with *Mycobacterium tuberculosis*, with Southeast Asia contributing to a major chunk of the load. Though the World Health Organization (WHO) reports that incidence and death rates are showing a falling trend in most parts of the world, the menace of drug-resistant TB is still an uphill challenge to be overcome.

The genus *Mycobacterium* has over 140 species of which >25 are responsible for causing infection in humans.[1] Apart from those belonging to the *M. tuberculosis* complex [including *M. tuberculosis, Mycobacterium bovis, M. bovis* bacillus Calmette-Guérin (BCG) and related species] and *Mycobacterium leprae,* other mycobacteria are commonly referred to as nontuberculous mycobacteria (NTM) or atypical mycobacteria. The terms environmental or opportunistic mycobacteria and mycobacteria other than tuberculosis (MOTT) are synonymous.[2] Though *M. tuberculosis* and *M. leprae* are the most common pathogens in humans, NTM such as *Mycobacterium ulcerans* and *Mycobacterium avium* complex (MAC) (*M. avium* and *Mycobacterium intracellulare*) constitute a significant proportion of the burden, especially in the clinical setting of immunosuppression.

CUTANEOUS TUBERCULOSIS

Despite TB being one of the most common and most widespread diseases, especially in developing countries, cutaneous disease is considered uncommon. It is rather difficult to estimate the actual incidence of cutaneous tuberculosis (CTB) short of reliable, long-term data. The problem is compounded by the fact that CTB has myriad of different clinical variants and presentations, the diagnosis of which requires a sharp and well-rounded clinical acumen apart from a good backup of ancillary investigational facilities. Given the global prevalence of TB, it is important for clinicians to accurately diagnose and differentiate the many clinical variants of CTB and its mimickers—especially subcutaneous fungal infections, syphilis, sarcoidosis, mycetoma, among the common ones—to avoid misdiagnosis.

Classification and Variants of CTB

The clinical presentation of CTB depends primarily on the route of infection (endogenous or exogenous), the immune status of the host, and previous exposure and sensitization with TB. Based on this, CTB can be classified into the following broad categories:[3,4]

- Exogenous inoculation
- Direct spread from endogenous tuberculosis
- Tuberculosis spread through hematogenous route

Tuberculosis due to Exogenous Inoculation

Tuberculous chancre: In a nonimmune or pauci-immune host, primary inoculation of the skin, most commonly following trauma or surgical procedures, results in a tuberculous chancre. Lesions begin as a firm, painless, slow-growing reddish-brown papule, or nodule and progress over 2–4 weeks into ulcers which often bleed.[5] The bacilli can further disseminate to regional lymph nodes as well.

Tuberculosis verrucosa cutis: Exogenous inoculation in a host with moderate-to-high immunity, perhaps as a result of previous exposure to mycobacteria, results in tuberculosis verrucosa cutis (TBVC/TVC), a localized variant, also sometimes called "prosector's wart" or warty tuberculosis.[3] It is commonly encountered in physicians, anatomists, and nursing professionals as an occupational hazard. Inoculation of mycobacteria can occur through various ways, such as unsterilized needles, or procedures such as tattooing, circumcision, and piercings.[3] Lesions most commonly occur on the fingers or other acral areas in the form of painless, erythematous, verrucous papules, and plaques often extending peripherally. They are frequently found to have a sporotrichoid pattern of distribution.

Tuberculosis from an Endogenous Source

Lupus vulgaris: The most common type of CTB in children and adults, lupus vulgaris (LV) is another chronic, progressive, paucibacillary form that usually occurs in an already sensitized individual with a high degree of immunity. It develops following direct inoculation or through hematogenous, lymphatic, or contiguous spread from an underlying focus of TB, in the form of a soft-to-firm plaque, composed of reddish-brown papules, and commonly occurs solitary. Gradual extension of the lesion at certain places and healing with scarring at others are particularly notable clinical features, often giving away the diagnosis. Trunk, buttocks, and lower limbs are the most common sites of involvement and as with other variants of CTB, sporotrichoid spread has been noted. Different clinical variants such as plaque form; vegetating, ulcerative, and mutilating forms; and tumoral and papulonodular forms have been described. Lesions often heal with scarring and deformities and show an apple jelly appearance on diascopy.

Scrofuloderma: A multibacillary form, scrofuloderma, also known as tuberculosis colliquativa cutis, is the most common type of CTB in the world.[2] Commonly seen in children, it results from contiguous involvement and breakdown of the skin overlying an underlying deeper focus of tuberculosis, most commonly lymph node, bone or joint disease, and testes or epididymis. Neck, axilla, and groin are the most common sites of involvement. It usually begins as asymptomatic, subcutaneous swellings, which break down to form ulcers with undermined edges. Sporotrichoid spread has been reported.[2] Lesions commonly heal, often spontaneously, with characteristic puckered scarring or atrophy.

Tuberculosis Spread through a Hematogenous Route

Tuberculous gumma: A relatively rare multibacillary form of CTB, tuberculous gumma, or metastatic tuberculous abscess results from hematogenous spread from a preexisting focus. Immunocompromised hosts are predisposed; though rarely, it may affect immunocompetent individuals as well. It presents as single or multiple, firm, subcutaneous nodule which may become fluctuant abscess or break down to form undermined ulcers. However, unlike scrofuloderma, underlying structures are not involved.

Orificial tuberculosis: Orificial TB, another rare form of CTB, presents as ulcers at mucocutaneous junctions including mouth, nose, and perianal and perineal regions in an immunocompromised patient, usually afflicted with advanced systemic TB, pulmonary, intestinal, or genitourinary.[5] It occurs due to autoinoculation from an underlying focus of infection. Lesions occur in the form of painful, friable, erythematous papules, and nodules, progressing to painful ulcers varying in size from 1 to 3 cm, usually never healing spontaneously.[5]

Acute cutaneous miliary tuberculosis: It is another rare form of CTB seen predominantly in severely immunocompromised hosts, due to the hematogenous spread of mycobacteria into the skin. It is usually seen in advanced pulmonary, meningeal or disseminated TB or those coinfected with HIV, and in infants and children, in whom it can also follow viral infections such as measles or malnutrition. Though rare, its incidence has been increasing primarily due to coinfection with HIV.[5] Clinically, crops of minute papules, vesicles, pustules or hemorrhagic lesions appear which break to form ulcers.[5]

Tuberculids: Tuberculids are considered to be the result of a cutaneous hypersensitivity response to hematogenously transmitted antigenic components of mycobacteria in a patient with high cell-mediated immunity to the TB bacilli, possibly with an extracutaneous source of *M. tuberculosis*. They have polymorphous clinical presentations and are grouped as follows:

True tuberculids:

- *Micropapular—lichen scrofulosorum*: It presents as asymptomatic, 0.5–3.0 mm diameter, closely grouped, skin-colored to lichenoid papules which are often perifollicular, mainly on the trunk and proximal limbs, but may occur on the face. Rarely, they can occur in an annular fashion or coalesce to form plaques. Children and adults with underlying diseases of bone and lymph nodes are often affected.[2,5]
- *Papular—papulonecrotic tuberculid*: These are seen more commonly in children and young adults as asymptomatic, symmetrical erythematous, papulonodular lesions which develop pustules or necrotic ulcers at the center. Lesions are particularly noted around the face, ears, extensor areas of the trunk, extremities, and buttocks, and heal over a period of weeks with varioliform scarring.
- *Nodular—erythema induratum of Bazin or nodular tuberculid*: The most commonly reported tuberculid, erythema induratum of Bazin is a type of lobular panniculitis associated with TB.[2] It presents usually in middle-aged females on the calves as tender, erythematous-purplish subcutaneous nodules which ulcerate. Tuberculin test is usually strongly positive.

The discrete relationship between tuberculids and TB continues to be speculated as *M. tuberculosis* complex DNA has been identified by polymerase chain reaction (PCR) only in some instances.[5] The diagnostic criteria include tuberculoid histology on skin biopsy, a strongly positive Mantoux reaction, absence of *M. tuberculosis* in smear and negative culture, and resolution of the skin lesions with antituberculous therapy.

Table 1 shows the most commonly followed classification of CTB.

Diagnosis

Cutaneous tuberculosis is often misdiagnosed or underdiagnosed because of the myriad of clinical presentations and frequent absence of an internal focus of infection. A constellation of investigational modalities are necessary to arrive at a diagnosis in most cases since the clinical picture might not always be very telling. The most important diagnostic modalities include a skin biopsy for histopathology, culture and PCR. Other ancillary investigations often include

TABLE 1: Classification of cutaneous tuberculosis (CTB).[2]

Host immunity	*Method of inoculation*	*Disease*
Multibacillary forms		
Naïve	Direct inoculation	Tuberculous chancre (primary inoculation)
Low	Contiguous spread	Scrofuloderma
Low	Autoinoculation	Orificial tuberculosis
Low	Hematogenous spread	Acute miliary cutaneous tuberculosis
Low	Hematogenous spread	Tubercular gumma (abscess)
Paucibacillary forms		
High	Direct inoculation	Warty tuberculosis (verrucosa cutis)
High	Direct inoculation	Lupus vulgaris (some)
High	Hematogenous spread	Lupus vulgaris
High	?Hematogenous spread	• Tuberculids • Lichen scrofulosorum • Papulonecrotic tuberculid • Erythema induratum (Bazin's)

a chest radiograph, an ultrasonography of the abdomen and a urine examination for the presence of acid-fast bacilli (AFB), among others. Subtle pointers which can aid the diagnosis, but are not sufficient for diagnosis alone include the presence of an active focus of TB elsewhere in the body, positive Mantoux test or interferon-γ (IFN-γ) release assay. Often, a therapeutic trial of antituberculous therapy gives satisfying outcome almost confirming the initial diagnosis.

Table 2 enlists the salient clinical features and differential diagnoses for the individual types of CTB.

Tuberculin Skin Test

The Mantoux test or the tuberculin skin test (TST), though one of the earliest known tests in the diagnosis of TB, has limited value as a diagnostic modality and at best serves as an ancillary or supportive evidence of current or past exposure to the bacilli. It is a reflection of delayed type hypersensitivity to mycobacterial antigens, in a person previously exposed to infection following an intradermal injection of 0.1 mL of purified protein derivative (PPD) (0.1 mL = 5 tuberculin units); PPD derived from attenuated strain of *M. tuberculosis*, and read after 48–72 hours. Induration along with erythema exceeding 10 mm is considered a positive result. However, in a TB-endemic country such as India, clinical or latent infection due to *M. tuberculosis*, BCG vaccination or contact with environmental mycobacteria can produce a positive result. This nonspecificity is one of the major drawbacks of this test. Being a lymphocyte-based delayed hypersensitivity (type 4) reaction, its sensitivity is low in immunocompromised patients like individuals with HIV or those with active TB or on immunosuppressive treatment, who often give false-negative results.[1] Hence, a positive test is not confirmatory of active infection nor is a negative result indicative of the absence of infection.

Interferon-γ Release Assays

These T cell-based assays measure the amount of IFN-γ released by lymphocytes in response to *M. tuberculosis* antigens. It is far more specific than tuberculin test, though sensitivity is comparable.[2] Unlike TST, they can also detect disease in BCG-vaccinated individuals (latent infection) as well as those with active infection. However, these tests are still not part of the routine workup of patients, primarily because of high cost and laborious techniques.

Histopathology

Histopathology of a skin biopsy shows granulomatous tissue response akin to other granulomatous cutaneous diseases such as cutaneous sarcoidosis, lupus miliaris disseminatus faciei, and subcutaneous fungal infections, among others. Though exact diagnosis of the type of CTB based on histopathological findings alone is near impossible, it is characterized by epithelioid cell granulomas in the dermis. The tubercular granulomas are well-formed, admixed with Langhans-type giant cells and surrounded by collarette of mature lymphocytes. They can be associated with variable amount of caseous necrosis at the center of the granulomas, along with neutrophilic infiltrate. The granulomas in tuberculosis verrucous cutis (TBVC), scrofuloderma, and tuberculous gumma are usually associated with large areas of necrosis compared to LV. The epidermis shows mild acanthosis in LV, whereas in TBVC, marked acanthosis and hyperkeratosis are observed. Granulomas are usually located in the upper and mid-dermis in TBVC and LV, and they are usually situated in the deeper dermis or subcutaneous tissue in scrofuloderma. Tuberculous bacilli are identified in 15–20% cases of CTB.

Culture and Nucleic Acid Amplification (PCR) Studies

Clinical features and histological findings might be corroborative but the only absolute confirmation of diagnosis comes from isolation or demonstration of *M. tuberculosis* in either tissue culture from skin biopsy, discharge or cytological smear, or isolation of mycobacterial DNA by PCR.[2,5] This is however, especially difficult in paucibacillary forms such as LV. Culture of *M. tuberculosis* on specific solid or liquid media still remains the gold standard for diagnosing as well as determining drug sensitivities. However, the long generation

TABLE 2: Salient clinical features and differential diagnoses for the individual types of cutaneous tuberculosis (TB).

Type of cutaneous TB	*Salient clinical features*	*Differential diagnosis*
Tuberculous chancre	Firm, reddish-brown papule, or nodule, gradually progressing to painless, shallow ulcer with undermined edges; regional lymphadenopathy, sporotrichoid pattern	Other infections showing sporotrichoid pattern such as sporotrichosis, leishmaniasis, atypical mycobacterial infection, cat scratch disease, syphilis, among others
Tuberculosis verrucosa cutis	Painless, verrucous papules and plaques, most common on extremities; sporotrichoid pattern, no adenopathy	Sporotrichosis, leishmaniasis, atypical mycobacterial infection (*Mycobacterium marinum*), verruca vulgaris, verrucous carcinoma, chromoblastomycosis, lichen planus hypertrophicus (LPH)
Lupus vulgaris	Soft-to-firm plaque, composed of reddish-brown papules, commonly solitary. Gradual extension at one edge and healing with scarring at other is characteristic. Trunk, buttocks, and lower limbs most common sites; sporotrichoid spread	Borderline tuberculoid leprosy is a commonly confused differential diagnosis; sporotrichosis, leishmaniasis recidivans, sarcoidosis, psoriasis, Bowen's disease, deep fungal infections such as sporotrichosis and chromoblastomycosis, lupoid leishmaniasis
Scrofuloderma	Begins as subcutaneous swellings, break down to form ulcers with undermined edges. Sporotrichoid spread; healing with characteristic puckered scarring or atrophy	Tertiary syphilis, paracoccidioidomycosis, actinomycoses, hidradenitis suppurativa, and lymphogranuloma venereum
Tuberculous gumma	Single or multiple, firm, subcutaneous nodule; may become fluctuant abscess or break down to form undermined ulcers; no involvement of underlying structures unlike scrofuloderma	Sporotrichosis, chromoblastomycosis, atypical mycobacterial infection, leishmaniasis, syphilis, leprosy, nocardiosis, staphylococcal abscess
Orificial TB	Painful, friable, erythematous papules and nodules, progressing to painful ulcers	• *Perioral*: Leishmaniasis, oral paracoccidioidomycosis, rhinoscleroma • *Anogenital*: Malignancy, Crohn's disease, cutaneous amoebiasis, anal paracoccidioidomycosis, chronic herpes simplex virus (HSV) infection, syphilis
Acute cutaneous miliary TB	Crops of minute papules, vesicles, pustules or hemorrhagic lesions breaking down to form ulcers	Cutaneous small vessel vasculitis, secondary syphilis
Tuberculids		
Lichen scrofulosorum	0.5–3.0 mm diameter, closely grouped, skin colored to lichenoid papules, often perifollicular, mainly on the trunk and proximal limbs	Lichen nitidus, lichen planus, micropapular sarcoid, lichenoid lesions of secondary syphilis, keratosis pilaris, keratosis spinulosa, popular/lichenoid sarcoidosis, pityriasis rubra pilaris (PRP)
Papulonecrotic tuberculid (PNT)	Symmetrical erythematous, papulonodular lesions with pustules or necrotic ulcers at the center. Face, ears, extensor trunk, extremities, and buttocks are common sites. Lesions heal with varioliform scarring	Pityriasis lichenoides et varioliformis acuta (PLEVA), nodular prurigo
Erythema induratum of Bazin or nodular tuberculid	Tender, erythematous-purplish subcutaneous nodules which ulcerate. Calves of "middle-aged females" most common site	Other small vessel vasculitis such as Wegener's granulomatosis, erythema nodosum (does not usually ulcerate), cutaneous PAN, LE profundus, cutaneous T-cell lymphoma

(LE: lupus erythematosus; PAN: polyarteritis nodosa)

time and low sensitivity are major drawbacks. Amplification of mycobacterial DNA by PCR studies is another useful modality as it can demonstrate the organism across different spectra of CTB including tuberculids, though it is still more useful for multibacillary forms. It is also less time consuming than culture along with higher sensitivity. Additionally, it is useful in a variety of specimens, including fresh biopsy, needle aspirate, formalin fixed, paraffin embedded tissue sections, etc. However, high cost, false-positive and -negative results, and possible contamination remain major drawbacks.

Treatment

A careful search has to be made for systemic focus of infection and rule out coinfection with HIV, with preferable bacteriological confirmation and testing for drug sensitivities as multidrug-resistant TB is on the rise. A multispecialist team may be essential if there is coexistent internal focus of infection. According to the Revised National Tuberculosis Control Programme's "National strategic plan for TB elimination 2017–2025," all patients are to be screened for drug resistance, especially for rifampicin. For drug sensitive disease, daily fixed-dose combinations (FDCs) of first-line antituberculosis drugs [isoniazid (H), rifampicin (R), pyrazinamide (Z), and ethambutol (E)] are to be administered in appropriate weight bands for all forms of TB and in all ages, including four drug FDC in the intensive phase for 8 weeks.[6] Only pyrazinamide is stopped in the maintenance phase and remaining three drug FDCs are continued in the continuation phase for 12 weeks. In cases where the diagnosis is uncertain, a therapeutic trial of antituberculous treatment can be initiated for at least 6 weeks and then judging by the response, can be continued for the entire duration of 6 months.

CUTANEOUS INFECTIONS CAUSED BY NONTUBERCULAR MYCOBACTERIA

Skin and soft-tissue infections (SSTIs) caused by NTM or atypical mycobacteria are steadily on the rise. Also called environmental mycobacteria, NTM are a diverse group of ubiquitous organisms, usually acquired from the environment. More than 180 species of NTM have been recognized, most of which affect soft tissue and skin.[7] NTM infections can pose diagnostic challenge due to their clinical diversity. They can produce localized as well as disseminated disease, especially in immunocompromised patients.

Traditionally, NTM are classified based on their morphology, rate of growth, and ability to produce pigment. The two major groups are rapidly growing mycobacteria (RGM) and slowly growing mycobacteria (SGM), which form mature colonies in culture within 7 days and >7 days, respectively.[8] RGM groups *Mycobacterium fortuitum*, *Mycobacterium chelonae*, and *Mycobacterium abscessus* and SGM species *Mycobacterium marinum* and *M. ulcerans* most commonly cause SSTI, though other NTM are implicated as well.[8] In fact, *M. ulcerans* is said to be the third most prevalent mycobacterial infection after TB and leprosy.[2,8]

The major risk factors for NTM infections include HIV infection and other immunocompromised states, although immunocompetent individuals can also acquire this infection following interventions such as surgical or cosmetic procedures including punch biopsy and filler injections, among others. Nosocomial outbreaks are mostly caused by the rapid growers as they resist common disinfectants such as glutaraldehyde and chlorine, possibly owing to the presence of biofilms.[7] Tap water is another common reservoir of NTM infection, particularly rapid growers, *Mycobacterium gordonae*, *Mycobacterium kansasii*, and MAC.

Clinical Features

Cutaneous infections caused by NTM present mostly as nonspecific, polymorphous lesions such as papules, plaques, nodules, abscesses, cellulitis, ulcers, and draining sinuses. As a result, a high index of suspicion is desirable in order to diagnose such infections. In fact, it is said that NTM infections must be evaluated for in those with SSTIs not responding to conventional treatment.

However, there are two particular presentations caused by two distinct species: (1) "fish-tank" granuloma caused by *M. marinum* and (2) Buruli ulcer (BU) caused by *M. ulcerans*.

Mycobacterium marinum

Commonly known as "fish-tank granuloma," "swimming pool granuloma" or "aquarium granuloma," the main risk factors for *M. marinum* infection include exposure to aquatic environments. It is a slow-growing NTM with an incubation period of about 16 days.[9] Lesions occur as a solitary, erythematous papule or nodule at the site of inoculation progressing to plaque which can be verrucous and/or may ulcerate with serosanguinous discharge. The upper extremity is the most common site of infection. Lymphatic spread often occurs with proximal extension of the infection resulting in sporotrichoid distribution.[7] Infection might also extend to involve deeper structures, such as bones and joints, though systemic dissemination is rare and mostly encountered in the immunocomprmised.[7]

Diagnosis requires a comprehensive history in addition to supportive investigations. Routine histological examination and tissue cultures are imperative for accurate diagnosis, with corroborative PCR studies, if available. A positive culture can be obtained in about 70–80% of cases if incubated between 30 and 33°C.[1] Colonies are usually seen after 2–4 weeks,[10] however, at least 6 weeks observation of cultures is necessary before declaring as negative. Skin biopsy reveals acanthosis, pseudoepitheliomatous hyperplasia, and exocytosis, in addition to granulomatous inflammatory infiltrate. AFB are rarely detected on routine microscopy. PCR studies may provide more rapid diagnosis, though culture is still desirable.

Mycobacterium ulcerans

Mycobacterium ulcerans, responsible for causing BU, is the third most important human pathogen after *M. tuberculosis* and *M. leprae*. It is a slow-growing NTM that begins as papules, plaques or nodules progressing to large ulcers with undermined edges. Children (5–15 years old) have the highest incidence of BU, with lower extremities being the most common site of infection. It is transmitted most commonly by local, minor, often unnoticed, skin trauma causing inoculation of *M. ulcerans,* mainly acquired from its aquatic niches; most commonly tropical wetlands, especially areas with stagnant water, though BU can also occur without wetland exposure.[1] Transmission from person to person is rare. Exposure to natural water sources, absence of protective gear, and negligence of minor wounds, and trauma are the major predisposing factors. The infection usually remains asymptomatic unless complicated by secondary infection.[7] Multiorgan involvement is rare, though up to 15% cases have been reported to develop osteomyelitis.[7]

Buruli ulcers are diagnosed mainly on the basis of their clinical presentation. PCR is the most common method for confirmation of diagnosis with a sensitivity of 70–80%.[7] Culture sensitivity is low (40–60%) and at least 6 weeks of incubation is required before deeming them negative. Samples should be obtained from the edge of an ulcer or center of a nonulcerated lesion.[7] Histopathology of BU reveals large numbers of extracellular AFB with marked necrosis and subcutaneous edema. Vascular occlusion, hemorrhage, and absence of well-defined granulomatous inflammation are the other biopsy findings in the initial stages. In later stages, however, granulomas can be formed.

Rapid Growers

The incidence of SSTI caused by rapid growers is steadily on the rise, especially in cases associated with trauma, and interventions, including surgery and cosmetic procedures. They are primarily caused by three species: *M. fortuitum*, *M. abscessus*, and *M. chelonae*, a common source of infection being contaminated water. In general, patients afflicted by *M. fortuitum* are younger and immunocompetent with often limited involvement and low incidence of mortality. However, *M. fortuitum* is growingly becoming an opportunistic pathogen causing disseminated infection, especially in patients with impaired cellular immunity. It is also often associated with history of trauma or intervention at the site of infection, while disease due to *M. chelonae* is strongly associated with concomitant corticosteroid therapy.[2]

Clinical presentation is usually nonspecific; therefore, a high index of suspicion is necessary. Cutaneous presentations include abscesses, subcutaneous nodules, ulcers, sinus tracts, and nonhealing wounds. These are variable depending on the causative RGM species. Multifocal lesions can often be seen in immunosuppressed patients. Culture and antibiotic sensitivity studies from tissue biopsy or discharge are necessary for accurate diagnosis, especially because treatment depends on the causative organism and its sensitivities. All three species are resistant to conventional antituberculosis drugs, but variably vulnerable to a number of other antibiotics.[7]

Mycobacterium avium Complex

Mycobacterium avium complex infection primarily involves pulmonary system. Cutaneous involvement is rare and usually occurs in immunocompromised individuals, especially those suffering from HIV with a CD4 count below 50 cells/μL.[2] In the latter, it usually causes dissemination of disease from the primary site of involvement due to mycobacteremia, though incidence is decreasing due to antiretroviral therapy (ART) and timely initiation of antibiotic prophylaxis. Infection can occur following traumatic inoculation, as in cervical lymphadenitis, simulating scrofuloderma. Skin lesions are polymorphous as in other NTM infections in the form of ulcers, nodules, abscesses as well as showing sporotrichoid spread.

Infections Caused by Other NTM (Mycobacterium kansasii, Mycobacterium haemophilum, Mycobacterium scrofulaceum, Mycobacterium szulgai)

Mycobacterium kansasii and *M. szulgai* typically cause pulmonary disease resembling TB. Exposure to contaminated water, especially after minor trauma predisposes a patient to primary cutaneous infection with *M. kansasii*. Lesions are localized and indolent in the immunocompetent patient, though disseminated disease can occur in the immunosuppressed.

Mycobacterium haemophilum infections occur commonly in the clinical setting of severe immunosuppression and sometimes in healthy children as lymphadenopathy.[7] Clinical spectrum of disease varies from localized disease to systemic involvement, with skin lesions usually confined to the extremities.

Mycobacterium scrofulaceum, like *M. haemophilum*, also primarily presents as cervical lymphadenopathy in children, though it can rarely cause cutaneous lesions and disseminated infection.

Diagnosis and Management of NTM Infections

Given the often nonspecific clinical presentations, the diagnosis of NTM infections mandates a detailed history, including that of trauma or any kind of intervention, an examination including that for lymphadenopathy, and investigative modalities such as skin biopsy for routine histopathology, smear for AFB, and tissue cultures, including bacterial, fungal, and AFB. Punch biopsy samples for tissue cultures should always be obtained from the edge of an ulcer or the center of a nonulcerative lesion.

Histopathology

Ill-defined granulomas surrounded by chronic inflammation and suppuration should always arouse concern for NTM infection, though many different types of granulomatous tissue reaction patterns may be found, including tuberculoid, palisading or sarcoidal granulomas, spindle cell pseudotumors, and rheumatoid-like nodules.[8] For rapidly growers, suppurative inflammation may be more prominent. AFB can be identified using AFB stains such as the Ziehl–Neelsen, Fite, Kinyoun or auramine-rhodamine fluorochrome stains, however, rate of positivity is low.

Tissue Culture

Growth in tissue culture in most NTM species is observed within 2–3 weeks, though cultures should be incubated for at least 6 weeks before being considered negative; exception being *M. ulcerans* which needs incubation for at least 8–12 weeks.[2,7,8] RGM species grow rapidly on subculture taking about a week, while growth in primary culture may take longer.

TABLE 3: Treatment for skin and soft-tissue infections caused by nontuberculous mycobacteria (NTM).[2,7,8]

Type of cutaneous NTM	*Source/predisposing factor(s)*	*Treatment regimen(s)*
Mycobacterium marinum	Aquatic niches including fresh and marine water sources, especially fish tanks and swimming pools	• *Limited skin and soft-tissue infections*: Monotherapy with clarithromycin, doxycycline/minocycline, and trimethoprim-sulfamethoxazole • *Severe infections*: Combination of clarithromycin and ethambutol ± rifampicin (10 mg/kg/day)
Mycobacterium ulcerans	Aquatic niches	• Combination of oral rifampicin and intramuscular streptomycin for 8 weeks • Surgical treatment for lesions progressing in spite of 4 weeks of antibiotic therapy and those >5 cm in diameter
Rapid growers *Mycobacterium fortuitum* *Mycobacterium abscessus* *Mycobacterium chelonae*	Often following a surgical or cosmetic procedure	• Single lesions may respond to monotherapy but disseminated cutaneous or pulmonary disease require multidrug therapy • Both localized and widespread infections require prolonged treatment • Culture studies and antimicrobial susceptibility testing are required to guide treatment • *Limited skin and soft-tissue infection*: Oral therapy with two susceptible agents for at least 4 months, such as clarithromycin or azithromycin in combination with ciprofloxacin, levofloxacin, doxycycline, minocycline, or trimethoprim-sulfamethoxazole • *For severe or disseminated disease*: Initial parenteral treatment with 2–3 agents to which the isolate is susceptible, followed by oral treatment for 6–12 months
Mycobacterium avium complex (MAC)	Immunosuppression	Surgical excision for localized cutaneous lesions. Macrolides mainstay agents for systemic disease
Mycobacterium kansasii *Mycobacterium haemophilum* *Mycobacterium scrofulaceum* *Mycobacterium szulgai*		No standard regimens; multidrug regimen guided by susceptibility studies

The optimum temperature for growth of most NTM species is between 28 and 37°C.[8] *M. haemophilum* requires iron or hemin as a cofactor for growth; hence iron supplementation of culture media is pertinent.

Molecular diagnostic tests, such as PCR, and other commercially available DNA probe-based assays can enable a relatively quicker diagnosis, though growth in tissue culture remains the gold standard. Tuberculin skin test is usually not specific or reliable as it is often positive in NTM infection because of antigens shared with *M. tuberculosis*, thereby leading to spurious results. IFN-γ release assays can be helpful to distinguish NTM from *M. tuberculosis*, being more specific than TST.[8]

Treatment

There have been no comparative trials of treatment regimens for infections with NTM of sufficient power to guide optimal management. Treatment decisions must therefore always be made on the basis of susceptibility testing, as far as possible. **Table 3** summarizes the various treatment strategies for NTM infections based on anecdotal reports and series.

KEY POINTS

- Cutaneous tuberculosis has several variants and polymorphic clinical presentation.
- Lupus vulgaris and scrofuloderma are the most common variants, while orificial TB and other multibacillary forms are rare and mainly seen in immunocompromised patients or those with a focus of severe systemic TB.
- Cutaneous tuberculosis can be classified based on exogenous source, endogenous source, and spread through a hematogenous route.
- Histopathology is characterized by well formed, epithelioid cell granulomas in the dermis, associated with variable amount of caseous necrosis at the center of the granulomas, along with neutrophilic infiltrate.
- Absolute confirmation of diagnosis comes from isolation or demonstration of *M. tuberculosis* or isolation of mycobacterial DNA by PCR.
- Tuberculin skin testing and IFN-γ release assays are useful as corroborative evidence.
- Daily fixed dose combinations of first-line antituberculosis drugs [isoniazid (H), rifampicin (R), pyrazinamide (Z),

and ethambutol (E)] are administered in the intensive phase for 8 weeks. Only pyrazinamide is stopped in the maintenance phase and remaining three drug FDCs are continued in the continuation phase for 12 weeks.

- In cases, where the diagnosis is uncertain, a therapeutic trial of antituberculous treatment can be initiated for at least 6 weeks.
- Water is a common source of NTM infections. Use of contaminated tap water in surgical procedures is frequently responsible for nosocomial infections.
- History of traumatic inoculation or surgical or cosmetic intervention extremely important in SSTIs caused by NTM species.
- *Mycobacterium fortuitum* commonly causes disseminated infection, mainly in patients with impaired cellular immunity, while disease due to *M. chelonae* is strongly associated with concomitant corticosteroid therapy.
- Skin lesions are polymorphous and histopathology often nonspecific; hence index of suspicion should be high. AFB staining is often negative.
- *Mycobacterium marinum* causes "fish-tank granuloma."
- *Mycobacterium ulcerans* causes the slow-growing, painless, and destructive BU.
- Rapid growers that include three main species (*M. fortuitum*, *M. abscessus*, and *M. chelonae*) are responsible for increasing number of SSTIs.
- *Mycobacterium fortuitum* generally causes a single nodule at the site of trauma or surgery, in a young, immunocompetent patient and is responsive to many oral antibiotics.
- *Mycobacterium abscessus* and *M. chelonae* are more likely to occur in older, immunosuppressed patients, present with multiple nodules or abscesses, and are more difficult to treat.
- Culture and molecular studies are diagnostic; however, negative results do not exclude infection by NTM. Often a therapeutic trial of anti-NTM therapy is useful.
- No definite guidelines for treatment of NTM infections. Treatment decisions must therefore always be made on the basis of susceptibility testing, as far as possible.

REFERENCES

1. European Centre for Disease Prevention and Control/WHO Regional Office for Europe. Tuberculosis Surveillance and Monitoring in Europe 2012. Stockholm: European Centre for Disease Prevention and Control, 2012.
2. Yates VM, Walker SL. Mycobacterial infections. In: Griffiths CEM, Baker J, Bleiker T, Chalmers R, Creamer D (Eds). Rook's Textbook of Dermatology, 9th edition. West Sussex: Wiley Blackwell; 2016.
3. van Zyl L, du Plessis J, Viljoen J. Cutaneous tuberculosis overview and current treatment regimens. Tuberculosis (Edinb). 2015;95(6):629-38.
4. Dias MF, Bernardes Filho F, Quaresma MV, Nascimento LV, Nery JA, Azulay DR. Update on cutaneous tuberculosis. An Bras Dermatol. 2014;89(6):925-38.
5. Khadka P, Koirala S, Thapaliya J. Cutaneous tuberculosis: clinicopathologic arrays and diagnostic challenges. Dermatol Res Pract. 2018;2018:7201973.
6. National Health Portal (2016). Revised National Tuberculosis Control Programme: National Strategic Plan for Tuberculosis Elimination 2017–2025. [online] Available from: https://www.nhp.gov.in/revised-national-tuberculosis-control-programme_pg [Last accessed January, 2021].
7. Gonzalez-Santiago TM, Drage LA. Nontuberculous mycobacteria: skin and soft tissue infections. Dermatol Clin. 2015;33(3):563-77.
8. Chung J, Ince D, Ford BA, Wanat KA. Cutaneous infections due to nontuberculosis *Mycobacterium*: recognition and management. Am J Clin Dermatol. 2018;19(6):867-78.
9. AlKhodair R, Al-Khenaizan S. Fish tank granuloma: misdiagnosed as cutaneous leishmaniasis. Int J Dermatol. 2010;49(1):53-5.
10. Gluckman SJ. *Mycobacterium marinum*. Clin Dermatol. 1995;13(3):273-6.

EXAMINATION QUESTIONS

1. How will you approach to a case of mycobacterial infection?
2. Explain atypical mycobacterial infection.
3. Explain cutaneous tuberculosis.
4. Write a short note on lupus vulgaris.

42 CHAPTER

Superficial Fungal Infections

Neha Bhardwaj, Ashish Amrani, Anupam Das

INTRODUCTION

Superficial fungal infections are infections of skin and its appendages, caused by fungus and limited to stratum corneum, hair, and nails.[1] Classification of superficial fungal infections of skin has been shown in **Table 1**.

PITYRIASIS VERSICOLOR

(*Synonyms*: Tinea versicolor, tinea flavea, chromophytosis)[1-3]

Pityriasis versicolor (PV) is a mild superficial fungal infection of the skin caused by *Malassezia* species. It is characterized by discrete or confluent, scaly discoloration the skin. *M. furfur* is most commonly implicated to cause PV but other species like *M. sympodialis*, *M. globosa*, *M. obtusa*, and *M. dermatis* have also been isolated from the clinical scenarios.

Epidemiology: It is more common in tropical countries. The condition is more prevalent in late teens and early twenties. Both sexes are equally prone to the condition. It is seen to be closely associated dermatosis with Cushing's disease and malnutrition.

Clinical features: PV presents with asymptomatic or mildly pruritic patches, with varying degree of change in skin color. The early lesion may be discrete, slightly erythematous and may evolve to form confluent skin lesions having fine scales over the surface. The color varies from mild hypopigmentation, thick dark hyperpigmented to salmon colored skin lesions. The scales can be attenuated by scratching the skin (coup d'ongle sign, Besnier's sign).[4] The lesions are distributed along neck, chest, back, face and upper arms and less commonly on scalp and groin.

Diagnosis: On KOH preparation from the scales, the typical picture of coarse mycelium with short filaments (2–5 microns wide) and up to 25 microns long along with spherical, thick-walled yeasts of 2–8 microns in diameter usually confirms the condition. The microscopic appearance has classically been described as "spaghetti and meatball" appearance or "bananas and grapes." Culture is usually not required. MALDI-TOF and other recent molecular techniques are useful for research purposes.

Differential diagnosis:
- Vitiligo
- Seborrheic dermatitis
- Pityriasis rosea
- Secondary syphilis
- Tinea corporis
- Erythrasma
- Pinta

Treatment: Treatment of PV has been shown in **Table 2**.

Malassezia Folliculitis[2,3]

It is an inflammatory condition of hair follicles, caused by *Malassezia* species. It presents as pruritic, erythematous, monomorphic papules and pustules on the face, trunk, and upper arms. Absence of comedones distinguishes it from acne vulgaris. Diagnosis is by KOH preparation which shows typical picture of *Malassezia* species. Treatment is by oral itraconazole or fluconazole along with topical azoles and keratolytics.

TINEA NIGRA

(*Synonyms*: Pityriasis nigra, keratomycosis nigricans palmaris)[3,5]

Tinea nigra is a superficial cutaneous mycosis, caused by *Hortaea werneckii* (also known as *Exophiala werneckii*, a darkly pigmented, dematiaceous fungus).

TABLE 1: Classification of superficial fungal infections of skin.[1]

Producing none to minimal inflammation	*Producing significant inflammation*
• Pityriasis versicolor • Tinea nigra • Piedra	• Dermatophytoses (Tinea corporis, tinea cruris, tinea manuum, tinea pedis, tinea barbae, tinea faciei, tinea unguium) • Cutaneous candidiasis

TABLE 2: Treatment algorithm for pityriasis versicolor.

First line	*Second line*
Topical azoles twice daily for 2–4 weeks	Oral fluconazole
Selenium sulfite or zinc pyrithione shampoos on alternate days for 3–4 weeks	Oral itraconazole
Topical terbinafine	
Propylene glycol in aqueous solution	

Epidemiology: Tinea nigra mainly occurs in tropical and subtropical areas of Asia, Africa, and Latin America. It is less prevalent in Europe and North America. It affects both sexes equally and can occur at all ages.

Clinical features: Tinea nigra typically presents as asymptomatic brownish-black macule or patch with no scales and other secondary changes, on the palms and soles. The lesion has irregular outlines and is usually darker at the advancing borders.

Diagnosis: KOH examination of the scrapings from the lesion reveals brownish to tan, thick branching septate hyphae, with oval to spindle-shaped yeast cells that may occur singly or in pairs with a central transverse septum. *Hortaea werneckii* yields slow growing brown to black colored colonies under Sabouraud dextrose agar (SDA) and incubation at 30°C within a week.

Differential diagnosis:
- Acral lentiginous melanoma
- Junctional nevus
- Dysplastic nevus
- Yaws
- Pinta
- Addisonian pigmentation.

Treatment: The first choice for treatment of tinea nigra is a topical azole preparation such as ketoconazole or clotrimazole. Other topical agents effective are butenafine, Whitfield's ointment tincture of iodine, and 2% salicylic acid. Topical treatment is continued for 2–4 weeks. Oral antifungal agents are rarely required.

PIEDRA

(*Synonym*: Trichomycosis nodularis)[3,5]

Piedra is an asymptomatic superficial fungal infection of the hair shaft. There are two variants of piedra—black piedra and white piedra.

Black Piedra

(*Synonym:* Tinea nodosa)
- It is caused by *Piedraia hortae* and is characterized by formation of hard and dark nodules on hair shaft.
- A rare infection, which occurs mainly in tropical regions of Americas and South East Asia and males are more affected than females.
- It is characterized by formation of black, hard, gritty nodules on hair shaft of the scalp and sometimes also on beard, moustache, and pubic areas. The nodules may be microscopic to around 1 mm in diameter.
- Growth of fungus may make the hair shaft fragile and they may fracture easily.

White Piedra

(*Synonym:* Trichosporosis nodosa)
- It is caused by *Trichosporon* species and occurs mainly in semitropical and temperate areas of South America, Asia, Middle East, and Africa.
- It affects facial, axillary and groin hair (*T. inkin*, *T. asahii* more common) more than scalp hair (*T. ovoides*).
- It presents with softer and less adherent whitish to cream colored discrete to large sleeve-like structures along the hair shaft, which can be easily detached.
- Compared to black piedra, hairs are less fragile and do not break easily.

Diagnosis: On KOH preparation, black piedra shows regularly aligned hyphae and arthroconidia 4–8 microns in diameter along the edge of the nodules. Club-shaped asci containing eight elongated ascospores may be formed. In white piedra, *Trichosporon* species show the presence of hyphae, arthroconidia 2–4 microns in diameter and budding blastoconidia. Culture is not recommended routinely in piedra.

Differential diagnosis:
- Pediculosis
- Trichomycosis axillaris
- Tinea capitis
- Monilethrix
- Trichorrhexis nodosa.

Treatment: Shaving the infected hair is considered the best treatment for both white and black piedra. It is often combined with topical azole application. Systemic azoles can be considered for recurrent infection.

DERMATOPHYTOSES

Nomenclature[1]: "Tinea" before Latin name of the involved body part (e.g., Tinea faciei is dermatophytosis involving face).

Pathogenesis[1,6]
- Caused by fungi belonging to three genera—*Trichophyton, Microsporum*, and *Epidermophyton*.
- Transmission to human by human (anthropophilic), animal (zoophilic), or soil (geophilic) **(Table 3)**.
- Pathogenic fungus comes in contact with the skin, produces enzyme keratinase which breaks down keratin and gives way to the entry of fungus into stratum corneum. The mannans in fungal cell wall inhibit the host immunity.
- In *Trichophyton rubrum*, the mannans have property to decrease epidermal proliferation, in addition to immuno-inhibition. This reduces the chances of the fungus being sloughed off before invasion into stratum corneum. This may explain the chronicity of *T. rubrum* infection.
- *Predisposing factors*: Immunosuppression (diabetes, AIDS, iatrogenic etc.), impaired skin barrier (atopic dermatitis,

TABLE 3: Different species of dermatophytes based on the source of infection.

Dermatophyte type	*Species*
Anthropophilic	• *Trichophyton rubrum* • *Trichophyton tonsurans* • *Epidermophyton floccosum* • *Trichophyton interdigitale*
Zoophilic	• *Trichophyton mentagrophytes (Reservoir-rats)* • *Trichophyton verrucosum (cattle)* • *Microsporum canis (cats, dogs)*
Geophilic	*Microsporum gypseum*

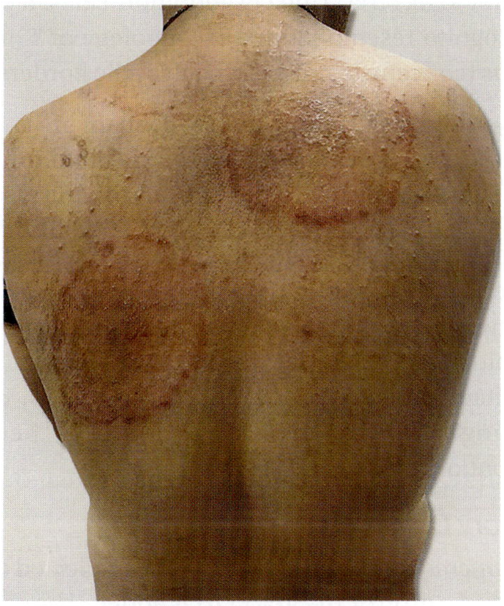

Fig. 1: Tinea corporis.
Courtesy: Dr Aarti Sarda.

ichthyosis), warm and humid environment, occlusive clothes, and footwear.
- Sebum has a protective role against dermatophytic infection.

Clinical Features[1,7,8]

Tinea Corporis (Synonym: Tinea Circinata) ***(Fig. 1)***
- It includes all superficial dermatophytoses of skin except those involving hair, face, palms, soles, nails, and groin.
- *T. rubrum* is the most common causative fungus worldwide, followed by *T. mentagrophytes*.
- *Incubation period*: 1–3 weeks
- Annular, sharply circumscribed, erythematous, scaly plaques with central clearing, and raised borders. Spread centrifugally, hence central clearing seen. Pustules may be present on the border.
- Associated with itching and burning.
- *Clinical variants:*
  - *Tinea profunda*: Widespread granulomatous or verrucous appearance of the lesions due to exaggerated inflammatory response to the fungus.
  - *Nodular perifolliculitis/Majocchi granuloma:* Deep pustular lesions such as kerion, resulting from disruption of follicular wall due to dermatophyte infection. Mostly seen on wrists, shins, areas of shaving, and occlusion.
  - *Tinea imbricata (Tokelau):* Caused by *T. concentricum*. Characterized by concentric rings of erythematous scaly plaques with polycyclic borders.

Tinea Cruris (Synonym: Jock itch, crotch itch)
- Dermatophytic infection of inguinal region. Usually upper medial thighs and may extend posteriorly to involve perineum and buttocks. Scrotum involvement is rare. (If scrotum involved, suspect candidiasis).
- *Common causes*: *T. rubrum, T. mentagrophytes, E. floccosum*
- Morphology same as *T. corporis* but with less scaling. In chronic cases, the lesions may become leathery and lichenified.

Tinea Manuum and Tinea Pedis
- Dermatophyte infection of palms and interdigital spaces—*T. manuum*. Dermatophyte infection of soles and webspaces between toes—*T. pedis*.
- These entities have some distinct characteristics believed to be because of lack of sebaceous glands on palms and soles.
- Athlete's foot (T. pedis) is the most common fungal disease of the feet.
- *Common causes*: *T. rubrum* (most common), *T. interdigitale, T. mentagrophytes, E. floccosum*
- May be limited to small lesion adjacent to an onychomycotic nail.
- *Two feet one hand syndrome*: When both feet and one hand are involved (usually dominant hand which is used by the patient to scratch the feet).
- Hyperhidrosis is usually present. Damp keratin acts as a great culture medium for fungi.
- *Clinical variants of T. pedis:*
  - *Moccasin:* Relatively less inflammation. Diffuse dull erythema and more pronounced silver scales.
  - *Interdigital:* Most common type, two lateral webspaces are usually involved.
  - *Inflammatory:* Caused by *T. mentagrophytes*. Vesicles and multilocular bullae are formed on the medial foot, often associated with dermatophytid reaction.
  - *Ulcerative:* Mostly seen in cases of immunosuppression and uncontrolled diabetes.

Tinea Barbae
- Beard ringworm, tinea sycosis, barber's itch.
- Typically caused by zoophilic dermatophytes—*T. mentagrophytes, T. verrucosum*
- Usually unilateral face or neck involvement.

- *Clinical variants:*
  - *Deep nodular suppurative*: Caused by *T. mentagrophytes, T. verrucosum*. Slow progression. Characterized by nodular kerion-like boggy swelling with abscesses. Hairs on the lesion are loose or absent.
  - *Superficial crusted*: Caused by *T. violaceum* or *T. rubrum*. Less inflammatory widespread pustular folliculitis.
  - *Verrucous epidermophytosis*: Extremely rare. Caused by *E. floccosum*. Characterized by diffusely spread verrucous lesions.

Tinea Faciei ***(Fig. 2)***

- Dermatophytic infection of the glabrous skin of the face.
- Causative fungi: *T. rubrum, T. mentagrophytes, M. canis*
- Suspect *T. faciei* for any inflammatory scaly lesion on the face.

Tinea Capitis

- Can be caused by all the pathogenic dermatophytes except *E. floccosum* and *T. concentricum*.

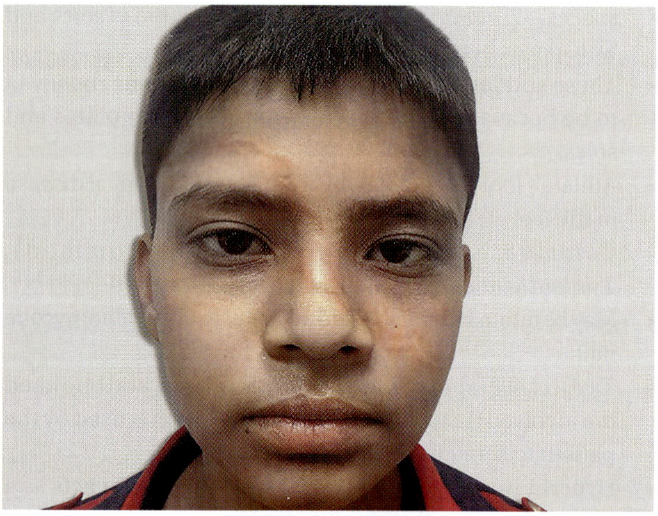

Fig. 2: Tinea faciei.
Courtesy: Dr Aarti Sarda.

- Mostly seen in children, but adults can be the carriers.
- Three clinical patterns as shown in the **Table 4**.
- *Kerion*: Advanced stage of T. capitis. Deep tender boggy swelling exuding pus. May lead to scarring alopecia.
- May be accompanied by posterior cervical and posterior auricular lymphadenopathy.

Tinea Incognito

- Atypical clinical morphology of tinea lesions due to prolonged treatment with topical corticosteroids.
- Usually widespread.
- Ask for history of steroid application.
- Look for signs of steroid abuse—inflammation, thin atrophic skin, stria, Tinea pseudoimbricata—a pattern of T. incognito resembling the morphology of T. imbricata lesions (concentric rings with polycyclic borders).

Approach to Diagnosis[1,3,5]

History and Clinical Examination

- Typical erythematous scaly annular plaques with raised margins, associated with itching and burning, usually located in warm and moist areas like body folds.
- Patches of alopecia in children—always rule out T. capitis.
- May have a history of immunosuppression, diabetes, wearing occlusive clothing or footwear because of occupation, etc.

Laboratory Diagnosis

- *KOH microscopy*: Skin scraping or hair collected on a glass slide and a drop of 10–30% KOH is added. The coverslip is placed. Gentle heat can be applied to dissolve the keratin faster. Then the slide is viewed under the microscope. Chlorazol black E stain can be used to highlight the fungal elements. Calcofluor stains the chitin in the fungal wall and gives apple green fluorescence under fluorescent microscope.
- *Dermatophytes*: Fungal hyphae can be demonstrated.
- *T. capitis*: The ectothrix and endothrix pattern as described in **Table 4**.

TABLE 4: Clinical patterns of tinea capitis.

Pattern	*Endothrix*	*Ectothrix*	*Favus*
Synonyms	Black dot ringworm	Grey patch ringworm	Most severe form of dermatophytic hair infection
Causative fungus	*T. tonsurans* *T. violaceum*	*M. canis*	*T. schoenleinii*
Clinical finding	The broken stubs of hair appear as black dots	Patchy scaly alopecia	• Thick yellow crusts composed of hyphae and skin debris—scutula • Mousy odor
Hair shaft examination	Produce chains of large spores within the hair shaft	Produce small spores visible on the outside of hair shaft	Hyphae and air spaces are observed within the hair shaft
Wood's light examination	Do not produce fluorescence	Produces yellow fluorescence	Produces bluish white fluorescence

TABLE 5: Summary of differential diagnoses of dermatophytosis.

Tinea corporis	*Tinea cruris*	*T. manuum and T. pedis*	*T. barbae*	*T. faciei*	*T. capitis*
• Psoriasis • Nummular eczema • Seborrheic dermatitis • Pityriasis rosea • Syphilis • Erythema annulare centrifugum	• Candidiasis—moist with collarette scales and satellite pustules • Erythrasma—copper colored, coral red fluorescence on Wood's light • Seborrheic dermatitis—may also involve scalp, axilla, central chest • Pemphigus vegetans • Inverse psoriasis	• Contact dermatitis • Psoriasis • Syphilis	• Sycosis vulgaris—Folliculitis caused by *Staphylococcus* (In T. barbae, upper lip area is usually spared and it is unilateral) • Herpes simplex—umbilicated vesicles, Tzanck positive • Acne vulgaris • Seborrheic dermatitis	• Rosacea • Lupus erythematous • Psoriasis	• Chronic staphylococcal folliculitis • Pediculosis capitis—Knits and eggs present • Seborrheic dermatitis • Alopecia areata—no inflammation or scaling • Psoriasis • Trichotillomania

- *T. concentricum*: Skin scrapings show interlacing, septate, mycelial filaments that branch dichotomously. Polyhedral spores are also present.
- *Culture*: Can be done for identification of species. Media used are SDA, Mycosel agar, or dermatophyte test medium.
- *Biopsy*: Rarely needed. Fungal hyphae are seen within stratum corneum. PAS or silver stains can be used to make the fungal elements stand out.
- Wood's light examination
- Fluorescence is demonstrated by *M. canis, M. audouinii, T. schoenleinii*: Infected hairs fluoresce due to the presence of pteridine.
- *Do not fluoresce*: Endothrix organisms (*T. tonsurans, T. violaceum*) and *T. verrucosum* (ectothrix, exception).
- *Dermoscopy*: Can be helpful in cases of patchy alopecia. In T. capitis, comma hair, corkscrew hair and dystrophic broken hair are seen.

Differential Diagnosis[1,3]

Differential diagnosis of dermatophytosis has been shown in **Table 5**.

Management[1,3,5]

General Measures

- Properly dry the body before wearing clothes, socks, shoes, etc.
- Keep the areas dry. Use antifungal powder in body folds.
- Avoid occlusive clothing. Wear loose cotton clothes.
- Wash all the clothes, towels and linen in hot water and dry in sunlight.
- Good glycemic control, if diabetic.
- Weight reduction, if obese.
- T. pedis—disinfect or discard shoes. Control hyperhidrosis by using powder, cotton socks, open footwear and aluminum chloride 10% solution.
- T. capitis—disinfect or discard combs, hair brushes, hats, etc.
- In T. capitis, all the household contacts are considered carriers and should be treated with ketoconazole or selenium sulfide shampoo.

Treatment[1,3,5]

Treatment of dermatophytosis has been shown in **Boxes 1 to 6**.

BOX 1: Treatment of tinea corporis.

Localized:
Topical terbinafine twice daily for 2 weeks
OR
Topical azoles (clotrimazole, luliconazole, etc.) once or twice daily for 2–4 weeks
Widespread:
Oral terbinafine 250 mg per day for 2–3 weeks
OR
Itraconazole 100 mg per day for 2–4 weeks

BOX 2: Treatment of tinea capitis.

Griseofulvin 10 mg/kg/day for 6 weeks or at least till 2 weeks after negative lab test
OR
Terbinafine: <10 kg – 62.5 mg, 10–20 kg – 125 mg, >20 kg – 250 mg. Given daily for 4 weeks
Adjunctive treatment: Ketoconazole 2% or selenium sulfide 2.5% shampoo to be used for a contact period of 5 minutes thrice weekly

Hairy areas like scalp are more resistant to treatment because hair follicles act as reservoirs for infection. Hence, longer treatment duration

BOX 3: Treatment of tinea barbae.

Systemic itraconazole or terbinafine for 4–6 weeks in addition to topical antifungals such as clotrimazole, sertaconazole

BOX 4: Treatment of tinea faciei.

- Single lesion with no folliculitis—topical antifungals
- Multiple lesions OR folliculitis—systemic plus topical antifungals

BOX 5: Treatment of tinea pedis and tinea manuum.

Oral terbinafine 250 mg/day for 2 weeks
OR
Itraconazole 200 mg/day for 2 weeks
Add topical antifungal twice daily

BOX 6: Treatment of tinea cruris.

Recent onset—topical imidazoles or terbinafine twice daily for 2 weeks
Chronic or widespread—oral terbinafine 250 mg/day for 2 weeks
OR
Itraconazole 100 mg/day for 2–4 weeks

MUCOCUTANEOUS CANDIDIASIS[1,7]

Introduction

- *Candida albicans* is normally present in human gastrointestinal tract, genitourinary tract, and skin.
- It is an opportunistic infection when there is impaired immunity (diabetes, antibiotic therapy, HIV, etc.) or presence of local conditions favoring its growth (warm, moist skin with higher pH, i.e., intertriginous areas).

Diagnosis

- *KOH examination*: Shows spores and pseudohyphae.
- *Culture*: SDA-creamy gray white colonies. Upon microscopic examination of colonies, clusters of budding cells are seen. When inoculated into cornmeal agar culture, round thick-walled chlamydospores are produced—characteristic of *C. albicans*.
- *Biopsy*: Dermatophyte hyphae run parallel to the skin surface whereas candida pseudohyphae are more likely to be oriented vertically.

Clinical Variants

- *Oral candidiasis/Thrush:*
  - Involvement of mucous membrane of the mouth.
  - In newborn, it is acquired from coming in contact with mother's vaginal flora. In children and adults, usually seen after antibiotic therapy, immunosuppression state, use of steroid inhalers.
  - Dry mouth is a predisposing factor because saliva inhibits the growth of candida.
  - *Types:*
    - *Pseudomembranous*: Cottage cheese like exudate seen.
    - *Chronic atrophic*: A patch of erythematous raw area of oral mucosa seen.
    - *Chronic hyperplastic*: Grayish white adherent membranous plaques, base of which is moist, red, and macerated.
    - *Glossitis*: Red painful smooth dorsal tongue.
  - Sometimes the infection extends to the corners of the mouth to form perlèche—first manifestation of AIDS and must be investigated further.
  - *Treatment*: In infants, oral nystatin suspension. In adults, a single dose of 150 mg fluconazole effective.
- *Perlèche/Angular cheilitis:*
  - Maceration and fissuring of the oral commissures, usually bilateral.
  - May also be due to riboflavin deficiency, drooling of saliva due to ill-fitting dentures, older people with atrophy of alveolar ridges.
  - *Treatment*: Antifungal creams like clotrimazole, dental intervention if required.
- *Candidal vulvovaginitis:*
  - *Clinical findings*: Erythematous, moist, swollen labia; vaginal discharge can vary from watery to thick curd like. Associated with itching and burning.
  - *Treatment*: Oral fluconazole 150 mg single dose with topical antifungals like clotrimazole, miconazole or nystatin. Pre- and probiotics also help.
- *Candidal intertrigo:*
  - Involvement of folds of genitals, groin, axilla, between buttocks, under breasts.
  - Erythematous moist patches surrounded by collarette scales and satellite pustules.
- *Diaper candidiasis:*
  - Involvement of folds and appearance of small satellite lesions (in contrast to diaper rash)
  - Topical anticandidal ointments with zinc oxide (which acts as a barrier against urine irritation)
- *Candidal paronychia:*
  - Infection of the nail folds, usually chronic. Associated with redness, edema, and tenderness.
  - Seen usually in diabetics, and due to chronic exposure to water, irritants, etc.
- *Erosio interdigitalis blastomycetica:*
  - A form of candidiasis presenting with macerated white skin with fissures on webspaces.
  - On hands, mostly seen in third webspace between middle and ring finger due to skin maceration beneath the ring.
  - On feet, usually 4th webspace is involved.
- *Chronic mucocutaneous candidiasis:*
  - Heterogeneous group of patients who have chronic candidal infection but it is limited to mucosa, skin, and nails.
  - Onset is usually before 6 years of age.

- Could be inherited or sporadic. Associated with multiple endocrinopathies.

ONYCHOMYCOSIS[1,3,5,9]

Onychomycosis (OM) is the fungal infection of the nails of fingers and toes. It can be caused by dermatophytes (tinea unguium), nondermatophytic molds, candida species, and other yeasts. It is the most prevalent nail disease.

Epidemiology

- OM can affect up to 14% of the population and can account for approximately 50% of all cases of onychodystrophy.
- It is prevalent in all the regions of the world.
- There is higher prevalence among older age groups and males being affected slightly higher than females. Other risk factors for developing OM include nail trauma, immunosuppression (e.g., HIV and diabetes), and peripheral vascular disease.

Clinical features: Various clinical variants of OM have been shown in **Table 6**.

Diagnosis: Common diagnostic modalities for OM have been shown in **Table 7**.

Differential diagnosis: Differential diagnosis for OM has been shown in **Table 8**.

Treatment: Treatment of OM has been shown in **Table 9**.

TABLE 6: Various clinical variants of onychomycosis (OM).

Clinical variant of OM	*Description*	*Common causes*
Distal and lateral subungual OM (DLSO)	• MC clinical variant • Invasion of stratum corneum of hyponychium of distal and lateral nail band • The infection spreads proximally along ventral nail plate and nail bed • Clinically presents with brownish yellow discoloration of the nail • Subungual hyperkeratosis and onycholysis can be seen	• *Trichophyton rubrum* • *Trichophyton interdigitale* • *Trichophyton tonsurans* • *Epidermophyton floccosum*
Proximal subungual OM (PSO)	• Relatively uncommon • The fungus first invades proximal nail fold and spreads distally • Clinically presents with subungual hyperkeratosis, transverse leukonychia and proximal onycholysis • Paronychia is common	• *Trichophyton rubrum* (most common cause) • *Trichophyton megnini* • *Trichophyton schoenleinii*
Superficial white OM (SWO)	• Distinctive pattern mainly affecting toenails • Invasion of fungus via nail plate • Clinically presents with well delineated whitish lesions on nail plate	• *Trichophyton interdigitale* (most common cause) • Acremonium species • *Aspergillus terreus* • *Fusarium oxysporum* • *Candida albicans*
Endonyx	• Invasion of fungus from distal and lateral nail fold but instead of involving nail bed, infection involves the nail plate only • Clinically presents with milky white patches spreading proximally without subungual hyperkeratosis and onycholysis	• *Trichophyton soudanense* • *Trichophyton violaceum*
Total dystrophic OM (TDO)	• Most severe variant • Total destruction of nail plate due to fungal invasion • Clinically there is thickened abnormal nail plate and keratotic debris • Often painful • More seen in immunodeficient states	*Candida* species (often occurs in chronic mucocutaneous candidiasis)

TABLE 7: Common diagnostic modalities for onychomycosis (OM).

Investigation	*Method*	*Findings*
Potassium hydroxide (KOH) preparation	Taking scales from advancing border, affected nail plate, or subungual debris and putting it in 10–30% KOH solution followed by gentle heating	Fungal hyphae, arthrospores or yeast forms depending upon the causative agent
Fluorescent microscopy using calcofluor white	Taking scales from advancing border, affected nail plate, or subungual debris	The dye stains chitin in the fungal cell wall which fluoresces blue under the fluorescent microscope
Culture	The clinical specimen collected as described above is used for culture with Sabouraud dextrose agar and modified Sabouraud's medium	Different culture features depending upon the causative agent isolated
Histopathology	Tissue obtained by nail plate or nail bed biopsy	Positive infection can be confirmed by PAS (pink) or GMS (black) staining of fungal cell wall

TABLE 8: Differential diagnoses for onychomycosis (OM).

More common differential diagnoses	*Less common differential diagnoses*
Nail psoriasis	Pachyonychia congenita
Nail lichen planus	Acquired and congenital leuckonychias
Chronic nail trauma	Darier-White disease
Chronic nail paronychia	Yellow nail syndrome
Onychogryphosis	Melanoma

TABLE 9: Treatment for onychomycosis (OM).

Topical therapy	*Systemic therapy*
Amorolfine 5% nail lacquer (once a week application) or ciclopirox 8% nail lacquer (daily application) for 4–6 months	• Oral terbinafine 250 mg/day for 6 weeks for fingernails and 3 months for toenails, OR • Oral itraconazole 400 mg/week for 2–3 months for fingernails and 3–4 months for toenails

KEY POINTS

- The cutaneous fungal infections include pityriasis versicolor, tinea nigra, piedra, dermatophytosis, and candidiasis.
- Dermatophytosis has presently acquired an epidemic-like scenario.
- Topical steroid misuse and abuse, rising prevalence of *Trichophyton mentagrophytes* Type VIII (ITS genotype) and resistance to terbinafine are the common causes of recalcitrant dermatophytosis.
- As of now, conventional dosage and duration of treatment of antifungals is not sufficient for the management of dermatophytosis.

REFERENCES

1. Elewski BE, Hughey LC, Hunt KM, Hay RJ. Fungal diseases. In: Bolognia JL, Schaffer JV, Cerroni L (Eds). Dermatology, 4th edition. Philadelphia: Elsevier; 2018. pp. 1329-62.
2. Ahronowitz I, Leslie K. Yeast infections. In: Kang S, Amagai M, Bruckner AL, Erik AH, et al. (Eds). Fitzpatrick's Dermatology, 9th edition. New York: McGraw Hill; 2019. pp. 2952-64.
3. Hay RJ, Ashbee HR. Fungal infections. In: Griffiths CEM, Barker J, Bleiker T, Chalmers R, et al. (Eds). Rook's Textbook of Dermatology, 9th edition. Oxford: Wiley-Blackwell; 2016. pp. 32.1-32.96.
4. Madke B, Nayak C. Eponymous signs in dermatology. Indian Dermatol Online J. 2012;3(3):159-65.
5. Craddock LN, Schieke SM. Superficial fungal infections. In Kang S, Amagai M, Bruckner AL, Erik AH, et al. (Eds). Fitzpatrick's Dermatology, 9th edition. New York: McGraw Hill; 2019. pp. 2925-51.
6. Dahl MV. Dermatophytosis and the immune response. J Am Acad Dermatol. 1994;31:S34-41.
7. Diseases resulting from fungi and yeasts. In: James WD, Berger TG, Elston DM (Eds). Andrew's Diseases of the Skin, 12th edition. Philadelphia: Elsevier; 2016. pp. 285-318.
8. Ilkit M, Durdu M, Karakaş M. Majocchi's granuloma: a symptom complex caused by fungal pathogens. Med Mycol. 2012;50(5):449-57.
9. Singal A, Khanna D. Onychomycosis: diagnosis and management. Indian J Dermatol Venereol Leprol. 2011; 77(6):659-72.

EXAMINATION QUESTIONS

1. Write short note on pityriasis versicolor.
2. Write short note on piedra.
3. Classify and describe management of candidiasis.
4. Explain current trends in dermatophytosis.
5. Describe antifungal resistance and its management.

43 CHAPTER

Deep Fungal Infections

Madhu Rengasamy, Janaki Chellam, Sentamilselvi Ganapathi

INTRODUCTION

Fungal infections affecting human beings may be broadly classified into superficial, cutaneous, and deep mycoses. Deep mycoses, encompass subcutaneous mycoses and systemic mycoses, which include the endemic mycoses and the opportunistic mycoses. These infections, which are rare, compared to the superficial mycoses, account for about 1% of all fungal infections.

SUBCUTANEOUS MYCOSES

Subcutaneous mycoses also referred to as, "implantation mycoses", are chronic granulomatous infections of the skin and the subcutaneous tissue caused by inoculation of the fungi following a trivial trauma, which is most often not recalled by the patients. These infections, which are more prevalent in the tropical and subtropical climate, with a characteristic long incubation period that ranges from months to years, are less common, compared to the superficial mycoses. Subcutaneous mycoses include mycetoma, phaeohyphomycosis, chromoblastomycosis, rhinosporidiosis, entomophthoromycosis and sporotrichosis, which occur in India with a varied prevalence in the different geographic regions of the country and lobomycosis which is endemic in the Brazilian Amazon region. Confirmation of the clinical diagnosis is by the direct demonstration of the fungi in the potassium hydroxide (KOH) wet mount, isolation of the etiological agent by culture and by mycopathological examination in hemotoxylin and eosin stain and special stains such as periodic acid-Schiff (PAS) stain and Gomori methenamine silver (GMS) stain.

MYCETOMA[1-3]

Mycetoma is a chronic progressive granulomatous exogenous infection of subcutaneous tissue caused by fungi (deuteromycetes and ascomycetes) and aerobic bacteria (actinomycetes). It is characterized by the presence of *swelling*, multiple draining *sinuses*, and discharge of *grains* (microcolonies of causal organisms).

History[1]

Atharvaveda: Mycetoma referred to as "Padvalmicum" which means "Anthill foot."

1842: John Gill, first described mycetoma in Madurai, Tamil Nadu.

1846: Colebrook coined the name, "Madura foot."

1860: Henry Vandyke Carter coined the term, "Mycetoma" and established the fungal etiology.

1871: Bristowe established the actinomycotic etiology of pale grains.

1913: Pinoy subdivided mycetoma into two etiological types as Eumycetoma caused by eumycetes, the true fungi and actinomycetoma caused by gram-positive filamentous bacteria.

Etiologic Agents

Etiologic agents of Eumycetoma	
Black grain	*Pale (White) grain*
Madurella mycetomatis *Trematosphaeria (Madurella) grisea* *Exophiala jeanselmei* *Leptosphaeria senegalensis* *Leptosphaeria tompkinsii* *Curvularia lunata* *Curvularia geniculata*	*Pseudallescheria boydii* *Neotestudina rosatt* *Aspergillus nidulans* *Aspergillus flavus* *Acremonium falciforme* *Fusarium* species

Etiologic agents of actinomycetoma	*Grain color*
Actinomadura madurae	White, yellow
Actinomadura pelletieri	Red
Nocardia asteroides	White to yellow
Nocardia brasiliensis	Yellowish white
Nocardia caviae	White to yellow
Nocardiopsis dassonvillei	Yellowish cream
Streptomyces somaliensis	

Geographic distribution: More prevalent in regions with annual rainfall between 50 and 500 mm, i.e., Africa, Asia, Central and South America. *Mycetoma belt*—area between latitudes 15°S and 30°N.

Epidemiology: Common age group—20–40 years; Male:Female = 3.5:1.

Predisposing factors: Barefoot walking, occupations that predispose to trivial trauma and contact with soil and thorny vegetation.

Pathogenesis

Organism in soil enters host subcutaneous tissue by accidental trauma by thorn prick/splinter injury → slow evolution → firm, painless swelling → fibrosis, localized subcutaneous nodules, discharging sinuses (serous, serosanguineous or purulent). Within host tissue, organisms form compact mass of colonies—"grain" is a vegetative aggregate of the fungal mycelia embedded in a hard, brown matrix which consists of extracellular cement substance (1,8-dihydroxynaphthalene melanin) in combination with host tissue debris.

Rigid matrix might act as a barrier protecting the fungus from the natural immunity of the host and antifungal agents. Melanin is thought to be protective to the fungus, in circumstances of host-induced oxidative stress.

Mycetoma spreads by contiguity and continuity to the deeper tissues, sparing tendons and nerves. Lymphatic spread may occur. Hematogenous spread may be seen in patients infected by *Nocardia* and *Streptomyces* species. Both cell-mediated and humoral immunity play a role. Evolution depends on ability of organism to evade or resist the host defense mechanism and alteration of host resistance.

Clinical Features

- Any site of the body, subjected to traumatic implantation of soil saprotrophs into subcutaneous tissue. Site often reflects the occupation.
- *Mainly exposed sites*: Foot (70%) and hand. *Other sites*: Leg, knee, gluteal region, thigh, perineum, arm, shoulder, chest, abdominal wall.
- *Rare*: Head, neck, face, paranasal sinuses, eyelid, orbit, vulva, scrotum, surgical incisions.
- *Characteristic clinical triad*: Painless swelling, draining sinuses with discharge of grains. Discharge is serous or serosanguinous in eumycetoma and purulent in actinomycetoma.
- Pain indicates secondary bacterial infection or bone involvement.
- One has to look for surface pigmentation, prominence of veins, deformity, mobility of the joint in the vicinity and disuse atrophy. Actinomycetoma is diffuse, rapidly progressive and aggressive while eumycetoma is localized, slow progressive, and less destructive **(Figs. 1 and 2)**.

Differential Diagnosis

- Osteomyelitis (Pyogenic, tuberculous, leprous)
- Actinomycosis, botryomycosis
- Tuberculosis, leishmaniasis, leprosy, syphilis, yaws, atypical mycobacterial, elephantiasis
- Coccidioidomycosis, blastomycosis, chromoblastomycosis, sporotrichosis
- Deep dermatophytosis, neoplasms, Kaposi's sarcoma.

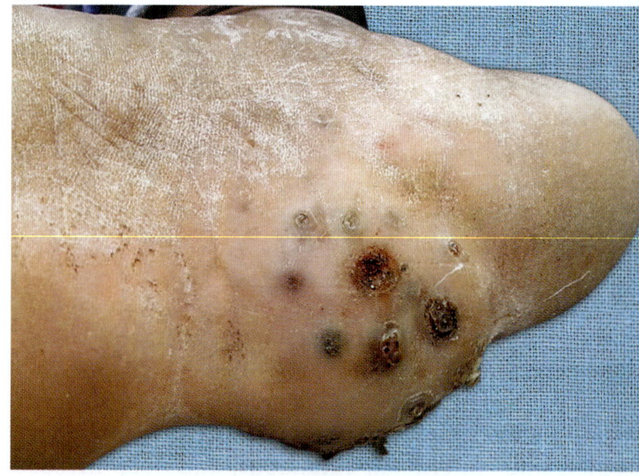

Fig. 1: Eumycotic mycetoma.

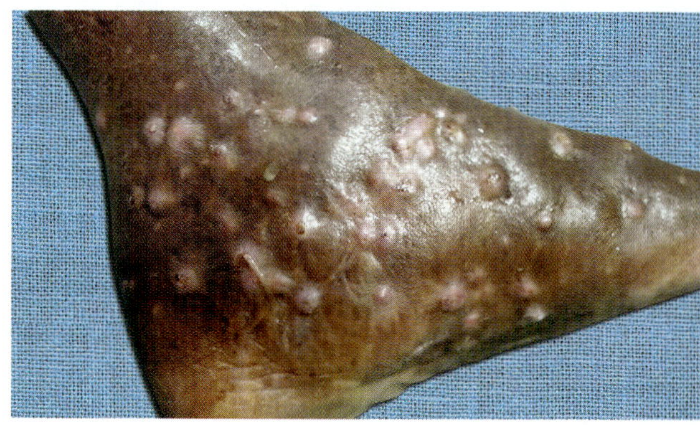

Fig. 2: Actinomycetoma.

Laboratory Diagnosis

Routine blood investigations: Complete blood count (CBC), blood sugar, renal function test (RFT), liver function test (LFT), and audiogram in patients with actinomycetoma if Welsh regimen planned.

Specimen: Grain, discharge, biopsy tissue (Grain to be crushed between glass slides; Touch smear from the discharging sinus after cleaning with spirit; Tissue to be smeared on the slide). In the absence of extrusion of grain, overnight saline gauze will help.

Microscopic appearance: Texture—hard in *Madurella mycetomatis, Curvularia geniculata*

- *Size:* Smallest is *Nocardia* grain <0.5 mm
- *Color:* Black → Eumycotic
    - White → Pale grain of eumycetoma/actinomycetoma
    - Red → *Actinomadura pelletieri*
    - Yellow → *Streptomyces somaliensis*
- Direct microscopy of the grain to be done in:
    - 10% KOH
    - Grain with wide fungal hyphae and chlamydospores:
        - Hyaline → white eumycotic

    - Brown→ black eumycotic **(Fig. 3)**
    - Pale grain with scalloped border → actinomycotic grain **(Fig. 4)**
- *Gram's stain:* Gram positive fine, thin branching filaments of bacterial dimension → *Actinomadura* species/*Nocardia* species
- *Ziehl-Neelsen (ZN) staining: Nocardia* species (acid fast)
- *Leishman stain:* Cellular reaction.

Mycopathology

Deep biopsy of a nodule (closed) is to be done. Grains are seen amidst a suppurative granulomatous inflammatory infiltrate consisting of neutrophils surrounded by histiocytes, lymphocytes, and multinucleated giant cells. Eosinophilic fringe of Splendore-Hoeppli phenomenon will be present around the grain. Fibrosis may be present in old lesions.

Appearance in Hematoxylin and Eosin

Actinomycotic grain: Multilobulated grain, scalloped border, dark basophilic mantle in the periphery, and pale amorphous center **(Fig. 5)**.

Eumycetoma: *Madurella mycetomatis*—brown to black large grain with intertwining septate hyphae embedded in interstitial brownish cement—radial, parallel hyphae in the periphery with or without chlamydospores and irregularly arranged hyphae in the center **(Fig. 6)**. Grains may be compact or vesicular. Special stains—PAS and GMS are confirmatory.

Culture Media

- *Actinomycetoma*: Sabouraud's dextrose agar (SDA) without antibiotics, blood agar, Lowenstein-Jensen media, and brain-heart infusion agar.
- *Eumycetoma*: SDA with chloramphenicol and without cycloheximide.

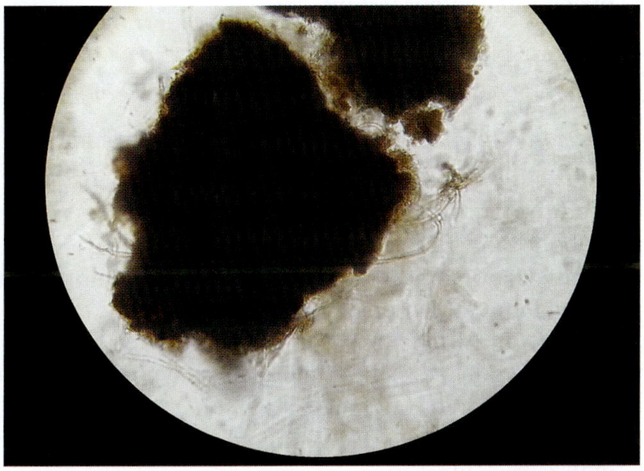

Fig. 3: Potassium hydroxide wet mount of a eumycotic black grain with hyphae in the periphery of the grain.

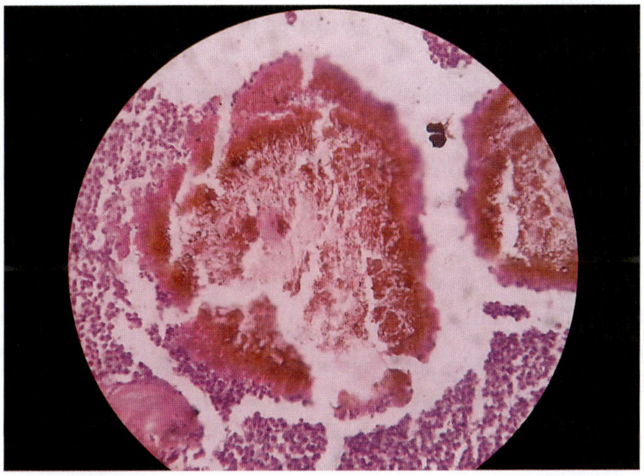

Fig. 5: High power view of histopathology of eumycotic grain in H&E showing parallel, radially arranged hyphae in the periphery with chlamydospores and irregularly arranged hyphae in the center.

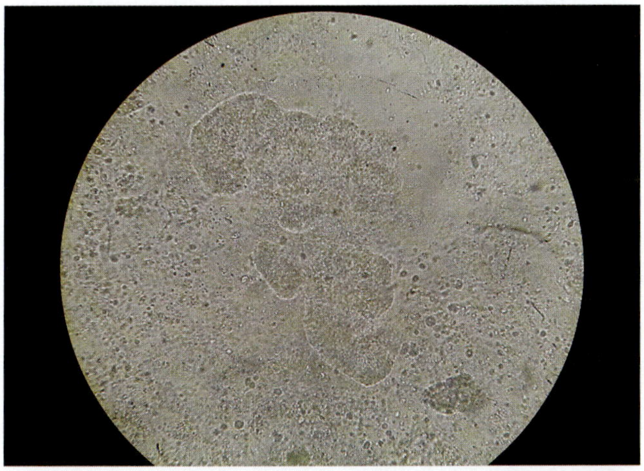

Fig. 4: Potassium hydroxide wet mount of an actinomycotic grain—pale grain with scalloped border.

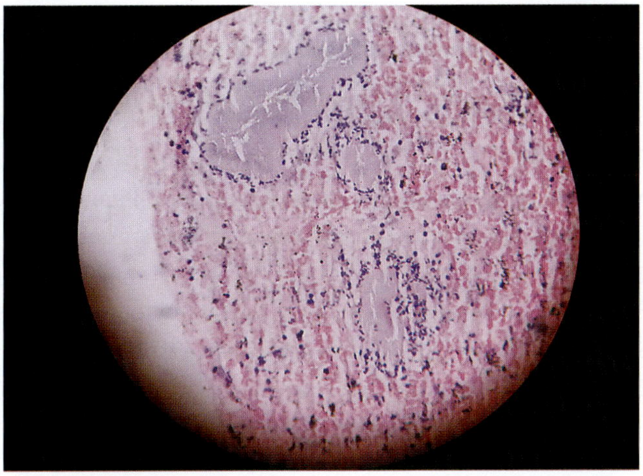

Fig. 6: High power view of histopathology of actinomycotic grain in H&E surrounded by Splendore-Hoeppli phenomenon.

Radiological Imaging

- *X-ray*: Swelling of soft tissue, widening of intermetatarsal spaces, periosteal reactions, osteolytic and osteosclerotic lesions, and ragged cortex. Sequestrum and pathological fracture absent.

Imaging	*Eumycetoma*	*Actinomycetoma*
X-ray	Localized, late, osteolytic changes nonrecoverable	Diffuse; early changes; osteosclerotic and osteolytic; recoverable
USG	• Grains seen as numerous sharp bright hyper-reflective echoes • Single or multiple thick-walled cavities with absent acoustic enhancement	• Similar findings but less distinct • Grains produce fine echoes—found at the bottom of the cavities

- *CT scan*: For early detection of bone involvement
- *MRI scan*: "Dot in the circle sign" (highly specific—dot is the grain)
- *Serodiagnosis*: ELISA, counterimmunoelectrophoresis (CIE)
- PCR/gene sequencing helps in rapid identification of the fungus.

Treatment: Actinomycotic—Welsh/Modified Ramam regimens, nocardiosis - cotrimoxazole; Eumycetoma—*no bone involvement*; surgical excision followed by itraconazole.

Bone affected: Itraconazole 200 mg *BD* with debulking; prolonged treatment; itraconazole and terbinafine combination in refractory cases. Potassium iodide can be used to reduce fibrosis.

PHAEOHYPHOMYCOSIS[4,5]

Rare subcutaneous and systemic fungal infection caused by phacoid (dematiaceous) fungi—saprotrophic which are ubiquitous in nature, found in soil, decaying vegetation, rotten woods, thorn, splinter. Increased occurrence in this era of increased solid organ transplantation and immunocompromised state; also in immunocompetent individuals; characterized by the presence of different types of melanized fungal elements—hyphae, pseudohyphae, yeast cells in the invading tissue.

Nomenclature: Term is derived from Greek word "Phaios" - gray.

History: De Beurman and Gougerot in France reported the first case in 1907. Dr Libero Ajello in 1974 coined the term Phaeohyphomycosis to include superficial, cutaneous, corneal, subcutaneous, and systemic infections.

Etiology: More than 120 species of 60 genera worldwide:

Bipolaris, Curvularia — *Phialophora verrucosa*
Alternaria alternata — *Phialophora compacta*
Exserohilum spp. — *Exophiala jeanselmei*
Wangiella dermatitidis — *Exophiala dermatitidis*
Cladosporium bantiana (*Cladophialophora bantiana* earlier)—CNS phaeohyphomycosis

Pathogenesis: Localized skin and soft tissue infections result from trauma with contaminated objects such as needles, thorns/splinters, or even medical instruments such as needles or catheters in transplant patients. Dark pigmentation of the molds is caused by the cell wall deposition of dihydroxynaphthalene melanin, which is the virulence factor.

Risk factors: Trauma, solid organ/bone marrow transplantation, immunosuppression. It may occur in immunocompetent individuals.

Clinical Features

- *Common sites*: Feet, legs, hand, arm, fingers, back. Less common—scalp, face, buttock
- Papulonodules, cysts (most common) **(Fig. 7)**, abscess, nonhealing ulcers
- Verrucous, hyperkeratotic, crusted or ulcerated plaques, pyogranulomatous lesions.

Differential Diagnosis

- *Cyst*: Ganglion, fibroma, lipoma, bursitis
- *Vegetative plaques*: Cutaneous tuberculosis, leishmaniasis, chromoblastomycosis

Laboratory Diagnosis

- *Specimen*: Aspirate from the cyst, touch smear or scraping from plaque
- *Direct microscopy in 10% KOH:* Pigmented/brown or hyaline branched, septate, moniliform hyphae, yeast-like cells, single or in short chains **(Fig. 8)**.
- Culture in SDA with cycloheximide—grayish black colony with reverse black pigmentation.
- Fine needle aspiration cytology
- (FNAC).

Mycopathology: Phaeohyphomycotic cyst presents as large cavity with fibrous capsule. Center filled with granulomatous

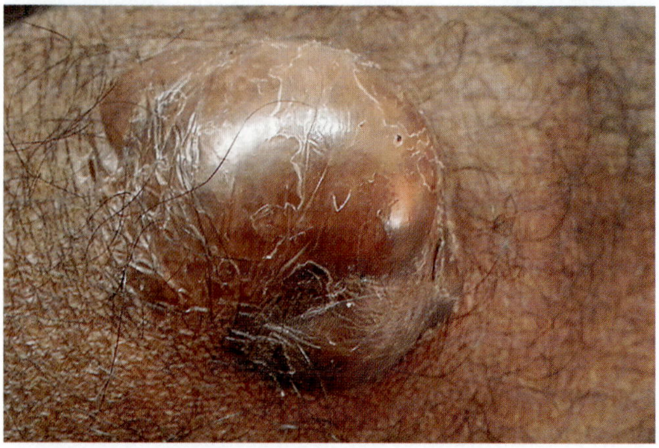

Fig. 7: Phaeohyphomycotic cyst in a renal transplant patient.

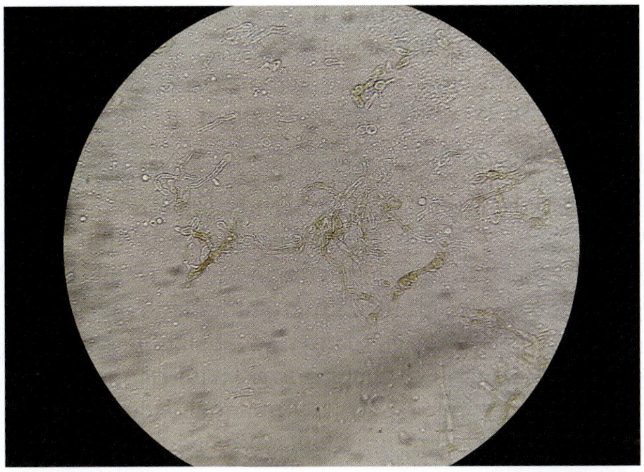

Fig. 8: Potassium hydroxide wet mount of phaeohyphomycosis showing pigmented septate irregular hyphae and thin-walled yeast cells.

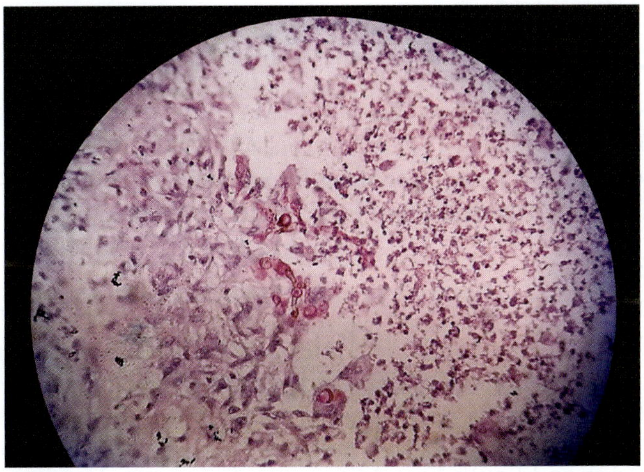

Fig. 9: High power view of histopathology of phaeohyphomycosis in H&E showing irregular, septate hyphae.

inflammatory infiltrate. Fungal hyphae may be seen in wall/cavity/within giant cells. They may not always be pigmented **(Fig. 9)**.

Special stains: PAS, GMS, and Masson–Fontana confirmatory.

Treatment

Cyst: Excision in immunocompetent; excision followed by chemotherapy in immunocompromised patients.

Systemic antifungals: Itraconazole is the mainstay (long duration); voriconazole, terbinafine, IV amphotericin B and 5-flucytosine in widespread lesions.

CHROMOBLASTOMYCOSIS[6]

Chromoblastomycosis is a chronic fungal infection of the skin and subcutaneous tissues caused by dematiaceous, i.e., pigmented fungi, which produce thick-walled single- or multicelled clusters (sclerotic or muriform bodies) in the tissue.

Nomenclature: Greek *Chroma*, ~atos = complexion, skin color; Greek *blastós* = sprout, bud; *mykes* = fungus *osis* Greek suffix denoting the state of something.

History

- Alexandrino Pedroso described in 1911.
- H Rudolph published the first clinical description in 1914.
- Medlar and Lane reported the first case in 1915 in Boston.
- The term "chromoblastomycosis" was proposed by Terra and colleagues in 1922.

Etiology

Fonsecaea pedrosoi (Phialophora pedrosoi), F. compacta (Phialophora compacta) Phialophora verrucosa, Cladosporium carrionii (earlier *Cladophialophora carrionii*), *Exophiala jeanselmei, Exophiala spinifera, Rhinocladiella aquaspersa, Exophiala dermatitidis*—less common.

Geographic distribution: Tropical and subtropical regions of Central and South America and Africa, Cuba, Jamaica, India, Madagascar.

Epidemiology: These are saprophytic fungi found in soil, decaying vegetation, pulp, paper. Common age group—30–50 years; Male:Female = 4:1. In Japan, M = F.

Predisposing factors: Outdoor occupations that predispose to contact with soil and plants affected by these fungi. Noncontagious, infective form is the mycelial form; sclerotic cells seen in man.

Pathogenesis

Early lesions start as a papule or nodule → slowly progress to form plaques with verrucous appearance over years. Usually localized, but satellite lesions may develop as a result of autoinoculation during scratching or lymphatic dissemination. Both humoral and cell-mediated immunity implicated.

Clinical Features

Site: Feet and shin (most common); shoulder, arms, gluteal regions, hands, chest, abdomen, face reported.

Clinical forms: Nodules, tumoral lesions, verrucous, scaly plaques, plaque with central scarring, cicatricial atropic skin lesions with sparing at the center. Single, multiple/disseminated **(Fig. 10)**. The black dots are seen on the surface = transepidermal elimination of fungi.

Complications: Secondary bacterial infection, ulceration, elephantiasis, keloid, squamous cell carcinoma (SCC).

Differential diagnosis: Verruca, tuberculosis verrucosa cutis (TbVC), verrucous carcinoma, SCC, leishmaniasis, syphilis, yaws, sporotrichosis, paracoccidioidomycosis, lobomycosis, sarcoidosis.

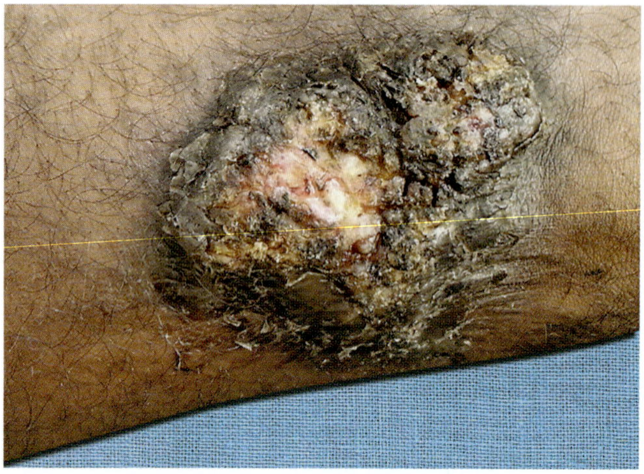

Fig. 10: Chromoblastomycosis.

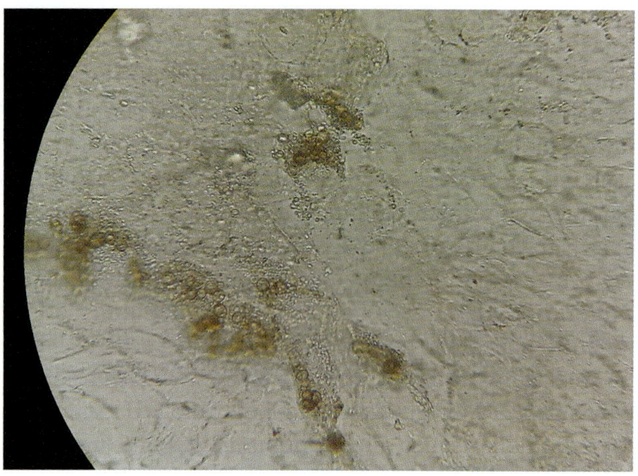

Fig. 11: Potassium hydroxide wet mount of chromoblastomycosis showing sclerotic cells.

Laboratory Diagnosis

- *Skin scraping or biopsy specimen in 10% KOH:* Characteristic sclerotic/muriform/medlar/copper penny bodies **(Fig. 11)**. Culture in SDA with chloramphenicol and cycloheximide to isolate the organism. Slow growing colony - dark green to black in color with reverse black.
- *Mycopathology* in H&E: Pseudoepitheliomatous hyperplasia, fibrosis, microabscess formation with sclerotic cells in the stratum corneum, dermis (single or in clusters) or in giant cells. Special stains not required. Other stains useful—Giemsa, Masson-Fontana, Ziehl-Neelsen, and Wade-Fite.

Treatment

- Cryotherapy/electrocautery/local application of heat/ surgical excision
- Itraconazole 400 mg/day, terbinafine 500 mg/day. voriconazole, posaconazole
- *Combination therapy:* Itraconazole and terbinafine
- *Disseminated lesions:* Inj. amphotericin B
- Treatment to be continued for several months following resolution of lesions.

ENTOMOPHTHOROMYCOSIS[7-9]

Chronic granulomatous (eosinophilic), subcutaneous, mucocutaneous and visceral infection that occurs predominantly in immunocompetent individuals caused by Entomophthorales, which along with Mucorales belong to the class, glomeromycota, which was earlier referred to as Zygomycota.

Two types: Basidiobolomycosis mostly seen in immunocompetent children and conidiobolomycosis is an infection of the adults, most common presentation being rhinoentomophthoromycosis. In the recent times, disseminated conidiobolomycosis has been reported in immunocompromised patients.

Nomenclature: Greek word, "*Entomon*" means insect; "*entomophthora*" means insect destroyer.

History

The first case of Basidiobolomycosis in humans was described by Lei-Kian Joe in 1956 in Indonesia. In India, first case was reported by Mukerji et al. in Bombay (Mumbai) in 1962. *Conidiobolus* infection was reported in humans in 1965.

Etiology

Basidiobolomycosis caused by *Basidiobolus ranarum* (Synonyms *B. haptosporus, B. meristosporus).*

Conidiobolomycosis caused by *Conidiobolus coronatus, C. incongruus, C. lamprauges. Geographic distribution*: Tropical and subtropical regions of Central and South America, Africa and South East Asia (India, Indonesia, Myanmar, Pakistan), and Northern Australia.

Epidemiology

Entomophthorales are found in soil, decaying vegetation, insects, and gastrointestinal tracts of amphibians.

Basidiobolomycosis: More common in children <10 years; M > F.

Conidiobolomycosis: Adults, 8 times more common in males.

Pathogenesis

Basidiobolomycosis is acquired through traumatic inoculation of the organism via minor cuts, abrasions, and insect bites. Gastrointestinal basidiobolomycosis results from ingestion.

Infection by *Conidiobolus* species is acquired through inhalation of spores and traumatic inoculation of the organism in the nasal mucosa. In both infections, infection starts as a subcutaneous nodule → expands → local spread. Lymphadenopathy may be present. There is no hematogenous spread. It has been postulated that these organisms cause infection in those patients who tend to have a subtle defect in immunity to these organisms.

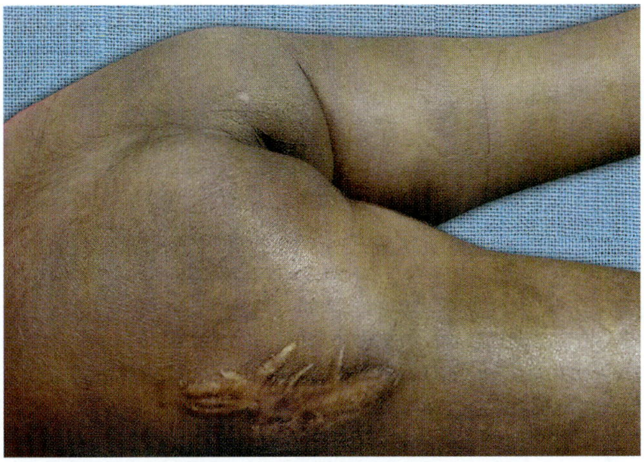

Fig. 12: Basidiobolomycosis.

Clinical Features

Basidiobolomycosis

- *Site*: Thighs, gluteal regions, arms, and trunk
- *Characteristic clinical presentation*: Painless, well defined, sharply circumscribed swelling with firm (Indian rubber) consistency, and finger insinuation possible beneath the margins of the mass. Sometimes, the involved limb may be swollen 2–3 times the normal size. Skin surface may be normal, tense or hyperpigmented. Small satellite lesions may occur in the circumscribed area **(Fig. 12)**.

Conidiobolomycosis

- *Site*: Nose, paranasal sinuses, cheeks, upper lip, eyelids, forehead. Intraoral involvement—hard and soft palate, pharynx and larynx.
- Painless, firm swelling which gradually progresses in size, firmly fixed to the underlying structures to produce disfigurement. Patients may suffer from nasal obstruction, rhinorrhea, epistaxis, and dysphagia. Ulceration may occur rarely in both the infections.
- Disseminated basidiobolomycosis and conidiobolomycosis have been reported.

Complications

Basidiobolomycosis: Reversible obstructive hydronephrosis, persistent lymphedema, bone, and muscle invasion.

Conidiobolomycosis: Bones, vessels and muscle are rarely involved.

Differential Diagnosis

Basidiobolomycosis	*Conidiobolomycosis*
• Chronic abscess, cellulitis, elephantiasis, sporotrichosis • Localized morphea, keloid, neurofibroma, soft-tissue tumor • Synovial sarcoma, lymphosarcoma, Burkitt's lymphoma, sarcoidosis, fibrosing panniculitis	• Midline lethal cyst • Lymphatic edema, leishmaniasis • Lymphoma, sarcoma

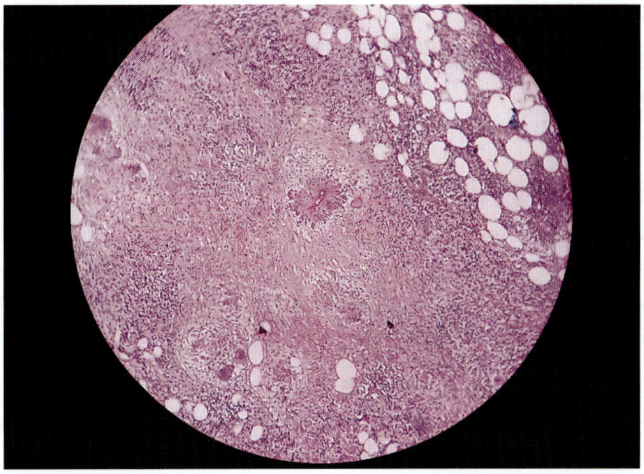

Fig. 13: High power view of histopathology of basidibolomycosis in H&E showing fungal hyphae surrounded by Splendore–Hoeppli phenomenon.

Laboratory Diagnosis

Gently teased biopsy specimen in 10% KOH: Broad, coenocytic (sparsely septate) hyphae with thin walls and right angle branching.

Mycopathology in H&E: Eosinophilic granuloma with foreign body and Langhans giant cells, moderate or few lymphocytes, and plasma cells. Fungal elements are visualized as unstained tubes and haloes with eosin stained thin walls surrounded by eosinophilic sleeve of Splendore–Hoeppli material **(Fig. 13)**.

Culture in SDA agar without cycloheximide: *B. ranarum* grows as flat, yellow-to-gray colony with radial folds and pale reverse. Microscopic in Lactophenol cotton blue (LPCB)—Beak-shaped zygospores is characteristic.

C. coronatus: Similar to *B. ranarum* but shows rapid growth. Microscopic in LPCB—characteristic papillated and villose conidia.

Treatment

Oral potassium iodide (KI): Mixture or supersaturated solution is the gold standard for both types. Combination of KI and trimethoprim-sulfamethoxazole/itraconazole is in vogue.

Conidiobolomycosis: Combination of KI and itraconazole is preferable. Itraconazole + terbinafine have also been successful. In addition, surgical intervention if feasible. Long duration of treatment—at least 1 month beyond complete resolution.

SPOROTRICHOSIS[10,11]

Synonyms: *Rose Gardener's disease, Rose handler's disease, Rose Thorn disease, Schenck's disease, Beurmann's disease.*[12]

Sporotrichosis is an acute or chronic granulomatous mycosis of the cutaneous and subcutaneous tissues of human and animals with lymphatic spread.

History

Benjamin Schenck, a medical student described the first case in 1898.

Lutz and Splendore observed asteroid body in 1907.

Etiology

Sporotrichosis is caused by dimorphic fungus, *Sporothrix schenckii* species complex [6 species—*S. albicans, S. brasiliensis, S. globosa* (worldwide), *S. luriei, S. mexicana, S. pallida,* and *S. schenckii*].

Geographic distribution: Sporotrichosis occurs worldwide with focal areas of endemicity in tropical, subtropical, and temperate zones.

Epidemiology

Sporothrix species are saprophytes present in soil, decaying vegetation—wood, hay, sphagnum moss, thorny plants, and splinters in the mold form.

It is predominantly seen in young population exposed to the above-mentioned sources of infection. M: F = 3:1; recently almost equal.

Zoonotic (dog, cat, cattle, horse, donkey, pig, birds) and man-to-man transmission has been reported.

Pathogenesis

Sporothrix species (mold form) enters following injury by thorn/splinter → thermal dimorphism → converts into yeast form in tissue → papulonodule → ulcerates → nodules along the lymphatic drainage. Organisms produce proteinase I and proteinase II which help in fungal invasion and growth.

Clinical Features

- *Incubation period*: Few days to few weeks; average—3 weeks
- *Three clinical forms*: Lymphocutaneous, fixed cutaneous, and extracutaneous. *Lymphocutaneous*—most common (70–80%).
    - *Site:* Extremities most common.
    - *Inoculation site:* Noduloulcerative lesion (Primary lesion—sporotrichotic chancre) → lymphatic drainage → secondary lesions occur in a linear form—string of nodules along the lymphatic chain (*Sporotrichoid*) which becomes indurated and cord-like.
- *Fixed cutaneous*: It is less common. Site—face, neck, trunk, arm. No lymphatic or systemic spread. Variable asymptomatic lesions—papulopustules, nodules, acniform, verrucous/erythematous plaques, nonhealing ulcers, abscess.
- *Extracutaneous* form is associated with immunosuppression. Five types are osteoarticular (knee, wrist, elbow, and ankle joints), pulmonary, mucocutaneous, ocular, and disseminated type.

Differential Diagnosis

Lymphocutaneous/ Fixed cutaneous	*Extracutaneous/ Disseminated*
• Cutaneous anthrax	• Osteoarticular
• Leishmaniasis	• Tuberculous arthritis
• Tuberculosis verrucosa cutis	• Rheumatoid arthritis
• Atypical mycobacterial infection	• Gout
• Nocardiosis	• Sarcoidosis
• Chromoblastomycosis	• *Pulmonary*
• Blastomycosis	• Tuberculosis
• Coccidioidomycosis	• Sarcoidosis
• Foreign body granuloma	• Blastomycosis
• Pyoderma gangrenosum	• Histoplasmosis
• Tularemia, syphilis chancre	• Paracoccidioidomycosis
• Cat-scratch disease	

Laboratory Diagnosis

- *KOH wet mount*: Very small, elongated yeast cells, and hence often negative.
- *Gram stain*: Gram positive yeast cells.
- Culture in SDA, blood agar, brain-heart infusion agar—moist cream colored colony evolves into gray or brown color. Microscopic—flower-like and palm tree-like sporulation.
- *FNAC/Mycopathology*: Three concentric zones (*STS zones*) is characteristic—central **S**uppurative (neutrophils); Middle **T**uberculoid (epithelioid cells, Langhans' giant cells) and outer **S**yphiloid zone (plasma cells) asteroid bodies, yeast cells seen within the giant cells and cigar-shaped bodies. This delineation is not seen in old lesions. Yeast cells (globose or cigar-shaped) well visualized in PAS/GMS stains while asteroid bodies (Splendore-Hoeppli phenomenon) in H&E.

Treatment

- Saturated solution of potassium iodide, itraconazole (ITC) terbinafine.
- *Disseminated sporotrichosis*: Amphotericin B for 4–6 weeks followed by ITC for 12 months.

RHINOSPORIDIOSIS[13,14]

Rhinosporidiosis, which is a chronic granulomatous infection of mucocutaneous tissues, is considered as pseudofungal infection, as the causative organism, *Rhinosporidium seeberi,* earlier thought to be fungus, is now considered to be a hydrophilic, protistan parasite.

Nomenclature: *"rhino"* – nose; "sporidiosis" – sporozoan.

History

- Carlos Malbran first observed this infection in Argentina in 1892.
- Guillermo Seeber first reported in 1900.
- Ashworth coined the term, "*Rhinosporidium seeberi.*"

Etiology

Rhinosporidiosis is caused by *"Rhinosporidium seeberi,"* a eukaryotic organism—protistan parasite that infects fish and amphibians, which is included under, "Mesomycetozoea".

Geographic distribution: Endemic in Southeast Asian countries (especially Sri Lanka and Southern India). Sporadic in South America, southern United States, South Africa, and Europe.

Epidemiology: *R. seeberi* is believed to be hydrophilic. Water acts as a reservoir. People who take bath in ponds and tanks are at risk. M:F = 3:1 to 4:1; 2nd and third decade of life.

Life cycle (3 stages): Trophozoite maturation → sporangia → 12,000–16,000 endospores.

Pathogenesis

Exact method of transmission is unknown—postulated—through inhalation of aerosols/dust particles, infected clothing and through swimming in stagnant water. Autoinoculation after trivial trauma. Hematogenous and lymphatic spread may also occur.

Clinical Features

The clinical features of rhinosporidiosis are described in **Table 1**.

Complications: Profuse bleeding, recurrence.

Laboratory Diagnosis

KOH wet mount: Touch smear from the lesion or biopsy tissue will show sporangia and endospores **(Fig. 15)**.

Culture: *R. seeberi* not cultivable.

HPE—Papillomatosis, sporangia in different stages, mixed granulomatous inflammatory infiltrate **(Fig. 16)**. PAS, Mucicarmine—well visualized.

Differential diagnosis: Coccidioidal sporangia is smaller.

Treatment

Surgical excision and electrodesiccation.

- *Medical*: Dapsone effective.
- *Other drugs*: Ketoconazole, cycloserine, pentavalent compounds of antimony.

LACAZIOSIS (LOBOMYCOSIS)[15]

Synonyms: *Jorge Lobo disease, Jorge Lobo blastomycosis, Keloidal blastomycosis, Caiabi leprosy.*

Chronic granulomatous fungal infection of slow progression that affects the skin and subcutaneous tissue, caused by *Lacazia loboi.*

History

- First observed by Brazilian dermatologist, Jorge Lobo in 1931.
- Borelli proposed the name, "Lobomycosis" and the agent as "Loboa loboi" in 1958.
- Taborda redesignated the genus as, "Lacazia."

Etiology: *Lacazia loboi.*

Geographic distribution: South and Central America; imported cases in North America and Europe.

TABLE 1: Clinical features of rhinosporidiosis.

	Nasal: 70%	*Ocular: 15%*	*Cutaneous rare* ***(Fig. 14)***	*Disseminated rare*	*Miscellaneous*
Site	• Anterior nares, nasal septum, inferior turbinate, nasopharynx, soft palate, larynx • Unilateral or bilateral	Bulbar and palpebral conjunctiva, corneal limbus lacrimal sac	Face, trunk, extremities	• Skin, bones, liver, lungs, spleen, brain • Bone involvement shows extensive bone destruction	Buccal cavity, lips, vagina, vulva, urethra, penis
Symptoms	• Epistaxis • Unilateral nasal obstruction, mucopurulent nasal discharge, pain if large polyp, discomfort	Foreign body sensation, red eye, photophobia, lid eversion conjunctivitis	Bleeding, pain if infected		Polyp from urethra: Hematuria, discharge
Clinical morphology	• Highly vascular, pedunculated or sessile polyps, lobulated cauliflower-like appearance • White spots on surface represent sporangia	Soft, reddish fleshy polyp With pin head sized grayish white spots on the surface	Sessile fleshy mass, wart-like, papillomatous, friable		Painless, friable reddish polyp protruding from urethral meatus
Differential diagnosis	• Rhinoscleroma, • Nasal polyposis • Syphilis • Leishmaniasis • Hemangioma • Angiofibroma sarcoma	• Chalazion • Dacryocystitis • Neoplasia	• Verruca • Cryptococcus • Coccidio-idomycosis • Adiaspiromycosis	Bone chondrosarcoma	• Penile: SCC • Anal: Condyloma, hemorrhoids

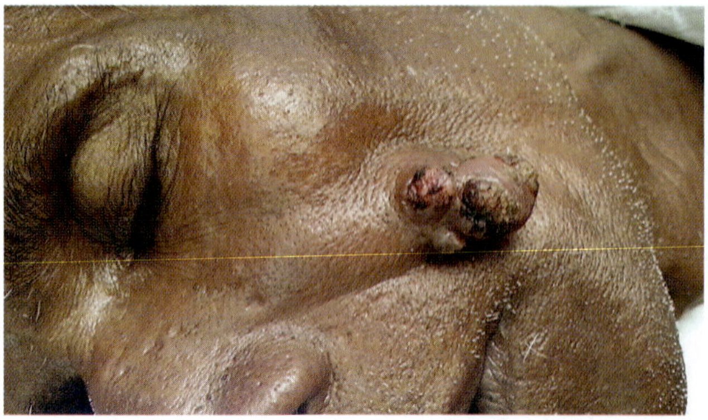

Fig. 14: Rhinosporidiosis.

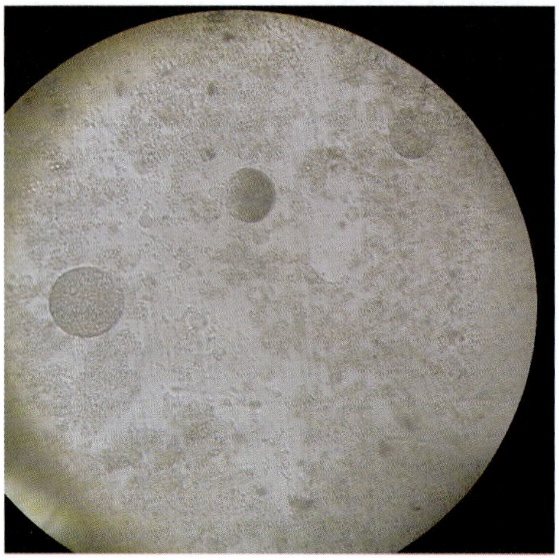

Fig. 15: Potassium hydroxide wet mount of rhinosporidiosis showing the sporangia.

Epidemiology

Lacazia loboi is said to be present in soil/vegetation and aquatic environment. It affects dolphins also. Farmers, miners, rubber workers, fishermen are at risk. It prefers cool sites in body.

M:F = 20:1

Pathogenesis

Trivial trauma - organism enters → long incubation period → papule → slow progression → plaque/nodule → Keloid/ scarring.

Clinical Features

Site (exposed)—lower limbs, ear, upper limbs, and face. Pruritus may be present.

Morphological types: Single or multiple nodules, macules, hypo- or hyperpigmentation, infiltrative, gummatous, verrucous, keloidal, and ulcerative.

Complications: Deformity, squamous cell carcinoma.

Differential diagnosis: Other mycoses—chromoblastomycosis, sporotrichosis, paracoccidioidomycosis, leishmaniasis, leprosy, keloid, cutaneous tuberculosis.

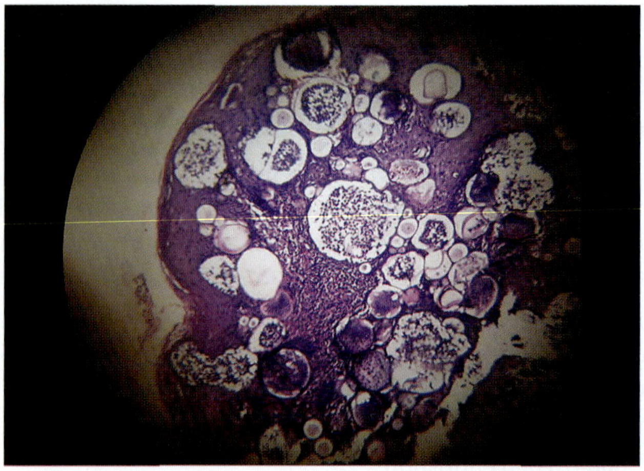

Fig. 16: High power view of histopathology of rhinosporidiosis in H&E showing sporangia in varying stages of maturation.

Laboratory Diagnosis

KOH: Scraping from lesion or smear from biopsy specimen—globose or lemon shaped, doubly refractile narrow-based budding yeast cells in chains

Culture: *L. loboi* not cultivable. HPE—atrophic epidermis, Grenz zone may be present, granulomatous inflammatory infiltrate with multinucleate and Langhans giant cells. Yeast cells are usually intracellular seen within the giant cells and may be seen in the dermis. Asteroid bodies may be seen. Special stains—PAS, GMS, Gridley stain for better visualization.

Treatment

Surgical excision. No effective therapy. Itraconazole, posaconazole can be tried.

SYSTEMIC MYCOSES

Systemic mycoses are classified as endemic respiratory mycoses and opportunistic mycoses. Endemic mycoses are caused by dimorphic fungi, which exist as hyphal form in the environment and as yeast in the host (in vivo). These infections are primarily endemic in certain regions of North and South America, with imported infection being reported in individuals who travel to these areas and the immigrants. They are acquired by inhalation of air borne conidia, resulting in an asymptomatic infection in 95% of the patients and dissemination to various organs including skin by hematogenous or lymphatic spread in the rest of the patients. The four major endemic mycoses are histoplasmosis, blastomycosis, coccidioidomycosis, and paracoccidioidomycosis, which occur in immunocompetent individuals and immunosuppressed patients.

Histoplasmosis[16,17]

Synonyms: Darling's disease, Cave disease, Ohio valley disease, histoplasmosis capsulati.

Nomenclature: Organisms seen in *Histiocyte* resembled *plasmo*dium with *capsule* and hence *Histoplasma capsulatum (H.c).*

History: First reported by Samuel Taylor Darling in 1905, he thought it was a parasite.

Henrique da Rocha-Lima first suspected yeast in 1934.

Etiology: *H.c.var.capsulatum* (Classic histoplasmosis), *H.c.var. duboisii (African histoplasmosis), H.c.var.farciminosum (epizootic). Histoplasma* spps exhibit thermal dimorphism-Mycelial phase between 25 and –30°C and Yeast form at 37°C.

Geographic distribution: Endemic in Central and South-Eastern USA, certain areas in South America, Africa. It is reported in 60 countries [Southeast Asia - Thailand and India (high prevalence in the north-eastern states)]. Sporadic cases reported elsewhere.

Epidemiology

Histoplasma capsulatum grows in soil mixed with bird droppings and bat guano. Risk - farmers, A/c Mechanics, demolition/construction workers in endemic areas. M>F; infants and children frequently affected.

Pathogenesis

Air borne microconidia → inhalation → lung converts into yeast form → survives within the macrophage → transported to the hilar and mediastinal lymph nodes and subsequently disseminates hematogeneously throughout the reticuloendothelial system. CMI important role. Hence, HIV patients are more susceptible to develop dissemination.

Clinical Features

- Asymptomatic in 90–95%. Reactivation occurs with immunosuppression.
- *Four types*: Acute pulmonary, chronic pulmonary, cutaneous/mucocutaneous, and disseminated.
- *Skin*: Primary very rare. Occurs through direct inoculation. Secondary through hematogenous dissemination.
- Papules, pustules, plaques, ulcers, nodules, ulcers, abscesses or MC/wart/cellulitis such as lesions, purpura, petechiae, EN, scars, fistulae, pigmentation. Nodules may be found on the tongue, lips buccal/gingival mucosa, and larynx. Oral ulcers - 50% of disseminated.
- *Disseminated*: Liver, spleen, lymph nodes, bone marrow, CNS, adrenal glands, endocarditis, bones, eyes.
- Skin and bone are more involved in African histoplasmosis.

Differential Diagnosis

- *Pulmonary*: Tuberculosis (TB)
- *Skin*: other systemic mycoses, phaeohyphomycosis
- *Disseminated*: Sarcoidosis, lymphoma, mycobacterial

Laboratory diagnosis and treatment are given in **Table 2**.

Blastomycosis[18,19]

Synonyms: Gilchrist's disease North American Blastomycosis.

Nomenclature: Greek, *blastós* bud; *Mykes* fungus *osis*-condition.

History: Thomas Casper Gilchrist first reported in 1894.

Etiology: *Blastomyces dermatitidis, B. gilchristii, B. percursus.*

Geographic distribution: Endemic in USA, Canada extended to Africa. Sporadic in India, Middle East.

Epidemiology: Exact reservoir unknown - moist soil with animal droppings/water bodies.

Risk: Outdoor/recreational exposure to above in endemic area; M>F; in outbreaks, males, females and children affected alike.

Pathogenesis

Inhalation of spores → Lungs → Yeast form → hematogenous dissemination - skin is the most common extrapulmonary site.

Clinical Features

- *Varied spectrum*: Asymptomatic/acute or chronic pneumonia/extrapulmonary
- *Four clinical forms*: Pulmonary, cutaneous, osseous, disseminated (skin, bone, CNS, genitourinary tract, orbit, sinuses, adrenal gland)
- *Skin*: Primary rare; occurs post-trauma → erythema, chancre, lymphadenopathy within 2 weeks. Spontaneous resolution may occur over several months
- *Secondary*: Through hematogenous; single or multiple; papules, nodules, ulcer, fistulae, abscess, verrucous lesions; lymphadenopathy, lymphangitis.

Differential Diagnosis

- *Pulmonary*: TB, carcinoma
- *Skin*: Cutaneous tuberculosis, pyoderma, leprosy, keratoacanthoma, tertiary syphilis
- Other systemic mycoses, SCC, blastomycosis-like pyoderma vegetans, pyoderma gangrenosum.

Laboratory diagnosis and treatment are given in **Table 2**.

Coccidioidomycosis[20,21]

Synonyms: Valley fever, San Joaquin valley fever, desert fever, desert rheumatism, Posadas Wernicke disease, coccidioidal granuloma.

Nomenclature: *Coccidia*—Protozoan parasite (Greek *Kokkis-little berry)* ***Oidis*** *- similar to.*

Coccidioides*—coccidia like; Latin* ***immitis*** harsh *im*-not; *mitis*-mild.

History: First case reported by Alejandro Posades in 1892.

Etiology: *Coccidioides immitis, C. posadasii.*

TABLE 2: Laboratory diagnosis and treatment of endemic mycoses.[16-21]

Title	*Histoplasmosis*	*Blastomycosis*	*Coccidioidomycosis*	*Paracoccidioidomycosis*
Specimen	Touch smear from skin lesion/biopsy tissue, sputum, lymph node aspirate, blood, bone marrow	Pus, skin scraping, biopsy (Bx) tissue, sputum, BAL fluid	Skin scrapings, Bx tissue, exudates, sputum, BAL fluid, CSF	Crust, Bx tissue, pus, sputum, BAL fluid, CSF
Direct microscopy KOH	Small oval, yeast cells within PMN/ lymphocytes May be missed; Giemsa, Wright, Calcofluor white useful	• Double contoured, thick walled, multi-nucleated with single broad-based budding yeast cells • Giemsa, Wright staining can be done	Refractile thick walled spherules filled with endospores. Hyphae may occasionally be present	Refractile, thick walled, rounded yeast cells with multipolar budding
Culture				
Media	SDA without actidione at 25°C and 37°C	SDA without actidione at 25°C and 37°C	SDA, blood agar, brain-heart infusion agar with actidione	SDA with antibiotics and actidione
Growth	White or tan, cottony colonies	White cottony colony that becomes tan later	Creamy white colony with glistening glabrous growth	Creamy, wrinkled pasty yeast colony
Microscopy	2 types of Conidia—large tuberculate macroconidia and small, oval, smooth or roughened microconidia	Smooth, thick walled, spherical conidia with single, broad based budding	Thin, hyaline branching, septate hyphae with alternate thick walled, barrel-shaped arthroconidia and empty cells—*Box car appearance*	Oval or globose yeast cells with multiple budding; daughter buds encircle the mother yeast cell attached by narrow neck—*Mariner wheel*
Histopathology	Suppurative granuloma with narrow-based yeast cells with clear halo within histiocytes/ giant cells (Parasitized macrophages) and extracellularly in the tissues	• Pseudoepitheliomatous hyperplasia with intraepidermal microabscess • Broad-based, thick-walled yeast cells are seen in clusters of neutrophils or within multinucleated giant cells	• Primary cutaneous—small abscesses; dense dermal inflammatory infiltrate. Spores present • Secondary cutaneous less tendency for abscess formation. Large, round, thick walled spores seen freely in the tissue and within giant cells	• Pseudoepitheliomatous hyperplasia with microabscess formation and mixed dermal inflammatory infiltrate • Yeast cells in the tissue may present as single cells with narrow based budding or multiple budding
HPE differential diagnosis	Rhinoscleroma, granuloma inguinale, leishmaniasis, talaromycosis, lepromatous leprosy	TbVC, halogenoderma, other deep mycoses, SCC	Spores of *C. immitis* larger than that of *Blastomyces*, *Cryptococcus*	Single budding yeast cells when present has to be differentiated from *B. dermatidis*, *C. immitis* and *C. neoformans*
Spores are best demonstrated in special stains such as PAS, GMS				
Treatment	Cutaneous—Itraconazole; Disseminated—Amphotericin B	• Immunocompetent/ nonthreatening—Itraconazole • Life-threatening/severe/ CNS—Amphotericin B	• *Rapid progression*—Amphotericin B/ amphotericin B and itraconazole • *Subacute/chronic*—Itraconazole, fluconazole	*Severe:* Amphotericin B *Others:* Itraconazole, sulfonamides with/without trimethoprim

(BAL: bronchoalveolar lavage; CNS: central nervous system; CSF: cerebrospinal fluid; GMS: Gomori methenamine silver; PAS: periodic acid-Schiff; PMN: polymorphonuclear leukocytes; SDA: Sabouraud's dextrose agar; SCC: squamous cell carcinoma)

Geographic distribution: Central valleys of California (*C. immitis*; Parts of Central and South America (*C. posadasii*). Imported cases in Indian patients who travel to endemic zones.

Epidemiology: *Coccidioides* spps inhabit sandy and alkaline soil in areas with semi-arid, very hot summers and little rainfall—10–50 cm/year.

Risk: Construction/agricultural workers, archeological students, HIV, diabetes, immune-suppression, pregnant women, laboratory exposure.

Pathogenesis

Inhalation of dust laden with arthroconidia → Swells in alveoli → Spherules → enlarge and nuclear division to form endospores. Spherule ruptures → endospores released

→ local spread/hilar lymph nodes and hematogenous dissemination—skin, bones, joints, meninges, upper GIT, adrenal glands. 17 β-estradiol, progesterone and testosterone stimulate spherule maturation, and release of endospores.

Clinical Features

- Incubation period of 1–4 weeks → primary pulmonary infection. Asymptomatic in 60%.
- *Four clinical forms*: Acute primary pulmonary (flu-like), persistent pneumonia, chronic fibrocavitory pneumonia and disseminated—1% skin, bones, joints, meninges.
- *Skin*: Primary rare; Postinoculation → transient lymphangitis/lymphadenopathy.
    - Skin lesions associated with primary pulmonary—transient morbilliform or scarlatiniform rash, erythema nodosum, EM, nonmigratory arthralgia (desert rheumatism)
    - Skin lesions in disseminated: About 15–20% of patients—papules, verrucous nodules/plaques, ulcerated plaques, subcutaneous abscess, scars, fistulae. Rare—widespread small pustules on an erythematous base.

Differential Diagnosis

- *Pulmonary*: Influenza, bronchitis.
- *Skin*: Cutaneous TB, atypical mycobacterial infection, other deep mycoses, syphilis.

Laboratory diagnosis and treatment are given in **Table 2**.

Paracoccidioidomycosis[21,22]

Synonyms: South American blastomycosis, Lutz-Splendore-Almeida's disease, Brazilian blastomycosis, paracoccidioidal blastomycosis or paracoccidioidal granuloma, Lutz's mycosis.

Nomenclature: *Para* - near/similar to. Initially it was thought to be similar to *Coccidioides spp.*

History

Adolfo Lutz in 1908 identified the organism and demonstrated dimorphism. Alfonso Splendore isolated the organism in new cases and described the clinical and histopathological characteristics.

In 1930, Floriano Paulo de Almeida designated the organism as *Paracoccidioides brasiliensis.*

Etiology: *Paracoccidioides brasiliensis, P. lutzii.*

Geographic distribution: Central and South America, Southern Brazil has the highest incidence of infection. It has not been reported in India.

Epidemiology: Ecological niche uncertain. It has been isolated from armadillos.

Risk: Farmers, coffee plantation workers, etc., with outdoor exposure. Malnutrition, alcohol, and smoking increase the risk of infection.

M>F = 15:1 in adults; Reason—estrogen prevents the conversion of mycelia to the yeast form. Not communicable between human beings or from animals to humans.

Pathogenesis

Inhalation of conidia → Primary pulmonary infection → dissemination—mucocutaneous lesions, CNS, bones, joints, eyes and endocrine system.

Clinical Features

- *Primary pulmonary form*: Benign infection
- *Five clinical forms*: Acute pulmonary in immunosuppression; chronic pulmonary; acute/subacute (juvenile form); chronic mucocutaneous (adult) and disseminated.
- *Acute/subacute (Juvenile) form:* M:F = 5.5:1 in children >12 years; lymphadenopathy is the most common feature. Hepato- and splenomegaly present. Pulmonary symptoms rare.
- *Chronic mucocutaneous (adult):* Mostly men 29–50 years; patients c/o dysphagia/hoarseness of voice. Pulmonary involvement is more common than oropharynx and lymph nodes; 50% patients: oral lesions, often with nasal and pharynx ulcers; sites—lip, tongue, gingival, buccal mucosa, floor of mouth.
- *Oral ulcers*: Swelling → Granulomatous, exuberant, mulberry-like surface with pin point hemorrhages.
- *Skin*: Polymorphic lesions; papule/nodule → hyperkeratotic/warty/crusted/ulcerative plaques. Common sites—nose, near mouth, anus, genitalia. Periorificial granulomatous plaques may progress with tissue destruction of adjacent structures. Cervical lymphadenopathy/sinus tracts.

Differential Diagnosis

- *Pulmonary*: Tuberculosis, other systemic mycoses.
- *Skin*: Mucocutaneous leishmaniasis, sporotrichosis, rhinoscleroma, actinomycosis, malignancy
- *Lymph nodes*: TB, Hodgkin's disease.

Laboratory diagnosis and treatment are given in **Table 2**.

OPPORTUNISTIC MYCOSES

Systemic opportunistic fungal infections are caused by fungi with low pathogenicity, which tend to produce severe infection in patients with immunosuppression and severe debilitating illness. These infections, unlike endemic mycoses, occur worldwide and are more common in the developing countries. Infection is through inhalation or skin inoculation. Candidiasis and cryptococcosis are opportunistic mycoses caused by yeasts while mucormycosis, aspergillosis and fusariosis are caused by molds. Penicilliosis is an opportunistic mycosis caused by dimorphic fungus.

Mucormycosis (Figs. 17 and 18)[23,24]

Synonyms: Formerly Zygomycosis

Nomenclature: Latin *mūcor* - "mouldiness, mustiness". *Mykes* fungus Greek *osis* - condition.

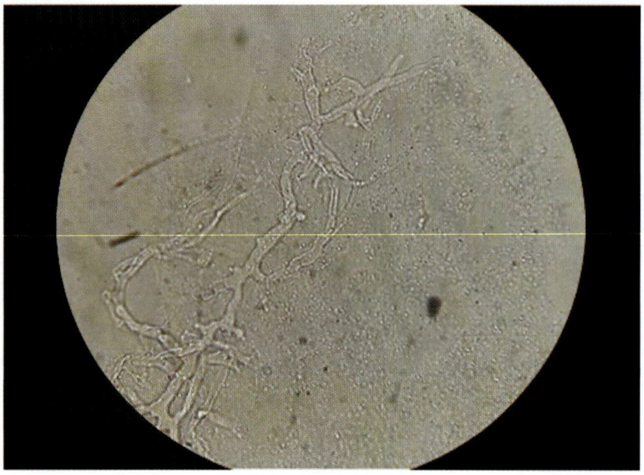

Fig. 17: Potassium hydroxide wet mount of mucormycosis showing broad, ribbon-shaped sparsely septate hyphae.

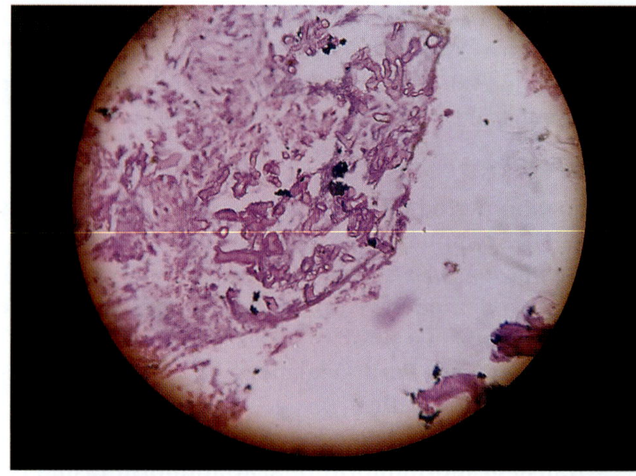

Fig. 18: High power view of histopathology of mucormycosis in H&E showing broad sparsely septate hyphae.

History: Kurchenmeister described the first case in 1855.

Etiology: Classified under phylum Zygomycota which is now termed as Glomeromycota (Order Mucorales). Rapid growers and thermotolerant; *Rhizopus arrhizus*- most common; *Mucor racemosus, Rhizoucor pusillus, Lichtheimia corymbifera, Apophysomyces spp, Saksenaea spp.*

Geographic distribution: Worldwide

Epidemiology: Saprophytes often isolated from soil, decaying organic matter and rotten fruits.

Risk factors: Uncontrolled diabetes mellitus, DKA, stem cell/solid organ transplant, neutropenia, cancer chemotherapy, deferoxamine therapy, trauma, burns, neonates.

Pathogenesis

Inhalation of spores → Paranasal sinuses → germinate → rapid invasion; Bronchoalveolar macrophages in immunosuppression unable to kill the organisms; Impaired chemotaxis and phagocytosis dysfunction in hyperglycemia. In the presence of acidosis/deferoxamine therapy → ferric iron is released from transferrin → rapid growth of molds and invasion of blood vessels → thrombosis → ischemia → tissue necrosis.

Cutaneous—Trauma/Burns/contaminated wound dressings → inoculation in primary; hematogenous dissemination → secondary.

Clinical Features

- *Six types*: Rhinocerebral, pulmonary, gastrointestinal, cutaneous, disseminated and miscellaneous
- *Rhinocerebral*: Most common
- *Symptoms*: Unilateral headache, soft tissue swelling, pain, pus/bloody discharge, fever, blurred vision/diplopia, rarely convulsion
- *Signs*: Periorbital cellulitis, proptosis, ptosis, ophthalmoplegia, necrotic ulcer with eschar, palatal perforation

Cutaneous

- *Primary*: Acute onset; swelling, pus discharge, tissue necrosis → black eschar → deeper invasion into fat, muscle, bone.
- *Secondary*: More common than primary. Most often seen in rhinocerebral; presents as cellulitis, necrotic ulcer with Eschar over eyelid/cheek/palate.

Differential Diagnosis

- *Rhinocerebral*: Bacterial orbital cellulitis, cavernous sinus thrombosis, aspergillosis
- *Cutaneous*: Ecthyma, necrotizing fasciitis, gangrene.

Laboratory diagnosis and treatment are given in **Table 3**.

Aspergillosis[23,25]

Nomenclature: Latin "*aspergo*" - to sprinkle. Sporing head of *Aspergillus* species resembles an aspergillum used to sprinkle holy water.

History: Micheli first defined the genus Aspergillus in 1729. John Hughes Bennett first described Aspergillosis in 1842. Fresenius introduced the term, aspergillosis in 1863.

Etiology: There are 339 species of which *A. fumigatus* is the most common, followed by *A. flavus, A. terreus and A. niger.*

Geographic distribution: Worldwide.

Epidemiology: Saprobes present in soil, water, dead and decaying organic matter, rotten vegetables and fruits, etc.

Risk factors: Organ transplants, hematological malignancy, neutropenia, radiation therapy, chemotherapy, diabetes mellitus, surgical wounds.

Pathogenesis

Inhalation/oral or local exposure; Inhalation of conidia → escape the ciliary clearance → alveoli → if immunosuppressed/neutropenia → alveolar macrophages are unable to kill conidia → germination → impaired neutrophil killing of

TABLE 3: Laboratory diagnosis and treatment of opportunistic mycoses caused by molds.[23]

Title	*Mucormycosis*	*Aspergillosis*	*Talaromycosis*
Direct microscopy KOH wet mount	Hyaline, sparsely septate, broad, ribbon-like hyphae with wide angle or right-angle branching **(Fig. 17)**	Hyaline, closely septate, hyphae with dichotomous branching at acute angle	Wright/Giemsa—intracellular or extra-cellular basophilic, spherical, oval/elliptical yeast-like cells with a central septum (multiply by transverse fission and not by budding)
Culture in modified SDA with antibiotics and without actidione	Rapidly growing, white/gray/gray-brown cottony growth; hence mucorales known as "lid-lifters"	Fast growth. Colony color varies in different species. *A. fumigatus*-velvety, blue/gray-green to olive green. Reverse—pale to light yellow	Rapid growth. At 25°C, grayish-green downy to granular colony with white periphery and a brown-red reverse due to red pigment diffusion At 37°C, no pigment production
Microscopy in Lacto Phenol cotton blue	• Hyaline, broad aseptate hyphae are present in all species • *Rhizopus spp.*—Rhizoids (roots) at the point where sporangiophore develops. Globose sporangia • *Mucor spp.*—Branched sporangiophores with no rhizoids	Smooth conidiophores with single row of phialides covering the upper half of vesicle	• 25°C—short, smooth conidiophores, smooth oval lemon shaped conidia • 37°C—ovoid or elongate yeast cells with a transverse septum
Histopathology	Hallmark is angioinvasion. Thin walled, aseptate broad hyphae amidst necrosis. As hyphae are fragile, collapse and appear as ring or oval shaped in cross sections **(Fig. 18)**	• Primary cutaneous in immuno-competent—well-developed granulomatous reaction with less number of hyphae • Severe/invasive forms—numerous hyphae seen in the dermis around necrotic foci • Hyphae are septate with acute angle branching. Angioinvasion seen	• In immunocompetent—granulomatous and suppurative reaction—yeast-like cells are seen within macrophages • Immunosuppressed—no granuloma formation, necrotizing reaction • Yeast cells are seen in plenty within foamy macrophages and extracellularly in sausage forms
	HPE differential diagnosis—Basidiobolomycosis, conidiobolomycosis—absent angioinvasion; presence of Splendore–Hoeppli phenomenon	HPE differential diagnosis—mucormycosis, Fusariosis, penicilliosis, Scedosporiosis	HPE differential diagnosis—lepromatous leprosy, leishmaniasis, histoplasmosis
Treatment	Early diagnosis and prompt treatment with multi-disciplinary approach. Surgical debridement with correction of the underlying predisposing factors. IV Amphotericin B, posaconazole, isavuconazole	• Liposomal amphotericin B, Voriconazole, posaconazole, itraconazole • Second-line choice in invasive aspergillosis—Caspofungin	Amphotericin B, Itraconazole

hyphae→ hematogenous dissemination to kidneys, brain, liver, spleen, skin, eyes, heart, and bone.

Allergic or noninvasive forms—pathogenesis not well-defined.

Inoculation post-trauma/burns/surgical wounds/contact with infected arm boards, external catheter sites.

Clinical Features

- Superficial, allergic, noninvasive and invasive aspergillosis can occur.
- *Superficial*: Onychomycosis, otomycosis
- *Various clinical presentations*: Pulmonary, cutaneous, other systems (sinusitis, cerebral, endocarditis, septic arthritis/osteomyelitis, endophthalmitis
- *Pulmonary*: Allergic bronchopulmonary aspergillosis (ABPA), aspergilloma, invasive aspergillosis
- *Cutaneous*:
  - Primary—papules, nodules, plaques, necrotic ulcers, Molluscum contagiosum like umbilicated papules have been described in patients with AIDS.
  - Secondary—result from hematogenous dissemination – often associated with pulmonary aspergillosis; necrotic ulcers seen.

Differential Diagnosis

Cutaneous: Ecthyma gangrenosum, mucormycosis, cryptococcosis, phaeohyphomycosis.

Laboratory diagnosis and treatment is given in **Table 3**.

Talaromycosis[26]

Synonyms: Earlier penicilliosis

Nomenclature: New Latin, equivalent to Latin *penicill(us)—brush,* Greek *osis*—condition

History: *Penicillium marneffi* was isolated from bamboo rats in 1956. First human infection was seen in Gabriel Segretain, a researcher at Pasteur Institute of Paris, due to accidental inoculation in 1959. He named the organism as "*Penicillium marneffi*" in honor of the Director, Dr Hubert Marneffe. First natural human infection was reported in 1973.

P. marneffi has been transferred to Talaromyces recently and is now called as "*Talaromyces marneffi.*"

Etiology: *Talaromyces marneffi* is the only known thermally dimorphic species of "Penicillium."

Geographic distribution: Endemic in Southeast Asia, Southern China, Thailand, Hong Kong, northeastern India. It is an AIDS-defining illness. Third most frequent opportunistic pathogen in endemic regions.

Epidemiology: Ecologic niche is uncertain. It has been found in the feces, liver, lung, and spleen of bamboo rats. Soil exposure is considered as risk factor. However, has not been isolated from soil. Males > Females.

Risk factors: Persons with AIDS with CD4 <200/μL, hematological malignancy/solid organ transplant/collagen vascular disease on immunosuppression.

Pathogenesis

- Inhalation of conidia, inoculation, and ingestion are modes of transmission
- Inhalation of arthroconidia → alveoli → conversion to yeast → macrophages engulf → reticuloendothelial system → affects lymph nodes, liver, spleen, bone marrow, bone, skin, and lungs.

Clinical Features

- Clinical manifestations may be due to primary infection, reinfection or reactivation of latent infection.
- *Pulmonary disseminated penicilliosis*: Fever, cough, weight loss, anemia, lymphadenopathy, hepatosplenomegaly.
- *Cutaneous*: Lesions seen in 85% of patients.
- Papules with and without umbilication/necrotic papules found on the face - forehead, pinnae, trunk and upper extremities. Nodules, pustules may be present.
- *Bone*: Osteolytic lesions
- *Multiorgan dissemination*: Bone, bone marrow, adrenals, liver, lung, kidney, meninges, pericardium, skin.

Differential Diagnosis

- *Cutaneous*: MC-like lesions in histoplasmosis, cryptococcosis, histoid Hansens, aspergillosis
- *Systemic*: Tuberculosis, histoplasmosis, pneumocystosis, cryptococcosis.

Laboratory diagnosis and treatment are given in **Table 3**.

Cryptococcosis[27]

Synonyms: European blastomycosis, Torulopsis, Busse-Buschke disease

Nomenclature: Greek, *Kruptos* - hidden; modern Latin- *coccus* from *Kokkos*-berry; Greek—*osis*—condition

History: 1894—organism was first reported by Sanfelice; first reported as pathogenic organism in human beings by Otto Busse and Buschke.

Etiology: 37 species. Most common is *Cryptococcus neoformans. C. neoformans var. grubbi* is the main cause of cryptococcosis associated with AIDS. *C. neoformans var neoformans* is less common. Others—*C. gatti, C. albidus, C. laurentti.*

Geographic distribution: Worldwide.

Epidemiology: *C. neoformans* is found in soil mixed with pigeon droppings. *C. gatti* is seen in the decayed Eucalyptus trees. Males >Females.

Risk factors: AIDS, Hodgkin's lymphoma, solid organ transplantation, systemic corticosteroid therapy for collagen vascular disease, sarcoidosis, etc.

Pathogenesis

Incubation period: 2–4 weeks; Desiccated yeast cells → inhalation → alveoli → localized in immunocompetent → dormant → weak immunity → reactivation. Immunosuppression → dissemination to CNS, eye, skin, bone - AIDS defining illness

Clinical Features

Five forms—pulmonary, CNS, visceral, cutaneous, and osseous.

Cutaneous: Primary due to traumatic inoculation is rare - solitary, exposed site; Secondary in disseminated cryptococcosis. Asymptomatic papules, molluscum contagiosum such as umbilicated papules, nodules, pustules, abscess, plaques, ulcer, grouped vesicles, cellulitis.

Most common sites: Scalp, face and neck.

CNS: Most common clinical form—meningitis, cryptococcoma.

Differential Diagnosis

Cutaneous—histoplasmosis, histoid Hansen, penicilliosis, other deep mycoses, Kaposi's sarcoma

Laboratory diagnosis and treatment are given in **Table 4**.

Candidiasis[28]

Synonyms: Moniliasis

TABLE 4: Laboratory diagnosis and treatment of opportunistic mycoses caused by yeasts.

Title	*Cryptococcosis*	*Candidiasis*
Specimen	Touch smear—exudates, pus, skin lesion, Bx tissue, sputum, BAL fluid, CSF, blood, urine	Touch smear/skin scraping, CSF, urine
Direct microscopy	• Indian Ink—budding yeast cells with the refractile capsule seen as a distinct clear halo • Gram stain—crystal violet yeast cells with the capsule seen as a faint red halo • Mucicarmine stain, Alcian blue stain	• KOH—budding yeast cells and pseudohyphae • Gram stain, Wright's stain, Giemsa stain
Culture in modified SDA with antibiotics and without actidione	• Yeast like, mucoid , cream colony • Microscopy in LPCB—budding yeast cells	• *C. albicans*—cream colored, glistening smooth, pasty colony • Species identification is based on germ tube formation, sugar fermentation and assimilation tests
Histopathology	• Two types —*Granulomatous* reaction with less number of yeast cells and *Gelatinous* reaction—numerous organisms with very little tissue reaction • Capsule does not stain with H&E/PAS. It contains acid mucopolysaccharides • Methylene blue—stains metachromatic purple; Alcian blue—blue, Mucicarmine—red	Organisms are better visualized in special stains—PAS and GMS. Aggregates of hyphae and spores seen in the dermis at sites of vascular damage/within microabscess
Treatment	Amphotericin B, fluconazole	Amphotericin B, voriconazole, itraconazole, caspofungin

(BAL: bronchoalveolar lavage; CSF: cerebrospinal fluid; GMS: Gomori methenamine silver; LPCB: lactophenol cotton blue; PAS: periodic acid-Schiff)

Nomenclature: Latin *Candidus*—white; Greek—asis to mean disease/morbid condition

History: 4th Century BC—First description as oral thrush by Hippocrates

1839—Lagenbeck described yeast-like organism

Etiology: 163 species—7 are common.

Candida albicans (most common*), C. krusei C. tropicalis, C. glabrata, C. parapsilosis, C. dubliniensis, C. guilliermondii.*

Geographic distribution: Worldwide

Epidemiology: *Candida* species are endogenous commensals present in the skin and mucosa. Some are present in the environment—Soil, water, plants, and sewage sludge.

Risk factors for invasive candidiasis: ICU patients—Burns, major surgeries (GIT/Cardiothoracic/sold organ transplants), prematurity/low birth weight <1.500 g.

Systemic steroids, cytotoxic therapy, profound neutropenia, intravascular catheters for TPN, mechanical ventilation, prolonged broad-spectrum antibiotics.

Pathogenesis: Invasive candidiasis is mainly nosocomial. Commensal strain → immunocompromised host status → pathogenic-colonization → hematogenous dissemination.

Clinical Features

Acute/chronic disseminated candidiasis: Triad of fever, rash and muscle tenderness; candidemia, urinary tract candidiasis, CNS candidiasis, endocarditis, endophthalmitis, peritonitis, osteomyelitis, pancreatitis, pulmonary.

Skin: Erythematous to violaceous papules, nodules—single or grouped on the trunk and extremities.

Differential Diagnosis

Tuberculosis, malignancy.

Laboratory diagnosis and treatment are given in **Table 4**.

KEY POINTS

- Deep mycoses include subcutaneous mycoses and systemic mycoses which is further divided into endemic mycoses and the opportunistic mycoses.
- Clinical morphology, characteristic KOH wet mount findings and histopathology in H&E and special stains help to arrive at the diagnosis of deep mycoses. At times, a high degree of clinical suspicion is essential.
- Subcutaneous mycoses or implantation mycoses, which occur after trivial trauma, are characterized by long incubation periods. Mycetoma, phaeohyphomycosis, chromoblastomycosis, rhinosporidiosis, entomophthoromycosis and sporotrichosis occur in India with a varied prevalence in the different geographic regions of the country.
- Endemic mycoses are rare in India. Sporadic or imported cases have been reported. Histoplasmosis is more common than blastomycosis and coccidioidomycoses. Paracoccidioidomycosis has not been reported in India.
- Opportunistic mycoses caused by molds and yeasts are on the rise due to the increase in the immunosuppressive states. Early diagnosis and prompt treatment would help to save the life and decrease the morbidity in these patients.

REFERENCES

1. Chander J. Mycetoma. In: Textbook of Medical Mycology, 4th edition. New Delhi: Jaypee Bothers Medical Publishers; 2018. pp. 203-28.
2. Fahal HA. Mycetoma. Khartoum Med J. 2011;4(1):514-23.
3. Relhan V, Mahajan K, Agarwal P, Garg VK. Mycetoma: an update. Indian J Dermatol. 2017;62:332-40.
4. Perfect JR, Schell WA, Cox GM. Phaeohyphomycosis. In: Dismukes WA, Pappas PG, Sobel JD (Eds). Clinical Mycology. New York: Oxford University Press; 2003. pp. 571-82.
5. Binesh F, Ayatollahi J, Behniafard N, Moghimi M, Vajihinejad M. Phaeohyphomycosisin an immunocompetent host: case report and literature review. Br JMed Med Res. 2016;14(7):1-5.
6. Krzyściak PM, Piaszczyńska MP, Piaszczy M. Chromoblastomycosis. Postep Derm Allergol. 2014;31(5):310-21.
7. Madhu R. Basidiobolomycosis. Indian J Pract Pediatr. 2012;14(3):351-7.
8. Ibrahim AS, Edwards Jr JE, Filler SG, Spellberg B. Mucormycosis and entomophthoramycosis (zygomycosis). In: Kauffman CA, Pappas PG, Sobel J, Dismukes WE (Eds). Essentials of Clinical Mycology, 2nd edition. New York: Springer Science Business Media; 2011. pp. 265-80.
9. Sentamilselvi G. Entomophthoromycosis. In: Sentamilselvi G, Janaki VR, Janaki C (Eds). The Handbook of Dermatomycology and Colour Atlas, 1st edition. Chennai: Dr. G. Sentamilselvi; 2006. pp. 31-41.
10. Reiss E, Shadomy JH, Lyon GM. Sporotrichosis. In: Fundamentals of Medical Mycology. New Jersey: Wiley-Blackwell; 2012. pp. 215-32.
11. Mahajan VK. Sporotrichosis: an overview and therapeutic options. Dermatol Res and Pract. 2014;2014:272376.
12. Geoffrey S Gottlieb, Cammie F. Lesser King K. Holmes, Anna Wald. Disseminated Sporotrichosis associated with treatment with immunosuppressants and tumor necrosis factor-α antagonists. Clinical Infectious Diseases. 2003;37(6):838-40.
13. Chander J. Rhinosporidiosis. In: Textbook of Medical Mycology, 4th edition. New Delhi: Jaypee Brothers Medical Publishers; 2018. pp. 811-27.
14. Tiwari R, Karthik K, Dhama K, Shabbir MZ, Khurana SK. Rhinosporidiosis: a riddled disease of man and animals. Adv Anim Vet Sci. 2015;3(2s):54-63.
15. Francesconi VA, Klein AP, Ana Paula Botelho Gualda Santos, Ramasawmy R, Francesconi F. Lobomycosis: epidemiology, clinical presentation, and management options. Ther Clin Risk Manag. 2014;10:851-60.
16. Raina RK, Mahajan V, Sood A, Saurabh S. Primary cutaneous histoplasmosis in an immunocompetent host from a nonendemic area. Indian J Dermatol. 2016;61:46-71.
17. Malhotra S, Dhundial R, Kaur NJK, Kaushal M, Duggal N. Cutaneous histoplasmosis and role of direct microscopy: a case report. Clin Microbiol. 2017;6(2):276.
18. Bradsher RW, Bariola JR. Blastomycosis. In: Kauffman CA, Pappas PG, Sobel JD, Dismukes WE (Eds). Essentials of Clinical Mycology, 2nd edition. New York: Springer Science Business Media. 2011; pp. 336-48.
19. Balasaraswathy P, Theerthanath. Cutaneous blastomycosis presenting as non-healing ulcer and responding to oral ketoconazole. Dermatol Online J. 2003;9(5):19.
20. Garcia SC, Alanis JC, Flores MG, Gonzalez SE, Cabrera LV, Candiani JO. Coccidioidomycosis and the skin: a comprehensive review. An Bras Dermatol. 2015;90(5):610-21.
21. Norton SA. Deep fungal skin diseases. In: James WD (Specialty Editor, MilitaryDermatology), Brigadier General Zajtchuk (Editor-in-Chief). Textbook of Military Medicine, Part III Disease and the Environment, 1st edition. Washington DC: TMM Publications; 1994. pp. 453-92.
22. Reiss E, Shadomy JH, Lyon GM. Paracoccidioidomycosis. In: Fundamentals of Medical Mycology. New Jersey: Wiley-Blackwell; 2012. pp. 187-200.
23. María Perusquía-Ortiz A, Vázquez-González D, Bonifaz A. Opportunistic filamentous mycoses: aspergillosis, mucormycosis, phaeohyphomycosis and hyalohyphomycosis. Journal der Deutschen Dermatologischen Gesellschaft. 2012;10:611-21.
24. Castrejon-Perez A, Welsh EC, Miranda I, Ocampo-Candiani J, Welsh O. Cutaneous mucormycosis. An Bras Dermatol. 2017;92(3):304-11.
25. Bernardeschi C, Foulet F, Ingen-Housz-Oro S, Ortonne N, Sitbon K, Quereux G, et al. Cutaneous invasive aspergillosis: retrospective multicenter study of the French Invasive-Aspergillosis Registry and Literature Review. Medicine (Baltimore). 2015;94(26):e1018.
26. Duong TA. Infection due to *Penicillium marneffei*, an emerging pathogen: review of 155 reported cases. Clin Infect Dis. 1996; 23(1):125-30.
27. Negroni R. Cryptococcosis. Clin Dermatol. 2012;30(6):599-609.
28. Sobel JD, Revanker SG. Systemic candidiasis: symptoms, diagnosis and treatment. BMJ Best Pract. 2018:2-9.

EXAMINATION QUESTIONS

Write short notes on the following:

1. Management of mycetoma.
2. Actinomycetoma vs. eumycetoma.
3. Mucormycosis.
4. Subcutaneous zygomycosis.
5. Approach to a case of mycetoma.

44 CHAPTER

Overview of Common Dermatologic Viral Diseases and their Causative Agents

Sudip Das, Yashpal Manchanda, Loknath Ghosal

INTRODUCTION

Viruses are a type of microorganism made of deoxyribonucleic acid (DNA) and ribonucleic acid (RNA), which basically consist of long protein molecules.[1,2] These are enclosed in a protein envelope known as capsid. They are capable of rapidly multiplying within living cells of not only plants and animals, but even in microorganism such as bacteria and parasites. These are known to cause several illnesses called viral infections. There are two main groups of viruses: (1) DNA, and (2) RNA. DNA viruses include adenovirus, herpes virus, pox, papova, and parvovirus. RNA viruses comprise arenavirus, coronavirus, orthomyxovirus, picornavirus, paramyxovirus, reovirus, and others. The virus groups involved in the causation of dermatological disease are summarized in **Table 1**.

Transmission: The skin can be affected mainly by three ways:

1. Direct inoculation
2. Systemic infection
3. Spread from internal focus

Viruses may also be classified according to their mode of transmission as: arthropod-borne viruses, fecal-oral viruses, respiratory viruses, venereal viruses, and contact (penetrating wound) viruses.

Pathogenesis: There are three ways by which the body handles a viral infection:

1. The most common mechanism is an acute infection followed by immune mechanism and viral clearance, e.g., measles.
2. Second mechanism is that of acute infection followed by latent infection. From time to time, a latent virus can become active (reactivation), new virions are produced, and other cells are infected, e.g., herpes virus infection.
3. A third mechanism is that of chronic infection as with human immunodeficiency virus (HIV).

Virus groups causing dermatological diseases:[3,4] The virus groups involved in causation of dermatological disease are enumerated in **Table 1**.

VIRAL EXANTHEMS

Widespread exanthems can be a manifestation of viral infections that cause a viremia.[5] The process starts with the arrival of blood-borne virus particles into the skin, where they lodge in dermal capillary loops. In the dermal capillaries, these viruses can replicate in capillary endothelium, causing direct

TABLE 1: Common virus groups involved in dermatological disease.

Pox virus	Variola virus	Smallpox
	Para-vaccinia	Milker's nodule
	Parapox virus	Orf
	Molluscum contagiosum virus	Molluscum contagiosum
Herpes virus	Herpes simplex (1, 2)	Herpes simplex
	Varicella zoster virus	Varicella (chickenpox), herpes zoster
	Human cytomegalovirus	Gianotti–Crosti syndrome, severe disease in immunocompromised
	Epstein–Barr virus	Infectious mononucleosis, Gianotti–Crosti syndrome
	Human herpes virus 6	Exanthema subitum
	Human herpes virus 8	Kaposi sarcoma
Picorna virus	Coxsackie virus	Hand-foot-and-mouth disease, herpangina, exanthematous fever
	Echo virus	Various exanthems
Paramyxovirus	Measles virus	Measles
	Mumps virus	Mumps
Togavirus	Rubella virus	Rubella (German measles)
Hepadnavirus	Hepatitis B virus	Gianotti–Crosti syndrome
Flavivirus	Hepatitis C virus	Lichen planus, porphyria cutanea tarda and cryoglobulinemia
Parvovirus	Parvovirus B19	Erythema infectiosum
Papillomavirus	Human papillomavirus	Warts (common and anogenital), cervical carcinoma
Retrovirus	HIV 1, 2	HIV/AIDS
	HTLV1	Adult T-cell leukemia, lymphoma

damage, or by inducing a type III hypersensitivity reaction that results in infarcts and hemorrhages. However, most of the viruses act as inert foreign particles, which react with circulating antibodies and sensitized lymphocytes to cause inflammation. The circulating immune complexes formed by the antibody and viral antigens also localize in dermal blood vessels, and are responsible for skin rashes. The types of exanthems[6,7] commonly seen are as follows:

- *Macular/maculopapular*: Rubella, Epstein–Barr, echovirus, coxsackievirus (especially A5, A9, A16, and B5), human herpesvirus 6 (HHV-6), rubeola virus, arbovirus (dengue fever), parvovirus B19, hepatitis B and C virus, HIV-1
- *Papular:* Human papillomavirus (HPV), Orf, HHV-8, milker's nodule, molluscum contagiosum (MC), HIV-1
- *Patches:* Epstein–Barr virus (EBV) [oral hairy leukoplakia (OHL)]
- *Petechial/purpura:* Hemorrhagic fever viruses, rubella, cytomegalovirus (CMV), Ebstein–Barr

Vesicular/vesiculopustular: Varicella-zoster virus (VZV), vaccinia, variola, herpes simplex virus (HSV-1 and -2), coxsackievirus [hand-foot-and-mouth disease (HFMD)], vesicular stomatitis virus, echovirus.

Viral exanthems: Classical clinical presentations are:

- *Measles*: Gray-white papules—Koplik's spots on buccal mucosa
- *Rubella*: Red macules on soft palate—Forchheimer's spots
- *Human herpesvirus 6 and 7*: Red papules on soft palate/uvula—Nagayama spots, uvulopalatoglossal spots
- *Enterovirus*: Painful posterior pharyngeal erosions

Pharyngeal congestion and pain are seen in Epstein–Barr, adenovirus, enterovirus infections.

Lymphadenopathy:

- *Generalized*: Measles, Epstein–Barr
- *Localized*:
  - Occipital, posterior cervical.
  - Seen in cervical lymph nodes in Epstein-Barr, enterovirus, CMV.
  - Arthralgia is seen in rubella, parvovirus (B19), enterovirus.

Eye findings:

- *Conjunctivitis*: Measles, rubella
- *Hemorrhagic conjunctivitis*: Enterovirus
- *Follicular keratoconjunctivitis*: Adenovirus

Hepatosplenomegaly: Measles, Epstein–Barr virus, CMV

Central nervous system (CNS) findings:

- *Encephalitis*: Measles, rubella, HHV-6 and HHV-7, adeno- and enterovirus
- *Seizures*: Human herpesvirus 6 and 7
- *Meningitis*: Human herpesvirus 6 and 7

Cardiovascular system: Myocarditis seen in measles, rubella, and enterovirus.

DESCRIPTION OF THE MOST COMMON DERMATOLOGICAL DISEASES CAUSED BY VIRUSES

Varicella

Also known as chickenpox, varicella is the primary infection with VZV.[1,2,5,6] In tropical climates, varicella involves the teenage population mainly.

Incubation period ranges from 10 to 21 days; transmission is commonly via the respiratory route but transmission by direct contact may occur.

Infected persons are most infectious from 5 days before the appearance of the rash, most infectious 1–2 days prior to the appearance of the rash and infectivity ceases 5–6 days after the onset of the rash. The intensity of the rash is age dependent, being most severe in the aged and in the pregnant. One infection confers lifelong immunity and second episodes generally denote immunosuppression or infection with coxsackievirus.

Chickenpox is characterized by a generalized vesicular rash with delicate teardrop-shaped lesions on an erythematous base (dewdrop on rose petal). Crops appear successively on the trunk, face, and oral mucosa. Vesicles may also develop on the mucous membranes of the mouth, nose, pharynx, larynx, trachea, gastrointestinal tract, urinary tract, and vagina. A characteristic feature of the varicella rash is centripetal distribution, the polymorphic nature, and rapid progression of the individual lesion from vesicle to crust.

Differentials include exanthems by coxsackie and echoviruses, impetigo, disseminated herpes zoster, small pox, and other pox virus infections.

The diagnosis is mostly made clinically. However, in some atypical cases,[8] laboratory support may be required for confirmation. The fastest and most reliable way to confirm the diagnosis is by doing polymerase chain reaction (PCR) of vesicle fluid or from a scraping taken from the base of a blister.

It can be prevented effectively by pre-exposure vaccination with live-attenuated vaccine, postexposure specific zoster immunoglobulin administered within 10 days of exposure, and antiviral prophylaxis with acyclovir given orally for 7 days starting again before 10 days of exposure.

Treatment of healthy children requires only symptomatic management with soothing topical antiseptic preparations, antipyretics for fever, and antihistamines for itching if present. Antibiotics are required only in cases presenting with secondary bacterial infection. Systemic antiviral agents are used generally in adult cases or in immunocompromised patients of any age.[9] It includes oral acyclovir given in the divided daily dose of 10 mg/kg up to maximum of 4 g for 5–7 days. Valacyclovir, a prodrug of acyclovir requires less frequent dosing and is given in 1 g thrice a day for 7 days.

Gianotti–Crosti Syndrome[10]

This syndrome (papular acrodermatitis of childhood[1]) is characterized by an acute onset of a symmetric erythematous papular eruption on extremities, face and buttocks, said to be caused by EBV most commonly. Other viruses implicated are adenovirus, CMV, enteroviruses, vaccinia, rotavirus, hepatitis A, B, and C virus, and others.

Most commonly affected cases are children between ages 6 months and 14 years (>90% occurring before age of 4 years). Proposed diagnostic features include: monomorphous flat-topped pink-brown papules or papulovesicles, involvement of at least three sites (face/buttocks–forearms/extensor legs), symmetry, and duration of 10 days in minimum. The exanthem can last anywhere from 2 weeks to 6 months, but typically resolves within 2–8 weeks. Negative diagnostic points include scaly lesions and extensive truncal lesions.

Pruritus is variable and mucous membranes are spared except when involved by the primary viral agent. Lymphadenopathy is variable in occurrence and nodes may remain moderately enlarged for 2–3 months.

The condition is self-limited and no treatment usually is required. Systemic antihistamines are used in case of pruritus.

Molluscum Contagiosum[11-14] (Fig. 1)

Molluscum contagiosum is caused by the pox virus known as *Molluscum contagiosum virus* (MCV) 1-4 and their variants. MCV-1 is the most common type causing MC worldwide particularly in children. In HIV-infected individuals, however, MCV-2 is the most common type. Three groups of population are mainly affected: (1) young children, (2) sexually active adults, and (3) immunosuppressed individuals.

Transmission is through direct skin contact, including sexual activity, contact sports, contact with fomites, or autoinoculation by scratching or touching an infected lesion.

Molluscum contagiosum virus contains an interleukin-18 (IL-18) binding protein, this blocks the host initial effective Th1 immune response against the virus by releasing viral interferon-γ. Lesions are monomorphic, and individual lesion is seen as dome-shaped smooth surfaced pearly firm papule about 3–5 mm; those 1.5 cm or more are known as "giant" lesions. However, a central dimple ("umbilication") is a characteristic finding. The pattern of involvement depends on the patient pattern.

Children are afflicted by numerous lesions ranging from a few to a hundred. Lesions tend to occur on the face, trunk, and extremities. If genital lesions are present, it is considered a sexually transmitted disease (STD), and in the case of children, when present exclusively on genital area, the chances of sexual abuse should be strongly investigated.

Molluscum contagiosum has a distinguishing histopathology. The follicular epithelium is involved—there is acanthosis with numerous small eosinophilic and later basophilic inclusion bodies (molluscum bodies or Henderson–Paterson bodies).

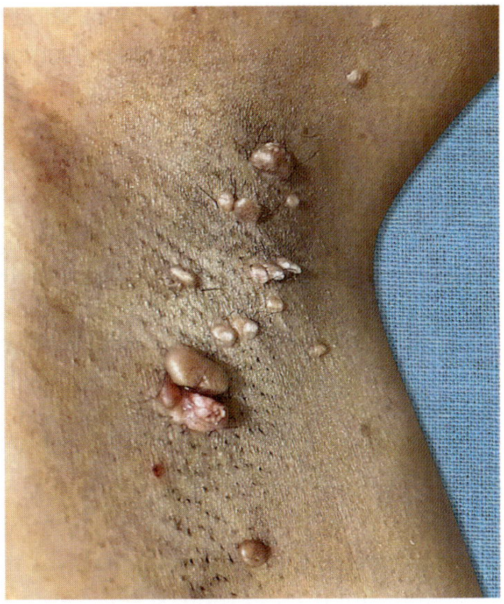

Fig. 1: Molluscum contagiosum.
Courtesy: Dr Aarti Sarda.

Treatment is usually local and involves destruction of lesions by any of the methods such as cryotherapy, curettage, podophyllotoxin, or cantharidin as first-line options based on the rapid, clinically evident response associated with their use.[14,15]

Herpes Simplex[2,3,6,7]

Herpes simplex refers to infections caused by HHV-1. There are two major antigenic types: herpes simplex virus 1 or 2 (HSV-1 or -2).

HSV-1 or 2 enters the body through small discontinuities in the skin or mucous membranes, replicates locally and affects the sensory ganglia through axons. Here, further replication occurs and the virus remains latent for indefinite periods.

After the initial infection, reactivation of the latent virus may occur during periods of local or systemic immunosuppression or stimuli (as UV light, fever). This leads to spread of the virus into areas supplied by the sensory nerve so infected previously. This is clinically apparent as herpetic "episodes." HSV infections may be classified as either "first episode" or "recurrent."

The process of infection in HSV-1 starts in childhood. Whereas, in case of HSV-2, only after sexual activity has started. Both HSV-1 and 2 can be shed when the patient is asymptomatic, unfortunately favoring enhanced transmission.

Both HSV-1 and 2 may cause oral and genital infection interchangeably; clinical presentation is also similar. However, chances of recurrence in the genital area are 10 times more often in HSV-2 than in HSV-1. In the oral area on the other hand, recurrence is more in case of infection by HSV-1.

Rapid diagnosis can be made by identification of viral antigen by either immunofluorescence in scrapping from the lesion, or by HSV DNA detection by PCR method. Electron microscopy can also be used for direct visualization of virus from the vesicle fluid.

Orofacial (orolabial) HSV infection is generally heralded with herpetic gingivostomatitis in infants. Clinically, extensive erosions with hemorrhagic crusts on the lips and oral mucosa are seen often with presence of systemic signs and symptoms. It is associated with enlarged tender draining regional lymph nodes. Fever subsides in 3–5 days, and usually complete recovery takes place in about 2 weeks' time. Recurrences of the same may occur as small grouped blisters on an erythematous base. These are often painful with evolution into pustules and erosions.

Milder and uncomplicated cases do not require any treatment. Prescribing topical antiseptics may help in reducing the chances of secondary bacterial infection. Systemic antivirals are used in more severe cases. Acyclovir 200 mg orally five times a day or 800 mg twice daily for 5–7 days is most commonly used agent. Shorter course with higher dose of valacyclovir[16] and single high dose (1.5 g) of famciclovir[17] given at the first sign of infection is helpful in thwarting the infection altogether. However, in severe cases with impairment in swallowing, acyclovir is given intravenously 5 mg/kg every 8 hours. In cases with frequent recurrences, prolonged course of acyclovir is given in the dose of 200–400 mg twice daily for 4–6 months (suppressive therapy).[18-20]

Genital HSV infections occur initially as rapidly eroded disseminated vesicles resulting in painful ulceration with lymphadenopathy in the genital area. Dysuria occurs often with malaise and fever. Healing generally occurs within 2–3 weeks. In STD clinics, the infection rate is 30–50%.

It responds well to oral antivirals such as acyclovir, valacyclovir, and famciclovir. The doses used are acyclovir 200 mg five times or 400 mg thrice a day for 5 days; Valacyclovir 500 mg twice daily for 3 days; famciclovir 125 mg twice a day for 5 days. In cases with frequent recurrences, suppressive dosages are used as follows: acyclovir 400 mg twice daily; valacyclovir 500 mg twice daily; famciclovir 250 mg twice daily.[19,21]

Herpes Zoster (Fig. 2)[2,3,5,6]

Herpes zoster is a segmental/zosteriform eruption as a result of reactivation of latent VZV lying latent in the sensory ganglia of affected cranial or spinal nerves in individuals who have previously had clinical or subclinical varicella infection. It affects both the nerve and the supplied skin. Maximum occurrence is seen in the ages between 50 and 70 years. Less frequently it occurs in younger population, especially in the immune suppressed.

Clinical onset is heralded by a prodromal phase in which dysesthesia or pain in the distribution of the nerve is appreciated. At times, it may be accompanied by systemic complaints such as fever, malaise, and headache.

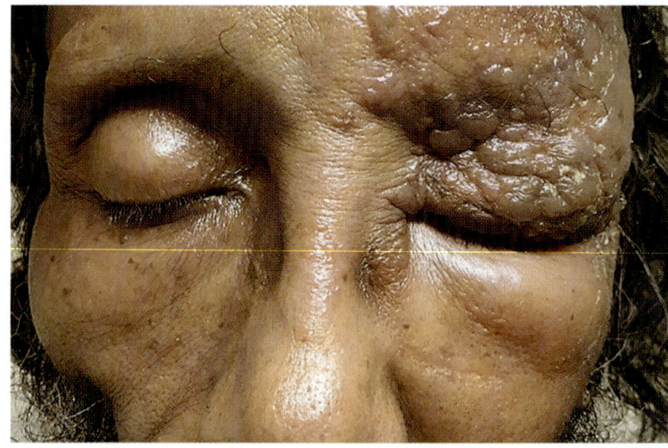

Fig. 2: Herpes zoster ophthalmicus.
Courtesy: Dr Aarti Sarda.

The prodrome is followed in 1–5 days (depend on the nerve involved) by eruption of grouped vesicles on erythematous base on the skin supplied by the involved nerve. The distribution of the rash respects the midline except in few places where nerve twigs may cross over to the other side. Regional lymph nodes are enlarged and tender. Widespread disease may represent disseminated herpes zoster and suggest immunosuppression. Healing occurs with drying, crusting and some scarring.

In uncomplicated cases, usually complete recovery occurs in 2–4 weeks depending upon the age of patient. With younger patients recovering faster when compared to older patients. Complications include ocular involvement, otic involvement (8th cranial nerve), Ramsay Hunt syndrome (7th and 8th cranial nerves), and sacral involvement (urinary or fecal retention). Postherpetic neuralgia[22] is the most common and most feared complication, it may at times last much >6 weeks.[23] Zoster in pregnancy generally is uneventful.

Preventive vaccine is recommended for individuals above 60 years of age.[24] It is usually given in the form of single a single dose with high tire of virus. Also useful in patients to be started on immunosuppressive treatment (to be given at least 2 weeks before).[25]

Treatment is usually rest and pain killers for milder cases in younger age groups. Antivirals are indicated for facial lesions affecting any age, or adults with painful lesions. The antiviral therapy has to be instituted within a day or 2, and most commonly involves acyclovir 800 mg given orally five times a day for 7–10 days. Other antiviral agents such as valacyclovir 1 g or famciclovir 250 mg thrice a day for 7 days are also effective. In immunosuppressed cases, acyclovir is used parenterally 10 mg/kg every 8 hours for up to 10 days.

Epstein–Barr Virus Infection[26]

Epstein–Barr virus (EBV, HHV-4) infects B lymphocytes and oro- and nasopharyngeal epithelial cells. In underprivileged societies, this infection is acquired in early childhood and spreads from saliva and fomites. Whereas, in developed communities, primary infection occurs in adults and spreads usually by kissing. Following a clinical or subclinical primary infection, the virus stays in latent form in memory B lymphocytes for lifelong.

Infectious mononucleosis is the most common implicated disease condition. This is characterized by initial pharyngitis. Lesser involvements include mucosal ulcerations and facial edema. Gianotti-Crosti syndrome is another childhood condition connected with EBV. Oral hairy leukoplakia in HIV-positive patients, Burkitt's lymphoma and nasopharyngeal carcinoma are other less common conditions linked with EBV. Diagnosis is by serology and examination of peripheral smear of blood.

Treatment includes symptomatic supportive therapy and antiviral agents are not effective.

Hand-Foot-and-Mouth Disease[27-29]

Hand-foot-and-mouth disease also called as enteroviral vesicular stomatitis with exanthem is generally a disease of children below 10 years of age. Causative agent is coxsackievirus A (types 5, 9, 10, and 16) and B (types 2 and 5).

Clinical features include small papule—papulovesicles located on the hands, feet, and buttocks. Associated with intraoral blisters or may be ulcerative stomatitis, especially on the hard palate.

Patients generally remain well with no serious complications, and the infection clears within a week in most cases.

Diagnosis is primarily clinical; serological tests may be employed chiefly for research purposes.

Treatment (other than mouth rinses and topical antibiotic) is not generally needed, but if severe cough or diarrhea sets in caution must be exercised.

Herpangina[2,3,5,6]

It is an illness chiefly involving children. This is caused by coxsackievirus A, B and echovirus.

After an incubation period of 3–4 days, the child is ill with sudden fever, malaise, headache, myalgia, and sore throat. Typical tiny ulcerations on the hard palate are visible which rapidly ulcerate to often become linear. The illness resolves within 4–5 days.

Diagnosis is clinical; virus may be isolated from the pharynx or stool.

Treatment is mainly supportive and usually includes topical anesthetic for painful ulcers causing problem in swallowing.

Common Warts[2,3,5,6]

These are also known as verruca vulgaris. These are hyperkeratotic papillomatous tumors caused by HPV. The lesions are characterized by loss of skin markings with a rough (warty) surface and hemorrhagic dots on paring.

The common sites involved are trauma-prone areas such as hands and feet. Periungual lesions are common on the hands. They spread by direct or indirect contact. But, to cause infection the virus needs to come in contact with cells in basal layer of epidermis. Thus, loss of epidermal barrier function due to trauma or maceration or both is a required prerequisite.

The incubation period is highly variable, and can vary from 1 week to more than a year.

The differential diagnosis of warts includes other keratotic lesions in adults such as seborrheic keratosis, stucco keratoses, and actinic keratoses. In children, they may mimic molluscum contagiosum. Other diseases caused by HPV (including types) are summarized in **Table 2**.

Warts, especially in children may resolve spontaneously. Also, procedures that are painful or cause scarring may be best avoided. Advice given on simple measures to prevent the spread of warts are turn out to be most beneficial.

Most forms of therapy have almost 50% recurrence rate. Therapy generally involves the destruction of the involved epidermis, and includes measures such as electrosurgery, cryosurgery, and application of salicylic acid plaster or collodions.[31] Laser destruction of painful or resistant cases may be tried using CO_2, erbium:YAG or Nd:Yag lasers; Imiquimod may also be tried in resistant cases.[32]

Genital Warts[2,3,5,6,33]

Genital warts (condylomata acuminata) are considered to be the most common sexually transmitted infection (STI), caused by HPV and affecting the anogenital area. These are most commonly seen in young adults between 16 and 24 years of age.

Transmission is by sexual intercourse—both homo- and heterosexual; vertical transmission in utero or during birth may occur when delivery occurs through an infected genital tract.

TABLE 2: Human papilloma viruses (HPVs) and diseases.[30]

Clinical condition	*Type*
Plantar warts	1, 2, 4, 60 ,63
Common, filiform, and plantar mosaic warts	1, 2, 3, 4, 7, 54
Plane warts + epidermodysplasia verruciformis	3, 10, 28
Epidermodysplasia verruciformis (macules and papules)	5, 8, 14, 17, 20, 38
Squamous cell carcinomas in immunosuppressed patients	5, 8, 38
Condylomata acuminate	6, 11 less often 16, 18, 31, 33
Bowenoid papulosis, Bowen disease (especially genital)	16, 18
Carcinoma of the cervix	16 (60%), 18 (20%) rarely 11, 31, 33, 35
Butcher's warts	7
Focal epithelial hyperplasia (Heck disease)	13, 32

Though the most common types involved are HPV-6 and 11, it is important to rule out infections by types 16 and 18 which have oncogenic potential.

Incubation period ranges from 1 to 6 months; clinical disease is heralded by appearance of white papules which enlarge slowly. They most commonly present as multiple asymptomatic soft, pinkish elongated papule with verrucous surface. They are most commonly seen around frenulum, corona, and glans in men, and posterior fourchette in women.

Condyloma lata, a lesion of secondary syphilis, may look similar, but are large, moist, and broad-based papules.

Prophylactic treatment with tetravalent anti-HPV vaccine early on in the life leads to reduced incidence of anogenital warts later in the life.[34-37]

Treatment includes application of 0.5% solution of podophyllotoxin twice daily for 3 days. Podophyllin tincture is cheap but is more irritating and contains various mutagenic and carcinogenic compounds. It should not be applied to the urethra or be used during pregnancy.[38]

Application of trichloroacetic acid tincture weekly is acceptable during pregnancy. Electrocautery, cryotherapy, and laser are other preferable methods during pregnancy. Imiquimod is another effective therapy.

Bowenoid Papulosis[2,3,5,6]

It is considered as an early carcinoma in situ or a pseudo-malignancy histologically resembling Bowen's disease. Bowenoid papulosis presents as multifocal pigmented macule—papules on the genital skin. It often progresses to involve the perineum or the penile shaft.

It may be mistaken for seborrheic keratosis on the genital skin. Histology is required for the confirmation of diagnosis.

Treatment involves 5-fluorouracil 5% cream, other modalities used are cryotherapy, excision, electrocautery, laser, and photodynamic therapy. Topical imiquimod is also helpful.

Epidermodysplasia Verruciformis[2,3,5,6]

Epidermodysplasia verruciformis (EDV) is a rare, autosomal recessive skin disorder characterized by eruptions of multiple and large wart on the body. These lesions are caused by infection with different HPV types among which some are known to be carcinogenic.

A specific immune defect caused by mutations in *EVER* genes on chromosome 17 causes susceptibility to infection by a series of different HPV types.[39]

Clinical presentation is in childhood when patients tend to develop widespread multiple plane warts and large flat lesions resembling pityriasis versicolor and erythematous plaques with no spontaneous regression.

Diagnosis is by biopsy and HPV typing; genetic studies are required for the assessment of prognosis. The histological findings are similar in different clinical lesions associated with EDV.

Complications include dysplastic and malignant changes in the lesions, most often located on the sun-exposed areas with up to one-third of the cases developing at least on squamous cell carcinoma.

Treatment: The patient is kept under regular supervision. General methods for wart treatment are used; Imiquimod[40] and topical 5-fluorouracil cream are useful. Systemic retinoids are helpful in preventing recurrence. Carcinomas are handled in usual ways.

HIV Infection and AIDS[2,3,5,6]

HIV infection denotes epidemic infection with human immunodeficiency virus (HIV types 1 or 2). Acquired immunodeficiency syndrome (AIDS) refers to an advanced stage of HIV infection defined by characteristic illnesses and reduction of T-cells bearing CD4+ marker (helper T-cells).

HIV-1 and HIV-2 are single-stranded RNA viruses being retroviruses in the lentivirus group. They employ reverse transcriptase with an affinity for CD4 cells, and thus wield cytopathic and cytolytic effects. Initial human infections began in Africa,[41] the Caribbean and the US during the 1970s. HIV-2 started in Western Africa and spread to India in the 1990s. AIDS has changed from being a disease of male homosexuals in the Western countries to become a demolishing disease affecting heterosexuals in India, Southeast Asian countries and later on in China.

Routes of transmission include sexual intercourse as the main pathway. With men are more likely to infect women than the reverse because of the anatomically larger surface area involved in intercourse. Blood and blood products form another important way of transmission of this virus. And, this type of transmission is commonly seen in IV drug abusers (due to needle sharing), recipients of blood/blood product transfusion, and healthcare workers (due to accidental needle prick). Also, it can be transmitted vertically from an infected mother during pregnancy, birth and in the nursing period—this is a burning problem in developing countries such as India. Organ transplantation also carries small risk.

The Centers for Disease Control and Prevention (CDC) staging recognizes categories A, B, and C.

Cutaneous disorders occurring in HIV include pruritus and pruritic eruptions as popular pruritic eruption of HIV, eosinophilic folliculitis, prurigo nodularis, atopic dermatitis, psoriasis, and seborrheic dermatitis. These are common complains with late and advanced HIV disease, especially in patients with CD4+ counts of 50/μL.

Erythroderma in HIV disease may be caused by drug hypersensitivity, atopic dermatitis, psoriasis, photosensitive allergic dermatitis, hypereosinophilic syndrome, coexisting human T-cell leukemia virus type 1 (HTLV-1) infection or cutaneous T-cell lymphoma.

Pigmentary disorders include postinflammatory hypopigmentation and hyperpigmentation, especially in visible areas. Idiopathic photosensitivity is infrequent, but might herald advanced disease. Cutaneous and systemic vasculitis has been seen to occur in HIV disease from several causes such as adverse drug reaction, CMV infection, polyarteritis nodosa, Kawasaki disease, and may be HIV itself. Systemic immunosuppressive agents are indicated in treatment.

Oropharyngeal disorders may be seen to be the presenting sign of HIV and their presence may be indicative of serotesting. Other than candidiasis (which the most common), other disorders of the lips and oropharynx include herpetic ulcers, xerostomia, cheilitis exfoliativa, OHL, Kaposi sarcoma, and papillary atrophy of the tongue.[42,43]

HIV-positive individuals are susceptible to a variety of adverse cutaneous drug eruptions (almost 100 times the general population) and prevalence increases with disease progression and immune deficiency. The onset of most drug eruptions occurred within 1–2 weeks of initiation of therapy. Co-trimoxazole and penicillin derivatives were causative agents in most cases. Systemic symptoms include fever, headache, and myalgia.

The diagnosis of HIV infection can be made by various tests done on either blood, saliva, and urine which detect the presence of either viral RNA, antigen, or antibodies against the virus. Antibody-detecting tests most commonly employed are enzyme-linked immunosorbent assay (ELISA) and Western blot test. Various PCR tests are based on the detection of viral antigens.[44,45]

The infection can be prevented by certain measures such as behavioral interventions, adoption of universal precautions in healthcare industry, pre- and postexposure antiretroviral prophylaxis, use of barrier methods, zidovudine prophylaxis in pregnant females during last trimester and at the time of childbirth.[46,47]

Treatment of HIV infection involves HAART (highly active antiretroviral therapy) and cART (combination antiretroviral therapy).[48-50]

Chikungunya Virus[51]

Chikungunya virus is transmitted by *Aedes* mosquito. Incubation period is 2–7 days. Patient presents with abrupt onset of high fever with joint pains in 40% of patients. Most patients complain of headache and severe nausea. Neuropathic acral findings such as Raynaud's phenomenon, acral coldness, and erythromelalgia are seen. Pruritic rash develops in 50–70% of patients and majority on second day. Morbilliform rash affects arm, upper trunk, and face and the rash has islands of sparing. Apthous-like ulceration can occur in oral, penoscrotal and axillary region preceded by erythema and pain. The lesions may heal with hyperpigmentation. Pediatric patients can present with bullous eruption. Virus-specific IgM is diagnostic. PCR from blister fluid also can help.

REFERENCES

1. Kliegman RM, Nelson WE. Nelson's Textbook of Pediatrics. Philadelphia: Elsevier Saunders; 2011.
2. Griffiths C, Barker J, Bleiker T, Chalmers R, Creamer D. Rook's Textbook of Dermatology, 9th edition. Chichester, West Sussex; Hoboken, NJ: John Wiley & Sons, Ltd; 2016.
3. Keighley CL, Saunderson RB, Kok J, Dwyer DE. Viral exanthems. Curr Opin Infect Dis. 2015;28(2):139-50.
4. Biesbroeck L, Sidbury R. Viral exanthems: an update. Dermatol Ther. 2013;26(6):433-8.
5. Habif TP. Clinical dermatology: a color guide to diagnosis and therapy, 5th edition. Philadelphia: Elsevier; 2010.
6. Bolognia JL, Jorizzo JJ, Schaffer JV, Callen JP, Cerroni L, Heymann WR, et al. Dermatology, 3rd edition. London: Elsevier Saunders; 2012.
7. Ramdass P, Mullick S, Farber HF. Viral Skin Diseases. Prim Care. 2015;42(4):517-67.
8. Gnann JW Jr. Varicella-zoster virus: atypical presentations and unusual complications. J Infect Dis. 2002;186(Suppl 1):S91-8.
9. Klassen TP, Hartling L, Wiebe N, Belseck EM. Acyclovir for treating varicella in otherwise healthy children and adolescents. Cochrane Database Syst Rev. 2005;(4):CD002980.
10. Jindal T, Arora VK. Gianotti–crosti syndrome. Indian Pediatr. 2000;37:683-4.
11. Chen X, Anstey AV, Bugert JJ. Molluscum contagiosum virus infection. Lancet Infect Dis. 2013;13:877-88.
12. Dohil MA, Lin P, Lee J, Lucky AW, Paller AS, Eichenfield LF. The epidemiology of molluscum contagiosum in children. J Am Acad Dermatol. 2006;54(1):47-54.
13. Lee R, Schwartz RA. Pediatric molluscum contagiosum: reflections on the last challenging poxvirus infection, Part 1. Cutis. 2010;86:230-6.
14. van der Wouden JC, van der Sande R, Kruithof EJ, Sollie A, van Suijlekom-Smit LW, Koning S. Interventions for cutaneous molluscum contagiosum. Cochrane Database Syst Rev. 2017;5:CD004767.
15. Forbat E, Al-Niaimi F, Ali FR. Molluscum contagiosum: review and update on management. Pediatr Dermatol. 2017;34(5):504-15.
16. Spruance SL, Jones TM, Blatter MM, Vargas-Cortes M, Barber J, Hill J, et al. High-dose, short-duration, early valacyclovir therapy for episodic treatment of cold sores: results of two randomized, placebo-controlled, multicenter studies. Antimicrob Agents Chemother. 2003;47:1072-80.
17. Spruance SL, Bodsworth N, Resnick H, Conant M, Oeuvray C, Gao J, et al. Single-dose, patient-initiated famciclovir: a randomized, double-blind, placebo-controlled trial for episodic treatment of herpes labialis. J Am Acad Dermatol. 2006;55:47-53.
18. Cernik C, Gallina K, Brodell RT. The treatment of herpes simplex infections: an evidence-based review. Arch Intern Med. 2008;168:1137-44.
19. Gilbert SC. Management and prevention of recurrent herpes labialis in immunocompetent patients. Herpes. 2007;14: 56-61.
20. Tyring SK, Baker D, Snowden W. Valacyclovir for herpes simplex virus infection: long-term safety and sustained efficacy after 20 years' experience with acyclovir. J Infect Dis. 2002;186 (Suppl 1): S40-6.
21. Patel R, Kennedy OJ, Clarke E, Geretti A, Nilsen A, Lautenschlager S, et al. 2017 European Guidelines for the Management of Genital Herpes. Int J STD AIDS. 2017;28(14):1366-79.

22. Argoff CE. Review of current guidelines on the care of postherpetic neuralgia. Postgrad Med. 2011;123:134-42.
23. Nalamachu S, Morley-Forster P. Diagnosing and managing postherpetic neuralgia. Drugs Aging. 2012;29:863-9.
24. Cunningham AL, Lal H, Kovac M, Chlibek R, Hwang SJ, Díez-Domingo J, et al. Efficacy of the Herpes Zoster Subunit Vaccine in Adults 70 Years of Age or Older. N Engl J Med. 2016;375: 1019-32.
25. Dooling KL, Guo A, Patel M, Lee GM, Moore K, Belongia EA, et al. Recommendations of the Advisory Committee on Immunization Practices for Use of Herpes Zoster Vaccines. MMWR Morb Mortal Wkly Rep. 2018;67:103-8.
26. Hall LD, Eminger LA, Hesterman KS, Heymann WR. Epstein-Barr virus: dermatologic associations and implications: part I. Mucocutaneous manifestations of Epstein-Barr virus and nonmalignant disorders. J Am Acad Dermatol. 2015;72(1): 1-19.
27. Flett K, Youngster I, Huang J, McAdam A, Sandora TJ, Rennick M, et al. Hand, foot, and mouth disease caused by coxsackievirus A6. Emerg Infect Dis. 2012;18:1702-4.
28. Hubiche T, Schuffenecker I, Boralevi F, Léauté-Labrèze C, Bornebusch L, Chiaverini C, et al. Dermatological spectrum of hand, foot and mouth disease from classical to generalized exanthema. Pediatr Infect Dis J. 2014;33:e92-8.
29. Feder HM Jr, Bennett N, Modlin JF. Atypical hand, foot, and mouth disease: a vesiculobullous eruption caused by Coxsackie virus A6. Lancet Infect Dis. 2014;14:83-6.
30. Carr J, Gyorfi T. Human papillomavirus: epidemiology, transmission, and pathogenesis. Clin Lab Med. 2000;20: 235-55.
31. Kwok CS, Gibbs S, Bennett C, Holland R, Abbott R. Topical treatments for cutaneous warts. Cochrane Database Syst Rev. 2012;(9):CD001781.
32. Sterling JC, Gibbs S, Haque Hussain SS, Mohd Mustapa MF, Handfield-Jones SE. British Association of Dermatologists' Guidelines for the Management of Cutaneous Warts 2014. Br J Dermatol. 2014;171:696-712.
33. Yanofsky VR, Patel RV, Goldenberg G. Genital warts: a comprehensive review. J Clin Aesthet Dermatol. 2012;5: 25-36.
34. Lowy DR, Schiller JT. Prophylactic human papillomavirus vaccines. J Clin Invest. 2006;116:1167-73.
35. Castle PE, Fetterman B, Akhtar I, Husain M, Gold MA, Guido R, et al. Age-appropriate use of human papillomavirus vaccines in the U.S. Gynecol Oncol. 2009;114:365-9.
36. Tabrizi SN, Brotherton JM, Kaldor JM, Skinner SR, Cummins E, Liu B, et al. Fall in human papillomavirus prevalence following a national vaccination program. J Infect Dis. 2012;206: 1645-51.
37. Donovan B, Franklin N, Guy R, Grulich AE, Regan DG, Ali H, et al. Quadrivalent Human Papillomavirus Vaccination and Trends in Genital Warts in Australia: Analysis of National Sentinel Surveillance Data. Lancet Infect Dis. 2011;11:39-44.
38. Scheinfeld N, Lehman DS. An evidence-based review of medical and surgical treatments of genital warts. Dermatol Online J. 2006;12:5.
39. Sun XK, Chen JF, Xu AE. A homozygous nonsense mutation in the *EVER2* gene leads to epidermodysplasia verruciformis. Clin Exp Dermatol. 2005;30:573-4.
40. Berthelot C, Dickerson MC, Rady P, He Q, Niroomand F, Tyring SK, et al. Treatment of a patient with epidermodysplasia verruciformis carrying a novel EVER2 mutation with imiquimod. J Am Acad Dermatol. 2007;56:882-6.
41. Robb ML, Eller LA, Kibuuka H, Rono K, Maganga L, Nitayaphan S, et al. Prospective Study of Acute HIV-1 Infection in Adults in East Africa and Thailand. N Engl J Med. 2016;374:2120-30.
42. Braun DL, Kouyos RD, Balmer B, Grube C, Weber R, Günthard HF. Frequency and spectrum of unexpected clinical manifestations of primary HIV-1 Infection. Clin Infect Dis. 2015;61:1013-21.
43. Daar ES, Pilcher CD, Hecht FM. Clinical presentation and diagnosis of primary HIV-1 infection. Curr Opin HIV AIDS. 2008;3:10-5.
44. Centers for Disease Control and Prevention (CDC). Detection of Acute HIV Infection in Two Evaluations of a New HIV Diagnostic Testing Algorithm—United States, 2011-2013. MMWR Morb Mortal Wkly Rep. 2013;62:489-94.
45. Owen SM. Testing for acute HIV infection: implications for treatment as prevention. Curr Opin HIV AIDS. 2012;7:125-30.
46. Cohen MS, Hellmann N, Levy JA, DeCock K, Lange J. The spread, treatment, and prevention of HIV-1: evolution of a global pandemic. J Clin Invest. 2008;118:1244-54.
47. Simon V, Ho DD, Abdool Karim Q. HIV/AIDS epidemiology, pathogenesis, prevention, and treatment. Lancet. 2006;368: 489-504.
48. Walker BD. Elite control of HIV Infection: implications for vaccines and treatment. Top HIV Med. 2007;15:134-6.
49. Aberg JA, Gallant JE, Ghanem KG, Emmanuel P, Zingman BS, Horberg MA, et al. Primary care guidelines for the management of persons infected with HIV: 2013 update by the HIV medicine association of the Infectious Diseases Society of America. Clin Infect Dis. 2014;58:e1-34.
50. AIDSETC. (2019). Panel on Antiretroviral Guidelines for Adults and Adolescents. Guidelines for the use of Antiretroviral Agents in HIV-1-infected Adults and Adolescents. Department of Health and Human Services. [online] Available from https://aidsetc.org/resource/guidelines-use-antiretroviral-agents-hiv-1-infected-adults-and-adolescents [Last accessed January, 2021].
51. Weaver SC, Lecuit M. Chikungunya virus and the global spread of a mosquito-borne disease. N Engl J Med. 2015;372(13):1231-9.

EXAMINATION QUESTIONS

Write short notes on the following:

1. HFMD
2. Herpangina
3. Viral maculopapular exanthem
4. Approach to case of pediatric fever with rash

45 CHAPTER Leishmaniasis and Other Protozoal Infection

Kingshuk Chatterjee

INTRODUCTION

Involvement of skin and subcutaneous tissues by protozoal infections has significant impact on public health, especially in tropical countries. Among all the infections, leishmaniasis continues to be the most common protozoal infection around the world with approximately 1.5 million new cases detected annually [World Health Organization (WHO)]. Trypanosomiases are prevalent in Africa and Latin America. Toxoplasmosis and pneumocystosis (formerly perceived to be caused by a protozoa), although have a high incidence in immunosuppressed population but not exclusively restricted to them. Less commonly, amoebiasis may cause significant morbidity. Widespread tourism has made these infections break through the confines of their geographic areas and natural reservoirs.

LEISHMANIASIS

Initial descriptions of cutaneous leishmaniasis can be traced back to first century AD. In 1985, the organisms were found within macrophages by Cunningham during his study on "Delhi boil", later identified by Leishman, in the spleen of a patient who succumbed to Dumdum fever in 1903. In 1922, Henrique Aragão described the transmission of *Leishmania* by sandflies of *Phlebotomus* genus. Cutaneous leishmaniasis forms a group of diseases due to wide spectrum of clinical manifestations ranging from cutaneous nodules to gross mucosal destruction.[1]

Classification

Flowchart 1 presents classification of leishmaniasis.

Flowchart 1: Classification of leishmaniasis.

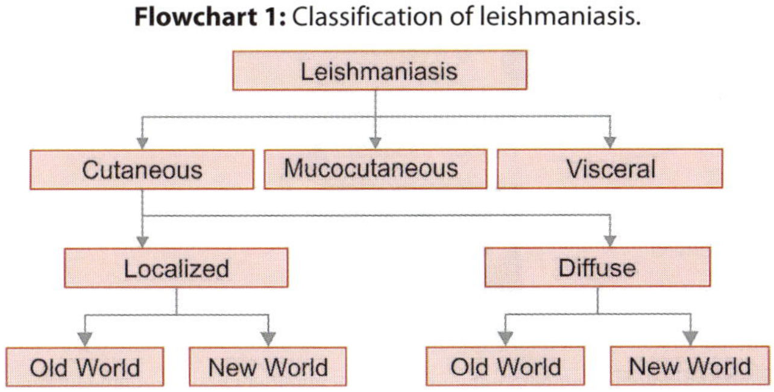

Causative Organism

It is caused by an intracellular protozoon belonging to the genus *Leishmania*. The species vary according to clinical types and geographic locations **(Table 1)**. Organisms prevalent

TABLE 1: Causative organisms according to clinical types and geographic locations of leishmaniasis.

Type of leishmaniasis	*Location*
Cutaneous leishmaniasis: Old World	
L. tropica	Eastern Mediterranean, India, and the Middle East
L. aethiopica	Ethiopia, Kenya, and Yemen
L. major	Africa, China, Pakistan, India, China, and the Middle East
L. infantum	Mediterranean
L. donovani	Sudan, Kenya, and Tanzania
Cutaneous leishmaniasis: New World	
L. mexicana	Mexico, Central America, and Texas
L. amazonensis	Brazil
L. braziliensis	Central America and Northern South America
L. guyanensis	Northern South America
L. peruviana	Peru (and neighboring countries)
L. panamensis	Panama (and neighboring countries)
L. pifanoi, L. gambami, L. venezuelensis	Venezuela
L. columbiensis	Colombia (and neighboring countries)
L. chagasi	Central America and Northern South America
Mucocutaneous leishmaniasis	
L. braziliensis	Central America and Northern South America
Diffuse cutaneous leishmaniasis: Old World	
L. aethiopica	Ethiopia, Kenya, and Yemen
Diffuse cutaneous leishmaniasis: New World	
L. amazonensis	Brazil
L. mexicana	Mexico and Central America
L. pifanoi	Venezuela
Visceral leishmaniasis	
L. chagasi	Central America and Northern South America
L. donovani	India, China, Pakistan, Nepal, Sudan, Kenya, and Ethiopia
L. infantum	Mediterranean, the Middle East, China, and Africa
L. amazonensis	Brazil
L. tropica	The Middle East and India

in America and adjoining countries are known to cause New World leishmaniasis whereas those found in non-American countries cause Old World leishmaniasis.

Vector

Sandflies (arthropods) from the genus *Phlebotomus* (Old World) or Lutzomyia (New World). Apart from human, domestic animals, i.e., dogs and horses are important sources of infection. Wild animals, i.e., tree-living anteaters, wild rats, opossums, and foxes also act as important reservoirs.[2] Life cycle of *Leishmania* has been shown in **Figure 1**.

Clinical Features

- *Old World cutaneous leishmaniasis*:
  - Starts with an erythematous papule or nodule (oriental button) at the site of insect feeding (face, neck, and arms).
  - Over several weeks, the papule turns into an ulcer with violaceous border. Subcutaneous nodules involving proximal lymphatics may be seen.
  - A depressed and sometimes disfiguring scar marks healing after several weeks to months.
  - Depending upon onset of ulceration, the disease is classified as zoonotic cutaneous leishmaniasis (ZCL/rural/early ulcerative form) and Anthroponotic cutaneous leishmaniasis (ACL/urban/late ulcerative form). The latter tends to be more chronic and lead to recidivans leishmaniasis, a prolonged, destructive, and difficult to treat form.
- *New World cutaneous leishmaniasis*:
  - Polymorphous disease with a wide spectrum of clinical manifestations.
  - Round ulcer with infiltrated border over exposed area is a typical lesion. Round, nonulcerated nodules are seen in immunocompromised patients.
  - Ulcer over the pinna of ear (Chiclero ulcer) or lower limbs (Bauru ulcer) are common in Central America and Brazil, respectively.
  - Papulotuberous, verrucous, and lymphatic lesions may also be seen.
  - A typical scar, characterized by thin and pale skin, overlying the ulcer, surrounded by a pigmented halo marks healing. Development of ulcers/papules surrounding the scar suggest recurrence.
  - Uncommon forms include—pustular, impetiginous, eczematous like, lupoid, sarcoid like, and erysipeloid.
- *Mucocutaneous leishmaniasis*:
  - Due to hematogenous dissemination of *Leishmania braziliensis*.
  - The initial lesion is followed by progressive swelling of the upper lip and nasal septum within 1–2 years.
  - A massive infiltration of the face, complete destruction of the nasal septum, and development of typical tapir face may be the end results.

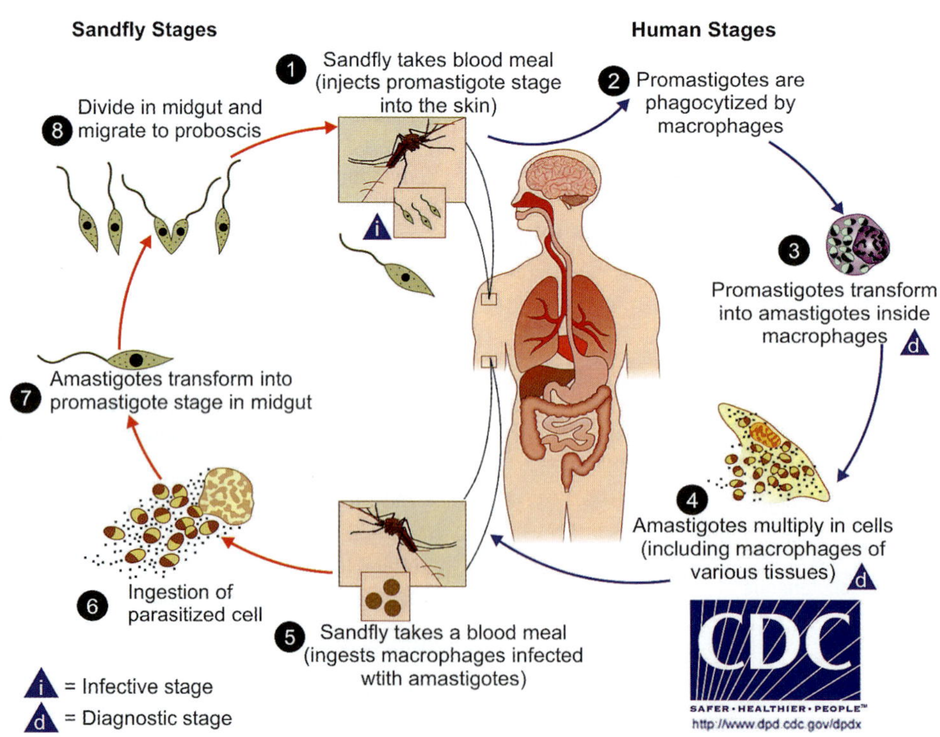

Fig. 1: Life cycle of *Leishmania*.

- Ulceration and infiltration of nose, mouth, pharynx, and lips are characteristic. Mucosae of eye and genitalia are rarely affected.
- *Diffuse cutaneous leishmaniasis*:
  - Aka anergic, lepromatous, or pseudolepromatous leishmaniasis.
  - Diffuse skin-colored papulonodules and tuberous lesions over face and the limbs, sparing the trunk are characteristic. Massive facial infiltration and mimicking leonine facies can be seen.
  - An intermediate form, known as borderline disseminated cutaneous leishmaniasis is characterized by an infiltrated, erythematous plaque over face and limbs, associated with lymphadenopathy.
- *Visceral leishmaniasis*:
  - Continuous or intermittent febrile episodes associated with splenomegaly and pancytopenia are characteristic systemic features.
  - Specific skin lesions are papules ore nodules at the inoculation site.
  - Nonspecific lesions include yellowish, fine brittle hair, purpura, and xeroderma.
  - Post-kala-azar dermal leishmaniasis (PKDL) is a sequela of untreated, treated, or asymptomatic visceral leishmaniasis (kala-azar), presenting as depigmented macules, malar erythema, nodules, and rarely ulcerations.

Investigations

- *Tissue smear*: Demonstration of amastigotes is the most important diagnostic method. They appear as pale violet oval bodies inside macrophages, in the tissue smear, collected from the edge of an ulcer followed by Giemsa staining.
- *Biopsy*: Parasites can also be found in skin biopsies or culture from biopsy sample in biphasic medium, i.e., Novy-MacNeal-Nicolle (NMN). For both tissue smear and culture, positive results are likely if samples are taken within first few weeks of infection.
- *Montenegro skin test*: A papule >5 mm after 72 hours of injection of phenol killed promastigotes into the dermis signifies cell-mediated immune response. It is not diagnostic but only indicates contact with *Leishmania* organisms.
- Enzyme-linked immunosorbent assay (ELISA) and western blot are useful to assess treatment response.
- Flow cytometric analysis of anti-live promastigote antibody (FC-ALPA).
- Polymerase chain reaction (PCR).[3]

Treatment[4]

Treatment of leishmaniasis has been summarized in **Table 2**.

TABLE 2: Treatment of leishmaniasis.

Agent	*Indication*	*Dosage*
Pentavalent antimonies: • Sodium stibogluconate • Meglumine antimonate • Urea stibamaine	Cutaneous leishmaniasis	Intramuscular (20 mg/kg for 20 days) and intralesional injections
Amphotericin B	Second line drug for cutaneous leishmaniasis	0.5–1.0 mg/kg daily or on alternate day, for total cumulative dose of 15–30 mg/kg (for liposomal formulations, 3 mg/kg/day on days 1–5 and 10; total 18–21 mg/kg)
Physical treatment (cryotherapy, thermotherapy, and curettage)	Simple lesions of Old and New World type	
Oral medications		
Fluconazole	Off-label for cutaneous leishmaniasis	200 mg daily for 6 weeks
Ketoconazole	Do	600 mg daily for 28 days
Miltefosine	Cutaneous leishmaniasis	50 mg twice daily for 28 days (between 30 and 44 kg); 50 mg thrice daily for 28 days (≥45 kg)

TRYPANOSOMIASIS

The infection is caused by the protozoa of the genus *Trypanosoma*. Depending upon endemicity, African and American forms have been described.[5]

African Trypanosomiasis

Human African trypanosomiasis, aka sleeping sickness, is an acute and chronic, potentially fatal disease.

Geographic Distribution

Southern Mali, Niger, Chad, Senegal, Ethiopia, Angola, Botswana, Zimbabwe, and Mozambique.

History

Atkins described the tale of death, dementia, and somnolence from Western Africa in 1734. Trypanosomes were detected in blood for the first time by Nepvue in 1890. Transmission of the disease by flies of genus *Glossina* was discovered by Bruce and Nabarro in 1903.

Causative Organism

They are hemoflagellates, which belong to Salivaria family, genus *Trypanosoma* and *Trypanosoma brucei* organisms of *brucei* species **(Table 3)**.

TABLE 3: Causative organisms of trypanosomiasis.

Human African trypanosomiasis	*Animal trypanosomiasis*
Trypanosoma brucei gambiense	Trypanosoma brucei brucei
Trypanosoma brucei rhodesiense	

Reservoirs

Human as well as pigs, dogs, and sheep.

Vector

Three species of tsetse flies:

1. *Glossina palpalis*
2. *Glossina tachinoides*
3. *Glossina fuscipes*

Clinical Features

- Local, pruritic, and painful indurated red or violaceous nodule, develops at the site of inoculation after 48 hours of bite by a tsetse fly—trypanosomal chancre (accompanied by regional lymphadenopathy).
- It desquamates within 2–3 weeks after a central necrotic eschar may form.
- Trypanids develop after 6–8 weeks as erythematous, urticarial, or macular targetoid lesions over the trunk. These indicate early stage of the disease.
- Dissemination of the organism in circulation leads to hemolymphatic stage, 3–10 days after the onset of chancre. It is characterized by high fever, headache, malaise, and joint pain, recurring at irregular intervals, corresponding to waves of parasitemia.
- Indolent, rubbery lymphadenopathy with hepatosplenomegaly, ascites, and peripheral edema are characteristic in this phase.
- Petechiae, intense generalized pruritus, erythema nodosum, and ichthyosis are rare complications before the onset of fatal meningoencephalic stage.

Diagnosis

- Identification of the parasite in buffy coat of centrifuged heparinized blood, stained by Giemsa or Wright stain
- Ion exchange chromatography
- Animal inoculation
- Indirect fluorescent antibody test
- ELISA

Treatment

- *Suramin*: 15–20 mg/kg intravenous (IV) per week, up to maximum 1 g in a single dose. A single course for an adult is 5 g, never to exceed 7 g.
- *Pentamidine*: 4 mg/kg on alternate days by intramuscular (IM) route for 10 doses.
- *Melarsoprol*: 3.6 mg/kg/day IV for three courses of 3 days each.
- *Nitrofurazone*: 30 mg/kg three to four times a day for 5–7 days.
- *Difluoromethylornithine*: 400 mg/kg/day IV in four divided doses for 2 weeks followed by 300 mg/kg/day orally in four doses for 30 days.[6-8]

American Trypanosomiasis

It is an arthropod borne infectious disease, also known as Chagas disease.

Geographic Distribution

Latin America (Argentina, Bolivia, Brazil, Chile, Paraguay, and Uruguay), Mexico, and United States.

History

In 1909, the Brazilian Physician Carlos Chagas first described the agent, vector, and clinical presentation of the disease.

Causative Organism

Flagellated trypanosome *Trypanosoma cruzi*.

Reservoirs

Human, domestic animals, armadillos, opossums, raccoons, rodents, sloths, monkeys, porcupines, capybaras, coatimundis, and marsupials.

Vector

Reduviid or kissing bugs of *Triatoma* species. *Triatoma infestans, Triatoma dimidiate, Triatoma sanguisuga, Triatoma lecticularia,* and *Triatoma gerstaekeri* are the principal vectors. *Panstrongylus* and *Rhodnius* are other genera of reduviid species.

Clinical Features

- Acute Chagas disease may remain asymptomatic. Symptomatic cases present with influenza-like syndrome with nonspecific symptoms such as fever, malaise, nausea, anorexia, vomiting, and diarrhea.
- Immunocompromised individuals, children with congenital disease, and acute disease present with generalized lymphadenopathy, myocarditis, hepatosplenomegaly, and meningoencephalitis.
- Cutaneous lesions in acute stage include furuncle-like violaceous lesions, accompanied by regional lymphadenopathy, induration, and discrete central edema (chagoma: cutaneous adenopathy complex), corresponding to the entry point of parasite on the skin.
- Unilateral painless bipalpebral edema, conjunctivitis, inflammation of the lacrimal gland, and local lymphadenopathy (*Romaña's sign:* Ophthalmoganglionar complex) develops when *T cruzi* penetrates the conjunctiva. Periorbital cellulitis and metastatic chagomas are seen sometimes with necrosis of fatty tissue.
- Transient skin rash (schizotripanides) is another sign of acute stage of the disease.

- A latent or indeterminate stage is mostly asymptomatic with seropositivity and one-third of them will develop chronic disease, characterized by chagasic heart disease and gastrointestinal manifestations.

Diagnosis

- *Direct detection*: Light microscopy, thick and thin blood smears, and centrifugation blood culture
- *Indirect (serologic) methods:* ELISA [immunoglobulin (IgG)] and radioimmunoassay precipitation assay
- Hemagglutination
- The WHO recommends at least two antigen detection tests for making a confirmed diagnosis.

Treatment

- Nifurtimox or benznidazole have been used in cases of acute and reactivation diseases, especially in children and immunocompromised. Nifurtimox is yet to get United States Food and Drug Administration (USFDA) approval.
- For chronic infections, allopurinol at 600 mg/day and itraconazole have been evaluated for treatment.
- The indeterminate stage requires no treatment.
- Mainstay of treatment is prevention involving sanitary education and use of insecticides.[9]

TOXOPLASMOSIS

Introduction

Toxoplasmosis is a global infection caused by *Toxoplasma gondii,* and in human, the infection is acquired by ingestion of contaminated food and water. The infection may also be acquired during pregnancy.

Organism

Toxoplasma gondii is a protozoan parasite that belongs to phylum Apicomplexa and subclass Coccidia. Three genetically similar strains of *T. gondii* have been identified, which differ in virulence and epidemiologic pattern of occurrence. They are referred to as types I, II, and III. While types I and II have been associated with congenital disease, type III has been primarily isolated form animals. Type II is most commonly found in human immunodeficiency virus (HIV) patients.

Vector

Toxoplasma gondii is an intestinal coccidian parasite of cats but readily infects virtually all warm-blooded vertebrates.

Clinical Features

- Hemorrhagic or necrotic papules over the trunk are seen in congenital toxoplasmosis.
- In acquired infections, patients present with polymorphous lesions viz. telangiectatic macules, papules, and vesicles. Lesions might resemble roseola, erythema multiforme and papular urticaria. Erythroderma and scleroderma are uncommon presentations.
- Cases of acute dermatomyositis-like syndrome have been reported.
- Toxoplasmosis can be broadly divided into congenital and acquired disease. In a typical case, isolated cervical or occipital nontender lymphadenopathy is accompanied by nonspecific flu-like self-limiting illness. Chronic lymphadenopathy along with myocarditis, polymyositis, pneumonitis, and encephalitis indicate chronicity.
- Chorioretinitis is seen in all stages of the disease.

Diagnosis

- *Histopathology*: Superficial and deep perivascular dermal infiltrates, composed of lymphocytes, eosinophils, plasma cells, and macrophages. In addition, capillary dilatation, dermal hemorrhagic foci, lymphatic gaps, and occasionally small vessel allergic vasculitis is seen.
- Immunoperoxidase stains for specific diagnosis.

Treatment

- Sulfadiazine (500 mg four times daily in adults and 25 mg/kg four times daily in children)
- Pyrimethamine (75 mg once daily in adults and 1 mg/kg/day in children)
- Clindamycin is used in patients sensitive to sulfonamides[10]

KEY POINTS

- Leishmaniasis is the most common protozoal infection all around the world.
- Cutaneous leishmaniasis depicts a wide range of manifestations on skin and/or mucosa.
- According to the geographic distribution of causative organisms, cutaneous leishmaniasis has been classified as Old World and New World types.
- Visceral leishmaniasis is followed by PKDL, an important entity.
- The Old World type and PKDL have been documented in India.
- Sandflies and domestic animals are important sources of infection.
- Demonstration of amastigotes from tissue smear is the most important diagnostic method for leishmaniasis.
- Sodium stibogluconate is the most commonly used parenteral and miltefosine is the most commonly used oral drug for leishmaniasis.

REFERENCES

1. Lupi O, Bartlett BL, Haugen RN, Dy LC, Sethi A, Klaus SN, et al. Tropical dermatology: tropical diseases caused by protozoa. J Am Acad Dermatol. 2009;60:897-925.
2. World Health Organization. Leishmaniasis. [online] Available from https://www.who.int/health-topics/leishmaniasis#tab=tab_1. [Last accessed January, 2021].

3. Dowlati Y. Cutaneous leishmaniasis: clinical aspects. Clin Dermatol. 1996;14:425-31.
4. Aronson N, Herwaldt BL, Libman M, Pearson R, Lopez-Velez R, Weina P, et al. Diagnosis and Treatment of Leishmaniasis: Clinical Practice Guidelines by the Infectious Diseases Society of America (IDSA) and the American Society of Tropical Medicine and Hygiene (ASTMH). Am J Trop Med Hyg. 2017; 96:24-45.
5. Semenovitch I, Lupi O. Trypanosomiasis. In: Tyring SK, Lupi O, Hengge UR (Eds). Tropical Dermatology. New York: Elsevier Inc.; 2006. pp. 29-39.
6. Sternberg JM. Human African trypanosomiasis: clinical presentation and immune response. Parasit Immunol. 2004; 26:469-76.
7. Stich A, Barrett MP, Krishna S. Waking up to sleeping sickness. Trends Parasitol. 2003;19:195-7.
8. Welburn SC, Odiit M. Recent developments in human African trypanosomiasis. Curr Opin Infect Dis. 2002;15:477-84.
9. Morel CM. Chagas disease, from discovery to control—and beyond: history, myths and lessons to take home. Mem Inst Oswaldo Cruz. 1999;94(suppl 1):3-16.
10. Montoya JG, Liesenfeld O. Toxoplasmosis. Lancet. 2004; 363:1965-76.

EXAMINATION QUESTIONS

1. Describe the cutaneous manifestations of leishmaniasis.
2. Write a short note on cutaneous leishmaniasis.
3. How do you manage a case of leishmaniasis?
4. How will you approach to a case of cutaneous leishmaniasis?

46 CHAPTER

Scabies, Pediculosis, and Other Infestations

Varsha Vaidyanathan

INTRODUCTION

Infestation is the state of being invaded by pests or parasites. These parasites can live on or inside the host organism. Infection is caused by microorganisms that enter the body tissues, multiply, and disrupt the normal functioning of the cells whereas infestation is caused by larger and more complex organisms which tend to replicate on the body surfaces, especially the skin. However, the term infestation can also refer to the invasion of the gastrointestinal tract by parasitic worms.

In this chapter, we will focus on the main infestations affecting the skin, viz., scabies, pediculosis, and demodicidosis.

SCABIES[1]

Epidemiology

There is a worldwide distribution of this intensely pruritic condition. Overcrowding, lack of hygiene, institutional settings, war-time, and hot humid climates are predisposing factors. Males and females are equally affected. Children and adolescents are more likely than adults to develop scabies. It has been noted to appear cyclically (7-year itch) possibly due to herd immunity.

Causative Organism (Fig. 1)

Scabies is caused by the itch mite *Sarcoptes scabiei var. hominis*. The adult mite is spherical, dorsoventrally flattened with four pairs of legs—two pairs in front and two behind. The front legs end in suckers and the rear legs in bristles. In males, only the third pair ends in bristles. The female mite measures around 0.4 mm, roughly double the size of the male mite.

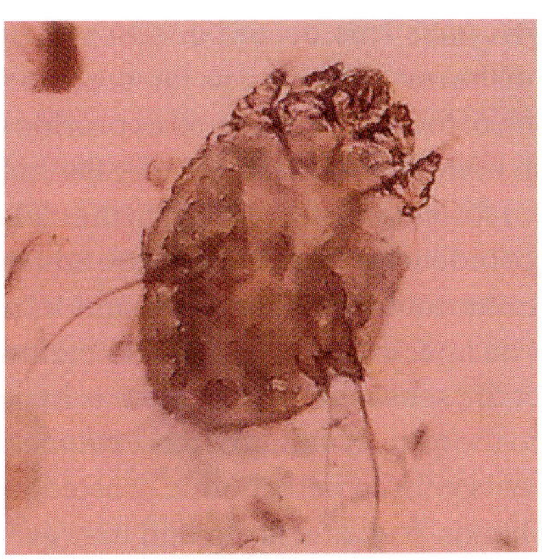

Fig. 1: Scabies mite.
Courtesy: Dr Deepali Tarate

Life Cycle

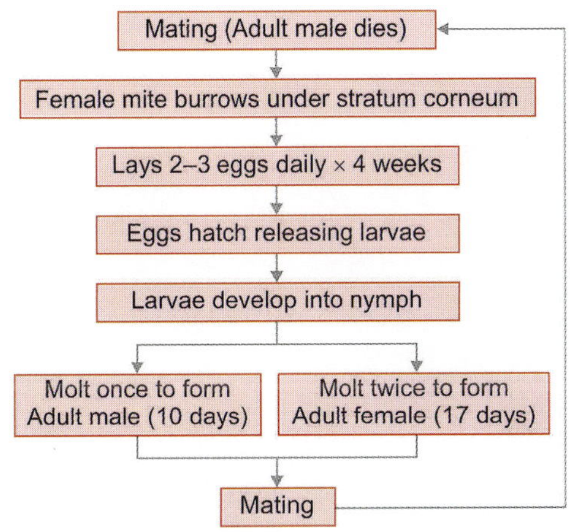

Pathogenesis

The scabies mite present in the skin (around 10–12 in the average individual) produces a type IV hypersensitivity reaction which takes approximately 4 weeks to manifest as a cutaneous rash. The second exposure may elicit a similar rash within a few days.

Clinical Features

Classically, scabies presents as a severely itchy rash worse at night. As it is highly contagious, invariably there will be a similar history among family members and close contacts.

The typical lesions are excoriated papules and papulovesicles distributed in the circle of Hebra—an imaginary circle joining the finger webspaces **(Fig. 2)**, wrist and elbow flexures, anterior axillary folds, nipples, umbilicus **(Fig. 3)**, buttocks, and genitals **(Fig. 4)**. These lesions may get secondarily infected **(Figs. 5A and B)** leading to pustular discharge and crusting. The pathognomonic feature of scabies is the burrow which is an S-shaped tunnel formed by the female mite and is blind in one end and usually seen in the finger and toe webspaces but rarely observed due to excoriations or secondary infection.

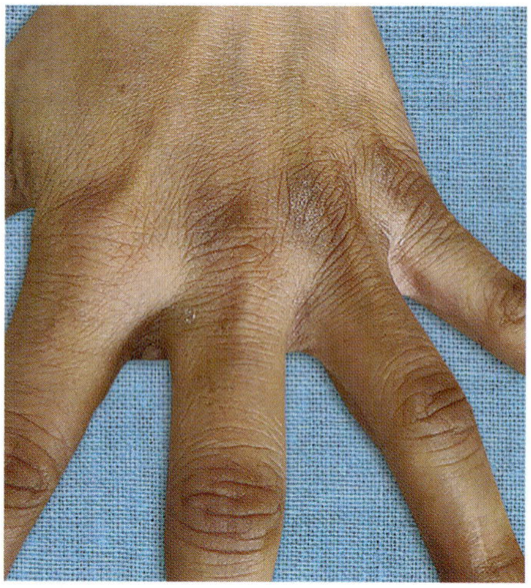

Fig. 2: Involvement of webspaces in scabies.
Courtesy: Dr Varsha Vaidyanathan

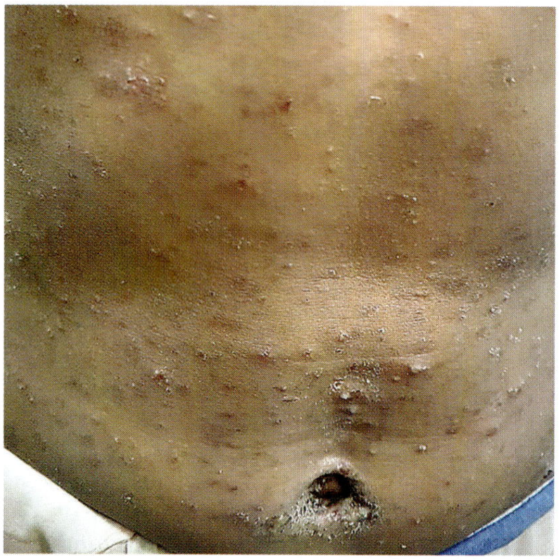

Fig. 3: Excoriated papules on trunk and periumbilical area.
Courtesy: Dr Smriti Kumar

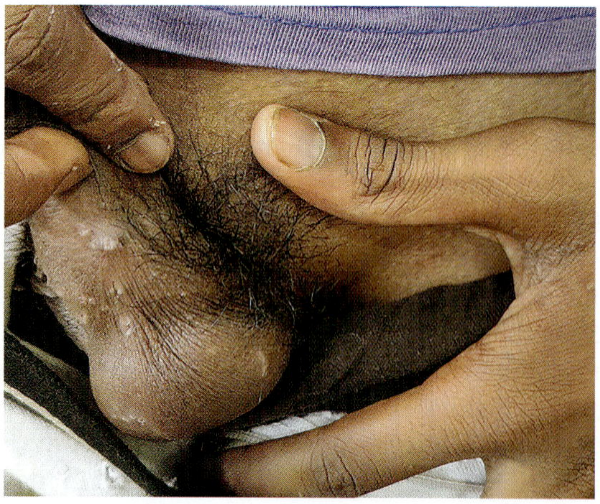

Fig. 4: Excoriated papules on the scrotum.
Courtesy: Dr Varsha Vaidyanathan

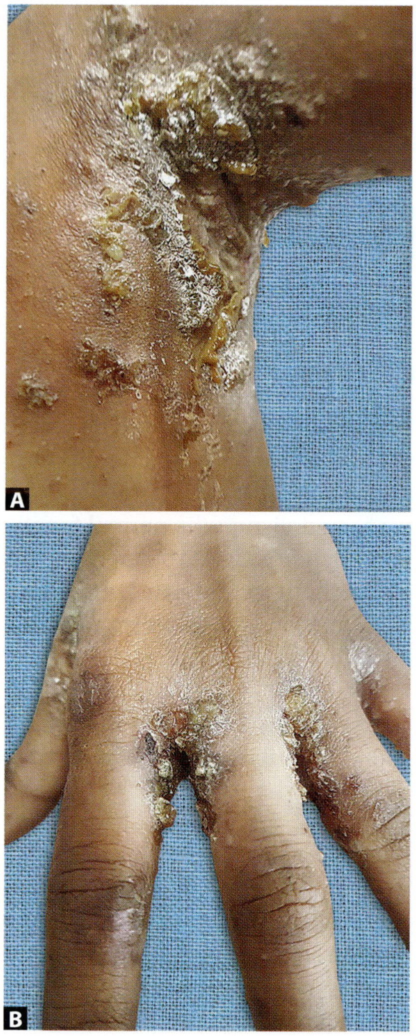

Figs. 5A and B: (A) Scabies with secondary infection; (B) Scabies with secondary infection.
Courtesy: Dr Smriti Kumar

The various clinical types of scabies are as follows:

- *Infantile scabies*: Unlike the classical type in adults and older children, there is frequent involvement of the face, palms, and soles. Papulopustular lesions in palms and soles in an infant should raise suspicions of scabies.
- *Nodular scabies*: This occurs due to a hypersensitivity reaction to the mite and persists for weeks to months after eradication of the mite. It presents as pruritic skin-colored to reddish nodules in the scrotum, axillae, and nipples.
- *Norwegian scabies/crusted scabies*: In the classical scabies, an average individual has 10–12 mites. Sometimes, in the elderly, in immunocompromised, and in physically or mentally incapacitated patients who cannot scratch or do not get the sensation of itch, there is hyperinfestation of mites to the tune of millions. It is extremely contagious and presents with hyperkeratotic crusted lesions in the flexures, hands, feet, and scalp and may even present as erythroderma. Secondary infections can cause the lesions to become malodorous.

- *Scabies incognito*: As in tinea incognito, topical steroid application leads to an alteration in the appearance of lesions and is thus harder to diagnose.
- *Bullous scabies*: Presence of large bullae—flaccid or tense—in the usual sites of scabies can be a rare form of scabies.
- *Genital scabies*: This occurs due to sexual transmission and has mainly genital lesions which are similar to that of the classical presentation.
- *Animal scabies/mange*: This occurs after contact with affected dogs and cats. Areas which come in contact with the pet (forearms, thighs, and trunk) are affected. One of the causative organisms is sarcoptes scabies var. canis.

Diagnosis

- *Clinical*: Most diagnoses are based on clinical history and examination.
- *Scraping*: Mites, eggs, or fecal pellets (scybala) may be visible on skin scraping in 10% KOH.
- *Dermatoscopy*: A noninvasive technique that reveals "jet with contrail" sign or "hang glider" sign or "delta" sign.[2]

Treatment[3,4]

Topical treatment is summarized in **Table 1**.

Ivermectin: Ivermectin belongs to the avermectin family, isolated from *Streptomyces avermitilis*. It binds selectively to glutamate-gated chloride channels in the nervous system of mites and brings about their death. It is given in a single dose of 0.2 mg/kg repeated after 1 week. Tablets are available in strengths of 3, 6, and 12 mg. It is not given in children below 5 years or weighing <15 kg.

Other Measures

- Topical treatment should be applied all over the body (excluding face and scalp in adults and older children) with special attention given to groin, navel, webspaces, axillae, and ends of nails and should be left in place overnight or for 8–12 hours.
- The patient's close contacts should be treated simultaneously to prevent "ping-pong effect" of various family members getting affected at different times from each other.
- Clothes, bedding, and towels used within the last 3 days should be washed in hot water (50°C or more) and sun-dried or sealed in a plastic bag for 1 week.
- Postscabetic itch may persist for up to a month and can be treated with antihistamines, emollients, and mild topical steroids.
- *Crusted scabies*: Permethrin is applied daily for 7 days and then twice a week until resolution. Oral ivermectin is given on days 1, 2, and 8. If live mites are still found on skin scrapings, it can be repeated on days 9 and 15.

Key Points

- Scabies is caused by the itch mite *Sarcoptes scabiei var hominis*.
- Nocturnal itching and positive family history point to the diagnosis.
- Lesions are seen in circle of Hebra.
- Dermatoscopy shows jet with contrail/hang glider/delta sign.
- Patient as well as close contacts are to be treated.

PEDICULOSIS[5]

Pediculosis is the infestation of head, body, or pubic louse in humans.

TABLE 1: Topical treatment in scabies.

Drug	*Strength*	*Method of application*	*Other remarks*
Permethrin	5%	8–14 hours continuously. Usually applied overnight. Repeat after 7 days	• Pyrethroid compound • Binds to voltage-gated sodium channels and causes paralysis of mite • Treatment of choice above 2 months of age • Pregnancy category B • Ovicidal
Gamma benzene hexachloride (GBH) (lindane)	1%	Applied overnight for 3 consecutive nights	• Organochlorine with neurotoxic effects • Inhibits GABA-gated chloride channels • Contraindicated in pregnancy, lactation and in infants • Risk of seizures so no longer recommended
Benzyl benzoate	25%	Applied overnight on days 1, 2, and 7	• Neurotoxic • Contraindicated in children <2 years of age
Crotamiton	10%	Applied on 2 consecutive nights. Rinsed 48 hours after last application	• Mainly used in infants in whom permethrin cannot be used • Has an antipruritic effect as well
Precipitated sulfur in petrolatum base	6%	Applied overnight on 3 consecutive nights	• Safe in pregnancy and lactation • Stains clothing • Malodorous
Ivermectin	1%	Applied overnight and repeated after 7 days	• Reportedly as effective as permethrin

(GABA: gamma-aminobutyric acid)

PEDICULOSIS CAPITIS

Epidemiology

It is seen commonly in unhygienic, poor, and overcrowded settings. Prisons, schools, and hostels are hotbeds for pediculosis infestations. It is more common in girls, perhaps due to a tendency for longer hair. It is usually spread via direct head-to-head contact but fomites such as combs, hairbrushes, hair clips, caps, headbands, and towels are known routes of transmission.

Causative Organism (Fig. 6)

Pediculus humanus var. capitis (head louse).

This is a small wingless insect approximately 1–4 mm in size. This has three pairs of short legs attached to a small thorax and each leg ends in a claw which can hold firmly to the hair shaft. The head has a pair of antennae and mouth parts adapted for blood-sucking. The body is translucent except after blood-sucking when it turns red.

Life Cycle of a Louse (Head/Body/Pubic)

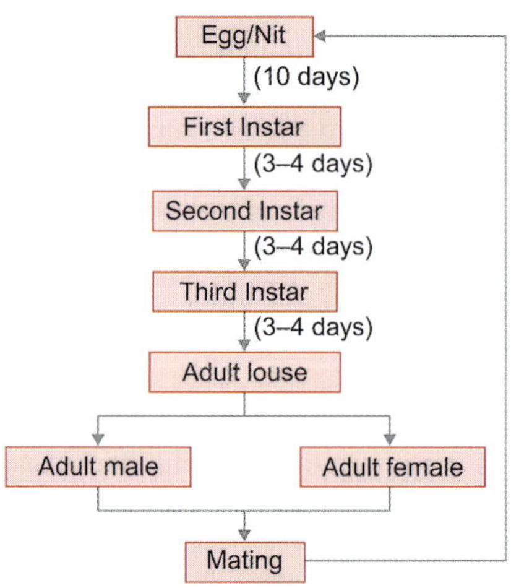

Clinical Features

Pruritus is the main feature and occurs due to hypersensitivity to the louse antigen. Excoriated papules, pustules, and scaling are seen, especially in the occipital and temporal areas. Enlargement of the occipital, postauricular, and cervical lymph nodes may be present. Sometimes due to secondary infection, the hair can get matted together to form plica polonica. Adult lice may be seen crawling on the hair. Nits can be seen attached to the hair shaft at an angle and close to the scalp (1–2 mm). A viable nit is tan in color with an operculum or opening at the free end **(Figs. 7 and 8)**.

Diagnosis

- *Clinical*: Presence of lice and nits. In a child with occipital lymphadenopathy, pruritus, and pustules on scalp, presumptive treatment can be started even without direct observation of lice.
- *Dermatoscopy* ***(Fig. 9)***: It can show lice and nits. Viability of nits can be determined by presence or absence of operculum. Dermatoscopy can differentiate between nits and pseudonits.

Treatment

- *Topical pediculocides*: These are summarized in **Table 2**.
- *Oral pediculocides*:
  - *Co-trimoxazole (Septran)*: It acts by killing the bacteria in the gut of the louse
  - *Ivermectin*: 0.2 mg/kg 2 doses 7 days apart
  - *Albendazole*: An antiparasitic drug given as a single dose of 400 mg.
- *Other measures*:
  - Wet combing with a fine-toothed comb daily
  - Petroleum jelly applied to hair and scalp and occluded with a shower cap overnight

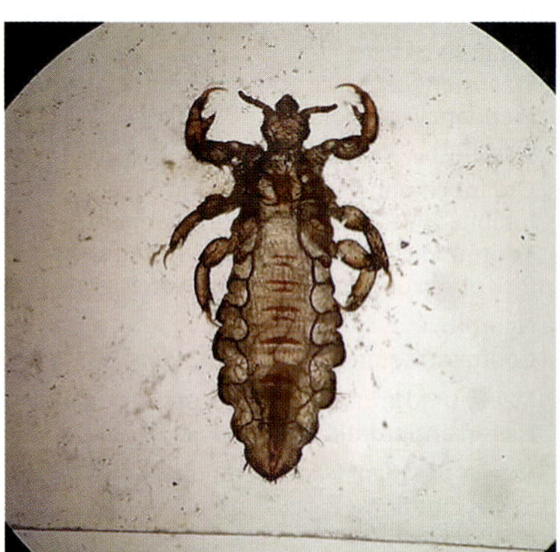

Fig. 6: Head louse.
Courtesy: Dr Divya Arora

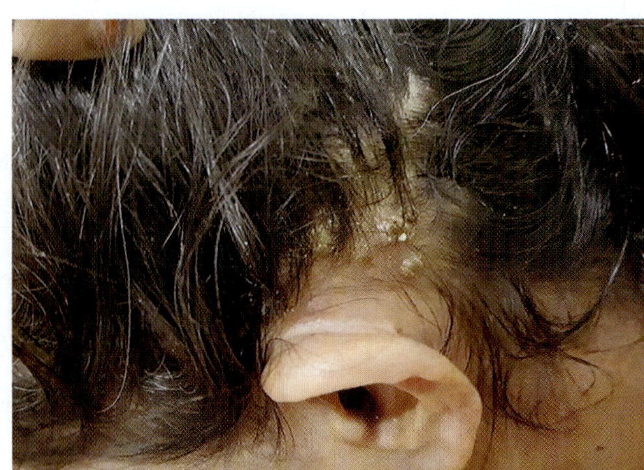

Fig. 7: Nits and pustules.
Courtesy: Dr Divya Arora

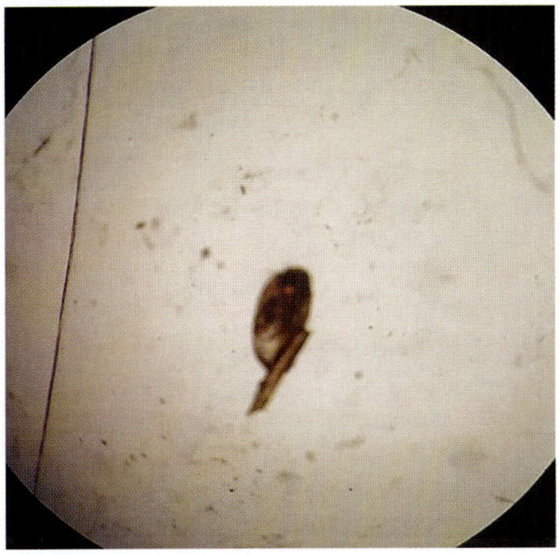

Fig. 8: Louse nit.
Courtesy: Dr Divya Arora

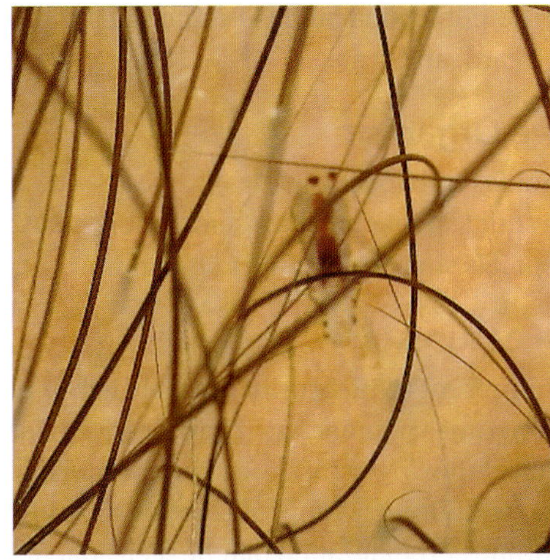

Fig. 9: Dermoscopy of louse. Translucent and engorged with blood.
Courtesy: Dr Varsha Vaidyanathan

TABLE 2: Topical pediculocides.

Agent	*Strength*	*Mode of application*	*Other remarks*
Permethrin	1%	Apply to clean dry hair for 10 minutes followed by rinsing and wet combing	• Not to be used below 2 months of age • Safe in pregnancy
Malathion	0.5%	Apply to clean dry hair for 8–12 hours	Safe in pregnancy
Ivermectin lotion	1%	Apply to clean dry hair for 10 minutes followed by rinsing and wet combing	Uncertain status in pregnancy
Lindane shampoo	1%	Apply to clean dry hair for 5 minutes followed by rinsing and wet combing	Contraindicated in pregnant women and children
Spinosad cream	0.9%	Apply for 10 minutes to clean dry hair then rinsed and wet combed	Safe in pregnancy and in children above 4 years of age

- Natural products such as tea tree oil, apple cider vinegar, and olive oil reportedly have some effect
- Maintaining head hygiene by regular shampooing
- Avoid sharing of caps, headbands, hair clips, and combs
- Pillow cases and caps should be washed in hot water
- Citronella spray can act as a louse repellant.

PEDICULOSIS CORPORIS

It is also known as vagabond's disease.

Epidemiology

It is seen in developing countries in populations with poor standard of hygiene. It affects homeless individuals and those living in prisons and refugee camps.

Causative Organism

Pediculus humanus var. corporis (body louse).

It is similar in appearance to the head louse.

Historically, the body louse is important as it is responsible for certain diseases where it acts as the vector:

- *Relapsing fever*: *Borrelia recurrentis*
- *Trench fever*: *Bartonella quintana*
- *Typhus*: *Rickettsia prowazekii*

Clinical Features

The patient presents with pruritus, especially in the areas where clothing seams touch the body. Excoriated papules, scaling, and eczematization are seen in parallel lines along the seams. The body louse lives in the clothing rather than on the skin. It crawls out only to feed.

Diagnosis

Clinically, diagnosis is based on history, examination, and finding of lice in the clothing seams.

Treatment

- Topical and oral pediculocides
- Maintain hygiene, daily change of clothes
- Laundering clothes in hot water followed by sun drying or ironing
- Permethrin spray or malathion powder to treat the clothing.

PEDICULOSIS PUBIS

It is also known as crabs since the mite physically resembles a crab. Since it is spread by close, sexual contact, it is deemed to be a sexually transmitted disease. It infests the hairy areas, especially the pubic area but also sometimes the eyelashes, eyebrows, beard, and scalp.

Causative Organism

Phthirus pubis (crab louse).

It has a squat appearance. It resembles the head and body louse except it is shorter and wider (1–2 mm).

Clinical Features

The patient presents with pruritus, mainly in the pubic area but also sometimes in other hair-bearing areas. The lice can be seen slowly moving across the skin but more often than not, they are stationary and resemble crusts. Erythema, excoriation, and eczematization may be seen. Maculae cerulea or taches bleuatres may be seen as bluish macules on the thighs and lower abdomen. These are breakdown products of blood due to louse saliva.

Diagnosis

Diagnosis is based on clinical history and examination and presence of lice.

Treatment

- Topical and oral pediculocides.
- Use of occlusive petroleum jelly which suffocates the louse by blocking respiratory spicules. It is the treatment of choice when the eyelashes are affected.
- Shaving of the area is unnecessary.

Key Points

- Head louse (Pediculus humanus var. capitis) and body louse (Pediculus humanus var. corporis) are similar in appearance. Pubic louse (Phthirus pubis) is shorter and wider.
- Body louse is found on clothing rather than on the skin.
- Pubic louse is a sexually transmitted disease.

DEMODICIDOSIS[6]

Epidemiology

The demodex mite is present on the face in most of the older adults although the density is low. More than five mites per follicle is considered pathogenic. Prevalence is low in infants and young children since they have less sebum secretion. People with oily skin have greater propensity for infestation.

Causative Organism

Demodex folliculorum and *Demodex brevis*: They infest humans exclusively. *D. folliculorum* measure 0.4 mm and occupies the hair follicle whereas *D. brevis* is smaller (0.2 mm) and lives in the sebaceous gland.

Life Cycle

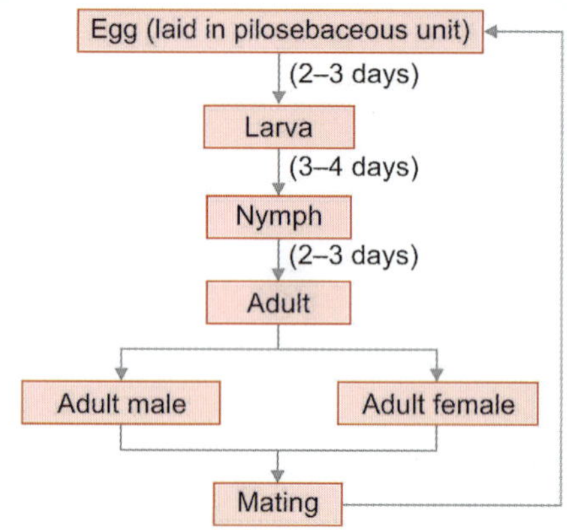

Clinical Features[7]

Primary Demodicidosis

- Abnormal increase in mite density with no preexisting skin or systemic disease.
- Occurs later in life with asymptomatic lesions seen in following patterns:
    - *Spinulate demodicido*sis: Discrete spiny lesions with mild erythema on sebaceous areas
    - *Demodex folliculitis*: Papulopustules or nodulocystic lesions in perioral and perifollicular areas
    - *Ocular demodicidosis*: Blepharitis, chalazia, kerato-conjunctivitis
    - *Demodex rosacea*: Erythema, papules, and pustules.

Secondary Demodicidosis

- Abnormal increase in mites in patients with known prior skin or systemic diseases
- Occurs earlier in life
- Immunocompromised patients.

Diagnosis

- Demodex mites identified on skin scrapings in 10% KOH.
- Demodex tails may be visualized on dermatoscopy.

Treatment

There is no consensus on effective treatment modalities:

- *Topical*: 20% azelaic acid, 1% metronidazole, and 5% permethrin have been used.
- *Oral*: Metronidazole, tetracyclines, and ivermectin.
- General measures such as regular washing of face, avoidance of greasy and oily makeup.

KEY POINTS

- Demodex folliculorum is larger and lives in the hair follicles whereas *D. brevis* is smaller and lives in the sebaceous gland.

- It is a normal resident of the human face but can become pathogenic depending on age and oiliness of skin.
- Primary demodicidosis does not have preexisting skin or systemic disease whereas secondary demodicidosis does.

REFERENCES

1. Hicks MI, Elston DM. Scabies. Dermatol Ther. 2009;22(4): 279-92.
2. Park JH, Kim CW, Kim SS. The diagnostic accuracy of dermoscopy for scabies. Ann Dermatol. 2012;24(2):194-9.
3. Panahi Y, Poursaleh Z, Goldust M. The efficacy of topical and oral ivermectin in the treatment of human scabies. Ann Parasitol. 2015;61(1):11-6.
4. Salavastru CM, Chosidow O, Boffa MJ, Janier M, Tiplica GS. European Guideline for the Management of Scabies. J Eur Acad Dermatol Venereol. 2017;31(8):1248-53.
5. Burkhart CN, Burkhart CG, Morrell DS. Infestations. In: Bolognia JL, Joseph JL, Schaffer JV (Eds). Dermatology, 3rd edition. Philadelphia: Elsevier Saunders; 2012. pp. 1426-30.
6. Rather PA, Hassan I. Human demodex mite: the versatile mite of dermatological importance. Indian J Dermatol. 2014;59(1):60-6.
7. Chen W, Plewig G. Human demodicosis: revisit and a proposed classification. Br J Dermatol. 2014;170(6):1219-25.

EXAMINATION QUESTIONS

1. Explain the treatment of scabies and complications of treatment.
2. Discuss the treatment of scabies in infancy and pregnancy.
3. Write a short note on demodex mite.

47 CHAPTER

Bites and Stings

Surajit Gorai, Preethi B Nayak, Vivek M Pai

INTRODUCTION

"Bites and strings" is a broad term, this chapter would cover topics of dermatological importance only.

Bites and stings are common and cause human disease through direct toxic effects of the venom, immune responses, and vector-borne infections.[1]

INSECTS[1,2]

Introduction: Insects are important disease vectors worldwide, and many emerging infectious diseases are linked to arthropod vectors.

Epidemiology: While some diseases have a single arthropod vector, others have multiple vectors along with additional means of transmission. Vector-borne diseases often become epidemic during war or following natural disasters, and poverty and homelessness contribute to the spread of vector-borne disease.

Clinical features: Characteristic insect bite reactions are grouped or disseminated, 2–8 mm, erythematous urticarial papules that are markedly pruritic and often excoriated, typically resolve over 5–10 days. Evanescent wheals or longer-lasting "papular urticaria," edematous plaques, targetoid lesions, purpuric papules, nodules, and vesiculobullous reactions can occur. They tend to involve exposed areas of the head, neck, and extremities. Commonly, only one member of a family is affected, as most clinical manifestations relate to the individual's immune response rather than the bite itself.

Bee and wasp stings typically produce immediate burning pain, which is followed by the development of local erythema and swelling that usually subsides within a few hours to days. Atrial arrhythmias have been reported after bee stings in the absence of anaphylaxis.

Histopathology: A wedge-shaped perivascular lymphocytic infiltrate with eosinophils, endothelial prominence, and overlying spongiosis or focal epidermal necrosis.

Treatment: Camphor and menthol lotion and gel formulations may be useful in the control of pruritus. Topical anesthetic preparations can also be helpful. For more persistent bite reactions, topical corticosteroids are often required. When topical agents fail, intralesional corticosteroid injection or excision of the pruritic nodule may be necessary. Prevention of bites is best accomplished through the use of protective clothing and repellents. DEET (N,N-diethyl-m-toluamide) remains the most widely used repellent for the prevention of bites.

BEDBUGS[1,3]

Introduction: Bedbugs belong to the family Cimicidae and are blood-sucking mammalian and avian ectoparasites. They have a flattened oval body, a segmented abdomen, a retroverted labium (sucking mouthpiece), a semicircular to triangular scutellum (dorsal sclerotic plate), and antennae with four segments.

Epidemiology: Cimex lectularius and *C. hemipterus* affect humans most frequently. Bedbugs are nocturnal. Red-brown fecal staining and nit-like ova are commonly visible in mattress seams.

Clinical features: Bedbug bites typically present as pruritic, erythematous, edematous papules, sometimes with a visible central hemorrhagic punctum. Three lesions in a row (referred to as "breakfast, lunch and dinner") are characteristic of, but not specific to, bedbug bites.

Treatment: Symptomatic treatment and treatment with topical steroids are preferred. Eradication of bedbugs from infested homes with integrated pest management strategies utilizing both insecticides and nonchemical methods (e.g., heating/steaming, freezing, elimination of cracks, and crevices) are most effective.

BLISTER BEETLES

Introduction: Blister beetles (order Coleoptera) belong to the family Meloidae. These insects produce the blistering agent cantharidin. Members of the family Oedemeridae are classified as "false" blister beetles but also produce cantharidin, whereas rove beetles of the family Staphylinidae make another vesicant, pederin.

Epidemiology: When threatened, larvae protect themselves by exuding cantharidin in a milky oral fluid, rather than in the hemolymph that adult beetles discharge from leg joints.

Clinical features: Contact with blister beetles typically results in the development of vesicles and bullae within 12–24 hours. Contact with pederin leads to inflamed skin with erythema and often pustules as well as vesicles.

Histopathology: Acantholysis in suprabasal keratinocytes.

Treatment: Avoidance is the best measure, but immediate washing with soap and water may be of some benefit.

FLEAS

Introduction: Fleas (order Siphonaptera) are ubiquitous pests and show little host specificity. The most common flea on dogs is *Ctenocephalides felis*, the cat flea.

Epidemiology: Serve as vectors for endemic (murine) typhus, flea-borne spotted fever, and plague.

Clinical features: Flea bites present as intensely pruritic papulovesicles, usually located on the lower legs. Flea allergy is common, and allergic patients tend to react to a wide range of fleas. Tungiasis (caused by sand flea, *Tunga penetrans*) usually presents with papular necrotic lesions on the feet, often located adjacent to the great toenail.

Treatment: Lufenuron, available in oral and injectable formulations, prevents fleas from reproducing and is an effective treatment for infested animals. Topical fipronil can then be used to prevent flea infestation in animals. Tungiasis is usually treated surgically.

LEPIDOPTERISM[1,4]

Lepidopterism refers to the broad spectrum of adverse reactions to caterpillars, cocoons, butterflies, and moths. Erythematous urticarial papules and macular erythema with pruritus are commonly localized to the flanks, feet, inner aspects of the arms and legs, and collar region. Ocular lesions are caused by caterpillar hairs.

Arachnids

Tick Bites[1,5]

Introduction: Patients with tick bites often present with the tick still attached. Hard ticks are important disease vectors (e.g., Lyme disease, Rocky Mountain spotted fever). Ornithodoros soft ticks transmit borrelial relapsing fever. Dermacentor ticks hidden in the scalp represent an occasional cause of paralysis. Ixodes scapularis, the eastern black-legged tick, is the best known of the Ixodes ticks, these are vectors for Lyme disease, human granulocytic anaplasmosis, babesiosis, viral encephalitis, and other borrelial and rickettsial infections.

Clinical features: Once the tick has been removed, hypersensitivity reactions at the site are common. Papular, nodular, and vesiculobullous lesions can occur and are typically pruritic.

TABLE 1: Tick control measures.

Personal	*Environmental*
Protective clothing tightly laced, snapped, or tied	Removal of leaf debris
Clothing treated with permethrin	Area acaricide application
Clothing treated with repellents such as DEET	Exclusion of animal hosts
Regular tick inspections	Acaricide-treated feed corn

Treatment: Milder tick bite reactions may respond to application of a potent topical corticosteroid; occlusion of these agents can increase efficacy. More intense reactions may require intralesional corticosteroid injection or surgical excision. Most tick-borne diseases respond readily to tetracyclines (drug of choice—doxycycline). Permethrin has been marketed as a tick repellent. The spray formulation is the most widely available form. Once applied to clothing, it is stable through several wash cycles. The combination of a DEET-containing repellent and permethrin-treated clothing is generally highly effective against a wide range of biting arthropods **(Table 1)**.

Mites

Introduction: Mites are small arachnids that range from 0.1 to 2 mm in length. The majority of mites are free-living, but thousands of species parasitize animals or plants. Like fleas, most mites lack host specificity.

Clinical features: Cutaneous reactions to mites are common and include papular, papulovesicular, bullous, urticarial, and morbilliform eruptions. Chigger bites most often affect the lower legs, skin at the edges of underwear, and the genital region. Larvae of trombiculid mites in Asia are vectors for scrub typhus, while house mouse mites transmit rickettsialpox. Eschars at the site of the bite are a clue to rickettsial disease. Seasonal penile swelling associated with pruritus and dysuria in children, referred to as "summer penile syndrome," appears to represent a hypersensitivity response to chigger bites.

Treatment: Mites inflict a "bite and run" injury, while others remain attached for a prolonged meal. Scraping, tape stripping, or vigorous washing with soap and water are all effective in removing. Definitive treatment requires avoidance or treatment of the infested source. The topical antipruritics and anesthetics, potent topical, or intralesional corticosteroid therapy may be helpful.

Spider Bites[1,6]

Widow Spider

Introduction: Widow spiders (*Latrodectus* spp.) are found worldwide. Black widows are large, shiny black spiders with a round abdomen.

Epidemiology: Widow spiders are typically found in woodpiles, in shoes, and under outhouse seats. Human envenomation usually occurs when the spider's environment is disturbed, and the spider is inadvertently trapped or pressed against the skin. Black widow venom contains latrotoxins that act by depolarizing neurons.

Clinical features: Local skin reactions are usually limited to transient erythema, edema, sweating, and piloerection. Extracutaneous manifestations are often prominent and can include painful muscle spasms (initially around the bite site, then more widespread). The symptoms of brown widow bites tend to be milder and restricted to the tissues near the bite.

Treatment: Benzodiazepines and intravenous calcium gluconate can be helpful for associated tetany.

Loxosceles Spiders

Introduction: Brown recluse spiders (Loxosceles spiders) are found throughout the world and classically have a dark brown, violin-shaped marking on the dorsal cephalothorax.

Epidemiology: The venoms of geographically diverse spiders such as *L. reclusa*, *L. laeta*, *L. deserta*, *L. gaucho*, and *L. intermedia* have similar sphingomyelinase activity and electrophoretic profiles, with a major protein band at 32–35 kDa. All contain hyaluronidase as well as metalloproteinases with fibrinogenolytic activity.

Clinical features: Local pain is frequently delayed until several hours after the bite, which most often occurs on an extremity. Cutaneous reactions typically begin with erythema and then develop central vesiculation or duskiness with a blanched halo, which may evolve into hemorrhagic bullae and necrosis. Dermonecrotic reactions can eventuate in dry, necrotic eschars or ulceration.

Treatment: Optimal treatment to prevent dermonecrotic reactions remains elusive. Most bites can be treated with rest, ice, and elevation. Intradermal injection of polyclonal anti-Loxosceles Fab fragments can attenuate necrosis in an animal model up to 4 hours after envenomation, and antivenin may reduce the ultimate size of the necrotic area even when administered up to 48 hours after envenomation. Hyperbaric oxygen therapy may decrease the final size of ulceration.

Scorpions[1,7]

Introduction: Many toxic scorpions exist worldwide. Scorpions are typically found under tabletops, in woodpiles, and in shoes.

Clinical features: Local and systemic symptoms (e.g., pain, paresthesia) are typically out of proportion to cutaneous signs such as erythema and edema, which are not usually prominent at the site of the sting. Most fatalities are related to cardiorespiratory manifestations.

Treatment: Antivenin is available in endemic areas and, along with supportive care helps. Application of ice is sufficient for most minor scorpion envenomation. Prazosin reverses the autonomic storm characteristic of Indian red scorpion (*Mesobuthus tamulus*) envenomation.

Centipedes (Chilopoda) and Millipedes (Diplopoda)[1,8]

Introduction: Centipedes are fierce hunters. They inject a neurotoxic venom through ducts in their jaws. Millipedes do not bite but can cause burn-like reactions.

Clinical features: Centipede bites may produce pain, erythema, and edema. The bites can bleed profusely and are frequently associated with paresthesia. Centipede ingestion by children can result in systemic toxicity. Millipedes do not bite, but they can secrete noxious substances that result in chemical irritant contact dermatitis.

Treatment: Centipede bites seldom require more than symptomatic treatment. Ice packs, analgesics, and hot water immersion provide similar improvements in pain after centipede envenomation.

Snake Bites

Introduction: Snake bites occur primarily in individuals who engage in outdoor activities.

Clinical features: Snake bites are typically associated with marked edema within an hour of the envenomation. Hemorrhage and necrosis are common. The presence of paired bite marks is often noted.

Treatment: Antivenin therapy is an important part of management and may be of benefit even when administration is delayed. Tourniquets to limit systemic toxicity from the venom may lead to tissue ischemia if improperly applied.

Leeches[9]

Introduction: Leech attachments occur after contact with bodies of fresh water such as ponds or rivers.

Clinical features: Leech attachment sites often become purpuric and may bleed freely when the leech is removed.

Treatment: Saturated salt solutions have been used to facilitate leech removal.

MARINE INJURY[1,10]

Marine organisms contain some of the most potent toxins known. Drowning can occur after loss of consciousness following envenomation. Penetrating injuries are prone to secondary infection. Marine Vibrio infections are more common in patients with liver disease. Sea urchins are echinoderms with fragile spines that break easily in the skin. Pigment from the spine often diffuses into the wound, making it difficult to find and remove the spine. Jellyfish stings result in immediate pain as well as delayed and occasionally recurrent cutaneous reactions. Erythematous, urticarial, or hemorrhagic streaks may be observed. First aid for most marine venoms includes immersion in hot water.

KEY POINTS

- Papular urticaria may be either localized to the sites of bites or generalized.
- Bedbugs are blood sucking insects that usually feed at night and leads to rows of edematous pruritic papules.
- Cantharidin produced by blister beetle is results in vesicles and bullae.
- Fleas serve as vectors for endemic (murine) typhus, flea-borne spotted fever, and plague.
- House mouse mite is a vector for rickettsialpox.
- Most fatalities due to scorpions are related to cardio-respiratory manifestations.
- Millipedes do not bite (biting jaws are absent), but can cause chemical irritant contact dermatitis.
- Marine organisms contain some of the most potent toxins known.

REFERENCES

1. Elston DM. Bites and stings. In: Bolognia JL, Schaffer JV, Duncan KO, Ko CJ (Eds). Dermatology Essentials (E-book). Gurugram: Elsevier Health Sciences; 2014. pp. 1720-37.
2. Asada H. Hypersensitivity to mosquito bites: a unique pathogenic mechanism linking Epstein Barr virus infection, allergy and oncogenesis. J Dermatol Sci. 2007;45:153-60.
3. Salazar R, Castillo-Neyra R, Tustin AW, Borrini-Mayorí K, Náquira C, Levy MZ. Bed bugs (*Cimex lectularius*) as vectors of *Trypanosoma cruzi*. Am J Trop Med Hyg. 2015;92:331-5.
4. Hossler EW. Caterpillars and moths. Dermatol Ther. 2009; 22:353-66.
5. Wikel S. Ticks and tick-borne pathogens at the cutaneous interface: host defenses, tick counter measures, and a suitable environment for pathogen establishment. Front Microbiol. 2013;4:337.
6. McDade J, Aygun B, Ware RE. Brown recluse spider (*Loxosceles reclusa*) envenomation leading to acute hemolytic anemia in six adolescents. J Pediatr. 2010;156:155-7.
7. Pandurang KS, Singh J, Bijesh S, Singh HP. Effectiveness of antiscorpion venom for red scorpion envenomation. Indian Pediatr. 2014;51:131-3.
8. Chaou CH, Chen CK, Chen JC, Chiu TF, Lin CC. Comparisons of ice packs, hot water immersion, and analgesia injection for the treatment of centipede envenomations in Taiwan. Clin Toxicol (Phila). 2009;47:659-62.
9. Sartor C, Bornet C, Guinard D, Fournier PE. Transmission of *Aeromonas hydrophila* by leeches. Lancet. 2013;381:1686.
10. Balhara KS, Stolbach A. Marine envenomations. Emerg Med Clin North Am. 2014;32:223-43.

EXAMINATION QUESTION

1. Write short note on the Spanish fly/blister beetle dermatitis.

5 SECTION | Autoimmune Skin Diseases

48 CHAPTER

An Introduction to the Autoimmune Blistering Diseases

Dipankar De, Anuradha Bishnoi

INTRODUCTION

Skin comprises epidermis, dermis, and subcutaneous tissue. Like any organ, the integrity of skin and its functions are dependent on the cohesion and cross-talk between the individual components.

DESMOSOMES/STICKY GLUES

The individual keratinocytes in the epidermis adhere to each other by the means of desmosomes (macula adherens). The desmosomes are further composed of transmembrane and intracellular proteins *desmogleins* (types 1 and 3 predominate in the skin), *desmocollins* (both desmogleins and desmocollins are cadherins, which are calcium-dependent adhering proteins), *armadillo family-associated proteins* (plakoglobins/plakophilins), and *plakins* (envoplakin/periplakin and desmoplakin). Desmogleins (four isoforms, 1–4) and desmocollins (three isoforms, 1–3) are always present in pairs.

The scaffolding formed by the desmosomal proteins extends all the way from the cell membrane to the nuclear envelope. Desmosomal attachments are stronger than the other type of intercellular connections, i.e., the adherens junction (formed by classical cadherins E, P, and N; alpha/beta catenins; and actin microfilaments). Over the years, it has been realized that desmosomes are as important functionally as they are structurally, and the key components of desmosomes have been identified to play a significant part in cellular signaling.

HEMIDESMOSOMES

The epidermis adheres to the dermis by means of hemidesmosomes. The hemidesmosomes are further composed of intracellular plectin and bullous pemphigoid antigen 1 (BPAg1, 230 kDa), transmembranous BPAg2 (collagen XVII, 180 kDa), laminin 332 (*anchoring filaments*) and integrin alpha6beta4, and dermal collagen VII (*anchoring fibrils*). Plectin and BPAg1 form the hemidesmosomal inner plaque. Anchoring filaments are formed by the ectodomain of BPAg2 and predominantly laminin 332. *Anchoring plaques* are amorphous electron-dense structures that are composed of collagen IV (the predominant component of basement membrane) and act as welding points for the attachment of the ends of loop-shaped collagen VII (anchoring fibrils).

The hemidesmosomes are embedded in the basement membrane that is composed predominantly of collagen IV. Ultrastructurally, the basement membrane has three components: (1) lamina lucida, (2) lamina densa, and (3) sublamina densa. Various components of the hemidesmosomes described above span these basement membrane components/zones in a way that anchoring filaments are seen to span the lamina lucida and anchor into the lamina densa whereas anchoring fibrils and plaques are present in the sublamina densa.

BPAg2 is a complex molecule that weighs 180 kDa and spans the entire cellular membrane, forming important interactions with the surrounding laminin 332 and alpha6 beta4 integrins. It has an intracellular N-terminal and an extracellular C-terminal ectodomain. The C-terminal ectodomain has both collagenous and noncollagenous areas. When this extracellular C-terminal ectodomain is cleaved off, a 120-kDa shorter segment is formed. Further degradation of the 120-kDa fragment leads to the formation of a 97-kDa molecule. The 180-kDa molecule is the antigenic target for autoantibodies in bullous pemphigoid (BP) whereas the 120- and 97-kDa cleaved chains are the antigenic targets in linear immunoglobulin A (IgA) disease of adults (LAD).

Both the desmosomes and the hemidesmosomes are attached to the cytoskeletal network and scaffolding, intricately formed by keratin intermediate filaments (basal layer keratins 5 and 14 in the case of hemidesmosomes, and keratins 10, 2 and 1 in suprabasal keratinocytes for desmosomes).

AUTOIMMUNE BLISTERING DISEASES

Understanding the mechanism of blister formation is important. A blister results from accumulation of fluid inside the epidermis or dermoepidermal junction (DEJ). Various mechanisms can cause this accumulation and include spongiosis (accumulation of extracellular fluid, seen in contact dermatitis), acantholysis (loss of cell–cell contact, seen in pemphigus group), ballooning degeneration (herpes), cytolysis (erythema multiforme), and the basement membrane zone (BMZ) destruction (pemphigoid group).

The integrity of the complex structure of the skin described above is crucial for its well-being. Either genetic or acquired defects in the epidermal–epidermal or epidermal–dermal cohesion can lead to skin fragility and formation of blisters. The autoimmune blistering diseases belong to a group of disorders wherein the above-mentioned cohesion molecules are targeted by the immune system. The formation of antibodies against these molecules leads to loss of their function and cohesion between the individual components and manifests as blisters on the skin and mucosae.

The type of antibodies (IgG1/IgG4/IgA) involved and their complement affinity further define subtle clinical features of the disease such as associated erythema, inflammation, presence of urticarial lesions, and the type of inflammatory infiltrate seen on histopathology. Also, the location of the targeted antigen determines the depth of the blisters and the extent and definition of erosions at the margin, scarring, pigmentary changes, milia formation, etc. Chiefly, the autoimmune blistering diseases can be classified as intraepidermal (antigens targeted are components of desmosomes) or subepidermal (antigens targeted are components of hemidesmosomes).

Pemphigus is the prototype of intraepidermal autoimmune blistering disorders. The group further comprises pemphigus vulgaris (PV; variant: pemphigus vegetans), pemphigus foliaceous (variants: pemphigus erythematosus, pemphigus herpetiformis, and endemic pemphigus), drug-induced pemphigus (usually of the pemphigus foliaceous type), IgA pemphigus, and paraneoplastic pemphigus. The pemphigus group as a whole is characterized by intraepidermal deposition of immunoglobulins directed against desmosomal components. The histopathological level of split is therefore intraepidermal in pemphigus. Further, subcorneal split is seen in pemphigus foliaceous and erythematosus, and subcorneal pustular dermatosis type of IgA pemphigus. Suprabasal split is classically observed in PV, pemphigus vegetans, intraepidermal neutrophilic type of IgA pemphigus, and paraneoplastic pemphigus. Eosinophilic spongiosis is additionally seen in pemphigus vegetans whereas IgA pemphigus features predominantly neutrophils.[1]

The subepidermal autoimmune blistering diseases include BP, pemphigoid gestationis (PG), mucous membrane pemphigoid (MMP), LAD, chronic bullous disease of childhood (CBDC), dermatitis herpetiformis (DH), epidermolysis bullosa acquisita (EBA), and bullous systemic lupus erythematosus (BSLE).[2] These diseases feature a subepidermal blister in histopathology, and immunoglobulins/complements are deposited in the BMZ leading to significant influx of inflammatory cells, notably granulocytes. Eosinophils are seen in BP and PG. Eosinophils and neutrophils are present in BP, PG, and MMP. Neutrophils are predominantly observed in bullous LE, DH, LAD, and CBDC.

Overall, there is a significant degree of overlap in the histopathological features of subepidermal immunobullous diseases and it is not a good tool for adequate characterization of these disorders. It just suggests that the level of split is in the DEJ, and the presence of inflammatory infiltrate suggests that the cause for the split in DEJ is an inflammatory reaction. The enzymes released by accumulated granulocytes (elastase) cause the disintegration of BMZ, which leads to the formation of blisters. The level of split in the subepidermal disorders is inside the basement membrane. It is inside lamina lucida/lamina densa in BP, MMP, PG, LAD, CBDC, and DH and inside sublamina densa in EBA and BSLE. **Table 1** describes the major autoimmune blistering diseases and the antigenic targets described in them.

Pemphigus

Pemphigus vulgaris (PV) is a chronic autoimmune blistering disorder characterized by flaccid blisters and painful erosions involving skin and/or mucosal surfaces **(Fig. 1)**.[6] PV is the most common autoimmune blistering disorder in India and can be clinically classified as mucosal predominant or mucocutaneous. It has equal prevalence in both genders, and the affected patients are usually in the age group of 40–60 years. Indian patients having pemphigus were found to be even younger than 40 years. Nearly 80% of PV patients have oral erosions, and 60% of patients have oral mucosal involvement as the initial/presenting feature.[7] In a study conducted in south India on 71 cases of PV of oral cavity,[8] the most commonly affected sites were buccal mucosa (90%) followed by palate (51%) and lips (51%). Patients with erosions extending to throat also complain of dysphagia, odynophagia, and dysphonia. A coexisting cutaneous component is present in almost half of the patients and presents clinically with fragile blisters (may become tense after treatment with oral corticosteroids) on normal or erythematous skin, which rupture rapidly to form raw erosions that spread centrifugally. Pustules as the primary lesions can be seen in IgA pemphigus.

Pemphigus vegetans is a variant of PV characterized clinically by vegetative, hypertrophic lesions with erosions localized to large flexures and histopathologically by pseudoepitheliomatous epidermal hyperplasia. Pemphigus foliaceous presents with cutaneous erosions that are associated with significant superficial scaling and crusting. Extensive involvement can also present with erythroderma. Pemphigus erythematosus (Senear–Usher syndrome) is a variant of pemphigus foliaceous, which features prominent facial involvement (in a malar distribution). Direct immunofluorescence (DIF) features both intercellular and DEJ deposits of immunoreactants, an immunofluorescence finding similar to paraneoplastic pemphigus. Pemphigus herpetiformis is a rare variant of pemphigus that presents with grouped itchy vesicles, clinically reminiscent of DH, but reveals a DIF pattern akin to pemphigus. Endemic pemphigus (fogo selvagem, meaning a wildfire) occurs in few selected geographical terrains in rural Brazil, Tunisia, and elsewhere that have abundance of black flies (*Simulium* species) and other hematophagus insects. The clinical manifestations of endemic

TABLE 1: Major autoimmune blistering disorders and the antigenic targets described in them.[1,3-5]

Disease	*Antigen*
Intraepidermal Autoimmune Blistering Disorders	
Pemphigus vulgaris	Desmoglein 3 (130 kDa), desmoglein 1 (160 kDa)
Pemphigus foliaceous	Desmoglein 1 (160 kDa)
Paraneoplastic pemphigus	Plakins (desmoplakins), desmogleins 1 and 3, BPAg1, BPAg2 (Note the presence of autoantibodies against antigens in both keratinocytes and DEJ. This is reflected in DIF, which features both intercellular and dermoepidermal deposits of immunoreactants)
IgA pemphigus	Desmocollin 1
Drug-induced pemphigus	Desmoglein 1
Subepidermal Autoimmune Blistering Disorders	
Bullous pemphigoid	BPAg1, BPAg2
Pemphigoid gestationis	BPAg2
Mucous membrane pemphigoid	BPAg2, alpha6beta4 integrin, laminin 332
Linear IgA disease	120- and 97-kDa antigens (shed ectodomains of BPAg2)
Chronic bullous disease of childhood	Similar, as above
Dermatitis herpetiformis	Epidermal transglutaminases
Epidermolysis bullosa acquisita	Collagen VII
Bullous lupus erythematosus	Collagen VII

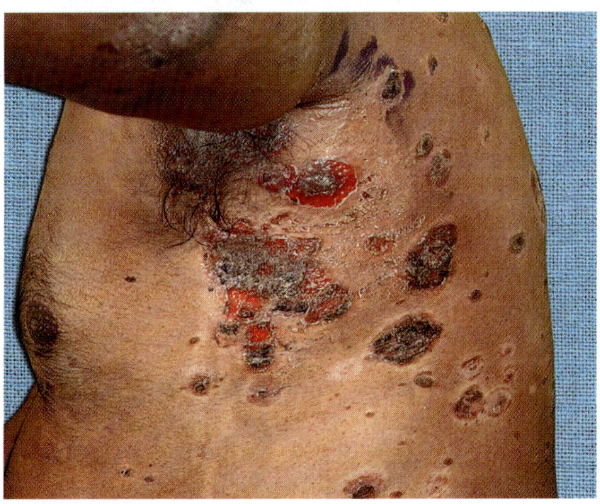

Fig. 1: Superficial crusted irregular erosions of pemphigus vulgaris. Note vegetating erosions in the axilla.

pemphigus are similar to pemphigus foliaceous. Endemic pemphigus is noncontagious but shows familial clustering and predominantly affects the younger individuals and children. The ecology plays an important part. Anti-desmoglein 1 antibodies are found in around 50% of the normal inhabitants of these geographic locations and pemphigus foliaceous-like presentation outnumbers PV by a staggering 17:1 ratio in the affected areas. Neonatal pemphigus is a transient disorder seen in the babies of the mothers affected by pemphigus and occurs due to the transfer of maternal autoantibodies through the placenta (without the antibodies being produced in the neonate itself). The resolution occurs after the neonate metabolizes the antibodies.[9]

Pemphigus is characterized by formation of autoantibodies against the desmosomal antigens in the epidermis. The induction of blisters by these autoantibodies does not require the presence of complement. The mechanism of vesicle formation in pemphigus is called acantholysis. The histopathology of pemphigus blisters consistently demonstrates separation of keratinocytes from each other resulting in the formation of round cells with a high nuclear/cytoplasmic ratio and peripheral condensation of cytoplasm. Similar cells can also be demonstrated on Tzanck smear. These cells are called acantholytic cells, and the process is labeled as *acantholysis.* To understand acantholysis, it is first essential to understand how individual keratinocytes are attached to each other. On light microscopic examination of a normal skin biopsy specimen, individual keratinocytes are seen attached to each other by spinous structures, which are nothing but desmosomes. Since the Greek work "acantha" means spinous process, the dissolution of these spinous structures/desmosomes is labeled as acantholysis.

Various theories have been proposed regarding the pathogenesis of pemphigus. Important ones include desmoglein compensation theory, basal cell shrinkage theory, multiple hit theory, and apoptolysis theory. Both *desmoglein compensation theory*[10] and *basal cell shrinkage theory*[11] rely on the fact that autoantibodies produced in the pemphigus are primarily directed against desmogleins and their major flaw lies in the assumption that the integrity of the epidermis lies entirely on desmosomes.

Besides desmosomes/desmogleins, the integrity of complex epithelia like skin depends upon multiple other factors.[12] Autocrine and paracrine acetylcholine (ACh) signaling is one such important factor that maintains the shape and cohesion of keratinocytes (via increased expression of both desmosomal cadherins and nondesmosomal cadherins in adherens junctions). Human keratinocytes express enzymes for synthesis and degradation of ACh. They also express receptors for ACh (AChRs), which are of both muscarinic (mAChR, G protein-coupled receptors) and nicotinic (nAChR) types.

Acantholysis is an active process that appears to be having a more complex mechanism than a mere interaction of anti-desmoglein antibodies with adhesion molecules. Apart from anti-desmoglein antibodies,[13] proteomics studies have demonstrated pemphigus autoantibodies that target the M_1 subtype of keratinocyte mAChRs. *Multiple hit hypothesis*[13] states that pemphigus results from a synergistic effect of multiple types of autoantibodies (not only anti-desmoglein antibodies) that target various kinds of cell membrane antigens and molecules including ones that *regulate* cell homeostasis (e.g., AChRs) and those that *mediate* cell–cell adhesion (e.g., desmosomal cadherins).

When hit primarily by anti-AChR autoantibodies, affected keratinocytes shrink and desmosomes get sloughed in the intercellular space that brings about production of secondary antibodies against the desmosomes themselves that saturate epidermis and inhibit adhesion by virtue of steric hindrance. The fact that the acantholysis and apoptosis of the keratinocytes in PV are mediated by the same set of signal effectors has led to the introduction of a new term called "*apoptolysis*".[14] It is initiated by binding of autoantibodies to antigens such as AChRs that transduce apoptolytic signals like executioner caspases and phosphorylases.

In a nutshell, desmosomes and adherens junctions keep keratinocytes glued together and the keratinocyte ACh axis maintains normal functioning of these structures by increasing their expression and minimizing their phosphorylation. In the presence of antibodies against ACh receptors, this axis is not maintained and the resulting phosphorylation causes disassembly of desmosomes causing separation of cells. Separation results in exposure of sloughed intercellular desmogleins to the immune system causing formation of secondary antibodies against desmogleins too, which causes further separation of cells by steric hindrance and other mechanisms. Pemphigus patients rarely develop myasthenia gravis, (an anti-nAChR autoimmune disease) that can be explained based on the subsequent production of secondary antibodies against nAChR after initial response against mAChR (epitope-spreading).[15,16] Many studies have observed negative association between pemphigus and cigarette smoking[17] (cigarette smoke contains nicotine that is a cholinergic agonist for nAChRs).

Pemphigoid Group of Disorders

This group of disorders is characterized by tense vesicles and bullae, usually present on an erythematous/urticarial or eczematous background.[5] BP is the most common disorder in this group and usually affects the elderly population.[18] It usually presents with large, tense bullae filled with serous or hemorrhagic fluid, on a background of urticarial lesions, classically located on the lower abdomen and thighs. The lesions are usually itchy and heal with characteristic hypopigmented patches with perifollicular hyperpigmentation. This is in contrast to pemphigus, where the healing is almost always accompanied with hyperpigmentation. The association between malignancy and BP is controversial, to say the best.[19] PG classically presents in the third trimester of pregnancy with intensely itchy vesicles that characteristically involve the umbilical area (unlike the pruritic urticarial papules and plaques of pregnancy) and spread to involve the rest of the body. It has been associated with adverse pregnancy outcomes including anhydramnios and fetal loss.[20] The risk of occurrence in future pregnancies is significant and might initiate at an even earlier gestational age. MMP presents with painful erosions of ocular, oropharyngeal, and genital mucosae. The involvement is usually painful and results in scarring of involved mucosae (cicatricial pemphigoid) **(Fig. 2)**. Erosive lichen planus can also exclusively involve mucosae and forms an important differential.

Linear IgA disease of adults and CBDC are characterized by their clinical morphology that resembles a string of pearls, referring to an annular arrangement of tense vesicles around central bullae/crust **(Fig. 3)**. DH is characterized by the formation of intensely itchy and usually grouped vesicles, erosions and excoriations that are present on shoulders, upper back, lower back, buttocks, and extensors of elbows and knees and rarely involves ears, hair margins, and forehead.[21] Tiny vesicles with angulated margins, when present, are characteristic of DH. The disease has a significant association with celiac disease that can predispose the patients to develop intestinal lymphomas.

Bullous SLE occurs usually in patients having SLE and presents as vesicles and bullae chiefly present (but not exclusively limited to) on photodistributed sites. EBA is characterized by skin lesions similar to hereditary epidermolysis bullosa with major involvement of extensors and trauma-prone sites and formation of atrophic scars,

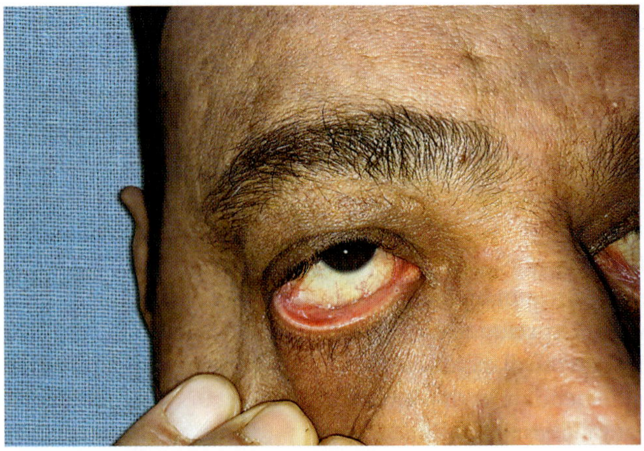

Fig. 2: Conjunctival erythema, erosion, and fibrotic bands of ocular mucous membrane pemphigoid.

milia, and nail dystrophy. **Table 2** enlists salient clinical, histopathological, and immunofluorescence findings of subepidermal blistering disorders.

Laboratory Diagnosis in Immunobullous Dermatoses

The laboratory diagnosis of immunobullous dermatoses involves simple laboratory procedures such as Tzanck smear to complex immunodiagnostic techniques.[24] Tzanck smears are performed on the scrapings from the floor of fresh blisters and demonstrates large, round keratinocytes with a hypertrophic nucleus, hazy or absent nucleoli, abundant basophilic cytoplasm showing perinuclear halo and condensed peripheries (*"mourning edge"* cells). The sensitivity and specificity of the Tzanck smear in pemphigus are 100% and 43.4%, respectively.

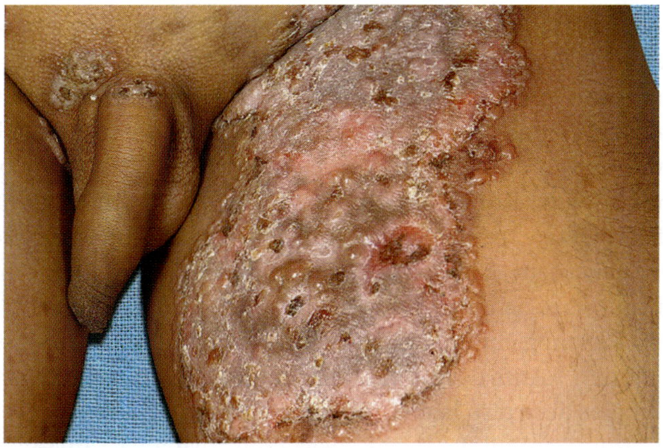

Fig. 3: Tense variable-sized blisters with a string of pearls appearance at the margin of the erosion in a young boy of chronic bullous disease of childhood.

Histopathology and DIF require a punch or elliptical biopsy. Additionally, for diagnosis of pemphigus, DIF can also be performed on plucked anagen hair. Specimens are preserved in 10% formalin for histopathology and in Michel's medium for DIF. Specimens stored in Michel's medium should not be immediately frozen. Till these are transported to the laboratory, these should preferably be maintained at room temperature. On histopathology, *PV* shows a suprabasal cleft leaving a monolayer of cuboidal basal keratinocytes attached to the basement membrane (*tombstone pattern*). *Paraneoplastic pemphigus* features upper dermal interface dermatitis with apoptotic (dyskeratotic) keratinocytes, and basal cell vacuolization in association with suprabasal acantholysis and clefting. Multilocular subepidermal vesicles are seen in DH. Teardrop-like subepidermal vesicles are seen in PG.

TABLE 2: Salient clinical, histopathological, and immunofluorescence findings of subepidermal blistering diseases.[1,3,5,22]

Disease	*Histopathology*	*DIF*	*Salt-split skin*
Bullous pemphigoid	Subepidermal split with eosinophils and neutrophils in dermis and blister cavity	Linear (wavy, tubular, granular) deposition of IgG and C3 (C3 > IgG) at DEJ	Roof (except anti-laminin-gamma1 pemphigoid targeting 200-kDa antigen)
Pemphigoid gestationis	Subepidermal teardrop vesicles containing eosinophils and neutrophils, dermal edema	Linear deposition of C3 and/or IgG at DEJ (C3 > IgG); sometimes C3 can be the only immunoreactant	Roof
Mucous membrane pemphigoid	Subepidermal split with sparse infiltrate comprising lymphocytes, neutrophils, and eosinophils[23]	Linear deposition of IgG, C3 at DEJ (C3 > IgG)	Roof or floor (anti-epiligrin/laminin cicatricial pemphigoid)
Dermatitis herpetiformis	Multilocular subepidermal vesicles, and papillary dermis tips containing neutrophils and eosinophils (papillary microabscess)	Granular IgA deposits on papillary dermis tips and along basement membrane zone, less frequently C3, IgG, and IgM	–
Linear IgA disease of adults, chronic bullous disease of childhood	Subepidermal blister with neutrophils in the blister cavity and dermis	Linear deposition of IgA at DEJ	Roof
Epidermolysis bullosa acquisita	Histopathology can be like bullous pemphigoid, mucous membrane pemphigoid, or linear IgA disease	• Usually multiple immunoreactants in a thick, homogeneous, and broad pattern at DEJ • Usually IgG (intense) > C3 (faint), IgM and IgA are also present concomitantly in multiple cases	Floor
Bullous lupus erythematosus	Subepidermal blister containing neutrophils	• Usually multiple immunoreactants in a thick, homogeneous, and broad pattern at DEJ • Usually IgG (intense) > C3 (faint), IgM and IgA are also present concomitantly in multiple cases	Floor

(Ig: immunoglobulin; C3: complement C3; DEJ: dermoepidermal junction; DIF: direct immunofluorescence)

Direct immunofluorescence identifies in vivo immunoglobulins and complement bound to tissue antigens. It is performed using perilesional skin/mucosa (few mm to 2 cm from blister edge). Immune deposits are partially or completely utilized in an already blistered skin and DIF may sometimes be falsely negative, if the biopsy was obtained from a relatively older blister, a fact that holds true while performing biopsy in immune complex-mediated vasculitis.

Primary site, class, and quantity of immune deposits are the chief parameters to be looked upon in DIF. If multiple, the identity of the most intense deposits should be sought. Immunoglobulin G1 (IgG1) and IgG4 are the subclasses of IgG present most commonly in patients having active lesions of PV. Complement C3 (C3), IgM, and IgA are present less commonly. In active pemphigus, intercellular staining is seen in the outer root sheath of plucked anagen hair on DIF. Pemphigus erythematosus and paraneoplastic pemphigus demonstrate IgG and/or complement (C3), both in the intercellular spaces and at the DEJ. IgA deposition in the intercellular space is characteristic of IgA pemphigus. The subclass of IgA autoantibodies is exclusively IgA1. The positive predictive value for DIF in pemphigus is 100% and the negative predictive value is 85–90%. Moreover, DIF can be used to differentiate erosive oral lichen planus from MMP and PV.[25]

C3 can be the exclusive immunoreactant at the BMZ in patients with PG. The patterns of DIF described in BP and PG include linear, wavy, tubular, and granular. A homogeneous, thick, and broad pattern of deposition favors EBA and bullous SLE. In EBA, intense IgG and less intense C3 deposition are almost consistently present. Deposition of IgA and IgM is present in approximately two-thirds and one-half of the cases, respectively. Compared with nonbullous SLE, bullous SLE more commonly features deposition of IgA. Almost all patients of DH demonstrate deposition of IgA.

For salt-split technique in DIF, punch biopsy samples are incubated in 5 mL of sodium chloride (NaCl, 1 mol/L) at 4°C for 24 hours (up to 72 hours) and then processed in the same manner as in DIF. Floor deposition is seen in EBA, bullous SLE, and anti-laminin gamma-1 pemphigoid.

Indirect immunofluorescence (IIF) is a two-step serological technique to detect circulating antibodies. For IIF, multiple substrates can be used. Normal human skin (rich in desmoglein 1), rabbit esophagus/lip, and monkey esophagus (rich in desmoglein 3) are used to see intercellular staining. Guinea pig esophagus is a substrate preferred in subepidermal disorders, and rat bladder (rich in desmoplakins) is preferred in paraneoplastic pemphigus. IgA anti-intercellular substance (ICS) antibodies are present in approximately 50% of patients having IgA pemphigus. IIF is positive in approximately 90% of patients with active PV resulting in a high predictive value. IgA anti-BMZ antibodies are present in one-third to one-half of patients having LAD. IgG anti-BMZ antibodies are seen in 75, 10, 25, and 50% cases of BP, PG, MMP, and EBA, respectively. The positive predictive value of IIF is therefore quite low in EBA, LAD, and IgA pemphigus. The negative predictive value of IIF for all bullous diseases is low.

Antibody detection can also be done by in vitro systems (membranes or cuvettes) that integrate the target antigens. Their reaction with the patient's serum-containing antibodies can be detected by immunoblotting, immunoprecipitation, and enzyme-linked-immunosorbent assay (ELISA). Immunoprecipitation and immunoblotting employ denatured antigens and are usually available in higher centers with research facilities. Immunoprecipitation is able to detect both linear and conformational epitopes whereas western blotting/immunoblotting detects only the linear epitopes. Since most epitopes on desmoglein 1 and 3 are conformational, immunoprecipitation is more useful in the diagnosis of pemphigus. ELISA kits for diagnosis of immunobullous disorders are available at quite a few centers, though these are also costly. The sensitivity of anti-desmoglein ELISA for diagnosis of pemphigus has been reported to be around 97%. Anti-desmoglein 1 ELISA additionally correlates with disease severity.[26] Anti-desmoglein antibodies ELISA on salivary samples have also been used in pemphigus patients.[27]

Immunobullous dermatoses comprise a vast diversity of diseases. Extensive research is undergoing in this field to enhance our understanding regarding their pathogenesis, diagnosis, and treatment. In this write-up, we have tried to introduce the postgraduate students to this interesting group of skin diseases. An extensive discussion including their treatment is beyond the scope of this chapter.

KEY POINTS

- Skin is the first barrier to the environment.
- Individual keratinocytes are attached to each other. The basal keratinocytes are also attached to the basement membrane through a variety of connections.
- Important connections between the *individual keratinocytes* include tight junctions (zonula occludens), adherens junctions (zonula adherens, belt desmosomes), desmosomes (macula adherens, spot desmosomes), and gap junctions (connexins).
- Important connections between *keratinocytes and the basement membrane* include hemidesmosomes and integrins/laminins.
- The autoimmune blistering diseases belong to a group of disorders wherein the above-mentioned cohesion molecules are targeted by the immune system and include pemphigus and pemphigoid group of disorders.
- Pemphigus is the prototype of *intraepidermal autoimmune blistering disorders*. The group further comprises pemphigus vulgaris (variant, pemphigus vegetans), pemphigus foliaceous (variant, pemphigus erythematosus, pemphigus herpetiformis, and endemic pemphigus), drug-induced pemphigus (usually of the pemphigus foliaceous type), IgA pemphigus, and paraneoplastic

pemphigus. The pemphigus group is characterized by intraepidermal deposition of immunoglobulins directed against desmosomal components.

- The *subepidermal autoimmune blistering diseases* include BP, PG, MMP, LAD, CBDC, DH, EBA, and BSLE. These diseases feature a subepidermal blister in histopathology, and immunoglobulins/complements are deposited in the basement membrane zone leading to significant influx of inflammatory cells, notably granulocytes.
- Both pemphigus and pemphigoid group of disorders have salient clinical, histopathological, and immunofluorescence findings.

REFERENCES

1. Hammers CM, Stanley JR. Mechanisms of disease: pemphigus and bullous pemphigoid. Annu Rev Pathol. 2016;11:175-97.
2. De D, Khullar G, Handa S, Saikia UN, Radotra BD, Saikia B, et al. Clinical, demographic and immunopathological spectrum of subepidermal autoimmune bullous diseases at a tertiary center: a 1-year audit. Indian J Dermatol Venereol Leprol. 2016;82:358.
3. Bieber K, Koga H, Nishie W. In vitro and in vivo models to investigate the pathomechanisms and novel treatments for pemphigoid diseases. Exp Dermatol. 2017;26:1163-70.
4. Toyonaga E, Nishie W, Izumi K, Natsuga K, Ujiie H, Iwata H, et al. C-Terminal processing of collagen XVII induces neoepitopes for linear IgA dermatosis autoantibodies. J Invest Dermatol. 2017;137:2552-9.
5. Kershenovich R, Hodak E, Mimouni D. Diagnosis and classification of pemphigus and bullous pemphigoid. Autoimmun Rev. 2014;13:477-81.
6. Kridin K. Pemphigus group: overview, epidemiology, mortality, and comorbidities. Immunol Res. 2018;66:255-70.
7. Rosenberg FR, Sanders S, Nelson CT. Pemphigus: a 20-year review of 107 patients treated with corticosteroids. Arch Dermatol. 1976;112:962-70.
8. Kumar KA. Incidence of pemphigus in Thrissur district, south India. Indian J Dermatol Venereol Leprol. 2008;74:349-51.
9. Kushner CJ, Concha JSS, Werth VP. Treatment of autoimmune bullous disorders in pregnancy. Am J Clin Dermatol. 2018; 19:391-403.
10. Amagai M. Autoimmunity against desmosomal cadherins in pemphigus. J Dermatol Sci. 1999;20:92-102.
11. Cirillo N, Femiano F, Gombos F, Lanza A. Serum from pemphigus vulgaris reduces desmoglein 3 half-life and perturbs its de novo assembly to desmosomal sites in cultured keratinocytes. FEBS Lett. 2006;580:3276-81.
12. Grando SA. Biological functions of keratinocyte cholinergic receptors. J Investig Dermatol Symp Proc. 1997;2:41-8.
13. Grando SA. Autoimmunity to keratinocyte acetylcholine receptors in pemphigus. Dermatology. 2000;201:290-5.
14. Grando SA. Pemphigus autoimmunity: hypotheses and realities. Autoimmunity. 2012;45:7-35.
15. Grando SA. New approaches to the treatment of pemphigus. J Investig Dermatol Symp Proc. 2004;9:84-91.
16. Didona D, Di Zenzo G. Humoral epitope spreading in autoimmune bullous diseases. Front Immunol. 2018;9:779.
17. Valikhani M, Kavusi S, Chams-Davatchi C, Hallaji Z, Esmaili N, Ghandi N, et al. Impact of smoking on pemphigus. Int J Dermatol. 2008;47:567-70.
18. Bagci IS, Horvath ON, Ruzicka T, Sardy M. Bullous pemphigoid. Autoimmun Rev. 2017;16:445-55.
19. Bishnoi A, Narang T, Handa S, Vishwajeet V, Saikia UN, Kapoor R, et al. Paraneoplastic bullous pemphigoid associated with penile squamous cell carcinoma. J Eur Acad Dermatol Venereol. 2018;32:e140-1.
20. Dabas G, Afra TP, De D, Mahajan R, Handa S, Arora A, et al. Anhydramnios in patients with pemphigoid gestationis. JAMA Dermatol. 2018;154:484-6.
21. Handa S, Dabas G, De D, Mahajan R, Chatterjee D, Saika UN, et al. A retrospective study of dermatitis herpetiformis from an immunobullous disease clinic in North India. Int J Dermatol. 2018;57(8):959-64.
22. Goyal N, Rao R, Shenoi SD, Pai S, Kumar P, Bhogal BS, et al. Epidermolysis bullosa acquisita and anti-p200 pemphigoid as major subepidermal autoimmune bullous diseases diagnosed by floor binding on indirect immunofluorescence microscopy using human salt-split skin. Indian J Dermatol Venereol Leprol. 2017;83:550-5.
23. Rose C, Schmidt E, Kerstan A, Thoma-Uszynski S, Wesselmann U, Kasbohrer U, et al. Histopathology of anti-laminin 5 mucous membrane pemphigoid. J Am Acad Dermatol. 2009;61:433-40.
24. Mihai S, Sitaru C. Immunopathology and molecular diagnosis of autoimmune bullous diseases. J Cell Mol Med. 2007;11:462-81.
25. Yamanaka Y, Yamashita M, Innocentini LMA, Macedo LD, Chahud F, Ribeiro-Silva A, et al. Direct immunofluorescence as a helpful tool for the differential diagnosis of oral lichen planus and oral lichenoid lesions. Am J Dermatopathol. 2018;40:491-7.
26. Abasq C, Mouquet H, Gilbert D, Tron F, Grassi V, Musette P, et al. ELISA testing of anti-desmoglein 1 and 3 antibodies in the management of pemphigus. Arch Dermatol. 2009;145: 529-35.
27. Hallaji Z, Mortazavi H, Lajevardi V, Tamizifar B, Amir Zargar A, Daneshpazhooh M, et al. Serum and salivary desmoglein 1 and 3 enzyme-linked immunosorbent assay in pemphigus vulgaris: correlation with phenotype and severity. J Eur Acad Dermatol Venereol. 2010;24:275-80.

EXAMINATION QUESTIONS

1. Ultrastructure of desmosomes.
2. Ultrastructure of basement membrane zone.
3. Pathogenesis of pemphigus.
4. Pathogenesis of bullous pemphigoid.
5. Variants of bullous pemphigoid.
6. Outline of diagnosis of suspected autoimmune bullous disease.
7. Treatment algorithm for pemphigus vulgaris/foliaceous.
8. Treatment algorithm for bullous pemphigoid.

49 CHAPTER

Pemphigus

Varsha M Shetty, Raghavendra Rao

INTRODUCTION

The term pemphigus is derived from a Greek word *pemphix* meaning "a blister" or "a bubble". Pemphigus is a chronic autoimmune blistering disorder, characterized by the presence of autoantibodies against desmogleins 1 and 3 (Dsg1 and Dsg3) resulting in acantholysis. Dsgs are glycoproteins responsible for intercellular adhesion in stratified squamous epithelia such as skin and mucosa.[1,2] **Table 1** depicts classification of pemphigus.

TABLE 1: Classification of pemphigus.[2]

Type of pemphigus	*Predominant antibody*
Pemphigus vulgaris (PV) Variant—Pemphigus vegetans	Antidesmoglein 3 (anti-Dsg3)
Pemphigus foliaceus (PF) Variant—Pemphigus erythematosus (PE)	Antidesmoglein 1 (anti-Dsg1)
IgA pemphigus	Antidesmocollin 1 (anti-Dsc1) and antidesmocollin 3 (anti-Dsc3)
Pemphigus herpetiformis (PH)	Anti-Dsg1
Paraneoplastic pemphigus (PNP)	Antibodies to desmoplakin 1, desmoplakin 2, envoplakin, periplakin, Dsg3 and Dsg1, and bullous pemphigoid (BP) 180 and 230

EPIDEMIOLOGY

The incidence of pemphigus in India ranges from 0.09 to 1.8% with pemphigus vulgaris (PV) accounting for 75–92% of all pemphigus patients followed by pemphigus foliaceus (PF), pemphigus erythematosus (PE), and pemphigus vegetans in the decreasing order of frequency.

Age Group

More commonly seen in 4th to 6th decade, however, a significant number of Indian patients with pemphigus are below 40 years of age.

Gender predilection: Seen equally in both sexes.

TABLE 2: Autoantibody profile in pemphigus.[1]

Antibody profile	*Mucosal dominant PV*	*Mucocutaneous PV*	*PF*
Anti-Dsg1	–	+	+
Anti-Dsg3	+	+	-

(Dsg: desmoglein; PF: pemphigus foliaceus; PV: pemphigus vulgaris)

ETIOLOGY

Genetic Factors

The increased prevalence of pathogenic autoantibodies in first degree relatives of pemphigus patients indicates the role of genetic factors in causation of the disease. It is commonly encountered in people of Jewish or Mediterranean descent.

A strong association of PV with HLA-DRB1*1404, HLA-DQA1*0101, and HLA-DQB1*0503 has been reported.[2]

Environmental Factors

Factors such as drugs containing the thiol group of drugs such as penicillamine and captopril can promote acantholysis by interfering with the biochemistry of keratinocyte membrane or immune balance.

Other triggers for pemphigus include viral infections, dietary factors and psychological stressors.

Immunological Factors

The expression of Dsg1 and 3 varies in skin and mucosa. In skin, Dsg1 is seen throughout the epidermis but more in the upper layers whereas Dsg3 is exclusively located in the basal and parabasal layers. However, in mucosa both Dsg1 and Dsg3 are expressed but Dsg1 levels are low. Hence, the autoantibody profile largely determines the clinical features as depicted in the **Table 2**.

PATHOGENESIS

The autoantibodies in pemphigus are predominantly of immunoglobulin G4 (IgG4) subclass, which does not require complement activation to bring about acantholysis.

Mechanisms by which autoantibodies induce acantholysis:

- Steric hindrance of desmosomal adhesion.

- Interference with desmosomal assembly by causing internalization and degradation of Dsgs.
- Cellular signaling pathways such as p38 mitogen-activated protein kinase (MAPK) pathway.[1]

CLINICAL FEATURES

Pemphigus Vulgaris

Pemphigus vulgaris can manifest as mucosal dominant, mucocutaneous, or less frequently as purely cutaneous form. Oral mucosa is the initial site of involvement in majority of PV patients with 53.52% of patients having the disease onset in oral mucosa and 23.94% presenting with oral and skin lesions occurring simultaneously **(Fig. 1)**. Erosions or ulcers in the buccal mucosa and hard palate are frequently seen. Other mucosae such as larynx, esophagus, conjunctiva, urethra, cervix, and anal canal may also be affected.[2]

Lesions on the skin are frequently encountered in the head, upper trunk, and groin and can manifest with flaccid bullae and crusted erosions **(Fig. 2)**.

Blisters or epidermal splitting may be induced by lateral pressure onto the normal appearing skin either perilesionally or on bony prominences (known as positive Nikolsky sign). Nikolsky sign is a marker of activity of the disease.[1]

Pemphigus Vegetans

It is a rare variant of PV accounting for less than 5% of total pemphigus cases. It is of two types:

1. *Neumann type*: Presents with periorificial papillomatous vegetations
2. *Hallopeau type*: Presents with pustules evolving into vegetations affecting the intertriginous areas.[3]

Pemphigus Foliaceus

Pemphigus foliaceus is of two types:

1. Sporadic—seen in middle aged and elderly
2. Fogo selvagem—endemic form of PF seen in children and young adults

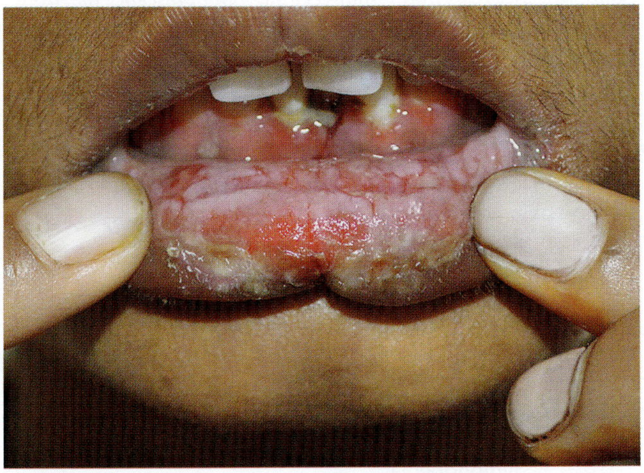

Fig. 1: Erosions in the lip and gingiva in pemphigus vulgaris.

It usually presents with multiple pruritic crusted erosions confined to the seborrheic areas that may progress to exfoliative dermatitis **(Fig. 3)**. Blisters are rarely seen as they easily rupture owing to their superficial location. Mucosa is characteristically spared in PF.

In fogo selvagem which is an endemic form of PF rampant in Brazil, cross-reactivity with blackfly (*Simulium nigrimanum*) salivary antigen with Dsg1 triggers the disease. It differs from sporadic PF by its geographical distribution, familial clustering of cases, and early age of onset.[1,4]

Pemphigus Erythematosus

It is also known as Senear–Usher syndrome; these patients tend to have serological findings suggestive of systemic lupus erythematosus (SLE), especially the antinuclear antibodies. The clinical features are similar to PF but restricted to photoexposed areas such as upper trunk, head, and neck.[4]

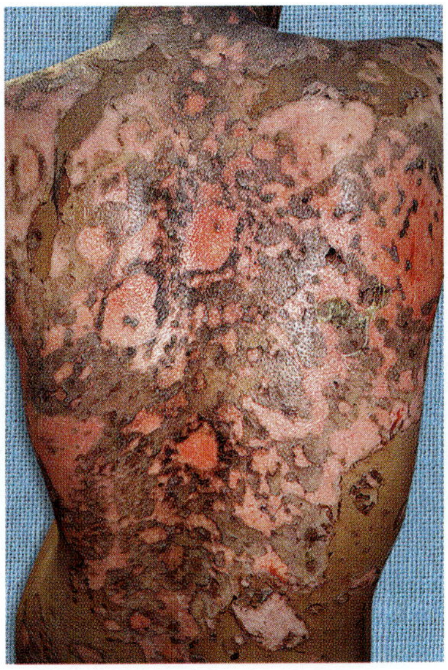

Fig. 2: Extensive erosions on the back in pemphigus vulgaris.

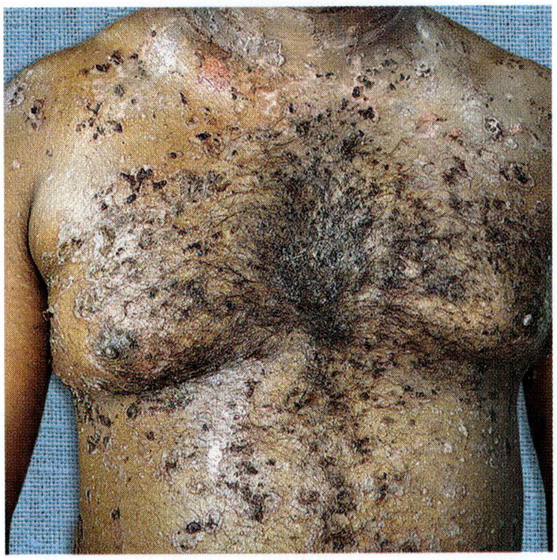

Fig. 3: Scaling and crusting of the chest and abdomen in pemphigus foliaceus.

DIAGNOSIS

Tzanck smear shows acantholytic cells. It is positive in 40% of cases with positivity rate increasing if the sample is taken within 3 months of disease onset.[2]

Histopathological and immunofluorescence findings **(Fig. 4)** are shown in **Table 3**.

Pemphigus erythematosus is identical to PF histopathologically whereas on direct immunofluorescence (DIF) shows linear basement membrane zone (BMZ) deposits of IgG and C3 in addition to intercellular space (ICS) staining.[4]

Serological Tests

Enzyme-linked immunosorbent assay (ELISA) can be used to detect anti-Dsg antibodies in the sera of the patients with pemphigus and has a high sensitivity of 96–100%. As the titers of autoantibodies correlate with disease activity, they can be used to monitor the immunological activity of the disease.[1]

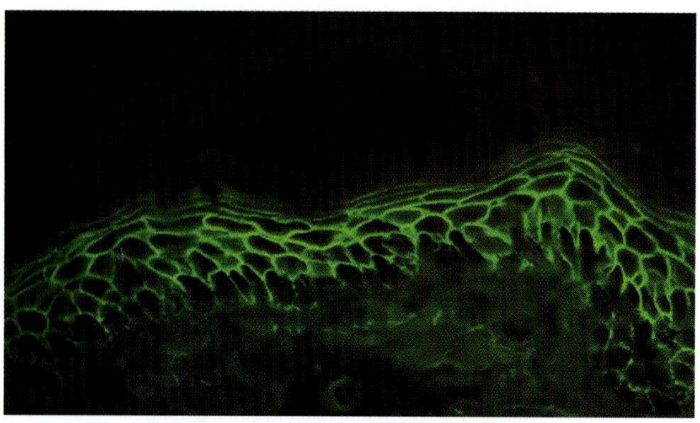

Fig. 4: Intercellular staining of epidermis with immunoglobulin G (IgG) in a fish-net pattern.

TREATMENT

First-line of Treatment

Systemic Corticosteroids

Prednisolone in the dose of 0.5–2.5 mg/kg/day is given depending on the severity of the disease. Once remission is attained and maintained, dose is tapered biweekly till 20 mg/day after which slow tapering is done.

When the daily dosage exceeds 100 mg, intravenous (IV) formulations of betamethasone or dexamethasone is given either daily or as pulses. IV dexamethasone 100 mg for 3 days every 3 weeks either alone or in combination with other agents such as cyclophosphamide or azathioprine is one such option.

Corticosteroids can be combined with other immunosuppressive agents when complications due to prolonged use of steroids are encountered.[5]

The various immunosuppressive agents used in pemphigus are depicted in **Table 4**.

Rituximab

It is an anti-CD20 humanized monoclonal antibody.

Mechanism of action in pemphigus: Depletes the B cells hence reducing the pathogenic anti-Dsg antibodies.[5]

Dose:

- Lymphoma protocol—4 weekly infusions of rituximab (RTX) at a dose of 375 mg/m^2
- Rheumatoid arthritis (RA) protocol—two infusions of 1,000 mg of RTX at an interval of 2 weeks
- Low-dose RTX—Two infusions of 500 mg of RTX at an interval of 2 weeks with or without IV immunoglobulin (IVIg)

A complete remission rate of 76% and a relapse rate of 40% have been reported. No significant difference in outcome was observed between lymphoma and RA protocol. However, high

TABLE 3: Histopathology and immunofluorescence.[1,4,5]

Disease	*Histopathology (lesional skin)*	*Direct immunofluorescence (DIF) from perilesional skin*	*Indirect immunofluorescence (IIF) from patients sera*
Pemphigus vulgaris (PV)	Suprabasal split with acantholytic cells and "row of tomb-stone appearance"	Immunoglobulin G (IgG) and C3 deposits in the intercellular space (ICS) referred to as "fish net" or "chicken-wire" appearance	IIF using monkey esophagus or normal human skin shows ICS deposits with IgG and C3, the titers of which correlate with disease severity
Pemphigus foliaceus (PF)	Acantholysis seen subcorneally with blister cavity containing acantholytic cells and occasionally neutrophils	IgG and C3 deposits in ICS with intensity of staining being more in upper layers of epidermis	IgG and C3 deposits in ICS

TABLE 4: Various immunosuppressive agents used in the treatment of pemphigus.[1,2,5]

Agent	*Dose*	*Adverse effects*
Azathioprine	1–3 mg/kg/day	Bone marrow suppression
Cyclophosphamide	2 mg/kg/day oral or as 500 mg intravenous (IV) infusion monthly	Infertility, genitourinary complications, and lymphopenia
Mycophenolate mofetil	2 g/day	Gastrointestinal side effects

dose of RTX (>2,000 mg) was associated with longer duration of remission.

Adverse effects:
- Infections as RTX causes hypogammaglobulinemia.[6]
- RTX can be combined with IVIg which works synergistically as well as overcomes the risk of depletion of B cells induced by RTX.[1]

Intravenous Immunoglobulin

Intravenous immunoglobulin is nothing but pooled plasma containing >95% IgG antibodies.

Mechanism of action in pemphigus:
- Saturates the Fc receptor of IgG antibody causing its disintegration and inhibits antigen presentation
- Upregulates the inhibitory gamma Fc receptors thereby inhibiting autoantibody mediated inflammation[1]

Dose: 2 g/kg/day IV over 2–5 days monthly[5]

Baseline investigations: Serum creatinine and immunoglobulin A (IgA) levels need to be checked before starting the therapy.

Adverse effects: Thrombotic complications, aseptic meningitis[1,5]

VARIANTS OF PEMPHIGUS

Pemphigus Herpetiformis

Definition and Epidemiology

The term "pemphigus herpetiformis (PH)" was first coined by Jabłońska et al. in 1975 to describe a group of disorders presenting with clinical features resembling dermatitis herpetiformis and immunopathological features consistent with pemphigus. It is a rare variant of pemphigus accounting for 6–7% of cases with equal gender predilection. It commonly affects the adults between the ages of 31 and 83 years.

Pathogenesis

Pemphigus herpetiformis is characterized by autoantibodies against epidermal components usually Dsg1 and less frequently Dsg3, desmocollin 1 (Dsc1), desmocollin 3 (Dsc3) and an unknown 178 kDa antigen.

The PH autoantibodies bind to minor epitopes of Dsg1 and 3, hence do not cause direct acantholysis. These autoantibodies are known to stimulate production of interleukin-8 (IL-8) by keratinocytes which in turn attracts inflammatory cells resulting in eosinophilic spongiosis and intercellular edema.

Clinical Features

Patients present with pruritic erythematous, gyrate, or annular edematous lesions with groups of vesicles and/or pustules.

Mucosal involvement is not frequently seen in PH, and patients with PH can eventually develop classical features of PF or PV.

Differential Diagnosis

- Dermatitis herpetiformis
- Bullous pemphigoid
- Linear IgA dermatosis
- Pemphigus vulgaris
- Pemphigus foliaceus

Diagnosis

Histopathology and immunofluorescence findings of PH are illustrated in **Table 5**.

TABLE 5: Histopathology and immunofluorescence findings in PH.[7]

Histopathology	*Immunofluorescence*
• Subcorneal and/or intraepidermal vesicles filled with neutrophils and/or eosinophils • Neutrophilic and/or eosinophilic spongiosis • Acantholysis is minimal or absent	• *DIF*: Intercellular deposits of IgG and C3 similar to classical forms of pemphigus • *IIF and ELISA*: Autoantibodies against Dsg1 or Dsg3 and less frequently against Dsc1, 3 and unknown 178 kDa antigen

(DIF: direct immunofluorescence; Dsc: desmocollin; Dsg: desmoglein; ELISA: enzyme-linked immunosorbent assay; IgG: immunoglobulin G; IIF: indirect immunofluorescence; PH: pemphigus herpetiformis)

Treatment

Pemphigus herpetiformis responds reasonably well to treatment with most patients achieving complete remission.

Dapsone can be used as monotherapy or in combination with systemic steroids. Immunosuppressants such as azathioprine and cyclophosphamide can be tried in patients evolving into the classical forms of pemphigus.[7]

Immunoglobulin A Pemphigus

Definition and Epidemiology

Wallach, Foldes, and Cottenot were the first to describe this entity in the year 1982.[1] IgA pemphigus is a rare autoimmune blistering disease characterized by epidermal IgA deposits. It commonly occurs in middle aged and elderly individuals with average age of onset being 48 years.[8,9]

Pathogenesis

Presently, IgA pemphigus is classified based on immunological and histopathological features into two subtypes:

1. *Subcorneal pustular dermatosis (SPD) type*: Here the IgA antibodies are directed against Dsc 1 strongly expressed in the upper layers of epidermis.
2. *Intraepidermal neutrophilic (IEN) dermatosis type*: In this type, IgA antibodies are directed against a wide range of proteins such as Dsg1, Dsg3, Dsc3 as well as nondesmosomal cell surface proteins. Hence, the target antigen in IEN needs further elucidation.[10]

Flowchart 1: Role of immunoglobulin A (IgA) antibodies in the pathogenesis.[7]

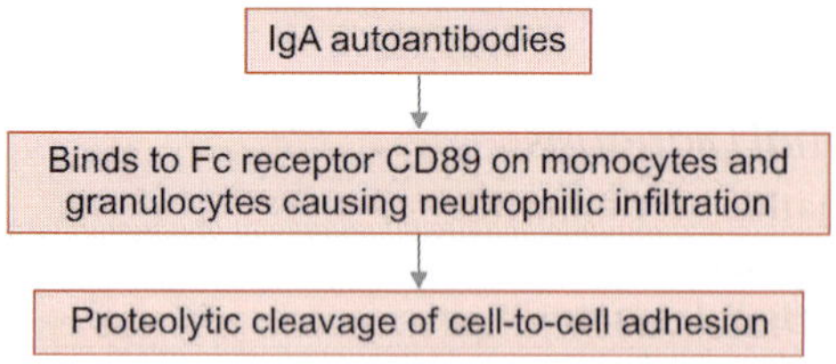

TABLE 6: Diagnosis of IgA pemphigus.[7,8]

Histopathology	*Immunofluorescence*
• Neutrophilic infiltration in the epidermis with minimal acantholysis • *SPD type*: Pustules are located subcorneally • *IEN type*: Suprabasilar cleavage confined to the lower epidermis or involving the entire epidermis	• *DIF*: Shows IgA deposition in the intercellular space • *SPD type*: IgA deposits mainly located in the upper epidermis • *IEN type*: IgA deposits concentrated in the lower epidermis or throughout the entire epidermis • *IIF*: Antibodies can be detected in less than 50% of the cases and are found in low titers

(DIF: direct immunofluorescence; IEN: intraepidermal neutrophilic; IgA: immunoglobulin A; IIF: indirect immunofluorescence; SPD: subcorneal pustular dermatosis)

Flowchart 1 depicts the role of IgA antibodies in the pathogenesis.

Clinical Features

Both the types of IgA pemphigus present with flaccid vesicles or pustules arranged in an annular or circinate pattern with central crusted area resembling a "sunflower-like configuration". The lesions commonly favor the flexures such as axilla and groins. Pruritus is generally present with sparing of the mucosa.[1]

The diagnostic features of IgA pemphigus is illustrated in **Table 6**.

Treatment

Dapsone is considered to be the drug of choice. Other treatment modalities include colchicine, systemic steroids, retinoids, tetracycline, sulfamethoxazole, cotrimoxazole, methotrexate, cyclosporine, adalimumab, azathioprine, and psoralen with ultraviolet A (PUVA) therapy.[9]

The clinical presentation of IgA pemphigus is milder and it runs a benign course compared to PV. However, IgA pemphigus especially the SPD type may be associated with malignant IgA gammopathy, in which case the prognosis was related to the malignancy.[7]

Paraneoplastic Pemphigus

Definition and Epidemiology

Paraneoplastic pemphigus (PNP) is an atypical pemphigus, first described by Anhalt et al. in 1990. Patients with PNP have an underlying malignancy, both benign and malignant **(Table 7)**.[11]

TABLE 7: Concomitant malignancies associated with paraneoplastic pemphigus (PNP).[11]

Associated malignancy	*Frequency*
Non-Hodgkin lymphoma	39%
Chronic lymphocytic leukemia	18%
Castleman disease	18%
Carcinoma	9%
Thymoma	6%
Sarcoma	6%
Waldenstrom macroglobulinemia	1%
Hodgkin lymphoma, monoclonal gammopathy, and melanoma each	<1%

It mostly affects adults between 45 and 70 years of age and its incidence is not fully known with only 450 cases reported in literature.[7]

Pathogenesis

The proposed theories for immune response in PNP include:

- The production of antibodies to tumor antigens which cross-react with epithelial antigens.
- The production of autoantibodies by the tumor or tumor-synthesizing cytokines such as IL-6 which promote B-cell differentiation ultimately resulting in autoimmunity.[7,11]

Clinical Features

The patient with PNP initially presents with severe refractory stomatitis with polymorphic lesions such as blisters, erosions, papules, and plaques. The skin manifestations usually follow the mucosal lesions with the upper body being frequently affected. **Box 1** depicts cutaneous features of PNP.

Paraneoplastic pemphigus can also affect other mucosa such as esophagus, stomach, duodenum, and colon. It can be associated with other systemic features such as bronchiolitis obliterans, glomerulonephritis, and neurological involvement, and hence PNP is often addressed as paraneoplastic autoimmune multiorgan syndrome (PAMS).[7]

Nikolsky's sign is usually positive in PNP.

Differential Diagnosis

- Pemphigus vulgaris
- Mucous membrane pemphigoid
- Bullous pemphigoid
- Lichen planus
- Aphthous stomatitis
- Herpes simplex virus infection
- Erythema multiforme
- Graft-versus-host disease
- Stevens–Johnson syndrome/toxic epidermal necrolysis

Diagnosis **(Box 2)**

Histopathology: PNP is chiefly characterized by vacuolar or lichenoid interface dermatitis. Acantholysis with

BOX 1: Cutaneous features of paraneoplastic pemphigus (PNP).[7]

- Pemphigus like lesions such as flaccid vesicles, erosions and crust
- Bullous pemphigoid like scaly erythematous papular lesions with or without tense bullae
- Erythema multiforme-like lesions
- Graft-versus-host disease like disseminated dusky red papules
- Lichen planus like lesions with severe mucosal involvement

BOX 2: Diagnostic criteria by Anhalt.[7,11]

- Painful mucosal erosions and polymorphous skin eruptions in association with malignancy
- Histopathological features of acantholysis, keratinocyte necrosis, and interface dermatitis
- DIF shows IgG and C3 deposition in ICS and along BMZ
- IIF showing same pattern as DIF in skin, mucosa, simple, columnar, and transitional epithelium
- Immunoprecipitation demonstrating antibodies against desmoplakin-1, desmoplakin-2, envoplakin, and periplakin

(BMZ: basement membrane zone; DIF: direct immunofluorescence; ICS: intercellular space; IgG: immunoglobulin G; IIF: indirect immunofluorescence)

intraepidermal cleft can be seen and very rarely subepidermal blisters may also be encountered. The different clinical variants can have their respective histopathological findings.

Immunofluorescence: DIF shows ICS staining with IgG and C3 along with linear deposits of IgG and C3 along the BMZ. Indirect immunofluorescence (IIF) shows binding of IgG antibodies to simple, columnar, and transitional epithelium with the rat bladder epithelium showing highest sensitivity and specificity. Immunoblotting and immunoprecipitation can demonstrate antibodies against Dsg3, desmoplakin-1, desmoplakin-2, envoplakin, plectin, periplakin, epiplakin, BP230, and occasionally Dsg1.

Enzyme-linked immunosorbent assay: The sera of patients with PNP are known to react with Dsc 1–3 in various patterns. ELISA may also exhibit antibodies against Dsg3 and less often Dsg1. Some of the novel ELISA kits capable of detecting antibodies against envoplakin have increased sensitivity and specificity, and hence are superior to the presently employed immunofluorescence testing.

Extensive work-up for malignancy is required in a suspected case of PNP such as blood counts, serum protein electrophoresis, biopsy of lymph nodes as well as bone marrow, and computed tomography of chest, abdomen, and pelvis. In one-third cases of PNP, malignancy was detected after the onset of symptoms of PNP.

Treatment

The prognosis of PNP depends on the underlying malignancy. The resection of benign tumor causes near total remission of the disease whereas the response to treatment is very poor in those with malignant tumors.

Systemic steroids (0.5–1 mg/kg) form the mainstay of treatment. Steroid-sparing agents such as cyclophosphamide, cyclosporine, and mycophenolate mofetil may be used but these agents carry an inherent risk of malignancy.

Rituximab is more often used in PNP, perhaps due to its reduced tumorigenicity potential and its beneficial role in lymphomas. Even IVIg has proven to be a good choice in these patients due to its safety profile.

However unfortunately, PNP is highly refractory to treatment with mortality rates as high as 75–90%, the main cause being respiratory failure.[7,11]

KEY POINTS

- Pemphigus is a chronic autoimmune-blistering disorder, characterized by the presence of autoantibodies against Dsg1 and 3 resulting in acantholysis.
- It is commonly known to affect people of 4th to 6th decade with a significant number of Indian patients with pemphigus below 40 years of age.
- Pemphigus vulgaris accounts for 75–92% of all pemphigus patients followed by PF, PE, and pemphigus vegetans in the decreasing order of frequency.
- Genetic, environmental, and immunological factors play a key role in its pathogenesis with the autoantibody profile determining the clinical features.
- Diagnostic tests include Tzanck smear, histopathology, immunofluorescence, and serological assays.
- Systemic steroids are the mainstay in the treatment of pemphigus group of disorders except PH and IgA pemphigus where dapsone is considered as the drug of first choice.

REFERENCES

1. Kasperkiewicz M, Ellebrecht CT, Takahashi H, Yamagami J, Zillikens D, Payne AS, et al. Pemphigus. Nat Rev Dis Primers. 2017;3:17026.
2. Kanwar AJ, De D. Pemphigus in India. Indian J Dermatol Venereol Leprol. 2011;77:439-49.
3. Mergler R, Kerstan A, Schmidt E, Goebeler M, Benoit S. Atypical clinical and serological manifestation of pemphigus vegetans: a case report and review of the literature. Case Rep Dermatol. 2017;9:121-30.
4. Khachemoune A, Guldbakke KK, Ehrsam E. Pemphigus foliaceus: a case report and short review. Cutis. 2006;78:105-10.
5. Gregoriou S, Efthymiou O, Stefanaki C, Rigopoulos D. Management of pemphigus vulgaris: challenges and solutions. Clin Cosmet Investig Dermatol. 2015;8:521-7.
6. Wang HH, Liu CW, Li YC, Huang YC. Efficacy of rituximab for pemphigus: a systematic review and meta-analysis of different regimens. Acta Derm Venereol. 2015;95:928-32.
7. Porro AM, Caetano Lde V, Maehara Lde S, Enokihara MM. Non-classical forms of pemphigus: pemphigus herpetiformis, IgA pemphigus, paraneoplastic pemphigus and IgG/IgA pemphigus. An Bras Dermatol. 2014;89:96-106.
8. Düker I, Schaller J, Rose C, Zillikens D, Hashimoto T, Kunze J. Subcorneal pustular dermatosis type IgA pemphigus with

autoantibodies to desmocollins 1, 2, and 3. Arch Dermatol. 2009;145:1159-62.
9. Neethu KC, Rao R, Balachandran C, Pai S. Juvenile IgA pemphigus: a case report and review of literature. Indian J Dermatol Venereol Leprol. 2016;8:439-42.
10. Geller S, Gat A, Zeeli T, Hafner A, Eming R, Hertl M, Sprecher E. The expanding spectrum of IgA pemphigus: a case report and review of the literature. Br J Dermatol. 2014;171:650-6.
11. Wieczorek M, Czernik A. Paraneoplastic pemphigus: a short review. Clin Cosmet Investig Dermatol. 2016;9:291-5.

EXAMINATION QUESTIONS

1. Discuss the etiopathogenesis of pemphigus and write a note on clinical features of pemphigus foliaceus.
2. Write a short note on acantholysis.
3. Describe the clinical features, pathogenesis, and management of IgA pemphigus.
4. Discuss the role of rituximab in the management of pemphigus vulgaris.
5. Discuss the diagnostic utility of Tzanck smear in dermatology.
6. Discuss the management of severe pemphigus.
7. Explain recent advances in management of pemphigus vulgaris.

50 CHAPTER Autoimmune Subepidermal Blistering Diseases

Sonal Singh, Abhishek De, Aarti Sarda

INTRODUCTION

- Autoimmune subepidermal blistering diseases of the skin and mucosae constitute a large group of sometimes devastating diseases, such as encompassing bullous pemphigoid, gestational pemphigoid, mucous membrane pemphigoid, epidermolysis bullosa acquisita (EBA), dermatitis herpetiformis, and anti-p200 pemphigoid.[1]
- These conditions show substantial clinical and immunopathological overlap **(Box 1, Table 1)**.

BULLOUS PEMPHIGOID

Introduction

- Bullous pemphigoid (BP) is the most common autoimmune subepidermal blistering disorder, representing 80% of subepidermal immunobullous cases.[2]
- This chronic autoimmune disease is characterized by tense bullae associated with pruritus and elderly age group.
- Atypical variants of BP present with either localized bullous lesions or nonbullous presentations and represent a diagnostic challenge.

History

- Walter Lever coined the term bullous pemphigoid in 1953.
- Jordan, Beutner and colleagues demonstrated the autoimmune nature of the disease.

Epidemiology

- *Age group:* BP typically affects elderly subjects above 70 years; however, it may rarely present in childhood also.

BOX 1: Autoimmune subepidermal blistering.

- Bullous pemphigoid
- Mucous membrane/cicatricial pemphigoid
- Gestational pemphigoid
- Linear IgA bullous disease
- Dermatitis herpetiformis
- Anti p-200 pemphigoid
- Bullous SLE
- Lichen planus pemphigoides
- Anti-type IV collagen pemphigoid
- Anti-105 kDa antigen pemphigoid
- EBA (mechanobullous disease)

- Annual incidence is 6–13 new cases per million.
- *Sex:* It has an equal incidence in both males and females
- There is no known ethnic, racial, or sexual predilection for developing bullous pemphigoid.
- *HLA class II association:* DQB1*0301 (white races), DRB1*04, DRB1*1101, DQB1*0302 (Japanese races).
- Bullous pemphigoid carries a significantly elevated mortality risk compared to the age-matched population with a 1-year mortality ranging from 13 to 38%.
- *Disease associations:*
  - *Neurological and psychiatric:* Parkinson disease, stroke, epilepsy, multiple sclerosis, uni/bipolar disorders, cognitive impairment
  - Psoriasis, lichen planus, lupus erythematosus
  - Diabetes mellitus, rheumatoid arthritis, autoimmune thrombocytopenia, pernicious anemia
  - *Malignancy:* Gastric cancer (most common), renal cell cancer, lung, lymphomas, myeloid leukemia, gallbladder, colon cancer
  - *Others:* Elevated IgE, eosinophilia.[1,3]

Etiopathogenesis

Predisposing Factors

- *External factors:* Psoralen and UV light, radiation (radiotherapy for breast cancer), thermal and electrical burns, skin grafting
- *Infections:* Cytomegalovirus, Epstein–Barr virus, HHV6, HHV8, hepatitis B and C viruses, *Helicobacter pylori, Toxoplasma gondi*, influenza vaccination
- *Drugs (drug-induced BP more common in younger age group):*
  - *Loop diuretic:* Furosemide
  - *Antihypertensives:* Enalapril, bumetanide, spironolactone
  - *Anti-inflammatory drugs:* Phenacetin, ibuprofen
  - *Antibiotics:* Ampicillin, penicillin, sulfapyridine, cephalexin
  - *Antidiabetic:* Gliptins
  - *Others:* Fluoxetine, penicillamine
  - *Topical drugs:* Benzyl benzoate, 5FU, anthralin.[2,4]

Pathogenesis

Pathogenesis of bullous pemphigoid has been shown in **Flowchart 1** and pathogenic mechanisms of blistering

TABLE 1: Autoimmune subepidermal blistering.

Characteristics	*Bullous pemphigoid*	*Linear IgA bullous disorder*	*Dermatitis herpetiformis*	*Epidermolysis bullosa acquisita*	*Mucous membrane pemphigoid*	*Pemphigoid gestationis*	*Lichen planus pemphigoides*
Age of onset	Elderly (60–75 years)	Before 5 years and after 60 years	Adult		60–65 years	Pregnancy	35–44 years
Cutaneous lesions	Tense, large bulla, urticarial plaques, milia	Vesicles/bullae—string of pearl pattern	Grouped vesicles and papules a/w excoriations	Skin fragility, tense blisters	Tense vesicles and erosions (20–25%) (involvement in cicatricial pemphigoid > MMP)	Urticarial papules, annular plaques, targetoid lesions, bulla	Vesicles both on pre-existing lichen planus lesions and uninvolved skin
Distribution pattern	Trunk > extremities	Trunk, extremities	Extensor surfaces, symmetrical	Trauma prone sites	Head and upper body	Periumbilical (face-spared)	Extremities > trunk
Mucosal lesions	Mild, transient (10–40%)	80%	Rare	50%	Predominant involvement (80–100%) Oral > conjunctiva > others	Spared	Spared
Histopathology	Subepidermal bulla (SEB) with eosinophilic infiltrate	SEB with neutrophilic > eosinophilic infiltrate	SEB with neutrophilic infiltrate	SEB	• SEB with infiltrates—eosinophils and especially plasma cells • Fibrosis in later stages	SEB with infiltrates especially eosinophils	Both features of BP and lichen planus
Antigen affected	BP 230, BP180 (membrane proximal region of NC16A)	LABD antigen 1 (LABD 97) and LAD-1 (derived from BP180)	Epidermal transglutaminase	Collagen 7	BP180 (C terminal epitope > NC16A) > BP230, collagen 7, laminin 332, α-6 integrins (ocular pemphigoid), β-4 integrin (oral pemphigoid)	BP180	BP 180 (N terminal NC16A), BP230, 200 kD of keratinocyte derivative
Direct IF	Linear IgG, C3 at BMZ (n-serrated pattern)	Linear IgA at BMZ > IgG	Granular IgA in dermal papillae	Linear IgG, C3 at BMZ (u-serrated pattern)	Linear IgG, C3 at BMZ	Linear IgG, C3 at BMZ	Lesional—Civatte body. Perilesional—linear IgG, IgM, IgA, C3 at BMZ
Indirect IF	Linear IgG at BMZ	Linear IgA at BMZ	Negative	Linear	Same as BP but lower titers	Linear C3 > IgG (HG factor)	Linear IgG at BMZ
Biopsy site for direct IF	Perilesional	Perilesional	Adjacent to normal appearing skin	–	Perilesional	Perilesional	Lesional and perilesional
Enteropathy	None	Rare	Common >90%	–	–	–	–
HLA association	Rare HLA DQ2 (20%)	HLA DQ2 (30%)	HLA DQ2 (>90%)	–	HLA DQB1	HLA DR3, HLA DR4	HLA B8, HLA CW7, HLA DR3
Dapsone responsiveness	Minimal – moderate	Good	Excellent	Nil	Good	Anecdotal	–

Flowchart 1: Pathogenesis of bullous pemphigoid (BP).

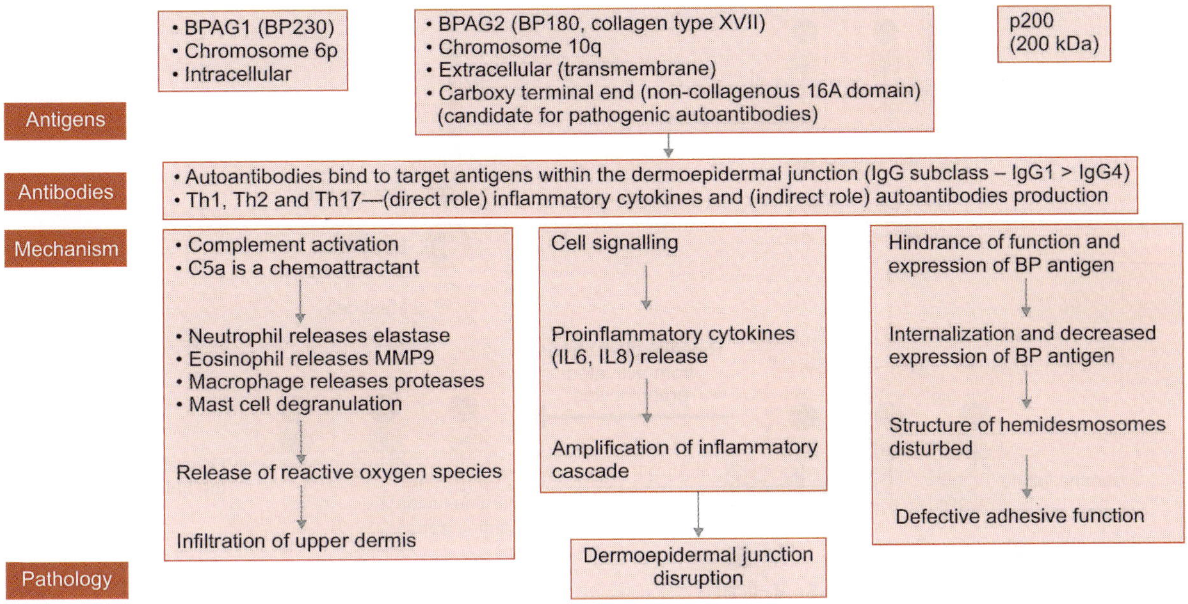

in bullous pemphigoid has been shown in **Figures 1A and B.**[2,4]

Clinical Features

- The classic form of BP is characterized by large, tense blisters arising **(Fig. 2)** on normal skin or on an erythematous or urticarial base.
- *Early nonbullous phase of BP:*
  - Nonbullous lesions are the first manifestation of bullous pemphigoid in almost half of patients.
  - It is a prodromal phase in which cutaneous lesions may be polymorphic. Signs and symptoms are usually nonspecific. These nonspecific findings may remain as the only signs of the BP. It can present either with urticaria like lesions or eczematous lesions **(Fig. 3)**.
  - *Urticaria-like presentation:* Mild-to-severe intractable pruritus alone or in association with erythematous presentation; lasts 1–3 weeks before blisters occur.
  - *Erythematous presentation:* Excoriated, eczematous, papular lesions which precede blisters by several months.
  - Other early nonbullous findings include serpiginous, or targetoid erythema multiforme-like lesions.
- *Bullous phase of BP:*
  - Prodromal phase can translate to generalized eruption blisters of BP even within weeks.
  - *Evolution of lesions:* Vesicles and bullae develop on apparently normal or erythematous skin together with urticarial and infiltrated papules and plaques that can be arranged in annular or figurate pattern. The noninflammatory form of bullous pemphigoid may be associated with a sparser inflammatory infiltrate histologically.
  - *Site:* Predominantly lower abdomen, inner or anterior thighs, flexural aspect of forearm are involved usually in symmetrical distribution.
  - *Mucosal lesions:* Mucous membrane lesions occur in approximately 10–30% of patients and are almost always limited to the oral mucosa. Lesions present with small blisters which can remain intact or rupture to heal rapidly (unlike pemphigus vulgaris). Other mucosal sites (eye, nasopharynx, esophagus or anogenital) are rarely involved.
  - *Morphology of lesions:* BP classically presents as tense and dome-shaped blisters (diameter in centimeters); blister walls are tough and may remain intact for several days. Blister cavity usually contains clear serous exudate (rarely hemorrhagic) which later may become jelly like content due to presence of coagulated fibrin. In some blisters, fluid is reabsorbed and epithelium settles back in place like a skin graft.[2-4]
  - The Nikolsky and Asboe-Hansen signs are negative **(Box 2)**.
  - The ruptured blisters form erosions which heal rapidly with postinflammatory pigmentary changes or milia. Erythema may even persist for weeks and months at the site of previous blisters.
  - Fresh crops of small blisters may continue to occur even with the achievement of apparent control of disease.
  - *Systemic association:* Acute phase is usually accompanied by eosinophilia and leukocytosis; fever is uncommon. The general condition of the patient is usually good in spite of extensive blistering.
- *Variants of BP:* Atypical variants of BP can be seen in up to 20% of BP patients **(Box 3)**.

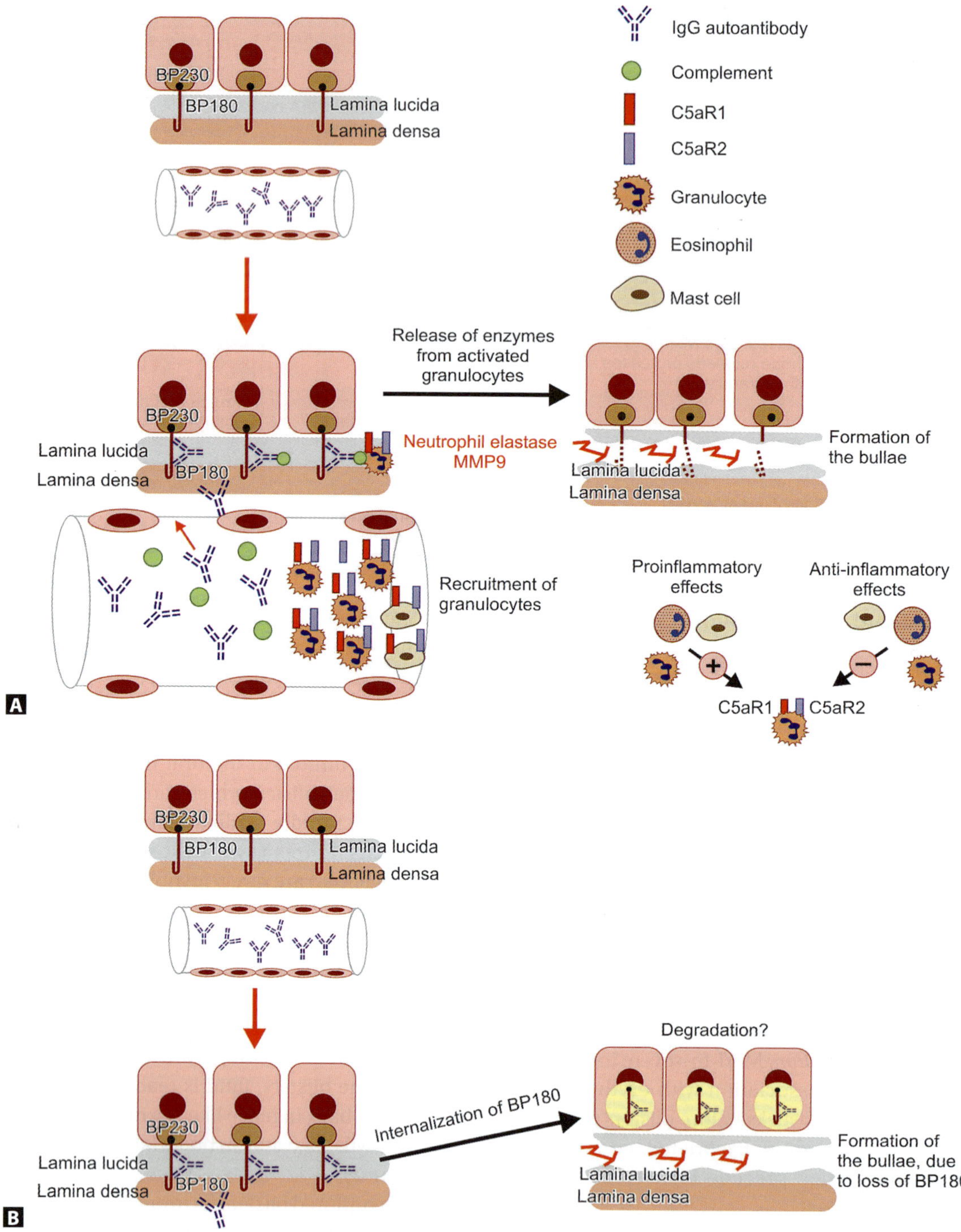

Figs. 1A and B: Pathogenic mechanisms of blistering in bullous pemphigoid. (A) Complement dependent pathways of bullae formation. Binding of IgG autoantibodies at the dermal epidermal junction leads to complement activation and recruitment of neutrophils. Activated neutrophils release proteolytic enzymes, inducing dermal-epidermal separation; (B) Complement-independent pathways of bullae formation. Binding of IgG autoantibodies to BP180 leads to depletion of the protein by internalization.

Differential Diagnosis of Bullous Lichen Planus

- *Investigations:*
  - *Histopathology:* Histopathology of a bullous lesion shows the typical feature of BP and shows a subepidermal separation with multiple eosinophils in the blister fluid and an eosinophilic infiltrate. On the other hand, histopathology of a lichenoid lesion shows the typical features of lichen planus with interface dermatitis with vacuolar change at the dermal-epidermal junction.
  - *Direct immunofluorescence (DIF):* IgG and C3 deposition at the dermal-epidermal junction zone can be detected using direct immunofluorescence of perilesional biopsies.

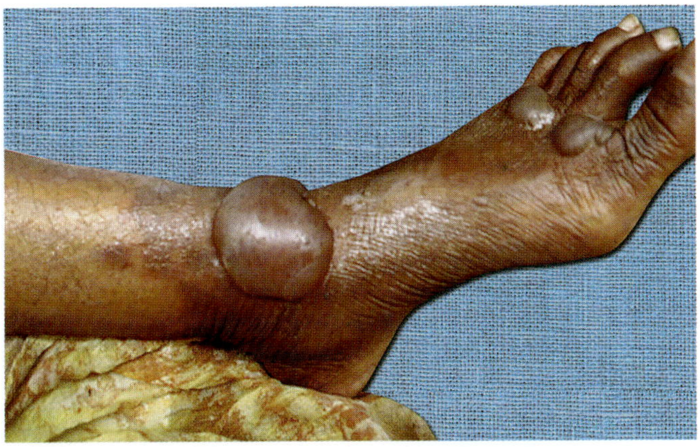

Fig. 2: Large tense blister in a patient of bullous pemphigoid.

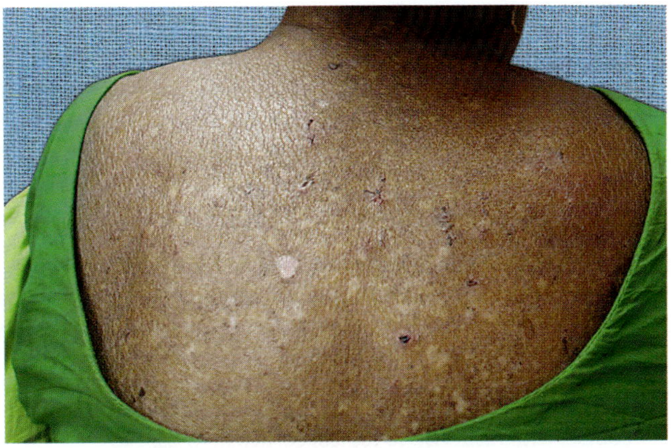

Fig. 3: Eczematous bullous pemphigoides.

BOX 2: Eponymous dermatological signs in bullous dermatoses.

- *Asboe Hansen sign or "bulla spread sign":*
  - This "bulla spread sign" refers to the extension of a blister to adjacent nonblistered skin when pressure is put on the top of the bulla
  - This sign is named after Gustav Asboe-Hansen.
  - In the traditional "bulla spread" sign also called Lutz sign, the margin of an intact bulla is first marked by a pen. Slow and careful unidirectional pressure applied by a finger to the bulla causes the bulla to extend beyond the marked margin.
  - While a regular rounded border is observed in bullous pemphigoid and other subepidermal blistering disorders irregular angulated border is seen in pemphigus vulgaris.
- *Nikolsky's sign:*
  - This sign is named after Pyotr Nikolsky, though the credit of first describing this finding should also go to his teacher MI Stukovenkov.
  - The sign is present when slight rubbing of the skin results in exfoliation of the outermost layer, forming a blister within minutes
  - Nikolsky's sign is useful in differentiating pemphigus vulgaris (where it is present) from bullous pemphigoid (where it is absent)
  - When the sign is elicited in the normal looking skin in the vicinity of the blister, then it is called marginal Nikolsky's sign and if it is elicited away from the blister it is called direct Nikolsky's sign.
  - Pseudo-Nikolsky's sign or epidermal peeling sign is positive in Stevens-Johnson syndrome, toxic epidermal necrolysis, in some cases of burns and bullous ichthyosiform erythroderma.
  - There is a phenomenon associated with this sign called "Nikolsky phenomenon." Here the superficial epidermis is felt to move over the deeper layers, and instead of an immediate reaction to form erosion as in Nikolsky's sign, the blisters develop after some time.
- *"False Nikolsky's sign" or "Sheklakov's sign":*
  - The "false Nikolsky's sign" is elicited and positive for subepidermal blistering disorders. It is seen in disorders such as bullous pemphigoid, cicatricial pemphigoid, dermatitis herpetiformis, epidermolysis bullosa, porphyrias, bullous systemic lupus erythematosus (SLE).
  - It is elicited by pulling the peripheral remnant roof of a ruptured blister, thus extending the erosion on the surrounding normal skin.
- *Premalatha sign:*
  - The term "cerebriform tongue" was coined by Premalatha.
  - Cerebriform tongue showing the typical sulci and gyri pattern over the dorsum of the tongue is a characteristic clinical sign in pemphigus vegetans which can precede, coincide or follow the skin lesions of pemphigus vegetans.

BOX 3: Atypical presentations of bullous pemphigoid (BP).

- *Dyshidrosiform/dyshidrotic eczema-like BP:* It is characterized by the presence of dyshidrosiform and pompholyx-like palmoplantar lesions and may represent an early localized presentation of BP. In most cases, lesions become generalized.
- *Vesicular/dermatitis herpetiformis-like BP:* Small vesicles seen instead of large bullae.
- *Prurigo nodularis-like BP:* This may create difficulty in diagnosis; this rare variant presents with itchy nodules. Shin is a common site for this type of BP. Blisters are rare but diagnostic. This condition can be more difficult to treat.
- *Erythrodermic BP:* Rarely BP can present as erythroderma.
- Ecthyma gangrenosum-like BP
- *Intertrigo-like, papular, eczematous, lymphomatoid papulosis-like, vegetating:* This rare form of BP presents with circumscribed hypertrophic lesions with crusts/erosions/pustules or vesicles at periphery.
- *Pemphigoid vegetans:* Intertriginous site involvement is seen with vegetating cutaneous lesions. Pemphigoid vegetans presents akin to pemphigus vegetans, but demonstrates histologic and immunopathologic changes seen in bullous pemphigoid.
- *Seborrheic pemphigoid:* It was first described in 1969. This form of BP resembles pemphigus erythematosus, with reputed bullae, erosions, and crusts involving the seborrheic areas

Contd...

Contd...

- Toxic-epidermolysis-like BP
- *Localized BP:* This form can be seen in about 5–30% of patients. It commonly affects the lower limb including the pretibial area, flexures, palms, soles, genital area, umbilicus, stomata and within sites of irradiation, hemodialysis fistulae. It may progress to generalize form.
- *Childhood BP:* Though BP is mostly a disease of elderly, it sometimes can affect children also with a bimodal (infantile and age of around 8 years) age of onset. In children, onset can be vaccination related. In childhood BP, facial involvement is more common. In infants, it predominantly affects acral skin; in relatively older children anogenital site is more commonly involved. One peculiar variant is vulvar childhood pemphigoid in girls. Overall childhood BP has a good prognosis; it is usually short lived and has a benign course. Childhood BP is treated with erythromycin, topical steroids and dapsone.
- *Lichen planus pemphigoides (LPP):* BP can occur in the background of lichen planus in both adults and children. LPP more often presents in middle-aged patients (mean age of onset, 35–45 years of age). Subepidermal blisters arise on both the lesions of lichen planus and also on normal skin. LPP is more localized to the extremities. This variant has a less severe clinical course compared with classic BP and it responds rapidly to treatment. Antibodies are demonstrated against the antigenic epitope of BP180 **(Box 4)**.
- *Stomal pemphigoid:* Patients demonstrate limited BP around the site of their stoma. This presentation appears to carry a milder clinical course, with response to topical corticosteroids.
- *Induced BP:* BP can be triggered by drugs, external factors as discussed as above. This group usually involves a younger population than classical BP.
- *Radiation aggravated pemphigoid:* The lesions in this type of BP are limited to the site of radiation therapy. This is particularly seen in patients treated with radiotherapy for breast cancer. Upon rechallenge, localized bullous pemphigoid will recur. Like other localized forms, this form demonstrates a good prognosis with response to topical therapy. However, radiation can lead to generalized development of BP.
- *Pemphigoid incipiens:* This rare variant is seen in elderly patients with generalized pruritus with or without skin lesions. These patients have circulating autoantibodies to the basement membrane zone with most commonly demonstrating reactivity against BP180 with or without anti BP230 antibodies. However, the patients usually have negative IF microscopy. This condition eventually translates to the BP and early treatment institutions may influence the clinical course of disease.
- *Hemiplegic pemphigoid:* The lesions of BP are limited to the area of neurologic deficit.
- *Stump pemphigoid:* The inflammatory lesions may only arise in a stump.

BOX 4: Lichen planus pemphigoides (LPP) **(Fig. 4)**.

- *Introduction:* LPP is a rare autoimmune subepidermal blistering disorder which was initially thought to be a variant of BP with cooccurrence of lichen planus. However, there is now a growing body of evidence suggesting that it is a disease entity in its own right. LPP can now be best defined as an autoimmune dermatosis, the hallmarks of which are lichenoid and bullous skin lesions, which develop in the context of autoantibodies targeting type XVII collagen.
- *History:* Kaposi was the first person to describe it in 1892.
- *Epidemiology:* The exact prevalence of LPP is unknown. However, it is seen in younger patients than BP (35–44 years). There is no specific gender predilection.
- *Pathogenesis:* LPP is characterized by autoantibodies against type XVII collagen (COL17, BPAG2) at the dermal-epidermal junction. The development of autoantibodies against COL17 in LP appears to be a primary event in the development of LPP. Both complement-dependent and complement-independent mechanisms may be relevant and the final pathogenic mechanisms result in the subepidermal cleavage.
- *Risk factors of developing LPP are:*
  - PUVA
  - Drugs like simvastatin, captopril, ramipril, cinnarizine, and anti-tubercular drugs.
- *Clinical features:*
  - In LPP, two discrete primary skin lesions occur: lichenoid papules/plaques and tense blisters.
  - The lichenoid eruption consists of pruritic violaceous polygonal papules and plaques with a shiny surface
  - On the mucosa, patterned white streaks may be found, most prominently on the buccal and the outer genital mucosa.
  - In childhood lichen planus pemphigoid palms and soles are also involved unlike adult counterparts.

Difference between LPP and BLP

Feature	*Lichen planus pemphigoid*	*Bullous lichen planus*
Site	Extremities (distal limbs) > trunk; bullae on lichenoid plaques as well as on normal skin	Extremities (shin > upper limb > thighs) (trunk is rarely involved); bullae on lichenoid plaques only
Etiology	Autoimmune disease precipitated by lichen planus	Due to severe liquefactive degeneration of basal layer (exaggerated max joseph space)
Histopathology	Subepidermal bulla similar to BP but with Neutrophil predominance	Subepidermal bulla with other features of lichenoid interface dermatitis)
Direct immunofluorescence (DIF)	Positive (linear deposits of IgG, C3 along DEJ)	Negative
Prognosis	Comparatively longer course	Shorter course

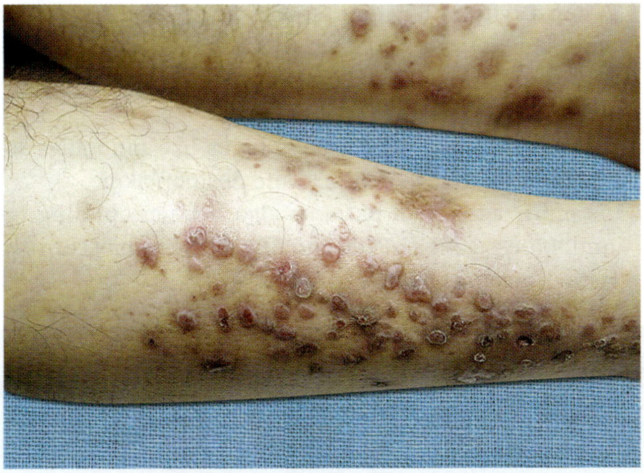

Fig. 4: Lichen planus pemphigoides.

- *Salt-split study:* Epidermal side binding of autoantibody I on salt-split study is seen.
- *Treatment:*
  - Management is usually in the line of BP.
  - Systemic corticosteroids are the most commonly used drug.
  - Other treatment options include topical corticosteroids, and dapsone.
  - Acitretin can be used to suppress the lichenoid reaction.[5]

Differential Diagnosis of Bullous Pemphigoid[2,3]

- Both intraepidermal (e.g., pemphigus vulgaris) and subepidermal (e.g., linear IgA disease, EBA) immunobullous conditions as well as bullous drug eruptions have to be considered in the differential diagnosis.
- *Non-bullous stage differentials:*
  - Prurigo
  - Scabies
  - Urticaria, urticarial vasculitis
  - Contact dermatitis
  - Drug reactions
  - Arthropod reactions
  - Ecthyma
- *Bullous stage differentials:*
  - *Subepidermal bullous disease:*
    - Cicatricial pemphigoid
    - Dermatitis herpetiformis
    - EBA
    - Linear IgA disease
    - Bullous systemic lupus
    - Porphyria cutanea tarda
    - Epidermolysis bullosa, hereditary
    - Erythema multiforme
    - TEN
  - *Intraepidermal bullous disease:*
    - Pemphigus **(Table 2)**
    - Hailey–Hailey disease
    - Incontinentia pigmenti
    - Allergic contact dermatitis
    - Bullous impetigo, staphylococcal scalded skin syndrome
    - Friction blisters

Diagnosis of Bullous Pemphigoid

Histopathology

- Early lesions show subepidermal cleft, roof of cleft formed by epidermis, papillary dermal edema with cell poor or cell rich perivascular lymphocytic and eosinophilic infiltrate.

TABLE 2: Differentiation between pemphigus vulgaris (PV) and bullous pemphigoid (BP).

	Pemphigus vulgaris	*Bullous pemphigoid*
Age group	Relatively in younger age	Common in elderly
Nature of blister	Flaccid	Tense
Peripheral extension of the erosion	Characteristic	Does not occur
Distribution	Scalp, seborrheic areas of trunk, axillae, groin	Abdomen, thigh, axillae and groin
Mucosal involvement	• Seen in 100%; starts with oral erosion in 50% • More severe	• Occurs only in 10–30% • Less severe
Course	Waxing and waning course, occasional spontaneous emission	Fatal if untreated
Nikolsky's sign	Positive	Negative
Tzanck test	Acantholytic cells	Eosinophil
Histopathology	Suprabasal blister with row of tombstone appearance	Subepidermal blister
Immunofluorescence (direct/DIF and indirect/IIF)	IgG +/– C3 in the intercellular space (ICS)	C3+/– IgG in a linear fashion along the BMZ
Indirect immunofluorescence (IIF)	Positive in 90% of patient with active disease; correlate with disease activity	Positive in 70%; does not correlate with disease activity

- Inflammatory BP (corresponds with blisters on erythematous skin) shows a cell rich pattern. The biopsy from such lesions demonstrates an eosinophilic papillary abscess with perivascular and interstitial mixed infiltrate (eosinophil, lymphocyte and neutrophil) with or without eosinophilic spongiosis.
- Noninflammatory BP (corresponds to blisters on relatively normal skin) shows a cell poor pattern. In such a scenario, dermis is acellular with scant perivascular infiltrate.
- Old blisters may demonstrate re-epithelialization along the base giving an artifactual intraepidermal blister.
- In pemphigoid vegetans, it also shows hypertrophic epidermis with papillomatosis **(Box 5)**.[2]

*Direct Immunofluorescence **(Fig. 5)***

- *Site:* A perilesional biopsy (within 2 cm of lesion) is taken. Lesional biopsy is avoided as immunoreactants are often lost from the roof.
- *Finding:* Direct IF of perilesional skin shows linear IgG and C3 along the basement membrane.
- DIF of BP needs to be differentiated from EBA by its n-serrated pattern (u-serrated pattern in EBA).[2,3,5]

*Salt-split Skin Study **(Fig. 6)***

- Biopsy sample incubated in 1 mol/L NaCl for localization of target antigen.
- Deposition of immune reactants is seen in the epidermal side of split (roof of artificial blister) unlike EBA where dermal side deposition is seen **(Table 3)**.

Indirect Immunofluorescence

- *Specimen used:* Usually blood is used but rarely blister fluid and urine are taken (less sensitive) in uncooperative patients/child.
- In approximately 70% of patients, there are circulating IgG autoantibodies that bind the basement membrane zone (BMZ) on normal human skin or monkey esophagus by indirect IF.

Enzyme-linked Immunosorbent Assay (ELISA)

- Commercial kits are available for detection of both BP180 (NC16A and total) and BP230 IgG antibodies.
- In the early stages of skin disease, only C3 may be present.
- A sensitivity of 89% and specificity of 98% have been reported.
- Transition from IgG1 to IgG4 marks diminution in disease activity.
- BP patients may also have pemphigus-like antibodies due to homology between BP230 and desmoplakin.
- As many as 75% of patients also have circulating IgE antibodies against BP180 and BP230; these may correlate with disease severity.

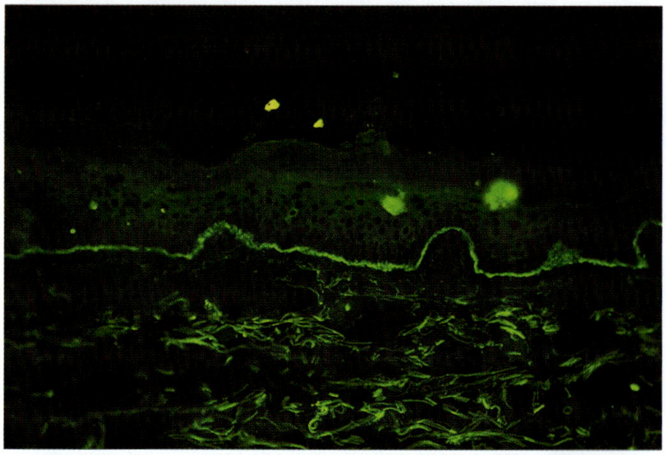

Fig. 5: DIF findings of BP showing linear deposition of IgG at basement membrane zone.

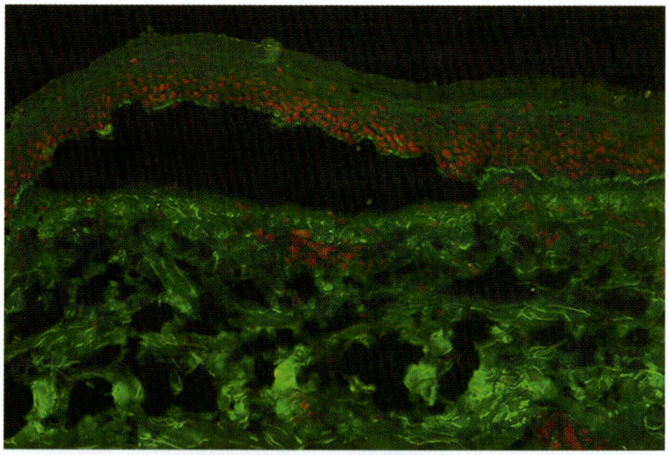

Fig. 6: Salt-split study showing epidermal staining in BP.

BOX 5: Histological differential diagnosis of subepidermal bullae.

- *Cell rich dermis (based on cell type of inflammatory infiltrate):*
  - *Lymphocyte rich:* Erythema multiforme
  - *Mast cell rich:* Mastocytosis
  - *Polymorphonuclear cells rich:* Dermatitis herpetiformis, chronic bullous disease of childhood
  - *Eosinophil rich:* Bullous pemphigoid, herpes gestationis
  - *Mixed:* Bullous pemphigoid, EBA, linear IgA disease
- *Cell poor dermis:*
  - *Congenital:* Epidermolysis bullosa dystrophica
  - *Acquired:* EBA, bullous SLE
  - *PAS-specific material:* Porphyria cutaneous tarda

TABLE 3: Step-wise approach to acquired blistering diseases.

Approach	*Results*
Tzanck test	• Shows plenty of eosinophils • Neutrophil rich inflitrate—consider other subepidermal blistering diseases
Histopathology	Subepidermal blister
Immunofluorescence (IF)	• Direct IF—presence of C3 +/– IgG in a linear distribution along the basement membrane zone • Indirect IF—detects the circulating autoantibodies; positive in 70% of patients with BP

- Approximately 7% of the normal population has anti-BP180 antibodies detectable by ELISA; the clinical significance of this positivity is not known.[5]

Fluorescence Overlay Antigen Mapping (FOAM)

Computer-aided fluorescence overlay antigen mapping can also differentiate BP and EBA on DIF.

Immunoelectron microscopy:

- *In vivo:* Autoantibodies are deposited in lamina lucida.
- *In vitro:* Antibodies bind to target antigens in association with dense plaque (BP230) and hemidesmosome (BP180).

Immunoblotting

- Circulating antibodies detected that react with BP230 and BP180 antigens.
- Autoantibodies against BP180 are associated with severe/prolonged disease.

Clinical Course and Prognosis

- Course of untreated BP is chronic, remitting, relapsing and ultimately self-limiting **(Flowchart 2)**.
- Localized disease is more likely to resolve spontaneously.
- High ELISA titers and positive direct IF at the time of therapy cessation has been associated with a high risk of relapse within the first year after cessation of therapy.
- *Duration:* Usually lasts for 3–6 years (remission can even occur within months)
- *Mortality:* Fatal especially in the active blistering stage in elderly (1/3rd in untreated BP).[2,5]
- *Poor prognostic indicators:*
  - Age more than 80
  - Daily dose of prednisolone more than 37 mg at discharge from hospital
  - ESR more than 30 mm/hour
  - Serum albumin less than 3.6 g/dL
  - Karnofsky Performance Status Scale score less than 40

Disease monitoring:

- *ELISA:* Anti-BP180 NC16A antibody levels (+ in 75–90%) correlates with the disease activity
- *Moderate titer ELISA:* BP180-NC16A score (3 times higher than the cut-off; >27 U/mL) and positive DIF findings at cessation of treatment is an independent predictor of increased relapse risk of BP in future (especially within 1 year of stopping the treatment)
- *ELISA at day 0 and day 60:* <20% decrease in serum autoantibodies is also associated with BP relapse within first year of treatment.

Management

Diagnostic Criteria of BP

- With 95% positive predictive value
- Linear IgG ± C3 deposits along the DEJ along with presence of 3 out of 4 criteria:
  - Age of patient >70 years

Flowchart 2: Algorithm to a patient with subepidermal autoimmune blistering diseases.

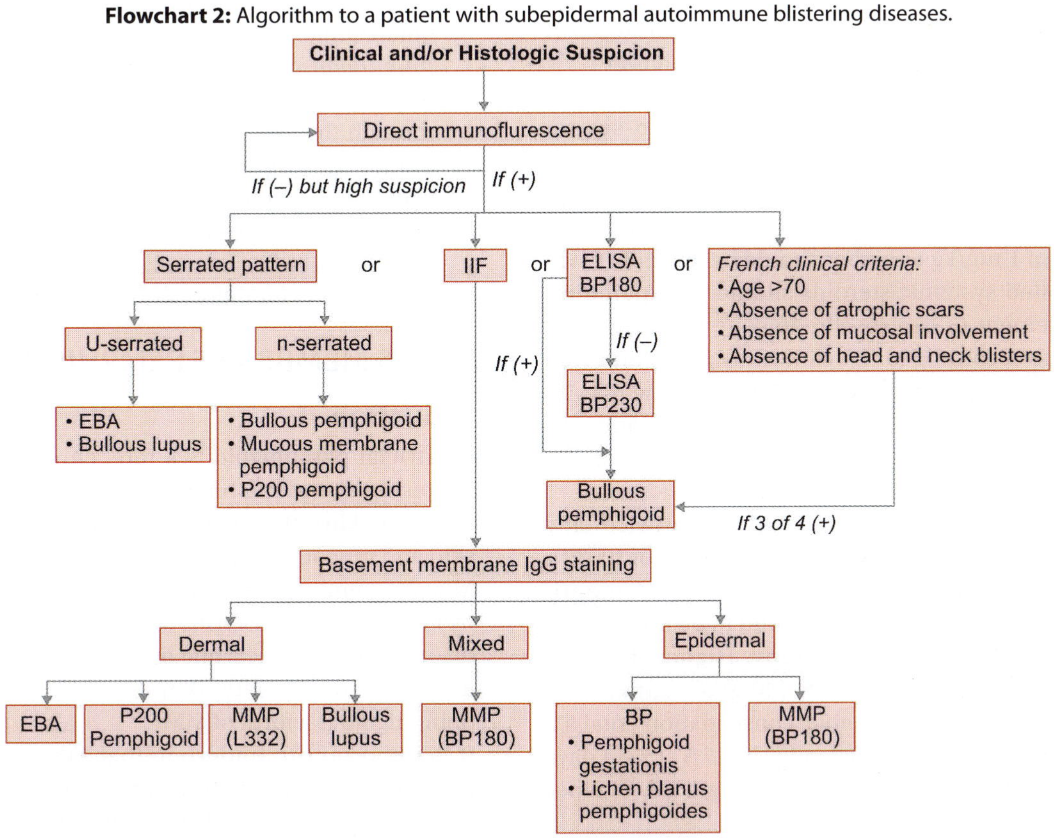

- Absence of mucosal involvement
- Absence of atrophic scars
- Sparing of predominant lesions on head and neck

Treatment Aim

- To suppress disease activity with minimum dose of necessary drugs (as elderly BP patients are commonly on many drugs, hence susceptible to adverse drug reactions).
- During prolonged treatment, it is advisable to aim for the presence of a blister once every few weeks to avoid overtreatment of elderly patients.

General Treatment

- Maintain nutrition
- *Oral mucosal care:* Chlorhexidine mouthwash, topical steroid, emollient
- *Genital and ocular mucosa:* Topical steroid, emollient
- *Eye care:* Ophthalmologist advice, topical artificial tear, antibiotic eye drops
- *Infection control:* Antibiotics
- Fluid electrolyte balance

Specific Treatment

- *Localized or mild disease:*
  - *Topical:* Very potent topical steroid such as clobetasol propionate. Applied to lesional skin.
  - *Systemic:* Corticosteroids 0.3 mg/kg daily, weaning on achievement of control ± very potent topical steroids
  - *Anti-inflammatory antibiotics:* Doxycycline 200 mg/day, oxytetracycline 1 g/day, minocycline 100 mg/day, erythromycin 1–2 g/day ± potent topical steroid
- *Moderate:* Severe disease
  - *Systemic:* In patients with moderate-to-severe disease, in which topical steroids cannot be used, oral corticosteroids are required. Corticosteroids are given at 0.5–1 mg/kg prednisolone equivalent daily. Doses of 1 mg/kg or higher should be avoided. Once controlled systemic steroids should be tapered on achievement of control. Prednisone tapering must be done according to the clinical response and side effects of the patient. The majority of disease may be controlled with small amounts of prednisone and immunosuppressive drugs. The maintenance can be continued on potent topical steroids.[6,7]
  - *Topical:* Very potent topical steroids 5–15 g twice daily to the whole skin surface. Daily application of 10–30 g of topical clobetasol propionate with a 4-month taper of oral prednisone was found to be noninferior to traditional systemic therapy. Higher doses of topical clobetasol propionate (40 g) are superior to oral prednisone. Once stable, consolidation entails a dose reduction of corticosteroids by 25% at 7–14 days interval until reaching 20 mg. At 20 mg, a slower taper every 2–4 weeks is recommended.[6,7]
  - Doxycycline or minocycline at 100 mg twice daily and niacinamide (1–2 g/day) may be of clinical benefit in controlling bullous pemphigoid with or without topical steroids.
- *BP refractory to or relapse on above-mentioned treatment:*
  - *Dapsone:* Dapsone has also been used in combination with topical steroids with variable success in mild-to-moderate disease at a dose of 50–200 mg daily.
  - *Steroid sparing immunosuppressants:* An adjuvant immunosuppression is added if either systemic corticosteroids are contraindicated or there is no adequate response.
    - Azathioprine 1–2.5 mg/kg daily
    - Methotrexate 5–15 mg weekly
    - MMF 0.5–1 g twice daily
    - Chlorambucil 0.05–0.1 mg/kg daily
    - Cyclophosphamide
  - *IVIG:* Patients refractory to conventional treatment or those with significant therapy-related side effects can be treated with IVIG as a monotherapy with clinical benefit.
  - *Rituximab:* While less well described in BP than in pemphigus, rituximab has demonstrated some efficacy in the treatment of BP. Rituximab can be combined with intravenous immunoglobulin also.
  - *Omalizumab:* The presence of anti-BP180 IgE and its correlation with disease activity has sparked interest in targeting IgE. Few cases have reported therapeutic benefit with targeting of IgE through the use of omalizumab.[6,7]
  - *Immunoadsorption:* Immunoadsorption refers to the removal of particular autoantibodies in patient serum through the use of different technologies. The use of immunoadsorption in BP resulted in rapid decreases of circulating autoantibodies.
  - *Future trends:* Current clinical trials are underway of the IL-5 inhibitor mepolizumab (NCT01705795) and the eotaxin-1 inhibitor bertilimumab (NCT02226146).

MUCOUS MEMBRANE PEMPHIGOID

Introduction

- Cicatricial pemphigoid is a rare, chronic autoimmune blistering disorder which can produce scarring. It can affect the skin only, mucous membranes only, or both the skin and mucous membranes.
- Mucous membrane pemphigoid (MMP) is the term agreed by international consensus for an autoimmune blistering disorder, which affects one or more mucous membranes and may involve the skin. Thus, ocular cicatricial pemphigoid is a form of MMP.
- It is important to underline that MMP should not be regarded as a single clinical entity but rather as a clinical phenotype shared by distinct autoimmune-mediated

diseases with lesions that favor the mucosal surfaces and show a tendency for scarring.

- Due to the risks of serious complications, such as blindness and airway compromise, early and aggressive treatment initiation may be warranted.[8]

History

- In 1794, Wichmann described a chronic blistering disorder characterized by ocular involvement.
- In 1949, Civatte separated this disorder from pemphigus on the basis of histopathologic findings.
- Lever coined the name "benign mucous membrane pemphigoid."
- In 2002, an international consensus conference agreed upon the designation of this disorder as MMP.[8,9]

Epidemiology

- MMP is extremely rare, with an incidence of up to 2 cases per million population in studies in Europe
- *Age:* MMP has a mean age of onset in the early to middle 60s.
- *Gender:* Females are affected 1.5–2.0 times as often as males
- HLA-DQB1*0301 is a disease susceptibility marker.[8,9]

Etiopathogenesis

- MMP is an antibody-mediated blistering disorder. Autoantibodies directed against antigens in the BMZ are responsible for the disease pathogenesis.
- BP180 appears to represent a major MMP autoantigen. BP180 is a transmembrane collagen, the noncollagenous portion of the domain (N-terminus) of BP180 is located near the cellular membrane and the collagenous portion of the domain (C-terminus) spans the lamina lucida and projects into the lamina densa. Sera from patients with bullous pemphigoid mainly target the N-terminus of BP180 whereas sera from cicatricial pemphigoid patients target the C-terminus. The variability in the target may explain the clinical differences seen among bullous pemphigoid and cicatricial pemphigoid patients.
- Other important antigens in MMP/Cicatricial pemphigoid are laminin 332, integrin subunit 4, integrin subunit 6, type VII collagen, and BP230 **(Table 4)**.
- As scarring is a major pathologic manifestation of MMP, profibrotic factors such as serpin h1; transforming growth factor-beta; interleukins 4, 5, and 13; and connective tissue growth factor plays an important role in the disease pathogenesis. Ocular scarring in MMP is associated with the "pro-fibrotic" phenotype of conjunctival fibroblasts.
- Epitope-spreading phenomenon where prior inflammatory process exposes hidden epithelial DEJ components to autoreactive T-cells leading to secondary autoimmune phenomenon, is involved in the disease process.

TABLE 4: Autoantigens involved in mucous membrane pemphigoid.

MMP antigen	*Site*	*Predominant involvement*
BP180 (C-terminal epitope > NC16A domain)	Epidermis, hemidesmosome	Mucosal > skin involvement
BP230	Epidermis, hemidesmosome	
Laminin 332 (antilaminin MMP/anti-epiligrin CP)	Lamina lucida–lamina densa interface	Only mucosal involvement; association with solid cancers (30%)
β-4 integrin	Epidermis, hemidesmosome	Ocular MMP
α-6 integrin	Epidermis, hemidesmosome	Oral MMP
Type VII collagen	Dermis, anchoring fibril	

BOX 6: Stages of ocular mucous membrane.

Stage 1: Subepithelial fibrosis/subconjunctival scarring
Stage 2: Fornix foreshortening
Stage 3: Symblepharon
Stage 4: Ankyloblepharon

- Dual antibody response (IgG ± IgA) is a marker for severe MMP.[8,10]

Clinical Features

- *Sites:* Oral mucosa (85%) is most commonly involved followed by conjunctiva (65%), skin (particularly head and upper body) (25–30%), nasal mucosa(20–40%), anogenital area (20%), pharynx, larynx, and esophagus
- *Oral lesions:*
    - *Morphology:* Painful erosions with or without tense blisters, sometimes leading to pseudomembrane formation. Oral MMO presents with desquamative gingivitis with eroded bleeding gums which may lead to reticulated scarring
    - *Involved areas:* Gingiva, buccal mucosa, and palate are more commonly involved than tongue, lips, alveolar ridge.
    - *Complications:* Adhesions form between tongue and the floor of mouth, uvula and tonsils. Dental caries are common. Other complications are periodontal ligament damage, loss of teeth, and bone mass.
- *Ocular lesions:*
    - *Prodromal symptoms:* Dryness, burning, photophobia, and foreign body sensation may precede ocular involvement.
    - Stages of ocular MMP (based on severity of scarring) **(Box 6)**
    - *Complications:*
        - Eyelid scarring leads to lagophthalmos, entropion, trichiasis, and secondary keratitis.

    - *Statue eye:* Corneal neovascularization and opacification leads to severe visual loss.
    - Glaucoma
  - *Pharynx and esophagus:* Dysphagia and structure leads to weight loss.
  - *Nasopharynx:* Nasal discharge, epistaxis, airway congestion, sore throat are seen.
  - *Middle ear:* Deafness may be caused by middle ear involvement.
  - *Genitalia:* Blisters, erosions and scarring may lead to labial fusion, introital shrinkage in females; and adhesion between prepuce and glans in male.
- *Skin lesions:* In about 30% patients of MMP cutaneous, lesions are seen in the form of tense vesicles, erosions, atrophic scars, milia, permanent scarring alopecia.
- *Brunsting–Perry pemphigoid:*
  - In 1957, Brunsting and Perry described this condition with recurrent scarring subepidermal blistering lesions on the head or neck.
  - The Brunsting–Perry pemphigoid is thought to be a rare variant of cicatricial pemphigoid characterized by blisters, hemorrhagic crusts, atrophic scars confined to head and neck without or with minimal mucosal involvement.
  - This variant is predominantly seen in men, and only in selected cases is associated with IgG autoantibodies against BP230 or BP180. Some patients of Brunsting–Perry have autoantibodies against collagen VII; suggesting it can also be a localized variant of EBA.[8,11]

Differential Diagnosis

- *Oral lesions:* Erosive lichen planus, pemphigus vulgaris, erythema multiforme
- *Conjunctival scarring:* Infective conjunctivitis, chronic allergy, erythema multiforme, TEN, burns
- *Genital scarring:* Lichen sclerosus, erosive lichen planus
- *Skin lesions:* BP, linear IgA disease, EBA.

Prognosis

- Course is chronic and progressive.
- Predictors of severe disease are:
  - Frequent relapses
  - Progressive course
  - Early permanent ocular lesions
  - Presence of both IgG and IgA antibodies against DEJ antigens.
  - *Presence of antiepiligrin antibodies:* Associated with risk of solid organ cancer especially adenocarcinoma.[11]

Investigations

The diagnosis of MMP should be based on correlation of all clinical, histopathological, and immunopathological findings.

Histopathology

- Subepidermal blisters with inflammatory infiltrates are rich in plasma cells, lymphocytes, histiocytes, eosinophils (less than in BP), and neutrophils.
- Plasma cells are seen more in mucosal lesions, whereas eosinophils and neutrophils are more commonly seen in skin lesions.
- Later stages show fibroblast proliferation and lamellar fibrosis.

Immunofluorescence

- *Direct immunofluorescence (DIF):*
  - DIF is positive in 80–100% cases of MMP.
  - In case perimucosal biopsy is not accessible, uninvolved skin and inner surface of lower lip (oral mucosa preferred over ocular mucosa)
  - Linear deposition of IgG and C3 with or without IgA along DEJ. In situ deposits of IgM, and/or fibrin are found in some patients.[12]
- *Indirect immunofluorescence (IIF):*
  - More than 50% patients shows positivity in IIF
  - Sensitivity can further increase by studying salt-split IIF.
  - Some studies suggest that the use of human mucosal tissue as substrate increases the sensitivity of IIF in patients with MMP.[8]
- *Salt-split IF:*
  - In salt-split studies IgG (and/or IgA) binding is usually directed against the epidermal side of 1 M NaCl split-skin, although combined epidermal and dermal or exclusively dermal binding can occur.
  - Epidermal side binding suggests circulating antibodies to BP180, α6 integrin, and β4 integrin.
  - Dermal side binding suggests antibodies to laminin 332 and collagen VII.[12]

ELISA/Western Blotting

Circulating antibodies (IgG4 is most common, followed by IgG1 and IgA) to the NC16A domain of BP180 may be positive.

Electron Microscopy

MMP blisters typically develop within the lamina lucida; blisters in the sublamina densa region are thought to represent mucosa-predominant forms of EBA.

Direct Immunoelectron Microscopy (IEM)

Sometimes the levels of these antibodies are below the detection threshold with standard IF and a more sensitive IEM, the gold standard for making the diagnosis, typically shows IgG and or C3 deposits in the lower part of the lamina lucida and in the lamina densa.[12]

Management

- Multidisciplinary approach involving dermatologist, ophthalmologist, otolaryngologist, gastroenterologist is required.

- It is preferable not to start systemic immunosuppressive therapies until the diagnosis of MMP has been confirmed with the specialist tests that are required.
- The goal of treatment is to stop disease progression and prevent scarring.
- All patients of MMP require long-term follow-up because of the possibility of relapse.[13]
- *General measures:*
    - *Oral:* Maintain hygiene, oral anesthetic rinses
    - *Nose:* Irrigation with isotonic saline, nasal lubricant
    - *Ocular:* Lubrication with artificial tears
    - Psychological support.
- Specific treatments **(Table 5)**

TABLE 5: Specific treatments for mucous membrane pemphigoid.

Mild disease	
Site	*Management*
Oral	Topical moderate-to-potent corticosteroid 2–4 times daily; topical corticosteroids under occlusion; topical calcineurin inhibitors; intralesional corticosteroids
Nose	Topical corticosteroids sprays or inhalers
Anogenital region	Topical corticosteroids; topical calcineurin inhibitors
Skin	Topical corticosteroids; topical calcineurin inhibitors
Moderate disease	
Moderate involvement of mouth, eyes, nose, larynx, esophagus, anogenital region Or Widespread MMP without rapid progression	Topical corticosteroids; topical calcineurin inhibitors PLUS Dapsone (1–2 mg/kg/day) OR Prednisolone 0.5–1 mg/kg/day (tapering) OR Anti-inflammatory antibiotics (Doxycycline/Minocycline) ± Nicotinamide
Severe disease	
Severe involvement of mouth, eyes, nose, larynx, esophagus, anogenital region Or Generalized MMP with rapid progression	Topical corticosteroids; topical calcineurin inhibitors PLUS Prednisone [1–2 mg/kg/day (tapering)] AND/OR Intravenous immunoglobulin (2 g/kg body weight over 2–3 days OR Mycophenolate mofetil (1–2.5 g/day) OR Azathioprine (2–2.5 mg/kg/day) OR Cyclophosphamide (1–2 mg/kg/day) OR Rituximab (1,000 mg on days 1 and 15)

PEMPHIGOID GESTATIONIS

Synonyms

- Gestational pemphigoid
- Dermatitis multiformis gestationis
- Herpes gestationis.

Introduction

- Pemphigoid gestationis (PG) is a rare autoimmune subepidermal blistering disease typically associated with pregnancy.
- PG is regarded as a specific pruritic dermatosis of pregnancy, although some rare cases have been associated with a hydatidiform mole, choriocarcinoma, or trophoblastic tumors.

History

- *1872:* Dr John Milton coined the term "herpes gestationis".
- *1973:* Complement deposition in PG was demonstrated by IF study.[14]

Epidemiology

- *Incidence:* 1 in 50,000 pregnancies
- *HLA:* HLADR4, HLADR3
- Multigravidae are more susceptible to develop PG than primigravidae with an earlier onset of symptoms.
- *Occurrence:* It occurs during the third trimester and less commonly in the second trimester or even after delivery, but it can manifest in principle during all three trimesters. It recurs in subsequent pregnancies earlier and as a more serious course.
- *Associations:* Hydatidiform mole, trophoblastic tumors, choriocarcinoma.
- Also associated with increased risk of Grave's disease.

Etiopathogenesis

- PG is associated with the presence of IgG autoantibodies against the NC16A domain of BP180.
- In the first trimester of pregnancy in the cytotrophoblast and syncytiotrophoblast of placenta and the epithelial cells of the amniotic membrane.
- Autoimmunization may occur due to loss of tolerance to this 180 kDa placental antigen, resulting in a local allogeneic reaction against the fetoplacental unit.
- This process, which is promoted by abnormal expression of placental HLA class II antigens, is accompanied by alterations in the placental basement membrane.
- After that, there is an immune response in the skin **(Flowchart 3)**
- *Role of hormones in the pathogenesis of PG:*
    - Progesterone suppresses antibody response (PG improves just before delivery when progesterone levels are high)
    - Estrogen enhances antibody production (oral contraceptives flares up disease).[15]

Clinical Features

- *Onset:* PG classically presents during the second trimester of pregnancy, though presentation from as early as the

Flowchart 3: Pathogenesis of pemphigoid gestationis (PG).

Aberrant expression of MHC II antigens (of paternal haplotype) in amniochorionic stromal cells and trophoblast
↓
Allogeneic response to placental DEJ
↓
Autoantibodies (IgG1, IgG4 called as HG factor) against self-antigen BP180 > BP230
↓
Immune complex formation
↓
Complement activation
↓
Recruitment of inflammatory cells
↓
Tissue damage and blister formation

second week of gestation to early postpartum has been described.

- *Course:* The disease usually improves in the last 6 weeks of pregnancy. It flares up again in the immediate postpartum period. PG usually resolves within 2 months after delivery. However, it may persist or exacerbate after pregnancy due to a sudden increase in the level of antibodies. Recurrence may occur with subsequent pregnancies, menstruations, or with oral contraceptives.
- *Lesions:* It manifests with inflammatory skin lesions and severe pruritus. The eruption of PG is polymorphic and may vary from pruritic urticated papules, annular plaques, eczematous lesions, targetoid lesions, and herpetiform vesicles. These progress to form tense blisters and bullae in about 65% of cases.
- *Main symptom:* Intense itching is the main symptom, and it may precede the manifestation of skin lesions in some cases.
- *Site:* Periumbilical area → abdomen → thighs, palms, soles (spared—face, mucosal areas)
- At first, the lesions erupt in the periumbilical area and subsequently spread to the abdominal region and the extremities involving mostly thighs, palms, and soles. The lesions may extend to the entire body, but spares face, mucosal areas.
- *Neonatal pemphigoid (3% of neonates):* Transfer of maternal antibodies can very rarely lead to bullous or papular rash in newborn.[14,16]

Prognosis

- The mean duration of disease is 6 months postpartum. About 5% may convert to BP and have a prolonged course. Active disease lasting 12 years postpartum has been described.
- Poor prognostic factors are:
  - Older maternal age group
  - Mucosal involvement
  - Multiparity
- Relapses can occur with the use of combined oral contraceptive pills or menstruation in a minority of women
- Skip pregnancies occur in a small subset (8%) of mothers, who may have an unaffected pregnancy following a previously affected pregnancy.
- *Fetal outcome:* Fetal risks observed in PG are low birth weight baby, prematurity, and temporary skin lesions which resolve several weeks after the birth, but there is no increased risk of stillbirth and abortion. This risk may be correlated with disease severity and early onset.
- Increased risk of Grave's disease.

Investigations

Histopathology

- Histopathologic studies are helpful; the findings during examination depend on the phase of the disease.
- Early lesions show eosinophilic spongiosis, dermal papilla edema, perivascular mixed inflammatory infiltrate
- Bullous lesions show basal layer necrosis leading to subepidermal bulla with eosinophil and tear drop appearance of papillary dermis.[15,17]

Immunofluorescence

- *Direct immunofluorescence:* Direct immunofluorescence is the most sensitive and specific examination used for confirming the diagnosis. It shows a positive linear C3 in 100% of the cases, and occasionally IgG in 30%, depositions along the dermal-epidermal junction. In salt-split skin, there is deposition on the epidermal side.
- *Indirect immunofluorescence:* Indirect immunofluorescence allows the detection of circulating IgG antibodies (circulating HG factor) in the patient's serum in 30–100% of cases.[15,17]

ELISA

ELISA-BP180 is very sensitive and specific (approximately 95%) for the diagnosis of PG. This allows to differentiate PG from other pruriginous dermatoses of pregnancy.

Other Tests

Other tests such as immunoblotting (circulating antibodies) and immunoelectron microscopy (localization of antibodies to anchoring filament) may be helpful in certain cases.

Treatment

Mild disease (localized disease with minimal blistering):

- Moderately potent topical corticosteroids and emollient
- Antihistamines

Moderate disease (exceeding 10% of the body surface): Oral corticosteroids at a dose of 0.3–0.5 mg/kg (20 mg to 40 mg/day) of prednisolone

Severe disease or refractory cases:

- Oral corticosteroids at a dose of 1–2 mg/kg body weight/day
- Immunosuppressant agents such as cyclosporine or azathioprine
- Intravenous immunoglobulins (IVIG)
- Immunophoresis
- Postpartum other drugs such dapsone, cyclosporine, cyclophosphamide, IVIG, or rituximab may be initiated.[18]

ANTI–P200 PEMPHIGOID

Introduction

- A very rare autoimmune subepidermal blistering disorder.
- This novel disease, presumed to be a subset of pemphigoid, was characterized by autoantibodies targeting a 200-kDa protein localized within the lower lamina lucida of the BMZ.

History

Anti-p200 pemphigoid was initially reported in 1996 by Zillikens and Hashimoto.[19]

Etiopathogenesis

- *The target antigen(s):*
  - The term anti-p200 pemphigoid was coined due to the reactivity of serum autoantibodies against a 200-kDa protein.
  - The true molecular identity of the p200 protein has not yet been fully unraveled.
  - The p200 protein was shown to be an acidic non-collagenous N-linked glycoprotein localized within the lower lamina lucida outside of hemidesmosomes by electron microscopy.
  - The C-terminus of laminin $\gamma1$ has been identified as an immunodominant region in anti-p200 pemphigoid.
  - Since then, some authors use the term anti-laminin $\gamma1$ pemphigoid when anti-laminin $\gamma1$ reactivity is detected in anti-p200 pemphigoid, while others prefer the original designation.
- Autoantibodies formed against this antigen, i.e., 200 kDa protein molecule (p200) is believed to cause the disease.[20]

Epidemiology

- Age group is somewhat younger than BP. The mean age of patients at disease onset is 69 years, ranging from 50 to 91 years
- The majority of the patients are males and of Asian ancestry.

Clinical Features

- The clinical presentation of anti-p200 is polymorphic and nonspecific.
- It may mimic bullous pemphigoid BP, MMP, DH, and other subepidermal AIBD
- Typically, patients present with tense blisters on erythematosus or normal skin resembling BP.
- Like in BP the clinical picture may be variable with erythema, erythematous plaques, erythematous papules, crusts, and vesicles.
- Mucosal involvement was reported in 39% of patients, with the oral mucosa (32%) being the most frequently involved.
- The extremities were the most frequently involved followed by the trunk, and palmoplantar involvement.
- When lesions are confined to hand and feet, pompholyx should be in the differential diagnosis.
- Lesions usually heal without scarring; milia formation has rarely been observed.
- *Association:* In the Japanese population, one-third of the patients also suffered from psoriasis, an association not found in Caucasians.[21]

Investigations

- Histopathology reveals subepidermal split accompanied by the accumulation of predominantly neutrophils in the upper dermis. In some patients, eosinophils can be admixed, and sometimes, microabscesses at the tips of dermal papillae can be found.
- DIF of a perilesional skin biopsy reveals linear deposits of IgG and/or C3 at the DEJ in an n-serrated pattern. In some patients, additional IgA deposits are detected at the DEJ.
- By indirect IF microscopy on 1 M NaCl-split normal human skin, autoantibodies label the floor of the artificial split.
- For definite diagnosis, circulating autoantibodies against the p200 antigen are detected by immunoblotting.[22]

Prognosis

Good prognosis and rapid response to treatment.

Treatment

- Management is on the same treatment ladder as that of BP.
- Very potent topical corticosteroids or tapering doses of prednisolone 0.5 mg/kg/day are often used.
- Dapsone, tetracyclines, azathioprine, and cyclosporine are also used.
- IVIG, plasmapheresis, and immunoadsorption are rarely used.[23]

EPIDERMOLYSIS BULLOSA ACQUISITA (FIG. 7)

Synonyms

- Acquired epidermolysis bullosa
- Dermolytic pemphigoid

Introduction

- EBA is a rare, sporadic autoimmune bullous disease of unknown etiology.

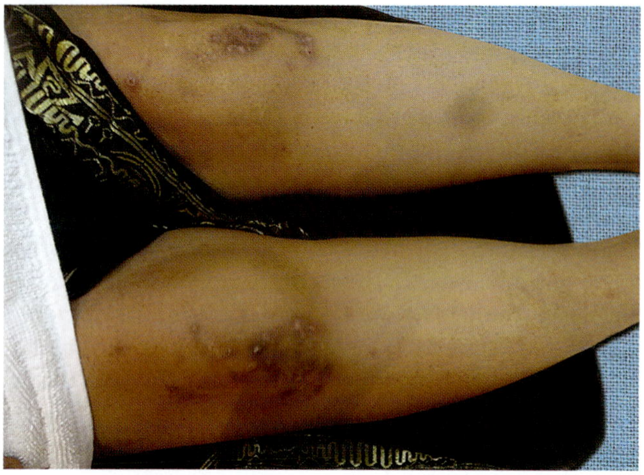

Fig. 7: EBA skin lesion involving extensors and healing with scarring.

- EBA is characterized by acquired, trauma-induced (mechanobullous) subepidermal blisters which usually heal with scarring and milia formation.
- It is specifically associated with autoantibodies against type VII collagen of the anchoring fibrils.[24]

Epidemiology

- EBA is a rare disease with an annual incidence of less than 0.5/million and a prevalence of about 3/million.
- EBA may occur at any age from neonate to old age with two peaks of onset, i.e., in the second and third decade and in the eighth and ninth decade.
- EBA is 1.5 times more likely to occur in females.
- It occurs in all races but has increased prevalence in individuals with a particular HLA types, notably HLA-DR2 in African-Americans and HLA-DRB1*15:03 in African Europeans.[24]

Etiopathogenesis

- EBA has circulating IgG autoantibodies against type VII collagen, within anchoring fibril structures that are located at the dermal–epidermal junction.
- The IgG autoantibodies most commonly binding to the noncollagenous 1 (NC-1) domain of type VII collagen chains result in decreased anchoring fibrils, but the pathway leading to this reduction is unknown.
- Experimental mouse models and in-vitro studies of EBA have demonstrated that autoantibodies to type VII collagen can induce dermal-epidermal separation.
- These antibodies may also directly interfere with the assembly of type VII collagen into anchoring fibrils or impede the interactions of type VII collagen with other matrix proteins such as laminin 332, fibronectin, or type IV collagen.[24,25]

Clinical Features

- Clinically, at least five phenotypes of EBA have been described.
  - A classic presentation (most common presentation)
  - A BP-like presentation, (most common inflammatory EBA presentation)
  - A MMP-like presentation
  - A Brunsting–Perry pemphigoid like presentation with scarring lesions and a predominant head and neck distribution
  - A linear IgA bullous dermatosis (LABD) or chronic bullous disease of childhood-like presentation
- *The classic noninflammatory presentation:*
  - This presentation is like that of porphyria cutanea tarda when it is mild and of the recessive dystrophic EB when it is severe.
  - The classic presentation is a noninflammatory mechanobullous disease characterized by skin fragility, tense blisters, erosions, scarring, milia formation, and postinflammatory dyspigmentation.
  - These findings are localized to trauma-prone sites and extensor surfaces, such as the elbows, knees, dorsal hands, and feet.
  - Severe acral involvement may be disfiguring with pseudosyndactyly, "mitten deformity" of digits, and nail dystrophy.
  - Scalp involvement can lead to nonhealing erosion with scarring alopecia.
- *Inflammatory variants of EBA:*
  - Inflammatory EBA may resemble BP, MMP, LABD, and Brunsting–Perry cicatricial pemphigoid.
  - BP-like EBA presents with widespread pruritic tense vesicles and bullae on an erythematous base, commonly involving the trunk, intertriginous areas, and extremities. Oral mucosa may be involved in approximately 50% of cases. The lesions heal without milia or scars.
  - MMP-like EBA predominant involves mucous membranes, with erosions and scarring of the oral cavity, esophagus, conjunctivae, anus, and vagina. Cases with ocular involvement may lead to blindness.
  - LABD-like EBA presents with tense vesicles, blisters, and urticarial plaques in an annular or polycyclic pattern, with mucous membrane involvement.
  - A Brunsting–Perry pemphigoid like EBA presents with vesiculobullous eruption and scarring lesions usually limited to head and neck area.[24,26]
- *Associations:*
  - Inflammatory bowel disease (Crohn's disease more than ulcerative colitis)—most common association
  - Thyroiditis
  - Rheumatoid arthritis, SLE
  - Multiple endocrinopathy syndrome
  - Multiple myeloma, lymphoma, chronic lymphocytic leukemia
  - Amyloidosis
  - Drug-induced EBA[24,26]

Differential Diagnosis

- Epidermolysis bullosa dystrophica (DEB) can be differentiated from EBA by the presence of family history, early onset, and negative DIF).
- Porphyria cutanea tarda (PCT) can be differentiated from EBA by the photodistribution, hypertrichosis, and porphyrin studies.
- Bullous pemphigoid **(Table 6)**
- Cicatricial pemphigoid
- Linear immunoglobulin A bullous disease (LAD)
- Brunsting–Perry pemphigoid
- Bullous systemic lupus erythematosus

Prognosis

- EBA is a chronic disease with periods of exacerbations and remissions.
- Prognosis and response to treatment may be better in children compared to adults.

Investigations

Histopathology ***(Figs. 8A and B)***

- Histologic examination of lesional skin obtained from EBA patients shows a subepidermal blister with varying degrees of inflammatory infiltrate depending on the clinical variant.
- The classic EBA presentation shows sparse neutrophilic inflammatory infiltrates in the papillary dermis.
- BP-like EBA presents with a dermal inflammatory infiltrate of neutrophils, lymphocytes, monocytes, and eosinophils. The histology of EBA skin specimens obtained from BP-like lesions may be difficult to distinguish from BP itself.[24,27]

TABLE 6: Differentiation between bullous pemphigoid (BP) and epidermolysis bullosa acquisita (EBA).

	BP	*EBA*
Clinical	• Tense vesicles and bullae on an erythematous base mainly over the chest, abdomen, axillae, back, groin and arm; the blisters contained clear fluid • The Nikolsky's sign and bulla spreading sign were negative	• Classic "noninflammatory" form of EBA is quite distinctive and presents with mechanobullous lesions, i.e., blisters at the trauma prone areas which heals with milia and scar • The "inflammatory" form closely mimics BP. This variants presents with vesicles and bullae involving flexures and intertriginous areas that heals without milia and scar formation
Histopathology	• Histopathology reveals subepidermal blister in both these conditions • BP can be: pauci-immune, eosinophil rich or mixed	• In EBA is usually pauci-immune • The predominant inflammatory cells are neutrophils; while that in BP is eosinophils
Direct immunofluorescence (DIF)	C3 is usually more stronger than IgG	Stronger BMZ band with IgG. Presence of IgA positivity suggests more of EBA
Pattern of BMZ band	"n" serrated	"u" serrated
Salt-split study using perilesional skin (direct salt split) or serum (indirect salt split)	Linear BMZ band is seen either on the epidermal side (roof pattern) or on either side of the split (mixed pattern)	Linear BMZ band is seen on the dermal side of the split (floor pattern)
Indirect immunofluorescence (IIF) study using toad skin as a substrate	Positive in BP	Negative

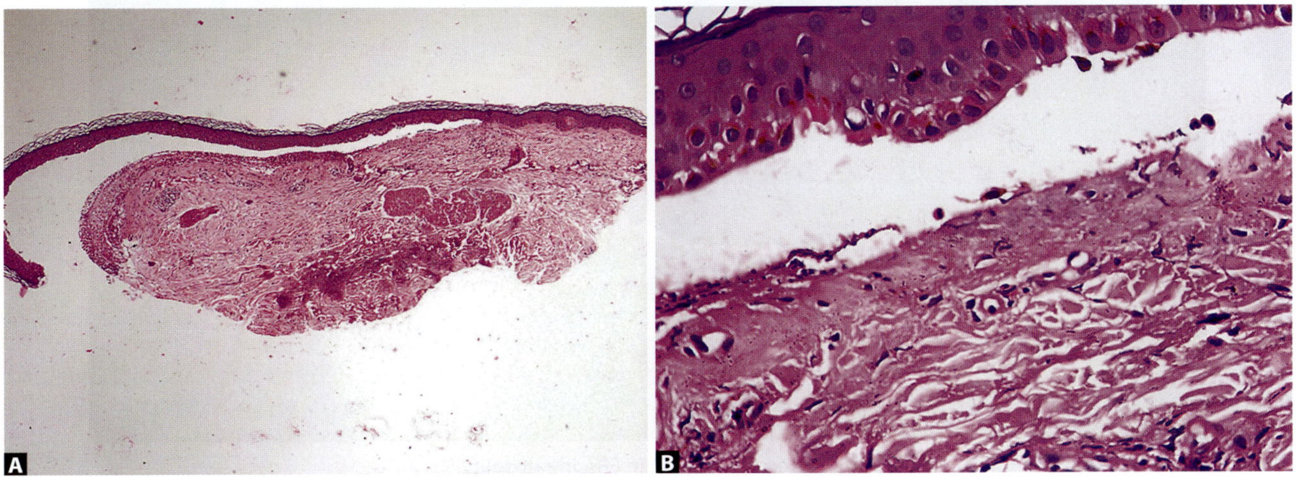

Figs. 8A and B: Epidermolysis bullosa acquisita histopathology.
Courtesy: Dr Subhra Dhar, Wizdermpathlab.

Immunofluorescence

- *Direct immunofluorescence:*
    - DIF of a biopsy specimen obtained from a perilesional site shows linear deposits of IgG along the epidermal BMZ.
    - Less commonly, linear deposits of C3, IgA, or IgM may also be detected.
    - A "u-serrated" immune deposition pattern at the BMZ helps differentiate EBA from BP, which has an "n-serrated" pattern **(Table 6)**.
- *Indirect immunofluorescence:*
    - Approximately 50% of patients with EBA have detectable anti-BMZ IgG antibodies in their serum, which would result in a linear fluorescent band along the DEJ on IIF.
    - Human skin or rat or monkey esophagus can be used as a substrate.
    - Knockout analysis—substrate as basement membrane from donors of inherited RDEB can be used to distinguish BP from EBA.
    - *Toad skin study:* Toad skin lacks EBA antigen but has BP antigen, hence it can be used as a substrate to distinguish BP from EBA.
- *Salt-split IF **(Fig. 9)**:* Salt-split skin IF preparations show immune deposits located on the dermal side of the cleavage, in contrast to BP, which has deposits located on the epidermal side of the separation.[24,27]

Transmission Electron Microscopy of the DEJ

Transmission electron microscopy shows cleavage in the sublamina densa zone, a decreased number of anchoring fibrils, and deposition of an amorphous, electron-dense material corresponding to the IgG, beneath the lamina densa in EBA skin.

Immunoblotting

- Electrophoretic membrane with immobilized proteins is incubated with EBA serum.
- Antibodies in EBA bind to 290-kD band (α-chain of collagen VII), 145-kD (N-terminal globular NC1 domain of collagen VII.

Immunoelectron Microscopy

- IEM is the traditional "gold standard" for the diagnosis of EBA.
- It can reveal immune deposits localized to anchoring fibrils within the sublamina densa.

FOAM

It distinguishes BP from EBA (IgG deposited above and below lamina densa respectively).

ELISA

- It is a quick and efficient test with high specificity (>96%).
- It uses recombinant NC1 and NC2 domains of type VII collagen to detect EBA autoantibodies.
- It can detect levels of autoantibodies, which correlate with disease severity.

Western Blot

Serum from EBA patients demonstrates binding of circulating autoantibodies to a 290 kDa protein or less frequently to a 145 kDa protein in western blot, which corresponds to the alpha-chain of type VII collagen and its NC1 domain, respectively.

Diagnostic Criteria of EBA

- Bullous disease with appropriate clinical features
- Absent family history

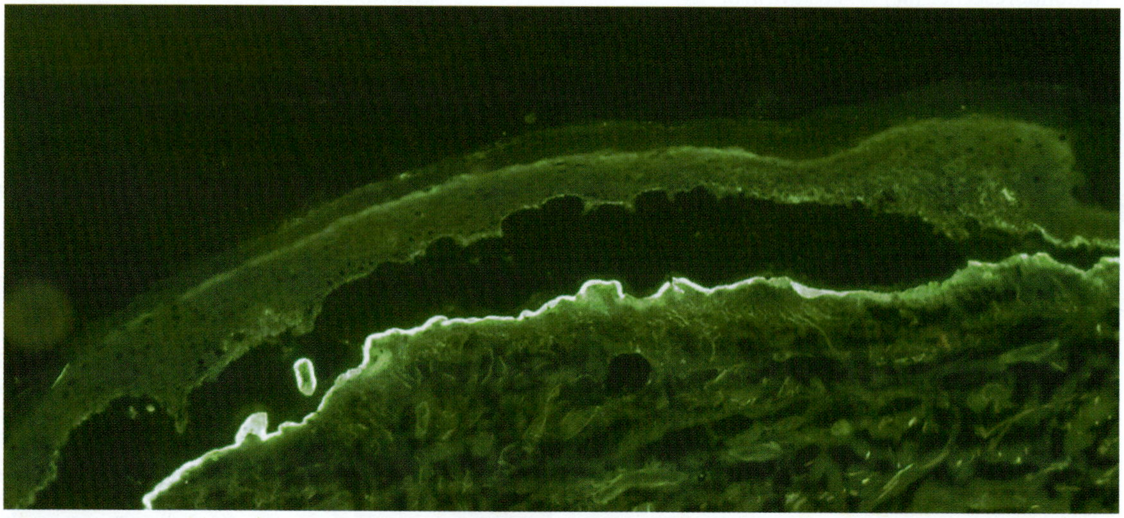

Fig. 9: Dermal staining in EBA in salt-split DIF.
Courtesy: Dr Subhra Dhar, Wizdermpathlab.

- *Histopathology:* Subepidermal blister
- *DIF (perilesional):* IgG deposition within DEJ
- *IEM (perilesional):* IgG localization within the lower lamina densa ± sublamina densa zone.
  Or
  Alternatively, salt-split IMF (direct/indirect), IIF using substrate deficient in molecules of basement membrane, western blotting, FOAM, ELISA **(Flowchart 4)**.[24,28]

Treatment

The treatment of EBA is challenging and requires a multidisciplinary approach involving dermatologist, ophthalmologist, otolaryngologist, and gastroenterologist.

General Measures

- Risk of complications need to be reduced by avoiding trauma, use of protective padding, proper wound care, and skin care.
- Persistent bulla needs to be ruptured under sterile precautions.
- A nonstick dressing (silicone/petroleum jelly gauze/hydrogel/foam dressing/absorptive/silver containing dressing/nonadherent lipidocolloid dressing/antimicrobial dressing) needs to be used.
- Further injuries need to be reduced by avoiding vigorous rubbing, over washing, and use of hot water, or harsh soap.
- Prolonged sun exposure needs to be avoided and use of sunscreen and other photoprotective measures should be promoted.
- Psychological and psychiatric support.
- Nutritional support.

Supportive care of mucosal sites:

- *Oral:* Oral hygiene needs to be maintained with the use of antiseptic, fluoride mouthwashes, topical antibiotics, topical NSAIDs, sucralfate suspensions, and mouth expanding devices.
- *Esophageal:* Dietary modification, balloon dilatation, colonic interposition may be required in certain cases.
- *Gastric:* Proton-pump inhibitors, prokinetics, osmotic laxatives (polyethylene glycol), and mineral oil may be required in some cases.
- *Ocular:* Surgical procedures such as division of symblepharon, or amniotic membrane transplantation may be required in specific cases.
- *Genitourinary:* Dilatation procedures to treat obstruction is done on select cases.[24,29]

Specific Treatment

- *Colchicine:* High doses of colchicine may be effective in the milder forms of both classic EBA and inflammatory EBA. The mechanism is unknown, but it is thought to reduce the production of antibodies and inhibit antigen presentation to T-cells.
- *Dapsone:* Dapsone may be especially beneficial in EBA patients with neutrophilic dermal infiltrates. A combination of dapsone and prednisolone may be tried for childhood EBA.
- *Oral corticosteroids:* Unlike other AIBD, oral corticosteroids do not usually have a dramatic effect in EBA. Systemic corticosteroids (0.5–1 mg/kg/day) may be effective in BP-like EBA and other inflammatory variants. For more severe cases, systemic steroids may be tried at 1 mg/kg/day

Flowchart 4: Approach to a patient with epidermolysis bullosa acquisita (EBA).

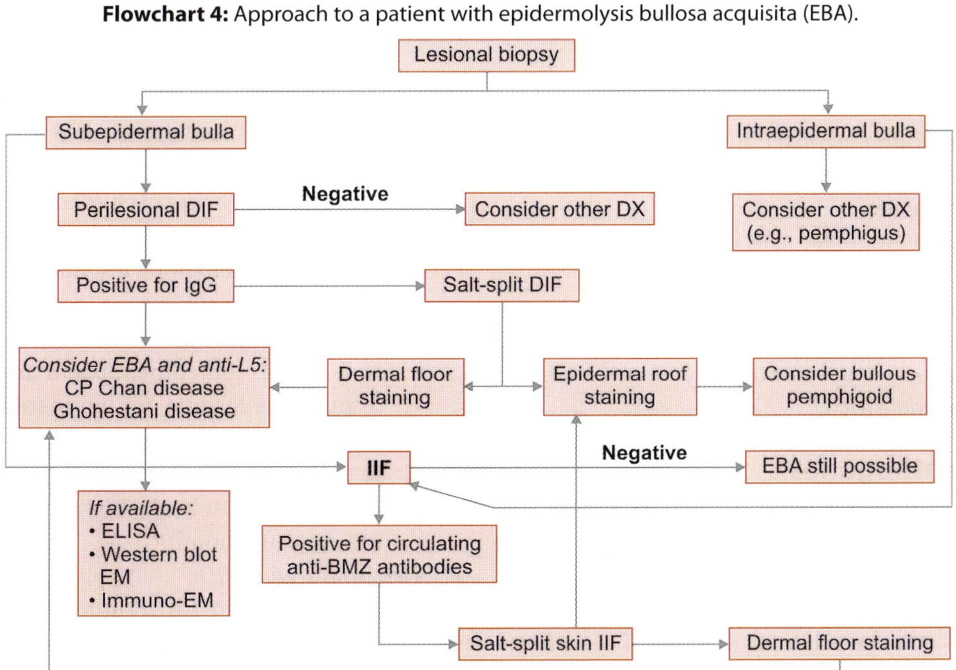

along with immunosuppressive medications, including azathioprine, cyclophosphamide, cyclosporine, methotrexate, or mycophenolate mofetil.

- *Cyclosporine:* High doses of cyclosporine may be needed (6 mg/kg) to control the disease in some patients, however, its long-term use must be avoided because of its side effects on the kidneys, blood pressure, and overall immune system.
- *Mycophenolate mofetil:* MMF in conjunction with systemic steroids has been reported in a few cases.
- *Rituximab:* Rituximab is reported to have dramatic results for some severe EBA patients.
- *Intravenous immunoglobulins:* IVIG have been used successfully in case reports.
- *Photopheresis or plasmapheresis:* These may improve the clinical features of EBA.[24,30]

LINEAR IGA BULLOUS DERMATOSIS

Introduction

- LABD is a rare immune-mediated, subepidermal blistering disease that occurs in both adults and children.
- *Chronic bullous disease of childhood* is a rare blistering disease that occurs predominantly in children younger than 5 years of age. It tends to have a distinct clinical appearance, but the underlying pathogenesis of the disease remains the same.

History

- Chorzelski and Jablonska in 1975 first described LABD as an individual entity based on immunopathological studies.
- Jordan et al. in 1970 coined the term benign chronic bullous disease of childhood.[31]

Epidemiology

- *Age group:* It has bimodal onset. In children, it is seen in preschool age (<5 years) and in adults, it is seen mostly in the sixth decade of life.
- A slight predominance of females is seen.
- *Incidence:* 0.5/million
- There may be increased frequency of HLA-B8 has been noted.
- *Geographic areas:* Most commonly seen in China, Southeast Asia, and Africa.[31,32]

Etiology and Pathogenesis

- *Genetic predisposition:* LA-B8, HLA-DR3, HLA-DQ2, and HLA-cw7 can be associated with both the childhood and adult variants of LABD.
- LABD is caused by circulating IgA antibodies directed against the 97-kDa extracellular domain of the BPAG2 or collagen XVII which is essential in anchoring basal keratinocytes to the epidermal basement membrane. The 97-kDa subunit lies within the well-known NC16A domain of the BPAG2 molecule. Additionally, some patients may display autoantigens toward LAD-1 (a 120-kDa truncated domain of BPAG2).
- Patients usually have relatively low titers of circulating IgA autoantibodies. Various theories regarding potential causative factors in the production of the offending IgA antibodies exist and include infectious etiologies, autoimmune disease, induction secondary to malignancy, or gastrointestinal disease.
- Rarely antibodies can be formed against other BMZ antigens such as BPAG1, LAD 285, type VII collagen.
- *Drug-induced LABD:* LABD is frequently caused by drugs in adults. The most frequently incriminated drug is vancomycin, which is responsible for nearly 50% of the cases of drug-induced LABD. Other frequently implicated medications include antibiotics (e.g., penicillins, cephalosporins, and rarely, sulfonamides antibiotics), ACE inhibitors (specifically, captopril), NSAID (e.g., diclofenac, naproxen), and phenytoin.
- *Other associations:* Autoimmune diseases (celiac disease, Crohn's disease, ulcerative colitis, systemic lupus erythematosus, rheumatoid arthritis, dermatomyositis, and multiple sclerosis) or malignancies (lymphoproliferative disorders, and thyroid, bladder, colon, renal, or esophageal cancers).[31,33]

Clinical Features

- *LABD in adults:*
  - LABD in adults can have heterogeneous presentation with combinations of annular or herpetiform papules, vesicles, and bullae.
  - Typically, the lesions atypically have a widespread symmetric distribution most commonly involving the extensor surfaces, including elbows, knees, and buttocks, but can also involve the scalp, genital area or face.
- *Chronic bullous disease of childhood:*
  - The classic clinical presentation of CBDC includes annular erythematous lesions with a ring of vesicles, commonly referred to as a "crown of jewels" or "string of pearls **(Fig. 10)**."
  - New lesions sometimes appear around the periphery of previous lesions, with a resulting "collarette" of blisters.
  - In children, the lesions most commonly occur on the abdomen, lower back, thighs, groin area, and around the eyes and mouth.
- *Drug-induced LABD:*
  - Drug-induced LABD may present as erythema multiforme–like lesion, toxic epidermal necrolysis–like lesion, localized palmar, and morbilliform variants.

- Drug-induced LABD may show the Koebner phenomenon, may even have a positive Nikolsky sign.

- *Mucous membrane involvement:*
  - LABD can also have mucous membrane involvement in about 70% of patients.
  - This involvement can range from largely asymptomatic oral ulcerations and erosions to severe oral or conjunctival disease.
  - Oral mucosa, conjunctivae, nares, and genital areas can be involved.
  - CBDC differs from LABD of adults in its relative paucity of serious mucosal involvement.
- *Pruritus:* LABD can vary symptomatically from completely asymptomatic, to mild or severe pruritus or burning sensation in both the adult and childhood form **(Table 7)**.[31,33,34]

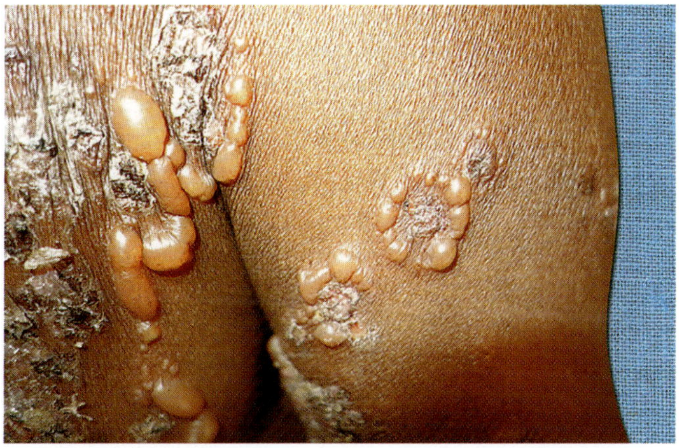

Fig. 10: String of pearl appearance in a case of LABD.

Investigations

Histopathology

- Subepidermal blisters are observed with a predominantly neutrophilic infiltrate.
- Early in the disease process, this neutrophilic infiltrate may be mainly localized to the dermal papillae, when it may be confused with dermatitis herpetiformis.
- Later in the disease process, eosinophils may be mixed with the neutrophilic infiltrate in the dermis, when it may be confused with BP.
- One clue to the diagnosis of LABD, over DH or BP, is the manner in which the neutrophils "line up" at the basement membrane.[31,35]

Immunofluorescence

- *Direct immunofluorescence:*
  - DIF is gold standard for diagnosis
  - In LABD, there is a homogeneous linear band of IgA at the dermal-epidermal BMZ occasionally along with IgG or C3.
- *Indirect immunofluorescence:*
  - Circulating IgA antibasement membrane zone antibodies are detected in up to 70% of LABD patients.
  - This can be helpful to differentiate from DH as circulating IgA antibasement membrane zone antibodies are not found in patients with DH.
- *Salt-split skin:* In the lamina lucida subtype of LABD, these antibodies will adhere to the roof of a salt-split skin test (epidermal side), while in the sub-lamina densa variant the antibodies will adhere to the floor (dermal side).[31,35]

TABLE 7: Clinical characteristics of CBDC and LABD of adults.

Features	*CBDC of adults*	*LABD of adults*
Age	6 months–10 years (4.5 years average)	Later teens–9th decade (around 60 years)
Onset	More abrupt	Less abrupt ± insidious
Sites	• *Younger children:* Face (perioral, periocular), genital area • *Older children:* Lower trunk, medial thigh (generalized eruption)	Trunk, limb > face, scalp
Evolution of skin lesions	• Asymptomatic/itchy/burning sensation • Tense, clear, hemorrhagic vesicles/bulla on normal/erythematous skin • String of pearl/cluster of jewels/rosette pattern (more common) central crust surrounded by new lesions arising around resolving lesions in arciform/annular pattern	• Insidious ± pruritus/burning sensation • Urticated plaques and papules • Blisters arising from normal/urticated skin
Mucosal lesions	• Common (60–80%) • Oral erosions, ulcers, hoarseness, nasal stuffiness, sore eyes, conjunctivitis	• Common (60–80%) • May be more severe than CBDC
Associations	Nil	Lymphoproliferative disorders, bladder and renal cancer, inflammatory bowel disease
Differentials	• Bullous impetigo • Sexual abuse • Bullous papular urticaria	• BP • Atypical erythema multiforme • Prurigo nodularis • DH
Prognosis	• Remits spontaneously (may last from a few months to up to 4 years) • Waxing and waning course • No scarring	Remits within 3–6 years

Differential Diagnosis

- Dermatitis herpetiformis
- Bullous pemphigoid
- EBA
- Bullous systemic lupus erythematosus
- Cicatricial pemphigoid
- Toxic epidermal necrolysis.

Prognosis

- CBDC is most often a self-limited disease, with most children going into remission within 2 years.
- Spontaneous remission may occur in 30–60% of adult patients after years of active disease.
- Drug-induced LABD also has a good prognosis with most cases remitting within 2–6 weeks after withdrawal of the inciting medication.
- *Poor prognostic factors:*
  - HLA-association (HLA-B8, HLA-CW7, HLA-DR3)
  - LABD associated with pregnancy remits from 2nd trimester onwards but relapse after 3 months postpartum (not associated with fetal damage).[31,36]

Treatment

- Potent steroids alone may be useful for mild disease **(Box 7)**.
- *Dapsone:*
  - Patients with linear IgA disease most often respond dramatically to dapsone.
  - Improvement may be seen as early as 2–3 days of drug initiation.
  - Relatively low doses of dapsone are usually required with an average of 100 mg daily for adults, while in CBDC, 1–2 mg/kg per day is given.
- Sulfapyridine can be another treatment option.
- *Oral corticosteroids:* Some patients may require adjunctive administration of low-dose prednisone therapy.
- *Mycophenolate mofetil:* It is useful as a steroid-sparing agent
- *Antibiotics:* Anti-inflammatory antibiotics such as tetracyclines, and trimethoprim-sulfamethoxazole, have also proven to be beneficial.
- Nicotinamide 1.5 g/day may be an effective adjunctive treatment.[31,37]

BOX 7: Pharmacological treatment ladder.

- *First line:*
  - Dapsone is the drug of choice in LABD. It is started at a lower dose of 0.5 mg/kg and slowly increased up to 2 mg/kg/day until blistering is controlled.
    PLUS
  - Potent topical corticosteroid
- *First line adjuvant:*
  - Low-dose prednisone (0.25–0.5 mg/kg/day)
- *Second line:*
  - Sulfapyridine (15–60 mg/kg/day)
    OR
  - Anti-inflammatory antibiotics (erythromycin, dicloxacillin, oxytetra-cycline, doxycycline) ± Nicotinamide
    OR
  - Colchicine (especially given in patients with G6PD deficiency where dapsone and sulfapyridine are contraindicated in patients; at a dose 0.5 mg twice daily)
- *Third line:*
  - Mycophenolate mofetil
  - Intravenous immunoglobulin
  - Immunoadsorption

DERMATITIS HERPETIFORMIS (FIG. 11)

Synonym

Duhring–Brocq disease

Introduction

Dermatitis herpetiformis (DH) is a rare, intensely pruritic, chronic, recurrent, papulovesicular disease associated with underlying gluten sensitive enteropathy and granular IgA deposition at dermoepidermal junction.

History

- *1884:* Louis Adolphus Duhring described DH.
- *1888:* Louis-Anne-Jean Brocq of Paris described a very similar disorder and called it dermatite polymorphe prurigineuse.
- *1966:* Marks described connection between DH and intestinal abnormalities were demonstrated.
- *1969:* van der Meer demonstrated IgA deposits at dermal papillae of uninvolved skin in DH.
- *2002:* Epidermal transglutaminase was identified as autoantigen in DH.
- *2016:* Görög demonstrated circulating transglutaminase 3–IgA immune complexes in DH patients.[38]

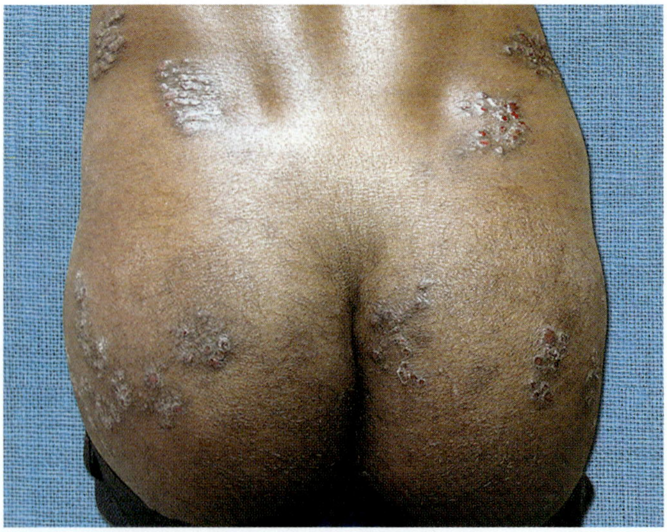

Fig. 11: Grouped vesicular lesions in extensors in a patient of dermatitis herpetiformis.

Epidemiology

- It is most common in people of northern European descent and is most uncommon in Asian and African populations.
- Prevalence of DH in various populations varies between 10 and 75 in 100,000.
- *Age group:* Onset is commonly in adult life, typically in the fourth decade, however, It may start at any age, including in childhood.
- *Gender:* The disease is more common in men than women
- Both concordant and discordant monozygotic twins are affected. Family history may be positive.
- *HLA:* There is a close association between DH and certain HLA types, particularly HLA-DQ2, and to a lesser extent, HLA-DQ8.
- *Season:* Onset of symptoms mostly reported during warmer months of year.[38,39]

Etiopathogenesis

Etiologic Factors

- *Gluten sensitive enteropathy:*
  - The principal environmental factor involved in the pathogenesis of the disease is dietary gluten and its constituent gliadin.
  - Tissue transglutaminase (tTG) is responsible for the modification of gliadin in the gut mucosa into a more immunogenic form.
  - Gluten-sensitive enteropathy is present in all patients but it is usually asymptomatic. Celiac disease is present in 10.5% of patients.
  - Gluten-rich foods are wheat, rye, barley, millet, oats.
  - Gluten-free diet not only treats enteropathy but also has a protective effect against the development of lymphoma.
- *Iodine:* Iodine exposure can precipitate flares of the disease.
- Adenovirus has a role in Celiac disease.
- Smoking has a protective role in both DH and CD.
- *Genetics:*
  - There is a close association between DH and certain HLA types, particularly HLA-DQ2, and to a lesser extent, HLA-DQ8.
  - First degree relatives of patients with gluten-sensitive enteropathy or dermatitis herpetiformis are characteristically more likely to be affected by one or other disorder.
  - Monozygotic twins have a disease concordance rate of over 0.9.
- *Role of transglutaminase:*
  - Tissue transglutaminase (tTG/TG2) is calcium-dependent enzyme which is expressed ubiquitously including basal keratinocytes and dermal capillaries.
  - tTG/TG2 is the autoantigen in Celiac disease.
  - Epidermal transglutaminase (Etg/TG3), unlike tTG, is restricted only to epidermis, small intestine, renal basement membrane, testes, and brain. It is involved in maintaining integrity of keratinocytes.
  - Etg/TG3 is the autoantigen in DH.
  - Both TG2 and TG3 share common conserved epitope for IgA autoantibody.
- *Role of trauma:* Trauma can release of eTG from keratinocytes and allows it drop to basement membrane.
- *Role of circulating IgA anti-eTG antibodies:* Epitope spread over time results in the development of IgA anti-eTG and this late onset of IgA anti-eTG antibodies play a role in the typical development of DH.[38,40,41]

Pathogenesis

- Dietary wheat, barley, or rye is processed by digestive enzymes into antigenic gliadin peptides, which are transported intact across the mucosal epithelium **(Fig. 12)**.
- Within the lamina propria, tissue transglutaminase (TG2): (1) deamidates glutamine residues within gliadin peptides to glutamic acid, and (2) becomes covalently crosslinked to gliadin peptides via isopeptidyl bonds (formed between gliadin glutamine and TG2 lysine residues).
- CD4+ T-cells in the lamina propria recognize deamidated gliadin peptides presented by HLA-DQ2 or -DQ8 molecules on antigen-presenting cells, resulting in the production of Th1 cytokines and matrix metalloproteinases that cause mucosal epithelial cell damage and tissue remodeling.
- In addition, TG2-specific B-cells take up TG2–gliadin complexes and present gliadin peptides to gliadin-specific helper T-cells, which stimulate the B-cells to produce IgA anti-TG2.
- Over time, IgA directed against TG3 (IgA anti-TG3) forms as a result of epitope spreading and both IgA anti-TG2 and IgA anti-TG3 circulate in the bloodstream.
- When IgA anti-TG3 antibodies reach the dermis, they complex with TG3 antigens which have been produced by keratinocytes (epidermal TG), and then have diffused into the dermis.
- That is, IgA/TG3 immune complexes are formed locally within the papillary dermis. This leads to neutrophil chemotaxis (with formation of neutrophilic abscesses), proteolytic cleavage of the lamina lucida, and subepidermal blister formation.[38,42]

Clinical Features

- *Onset:* Acute or gradual
- *Morphology of cutaneous lesions:*
  - The first and predominant symptom is usually pruritus.
  - Early lesions are erythematous papules, urticarial wheals or grouped vesicles grouped erythematous papules and vesicles located over extensor sites. Because the condition is so pruritic, intact vesicles are rarely seen and the patient may simply present with excoriations. These grouped vesicles are mostly seen on erythematous plaques.

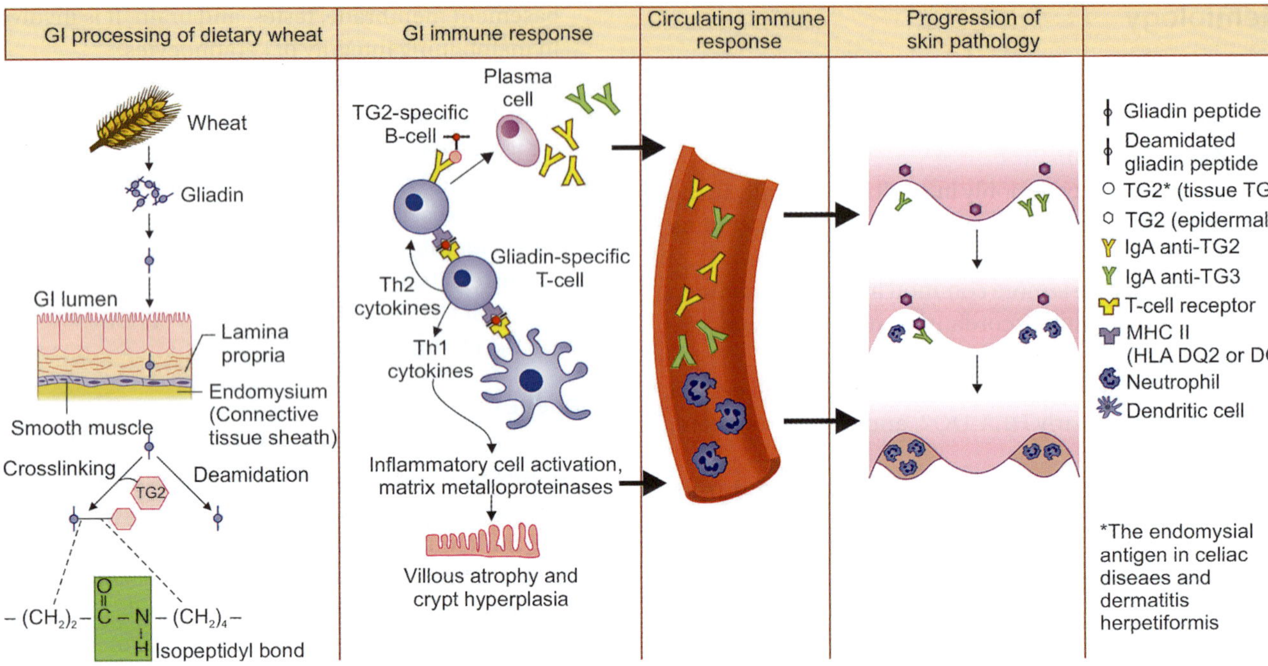

Fig. 12: Proposed pathogenesis of dermatitis herpetiformis and celiac disease.

- Rarely 1–2 cm in diameter blisters can occur (common in repalse).
- Papules can even occur without blistering.
- Lesions tend to be symmetrical and heal without scarring.
- Later lesions show eczematous changes which may lead to lichenification.

- *Distribution:*
  - Lesions are characteristically symmetrical in distribution.
  - Classically extensor surface of limbs including knees, elbows, shoulder, middle line of the back, buttocks, and natal cleft. Less commonly axillary folds, trunk, scalp, and face are involved.
  - Scalp and chin are involved in partially suppressed disease.
  - Oral lesions are common but are usually asymptomatic.
- *Complications:*
  - Risk of small bowel lymphoma
  - Anemia
  - Weight loss
  - Dental abnormalities such as enamel pits may be present.
  - Alopecia (due to zinc deficiency)
  - Early osteoporosis
  - Neurological diseases such as ataxia and neuropathy.
- *Atypical presentations:*
  - Patients may develop punctate purpura on the palms and soles more commonly in children.
  - Palmoplantar keratosis
  - Chronic urticaria-like lesions
- *Constitutional symptoms:*
  - Malaise is common in the acute phase.
  - Gluten-sensitive enteropathy presents with bouts of bloating, abdominal pain, constipation, diarrhea, and undernourishment.
  - Patients may feel tired because of associated anemia due to iron, folate and vitamin B_{12} deficiency.
- *Chances of malignancy:*
  - There is a significant increase in non-Hodgkin lymphomas in patients with DH and an occasional GI lymphoma. Risk of GI lymphoma is about 6–10-fold at diagnosis.
  - There can be a protective role for a gluten-free diet against GI lymphomas.[38,42,43]

Associated Diseases

- Gluten-sensitive enteropathy
- T-cell lymphoma (poor prognosis), B-cell lymphoma, small bowel adenocarcinoma
- Autoimmune thyroid disease (Hashimoto's thyroiditis)
- Insulin-dependent diabetes mellitus
- Pernicious anemia
- *Others:* SLE, Sjögren syndrome, vitiligo, alopecia areata, Down and Turner syndrome
- *Neurological disorders:* Gluten ataxia, demyelinating neuropathy, myopathies, epilepsy, dementia, multifocal leukoencephalopathy

Prognosis

- DH persists indefinitely in most patients, with exacerbations and remissions.

- But it is a treatable disease with favorable prognosis.
- Strict adherence to a gluten-free diet from 4 months to 1 year, reduces or eliminates the requirement for medication in the majority of patients.
- Intestinal lesions also respond to the dietary gluten withdrawal.

Differential Diagnosis

- Scabies
- Eczema, atopic dermatitis, papular urticaria, and prurigo
- Neurotic excoriations
- Erythema multiforme
- Bullous lupus erythematosus
- Bullous pemphigoid
- Linear IgA bullous disease
- Wegener's granulomatosis
- Churg-Strauss syndrome

Cutaneous Investigations

Histopathology

- The histology of an early clinically nonvesicular lesion is characterized by dermal papillary collections of neutrophils, neutrophilic fragments, varying numbers of eosinophils, fibrin, and, at times, separation of the papillary tips from the overlying epidermis.
- The histopathology of an intact vesicle in dermatitis herpetiformis demonstrates subepidermal blister formation with neutrophils located at the tips of the dermal papillae.
- There is frequently perivascular lymphohistiocytic infiltrate, as well as some neutrophils and an occasional eosinophil.
- There may be microabscess formation between dermal papilla and epidermis. Apoptotic keratinocytes may be seen above papillary microabscess.
- Initially, the blisters may be multiloculated blisters, and later these become unilocular as the rete ridges lose their attachment to dermis.
- Papilla may appear bluish due to fibrin deposition.[38,44,45]

Immunofluorescence

- *Direct immunofluorescence:*
  - Characteristically, there is granular deposition of IgA in the papillary dermis.
  - Occasionally, there may be C3 deposition associated with IgA.
  - Finding granular IgA deposits in normal skin is the most reliable criterion for the diagnosis of DH. These IgA deposits are unaffected with treatment, but may disappear after a gluten-free diet.
- *Indirect immunofluorescence*—is routinely negative.[38,44,45]

Serology

- ELISA-based IgA-class TG2 antibody test should be the first line serological test used when DH is suspected. Family members can be screened with IgA anti-TG3 for gluten-sensitive enteropathy.
- Antigliadin antibodies are no longer used because of their lack of specificity.
- Though endomysial antibodies have comparable reliability for DH as TG2 antibodies, the indirect immunofluorescence-based endomysial antibody test is more laborious and subjective in the interpretation.[38,46]

Electron Microscopy

- Subepidermal blister
- Basal lamina can be fragmented in the lesions; it can be thickened and reduplicated in adjacent skin.
- Basal cells can show cytolysis secondary to the effects of inflammatory cells.

Immunoelectron microscopy: IgA deposits associated with dermal microfibrillar bundles.

Gastrointestinal Investigations

- All the abnormalities of Celiac disease can be found.
- Blood counts reveal anemia (due to iron or folate deficiency); Howell–Jolly bodies may also be found indicative of splenic atrophy.
- Jejunal biopsy shows signs of gluten-sensitive enteropathy with raised intraepidermal lymphocyte count **(Box 8)**.[38,47]

Management

- *Gluten-free diet:* The treatment of choice for all patients with DH is a strict life-long gluten-free diet. Patients are best managed in consultation with an experienced dietitian. The rash in DH responds slowly to the diet, and it usually takes several months (from 4 months to 1 year) to improve. This is also important in the management of associated gluten-sensitive enteropathy. Adherence to GFD for >5 years seems to protect against lymphoma. Wheat, rye and barley are excluded from the diet, but the majority of patients with DH tolerate oats. About 2% of

BOX 8: Therapeutic algorithm of dermatitis herpetiformis (DH).

First line:
- *Gluten-free diet:* Wheat, rye, and barley can be replaced by corn, rice, and oat
- *Dapsone:* May be started with 25–50 mg/day and then slowly increase to 100–200 mg/day
- *Potent topical steroids:* Systemic steroids are usually ineffective and not indicated in DH

Second line (along with a gluten-free diet): Sulphamethoxypyridazine: Can be given at a dose of 0.5–1.5 g daily

Third line (along with a gluten-free diet):
- *Sulphapyridine:* Can be given at a dose of 250–750 mg daily
- *Sulfasalazine:* Can be given at a dose of 1–2 g daily

Others: May be used in certain refractory cases. Cyclosporine, colchicine, heparin, tetracycline, nicotinamide

Adjunctive treatment: Vitamin C supplementation

DH may be refractory DH who do not respond to strict gluten-free diets.[38,48]

- *Dapsone:* Dapsone is known to relieve the itch and the rash in DH in a few days; however, it has no effect on the enteropathy. The mechanism of action of dapsone in DH is through its effects on neutrophil function and recruitment. It is generally started with a dose of 25–50 mg/day and then slowly increased to 100–200 mg/day depending on the response. Dapsone is usually well tolerated, but it has some potential dose-dependent hematological adverse effects, including hemolysis, methemoglobinemia, and agranulocytosis. Nonhematological adverse effects include dapsone hypersensitivity syndrome and peripheral neuropathy. Patients with a G6PD deficiency are more prone to adverse effects of dapsone.
- *Other sulfonamide drugs:* Sulphamethoxypyridazine, sulphapyridine, and sulfasalazine may be of utility in patients intolerant of dapsone.
- *Corticosteroids:* Systemic corticosteroids are of little benefit, though potent topical corticosteroids may be of use in the short term to lessen pruritus.[38,49]

BULLOUS SYSTEMIC LUPUS ERYTHEMATOSUS

Synonyms

- Vesiculobullous SLE
- Bullous eruption of SLE.

Introduction

- Bullous systemic lupus erythematosus (BSLE) is clinically and immunopathologically distinct autoimmune blistering disease which is a rare manifestation of systemic lupus erythematosus.
- BSLE is typically a subepidermal, transient, tense, vesiculobullous eruption, which normally heals without scarring or milia.

Epidemiology

- *Incidence:* Approximately 1–2% of patients of SLE may have bullous manifestation. The reported incidence is limited but estimated at 2% of all subepidermal autoimmune bullous cutaneous conditions.
- *Age:* BSLE is seen most commonly in the second to fourth decade of life.
- *Sex:* BSLE affects more females than males.
- *Ethnicity:* More common in patients of African descent.

Pathophysiology

- *Types of BSLE:* BSLE can be divided into two major types depending on the antigen involved.
  1. Type I BSLE involves the NC1 domain of type VII collagen.
  2. Type II BSLE may involve BP180, BP230, or laminin 332 antigen.
- The primary autoimmune process is systemic lupus characterized by the interface dermatitis which leads to the unmasking of DEJ proteins (antigens). This subsequently leads to a secondary autoimmune cascade resulting in a weakened basement membrane-dermal adhesion, which appears as subepidermal blistering.[50,51]
- Predisposing factors of developing BSLE can be:
  - UVB radiation
  - Drugs such as hydralazine, penicillamine, or methimazole.

Clinical Features

- BSLE often has an acute onset of presentation with generalized eruption of blisters in SLE. Most patients with BSLE have an existing diagnosis of SLE, although there are several reports of BSLE as an initial presentation of SLE.
- Pruritus may be present but is usually mild. There can be a burning sensation associated.
- BSLE presents with tense bullae and vesicles with clear or hemorrhagic blister content on otherwise normal or erythematous skin. Sometimes, there can be annular or targetoid configuration.
- Oral mucosa involvement may be seen.
- Lesions heals with hypo/hyperpigmentation of the affected skin, milia or scar formation are rare.
- Erythema gyratum repens kind of lesions were reported rarely.
- Blisters often have a predilection for sun-exposed areas but can be seen in nonsun-exposed skin and mucosa.
- Most commonly involved areas are trunk, face, neck, vermillion border, upper extremities-extensor surfaces, supraclavicular region, and oral mucosa. Extensor surface involvement, in contrast to DH, is much less common.[50,52]

Associations

- Several reports have shown an association with BSLE and active lupus nephritis.
- Pemphigus
- Dermatitis herpetiformis.

Differential Diagnosis

- Drug eruption
- *Bullous pemphigoid:* It can be differentiated with the aid of immunofluorescence antibody deposition is found on the epidermal side of salt-split skin.
- DH has a skin distribution different from BSLE. The pruritic lesions have a predilection to the extensor surfaces, elbows, knees, and buttocks.
- *LABD:* Immunofluorescence shows IgA deposition on the epidermal side of split skin.
- EBA exhibits similar antibodies against type VII collagen. It is more likely to heal with scarring and milia formation compared to BSLE.

- Anti-p200 pemphigoid
- Systemic lupus erythematosus with blisters

Prognosis

Prognosis is usually good for BSLE. It has a self-limited course usually with no recurrence irrespective of systemic disease activity.

Investigations

Histopathology

- The histopathology of BSLE shows subepidermal split neutrophil-rich infiltrate in upper dermis concentrated on the papillary tip with the association of nuclear dust and fibrin resembling DH. A microabscess may or may not be present at papillary dermis.
- A distinguishing feature from DH mucin deposition in reticular dermis. However, basal layer vacuolar degeneration is not seen unlike cutaneous LE.

Immunofluorescence

- DIF staining of perilesional skin demonstrates a linear or granular IgG deposition with or without IgA, IgM, or C3 deposits at DEJ.
- It usually reveals a u-serrated staining pattern in type I BSLE.
- DIF studies on salt-split skin samples from BSLE patients show immune reactant deposition along the dermal side of the blister cavity.
- IIF is positive on intact skin, salt split is the preferred method to carry out confirmatory IIF studies.

Immunoelectron Microscopy

IEM reveals localization of immunoreactants beneath lamina densa.

Diagnostic Criteria

- The diagnostic criteria of BSLE were first described by Camisa and Sharma in 1983 and were revised in 1988.
- These criteria are:
  - Diagnosis of SLE based on ACR criteria
  - Vesicles and/or bullae
  - Histopathologic features similar to DH
  - DIF with IgG and/or IgM and often IgA at the BMZ; and
  - IIF testing that can be negative or positive for circulating autoantibodies against the BMZ via the salt-split skin technique.[50,52]

Subtypes of BSLE

- BSLE is divided into three groups based on the antibodies against the BMZ
  - Type I, the most common type, requires evidence of autoantibodies to type VII collagen, either circulating as determined by IIF or deposited via direct IEM.
  - Type II is characterized by the lack of autoantibodies to type VII collagen entirely.
  - Type III, the most recently proposed subgroup, is based on the presence of autoantibodies that bind either epidermal or both dermal and epidermal epitopes.[52]

Management of BSLE

First line: Dapsone at a dose of 1.0–1.5 mg/kg/day

Second line: Systemic corticosteroids (prednisolone at a dose of 0.5–1 mg/kg/day) with or without azathioprine (dose 2.5 mg/kg/day) or MMF (dose 2 g/day)

Third line:

- Methotrexate at a dose of 10–15 mg/week
- Rituximab 2 cycles of 1 g at 2 weeks apart

Management

- Dapsone is considered the first line of treatment for BSLE; however, the response may be variable. The use of dapsone may be limited by side effects such as anemia, hepatitis, or hypersensitivity syndrome.
- In case of dapsone intolerance or extensive skin involvement, the use of steroids may be considered.
- Steroid-sparing agents such as cyclophosphamide, azathioprine, mycophenolate mofetil, and methotrexate may be used with or without prednisolone.
- Rituximab can be used in more refractory cases.[50,52,53]

REFERENCES

1. Basu K, Chatterjee M, De A, Sengupta M, Datta C, Mitra P. A clinicopathological and immunofluorescence study of intraepidermal immunobullous diseases. Indian J Dermatol. 2019;64(2):101-5.
2. Baigrie D, Nookala V. Bullous Pemphigoid. In: StatPearls [Internet]. Treasure Island (FL): StatPearls Publishing; 2021.
3. Paul A, Basu K, Bandhopadhyay R, De A, Dutta A. Clinico-pathological study of immunobullous disorders with special reference to immunofluorescence. Int J Res Rev. 2021;8(3): 742-50.
4. Genovese G, Di Zenzo G, Cozzani E, Berti E, Cugno M, Marzano AV. New insights into the pathogenesis of bullous pemphigoid: 2019 update. Front Immunol. 2019;10:1506.
5. Hübner F, Langan EA, Recke A. Lichen planus pemphigoides: from lichenoid inflammation to autoantibody-mediated blistering. Front Immunol. 2019;10:1389.
6. Bağcı IS, Horváth ON, Ruzicka T, Sárdy M. Bullous pemphigoid. Autoimmun Rev. 2017;16(5):445-55.
7. De A, Ansari A, Sharma N, Sarda A. Shifting focus in the therapeutics of immunobullous disease. Indian J Dermatol. 2017;62(3):282-90.
8. Tolaymat L, Hall MR. Cicatricial pemphigoid. In: StatPearls [Internet]. Treasure Island (FL): StatPearls Publishing; 2021.
9. Carey B, Setterfield J. Mucous membrane pemphigoid and oral blistering diseases. Clin Exp Dermatol. 2019;44(7): 732-9.
10. Kamaguchi M, Iwata H. The diagnosis and blistering mechanisms of mucous membrane pemphigoid. Front Immunol. 2019;10:34.

11. Schmidt E, Zillikens D. Pemphigoid diseases. Lancet. 2013;381(9863):320-32.
12. Buonavoglia A, Leone P, Dammacco R, Di Lernia G, Petruzzi M, Bonamonte D, et al. Pemphigus and mucous membrane pemphigoid: an update from diagnosis to therapy. Autoimmun Rev. 2019;18(4):349-58.
13. Patel PM, Jones VA, Murray TN, Amber KT. A review comparing international guidelines for the management of bullous pemphigoid, pemphigoid gestationis, mucous membrane pemphigoid, and epidermolysis bullosa acquisita. Am J Clin Dermatol. 2020;21(4):557-65.
14. Fong M, Gandhi GR, Gharbi A, Hafsi W. Pemphigoid gestationis. In: StatPearls [Internet]. Treasure Island (FL): StatPearls Publishing; 2021.
15. Sävervall C, Sand FL, Thomsen SF. Pemphigoid gestationis: current perspectives. Clin Cosmet Investig Dermatol. 2017; 10:441-9.
16. Cohen S, Strowd LC, Pichardo RO. Pemphigoid gestationis: a case series and review of the literature. J Dermatolog Treat. 2018;29(8):815-8.
17. Lipozenčić J, Ljubojevic S, Bukvić-Mokos Z. Pemphigoid gestationis. Clin Dermatol. 2012;30(1):51-5.
18. Genovese G, Derlino F, Berti E, Marzano AV. Treatment of autoimmune bullous diseases during pregnancy and lactation: a review focusing on pemphigus and pemphigoid gestationis. Front Pharmacol. 2020;11:583354.
19. Goletz S, Hashimoto T, Zillikens D, Schmidt E. Anti-p200 pemphigoid. J Am Acad Dermatol. 2014;71(1):185-91.
20. Kridin K, Ahmed AR. Anti-p200 pemphigoid: a systematic review. Front Immunol. 2019;10:2466.
21. Holtsche MM, Goletz S, Zillikens D. Anti-p200-pemphigoid [Anti-p200 pemphigoid]. Hautarzt. 2019;70(4):271-6.
22. Meijer JM, Diercks GF, Schmidt E, Pas HH, Jonkman MF. Laboratory diagnosis and clinical profile of anti-p200 pemphigoid. JAMA Dermatol. 2016;152(8):897-904.
23. Drerup KA, Wehkamp U. Anti-p200-Pemphigoid: Klinik, Diagnostik, Therapie [Anti-p200 pemphigoid: clinical, diagnostic and therapeutic aspects]. Hautarzt. 2020;71(2):130-3.
24. Xiao A, Tsuchiya A. Epidermolysis bullosa acquisita. In: StatPearls [Internet]. Treasure Island (FL): StatPearls Publishing; 2021.
25. Kridin K, Kneiber D, Kowalski EH, Valdebran M, Amber KT. Epidermolysis bullosa acquisita: a comprehensive review. Autoimmun Rev. 2019;18(8):786-95.
26. Koga H, Prost-Squarcioni C, Iwata H, Jonkman MF, Ludwig RJ, Bieber K. Epidermolysis bullosa acquisita: the 2019 update. Front Med (Lausanne). 2019;5:362.
27. De A, Rao R, Balachandran C. Salt split technique: a useful tool in the diagnosis of subepidermal bullous disorders. Indian J Dermatol. 2010;55(4):334-6.
28. Prost-Squarcioni C, Caux F, Schmidt E, Jonkman MF, Vassileva S, Kim SC, et al. International Bullous Diseases Group: consensus on diagnostic criteria for epidermolysis bullosa acquisita. Br J Dermatol. 2018;179(1):30-41.
29. Cobos G, Mu E, Cohen J, Beasley J, Brinster N, Femia A. Epidermolysis bullosa acquisita. Dermatol Online J. 2017; 23(12):13030.
30. Kim JH, Kim SC. Epidermolysis bullosa acquisita. J Eur Acad Dermatol Venereol. 2013;27(10):1204-13.
31. Bernett CN, Fong M, Rosario-Collazo JA. Linear IGA dermatosis. In: StatPearls [Internet]. Treasure Island (FL): StatPearls Publishing; 2021.
32. Juratli HA, Sárdy M. Lineare IgA-Dermatose [Linear IgA bullous dermatosis]. Hautarzt. 2019;70(4):254-9.
33. Lammer J, Hein R, Roenneberg S, Biedermann T, Volz T. Drug-induced linear IgA bullous dermatosis: a case report and review of the literature. Acta Derm Venereol. 2019;99(6):508-15.
34. Genovese G, Venegoni L, Fanoni D, Muratori S, Berti E, Marzano AV. Linear IgA bullous dermatosis in adults and children: a clinical and immunopathological study of 38 patients. Orphanet J Rare Dis. 2019;14(1):115.
35. Vico-Alonso C, Palencia-Pérez S. Linear IgA bullous dermatosis. N Engl J Med. 2020;382(23):2248.
36. Díaz MS, Morita L, Ferrari B, Sartori S, Greco MF, Sobrevias Bonells L, et al. Linear IgA bullous dermatosis: a series of 17 cases. Actas Dermosifiliogr. 2019;110(8):673-80.
37. Vale ECSD, Dimatos OC, Porro AM, Santi CG. Consensus on the treatment of autoimmune bullous dermatoses: dermatitis herpetiformis and linear IgA bullous dermatosis. An Bras Dermatol. 2019;94(2 Suppl 1):48-55.
38. Mirza HA, Gharbi A, Bhutta BS. Dermatitis herpetiformis. In: StatPearls [Internet]. Treasure Island (FL): StatPearls Publishing; 2021.
39. Salmi TT. Dermatitis herpetiformis. Clin Exp Dermatol. 2019;44(7):728-31.
40. Antiga E, Maglie R, Quintarelli L, Verdelli A, Bonciani D, Bonciolini V, et al. Dermatitis herpetiformis: novel perspectives. Front Immunol. 2019;10:1290.
41. Mendes FB, Hissa-Elian A, Abreu MA, Gonçalves VS. Review: dermatitis herpetiformis. An Bras Dermatol. 2013;88(4): 594-9.
42. Salmi T, Hervonen K. Current concepts of dermatitis herpetiformis. Acta Derm Venereol. 2020;100(5):adv00056.
43. Collin P, Salmi TT, Hervonen K, Kaukinen K, Reunala T. Dermatitis herpetiformis: a cutaneous manifestation of coeliac disease. Ann Med. 2017;49(1):23-31.
44. Jakes AD, Bradley S, Donlevy L. Dermatitis herpetiformis. BMJ. 2014;348:g2557.
45. Dmochowski M, Gornowicz-Porowska J, Bowszyc-Dmochowska M. An update on direct immunofluorescence for diagnosing dermatitis herpetiformis. Postepy Dermatol Alergol. 2019;36(6):655-8.
46. Reunala T, Salmi TT, Hervonen K, Kaukinen K, Collin P. Dermatitis herpetiformis: a common extraintestinal manifestation of coeliac disease. Nutrients. 2018;10(5):602.
47. Plotnikova N, Miller JL. Dermatitis herpetiformis. Skin Therapy Lett. 2013;18(3):1-3.
48. Al-Toma A, Volta U, Auricchio R, Castillejo G, Sanders DS, Cellier C, et al. European Society for the Study of Coeliac Disease (ESsCD) guideline for coeliac disease and other gluten-related disorders. United European Gastroenterol J. 2019;7(5):583-613.
49. Kárpáti S. Dermatitis herpetiformis. Clin Dermatol. 2012; 30(1):56-9.

50. Odonwodo A, Vashisht P. Bullous systemic lupus erythematosus. In: StatPearls [Internet]. Treasure Island (FL): StatPearls Publishing; 2021.
51. Ghosh AP, Nag F, Biswas S, Rao R, De A. Clinicopathological and immunological profile of patients with cutaneous manifestations and their relationship with organ involvement in systemic lupus erythematosus attending a tertiary care center of Eastern India. Indian J Dermatol. 2020;65(1):22-8.
52. Contestable JJ, Edhegard KD, Meyerle JH. Bullous systemic lupus erythematosus: a review and update to diagnosis and treatment. Am J Clin Dermatol. 2014;15(6):517-24.
53. Grover C, Khurana A, Sharma S, Singal A. Bullous systemic lupus erythematosus. Indian J Dermatol. 2013;58(6):492.

EXAMINATION QUESTIONS

Write short notes on the following:

1. LABD
2. Mucus membrane pemphigoid
3. CBDC
4. Direct immunofluoroscence
5. Classify subepidermal bullous disorders and explain the pathogenesis of bullous pemphigoid.
6. Illustrate the treatment algorithm for bullous pemphigoid.

51 CHAPTER

Antinuclear Antibodies and Introduction to Connective Tissue Disorders

Maitreyee Panda, Akash Agarwal

ANTINUCLEAR ANTIBODIES

Introduction

Antinuclear antibodies (ANA) are a heterogeneous group of autoantibodies that act against the self-proteins present within the cell nucleus. Positive titers in serum are of value in diagnosing connective tissue disorders (CTDs); however, in some chronic infectious diseases, cancers, medications or even healthy people, it may also be positive.

Correctly correlating clinical features along with ANA titers and its subtypes forms an integral part in diagnosing patients with CTDs.

History[1]

- In 1948, Malcom Hargrave, Helen Richmond, and Robert Morton discovered LE cell (mature leucocytes engulfing nuclear material of another leucocyte) in bone marrow of a systemic lupus erythematosus (SLE) patient.
- In 1957, Holboro et al. demonstrated specific nuclei florescence in all tissues exposed to LE cell-positive sera on staining with antiglobulin antibody.
- In 1958, Friou et al. created an indirect immunofluorescence assay (IFA) with specific end points for detection of ANAs.
- Swanson introduced concept of ANA immunofluorescence patterns and its diagnostic importance in clinical medicine.

Enigma of Antinuclear Antibodies[2]

- *ANA positivity in various other pathological conditions* ***(Table 1)***: Although classically ANA is related to autoimmune CTDs, it is also positive in other diseases summarized in **Table 1**.
- *ANA in healthy individuals:*
  - ANA are commonly found to be positive in up to 20% of healthy population, but significant high titers are observed in 2.5% cases.
  - Comparable prevalence all CTDs from 5 to 7% among populations of different ethnicity and race.
  - *Possible etiologies:* Increasing age (decreased self-regulatory mechanisms, presence of thyroglobulin, antibodies to cartilage proteoglycan, up regulation of some genes such as MX-1 or type 1 interferon)

TABLE 1: Antinuclear antibodies (ANA) positivity in diseases apart from autoimmune connective tissue disorders.

Liver diseases	• Chronic hepatitis • Primary biliary cirrhosis • Autoimmune hepatitis
Infections	• Tuberculosis • Viral hepatitis • Parasitic infections • Syphilis
Skin diseases	• Atopic dermatitis • Psoriasis
Neoplasms	• Breast cancer • Prostate cancer • Hodgkin lymphoma • Leukemia
Other autoimmune diseases	• Type 1 diabetes • Addison's disease • Autoimmune anemia • Hashimoto's thyroiditis

- *ANA and female gender:*
  - Estrogens induce Th2 immune response thereby interacting through receptors present on many immune system cells.
  - They are responsible for local concentration and inflammation which may induce ANA formation
  - On a genetic level, break in immune tolerance of some gene products present on inactivated X chromosome may cause autoimmunity
  - Extensive exposure to nuclear antigens during pregnancy along with increased inflammatory activity might cause ANA positivity in healthy females.
- *ANA and xenobiotics:*
  - Sulfasalazine, Gold salts, IVIg, TNF-α blockers (infliximab), and procainamide are notoriously known to induce ANA productivity.
  - Environmental allergens such as smoke, silica, and tobacco are also known triggers.
  - Triclosan in antibacterial soaps and toothpastes also proven to cause rise in ANA.
- *ANA in patients of atopic dermatitis:*
  - Severe keratinocyte apoptosis in patients of atopic dermatitis along with high IgE levels is postulated in ANA induction.
  - Specific autoantibodies associated are against human Homs 1-5 (Homo sapiens allergen 1-5) and DFS70.

Types of Antinuclear Antibodies[3]

1. *Antibodies against DNA and histones:*

dsDNA	Diagnostic of SLE
Histones	Indicates drug-induced SLE

2. *Antibodies against extractable nuclear antigens (ENAs):*
   - Most of ENA are disease specific but overlap is commonly seen.

Smith	*Specific for SLE*
Anti-SS-A/Ro and anti-SS-B/La	Specific for Sjögren, subacute cutaneous LE, and neonatal LE
Anticentromere	Specific for limited cutaneous systemic sclerosis
Jo-1	Specific for polymyositis
Anti-U3-RNP and Scl-70	Specific for systemic sclerosis
Topoisomerases-1, centromere protein B and RNA polymerase I-III	Newer antigens recently described

Detection of Antinuclear Antibodies

- Indirect immunofluorescence antinuclear antibody test (IF-ANA) and enzyme-linked immunosorbent assay (ELISA) are most commonly used techniques. The advantages and disadvantages of each technique have been discussed in **Table 2**.
- *IFA:* Gold standard test
  - Parameters while reporting ANA report [International Autoantibody Standardization (IAS) and International Consensus on ANA Patterns (ICAP)][4]:
    - Pattern of fluorescence
    - Substrate used
    - Titer of a positive test.
  - *Substrate:*
    - Hep-2 cell line from human laryngeal carcinoma most commonly used.
    - It comprises an "antigenic array" with more than 100 autoantibody targets
    - Nowadays, transfection with human 60 kDa Ro/SS-A protein (common nuclear antigen found in different autoimmune systemic diseases) to improve testing performance is being carried out.
  - *Technique:*
    - Microscopic slides are first coated with single layer of Hep-2 cells and then incubated with blood specimens containing autoantibodies.
    - Fluorescence-labeled antibody is added and visualized under fluorescent microscope for the distinct immunofluorescence patterns.
    - ANA titers are determined by dilution of specimens in buffered solution till staining can no longer be seen which marks end dilution titers.
  - A titer of 1:160 is taken as significant for the diagnosis of CTDs.
  - A negative IFA result rules out possibility of active CTD.
- *ELISA:* Most widely used test
  - *Technique:*
    - Purified autoantigen panel is prepared, and each antigen is immobilized on a solid surface.
    - It is incubated with diluted human serum and an antiglobulin antibody is used to detect bound autoantibodies
  - *Types:*
    - *Generic assay:* Detects ANA of broad specificity like IFA.
    - *Antigen-specific assay:* Detects ANA and reacts with single auto-antigen.
  - Results can be positive, equivocal, or negative, based on the determination of the optical density value of the solution.

TABLE 2: Advantages and disadvantages of indirect immunofluorescence and ELISA technique.

Techniques	*Advantages*	*Disadvantages*
Indirect immunofluorescence method	• Easy to perform • High sensitivity (95%) and specificity (human origin) • Possibility to identify many patterns • Cost effective	• Time consuming • Extractable nuclear antigen categorization is difficult • Labor and skill intensive • Possibility of false positive reports
Enzyme-linked immunosorbent assay	• Automation • Allows quantification • High sensitivity	• False positive reports • Expensive • Requires purified antigen

Staining Patterns

- Three distinct clinical patterns of immunofluorescence has been described[5]
  1. *Nuclear patterns*: Homogeneous, speckled (fine and coarse), peripheral/rim, nucleolar, centromeric, proliferating cell nuclear antigen, nuclear dots, nuclear membrane, and diffuse grainy.
  2. *Cytoplasmic patterns*: Speckled, mitochondrial-like, ribosomal-like, Golgi apparatus, lysosomal-like, cytoskeletal filaments(actin, vimentin, cytokeratin)
  3. *Mitotic patterns*: Mitotic spindle, centrosomes, nuclear mitotic apparatus, mid body, and centromere protein.
- Homogeneous, speckled, peripheral, and nucleolar patterns are more common and are clinically important.
- Intensity of fluorescence from 0 to 4+ depicts antibody concentration and severity of CTD.
- A summary of most commonly observed nuclear staining patterns, its characteristics, antigens, and diseases associated is given in **Table 3**.

TABLE 3: Commonly observed nuclear staining patterns, its characteristics, antigens, and diseases associated.

IF pattern	*Characteristics*	*Antigens*	*Diseases*
Smooth nuclear membrane	• Intense linear fluorescence along nuclear membrane and less intense homogeneous fluorescence of nucleus • Nucleoli not visible	• Lamins A, B1, B2, C • Lamin-associated proteins LAP 1A and 2	• SLE • Systemic sclerosis • Seronegative arthritis • Chronic fatigue syndrome
Punctate nuclear membrane	Granular pores present in nuclear membrane	• Glycoprotein 210 • Nucleoporin p62	• Polymyositis • Primary biliary cirrhosis
Homogeneous nuclear	• Uniform staining of all nucleoplasm • Nucleolar staining may be positive/ negative	• dsDNA • Histones • Nucleosome	• SLE • RA • Drug-induced SLE • Systemic sclerosis • Juvenile chronic arthritis
Nuclear matrix/large speckled pattern	• Large speckles with sponge-like aspect • Nucleoli can be stained or unstained	hnRNPs A1, A2, B1, B2	SLE, MCTD, and RA
		hnRNPs C1, C2, I	Systemic sclerosis
Nuclear coarse speckled	• Dense, intermediate sized speckles and large speckles • Nucleoli are unstained	Sm and U1-snRNP	SLE and MCTD
		U2-RNPs	Systemic sclerosis-Polymyositis overlap, MCTD, SLE, psoriasis, and Raynaud's
		U4-sn RNP	Systemic sclerosis and SJS
Nuclear fine specked	• Fine, tiny speckles uniformly distributed • Nucleoli are unstained	• SSA • SSB • Ku • Ki • RNA polymerases II and III • Mi-2	• SLE • SjS • Myositis • MCTD • Systemic sclerosis
Densely fine speckled	• Speckles of varying sizes, distribution and brightness • Areas of some denser and looser areas of freckles • Nucleoli unstained	Lens epithelium-derived growth factor p75	Exclusive positivity helps identify patients with no rheumatological disease
Few nuclear dots	1-6 discrete dots known as colloid bodies or Cajal bodies are visualized	p80-collins	Primary biliary cirrhosis
Multiple nuclear dots	6–20 dots of variable size per cell	• Promyelocytic leukemia protein (PML) • Sp-100 protein • NDP52	• Primary biliary cirrhosis • SJS
Centromere	Discrete coarse speckles (40–60/cell) spread over entire nucleus	CENP-A, B, C, D, E, G and H	• Limited cutaneous systemic sclerosis—CREST • Primary biliary cirrhosis
Nucleolar homogeneous	Diffuse homogeneous florescence of nucleolus with fine granular weak staining of surrounding neoplasm	• PM-Scl 75 • PM-Scl 100	Myositis-scleroderma overlap
		Rpp25	• Systemic sclerosis • SLE • RA • Polymyositis
Nucleolar speckled	Distinct dense grains in nucleolus with fine speckled nucleoplasm	RNA polymerase I-III	• Systemic sclerosis (4–20%). • SLE • MCTD • RA
Clumpy nucleolar	Irregular staining of the nucleoli and Cajal bodies with a perichromosomal staining	Antifibrillin	Systemic sclerosis

(IF: immunofluorescence; MCTD: mixed connective tissue disease; RA: rheumatoid arthritis; SjS: Sjögren's syndrome; SLE: systemic lupus erythematosus)

Interpretation of Antinuclear Antibodies[5]

- ANA positive result alone has no diagnostic value.
- When ANA value exceeds 1:160 and clinical signs are present, systemic connective tissue diseases may be suspected.
- ANA profile for specific ENA should be ordered after high titers of ANA in a setting of CTD suspicion is obtained.
- Although presence of autoantibodies may be present many years prior to diagnosis of CTD, positive ANA in itself should not warrant extensive search in healthy individuals nor a need for periodic checkups.
- In an ANA negative patient, repeat checkup is done only in cases of high degree of suspicion. If ANA is negative again, Anti-SSA antibody positivity may help diagnose ANA-negative SLE.

When Not to Test for ANA[6]

- In patients with rheumatoid arthritis and osteoarthritis
- Evaluation of fatigue, back pain or musculoskeletal pain unless associated with CTD-related clinical features
- Screening of asymptomatic individuals
- Repeat ANA is of no value as they do not help in monitoring disease activity.

INTRODUCTION TO CONNECTIVE TISSUE DISORDERS

Autoimmune CTDs represent a group of disease affecting multisystem target organs sharing similar immunopathogenic mechanisms linked to genetic polymorphism and are characterized by presence of antinuclear antibodies and its subtypes in the blood. Cutaneous manifestations often lead to initial suspicion of underlying CTD and thus a dermatologist plays an important role in the initial diagnosis and management of such conditions.

The classic autoimmune CTDs include SLE, dermatomyositis/polymyositis (DM/PM), systemic sclerosis (SSc), Sjögren's syndrome (SS), undifferentiated CTD (UTCD), and overlap syndromes (MCTD).

Etiopathogenesis[7]

- Immune tolerance refers to inactivity toward specific antigens of the body be it foreign or self (autotolerance).
- Failure of various immune tolerance mechanisms have been implicated in the possible etiopathogenesis of CTDs. They are discussed as follows :
  - *Antigen sequestration*: Anatomical barrier preventing interaction between naïve auto-Ag is lost due to traumatic event leading to autoimmune response.
  - *Clonal detection*: Failure of self-regulatory apoptosis of lymphocytes which might be capable of recognizing autoantigens.
  - *Clonal anergy*: Failure of functional inactivation of autoreactive lymphocytes not subjected to clonal deletion.
  - *Regulation of Th1/Th2 balance:* Bacterial, viral infections, and sex hormones (estrogens) are factors that cause immune system dysregulation affecting functional status of subpopulation of T-cells.

Approach to a Patient with CTD[8]

- *History:*
  - *Age of onset and sexual predilection:* Common in 2nd–3rd decade with female preponderance.
  - *Constitutional symptoms:* Unexplained fever and fatigue, cough and dyspnea, pain abdomen, photosensitivity, weight loss, joint complaints, altered bowel bladder habits, dysphagia, peripheral neuropathy, psychosis, etc.
  - *Precipitating factors:* Sunlight exposure, seasonal variation, stress, infections
  - *History of drug intake:* Temporal association with drugs and specific autoimmune CTD exist.

SLE	Isoniazid, minocycline, penicillamine, griseofulvin, dapsone, procainamide, hydralazine
Dermatomyositis	Hydroxycarbamide
Systemic sclerosis	Paclitaxel, pentazocine, cocaine, D-penicillamine

  - Raynaud's phenomenon, history of gangrene, and autoamputation should arouse suspicion of scleroderma.
  - *Vaccination history:* Multiple case reports linking vaccination against infections leading to autoimmune diseases have been described.
  - *Underlying malignancy and ongoing chemotherapy:* Increased risk of developing malignancy especially lymphoproliferative disorders. Immunosuppressive drugs may have carcinogenic potential.
  - *History of recurrent abortions:* Arouses suspicion of antiphospholipid antibodies (APLA).
- *Clinical examination:* Clinical clues
  - *General examination:*

Clinical findings	*Possible etiology*
Pallor, icterus, lymphadenopathy, edema	SLE
Peripheral cyanosis (as part of Raynaud's phenomenon), high blood pressure	Systemic sclerosis
Decreased salivation and tear formation	Sjögren's syndrome

  - *Systemic examination:*
    - Hepatomegaly, splenomegaly, pleurisy, and altered higher mental functions: SLE
    - Restrictive lung pattern of interstitial lung disease: Systemic sclerosis and dermatomyositis

- *Musculoskeletal examination:*
  - Proximal muscle weakness is classical of dermatomyositis
  - Tendon friction rubs, muscle weakness is seen in systemic sclerosis.
- *Cutaneous examination:*

Cutaneous findings	*Nail findings*	*Disease associated*
Malar rash, lupus hair, painless oral ulcers, discoid rash, Raynaud's phenomenon, cutaneous vasculitic lesions, chilblain lesions	Nail fold erythema, splinter hemorrhages, red lunulae, nail-fold hyperkeratosis	SLE
Heliotrope rash, Gottron's papules, Shawl's sign, Holster's sign, V sign, flagellate erythema, poikilodermatous changes, calcinosis cutis	Periungual erythema, hypertrophic ragged cuticles	Dermatomyositis
Raynaud's phenomenon, salt pepper pigmentation, sclerodactyly, mask-like facies, nasal beaking, calcinosis	Digital pitting, digital gangrene, paronychia, and ragged cuticles	Systemic sclerosis
Thrombophlebitis, purpura, livedo reticularis, leg ulcers , gangrene with clinical history of recurrent abortions	–	APLA

- *Investigations*
  - *Complete hemogram:* To look for anemia, leukocytopenia and thrombocytopenia
  - *Erythrocyte sedimentation rate:* Marker of inflammation
  - C-reactive protein
  - *Urine routine and microscopy:* To look for hematuria, proteinuria, casts
  - Liver function test
  - Renal function tests
  - *Muscle enzymes:* Serum creatine phosphokinase (CPK), lactic dehydrogenase (LDH).
  - ANA titer followed by ANA profile if warranted
  - *APLA levels:* Suspected APLA syndrome
  - Radiological investigations as per relevant indications
  - Skin biopsy if needed for diagnosis
  - Muscle biopsy is warranted in cases of suspected dermatomyositis
- *Treatment:*
  - Identifications of triggers and counseling regarding the same is of paramount importance.
  - Immunosuppressive therapy forms basis of therapy in CTDs.
  - Mild-to-moderate disease without internal organ involvement can be managed by low-dose oral corticosteroids.
  - Severe disease or internal organ involvement requires higher degree of immunosuppression along with multi-disciplinary treatment.

Connective Tissue Disorders in Children[9]

A summary of how various juvenile autoimmune connective disorders are different from adult disease has been tabulated in **Table 4**.

Connective Tissue Disorders in Pregnancy[10]

A summary of special pregnancy considerations in autoimmune CTDs has been provided in **Table 5**.

TABLE 4: Differences of various juvenile CTDs from adult CTDs.

	Juvenile SLE	*Juvenile DM*	*Juvenile SSc*
Epidemiology	Accounts for 15–20% of SLE cases having a more severe disease course	• Rarer than adult DM • Mean age of presentation is 7 years with 25% patients below 5 years	3% of all cases of systemic sclerosis
Clinical features	Malar rash, mucocutaneous involvement, hematological abnormalities, seizures, renal involvement, urinary casts and proteinuria, adenopathy and fever more common in children	• Not considered to have increased risk of malignancy like adult DM • Calcinosis and acquired lipodystrophy are common findings	• Raynaud's phenomenon is first presenting features followed years later by skin tightening • Cardiac abnormalities like pericarditis, left or biventricular failure or arrhythmias are common • Delphi classification criteria used for early diagnosis
Investigations	• Similar along lines of adult SLE • Upto 10% healthy children may have ANA positivity, which may confuse the clinician	• Less association with adult myo-specific Ab (Anti Jo-1 and anti Mi-2) • Anti-TIF-1γ associated with ulcerative skin lesions in children	Less specific autoantibodies as compared to adults

Contd...

Contd...

	Juvenile SLE	*Juvenile DM*	*Juvenile SSc*
Treatment	• Judicious use of immunosuppressants is advocated • Flares to be treated aggressively to prevent organ damage	Early high-dose corticosteroids to halt or slow down disease progression	Aggressive therapy to prevent progression of skin tightness and joint contractures
Prognosis	• Poor due to long-term disease period and longer duration of immunosuppressive therapy • 40% children at onset and 60–70% children develop renal involvement: Single most important predictor of poor outcome	• One-third patients go into remission in 2-year time • Two-thirds patients have chronic relapsing course with high risk of developing calcinosis, progressive muscular difficulties and respiratory failure	• Depends on functional impairment and the course of visceral disease • Usually better outcome as internal organ involvement is less common • Skin eventually softens after years of disease initiation • Most common causes of death in children are due to cardiac, renal, and pulmonary systems

(DM: dermatomyositis; SLE: systemic lupus erythematosus; SSc: systemic sclerosis; SS: Sjögren's syndrome)

TABLE 5: Special considerations of various autoimmune diseases in pregnancy.

Disease	*Special considerations*
SLE	• Fertility is unaffected if renal function remains normal • Flare of SLE is uncommon if adequate immunosuppression is maintained • Increased rates of intrauterine growth restriction (IUGR), preterm birth and fetal loss, as well as neonatal lupus • Higher rates of hypertensive disorders and cesarean deliveries with 20-fold increased mortality risk • Oral corticosteroids (prednisolone) is considered safe along with hydroxychloroquine
APLA	• Recurrent pregnancy losses if untreated • Treatment recommended is prophylactic low molecular weight heparin and low dose aspirin
Systemic sclerosis	• Disease activity is stable during pregnancy • Increased risk of hypertensive disease of pregnancy, including preeclampsia, IUGR, premature births, and low birth weight for babies • Use of folic acid and the presence of antitopoisomerase is considered protective • Raynaud's phenomenon and digital ulcers improved temporarily during second trimester
Dermatomyositis	• DM improves during pregnancy with relapse postdelivery • Neonatal outcome is good with preterm delivery and small for gestational age babies seen less commonly • Maternal pregnancy-related complications are uncommon
Sjögren's	• Pregnancy resulting in neonatal lupus could indicate primary Sjögren's associated with anti-Ro/La antibodies • Literature lacking with regards to pregnancy outcomes • In small studies, lower birthweights, older maternal age, and more assisted common delivery was observed • In association with SLE, higher rates of abortion and premature deliveries were noted

(DM: dermatomyositis; SLE: systemic lupus erythematosus)

KEY POINTS

- ANA are commonly found to be positive in up to 20% of healthy population, but significant high titers are observed in 2.5% cases. So, ANA positive result alone has no diagnostic value.
- Indirect immunofluorescence antinuclear antibody test (IF-ANA) and enzyme-linked immunosorbent assay (ELISA) are most commonly used techniques for detection of ANA.
- An ANA titer of 1:160 is taken as significant for the diagnosis of connective tissue disorders.
- ANA profile for specific ENA should be ordered after high titers of ANA in a setting of CTD suspicion is obtained.
- Homogeneous, speckled, peripheral, and nucleolar patterns are most common immunofluorescence staining that are clinically important.
- Although presence of autoantibodies may be present many years prior to diagnosis of CTD, positive ANA in itself should not warrant extensive search in healthy individuals nor a need for periodic checkups
- Repeat ANA test is of no value as they do not help in monitoring disease activity.
- Failure of various immune tolerance mechanisms such as antigen sequestration, clonal detection, clonal anergy, and Th1/Th2 balance regulation have been implicated in the possible etiopathogenesis of CTDs.

- Identifications of triggers in CTDs and counseling regarding the same is of paramount importance.
- Immunosuppressive therapy forms basis of therapy in all CTDs.

REFERENCES

1. Moschou D, Pipi E, Tsirogianni A. The history and recent advancements in antinuclear antibody testing. J Res Pract Musculoskelet Syst. 2017;01(02):50-4.
2. Grygiel-Górniak B, Rogacka N, Puszczewicz M. Antinuclear antibodies in healthy people and non-rheumatic diseases: diagnostic and clinical implications. Reumatologia/ Rheumatology. 2018;56(4):243-8.
3. Sur LM, Floca E, Sur DG, Colceriu MC, Samasca G, Sur G. Antinuclear antibodies: marker of diagnosis and evolution in autoimmune diseases. Lab Med. 2018;49(3).
4. Chan EK, Damoiseaux J, Carballo OG, Conrad K, de Melo Cruvinel W, Francescantonio PL, et al. Report of the First International Consensus on Standardized Nomenclature of Antinuclear Antibody HEp-2 Cell Patterns 2014-2015. Front Immunol. 2015;6:412.
5. Moschou D, Pipi E, Tsirogianni A. The history and recent advancements in antinuclear antibody testing. J Res Pract Musculoskelet Syst. 2017;01(02):50-4.
6. Santhosh P, Ajithkumar K. Anti-nuclear antibodies: a practical approach to testing and interpretation. J Skin Sex Transmitted Dis. 2020;1-5.
7. Grygiel-Górniak B, Rogacka N, Rogacki M, Puszczewicz M. Antinuclear antibodies in autoimmune and allergic diseases. Reumatologia. 2017;55(6):298-304.
8. Fernandez AP. Connective tissue disease. Dermatol Clin. 2019; 37(1):37-48.
9. Kumar TS, Aggarwal A. Approach to a patient with connective tissue disease. Indian J Pediatr. 2010;77(10):1157-64.
10. Marder W, Littlejohn EA, Somers EC. Pregnancy and autoimmune connective tissue diseases: best practice and research. Clin Rheumatol. 2016;30(1):63-80.

EXAMINATION QUESTIONS

1. Write a short note on antinuclear antibodies.
2. What are the different types of antinuclear antibodies? Mention their significance in dermatological conditions.
3. Distinguish between different staining patterns of ANA and mention their diagnostic implications.

52 CHAPTER Lupus Erythematosus

Surajit Gorai, Adhyatm Bhandari

INTRODUCTION

Lupus erythematosus (LE) is a group of heterogeneous autoimmune illnesses with development of immunity to self-nucleic acids and associated proteins (nucleosomes and ribonucleoproteins), encompasses a spectrum with skin-only disease at one end and severe life-threatening systemic manifestations at the other.[1]

GILLIAM CLASSIFICATION

- LE-specific (shows characteristic histopathology of lupus erythematosus displaying interface dermatitis).
- LE-nonspecific (associated phenomenon, without any histopathologic changes of LE, may be seen in other autoimmune diseases).

  Gilliam classification has been listed in **Table 1**.

TABLE 1: The Gilliam classification.

LE-specific skin disease
Acute cutaneous LE (ACLE) (15%): • Localized ACLE (malar rash; butterfly rash)(90–95%) • Generalized ACLE (morbilliform)(5–10%) • Toxic epidermal necrolysis (TEN) like ACLE (rare)
Subacute cutaneous LE (SCLE): • Annular SCLE (42%) • Papulosquamous/psoriasiform SCLE (39%) • Vesiculobullous annular SCLE • TEN-like SCLE

Chronic cutaneous LE (CCLE):
• *Classic discoid LE (DLE) (85%):*
  – Localized DLE (70%)
  – Generalized DLE (30%)
• Hypertrophic/verrucous DLE
• Lupus profundus/lupus panniculitis
• *Mucosal DLE:*
  – Oral DLE
  – Conjunctival DLE
• Lupus tumidus (urticarial plaque of LE)
• Chilblain LE (chilblain lupus)
• Lichenoid DLE (LE/lichen planus overlap, lupus planus)

LE-nonspecific skin disease

• *Cutaneous vascular disease:*
  – *Vasculitis:*
    - Leukocytoclastic
      ▪ Palpable purpura
      ▪ Urticarial vasculitis
    - Periarteritis nodosa-like cutaneous lesions
  – *Vasculopathy:*
    - Degos disease-like lesions
    - Secondary atrophie blanche
  – Periungual telangiectasia
  – Livedo reticularis
  – Thrombophlebitis
  – Raynaud phenomenon
  – Erythromelalgia (erythermalgia)
• *Nonscarring alopecia:*
  – "Lupus hair"
  – Telogen effluvium
  – Alopecia areata
• Sclerodactyly
• Rheumatoid nodules
• Calcinosis cutis
• LE-nonspecific bullous lesions
• Urticaria
• Papulonodular mucinosis
• Cutis laxa/anetoderma
• Acanthosis nigricans (type B insulin resistance)
• Erythema multiforme
• Leg ulcers
• Lichen planus

PATHOGENESIS OF LUPUS ERYTHEMATOSUS

Multifactorial: Genetic susceptibility, environmental factors, and hormonal influences.

High frequency is seen among first degree relatives.

- *Genetic:* Supported by increase concordance rate in monozygotic twin (65%) in systemic lupus erythematosus (SLE)
  - SLE- HLA -DR2, -DR3
  - Subacute cutaneous LE (SCLE)- HLA -B8, -DR3
  - Chronic cutaneous LE (CCLE)- HLA -B7,-B8,- DR3
  - *Genetic deficiency:* Complement gene- C1q, C2, and C4.
- *UV radiation:* Induce apoptosis of keratinocyte, which makes previously cryptic peptides available for immune surveillance breaking tolerance to self-antigen and also causes exaggerated release of immune mediators. ACLE, SCLE, and tumid LE highly photosensitive.
- *Infection and stress*

  Virus: Epstein–Barr virus (EBV) and cytomegalovirus (CMV): EBV-induce cell surface expression of SS A and related autoantigens in apoptotic cells, thus triggering a flare.
- *Hormonal factor:*
  - F:M 9:1
  - Premenstrual flare up

- Drugs precipitated by isoniazid, procainamide, hydralazine, minocycline, anti-TNFα biologics, etc.
- *Tobacco:* It alters endogenous proteins and DNA, making them more immunogenic. These altered adducts are found at high concentration within immune complexes. Reactive oxygen species (ROS) generated from tobacco triggers the production of autoantigen and autoreactive T-cells.
- *Role of T-cell and B-cell:* When a T-lymphocyte to an antigen-presenting cell (APC) is introduced, the T-cell receptor binds to the MHC portion of the APC, which leads to cytokine release, inflammation, and B-cell stimulation. Now these B-cells produce IgG autoantibodies against antigens that are exposed on the surface of apoptotic cells. It is believed that the removal of these apoptotic cells is compromised because of the impaired functioning of phagocytic cells, resulting in suboptimal disposal of dying cells and antigen recognition in patients with SLE.[2]
- *Interferon-alpha (IFN-α):* High levels of IFNα lead to immune dysregulation.
- *Role of autoantibodies in tissue damage:*
  - Immune complex deposition activates complements which initiate the tissue damage
  - Anti-ds DNA antibody cross-react with proteins in various organs, explained with direct pathogenic effect on renal cells

CHRONIC CUTANEOUS LUPUS ERYTHEMATOSUS/DISCOID LUPUS ERYTHEMATOSUS

- CCLE patients most often have skin-only or skin predominant disease
- Up to 3 times more common than SLE
- *Localized*: Head and neck (70%)
- *Disseminated*: Affecting below neck also (30%)
- *Risk of developing SLE:* 5% in localized and 20% in generalized
- *Sex:* F:M = 2:1
- *Age of onset:* Mostly fourth decade

Morphology:
- Erythematous, discoid plaque with follicular plugging and adherent scaling.
- Later develops central depigmentation and scarring with peripheral hyperpigmentation and erythema.
- Heals with pigmentary change, atrophy, and scarring.

Most common site: Sun-exposed areas—face, ear, scalp.

Scalp is involved in 60% of cases and one-third develops scarring alopecia.

Photosensitivity occurs in 70% of patients with DLE.

Shuster sign: Wide follicular pits often containing scales or blackheads seen in concha of the ear.

Tin-tack sign/carpet tack sign: Adherent scale undersurface shows horny plugs which have occupied dilated pilosebaceous canals.

Mucous membrane involved in 25% cases
- Lips and buccal mucosa
- Sharply marginated plaque with scalloped border, surrounded by radiating white striae and telangiectasia.

Histopathology

Presence of at least two of these is essential for histological diagnosis of LE:

1. Liquefactive degeneration of the basal cell layer of the epidermis.
2. Degenerative changes in the connective tissue, consisting of hyalinization, edema and fibrinoid change, most marked immediately below the epidermis.
3. Patchy dermal lymphocytic infiltrate with few plasma cells and histiocytes, particularly around the appendages, which may be atrophic.

Epidermis:
- Focal hyperkeratosis/parakeratosis
- Follicular plugging
- Atrophy of stratum Malpighi
- Focal liquefactive degeneration of basal cells
- Thick band like periodic acid-Schiff (PAS) positive basement membrane.

Dermis:
- Edema in upper dermis
- Destruction of elastic fibers
- Vasculitis with fibrinoid deposit and extravasation of RBCs
- Mucin deposition rarely.

Prognosis:
- Patients with active DLE seldom develop severe renal disease.[3]
- Rarely, DLE scars develop squamous cell carcinoma (SCC).

Hypertrophic or Verrucous LE

- Rare (2% of CCLE)
- Affects the extensor surface of the arms and legs, upper back, and face
- Dull red indurated lesions covered by keratotic multilayered horny white or yellow scales with a central crateriform atrophy
- Less chance of progression to SLE
- Histopathology shows marked acanthosis, hyperkeratosis, and hypergranulosis.
- Resistant to therapy, systemic isotretinoin effective

Mucosal DLE

- Oral mucosa more frequently involved—buccal mucosa > palate > alveolar process > tongue
- Morphology—painless erythematous patches with a depressed center and superficial ulceration, have irregular white borders with radiating striae

- Lesions on the palate often have honeycomb appearance.
- Heals with scarring
- Rarely develop SCC
- Histopathology—lymphocyte-rich interface mucositis.
- Direct immunofluorescence (DIF)—similar to cutaneous LE
- Treatment—topical high-potency corticosteroids and tacrolimus

Chilblain Lupus

- Rare
- Cold-induced lesions localized to acral areas without cold agglutinins and cryoglobulins
- Predominant in females
- *C/F:* Located on fingers, toes, calves, heels, knees, elbows, nose, and ears
- Represented by papuloerythematous purplish, sometimes infiltrated, pruriginous or painful elements and may ulcerate rarely
- 15% of patients develop SLE
- Usually Ro antibody positive
- *Histopathology:* Atrophic epidermis, vacuolated dermal-epidermal junction (DEJ) and dermal mononuclear infiltrate of variable intensity around blood vessels and pilosebaceous appendages
- *Treatment:* Topical or oral corticosteroids, pentoxifylline, dapsone, etretinate, vasodilators, and mycophenolate mofetil. Warm environment and suitable clothes are more important

LE Profundus

- Rare
- Inflammatory lesion in lower dermis and subcutaneous tissue
- LE profundus—lupus panniculitis and DLE lesion
- LE panniculitis—only subcutaneous tissue involvement
- Female predominance (F:M 2:1)
- Predilection for the face, proximal extremities, buttocks, breasts, and trunk
- Presents as indurated, subcutaneous nodules that are usually firm, rubbery, sharply defined, and persistent
- Heals with depression of overlying skin
- Positive antinuclear antibodies (ANA) (70–75%), higher incidence of SLE
- *Histopathology:* Typical lobular lymphocytic panniculitis with hyaline necrosis of fat, lymphocytic aggregates or lymphoid nodules associated with lymphocytic nuclear dust. Calcification is common, thickened, and hyalinized vessels in the subcutaneous fat and septal regions
- *Treatment:* Corticosteroids (systemic/topical) and antimalarials. Dapsone and thalidomide in resistant cases

Tumid LE

- Highly photosensitive
- Predominantly affects male
- Good prognosis
- Mean age at onset—40 years
- Affects face, upper back, V-area of neck, extensor aspects of the arms, and shoulders
- Manifests as single or multiple raised polycyclic erythematous, edematous plaques with bright reddish or violaceous, smooth surface
- Borders are sharply limited, tendency of swelling in the periphery, and flattening in the center of plaque
- No scarring, no pigmentary changes
- DIF—mostly negative
- ANA positive in 10% of patients
- *Histopathology:* Minimal follicular hyperkeratosis with basal layer vacuolization, considerable dermal lymphocytic infiltrate, and interstitial mucin deposition
- Systemic involvement—very rare
- Rapid and effective response to systemic antimalarials, photoprotection recommended

Lupus Band Test

Deposition of immunoglobulins and complement components in the skin of patients with LE, demonstrable as a linear band at the basement membrane zone (BMZ) by DIF. Considered positive when one or more immunoreactants (Ig G, A, M, C3) are found. Has both, diagnostic and prognostic value.[4]

Lesional LBT and nonlesional LBT are used to denote biopsy from involved and uninvolved skin.

- *Lesional:* Skin lesion
- *Nonlesional:* UV exposed, uninvolved—forearm
  - UV protected, uninvolved- buttocks (highly specific for LE if ≥3 immunoreactants are seen in the nonlesional UV protected skin).

Uses:

- *Highly sensitive and specific test for LE:*
  - Approximately 90–95% of the patients with systemic or discoid LE have positive LBT in involved skin
  - The sensitivity of the LBT for active disease is higher than that of other laboratory variables such as serum C3 and C4 levels, anti-DNA antibody, LE cell test, lymphocyte count, and erythrocyte sedimentation rate (ESR)
- *Differentiation of systemic LE from discoid LE:* LBT is positive in systemic LE in both involved and uninvolved skin, and only in involved skin in discoid LE
- *Diagnosing systemic LE in patients without cutaneous lesions:* A positive LBT in clinically normal skin provides early confirmation of SLE in patients without LE lesions.
- Diagnosis of SLE from other ANA positive collagen diseases

Prognostic significance:

- Positive LBT from sun-protected normal skin indicates decreased long-term survival.
- Correlates positively with risk of developing nephritis.

Subacute Cutaneous Lupus Erythematosus

SCLE includes patients with clinically erythematous, non-scarring lesions, pronounced photosensitivity, musculoskeletal complaints, serologic abnormalities, and a variety of relatively mild systemic symptoms.

- Forms 7–27% patients of LE
- F:M 4:1

Morphology:

- Papulosquamous (2/3)
- Annular polycyclic (1/3) (primary lesions expand and clear centrally to produce annular lesions that merge into polycyclic lesions)

Rarely vesiculation and crusting at the active border with hypopigmentation and telangiectasias at center may be seen in annular SCLE.

- Site—above the waist, around the neck, trunk, and outer aspect of arm
- May cause pigmentary changes and telangiectasia
- No atrophy, no scarring
- Drugs such as hydrochlorothiazide, antiepileptics, NSAIDs, calcium channel blockers, ACE inhibitors, terbinafine, anti-TNFα inhibitors are associated with onset or exacerbation of SCLE
- 50% of SCLE patients fulfill the American Rheumatism Association (ARA) criteria for SLE
- 20–30% of patients develop features of ACLE or DLE
- Risk factors for development of SLE—papulosquamous type, leukopenia, ANA titer > 1:640, anti-dsDNA antibody

Histopathology: SCLE has less hyperkeratosis, basement membrane thickening, follicular plugging, inflammatory infiltration, and more epidermal atrophy compared to DLE. Colloid bodies and epidermal necrosis present in more than 50%, especially in those with Ro/SS-A antibodies.

Antibodies positive:

- ANA in 60–80%
- Anti-Ro/SS A— 80–90%
- Anti-La/SS B—30–50%.

Neonatal LE

Etiology:

- Transplacental passage of maternal Ab.
- Mostly associated with Ro/SS-A antibody (100%) - La/SS-B (50%).

C/F: Skin and cardiac involvement most frequent

Skin lesion:

- Appears within 4–6 weeks of life
- Resembles SCLE, frequent around eyes
- Erythematous slightly scaly eruption over face and periorbital area (raccoon sign, owl eye, eye mask sign), scalp, trunk
- Photosensitive
- Resolve with clearance of maternal antibody by 6 months

Cardiac lesion:

- Heart block (most common), myocarditis, and cardiomyopathy

Other—thrombocytopenia, hemolytic anemia, neutropenia, hepatomegaly, and splenomegaly

- *Treatment:*
  - *Skin lesion:* Photoavoidance, mild topical steroid
  - *Cardiac:* Systemic steroids within 16 weeks of birth

Systemic Lupus Erythematosus

A systemic disease characterized by multisystem organ inflammation, most commonly the skin, joints and vasculature with immunological abnormalities. Skin involvement is second to joint involvement. Approximately 80% patients have a rash at some stage, and presenting sign in up to 25%.

The new 2019 European League Against Rheumatism (EULAR)/ American College of Rheumatology (ACR) classification criteria for SLE require a positive ANA as obligatory entry criterion. Other criteria were chosen from 7 clinical (constitutional, hematologic, neuropsychiatric, mucocutaneous, serosal, musculoskeletal, and renal) and 3 immunologic (antiphospholipid antibodies, complement proteins, and SLE-specific antibodies) categories, and weighted from 2 to 10. These new criteria have a sensitivity of 98% and specificity of 96%. Patients with ≥10 points are classified as having SLE.[5]

Entry criterion

Antinuclear antibodies (ANA) at a titer of ≥1:80 on HEp-2 cells or an equivalent positive test (ever)

↓

If absent, do not classify as systemic lupus erythematosus (SLE). If present, apply additive criteria

↓

- Additive criteria do not count a criterion, if there is a more likely explanation than SLE.
- Occurrence of a criterion on at least one occasion is sufficient.
- SLE classification requires at least one clinical criterion and ≥10 points.
- Criteria need not occur simultaneously.
- Within each domain, only the highest-weighted criterion is counted toward the total score.

Clinical domains and criteria weight		*Immunology domains and criteria weight*	
Constitutional		*Antiphospholipid antibodies*	
Fever	2	Anticardiolipin antibodies OR Hematologic anti-β2GP1 antibodies OR Lupus anticoagulant	2
Hematologic		*Complement proteins*	
Leukopenia	3	Low C3 OR low C4	3
Thrombocytopenia	4	Low C3 AND low C4	4
Autoimmune hemolysis	4		

Contd...

Contd...

Clinical domains and criteria weight		*Immunology domains and criteria weight*	
Neuropsychiatric		*SLE-specific antibodies*	
Delirium	2	Anti-dsDNA antibody OR	
Psychosis	3	Anti-Smith antibody	6
Seizure	5		
Mucocutaneous			
Nonscarring alopecia	2		
Oral ulcers	2		
Subacute cutaneous OR			
Discoid lupus	4		
Acute cutaneous lupus	6		
Serosal			
Pleural or pericardial effusion	5		
Acute pericarditis	6		
Musculoskeletal			
Joint involvement	6		
Renal			
Proteinuria >0.5 g/24 h	4		
Renal biopsy Class II or V lupus nephritis	8		
Renal biopsy Class III or IV lupus nephritis	10		
Total score ↓ Classify as SLE with a score of 10 or more if entry criterion fulfilled.			

Acute Cutaneous Lupus Erythematosus

Localized ACLE (Malar rash/Butterfly rash):

- Confluent symmetric fixed erythema and edema centered over the malar area and bridge of the nose. Nasolabial fold spared. Forehead, chin, and V area of neck may be involved.
- This butterfly rash is present at diagnosis in 40–52% of SLE patients.

Generalized ACLE (Photosensitive lupus dermatitis/lupus maculopapular rash/SLE rash):

- Discrete maculopapular rash involving the photoexposed area. There is often erythema and edema of hands, particularly over the dorsal and interphalangeal areas, sparing the skin over knuckles.
- It may be present in about one-third of patients with SLE.
- Postinflammatory hyperpigmentation/hypopigmentation can persist long after active inflammation has subsided.

Typically precipitated by exposure to UV light (ACLE, SCLE, and tumid LE are highly photosensitive and non-scarring).

Histopathology—Similar to SCLE with more intense edema.

LBT performed on even noninvolved and nonexposed skin is mostly positive.

Immunologic abnormalities:

- ANA positive in 95% of SLE
- *Anti-dsDNA (70%):* Specific for SLE. High titers associated with renal lupus and clinical activity.
- Anti-Sm antibodies are specific for SLE.
- Hypocomplementemia is another common abnormality.

Both localized and generalized forms of ACLE flare and abate in parallel with SLE disease activity. ACLE is always associated with active SLE.[6]

Nonspecific Cutaneous LE Lesions

Cutaneous Vascular Disease

Telangiectasia:

- Reticulate telangiectasia and erythema involving thenar and hypothenar eminence, pulp, and dorsum of finger
- Dilated nail fold capillaries

Vasculitis:

All sizes of vessel may be affected.

- Small vessel vasculitis—infarcts along the lateral nail folds, elbows, and lower extremities
- Large vessel vasculitis—peripheral gangrene, painful subcutaneous nodule, chronic recurrent ulcer, polyarteritis-like cutaneous lesions.
- Urticarial vasculitis, due to:
  - C1 deficiency
  - Immune complex deposition

  About 10–20% of SLE patients have some form of vasculitis.

Livedo reticularis—outer aspect of arm

- Thrombophlebitis
- Raynaud's phenomenon
- Erythromelalgia
- Degos disease-like lesions
- Secondary atrophie blanche

Alopecia: Diffuse and nonscarring. Mostly in active stage.

- Telogen effluvium
- Alopecia areata
- *Lupus hair:* These are coarse, dry, brittle, broken off shortened unruly hair on the frontal margin. Usually persist longer, occurs in 30% patients.

Hair recovers once disease becomes inactive but the lupus hair tends to persist longer.

Nails:

- Show pitting, ridging, onycholysis, striate leukonychia, red lunula, and splinter hemorrhage
- Nail fold may show hyperkeratotic and ragged cuticles. It may be erythematous and capillaroscopy reveals glomerulization and telangiectasia.
- There may be small vascular necrosis on the tips of the fingers and alongside the nails

Mucous membrane lesions: In 25% cases of SLE

Palate, buccal mucosa, and gum:

- Erythematous
- Discoid
- Ulcerative

Other nonspecific skin findings:

- Sclerodactyly
- Rheumatoid nodules
- Calcinosis cutis
- LE-nonspecific bullous lesions
- Urticaria
- Papulonodular mucinosis
- Cutis laxa/anetoderma
- Acanthosis nigricans
- Erythema multiforme
- Leg ulcers
- Lichen planus

Bullous lesion in SLE:

- *Subepidermal bullae in SCLE and ACLE:*
  - Result of separation of the epidermis and dermis
  - Due to *severe liquefactive degeneration* of the basal layer and dermal edema (TEN-like ACLE and Rowell syndrome)
- *SLE-associated autoimmune bullous disease:* Dermatitis herpetiformis, pemphigus erythematosus, pemphigus foliaceus, paraneoplastic pemphigus, bullous pemphigoid, pseudoporphyria, epidermolysis bullosa acquisita and IgA disease
- *Bullous SLE:*
  - Rare
  - Young adults
  - Autoantibodies to VII collagen
  - Upper trunk, face, neck
  - May arise on erythematous or normal skin

Three types:

1. Pruritic large tensed bulla—bullous pemphigoid like
2. Small grouped vesicles-like dermatitis herpetiformis
3. Mechanobullous-like epidermolysis bullosa acquisita

Generalized blistering seen in patients who meet ARA criteria.

Histopathology: Subepidermal blister with neutrophil-predominant inflammation in the papillary dermis *without* liquefactive degeneration.[7]

- LBT positive
- Hydralazine and IFN α may precipitate
- R_x- Dapsone ± prednisolone.

Rowel syndrome: ACLE/SCLE/DLE + erythema multiforme like lesion

Adult females affected:

- Anti SS-B or Anti SS-A +ve
- Speckled ANA +ve
- Rheumatoid factor +ve

Drug-induced lupus:

- Autoimmune phenomenon.
- Drug exposure leads to the development of SLE-like clinical features.
- Most common systemic complaint is arthralgia.
- Anti-histone antibodies—95% (in SLE = 70%).
- Anti-DNA antibodies—absent.
- Serum complements—normal.
- Renal and CNS involvement is uncommon.
- Drugs such as hydralazine, procainamide, hydrochlorothiazide, chlorpromazine, isoniazid, quinidine, penicillamine, anti-TNF agents responsible

SLE in childhood:

- Approximately 15–20% of SLE has its onset in childhood.
- Children have more acute and severe disease.
- Malar rash, fever, adenopathy, mucocutaneous involvement, hematological abnormalities, seizures, renal involvement, urinary cellular casts, and proteinuria are more common in children.[8]
- Isolated DLE is uncommon in children

SLE in pregnancy:

- Fertility is not affected if renal function is good.
- Active lupus nephritis increases the risk of stillbirth, preterm birth, low birth weight, and pre-eclampsia.
- SLE flare is uncommon during pregnancy if patient is receiving immunosuppressive therapy.
- Patients having clinical remission 6 months prior to conception have lower chances of SLE flare.

Antiphospholipid syndrome:

- Characterized by the presence of antiphospholipid antibodies (APAbs) + vascular thrombosis/recurrent pregnancy complications
- Fetal loss in 45–90% of untreated pregnancies
- Female with APAbs and a history of pregnancy complications needs prophylactic low-molecular-weight heparin (LMWH) and low-dose aspirin
- Neonatal lupus can occur in the babies of mothers with anti-Ro/SSA or anti-La/SSB antibodies

Kikuchi Fujimoto disease (KFD) and SLE: KFD is a benign, self-limiting histiocytic necrotizing lymphadenitis of unknown etiology. SLE can present concurrently or follow a diagnosis of KFD.

Systemic manifestation of SLE:

- *General:* Fever, fatigue, malaise, weight loss
- *Musculoskeletal:*
  - Arthralgia and nonerosive arthritis
  - Avascular bone necrosis
  - Myalgia, myositis
- *Hematological:*
  - *Anemia:*
    - Hemolytic
    - Normocytic normochromic
  - Leukopenia
  - Thrombocytopenia
- *Heart:*
  - Pericarditis
  - Endocarditis (Libman-Sacks)

- Heart block
- Myocardial infarction (MI)

- *Lung:*
  - Pleurisy
  - Pleural effusion
- *Renal change:*
  - Common cause of death
  - *Lupus glomerulonephritis (LN):*
    - *Class 1:* minimal mesangial LN
    - *Class 2:* mesangial proliferative LN
    - *Class 3:* focal LN
    - *Class 4:* diffuse LN
    - *Class 5:* membranous LN
    - *Class 6:* advanced sclerosis LN
  - Malignant hypertension
- *Neuropsychiatric:*
  - Seizure
  - Psychosis
  - Headache
- *Gastrointestinal:*
  - Ascites
  - Anorexia, nausea, vomiting, abdominal pain, diarrhea
  - Hepatitis, hepatomegaly
- *Ocular:*
  - Conjunctivitis, episcleritis, uveitis
  - Blindness secondary to retinal artery occlusion
  - Keratoconjunctivitis sicca

SLE Investigations:

- Complete blood count (CBC) with differential count
- ESR, C-reactive protein (CRP)
- *Urine:*
  - R/E
  - 24 hours urinary protein
- Liver and renal function
- Complement—C3 and C4
- LE cell
- ANA (>1:64) (using hep cell SLE 98%, SCLE 60–80%, CCLE 30–40%) (most common- homogenous type)
- Antibody to DsDNA—correlate with disease activity
- *Other Ab:*
  - Antihistone Ab drug-induced SLE
  - Anti-Sm Ab- specific for SLE
  - Anti-Ro (SS-A)—associated with tumid LE, SCLE, neonatal LE, high risk for vasculitis, lower risk for renal involvement
  - Anti-La (SS-B)—associated with anti-Ro, lower risk for renal involvement
  - Anti-U_1 ribonucleoprotein (RNP)—mixed connective tissue disease (MCTD)
  - *Antiphospholipid Ab:* Thrombosis, recurrent fetal loss
- Chest X-ray (CXR)
- USG abdomen

LE cell phenomenon:

- Seen in 80% of SLE
- Polymorphonuclear leukocytes (PMNs) which have ingested nuclear material from degenerative white blood cells (WBCs), in the presence of antibody to deoxyribonucleoprotein (LE cell factor)
- Also positive in drug-induced LE, DLE, systemic sclerosis, RA.

Treatment:

Photoprotection:

- Avoidance of sun exposure
- Physical protection
- Broad-spectrum sunscreen
- Elimination of photosensitizing drugs

Experimental UV protection:

- Antioxidants
- Alpha-MSH
- Thymidine dinucleotide
- Oral polypodium leucotomos

First line	*Second line*	*Others*	*New drugs*
Topical Topical steroids Systemic Antimalarials Steroids	Topical Calcineurin inhibitors Systemic Retinoids Methotrexate	Azathioprine Mycophenolate mofetil (MMF) Dapsone Thalidomide Extracorporeal photopheresis Sulfasalazine Danazol	Imiquimod R-salbutamol Intravenous immunoglobulins (IVIG) Efalizumab

Patients who smoke are less responsive to antimalarial treatment.

Newer biologicals:

- B-lymphocyte stimulator (BLyS) inhibitor-Belulimab (FDA approved)[9]
- Tocilizumab
- Eculizumab
- Rituximab.

IFNα-related therapies:

- Sifalimumab
- Rontalizumab

Janus kinase (JAK) inhibitors:

- Baricitinib
- Ruxolitinib

KEY POINTS

- Gilliam's classification of lupus includes specific as well as non-specific cutaneous lesions.
- Exact pathomechanism of autoimmunity lupus is still an enigma; UV radiation, viral infection, hormonal factors, drugs are thought to be involved.
- Classical cutaneous lesion of LE is DLE (discoid lupus erythematosus), 3 times commoner than SLE.

- These disorders are more common in females.
- Neonatal LE is due transplacental passage of maternal ab.
- 2019 ACR criteria require a positive ANA as obligatory entry criteria.
- Early identification of systemic features of SLE is important to prevent serious sequalae.
- Treatment is mainly with steroid or steroid-sparing agents.

REFERENCES

1. Ali A, Sayyed Z, Ameer M, Arif A, Kiran F, Iftikhar A, et al. Systemic lupus erythematosus: an overview of the disease pathology and its management. Cureus. 2018;10(9):e3288.
2. Bernatsky S, Boivin JF, Joseph L, Manzi S, Ginzler E, Gladman DD, et al. Mortality in systemic lupus erythematosus. Arthritis Rheum. 2006;54(8):2550-7.
3. Merola JF, Chang CA, Sanchez MR, Prystowsky SD. Is chronic cutaneous discoid lupus protective against severe renal disease in patients with systemic lupus erythematosus? J Drugs Dermatol. 2011;10(12):1413-20.
4. Zečević RD, Pavlović MD, Stefanović D. Lupus band test and disease activity in systemic lupus erythematosus: does it still matter? Clin Exp Dermatol: Clin Dermatol. 2006;31(3): 358-60.
5. Aringer M, Costenbader K, Daikh D, Brinks R, Mosca M, Ramsey-Goldman R, et al. 2019 European League Against Rheumatism/American College of Rheumatology classification criteria for systemic lupus erythematosus. Arthritis Rheum. 2019;71(9):1400-12.
6. Grönhagen CM, Nyberg F. Cutaneous lupus erythematosus: an update. Indian Dermatol Online J. 2014;5(1):7.
7. Contestable JJ, Edhegard KD, Meyerle JH. Bullous systemic lupus erythematosus: a review and update to diagnosis and treatment. Am J Clin Dermatol. 2014;15(6):517-24.
8. Livingston B, Bonner A, Pope J. Differences in clinical manifestations between childhood-onset lupus and adult-onset lupus: a meta-analysis. Lupus. 2011;20(13):1345-55.
9. Espinosa G, Cervera R. Belimumab. A BLyS-specific inhibitor for the treatment of systemic lupus erythematosus. Drugs Today (Barc). 2010;46(12):891-9.

EXAMINATION QUESTIONS

1. What is pathogenesis of SLE?
2. Write a short note on tumid LE.
3. Write a short note on neonatal lupus.
4. Discuss SLE in pregnancy.
5. What are EULAR/ACR 2019 criteria of SLE?
6. Discuss newer treatment in LE.
7. How will you approach a case of SLE in a 21-year-old female?
8. Discuss cutaneous manifestations of SLE.
9. Explain LE panniculitis.
10. Write a short note on Lupus band test.
11. What is antiphospholipid syndrome.

53 CHAPTER Lichen Sclerosus and Morphea

Resham Vasani, Kapisha Shah

LICHEN SCLEROSUS

Introduction

Lichen sclerosus (LS) is a chronic inflammatory scarring mucocutaneous disorder of unknown etiology characterized by a lymphocytic response. The old terms balanitis xerotica obliterans and kraurosis vulvae are now no longer used and the suffix "et atrophicus" has been dropped, as some cases of LS are associated with a hypertrophic rather than atrophic epithelium.

Etiopathogenesis

Women are 6–10 times more commonly affected by genital LS compared to men. LS has a bimodal peak of presentation in women, prepubertal and postmenopausal, suggesting a hormonal factor. Pregnancy is known to improve the disease and normal vaginal delivery is possible.

Men are usually diagnosed between 30 and 40 years of life.[1] There is an increased association of increased body mass index, coronary artery disease, diabetes mellitus, smoking, and tobacco use.[2] The dysfunctional performance of the naviculo-meatal fossa and meatal lips acting as a low pressure valve causes microincontinence of urine, which leads to a moist environment under the foreskin, which in turn predisposes to LS.[3] The association of LS with urostomy and ileostomy suggests moisture and irritation may play a role in the etiology of LS.[4]

HLA DQ7 is commonly associated with LS. It is also associated with other autoimmune diseases including autoimmune thyroid disease, alopecia areata, vitiligo, pernicious anemia, and diabetes.[1] An infective etiology has been postulated and the spirochete *Borrelia burgdorferi* has been implicated.

Clinical Features

15–20% of patients with genital LS also have extragenital manifestations, while only 6% of LS patients have extra-genital lesions exclusively.[1]

Genital Lesions in Adult Females

- In females, itching is the predominant symptom, but pain may be a consequence of erosions and fissures. Dyspareunia occurs in presence of erosions, fissures, or introital narrowing. Rarely lesions can be completely asymptomatic and can be an incidental finding on examination. Urinary symptoms and urinary incontinence are reported by women having LS.
- The typical findings are porcelain white papules and plaques, often associated with areas of ecchymosis with follicular delling and hyperkeratosis being a predominant feature in some cases. The interlabial sulci, labia minora, clitoral hood, clitoris, and perineal body are the characteristic sites of involvement. In late stages, it can cause atrophy of the labia minora, scarring of the clitoral hood, and labial and/or clitoral hood adhesions **(Fig. 1)**. The plaques may extend to the anogenital region causing a "figure of eight appearance" **(Fig. 2)**.
- Genital LS spares the mucosa, and thus the vagina and cervix are almost always spared thus differentiating it from lichen planus.
- Involvement of mucocutaneous junction leads to introital narrowing giving a "key hole appearance."

Genital Lesions in Prepubertal Girls

- In prepubertal girls, pruritus and soreness are the most common presenting features.

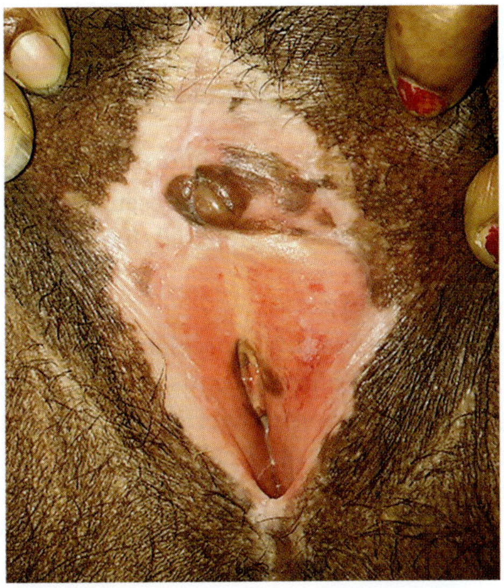

Fig. 1: Lichen sclerosus with atrophy and scarring of the labia minora and resorption of the clitoral hood.

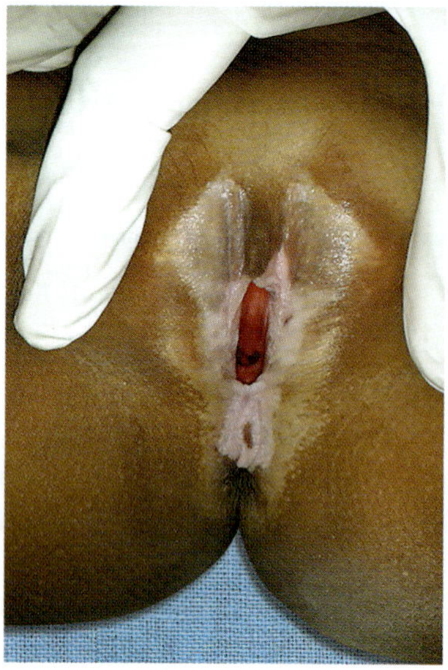

Fig. 2: Lichen sclerosus in a figure-of-eight pattern in a child.

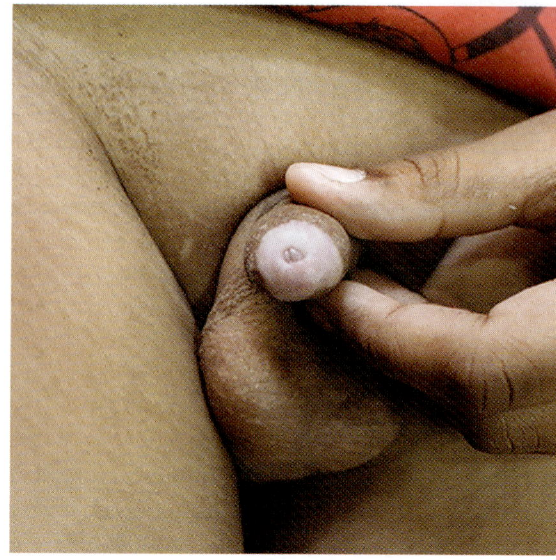

Fig. 3: Lichen sclerosus with phimosis.

- In children, ecchymoses can be very striking and can be mistaken as child abuse. Perianal involvement is more common and can lead to constipation because of painful fissuring. Anogenital LS usually resolves by menarche in approximately two-thirds of prepubertal cases; the remaining one-third develop chronic atrophy. After puberty resolution of lesions is unlikely.

Genital Involvement in Adult Males

In men, the glans and prepuce are most commonly affected, which can be asymptomatic or presenting as tightening of the foreskin which may lead to painful erection, paraphimosis, phimosis, and painful intercourse **(Fig. 3)**. The perimeatal area can be involved and the postinflammatory scarring may lead to stenosis and obstruction. Initial meatal involvement may lead to problematic voiding and further the involvement can progress to involve the urethra leading to urethral strictures and subsequent poor urinary stream and decreased penile sensitivity. Extragenital lesions in male are rare.

Genital Involvement in Male Children

In male children, the most frequent presentation is phimosis and it can be complicated by preputial stones.

Extragenital Lesions

The lesions present as tiny, porcelain white macules or papules with dilated pilosebaceous duct openings which contain yellow-brown horny plug **(Fig. 4)**. In the later stage, they become atrophic with a wrinkled depressed appearance. The common sites are the trunk, pressure sites, flexor aspect of wrist, neck, buttocks, and thighs. Koebner phenomenon is present. The clinical types of extragenital LS include an extensive bullous form and annular, Blaschkoid, and keratotic variants.

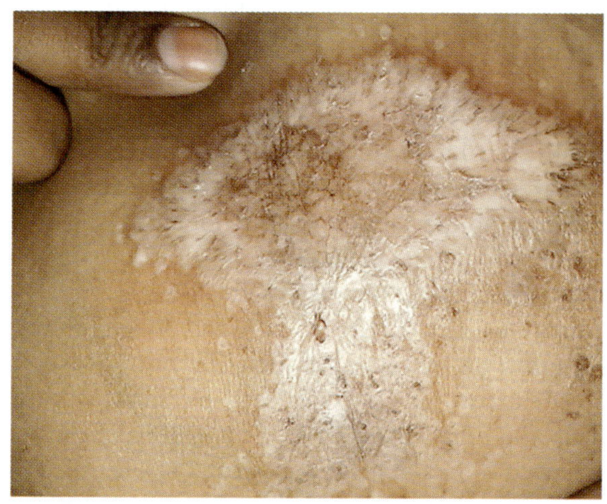

Fig. 4: Extragenital lichen sclerosus on the breast.

Histopathology

Lichen sclerosus is a clinical diagnosis, and biopsy is not always necessary when typical features are present. However, a biopsy must be considered if:[5]

- *Suspicion of neoplastic change*: Persistent area of hyperkeratosis, erosion, erythema, or new verrucous or papular lesions.
- No or inadequate response to treatment.
- Cases of extragenital LS mimicking morphea.
- After circumcision is performed, foreskin should be sent for confirmation of diagnosis and ruling out penile intraepithelial neoplasia.
- In case of pigmented areas, to rule out abnormal melanocytic proliferation.
- Before urological surgery for urethral disease for confirmation of diagnosis.

The histopathological features include "trilayered" or "striped" appearance consisting of **(Fig. 5)**:

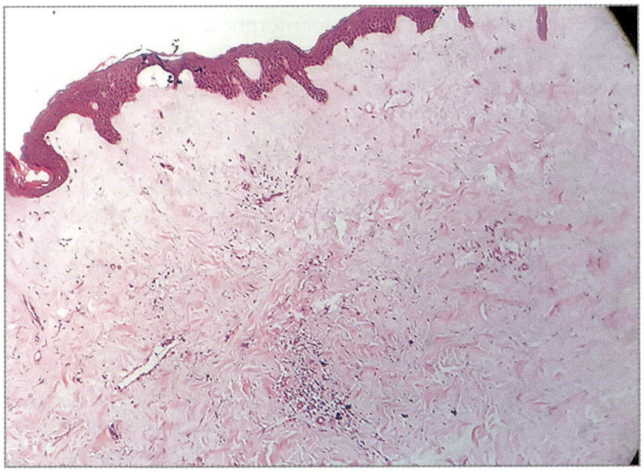

Fig. 5: Trilayered or striped appearance of lichen sclerosus (LS).

- *Epidermal changes*: Hyperkeratosis with follicular plugging, atrophy of the stratum malpighii with hydropic degeneration of basal cells.
- *Dermal changes*: Pronounced edema and homogenization of the collagen in the upper dermis with inflammatory, lymphohistiocytic infiltrate in the mid-dermis.

Differential Diagnosis

Extragenital

- Guttate morphea
- Lichen planus
- Vitiligo

Genital

- *In female*:
  - Vitiligo
  - Genital lichen planus
  - Lichen simplex chronicus
  - Vulvar intraepithelial neoplasia
  - Extramammary Paget's disease
- *In male*:
  - Balanoposthitis
  - Idiopathic phimosis
  - Erosive lichen planus

Complications

- *Malignancy*: In females, the risk of developing malignancy is approximately 3.5–5% and that in males is 4–5%. Squamous cell carcinoma of the usual and verrucous type has been described in genital LS. In addition, melanoma, basal cell carcinoma, and Merkel cell carcinoma have been described in female genital LS. Melanoma has been described in male genital LS.
- Scarring leading to complications such as introital narrowing and pseudocyst of the clitoris in females while phimosis, adhesions, meatal stenosis, and urethral strictures can occur in males.
- Sensory abnormalities such as vulvodynia and penile dysesthesia can be persistent issues despite objective clinical improvement and do not respond to topical corticosteroids.
- Psychosexual disorders such as lack of interest in sexual activity and sexual dysfunction can be encountered.

Management

- Counselling should emphasize on the permanent nature of the scarring, if present. Compliance to maintenance treatment is emphasized upon to avoid recurrences as well to screen for malignant changes. Emphasis should be laid on the need for monthly self-examination and yearly follow-ups in high-risk cases of LS such as ulcerative LS.
- Use of soap-free cleansers, bland emollients, and avoidance of irritants is advisable.[6]
- *Ultrapotent topical corticosteroids*: It is the treatment of choice in adults. Topical clobetasol propionate 0.05% ointment 0.5 g (1 FTU) can be given once at night for 1–3 months with no >10 g used monthly. For meatal involvement, it can be applied via a cotton wool bud or meatal dilator. Maintenance treatment is essential with applications ranging from thrice weekly to twice monthly depending upon the clinical scenario. If daily use is needed, addition of calcineurin inhibitor is recommended.
- Intralesional steroids such as triamcinolone are effective alternative to topical steroids for thick indurated plaques.
- Topical tacrolimus or pimecrolimus is recommended as a second agent for maintenance and tacrolimus works better than pimecrolimus. The main limiting factor with this class being the adverse effect of burning.
- Short contact topical retinoid is efficacious but limited by irritation. Oral acitretin has been used in some cases.
- Case reports for psoralen plus ultraviolet A (PUVA), narrowband UVB, and photodynamic therapy have been reported.
- Oral antimalarials have been tried.
- Oral methotrexate, cyclosporine, and acitretin in combination with oral steroids have been used.
- Other modalities which have been tried are topical estrogen, cryosurgery, CO_2 laser, potassium para-aminobenzoate, oral stanozolol, and tangential excision.
- *Surgical treatment*: Circumcision will benefit male patients with LS and phimosis. Vulvar surgery has not been recommended unless an associated malignancy is present.

MORPHEA

Introduction

Morphea is a type of localized scleroderma caused due to excessive deposition of collagen leading to thickening of the dermis and subcutaneous tissues. It is characterized by sclerosis, fibrosis, atrophy in skin and subcutaneous tissue and sometimes extending to the muscle, bone, and brain. Extracutaneous manifestations can occur in 25% of the cases. In contrast to the systemic counterpart, the chances of internal involvement are lesser, there is no vascular involvement, negative Scl-70 antibody, and no increase in mortality. Morbidity can occur in the form of joint contractures, facial and limb asymmetry, extracutaneous manifestations, association with other connective tissue disorders, and psychological impact of the condition.

Epidemiology

The annual incidence of morphea is 3.4–27 cases per 1,000,000. It is more common in females as compared to males with a female-to-male ratio of 2.4–5:1.[7] It has a bimodal age presentation and is common in children and adults. The mean age of children presenting with morphea is between 7 and 11 years and adults between 44 and 47 years.[7]

Pathogenesis

Exact pathogenesis is unknown. Vascular dysfunction with immune dysregulation signified by the development of antibodies and concomitant autoimmune disease is implicated.[8]

Increased serum levels of vascular cell adhesion molecule 1 (VCAM-1) and intercellular adhesion molecule 1 (ICAM-1) with predominance of Th1 and Th17 in the early active disease with Th2 predominance in the sclerotic phase of the disease are postulated.[8]

Excessive extracellular matrix formation on account of increased expression of transforming growth factor beta 1 (TGF-β1) and several other collagen types combined with an inhibitory effect on matrix degradation are thought to be responsible.[8]

Development of morphea has been associated with local tissue factors such as friction, long-term pressure, vaccination, trauma including radiation, surgery, insect bites, and intramuscular injections. Certain medications such as bisoprolol, bleomycin, peplomycin, D-penicillamine, bromocriptine, carbidopa, and pentazocine have been associated with morphea. *Borrelia* has also been implicated as a possible infectious cause of morphea.

Classification

Multiple classification systems exist, a summary of which has been mentioned in **Table 1**. As per the classification system outlined by Laxer and Zulian, there are five subtypes of morphea which will be further discussed in detail in this chapter:

1. *Circumscribed morphea:* Superficial and deep
2. Linear morphea (including the limb/trunk and head variant)
3. Generalized morphea
4. Pansclerotic morphea
5. Mixed subtype

TABLE 1: Classification systems for morphea.

Peterson et al. 1995	*Laxer and Zulian 2006*	*Kreuter et al. 2009*
Plaque morphea	*Circumscribed morphea*	*Limited type*
• Morphea en plaque • Guttate morphea • Atrophoderma of Pasini–Pierini • Lichen sclerosus • Keloidal morphea	• Superficial • Deep	• Morphea (plaque type) • Guttate morphea • Atrophoderma of Pasini–Pierini
Generalized morphea (lesions at three or more anatomical sites)	*Generalized morphea*	*Generalized type* • Generalized scleroderma (three or more anatomical sites morphea) • Disabling pan-sclerotic • Eosinophilic fasciitis
Linear morphea	*Linear morphea*	*Linear type*
• Linear morphea of the limbs or trunk • En coup de sabre morphea • Progressive hemifacial atrophy/ Parry–Romberg syndrome	• Trunk/limb variant • Head variant	• Linear localized scleroderma (usually of the extremities) • Linear localized scleroderma "en coup de sabre" type • Progressive facial hemiatrophy
Bullous morphea	*Pansclerotic morphea*	*Deep type*
Deep morphea • Subcutaneous morphea • Morphea profunda • Eosinophilic fasciitis • Disabling pan-sclerotic morphea	*Mixed morphea*	

Other classification systems include guttate and bullous variants and also variants that are debated to be a part of the morphea spectrum including atrophoderma of Pasini and Pierini, extragenital lichen sclerosus et atrophicus, and eosinophilic fasciitis.

Origin and Progression of Morphea

Morphea lesions have an initial active stage of erythematous to violaceous plaques. Over time, the center becomes white and sclerotic and the borders have a characteristic violaceous border or "lilac ring" **(Fig. 6)**. As the active stage subsides, it presents as a white sclerotic plaque with postinflammatory hyperpigmentation. There is associated destruction of lesional hair follicle and adnexal structures, resulting in an atrophic anhidrotic hairless patch. It is usually self-limiting

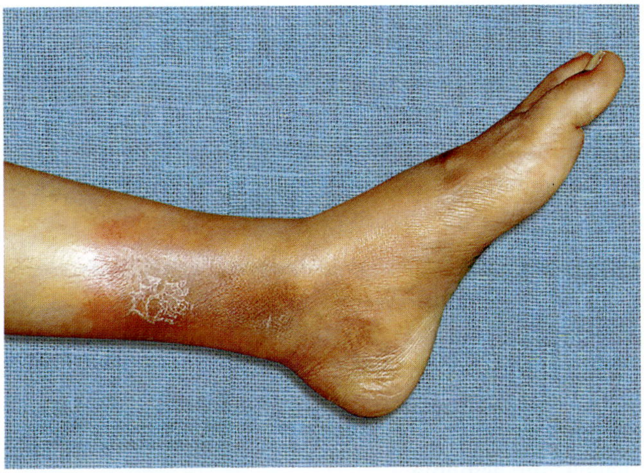

Fig. 6: Active morphea with lilac border.

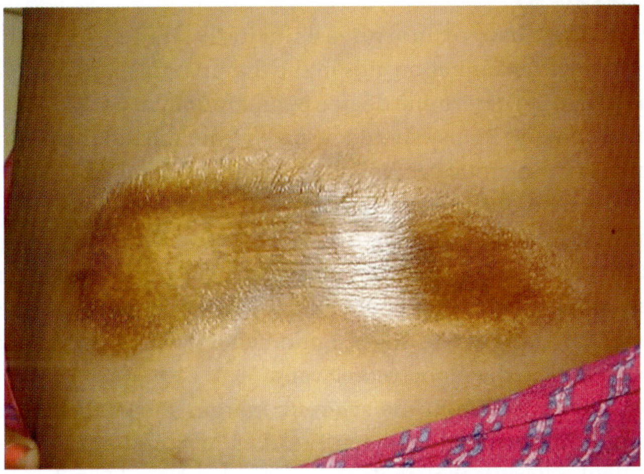

Fig. 7: Circumscribed superficial morphea.

in 3–5 years with softening of the skin in months to years with residual damage such as pigment alteration and subcutaneous atrophy. An early age of onset would allow the disease to generally remain progressive for many years with flares of the disease occurring frequently.

Clinical characteristics of each subtype are enumerated in the following text.

Circumscribed superficial morphea also known as morphea en plaque is the most common subtype of morphea **(Fig. 7)**. Involvement is usually limited to the dermis. Solitary or few plaques affecting the trunk, waist, and the submammary area are seen. It causes few problems besides local discomfort and visible disfigurement.

Circumscribed deep morphea (Morphea Profunda): Rare subtype where the sclerosis reaches the subcutaneous tissue and may also extend to the fascia and muscle. It appears as an ill-defined sclerotic plaque with a "pseudo-cellulite" appearance, fixed to the underlying structure. The induration merges with the normal skin without any definite margin. Lower extremities are often affected symmetrically and it leads to contractures and subcutaneous atrophy.

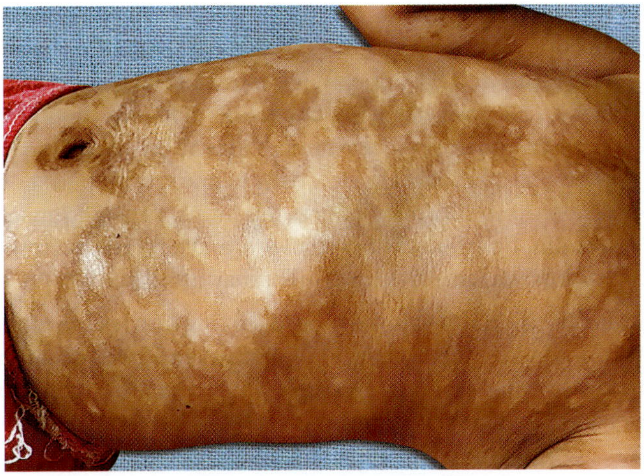

Fig. 8: Generalized morphea.

Generalized morphea is a rare variant occurring in 7–9% of morphea patients. It is defined as >4 indurated plaques larger than 3 cm and/or involving two or more body sites **(Fig. 8)**. It is usually limited to the dermis but deeper involvement is often present. Patients with generalized morphea may have systemic symptoms such as myalgias, arthralgias, and fatigue. They are more likely to have positive serology for autoantibodies particularly antinuclear antibody (ANA).

In contrast to systemic sclerosis, there is lack of Raynaud's phenomenon, digital ulceration, phalanx resorption or change in the nail-fold capillaries. Pulmonary, esophageal, renal, or cardiac abnormalities are only occasionally present.

Linear morphea is the most common subtype in childhood onset morphea. It presents as a single unilateral linear band of cutaneous induration that may involve the dermis/subcutaneous tissue/muscle/bone. The lower limbs are more commonly affected than the upper limbs and occasionally may follow the lines of Blaschko. It follows a chronic disease course as disease may remain active for many decades and recurrences occur.

The three most common variants are: (1) en coup de sabre, (2) progressive hemifacial atrophy, and (3) linear limb involvement:

- *En coup de sabre (which means "cut of the sword" in French)*: Linear atrophic depressed groove appears on the frontoparietal region and can extend onto the scalp, giving rise to cicatricial alopecia **(Fig. 9)**. Frontoparietal lesions may be associated with headaches and seizures. Ocular abnormalities such as ptosis, anterior uveitis, episcleritis, keratitis, and xerophthalmia and odontostomatological abnormalities such as altered dentition, malocclusion, and asymmetry of tongue may also present with frontoparietal lesions.
- Progressive hemifacial atrophy, also known as Parry–Romberg syndrome (PRS), is a progressive, unilateral,

primary atrophic disorder of the skin, subcutaneous tissue, muscle and underlying cartilage and bone **(Figs. 10A and B)**. Possibly, it is a part of en coup de sabre since 71% have overlying cutaneous sclerosis though in some cases there is no apparent change on the skin.[9] Disease evolution takes place in a few years followed by stabilization.

- Linear limb morphea affects the limbs, causing muscle atrophy, limb length discrepancies, and joint contractures. In children, growth impairment may be present.

Pansclerotic morphea is the most disabling form of morphea which affects the subcutaneous tissue and deeper, often including the underlying bone **(Fig. 11)**. It results in significant morbidity due to severe muscle atrophy, joint contractures, and nonhealing ulcers. Patients of pansclerotic morphea with chronic nonhealing ulcers are at an increased risk of squamous cell carcinoma of the skin.

Mixed morphea: Combination of two or more of the previous subtypes would qualify as a mixed subtype.

Bullous morphea presents as tense subepidermal bullae that occur within affected sclerotic plaque that may lead to overlying erosions.

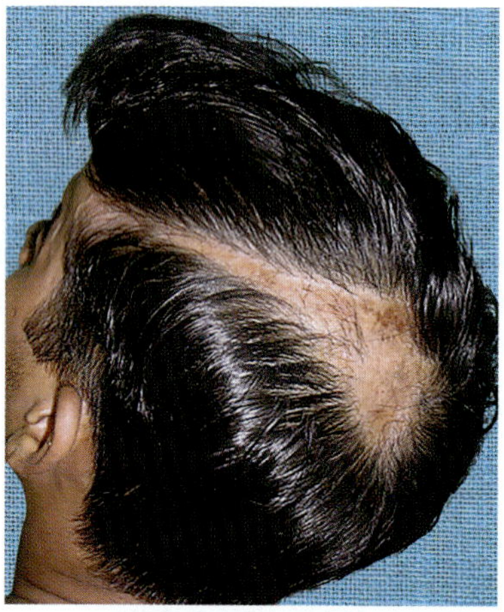

Fig. 9: En coup de sabre.

Atrophoderma of Pasini–Pierini: There are controversial opinions as to whether it represents a separate entity or is a superficial atrophic variant of morphea. It is a rare condition that usually occurs in young adults. The typical lesions are nonindurated, blue-gray to brown, hyperpigmented, and sharply demarcated depressed patches present symmetrically over the trunk and extremities, with a "cliff-drop" border.

Eosinophilic fasciitis or Shulman syndrome: It is characterized by acute or subacute pitting edema with erythema. The extremities are affected bilaterally symmetrically with exclusion of hands and feet. The edema is gradually replaced by a "peau d'orange" appearance as deep sclerosis gradually sets in. There are associated symptoms such as weight loss, myalgia, and asthenia.

Histology

The diagnosis of morphea is usually made clinically. Histologic examination aids in the therapeutic management as it helps to determine degree of inflammation and depth of involvement. Biopsy should be taken from the inflammatory border or sclerotic center including the subcutaneous fat.

In case of the early lesions, when the biopsy is taken from an inflamed border, it shows a perivascular and interstitial infiltrate of lymphocytes, plasma cells, and occasional eosinophils and focal panniculitis. The epidermis is normal with flattening of rete ridges. Endothelial swelling and edema is present in the blood vessel walls.

The biopsy from the sclerotic margin shows thickened and homogenized collagen bundles at the papillary and reticular dermis that enclose eccrine glands and few dermal vessels with fibrotic walls and narrow lumina. Appendages have a "pulled up appearance" **(Figs. 12A and B)** with the replacement of the subcutaneous tissue with collagen. In the late sclerotic stage, there is increased collagen with few visible blood vessels and the adnexal structures are progressively lost **(Fig. 12C)**.

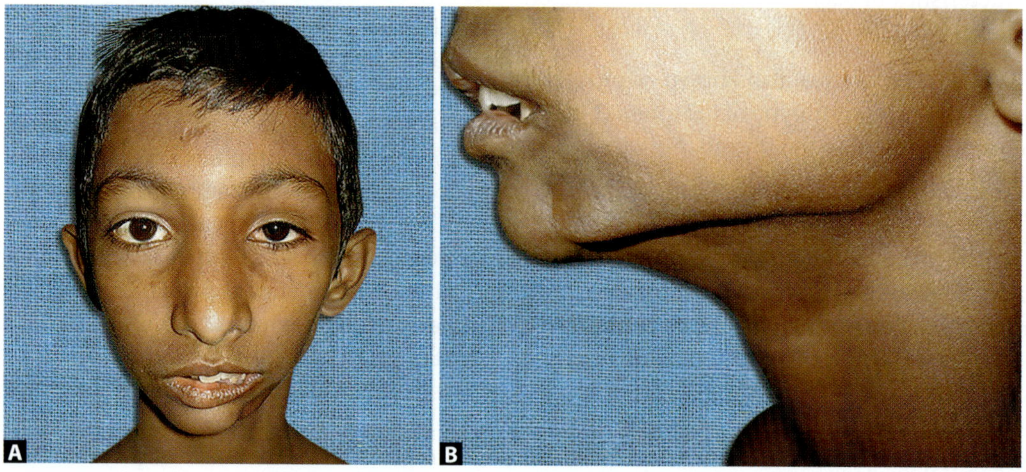

Figs. 10A and B: Parry–Romberg syndrome.

Laboratory Tests

Peripheral eosinophilia, hypergammaglobulinemia, and raised erythrocyte sedimentation rate/C-reactive protein (ESR/CRP) may occur with active disease.

Serum antibodies: The autoantibodies reported in morphea are ANAs, anti-single-stranded DNA, anti-double-stranded DNA, antihistone, antitopoisomerase II, antiphospholipid, anticentromere, anti-Scl-70, and rheumatoid factor. ANA occur in 39–80% of patients are more common in linear or generalized disease.[10] The clinical significance of these antibodies remain unclear and hence no testing of autoantibodies is recommended for diagnosis or for disease monitoring purposes.

Imaging: High-frequency ultrasonography evaluates tissue thickness, loss of subcutaneous fat, or other architectural changes.

Magnetic resonance imaging helps to assess the extent of disease including depth of involvement and disease activity and should be done when indicated and not as a routine.

Infrared thermography is another useful imaging modality.

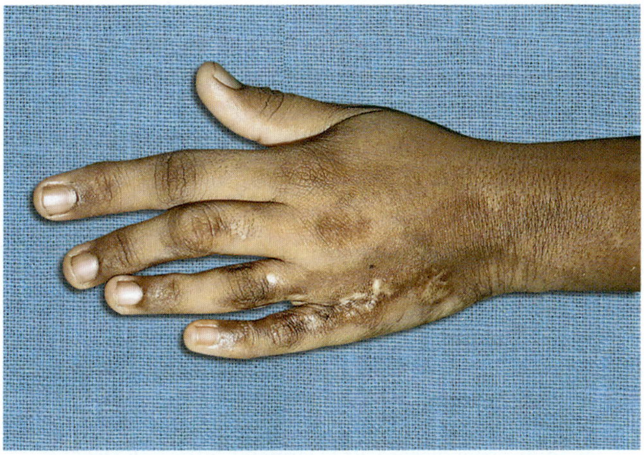

Fig. 11: Linear morphea causing bone deformity.

Complications

Complications of morphea are given in **Box 1**.

Differential Diagnosis

- Systemic sclerosis
- Lipodermatosclerosis
- Eosinophilic fasciitis
- Trauma-induced fat necrosis
- Nephrogenic systemic fibrosis
- Chronic graft versus host disease

Treatment

Considerations before starting treatment are the disease severity, disease activity, depth of involvement, and quality-of-life of the patient **(Table 2)**.

General Guidelines in Treatment of Morphea

In the active stage of the disease, the aim of treatment is stabilizing the size of the current lesions and preventing occurrence of new lesions. Anti-inflammatory and immunosuppressive agents are unlikely to improve burnt out phase of morphea and hence should not be used for the burnt out stage of the disease.

In cases of circumscribed superficial plaque type, morphea topical therapy should be the treatment of choice. Topical therapy includes topical corticosteroids alone or in combination with topical tacrolimus or topical vitamin D analogs under occlusion. Imiquimod and topical pirfenidone creams have been tried. In widespread superficial disease, phototherapy such as systemic and bath PUVA, UVA1 therapy, narrowband UVB therapy, and extracorporeal photochemotherapy should be considered or methotrexate should be tried. In cases of deep involvement, methotrexate should be the early consideration. If severe disease with rapid progression or with looming contractures, systemic corticosteroids are a valuable addition.

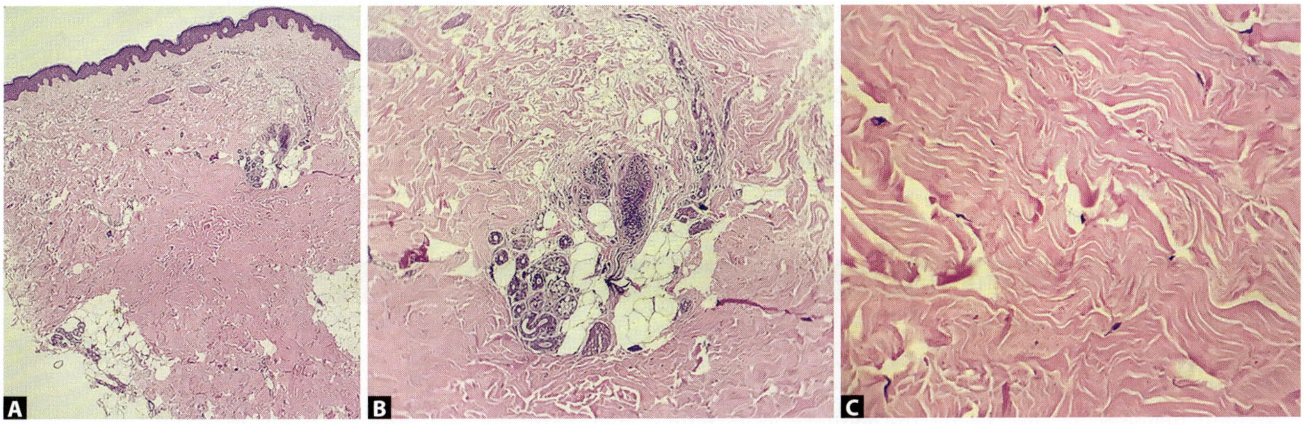

Figs. 12A to C: (A) Thickened and homogenized collagen bundles at the papillary and reticular dermis with few blood vessels and adnexal structures; (B) "Pulled up appearance" of the appendages with replacement of the subcutaneous tissue with collagen; and (C) Thickened and homogenized collagen present in the late sclerotic stage.

Courtesy: Dr Chirag Desai, Consultant Dermatologist, Divyasparsh Clinic, Mumbai, Maharashtra, India

BOX 1: Complications of morphea.

- Myalgia, arthralgia, and fatigue seen in generalized morphea
- Neurologic manifestations—seizures, headaches, peripheral neuropathy, vascular malformations, and CNS vasculitis seen in en coup de sabre or progressive hemifacial atrophy
- Ocular complications—sclerosis of adnexal structures, anterior segment inflammation, and anterior uveitis
- Eyelid lesions, exophthalmos, uveitis, episcleritis, xerophthalmia, papilledema, and glaucoma
- Squamous cell carcinoma—pansclerotic morphea has been associated with an increased risk due to chronic ulcers
- Compartment syndrome, bullae, and ulcers due to circumferential sclerosis

TABLE 2: Severity of morphea and its variants.

Severity of morphea	*Morphea variants*
Severe morphea	Pansclerotic
	Generalized
	Linear scleroderma of face
	Subtypes with high morbidity such as CNS involvement, extremity shortening, and joint contractures
Moderately severe morphea	Circumscribed deep morphea
	Linear scleroderma of trunk and feet
Low severity morphea	Superficial circumscribed morphea (plaque type)

(CNS: central nervous system)

KEY POINTS

Lichen sclerosus:

- Lichen sclerosus is a chronic inflammatory scarring mucocutaneous disorder with a lymphocytic response. Genital region is more commonly affected than extragenital region.
- In females, itching is the predominant symptom whereas in males it can be asymptomatic or present as phimosis. Typical findings are porcelain white shiny papules and plaques.
- Complications include malignancy, scarring, sensory disorders of genitalia, and psychosexual disorders.
- Treatment aims at reducing symptoms, decreasing chances of recurrences, and preventing scarring and malignant changes.

Morphea:

- It is a type of localized scleroderma which leads to thickening of the dermis and subcutaneous tissue. The variants include circumscribed, generalized, linear, deep, pansclerotic, bullous, or mixed types.
- It is characterized by sclerosis, fibrosis, atrophy in skin and subcutaneous tissue and sometimes extending to the muscle, bone, and brain.
- The diagnosis is usually clinical; however, histopathological evaluation helps in therapeutic management of the disease.
- In case of circumscribed superficial morphea, topical therapy is the treatment of choice and in case of widespread lesions or deeper involvement or impending complications, phototherapy or methotrexate can be used.

REFERENCES

1. Fistarol SK, Itin PH. Diagnosis and treatment of lichen sclerosus: an update. Am J Clin Dermatol. 2013;14:27-47.
2. Hofer MD, Meeks JJ, Mehdiratta N, Granieri MA, Cashy J, Gonzalez CM. Lichen sclerosus in men is associated with elevated body mass index, diabetes mellitus, coronary artery disease and smoking. World J Urol. 2014;32:105-8.
3. Bunker CB, Patel N, Shim TN. Urinary voiding symptomatology (micro-incontinence) in male genital lichen sclerosus. Acta Derm Venereol. 2013;93:246-8.
4. Al-Niaimi F, Lyon C. Peristomal lichen sclerosus: the role of occlusion and urine exposure? Br J Dermatol. 2013;168:643-6.
5. Lewis FM, Tatnall FM, Velangi SS, Bunker CB, Kumar A, Brackenbury F, et al. British Association of Dermatologists Guidelines for the Management of Lichen Sclerosus, 2018. Br J Dermatol. 2018;178(4):839-53.
6. Kirtschig G. Lichen sclerosus: presentation, diagnosis and management. Dtsch Arztebl Int. 2016;113:337-43.
7. Mertens JS, Seyger MM, Kievit W, Hoppenreijs EP, Jansen TL, van de Kerkhof PC, et al. Disease recurrence in localized scleroderma: a retrospective analysis of 344 patients with paediatric- or adult-onset disease. Br J Dermatol. 2015;172(3):722-8.
8. Mertens JS, Seyger MMB, Thurlings RM, Radstake TRDJ, de Jong EMGJ. Morphea and eosinophilic fasciitis: an update. Am J Clin Dermatol. 2017;18(4):491-512.
9. Tollefson MM, Witman PM. En coup de sabre morphea and Parry-Romberg syndrome: a retrospective review of 54 patients. J Am Acad Dermatol. 2007;56:257-63.
10. Falanga V, Medsger TA Jr, Reichlin M. Antinuclear and anti-single-stranded DNA antibodies in morphea and generalized morphea. Arch Dermatol. 1987;123:350-3.

EXAMINATION QUESTIONS

Write short notes on the following:

1. Histopathological features of morphea.
2. Management of morphea.
3. Explain lichen sclerosus. Discuss the genital manifestations, histopathological features, complications and management of lichen sclerosus.
4. Describe eosinophilic fasciitis.

54 CHAPTER

Sclerodermaand Other Sclerodermatous Skin Changes

Imran Majid, Sameena Batool

INTRODUCTION

The term scleroderma is an umbrella term that is used for any cutaneous condition causing binding down or "sclerosis" of the skin. The condition may or may not be associated with systemic involvement. When there is involvement of the internal organs along with sclerosis of skin, it is called systemic sclerosis. When there is localized sclerosis of skin with no internal organ involvement, it is called morphea (cutaneous or localized scleroderma).[1,2]

SYSTEMIC SCLEROSIS

It is an autoimmune disease, which causes sclerosis of the skin along with internal organ involvement. The disease has an early vascular and inflammatory component that manifests typically in the form of Raynaud's phenomenon. In addition to sclerosis, patients also show varying degrees of scarring or ulceration of fingertips, calcinosis, vascular abnormalities such as telangiectasias and even gangrenous changes at times. Pigmentary abnormality of diffuse hyperpigmentation and hypopigmentation may also be present, known as salt and pepper pigmentation. Internal organ manifestation can affect the gastrointestinal system, respiratory system, cardiovascular system, kidneys, and other organs.[3,4]

It has two main subtypes:

1. Limited systemic sclerosis
2. Diffuse systemic sclerosis

- In limited systemic sclerosis, the skin sclerosis is limited to extremities and face and there is low risk of organ-based complications. The autoantibody specific for this type is anticentromere antibody. The acronym CREST (calcinosis, Raynaud's phenomenon, esophageal dysfunction, sclerodactyly, and telangiectasia) syndrome is included in the subtype of limited systemic sclerosis.[5]
- In diffuse systemic sclerosis, the skin sclerosis extends to the trunk, proximal limbs, and face and there is a high risk of organ-based complications. The autoantibody specific for this type is antitopoisomerase antibody (ATA, Scl-70).[6]

Clinical Features

Clinical features of systemic sclerosis can be divided into cutaneous and extracutaneous manifestations **(Table 1)**.

Cutaneous Manifestations

One of the earliest features of systemic sclerosis is Raynaud's phenomenon. It is the change in the color of digits on exposure to cold. It may be triphasic meaning that it is whitish initially due to vasospasm, then changes to blue, and then red on rewarming and is often associated with pain. At times, it may be biphasic too without red or erythematous component. Patients with Raynaud's phenomenon are prone to complications such as fingertip ulcerations, fingertip scars, paronychia, and loss of pulp of fingers. In fact, disappearance of the conical contour of fingerpads is one of the earliest signs of scleroderma or systemic sclerosis as these fingerpads assume a hemispheric shape. This is also known as round finger pad (RFP) sign or Mizutani sign.[7] Long history of Raynaud's phenomenon is associated with limited systemic sclerosis **(Fig. 1)**.[8]

Cutaneous manifestations start with puffiness and nonpitting edema, which is first noticed in fingers and face. The skin over these areas is thickened indurated and tight leading to sclerodactyly.[9] Later, these patients develop the typical scleroderma facies which is basically an expressionless "mask"-like facies **(Fig. 2)**.

It is really difficult to retract the lower eyelid in established cases of systemic sclerosis. This inability of retracting the lower eyelid is known as "Ingram's sign" and this is seen in combination with beaking of the nose, prominent perioral

TABLE 1: Features of cutaneous and extracutaneous manifestations.

Cutaneous manifestations	*Extracutaneous manifestations*
• Raynaud's phenomenon • Tightening and binding down of skin over fingers, hands, feet, and face • Sclerodactyly • Digital pitted scars • Diffuse pigmentation of skin, especially on exposed parts • Telangiectasia • Fish-mouth appearance • Microstomia • Digital deformities and gangrene in late stages	• Dysphagia • Gastroesophageal reflux • Dyspnea and cough • Arrhythmias • Scleroderma renal crisis • Muscle weakness and myalgias

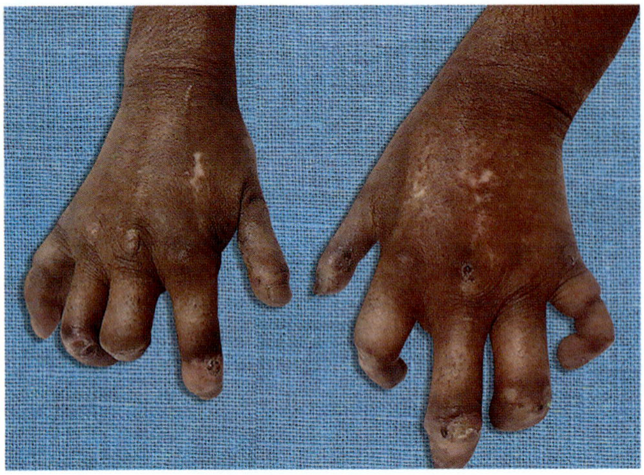

Fig. 1: Resorption of digits and digital ulcers in systemic sclerosis.
Courtesy: Dr Aarti Sarda.

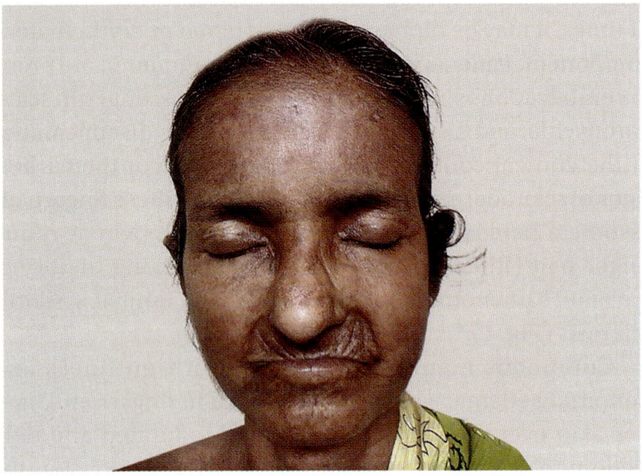

Fig. 2: Tightening of the skin and purse-string mouth in systemic sclerosis.
Courtesy: Dr Aarti Sarda.

wrinkling, and decreased oral aperture giving a fish-mouth appearance.

The degree of skin sclerosis can be assessed by a scoring system known as "modified Rodnan score."

Extracutaneous Manifestations

Gastrointestinal manifestations: The basic abnormality in systemic sclerosis is a motility disorder that has been attributed to reduced neuromuscular coordination. Due to this, there is dysphagia and symptoms of gastroesophageal reflux. Involvement of small intestine leads to features of pseudo-obstruction such as bloating, diarrhea, and malabsorption. Involvement of the large intestine leads to constipation.[10]

Cardiopulmonary manifestations: Interstitial lung disease, pulmonary fibrosis, and pulmonary artery hypertension (PAH) are the cardiopulmonary manifestations of systemic sclerosis. Cardiac myositis and interstitial fibrosis cause cardiomyopathy and arrhythmias. Interstitial lung disease and PAH are the major causes of deaths in systemic sclerosis.[11,12]

Renal manifestations: Scleroderma renal crisis is a complication of systemic sclerosis, which occurs in first few years of onset of the disease. Patients who have RNA polymerase 3 autoantibody positive are susceptible to renal crisis. Timely treatment with angiotensin-converting enzyme inhibitors has helped in combating the hypertensive renal crisis and has brought down the mortality rates associated with this disease.[13,14]

Musculoskeletal manifestations: Muscle involvement manifests in the form of mild muscle weakness, raised creatine kinase levels, and mild electromyographic changes. Due to the infiltration of the connective tissue that surrounds the tendon retinacula of the wrist elbow knees and ankle, there is thickening of these tendons. As a result, when the movement is done at these joints, there is a coarse cracking crepitus heard which is called tendon friction rubs. Their significance is that it is the indicator of the diffuse nature of the disease and it decreases the survival rate by 5–10%.[15,16]

Laboratory Investigations

Laboratory investigations of systemic sclerosis are given in **Table 2**.

Management

The management of this disease depends upon the extent of involvement of the skin and organs. The treatment is mainly aimed to slow down the progression of the disease and to prevent the complications associated with the disease.

General Management of the Common Morbidities

The treatment of the most common morbidities associated with systemic sclerosis is done symptomatically.

- Raynaud's phenomenon is treated by angiotensin receptor blockers (ARBs), calcium channel blockers (CCBs), selective serotonin reuptake inhibitors (SSRIs), and iloprost.
- Losartan in a dose of 25–50 mg/day is given in the class of ARBs. In the class of CCBs, nifedipine at a dose of

TABLE 2: Laboratory investigations of systemic sclerosis.

General baseline tests	*Specific tests*
• Complete hemogram • Kidney function test • Liver function test • Chest X-ray • Pulmonary function test • HRCT chest • Upper GI endoscopy • Electrocardiogram • Echocardiograph • Electromyography (in cases of muscle weakness)	ANA, anticentromere antibodies, antitopoisomerase antibodies, nailfold capillaroscopy, investigations to rule out other autoimmune rheumatic disease

(ANA: antinuclear antibody; GI: gastrointestinal; HRCT: high-resolution computed tomography)

10 mg thrice a day and diltiazem at a dose of 60 mg twice a day is given.

- In SSRIs, fluoxetine at a dose of 20 mg/day is given.
- Iloprost is given at a dose of 0.5–2 ng/kg/min for 3–5 days.
- Gastroesophageal reflux disease (GERD) is treated by proton-pump inhibitors such as omeprazole and lansoprazole or H_2 receptor blockers such as ranitidine 150–300 mg daily.
- Erectile dysfunction is another problem seen in men with systemic sclerosis. Phosphodiesterase-5 (PDE5) inhibitor, sildenafil is often given to treat the condition.
- For telangiectasia vascular, lasers such as pulsed dye laser or even intense pulse light (IPL) are used.
- Calcinosis is treated by excision or curettage.
- In hypertensive renal crisis, we have to avoid high-dose steroids. ARBs and ACE inhibitors are used to treat the condition. In additional antihypertensives, CCBs and α-blockers are used.[17] Intravenous iloprost is also used.
- In limited systemic sclerosis, treatment is directed at vascular complications.

Disease Modifying Agents

In diffuse or progressive skin sclerosis, methotrexate at a dose of 15–25 mg/week or mycophenolate mofetil at a dose of 2–3 g/day can be used.[18-20] If diffuse disease is associated with pulmonary involvement, a monthly dose of intravenous cyclophosphamide at a dose of 600 mg/m^2 for 6 months is given along with oral cyclophosphamide up to 2 mg/kg/day for 1 year in usual cases.

The treatment of systemic sclerosis is usually multimodal depending upon the extent of cutaneous and internal organ involvement. Progress is going on with clinical trials targeting newer drugs for this disease.

Treatment

Treatment of systemic sclerosis is given in **Table 3**.

TABLE 3: Treatment of systemic sclerosis.

Treatment of symptoms and signs	*Disease-modifying agents*
• Vasodilators • Ca-channel blockers • ARBs • Fluoxetine • Iloprost • Topical minoxidil • Proton-pump inhibitors • Sildenafil	• Immunosuppressants • Methotrexate • Mycophenolate mofetil • Cyclophosphamide • Steroid pulses • Hydroxychloroquine

(ARBs: angiotensin receptor blockers)

MORPHEA

It is also known as "cutaneous scleroderma" as in this variant, the disease process usually remains localized to the skin only. The cardinal features are sclerosis, atrophy, and fibrosis of the skin. In some rare cases, the disease process can also affect the underlying structures such as subcutaneous tissue, muscle, and bone. As compared to systemic sclerosis, there is no internal organ fibrosis and vascular changes.

Morphea is associated with significant morbidity and negative impact on quality of life.[21-24] Localized scleroderma is an umbrella term that has been used to describe various types of morphea such as limited type, generalized type, and linear and mixed variants.[25]

The subtypes of limited morphea are:

- Limited plaque morphea
- Guttate morphea
- Atrophoderma of Pasini and Pierini
- Keloidal morphea
- Limited deep morphea

The subtypes of generalized morphea are:

- Disseminated plaque morphea
- Pansclerotic morphea
- Eosinophilic fasciitis

The subtypes of linear variant are:

- Linear morphea
- Linear atrophoderma of Moulin
- Linear deep atrophic morphea
- Morphea en coup de sabre
- Progressive hemifacial atrophy

In addition to the above types, there is a mixed variant as well:
Morphea lichen sclerosus overlap: Morphea is often considered a self-limiting disease. As compared to systemic sclerosis, there are no internal organ-related complications such as pulmonary fibrosis, gastrointestinal tract fibrosis, pulmonary hypertension, and renal crisis in morphea. The systemic sclerosis-related autoantibodies are rarely raised and there is normal nailfold capillaroscopy study. Sclerodactyly is not seen in morphea.[26-28]

Morphea can be associated with other autoimmune conditions such as psoriasis, vitiligo, alopecia areata, autoimmune hepatitis, autoimmune thyroid disease, primary biliary cirrhosis, inflammatory bowel disease, rheumatoid arthritis, and mixed connective tissue disease.[29-31]

Clinical Features

Presentation: Onset of the disease is usually insidious. Morphea can start as skin discoloration associated with pruritus and pain. When the disease spreads across joints, it results in contractures and leads to limb asymmetry. Morphea begins with erythema, edema, and inflammation of the skin. After this phase, there is sclerosis of the skin, which results in the change in color and texture of the skin. The skin gets thickened and yellowish in color. Then in a span of months or years, these plaques become atrophic with hypo- or hyperpigmentation.[32,33] The severity of the disease is determined by the type of disease and extent of involvement of the subcutaneous tissues.

Clinical Features of the Individual Subtypes of Morphea

- *Limited plaque morphea*: This type of morphea is superficial and does not extend beyond dermis. The plaques are mostly seen over trunk and they are >1 cm in diameter in size and round to oval in shape.[34]
- *Guttate morphea*: The plaques in this type of morphea are <1 cm in diameter and they are also superficial plaques. The surface of the lesion gives shiny and crinkled appearance. These lesions heal with hyperpigmentation.[35]
- *Atrophoderma of Passini–Pierini*: This variant of morphea is still under consideration whether to include this as a subtype of morphea or an isolated entity. There are well-defined depressed plaques with a "cliff drop" border often with bluish-brown hyperpigmentation. It is also a superficial and atrophic variant of morphea.[36,37]
- *Keloidal/nodular morphea*: This is a rare subtype of morphea and it occurs as a keloid over a sclerodermatous skin. The lesions are most commonly seen on the trunk where they can coalesce to give a linear appearance. Sometimes, there can also be the occurrence of nodules over the normal skin and it usually occurs in patients predisposed to keloid formation.[38]
- *Limited deep morphea*: This is a variant of morphea in which the inflammation and sclerosis is deep down in the dermis affecting the muscle and the fat. There is a diagnostic criterion by Person and Su, which includes "presence of diffuse, taut, bound down, deep cutaneous sclerosis and significant hyalinization and thickening of collagen bundles in the deep dermis and in the septa of subcutaneous fat and fascia."[39,40]
- *Disseminated plaque morphea*: This type of morphea includes multiple plaques commonly over trunk and thighs. They are present symmetrically and multiple plaques can also coalesce. They are present over areas of frictions such as waistband, under the breast and groins. They are particularly seen in middle-aged women.[41,42]
- *Pansclerotic morphea*: It is a rare variant of morphea and is characterized by extensive and circumferential involvement of the body. It spares the areola fingers and toes. In children, there occurs deep fibrosis affecting the muscle fascia and bone, which is referred as disabling pansclerotic morphea of childhood.[43-46]
- *Eosinophilic fasciitis*: It is also known as Schulman syndrome. It affects the extremities, especially the lower limbs sparing the fingers and face. In the early stages, there is burning, pitting edema, and painful erythema of the affected area. This is followed by induration and fibrosis giving a typical peau d'orange appearance of the skin. There is also tethering around the blood vessels, which produce guttering known as groove sign. Sclerosis involves the fibrous septa of the subcutis and muscle and fascia.[47-49] Eosinophilia is common and C-reactive protein levels are raised.
- *Morphea en coup de sabre*: It usually occurs in childhood and involves the frontoparietal area of the face and scalp in paramedian distribution and follows Blaschko's lines. Sclerosis is initially superficial but later involves the fascia and bone.[50,51]
- *Progressive hemifacial atrophy*: This is also called Parry–Romberg syndrome. It affects the area supplied by one or more branches of trigeminal nerve. It begins in childhood and it is unilateral progressive atrophic disorder of the skin affecting the deeper structures muscle fascia and bone. Mouth and nose can be deviated to one side as a result of unilateral atrophy of the structures. Pigmentary abnormalities such as brownish hyperpigmentation or hypopigmentation can also occur over these areas. Typically, there are bruise-like changes over the skin; neurological and ocular complications in this disease often occur.[52-56]
- *Linear atrophoderma of Moulin*: Unilateral, hyperpigmented, and depressed plaques are present over trunk and limbs in this type of morphea.
- *Mixed types*: In this, there is often existence of more than one subtype of morphea.

Extracutaneous Manifestations in Morphea

- Arthralgias
- Dysphagia
- Raynaud's phenomenon
- Neurological complications, e.g., headache and seizures
- Peripheral neuropathy, central nervous system (CNS) vasculitis
- Dental problems, e.g., malocclusion
- Ocular complications, e.g., anterior uveitis, episcleritis, and keratitis.

Management of Morphea

Investigations

- Full blood count, serum antinuclear antibody (ANA), eosinophils, immunoglobulins, erythrocyte sedimentation rate (ESR) and C-reactive protein levels, and rheumatoid factor
- *Skin biopsy*: Deep incisional biopsy is taken to include the fascia and muscle if deep involvement is suspected
- Creatine kinase and aldolase levels are done to rule out the muscle involvement
- MRI and CT scans are done to image the brain and the linear lesions
- Borrelia serology
- Timely referral to concerned speciality units such as plastic surgery, orthopedics, ENT, and ophthalmology

TREATMENT

Limited and Superficial Disease

Treatment options include:

- Topical tacrolimus ointment 0.1% twice a day is used.
- Topical or intralesional steroids can also be used.
- Twice-daily application of vitamin D analogs that is calcipotriol alone or in combination with steroids has been used.
- Phototherapy such as narrowband ultraviolet B (NBUVB) and psoralen-ultraviolet A (PUVA) have been tried with varying results.

Disseminated Plaque Disease

Treatment options include:

- UVA1 phototherapy
- PUVA therapy
- NBUVB
- Broadband UVA
- Calcipotriol and low-dose UVA1

Pansclerotic, Linear or Deep Disease

Treatment options are:

- Methotrexate and intravenous corticosteroid pulses
- Methotrexate and oral corticosteroids
- Mycophenolate mofetil
- Combination therapies such as methotrexate mycophenolate and cyclosporine

Scleroderma Spectrum Disorders

These disorders are all those conditions that mimic scleroderma but are the result of some other causes. These are sometimes also known as "pseudoscleroderma".

The conditions are as follows:

- *Deposition disorders*: Amyloidosis, scleredema, scleromyxedema
- *Metabolic disorders*: Hypothyroidism, porphyria cutanea tarda, carcinoid syndrome, phenylketonuria
- *Genetic disorders*: Werner syndrome, progeria, acrogeria, GEMSS (glaucoma, lens ectopia, microspherophakia, stiffness of joints, short stature) syndrome, melorheostosis, poikilodermatous epidermolysis bullosa
- *Occupational causes*: Vinyl chloride disease, organic solvents, pesticides, epoxy resins, silicone
- *Chemically induced*: Eosinophilia myalgia syndrome occurs due to ingestion of L-tryptophan; toxic oil syndrome occurs due to ingestion of rapeseed oil contaminated with aniline
- *Drug induced*: Bleomycin, pentazocine, vitamin B_{12}, paclitaxel, bisoprolol, ibuprofen, D-penicillamine

The management of scleroderma should be aimed at arresting the active disease and improve the cosmetic appearance for the damage that has already occurred provided the disease is controlled and is inactive. We hope for the newer and better treatment options for this disease spectrum in future.

KEY POINTS

- The term scleroderma is used for any cutaneous condition causing binding down or "sclerosis" of the skin.
- When there is involvement of the internal organs along with sclerosis of skin, it is called systemic sclerosis.
- Systemic sclerosis is divided into two main types:
  1. Limited systemic sclerosis
  2. Diffuse systemic sclerosis
- Scleroderma limited to skin only is also known as morphea.
- Morphea has a number of morphological types but the most common type is plaque variant of morphea.
- Almost all the organ systems are involved in late systemic sclerosis but the three most important organ systems affected are the lungs, kidneys, and cardiovascular system.
- Treatment of systemic sclerosis is done on the basis of the presence and severity of specific organ system involvement.

REFERENCES

1. LeRoy EC, Black C, Fleischmajer R, Jablonska S, Krieg T, Medsger TA Jr, et al. Scleroderma (systemic sclerosis: classification, subsets and pathogenesis. J Rheumatol. 1988;15(2):202-5.
2. LeRoy EC, Medsger TA Jr. Criteria for the classification of early systemic sclerosis. J Rheumatol. 2001;28(7):1573-6.
3. Varga J. Systemic sclerosis: an update. Bull NYU Hosp Jt Dis. 2008;66(3):198-202.
4. Sticherling M. Systemic sclerosis—focus on dermatological aspects. Part 2: diagnostics, therapy. J Dtsch Dermatol Ges. 2012;10(11):783-91.
5. Pakozdi A, Nihtyanova S, Moinzadeh P, Ong VH, Black CM, Denton CP. Clinical and serological hallmarks of systemic sclerosis overlap syndromes. J Rheumatol. 2011;38(11):2406-9.
6. Walker JG, Fritzler MJ. Update on autoantibodies in systemic sclerosis. Curr Opin Rheumatol. 2007;19(6):580-91.
7. Steen V, Denton CP, Pope JE, Matucci-Cerinic M. Digital ulcers: overt vascular disease in systemic sclerosis. Rheumatology (Oxford). 2009;48 Suppl 3:iii19-24.
8. Pavlov-Dolijanovic S, Damjanov NS, Vujasinovic Stupar NZ, Radunovic GL, Stojanovic RM, Babic D. Late appearance and exacerbation of primary Raynaud's phenomenon attacks can predict future development of connective tissue disease: a retrospective chart review of 3,035 patients. Rheumatol Int. 2013;33(4):921-6.
9. Ferri C, Valentini G, Cozzi F, Sebastiani M, Michelassi C, La Montagna G, et al. Systemic sclerosis: demographic, clinical, and serologic features and survival in 1,012 Italian patients. Medicine (Baltimore). 2002;81(2):139-53.
10. Greydanus MP, Camilleri M. Abnormal postcibal antral and small bowel motility due to neuropathy or myopathy in systemic sclerosis. Gastroenterology. 1989;96(1):110-5.
11. Steen VD, Medsger TA. Changes in causes of death in systemic sclerosis, 1972–2002. Ann Rheum Dis. 2007;66(7):940-4.

12. Tyndall AJ, Bannert B, Vonk M, Airò P, Cozzi F, Carreira PE, et al. Causes and risk factors for death in systemic sclerosis: a study from the EULAR Scleroderma Trials and Research (EUSTAR) database. Ann Rheum Dis. 2010;69(10):1809-15.
13. Penn H, Howie AJ, Kingdon EJ, Bunn CC, Stratton RJ, Black CM, et al. Scleroderma renal crisis: patient characteristics and long-term outcomes. QJM. 2007;100(8):485-94.
14. Denton CP, Lapadula G, Mouthon L, Muller-Ladner U. Renal complications and scleroderma renal crisis. Rheumatology (Oxford). 2009;48(Suppl 3):iii32-5.
15. Dore A, Lucas M, Ivanco D, Medsger TA Jr, Domsic RT. Significance of palpable tendon friction rubs in early diffuse cutaneous systemic sclerosis. Arthritis Care Res. 2013;65(8): 1385-9.
16. Steen VD, Medsger TA Jr. The palpable tendon friction rub: an important physical examination finding in patients with systemic sclerosis. Arthritis Rheum. 1997;40(6):1146-51.
17. Steen VD. Kidney involvement in systemic sclerosis. Presse Med. 2014;43(10 Pt 2):e305-14.
18. Walker KM, Pope J, participating members of the Scleroderma Clinical Trials Consortium (SCTC), Canadian Scleroderma Research Group (CSRG). Treatment of systemic sclerosis complications: what to use when first-line treatment fails: a consensus of systemic sclerosis experts. Semin Arthritis Rheum. 2012;42(1):42-55.
19. Kowal-Bielecka O, Landewé R, Avouac J, Chwiesko S, Miniati I, Czirjak L, et al. EULAR recommendations for the treatment of systemic sclerosis: a report from the EULAR Scleroderma Trials and Research group (EUSTAR). Ann Rheum Dis. 2009; 68(5):620-8.
20. Frech TM, Shanmugam VK, Shah AA, Assassi S, Gordon JK, Hant FN, et al. Treatment of early diffuse systemic sclerosis skin disease. Clin Exp Rheumatol. 2013;31(2 Suppl. 76):166-71.
21. Fett N, Werth VP. Update on morphea: part I. Epidemiology, clinical presentation, and pathogenesis. J Am Acad Dermatol. 2011;64(2):217-28; quiz 29-30.
22. Fett N, Werth VP. Update on morphea: part II. Outcome measures and treatment. J Am Acad Dermatol. 2011;64(2):231-42; quiz 43-4.
23. Fett N. Scleroderma: nomenclature, etiology, pathogenesis, prognosis, and treatments: facts and controversies. Clin Dermatol. 2013;31(4):432-7.
24. Kreuter A. Localized scleroderma. Dermatol Ther. 2012;25(2): 135-47.
25. Kreuter A, Krieg T, Worm M, Wenzel J, Gambichler T, Kuhn A, et al. AWMF Guideline no. 013/066. Diagnosis and therapy of circumscribed scleroderma. J Dtsch Dermatol Ges. 2009;7(Suppl. 6):S1-14.
26. Marzano AV, Menni S, Parodi A, Borghi A, Fuligni A, Fabbri P, et al. Localized scleroderma in adults and children. Clinical and laboratory investigations on 239 cases. Eur J Dermatol. 2003;13(2):171-6.
27. Piram M, McCuaig CC, Saint-Cyr C, Marcoux D, Hatami A, Haddad E, et al. Short- and long-term outcome of linear morphoea in children. Br J Dermatol. 2013;169(6):1265-71.
28. Saxton-Daniels S, Jacobe HT. An evaluation of long-term outcomes in adults with pediatric-onset morphea. Arch Dermatol. 2010;146(9):1044-05.
29. Leitenberger JJ, Cayce RL, Haley RW, Adams-Huet B, Bergstresser PR, Jacobe HT. Distinct autoimmune syndromes in morphea: a review of 245 adult and pediatric cases. Arch Dermatol. 2009;145:545-50.
30. Zulian F, Vallongo C, Woo P, Russo R, Ruperto N, Harper J, et al. Localized scleroderma in childhood is not just a skin disease. Arthritis Rheum. 2005;52(9):2873-81.
31. Harrington CI, Dunsmore IR. An investigation into the incidence of auto-immune disorders in patients with localized morphoea. Br J Dermatol. 1989;120(5):645-8.
32. Zulian F, Athreya BH, Laxer R, Nelson AM, Feitosa de Oliveira SK, Punaro MG, et al. Juvenile localized scleroderma: clinical and epidemiological features in 750 children. An international study. Rheumatology. 2006;45:614-20.
33. Herrick AL, Ennis H, Bhushan M, Silman AJ, Baildam EM. Clinical features of childhood localized scleroderma in an incidence cohort. Rheumatology. 2011;50(10):1865-8.
34. Peterson LS, Nelson AM, Su WP. Classification of morphea (localized scleroderma). Mayo Clinic Proc. 1995;70(11):1068-76.
35. Tuffanelli DL. Localized scleroderma. Semin Cutan Med Surg. 1998;17(1):27-33.
36. Kencka D, Blaszczyk M, Jablonska S. Atrophoderma Pasini-Pierini is a primary atrophic abortive morphea. Dermatology. 1995;190(3):203-6.
37. Canizares O, Sachs PM, Jaimovich L, Torres VM. Idiopathic atrophoderma of Pasini and Pierini. AMA Arch Dermatol. 1958;77(1):42-58; discussion 60.
38. Rencic A, Brinster N, Nousari CH. Keloid morphea and nodular scleroderma: two distinct clinical variants of scleroderma? J Cutan Med Surg. 2003;7(1):20-4.
39. Su WP, Person JR. Morphea profunda: a new concept and a histopathologic study of 23 cases. Am J Dermatopathol. 1981;3(3):251-60.
40. Person JR, Su WP. Subcutaneous morphoea: a clinical study of sixteen cases. Br J Dermatol. 1979;100(4):371-80.
41. Grabell D, Hsieh C, Andrew R, Martires K, Kim A, Vasquez R, et al. The role of skin trauma in the distribution of morphea lesions: a cross-sectional survey of the Morphea in Adults and Children cohort IV. J Am Acad Dermatol. 2014;71(3): 493-8.
42. Ahn JG, Kim YT, Lee CW. Trauma-induced isomorphic lesions in morphea—a brief case report. J Korean Med Sci. 1995;10(2):152-4.
43. Wollina U, Buslau M, Heinig B, Petrov I, Unger E, Kyriopoulou E, et al. Disabling pansclerotic morphea of childhood poses a high risk of chronic ulceration of the skin and squamous cell carcinoma. Int J Low Extrem Wounds. 2007;6(4):291-8.
44. Parodi PC, Riberti C, Draganic Stinco D, Patrone P, Stinco G. Squamous cell carcinoma arising in a patient with long-standing pansclerotic morphea. Br J Dermatol. 2001;144(2): 417-9.
45. Wollina U, Buslau M, Weyers W. Squamous cell carcinoma in pansclerotic morphea of childhood. Pediatr Dermatol. 2002;19(2):151-4.
46. Petrov I, Gantcheva M, Miteva L, Vassileva S, Pramatarov K. Lower lip squamous cell carcinoma in disabling pansclerotic morphea of childhood. Pediatr Dermatol. 2009;26(1):59-61.
47. Lakhanpal S, Ginsburg WW, Michet CJ, Doyle JA, Moore SB. Eosinophilic fasciitis: clinical spectrum and therapeutic response in 52 cases. Semin Arthritis Rheum. 1988;17(4):221-31.
48. Barnes L, Rodnan GP, Medsger TA, Short D. Eosinophilic fasciitis. A pathologic study of twenty cases. Am J Pathol. 1979; 96(2):493-518.
49. Michet CJ Jr, Doyle JA, Ginsburg WW. Eosinophilic fasciitis: report of 15 cases. Mayo Clin Proc. 1981;56(1):27-34.
50. Weibel L, Harper JI. Linear morphoea follows Blaschko's lines. Br J Dermatol. 2008;159(1):175-81.

51. Soma Y, Fujimoto M. Frontoparietal scleroderma (en coup de sabre) following Blaschko's lines. J Am Acad Dermatol. 1998;38(2 Pt 2):366-8.
52. Tollefson MM, Witman PM. En coup de sabre morphea and Parry-Romberg syndrome: a retrospective review of 54 patients. J Am Acad Dermatol. 2007;56(2):257-63.
53. Sommer A, Gambichler T, Bacharach-Buhles M, von Rothenburg T, Altmeyer P, Kreuter A. Clinical and serological characteristics of progressive facial hemiatrophy: a case series of 12 patients. J Am Acad Dermatol. 2006;54(2):227-33.
54. Blaszczyk M, Krolicki L, Krasu M, Glinska O, Jablonska S. Progressive facial hemiatrophy: central nervous system involvement and relationship with scleroderma en coup de sabre. J Rheumatol. 2003;30(9):1997-2004.
55. Blaszczyk M, Jablonska S. Linear scleroderma en coup de sabre. Relationship with progressive facial hemiatrophy (PFH). Adv Exp Med Biol. 1999;455:101-4.
56. El-Kehdy J, Abbas O, Rubeiz N. A review of Parry-Romberg syndrome. J Am Acad Dermatol. 2012;67(4):769-84.

EXAMINATION QUESTIONS

1. How do we classify scleroderma? Describe the clinical presentation of different types.
2. What is the etiopathogenesis of scleroderma? Explain in detail.
3. How do we manage scleroderma?
4. What are the recent advances in the treatment of scleroderma?

55 CHAPTER Dermatomyositis

Arghyaprasun Ghosh

INTRODUCTION

Dermatomyositis (DM) is a rare connective tissue disorder classified under the idiopathic inflammatory myopathies/dermatomyopathies (IIMs/IIDMs—there is no conclusive consensus between these two terms). The term dermatomyositis was coined by Unverricht in 1891.[1] In its classic form DM presents with proximal extensor muscle weakness with a confluent macular violaceous erythematous rash which is characteristic in its morphology and distribution. It has both adult onset and juvenile onset forms with 18 years being the cut off. The adult onset disease has chances of associated internal malignancy and interstitial lung disease (ILD) while the juvenile onset form has increased chances of vasculopathy/vasculitis with consequent dystrophic calcinosis cutis.[2] There is a distinct subset of patients who present with classical skin changes of DM without any muscle involvement that are termed to be suffering from clinically amyopathic dermatomyositis (CADM) or have muscle disease detected only on muscle specific tests that are termed hypomyopathic dermatomyositis (HDM). In contrast, there is no skin involvement in polymyositis (PM).

CLASSIFICATION OF IDIOPATHIC INFLAMMATORY MYOPATHIES/IDIOPATHIC INFLAMMATORY DERMATOMYOPATHIES

- *Dermatomyositis*:
  - *Adult onset* (18 years or older):
    - Classic DM
      - Classic DM alone
      - Classic DM associated with malignancy
      - Classic DM as part of overlap connective tissue disorder
    - Clinically amyopathic dermatomyositis
      - Amyopathic DM
      - Hypomyopathic DM
  - *Juvenile onset:*
    - Classic DM
    - *CADM*:
      - Amyopathic DM
      - Hypomyopathic DM
- *Polymyositis*:
  - Isolated PM
  - PM as part of overlap connective tissue disorder
  - PM associated with? malignancy
- *Inclusion body myositis*

Adapted from Fitzpatrick's Dermatology in General Medicine, 8th edition.

The modified Bohan and Peter (1975) classification for PM and DM is depicted in **Table 1**.[3]

The latest classification criteria for PM and DM were put forward by Tanimoto K et al. in 1995 which is depicted in **Box 1**.[4]

EPIDEMIOLOGY

Onset of classic DM most commonly occurs between 40 and 60 years of age with a female preponderance (F:M = 2:1). In children, the disease is five times more common in girls.[3] It is rarely reported in infants. The onset of DM associated with malignancy depends on the latter although either can precede the onset of the other.

ETIOLOGY AND PATHOGENESIS

The probable triggering factors for DM are shown in **Table 2**.

TABLE 1: Bohan and Peter classification for PM and DM.

Features	*Polymyositis (PM)*	*Dermatomyositis (DM)*
Symmetric proximal muscle weakness	*Definite:* All of 1–4 *Probable:* Any three of 1–4 *Possible:* Any two of 1–4	*Definite:* 5 plus any three of 1–4 *Probable:* 5 plus any two of 1–4 *Possible:* 5 plus any one of 1–4
Muscle biopsy evidence of myositis		
Elevation of serum skeletal muscle enzymes		
Characteristic electromyographic pattern of myositis		
Typical rash of dermatomyositis		

BOX 1: Classification criteria for polymyositis and dermatomyositis.

1. *Skin lesions:*
   - *Heliotrope rash:* Violaceous edematous erythema on the upper palpebra
   - *Gottron's sign:* Violaceous keratotic, atrophic erythema or macules on the extensor surface of finger joints. Violaceous erythema on the extensor surface of extremity joints, slight raised violaceous erythema over extensors of elbows and knees
2. Proximal muscle weakness (upper or lower extremity and trunk)
3. Elevated serum creatine kinase or aldolase level
4. Muscle pain on grasping or spontaneous pain
5. Myogenic changes on electromyography
6. Positive anti-Jo-1 antibody test (histidyl-tRNA synthetase)
7. Nondestructive arthritis or arthralgias
8. Systemic inflammatory signs (temperature >37°C at axilla, raised CRP, ESR >20 mm/h)
9. Pathologic findings compatible with inflammatory myositis
   - *Dermatomyositis*: At least one finding from serial number 1+ four findings from serial numbers 2 through 9
   - *Polymyositis*: At least four findings from serial numbers 2 through 9

(CRP: C-reactive protein; ESR: erythrocyte sedimentation rate)

TABLE 2: Probable triggering factors of dermatomyositis (DM).

Infections (supported by seasonal variation)	• Coxsackievirus • Parvovirus B19 • Picornavirus • EB virus	• HIV • HTLV-1 • Echovirus	• Toxoplasmosis • Staphylococci • Streptococci • *Escherichia coli*
UV rays			
Drugs	• Hydroxyurea (≥2 years) • Penicillamine • NSAIDs (diclofenac sodium) • Statins		• Phenytoin • Alfuzosin • Tamoxifen • Practolol
Malignancy (only adults)	• Ovarian Ca (most common in females) • Breast Ca • Colonic Ca • Nasopharyngeal Ca • Lung Ca		• Gastric Ca • Pancreatic Ca • Melanoma • Mycosis fungoides • Kaposi's sarcoma
Preceding heavy muscular exercise			

(Ca: cancer; EB: Epstein-Barr; NSAIDs: nonsteroidal anti-inflammatory drugs; UV: ultraviolet)

There is a strong genetic predisposition supported by its occurrence in monozygotic twins[5] and family members of DM/PM patients showing antinuclear antibody (ANA) positivity.[3] Increased human leukocyte antigen (HLA)-DR3 and B8 association is seen in white children whereas HLA-DR3 is seen in adults.[3,5] HLA-B14 and B40 are seen in adults with DM overlap.[5]

The pathogenesis of DM progresses through four stages starting with the susceptibility phase in genetically predisposed individuals with HLA linkages. In the induction phase there is a loss of self-tolerance under the influence of UV light and/or infections. This is followed by the expansion phase where there is autoreactive T-cell expansion and autoantibody formation. This culminates in the injury phase mediated by autoantibody binding, complement fixation, cytotoxic T-cell and cytokine production leading to microvascular injury, dropouts and ischemia, clinical disease, weakness, and fatigue.[2]

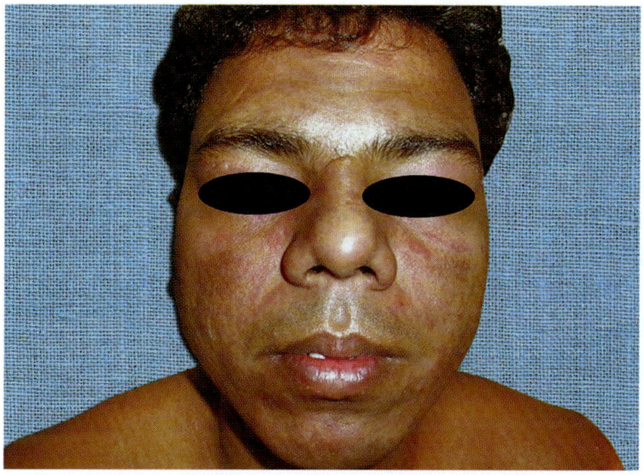

Fig. 1: Heliotrope rash with periorbital swelling.

The Th-1 cellular response causes the epidermal-dermal interface changes seen on histopathology.[2,5] The role of humoral immunity in addition is supported by the association of DM with other autoimmune diseases and the presence of specific antibodies. In contrast, only cell-mediated immunity (CMI) seems to play a role in the pathogenesis of PM.[3]

Myositis or skin-related antigens expressed by malignant tumors probably trigger an autoimmune response in DM/CADM.

CLINICAL FEATURES

The classical presentation of DM is a symmetric violaceous confluent macular erythema presenting over eyelids (heliotrope rash resembling heliotrope flower), forehead, cheeks, temples, extensors of limbs, and knuckles with or without periorbital edema and symmetric proximal extensor muscle weakness manifested as inability to comb hair or rise from a squatting position (**Fig. 1**).[2,3,5] In 60% of cases, onset of skin lesions and muscle weakness occur together; in 30% skin lesions, skin lesions precede muscle weakness, and in 10% cases, it is the opposite. A similar kind of rash can occur symmetrically over the extensor aspects of the inter-/metacarpo-phalangeal joints, olecranon processes, patellae, medial malleoli (Gottron's sign); over the dorsal aspects of fingers, hands, forearms, arms, neck, and back of shoulders (shawl sign); over the V area of neck and upper chest (V sign); and over the lateral aspects of hips and thighs (Holster sign).[2] These lesions are often associated with pruritus.[5]

The highly characteristic Gottron's papules over the dorsolateral aspect of interphalangeal and/or metacarpo-phalangeal joints, nailfolds, dorsa of toes, extensors of knees, and elbows present as skin colored or violaceous papules with mild atrophy at the center (**Fig. 2**). Mild scaling with telangiectasia may be seen.[2,3] Similar lesions over the finger creases are called inverse Gottron's papules.[3]

The violaceous hue in DM is both due to upper dermal edema pushing the dermal vessels deeper (Tyndall effect) and flow of deoxygenated blood through the abnormal vasculature. The shiny skin, in addition, is due to the dermal mucin deposit.[2]

Dermatomyositis patients can present with poikiloderma atrophicans vasculare similar to the one seen in cutaneous T-cell lymphoma (CTCL).

Dystrophic calcification in deep fascia or muscle, especially in juvenile dermatomyositis (JDM), can follow trauma or vasculopathy and panniculitis (**Fig. 3**). This is more common, if DM is associated with overlapping systemic sclerosis (sclerodermatomyositis). In DM, the calcification is seen throughout the muscle and soft tissue on X-ray. Calcinosis is a good prognostic sign for survival but functional disability is more.

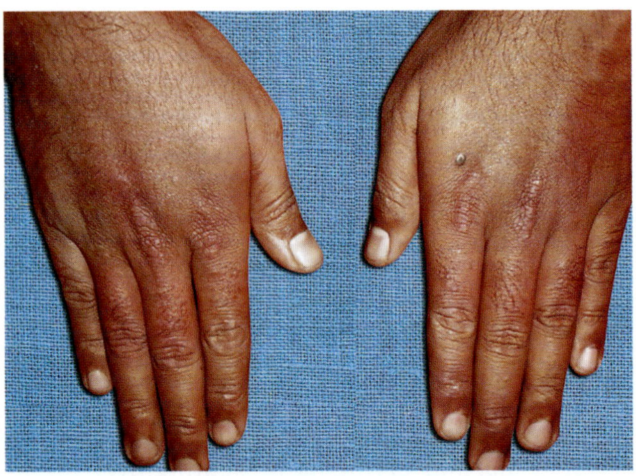

Fig. 2: Gottron's papules in linear streaks over dorsum of fingers extending on to hands.

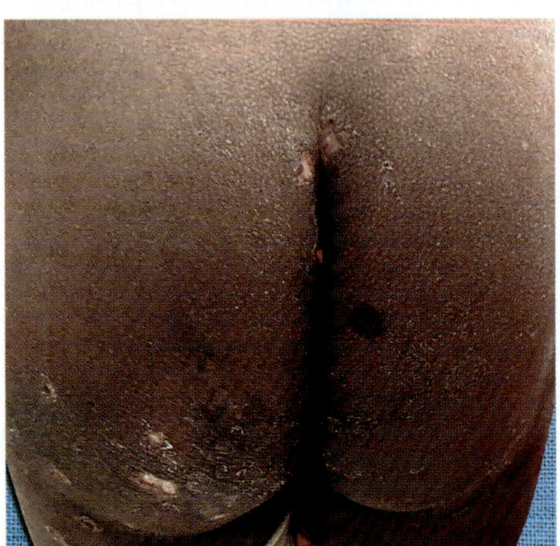

Fig. 3: Dystrophic calcification leading to ulcers over gluteal region of a child.

Dilated tortuous capillaries are seen over nail folds which look red and shiny. Ragged cuticles are also seen. Capillary changes are more marked in patients with the antisynthetase syndrome (Raynaud's phenomenon, nonerosive polyarthritis, ILD/pulmonary involvement, mechanic's hand, presence of antibodies to histidyl-tRNA synthetase or Jo-1, PL-7 and PL-12 occurring in both classic DM and CADM).[2,3] Improvement of periungual telangiectasia is a favorable sign for remission of disease.[2] Mechanic's hand presents with hyperkeratosis, fissuring, and linear hyperpigmentation over ulnar aspect of thumb and radial aspect and palmer surface of other fingers. A characteristic presentation, although rare, is the typical rash of DM occurring as linear streaks over the dorsum of fingers extending onto that of hands. Punched-out vasculopathic ulcers associated with anti-MDA5 antibodies (abs) are rarely seen over the extensor aspects of the interphalangeal and metacarpophalangeal joints, elbows, and knees.[3] Several centimeters long and a centimeter broad flagellate erythema are seen over the trunk and proximal limbs assuming a crisscross pattern. This is a rare presentation often associated with a rapidly progressing dyspnea and hypoxemia within a month of onset of ILD which is resistant to treatment.[2,3]

Less common changes encountered are bullous lesions, erythroderma, hypertrichosis, erythema over scalp with nonscarring alopecia, and PRP-like follicular keratosis (Wong-type DM) besides others.[3,6]

Besides the weakness and pain in the proximal extensor muscles of the limbs there may be tenderness and later atrophy. Depending on the involvement of various other muscles it might lead to difficulty in speech and swallowing, drooping of eyelids, respiratory difficulty, and even heart failure. Other systemic features include interstitial pneumonitis, cough and dyspnea, pulmonary hypertension with cor pulmonale, myocarditis, myocardial fibrosis, and conduction defects. The traditional muscle testing and grades from 0 to 5 has been replaced by International Myositis Assessment and Clinical Studies (IMACS) group 0 to 10 scale grading for all IIMs.[3]

Dermatomyositis/clinically amyopathic dermatomyositis and internal malignancy: The incidence of associated malignancy varies widely from <10 to >50% of adults with DM/CADM,[5] but is said to be between 15 and 34%.[3] DM precedes onset of malignancy in 40%, occurs together in 26%, and appears later in 34% of cases.[3] Risk of malignancy arises with older age; severe skin disease with erythema, necrosis, ulceration, and vesiculobullous lesions; dysphagia; diaphragmatic weakness; lack of extramuscular systemic features such as ILD; elevated creatine kinase (CK) levels; and antibodies to transcription intermediary factor-1γ (anti-TIF-1γ) or nuclear matrix protein 2 (anti-NXP-2).[2,3] Patients with DM/CADM with concurrent malignancy have sudden onset of severe cutaneous disease mostly over exposed parts mimicking other pruritic dermatoses. They are less responsive to therapy but skin lesions improve with treatment of malignancy. Features of internal malignancy should be sought every 3–6 months for at least 3 years from onset of DM/CADM.

Juvenile dermatomyositis/clinically amyopathic dermatomyositis: Dermatomyositis/clinically amyopathic dermatomyositis in children occurs due to microchimerism. Although the clinical features resemble that in adults the association with malignancy is almost not seen. Calcinosis is more common (>40%) and usually follows vasculopathy. The areas of vasculopathy can ulcerate. Systemic vasculopathy can lead to gastrointestinal (GI) ulceration and perforation, ocular, and central nervous system (CNS) manifestations in addition to cutaneous features.[2,3] Sclerodermatomyositis can occur in children. Acquired partial lipodystrophy is seen in 10% of cases and is associated with insulin-resistant type 2 diabetes and acanthosis nigricans.[3] Gingival telangiectasia is seen exclusively in children.

Dermatomyositis/clinically amyopathic dermatomyositis and pregnancy: Onset of DM may occur in pregnancy. The overall fetal loss is 50%. The outcome is worse during the first trimester. Premature birth occurs in considerable number of cases. Conversely, pregnancy exacerbates DM in 50% of cases and hence should be planned during remission. There is postpartum worsening of DM as is seen with all other autoimmune diseases.[2,3]

DIFFERENTIAL DIAGNOSIS

It depends on the clinical presentation and the presence or absence of myopathy. It is mostly confused with systemic lupus erythematosus (SLE) (violaceous erythema not seen) and overlap autoimmune connective tissue disorders and mixed connective tissue disease (MCTD), and various dermatitis including the photoaggravated ones and neuropathies.

HISTOPATHOLOGY

There are no telltale signs of DM on histology of the skin. There is a lichenoid tissue reaction pattern with sparse perivascular lymphocytic infiltrate. Epidermal atrophy with basal vacuolar degeneration mimics LE. Upper dermal edema with mucin deposition is more pronounced in DM. Poikilodermatous changes reflect with melanin incontinence and dilatation of superficial blood vessels. Calcinosis may be seen. There will be hyperkeratosis, in addition, in case of Gottron's papules. Vascular deposits of complement components C5b-9 are found in DM in contrast to LE.[6] Muscle biopsy from affected muscle or triceps reveals loss of transverse striations, hyalinization of sarcoplasm, and increase in sarcolemmal nuclei. The fibers fragment in later stages.[3]

INVESTIGATIONS

Routine blood tests are done both for monitoring disease and therapy. Raised erythrocyte sedimentation rate (ESR) with signs of cutaneous necrosis is a marker of internal malignancy.[3] Serum creatine phosphokinase (CPK/CK) level is the most sensitive and specific marker of muscle involvement and is most often raised in classic DM (CK levels are normal in steroid-induced myopathy). CK levels vary widely in case of malignancy associated DM. A less sensitive marker serum aldolase level may be raised in spite of normal CK levels, especially in JDM. The serological tests and their clinical significance are depicted in **Table 3**.[2,3,5]

TABLE 3: Serological tests and their clinical significance.

Antibodies	*Clinical significance*	*Remarks*
ANA		Will be negative when antisynthetase antibodies against cytoplasmic antigens are present
Anti-dsDNA		Negative. To rule out LE
Anti-histidyl-tRNA synthetase (Jo-1)	ILD	• PM—30%, overlap—15% • Treatment resistant
Anti-aminoacyl-tRNA synthetase	Myositis associated	
Anti-PM-Scl	Myositis associated	Overlap 10%
Anti-U_1RNP	Myositis associated	Overlap 30–40%
Anti-M_i 2	• Classic skin changes of DM • Myositis specific	DM 10–15%. Most specific
Anti-TIF-1γ	Severe skin disease. Highly specific for DM/CADM	Risk for internal malignancy
Anti-NXP-2 (nuclear matrix protein)	Associated with calcinosis in JDM	
Anti-SRP (signal recognition particle)	Skin lesions rare. Cardiac involvement	Treatment resistant
Anti-MDA5	Punched-out vasculopathic ulcers	

(ANA: antinuclear antibody; CADM: clinically amyopathic dermatomyositis; DM: dermatomyositis; ILD: interstitial lung disease; JDM: juvenile dermatomyositis; LE: lupus erythematosus; TIF-1γ: transcriptional intermediary factor-1γ; MDA5 = anti-melanoma differentiation-associated gene 5)

- Serial estimation of 24-hour urinary creatinine levels is helpful to monitor myopathy.
- Clinical examination of breast, pelvis, and rectum along with chest X-ray, USG of abdomen, stool for occult blood test (OBT), prostate-specific antigen (PSA), carcinoembryonic antigen (CEA), and CT scan of neck, thorax, abdomen, and pelvis are done in all adults to rule out internal malignancy.[3]
- Pulmonary function test is done if pulmonary involvement (ILD) is suspected.
- Electromyography (EMG) (sensitive in >90%), USG, and MRI of muscles are done as noninvasive techniques to rule out HDM along with muscle enzyme levels.
- ECG/echocardiography is done to detect cardiac defects.

Prognosis: Prognosis of DM/CADM is depicted in **Table 4**.

Patients with antisynthetase syndrome, cardiac involvement, and internal malignancy are treatment resistant.[2]

TREATMENT

Advise rest in the acute phase. Passive exercises are recommended in early active disease while active physiotherapy is advised during remission. Physical methods of sun protection along with sunscreens are advised. Emollients along with intermittent topical corticosteroids and tacrolimus are prescribed for skin disease. Poikiloderma can be treated with pulsed dye laser. Pruritus is somewhat controlled by sedating antihistamines. The medications used in the treatment of DM are summarized in **Table 5**.

TABLE 4: Prognosis of DM/CADM.

Children	Better prognosis. Death due to systemic vasculopathy, widespread dystrophic calcification and prolonged immunosuppressive-induced complications
Adults	Pulmonary and cardiac complications and respiratory infection most common causes of death. Malignancy-associated worse prognosis. Antisynthetase antibody—risk factor for chronicity and ILD. Mechanic's hand—risk factor for ILD. Ulcerative/necrotic lesions—associated with malignancy

(DM/CADM: dermatomyositis/clinically amyopathic dermatomyositis; ILD: interstitial lung disease)

TABLE 5: Medications used in the treatment of dermatomyositis (DM).

Mechanism of action	*Name of drugs*	*Dosage*
Immunosuppressant and immunomodulators	*Disease limited to skin:* • Hydroxychloroquine	6 mg/kg/day
	• Chloroquine	3.5 mg/kg/day
	Myopathy: • Prednisolone	*Adults*: 1–1.5 mg/kg/day *Children*: 1–2 mg/kg/day Taper slowly over 2–3 years
	• Methotrexate	7.5–25 mg/week
	• Azathioprine	1.5–3 mg/kg/day (especially for lung disease)
	• Cyclosporine	*Adults*: 5 mg/kg/day *Children*: 2.5–7.5 mg/kg/day
	• Cyclophosphamide	100 mg/day (lung disease)
	• Methylprednisolone	1 g IV × 3 days/month till response
	• IVIg	1 mg/kg × 2 days/month × 4–6 months
	• Dapsone	100 mg/day (after G6PD estimation)
	• Infliximab	5 mg/kg infusion at weeks 0, 2, 6, 14[7]
Tumor necrosis factor-α (TNF-α) inhibitors (in some subsets of refractory disease)	Etanercept	50 mg SC weekly × 52 weeks[8]
Anti-CD20+ B-cells (off-label use; validated criteria lacking)	Rituximab	(575–750 mg)/m^2 BSA at weeks 0 and 1[9]
Miscellaneous	Plasma exchange and extracorporeal photochemotherapy	Resistant cases
	Aspirin	Prevent platelet thrombosis
	Calcium supplements (with prednisolone) Diltiazem, bisphosphonates, aluminum oxide, ESWL (electric shock wave lithotripsy), surgical excision	In dystrophic calcinosis cutis

(BSA: body surface area; G6PD: glucose-6-phosphate dehydrogenase; IVIg: intravenous immunoglobulin)

If the disease is limited to the skin hydroxychloroquine (6 mg/kg/day) or chloroquine (3.5 mg/kg/day) can be prescribed in divided doses with ophthalmological checkups. Dapsone (100 mg/day) is sometimes effective.

For myopathy or systemic disease the patient is started with prednisolone (adults: 1–1.5 mg/kg/day; children: 1–2 mg/kg/day) for at least 1–3 months and then tapered to 50% of the dosage over a period of 6 months and to zero over 2–3 years. On the contrary, if the patient on prednisolone does not show any improvement after 2 months of commencement or is partially effective or there is worsening of myopathy, then alternatives such as methotrexate (7.5–25 mg/week), azathioprine (1.5–3 mg/kg/day, especially for pulmonary disease), cyclosporine (adults: 5 mg/kg/day; children: 2.5–7.5 mg/kg/day), and cyclophosphamide (100 mg/day—pulmonary disease) are used. Some centers use methylprednisolone (1 g IV on 2–3 consecutive days every month till response) or intravenous immunoglobulin (IVIg) (1 mg/kg for 2 days monthly for 4–6 months).

Biologics such as infliximab, etanercept, and rituximab are being used now but experience with these is less.

Plasma exchange and extracorporeal photochemotherapy are resorted to in resistant cases.

Aspirin or dipyridamole (to prevent platelet thrombosis), and calcium supplements (with corticosteroids) are frequently added.

Infections should be treated promptly if they are suspected early in the disease and during the course.

Calcinosis is treated with diltiazem, bisphosphonates such as alendronate, aluminum oxide (decrease intestinal absorption of phosphates), electric shock wave lithotripsy (ESWL), and surgical excision.[2,3,5]

There should be continuous follow-up to detect internal malignancy, especially in adults, and treat them as necessary.

SUMMARY

Dermatomyositis is an autoimmune inflammatory myopathy which in its classic form usually occurs in the age group of 40–60 years with a female to male ratio of 2:1. Juvenile dermatomyositis can affect children below 18 years and has a better prognosis. Both the adult and juvenile disease can present without muscle involvement and then is called CADM.

The predisposing factors range from a genetic predisposition to various infections, drugs, and internal malignancy although the latter is not associated with JDM.

The classical violaceous erythematous rash seen in DM/CADM is a heliotrope seen around the edematous eyelids and the Gottron's sign seen over the extensors of the finger joints extending onto the dorsum of the hands, extensors of the elbows, neck, upper back, extensors of the knees, and medial malleoli. This is associated with both the lower and upper limb proximal extensor muscle weakness and/or tenderness in the classical variety. Patients might have Raynaud's phenomenon, nail fold or widespread telangiectasia, and nondestructive arthritis.

Children often present with widespread scaly pigmented pruritic lesions which mimic other dermatoses. They might suffer from vasculopathy and dystrophic calcinosis cutis and the former if involves systemic vessels can even lead to mortality.

Sudden onset of pruritic dermatoses in sun-exposed sites with cutaneous ulceration in a middle aged or elderly person points toward an associated internal malignancy.

In addition, there might be ILD associated with the antisynthetase syndrome and cardiac ailments. These along with pulmonary infection and internal malignancy are important causes of mortality in adults.

Dermatomyositis is sometimes present with other autoimmune connective tissue disorders in an overlap syndrome. When associated with scleroderma it is called sclerodermatomyositis and is said to have a better prognosis.

Pregnancy should be planned during remission as advised with all autoimmune connective tissue disorders to avoid adverse outcome.

Routine blood parameters, relevant antinuclear and anticytoplasmic antibody profile, serum CPK, and 24-hour urinary creatinine clearance measures should be performed. Electromyography, MRI, or USG of affected muscles can be undertaken before muscle biopsy.

Malignancy screen should be performed in all suspected adult patients every 3–6 months for at least 3 years.

Clinically amyopathic dermatomyositis is treated with emollients, topical steroids or tacrolimus, and hydroxychloroquine. Systemic steroids are the first line of therapy for associated myopathy and systemic disease and should be continued for at least 2–3 years with slow tapering. The other medications used are methotrexate, azathioprine (for lung disease), cyclosporine, dapsone, infliximab, etanercept, and rituximab. Calcinosis is treated with bisphosphonates, aluminum oxide, and surgical excision. Passive exercises during active disease and active physiotherapy during remission should be stressed.

REFERENCES

1. Raychaudhuri SP, Mitra A. Polymyositis and dermatomyositis: Disease spectrum and classification. Indian J Dermatol. 2012;57:366-70.
2. Sontheimer RD, Hansen CB, Costner MI. Dermatomyositis. In: Goldsmith LA, Katz SI, Gilchrest BA, Paller AS, Leffell DJ, Wolff K (Eds). Fitzpatrick's Dermatology in General Medicine, 8th edition. New York: McGraw Hill; 2012. pp. 1926-42.
3. Gordon P, Creamer D. Dermatomyositis. In: Griffiths C, Barker J, Bleiker T, Chalmers R, Creamer D (Eds). Rook's Textbook of Dermatology, 9th edition. New Delhi: Wiley Blackwell; 2016. pp. 53.1-53.13.

4. Tanimoto K, Nakano K, Kano S, Mori S, Ueki H, Nishitani H, et al. Classification criteria for polymyositis and dermatomyositis. J Rheumatol. 1995;22(4):668-74.
5. Jorizzo JL, Vleugels RA. Dermatomyositis. In: Bolognia JL, Jorizzo JL, Schaffer JV (Eds). Dermatology, 3rd edition. Philadelphia, PA: Elsevier Saunders; 2013. pp. 631-41.
6. The lichenoid tissue reaction ('interface dermatitis'). In: Weedon D (Ed). Skin Pathology, 3rd edition. London: Churchill Livingstone Elsevier; 2010. pp. 36-70.
7. Schiffenbauer A, Garg M, Castro C, Pokrovnichka A, Joe G, Shrader J, et al. A randomized, double-blind, placebo-controlled trial of infliximab in refractory polymyositis and dermatomyositis. Semin Arthritis Rheum. 2018;47(6):858-64.
8. Brunasso AMG, Aberer W, Massone C. New onset of dermatomyositis/polymyositis during anti-TNF-α therapies: a systematic literature review. ScientificWorld Journal. 2014;2014:179180.
9. Fasano S, Gordon P, Hajji R, Loyo E, Isenberg DA. Rituximab in the treatment of inflammatory myopathies: a review. Rheumatology. 2017;56(1):26-36.

EXAMINATION QUESTIONS

1. Classify criteria for diagnosing DM.
2. Write a short note on calcinosis cutis.
3. Describe cutaneous manifestations of DM.
4. Explain the investigations and treatment in DM.

56 CHAPTER

Sjögren's and Other AICTD

Banashree Majumdar, Gobinda Chatterjee

PATHOGENIC AND CLINICAL FINDINGS

Sjögren's syndrome (SS) (Mikulicz syndrome) is a chronic autoimmune disease characterized by destruction and dysfunction of exocrine glands notably salivary and lacrimal glands. It predominantly affects middle-aged females with a worldwide prevalence of around 1–3%. It can occur alone (primary) or may be associated with other autoimmune diseases such as rheumatoid arthritis (RA) and systemic lupus erythematosus (SLE) (secondary). Even though it has an indolent course mostly confined to exocrine glands, however, one-third of patients experience a more generalized course. In a few patients, alarming signs of purpura, low C4 level or mixed monoclonal cryoglobulins demand stringent follow-up. This immune system disease is acknowledged largely by two common symptoms—dry eyes and dry mouth.[1,2] Presenting complains are usually a burning, itching or gritty sensation in eyes and difficulty in swallowing or speaking. Few patients may experience swollen salivary glands (front of ear and behind jaw). Systemic manifestations are noted in almost half of SS patients as mild extraglandular features which include easy fatigue, low-grade fever along with arthralgia, myalgia, morning stiffness, nonerosive rheumatoid-like symmetrical arthritis, vaginal dryness, and a dry skin.[3-5] Dry cough due to xerotrachea or bronchitis, dysphagia, and atrophic gastritis are also common. Raynaud's phenomenon is seen in more than one-third of patients with nail fold capillaroscopy revealing scleroderma-like picture. Recurrent urticaria and annular erythema of face are other presentation. Neurological manifestations include entrapment neuropathy, peripheral sensory-motor, and mononeuritis multiplex.

Risk factors include age > 40 years, female sex, and other associated autoimmune diseases such as RA. Both genetic as well as environmental factors play a role in pathogenesis. A delay in diagnosis and treatment is usually a common phenomenon due to its wide range of confusing clinical manifestations although the use of the definite criteria for diagnosis can support patient identification with SS early. Further the side effects of certain medications such as anticholinergics can also mimic few SS symptoms, thus adding to further confusions. Although a non-life-threatening benign disorder, an appropriate treatment is warranted to avoid complications and to improve quality of life. Among the most common complications, vision trouble attributed to dry eyes. Dental cavities and yeast infection of oral cavity are quite common presentations mainly due to loss of protective effects of saliva. Less commonly lungs, liver, and kidneys may be affected leading to pneumonia, bronchitis, hepatitis/cirrhosis, and deranged renal function. These patients are also prone to develop lymphomas[6] (malignant non-Hodgkin's lymphoma) as compared to general population with 4–6% of patients with primary SS developing lymphoproliferative changes in mucosa-associated lymphoid tissue (MALT) during course of illness. Major risk factors are persistent unilateral or bilateral parotid gland enlargement, splenomegaly, lymphadenopathy, and mixed monoclonal cryoglobulinemia.

DIAGNOSTIC INVESTIGATIONS

Although there are no specific tests for the accurate diagnosis of SS, still the relevant laboratory investigations include:

- Complete blood count
- Blood levels of inflammatory markers such as erythrocyte sedimentation rate (ESR), etc.
- Liver and renal function tests
- Specific antibodies such as anti-Ro/SSA and anti-La/SSB
- Rheumatoid factor assay
- Anti-alpha-fodrin antibody assay, which is considered as a reliable marker for juvenile SS
- Tests to assess the degree of dryness of eyes such as Schirmer's tear test whereby we place a filter paper in lower conjunctival sac to measure tear production.
- Rose bengal and lissamine green tests which are specific tests to examine the surface of eyes for presence of dry spots using dye containing eye drops.
- Imaging tests to monitor the function of salivary glands such as sialogram, which shows how much saliva flows into the oral cavity and salivary scintigraphy, which is a nuclear medicine test.
- Biopsy of minor salivary glands which is the single best test to establish the diagnosis of SS.
- Serum protein electrophoresis as these patients has a rare possibility of developing polyclonal gammopathy.

CLASSIFICATION CRITERIA

Although several classification criteria have been put forward from time to time, but the most widely accepted classification criteria for SS are as follows:[7]

American-European Consensus Sjögren's Classification Criteria

This criterion for SS is based on affirmation of subjective complaints about dryness of mouth and eyes along with objective evidence of salivary and lacrimal gland involvement supported by serum autoantibodies against SSA (Ro) and SSB (La) and presence of lymphocytic infiltration in salivary glands (sialadenitis).

I. *Ocular symptoms (at least one)*:
   - Dry eyes >3 months
   - Foreign body sensation in the eyes
   - Use of artificial tears >3 × per day

II. *Oral symptoms (at least one)*:
   - Dry mouth >3 months
   - Recurrent or persistently swollen salivary glands
   - Need liquids to swallow dry foods

III. *Ocular signs (at least one)*:
   - Schirmer's test (without anesthesia) ≤5 mm/ 5 minutes
   - Positive vital dye staining (van Bijsterveld ≥4)

IV. *Histopathology lip biopsy* showing focal lymphocytic sialoadenitis (presence of focal lymphocytic sialadenitis in minor salivary glands with a focus score >1 defined as a number of lymphocytic foci adjacent to normal appearing mucous acini and containing greater than 50 lymphocytes per 4 mm^2 of glandular tissue).

V. *Oral signs (at least one)*:
   - Unstimulated whole salivary flow (≤1.5 mL in 15 minutes)
   - Abnormal parotid sialography
   - Abnormal salivary scintigraphy

VI. *Autoantibodies (at least one)*:
Anti-SSA (Ro) or Anti-SSB (La)

For a primary Sjögren's diagnosis:
- Any four of the six criteria, must include either item IV (histopathology) or VI (autoantibodies)
- Any three of the four objective criteria (III, IV, V, and VI)

For a secondary Sjögren's diagnosis:
In patients with another well-defined major connective tissue disease, the presence of one symptom (I or II) plus two of the three objective criteria (III, IV, and V) is indicative of secondary SS.

Exclusion criteria include:
- Past head and neck radiation treatment
- Hepatitis C infection
- Acquired immunodeficiency syndrome (AIDS)
- Pre-existing lymphoma
- Sarcoidosis
- Graft versus host disease
- Current use of anticholinergic drugs

American College of Rheumatology Classification Criteria

Case definition requires at least two out of the following three:
1. Positive serum anti-SSA and/or anti-SSB or [positive rheumatoid factor and antinuclear antibody test (ANA) ≥ 1:320]
2. Ocular staining score ≥3
3. Presence of focal lymphocytic sialadenitis with focus score ≥1 focus/4 mm^2 in labial salivary gland biopsies.

TREATMENT

Patients should be well aware that no curative agents are available for this disease and the treatment is mainly symptomatic and not highly satisfactory. Organ-wise symptomatic management has been enumerated in **Tables 1 and 2**. Both nonpharmacological as well as pharmacological managements plays equally important role in improving the disease quality of life of these patients. For advanced disease

TABLE 1: Management for dry eyes, mouth, and nasal cavity.

Dry eyes	• Preservative free artificial tears drops and gel formulations • Serum tears (prepared from patients own serum) • Lifitegrast, an Food and Drug Administration (FDA) approved anti-inflammatory drug for dry eye symptom • Cyclosporine eye drops • For severe cases of xerophthalmia not responding to above measures punctual occlusion with silicon or collagen plugs • Cauterization as last resort only if trial of plugs have not given desired result
Dry mouth	• Medications which increase salivary production such as pilocarpine and cevimeline • Antifungals for oral cavity yeast infections
Nasal dryness	• Humidifiers • Saline nasal irrigation

TABLE 2: Symptomatic management for specific organ system involvement.

Recalcitrant gastric acid reflux	Proton pump inhibitors and H_2 blockers
Liver affection	Ursodeoxycholic acid
Neurologic involvement	Intravenous immunoglobulin
Arthritis	NSAIDs and hydroxychloroquine

(NSAIDs: nonsteroidal anti-inflammatory drugs)

requiring systemic management following points to be kept in mind:

- Oral or parenteral corticosteroids should be our first approach while addressing systemic or extraglandular major organ system affection.[8]
- Although none of the disease-modifying anti-rheumatic drugs (DMARDs) have been specifically approved for Sjögren but few trials suggests efficacy of methotrexate, cyclosporine, and cyclophosphamide and have been successfully employed as steroid sparing agents.
- No proven efficacy of tumor necrosis factor-alpha (TNF-α) inhibitors for Sjögren.

Other AICTDs Quick Glance

- *Overlap syndrome:* It manifests as a combination of at least two collagen vascular diseases with similar presentations like mixed connective tissue disease but without necessarily demonstrating antibody against U1 RNP.
- *Undifferentiated connective tissue disease (UCTD):* This condition is diagnosed when there is evidence of an existing autoimmune state which does not fulfil the diagnostic criteria for any known specific autoimmune disease, however in due course of time can evolve into more specific conditions. Latent lupus and incomplete lupus are alternative terms that have been used to describe this condition.

KEY POINTS

Although there are several criterias and laboratory tests available for the diagnosis of autoimmune connective tissue diseases, still clinical acumen is the single most relevant diagnostic aid in routine practice. Even though no single gold standard treatment option available still symptomatic management in mild cases and a more enthusiastic approach in moderate-severe cases play an important role in improving quality of life of these patients.

REFERENCES

1. Bron AJ, Tomlinson A, Foulks GN, et al. Rethinking dry eye disease: a perspective on clinical implications. Ocul Surf. 2014;12:1-31.
2. Villa A, Abati S. Risk factors and symptoms associated with xerostomia: a cross-sectional study. Aust Dent J. 2011;56: 290–95.
3. Kassan SS, Moutsopoulos HM. Clinical manifestations and early diagnosis of Sjögren syndrome. Arch Intern Med. 2004;164(12):1275-84.
4. Tincani A, Andreoli L, Cavazzana I, et al. Novel aspects Sjögren's syndrome in 2012. BMC Med. 2013;11:93.
5. Ramos-Casals M, Brito-Zeron P, Solans R, et al. Systemic involvement in primary Sjögren's syndrome evaluated by the EULAR-SS disease activity index: analysis of 921 Spanish patients (GEAS-SS Registry). Rheumatology (Oxford). 2014;53: 321-31.
6. Evans R, Zdebik A, Ciurtin C, Walsh SB. Renal involvement in primary Sjögren's syndrome. Rheumatology (Oxford) 2015; 549:1541-8.
7. Shiboski CH, Shiboski SC, Seror R, et al. 2016 American College of Rheumatology/European League Against Rheumatism classification criteria for primary Sjögren's syndrome: a consensus and data-driven methodology involving three international patient cohorts. Ann Rheum Dis. 2017;76:9-16.
8. Stefanski, Ana-Luisa et al. The diagnosis and treatment of Sjögren's syndrome. Deutsches arzteblatt International Vol. 114,20 (2017): 354-61. doi:10.3238/arztebl.2017.0354.

EXAMINATION QUESTIONS

Write short notes on the following:

1. Sjögren syndrome
2. Overlap syndrome
3. MCTD
4. Elaborate diagnosis and management of Sjögren syndrome.

6 SECTION | Papulosquamous Diseases

57 CHAPTER

Psoriasis

Manas Chatterjee, Surbhi Rajput

INTRODUCTION

Psoriasis is a chronic inflammatory papulosquamous disease characterized by epidermal hyperplasia and painful and destructive arthritis with multiple remissions and relapses. The etiopathogenesis of psoriasis is related with immunologic, autoimmune, and genetic attributes and extensive research has been done on treatment modalities involved.

The characteristic lesion is a well circumscribed erythematous plaque with silvery white scales and sharp demarcated margins predominantly involving the extensor surfaces. In surveys, the majority of psoriatic patients indicate a serious impairment in their quality of life and they also feel that the current treatments, although often effective, do not provide a satisfactory long-term solution. This, in turn poses a challenge to develop specific, safe, and effective long-term therapies.

HISTORY

During 129–99 BC, the word "psora" which means to itch was first used by Galen to describe a skin disorder characterized by a scaliness of the eyelids and was thought to be an eczematous process. Hippocrates used the term psora and lepra for the same condition that can be recognized as psoriasis. The confusion between leprosy and psoriasis continued for several centuries. Many psoriatic patients were misdiagnosed as lepers and received the same brutal treatment. It was in 19th century that psoriasis was recognized distinct from leprosy. Robert Wilan (1809) was the first to give an accurate description of psoriasis. Perhaps the oldest treatment for psoriasis has been exposure to sunlight. Until quite recently, new treatments for psoriasis were based on empiric observations.

EPIDEMIOLOGY

The prevalence of psoriasis rises during childhood and is said to be 2% of the world's population in Europe. Psoriasis can first appear at any age, from infancy to the eighth decade of life. It has been reported that there is a bimodal peak: one at 20–30 years of age and a second peak at 50–60 years. In approximately 75% of patients, the onset is before the age of 40 years. The epidemiological data published from India, mostly hospital based, vary from 0.8 to 5.6%, however it does not reflect the true prevalence of psoriasis.[1-3]

ETIOPATHOGENESIS[1,2]

Psoriasis is a chronic inflammatory, T-cell immune-mediated genetically determined disease affecting skin, nail and joints and has various systemic associations. The lesions show epidermal hyperplasia driven by T-cells being characterized by production of signature cytokines like lL-17A, IL-22, and IFN-γ. The various etiopathogenetic factors are listed as under:

- *Age:* Follows a bimodal distribution, first peak of onset is generally seen at 16–22 years of age and second peak at the age of 60 years, uncommon below 10 years of age, but the disease may affect any age. Individuals in possession of certain HLA class I antigen, particularly HLA Cw-6, are associated with earlier age of onset. Based on these findings two types of psoriasis have been proposed:
  1. *Type I psoriasis:* The onset is before the age of 40 years, severe form, generally shows HLA association and has positive family history.
  2. *Type II psoriasis:* The onset is after 40 years, less severe and lacks HLA association.
- *Sex:* Males and females are equally affected though early onset is seen in females. Risk is higher among fair skinned individuals.
- *Genetics:* Incidence of psoriasis is higher among first and second degree relatives.
  1. Risk is 2% if no parent/sibling affected, 6% if one sibling is affected, 14% and 41% if one parent and both parents are affected respectively.
  2. Concordance for psoriasis is 64% in monozygotic twins and 15% in dizygotic twins.
- Multiple HLA alleles have been associated with psoriasis particularly HLA-B13, B37, B46, B57, HLA CW1- CW6. HLA-C*06:02 has consistently demonstrated highest relative risk for psoriasis, psoriatic arthritis and early onset of disease. Only about 10% of HLA-CW6 carriers develop psoriasis and PSORS1 accounts for one half to one third variation in genetic liability to psoriasis. Other loci include PSORS2, PSORS4, PSORS5, PSORS8, and PSORS9 **(Table 1)**.
- HLA-C*06:02 defines early onset, severity, and familial clustering of psoriasis. Unlike HLA-class II-associated autoimmune diseases psoriasis shows no evidence of interactions between different HLA alleles. *HLA-C*06:02* contributes a nonadditive risk effect and represents a true HLA-class I risk gene.

TABLE 1: Genetic loci linked to psoriasis.[3]

Gene locus	*Chromosomal location*	*Gene locus*	*Chromosomal location*
PSORS1	6p21.3	*PSORS6*	19p13–q13
PSORS2	17q25	*PSORS7*	1p35–34
PSORS3	4q32–35	*PSORS8*	16q12–13
PSORS4	1cen–q21	*PSORS9*	4q31–34
PSORS5	3q21	*PSORASI*	16q12

- The predisposing HLA allele appears as an essential precondition for a tissue- and antigen-specific autoimmune response by its capacity for presentation of select autoantigens. By itself, however, autoantigen presentation is likely not sufficient for causing disease onset but requires the additive effects of common gene variants in genes which provide the costimulatory signals for activation of the actual autoimmune response.

Variation in the HLA genes are associated with various immune-mediated inflammatory diseases (IMIDS), e.g., HLA-C*06:02 is associated with psoriasis and HLA-B 27 with ankylosing spondylitis.

Many of the psoriasis-associated HLA-class I alleles are also significantly increased in Crohn's disease (*HLA-C*06:02, HLA-C*12:02*) and ulcerative colitis (*HLA-C*12:02, HLA-C*07:02*). *HLA-B27* predisposes for ankylosing spondylitis, inflammatory bowel disease, and psoriasis arthritis, creating an overlapping HLA-class I risk pattern although no autoantigens have been identified in these diseases. HLA-B27 is strongly associated with axial variant of psoriatic arthritis.

- *Environmental risk factors:*
  - Trauma-Koebner's phenomenon (KP) has been well documented in cases of psoriasis. The time interval between injury and onset of psoriasis varies from 7 to 14 days. The factors that contribute to Koebnerization **(Fig. 1)** include season (seen more frequently in winters than in summers) and disease severity (more in unstable or flaring disease). It has been suggested that trauma has to cause both epidermal cell injury and dermal inflammation to produce KP. The onset of KP may be a two-step process. The first step is of nonspecific inflammation, which initiates production of inflammatory mediators, including cytokines (especially IL-23), stress proteins (mainly nerve growth factor and basic fibroblastic growth factor), adhesion molecules and autoantigens and the second step is characterized by disease-specific reactions by T-cells, B-cells, autoantibodies, and immune deposits under the restriction of genetic backgrounds. *LCE3B* and *LCE3C* genes are also induced after minor skin trauma and deletion of these proteins leads to incomplete barrier repair after minor trauma which in turn causes induction of inflammatory response.
  - *Infection:* Guttate psoriasis is strongly associated with preceding/concurrent streptococcal infection commonly pharyngitis and other sites being dental abscess, perianal sinusitis and impetigo, whereas disease exacerbation has been linked with skin and/or gut colonization by *Staphylococcus aureus*, *Malassezia*, and *Candida albicans*. The superantigens from *S. aureus*, streptococci, and *Candida* can cause polyclonal activation of T-cells, responsible for its pathology. However, psoriatic lesions are characterized by an oligoclonal T-cell expansion, which points toward an antigen-specific T-cell response. It was suggested that streptococcal M protein may be this antigen, due to its mimicry with type 1 keratin. A few other autoantigens, such as peroxiredoxin 2 and heat shock protein 27, show homology to streptococcal antigens. Recently, it has been found that a molecule, ADAMTSL5, peptide derived from melanocytes acts as a HLA C*06: 02 restricted autoantigen and induces release of signature proinflammatory cytokines like IL-17A from epidermal CD8+ T-cells mediating the inflammatory process.[4] Baker et al. suggested that streptococcal peptidoglycan is more likely to be the candidate than M protein as it is a strong proinflammatory immunogen and the genes encoding the peptidoglycan recognition receptors are located within the linkage sites associated with psoriasis.[5] Tonsillectomy may improve chronic psoriasis because the palatine tonsils generate effector T-cells that recognize keratin determinants in the skin. HIV infection has also been shown to aggravate psoriasis. The frequency of psoriasis is not increased in HIV-positive patients, but the severity of the disease is greater in this population.
  - *Drugs:* Drugs can cause drug triggered psoriasis (i.e., induction of psoriatic lesions on clinically uninvolved skin in patients with psoriasis) as well as drug-induced psoriasis (i.e., precipitation of the disease in genetically predisposed individuals). Although a plethora of drugs have been implicated

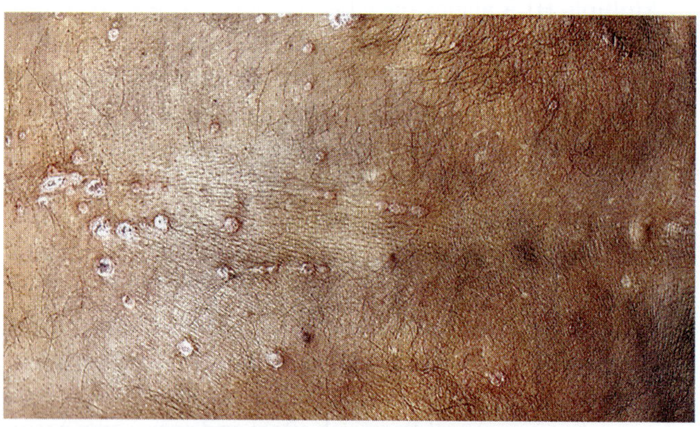

Fig. 1: Koebnerization in psoriasis.

in provoking psoriasis, the strongest evidence is for lithium, beta-blockers, antimalarials, nonsteroidal anti-inflammatory drugs and tetracyclines. In addition, angiotensin-converting enzyme inhibitors, interferons, imiquimod, digoxin, clonidine, carbamazepine, valproic acid, calcium-channel blockers, have been reported to exacerbate psoriasis. Exacerbation and onset of psoriasis have been described in patients receiving TNF inhibitor therapy. Rapid tapers of corticosteroids can induce pustular psoriasis as well as flares of plaque psoriasis.[6]

- *Sunlight:* It is generally beneficial but in few patients, psoriasis may be provoked by sunlight. Severely photosensitive psoriasis is predominantly seen in female, strongly associated with HLA-cw6, family history, and very early age of onset.
- *Metabolic factors:* Hormonal factors may lead to early onset of psoriasis in woman, peak around puberty, provoked by high dose of estrogen therapy. Hypocalcemia has been reported to be a triggering factor for generalized pustular psoriasis (GPP). During pregnancy the disease remains unaltered in 40%, improves in 40% and worsens in 14% women.
- *Psychogenic factors:* Stress is related to onset and exacerbation of disease. Psoriasis has detrimental effect on psychosocial quality of life. Patients who are pathologically worried less likely to clear with PUVA.
- Obesity, increased alcohol consumption, and an increased incidence of smoking have been associated with psoriasis. In a recent report, smoking appeared to have a role in the onset of psoriasis, while obesity appeared to be a consequence of psoriasis.[7]

Cardinal features of lesional psoriatic skin are:

- Epidermal proliferation with loss of differentiation
- Dilatation and proliferation of dermal vessels
- Accumulation of inflammatory cells

Epidermal Hyperproliferation

- It occurs due to increase in proliferating cell compartment in basal and suprabasal level and not due to shortened cell cycle time.
- Number of cycling cells is increased to approximately seven fold.
- TNF-α acts as an important autocrine mediator for epidermal hyperproliferation

Vascular Changes

- Vertical dermal capillary loops appear dilated, elongated and twisted and there is proliferation of vascular endothelium (angiogenesis).
- Epidermal keratinocytes act as primary source of angiogenic activity by producing mediators such as vascular endothelial growth factor (VEGF).
- Dermal capillaries contribute to inflammatory process actively through expression of surface molecules such as ICAM-1 and selectin.

Cellular Participants in Psoriasis

- *T-lymphocytes* play an important role in development of plaque psoriasis.
  - There is an early influx of T-cell in expanding lesions which is evidenced by strong association with MHC particularly HLA-Cw6.
  - Increased antigen presentation in psoriatic plaque.
  - CD4+(dermis) and CD8+ (epidermis) T-cells are mainly involved in the pathogenesis.
  - There is abundance of antimicrobial peptides such as cathelicidin and B defensin.
  - Dysregulated innate response leads to antigen-mediated T-cell expansion and activation which further releases IFN-γ.
  - Recent trials suggest that a subset of T-cells, TH17 cells play a role in the inflammation by production of IL-17
  - Several regulatory T-cells exist and have an impaired inhibitory function and hence leads to T-cell proliferation.
  - Natural killer cells are the main source of IFN-γ production.
  - Dendritic cells have a role in priming of adaptive immune response by antigen presentation and have increased expression of MHCII and factor XIII receptors
  - MasT-cells and macrophages are present below the basement membrane and cause damage by producing TNF-α.
- *Keratinocytes:* Lesional epidermal keratinocytes express the transcription factor STAT-3 which induces the upregulation of a number of genes such as ICAM-1 and TGF-α. As STAT-3 is activated by a variety of cytokines such as IL-6, IL-20, IL-22, and IFN-γ, this could be a link between keratinocyte activation and immunocytes in the development of psoriasis. They are major producer of innate immune response mediators such as cathelecidin and β-defensin.
- *Other cells:* The presence of neutrophils is prominent in active lesions and in the marginal zone, but, in contrast to T-cells, they are not a consistent feature of lesional skin. Endothelial cells get activated and cause increase in blood flow and increase in tortuous blood vessels. Fibroblasts support keratinocyte proliferation by producing various cytokines.
- *Signaling molecules in psoriasis:*
  Cytokines IFN-γ, TNF-α, IL-2, IL-6, IL-8, IL-15, IL-17, IL-22.
  Cytokines produced by TH1 cells are IFN-γ, TNF-α, IL-2.
  Cytokines produced by dendritic cells are IL-18, IL-12, IL-23

IFN-γ is released by activated T-cells and NK T-cells in the epidermis and activates members of the STAT transcription factor family, which drives the expression of a large number of immune-related genes in psoriasis. IL-23 supports chronic inflammation by maintaining subset of TH17 cells which produce IL-17 and IL-22.

Chemokines—CXCL8 is thought to mediate the often-prominent infiltration by neutrophils. CCL2, CCL5, CCL20, CCL27 and CXCL9 are implicated in attracting T-cells to the psoriatic plaque.

Innate Immune Response

β-defensin and various other mediators like LL-37 and elafin are produced by keratinocytes in response to TH1 cytokines. Keratinocytes express Toll-like receptors (TLRs) which secrete signaling molecules such as IL-1, IL-8, and TNF-α. The antimicrobial effector protein hβD2 was also shown to have chemotactic activity via CCR6 and binds to TLR-4. S100 proteins bind to calcium and exert chemotactic properties. Nitric oxide produced by dendritic cells also contribute to inflammation.

Growth Factors

Members of the EGF family induce their own production in the keratinocytes including TGF-β and amphiregulin.

This in-turn produces VEGF and NGF by keratinocytes.

Proteases and their Inhibitors

There is overexpression of proteinases by keratinocytes—like matrix metalloproteinases which release various cytokines such as TNF-α further augmenting the inflammation.

Signal Transduction

Multiple signals transduction mechanisms are dysregulated in psoriasis including tyrosine kinase pathway, STAT, and NF-κB pathways.

Clinical Features

It presents as well defined erythematous papule or plaque with white silvery scales. The white appearance of scales occurs due to entrapment of air between the layers.

Grattage test: Coherence of scales is seen as if one scratches a candle wax, also called as signe de la tache de bougie.

Auspitz sign: Removal of scales further shows a smooth, red, glossy membrane (membrane of Bulckeley) which on removal gives a wet surface with tiny bleeding points. It is a clinical reflection of elongated vessels in the dermal papillae, in addition to thinning of the suprapapillary epidermis.

Woronoffs ring: Appearance of a blanched halo of uniform width surrounding the psoriatic lesions is seen after treatment with topical corticosteroids or phototherapy and occurs due to depletion of PG E2.

Koebner phenomenon: Appearance of isomorphic lesions at the site of trauma in an uninvolved skin and is commonly seen during the florid phase.

Clinical Types

- Chronic plaque psoriasis
- Guttate psoriasis
- Erythrodermic psoriasis
- Palmoplantar psoriasis
- Nail psoriasis
- *Pustular psoriasis:*
  - Generalize pustular psoriasis (Von Zumbusch type)
  - Impetigo herpetiformis
  - Localized pustular psoriasis
  - Palmoplantar pustular psoriasis (Barber type)
  - Acrodermatitis continua of Hallopeau
- *Psoriatic arthritis:*
  - Peripheral oligoarthritis
  - Distal interphalangeal joint
  - Arthritis mutilans
  - Rheumatoid-like psoriatic arthritis
  - Axial arthritis
- *Regional variations in psoriasis:* Scalp, face, eyes, body flexures, scrotum, napkin area, palms, and soles.

Chronic Plaque Psoriasis

It is the most common type and presents as symmetrical multiple red scaly plaques which vary from coin sized to large sized lesions **(Figs. 2 and 3)**. Unstable forms refer to lesions showing sudden fluctuations in disease and is precipitated by infection, sudden withdrawal of systemic and topical medications, hypocalcemia, and mental stress.

Clinical Evaluation

The extent and involvement of different body surface area has a great impact on the quality of life and the prognosis of the disease. Psoriatic Area Severity Index (PASI) is an important tool to monitor the extent of the disease and response of therapy **(Table 2)**.[8] The scoring involves the following four areas viz head, upper limb, trunk and lower limbs with a different correlation factor for each site to allow for differing

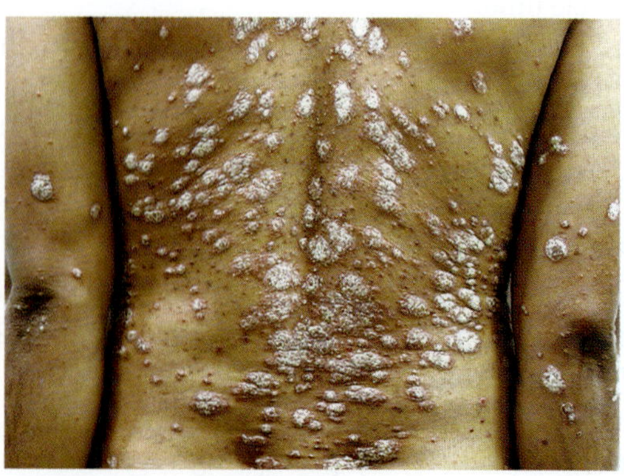

Fig. 2: Chronic plaque psoriasis.

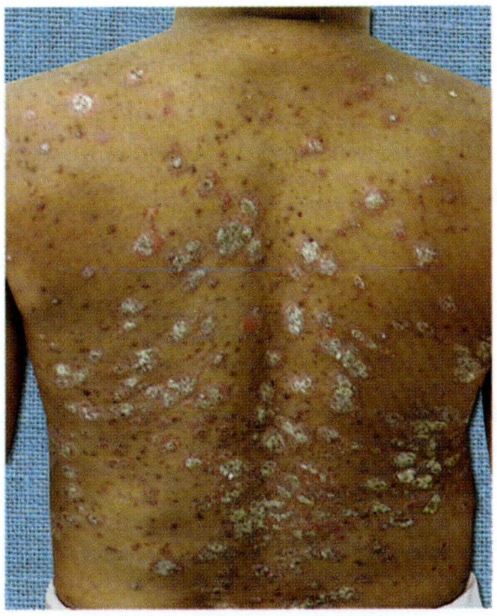

Fig. 3: Chronic plaque.

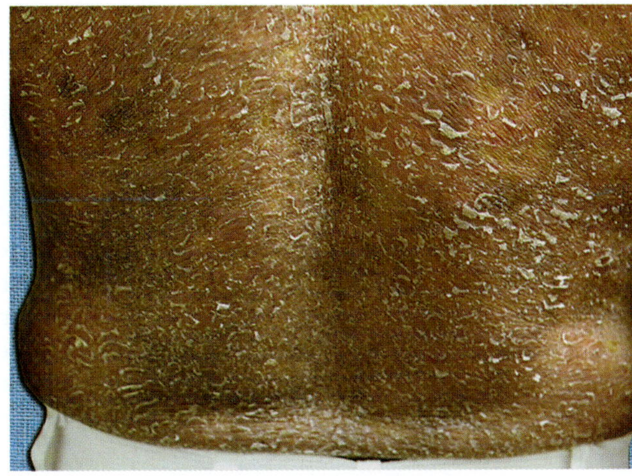

Fig. 4: Erythrodermic psoriasis.

TABLE 2: Calculation of the Psoriasis Area and Severity Index (PASI) (The PASI ranges from 0 to 72).

Calculation of the PASI				
Severity of psoriatic lesions (0: none; 1: slight; 2: moderate; 3: severe; 4: very severe)				
	Head	*Trunk*	*Upper limbs*	*Lower limbs*
Erythema	0–4	0–4	0–4	0–4
Induration	0–4	0–4	0–4	0–4
Scaling	0–4	0–4	0–4	0–4
Total score = 1	Sum of the above	Sum of the above	Sum of the above	Sum of the above
Area of psoriatic involvement (0: none; 1: <10%; 2: 10 to <30%; 3: 30 to <50%; 4: 50 to <70%; 5: 70 to <90%; 6: 90–100%)				
Degree of involvement = 2	0–6	0–6	0–6	0–6
Multiply 1 x 2	1 x 2	1 x 2	1 x 2	1 x 2
Correction factor for area of involvement = 3	0.10	0.30	0.20	0.40
1 x 2 x 3	A	B	C	D
A + B + C + D = Total PASI				

surface area. Erythema, scaling and induration is graded on a scale of 0–4. The score ranges from 0 to 72.

The other more convenient and comprehensive methods of assessment of severity is by DLQI which is a validated method. Other more recent methods to assess the severity are Skindex-17, Salford Psoriasis Index, Sf-36 and so on.

Acute Guttate Psoriasis

It is the appearance of tiny rain drop like erythematous papules diffusely present all over the body. Palms and soles are generally spared. This clinical form follows an upper respiratory tract infection, or tonsillitis due to B hemolytic streptococci. It has a strong association with HLA-Cw6 an prognosis is generally good. The prognosis of guttate psoriasis is excellent in children, with spontaneous remissions occurring over the course of weeks to months.

Erythrodermic Psoriasis

It appears as an involvement of more than 90% of body surface area with scaling, erythema, and induration **(Fig. 4)**. It can also be seen in unstable psoriasis precipitated by a focus of infection, withdrawal of systemic steroids or by overtreatment by dithranol. Patients are prone to develop secondary complications like transepidermal loss of water, hypoalbuminemia, secondary infections, hypothermia, and so on. There is increase in cutaneous blood flow which leads to high output cardiac failure manifesting as tachycardia, high volume pulse with raised JVP and cardiomegaly. There is decrease in renal blood flow which can lead to oliguria. There is dermatopathic enteropathy which can lead to malabsorption of various essential nutrients. There is generalized benign enlargement of lymph nodes called as dermatopathic lymphadenopathy.

Palmoplantar Psoriasis

In the palms and soles, psoriasis most often presents with less well-defined plaques resembling chronic hyperkeratotic eczema or lichen simplex chronicus **(Fig. 5)**. Mixed forms occur and it is sometimes difficult to distinguish psoriasis from eczema in this location. A sharply defined edge and absence of vesiculation are helpful but not sacrosanct. Localized hyperkeratosis of the knuckles occur on dorsum of hands. There may be a correlation to trauma or occupational irritants.

Pustular Psoriasis

Pustular psoriasis is an uncommon form consisting of widespread pustules on an erythematous background. It can occur primarily or can be precipitated by withdrawal of topical corticosteroids or overtreatment with irritants. It can occur in localized and generalized forms. The true localized forms affect the palms and soles and is called as palmoplantar pustulosis.

Generalized Pustular Psoriasis of Von Zumbusch

It is a rare form associated with sterile pustulosis in an acute, subacute or chronic psoriatic eruption **(Fig. 6)**. The pinhead sized pustules gradually coalesce to form lakes of pus. There may be systemic involvement in the form of fever, arthralgia, chills, and malaise. The buccal mucosa is involved in the form of red denuded areas with white margins. The nails become thickened or may get elevated by subungual collection of pus. The remission may occur within a few days but relapses are common.

Localized Type

Sometimes pustules appear within or at the edge of existing psoriatic plaques. This can be seen during the unstable phase of chronic plaque psoriasis and following the application of irritants, e.g., tars.

Impetigo Herpetiformis

It is a variant of GPP, first described by Hebra, which occurs generally in the last trimester of pregnancy and can persist after the child is born. There is appearance of sterile pustules usually on the flexors with a tendency to symmetry. The constitutional involvement is severe in the form of high-grade fever, chills, arthralgias, and death may occur due to cardiac failure. There is a risk of placental insufficiency leading to still birth, neonatal deaths, and fetal abnormalities. The disease may recur in subsequent pregnancies.

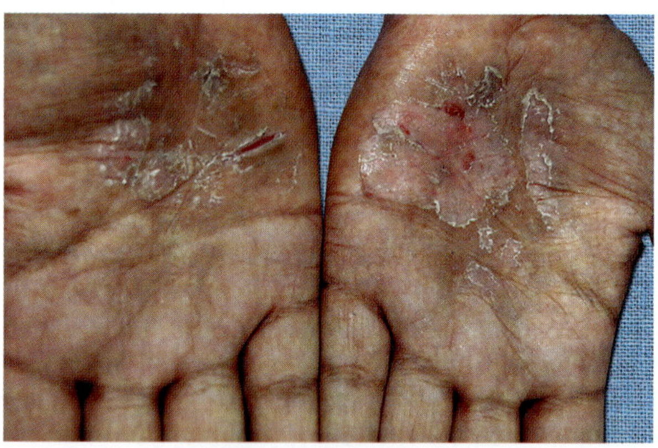

Fig. 5: Palmar psoriasis.

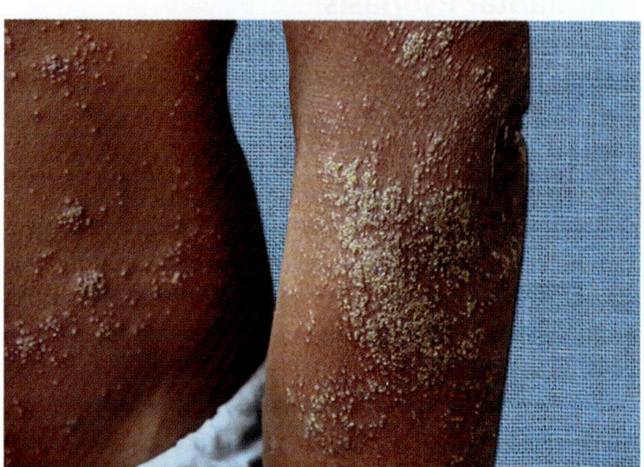

Fig. 6: Pustular psoriasis.

Infantile and Juvenile Pustular Psoriasis

Although GPP can occur at any age group, in 25% of the cases, onset occurs in the first year of life. The systemic features are absent in infantile GPP and spontaneous remission is common. Pustular psoriasis may be localized to flexural areas like neck in infants. The onset is at 2–10 years in majority of children and annular and circinate forms are more common.

Localized Pustular Psoriasis

Palmoplantar pustulosis: This is a common condition where in the sterile pustules appear only on palms and soles. It is also called as pustulosis palmaris et plantaris. There has been an association of thyroid diseases and SAPHO syndrome. Smoking is reported to be strongly associated with it. It presents with well-defined plaques mainly on palms and soles tending towards symmetry. This form may be associated with arthropathy and typical nail changes may be seen.

Acrodermatitis continua of Hallopeau: The eruptions start at the tips of fingers and toes and slowly extend locally or may evolve into GPP. The digits tend to become extremely painful and underlying bony changes in the form of osteolysis of distal phalanx. The digits at times resemble scleroderma and the disease worsens during cold weather due to circulatory dysfunction.

Psoriatic Arthritis

It is the arthritis which is seronegative and is seen in almost 40% of patients. It is destructive arthritis and can be differentiated from other forms by CASPAR criteria **(Table 3)**. It is associated with HLA-B27.

A classification of PsA is met if the final score is equal to or more than 3 points.

It has traditionally been divided into clinical subtypes according to the criteria[10,11] of Moll and Wright:

- *Peripheral mono or asymmetrical oligoarthritis*: It is the most common type of psoriatic arthritis involving usually a single joint or a few interphalangeal or metacarpophalangeal joints along with ongoing dactylitis.
- *Distal interphalangeal arthritis*: This is the classic form of psoriatic arthritis and involves the distal interphalangeal joint of fingers and toes. Usually the nails are also involved.
- *Rheumatoid-like arthritis*: This mainly involves the proximal interphalangeal joint-like the rheumatoid arthritis and is seen in almost 15% of the patients and is symmetrical in nature.

- *Axial arthritis*: This type of arthritis manifests in a few individuals and is associated with features of ankylosing spondylitis and sacroiliitis.
- *Arthritis mutilans*: This is a rare form affecting only 5% of the cases where there is gross resorption of the digits leading to foreshortening along with deformities.

Regional Variations

- *Scalp psoriasis* **(*Fig. 7*)**: There is appearance of well-defined erythematous plaques on scalp, sometimes becoming diffuse when associated with seborrheic dermatitis. The plaques generally extend beyond the hairline to give a characteristic pattern called as "corona psoriatica."
- *Nail psoriasis* **(*Fig. 8*)**: There is increase in the rate of growth of nails in psoriasis. Nail changes are seen in around 40% of patients of the disease. Psoriasis may involve any part of the nail including nail matrix, nail bed, and the hyponychium. The involvement of the nail matrix presents as pits and ridges which is the most common finding. The nail bed involvement appears as subungual oil drop sign which is highly specific for psoriasis. It may also cause distal onycholysis, splinter hemorrhages and subungual hyperkeratosis. Nail pitting is most common in finger nails and subungual hyperkeratosis is the most common finding in toe nails.
- *Flexural psoriasis:* Flexural lesions are characterized by shiny, pink to red, sharply demarcated thin plaques. There is much less scale than in untreated chronic plaque psoriasis. The most common sites of involvement are the axillae, the inguinal crease, the intergluteal cleft, the inframammary region, and the retroauricular folds. When flexural areas are the only sites of involvement, the term "inverse" psoriasis is used **(Fig. 9)**.
- *Follicular psoriasis:* Psoriasis affecting the hair follicles on the trunk and the limbs is called as follicular psoriasis. The lesions appear smaller than guttate psoriasis and may mimic as pityriasis rubra pilaris in children.
- *Genital psoriasis:* The genital skin is generally involved as part of inverse psoriasis. In males, the scrotum and penile shaft may be involved but glans has the maximum predilection. The vulva shows a well-defined erythematous and a nonscaly plaque with marked pruritus. It is a more common finding seen in children.
- *Mucosal lesions:* The mucosa in psoriasis is rarely involved. There may be fissuring of the tongue and sometimes geographical tongue may also be found. The association of geographical tongue with psoriasis is yet to be established.
- *Ocular lesions:* The eye can be involved directly in psoriasis or as a consequence of immunological reaction. Blepharitis is the most common ocular complication. There may be nonspecific conjunctivitis. Keratitis and xerosis are rare complications. Uveitis may be seen as an immunologically mediated reaction and is more commonly seen with psoriatic arthritis.
- *Atypical forms of psoriasis:* There are many atypical variants of psoriasis like interdigital psoriasis. Verrucous lesions appear on legs commonly. Rupioid, elephantine and ostraceous psoriasis are terms used for hyperkeratotic lesions. Linear or segmental psoriasis which is extremely

TABLE 3: Classification criteria for psoriatic arthritis (CASPAR).[9]

Entry criteria: Inflammatory articular disease of the joints, spine, or enthesis		
Psoriasis	Current psoriasis	2
	Personal history of psoriasis	1
	Psoriasis in a first- or second-degree relative	1
Typical psoriatic nail involvement	Onycholysis, pitting, hyperkeratosis	1
A negative test for rheumatoid factor	Any method except latex agglutination	1
Dactylitis	Current dactylitis or History of dactylitis	1
Radiological evidence of juxta-articular new bone formation		1

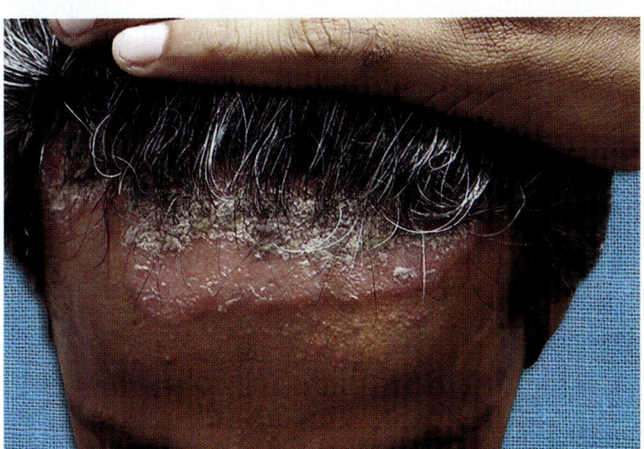

Fig. 7: Scalp psoriasis.

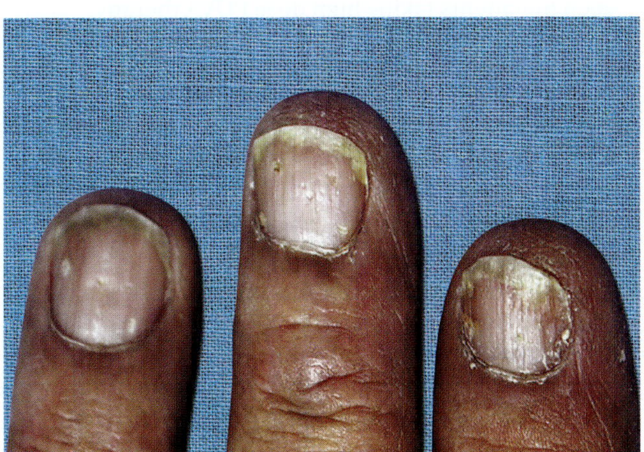

Fig. 8: Nail psoriasis showing coarse pitting.

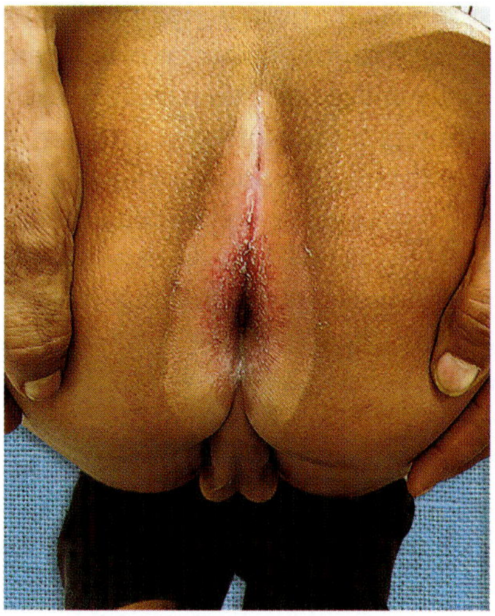

Fig. 9: Inverse psoriasis.
Courtesy: Dr Koushik Lahiri.

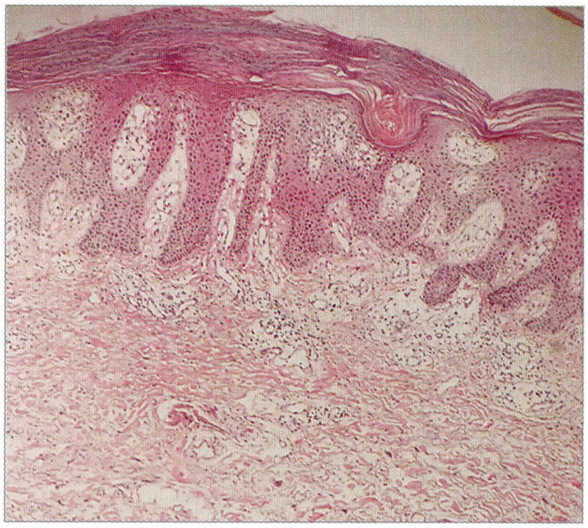

Fig. 10: Section of psoriasis showing hyperkeratosis, acanthosis and parakeratosis and uniform elongation of club-shaped rete ridges (H&E ×100).

uncommon occurs along the Blashko's line and appear in the younger age group.

Complications

- *Inflammatory disorders:* Psoriatic arthritis is the one of the most common inflammatory disorder associated with other immune-mediated diseases such as inflammatory bowel disease, type 1 diabetes and thyroid disorders.
- *Infection:* Infection is rarely seen in psoriasis and resistance is caused by endogenous cathelicidins and B-defensins.
- *Psychological distress:* It is associated with psychological stress and has a great impact on self-image. Alcohol consumption is more in patients with psoriasis and may be related to the psychological trauma associated with the disease.
- *Metabolic syndrome:* The syndrome consisting of truncal obesity, hyperlipidemia, hypertension, and insulin resistance is strongly associated with psoriasis.
- *Cancer:* Non-melanoma skin cancer appears to be frequent with psoriasis. Cutaneous squamous cell carcinoma is seen in patients taking high dose PUVA therapy.

Histopathological Findings

Epidermis

- The epidermis is acanthotic with focal accumulations of neutrophils and lymphocytes. The epidermis is variably spongiotic at these sites **(Figs. 10 to 13)**.
- Above these foci, the granular layer is absent and the stratum corneum still contains flattened nuclei called as parakeratosis.
- The accumulation of neutrophils within a spongiotic pustule is referred to as a 'spongiform pustule of Kogoj and the accumulation of neutrophil remnants in the stratum corneum, surrounded by parakeratosis, as a "microabscess of Munro." These findings are pathognomonic for psoriasis.

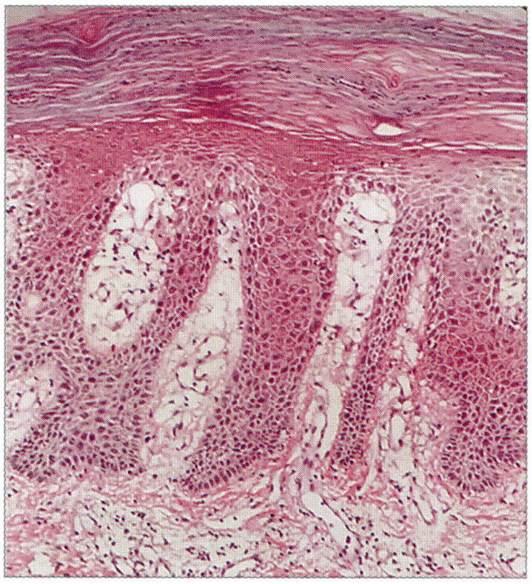

Fig. 11: Section of psoriasis showing hyperkeratosis, acanthosis and parakeratosis and uniform elongation of club-shaped rete ridges (H&E ×200).

Dermis

The capillaries are increased in number and in length and they have a tortuous appearance. Marked edema is seen especially at the tops of the papillae. There is a mixed perivascular infiltrate of lymphocytes, macrophages and neutrophils, and lymphocytes and neutrophils have migrated into the epidermis. Elongation of the rete ridges with camel foot like appearance is seen.

DIFFERENTIAL DIAGNOSIS (TABLE 4)

Treatment

General

Treatment depends upon many variables including age, gender, occupation, personality, general health, intelligence and resources, as well as the type, extent, site, duration, and natural history of the disease. Attention to the patients'

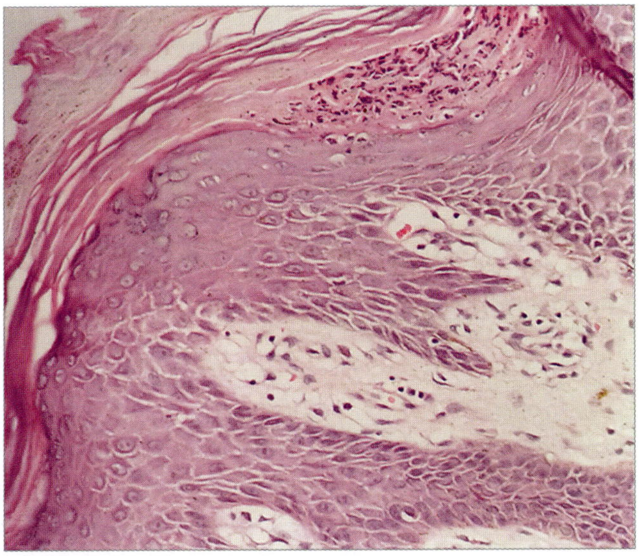

Fig. 12: High power view of thickened stratum corneum showing numerous neutrophils forming Munro's microabscess in the top (H&E ×400)

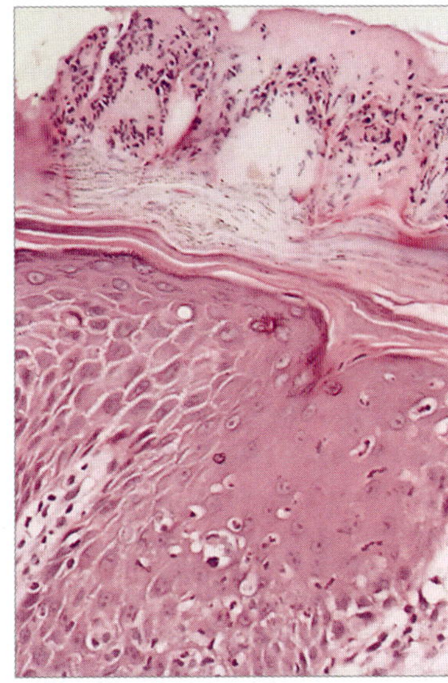

Fig. 13: Collection of neutrophils in the stratum spinosum (spongiform pustule of Kogoj) (H&E ×400).

TABLE 4: Differential diagnosis of psoriasis.

Chronic plaque	*Erythrodermic psoriasis*	*Inverse psoriasis*	*Guttate psoriasis*
Discoid eczema	Drug induced	Seborrheic dermatitis	Pityriasis rosea
Tinea corporis	Eczema	Tinea cruris	Lichen planus
Seborrheic dermatitis	Cutaneous T-cell lymphoma	Candidiasis	Secondary syphilis
Pityriasis rubra pilaris	Pityriasis rubra pilaris	Allergic contact dermatitis	Pityriasis lichenoides chronica
Lichen planus		Bacterial intertrigo	
Mycosis fungoides pilaris			

TABLE 5: Properties of topical treatments.

Treatment	*Relative efficacy*	*Suitability for inducing clearance*	*Suitability for maintenance of remission*	*Patient acceptability*
Topical corticosteroids	√√√√	√√√	√	√√
Vitamin D analog	√√√	√√√	√√√	√√
Outpatient dithranol	√√	√√	—	—
Refined coal tar	√	√	—	—
Tazarotene	√√	√√	√√	√√

general, physical and psychological health is always worthwhile. Known comorbidities like psoriatic arthritis and cardiovascular disease should be actively looked for and treated. Lifestyle and behavior that contribute to general health and treatment responsiveness such as weight management and smoking cessation should be addressed.

Topical Therapy[12]

Topical therapies are the mainstay of treatment for psoriasis of limited extent. Patients with more extensive psoriasis also often use topical therapies, at least for selected body areas. The main groups of topical therapies are emollients, corticosteroids, vitamin D and its analogues, coal tar, dithranol, and retinoids **(Table 5)**.

Phototherapy

Phototherapy with narrow-band UVB is the recommended first-line therapy for most patients with moderate-to-severe psoriasis, uses a wavelength of 311–313 nm. NBUVB works by antiproliferative and proapoptotic mechanisms and also plays a role in immunomodulation. NB-UVB can cause erythema and pruritus in the acute setting and rarely blisters can develop in the resolving plaques. The cutaneous carcinogenic potential is unknown.

PUVA Chemotherapy

PUVA is the combination of psoralens and long-wave ultraviolet radiation (UVA 320–400 nm). Psoralens bind to DNA and when activated by UVA cause permanent DNA damage with resulting cell death. This reduces keratinocyte hyperproliferation, decreases antigen-presenting cells in the dermis, causing apoptosis. The psoralens that are commonly used are 8-methoxypsoralen (8-MOP), 5-methoxypsoralen (5-MOP), and trioxypsoralen (T-MOP). Psoralens are used either topically or orally in combination with UVA.

Systemic Therapy[13]

The initiation of systemic therapy depends equally on the patient and the clinician after considering the risk–benefit ratio. In general, systemic treatment is used for more extensive disease that is not responsive to topical therapy or phototherapy.

Methotrexate: Methotrexate is used as the first-line systemic agent in plaque psoriasis, particularly if there is concomitant psoriatic arthritis. It is also used in localized severe psoriasis, GPP, and erythroderma. The slow onset of action makes it less suitable for rapid control of severe disease. The common side effects are nausea, bone marrow suppression, mucositis, and hepatotoxicity. Pulmonary fibrosis has only been reported rarely in psoriasis patients treated with methotrexate.

Cyclosporin: Cyclosporin inhibits IL-2 production by lymphocytes via calcineurin inhibition. This results in the reduction of NFκB and multiple cytokines including IL-2, TNF-α and IL-8. The major side effects are renal impairment, hypertension, hyperlipidemia, and risk of cutaneous malignancies.

Acitretin: Acitretin binds to nuclear receptors of the steroid superfamily like the vitamin D receptor. It reduces keratinocyte proliferation and also reduces Th17 cells with a concomitant increase in regulatory T-cells. Acitretin is not immunosuppressant and therefore can be considered in situations where other systemic medications are contraindicated, such as active malignancy. It can cause hyperlipidemia and rarely hepatitis. Acitretin is teratogenic and is contraindicated in pregnancy and due to its lipophilic nature can persist in adipose tissue for up to 2 years. Women of childbearing age must not become pregnant for 3 years after cessation of acitretin.

Apremilast: Apremilast is a small molecule inhibitor of phosphodiesterase 4, which modulates proinflammatory mediator production.

Biologics: Biological treatments are now well-established modality for moderate-to-severe psoriasis. Currently licensed treatments in this category are TNF-α inhibitors (TNFi), an IL-12/IL-23 p40 inhibitor and an IL-17 inhibitor. The discussion of biologics is beyond the scope of this chapter.

Treatment ladder

Mild Plaque Psoriasis without Psoriatic Arthritis

First line:
- Potent topical corticosteroid
- Vitamin D analog
- Coal tar
- Dithranol

Second line:
- Local NB–UVB or PUVA
- Excimer laser

Contd...

Contd...

Moderate-to-severe Plaque Psoriasis without Psoriatic Arthritis

First line:
- NB–UVB or PUVA

Second line:
- Methotrexate
- Cyclosporin
- Acitretin
- Apremilast

Third line:
- Adalimumab
- Etanercept
- Infliximab
- Secukinumab
- Ustekinumab

Moderate-to-severe Plaque Psoriasis with Psoriatic Arthritis

First line:
- Methotrexate
- Apremilast

Second line:
- Adalimumab
- Etanercept
- Infliximab
- Ustekinumab
- Secukinumab

Third line:
- Combination therapy

CONCLUSION

One of the most common dermatological conditions and is still one of the most difficult to manage, especially the more severe forms of the disease. Its systemic nature is now proven and the condition needs to be managed as such with drugs that not only treat the skin but also the systemic inflammation, which is a common concomitant, especially in the more severe forms of the disease. To this extent, one needs to assess the type and severity of disease and look for involvement of the joints, which, if not treated in time, lead to crippling deformities. Features of systemic inflammation need to be addressed in addition to the skin to ensure holistic management of the condition.

KEY POINTS

- A chronic inflammatory disorder with genetic predisposition and triggering environmental factors such as trauma, infections and drugs.
- Affects 2–3% of the world.
- Association of psoriasis is seen with metabolic syndrome and stress disorders.
- Erythematous scaly papules and plaques can have pustular and erythrodermic morphology also.
- Most common sites of involvement are extensor surfaces such as the scalp, elbows, knees, hands, feet, trunk and nails.
- Psoriatic arthritis is seen in 10–25% of patients.
- Histopathologically, it is characterized by elongation of rete ridges with dilated capillaries with intermittent

parakeratosis and epidermal and dermal infiltrates of lymphocytes and neutrophils.

- Treatment varies depending on individual variables such as age, gender, body surface area, and comorbid illness. Active search for comorbidities such as cardiovascular disease should be looked for.
- The main groups of topical therapies are emollients, corticosteroids, vitamin D and its analogs, coal tar, dithranol, and retinoids.
- Narrow band UVB is the first-line treatment modality for moderate-to-severe psoriasis.
- Methotrexate remains first-line systemic agent for moderate-to-severe psoriasis. The various others are cyclosporin, oral retinoids, apremilast, and biologics.

REFERENCES

1. Mahajan R, Handa S. Pathophysiology of psoriasis. Indian J Dermatol Venereol Leprol. 2013;79:1-9.
2. Prinz JC. Human leukocyte antigen-class I alleles and the autoreactive T-cell response in psoriasis pathogenesis. Front Immunol. 2018;9:954.
3. Nair RP, Stuart PE, Nistor I, Hiremagalore R, Chia NVC, Jenisch S, et al. Sequence and haplotype analysis supports HLA-C as the psoriasis susceptibility gene. Am J Hum Genet. 2006;78:827-51.
4. Arakawa A, Siewert K, Stöhr J, Besgen P, Kim SM, Rühl G, et al. Melanocyte antigen triggers autoimmunity in human psoriasis. J Exp Med. 2015;212(13):2203-12.
5. Baker BS, Ovigne JM, Fischetti VA, Powles A, Fry L. Selective response of dermal Th-1 cells to 20-50 kDa streptococcal cell-wall proteins in chronic plaque psoriasis. Scand J Immunol. 2003;58:335-41.
6. Tsankov N, Angelova I, Kazandjieva R. Drug-induced psoriasis: Recognition and management. Am J Clin Dermatol. 2000;1: 159-65.
7. Herron MD, Hinckley M, Hoffman MS, Papenfuss J, Hansen CB, Callis KP, et al. Impact of obesity and smoking on psoriasis presentation and management. Arch Dermatol. 2005;141: 1527-34.
8. Van de kerkhof PC. On the limitations of the psoriasis area and severity index (PASI). Br J Dermatology.1992;126: 205-6.
9. Taylor W, Gladman D, Hellliwell P, Maechesoni A, Mease P, Milelants H, CASPAR study Group. Classification criteria for psoriatic arthritis: development of new criteria from a large international study. Arthritis Rheum. 2006;54:2665-73.
10. Lassus A, Mustakallio KK, Laine V. Psoriasis arthropathy and rheumatoid arthritis. Acta Rheum Scand. 1964;10:62-8.
11. Moll JMH, Wright V. Psoriatic arthritis. Semin Arthritis Rheum. 1973;3:55-78.
12. Menter A, Korman NJ, Elmets CA, Feldman SR, Gelfand JM, Gordon KB, et al. Guidelines of care for the management and treatment of psoriasis and psoriatic arthritis with topical therapies. J Am Acad Dermatol. 2009;60(4):643-59.
13. Menter A, Korman NJ, Elments CA, Feldman SR, Gelfand JM, Gordon KB, et al. Guidelines of care for the management and treatment of psoriasis with traditional systemic agents. J Am Acad Dermatol. 2009;61(3):451-85.

EXAMINATION QUESTIONS

1. Describe the etiopathogenesis of psoriasis with various targets of therapeutic modalities.
2. Discuss pathology, clinical features, and treatment of psoriasis.
3. Describe the clinical features, complications and management of psoriasis-induced erythroderma.
4. Outline the classification, risk factors, and treatment of pustular psoriasis.
5. Draw a well-labeled diagram of nail unit and discuss features of nail psoriasis.

Write short notes on the following:

6. Psoriatic arthritis.
7. Biologicals in psoriasis.
8. Recent treatment advances in psoriasis.

58 CHAPTER Pityriasis Rubra Pilaris and Related Disorders

Abhijit Saha, Maitreyee Sengupta

INTRODUCTION

The disorders of cornification are a heterogeneous group of disorders characterized by epidermal dysregulation and impaired keratinization. They include various groups of diseases: psoriasiform disorders such as pityriasis rubra pilaris; the various inherited and acquired ichthyoses; the inherited palmoplantar keratodermas (epidermolytic, diffuse nonepidermolytic, Mal de Meleda, Olmsted syndrome, etc.); the acantholytic disorders (Darier's disease, Hailey–Hailey disease, Grover's disease, etc.); and porokeratosis. Since discussion of all these disease is beyond the scope of this chapter, this chapter will focus on the diseases which are important from an MD examination point of view, viz., pityriasis rubra pilaris, Darier's disease, and Hailey–Hailey disease.

PITYRIASIS RUBRA PILARIS

Introduction

Pityriasis rubra pilaris (PRP) is a rare papulosquamous disorder of unknown etiology that presents with erythematous hyperkeratotic perifollicular papules which tend to coalesce into plaques but may progress to erythroderma, particularly in adults. PRP was first described by Claudius Tarral in 1828 and given its present name by Besnier in 1889.[1] Griffith classified it into five clinical types.[2]

Epidemiology

- PRP shows no gender bias, affecting both men and women equally and all races.
- The incidence ranges from 1 in 5,000 to 1 in 50,000.
- PRP has a bimodal distribution with peaks in the first and fifth decades.
- Nearly all cases are acquired, with occasional reports of a familial form.

Pathogenesis

- The pathogenesis of PRP is unknown.
- The therapeutic success of systemic retinoids has suggested a possible dysfunction in keratinization or vitamin A metabolism. However, attempts to produce keratotic lesions by vitamin A deprivation have been unsuccessful.
- Various minor traumas to the skin, UV exposure, or infections have been reported to precede the onset of PRP, implicating a physical trigger or superantigen.[3]
- An abnormal immunologic response has been suggested by the coexistence of PRP with HIV infection as well as internal malignancies (e.g., renal cell, bronchogenic, and hepatocellular carcinomas).[4]
- The rare genetic form has been linked in some to gain-of-function mutations in the *CARD14* gene, an activator of nuclear factor kappa light chain enhancer of activated B-cells (NF-κB).[5] The familial form of PRP is inherited as an autosomal dominant trait mapped to chromosome 17q25.3.

Clinical Features

- Patients typically show an eruption of follicular hyperkeratotic papules. These are prominent on the elbows, wrists and the backs of the fingers, giving a "nutmeg grater" appearance.[1]
- The papules are also seen on the trunk where they can coalesce to form large red to orange-red plaques with distinctive "islands of sparing" **(Fig. 1)**.[1,6]
- The disease often starts on the scalp before spreading down over the rest of the body. Some patients may become erythrodermic. Pruritus may be present in the early stages.

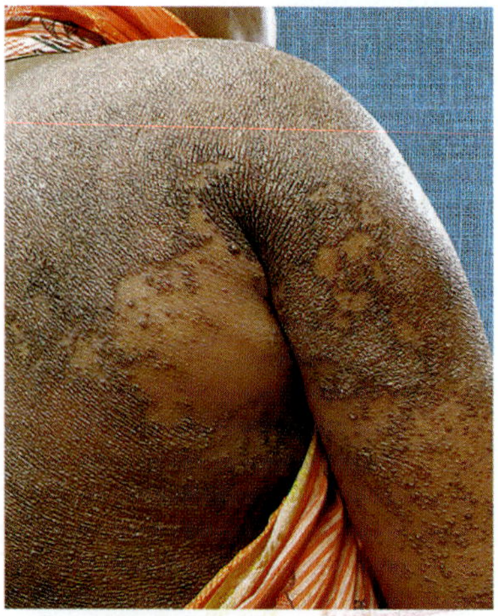

Fig. 1: Classical adult onset PRP with follicular hyperkeratotic papules and "Island of sparing".
Courtesy: Dr Abhijit Saha.

- The palms and soles are commonly involved with a distinctive orange-red waxy keratoderma.[6]
- Nail changes include distal yellow-brown discoloration, nail plate thickening, splinter hemorrhages, and subungual hyperkeratosis.
- Mucous membrane involvement is rare, but may show a diffuse whitish appearance of the buccal mucosa with lacy white plaques and erosions, similar to lichen planus.

Clinical Variants

- PRP has been divided into five clinical types by Griffiths and a sixth type related to HIV infection has been described more recently.[2,5]
- *Type I—Classical adult-onset PRP:*
  - This is the most common and recognizable form, representing over 50% of all cases.
  - The eruption usually starts with erythematous perifollicular papules, each with a central acuminate keratotic plug, on the head or neck and then proceeds in a cephalo-caudal distribution **(Fig. 2)**.
  - Interfollicular erythema appears and the follicular lesions are gradually submerged in sheets of erythema of a slight orange hue, with interspersed sharply demarcated "islands of sparing." The scalp shows diffuse bran-like scaling.
  - Prolonged erythema may give rise to peripheral edema and, in the elderly, may precipitate high-output cardiac failure.
  - Erythroderma frequently develops within 2–3 months. The face becomes uniformly erythematous and mild ectropion may follow.
  - The palms and soles become hyperkeratotic and yellow. The nails are thickened and discolored distally, showing splinter hemorrhages.
  - The disease generally resolves within 3 years in a majority of untreated patients.

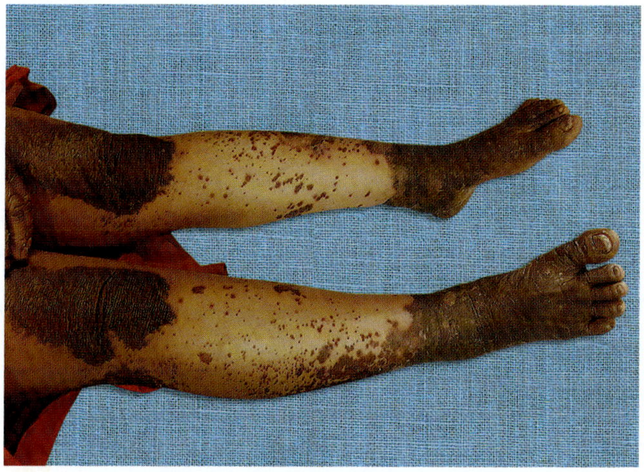

Fig. 2: PRP in dark skin over knee and ankel, difficult to appreciate erythema and orange hue.
Courtesy: Dr Abhijit Saha.

- *Type II—Atypical adult-onset PRP:*
  - This is a much more chronic form, which may last many years, accounting for 5% of cases.
  - Many patients show eczematous features and coarser keratoderma along with the perifollicular scaly papules.
  - Ichthyosiform scale on the legs and variable alopecia of the scalp may be present.
- *Type III—Classical juvenile-onset PRP:*
  - Type III is the most common childhood form of PRP with an onset between the ages of 5 and 10 years.[6,7] It has a generalized distribution and is clinically similar to type I PRP.
  - This form of PRP usually undergoes spontaneous resolution in 1–2 years.
- *Type IV—Circumscribed juvenile PRP:*
  - This type represents about 25% of cases and occurs in prepubertal children, usually under 12 years of age.[7]
  - Clinically, well-circumscribed plaques of erythema and follicular hyperkeratosis confined to the elbows and knees are seen, reminiscent of localized psoriasis.
  - The prognosis of type IV PRP is uncertain.
- *Type V—Atypical juvenile PRP:*
  - This type accounts for 5% of cases. It is a chronic form that presents at birth or start in early childhood with erythema and hyperkeratosis.[7]
  - Familial PRP is most often of this type, which may be genetically heterogeneous and may be difficult to distinguish from ichthyoses and erythrokeratoderma.
  - Follicular hyperkeratosis is a prominent feature and keratoderma is common.
- *Type VI—HIV-related PRP:*
  - This form of PRP became apparent with the onset of the HIV epidemic. It tends to resemble type I PRP and to be resistant to treatment. It may, however, respond to antiretroviral therapy.[4]
  - It may be associated with acne conglobata, hidradenitis suppurativa, or lichen spinulosus.

Histopathology

- The skin biopsy shows hyperkeratosis with follicular plugging.[6]
- Orthokeratosis and parakeratosis alternate in the skin both vertically and horizontally in a "checkerboard pattern." The follicles may show foci of parakeratosis in the perifollicular shoulder.
- There may be patchy or confluent hypergranulosis with dilated dermal capillaries and thick, shortened rete ridges.
- Acantholysis may be present, often restricted to adnexal epithelium.[8]
- There is a sparse lymphohistiocytic dermal infiltrate but no neutrophils.
- The histologic features are not pathognomonic but help to differentiate from psoriasis and other causes of erythroderma.

Differential Diagnosis

- The major differential diagnosis is psoriasis. Clinically, follicular plugging favors PRP while typical nail changes of onycholysis, pitting, oil drop sign favor psoriasis.
- A PRP-like eruption can be seen in patients with dermatomyositis (Wong type) and cutaneous T-cell lymphoma as can erythema and scaling of the scalp.
- Children with acute-onset PRP may be misdiagnosed as having Kawasaki disease, and, occasionally, PRP can be confused with symmetric progressive erythrokeratoderma.
- PRP should also be differentiated from seborrheic dermatitis and other causes of erythroderma.

Course and Prognosis

- In erythroderma, PRP may be complicated by dependent edema and high-output cardiac failure.
- Disease course and prognosis depends on the type of PRP.
- Classical adult PRP (type I) may progress from limited disease to erythroderma in a matter of weeks but eventually clears spontaneously in around 3 years.
- Classical juvenile PRP (type III) typically runs a shorter course with remission in an average of 1–2 years.
- Atypical PRP (types II and V) are chronic diseases with little tendency to resolve spontaneously.
- The prognosis of circumscribed juvenile PRP (type IV) is uncertain, but may resolve in late teens.
- Clinical manifestations in the HIV infection-associated type VI are severe and occasionally fatal with death occurring due to complications of cutaneous sepsis.

Treatment

- Patients with pityriasis rubra pilaris are often unresponsive to multiple therapies, both topical and systemic. As this is a relatively rare disease, large-scale controlled studies regarding treatment are lacking.
- Emollients should be applied liberally and form an important part of management for treating dry skin and restoring barrier function in all patients with PRP.
- Topical corticosteroids may provide symptomatic relief in patients with pruritus but have no long-term effect on the course of PRP.
- Oral retinoids are the mainstay of therapy. Emollients are essential and often, topical corticosteroids have to be added.[6] Isotretinoin, in doses of 1–1.5 mg/kg/day, can induce significant clearing within 3–6 months of instituting therapy. Higher doses (up to 2 mg/kg/day) are occasionally required. Acitretin is also beneficial in the treatment of PRP. The effect of retinoids on familial PRP appears less certain.
- Topical calcipotriol and topical tazarotene have both been used in type IV PRP.
- Methotrexate has also been reported to lead to significant clinical improvement. Weekly oral doses of 10–25 mg are usually employed, and responses are seen within 3–6 months.
- In patients with severe symptoms, effective amelioration of the disease may require extracorporeal photopheresis.
- Familial PRP may show dramatic response to the anti-IL-12/IL-23 antibody, ustekinumab. This agent suppresses activation of the NF-κB pathway, which is known to be overactive in individuals with familial PRP.
- In severe cases of PRP, the combination of methotrexate (5–30 mg/week) plus acitretin has been used. Ustekinumab and anti-TNF agents may be considered for severe type I PRP when acitretin or methotrexate have failed or cannot be used.
- Immunosuppressive agents are of inconsistent benefit. Cyclosporine, azathioprine, anti-TNF agents (infliximab, adalimumab, etanercept) have all been tried with variable success.
- Although UV light therapy runs the risk of exacerbating the disease, there are some reports of success with narrowband ultraviolet B (UVB), UVA1 or psoralens and ultraviolet A (PUVA) in combination with an oral retinoid.[9]
- Less toxic regimens are recommended for the classic juvenile form of PRP, given the high likelihood of spontaneous remission and the potential long-term effects of aggressive systemic therapies.[7]

DARIER'S DISEASE

Introduction

Darier's disease (DD) is a rare autosomal dominant genodermatosis, characterized by chronic and recurrent keratotic papules, generally of teenage or adult onset, predominantly in seborrheic areas. Histology of the keratotic lesions shows suprabasal acantholysis with overlying dyskeratosis. Other features include specific nail changes palmoplantar pits, papules on the dorsum of hands and feet. This disease was reported independently by Darier's and White in 1889.[10,11] It is also known as Darier–White disease or keratosis follicularis.

Epidemiology

- Darier's disease has a worldwide distribution; affecting both sexes equally and all ethnic groups. Its prevalence varies from 1:30,000 to 1:100,000 in Europe.[12]
- The mode of inheritance is autosomal dominant with complete penetrance.[12] However, novel mutations in hitherto unaffected families are fairly common.
- Variable expressivity is seen in affected members of the same family with some patients demonstrating nail changes only.
- The age of onset is typically early teenage, but some patients may not present till sixth or seventh decade.

Pathogenesis and Pathophysiology

- The gene for Darier's disease was mapped by linkage analysis to chromosome band 12q23-24 in 1993.
- The basic defect is a "loss of function" mutation in the intracellular calcium pump, *ATP2A2*, which encodes sarco/endoplasmic reticulum Ca^{2+} ATPase type 2 (SERCA2). SERCA2 is a transmembrane ion channel that pumps Ca^{2+} ions into the sarco/endoplasmic reticulum (ER) against a calcium gradient.[13,14]
- Although both SERCA2a and 2b isoforms are found in the epidermis, SERCA2b is the major product and its dysfunction alone can produce Darier's disease, suggesting that this isoform is essential.
- Defect in the pump leads to reduced ER calcium levels and increased cytoplasmic calcium levels, which interferes with intracellular calcium dependent signaling and transport of adhesion proteins (like desmoplakins), ultimately causing acantholysis.
- Increased intracellular calcium levels also activate calcineurin and calmodulin-dependent protein kinases, which regulate cell division and differentiation, resulting in apoptosis and dyskeratosis.
- Over 200 different pathogenic mutations in *ATP2A2* have now been reported, they include missense, nonsense, frameshift mutations, and in-frame deletions, or insertions.

Clinical Features

- The usual age of onset is between 6 and 20 years (peak onset being puberty between 11 and 15 years of age) but disease may present in infants or old age.[12]
- Discrete or confluent rough, greasy, skin-colored, or yellowish-brown papules are commonest on the seborrheic areas of the trunk, face, ears, scalp, neck, and flexures: The perineum, axillae and groin.
- The primary lesions are keratotic, sometimes crusted, red to brown papules. Despite its initial description as follicular dyskeratosis, the papules are not limited to hair follicles. Hair growth is unaffected.[12]
- The lesions tend to become confluent and may form papillomatous masses. The skin lesions can become vegetating in the folds and are often infected, malodorous, and responsible for major discomfort.
- Small (2–3 mm) hypomelanotic macules may be admixed with the keratotic papules and occasionally are the predominant feature.
- Acrokeratosis verruciformis, plane wart-like lesions, which are flat, skin-colored or brownish 2–4 mm papules, best seen by transverse illumination, are commonest on the dorsal hands but can be detected in other sites (feet, forearms, and legs).
- Focal palmoplantar lesions, pits or keratoses are common, occasionally causing a more diffuse keratoderma.
- Nail fragility, painful longitudinal splits or distinctive red and white longitudinal bands terminating in V-shaped nicks are typical.
- The hard palate, buccal mucosa, gingivae, esophagus, vulva and rectum may develop small whitish umbilicate or cobblestone papules, which may coalesce to resemble leukoplakia. Salivary duct occlusion and recurrent sialadenitis is recognized.[15]
- Ocular manifestations include hyperkeratotic plaques and seborrheic debris at the eyelid margin. Chronic blepharitis is associated with dry eye syndrome and corneal erosions.[12,15]
- Most patients complain of moderate itching. Extensive, malodorous and painful skin impacts social interaction. UV exposure, sweating, heat and occlusion are aggravating factors.
- *Course of the disease*: Darier's disease has a chronic, relapsing course, with unpredictable severity. It can both improve and deteriorate in old age.

Classification of Severity

The following grades are proposed:[16]

- *Grade 0*: Subclinical; the typical rash is absent or subtle but associated features like acrokeratoses or nail dystrophy are present. This grade is usually only recognized in the context of a family history.
- *Grade I*: Mild; localized keratotic papules occupy up to 10% of affected areas and may give rise to pruritus or mild irritation.
- *Grade II*: Moderate; extensive papular and subconfluent lesions with crusting or secondary infection affect 10–30% of the affected area, or there is extensive and symptomatic papular flexural involvement.
- *Grade III*: Severe; widespread confluent, crusted, eroded or bullous rash affects >30% of the trunk or confluent eroded or hyperkeratotic disease of the limbs or flexures.

Clinical Variants

- There is considerable variation in severity of disease, even within families, from subtle palmar or nail changes to widespread involvement.
- Reported variants include erosive or vesiculobullous disease, especially in flexures, and eroded or hyperkeratotic plaques, particularly of distal limbs.
- *Acral hemorrhagic type*: Palmoplantar hemorrhagic macules with irregular margins occur consistently within families and may be due to specific mutations.[17]
- *Segmental types 1 and 2*: Lesions of Darier's disease may occur in a unilateral distribution along Blaschko's lines due to genetic mosaicism. This may occur in an isolated form (type 1) or in a background of milder generalized Darier's disease (type 2).[16]
- Patients may have multiple comedones or nodulocystic acne with typical lesions, causing deeply pitted scars.

- Pigmented papular lesions of the trunk resembling Grover's disease have been described.
- In racially deeply pigmented skin, focal lesions also produce guttate leukoderma—confetti-like hypopigmented macules and papules.

Complications and Associated Manifestations

- The keratotic and papillomatous lesions in Darier's disease are prone to secondary infection with bacteria, yeast or dermatophytes, often leading to vegetating, malodorous lesions. Impetiginization and eczematization are common, and patients have an increased susceptibility to infection with herpes simplex, herpes zoster or cowpox; severe infections may be disseminated or fatal.
- Neuropsychiatric features, including depression, bipolar disorder, epilepsy, and intellectual difficulties have been reported.[18] The accumulation of mutant protein aggregates in neurons could provide a mechanism for these features. Lithium may exacerbate cutaneous disease, possibly by suppressing levels of epidermal SERCA2.
- There are reports of squamous cell carcinomas of the skin or mucosa and mammary Paget's disease. Bone cysts have been recorded.

Histopathology

- There are two prominent histologic features in Darier's disease: acantholysis and dyskeratosis.[13,19]
  - Acantholysis is due to a disturbance in cell adhesion that leads to suprabasilar cleft formation.
  - Dyskeratosis is due to apoptosis of keratinocytes and is characterized by nuclear condensation and perinuclear keratin clumping.
- Two types of dyskeratotic cells are observed in Darier's disease:[19]
  1. "Corps ronds"—acantholytic enlarged keratinocytes in the Malpighian layer with darkly staining and partially fragmented nuclei surrounded by a clear cytoplasm and encircled by a bright ring of collapsed keratin bundles.
  2. "Grains"—small, oval cells in the stratum corneum characterized by an intensely eosinophilic cytoplasm composed of collapsed keratin bundles containing shrunken parakeratotic nuclear remnants.
- "Grains" are likely derived from "corps ronds" but formal proof that they indeed represent different stages of the same pathologic process is lacking.
- The epidermis overlying acantholytic and dyskeratotic foci is thickened and shows papillomatosis and hyperkeratosis.
- In the superficial dermis, there is a mild-to-moderate perivascular inflammatory infiltrate.
- Immunohistochemistry shows desmosomal components diffusely distributed in the cytoplasm of acantholytic cells, and their intra- and extracellular domains are dissociated.
- Ultrastructurally, tonofilaments separate from the desmosomes with aggregation of keratin filaments around the cell nucleus.

Differential Diagnosis[3,20]

- Darier's disease may resemble seborrheic dermatitis, particularly in the scalp, nail, and hand signs help to distinguish these.
- Erosive, bullous or hypertrophic lesions of the flexures clinically and histologically overlap with Hailey–Hailey disease. Erosive or bullous flexural lesions may suggest pemphigus vulgaris/vegetans or pyoderma vegetans.
- Pigmented flexural lesions have to be differentiated from Dowling-Degos disease and acanthosis nigricans.
- Histologically, other acantholytic disorders such as Grover's disease and Galli–Galli disease may have to be differentiated.
- In acrokeratosis verruciformis of Hopf, multiple flesh-colored or lightly pigmented papules are seen, which are clinically identical to those seen in Darier's disease. Histology shows a "church spire" pattern of hyperkeratosis, but acantholysis is not usually found. In some, acrokeratosis verruciformis of Hopf has been found to be allelic to Darier's disease.

Diagnosis and Investigations

- The disorder is usually diagnosed clinically with histological confirmation.
- In symptomatic or overtly infected lesions, specimens should be taken for bacteriological culture, and virological or fungal investigations should be considered in exacerbations or treatment-resistant disease.

Treatment

- General measures include sunscreens and light garments to minimize both UV exposure as well as heat exposure. Daily skin care with urea or lactic acid-containing emollients and topical antiseptics is recommended. This may be sufficient for mild disease.[16,20]
- In acute, symptomatic and inflammatory disease, topical corticosteroids are commonly used. In general, potent or even highly potent steroids are necessary and are often combined with topical antimicrobials.[20] Chronic use of potent topical corticosteroids should be avoided, especially in the flexures.
- Topical retinoids are more effective, but also more irritant, than topical corticosteroids. Other topical agents that have been used include tacrolimus, tacalcitol, and topical 5-FU cream.
- Oral retinoids are the mainstay of treatment of severe disease.[14,20] Acitretin 0.25–0.5 mg/kg/day or isotretinoin 0.5 mg/kg/day reduce hyperkeratosis and malodor. Two forms of birth control are mandatory for women of

childbearing age treated with systemic retinoids, because of their teratogenic potential. Oral alitretinoin may provide an alternative to acitretin, and may be useful in women of child-bearing potential.

- Ciclosporin has no effect in chronic stable disease but has been reported to be effective in severe inflammatory or eczematized episodes and vulval disease.[20]
- Infected exacerbations are most commonly due to staphylococcal infection and short courses of appropriate oral antibiotics may be necessary. Long-term oral antibiotics are not generally recommended. Herpes simplex infection needs urgent oral or parenteral antiviral agents such as acyclovir.
- *Surgical therapy:* Physical therapies used to treat localized disease include excision and grafting, electrodessication, dermabrasion, and ablative laser therapy. Botulinum toxin can be considered to reduce maceration in flexural disease and breast reduction has been used for inframammary disease.

HAILEY–HAILEY DISEASE

Introduction

Hailey–Hailey disease is an autosomal dominant genodermatosis characterized by erosions and blistering, most prominently in the flexures and sites of friction or trauma.[21] In 1939, Howard and Hugh Hailey, brothers working in the Department of Dermatology at Emory University School of Medicine in Atlanta, Georgia, described a chronic erosive dermatosis in two sets of brothers.[22] Histologic sections from all four patients showed similar features, i.e., intraepidermal vesicles, mild dyskeratosis, hyperkeratosis, and a moderate dermal lymphocytic infiltrate. They coined the name "familial benign chronic pemphigus."

Epidemiology

- There are no data regarding the exact prevalence of Hailey–Hailey disease, although an incidence of one in 50,000 has been reported.[21]
- It is probably as frequent as Darier's disease, but is underrecognized.

Pathogenesis and Genetics

- Hailey–Hailey disease is an inherited disorder of keratinocyte adhesion. The mode of inheritance is autosomal dominant with complete penetrance, but the age of onset and expressivity varies greatly among the affected members of a family.
- It is caused by mutations in a gene encoding a Ca^{2+} ATPase, *ATP2C1*, whose protein product, hSPCA1 (human secretory pathway Ca^{2+}/Mn^{2+} ATPase), is localized to the Golgi apparatus. The *ATP2C1* gene is present on chromosome 3q21-24.[23,24]
- Hailey–Hailey disease is caused by loss-of-function mutations inactivating one *ATP2C1* allele leading to haploinsufficiency. These may be nonsense, missense, or frameshift mutations. There appears to be no consistent genotype/phenotype correlation.
- *ATP2C1* is most highly expressed in the basal layer of epidermis, but it is also present in suprabasal keratinocytes. Calcium sequestration into the Golgi is reduced in these keratinocytes.
- Trafficking of desmoplakin and desmoglein 3 to the cell membrane is reduced which inhibits cell-cell adhesion.
- In addition, Hailey–Hailey keratinocytes and epidermis demonstrate reduced cellular ATP levels, leading to impaired actin reorganization, which may result in abnormal formation of the adherens junctions required for normal keratinocyte cell-to-cell adhesion.
- Additional factors such as heat, friction or infection are clearly required to trigger the clinical disorder, as presentation is late and localized.

Clinical Features

- Hailey–Hailey disease typically presents between the second and fourth decade with painful, pruritic and often malodorous lesions of flexures (neck, axilla, submammary region, groin, and perineum) or other sites of friction.[21]
- Painful fissures (rhagades) in flexures are common and very suggestive of the disease. The scalp, the antecubital and popliteal fossae or trunk are less frequently involved. Inframammary lesions are common in women, whereas vulvar disease is unusual.[25]
- The initial lesion is a flaccid vesicle on erythematous or normal skin, which ruptures easily and therefore is often overlooked. The blisters give rise to macerated or crusted erosions, which tend to spread peripherally, producing a circinate border with crusts and small vesicles when examined carefully.
- Healing occurs without scarring, leaving postinflammatory hyperpigmentation. Common precipitating factors include heat, sweating, friction, and infection.
- Asymptomatic, longitudinal white bands in the fingernails (longitudinal leukonychia) may serve as a subtle diagnostic clue in patients with limited or atypical disease.[26]
- Mucosal involvement is rare. Even mild disease has been shown to reduce quality-of-life, and flexural or groin involvement can be particularly disabling.
- Complete remissions as well as flares are common, and the clinical course in an individual patient is difficult to predict. Some patients report attenuation of the disease at an older age, whereas others state that there is no change or a worsening with aging.

Complications and Comorbidities

- As in Darier's disease, colonization and secondary bacterial, fungal, and viral infections play an important role in disease exacerbation and persistence.[21,27]
- Recalcitrant intertriginous lesions have been described in association with herpes simplex virus (HSV) infections. Kaposi's varicelliform eruption due to HSV is a rare complication of Hailey–Hailey disease. It is characterized by fever and a rapidly spreading vesicular eruption, and should be promptly treated with an oral antiviral medication, e.g., valacyclovir.
- Human papillomavirus (HPV) may be present in verrucous perineal lesions. Squamous cell carcinoma reported in association may be related to HPV carriage.

Clinical Variants

- Papular acantholytic dermatosis of the genitocrural area without other features of Hailey–Hailey disease is in some cases allelic to Hailey–Hailey disease.
- Type 1 mosaicism presents with relapsing linear acantholytic dermatoses with histopathological and ultrastructural features of Hailey–Hailey disease, sometimes in childhood.
- Type 2 mosaicism, which is rarer, presents with more severe linear lesions on a background of milder, generalized disease.

Histopathology

- Widespread loss of intercellular bridges within the epidermis in Hailey–Hailey disease leads to large areas of dyscohesion with single or groups of acantholytic cells, which have been likened to a "dilapidated brick wall."[28]
- Dermal papillae, lined by a single layer of basal cells, protrude into the blister cavities and are referred to as "villi."
- Mild dyskeratosis may be present but unlike Darier's disease, necrotic keratinocytes are uncommon.
- In more chronic lesions, epidermal hyperplasia, parakeratosis and focal crusts are found. A moderate perivascular lymphocytic infiltrate is observed in the superficial dermis.
- Ultrastructural studies of acantholytic cells have shown perinuclear aggregates of keratin filaments that have retracted from desmosomal plaques.

Differential Diagnosis

- Hailey–Hailey disease shows considerable clinical and histologic overlap with Darier's disease, although acantholysis is more widespread in Hailey–Hailey disease, whereas dyskeratosis is a predominant feature of Darier's disease.[21,22]
- Intertriginous lesions may be mistaken for intertrigo or candidiasis or flexural seborrheic eczema.[21,27]
- The lesions of inverse psoriasis have sharper borders, fewer erosions, and less crusting.
- Vegetating intertriginous lesions in Hailey–Hailey disease may be identical to those of pemphigus vegetans (Hallopeau type). Histology, including immunofluorescence, may be necessary to exclude autoimmune pemphigus.[21,26]
- Severe bullous and erosive lesions can suggest erythema multiforme or even toxic epidermal necrolysis.

Treatment

- General measures include loose clothing, absorbent pads in flexures and, where appropriate, weight loss. Emollients and antimicrobial agents may help prevent exacerbations.[21]
- Colonization and secondary bacterial, fungal, and viral infections should be treated with appropriate topical and/or systemic antimicrobials. Painful, recalcitrant disease may indicate superinfection by herpes simplex and systemic antiviral treatment should be considered.[21,27]
- Potent or highly potent topical corticosteroids can be effective, especially combined with antibacterial/antifungal agents.[21,29] Their prompt and early use for exacerbations is recommended but extended treatment should be avoided because of the risk of cutaneous atrophy, especially in the flexures.
- Anecdotal reports have described a therapeutic benefit for topical tacrolimus, cyclosporine, calcipotriol, and tacalcitol.
- When the disease is refractory to topical preparations, it may respond to intralesional corticosteroids.
- The evidence base for systemic agents is limited, but systemic corticosteroids are useful for acute severe inflammatory disease. Oral acitretin, cyclosporine, methotrexate, dapsone, and calcitriol have all been reported to help.
- Physical interventions reported include ablative treatments such as cryosurgery, dermabrasion, electrodessication, various forms of laser therapy and argon plasma coagulation. Axillary or inframammary use of botulinum toxin can reduce sweating.
- Surgical excision of flexural disease, with or without grafting, and breast reduction for inframammary disease have been reported.

KEY POINTS

Pityriasis rubra pilaris

- PRP is a rare papulosquamous disease of unknown etiopathogenesis that is characterized clinically and histologically by follicular plugging. There is no race or sex predilection.
- Clinically, erythematous hyperkeratotic follicular papules are seen, with a "nutmeg grater" appearance. Over the

trunk, these papules coalesce to form large plaques with "islands of sparing." The rash spreads in a cephalo-caudal direction.

- Griffith classified PRP into five types. Types I and II are of adult onset while types III, IV and V have their onset in childhood. Later, a Type VI has been described in association with HIV infection.
- Histologically, follicular plugging is seen with prominent parakeratosis in the perifollicular shoulder. Alternating bands of parakeratosis in both vertical and horizontal directions give a "checkerboard pattern."
- The disease has to be differentiated from psoriasis, seborrheic dermatitis, and other forms of erythroderma.
- Types I and III spontaneously resolve within 1-3 years while the other types have a more chronic course.
- Treatment is not definitive. Oral retinoids with emollients are the mainstay. Other topical and systemic immunosuppressives as well as biologics have also been tried.

Darier's disease

- Darier's disease is an autosomal dominant disorder, characterized clinically by chronic, recurrent keratotic papules primarily in seborrheic areas, and histologically by suprabasal acantholysis with overlying dyskeratosis.
- "Loss of function" mutation in the *ATP2A2* gene, mapped to chromosome 12q23-24, which codes for SERCA2, that pumps Ca^{2+} ions into the endoplasmic reticulum against a calcium gradient, leads to loss of keratinocyte adhesion resulting in acantholysis.
- The onset is between 6 and 20 years of age characterized by multiple greasy, dirty, warty papules on the trunk, neck, face, scalp, and flexures which may later become confluent and infected to form papillomatous, malodorous masses.
- Other features include palmoplantar pits and keratoses, nail fragility with V-shaped nicking, and hypopigmented, confetti-like macules.
- Skin biopsy shows acantholytic dyskeratosis with the characteristic "corps ronds" (large acantholytic keratinocytes with small, pyknotic nuclei, clear cytoplasm, and encircled by a bright ring of collapsed keratin bundles) and "grains" (small, oval, apoptotic cells with brightly eosinophilic cytoplasm).
- Treatment includes use of sunscreens and avoidance of sun-exposure. Mild-to-moderate disease can be controlled by potent topical corticosteroids. Oral retinoids are mainstay of treatment of severe disease.

Hailey–Hailey disease

- Hailey–Hailey disease is an autosomal dominant disorder characterized by erosions and blistering, predominantly in the flexures.
- "Loss of function" mutation in the *ATP2C1* gene, mapped to chromosome 3q21-24, which codes for hSPCA1 that transports Ca^{2+} ions into the Golgi apparatus, leads to loss of keratinocyte adhesion.
- Hailey–Hailey disease typically presents between the 2nd and 4th decade with painful, pruritic and often malodorous, crusted or macerated erosions of flexures. Rhagades are frequent.
- Longitudinal leukonychia is common but nail fragility is not seen.
- Skin biopsy shows widespread acantholysis giving a "dilapidated brick wall" appearance. Dermal papillae with a single layer of basal cells project into the acantholytic spaces and are known as "villi."
- The disease has to be differentiated form Darier's disease, inverse psoriasis, seborrheic eczema, and pemphigus.
- Treatment includes control of secondary infections with topical or systemic antimicrobials. Mild-to- moderate disease may be treated with potent topical corticosteroids or other agents such as tacrolimus and cyclosporine. Severe, refractory disease may require systemic immunomodulating agents.

REFERENCES

1. Besnier E. Observations pour server a l'histoire clinique du pityriasis rubra pilaire (pityriasis pilaris de Devergie et de Richaud). Ann Dermatol Syphilol. 1889;10:253-87.
2. Griffiths WA. Pityriasis rubra pilaris: the problem of its classification. J Am Acad Dermatol. 1992;26:140-2.
3. Ferrandiz-Pulido C, Bartralot R, Bassas P, Bodet D, Repiso T, Aparicio G, et al. Acute postinfectious pityriasis rubra pilaris: a superantigen-mediated dermatosis. Acta Dermosifiliogr. 2009;100:706-9.
4. Miralles ES, Nunez M, De Las Heras ME, Pérez B, Moreno R, Ledo A. Pityriasis rubra pilaris and human immunodeficiency virus infection. Br J Dermatol. 1995;133:990-3.
5. Fuchs-Telem D, Sarig O, van Steensel MA, Isakov O, Israeli S, Nousbeck J, et al. Familial pityriasis rubra pilaris is caused by mutations in CARD14. Am J Hum Genet. 2012;91: 163-70.
6. Griffiths WAD. Pityriasis rubra pilaris. Clin Exp Dermatol. 1980;5:105-12.
7. Allison DS, El-Azhary RA, Calobrisi SD, Dicken CH. Pityriasis rubra pilaris in children. J Am Acad Dermatol. 2002;47: 386-9.
8. Howe K, Foresman P, Griffin T, Johnson W. Pityriasis rubra pilaris with acantholysis. J Cutan Pathol. 1996;23:270-4.
9. Kirby B, Watson R. Pityriasis rubra pilaris treated with acitretin and narrow-band ultraviolet B (Re-TL-01). Br J Dermatol. 2000;142:376-7.
10. Darier's J. De la psorospermose folliculaire vegetante. Ann Dermatol Syphilol. 1889;10:597-612.
11. White JC. A case of keratosis (ichthyosis) follicularis. J Cutan Dis. 1889;7:201-9.
12. Munro CS. The phenotype of Darier's disease: penetrance and expressivity in adults and children. Br J Dermatol. 1992;127: 126-30.
13. Foggia L, Hovnanian A. Calcium pump disorders of the skin. Am J Med Genet C Semin Med Genet. 2004;131C:20-31.

14. Dhitavat J, Dode L, Leslie N, Sakuntabhai A, Lorette G, Hovnanian A. Mutations in the sarcoplasmic/endoplasmic reticulum Ca^{2+} ATPase isoform cause Darier's disease. J Invest Dermatol. 2003;121:486-9.
15. Frezzini C, Cedro M, Leao JC, Porter S. Darier's disease affecting the gingival and oral mucosal surfaces. Oral Surg Oral Med Oral Pathol Oral Radiol Endod. 2006;102:e29-33.
16. Sakuntabhai A, Dhitavat J, Burge S, Hovnanian A. Mosaicism for ATP2A2 mutations causes segmental Darier's disease. J Invest Dermatol. 2000;115:1144.
17. Sanchez Salas MP, Latasa de Aranibar FJG, Oncins Torres R, Gambó Grasa P. Bullous hemorrhagic Darier's disease. Skinmed. 2011;9:65-6.
18. Gordon-Smith K, Jones LA, Burge SM, Munro CS, Tavadia S, Craddock N. The neuropsychiatric phenotype in Darier's disease. Br J Dermatol. 2010;163:515-22.
19. Douwes FR. On the histology and histochemistry of Darier's disease. Arch Klin Exp Dermatol.1968;233:309-22.
20. Cooper SM, Burge SM. Darier's disease: epidemiology, pathophysiology, and management. Am J Clin Dermatol. 2003;4:97-105.
21. Burge SM. Hailey-Hailey disease: the clinical features, response to treatment and prognosis. Br J Dermatol. 1992; 126: 275-82.
22. Hailey H, Hailey H. Familial benign chronic pemphigus. Arch Dermatol. 1939;39:679-85.
23. Sudbrak R, Brown J, Dobson-Stone C, Carter S, Ramser J, White J, et al. Hailey–Hailey disease is caused by mutations in ATP2C1 encoding a novel Ca^{2+} pump. Hum Mol Genet. 2000;9:1131-40.
24. Vanoevelen J, Dode L, Van Baelen K, Fairclough RJ, Missiaen L, Raeymaekers L, et al. The secretory pathway Ca^{2+}/Mn^{2+}-ATPase 2 is a Golgi-localized pump with high affinity for Ca^{2+} ions. J Biol Chem. 2005;280:22800-8.
25. Wieselthier JS, Pincus SH. Hailey–Hailey disease of the vulva. Arch Dermatol. 1993;129:1344-5.
26. Kirtschig G, Effendy I, Happle R. Leukonychia longitudinalis as the primary symptom of Hailey–Hailey disease. Hautarzt Z Fur Dermatol Venerol Verwandte Geb. 1992;43:451-2.
27. Mashiko M, Akiyama M, Tsuji-Abe Y, Shimizu H. Bacterial infection-induced generalized Hailey-Hailey disease successfully treated by etretinate. Clin Exp Dermatol. 2006; 31:57-9.
28. Burge SM, Millard PR, Wojnarowska F. Hailey–Hailey disease: a widespread abnormality of cell adhesion. Br J Dermatol. 1991;124:329-32.
29. Ikeda S, Suga Y, Ogawa H. Successful management of Hailey-Hailey disease with potent topical steroid ointment. J Dermatol Sci. 1993;5:205-11.

EXAMINATION QUESTION

1. Describe the classification and management of pityriasis rubra pilaris (PRP).

59 CHAPTER

Lichen Planus and Lichenoid Disorders

Vishal Chugh

INTRODUCTION

Lichen planus (LP) is an inflammatory, pruritic, papulosquamous disorder of unknown etiology affecting either or all of skin, mucous membrane, hair, and nail. First described by Hebra as lichen ruber; but, Erasmus Wilson in 1869 coined Lichen planus [Greek word "*leichen*" (tree moss); Latin word "*planus*" (flat)].[1] On the contrary "lichenoid" is used to describe an LP-like eruption clinically, or by pathologists to describe a consistent interface dermatitis phenotype of tissue reaction.

Lichen planus has <1% worldwide distribution, with incidence of 0.38% reported in India.[2,3] It appears initially during the fourth or fifth decade and affects women preferentially, rarely seen in childhood (familial cases observed).[1]

ETIOPATHOGENESIS

Four domains, which have significant role in pathogenesis are:

1. *Immunological dysregulation*: A milieu of up and down regulated adhesion molecules, inflammatory, proapoptotic mediators, cytokines and growth factors (IL-1α, IL-6,8, IFN-γ, TNFα, VEGF, TGFβ1, caspase 3, Bcl-2) with major histocompatibility complex II activate T helper cells; CD8+ principally and CD4+, eventually CD8+ cells infiltrate the epidermis, causing self-perpetuating basal keratinocyte damage.[4] The process involves three sequential stages: LP-specific antigen recognition, cytotoxic lymphocyte activation, and keratinocyte apoptosis.[1] Recently, accumulation of plasmacytoid dendritic cells, IFNα-inducible protein myxovirus resistance 1 protein, and transcription factor Brn2 has been implicated.[4]
2. *Infections*: HCV infection is well documented. IFN therapy for HCV also worsens LP. Pathogens implicated: Hepatitis B (also hepatitis B vaccination), varicella zoster, and human herpes virus 6 and 7.[4]
3. *Genetic predisposition*: The familial form is common among human leukocyte antigen (HLA) haplotypes-B7, -Aw19, -B18 and -Cw8.[1] Currently, genetic loci HLA-A5, A-3, A-28, B-8, DR-1, DR-10, DRB1*01:01 are reported.[4] Single nucleotide polymorphism and HLA-DQB1*05:01 haplotype previously implicated in vulvovaginogingival syndrome found to be strongly associated with LP.[4]
4. *Environmental factors*: Drugs, psychological factors like stress, depression, anxiety, etc.

CLINICAL FEATURES

Table 1 enumerates the clinical subtypes of LP.

Cutaneous LP

The traditional 6 Ps in classical cutaneous LP are purple, pruritic, polygonal, planar, papules, and plaques **(Fig. 1)**. A network of fine white lines or puncta referred as Wickham striae is present in well-developed papules. Lesions are distributed symmetrically, with predilection in flexural areas (wrists, arms, legs). Thighs, lumbar area, trunk, neck, and

TABLE 1: Clinical subtypes of lichen planus.

Cutaneous LP	*Mucosal LP*	*Appendageal LP*
Based on configuration and morphology: • Classical/papular • Hypertrophic • Vesiculobullous • Actinic • Atrophic • Linear • LP pigmentosus • LP pigmentosus-inversus • Palmoplantar LP	• Oral • Genital • Esophageal • Laryngeal • Ocular • Plurimucosal (Vulvovaginogingival syndrome) *Overlap syndromes:* • LP with lupus erythematosus • LP pemphigoids	• Lichen planopilaris • Nail

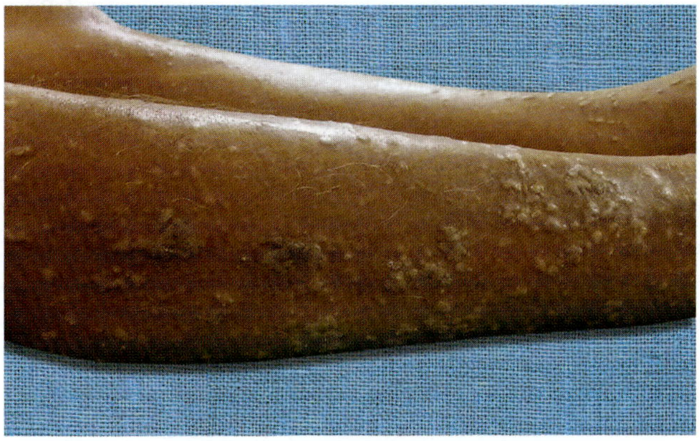

Fig. 1: Classical lichen planus (LP).

TABLE 2: Clinical characteristics of lichen planus (LP) variants.

Subtype	*Clinical characteristics*
Linear LP	Due to Koebnerization. True linear LP follows Blashko's line or is dermatomal (*Zosteriform LP*: De novo or at site of healed herpes zoster lesions- isotopic response)
Hypertrophic LP	Pruritic, lichenified, hyperpigmented plaques, symmetric; site: Shin and interphalangeal joints **(Figs. 2A and B)**
Atrophic LP	Site: Trunk and extremities, surface is atrophic
Annular LP	Site: Penis and scrotum, develop from a ring of typical LP papules that progress peripherally and produce central clearing
Actinic LP	Also known as lichen planus tropicus. Pigmented papular lesions on sun exposed areas (neck, dorsum of hands, forearm, and arms)
LP pigmentosus	Macular slate gray hyperpigmentation is diffuse; site: Face, neck and upper limbs **(Fig. 3)**
LP pigmentosus inversus	Diffuse macular slate gray hyperpigmentation in intertriginous and flexural areas[4]
Erosive/ Ulcerative LP	Chronic, painful vesicles and ulceration of feet, scalp and nails with mucosal lesions; definite risk of squamous cell carcinoma
Bullous LP	Bullae and vesicles restricted to areas of cutaneous LP
Palmoplantar LP	Erythematous scaly/hyperkeratotic plaques/ vesiculobullous. Symmetrical, pruritic. Site: Malleoli and internal plantar arch

dorsal surfaces of the hands and nails may also be affected. The face and scalp are usually spared. Absence of scratching, as patient rubs instead of scratching to gain relief is referred to as Brocq's phenomena. In Brocq's grattage test, careful scraping of classical lesion causes turgescence of papules and purpura due to subepidermal hemorrhage unlike pinpoint bleeding of psoriasis.

Table 2 enumerates the characteristic features of LP subtypes.

Mucosal LP

Mucosal involvement occurs with cutaneous LP, or independently. Oral cavity (common), glans penis, vulva, vagina, anus, nose, larynx, trachea, esophagus, urethra, and tympanic membrane lesions have been documented.

Oral LP: Present in 60–70% of cases; buccal mucosa and tongue commonly affected. The lesions consist of lacy, reticulated white streaks, white papules and plaques, and erythematous, atrophic or ulcerated patches with painful, burning sensations. Mucosal subtypes: Reticular (Common: Posterior buccal mucosa—**Fig. 4**), erosive [ulcerative, painful: Dorsum and lateral borders of the tongue and gingiva, pseudomembrane; 0.8% risk of squamous cell carcinoma (SCC[5])], atrophic (gingiva); bullous, and plaque.

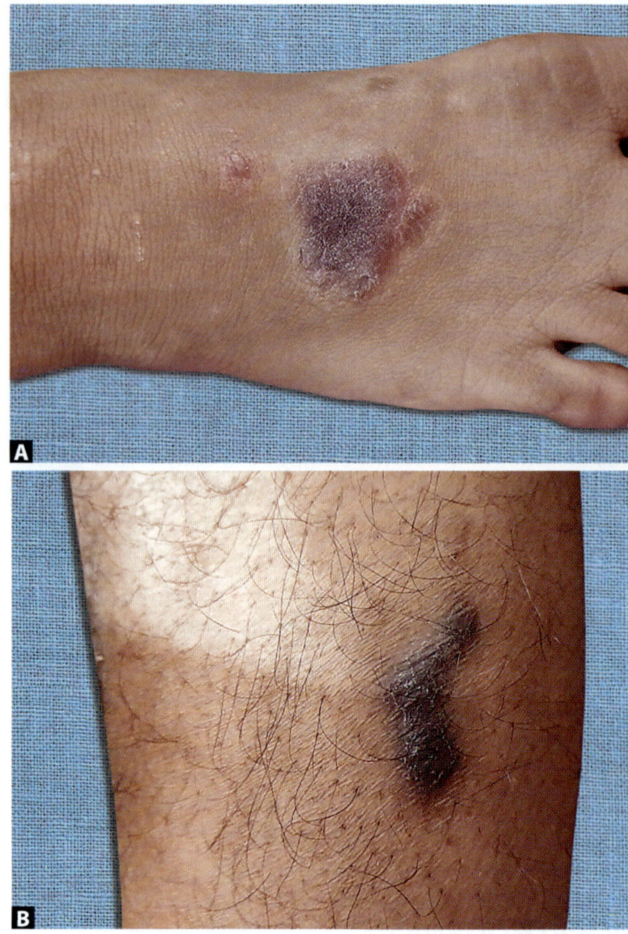

Figs. 2A and B: Hypertrophic lichen planus (LP).

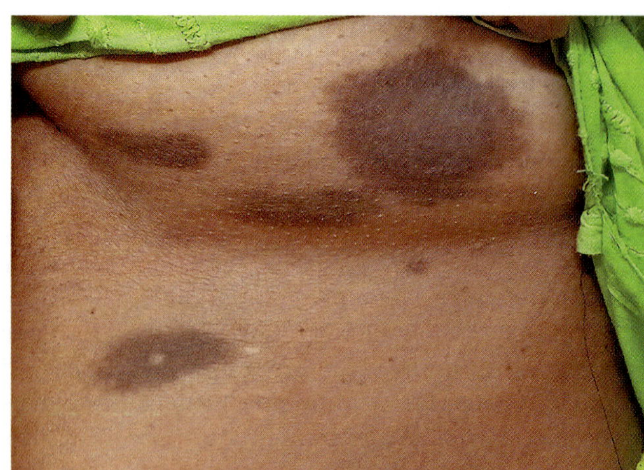

Fig. 3: Lichen planus pigmentosus.

Genital LP: In young men, genital lesions are seen on penile shaft, glans penis, prepuce, or scrotum. Annular LP is the most common morphology. Ulceration is very unlikely.

In females, occurs in the peri- and postmenopausal period. Painful vulval introital erosions with white, lacy, reticulate borders extending into the vagina are characteristic. Scarring is common; sequelae: Loss of labia minora, clitoral

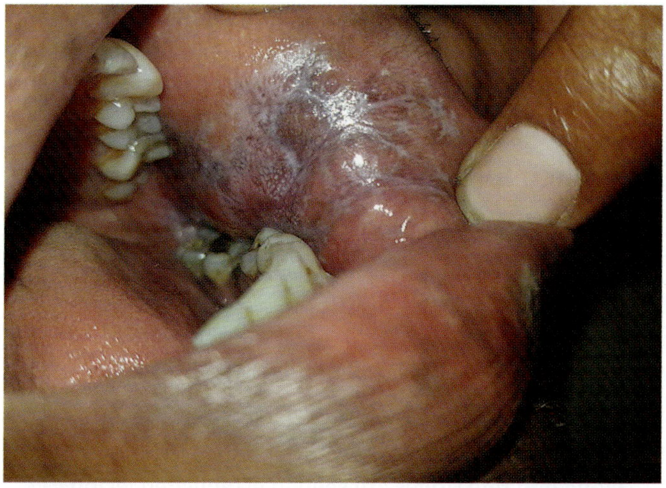

Fig. 4: Mucosal lichen planus (LP): Lacy reticular network.

burying, and narrowing of the introitus. Erosive LP of the vulva and vagina with desquamative gingivitis is termed vulvovaginal-gingival syndrome.

Ocular LP: Blepharitis, xerophthalmia, cicatricial conjunctivitis, keratouveitis, keratoconjunctivitis sicca, punctuate epithelial erosions, corneal ulceration, forniceal symblepharon, and subconjunctiva fibrosis have been reported.[6]

Laryngeal LP: Extremely rare, Kunelskaya Ya et al. reported largest case series, wherein epiglottis and aryepiglottic folds were involved more than vocal cords.[6]

Appendageal LP

Lichen planopilaris (LPP)/follicular LP: It appears as isolated or aggregated, pinhead-sized red papules, which carry a conical acuminated hyperkeratosis (LP acuminatus). Sites of predilection include the trunk, neck, sacral region, and proximal extremities. Scalp LPP leads to cicatricial alopecia. The symptom combination of follicular LP on the trunk and on the scalp with nail dystrophy has been described as Lassuerur-Graham-Little syndrome.

Nail LP: Nail changes in LP include longitudinal ridging and splitting of the nail plate, thinning of nail plate (Angel wing deformity), erythema of lunula, onycholysis, dorsal pterygium formation, onychodystrophy, trachyonychia or complete loss of the nail plate. Rarely, onychopapilloma, localized distal subungual hyperkeratosis with multinucleated cells can arise. Idiopathic atrophy of the nails can occur causing rapid diffuse nail atrophy and pterygium of the nails leading to permanent anonychia.[6]

In isolated nail LP, changes will be restricted to nail unit and characteristic pattern seen is longitudinal pattern of ridging over the nail plate.[7] The other changes as mentioned above can also occur. Finger nails are affected more than toe nails. In isolated nail LP, severity has been classified as shown in **Table 3**.[7] Nail biopsy is mandatory and biopsy site depends on clinical finding. The course of this type can be unpredictable causing nail dystrophy, high rates of relapse, recurrence, and treatment failure; however, prompt early intervention can give satisfactory results.[7]

TABLE 3: Severity grades of isolated nail lichen planus (LP).

Severity grades	*Features*
Mild	• Nail thinning • Longitudinal ridging • Distal splitting <3 mm length • Onycholysis <25% • No nailbed hyperkeratosis
Moderate	• Distal splitting 3–5 mm length • Onycholysis of 25–50% • Subungual hyperkeratosis • Partial fissuring • Longitudinal grooves • Mottled erythema of lunula
Severe	• Distal splitting >5 mm length • Onycholysis >50% • Complete fissuring • Deep grooves • Diffuse erythema of lunula • Pterygium and anonychia

TABLE 4: Drug-induced lichen planus and lichenoid eruptions.

Pattern of lichenoid reaction	*Drugs implicated*
Classic cutaneous lichenoid eruption	Angiotensin converting enzyme inhibitors (ACE inhibitors), antimalarials, β-blockers, penicillamine, methyldopa, gold, lithium, quinidine, sulfonylureas, thiazide diuretics, TNFα inhibitors, tyrosine kinase inhibitors
Photodistributed lichenoid eruption	Carbamazepine, chlorpromazine, diltiazem, ethambutol, quinidine, tetracyclines, thiazide diuretics
Cutaneous and oral LP	ACE inhibitors, allopurinol, anticonvulsants, gold, ketoconazole, NSAIDs

LICHENOID DISORDERS

They include drug-induced LP, lichenoid contact dermatitis or mucositis, chronic graft-versus-host disease (GVHD), keratosis lichenoides chronica, and lichen nitidus (LN).

Lichenoid Drug Eruptions

Clinically, the lesions are extensive, psoriasiform with a predilection for the face and upper trunk rather than the flexures; develop over weeks to months after initiation of therapy. Lichenoid drug eruptions (LDEs) are similar to LP lesions, but are more polymorphic, lack Wickham striae and oral involvement, tend to have psoriasiform or eczematous morphology.[4] Stoppage of the offending drug leads to slow resolution of the lesions over a period of 1–4 months.

Medications commonly implicated with development of LP and LDEs are enumerated in **Table 4**.

Lichenoid Cutaneous Graft-versus-Host Reaction

In early chronic GVHD, occurrence of disseminated lichenoid eruptions is clinically indistinguishable from classic LP involving skin, ears, trunk, thighs, oral mucosa, scalp, palms, soles, and nails. The skin lesions may be localized or diffuse. Localized lesions may be linear or Blaschkoid. Pigmentary changes, both hyper- and hypopigmentation, may be associated.[8]

Nekam's Disease (Synonym: Keratosis Lichenoides Chronica)

It is a rare and occur in young adults (20–40 years), occasionally children may be affected.[9] It is characterized by chronic progressive violaceous, hyperkeratotic, papulonodular lesions, arranged in a linear or reticulate pattern, especially on the buttocks and extremities. A seborrheic dermatitis-like presentation may be observed on the scalp, face, and neck. There may be oral and genital mucosal and palmoplantar involvement. Nail involvement takes the form of thickening, longitudinal ridging, and recurrent paronychia. It is treatment resistant though PUVA, etretinate, and calcipotriene have been tried.

Lichen Nitidus

Idiopathic lichenoid dermatosis characterized by a self-limiting monomorphic eruption of asymptomatic, minute, flesh-colored papules with flat shiny surface. Children and young adults are the usual sufferers. Common sites of involvement are the forearm, penis (glans and shaft), buttocks, lower abdomen, and chest. Some cases may have a generalized distribution. Koebnerization may be present. Linear,[10] spinous, vesicular, follicular, perforating, hemorrhagic, and actinic are rare morphological variants. Mucosal involvement is rare, with discrete, grouped, yellowish papules of 1 mm size, distributed on the hard palate and gum. Nail changes are longitudinal, beaded ridges, terminal splitting, and irregular pittings with a fine rippled. LN may occur in association with LP in 25–30% cases and also atopic dermatitis, Down's syndrome, Crohn's disease, and congenital megacolon.[4] Fluorinated topical/systemic steroids, phototherapy may be used in symptomatic/generalized cases.[11]

LP-like keratosis (LPLK): They appear as solitary, scaly pinkish-pigmented plaques on upper extremities, trunk and sun-exposed areas; misdiagnosed as superficial BCC. LPLK is believed to arise from regressing seborrheic keratosis or solar lentigo.[4]

Lichen striatus: They are asymptomatic self-limiting eruption common in children presenting as pinkish papules that coalesce into linear configuration in a Blaschkoid pattern seen on neck, limbs, abdomen, and buttocks.

Lichen sclerosis: It affects in a biphasic manner, common in women usually involves perianal and genital regions. It has been associated with alopecia areata, pernicious anemia, and thyroid disease.

Approach to Lichen Planus and Lichenoid Disorders

Clinical diagnosis of LP is easier with characteristic features. Differentials to be considered in common variants of LP **(Table 5)**.

Dermoscopy **(Table 6; Figs. 5A and B)**

Histopathology:

- Compact hyperkeratosis, wedge-shaped hypergranulosis, elongated rete ridges are seen in established lesion.
- Focal hypergranulosis (Wickham striae).
- Rete ridges flattened or effaced ("saw-tooth" appearance).
- Focal separation from dermis to Max-Joseph space.
- *Apoptotic basal cells:* Civatte bodies/colloid bodies/hyaline bodies at dermoepidermal junction and papillary dermis.
- A band-like, dense, lymphohistiocytic infiltrate at the papillary dermis impinges on the epidermis.
- Absent epidermal melanocytes with pigmentary incontinence and dermal melanophages is characteristic.

In hypertrophic LP: Epidermal changes are marked with thicker collagen bundles in the dermis. Rete ridges are more elongated and rounded as opposed to the typical saw-tooth pattern.

TABLE 5: Differentials to be considered in common variants of lichen planus (LP).

LP variants	*Differentials*
Classical LP	Psoriasis, pityriasis rosea, chronic cutaneous lupus erythematosus, lichen simplex chronicus, graft-versus-host disease, secondary syphilis, lichenoid mycosis fungoides
Annular LP	Granuloma annulare, dermatophytosis
Atrophic LP	Lichen sclerosus et atrophicus
Linear LP	Lichen striatus, inflammatory linear verrucous epidermal nevus, nevus unius lateris
Hypertrophic LP	Psoriasis, prurigo nodularis, lichenoid cutaneous amyloidosis, lichen simplex chronicus
Vesiculobullous LP	Lichen planus pemphigoids, bullous pemphigoid, pemphigus vulgaris
Lichen planopilaris	Lichen spinulosus
Oral LP	Leukoplakia, candidiasis, erythema multiforme, pemphigus vulgaris, bullous pemphigoid, lichen sclerosus, secondary syphilis, lichen sclerosus et atrophicus
LP pigmentosus	Ashy dermatosis, Riehl's melanosis

TABLE 6: Dermoscopic features of lichen planus (LP).

• Pink to violaceous papules with scaling • Radial, linear capillaries, blue-gray dots and globules (dermal pigmentary incontinence)	In hypertrophic LP, accentuated scaling at follicular opening, comedo-like structures (corn pearls)
Wickham striae patterns	• Reticular (common) • Circular • Radial streaming • *Leaf venation:* Secondary striae branching from the centered WS venation • Clustered, follicular white dots
Lichen planopilaris	Perifollicular whitish-gray scaling associated with erythema, arboriform vessels, absence of follicular openings and follicular plugging, pigment incontinence around follicular opening (target sign)
Lichen planus pigmentosus	• *Diffuse:* Characterized by diffuse, structureless, brownish areas—epidermal pigmentation • *Dotted:* Fine or coarse gray-blue or brown dots or globules related to dermal melanophages • *Mixed:* Combining diffuse brownish areas with dotted structures

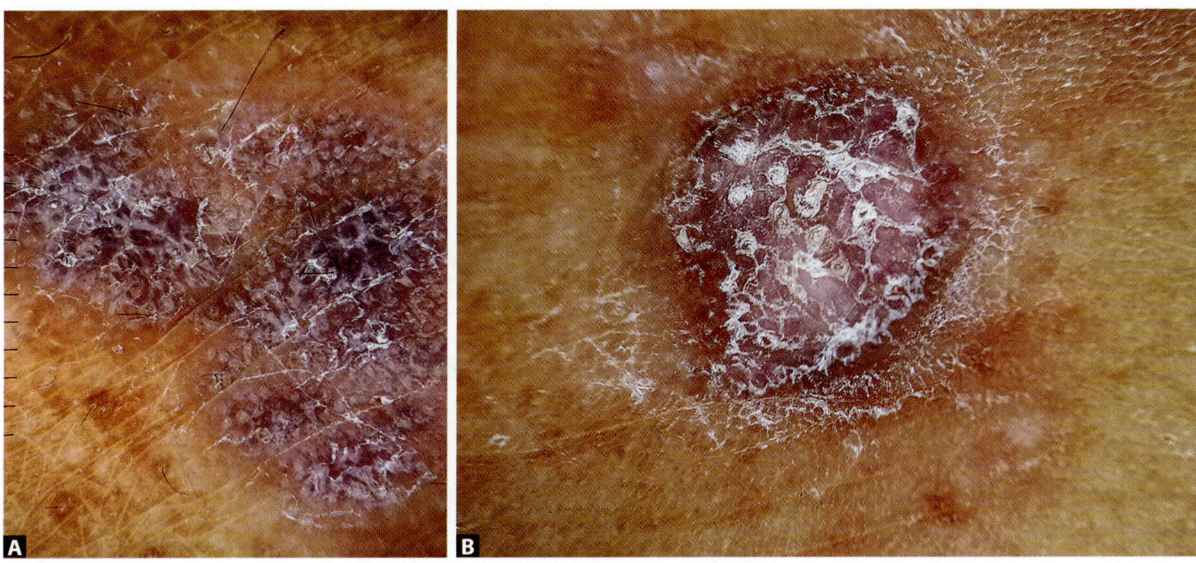

Figs. 5A and B: (A) Dermoscopy showing purplish background, linear streaks of scales (WS), blue-gray globules and dots; (B) Purplish background, with scaling at follicular orifices forming comedo-like structures (corn pearls) [Polarized × 10 view, digitally zoomed, DL3 dermoscope].

In atrophic LP: Rete ridges lost and dermal fibrosis is prominent.

In LPP: Interface dermatitis is initially contained in the peribulge area including the infundibulum and isthmus with sparing of the lower segment of the hair follicle with orthokeratosis, hypergranulosis, and follicular plugging. Fibrotic tissue progressively replaces the hair follicles.

Mucosal LP: Epithelial changes—less specific, atrophic, lacks saw-tooth pattern, parakeratosis, rarely exhibit orthokeratosis.

Histopathological features in lichenoid dermatosis are enlisted in **Table 7**.

Direct immunofluorescence (DIF): LP shows shaggy, ragged fibrin band at basement membrane zone (and clusters of colloid bodies with IgM and C_3; lesser extent with other classes of immunoglobulin).

Treatment

Treatment of lichen planus has been shown in **Table 8**.

In isolated nail LP, inflammation needs to be suppressed at the earliest. First line of therapy should include intralesional triamcinolone acetonide 2.5–10 mg/mL according to disease severity to nail matrix/nailbed.[7] Injections repeated every 4–5 weeks till clinical improved and tapering done by giving injection once in 6–8 weeks. If >3 nails involved intramuscular triamcinolone (0.5–1 mg/kg every month), oral immunosuppressants can be added.[7]

KEY POINTS

- LP is a chronic mucocutaneous inflammatory disease of unknown origin involving skin and mucosa.
- Myriad of clinical presentations and plurimucosal involvement.

TABLE 7: Histopathological features in lichenoid dermatosis.

Lichenoid variant	*Dermoscopic features*	*Histopathology*
LDEs	Absent WS	• *Epidermal changes:* Focal parakeratosis, acanthosis, cytoid bodies, satellite cell necrosis • Interface dermatitis with abundant eosinophils • Exocytosis of lymphoid cells into upper epidermis • Perivascular infiltrate, pigmentary incontinence
LN	• Keratin plug surrounded by annular cloud like areas • Mild scaling	• Thinned out epidermis with occasional basal cell degeneration • Focus of infiltrate, composed of lymphohistiocytes, plasma cells and Langhans giant cells encircled by elongated rete ridges ("claw clutching a ball")
LPLK	• Fissures and ridges • Milia like cysts, comedo like cysts • Cluster of gray dots	• Lichenoid inflammatory infiltrate with parakeratosis
Lichen sclerosus	• White structureless areas • Comedo like openings • Telangiectasia	• Lichenoid infiltrate with compact hyperkeratosis
Lichen striatus	• Well-delineated white structure • Yellow keratotic cerebriform structures • Red dots	• Acanthotic epidermis with lichenoid infiltrate • Melanophages in dermis • Apoptotic keratinocytes

(LDEs: lichenoid drug eruptions; LN: lichen nitidus; LPLK: lichen planus-like keratosis)

TABLE 8: Treatment of lichen planus.

Cutaneous LP		*Oral LP*	
Topical	*Systemic*	*General measures*	*Specific therapy*
Potent corticosteroids (First line) (Intralesional triamcinolone acetonide, 40 mg/mL in thick plaques)	Prednisolone (0.5–1 mg/kg body weight) *ACTH or tetracosactin:* Tapering dose over 6 weeks	Dental hygiene Removal of dental amalgam	Topical corticosteroid, betamethasone mouth washes, topical pimecrolimus, intralesional triamcinolone *Resistant/severe:* Oral glucocorticosteroids, cyclosporine and retinoids
Calcineurin inhibitors: Cyclosporine (5 mL to 100 mg/mL TID especially mouth wash or local massage), tacrolimus, pimecrolimus (oral and genital erosive LP)	Retinoids (Acitretin 0.2–0.3 mg/kg/day) Cyclosporine (1–6 mg/kg body weight per day) Azathioprine (100 mg/day) PUVA/NBUVB therapy	*Others:* Carbon dioxide and Nd:Yag laser therapy 308 nm UVB excimer laser	Griseofulvin, dapsone, hydroxychloroquine, itraconazole, metronidazole, low molecular weight heparin, thalidomide

- Significant association with hepatitis C.
- Potent corticosteroids are first line therapies.
- Cutaneous LP shows spontaneous resolution; mucosal tends to be resistant.
- Early identification and treatment essential in isolated nail LP.
- SCC tendency in hypertrophic LP and erosive LP.

REFERENCES

1. Daoud MS, Pittelkow MR. Lichen planus. In: Irwin MF, Eisen AZ, Wolff K, Austen KF, Goldsmith LA, Katz SI (Eds). Fitzpatrick's Dermatology in General Medicine, 6th edition. New York: McGraw-Hill; 2003. pp. 463-77.
2. Boyd AS, Neldner KH. Lichen planus. J Am Acad Dermatol. 1991;25:593-619.
3. Bhattacharya M, Kaur I, Kumar B. Lichen planus: a clinical and epidemiological study. J Dermatol. 2000;27:576-82.
4. Tziotzios C, Lee JYW, Brier T, Saito R, Hsu C-K, Bhargava K, et al. Lichen planus and lichenoid dermatoses. J Am Acad Dermatol. 2018;79:789-804.
5. Rajentheran R, McLean NR, Kelly CG, Reed MF, Nolan A. Malignant transformation of oral lichen planus. Eur J Surg Oncol.1999;25:520-3.
6. Gorouhi F, Davari P, Fazel N. Cutaneous and mucosal lichen planus: a comprehensive review of clinical subtypes, risk factors, diagnosis, and prognosis. Sci World J. 2014;1-22.
7. Lorizzo M, Tosti A, Starace M, Baran R, Daniel CR 3rd, Di Chiacchio N, et al. Isolated nail lichen planus: an expert consensus on treatment of the classical form. J Am Acad Dermatol. 2020;83(6):1717-23.
8. Breathnach SM, Black MM. Lichen planus and lichenoid disorders. In: Burns T, Breathnach S, Cox N, et al (Eds). Rook's Textbook of Dermatology, 7th edition. Oxford: Blackwell Science; 2004. pp. 42.1-32.
9. Masouye I, Saurat JM. Keratosis lichenoides chronic. The centenary of another Kaposi's disease. Dermatology. 1995;191:188-92.

10. Prigent F, Cavelier-Balloy B, Lemarchand-Venencie F, Civatte J. Lichen nitidus linéaire. Ann Dermatol Vénéréol. 1989;116; 814-5.

11. Daoud MS, Pittelkow MR. Lichen nitidus. In: Irwin MF, Eisen AZ, Wolff K, et al. (Eds). Fitzpatrick's Dermatology in General Medicine, 6th edition. New York: McGraw-Hill; 2003. pp. 478-81.

EXAMINATION QUESTIONS

1. Discuss approach and management of oral lichen planus.
2. How would you evaluate isolated nail lichen planus? How would you differentiate between lichen planus and lichenoid drug eruptions?

60 CHAPTER Porokeratosis

Rajesh K Mondal, Abhijit Saha

INTRODUCTION

- Porokeratosis is an uncommon cutaneous disorder of unknown origin, characterized clinically by keratotic papules and annular plaques with grooved keratotic borders and histopathologically by presence of cornoid lamellae.
- Numerous clinical variants are described with characteristic morphological presentation, distribution, and course. It mostly affects the sun-exposed skin and may be localized or widespread.
- The age and gender variations in occurrence of the disease depends on different clinical variants. Various genetic mutations are considered to give rise to this condition. Often there may be a familial predisposition which indicates a hereditary component.
- Ultraviolet (UV) radiation, immunosuppression, infections, and malignancy are usually considered to be associated with porokeratosis.
- Often it is considered as a premalignant condition so long-term follow-up is needed.
- Treatment is difficult and unsatisfactory.

EPIDEMIOLOGY

- The exact incidence and prevalence of the disease are not known.
- Usually, it affects adults mostly but certain types such as disseminated superficial porokeratosis (DSP) and porokeratosis of mibelli (PM) may also occur in childhood.[1]
- There is no known ethnic and racial variation.[2]
- Men and women are equally affected but certain data suggests that men are more commonly affected with PM and porokeratosis palmaris plantaris et disseminate (PPPD) whereas women are more affected by linear porokeratosis (LP) and disseminated superficial actinic porokeratosis (DSAP).[3]

PATHOGENESIS

- It is a disorder of keratinization which arises from clonal proliferation of keratinocytes. Though the exact etiology and pathogenesis are not known, it is considered to be multifactorial.
- *Genetic factor*:
  - Reports of multiple familial cases PM, DSAP, DSP, LP, and PPPD inherited as autosomal dominant trait with variable penetrance.[1,2]
  - Multiple genetic loci have been identified on different chromosomes, such as in DSAP five genetic loci on chromosomes 1, 12, 15, 16, and 18 are identified.[4-6]
  - Other genes identified are SSh1, SART3, and SLC17A9.[7]
  - Focal loss of heterozygosity through somatic mutation is considered to cause PM and LP variants.[8]
- *Ultraviolet radiation exposure*:
  - Sun-exposed sites are more involved, disease exacerbation is seen in summers.[1]
  - Also phototherapy-induced new lesions were observed in some studies.[9]
- *Immunosuppression*:
  - It is associated with hematologic malignancies, organ transplant, HIV infection, autoimmune diseases, and drugs.
  - Disseminated superficial actinic porokeratosis (DSAP) and PM variants are mostly associated with immunosuppression.[1,10]
- *Infections*: Hepatitis C (HCV), herpes simplex virus (HSV), human papillomavirus (HPV), and leishmania
- *Drugs*: Furosemide, hydrochlorothiazide, hydroxyurea, flucloxacillin, etanercept, and certolizumab are also reported to be associated with porokeratosis.[11,12]

CLINICAL FEATURES

Porokeratosis clinically presents as a keratotic papule or annular plaque with well-defined keratoticgrooved margin which may be atrophic and hyperpigmented. There are multiple clinical variants of porokeratosis **(Table 1)** with specific morphology, distribution, and clinical course and are summarized here.

Disseminated Actinic Superficial Porokeratosis

- It is the most common variant of porokeratosis and is directly associated with sunlight exposure.
- Females in third and fourth decade are affected more (M: F, 1:1.8).[1,2]

TABLE 1: Clinical variants of porokeratosis.

Clinical variant	*Age of onset*	*Triggering factor*	*Clinical feature*	*Malignant potential*	*Associations*
DSAP	Third to fourth decade, F > M	UV radiation	Numerous asymptomatic small annular papules, plaques with keratotic margin distributed symmetrically	Rarely associated with malignancy	
DSP	First decade (5–10 years)	Immuno-suppression	Numerous asymptomatic small annular papules, plaques with keratotic margin distributed symmetrically	Rare	Solid organ tumors
PM	Childhood	Immuno-suppression	Solitary to few in number, asymptomatic to pruritic annular plaques with keratotic margin with furrow affecting trunk or extremities	<10%	
EDP	Middle age, F > M	HCV, malignancy	Intensely pruritic Erythematous papules with keratotic margin	rare	Hepatic and hematological malignancy
LP	Childhood to adults, M > F		Asymptomatic small annular papules, plaques with keratotic margin arranged in a linear fashion following Blaschko lines	19%	
PPPD	Childhood to early adolescence, M > F	UV radiation	Small keratotic papules of 1–2 mm diameter over palms and soles, may affect mucosa and trunk	10%	
PP	Adolescent or young adults		Keratotic seed-like papules over palms and soles	Rare	
Porokeratosis ptychotropica	Middle age Mostly men	Trauma	Pruritic verrucous hyperkeratotic plaques on perianal area and buttocks	Rare	

(DSP: disseminated superficial porokeratosis; DSAP: disseminated superficial actinic porokeratosis; EDP: eruptive disseminated porokeratosis; LP: linear porokeratosis; PM: porokeratosis of mibelli; PPPD: porokeratosis palmaris plantaris et disseminate; UV: ultraviolet)

- It is characterized by small annular papules ranging from 2 to 7 mm which may coalesce to form plaques. The lesions progress slowly with radial expansion, the center becomes atrophic with well-demarcated thin elevated, furrowed, and keratotic rim.
- Lesions usually are on extensors and back and are bilaterally symmetrical.
- Palms, soles, and mucosa are spared.
- Lesions are mostly asymptomatic but there may be associated pruritus in about one-third of cases.

Disseminated Superficial Porokeratosis

- Disseminated superficial porokeratosis clinically resembles DSAP but UV radiation is not a triggering factor in DSP.
- Lesions may present over both exposed and nonexposed areas **(Fig. 1)**.
- The onset of disease is in 5–10 years of age.[1,2]

Porokeratosis of Mibelli

- Porokeratosis of mibelli is the next common type of porokeratosis.
- It usually occurs during infancy or childhood.
- Males are more commonly affected (M:F, 3:1).[1]
- The lesion starts as an asymptomatic skin-colored to brown keratotic papule which slowly enlarges to become an annular plaque of several centimeters in diameter **(Fig. 2)**. The margin is well-defined, elevated, and keratotic with a longitudinal furrow. Center of the lesion may be atrophic, hypopigmented, or hyperpigmented.
- The lesions usually involve extremities but may occur over any site involving mucosa and are unilateral and localized.
- Rarely, individual lesion may enlarge to exceed 20 cm and then known as giant porokeratosis which has the high malignant potential **(Fig. 3)**.[13]

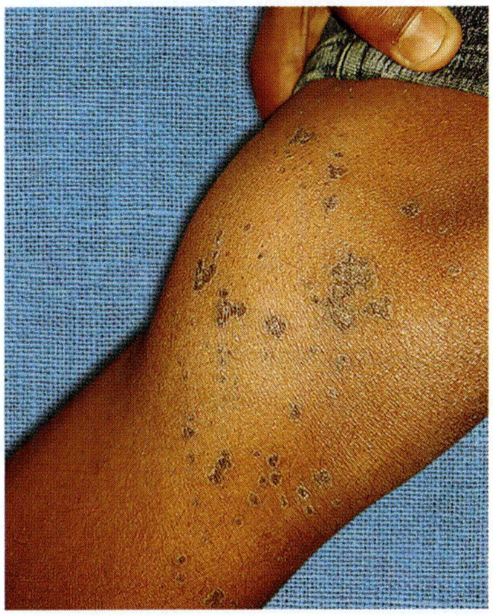

Fig. 1: Small keratotic papules and plaques in DSP.

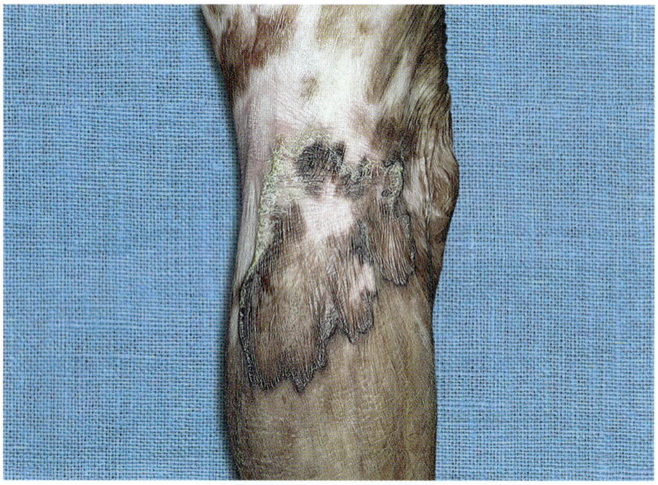

Fig. 2: Large annular plaque with grooved keratotic and hypertrophic margin and central atrophy in PM.

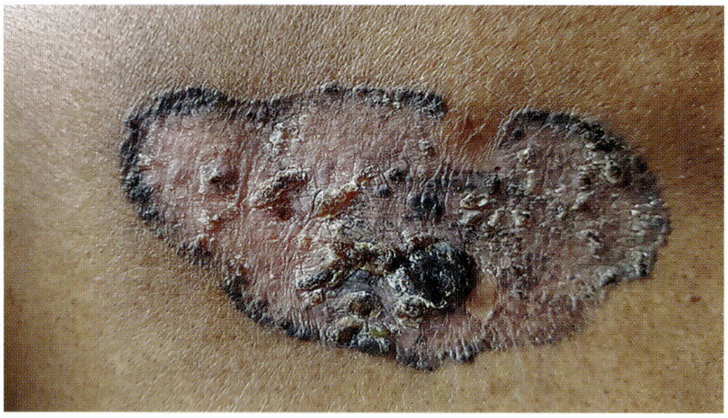

Fig. 3: Giant porokeratosis with malignant transformation. *Courtesy:* Dr Abhijit Saha.

Linear Porokeratosis

- Linear porokeratosis is an uncommon entity.
- It usually occurs in infancy and childhood.
- It is considered as a linear variant of PM by some authors.[14] The lesions are keratotic papules distributed in a linear pattern following Blaschko lines over extremities mostly **(Fig. 4)**.
- Individual lesions resemble PM morphologically.
- Sometimes, it may coexist with DSAP due to loss of heterozygosity.[14]

Eruptive Disseminated Porokeratosis

- It is rare variant of porokeratosis which is characterized by sudden onset of erythematous and pruritic papules and plaques with well-defined margin.
- It has been subdivided into paraneoplastic, immunosuppression-related and inflammatory forms by some authors.
- Eruptive disseminated porokeratosis mostly occurred in middle-aged men with half of them having other variant of porokeratosis previously.

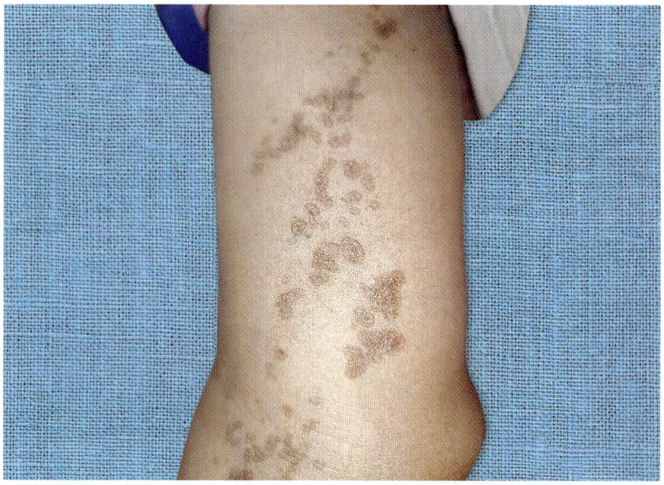

Fig. 4: Linearly arranged keratotic papules and plaques in linear variant of porokeatosis.

- Importantly one-third of patients with EDP had underlying hepatobiliary or hematologic malignancy,[15,16] so screening of every patient of EDP for underlying malignancy is important.
- 20% of EDP patients had associated viral infections suggesting immunosuppression.
- Mostly EDP resolves spontaneously.

Porokeratosis Palmaris Et Plantaris Disseminate

- It is a rare variant with autosomal dominant inheritance.
- It mainly affects adolescent males.
- Lesions resemble DSAP but are smaller (1–2 mm) in size and are distributed symmetrically. Mostly, it starts from palms and soles, and slowly affects other sites.[17]

Punctate Porokeratosis

- Punctate porokeratosis affects adolescents or young adults.
- It is characterized by multiple small seed-like keratotic papules over palms and soles sometimes resembling punctate keratoderma.
- This variant may occur in association of PM and LP variant of porokeratosis.[18]

Porokeratosis Ptychotropica

- It is a considered under genitogluteal variant of porokeratosis.
- It is very rare entity affecting middle-aged men.
- The lesions are characterized by pruritic, erythematous to brownish, verrucous, plaque distributed over perianal area, and the buttocks **(Fig. 5A)**. There may be satellite lesions. Sometimes genitalia may be affected **(Fig. 5B)**.[19,20]
- It is commonly confused with eczema or genital warts.

Other reported variants of porokeratosis **(Figs. 6A to C)** are:

- Follicular
- Pustular

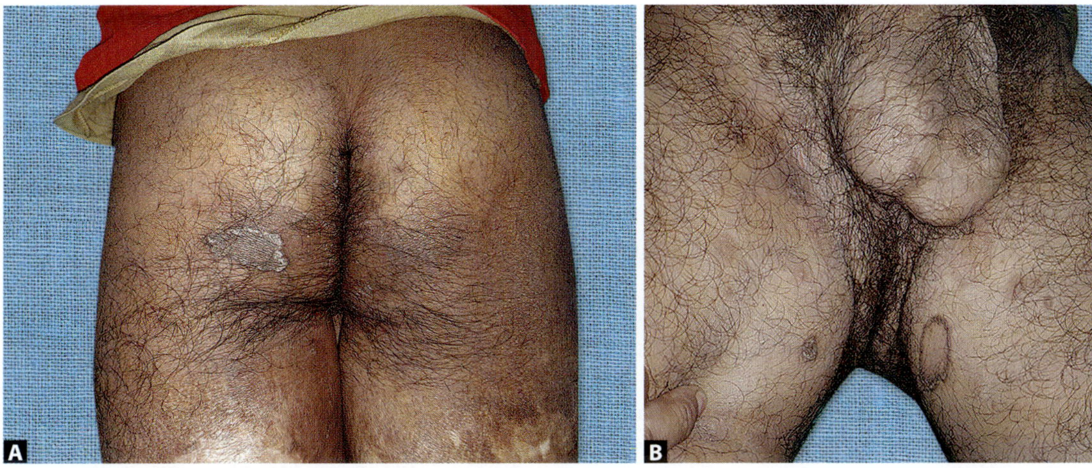

Figs. 5A and B: Annular plaqueswith keratotic grooved margin of porokeratoisiinvolving buttock and genitalia in Porokeratosisptychotropica.

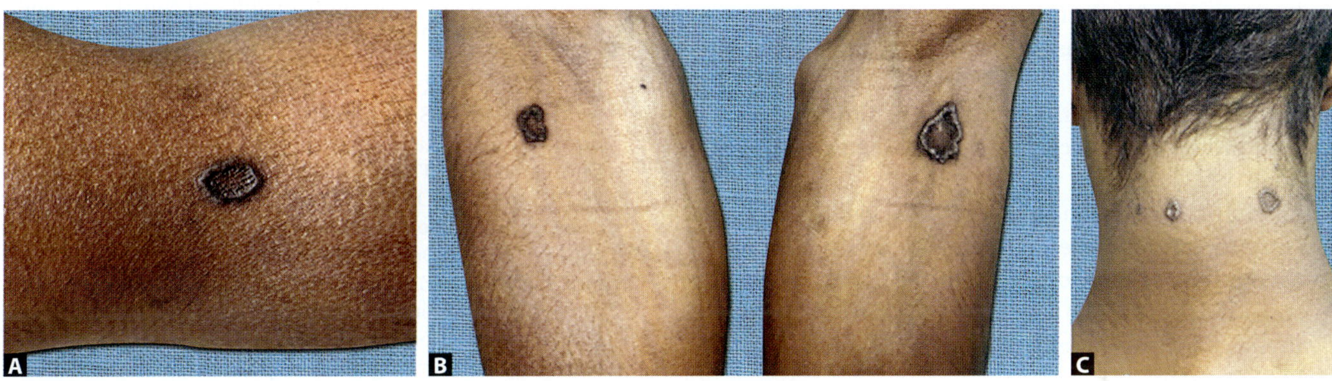

Figs. 6A to C: Porokeratosis.
Courtesy: Subhra Sankar Sahoo.

TABLE 2: Differential diagnoses of porokeratosis.

DSAP	*PM*	*LP*	*PPPD and PP*	*Porokeratosis ptychotropica*
• Lichen planus • Seborrheic keratosis • Guttate psoriasis	• Bowen's disease • Tinea corporis • Lichen simplex chronic	• Lichen striatus • Linear lichen planus • Inflammatory verrucous epidermal nevus	• Arsenical keratosis • Punctate palmoplantar keratoderma • Darier's disease	• Psoriasis • Viral wart • Acrodermatitis enteropathica
• Actinic keratosis	• Basal cell carcinoma	• Linear Darier's disease	• Gorlin's syndrome	• Necrolytic migratory erythema

(DSAP: disseminated superficial actinic porokeratosis; PM: porokeratosis of mibelli; LP: linear porokeratosis; PPPD: porokeratosis palmaris plantaris et disseminate)

- Bullous and reticulated
- Prurigo nodularis type
- Seborrheic dermatoses such as porokeratosis
- Porokeratotic eccrine ostial dermal duct nevus (PEODDN)
- Recently identified type porokeratoma.[21-25]

DIFFERENTIAL DIAGNOSIS

The differential diagnoses of porokeratosis are based on the different variants and are mentioned in the **Table 2**.

DIAGNOSIS

- The diagnosis of porokeratosis can be done clinically.
- Dermoscopy shows hyperkeratotic yellow or brown peripheral edge known as "double track sign" with homogeneous central scar like area. Irregular globular and linear vessels may be seen.
- In doubtful cases, skin biopsy is confirmative:
  - Biopsy should be done from the margin of the lesion.

- The "cornoid lamellae" is the sine qua non for histopathological diagnosis. It is characterized by column of tightly packed parakeratotic cells.
- There is hypogranulosis or agranulosis just below the cornoid lamellae.
- Dyskeratotic and pyknotic keratinocytes may be present in spinous layer.
- There may be perivascular lymphocytic infiltration in the dermis.
- Sometimes multiple cornoid lamellae may be present especially in porokeratoma and genitogluteal variants.
- Cornoid lamellae may also be seen in verruca vulgaris and actinic keratosis which should be considered as histopathological differentials.

TREATMENT

- Porokeratosis has a chronic course and is refractory to treatment. Only few cases (16%) show complete clearance of lesions.
- Counseling regarding the course and nature of the disease with proper avoidance of triggering factors should be done.
- Careful observation and regular follow-ups with adequate sun protection and emollients can be done in early, asymptomatic and localized cases. Special attention should be paid to large lesions, PM, LP, and PPPD variants. Investigating any underlying malignancy should be done in EDP variant.
- Topical therapy includes 5-FU, retinoids, imiquimod 5%, and vitamin D analog and is worth trying in localized cases.[26]
- Oral retinoid may be used in DSAP and other widespread lesions.[26]
- Other less common treatment modalities include cryotherapy, shaving, curettage, dermabrasion, electrodessication, photodynamic therapy (PDT), and laser.

PROGNOSIS

The prognosis of most variants is very good especially for DSP. Large lesions and linear variant should be carefully followed as there is chance of malignant transformation. PM involving any digit circumferentially may lead to pseudoainhum. Large lesions over face may involve soft tissue and cause disfigurement.

KEY POINTS

- Porokeratosis is an uncommon disease with clonal proliferation of keratinocytes.
- The etiopathogenesis is multifactorial, UV radiation exposure, genetic cause, infections, and immunosuppression are commonly associated factors.
- Various clinical variants are described; DSAP is the most common among them. LP variant is having highest malignant potentiality.
- Presence of cornoid lamellae is the histological hallmark of disease identification.
- Response to treatment is variable, avoiding the triggering factors and careful observation is important. Sometimes resolves spontaneously.

REFERENCES

1. Kanitakis J. Porokeratoses: an update of clinical, aetiopathogenic and therapeutic features. Eur J Dermatol. 2014;24:533-44.
2. Sertznig P, von Felbert V, Megahed M. Porokeratosis: present concepts. J Eur Acad Dermatol Venereol. 2012;26:404-12.
3. Leow YH, Soon YH, Tham SN. A report of 31 cases of porokeratosis at the National Skin Centre. Ann Acad Med Singapore. 1996;25:837-41.
4. Xia JH, Yang YF, Deng H, Tang BS, Tang DS, He YG, et al. Identification of a locus for disseminated superficial actinic porokeratosis at chromosome 12q23.2-24.1. J Invest Dermatol. 2000;114:1071-4.
5. Xia K, Deng H, Xia JH, Zheng D, Zhang HL, Lu CY, et al. A novel locus (DSAP2) for disseminated superficial actinic porokeratosis maps to chromosome 15q25.1-26.1. Br J Dermatol. 2002;147(4):650-4.
6. Wei S, Yang S, Lin D, Li M, Zhang X, Bu L, et al. A novel locus for disseminated superficial porokeratosis maps to chromosome 18p11.3. J Invest Dermatol. 2004;123:872-5.
7. FuX, Liu T, Wang Z, Zhou G, Yu M, Lu X, et al. Two novel SSH1 mutations in Chinese patients with disseminated superficial actinic porokeratosis and immunohistochemical analysis of anti-slings hot homolog 1 antibody in one typical patient. J Eur Acad Dermatol Venereol. 2019;33:e486-8.
8. Murase J, Gilliam AC. Disseminated superficial actinic porokeratosis co-existing with linear and verrucous porokeratosis in an elderly woman: update on the genetics and clinical expression of porokeratosis. J Am Acad Dermatol. 2010;63:886-91.
9. Marque M, Meunier L. Porokeratosis. Ann Dermatol Venereol. 2012;139:668-76.
10. Pini M, Balice Y, Tavecchio S, Crippa D. Eruptive disseminated porokeratosis following bone marrow transplantation for acute lymphoblastic leukemia in a child. J Dermatol. 2012;39:403-4.
11. Goulding JMR, Teoh JK, Carr RA, Humphreys F, Gee BC. Eruptive disseminated superficial porokeratosis with rapid resolution: a drug-induced phenomenon? Clin Exp Dermatol. 2009;34:895-7.
12. Mangas C, Espeli V, Blum R. A case of eruptive disseminated porokeratosis in a cancer patient after trastuzumab and exemestane treatment: cancer-related or drug-induced phenomenon? Actas Dermosifiliogr. 2018;109:559-60.
13. Vence L, Thompson CB, Callen JP, Brown TS. Giant porokeratosis with malignant transformation to squamous cell carcinoma. Dermatol Surg. 2018;44:580-1.
14. Schwarz N, Stadie V, Kreft B, Happle R, Marsch WCh, Fiedler E. Systematized linear porokeratosis: concept of type 2 segmental manifestation implies an increased cancer risk. J Dermatol. 2012;39:953-4.
15. Schena D, Papagrigoraki A, Frigo A, Girolomoni G. Eruptive disseminated porokeratosis associated with internal malignancies: a case report. Cutis. 2010;85:156-9.

16. Kono T, Kobayashi H, Ishii M, Nishiguchi S, Taniguchi S. Synchronous development of disseminated superficial porokeratosis and hepatitis C virus-related hepatocellular carcinoma. J Am Acad Dermatol. 2000;43:966-8.
17. Chinmay K, Prodip S, Sabyasachi B, Rabindranath B, Pallab D. Porokeratosis palmaris et plantaris disseminata: a rare entity. J Pak Assoc Dermatol. 2017;26:371-4.
18. Lanka P, Lanka LR, Manivachagam D. Punctate porokeratosis palmaris et plantaris. Indian J Dermatol. 2015;60:284-6.
19. Joshi R, Minni K. Genitogluteal porokeratosis: a clinical review. Clin Cosmet Investig Dermatol. 2018;11:219-29.
20. Miller DD, Ruben BS. Pustular porokeratosis. J Cutan Pathol. 2009;36:1191-3.
21. Watanabe T, Murakami T, Okochi H, Kikuchi K, Furue M. Ulcerative porokeratosis. Dermatology. 1998;196:256-9.
22. Ricci C, Rosset A, Panizzon RG. Bullous and pruritic variant of disseminated superficial actinic porokeratosis: successful treatment with grenz rays. Dermatology. 1999;199:328-31.
23. Helfman RJ, Poulos EG. Reticulated porokeratosis: a unique variant of porokeratosis. Arch Dermatol. 1985;121:1542-3.
24. Kang BD, Kye YC, Kim SN. Disseminated superficial actinic porokeratosis with both typical and prurigo nodularis-like lesions. J Dermatol. 2001;28:81-5.
25. Asawanonda P, Noppakun N, Huiprasert P. Seborrheic keratosis-like porokeratosis: a case report. Dermatol Online J. 2005;11:18. 84.
26. Weidner T, Illing T, Miguel D, Elsner P. Treatment of porokeratosis: a systematic review. Am J Clin Dermatol. 2017;18:435-49.

EXAMINATION QUESTIONS

1. Write a short note on porokeratosis.
2. Describe the classification, clinical features, diagnosis and treatment of porokeratosis.

61 CHAPTER

Perforating Disorders

Abhijit Saha, Maitreyee Sengupta

INTRODUCTION

The perforating disorders are a diverse group of conditions characterized by crusted keratotic papules sharing the common pathological feature of transepidermal elimination. Dermal connective tissue "perforates" or is eliminated through the epidermis.[1] There are four major perforating disorders. They include: Kyrle's disease, reactive perforating collagenosis (RPC), elastosis perforans serpiginosa (EPS), and perforating folliculitis. This classification is primarily based on the nature of the eliminated material and the type of epidermal disruption. Certain other papulonodular conditions are classified as secondary perforating disorders including perforating granuloma annulare, perforating calcinosis, perforating pseudoxanthoma elasticum, necrobiosis lipoidica, etc.

PATHOGENESIS

- The precise pathogenesis for the perforating disorders is unknown. However, trauma is a clear trigger of perforating disorders, although the molecular basis is unclear.
- It is unlikely that dermal connective tissue or hair shafts actively perforate into the epithelium, so some have argued that "transepidermal elimination" is a more accurate term.[1]
- Epithelium becomes hyperplastic and eventually surrounds the abnormal connective tissue, just as with foreign bodies. In Kyrle's disease and RPC, pruritus leads to chronic scratching, followed by an abnormal healing response after excoriation, where the regenerating epidermis forms epidermal tunnels through which the central necrotic mass and its associated collagen bundles are lifted.[1,2]
- The perforating diseases may be due to either genetic or acquired abnormalities of collagen or elastic fibers. In EPS, interactions between elastin and elastin receptors on keratinocytes have been observed. In Kyrle's disease, the primary event is claimed to be a disturbance of epidermal keratinization characterized by the formation of dyskeratotic foci and acceleration of the process of keratinization.
- Fibronectin levels have been shown to be increased in the serum of patients with diabetes mellitus and uremia, and it is also increased in the skin at sites of perforating lesions.[2,3] Fibronectin plays a role in epithelial cell signaling, locomotion, and differentiation. It binds to type IV collagen (found in basement membranes) and to keratinocytes, and may incite epithelial proliferation and perforation.
- Koebner's phenomenon has been demonstrated and lesions can be produced experimentally by traumatizing the skin and after laser hair removal. Evidence supports an underlying dermal microvasculopathy in some patients and aberrant epidermal migration in others.
- Other proposed pathomechanisms include abnormal vitamin D metabolism, vitamin A deficiency or excess, enzyme release from neutrophils, microangiopathy related to diabetes, elevated plasma silicon levels in patients on dialysis, salt water chemical burns, and an imbalance in the expression of metalloproteinases and their tissue inhibitors.[3]

The salient features of the four major perforating disorders are individually described here.

1. Kyrle's Disease

- In 1916, Kyrle reported a diabetic woman with generalized hyperkeratotic nodules, which he called hyperkeratosis follicularis et parafollicularis in cutem penetrans.[4]
- Kyrle's disease has two distinct forms: (1) An inherited form that presents in childhood and (2) an acquired form that usually develops in adulthood, more commonly in women between 30 and 50 years of age associated with some underlying systemic disorder (diabetes or renal disease and less commonly, with liver disease or internal malignancy).[5]
- *Clinical features*:
  - Lesions are characterized by umbilicated papules with central white, keratotic crusts that can become quite hyperkeratotic and can resemble prurigo nodularis.[4]
  - The lesions most often develop on the arms and legs, but any site can be affected, including the trunk and scalp.
  - Lesions are almost always pruritic and scratching can lead to koebnerization.
- *Histopathology*:
  - In all perforating disorders, there is an invagination of the epidermis with extrusion of altered dermal

substance into the necrotic basophilic tissue within the invaginated, cup-shaped epidermal depression.

- There is a plug of crusting or hyperkeratosis, with a variable column of parakeratosis, depending upon the stage of the lesion. A dense dermal inflammatory infiltrate with granulomatous reaction is present.
- In Kyrle's disease, amorphous dermal material and/or keratin perforates through the epidermis. The lesions may be follicular or extrafollicular. Masson trichrome stain has demonstrated collagen bundles at the base of the epidermal invagination, suggesting an overlap with RPC.[3,5]

- *Differential diagnosis*:
  - *Other perforating disorders*: RPC, perforating folliculitis
  - Prurigo nodularis, arthropod bites, multiple kerato-acanthomas
  - Perforating of exogenous foreign materials such as silica, wood, etc.

2. Reactive Perforating Collagenosis

- Mehregan, Schwartz and Livingood reported the first child with RPC in 1967. Like Kyrle's disease, RPC is also seen in two forms: Inherited and secondary.[6]
- *Clinical features*:
  - The inherited form of RPC is a rare familial disorder that begins during childhood. Acquired RPC begins during adulthood, especially in association with diabetes mellitus or renal insufficiency.[2,3]
  - After superficial trauma, patients develop pruritic keratotic umbilicated papules which reach a size of 5–8 mm over the following 3–4 weeks. The papules tend to spontaneously resolve over 6–8 weeks.
  - Arms and hands are the most common sites of involvement but any site like trunk or scalp may be involved.
  - Koebnerization is more commonly observed with RPC than with the other perforating disorders, leading to new lesions in a linear distribution.
  - Verrucous perforating collagenoma (*collagenome perforant verruciformé*) is a very rare nonfamilial variant of RPC in which severe trauma to the skin results in verrucous papules with transepidermal elimination of collagen.[6]
- *Histopathology*:
  - Microscopic examination of the keratotic papule shows a plug of hyperkeratosis with variable parakeratosis.
  - Collagen fibers are seen within the plug or within the epidermis while the dermal connective tissue adjacent to the plug appears unremarkable.[1,3,6]
  - The Verhoeff-van Gieson stain is helpful in differentiating RPC from EPS, because collagen fibers appear red and elastic fibers appear black.
- *Differential diagnosis*:
  - *Other perforating disorders*: Kyrle's disease, EPS, perforating pseudoxanthoma elasticum
  - *Excoriated dermal diseases*: Prurigo nodularis, prurigo simplex, arthropod bites
  - *Other conditions with Koebnerization*: Lichen planus, psoriasis

3. Perforating Folliculitis

- Perforating folliculitis was first described by Mehregan and Coskey as a perforating disorder in 1968.[7] However, some authorities do not consider it a specific entity, since rupture of follicles occurs in a wide variety of folliculitis, regardless of whether caused by bacteria, fungi, *Demodex* mites, physical trauma, or other mechanisms.
- Perforating folliculitis has overlapping features with Kyrle's disease. It is a relatively uncommon disorder usually observed in the 2nd to 4th decade.
- Clinically, it is characterized by umbilicated papules with central white, keratotic crusts centered on a hair follicle.
- Perforating folliculitis is characterized histologically by follicular perforation. A focal inflammatory infiltrate is seen adjacent to areas of perforation of the follicular epithelium.[1]
- Degenerating collagen and extracellular matrix tissues mixed with inflammatory cells and orthokeratotic and parakeratotic material fill the dilated hair follicle. Occasionally, a curled up hair is seen close to or within the area of perforation or even in the dermis, surrounded by a foreign body granuloma.
- Perforating folliculitis has to be differentiated from prurigo nodularis, other forms of folliculitis and Flegel disease (hyperkeratosis follicularis perstans).

4. Elastosis Perforans Serpiginosa

- Lutz first described EPS as keratosis follicularis serpiginosa in 1953, and, in 1955, Miescher described the histologic findings, naming it elastoma intrapapillare perforans verruciforme.[8]
- EPS is a unique perforating disorder characterized by transepidermal elimination of elastic fibers. Although most cases are sporadic, familial cases of EPS have been reported with different modes of inheritance.
- *Clinical features*:
  - EPS begins during childhood or early adulthood. It affects nearly four times more men than women.
  - A clear trigger for EPS appears to be D-penicillamine, which disrupts desmosine crosslinks within elastin. It is usually seen after long-term therapy of Wilson disease or cystinuria. Abnormal elastic fibers have been found in the lungs as well as the skin of penicillamine-treated patients.[8]

 - About 40% of cases occur in association with other genetic disorders and connective tissue diseases, including Down syndrome, Ehlers-Danlos syndrome, osteogenesis imperfecta, Marfan syndrome, pseudoxanthoma elasticum, cutis laxa, Rothmund-Thomson syndrome, and acrogeria.[8]
 - Cutaneous lesions are keratotic 2-5 mm papules arranged in a serpiginous or annular pattern, most commonly on the lateral neck, but also on the face, arms or other flexural areas. The rings of papules may reach several centimeters in size. Skin within these serpiginous arcs is often atrophic.
 - The lesions may be mildly pruritic, but are otherwise asymptomatic. They may spontaneously resolve, but they tend to persist longer, often for several years.
 - In rare instances, elastic tissue in the endocardium, bronchiolar walls, and arteries is involved. Rupture of the aorta has been reported.
- *Histopathology*:
 - Histologically, transepidermal elimination of elastic fibers is seen through the plug of hyperkeratosis. Elastic fibers are stained black with the Verhoeff-Van Gieson stain. However, higher up in the epidermis, the elastic fibers may lose their ability to stain black.[1]
 - The elastic tissue penetrates through straight or tortuous channels in the acanthotic epidermis. The channels also contain necrobiotic material with degenerated epithelial cells and parakeratotic nuclei of inflammatory cells.
 - A characteristic inflammatory infiltrate of lymphocytes, macrophages or multinucleated giant cells are present in the dermis at the site of perforation. Also, an increased amount of brightly eosinophilic elastic tissue is often present in the superficial dermis.
 - In penicillamine-induced EPS, characteristic *"lumpy-bumpy"* elastic fibers with lateral buds resembling a *"bramble bush"* are seen in both lesional and nonlesional skin.
- *Differential diagnosis*:
 - *Other perforating disorders*: RPC, perforating pseudoxanthoma elasticum
 - *Other annular diseases*: Tinea, sarcoidosis, granuloma annulare
 - Porokeratosis, discoid lupus erythematosus, actinic granuloma

TREATMENT

- The perforating disorders are difficult to treat. The prognosis is tied to the underlying diseases, so treatment of the underlying cause can be effective. Perforating disorders frequently resolve after renal transplantation in patients with underlying kidney failure.
- Topical corticosteroids and retinoids may be successful in some cases and are the first line of therapy. Patients with mild RPC may be satisfied to simply avoid trauma and wait for lesions to resolve spontaneously.[6]
- Phototherapy with narrow band ultraviolet B (UVB) or broadband UVB can result in substantial improvement, but is not as reliably effective as phototherapy for uremic pruritus.[9]
- Systemic agents include oral retinoids, allopurinol, doxycycline, and oral clindamycin (often combined with surgery).
- EPS may be treated with local cryotherapy, tangential excision, electrosurgical destruction, or cellophane tape stripping.[8] Aggressive treatment is more likely to result in scarring. Intralesional corticosteroids may be helpful.
- Treatment of generalized acquired perforating dermatosis or extensive perforating folliculitis is often difficult. Antihistamines are marginally helpful.

KEY POINTS

- The perforating disorders are a group of papulonodular conditions characterized by transepidermal elimination. They have classically been divided into four types: Kyrle's disease, RPC, perforating folliculitis, and EPS.
- The epidermis becomes hyperkeratotic and surrounds the abnormal connective tissue which is then lifted through the epidermal tunnel. The four disorders are differentiated depending on the type of material extruded.
- Kyrle's disease may present in childhood (inherited) or adulthood (acquired) with crusted, umbilicated papules on the extremities. Keratin and/or necrotic debris admixed with few collagen fibers is usually extruded through these papules.
- RPC may also be inherited or acquired and the keratotic papules usually appear following some minor trauma over the arms or hands. Koebnerization is common and histology shows collagen fibers being extruded.
- Perforating folliculitis lesions are centered on a hair follicle. Microscopy shows dilated follicles with or without a curled up hair.
- EPS presents in childhood or early adulthood with keratotic papules arranged in a serpiginous or annular pattern, most commonly on the lateral neck. Microscopically, elastic fibers are seen in the epidermal tunnel surrounded by a brightly eosinophilic chronic inflammatory infiltrate.
- Kyrle's disease and RPC are commonly seen in patients of diabetes mellitus and chronic renal insufficiency, while EPS has been linked to D-penicillamine.
- Sometimes, the lesions may resolve spontaneously, particularly if the underlying cause is stabilized, but treatment is often unsatisfactory.

REFERENCES

1. Naik NS, Nousari CH, Heilman ER, Friedman RJ. Degenerative diseases and perforating disorders. In: Elder DE (Ed). Lever's Histopathology of the Skin, 9th edition. Philadelphia: JB Lippincott Williams and Wilkins; 2005. pp. 401-17.
2. Bilezikci B, Seckin D, Demirhan B. Acquired perforating dermatosis in patients with chronic renal failure: a possible role for fibronectin. J Eur Acad Dermatol Venereol. 2003;17: 230-2.
3. Haftek M, Euvrard S, Kanitakis J, Delawari E, Schmitt D. Acquired perforating dermatosis of diabetes mellitus and renal failure: further ultrastructural clues to its pathogenesis. J Cutan Pathol. 1993;20:350-5.
4. Kyrle J. Hyperkeratosis follicularis et parafollicularis in cutem penetrans. Arch Derm Syph. 1916;123:466-93.
5. Viswanathan S, Narurkar SD, Rajpal A, Nagpur NG, Avasare SS. Rare presentation of Kyrle's disease in siblings. Indian J Dermatol. 2008;53:85-7.
6. Yancovitz M, Johnson H, Wang N, Pomeranz MK. Perforating collagenosis. Dermatol Online J. 2008;14:14.
7. Mehregan AH, Coskey RJ. Perforating folliculitis. Arch Dermatol. 1968;97:394.
8. Mehta RK, Burrows NP, Payne CM, Mendelsohn SS, Pope FM, Rytina E. Elastosis perforans serpiginosa and associated disorders. Clin Exp Dermatol. 2001;26:521-4.
9. Ohe S, Danno K, Sasaki H, Isei T, Okamoto H, Horio T. Treatment of acquired perforating dermatosis with narrowband ultraviolet B. J Am Acad Dermatol. 2004;50:892-4.

EXAMINATION QUESTIONS

1. Explain perforating disorders in dermatology.
2. Write the clinical features of various dermatoses due to transepidermal elimination.

62 CHAPTER Ichthyosis

Abhishek De, Aarti Sarda, Sachi Gupta

INTRODUCTION

Ichthyoses are disorders of cornification in which abnormal differentiation and/or desquamation of the epidermis result in a defective epidermal barrier. Ichthyoses represent a large genetically and phenotypically heterogeneous group of conditions that feature generalized scaling of the skin. Ichthyosis can be an inherited disease; or can be acquired from multiple infective or noninfective conditions. Inherited ichthyosis can present as a single entity or may be a part of more generalized syndromes involving multiple systems.[1]

NOMENCLATURE

Robert Willan introduced the term "ichthyosis," from the Greek word *"ichthy" meaning fish.*[1]

HISTORY

- A disease called Ekakushtha, with scales resembling that of fishes, was mentioned in an ancient Indian literature in 250 BC.
- In 1730, Porcupine man was described (Ichthyosis hystrix).
- Alibert mentioned the autosomal dominant inheritance of ichthyosis vulgaris (1806).
- Willan first used the terminology of ichthyosis as squamous disease (1808).
- Description of harlequin ichthyosis was found in the early 19th century.
- Brocq first recognized variants of congenital ichthyosis as bullous and nonbullous.
- Brocq also coined the name "congenital ichthyosiform erythroderma" (1902).
- Frost and Van Scott described autosomal recessive inheritance of "lamellar ichthyosis" (1966).[1]

CLASSIFICATION[2]

Ichthyosis can be congenital and acquired. Congenital ichthyosis can be divided into a nonsyndromic and syndromic form.

I. CONGENITAL ICHTHYOSIS		
A. Nonsyndromic Congenital Ichthyosis		
Common ichthyosis:		
Ichthyosis vulgaris	Autosomal semi-dominant	*(Filaggrin) FLG gene (1q21.3)*
X-linked recessive ichthyosis	XLR	*(Steroid sulfatase) STS gene (Xp22.32)*
Nonsyndromic autosomal recessive congenital ichthyoses:		
Lamellar ichthyosis	Autosomal recessive (AR)	*Type 1: Transglutaminase 1 gene (TGM1) (14q12)* *Type 2: ABCA12 (2q35)*
Harlequin ichthyosis	AR	*ABCA12 (2q35)* *[ATP-binding cassette (ABC) subfamily A member 12]*
Congenital ichthyosiform erythroderma (nonbullous)	AR	*TGM1 (14q12)* *12R-lipoxygenase gene (ALOX12B) (17p13.1)* *Lipoxygenase 3 gene (ALOXE3) (17p13.1)*
Keratinopathic ichthyoses:		
Epidermolytic ichthyosis (bullous CIE)	Autosomal dominant (AD)	*(Keratin 1) KRT1 (12q13.13),* *(Keratin 10) KRT10 (17q21.2)*
Superficial epidermolytic ichthyosis (ichthyosis bullosa of Siemens)	AD	*(Keratin 2) KRT2 (12q11–q13)*
Ichthyosis hystrix (Curth–Macklin)	AD	*(Keratin 1) KRT1 (12q11–q13)*

Contd...

Contd...

Rarer nonsyndromic ichthyosis:		
Acral self-healing collodion baby	AR	*(Transglutaminase 1) TGM1*
Bathing suit ichthyosis	AR	*(Transglutaminase 1) TGM1*
Congenital reticular ichthyosiform erythroderma (CRIE)	AD	*(Keratin 10) KRT10 (17q21–q22)*
Annular epidermolytic ichthyosis (AEI)	AD	*(Keratin 1, 10) KRT1, KRT10*
Epidermolytic nevi	Somatic mutations	*(Keratin 1, 10) KRT1, KRT10*
Erythrokeratodermias:		
Erythrokeratodermia variabilis	AD	*Connexin 31, Connexin 30.3* *Gap junction B3 (GJB3) (1p35.1)* *Gap junction B4 (GJB) (1p35.1)*
Progressive symmetric erythrokeratoderma	AD/AR	*Loricrin (LOR) (1q21.3)* *Gap junction B4 (GJB4) (1p34.3)*
B. Congenital Ichthyosiform Syndromes		
Netherton syndrome (Ichthyosis linearis circumflexa + Atopy + Trichorrhexis invaginata)	AR	*Serine protease inhibitor Kazal type 5 gene (SPINK5) (5q33.1)*
Sjögren–Larsson syndrome (*I*chthyosis+ *C*erebral palsy + *M*ental retardation + *R*etinopathy)	AR	*Fatty aldehyde dehydrogenase gene (ALDH3A2) (17p11.2)*
Refsum disease (Retinitis pigmentosa + Mixed sensory motor neuropathy + Ichthyosis vulgaris + Sensory-neural deafness + Ataxia + Anosmia)	AR	*Phytanoyl-CoA hydroxylase PHYH (10p13),* *Peroxisome biogenesis factor 7 PEX7 (6q23.3)*
IBID (*Syn*: Trichothiodystrophy/TAY syndrome) (Decreased sulfur contain in hair and DNA repair defect Ichthyosis + brittle hair + MR + decreased fertility + short stature) PIBID (with photosensitivity) SIBID (with scleroderma)	AR	*ERCC3 (19q13.32)* *GTF2H5 (2q14.3 6q25.3)*
KID (Keratitis + deafness + ichthyosis)	AD	*Connexin 26, (Gap junction b2)GJB2 (13q12.11)*
HID (Hystrix like ichthyosis + deafness)		
CHILD (Congenital hemidysplasia + IE + limb defect)	XLD	*NSDHL (Xq28)*
Conradi–Hünerman–Happle syndrome (Chondrodysplasia punctata + ichthyosis + cataract)	XLD	*Emopamil-binding protein (EBP) (Xp11.23)*
RUD syndrome (X-linked recessive ichthyosis + mental retardation + epilepsy + hypogonadism + obesity + endocrinopathy)		
IFAP (Ichthyosis follicularis + alopecia + photophobia)	XLR	*MBTPS2*
Neutral lipid storage disease (*Syn*: Chanarin–Dorfman syndrome)	AR	*Abhydrolase domain containing 5 gene (ABHD5) 3p21.33*
II. ACQUIRED ICHTHYOSIS		
Drugs	Clofazimine, statins, nicotinic acid, allopurinol, maprotiline,	
Malignancy	Hodgkin, non-Hodgkin, CTCL, CA (breast, lung, liver)	
Infection	HIV, leprosy	
Metabolic	Malabsorption, malnutrition, essential FA deficiency	
Connective tissue disease	SLE, DM, eosinophilic fasciitis	
Endocrine disease	CRF, thyroid, parathyroid, pituitary	
Granulomatous disease	Sarcoidosis	
Miscellaneous	Post-BM transplant	

Major Ichthyosis[3-5]

	Ichthyosis vulgaris (Fig. 1)	*X-linked recessive ichthyosis (Fig. 3)*	*Lamellar ichthyosis (Figs. 2A to C)*	*Bullous congenital ichthyosiform erythroderma*	*Nonbullous ichthyosiform erythroderma*
Introduction	• *Syn*: Autosomal dominant ichthyosis • Most common type • Least severe type	• *Syn*: Steroid sulfatase deficiency • Associated obstetrics and extra cutaneous manifestation	• *Syn*: Autosomal recessive congenital ichthyosis-1 (ARCI-1) • Lamella means Plate • Was described as Alligator baby	*Syn*: Epidermolytic hyperkeratosis (EI)	*Syn*: Autosomal recessive congenital ichthyosis-2 (ARCI-2)
Epidemiology	• *Prevalence*: 1:250 • Male = Female	• *Incidence*: <1:2,000 male birth • Affects male child • Females are carriers	• Autosomal recessive inheritance • 1 in 200,000 prevalence • Parental consanguinity	• Rare (prevalence 1 in 200,000) • Male = Female	• Autosomal recessive • Slightly more prevalent than lamellar ichthyosis • Affects 1 in 100,000 • Milder than those of classic lamellar ichthyosis • *Consanguinity*: Usually present
Pathogenesis	• Autosomal semi-dominant • Loss of function mutation in *FLG* gene (1q21.3) • *Animal model*: Flaky tail mouse • Retention hyperkeratosis is seen • FLG encodes profilaggrin • Decreased conversion of profilaggrin to filaggrin • Diminished granular layer • Filaggrin deficiency results in impaired squamous cell formation, transepidermal water loss and a propensity to develop allergic diseases	• X-linked recessive • Reduced or absent steroid sulfatase activity • Mutation of steroid sulfatase (*STS*) gene (Xp22.31) • STS deficiency results in impaired hydrolysis of cholesterol sulfate and dehydroepiandrosterone sulfate (DHEAS) with accumulation of cholesterol 3-sulfate in the epidermis • This inhibit transglutaminase-1; hampering formation of the cornified envelope and epidermal barrier	• Transglutaminase-1 deficiency (most patients) due to mutations in *TGM1* gene • *TGM1* mutations perturb cornification and desquamation • Mutations in the ATP-binding cassette subfamily A member 12 gene (*ABCA12*) were also reported. This affects energy-dependent transport of lipid substrates across membranes and function of lamellar bodies • Mutations in the *CYP4F22* gene are also described	• Autosomal dominant disorder with complete penetrance • Keratin 1 (*KRT1*) and keratin 10 (*KRT10*) gene mutation (chromosome 12 and 17) • Defective synthesis of keratin 1 and 10 keratin alignment, oligomerization and filament assembly is disturbed • Weakened cytoskeleton and compromised cellular integrity of the epidermis	• At least five different genes are reported • Transglutaminase-1 gene (minority of patients) • Type II—ATP binding Cassette *A12* gene (*ABCA12*) • Two lipoxygenase (*LOX*) genes— *ALOX12B* and *ALOXE3*
Histopathology	• Mild orthokeratotic hyperkeratosis • Attenuated/absent granular layer • Immunostaining demonstrates a reduced or absent filaggrin	• Hyperkeratosis or parakeratosis • Normal or slightly thickened granular layer • Follicular hyperkeratosis	• Orthokeratotic hyperkeratosis • Acanthosis	• Orthokeratotic hyperkeratosis • Acanthosis • Hypergranulosis • Suprabasal cytolysis • Intraepidermal blisters • Granular layer—perinuclear halo and split	• Prominent parakeratosis • Hypergranulosis • Pronounced acanthosis
Electron microscopy	Fragmented or absent KHG	• Increased keratohyalin granules • Abnormal persistence of desmosomes in the stratum corneum	• Variable numbers of translucent lipid droplets in the stratum corneum • Elongated cholesterol cleft • Thin or absent cornified cell envelope	• Fragmented, clumped keratin intermediate filament (KIF) in the lower epidermis • Perinuclear KIF shells in the upper epidermis	• Increased number of lamellar bodies • Accumulation of lipid droplets in the stratum corneum • Disorganized intercellular lipid lamellae

Contd...

Contd...

	Ichthyosis vulgaris (Fig. 1)	*X-linked recessive ichthyosis (Fig. 3)*	*Lamellar ichthyosis (Figs. 2A to C)*	*Bullous congenital ichthyosiform erythroderma*	*Nonbullous ichthyosiform erythroderma*
Onset	• Not evident at birth • Appear during infancy or early childhood	Within 1st week in 75% of patient	• Presents at birth and persists throughout life • Neonates are covered in a collodion membrane	• *At birth*: Generalized erythema, widespread erosion • Later hyperkeratosis	• Collodion baby at birth • Subsequent generalized mild erythroderma with fine white scale
Sites	• Extensor, back, palms and soles, scalp • Flexures are not involved	• Extensors, sides of neck, abdomen • *Neck*: Invariably involved (dirty neck disease) • *Face*: Spared except periauricular area • *Flexures*: Usually spared	• Generalized • Flexures ++ • Variable • Palmoplantar keratoderma • "Bathing suit ichthyosis" is a variant, that affects only the trunk and scalp	• Generalized • *Flexures*: Severe • Palm/soles ++	• Generalized • Flexures ++ • Palm/soles ++
Scales	Small, white-gray, branny or flaky, semi-adherent, pasted on	Polygonal, dark-brown, adherent scales	• Large, brown, plate-like malodorous scales that form a mosaic or bark-like pattern • Free at edge and adherent at center • *Erythroderma*: Minimal or absent	• Small, hard, shotty • Yellow brown • Ridged/corrugated	• Generalized white, small scales with a "powdery" consistency • Superficial • Semiadherent
Others	• *Leg*: Larger scales with an adherent center and detached, outward-turning edges • *Palms and soles*: Mild keratoderma • Hyperlinear palms and soles • *Soles*: Fissures • *Scalp*: Scaling	• *Scalp*: Fine scaling • Plam/sole are spared • Testicular maldescent, abnormal sperm, chances of testicular cancer Inguinal hernia • Unilateral renal agenesis • *Eye*: Comma-shaped corneal opacity deuteranopia (green color-blindness) (rare) • *Obstetric*: IUGR, prolonged labor	• Ectropion and eclabium • *Ear/Nose*: Hypoplasia of cartilage • Scarring alopecia • *Nails*: Stippled ridge/subungual hyperkeratosis • Flexion contracture	• Flaccid bulla • Rupture followed by rapid healing without scar • Ridged HK of flexures • Cobblestone hyperkeratosis over the extensor surfaces of the joints • *Palms/soles*: Keratoderma contracture, fissure, deformity • Pungent body odor • Nail, hair, teeth—unaffected	• Intense, bright red erythroderma • *Palms and soles*: Severely affected with a diffuse, fissuring keratoderma • *Scalp*: Scarring alopecia, T. amantacia • *Eye*: Ectropion • *Nose/Ear*: Hypoplasia of cartilage • *Nails*: Ridging and dystrophy
Associated features	• Pruritus • Atopic dermatitis (35–50%) • Keratosis pilaris	• RUD syndrome • Kallmann syndrome • Mental retardation		• Sepsis and electrolyte imbalances (neonatal age) • Mitral regurgitation, VSD, club feet, • Breast hypoplasia	• Hypohidrosis and heat intolerance • Most children have normal growth and development; rarely short stature and growth retardation • Risk of infection, digital flexion contracture and squamous cell carcinoma
Course	• Improves in summer • Improves with age	• Improves in summer • Does not improve with age • Periodic molting	• Periodic molting • Persistent throughout life	• Skin fragility, blistering and erythema improves with age • Severe hyper-keratosis prevails	Variable

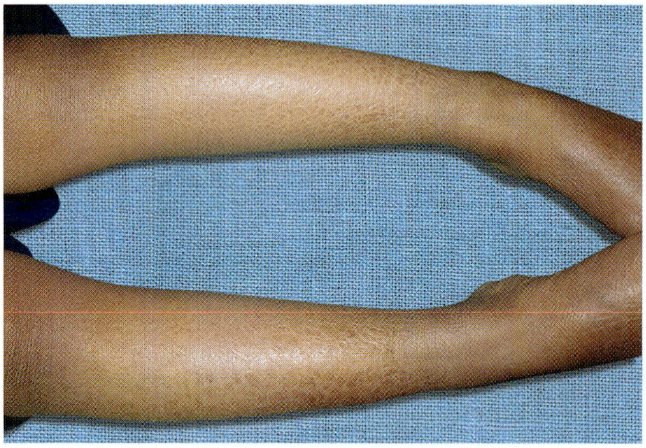

Fig. 1: Ichthyosis vulgaris.
Courtesy: Dr Rahul Ahar.

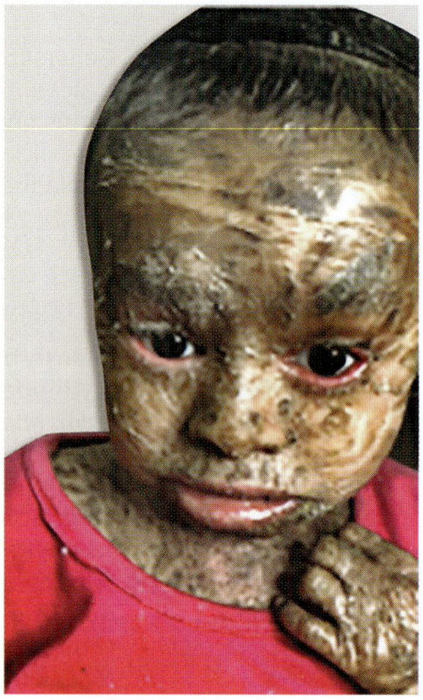

Fig. 2A: Lamellar Ichthyosis.
Courtesy: Dr Koushik Lahiri.

Ichthyosis Hystrix (Fig. 4)[6]

- *Synonym: Porcupine man*
- *Definition:* Group of rare disorder characterized by *spiny HK scales*
- *History:* First described by Curth and Macklin (1954)
- *Etiology:*
  - Keratin 1 gene (*KRT1*) defect in chromosome 12 and 17
  - *HID syndrome:* Connexin 26 autosomal dominant
- *Clinical features:*
  - May present at birth
  - Hyperkeratotic areas mimic EI, but there is no skin fragility
  - Generalized or *Nevoid* scaly erythema
  - *Hystrix (porcupine) like scaling*: Muddy brown
  - Nevoid forms follow lines of Blaschko
  - Functional impairment/contracture/nail dystrophy
- *HID syndrome: H*ystrix *I*chthyosis/*D*eafness
- *Differential diagnosis from bullous ichthyosiform erythroderma (BIE):* No bulla, more nevoid form, erythroderma is mild or absent
- *HPE:*
  - HK, PK, acanthosis, papillomatosis
  - Scattered vacuolated *bi-nucleate keratinocyte* in upper epidermis
- *Rx:* Emollient, retinoid, calcipotriol

Ichthyosis Bullosa of Siemens

- *Synonym:* Superficial epidermolytic ichthyosis
- *History:* Described by Siemens in Dutch Kindred, 1937
- *Etiology:*
  - Autosomal dominant
  - Abnormal expression of K_2e in upper stratum spinosum
  - Missense mutation of keratin 2 (*KRT2*) gene
- *HPE:*
  - Abnormality is confined to upper stratum spinosum and stratum granulosum

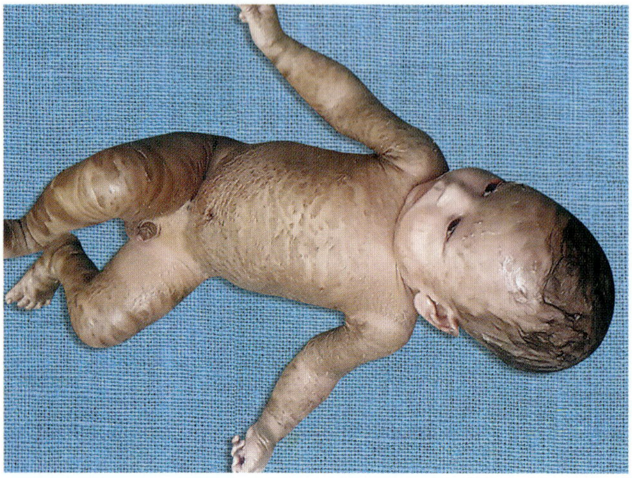

Fig. 2B: Lamellar Ichthyosis.
Courtesy: Dr Abhijit Saha.

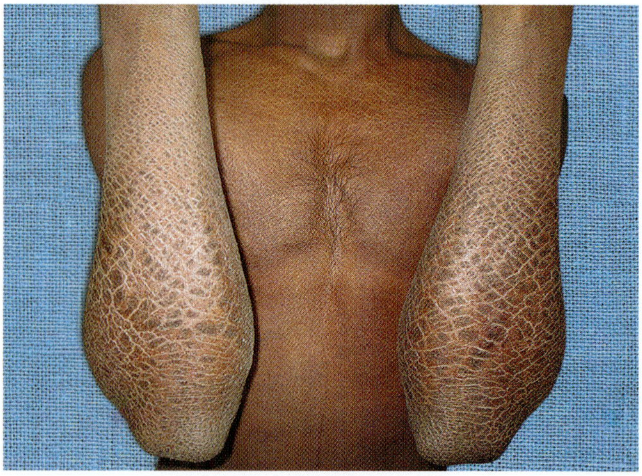

Fig. 2C: Lamellar ichthyosis.
Courtesy: Dr Rahul Ahar.

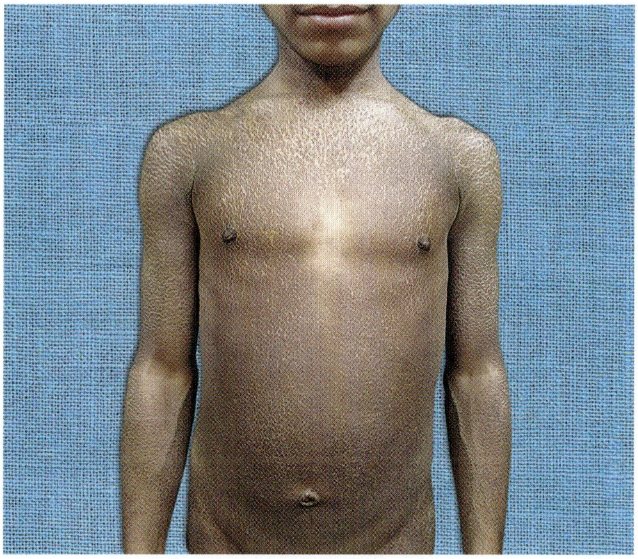

Fig. 3: X-linked recessive ichthyosis.
Courtesy: Dr Rahul Ahar.

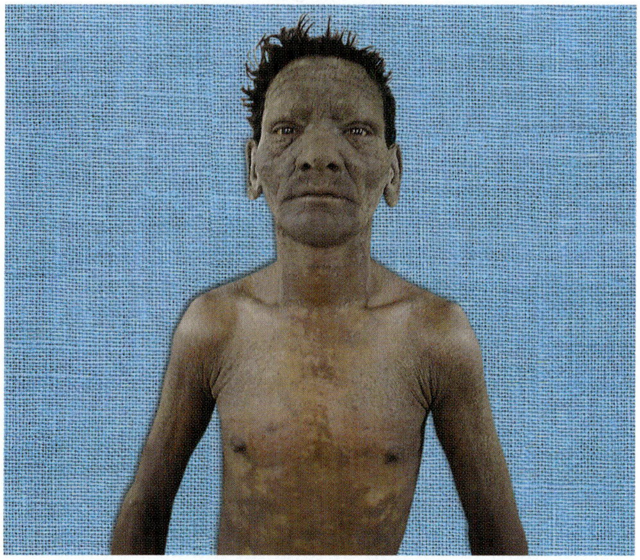

Fig. 4: Ichthyosis hystrix.

- At the site of "Mauserung" there is *intracorneal blister* with HK above and below
- *EM:* Clumping of tonofilaments is limited to the upper spinous and granular cell layers.
- *Clinical features:*
  - *At birth:* Appear normal or show mild blistering.
  - Mild; onset is at neonate or delayed within first 1 year
  - *Site:* Flexures, shin, abdomen
  - *Scales:* Variable, rippled, gray
  - No PPK, malodor
- *Evolution:* Superficial → blistering quick → rupture annular skin peeling
- *Mauserung:* Focal, circumscribed, annular desquamation
- *Differential diagnosis from BIE:* Less common, milder, no erythroderma
- *Complications:* Palmoplantar blistering, hyperhidrosis, infection

Harlequin Ichthyosis[7]

- *Introduction:*
  - Severest form of autosomal recessive congenital ichthyosis
  - Survival is difficult but reported
  - "Harlequin" refers to the chequered costume of the comic servant character in Italian comedy plays.
- *History:* First described by Oliver Hurt
- *Etiology:*
  - Autosomal recessive
  - Loss-of-function mutations in the ABC transporter gene *(ABCA12)*
- *HPE:* Ortho-HK, PK in type 3
- *EM:* Lipid droplet, vacuoles and cellular remnants
- *Clinical features:*
  - Usually prematurely stillborn
  - *Coat of Armour:* Rigid, taut, HK, adherent, skin covering whole body
  - *Cast split:* Producing fissures
  - *Distorted face:* Severe ectropion, boggy scalp
  - Mitten-like hand
- *Complications:* Restricted movement, respiratory insufficiency, hypoglycemia, hypothermia, dehydration, renal failure, infection.

Confetti Ichthyosis

- *Etiology:*
  - Autosomal dominant
  - Frameshift mutations in the Keratin 10 (*KRT10*) gene
- *Clinical features*:
  - *At birth:* Ichthyosiform erythroderma and palmoplantar keratoderma
  - *Infancy and childhood:* Develops hundreds of small, confetti-like "islands" of normal skin.

Collodion Baby

- *Introduction:* It is not a separate disease entity; many congenital ichthyoses (mostly recessive) present at birth with a collodion membrane.
- *Etiology:*
  - The two most common causes are nonbullous congenital ichthyosiform erythoderma and lamellar ichthyosis.
  - Transglutaminase-1 deficiency is often described as the cause of the collodion membrane in such conditions.
  - Milder phenotype of a self-healing (or self-improving collodion baby has been reported where transglutaminase-1 activity improves after birth).
  - Other rarer causes of collodion baby are Sjögren–Larsson syndrome, trichothiodystrophy, neutral lipid

storage disease, infantile Gaucher disease, Conradi–Hünermann–Happle syndrome and ectodermal dysplasias.

- *Clinical features*:
    - Often associated with premature birth and perinatal mortality and morbidity.
    - Babies, at birth, is covered with taut, shiny, transparent, plastic-wrap like membrane formed by the thickened stratum corneum.
    - It is often associated with ectropion, eclabium and hypoplasia of nasal and ear cartilage.
    - After birth, the parchment-like membrane cracks and breaks up leading to increased transcutaneous fluid and electrolyte loss and skin infections.
- *HPE:* Nonspecific, excessively thickened, orthokeratotic stratum corneum

Netherton Syndrome[8]

- *Introduction:*
    - Most common multisystem ichthyosiform syndrome
    - Described by Netherton, 1958
- *Etiopathogenesis:*
    - Autosomal recessive
    - *SPINK5* (*S*erine *P*rotease *I*nhibitor *K*azal Type 5) mutation (chromosome 5q32)
    - Premature LB secretion/abnormal lipid processing
    - Intermittent disruption of hair shaft and epidermal maturation
- *Clinical triad:*
    - *Skin:* Ichthyosiform dermatosis (ILC) + variable erythroderma
    - *Hair:* Trichorrhexis invaginata
    - Atopy
- *Clinical features:*
    - *Skin:*
        - *At birth:* Generalized erythroderma/no collodion membrane
        - *Infancy:* Erythroderma leading to complications such as infection, temperature instability, hypernatremia, failure to thrive, dermopathic enteropathy.
        - *Childhood:*
            - *Ichthyosis linearis circumflexa:* Scaly annular patches with advancing double edge-peeling scales
            - Fluctuating erythroderma (severe NS)
        - *Later:*
            - Gradual improvement with age
            - Chronic erythroderma followed by flexural edema (premalignant condition)
    - *Hair defect:*
        - Trichorrhexis invaginata
        - Others—pili torti, trichorrhexis nodosa
    - *Atopy:* Personal/family
- *Histopathology:*
    - *Skin:*
        - HK, PK, decreased granular layers.
        - Eosinophilic material in stratum corneum and stratum granulosum
    - *Hair:* Bamboo nodal dilatation, "golf tee" hair
- *Treatment:*
    - *ICU:* For erythroderma and complication
    - *Topical steroid:* Ineffective in neonate and should be avoided
    - *Older patients:* Emollient, topical steroid, antipruritic
    - *Retinoid:* Not effective
    - *Other treatment tried:* PUVA, methotrexate, and cyclosporine

Sjögren–Larsson Syndrome[9]

- *Introduction:*
    - Autosomal recessive
    - Described by Sjögren and Larsson in 1957
- *Triad:* Ichthyosis + spastic diplegia and MR + retinopathy
- *Etiology:* Fatty aldehyde dehydrogenase deficiency d/t mutation in of *FALDH* gene (chromosome 17) leading to defective FA metabolism
- *Clinical features:*
    - *Skin:*
        - *At birth:* Dry and mild erythrodermic skin
        - Scaling after 3 months
        - *Later:* Lamellar ichthyosis + periodic shedding
        - *Still later*: Velvety lichenification
    - *CNS:*
        - Nonprogressive spastic diplegia
        - Delayed milestones
        - *Seizures:* Grand mal
    - *Eye:* Glistening dots due to lipofuscin granules deposition in foveal and parafoveal retina
- *Treatment:* Reduction of total fat intake + supplement essential FA keratolytic/emollient

Refsum Disease[1]

- *Introduction:*
    - Autosomal recessive
    - Described by Refsum (Norway), 1946
- *Synonym:* Heredopathia atactica polyneuritiformis
- *Etiology:*
    - Impaired oxidation of phytanic acid (20 carbon branched FA)
    - Phytanic acid is derived from plant chlorophyll and animal fats
    - Chromosome 10p
- *Clinical features:*
    - *Onset:* Early adult life

- Cerebellar ataxia + mixed sensory-motor neuropathy + hypertrophied peripheral nerves
- *Retinitis pigmentosa:* Night blindness + decreased vision
- Sensorineural deafness
- Anosmia
- Ichthyosis vulgaris

- *Association:* Cardiomyopathy and skeletal defect
- *Treatment:*
  - Exclusion of green leafy vegetables and animal fat from diet
  - High carbohydrate diet

IBIDS Syndrome[1]

- *Synonym:* Tay syndrome/trichothiodystrophy
- *Pathogenesis:* Decreased level of sulfur containing AA in hair with normal circulating AA level
- *Clinical features:* Ichthyosis + impaired intelligence + decreased fertility + short stature
- *PIDIDS:* Photosensitivity + IBIDS
- *KIDS:* Keratitis + ichthyosis + deafness
- *HID:* Hystrix like ichthyosis + deafness
- *CHILD:* Congenital hemidysplasia + IE + limb defect
- *RUD:*
  - XLR ichthyosis
  - MR + epilepsy
  - Hypogonadism + obesity + endocrinopathy

X-linked Dominant Ichthyosis[1]

- *Synonym:* Conradi–Hünermann–Happle syndrome
- *Triad:* Chondrodysplasia punctate + ichthyosis + PPK
- *Clinical features:* XLD; females
  - *Skin:*
    - *At birth:* Collodian/IE
    - Ichthyosis improves with age
    - Nail dystrophy
    - PPK
  - *Skeletal:*
    - Asymmetric facies
    - Asymmetric limb shortening
    - Kyphoscoliosis
    - Supernumerary digits
    - Stippled calcification of bones
  - *Eye:* Mosaic lens involvement, asymmetric cataract

Neutral Lipid Storage Disease[1]

- *Synonym:* Chanarin–Dorfman syndrome
- *Clinical features:*
  - Non-BIE (± ectropion + nail dystrophy + PPK + alopecia)
  - Proximal myopathy
  - HSM + elevated liver enzymes
  - Cataract
  - Jordons' anomaly

APPROACH TO DIAGNOSIS OF A CASE OF ICHTHYOSIS[2-5]

History

- A thorough history of onset, evolution, progression, seasonal variation of the disease is elicited.
- Family history and consanguinity of marriage is important to establish dominant or recessive inheritance.
- Any temporal history of drug intake should be elicited.
- Some relevant history may give clinical clues for diagnosis such as:
  - *Anosmia:* Refsum disease
  - *Mental retardation:* Sjögren–Larsson syndrome, trichothiodystrophy, multiple sulfatase deficiency
  - *Photosensitivity:* Trichothiodystrophy
  - *Hearing impairment:* KID syndrome, Refsum disease, neutral lipid storage disease, CHILD syndrome

Examination

Thorough cutaneous and systemic investigation reveals important clues for diagnosis.

- *Bullae/blisters:* Epidermolytic ichthyosis, superficial epidermolytic ichthyosis (ichthyosis bullosa of Siemens)
- *Erythroderma:* Congenital ichthyosiform erythroderma, lamellar ichthyosis (mild), Harlequin ichthyosis (survivors), Netherton syndrome
- *Hair shaft abnormalities:* Trichothiodystrophy, Netherton syndrome
- *Hyperlinear palms and soles:* Ichthyosis vulgaris
- *Hystrix-like hyperkeratosis:* Ichthyosis hystrix
- *Ocular findings:* Cataracts (Refsum disease, trichothiodystrophy), corneal opacities (steroid sulfatase deficiency), keratitis (KID syndrome, IFAP syndrome)
- *Sensorineural hearing impairment:* KID syndrome, Refsum disease

Laboratories

- Complete blood count, electrolytes, liver function test, IgE
- Peripheral blood smear (to evaluate for vacuoles in leukocytes)
- Light microscopic examination of hairs (including eyebrow hairs)
- Testing for hearing ability
- Ophthalmologic examination
- Consider skin biopsy, especially if in case of presence of bullae (to assess for epidermolysis)
- Consider genetic mutation study

Differential Diagnosis[1,6]

- *Ichthyosis vulgaris:* X-linked ichthyosis, leprosy, sarcoidosis, lymphoma, malnutrition

- *X-linked ichthyosis:* Ichthyosis vulgaris, Kallmann syndrome, Rud syndrome, chondrodysplasia punctate
- *Lamellar ichthyosis:* Non-BIE

Treatment

- *Regular use of emollients and humectants:* Preparations containing ceramides together with other lipids may be especially effective. More severe dryness may need hydration like soaks.
- Urea or keratolytics, such as α-hydroxy, lactic and salicylic acids are effective. However, for infants and children care must be taken to prevent salicylate toxicity while using salicylic acid preparation.
- Topical retinoids may decrease scaling, but irritation potential is high.
- Systemic treatment with acitretin or isotretinoin may be done when necessary. However, systemic retinoid may make skin fragile; so, it is preferable to start with a low dose of retinoids and gradually increase over a period of time.
- More severe presentation especially in the neonatal ages needs intensive care. Thermoregulation should be ensured and electrolyte imbalance should be corrected.
- In case of clinical infection or sepsis, a course of systemic antibiotics may be required. However, long-term use of antibiotics should be avoided, as there is chance of developing resistance.
- Flexural and facial involved areas may be treated with topical vitamin D analogs.

KEY POINTS

- Ichthyoses are clinically and etiologically heterogeneous groups of disorders of cornification characterized by scaling of the skin in a widespread distribution.
- Ichthyosis can be inherited or can arise secondary to many infective and noninfective conditions.
- Most inherited ichthyoses are evident at birth or manifest in early infancy. Inherited ichthyosis can also manifest itself as a part of a syndrome affecting multiple systems.
- The two most common causes of collodion baby are nonbullous congenital ichthyosiform erythroderma and lamellar ichthyosis.
- Clinical features, pattern of inheritance and structural, biochemical and molecular abnormalities help to differentiate these disorders.
- The diagnosis is mostly clinical aided with thorough personal and family history; but can be supplemented with histopathology and molecular characterization.
- Therapy is symptomatic and primarily aimed at reducing hyperkeratosis. Topical management consists of emollients, keratolytics, and retinoids.
- Many, but not all, disorders respond well to oral retinoids. Treatment is initiated at low doses and titrated to response. Benefits and side effects must be careful.

REFERENCES

1. Takeichi T, Akiyama M. Inherited ichthyosis: nonsyndromic forms. J Dermatol. 2016;43(3):242-51.
2. Hernández-Martín A, González-Sarmiento R. Recent advances in congenital ichthyoses. Curr Opin Pediatr. 2015;27(4):473-9.
3. D'Alessio M, Fortugno P, Zambruno G, Hovnanian A. Netherton syndrome and its multifaceted defective protein LEKTI. G Ital Dermatol Venereol. 2013;148(1):37-51.
4. Dyer JA, Spraker M, Williams M. Care of the newborn with ichthyosis. Dermatol Ther. 2013;26(1):1-15.
5. Oji V, Tadini G, Akiyama M, Blanchet Bardon C, Bodemer C, Bourrat E, et al. Revised nomenclature and classification of inherited ichthyoses: results of the first ichthyosis consensus conference in Sorèze, 2009. J Am Acad Dermatol. 2010; 63(4):607-41.
6. Phadnis SV, Griffin DR, Eady RA, Rodeck CH, Chitty LS. Prenatal diagnosis and management strategies in a family with a rare type of congenital ichthyosis. Ultrasound Obstet Gynecol. 2007; 30(6):908-10.
7. Mazereeuw-Hautier J, Bitoun E, Chevrant-Breton J, Man SY, Bodemer C, Prins C, et al. Keratitis-ichthyosis-deafness syndrome: disease expression and spectrum of connexin 26 (GJB2) mutations in 14 patients. Br J Dermatol. 2007;156(5):1015-9.
8. Layton J. A review of Harlequin ichthyosis. Neonatal Netw. 2005;24(3):17-23.
9. Hernández-Martin A, Aranegui B, Martin-Santiago A, Garcia-Doval I. A systematic review of clinical trials of treatments for the congenital ichthyoses, excluding ichthyosis vulgaris. J Am Acad Dermatol. 2013;69(4):544-9.

EXAMINATION QUESTIONS

1. Classify ichthyosis.
2. Write a brief note on X-linked ichthyosis.
3. Write a brief note on harlequin ichthyosis.
4. Write a brief note on acquired ichthyosis.
5. How do you approach a case of congenital ichthyosis?
6. Explain nonbullous congenital ichthyosiform erythroderma.
7. Write a short note on collodion baby.
8. Describe epidermolytic hyperkeratosis.
9. Enlist types of ichthyosiform congenital dermatosis and discuss histological features in differentiation of ichthyosiform disorders.

63 CHAPTER Keratoderma

Fenil Patel

INTRODUCTION

Palmoplantar keratoderma (PPK) comprises a diverse entity of hereditary or acquired disorders of keratinization characterized by hyperkeratosis of palms and soles. Hereditary PPK can be associated with other ectodermal abnormalities and systemic involvement. Early age of onset and familial occurrence is suggestive of some genetic defect. Hereditary PPK may be present as an isolated condition, few are a part of other dermatosis. Some PPK have acquired causes.[1]

CLASSIFICATION[1,2]

Various classifications are described in literature.

- Palmoplantar keratoderma can be:
  - Inherited can be subclassified as:
    - Nonsyndromic, isolated PPK
    - Syndromic PPK
  - Acquired
- *Based on clinical pattern:*
  - Diffuse PPK—uniform involvement of palms and soles
  - Focal PPK—localized involvement of palms and soles
    - Focal PPK is subclassified as:
      - Areata or nummular—oval lesions
      - Striate type—longitudinal hyperkeratosis of palms over the volar surface of the fingers
  - Punctate PPK—multiple discrete and scattered keratotic papules over the palms and soles

If PPK hyperkeratosis extends on dorsal aspect of fingers and flexor aspects of wrist and heel, then it is called as "transgredient PPK."

The above classifications are not definite; in future, classification will be required on the basis of molecular defect.

HEREDITARY PALMOPLANTAR KERATODERMA

Nonsyndromic Palmoplantar Keratoderma

It is of two types:

1. Epidermolytic palmoplantar keratoderma (EPPK)
2. Nonepidermolytic palmoplantar keratoderma (NEPPK)

Epidermolytic Palmoplantar Keratoderma[1-5]

- *Synonyms*: Unna-Thost disease, Voerner disease
- *Type*: Diffuse PPK
- *Inheritance*: Autosomal dominant (AD)
- *Gene defect*: *KRT9*, *KRT1* (1B domain)
- *Protein defect*: Keratin 9, keratin 1
- *PPK features and key clinical features*: Starts in infancy
  - Diffuse, thick, yellow hyperkeratosis with erythematous borders
  - In adult, confluent keratoderma present
  - Blistering and fissuring are seen sometimes
- *Transgrediens*: Absent
- *Nail involvement*: Thickened nail present occasionally
- *Hyperhidrosis*: Absent
- *Other clinical findings*: Knuckle pad hyperkeratosis
  - Disabling pain indicates "tonotubular" PPK, pitted keratolysis
  - Fungal superinfection is seen in most of patients
- *Histopathological examination (HPE) and ultrastructure*: Epidermolytic hyperkeratosis, vacuolated suprabasal keratinocytes, round or oval eosinophilic inclusion body, whorls of keratin-containing tubular structures are seen on electron microscopy in "tonotubular" PPK.
- *Treatment*: Paring, topical keratolytics (urea, salicylic acid, lactic acid), occlusion with polythene increases the efficacy of keratolytics, oral retinoids in low dose, topical calcipotriol, if fungal superinfection is associated treat with topical antifungal agents.

Nonepidermolytic Palmoplantar Keratoderma

Mal de Meleda[1-6]

- *Synonyms*: Keratosis palmoplantaris transgrediens of Siemens, Meleda disease, Acroerythrokeratoderma
- *Type*: Diffuse PPK
- *Inheritance*: Autosomal recessive (AR)
- *Gene defect*: *SLURP1*
- *Protein defect*: Secreted lymphocytes antigen 6/urokinase-type plasminogen activator receptor (uPAR)-related protein 1
- *PPK features and key clinical features:* Starts in infancy
  - Severe PPK which progress to involve dorsal aspect of hand and feet ("glove and stocking keratoderma"), malodorous, maceration is seen because of hyperhidrosis
  - Reduced movement of hands and feet
- *Transgrediens*: Present
- *Nail involvement*: Koilonychias, dystrophy of great toe nail, subungual hyperkeratosis

- *Hyperhidrosis*: Present
- *Other clinical findings*: Fungal superinfection, sclerodactyly, pseudoainhum, amputation of digits, perioral erythema, hyperkeratotic or lichenoid lesions over elbow and knees, progressive conical tapering of finger tips which cause contracture of the fingers, corneal lesions, and high-arched palate
- *HPE*: Orthohyperkeratosis, hypergranulosis, acanthosis, and perivascular lymphohistiocytic infiltrates
- *Treatment*: Oral retinoids, paring, split-thickness skin grafting in functional impairment of hands and feet, patient with long-term history is screened for secondary malignancies.

Nagashima type NEPPK[1-5]

It is seen in Chinese and Japanese people.

- *Synonyms*: Keratosis palmoplantaris Nagashima
- *Type*: Diffuse PPK
- *Inheritance*: AR
- *Gene defect*: *SERPINB7*
- *Protein defects*: Serpin peptidase inhibitor family B member 7
- *PPK features and key clinical features*: Present at birth or starts in early infancy, diffuse, erythematous hyperkeratosis of palms and soles, white sponge-like appearance of hyperkeratosis after water exposure
- *Transgrediens*: Present
- *Nail involvement*: Not involved
- *Hyperhidrosis*: Present
- *Other clinical findings*: Hyperkeratotic lesions over knee, elbow and Achilles tendon, and fungal and bacterial superinfection
- *HPE*: Orthohyperkeratosis, acanthosis, hypergranulosis
- *Treatment*: Topical keratolytics (urea, salicylic acid, lactic acid), occlusion with polythene increases the efficacy of keratolytics, oral retinoids in low dose, topical tacrolimus, also treat fungal and bacterial superinfection

Bothnia type NEPPK[1-5]

- *Synonyms*: Nonepidermolytic palmoplantar tylosis
- *Type*: Diffuse PPK
- *Inheritance*: AD
- *Gene defect*: *AQP5*
- *Protein defect*: Aquaporin 5
- *PPK features and key clinical features*: Yellowish hyperkeratosis starts in early childhood, white sponge-like appearance of hyperkeratosis after water exposure.
- *Transgrediens*: Present
- *Nail involvement*: Curved nails, ragged cuticles
- *Hyperhidrosis*: Present
- *Other clinical findings*: Fungal and bacterial superinfection
- *HPE*: Orthohyperkeratosis, acanthosis
- *Treatment*: Topical keratolytics (urea, salicylic acid, lactic acid), occlusion with polythene increases the efficacy of keratolytics, oral retinoids in low dose, oral erythromycin

Kimonis type NEPPK[1,2]

- *Synonyms*: Nonepidermolytic keratinopathic PPK
- *Type*: Diffuse PPK
- *Inheritance*: AD
- *Gene defect*: KRT1 (V1 domain)
- *Protein defect*: Keratin 1
- *PPK features and key clinical features*: Diffuse hyperkeratosis of palms and soles, discrete papular lesions on dorsal aspect of fingers, hyperkeratosis over knuckles
- *Transgrediens*: Present
- *Nail involvement*: Not involved
- *Hyperhidrosis*: Present
- *Other clinical findings*: Mild keratosis and dryness of knees and elbows, hyperkeratosis of umbilicus and nipple areola, achilles tendon may be involved
- *HPE*: Orthohyperkeratosis, acanthosis
- *Treatment*: Topical keratolytics (urea, salicylic acid, lactic acid), occlusion with polythene increases the efficacy of keratolytics, oral retinoids in low dose

Greither keratoderma[1-5,7]

- *Synonyms*: Keratosis extremitatum hereditaria progrediens
- *Type*: Diffuse PPK
- *Inheritance*: AD
- *Gene defect*: *KRT1*
- *Protein defect*: Keratin 1
- *PPK features and key clinical features*: Onset after age of 2 years, may disappear in later life (usually in fifth decade), hyperkeratosis on ventral aspect of wrist, hyperkeratosis of palms and soles, erythematous border between hyperkeratotic and normal skin
- *Transgrediens*: Present
- *Nail involvement*: Not involved
- *Hyperhidrosis*: Present
- *Other clinical findings*: Blistering, autoamputation of digits, extending over Achilles tendon, hyperkeratosis over elbows and knees, if woolly hair present exclude Carvajal syndrome
- *HPE and ultrastructure*: Nonspecific, on electron microscopy—aggregates of tonofilaments around nuclei, cell-cell junctions showed imbricated pattern
- *Treatment*: Topical keratolytics (urea, salicylic acid, lactic acid), occlusion with polythene increases the efficacy of keratolytics

Loricrin keratoderma[1-4,8]

- *Synonyms*: Variant Vohwinkel syndrome, mutilating keratoderma with ichthyosis, Camisa syndrome
- *Type*: Diffuse PPK
- *Inheritance*: AD
- *Gene defect*: *LOR*
- *Protein defect*: Loricrin
- *PPK features and key clinical features*: Generalized desquamation and collodion babies are reported at birth, mild generalized ichthyosis, "honey-comb" pattern PPK develops in childhood, pseudoainhum

- *Transgrediens*: Present
- *Nail involvement*: Not involved
- *Hyperhidrosis*: Absent
- *Other clinical findings*: Knuckle pads, warty keratoses
- *HPE*: Hyperkeratosis, hypergranulosis, focal parakeratosis, agranulosis
  On immunoelectron microscopy—loricrin present in nuclei
- *Treatment*: Oral isotretinoin

Syndromic Palmoplantar Keratoderma

*Palmoplantar Keratoderma and Hearing Impairment (**Table 1**)*

- Vohwinkel syndrome[1,2,4,9,10]
- Bart–Pumphrey syndrome[1,2,4,9,11]
- Mitochondrial palmoplantar keratoderma with hearing impairment[1,2,9]

*Palmoplantar Keratoderma and Cardiomyopathy (**Table 2**)*

- Naxos disease[1,2,9,12]
- Carvajal-Huerta syndrome[1,2,9,13]

Arrhythmogenic right ventricular dysplasia, with diffuse mild palmoplantar keratoderma and woolly hair, is AR disorder which occurs due to *DSC2* gene mutation.

*Palmoplantar Keratoderma and Cancer (**Table 3**)*

- Huriez syndrome[1-4,14]
- Howel–Evans syndrome[1,2,4,9,15]
- Palmoplantar keratoderma, sex reversal, and cancer[1,2,9]

*Palmoplantar Keratoderma in Ectodermal Dysplasia and Related Diseases (**Table 4**)*

- Clouston syndrome[1,2,4,16]
- Odonto-onycho-dermal dysplasia[1,2,4]
- Papillon–Lefèvre syndrome[1,2,4,9,17]
- Haim–Munk syndrome[1,2,4,9,18]
- Olmsted syndrome[1-4,19]

Differential diagnosis of Olmsted syndrome: Mal de Meleda, acrodermatitis enteropathica, psoriasis inversa, Clouston syndrome, Papillon–Lefèvre syndrome, Vohwinkel syndrome, and pachyonychia congenital (PC).

TABLE 1: Palmoplantar keratoderma and hearing impairment.

	Vohwinkel syndrome	*Bart–Pumphrey syndrome*	*Mitochondrial palmoplantar keratoderma with hearing impairment*
Synonyms	• Keratoma hereditarum mutilans • Cicatrizing keratoderma with hearing impairment • Keratoderma with sensorineural deafness		Mitochondrial sensorineural hearing loss with PPK
Type of PPK	Diffuse, striate (rarely)	Diffuse, striate (rarely)	Diffuse or focal
Inheritance	AD	AD	Mitochondrial
Gene defect	*GJB2*	*GJB2*	*MT-TS1*
Protein defect	Connexin 26	Connexin 26	Mt tRNA serine 1
PPK features and key clinical features	PPK starts in childhood, "honeycomb"-like PPK, "Starfish"-like keratoses on knuckles, a high-toned nonprogressive sensorineural deafness	"Knuckle pads"—hyperkeratosis over interphalangeal, metacarpophalangeal joints, "honeycomb"-like PPK, mixed hearing loss (both sensorineural and conductive)	PPK starts in childhood, honeycomb-like PPK, callus on the heels and toes, progressive sensorineural deafness
Transgrediens	Present	Present	
Nail involvement	Not involved	Leukonychia	Not involved
Hyperhidrosis	Absent	Absent	Absent
Other clinical findings	Pseudoainhum, autoamputation, alopecia		Coincidence with warty linear epidermal nevi, ichthyosis vulgaris, cholesteatoma
HPE and ultrastructure	Nonspecific, orthohyperkeratosis, papillomatosis	Nonspecific, orthohyperkeratosis, papillomatosis	Hypergranulosis, moderate acanthosis without epidermolytic changes
Treatment	Oral retinoids, surgical correction of pseudoainhum, appropriate rehabilitation for deafness	Oral retinoids, surgical correction of pseudoainhum, appropriate rehabilitation for deafness	Appropriate rehabilitation for deafness

(AD: autosomal dominant; HPE: histopathological examination; PPK: palmoplantar keratoderma)

TABLE 2: Palmoplantar keratoderma and cardiomyopathy.

	Naxos disease	*Carvajal-Huerta syndrome*
Synonyms	Diffuse NEPPK with woolly hair and arrhythmogenic cardiomyopathy	Carvajal syndrome
Type of PPK	Diffuse, focal (rarely)	Striate
Inheritance	AR	AR > AD*
Gene defect	*JUP*	*DSP*
Protein defect	Junction plakoglobin	Desmoplakin
PPK features and key clinical features	Woolly hair present at birth, diffuse or striate PPK develops in infancy, right ventricular cardiomyopathy seen in adolescence	Striate PPK develops during infancy, woolly hair present at birth, left ventricular cardiomyopathy (represents at younger age then Naxos disease)
Transgrediens	Absent	Absent
Nail involvement	Nail dystrophy	Leukonychia (seen in AD variant)
Hyperhidrosis	Present	Present
Other clinical findings		Psoriasiform plaques on elbows, knees and flexural aspect, blisters or erosions at the site of friction, dental enemal defects
HPE and ultrastructure	Hyperkeratosis, hypergranulosis, acanthosis, widening of intercellular space of suprabasal keratinocytes Immunofluorescence—decrease plakoglobin expression	• Epidermolytic hyperkeratosis, widening of intercellular space of suprabasal keratinocytes • Electron microscopy—clumping of desmosomes
Treatment	Treatment of arrhythmia, topical keratolytics	Treatment of arrhythmia, topical keratolytics

(AD: autosomal dominant; AR: autosomal recessive; HPE: histopathological examination; NEPPK: nonepidermolytic palmoplantar keratoderma; PPK: palmoplantar keratoderma)

*In AD variant of Carvajal syndrome—Leukonychia and oligodontia are associated with striate PPK, woolly hair, and cardiomyopathy.

TABLE 3: Palmoplantar keratoderma and cancer.

	Huriez syndrome	*Howel–Evans syndrome*	*Palmoplantar keratoderma (PPK), sex reversal, and cancer*
Synonyms	Scleroatrophic and keratotic dermatosis of limbs	Tylosis esophageal cancer	Palmoplantar hyperkeratosis with SCC and 46, XX sex reversal
Type of PPK	Diffuse	Focal NEPPK	Diffuse
Inheritance	AD	AD	AR
Gene defect	Unknown	*RHBDF2*	*RSPO1*
Protein defect		Rhomboid 5 homolog 2	R-spondin protein 1
PPK features and key clinical features	Onset of disease in infancy, scleroatrophy of hands, sclerodactyly, absent dermatoglyphics	Focal PPK develops in childhood, mild involvement of palms, limited involvement of pressure areas of soles (callosities)	Diffuse NEPPK develops in infancy, sclerodactyly, early loss of teeth due to chronic periodontitis
Transgrediens	Present	Absent	Absent
Nail involvement	Hypoplastic nail changes	Not involved	Hypoplastic nail changes
Hyperhidrosis	Absent	Absent	Present
Other clinical findings	• Risk of SCC 100-fold increased—seen at young age, hypohidrosis • *Important D/D:* Kindler syndrome, dyskeratosis congenital, PPK with sex reversal and SCC	High risk of esophageal squamous cell carcinoma, keratosis pilaris, oral leukokeratosis, dry rough skin, oral leukoplakia, maxillary decalcification, chronic rhinitis, alveolysis	• High risk of developing SCC and laryngeal carcinoma • *Male patient:* Hypospadia, hypogonadism, gynecomastia • *Female patient:* True hermaphroditism, bilateral cataract, bilateral optic nerve coloboma
HPE and ultrastructure	Orthohyperkeratosis, hypergranulosis, acanthosis, absence of Langerhans cells	• Nonepidermolytic hyperkeratosis, hypergranulosis, acanthosis • Immunohistochemistry—reduced cyto-plasmic staining of iRhom2 in epidermis	Hyperkeratosis, hypergranulosis, vacuolar degeneration of keratinocytes in stratum spinosum
Treatment	Acitretin-reduced hyper-keratosis and chance of SCC	Topical keratolytics, careful selection of footwear, oral retinoids	

(AD: autosomal dominant; AR: autosomal recessive; D/D: differential diagnosis; HPE: histopathological examination; NEPPK: nonepidermolytic palmoplantar keratoderma; SCC: squamous cell carcinoma)

Palmoplantar Keratoderma and Ophthalmic Manifestation

Richner-Hanhart syndrome[1,2,4,9,20]

- *Synonyms*: Oculocutaneous tyrosinemia, tyrosinemia type II, tyrosine transaminase deficiency
- *Type of PPK*: Focal PPK
- *Inheritance:* AR
- *Gene defect*: *TAT*
- *Protein defect*: Tyrosine aminotransferase
- *PPK features and key clinical features*: Painful focal PPK develops in early childhood, yellow-white papular lesions, blistering
- *Transgrediens*: Absent
- *Nail involvement*: Not involved

TABLE 4: Palmoplantar keratoderma in ectodermal dysplasia and related diseases.

	Clouston syndrome	*Odonto-onycho-dermal dysplasia*	*Papillon–Lefèvre syndrome*	*Haim–Munk syndrome*	*Olmsted syndrome*
Synonyms	Hidrotic ectodermal dysplasia 2 (HED2)	• Schopf-Schulz-Passarge syndrome • PPK with cystic eyelids, hypodontia and hypotrichosis • Eccrine tumors with ectodermal dysplasia • Tricho-odonto-onychodermal dysplasia	Keratoderma with periodontitis	Keratoderma with periodontitis, onychogryphosis, arachnodactyly, and acro-osteolysis	Mutilating PPK with periorificial keratotic plaques
Type of PPK	Diffuse	Diffuse	Diffuse	Diffuse	Diffuse, striate on flexor aspect
Inheritance	AD	AR	AR	AR	Sporadic (most common) AD > AR XR
Gene defect	*GJB6*	*WNT10A*	*CTSC*	*CTSC*	TRPV3 (In autosomal inheritance) *MBTPS2* (In X-linked inheritance)
Protein defect	Connexin 30	Wnt 10A	Cathepsin C	Cathepsin C	Transient receptor potential vanilloid 3 (In autosomal inheritance) Membrane-bound transcription factor peptidase, site 2 (In X-linked inheritance)
PPK features and key clinical features	Diffuse PPK, nail dystrophy, hypotrichosis (progressive), pseudo-ainhum, "pebbled" appearance of hyperkeratotic skin seen over the dorsal aspect of digits, knees and elbows	Diffuse PPK develops due to multiple palmoplantar eccrine syringofibroadenoma, dental anomalies (small teeth, hypodontia), hydrocystomas of eyelids, hypotrichosis	Diffuse PPK with erythema, pseudoainhum, periodontitis, gingivitis	Diffuse PPK with erythema, pseudoainhum, periodontitis, gingivitis, onychogryphosis, arachnodactyly, acro-osteolysis	Starts in infancy, diffuse PPK with erythematous border, progressive PPK leads to flexion contracture, digital constriction and autoamputation, striate hyperkeratosis with perifollicular distribution develops on flexor aspect, erythema and warty hyperkeratotic plaques develops in perioral and perianal regions leads to pruritus and pain, intertriginous sites shows hyperkeratosis and fissuring
Trans-grediens	Present		Present	Present	Present
Nail involvement	Nail dystrophy, clubbing	Nail dystrophy	Not involved	Onychogryphosis	Nail anomalies
Hyperhidrosis		Present	Present	Present	Present

Contd...

Contd...

	Clouston syndrome	*Odonto-onycho-dermal dysplasia*	*Papillon–Lefèvre syndrome*	*Haim–Munk syndrome*	*Olmsted syndrome*
Other clinical findings	Pale and fine hair, sparse or absent eyebrows, hyperpigmentation over joints, eye defects, eccrine syringofibroadenomas, cataract, strabismus, oral leukoplakia	Follicular and adnexal tumors seen in older patients	Bacterial infection of internal organs, psoriasiform plaques on elbows and knees, loss of deciduous teeth in early childhood, intracranial calcification, mental retardation, high IgE level	Premature loss of deciduous teeth, flat foot, flexion contracture of joints, arthralgia	Pruritus, Alopecia, dental anomalies, ocular abnormalities, joint laxity, SCC and malignant melanomas are seen rarely, high IgE levels, eosinophilia, erythromelalgia, hearing loss, primary sclerosing cholangitis, hemangioma
HPE and ultrastructure	Orthohyperkeratosis, normal granular layer, ultrastructure examination of hair—loss of hair shaft cuticle, disorganized hair fibers	Slender, anastomosing epithelial cords of acrosyringeal cells with or without formation of lumina, embedded in fibrovascular stroma seen in biopsy	• Hyperkeratosis associated with irregular parakeratosis, acanthosis • Ultrastructure—lipid-like vacuoles in granulocytes and corneocytes, irregular keratohyalin granules, reduced tonofilaments	• Hyperkeratosis associated with irregular parakeratosis, acanthosis • Ultrastructure—lipid-like vacuoles in granulocytes and corneocytes, irregular keratohyalin granules, reduced tonofilaments	Psoriasiform hyperplasia, orthohyperkeratosis, parakeratosis, hypergranulosis with foci of hypogranulosis, perivascular inflammatory infiltrate, increased mast cell numbers
Treatment	Topical keratolytics, special hair and nail care	Topical keratolytics, treat follicular and adnexal tumors	Oral retinoids, antibiotics, dental care	Oral retinoids, antibiotics, dental care	Topical keratolytics, emollients, corticosteroids, calcineurin inhibitors gives temporary symptomatic relief, excision of lesions and skin grafting gives long-term symptomatic relief, erlotinib (EGFR inhibitor) therapy leads to thinning of hyperkeratosis

(AD: autosomal dominant; AR: autosomal recessive; EGFR: epidermal growth factor receptor; HPE: histopathological examination; NEPPK: nonepidermolytic palmoplantar keratoderma; IgE: immunoglobulin E; PPK: palmoplantar keratoderma; SCC: squamous cell carcinoma ; XR: X-linked recessive)

- *Hyperhidrosis*: Present
- *Other clinical findings*: Photophobia, redness of eyes, increased lacrimation and herpetiform corneal ulcer develops in infancy, behavioral problems occurs in untreated cases
- *HPE and ultrastructure*: Hyperkeratosis, hypergranulosis, acanthosis

  Electron microscopy—clumping of tonofilaments with adherent globoid keratohyalin granules and needle shape tyrosine crystalline inclusion in keratinocytes
- *Investigations*: Screening of tyrosine and its metabolites level in blood and urine, slit-lamp examination of eyes (tyrosine crystal deposition seen), gene analysis for tyrosine aminotransferase
- *Treatment*: Goal is to reduce plasma tyrosine by restricting natural protein intake, phenylalanine, and tyrosine-free diet.

Nonsyndromic Focal Palmoplantar Keratoderma (Figs. 1 and 2)

Striate Palmoplantar Keratoderma[1-4,21] *(Table 5 and Fig. 3)*

Synonyms: Brunauer–Fuhs–Siemens syndrome, keratosis palmoplantaris varians of Wachters, keratosis palmoplantaris areata et striata.

Nonsyndromic Punctate Palmoplantar Keratoderma

Punctate Palmoplantar Keratoderma[1-4,22]

- *Synonyms*: Palmoplantar keratoderma punctata type 1, keratosis punctata palmoplantaris type—Buschke-Fischer-Brauer, keratoma dissipatum, disseminated clavus

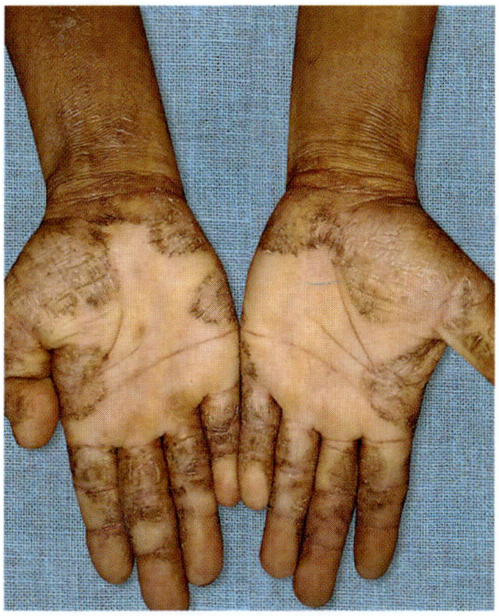

Fig. 1: Focal palmar keratoderma.

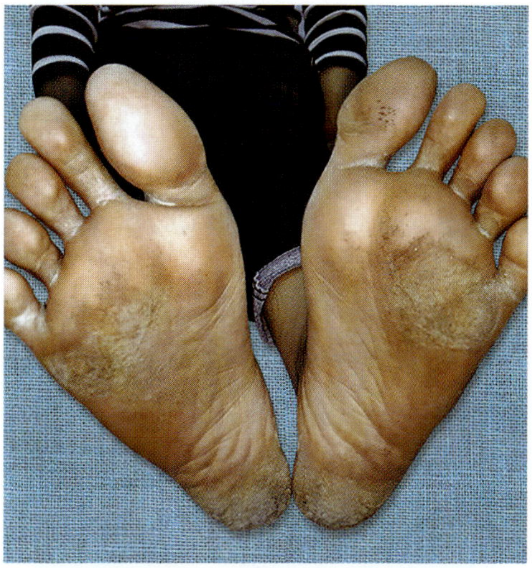

Fig. 2: Focal plantar keratoderma.

TABLE 5: Striate palmoplantar keratoderma.

	Type 1 (SPPK1)	*Type 2 (SPPK2)*	*Type 3 (SPPK3)*
Type of PPK	Focal	Focal	Focal
Inheritance	AD	AD	AD
Gene defect	*DSG1*	*DSP*	*KRT1* (V1 domain)
Protein defect	Desmoglein 1	Desmoplakin	Keratin 1
PPK features and key clinical features	Striate hyperkeratosis of fingers and palms on flexor aspect, soles shows diffuse and focal changes, lesions develops in adult age and aggravated by mechanical stress	Striate hyperkeratosis of fingers and palms on flexor aspect, soles shows diffuse and focal changes, lesions develops in adult age and aggravated by mechanical stress	Striate hyperkeratosis of fingers and palms on flexor aspect, soles shows diffuse and focal changes, lesions develops in childhood and aggravated by mechanical stress
Transgrediens	Absent	Absent	Absent
Nail involvement	Rarely seen (onycholysis)	Rarely seen (onycholysis)	Rarely seen (onycholysis)
Hyperhidrosis	Present	Absent	Absent
Other clinical findings	Pain, hyperkeratosis of knee and elbow	Woolly hair without cardiomyopathy	
HPE and ultrastructure	Orthohyperkeratosis, hypergranulosis, acanthosis, disadhesion of suprabasal keratinocytes, widening of the intercellular space	Orthohyperkeratosis, hypergranulosis, acanthosis, disadhesion of suprabasal keratinocytes, widening of the intercellular space	Ultrastructure—less electron dense intermediate filaments in stratum spinosum, normal desmosomes
Treatment	Oral acitretin, topical keratolytics	Oral acitretin, topical keratolytics	Oral acitretin, topical keratolytics

(AD: autosomal dominant; HPE: histopathological examination; PPK: palmoplantar keratoderma)

- *Type of PPK*: Punctate PPK
- *Inheritance*: AD
- *Gene defect*: *AAGAB*
- *Protein defect*: α- and γ-adaptin-binding protein p34
- *PPK features and key clinical features*: Multiple small keratotic papules develops on palms and soles during adolescence, papules are initially translucent with central indentation, later becomes opaque and verrucous, lesions are aggravated by manual work and after exposure to water
- *Transgrediens*: Absent
- *Nail involvement*: Not involved
- *Hyperhidrosis*: Absent
- *Differential diagnosis*: Verucca, punctate porokeratosis, Darier disease, Cowden disease, and acquired PPK secondary to arsenic
- *HPE and ultrastructure*: Orthohyperkeratosis, acanthosis, hypergranulosis, sometimes lesion shows hypogranulosis and parakeratosis

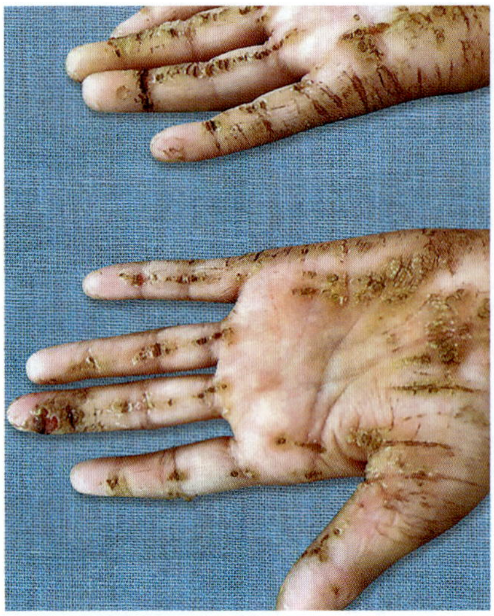

Fig. 3: Striate keratoderma.

- *Treatment*: Topical keratolytics, topical retinoids and topical calcipotriol are not effective, regular use of pumice stone and proper footwear selection are useful.

Spiny Keratoderma[1-4,23]

- *Synonyms*: Palmoplantar keratoderma punctata type 2, music box spine keratoderma, punctate porokeratotic keratoderma
- *Type of PPK*: Punctate PPK
- *Inheritance*: AD
- *Gene defect*: Unknown
- *Protein defect*: Unknown
- *PPK features and key clinical features*: Multiple small keratotic spiny papules projects from palms and soles, lesions can be start from first to fifth decade and gradually increase in numbers.
- *Transgrediens*: Absent
- *Nail involvement*: Not involved
- Hyperhidrosis: Absent
- *Differential diagnosis*: Darier disease, epidermodysplasia verruciformis, arsenic keratosis, filiform warts, paraneoplastic follicular hyperkeratosis.
- *HPE and ultrastructure*: Columns of parakeratosis over the hypogranular epidermis
- *Investigations*: Screen patient for liver and kidney disease, HIV, tuberculosis, malignancy to rule out associated condition
- *Treatment*: Dermabrasion, topical keratolytics and oral retinoids, topical 5-fluorouracil gives variable results

Marginal Papular Keratoderma: Acrokeratoelastoidosis and Focal Acral Hyperkeratosis[1-4,24]

- *Synonyms*: Palmoplantar keratoderma punctata type 3
- *Type of PPK*: Punctate PPK
- *Inheritance*: AD
- *Gene defect*: Unknown
- *Protein defect*: Unknown
- *PPK features and key clinical features*: Multiple hyperkeratotic papules along the margins of palms and soles, papules are skin colored to hyperpigmented in focal acral hyperkeratosis and yellow colored in acrokeratoelastoidosis
- *Transgrediens*: Present
- *Differential diagnosis*: Punctate keratosis of the palmar creases, keratoelastoidosis marginalis, mosaic acral keratosis
- *HPE and ultrastructure*: Orthohyperkeratosis, key differentiating features between acrokeratoelastoidosis and focal acral hyperkeratosis is elastosis, seen in acrokeratoelastoidosis and absent in other.

Syndromic Punctate Palmoplantar Keratoderma

Cole Disease[1,2,9]

- *Synonyms*: Guttate hypopigmentation, punctate PPK with or without ectopic calcification
- *Type of PPK*: Punctate PPK
- *Inheritance*: AD
- *Gene defect*: *ENPP1*
- *Protein defect*: Ectonucleotide pyrophosphatase/ phosphodiesterase 1
- *PPK features and key clinical features*: Onset of disease in infancy, mild focal or punctate PPK with sharply demarcated irregular macules with varying degree of hypopigmentation mainly over proximal extremities
- *Other clinical findings*: Early-onset calcific tendinopathy or calcinosis cutis
- *HPE and ultrastructure*: Orthohyperkeratosis, hypergranulosis, acanthosis, ultrastructure—reduction of melanin content in keratinocytes with large melanosomes, number of melanocytes is normal.
- *Differential diagnosis*: Epidermolysis bullosa simplex with mottled pigmentation, Naegeli–Franceschetti–Jadassohn syndrome

Transient Aquagenic Keratoderma[1,2,9,25]

- *Synonyms*: Transient reactive papulotranslucent acrokeratoderma, aquagenic syringeal acrokeratoderma, transient aquagenic keratoderma, acquired aquagenic palmoplantar keratoderma
- *Inheritance*: AR or AD
- *PPK features and key clinical features*: Onset in second decade of life, incidence rate is more in female. Patient develops thickening and white to translucent, "pebbly" changes on palms shortly after immersion in water ("hand-in-the-bucket" sign), edema and burning pain are also associated, soles involved rarely, these features disappear shortly after drying, leaving minimal hyperkeratosis.

- *Other clinical findings*: Onset associated after use of cyclooxygenase-2 inhibitor, also seen in half of the cystic fibrosis patients.
- *HPE and ultrastructure*: Dilated eccrine ostia and mild hyperkeratotic stratum corneum
- *Differential diagnosis*: Bothnia type NEPPK
- *Treatment*: 20% aluminum chloride hexahydrate followed by urea, botulinum toxin type A

Pachyonychia Congenita[1,2,4,26]

- *Types*:
    - *Type 1*: Jadassohn–Lewandowsky (due to keratin 6A/16 defects)
    - *Type 2*: Jackson–Lawler (due to keratin 6B/17 defects)
- *Type of PPK*: Focal PPK (thick yellow plantar keratoses on pressure sites)
- *Inheritance*: AD
- *Gene defect*: *KRT6A, KRT6B, KRT6C, KRT16, KRT17*
- *Protein defect*: Keratin 6A, 6B, 6C, 16, 17
- *PPK features and key clinical features*: Three cardinal features of PC—(1) toenail dystrophy, (2) focal keratoderma, and (3) plantar pain.

  Fissures, calluses, and blisters may present. Blisters develops on pressure sites in summer
- *Nail involvement*: "Omega" shape nail due to subungual hyperkeratosis and darkening of the nail plate, paronychia
- *Hyperhidrosis*: Present
- *Other clinical findings*: Type 1—severe PPK, oral leukokeratosis; type 2—pilosebaceous cysts and natal teeth

  Follicular hyperkeratosis on knees and elbows, pili torti, vellus hair cysts, steatocystoma multiplex, pilosebaceous cysts, laryngeal involvement causes hoarseness of voice and respiratory tract obstruction
- *HPE and ultrastructure*: Pale cytoplasm and eosinophilic inclusions seen in superficial keratinocytes, hyperkeratosis, with alternating ortho- and parakeratosis, acanthosis

  Ultrastructure—perinuclear condensation of mutated keratin filaments, vacuolization of peripheral cytoplasm
- *Differential diagnosis*: Clouston syndrome
- *Treatment*: Mechanical measures (i.e., cutting, grinding, filing, etc.) for symptomatic relief of hyperkeratosis and dystrophic nails, topical emollients and keratolytics, careful selection of footwear, treatment of hyperhidrosis reduces chance of blistering

Acquired Palmoplantar Keratoderma[27]

Keratoderma Climactericum

Synonyms: Haxthausen disease

Keratoderma climactericum mostly seen in menopausal women.

Clinical features: Hyperkeratotic lesions first starts on pressure points of the soles, followed by development of erythema and fissuring, which cause difficulty in walking due to pain. Pruritus is rare. Later lesions can involve palms also, first starts between thenar and hypothenar region and gradually become confluent to involve whole palm.

HPE: Orthohyperkeratosis, hypergranulosis

Differential diagnosis: Contact dermatitis, dermatophytic infection, altered vitamin A level in serum

Treatment: Oral etretinate, acitretin is treatment of choice. Topical estrogen can be given.

Palmoplantar Keratoderma Secondary to Infection

Human papillomavirus infection, Norwegian scabies, dermatophytosis, tuberculosis.

Palmoplantar Keratoderma Secondary to Dermatoses

Pityriasis rubra pilaris, psoriasis, keratoderma blennorrhagica, atopic dermatitis, chronic hand eczema, lichen planus, lupus erythematosus.

Drug-related Palmoplantar Keratoderma

Hydroxyurea, bleomycin, lithium, venlafaxine, quinacrine, glucan, fluorouracil.

Palmoplantar Keratoderma Secondary to Systemic Disease

Hypothyroidism, chronic lymphedema, myxedema.

Palmoplantar Kertoderma Secondary to Chemical Exposure

Arsenic, chloracnegens.

Palmoplantar Keratoderma Associated with Malignancy

Acrokeratosis paraneoplastica (Bazex syndrome), esophageal cancer, lung cancer, breast cancer, bladder cancer, stomach cancer, colon cancer, myeloma, mycosis fungoides, Sezary syndrome.

DIAGNOSTIC APPROACH

For diagnosis of PPK, history taking is very important.

- Age of onset of PPK
- Type of PPK (diffuse/focal/striate/punctate)
- Any systemic involvement (nonsyndromic/syndromic)
- Transgrediens
- Hyperhidrosis
- Family history of similar complaints
- Consanguinity of parents
- Any metabolic disorder
- Underlying malignancy
- Occupation (any improvement during vacation?)

- History of any medication/drug
- Any infection
- Any associated dermatosis

After proper history, histological, and genetic diagnosis should be consider.

KEY POINTS

Diffuse PPK with AD inheritance:

- *Nonsyndromic*:
  - *Epidermolytic PPK*:
    - Unna–Thost disease
  - *Nonepidermolytic PPK*:
    - Bothnia type NEPPK
    - Kimonis type NEPPK
    - Greither type NEPPK
    - Loricrin keratoderma
- *Syndromic:*
  - Vohwinkel syndrome } Hearing loss along with PPK
  - Bart–Pumphrey syndrome } Hearing loss along with PPK

  Huriez syndrome—cancer is a feature of Huriez syndrome along with PPK
  - Clouston syndrome } Ectodermal dysplasia related disease along with PPK
  - Olmsted syndrome (rarely present as AD inheritance)* } Ectodermal dysplasia related disease along with PPK

Diffuse PPK with AR inheritance:

- *Nonsyndromic*:
  - *Nonepidermolytic PPK*:
    - Mal de Meleda
    - Nagashima type NEPPK
- *Syndromic*:
  - Naxos disease—cardiomyopathy
  - Palmoplantar keratoderma, sex reversal, and cancer is seen along with PPK in this:
    - Odonto-onycho-dermal dysplasia } Ectodermal dysplasia related disease along with PPK
    - Papillon–Lefèvre syndrome } Ectodermal dysplasia related disease along with PPK
    - Haim–Munk syndrome } Ectodermal dysplasia related disease along with PPK
    - Olmsted syndrome (rarely present as AR inheritance) } Ectodermal dysplasia related disease along with PPK

Focal PPK with AD inheritance:

- *Nonsyndromic:*
  - Striate palmoplantar keratoderma
  - Punctate palmoplantar keratoderma
  - Spiny keratoderma
  - *Marginal papular keratoderma*: Acrokeratoelastoidosis and focal acral hyperkeratosis
- *Syndromic:*
  - Howel–Evans syndrome—esophageal squamous cell carcinoma
  - Pachyonychia congenita—nail changes, plantar pain
  - Cole disease—hypopigmented macules over proximal extremities

Focal PPK with AR inheritance:

- *Syndromic:*
  - Carvajal syndrome[#]—cardiomyopathy
  - Richner–Hanhart syndrome—ophthalmic manifestation

Acquired palmoplantar keratoderma:

- Haxthausen disease—seen in menopausal women
- PPK secondary to infection
- PPK secondary to dermatoses
- PPK secondary to systemic disease
- PPK secondary to chemical exposure
- Drug-related PPK
- PPK associated with malignancy

Mitochondrial PPK with hearing impairment—mitochondrial inheritance (diffuse or focal PPK)

[#]Carvajal syndrome can be AR > AD.
[*]Olmsted syndrome most cases are sporadic but AD > AR, XR can be seen.

REFERENCES

1. Griffiths C, Barker J, Bleiker T, Chalmers R, Creamer D (Eds). Rook's Textbook of Dermatology, 9th edition. New Delhi: Wiley Blackwell; 2016. pp. 65.42-65.66.
2. Bolognia JL, Schaffer JV, Cerroni L (Eds). Dermatology, 4th edition. Philadelphia: Elsevier; 2018. pp. 924-40.
3. Guerra L, Castori M, Didona B, Castiglia D, Zambruno G. Hereditary palmoplantar keratodermas. Part I. Non-syndromic palmoplantar keratodermas: classification, clinical and genetic features. J Eur Acad Dermatol Venereol. 2018;32(5):704-19.
4. Dev T, Mahajan VK, Sethuraman G. Hereditary palmoplantar keratoderma: a Practical approach to the diagnosis. Indian Dermatol Online J. 2019;10:365-79.
5. Sakiyama T, Kubo A. Hereditary palmoplantar keratoderma: clinical and genetic differential diagnosis. J Dermatol. 2016; 43(3):264-74.
6. Nath AK, Chaudhuri S, Thappa DM. Mal de Meleda with lip involvement: a report of two cases. Indian J Dermatol. 2012; 57:390-3.
7. Athanikar SB, Inamdar AC, Patil A, Sampagavi VV, Deshmukh NS. Griether's disease. Indian J Dermatol Venereol Leprol. 2003;69:292-3.
8. Rajashekar TS, Singh G, Naik CL, Okade R. Camisa disease: A rare variant of Vohwinkel syndrome. Indian J Dermatol Venereol Leprol. 2008;74:81.
9. Guerra L, Castori M, Didona B, Castiglia D, Zambruno G. Hereditary palmoplantar keratodermas. Part II. Syndromic palmoplantar keratodermas—Diagnostic algorithm and principles of therapy. J Eur Acad Dermatol Venereol. 2018; 32(6):899-925.
10. Choudhary N, Ahar R, De A, Biswas P. Vohwinkel's syndrome: A rare disorder of keratinisation. Indian J Dermatol. 2014; 59:619-21.
11. Gonul M, Gul U, Hizil P, Hizil O. A family of Bart-Pumphrey syndrome. Indian J Dermatol Venereol Leprol. 2012;78:178-81.
12. Rai R, Ramachandran B, Sundaram VS, Rajendren G, Srinivas CR. Naxos disease: a rare occurrence of cardiomyopathy with woolly hair and palmoplantar keratoderma. Indian J Dermatol Venereol Leprol. 2008;74:50-2.

13. Parvez Y, Al-Hassan AA. Carvajal syndrome: A variant of Naxos disease in two Saudi siblings. Niger J Exp Clin Biosci. 2013;1: 48-9.
14. Kharge P, Fernendes C, Jairath V, Mohan M, Chandra S. Poikiloderma a varied presentation—Huriez syndrome. Indian Dermatol Online J. 2015;6:27-30.
15. Ellis A, Risk JM, Maruthappu T, Kelsell DP. Tylosis with oesophageal cancer: diagnosis, management and molecular mechanisms. Orphanet J Rare Dis. 2015;10:126.
16. Khatter S, Puri RD, Mahay SB, Bhai P, Saxena R, Verma IC. Mutation-proved Clouston syndrome in a large Indian family with a variant phenotype. Indian J Dermatol. 2019;64: 143-5.
17. Muppa R, Prameela B, Duddu M, Dandempally A. Papillon-lefevre syndrome: a combined approach from the dermatologist and dentist—a clinical presentation. Indian J Dermatol. 2011;56:740-3.
18. Mohan RS, Verma S. Haim Munk syndrome: Report of two siblings of northern Indian treated with acitretin. Indian J Dermatol Venereol Leprol. 2011;77:252.
19. Tharini GK, Hema N, Jayakumar S, Parveen B. Olmsted syndrome: report of two cases. Indian J Dermatol. 2011;56: 591-3.
20. al-Hemidan AI, al-Hazzaa SA. Richner-Hanhart syndrome (tyrosinemia type II): case report and literature review. Ophthalmic Genet. 1995;16(1):21-6.
21. Tiwary AK, Chatterjee S, Mishra DK. Brunauer-Fuhs-Siemens palmoplantar keratoderma: a rare striate type of focal palmoplantar keratoderma. Indian J Paediatr Dermatol. 2016; 17: 246-8.
22. Jose S, Kamath KN, Pai GS, Pinto J. Punctate palmoplantar keratoderma. Indian J Dermatol Venereol Leprol. 2003;69 Suppl S1:70-1.
23. Torres G, Behshad R, Han A, Castrovinci AJ, Gilliam AC. "I forgot to shave my hands": a case of spiny keratoderma. J Am Acad Dermatol. 2008;58(2):344-8.
24. Rambhia KD, Khopkar US. Acrokeratoelastoidosis. Indian Dermatol Onine J. 2015;6:460-1.
25. Tchernev G, Semkova K, Cardoso JC, Ananiev JJ, Wollina U. Aquagenic keratoderma: two new case reports and a new hypothesis. Indian Dermatol Online J. 2014;5:30-3.
26. Agarwal P, Chhaperwal MK, Singh A, Verma A, Nijhawan M, Singh K, et al. Pachyonychia congenital: a rare genodermatosis. Indian Dermatol Online J. 2013;4:225-7.
27. Patel S, Zirwas M, English JC 3rd. Acquired palmoplantar keratoderma. Am J Clin Dermatol. 2007;8(1):1-11.

EXAMINATION QUESTIONS

1. Classify PPK.
2. Write a write short note on pachyonychia congenita.

7 SECTION | Skin and Systemic Disease

64 CHAPTER

Skin Changes in Diabetes Mellitus and Endocrine Disease

Surajit Gorai, Hemanta Kumar Nath

INTRODUCTION

The majority of endocrine diseases have skin manifestations. So, it is important for us to know about the skin changes in different endocrine diseases which will be very helpful in early diagnosis of the diseases. But among different endocrine disease, skin manifestations are more common in diabetes mellitus, thyroid disorders, adrenal disorders, and pituitary disorders. So, we will be discussing about these disorders in brief and will try to get an insight into different manifestations associated with different endocrine systems.

Skin manifestations could be specific to the disease or may be sometimes nonspecific. Nonspecific manifestations could be pruritus, dryness, keratosis pilaris, infections, psoriasis, vitiligo, eczema, and warts. Some of the common changes have been mentioned in **Table 1**.

TABLE 1: Some common skin changes and their clinical description.

Skin changes	*Clinical description*	*Comments*
Acanthosis nigricans[2]	Velvety hyperpigmentation of the intertriginous/flexural areas, neck, axilla, groin and, less often extensor surfaces	Commonly associated with insulin resistance in both adults and children. Activation in IGF-R which mediates proliferation of keratinocyte and fibroblast
Xanthomas	Red-yellow papules that appear over a period of weeks to months	Associated with elevated serum triglycerides in patients with poorly controlled diabetes. Control of the DM results in resolution of the xanthomas. Deposition of lipids in histiocytes
Gangrene	Necrosis of the toes > fingertips. May be wet or dry	Ischemia due to vascular disease in larger vessels
Acral erythema	Erysipelas-like erythema of the hands and/or feet. Well demarcated, painless and edematous	May be due to small vessel occlusive disease with compensatory hyperemia
Diabetic dermopathy	Brown atrophic macules and patches on the legs. More than 3 is necessary to term it dermopathy	Possibly precipitated by trauma and increased vascular permeability
Diabetic foot	• *Sensory neuropathy*—non-painful ulcerations at sites of pressure, most commonly on the foot. When the ulcer is on the plantar surface, a characteristic keratotic rim is seen • *Motor neuropathy*—pes cavus, hammer toe • *Autonomic neuropathy*—loss of sweating, cracking, fissure • Microangiopathy—poor perfusion and healing	Associated with neuropathy, vasculopathy, infections and poor healing
Diabetic bullae (bullosis diabeticorum)	Tense noninflammatory bullae on the lower extremities	Uncertain pathogenesis; microvascular angiopathy possible contributor
Necrobiosis lipoidica	Yellow atrophic patches, most often on the shins with translucent surface. A red-brown rim may indicate activity at the border. Ulceration can occur and is often slow to heal. It may precede the onset of DM	Develops in <1% of patients with DM; *diabeticorum* was dropped from its name because not always associated with DM
Perforating disorders (e.g., acquired perforating dermatosis)	Grouped pruritic keratotic papules, primarily on the extremities	Often occurs in diabetic patients with chronic kidney disease on dialysis. Transepidermal elimination of dermal constituents
Granuloma annulare	Erythematous annular lesions composed of papules Types—localized, generalized, subcutaneous	May occur spontaneously, after insect bite, photodamage
Scleredema (adultorum of Buschke)	Induration of the upper back and nape due to glycosaminoglycan deposition; may have overlying erythema	No relationship to control of the DM. Also referred to as type III scleredema

Contd...

Contd...

Skin changes	*Clinical description*	*Comments*
Infections[3]	• Bacterial—Staphylococcal and streptococcal infections causing folliculitis, furuncle, ecthyma. Malignant otitis externa caused by *Pseudomonas* • Fungal—candidiasis, rhinocerebral mucormycosis, phycomycetes	• Due to decreased chemotaxis, phagocytosis and WBC • Seen in diabetes
Diabetic cheiroarthropathy	Thickened skin and limited joint mobility of the hands and fingers, leading to flexion contractures (starting with the fifth digit and progressing radially) and an inability to approximate the palmar surfaces of the hands and fingers (Prayer sign)	• Postulated to result from increased glycosylation of collagen in the skin. Associated with retinopathy, nephropathy, and duration • Seen on diabetes/immunocompromised

DIABETES MELLITUS

Diabetes mellitus is caused due to disorder of the pancreas leading to problematic secretion of insulin or sometimes insulin is normally secreted but the body becomes nonresponsive to insulin. About 40–60% of patients have skin manifestations. Most of the persons having skin manifestations are elderly due to long-standing diabetes. Insulin-dependent diabetes has more skin manifestations. Mechanism of many cutaneous lesions remain unknown but pathogenesis is linked directly or through damage to vascular, neurological, or immune systems.[1]

Hyperglycemia → Nonenzymatic glycosylation of collagen → advanced glycosylation end-products → reduces acid solubility and enzymatic degradation → diabetic skin manifestations

In case of suspicion of associated diabetes mellitus in correlation with clinical features, we could advice for blood tests for FBS, PPBS, HbA1C, insulin levels.

Nonspecific features should be treated accordingly but some of the specific features may require different approach. Most important of all in foot ulcer:

- Foot ulcer should be treated with proper antibiotics, protective dressings, decrease pressure bearing, foot care advice and debridement
- Acanthosis nigricans require weight reduction, keratolytics
- Diabetic bullae usually resolves spontaneously.
- Cheiroarthropathy may require methotrexate, psoralen, and physiotherapy.
- Eruptive xanthomas usually resolve on control of glucose and lipid levels

THYROID DISEASES

Thyroid gland plays an important role in the human body. It secretes two hormones in our body tri-iodothyronine and thyroxine. They are mainly responsible for regulating the metabolism in the body. They are important for proper development of cells. They help in neural maturation. Its increased and decreased activity can easily be appreciated in the skin, hair, and nail of the person.

Skin, hair and nail changes in hypo- and hyperthyroidism are described in **Table 2**.

To confirm the diagnosis along with clinical features lab tests are also necessary to level it thyroid abnormality involvement, we can run test for TSH, T3, T4 levels in the blood.

If there is irregularities in their levels, proper management of thyroid hormone levels usually resolves the cutaneous symptoms in most of the cases.

Pretibial myxedema may require additional oral/topical/intralesional steroids, and compression stockings.

PITUITARY GLAND

It is the master gland which control other endocrine glands. It produces hormones that direct different glands to produce their respective hormones.[5]

It secretes growth hormones whose abnormality has been described in **Table 3**. It secretes thyroid stimulating hormone which act on thyroid gland, whose features has been described in **Table 2**. It secretes ACTH which act on adrenal and produce cortisol whose features has been described in **Table 3**. Classical appearance of hyperpituitarism-prognathism, frontal bossing, enlarged lower lips, widely spaced teeth, macroglossia, enlarged hands and feet, thick heel pad: Pituitary abnormality can be detected by blood levels of different hormones such as GH, ACTH, TSH, and radioimaging for suspected tumors.

Acromegaly improves either with surgical intervention/radiotherapy. Somatostatin analogue has been tried.

ADRENAL GLAND

These glands are present over the kidneys and are responsible for production of glucocorticoids, mineralocorticoids, and sex hormones. Out of which we are more concerned about cortisol function. It controls sleep-wake cycle. It is secreted at the time of stress to handle emergency situation. It regulates blood pressure and sugar. It controls metabolism carbohydrates, fats, and proteins **(Table 4)**.

To confirm the association of adrenal glands, we can test for serum adrenal hormone levels along with the clinical features.

TABLE 2: Different skin, hair and nail changes in thyroid disorders.

	Hyperthyroidism	*Hypothyroidism*
	It is a hypermetabolic state resulting from excess thyroid hormones (T4, T3)	It is a slow metabolic state due to decreased concentration of thyroid hormone in blood or target cell resistant to thyroid hormone
Etiology	Graves' disease, toxic multinodular goiter, drugs, adenoma, thyroiditis, pituitary tumor	Idiopathic, iatrogenic, iodine deficiency, cretinism, hypothalamic failure
Cutaneous changes	• Fine, reddish smooth skin • Warm and moist due to increased sweating and vasodilatation flushing, palmar erythema.[4] • Hyperpigmentation—localized or generalized • *Jellinek's sign*—hyperpigmented eyelids • *Pemberton sign*—facial suffusion provoked with substernal goiter	• Dry, rough, coarse skin • Cold and pale extremities due to reflex vasoconstriction • Decreased sweating • Puffy eyelids, swollen lips, large tongue due to dermal accumulation of mucopolysaccharide • Easy bruising due to loss of capillary support
Cutaneous diseases/ syndrome	• *Pretibial myxedema*—localized edematous plaque in the shins. Usually associated with opthalmopathy[1] • *Thyroid acropachy* (acral soft tissue swelling, periostitis, and clubbing of the digits) • *Diamond syndrome*—pretibial myxedema, thyroid acropachy, exophthalmos • *EMO syndrome*—exophthalmos, myxedema, osteoarthropathy	• Acquired ichthyosis and palmoplantar keratoderma due to decreased sweating • Eruptive and/or tuberous • Xanthomas • *Hertoghe sign*—alopecia of the lateral third of the eyebrows
Hair changes/ diseases	• Fine, thin • Mild, diffuse alopecia • Increased incidence of alopecia areata	• Dull, coarse, brittle • Slow growth • Increased incidence of alopecia areata
Nail changes	• Onycholysis—thin, brittle, striated • Koilonychia, fast growth • Clubbing from thyroid • Acropachy	• Thin, brittle, striated • Onycholysis (rare)

TABLE 3: Different skin, hair and nail changes in pituitary disorders.

	Hyperpituitarism	*Hypopituitarism*
Associated syndrome	*Nelson syndrome*—due to non-ACTH secreting pituitary tumor after a bilateral adrenalectomy in a patient with pituitary-dependent hypercorticism characterized by hyperpigmentation	*Sheehan syndrome*—hypopituitarism develop due to pituitary damage due to postpartum hemorrhage
Skin changes	Hyperpigmentation, increased sweating, cutis verticis gyrata	Hypopigmentation, dryness and premature aging
Hair	Hirsutism, loss of secondary sexual hair	Loss of secondary hair
Nail	Faster nail growth	Onycholysis, longitudinal ridging

TABLE 4: Different cutaneous changes in adrenal disorders.

Cushing syndrome/hypercorticism	*Adrenal insufficiency*
It is due to excess glucocorticoids can be exogenous, adrenal hypersecretion, pituitary hypersecretion or ectopic secretion	Due to decreased cortisol level
Altered subcutaneous fat distribution: • "Moon" facies[6] • Dorsal cervical fat deposition "buffalo hump" • Reduced fat in the arms and legs—lemon on sticks appearance *Skin atrophy:* • Multiple striae over abdomen, breasts—telangiectasia • Fragile skin • Prolonged wound healing • *Purpura from minor trauma:* – Cigarette paper-like wrinkling of skin – Cutaneous infections hyperpigmentation • Dermatophytosis and onychomycosis • Candidiasis • Acneiform eruptions	*Hyperpigmentation (MSH-like effect of ACTH):* • Photo-exposed skin elbow, knee • Palmar creases—genitals, perineum • Mucous membranes • Hair • Nails (longitudinal melanonychia) • Melanocytic nevi and lentigines Loss of androgen-stimulated (axillary, pubic) hair in postpubertal women

Most of the symptoms decrease with normalization of hormonal levels with treatment.

KEY POINTS

- Basic skin changes in different endocrine disorders.
- Skin, hair and nail changes in DM.
- Skin changes in thyroid disorder.
- Skin changes in altered cortisol level in blood.

REFERENCES

1. Parasramani SG, Oberoi C. Cutaneous manifestations in diabetes mellitus. In: Sacchidanand S, Oberoi C, Inamdar AC (Eds). IADVL Textbook of Dermatology, 4th edition. Mumbai: Bhalani Publishing House; 2013. pp. 1915-29.
2. Schwarzenberger K, Callen JP. Dermatologic manifestations in patients with systemic disease. In: Bolognia JL, Schaffer JV, Cerroni L (Eds). Dermatology, 4th edition. Elsevier Limited; 2018. pp. 827-30.
3. Gajula N, Pratheepa R, Rohit V, Vumma N. Cutaneous manifestations of diabetes mellitus. J Med Sci Clin Res. 2018;6.
4. Puri N. A study on cutaneous manifestations of thyroid disease. Indian J Dermatol. 2012;57(3):247.
5. Davidovici BB, Orion E, Wolf R. Cutaneous manifestations of pituitary gland diseases. Clin Dermatol. 2008;26(3): 288-95.
6. Jabbour SA. Cutaneous manifestations of endocrine disorders. Am J Clin Dermatol. 2003;4(5):315-31.

EXAMINATION QUESTIONS

1. Discuss the cutaneous manifestations of diabetes mellitus.
2. What are the skin changes in thyroid diseases?
3. What is diabetic dermopathy?
4. What is pretibial myxedema?

65 CHAPTER Skin Changes in Systemic Diseases

Sudip Kumar Ghosh, Satarupa Mondal

INTRODUCTION

Skin is the window of our body and an experienced clinician can perceive the internal organs through this window. Diseases of several organs often have prominent cutaneous features and not infrequently the cutaneous signs can be the presenting features of these diseases. Detailed discussion of all these manifestations is beyond the scope of this present chapter. So, the common mucocutaneous presentations of endocrine, gastrointestinal, hepatic, renal, cardiac, respiratory, and nervous systems are described here.

MUCOCUTANEOUS MANIFESTATIONS OF ENDOCRINAL DISORDERS

Dermatologists may commonly see mucocutaneous lesions that reflect an underlying endocrine disorder.[1] The common dermatological manifestations of endocrine disorders are discussed below.

Diabetes Mellitus[1-5]

Some of the mucocutaneous features of diabetes mellitus correlate with metabolic derangements; some correlate with degenerative complications; some are seen more commonly in diabetic patients; while other complications are iatrogenic in nature. Cutaneous infections including furunculosis, carbuncle, group B streptococcal infections, botryomycosis, necrotizing fasciitis, cellulitis, malignant otitis externa, candidiasis (particularly candidal balanoposthitis) **(Fig. 1)**, and dermatophytosis are more common in the setting of diabetes. Mucormycosis may be associated with diabetic ketoacidosis. Acanthosis nigricans and thickened indurated skin mainly over back and neck (scleredema) may be present.

Diabetic cheiroarthropathy is a recognized complication of diabetes mellitus and the resultant prayer sign is often present. Eruptive xanthomas **(Fig. 2)** and necrobiosis lipoidica are very important cutaneous markers of diabetes. Nonhealing ulcers (mostly over lower extremities) and diabetic dermopathy (small atrophic brown, scar-like macules on both shins) are also important cutaneous manifestation of diabetes. Generalized **(Fig. 3)** or perforating granuloma

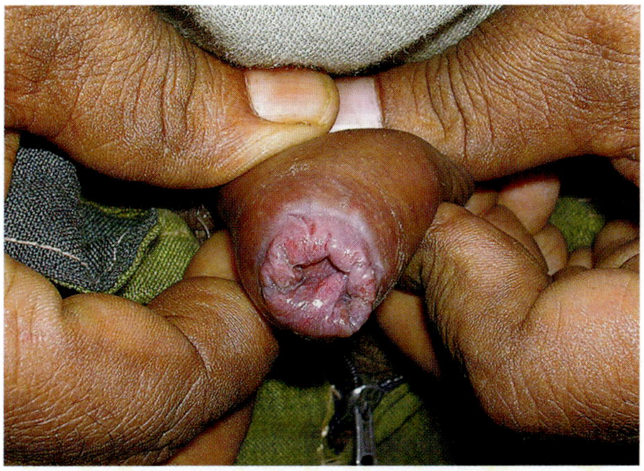

Fig. 1: Candidal balanoposthitis.

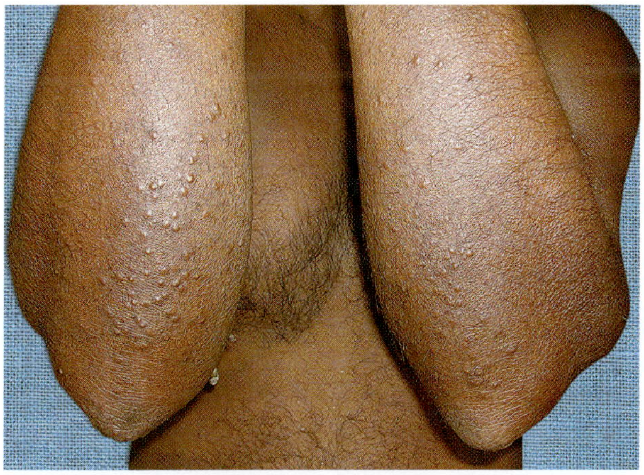

Fig. 2: Eruptive xanthoma.

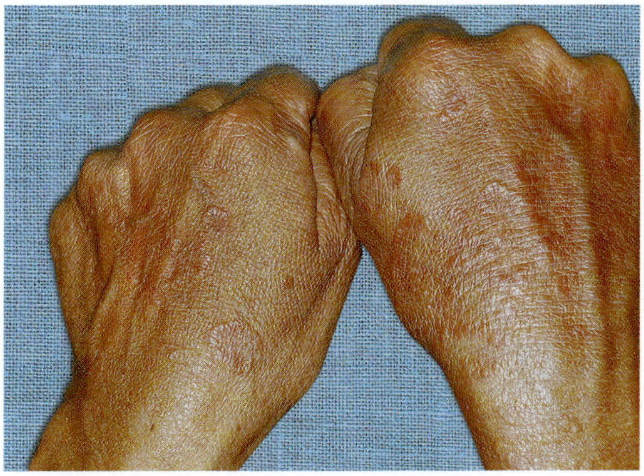

Fig. 3: Granuloma annulare on the dorsum of hands.

annulare and acquired perforating disorders are also rarely seen. Diabetic bullae are characterized by abrupt onset, noninflammatory, painless bullae on extremities, feet, toes, and shins. Glucagonoma may present with necrolytic acral erythema, typically annular or polycyclic skin lesions which may demonstrate confluence in severely affected areas. Other associated mucocutaneous findings include atrophic glossitis, cheilosis, onychoschizia, buccal mucosal inflammation, and rarely dyspareunia.

Thyroid Disorders[1,4,6]

Cutaneous manifestations of thyroid disease are protean in nature and involve all age groups. A brief account of the mucocutaneous manifestations of hypothyroidism and hyperthyroidism are given in **Table 1**.

Hashimoto's Thyroiditis

In addition, Hashimotos thyroiditis may be associated with acanthosis nigricans, alopecia areata, alopecia totalis, diffuse alopecia, chronic mucocutaneous candidiasis among others.

Adrenal Dysfunction[1,4,7]

Cutaneous manifestations of adrenal dysfunctions are summarized in **Table 2**.

Parathyroid Dysfunction[1,4]

Dermatologic manifestations of parathyroid-related disorders, though rarely present in sporadic cases, are not infrequent in familial syndromes.

Common cutaneous manifestations of hypoparathyroidism are puffy, hyperkeratotic, and scaly skin; coarse hairs with patchy alopecia or diffuse thinning and brittle nails with transverse ridges. Common cutaneous manifestations of hyperparathyroidism are subcutaneous calcification, violaceous mottled to reticulated patches, and plaques with occasional bulla. Painful necrotic indurated plaques, nodules, ulcers with thick dark eschar, and acral gangrene are also seen.

Miscellaneous

Mucocutaneous manifestations of other endocrinal disorders[1,4,7,8] are depicted in **Table 3**.

MUCOCUTANEOUS MANIFESTATIONS OF GASTROINTESTINAL DISEASES

Skin manifestations are frequently seen as a part of different gastrointestinal (GI) diseases.[8-11] Dermatologists play an important role in recognizing the symptoms, patient workup, and arriving at appropriate diagnosis, in consultation with gastroenterologists.

Different GI symptoms and its association with cutaneous disease are summarized in **Table 4**.

Cutaneous Manifestations According to the Site and Type of Pathology of the GI Tract[8-11]

Diseases of the Esophagus

Mucositis: Mucositis may occur in the setting of Stevens-Johnson syndrome, Behçet's disease and pemphigus.

Dysphagia: It is common feature of systemic sclerosis and dermatomyositis.

TABLE 1: Mucocutaneous manifestations of hypothyroidism and hyperthyroidism.

Features	*Hypothyroidism*	*Hyperthyroidism*
Temperature regulation	• Cold intolerance • Cold, pale skin	• Heat intolerance • Warm, moist, smooth skin
Other mucocutaneous changes	• Acquired ichthyosis **(Fig. 4)** • Palmoplantar keratoderma • Asteatotic eczema • Malar flush • Yellowish skin (carotenemia) • Xanthomatosis (hyperlipidemia) • Generalized myxedema with doughy, swollen, dry, pale, and waxy-to-touch non-pitting edematous skin • Delayed wound healing • *Facial appearance*: Broad nose, swollen lips, puffy eyelids, madarosis and flattening of affect • *Oral mucosal features*: Macroglossia, gingival swelling and oral candidiasis	• Generalized hyperhidrosis • Hyperpigmentation of skin • Generalized pruritus • Palmar erythema • *Pretibial thyroid dermopathy (Pretibial myxedema)*: Bilateral, localized non-pitting, firm, hyperpigmented nodules or plaques on legs and also over arms, shoulders, neck, and at sites of trauma and scars • *Thyroid acropachy*: Clubbing of the fingers and toes associated with soft tissue swellings of hand and feet
Nail changes	Slowly growing, brittle with prominent longitudinal ridges	Rapidly growing, soft, having concave contour, distal onycholysis (Plummer's nail)
Hair changes	• Coarse sparse scalp hair and loss of pubic, axillary, and facial hair • Association with alopecia areata	• Fine, soft, friable, and are often associated with diffuse nonscarring alopecia. • Association with alopecia areata
Associated diseases	• Bullous pemphigoid • Dermatomyositis	• Chronic urticaria • Vitiligo

Howel-Evans syndrome: It presents with tylosis in childhood and high risk of esophageal carcinomas in adults.

Acrokeratosis paraneoplastica (Bazex syndrome): It is characterized by the occurrence of hyperkeratotic lesions on the nose, ears, palms, and soles that appear in association with malignancies of the upper aerodigestive tract, most often a squamous cell carcinoma.

Diseases of the Pancreas

Table 5 summarizes different mucocutaneous features of pancreatic diseases.[8-10]

Diseases of the Small and Large Intestines[8-11]

Polyposis syndromes: There are two groups of hereditary polyposis; adenomatous syndromes (e.g., familial adenomatous polyposis, Gardner's syndrome) and hamartomatous syndromes (e.g., Peutz-Jeghers and Cronkhite-Canada syndromes). Adenomas have proven malignant potential. Hamartomatous polyps represent proliferation and malformation of connective tissue of the intestinal mucosa and have relatively less risk of malignancy. **Table 6** summarizes the diverse mucocutaneous features associated with different colonic polyposis.

Inflammatory bowel disease (IBD): IBD disease with its two main subtypes (Crohn's disease and ulcerative colitis) is not restricted to the GI tract. Several mucocutaneous manifestations associated with IBD are summarized in **Table 7**.[9-11]

Rectum: Extramammary Paget's disease may reflect underlying rectal carcinoma.

Cutaneous manifestations of gastrointestinal malignancy:[8-11] There are both syndrome-related and acquired cutaneous markers of GI malignancies. They include acanthosis

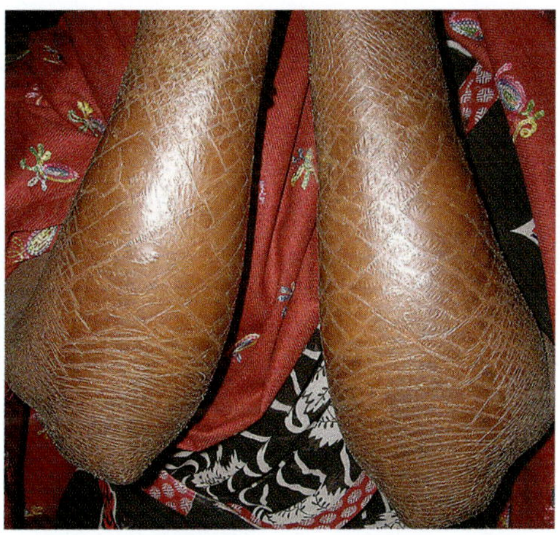

Fig. 4: Ichthyosis of skin.

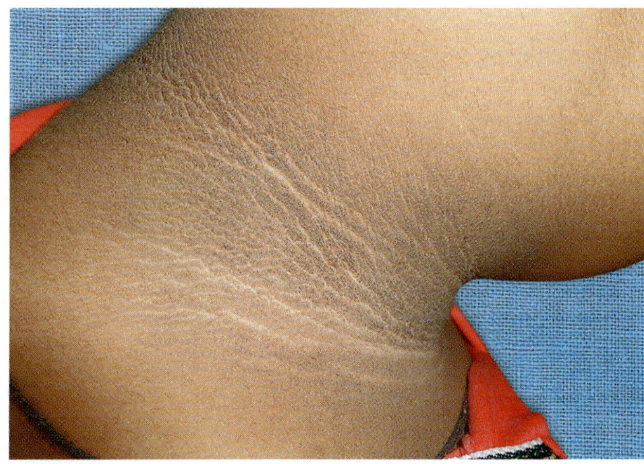

Fig. 5: Acanthosis nigricans.

TABLE 2: Cutaneous manifestations of adrenal dysfunctions.

Addison's disease	Skin changes	• Hyperpigmentation over photo-exposed areas, friction prone areas, highly pigmented areas, mucous membranes, and scars • Generalized xerosis
	Nail changes	Longitudinal melanonychia (pigmented bands)
	Hair changes	Decreased axillary and pubic hairs occur in women
	Others	• Fibrosis and calcification of pinna • Associated with polyglandular autoimmune disorders (vitiligo and chronic mucocutaneous candidiasis)
Cushing's syndrome	Skin changes	Atrophic, smooth, transparent, and paper-thin skin
	Changes on minor trauma	Tearing of skin, ulceration, purpura, and ecchymosis
	Striae	Broad purple with sufficient depth, breadth on the abdomen, thigh, arm, axilla
	Facial changes	Full and round (moon facies), plethoric with telangiectasia, hirsutism, and acneiform eruption
	Subcutaneous fat	Buffalo hump and full supraclavicular fossa
	Others	• Increased prevalence of dermatophytosis and yeast infections • Hypertrichosis • Acanthosis nigricans **(Fig. 5)** • Hyperpigmentation
Pheochromocytoma	Features and associations	• Association with neurofibromatosis (NF) type 1 • *Specific skin lesions*: Multiple cutaneous metastases in malignant pheochromocytoma • Increased prevalence of dermatomyositis, Behçet's disease, Sweet syndrome, and erythema nodosum

TABLE 3: Mucocutaneous manifestations of miscellaneous endocrinal disorders.

Endocrinal dysfunction	*Mucocutaneous features*	
Panhypopituitarism	Skin changes	• Paleness of the skin with a yellowish tinge • Xerotic and thin skin with fine wrinkling around the eyes and mouth • Older look • Generalized hypopigmentation
	Hair changes	Hypotrichosis with generalized thinning of scalp, axillary, pubic hairs, and beard
	Nail changes	• Slowly growing • Brittle • Opaque • Thin
Acromegaly	Facies	• Coarsening of facial features due to dermal thickening • Leonine facies • Gigantic hypertrophy of the chin, nose and supraorbital ridges with deep folds and furrows • *Lips*: Thickened and protruded • *Tongue*: Large and furrowed • *Eyelids*: Thickened
	Extremities	Hands and feet are swollen, doughy, and spade-like
	Hair	Coarse body hairs, hirsutism in females
	Pigmentary	Acanthosis nigricans
Posterior pituitary dysfunction		Langerhans cell histiocytosis (LCH) associated with diabetes insipidus (particularly in Hand-Schuller –Christian disease)
Androgen-related disorders	Male	• *Male hypogonadism*: Delay of puberty and reduced growth and/or function of genital organs, terminal hairs, male voice, and male sexuality • Smooth skin with fine wrinkles • Markedly reduced function of sebaceous glands • Hyperandrogenism in males may present with androgenetic alopecia and acne fulminans
	Female	Female hyperandrogenism presents with: • Sudden-onset acne • Treatment-refractory severe acne • Hirsutism **(Fig. 6)** • Temporal balding • Clitoromegaly
Estrogenic disorders	Estrogen excess	• Telangiectasia • Palmar erythema • Spider angioma • Hyperpigmentation • Acanthosis nigricans
	Estrogen deficiency	• Hot flushes • Atrophy of genital mucosa • Decreased breast size
Multiple endocrine neoplasias		• Neuroma • Lichen amyloidosis
Autoimmune polyendocrinopathy syndrome		Features of Addison's disease, hypoparathyroidism, and chronic mucocutaneous candidiasis

nigricans, Sister Mary Joseph nodule (metastasis to the umbilicus from an abdominal tumor), cutaneous features of Cowden syndrome (facial trichilemmomas, oral papillomas with cobblestoning, and acral keratosis), Muir—Torre syndrome (sebaceous neoplasms and keratoacanthomas), and Kaposi's sarcoma.

Several Multisystem Disorders Which have Both GI and Cutaneous Manifestations[8-11]

They include Fabry disease (lesions of angiokeratoma corporis diffusum), hereditary hemorrhagic telangiectasia, neurofibromatosis, pseudoxanthoma elasticum, several infections (strongyloidiasis, tuberculosis, typhoid fever), Behçet's disese, IgA vasculitis, polyarteritis nodosa, systemic lupus erythematosus (SLE), systemic sclerosis, several neoplastic conditions (carcinoid syndrome, glucagonoma, mastocytosis), angioedema, amyloidosis, scurvy, etc.

Stoma-related complications: Irritant or allergic contact dermatitis, erythema, maceration, erosions, parastomal ulcer, abscess, fistula, infections, and pyoderma gangrenosum may occur as part of stoma-related complications.

MUCOCUTANEOUS MANIFESTATIONS OF HEPATIC DISEASES

Patients with liver diseases can present with a number of cutaneous manifestations. Thorough knowledge of these

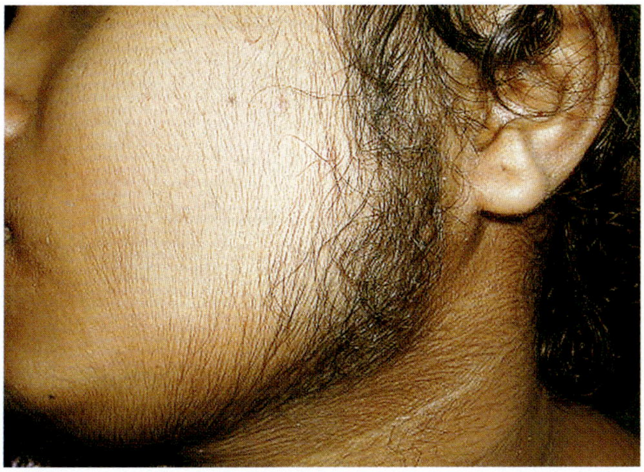

Fig. 6: Hirsutism.

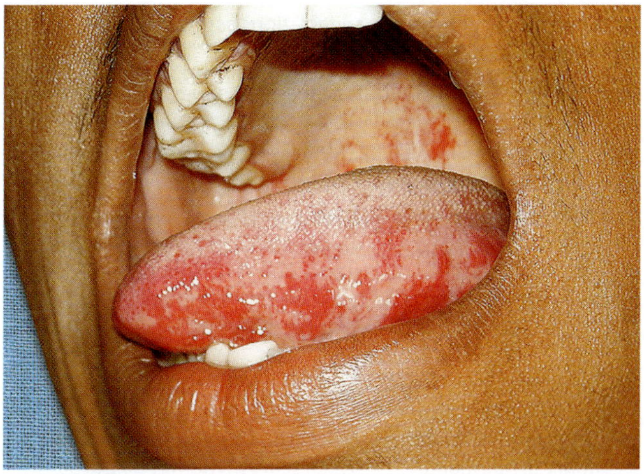

Fig. 7: Hereditary hemorrhagic telangiectasia.

TABLE 4: Different gastrointestinal (GI) symptoms and its association with cutaneous disease.[8-11]

GI symptoms	*Associated diseases which have cutaneous features/mucocutaneous manifestations*
GI bleeding	Vasculitis, hereditary hemorrhagic telangiectasia (**Fig. 7**), with perioral telangiectasia, pulmonary arteriovenous fistulas, vascular tumors: both benign (blue rubber bleb nevus) and malignant (Kaposi sarcoma), connective tissue defects such as vascular form of Ehlers Danlos syndrome, and pseudoxanthoma elasticum
Malabsorption/diarrhea	• Dry scaly skin, pruritus • Diffuse nonscarring alopecia • Slow growing, brittle nails • *Associated diseases*: Celiac disease with dermatitis herpetiformis, acrodermatitis enteropathica with zinc deficiency, and autoimmune connective tissue diseases
Pain abdomen	Herpes zoster, angioedema, carcinoid syndrome, glucagonoma, mastocytosis, strongyloidiasis, tuberculosis, typhoid fever, Behçet disease, IgA vasculitis, polyarteritis nodosa, inflammatory bowel disorders, pancreatitis

TABLE 5: Mucocutaneous features of pancreatic diseases.

Pancreatic diseases	*Mucocutaneous features*	
Acute pancreatitis	Ecchymosis at different sites	
	Periumbilical	Cullen sign
	Flank	Gray Turner sign
	Upper thigh	Fox's sign
	Scrotum	Bryant's sign
Pancreatic carcinoma	• Trousseau's sign (superficial migratory thrombophlebitis) • Other unexplained thrombosis • Liquefying predominantly lobular panniculitis • Metastatic nodules, especially to umbilicus (Sister Mary Joseph's nodule)	
Miscellaneous	• *Liquefying predominantly lobular panniculitis*: A sign of pancreatic inflammation and tumors • *Necrolytic migratory erythema along with stomatitis*: Glucagonoma	

TABLE 6: Mucocutaneous features associated with different colonic polyposis.

Type of polyposis	*Associated syndromes*	*Cutaneous features*
Adenomatous polyposis	Gardner's syndrome (Familial adenomatous polyposis)	Epidermoid cysts, fibromas, lipomas, desmoid tumors, pilomatricomas, and osteomas of the facial bones and skull
Hamartomatous polyposis	Peutz–Jeghers syndrome	Darkly pigmented macules on the lips, buccal mucosa, and digits
	Cronkhite–Canada syndromes	Patchy alopecia and characteristic nail changes
Vasoactive syndromes	Zollinger–Ellison syndrome	Flushing and diarrhea

TABLE 7: Mucocutaneous manifestations associated with inflammatory bowel disease (IBD).

Specific lesions	Fissures and fistulas, aphthous stomatitis, mucosal nodularity (cobblestoning), pyostomatitis vegetans, metastatic Crohn's disease
Reactive lesions	Erythema nodosum, pyoderma gangrenosum **(Fig. 8)**, aphthous stomatitis
Associated cutaneous disorders or dermatosis	Vitiligo, epidermolysis bullosa acquisita, psoriasis, secondary amyloidosis, bowel associated dermatosis-arthritis syndrome
Mucocutaneous features secondary to nutritional malabsorption	Acrodermatitis enteropathica (zinc), scurvy (vitamin C), purpura (vitamin C and K), pellagra (niacin), stomatitis, glossitis, and angular cheilitis (vitamin B complex), non-specific eczema and dry skin (essential fatty acids), abnormal hair and nails (protein)
Secondary to treatment of IBD	Drug eruption, peristomal dermatitis
Bowel associated dermatosis-arthritis syndrome	Erythematous macules with central vesicle or pustule, erythema nodosum, and panniculitis

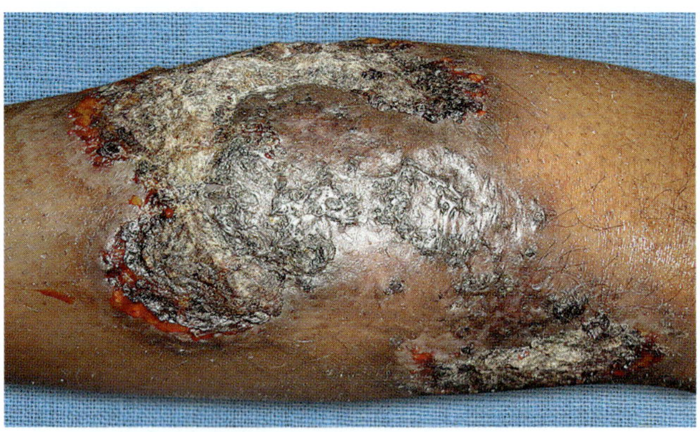

Fig. 8: Pyoderma gangrenosum.

TABLE 8: Mucocutaneous manifestations of hepatic malfunction.

Jaundice	Yellow skin and sclera
Pruritus	Persistent in nature
Vascular signs	• Spider angioma • Palmar erythema **(Fig. 9)** • Paper money skin • Corkscrew scleral vessels • Caput medusa • Purpuric lesions • Epistaxis, gingival bleeding • Bier spots
Xanthoma	Xanthoma of different types
Pigmentary changes	• Muddy gray hyperpigmentation, • Exaggerated in sun-exposed areas, perioral, peri-ocular areas, and palmar creases, around areola • Blotchy/diffuse in character
Hair changes	• Loss of forearm, axillary and pubic hair in both sexes • Decreased growth of facial hair and development of female pubic hair pattern of men
Nail changes	Terry's nail, Mee's line, clubbing, watch glass deformity (milder form of clubbing), koilonychia, ridging, brittleness, discoloration
Hormonal changes	Gynecomastia, striae distensae, and testicular atrophy
Nutritional deficiencies	Angular stomatitis, glossitis, brittle nails, alopecia, dermatitis over body and erosions over genital, perianal, and perioral areas

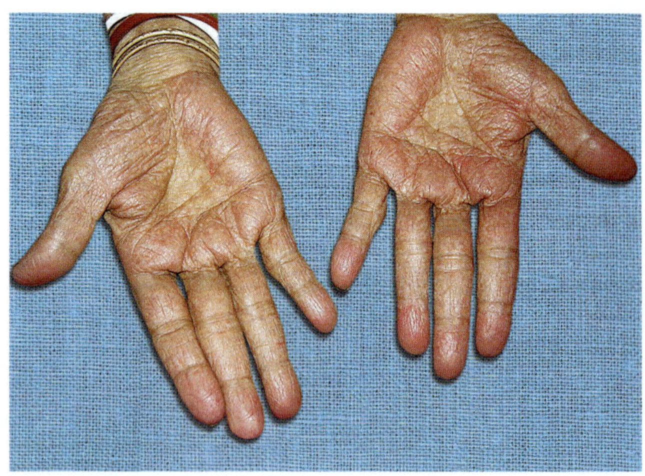

Fig. 9: Palmar erythema.

cutaneous changes is essential both for dermatologists and for hepatologists, so as to make a timely diagnosis aiding in prompt intervention.

Mucocutaneous Manifestations of Hepatic Malfunctions

Table 8 summarizes several mucocutaneous manifestations of hepatic malfunction.[8,9,12-14]

Cutaneous Signs of Specific Liver Diseases

Viral hepatitis: Mucocutaneous manifestations of viral hepatitis are summarized in **Table 9.**

Cirrhosis: Mucocutaneous features of cirrhosis are summarized in **Table 10.**[8,9,13,14]

Primary biliary cirrhosis:[8,9] It often presents with a combination of pruritus, jaundice, clubbing, and xanthomas; often associated with steatorrhea and bone pain.

Hemochromatosis: This is the most common genetic disorder with abnormal iron absorption and hepatic deposition causing cirrhosis, arthritis, diabetes mellitus, and skin discoloration.[8-10]

Wilson disease: In this autosomal recessive defect, deposition of copper occurs in the liver (cirrhosis, jaundice), brain, and eyes (Kayser Fleischer ring—a pigmented band around the iris). The skin often exhibits gray-brown discoloration and bluish discoloration of lunula (azure lunula).[8-10]

Hepatic neoplasms:[8-10] Skin changes are rarely seen in patients with hepatocellular carcinoma (HCC). Cutaneous metastasis presenting as single or multiple firm, painless, reddish-blue nodules are seen in only 1–5% cases. Pityriasis rotunda presenting as round to oval patches of dry ichthyotic skin has been found to be more common in patients with HCC. Hemangioendothelioma, leiomyosarcoma, and sarcomatoid carcinoma are other hepatic tumors which can present with cutaneous metastasis.

Primary Cutaneous Diseases with Hepatic Abnormalities

They are relatively rare and may include hepatic metastasis of cutaneous squamous cell carcinoma and melanoma.[8]

Multisystem Disorder with Hepatic and Cutaneous Manifestations

A wide variety of multisystem disorders may have prominent mucocutaneous and hepatic manifestations. Examples of such conditions include syphilis, sarcoidosis, Gaucher's disease, polyarteritis nodosa, and cytophagic histiocytic panniculitis among others.[8-10]

Iatrogenic

Drugs used for cutaneous conditions may cause hepatotoxicity (e.g., methotrexate, itraconazole, etc.). On the other hand, drugs used for liver disease may cause cutaneous adverse drug reactions (e.g., cutaneous side-effect of interferon includes transient alopecia, vasculitis, cutaneous necrosis, lichen planus, psoriasis, and most commonly injection-site reaction). Drug reaction with eosinophilia and systemic symptoms (DRESS) or drug hypersensitivity syndrome may affect both skin and liver.[8-10]

TABLE 9: Mucocutaneous manifestations of specific liver diseases.

Type of hepatitis	*Cutaneous features*
Hepatitis A	Jaundice, urticaria, exanthema, itching, purpura, and small vessel vasculitis
Hepatitis B	Polyarteritis nodosa, small vessel vasculitis, erythema multiforme, urticaria, urticarial vasculitis, pruritus, cryoglobulinemia, porphyria cutanea tarda , sarcoidosis after interferon/ribavirin, serum sickness-like reaction, erythema nodosum, Gianotti–Crosti syndrome
Hepatitis C	Necrolytic acral erythema (**Fig. 10**), small vessel vasculitis, urticaria, urticarial vasculitis, serum sickness-like reaction, sialadenitis, pruritus, erythema multiforme, cryoglobulinemia, porphyria cutanea tarda, antiphospholipid syndrome, sarcoidosis after interferon/ribavirin, erythema nodosum, Gianotti-Crosti syndrome, lichen planus–erosive oral disease, and vitiligo

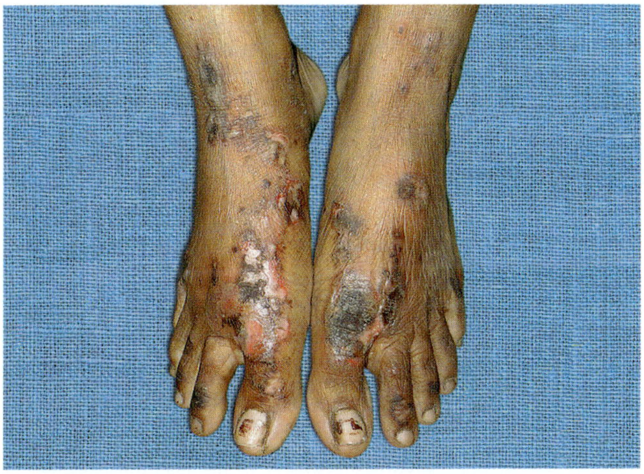

Fig. 10: Necrolytic acral erythema.

TABLE 10: Mucocutaneous features of cirrhosis.

Vascular changes	Telangiectasia (spider nevi), palmar erythema (liver palms), prominent abdominal veins (caput medusae), and vascular changes (mentioned in **Table 8**)
Madelung's disease	Large symmetrical subcutaneous lipomas affecting the neck
Sarcopenia	Loss of muscle mass and function
Dupuytren's contracture	Thickening of the palmar fascia
Miscellaneous changes	Gynecomastia, loss of body hair, ascites, leg edema, easy bruising, striae distensae
Nail changes	White finger nails, digital clubbing, hypertrophic osteoarthropathy

MUCOCUTANEOUS MANIFESTATIONS OF RENAL DISEASES

Patients with end-stage renal disease (ESRD) may develop a wide gamut of cutaneous features related to metabolic abnormalities, including anemia, calcium-phosphate dysregulation, and glucose intolerance.[8,9,15,16]

Mucocutaneous Features of Renal Failure and Dialysis

They are summarized in **Table 11**.[8,9,15,16]

Systemic Diseases which have Both Renal and Cutaneous Manifestations[8,9,15,16]

- *Autoimmune connective tissue diseases:* SLE, progressive systemic sclerosis, etc.
- *Vasculitis*: Polyarteritis nodosa, granulomatosis with polyangiitis, IgA vasculitis, microscopic polyangiitis, Behçet's disease, etc.

- *Genetic diseases:* Tuberous sclerosis, Reed syndrome, Birt–Hogg–Dube syndrome, Fabry disease, Von Hippel–Lindau disease, etc.
- *Infections:* Hepatitis B, Hepatitis C, loiasis
- *Inflammatory disease:* Drug reaction with eosinophilia and systemic symptoms (DRESS).
- *Metabolic diseases*: Diabetes, primary systemic amyloidosis, atherosclerotic/cholesterol emboli *Miscellaneous diseases*: Sarcoidosis, amyloidosis, graft versus host disease, cholesterol emboli.

Disease Associated with Renal Transplantation[15]

Numerous cutaneous complications, both from the immunosuppressive medications indispensable for allograft survival and from the state of immunosuppression can occur following renal transplantation. Cushingoid changes, acneiform eruption, and folliculitis may result from systemic steroid therapy. Gum hypertrophy and hypertrichosis may result from cyclosporine. There is an increased potential for bacterial, fungal, mycobacterial, parasitic, and viral infections also. In addition, there is also increased chance of actinic keratosis (precancerous), basal cell carcinoma (BCC), Kaposi sarcoma (KS), melanoma, Merkel cell carcinoma, and squamous cell carcinoma (SCC) in these patients.

TABLE 11: Cutaneous signs of renal failure and dialysis.

Dyspigmentation	Hyperpigmentation, pallor, a slate-grey discoloration, and a yellow skin hue
Pruritus	*Associated secondary changes*: Excoriations, skin lichenification, prurigo nodularis, and accentuation of perforating disorders
Xerosis	Dry skin, thick rhomboidal scales, and fissures
Abnormal calcium metabolism	Calcinosis cutis, calciphylaxis
Bullous diseases of hemodialysis	Porphyria cutanea tarda, pseudoporphyria
Acquired perforating dermatoses	Hyperkeratotic papules or nodules with a central crust filled plug **(Fig. 11)** on trunk and extensors
Nephrogenic systemic fibrosis	Cutaneous and systemic fibrosis due to gadolinium contrast material
Uremic frost	Eccrine deposition of urea crystals due to severe uremia
Nail changes	Beau's lines, half-and-half nails (Lindsay's nails), and nail fold capillary abnormalities
Hair changes	Alopecia due to systemic lupus erythematosus (SLE), malnutrition, or chronic telogen effluvium

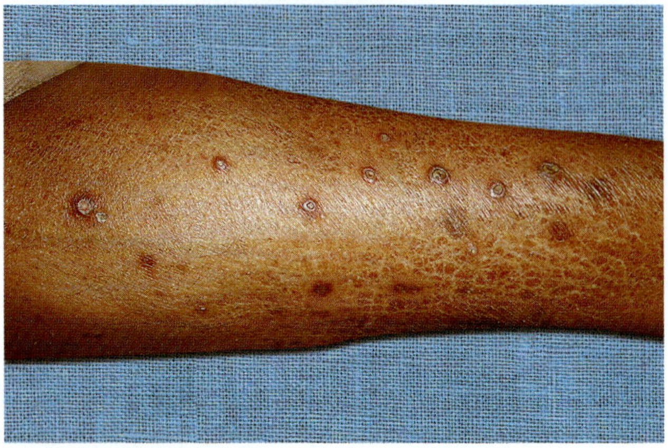

Fig. 11: Acquired perforating dermatosis.

MUCOCUTANEOUS MANIFESTATIONS OF CARDIAC DISEASES

Cardiovascular disorders and therapies are often associated with a variety of dermatologic manifestations. Often, these cutaneous signs can be used in enabling a diagnosis of the underlying cardiac disease.

Primary Cardiac Diseases

Table 12 displays the mucocutaneous manifestations of different primary cardiac diseases.[8,9,17,18]

TABLE 12: Mucocutaneous manifestations of different primary cardiac diseases.

Primary cardiac disease	*Cutaneous findings*
Coronary artery disease/ atherosclerosis	Diagonal earlobe crease, androgenetic alopecia, thoracic hairiness, hair in the ears, xanthomas, arcus juvenalis, skin tags, nicotine stains
Infective endocarditis	Osler's nodes, Janeway's lesions, petechiae, purpuric pustules, splinter hemorrhages, leukocytoclastic vasculitis, cutaneous infarct
Congenital cyanotic heart disease	Cyanosis, clubbing
Congestive heart failure	Dependent pitting edema
Embolic phenomenon (from atherosclerotic plaques, left atrial myxoma, subacute bacterial endocarditis, etc.)	Palpable purpura, livedo reticularis, ulcerations
Chronic venous insufficiency	Stasis dermatitis, peripheral edema, lipodermatosclerosis, lower leg ulcerations
Chronic arterial insufficiency	Muscular atrophy and absence of hair on extremity, ulceration
Dyslipidemia	Xanthelasma, plane xanthomas, palmar crease xanthoma, tendon xanthomas, and tuberous xanthomas **(Fig. 12)**
Postcardiac transplantation (from any cause)	Increased risk of skin cancers and cutaneous infections

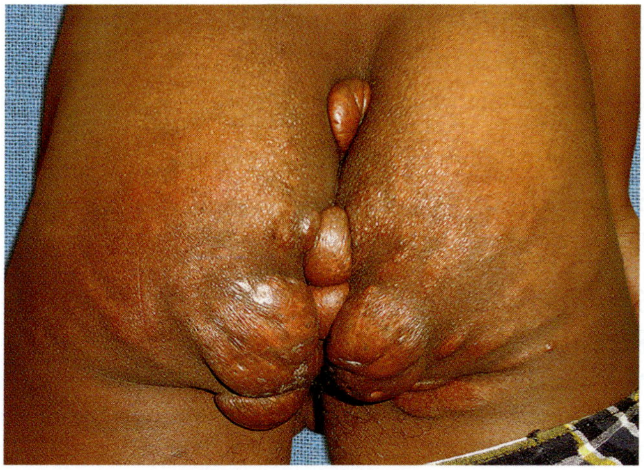

Fig. 12: Tuberous xanthomas.

Multisystem Disorders with Prominent Cutaneous and Cardiovascular Manifestations[8,9,17,18]

Genetic disorders: Carney complex (atrial myxoma, lentigines, coarse facies, blue nevi and cutaneous myxomas), cutis laxa (aortic dilation and rupture, pulmonary artery stenosis, loose skin), hemochromatosis (cardiomyopathy, slate-grey or brownish bronze hyperpigmentation of skin), tuberous sclerosis (cardiac rhabdomyomas, arrhythmias along with facial angiofibromas, periungual fibromas, ash-leaf macules and shagreen patch), Ehlers-Danlos syndrome (aortic dilation and dissection, MV prolapse along with hyperelastic, fragile skin, delayed wound healing and atrophic scars), Marfan syndrome (aortic dilation and dissection, MV and TV prolapse and regurgitation along with striae, arachnodactyly, elastosis perforans serpiginosa), Noonan syndrome (pulmonary stenosis, hypertrophic cardiomyopathy, webbed neck, keratosis pilaris atrophicans, keloids, lymphedema), LEOPARD syndrome (conduction abnormalities, PV stenosis, hypertrophic cardiomyopathy, lentigines, café-au-lait macules), Naxos disease (arrhythmogenic right ventricular cardiomyopathy, diffuse palmoplantar keratoderma, woolly scalp hair), and Carvajal syndrome (dilated left ventricular cardiomyopathy, woolly hair, focal palmoplantar keratoderma) are some of the important genetic conditions with prominent cardiac and cutaneous manifestations.[8,9,17,18]

Autoimmune/rheumatologic diseases: Rheumatic fever (pancarditis, valvulopathy, erythema marginatum and subcutaneous nodules), SLE/neonatal LE (pericarditis, myocarditis, conduction abnormalities, valvulopathy, complete heart block, and distinctive cutaneous features), systemic sclerosis (pericarditis, myocarditis, arrhythmias, pulmonary artery hypertension, Raynaud's phenomenon and other characteristic cutaneous features), dermatomyositis (myocarditis, conduction abnormalities, congestive cardiac failure and other characteristic cutaneous features), and Behçet's disease (pancarditis, coronary arteritis/aneurysm, arrhythmias, valvulopathy, thrombosis, oral and genital ulcers, pustular eruptions, pyoderma gangrenosum-like lesions) have several cardiocutaneous manifestations.[8,9,17,18]

Inflammatory conditions: Psoriasis (increased risk of cardiovascular disease, atherosclerosis), Kawasaki disease (coronary artery aneurysm, polymorphous exanthema, desquamation of palms, soles, and lips), and erythroderma (high-output cardiac failure) may have prominent cardio-cutaneous manifestations.[8,9,17,18]

Endocrine diseases: Cushing's syndrome (hypertension, atrophy and striae, ecchymoses, acne, telangiectasia), diabetes (coronary artery disease and a wide gamut of cutaneous diseases as discussed above), hypothyroidism (impaired cardiac contractility and diastolic function, increased systemic vascular resistance), and hyperthyroidism (palpitations, anginal chest pain, atrial fibrillation, systolic hypertension) have both cutaneous and cardiac manifestations.[8,9,17,18]

Infective conditions: Syphilis (aortitis), Lyme disease (heart block, myopericarditis, erythema migrans, borrelial lymphocytoma), and tuberculosis (constrictive pericarditis) may also have prominent cutaneous features.[8,9,17,18]

Miscellaneous Conditions

Primary systemic amyloidosis (heart failure, conduction abnormalities, syncope, sudden death, restrictive cardiomyopathy, purpura, periorbital ecchymosis, waxy papules and plaques), and sarcoidosis (conduction abnormalities, arrhythmias, cardiomyopathy, congestive cardiac failure, sudden cardiac death, cutaneous papules, nodules, plaques, etc.) involve both skin and heart.[8,9,17,18]

Iatrogenic

Several cutaneous manifestations may arise out of several diagnostic and therapeutic cardiac interventions.

Pacemakers implantation (pacemaker dermatitis), percutaneous coronary intervention (skin infections, allergic contact dermatitis and irritant contact dermatitis), and cardiac bypass surgery (infection, later donor site dermatitis, cellulitis or keloid formation) may lead to several dermatological complications.

Several drugs used in cardiovascular diseases may lead to cutaneous adverse drug reactions. For example, amiodarone (photosensitivity, resultant slate blue-gray pigmentation), ACE inhibitors (angioedema), β-adrenergic blockers (flaring of psoriasis, worsening of Raynaud's phenomenon), minoxidil (hypertrichosis), quinidine (petechiae, photosensitivity), procainamide (drug-induced SLE), spironolactone (gynecomastia), statins (xerosis), calcium channel blockers (pedal edema), and heparin (petechiae, skin necrosis) may have several cutaneous adverse drug reactions among others.[8,9,17,18]

MUCOCUTANEOUS MANIFESTATIONS OF RESPIRATORY DISORDERS

A wide range of mucocutaneous manifestations can occur in respiratory diseases.[9,19,20]

Primary Dermatological Diseases with Pulmonary Manifestations[9,19,20]

Staphylococcus aureus skin infection can lead to pneumonia by hematogenous spread of infection. Septic vasculitis can lead to pneumonia and septic pulmonary emboli.

Malignant melanoma or squamous cell carcinoma of the skin can metastasize to lung.

Kaposi sarcoma can have a multifocal origin in skin and lungs or can lead to pleural effusion.

Cutaneous larva migrans: Patients with cutaneous larva migrans rarely may have persistent dry cough and eosinophilic, migratory pulmonary infiltrates.

Primary Pulmonary Diseases with Cutaneous Manifestations[8,9,19,20]

Cyanosis: Central cyanosis is caused due to any severe respiratory diseases including pulmonary edema, thromboembolism, severe pneumonia, acute severe attack of asthma, chronic obstructive pulmonary disease (COPD), and others.

Clubbing: Digital clubbing is frequently seen in association with pulmonary diseases including lung cancer, interstitial pulmonary fibrosis, pulmonary tuberculosis, empyema, and bronchiectasis.

Superior vena cava obstruction: Patients present with markedly dilated veins often in vertical parallel clusters above the level of heart, facial edema, plethora of head and neck, conjunctival suffusion along with breathlessness, productive cough, hemoptysis, etc.

Erythema gyratum repens: Concentric erythematous lesions of erythema gyratum repens with wood grain appearance may occur with underlying lung carcinoma.

Congenital/Developmental Disorders with Cutaneous and Pulmonary Manifestations

They are summarized in **Table 13.**[8,9,19,20]

Systemic Diseases Affecting both Skin and Lungs[8,9,19,20]

They are depicted in **Table 14.**

Skin Changes due to Drugs Used to Treat Respiratory Diseases[8,9,19,20]

Antibiotics used to treat respiratory infection may cause different skin rashes, the most common drug being penicillin group. Antitubercular drugs can lead to skin rashes, purpura due to thrombocytopenia, and other hypersensitivity manifestations in the skin or acneiform eruption. Immunosuppressant drugs used to treat autoimmune diseases, anticancer drugs, and long-term use of systemic steroids can lead to fungal or bacterial skin infections.

Long-term use of systemic steroids can lead to the typical cushingoid appearance. Fluoroquinolones, tetracycline, and epidermal growth factor receptor inhibitors can lead to drug-induced photosensitivity.

MUCOCUTANEOUS MANIFESTATIONS OF NEUROCUTANEOUS DISORDERS

Several neurocutaneous diseases may occur as a result of developmental, metabolic, infectious, immunological, iatrogenic, and miscellaneous causes.[8,21,22]

Developmental Neurocutaneous Disorders

The features of some important developmental neurocutaneous disorders are summarized in **Table 15.**[8,21,22]

Metabolic Causes[8,21,22]

Fabry disease may present with acroparesthesia, cerebrovascular disease, dementia, depression, and angiokeratoma corporis diffusum.

TABLE 13: Congenital/developmental disorders with cutaneous and pulmonary manifestations.

Congenital/developmental disorders	*Cutaneous features*	*Pulmonary features*
Neurofibromatosis type1	Neurofibroma, café-au-lait macules, freckling	Lung cysts/bulla, pulmonary fibrosis and honeycombing
Hereditary hemorrhagic telangiectasia (HHT)	Telangiectasia over mucosa and skin	Pulmonary arteriovenous malformations
Yellow nail syndrome	Lymphedema, yellow dystrophic nail	Pleural effusion, bronchiectasis/chronic sinusitis
Birt–Hogg–Dubé syndrome	Fibrofolliculoma, trichodiscomas, acrochordons	Lung cyst, recurrent pneumothorax
Ehlers–Danlos syndrome	Stretchy skin, loose joints, abnormal scar	Emphysematous bulla, pneumothorax
Marfan syndrome	Dolichocephalic skull, high arched palate, arachnodactyly	Emphysema, lung cyst, pneumothorax, pectus excavatum, kyphoscoliosis
Generalized elastolysis (Cutis laxa)	Sagging, inelastic hanging loose skin	Progressive emphysema, cor pulmonale, chronic respiratory failure

TABLE 14: Systemic diseases affecting the skin and lungs.

Systemic disease	*Cutaneous features*	*Pulmonary features*
Progressive systemic sclerosis	Skin tightening, Raynaud's phenomenon, dyspigmentation, finger- tip ulceration/scarring	Interstitial lung disease, pulmonary hypertension, bronchiectasis
Systemic lupus erythematosus	Malar rash, photosensitivity, oral ulcers, discoid LE, subacute LE, etc.	Pleuritis, pneumonitis, diffuse alveolar hemorrhage, pulmonary hypertension
Dermatomyositis	Gottron papules, heliotrope rash, shawl sign, mechanic's hands	Interstitial lung disease, bronchiolitis obliterans, aspiration pneumonia, lung cancer
Granulomatosis with polyangiitis	Palpable purpura, friable gingiva, ulcers, papulonecrotic lesions	*Upper and lower airway involvement*: Sinusitis, epistaxis, nasal septal perforation, cough, hemoptysis
Eosinophilic granulomatosis with polyangiitis	Palpable purpura, subcutaneous nodule, urticaria	Allergic rhinitis, nasal polyp, asthma, pneumonia
Sarcoidosis	Papules, nodules, plaques **(Fig. 13)** with predilection for scars and tattoos	Hilar lymphadenopathy, parenchymal opacities
Rheumatoid arthritis	Rheumatoid nodules, palpable purpura, ulcers, neutrophilic dermatoses	Interstitial lung disease, bronchiolitis obliterans
Relapsing polychondritis	Erythematous edematous pinna (sparing ear lobes) / nasal tip	Hoarseness of voice, structural insufficiency, airway collapse
Sjögren's syndrome	Xerosis, pruritus, features of vasculitis	Sinusitis, bronchoalveolitis and interstitial lung disease
Mixed connective tissue disease	Hand edema, Raynaud's phenomenon	Pulmonary hypertension
Microscopic polyangiitis	Palpable purpura, livedo reticularis, ulcers	Pulmonary capillaritis, pulmonary infiltrate

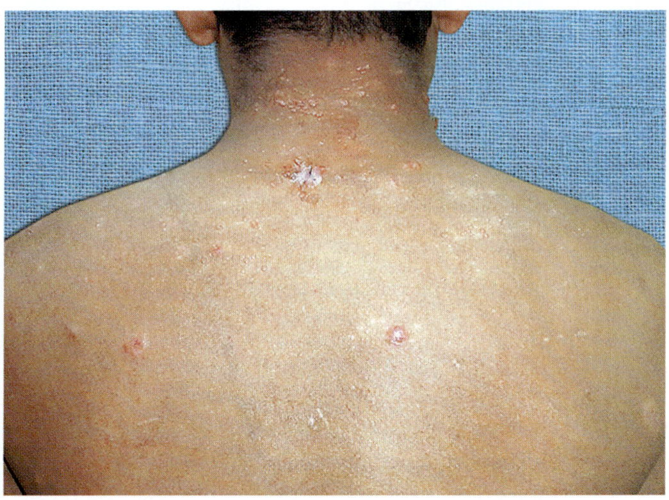

Fig. 13: Cutaneous lesions of sarcoidosis.

Congenital hypothyroidism may present with intellectual disability, hypotonia with delayed reflexes, developmental delay, mental retardation, and cutaneous features of hypothyroidism (discussed in **Table 1**).

Infections

Several infective conditions like herpes simplex, varicella-zoster, hand foot and mouth disease by enterovirus 71, dengue virus infection, *Neisseria meningitidis* infection, syphilis, rickettsial infection, and systemic fungal infections (cryptococcosis, histoplasmosis, paracoccidioidomycosis, penicilliosis, and mucormycosis, etc.) have both cutaneous and neurological manifestations.[8,21,22]

Immune Disorders

Vasculitis (both central and peripheral nervous systems may be involved), Behçet's disease (acute meningoencephalitis, cranial nerve palsy, brainstem lesions, pyramidal and extra-pyramidal features), and SLE (psychosis, seizures, headaches, acute confusional state, cognitive dysfunction, aseptic meningitis, chorea, etc.) have prominent cutaneous and neurological features.[8,21,22]

Miscellaneous

Apart from the above-mentioned causes, iatrogenic disorders and several other diseases like, dyschromatosis symmetrica hereditaria, vitamin B_{12} deficiency, xeroderma pigmentosum, etc., may have both neurological and cutaneous manifestations.[8,21,22]

KEY POINTS

- Skin signs often provide important clues which help diagnosing underlying systemic diseases.
- Sometimes, skin disease may be the only manifestation of the internal disease.
- There are several mucocutaneous features of primary systemic diseases.
- Primary skin diseases may also rarely affect different organ systems.

TABLE 15: Mucocutaneous features of developmental neurocutaneous disorders.

Disease	*Characteristic cutaneous features*	*Neurological/systemic features*
Neurofibromatosis type 1	• Six or more café-au-lait spots greater than 1.5 cm in adults and 0.5 cm in prepubertal children • Two or more neurofibromas of any type or one plexiform neurofibroma • Axillary or inguinal freckling	• Two or more Lisch nodules in the eyes • Optic glioma • Sphenoid dysplasia • Thickening of a long bone cortex with or without pseudoarthrosis
Tuberous sclerosis	• Facial angiofibromas **(Fig. 14)** • Ash leaf macules • Periungual fibromas (Koenen's tumors) • Shagreen patch • Confetti-like hypopigmented macules	• Renal angiomyolipoma • Cortical tumors and cysts • Cardiac rhabdomyoma • Pulmonary lymphangioleiomyomatosis
Sturge–Weber syndrome	Port wine stain (PWS) on the forehead and upper eyelids, in the area of the ophthalmic branch of the trigeminal (Vth cranial) nerve, either alone or in combination with the V2 and V3 distributions	• Seizures • Focal neurologic impairment • Ocular features include glaucoma and capillary-venous vascular malformations of the conjunctiva, choroid, and retina • Cognitive impairment
Cobb syndrome	Port wine stain or cavernous hemangioma with a vascular malformation	• Congenital cutaneous vascular malformation distributed in a dermatomal pattern with associated spinal angiomas or arteriovenous malformations • Pain, motor dysfunction, paresthesias, and paraplegia
Ataxia telangiectasia	Cutaneous telangiectasia	• Ocular telangiectasia • Cerebellar ataxia • Variable immune deficiency with susceptibility to sinopulmonary infections, impaired organ maturation
Waardenburg syndrome	• Heterochromia iridis • Achromia of the hair, skin	• Synophrys • Hypertelorism • Dystopia canthorum • Heterochromia iridis • Congenital hearing loss
Incontinentia pigmenti	• Scattered erythema and vesicles • Verrucous linear plaques • Hyperpigmented swirls along the lines of Blaschko	Anomalies of the CNS, eyes, teeth, hair, nails, and bones
Hypomelanosis of Ito (HI): A form of pigment mosaicism with hypopigmentation	• Hypopigmented streaks and whorls along the lines of Blaschko • Hypopigmentation tends to fade with age	• Seizures • Electroencephalogram abnormalities • Strabismus • Language impairment
Vogt–Koyanagi–Harada syndrome	Vitiligo-like depigmentation of the skin (especially of the eyebrows and eyelashes)	• Headache • Sterile meningitis • Uveitis • Optic neuritis
Epidermal nevus syndrome	Epidermal nevi	• Neurologic abnormalities • Musculoskeletal • Ocular
Sjögren–Larsson syndrome	• Lamellar ichthyosis • Palmoplantar keratoderma	• Seizures • Spastic diplegia or quadriplegia • Mental retardation • Macular degeneration with retinal crystals

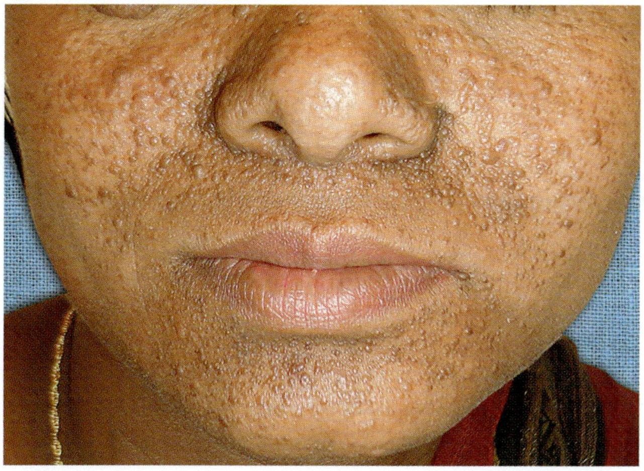

Fig. 14: Angiofibroma in a patient with tuberous sclerosis.

- A group of multisystem disorders may affect the skin and other internal organs.
- Several drugs and different therapeutic interventions used to treat systemic diseases often have prominent mucocutaneous manifestations.
- The knowledge of the relationship between dermatologic manifestations and disorders and internal diseases may expedite early identification of systemic diseases.

REFERENCES

1. Jabbour SA. Cutaneous manifestations of endocrine disorders: a guide for dermatologists. Am J Clin Dermatol. 2003;4:315-31.
2. Murphy-Chutorian B, Han G, Cohen SR. Dermatologic manifestations of diabetes mellitus: a review. Endocrinol Metab Clin North Am. 2013;42:869-98.
3. Lima AL, Illing T, Schliemann S, Elsner P. Cutaneous manifestations of diabetes mellitus: a review. Am J Clin Dermatol. 2017;18:541-53.
4. Schachtel A, Kalus A. Diabetes and other endocrine diseases. In: Kang S, Amagai M, Bruckner AL, Enk AH, Margolis DJ, Mcmichael AJ, et al. (Eds). Fitzpatrick's Dermatology, Ninth edition. New York: McGraw Hill; 2019. pp. 2493-2526.
5. Ahn CS, Yosipovitch G, Huang WW. Diabetes and the skin. In: Callen JP, Jorizzo JL, Zone JJ, Rosenbach MA. Piette WW, Vleugels RA (Eds). Dermatological Signs of Systemic Disease. Fifth edition. Edinburgh: Elsevier; 2017. pp. 205-14.
6. Ghazi E, Rosen T, Jorizzo JL, Heymann WR. Thyroid and the skin. In: Callen JP, Jorizzo JL, Zone JJ, Rosenbach MA. Piette WW, Vleugels RA (Eds). Dermatological Signs of Systemic Disease. 5th edition. Edinburgh: Elsevier; 2017. pp. 215-21.
7. Micheletti RG. Adrenal, androgen-related, and pituitary disorders. In: Callen JP, Jorizzo JL, Zone JJ, Rosenbach MA. Piette WW, Vleugels RA (Eds). Dermatological Signs of Systemic Disease. 5th edition. Edinburgh: Elsevier; 2017. pp. 228-34.
8. James WD, Elston DM, Treat JR, Rosenbach MA, Neuhaus IM (Eds). Andrews' Diseases of the Skin—Clinical Dermatology. Edinburgh: Elsevier; 2020.
9. Forrestel AK, Micheletti RG. Skin manifestations of internal organ disorders. In: Kang S, Amagai M, Bruckner AL, Enk AH, Margolis DJ, Mcmichael AJ, et al. (Eds). In: Fitzpatrick's Dermatology. 9th edition. New York: McGraw Hill; 2019. pp. 2425-40.
10. Herron MD, Zone JJ. Cutaneous diseases associated with gastrointestinal abnormalities. In: Callen JP, Jorizzo JL, Zone JJ, Rosenbach MA. Piette WW, Vleugels RA (Eds). In: Dermatological Signs of Systemic Disease. 5th edition. Edinburgh: Elsevier; 2017. pp. 243-54.
11. Trost LB, McDonnell JK. Important cutaneous manifestations of inflammatory bowel disease. Postgrad Med J. 2005;81:580-5.
12. Wieland C. Clinical examination: skin. Clin Liver Dis (Hoboken). 2016;7:119-25.
13. Dogra S, Jindal R. Cutaneous manifestations of common liver diseases. J Clin Exp Hepatol. 2011;1:177-84.
14. Jackson JM, Callen JP, Greer KE. Hepatic disease and the skin. In: Callen JP, Jorizzo JL, Zone JJ, Rosenbach MA. Piette WW, Vleugels RA (Eds). In: Dermatological Signs of Systemic Disease. 5th edition. Edinburgh: Elsevier; 2017. pp. 255-61.
15. Maiberger MP, Nunley JR. Renal disease and the skin. In: Callen JP, Jorizzo JL, Zone JJ, Rosenbach MA. Piette WW, Vleugels RA (Eds). Dermatological signs of systemic disease. Fifth edition. Edinburgh: Elsevier; 2017. pp. 323-29.
16. Van de Velde-Kossmann KM. Skin examination: an important diagnostic tool in renal failure patients. Blood Purif. 2018;45:187-93.
17. Femia A, Schwarzenberger K, Callen JP. Cardiovascular diseases and the skin. In: Callen JP, Jorizzo JL, Zone JJ, Rosenbach MA, Piette WW, Vleugels RA (Eds). Dermatological Signs of Systemic Disease. 5th edition. Edinburgh: Elsevier; 2017. pp. 315-22.
18. Annemarie U, Lebwohl M. Cutaneous manifestations of cardiovascular diseases. Clin Dermatol. 2008;26:243-54.
19. Moleyar VS, Noojibail A. Diseases with skin and lung involvement: Pulmonologist's perspective. Med J DY Patil Vidyapeeth. 2020;13:106-12.
20. Chew AL, Creamer D. Cutaneous manifestations of lung disease. Br J Hosp Med (Lond). 2006;67:141-7.
21. Cipriano SD, Zone JJ. Neurocutaneous disease. In: Callen JP, Jorizzo JL, Zone JJ, Rosenbach MA. Piette WW, Vleugels RA (Eds). In: Dermatological Signs of Systemic Disease. 5th edition. Edinburgh: Elsevier; 2017; pp. 345-58.
22. Little H, Kamat D, Sivaswamy L. Common neurocutaneous syndromes. Pediatr Ann. 2015;44:496-504.

EXAMINATION QUESTIONS

1. Briefly discuss the mucocutaneous manifestations of diabetes mellitus.
2. Briefly discuss the mucocutaneous manifestations of rheumatoid arthritis.
3. Briefly discuss the mucocutaneous manifestations of different endocrine disorders.
4. Briefly discuss the mucocutaneous manifestations of thyroid disorders.
5. Briefly discuss the mucocutaneous manifestations of renal diseases.
6. Briefly discuss the mucocutaneous manifestations of inflammatory bowel diseases.

66 CHAPTER Sarcoidosis

Chinmay Kar

INTRODUCTION

Sarcoidosis is a multisystem disease with a wide variety of clinical manifestations. It involves mainly lungs, reticuloendothelial system, eyes, skin, nervous system, and so on. It is a granulomatous disease without any specific identifiable cause. Cutaneous lesions can exhibit many different morphologies and seem very close to other skin diseases. It is a great mimicker and is diagnosed by exclusion of others.

HISTORY

As early as 1869, Jonathan Hutchinson observed a case which was most likely one of sarcoidoses and named it as "Mortimer's Malady" from the name of patient, "Mr. Mortimer." It was published in 1975. In 1889, Ernest Besnier described a skin condition, called "lupus pernio." In 1897, Caesar Boeck first demonstrated the disease and in 1899, it was published in American journal as "Multiple, Benign, Skin-sarcoid."

EPIDEMIOLOGY

Age

Sarcoidosis has been found in all age groups but highest incidence is found in 25–40 years of age and a smaller second peak (approximately 30%) in around 60 years of age.

Sex

The females are affected more than males (Female:Male—2:1).

Incidence and Ethnicity

The incidence rate of sarcoidosis varies in different geographic areas. In Sweden and Iceland, the reported incidence rates are about 60 cases per 100,000 population whereas in Japan, it is nearly 1.3 cases per 100,000 population. Interestingly, there are some reports about seasonal clustering of occurrence of this disease, mostly in March, April to June, July, and indicate some specific seasonal changes (microbial infection) in weather.

There are also some racial predilections on disease severity and clinical manifestations. The sarcoidosis of chronic, severe, and multiorgan involvement are mostly seen in African-Americans whereas ocular and cardiac lesions are mostly found in Japanese patients. Scandinavians and Spanish patients are more prone to Löfgren syndrome.

PATHOPHYSIOLOGY

The histopathological hallmark of sarcoidosis is the development of noncaseating granuloma. It affects multiple organs and widely distributed throughout the world with great variations. Geographical and racial variations indicate genetic predisposition. Sarcoidosis is a polygenic disease. A positive family history ranges from 2.7 to 17% with fivefold increased risk in first-degree relatives. Monozygotic co-twin is highly affected than dizygotic one. The aim of granuloma formation is to combat the offending antigen by immune system of our body and suggests immunopathogenesis of sarcoidosis. But there is a great confusion about antigen for which the excessive immune reaction happens to form granuloma. The antigens may be various microbes or their products or environmental factors. Due to high incidence of lung sarcoidosis (90%), almost all probable antigens may enter through respiratory tract. The presence of microbes and their proteins within the sarcoid granulomas were investigated at genomic level.[1] Very few current studies reported the "vimentin" as autoantigen and subsequently detected antibody and vimentin-specific T-cells. Still, there is a lack of animal model to confirm the autoimmune origin of this disease.[2]

Though there is no known exact etiological factor of sarcoidosis, there may be a combination of more than one factor for the excessive immune reaction to form sarcoid granuloma by immunopathogenic reaction pattern described here. Proposed etiopathological factors of sarcoidosis are described in **Table 1**.

IMMUNOPATHOLOGY

Three probable immunopathologic mechanisms may play conjointly or separately to form a noncaseating epithelioid cell granuloma. Firstly, invaded environmental antigens or microbes, described above, are taken up by dendritic cells. These dendritic cells migrate to lymph nodes to interact with particular T-cells and promoting differentiation and clonal proliferation of T helper cells (Th1 and Th17). These two activated T helper cells promote an inflammatory response to release various cytokines namely interferon-γ (IFN-γ), interleukin 2 (IL-2), interleukin 17 (IL-17), and interleukin 23 (IL-23) and contribute aggregation for granuloma formation. Secondly, the phagocytes such as monocytes and macrophages are directly engulfed the microbes (*Mycobacteria, C. acnes, Chlamydia,* etc.). They are unable to destroy the microbes properly and ultimately differentiated into epithelioid cells and giant cells. These active cells produce tumor necrosis factor-α (TNF-α) which takes part in formation and maintenance of granuloma. In addition, macrophages attract Th1 cells, Th17 cells, regulatory T-cells (Treg cells) and also monocytes by secreting monocyte chemoattractant protein-1 (MCP-1) and IFN-γ-induced protein-10 (IP-10). The Treg cells secrete transforming growth factor-β (TGF-β) that causes fibrosis and organization of granuloma. Lastly, the dysbiosis (altered composition of microbiota) of lungs or gut may act as source of microorganisms. They secrete pathogen-associated molecular patterns (PAMPs) that activate the monocytes, macrophages, or eosinophils by interacting with pathogen recognition receptors (PRRs), namely toll-like receptors (TLRs). By activation of various immune cells, they secrete various cytokines such as IL-6, IL-12, IL-18, IL-23, and TNF-α to promote further generation of epithelioid and giant cells. Thus, they further contribute to granuloma formation **(Fig. 1)**.

TABLE 1: Etiopathological factors of sarcoidosis.

Genetic factors	• HLA-DRB1*03, HLA-DRB1*11, HLA-DRB1*12, HLA-DRB1*14, HLA-DRB1*15—increased risk of developing sarcoidosis • HLA-DRB1*03—Lofgren syndrome • HLA-DRB1*1501, HLA-DQB1*0602—chronic course with pulmonary fibrosis • Butyrophilin-like 2 (*BTNL2*)—associated with sarcoidosis
Environ-mental factors	Inorganic particulate matters, insecticides, pesticides, metal particles, chemical fumes, pigment particles (tattoo), and even World Trade Center (WTC) disaster dust
Microbial factors	• Strong association with *Cutibacterium acnes* (previously known as *Propionibacterium acnes*) and *Cutibacterium* species, *Mycobacterium tuberculosis* and *Mycobacterium* species, *Borrelia* species, *Borrelia burgdorferi* • Doubtful association—*Rickettsia helvetica, Chlamydia* species, herpesvirus, Epstein–Barr virus, *Histoplasma*, and other fungi

HISTOPATHOLOGY

The classical histopathology of sarcoidosis is characterized by discrete collection of epithelioid cells with a few, if any, Langhans giant cells to form epithelioid cell granuloma or

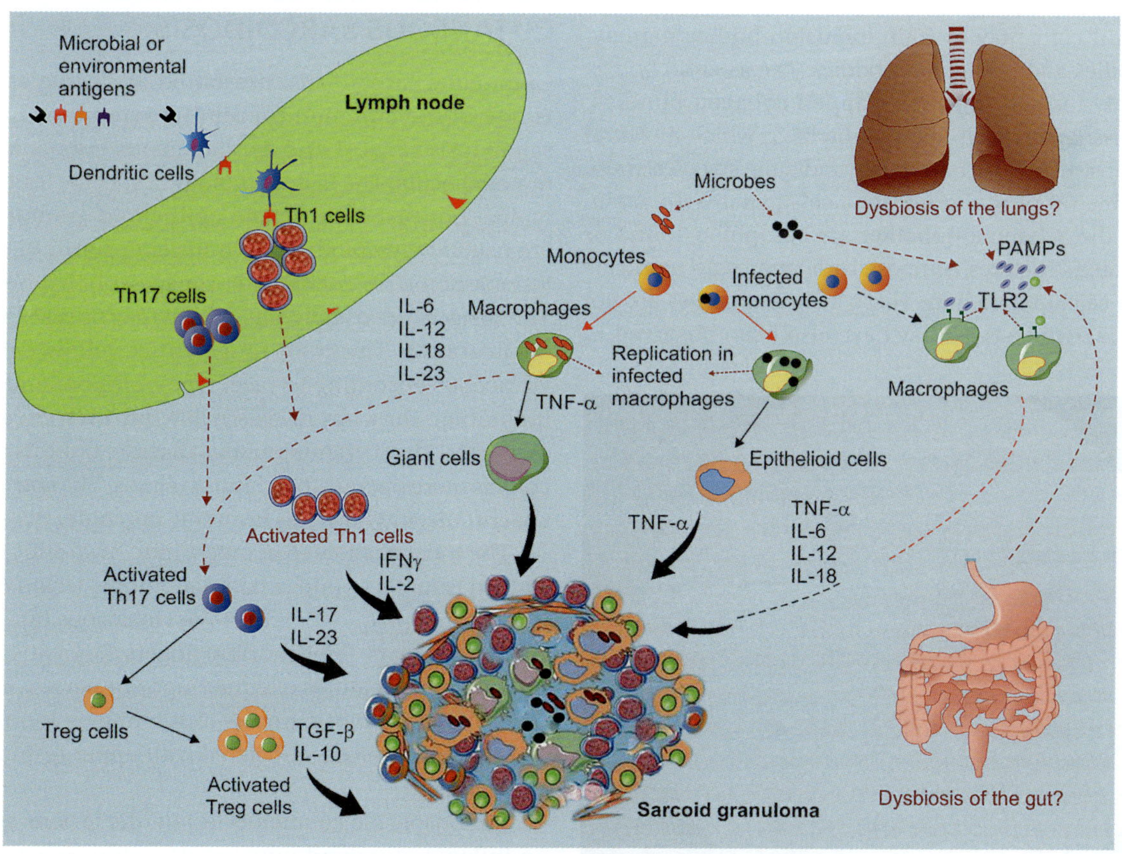

Fig. 1: A schematic model of sarcoid granuloma formation.[1]
(IFN-γ: interferon γ IL: interleukin; PAMPs: pathogen-associated molecular patterns; TGF-β: transforming growth factor-β; TNF-α: tumor necrosis factor-α; Treg cells: regulatory T-cells; TLR2: toll-like receptor 2)

epithelioid cell tubercle **(Fig. 2)**. Sparse lymphocytic infiltrates are found at the periphery of tubercle to designate it as "naked" tubercle. The periphery of granuloma is surrounded by a network of fibrous tissue. Central caseation is usually absent (noncaseating granuloma), though fibrinoid or coagulation necrosis may be observed in very few cases. This typical presentation of sarcoidosis is found in all involved organs. The granulomas are scattered throughout the dermis and occasionally may extend into subcutis. Actually, this classic representation has been altered on different types of lesions and in different stages of evolution. In erythrodermic sarcoidosis, numerous lymphocytes are found at periphery and within granulomas. In verrucous sarcoid, epidermis is hyperkeratotic and acanthotic, unlike uninvolved epidermis in classic one. Granuloma may occur around cutaneous nerves in hypopigmented type and difficult to differentiate from Hansen's infection. In old lesions, the giant cells may be in moderate number with large and irregular in shape. Subcutaneous sarcoid exhibits granuloma in subcutaneous fat. In involution stage of lesion, fibrosis extends from periphery to center with gradual disappearance of epithelioid cells. Marked fibrosis are also found in morpheaform sarcoid. Histopathology of erythema nodosum (EN) of sarcoidosis or idiopathic origin shows usually septal panniculitis with lymphocytes and mixed infiltrates *(no classical sarcoid granuloma)*.

The giant cells may contain inclusion bodies namely, asteroid bodies and Schaumann bodies. The asteroid bodies are probably formed from the trapped collagen bundles. It looks star-shaped or an open umbrella in which a central eosinophilic structure surrounded by radiating spicules, more clearly visible on phosphotungstic acid-hematoxylin stain. Contrarily, the Schaumann bodies are basophilic, round or oval, lamellated structures, composed of lipomucoglycoproteins mixed with calcium and iron. These inclusion bodies are not specific for sarcoidosis as they have also been observed in leprosy, tuberculosis, foreign body reactions, Crohn's disease, necrobiotic xanthogranuloma, etc.

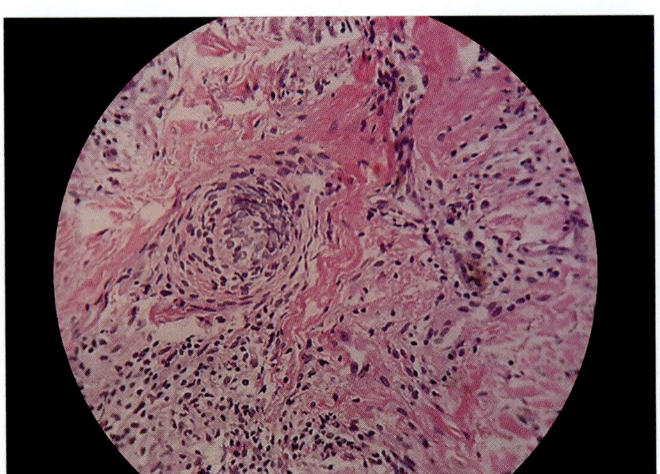

Fig. 2: Histopathology shows noncaseating granuloma.
Courtesy: Dr Prodip Sarkar, Kolkata.

So, sarcoidosis can be diagnosed only by exclusion due to many overlap features.

Granuloma is defined as organized collection of macrophages or histiocytes, usually arising in response to an infectious pathogen or foreign or unknown substance. Classification of granuloma is depicted in **Flowchart 1**.

Epithelioid cell granuloma without any identifiable pattern:

- *Leishmaniasis:* Loose epithelioid cell granuloma, few lymphocytes with or without plasma cells and LD bodies.
- *Post-kala-azar dermal leishmaniasis (nodular):* Nodular collection of epithelioid cells with dense diffuse infiltrate of lymphocytes, histiocytes, and plasma cells.
- *Papulonecrotic tuberculid:* Loose epithelioid granuloma with leukocytoclastic vasculitis, and epithelial necrosis.
- *Granulomatous syphilis:* Band-like epithelioid granuloma in superficial blood vessels and appendages, usually with plasma cells.

CLASSIFICATION

Classification of sarcoidosis is given in **Flowchart 2**.

CLINICAL MANIFESTATIONS OF CUTANEOUS SARCOIDOSIS

Cutaneous sarcoidosis, presented as visible skin lesion, is one of the common presenting symptoms of systemic sarcoidosis **(Figs. 3 and 4)**. Cutaneous lesions are specific or nonspecific. The histopathology of specific lesions reveals typical noncaseating, naked epithelioid granuloma. They are usually asymptomatic or transient pruritic elevated skin lesions. Some are erythematous macules or hypopigmented. The surfaces are usually smooth but may be scaly, verrucous, or ulcerative. The color ranges from yellow ochre to red violaceous according to race, type of lesion, and degree of infiltration. Diascopy reveals yellow-brown spot (apple jelly) characteristic of granulomatous disease, but this apple-jelly color is more opaque than lupus vulgaris. The specific lesions are chronic and have less favorable outcome.

The most distinctive manifestation of specific cutaneous sarcoid is lupus pernio, a pathognomonic lesion[3] **(Fig. 5)**. It is infiltrated plaques of reddish to violaceous hue over nose, cheeks, lips, ears, forehead, and fingers. It is a misnomer as it does not have features of either lupus or pernio. It is neither painful like perniosis nor as mutilating as lupus vulgaris. Most lupus pernio is associated with upper respiratory tract involvement.

In nonspecific cutaneous lesion, the lesions are actually an inflammatory and nongranulomatous reaction of skin. They are more acute, benign and have favorable outcome. The most common nonspecific skin lesion of sarcoidosis is

Flowchart 1: Classification of granuloma.

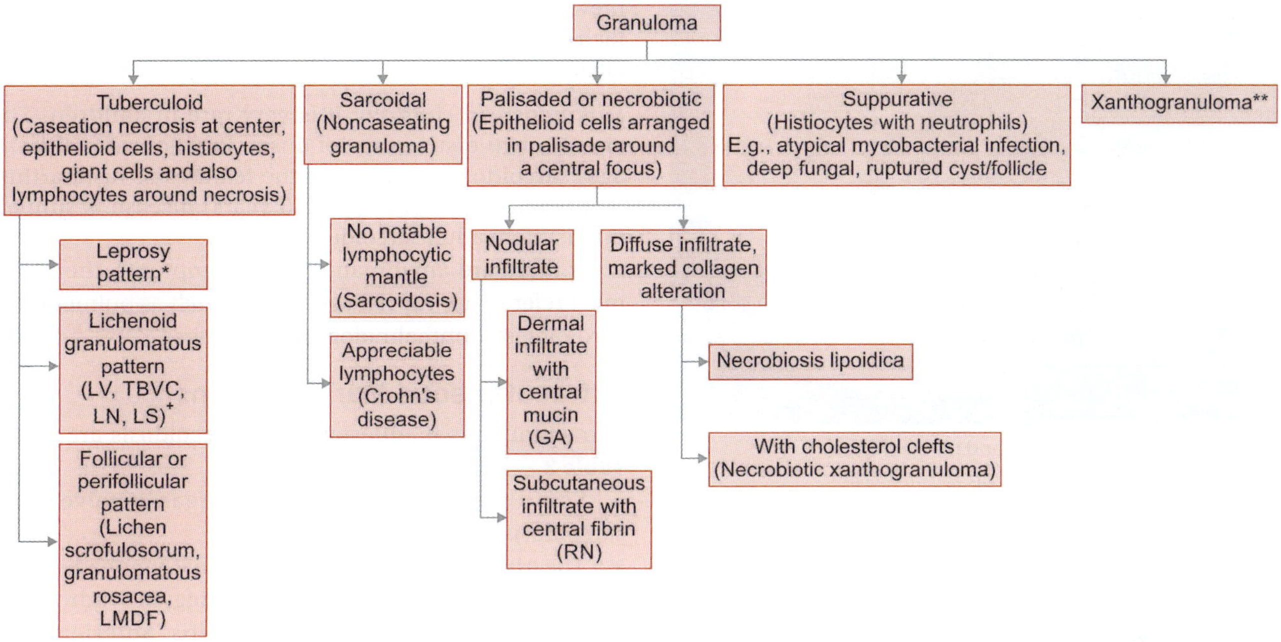

Note:

Foreign body granuloma: Well formed, often noncaseating granuloma consisting of histiocytes, usually epithelioid cells around the foreign body material and foreign body type giant cells. It is surrounded by variable amounts of lymphocyte, plasma cells, eosinophils and reactive dermal fibrosis.

* *Leprosy pattern:* Tuberculoid granuloma with characteristic silhouette. The silhouettes are perivascular and periappendageal, superficial and deep, curvilinear, sharply circumscribed, and lastly dermal aggregates.

+ *Lichenoid granulomatous pattern:* Usually epidermal changes with damage of basal layer with infiltrates. In lupus vulgaris (LV), there is occasional necrosis.

** *Xanthogranuloma:* Heterogeneous collection of macrophage cell types (vacuolated, xanthomatized, scalloped, spindle-shaped, and oncocytic), often with giant cells.

(GA: granuloma annulare; LMDF: lupus miliaris disseminata faciei; LN: lichen nitidus; LS: lichen striatus; RN: rheumatoid nodule; TBVC: tuberculosis verrucosa cutis)

Flowchart 2: Classification of sarcoidosis.

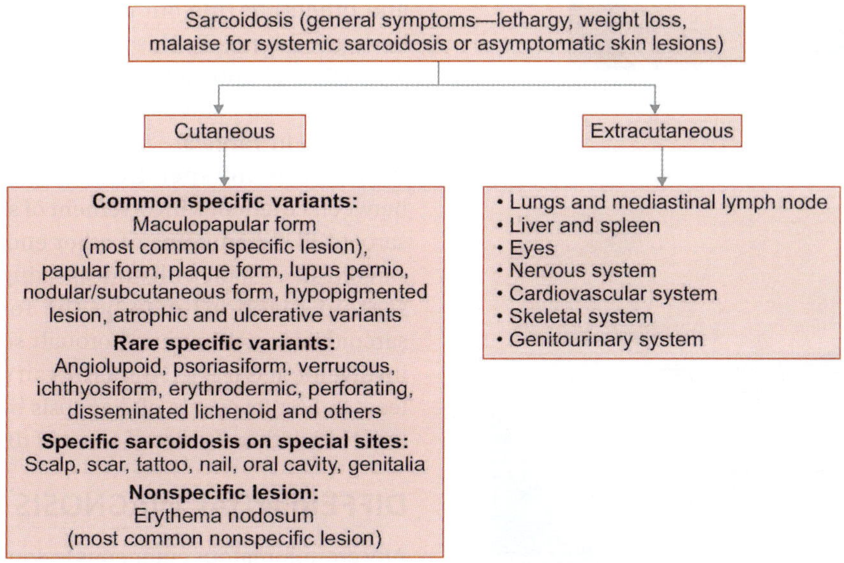

EN, presented as tender, painful, erythematous lesions over extremities preferably over shins in middle-aged patients. EN due to sarcoidosis is more common (16–30%) in western countries. In India, its prevalence due to sarcoidosis is very less. Other nonspecific lesions are erythema multiforme, prurigo, cutaneous calcinosis, and digital clubbing.

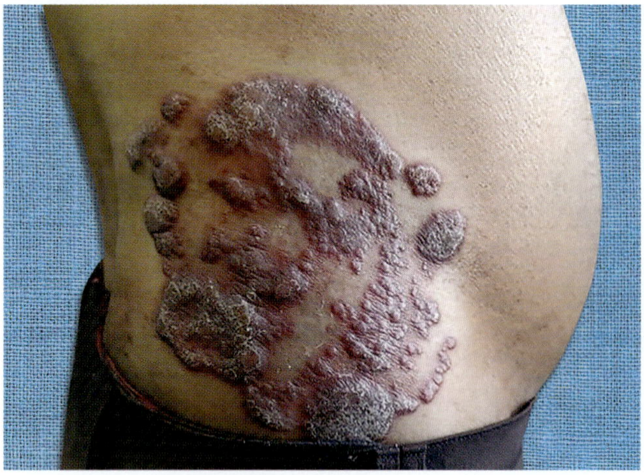

Fig. 3: Papule and plaque forms.
Courtesy: Dr Prodip Sarkar, Kolkata.

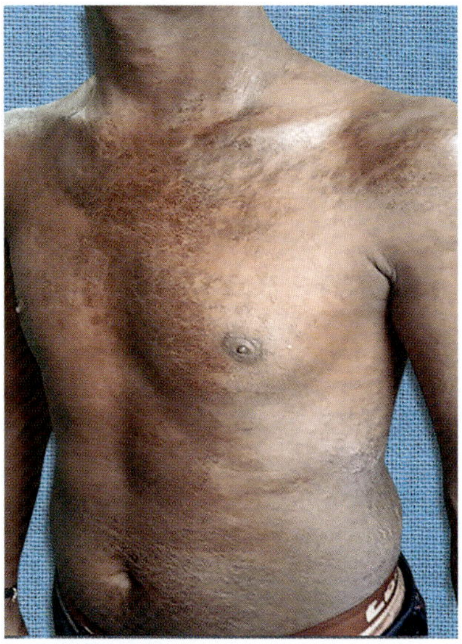

Fig. 4: Ichthyosiform sarcoidosis.
Courtesy: Dr Prodip Sarkar, Kolkata.

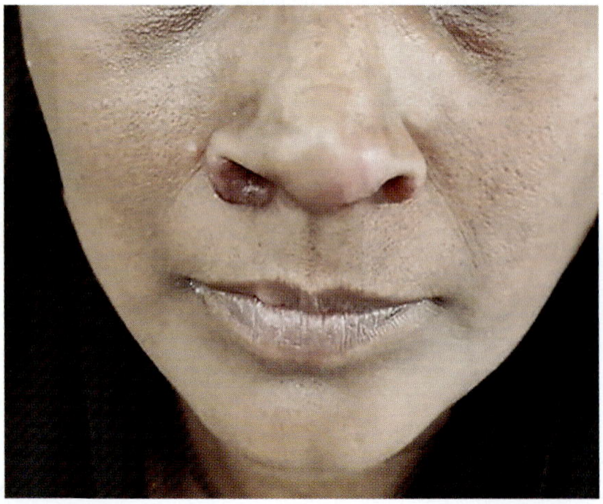

Fig. 5: Lupus pernio.

Sarcoidosis and pregnancy: Sarcoidosis generally does not prevent successful outcome of pregnancy and delivery because high estrogen level may have a beneficial immunomodulatory effect.

Sarcoidosis in children: It is very rare in children. There are also two distinct age of onset. Early-onset (<4 years of age) sarcoidosis usually has the features of rash, arthritis, and uveitis. Late-onset (13–15 years) disease is similar to multisystem adult sarcoidosis.

If there are any organ-specific symptoms, the patients must refer to appropriate specialists such as pulmonologist, cardiologist, ophthalmologist, and others.

Extracutaneous Manifestations

Extracutaneous manifestations of sarcoidosis are given in **Table 2**.

Some special constellation of organ involvement in sarcoidosis:

- The triad of ankle arthritis, mediastinal lymphadenopathy, and erythema nodosum is called Lofgren syndrome.
- The combination of fever, parotitis, anterior uveitis, mediastinal lymphadenopathy, and (sometimes) facial nerve palsy is called Heerfordt syndrome or uveoparotid fever.

INVESTIGATIONS

Though the cutaneous involvement occurs in 20–35% of systemic sarcoidosis cases, cutaneous manifestation solely occurs very little percentage of cases. In any granulomatous or suspected skin lesion of sarcoidosis, we first do skin biopsy to know any granulomatous histopathology along with special stains (modified Ziehl–Neelsen stain, Giemsa stain, PAS stain, and others) to rule out any infective pathology or foreign body granuloma. By this time, we investigate some primary tests **(Box 1)** and special investigations are given in **Box 2**. The pulmonary sarcoidosis staging on chest radiograph is described in **Table 3**.

There is no specific histopathological difference between cutaneous involvement of systemic sarcoidosis and sarcoid-like granuloma of other etiology. As, the cutaneous sarcoid-like lesion with noncaseating granuloma (idiopathic sarcoid reaction) may be the forerunner of systemic sarcoidosis, continuous thorough screening of other organ involvement is a rule. Annual organ screening is indicated at least in first few years of diagnosis because other organs are involved within 2 years of onset of disease.

DIFFERENTIAL DIAGNOSIS

Any granulomatous cutaneous lesion should be differentiated from cutaneous sarcoidosis because it is a great imitator. The clinical differential diagnosis of sarcoidosis is given in **Box 3**.

Sarcoidosis may be a differential diagnosis of some atypical hypopigmented, ichthyosiform, or psoriasiform lesions.

TABLE 2: Extracutaneous manifestations of sarcoidosis.

Lungs and mediastinal lymph nodes (>90%)	• Mediastinal lymphadenopathy • Parenchymal involvement (alveoli/interstitium) • Pulmonary fibrosis • Bronchial involvement (approximately 10%, often obstructive) • Pleural involvement (rare) • Pulmonary hypertension
Liver and spleen (15–20%)	• Nodular parenchymal involvement • Cirrhosis, portal hypertension • Involvement of the biliary pathways, cholestasis, biliary cirrhosis • Vascular involvement/stenosis due to lymphadenopathy (rare) • Hypersplenism
Eye (15–20%)	• Uveitis is the most frequent eye symptom • Anterior uveitis (iridocyclitis, trabeculitis with glaucoma) • Intermediate uveitis • Posterior uveitis (choroiditis, periphlebitis retinae) • Lacrimal gland involvement (may cause Mikulicz's syndrome) • Granulomatous conjunctivitis • Optic neuritis • Orbital granuloma
Nervous system involvement (both central and peripheral nervous systems) (approximately 10%)	• Nodular lesions lead to space-occupying lesion, epilepsy, brainstem and spinal syndromes • Pituitary involvement (often with diabetes insipidus) • Encephalopathy • Meningeal involvement • Facial nerve palsy (one of the common causes of bilateral facial nerve palsies) • Other cranial nerve deficits • Mononeuritis multiplex • Polyradiculitis, polyneuropathy
Kidney (approximately 5%) involved by sarcoid granuloma itself or secondary to hypercalcemia, hypercalciuria	• Nephrolithiasis • Renal failure of postrenal cause (hypercalcemia) • Interstitial nephritis
Heart (2–5%)—symptoms are dyspnea, palpitation, chest pain, syncope, etc.	• Conducting system (common; bundle branch block, AV block) • Myocardial involvement (danger of ventricular tachycardia) • Pericardial involvement (rare)
Bones of hands and feet mainly (approximately 1%)	• Nodular lesions • Cystic lesions involving the joints (Jüngling's disease) • Central necrotizing foci in the skull • Bone marrow involvement

(AV: atrioventricular)

BOX 1: Primary investigations for sarcoidosis.

- Complete blood count
- Serum urea, creatinine level
- Liver function test including gamma-glutamyl transferase
- Chest X-ray
- Tuberculin test, QuantiFERON-TB Gold test/IGRA
- Urinary and serum calcium levels, serum ACE level
- Tissue culture to rule out any infective pathology
- Abdominal ultrasonography
- Electrocardiography
- *Kveim test (now rarely done):* Particulate saline suspensions of sarcoid tissue injected at forearm intradermally to see any granulomatous reaction after 2–3 weeks

(ACE: angiotensin-converting enzyme; IGRA: interferon-gamma release assay)

BOX 2: Special investigations.

- Pulmonary function test, high-resolution CT, PET scan, MRI thorax, cytological and histological studies from bronchoalveolar lavage (BAL), and lung or mediastinal lymph node biopsy specimen, respectively, BAL CD4/CD8 ratio by pulmonologist
- Echocardiography, Holter ECG by cardiologist
- MRI brain, muscle by neurologist
- Whole body MRI to know any occult area involvement
- ^{18}F-FDG-PET if diffuse bone involvement is suspected, or to search for foci of involvement

(^{18}F-FDG-PET: 18F-fluordeoxyglucose positron emission tomography)

TABLE 3: Pulmonary sarcoidosis staging on chest radiograph.[4]

Stage 0	Normal chest radiograph (in 5–10% cases)
Stage 1	Hilar or mediastinal nodal enlargement only (in 45–65% cases)
Stage 2	Nodal enlargement and parenchymal disease (in 25–30% cases)
Stage 3	Parenchymal disease only (in 15% cases)
Stage 4	End-stage (pulmonary fibrosis)

BOX 3: Clinical differential diagnosis of sarcoidosis.

- Cutaneous tuberculosis mainly lupus vulgaris
- Hansen's infection
- Foreign body granulomas
- Atypical mycobacterial infection
- Deep fungal (sporotrichosis) or systemic fungal infections (histoplasmosis, coccidioidomycosis)
- Bartonellosis, toxoplasmosis
- Pseudolymphoma
- Sarcoid-like lesions due to cancer (nonmelanoma skin cancer, cutaneous T-cell lymphoma)
- Sarcoid-like lesions due to an immunodeficiency
- Heavy-metal-associated granulomatosis
- Cutaneous vasculitis

APPROACH TO DIAGNOSIS

Approach to diagnose a case of cutaneous sarcoidosis is shown in **Flowchart 3**.

Flowchart 3: Approach to diagnosis.

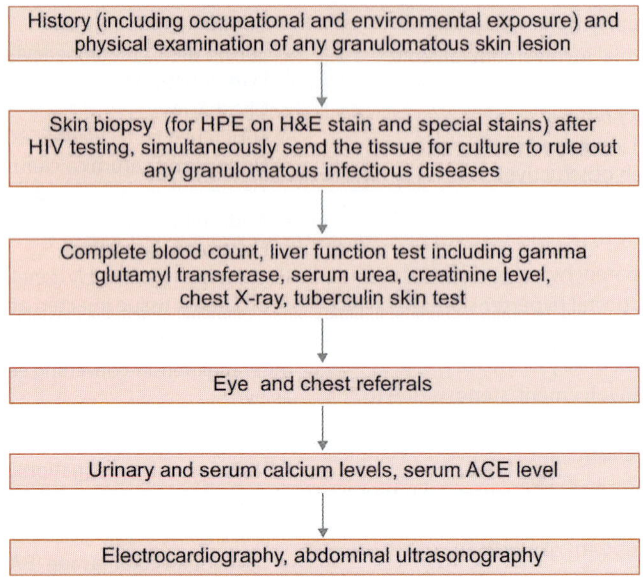

(ACE: angiotensin-converting enzyme; HPE: histopathological examination; HIV: human immunodeficiency virus)

Flowchart 4: Treatment guidelines of cutaneous sarcoidosis.

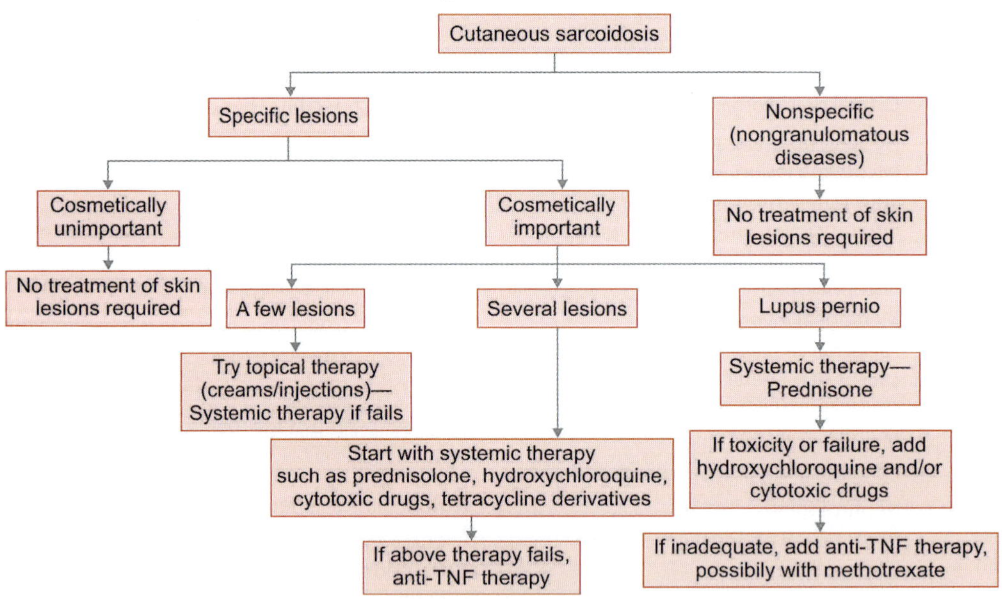

(TNF: tumor necrosis factor)

Source: Adapted from Sarcoidosis Treatment Guidelines by B Robert, C Dan, D Wonder, J Marc, M Lisa, M Dave, et al.

We should be very careful to diagnose sarcoidosis, if there is only one system involvement. We should also be very careful about confirmation of cutaneous sarcoidosis by rule out other infectious and noninfectious granulomatous skin lesions.

TREATMENT

For a few cutaneous, cosmetically important lesions, the initial recommended topical therapies are potent corticosteroid, calcineurin inhibitors, or intralesional triamcinolone acetonide (5–20 mg/mL in every 3–4 weeks interval).

Oral drugs are mainly used in multiple skin lesions or associated with other system involvement. The recommended systemic drugs are corticosteroid (prednisolone 20–40 mg/day or equivalent dose of methylprednisolone), hydroxychloroquine 200–400 mg/day (may also chloroquine 250–1,000 mg/day), tetracycline derivatives (doxycycline or minocycline 200 mg/day), cytotoxic drugs (methotrexate 10–25 mg/week, azathioprine 50–200 mg/day), mycophenolate mofetil (500–1,500 mg twice daily), leflunomide (10–20 mg/day), anti-TNF-α antibody therapy (infliximab 5 mg/kg every 6 weeks and adalimumab), and also thalidomide (50–200 mg/day). Recently for the treatment of sarcoidosis with neuropathic and autonomic symptoms, the innate repair receptor (IRR) activator ARA 290 (an erythropoietin derivative with tissue protective and healing properties without stimulating erythropoiesis) has been used to decrease pain in USA and European Union.[5]

The two biomarkers (soluble IL-2 receptor alpha and neopterin) are suitable for treatment monitoring of disease.

Flowchart 4 shows treatment guidelines of cutaneous sarcoidosis.

KEY POINTS

- Sarcoidosis is a chronic granulomatous disease with bimodal age of occurrence.
- Etiology is not clearly understood.
- It involves most commonly in lungs (90% of all cases). It also affects reticuloendothelial system, skin, eyes, nervous system, heart, bones, etc.
- Noncaseating, naked granuloma is the classic histological picture.
- Diagnosis is by exclusion of other diseases.
- Corticosteroid is the main stay of treatment.

REFERENCES

1. Inaoka PT, Shono M, Kamada M, Espinoza JL et al. Host-microbe interactions in the pathogenesis and clinical course of sarcoidosis. J Biomed Sci. 2019;26:45.
2. Starshinova AA, Malkova AM, Basantsova NY, Zinchenko YS, Kudryavtsev IV, Ershov GA, et al. Sarcoidosis as an autoimmune disease. Front Immunol. 2020;10:2933.
3. James WD, Berger TG, Elston DM, Andrews GC (Eds). Andrews' Diseases of the Skin: Clinical Dermatology, 12th edition. Philadelphia, PA: Saunders Elsevier; 2015.
4. Collins J, Stern EJ (Eds). Chest radiology, 3rd edition. Philadelphia: Wolters Kluwer Health/Lippincott Williams & Wilkins; 2014.
5. Van Velzen M, Heij L, Niesters M, Cerami A, Dunne A, Dahan A, Brines M. ARA 290 for treatment of small fiber neuropathy in sarcoidosis. Expert Opin Investig Drugs. 2014;23(4):541-50.

EXAMINATION QUESTIONS

1. Explain immunopathology of sarcoidosis.
2. Briefly discuss the extracutaneous manifestations of sarcoidosis.
3. How will you approach to a case of cutaneous sarcoidosis?
4. Describe the treatment of sarcoidosis.

67 CHAPTER

Cutaneous Markers of Internal Malignancies

Shekhar Neema

INTRODUCTION

Cutaneous manifestation of systemic diseases continues to provide a valuable insight into the functional status of the body. Identifying the underlying pathology by examining the skin continues to fascinate dermatologist's world over till date. Internal malignancies may be associated with myriad of cutaneous presentation in varying severity.

Cutaneous metastasis is a relatively uncommon phenomenon with a prevalence reported between 0.7 and 10% of all patients diagnosed with cancer.[1] The expertise in identifying these malignancies by its cutaneous manifestation continues to rise at rapid pace as number of cases diagnosed with malignancies are increasing.

HISTORY

Skin is the largest organ of the human body and a variety of pathological conditions affect it either directly or indirectly. A large number of systemic diseases and internal malignancies have cutaneous manifestations, which are highly varied and diverse.

In 1868, Hebra suggested that skin pigmentation could be indicative of underlying malignancy.[2] Ever since, more than 50 dermatological conditions have been documented as potential markers of internal malignancy.[3] Involvement of skin can be either direct or indirect. Direct invasion is characterized by presence of cancerous cells in the skin either due to extension or metastasis. Indirect involvement is a result of various inflammatory, proliferative, and metabolic factors from neoplasia. In these cases, there is no neoplastic cell in skin and this is considered as dermatological paraneoplastic syndrome.

Cutaneous markers of internal malignancies can be classified on the basis of etiology for better understanding, though the ideal classification is lacking **(Box 1)**.

MALIGNANT INVOLVEMENT OF SKIN

Metastasis to skin is the most specific marker of internal malignancy. It occurs either because of direct extension from underlying malignancy, or as a result of dissemination of cancerous cells via blood or lymphatic channels. This is most commonly seen in hematopoietic malignancies, and can have either malignant cells or histologically benign cells in lesions of the skin.

BOX 1: Classification—cutaneous markers of internal malignancies.

- Malignant involvement of skin
- Genodermatosis associated with increased risk of internal malignancy
- Paraneoplastic dermatoses
- Indirect cutaneous markers (i.e., environmental carcinogens)

Metastatic Carcinoma/Direct Tumor Extension/Metastasis from Tumors of Viscera

Cutaneous metastasis from internal malignancies is quite rare. Data from a meta-analysis done by Krathen et al. estimated the incidence of 5.3%.[4] Lung and colon are the most common site of origin in males while in females, breast and colon are more frequently associated. Patient presents with solitary or multiple, firm-to-hard, skin-colored to blue-brown nodules. The nodules may be subcutaneous or dermal. Most common age of presentation is 5th decade. Lesions are frequently seen around the area of primary site **(Fig. 1)**. However, unusual presentation such as periumbilical lesions is seen in gastric carcinomas (Sister Mary Joseph nodules) **(Fig. 2)**.

Carcinoma En Cuirasse

Presentation: Firm-to-hard, infiltrated, morphea-like plaque over the chest wall. It occurs due to fibrosis of skin resulting from blockage and stasis of lymphatics.

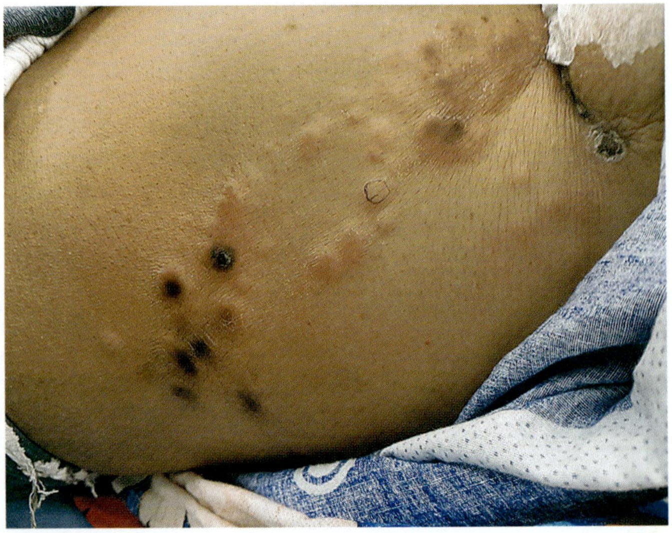

Fig. 1: Cutaneous metastases presenting as dermal nodules around primary site of carcinoma breast.

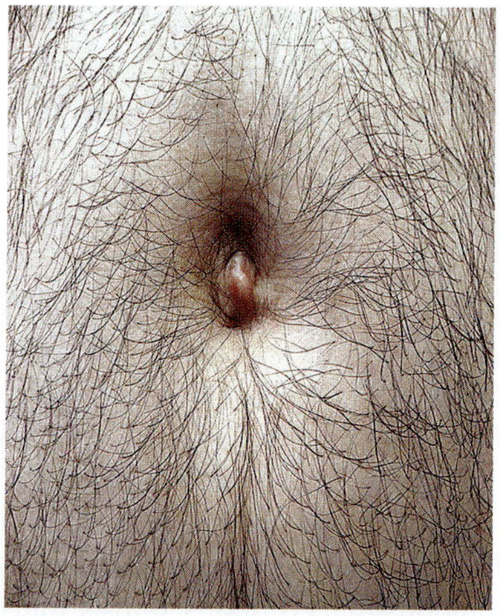

Fig. 2: Sister Mary Joseph nodule in a case of gastric carcinoma.

Associations: It is most commonly seen in breast malignancies; however, it may also be seen in lung, gastrointestinal, and renal malignancies.

Carcinoma Erysipeloides

Presentation: Erysipelas-like red, indurated skin with sharply marginated borders. It occurs due to migration of malignant cells into dermal lymphatics.

Associations: Most commonly associated with breast carcinoma. It may also be seen in lung, prostate, esophagus, bladder, colon, larynx, rectum, stomach, and pancreatic carcinoma.

Telangiectatic Metastatic Carcinoma

Presentation: Dilated vasculature on erythematous background along with papulovesicular lesions.

Associations: Typically associated with breast cancer. In cases of extensive vascular involvement, it can resemble angiosarcoma.

Paget's Disease

- Uncommon malignancy of breast.
- *Presentation*: Eczematous lesion over nipple and areola.
- Mostly unilateral, mass in the breast may be palpated.
- *Associations*: Associated with intraductal or infiltrating breast carcinoma. Histopathology reveals skin infiltration with tumor cells containing pale-staining cytoplasm and large vesicular to hyperchromatic nuclei with prominent nucleoli.

Extramammary Paget's Disease

- Rare disease
- Involves areas with high density of apocrine gland, e.g., vulva, anus, scrotum, penis, axilla, perianal area
- *Presentation*: Light-colored or eczematous lesion with oozing or bleeding
- Sharp raised margin and is characteristically progressive in nature
- May not be associated with a tumor
- Extramammary Paget's disease (EMPD) arises as primary cutaneous adenocarcinoma. Associated malignancies are cutaneous adnexal carcinoma, carcinoma of Bartholin's gland, bladder, vagina, cervix, endometrium, and prostate

Lymphoreticular and Hematological Malignancies

Leukemias and Lymphomas

- Skin involvement in systemic leukemia or lymphomas can be either specific or nonspecific.
- Lesions may have specific lesions called as leukemia cutis or lymphoma cutis or a benign dermatosis because of paraneoplastic phenomenon or systemic effects of the disease.
- Lesions of leukemia cutis are firm-to-hard papules, nodules, or plaques.

Multiple Myeloma

- Cutaneous involvement may be a result of metastasis or direct extension from underlying bone lesions.
- Lesions are mostly nontender, cutaneous or subcutaneous, can range from skin colored to violaceous.
- Crusting or ulceration of skin lesions may be seen.

Genodermatosis

Genodermatoses or genetic diseases of skin refer to group of inherited disorders with cutaneous and systemic symptoms. Many of these have an association with internal malignancy. An understanding of the cutaneous presentation can provide a valuable insight into the underlying systemic involvement. Mechanisms proposed in the pathogenesis of these conditions involves: Chromosomal instability, DNA repair default, abnormal lymphocyte function, and immune surveillance.[11]

Box 2 gives a list of such genodermatoses encountered by dermatologists. Common conditions will be discussed briefly in **Table 1**.

Paraneoplastic Syndrome

Paraneoplastic diseases can be defined as hormonal, neurological, or hematological disturbances and as clinical and biochemical imbalances associated with the presence of malignancies without direct association with primary tumor, invasion or metastasis **(Table 2)**.

Criteria that define paraneoplastic syndrome were given by Curth. They include:[12]

- Concurrent onset of cutaneous disease and malignancy
- Parallel course of the skin disease and internal malignancy
- A specific type or site of malignancy associated with the skin disease

- Sound statistical evidence that the malignancy is more frequent in patients with the skin disease than in age and sex-matched controls
- A genetic link between a syndrome with skin manifestations and an internal malignancy

Note: It is not necessary that all the criteria have to meet.

BOX 2: Genodermatosis.

- *Primary immunodeficiency disorders:*
  - Ataxia-telangiectasia
  - Wiskott-Aldrich syndrome
  - Common variable immunodeficiency
  - Severe combined immunodeficiency
  - Bruton's agammaglobulinemia
- *Gastrointestinal polyposis syndromes:*
  - Gardner's syndrome
  - Peutz–Jeghers syndrome
- Cowden's disease
- Muir–Torre syndrome
- Howel–Evans syndrome
- Multiple endocrine neoplasia, type III
- *Syndromes associated with chromosomal instability:*
  - Bloom's syndrome
  - Dyskeratosis congenita
  - Adult progeria
  - Fanconi's anemia
- Nevoid basal cell carcinoma
- Neurofibromatosis
- Hemochromatosis

CUTANEOUS MANIFESTATION OF CHEMOTHERAPY

Skin and its appendages very often bear the brunt of chemotherapeutic agents. These structures are most susceptible to these adverse effects as they have a very rapid rate of proliferation. Generalized hyperpigmentation, hand–foot syndrome, diffuse alopecia is seen with use of capecitabine **(Fig. 6)**. Epidermal growth factor inhibitor receptors inhibitors such as erlotinib, dasatinib, and imatinib can cause papulopustular eruptions, xerosis, mucosal changes such as dryness and pruritus, pyogenic granuloma, and paronychia. Flagellate pigmentation is noticed with the use of bleomycin. Diffuse alopecia is seen with agents such as vincristine, cyclophosphamide, adriamycin, paclitaxel, and carboplatin. Diffuse hyperpigmentation and longitudinal melanonychia can occur as a result of drugs such as vincristine, doxorubicin, bleomycin, cyclophosphamide,

TABLE 1: Common genodermatoses associated with internal malignancy.

Genodermatoses	*Transmission*	*Presentation*	*Cutaneous features*	*Associated malignancy*
Ataxia-telangiectasia	AR	Cerebellar ataxia, mental retardation	Ocular telangiectasia, café-au-lait macules, hypopigmented macules, hypertrichosis, bird-like facies	Leukemia, lymphoma
Wiskott–Aldrich syndrome	XR	Triad of immunodeficiency, thrombocytopenia and eczema	• Atopic dermatitis • Bacterial infections, thrombocytopenic purpura	Leukemia, lymphoma
Peutz–Jeghers syndrome[5,6]	AD	Gastrointestinal polyposis syndrome	Melanocytic mucocutaneous pigmentation and intestinal hamartomatous polyps	Gastrointestinal, breast, ovary, uterus, cervix, lung and testis
Muir–Torre syndrome[7]	AD	Mutation in DNA mismatch repair genes	Sebaceous neoplasm of skin including adenoma and carcinoma	Colorectal, breast, urogenital
Howel–Evans syndrome[8]	AD	Palmoplantar keratoderma (PPK)	PPK, oral leukoplakia	Esophageal carcinoma
Multiple endocrine neoplasia Type III[9]	AD	Multiple neuromas, medullary thyroid carcinoma, pheochromocytoma	Mucosal neuroma, marfanoid habitus	
Bloom syndrome	AR	Photosensitivity, conjunctivitis, growth retardation and immunological abnormalities	Malar erythema, telangiectasia	Lymphoreticular
Werner syndrome[10]	AR	Premature aging and increased risk of malignancy, short stature, early atherosclerosis, cataract, osteoporosis, diabetes and hypogonadism	Scleroderma-like skin, alopecia, premature canities	Sarcomas, melanomas, leukemia, meningiomas and a variety of epithelial-derived carcinomas
Fanconi anemia	AR	Congenital malformation, progressive pancytopenia and malignancies	Reticulated hyperpigmentation of neck, trunk and flexures	Leukemia, mucosal squamous cell carcinomas, breast tumors
Dyskeratosis congenita	XR, AR, AD	Cytopenia	• Reticulated hyperpigmentation of skin, nail dystrophy and leukoplakia • Poikiloderma, telangiectasia	Squamous cell carcinoma of mouth, nasopharynx, esophagus, rectum, vagina, cervix. Hodgkin lymphoma and adenocarcinoma of GIT

(AD: autosomal dominant; AR: autosomal recessive; GIT: gastrointestinal tract; XR: X-linked recessive)

TABLE 2: Paraneoplastic syndromes.

Dermatosis	*Clinical features*	*Systemic neoplasm*
Acanthosis nigricans	Velvety thickening and hyperpigmentation of flexures and axillae. Benign form is much more common than malignant	Gastrointestinal adenocarcinomas
Acquired pachydermatoglyphia **(Fig. 3)**	Yellowish, velvety, diffuse palmar hyperkeratosis, along with accentuated dermatoglyphic patterns "tripe palms"	Gastric and pulmonary carcinoma
Erythema gyratum repens	Diffuse, serpiginous, polycyclic and pruriginous erythema with desquamation around the edges and fast growing, about 1 cm/day, which produces concentric figures that resemble a wood surface	Pulmonary, esophageal and breast carcinoma
Bazex paraneoplastic acrokeratosis	Psoriasiform plaques, symmetrically distribution, acrally on helices of the ear, and nose. Nail dystrophy may be seen	Aerodigestive tract (oral cavity, larynx, pharynx, trachea, esophagus and lung)
Acquired hypertrichosis lanuginosa	Rapid growth of fine long, lanugo type hair around face, eyebrows, forehead and nose in adulthood	Colorectal, pulmonary and breast carcinoma
Necrolytic migratory erythema	Lesions, begins with erythematous macules which evolve centrifugally into circinate and polycyclic lesions. Painful glossitis, angular cheilitis, anemia, and weight loss	Glucagonoma
Leser–Trélat sign (eruptive seborrheic keratoses) **(Fig. 4)**	Sudden increase in size and number of seborrheic keratoses. Mostly on thorax followed by the extremities, face, abdomen, neck and axilla	Gastric and colorectal carcinoma
Paraneoplastic pemphigus	*Painful stomatitis:* Conjunctival and anorectal mucosa erosions. Cutaneous lesions may range from papules and plaques-like erythema multiforme, vesicles and blisters resembling pemphigus vulgaris or even pruritic plaques similar to lichen planus	Non-Hodgkin lymphoma, chronic lymphocytic leukemia, Castleman's disease, thymoma
Pityriasis rotunda	Round or oval scaly pigmented patches which mainly occurs on trunk, arms and legs	Hepatocellular carcinoma, gastric and esophageal carcinoma, prostate cancer, chronic lymphocytic leukemia and multiple myeloma
Dermatomyositis	Violaceous, photosensitive rash, proximal myopathy, elevated serum creatinine kinase and abnormal electromyogram, heliotrope rash, nail fold changes and Gottron papules	Ovarian carcinoma, bronchogenic carcinoma
Palmoplantar keratoderma	Abnormal thickening of palms and soles	Esophageal carcinoma
Pyoderma gangrenosum	Painful nodules and pustules with rapid progress to deep ulcerations and undermined edges. Pretibial area is the most affected	Myelodysplastic syndrome, myeloma, leukemia
Sweet syndrome **(Fig. 5)**	Characterized by painful, edematous, shiny erythematous nodules or plaques, mostly on head, neck and upper limbs	Acute myelogenous leukemia, myelodysplastic syndrome

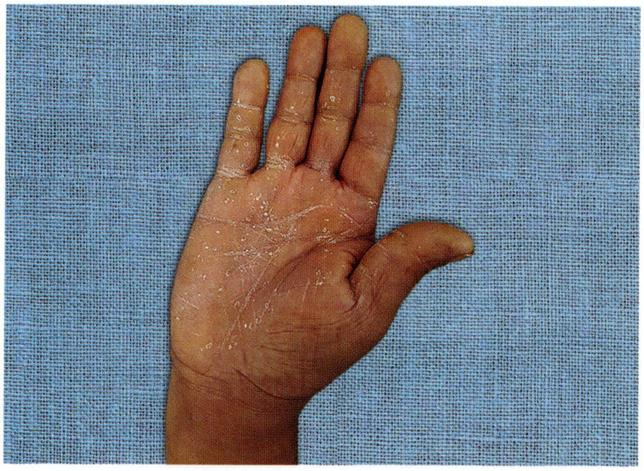

Fig. 3: Tripe palms seen in a case of gastric carcinoma.

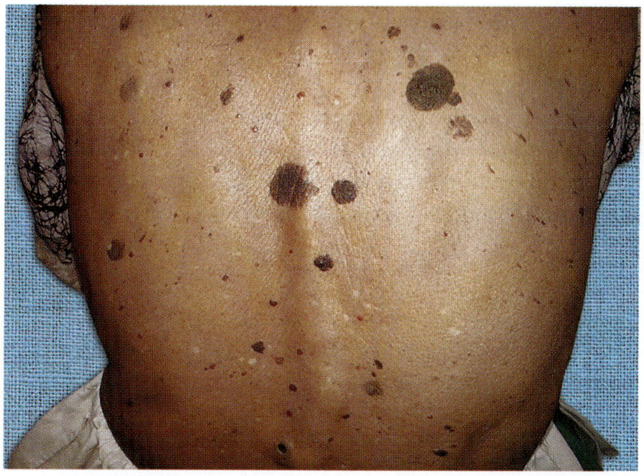

Fig. 4: Leser–Trélat sign in a case of colonic carcinoma.

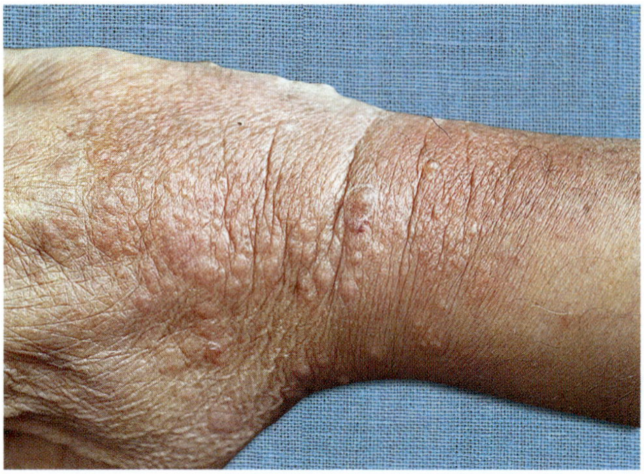

Fig. 5: Sweet syndrome in a case of multiple myeloma.

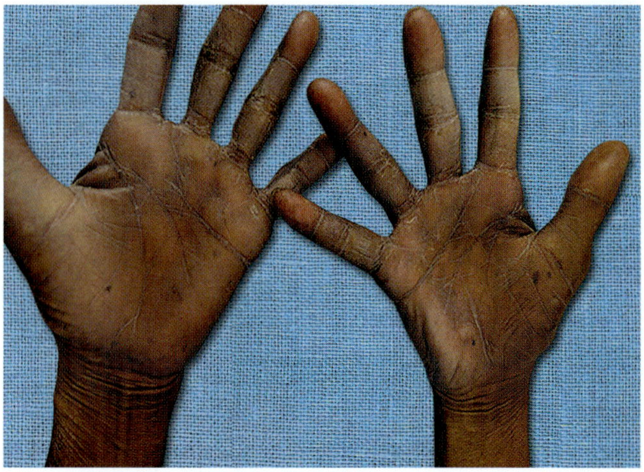

Fig. 6: Capecitabine-induced hand–foot syndrome.

and daunorubicin. Supravenous hyperpigmentation due to docetaxel and ichthyosis has been reported with hydroxyurea. Most of these adverse effects are self-limiting and are not reported by the patients. Role of the dermatologists in today's era is not only to manage these side effects but also to guide the treating physician to make the judgment on continuation or discontinuation of the therapy if required. Accordingly, the oncologist can either stop, substitute, or to continue the therapy.

KEY POINTS

- Internal malignancies can present with cutaneous manifestations.
- High index of suspicion is required for diagnosis of internal malignancies in patients presenting with dermal nodules.

REFERENCES

1. Lookingbill DP, Spangler N, Sexton FM. Skin involvement as the presenting sign of internal carcinoma: a retrospective study of 7316 cancer patients. J Am Acad Dermatol. 1990;22(1): 19-26.
2. Sneddon IB. Cutaneous manifestations of visceral malignancy. Postgrad Med J. 1970;46(541):678-85.
3. Poole S, Fenske NA. Cutaneous markers of internal malignancy. I. Malignant involvement of the skin and the genodermatoses. J Am Acad Dermatol. 1993;28(1):1-13.
4. Krathen RA, Orengo IF, Rosen T. Cutaneous metastasis: A meta-analysis of data. South Med J. 2003;96(2):164-7.
5. Schreibman IR, Baker M, Amos C, McGarrity TJ. The hamartomatous polyposis syndromes: a clinic and molecular review. Am J Gastroenterol. 2005;100(5):476-90.
6. Westerman AM, Wilson JH. Peutz-Jeghers syndrome: risks of a hereditary condition. Scand J Gastroenterol. 1999;230:64S-70S.
7. Serleth HJ, Kisken WA. A Muir-Torre syndrome family. Am Surg. 1998;64(4):365-9.
8. Clarke CA, McConnell RB, Howel-Evans W. Carcinoma of the esophagus in associated tylosis. Br Med J. 1957;1(5024):945.
9. Baum JL, Adler ME. Pheochromocytoma, medullary thyroid carcinoma, multiple mucosal neuroma. Arch Opthalmol. 1972; 87(5):574-84.
10. Thannhauser SJ. Werner's syndrome (progeria of adults) and Rothmund's syndrome: Two types of closely related heredo familial atrophic dermatoses with juvenile cataracts and endocrine features: critical study with 5 new cases. Ann Intern Med. 1945;23:559-626.
11. Xie J, Johnson RL, Zhang X, Bare JW, Waldman FM, Cogen PH, et al. Mutations of the *PATCHED* gene in several types of sporadic extracutaneous tumors. Cancer Res. 1997;57:2369-72.
12. Curth HO. Skin lesions and internal carcinoma. In: Andrade R, Gumport SL, Popkin GL, Rees TD (Eds). Cancer of the skin. Philadelphia: WB Saunders; 1976. pp. 1308-9.

EXAMINATION QUESTIONS

1. Discuss cutaneous features of internal malignancies.
2. Explain paraneoplastic dermatoses.

68 CHAPTER

Cutaneous Amyloidosis

Suneil Gandhi

INTRODUCTION

It is a heterogeneous group of diseases in which amyloid accumulates within various tissues and organs. Virchow introduced the term "amyloid" in 1854. Dermatologists come across this condition in two clinical scenarios: (1) Primary cutaneous amyloidosis, and (2) Systemic amyloidosis with cutaneous manifestations. Systemic amyloidosis is generalized and several organ systems are involved. In the localized form of amyloidosis, single organs (such as the skin) are involved. The clinical classification of amyloidosis is depicted in **Table 1**.

EPIDEMIOLOGY

The exact epidemiology is unknown as this diagnosis is frequently overlooked. Primary systemic amyloidosis is seen in 6–15% of patients suffering from multiple myeloma and in 5–11% of patients with rheumatoid arthritis. Primary cutaneous amyloidosis is more common in South-east Asian countries. Macular amyloidosis is also common in Central and South American countries. Lichen amyloidosis is more common in Chinese people. Macular and lichen amyloidosis occur most frequently in skin types 3 and 4.

TABLE 1: Clinical classification of amyloidosis.

	Localized Amyloidosis
Primary cutaneous	Macular, lichen, nodular, biphasic, dyschromic
Secondary cutaneous	Seen within various skin tumors and following PUVA therapy
Endocrine	Medullary carcinoma of thyroid, insulinoma
Cerebral	Alzheimer's disease
	Systemic Amyloidosis
Primary systemic amyloidosis	• Plasma cell dyscrasias • Multiple myeloma associated
Secondary systemic amyloidosis	• Chronic inflammatory disease • Chronic infection
	Hemodialysis-associated Amyloidosis
Genetic forms of hemodialysis	• Familial amyloid neuropathy • Muckle–Wells syndrome • Familial Mediterranean fever • TNF receptor-associated periodic syndrome • Finnish type familial amyloidosis

(PUVA: psoralen-ultraviolet A; TNF: tumor necrosis factor)

AMYLOID CHARACTERISTICS

Amyloid is an insoluble fibril protein. Characteristic properties include a cross β-pleated sheet configuration on X-ray crystallography and eosinophilic hyaline appearance with hematoxylin and eosin stain. Congo stain gives amyloid an orange-red color, which is doubly refractive and apple-green when examined in polarized light. Other special stains that reveal amyloid include crystal violet, methyl violet, periodic acid–Schiff (PAS), Sirius red, pagoda red, Dylon stain, and thioflavin T. On electron microscopy, amyloid appears as 7–10 nm wide, nonbranching and nonanastomosing fibrils. About 18 unique forms of amyloid proteins and precursors have been described. They include AL (amyloid light chains), AA (amyloid-associated), Aβ, amyloid transthyretin (ATTR), etc. The common types of amyloid proteins, their precursors, and associated clinical disease are depicted in **Table 2**.

Pathogenesis

The precise mechanism by which amyloid gets deposited in tissues is unknown. Destabilization or mutation of precursor proteins alters the stability and increases amyloidogenicity. They undergo changes leading to aggregation, polymerization, and fibril formation. These then get deposited in tissues. Accumulation of amyloid leads to pressure atrophy and interference with normal function. Genetic predisposition, friction, Epstein–Barr virus infection and environmental factors are proposed as etiological factors of primary cutaneous amyloidosis. The amyloid material is possibly derived from keratinocytes. The fibrillar theory proposes that the tonofilaments of keratinocytes undergo degeneration and pass into the dermis. An alternative theory suggests that amyloid material is produced around the dermoepidermal junction.

PRIMARY CUTANEOUS AMYLOIDOSIS

Clinical Features

This is classically divided into macular, papular (lichen amyloidosis), and nodular forms. However, macular and lichen amyloidosis represent the ends of a clinical spectrum. Both variants exist in some patients, which are called biphasic amyloidosis.

TABLE 2: Types of amyloid proteins and their associated diseases.

Precursor protein	*Amyloid protein*	*Clinical disease*
Apo serum AA	AA	Secondary systemic amyloidosis, cryopyrinopathies
Apolipoprotein AI	AApoAI	Familial amyloid polyneuropathy
Gelsolin	AGel	Finnish familial amyloidosis
Keratin	AKer	Primary localized cutaneous amyloidosis
Immunoglobulin light chain	AL	Primary systemic amyloidosis, primary cutaneous nodular amyloidosis
Transthyretin	ATTR	Familial amyloid polyneuropathy, senile systemic amyloidosis
Aβ precursor protein	Aβ	Alzheimer's disease
β_2 microglobulin	$A\beta_2M$	Chronic hemodialysis

(AL: amyloid light chains; AA: amyloid associated; AApoAI: apolipoprotein AI-derived; ATTR: amyloid transthyretin)

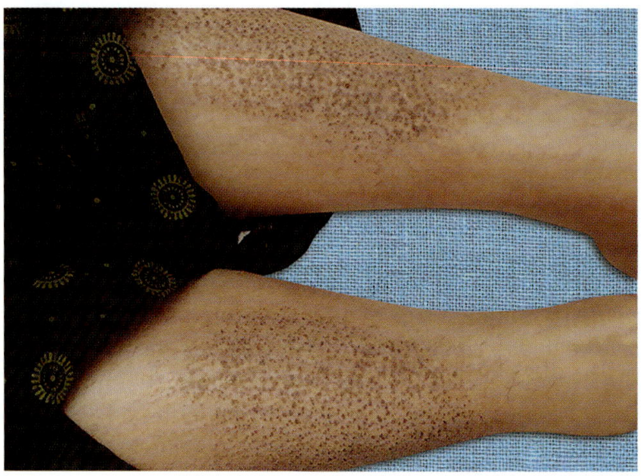

Fig. 1: Lichen amyloidosis.

Macular Amyloidosis

The lesions are hyperpigmented and distributed in a confluent or rippled pattern. It appears in early adulthood and affects both genders equally. The common sites of involvement include the upper back and extensor aspect of extremities. It can be pruritic or asymptomatic. Friction amyloidosis is the term used when the lesions are produced secondary to localized friction from bathing brushes, towels, and other materials.

Lichen Amyloidosis

This is the most common form of primary cutaneous amyloidosis. It presents as severely pruritic papules on the shins and other extensor aspects of extremities **(Fig. 1)**. The anosacral area can also be involved. The papules are closely grouped, firm, skin-colored to red-brown and slightly scaly. They may coalesce to form plaques. They are usually unilateral to begin with, but can then be bilateral in distribution. Bullous lesions have also been described in association with lichen amyloidosis.

Dyschromic Amyloidosis

This is a rare variant which has its onset before puberty. It is characterized by dotted reticular hyperpigmentation with hypopigmented macules distributed nearly all over the body. There is little or no itching at all.

Nodular Amyloidosis

This is a very rare variant, associated with paraproteinemia. Immunoglobulin-γ light chains are demonstrated in the lesions. It presents as red-brown waxy nodules and plaques. There is central thinning, so the underlying fat is seen with a yellow shimmer. The scalp, trunk, and extremities are the common areas involved. About 7% of such cases can progress to systemic involvement, so long-term follow-up is necessary.

Atrophic Cutaneous Nodular Amyloidosis

This is the rarest variant of nodular amyloidosis, with less than five cases being described in the literature so far. It appears as solitary or multiple brown or yellow nodules which are asymptomatic. They have an atrophic surface with a whitish-yellow color, and usually are present on photo-protected skin. Histopathology features include amyloid deposits in the dermis, subcutaneous fat, and blood vessel walls. Regular follow-up is necessary to check for disease progression and systemic involvement, just like nodular amyloidosis.

Pathology

The amyloid deposits are restricted to the upper papillary dermis. It may expand the papillae and displace the elongated rete ridges laterally. The overlying epidermis shows irregular acanthosis and hyperkeratosis. A few melanophages may be present, with sparse lymphohistiocytic infiltrate.

Differential Diagnosis

Macular amyloidosis needs to be differentiated from nostalgia paresthetica. The former lacks the amyloid deposits on biopsy, is usually unilateral, and presents as an intensely itchy hyperpigmented patch over the scapular area. The other differentials include postinflammatory hyperpigmentation, fixed drug eruption, pityriasis versicolor, erythema dyschromicum perstans, and photodermatitis. Lichen amyloidosis needs to be differentiated from lichen simplex chronicus, hypertrophic lichen planus, pretibial myxedema, papular mucinosis, prurigo nodularis, and epidermolysis bullosa pruriginosa. Nodular amyloidosis can resemble the cutaneous lesions of primary systemic amyloidosis and colloid milium. The other differentials include lymphoma cutis, pseudolymphoma, sarcoidosis, granuloma annulare, granuloma faciale, and reticulohistiocytosis.

Management

No treatment modality is effective in removing the amyloid deposits. Chronic friction, scratching or rubbing the areas must be avoided. High-potency topical corticosteroids are useful, and can be used in combination with a keratolytic such as salicylic acid, and under occlusion. Topical dimethyl sulfoxide (DMSO), topical calcineurin inhibitors may help. Topical psoralen-ultraviolet A (PUVA) therapy and ultraviolet B (UVB) phototherapy have shown to reduce pruritus. Dermabrasion helps to reduce the papules of lichen amyloidosis. Fractional, Q-switched, and pulsed dye lasers have been tried with variable success. Oral retinoids and cyclophosphamide have been reported effective in reducing the lesions and symptoms in a few studies. Excision, cryotherapy, and laser ablation have been used to treat nodular amyloidosis, but recurrences have been described.

SECONDARY CUTANEOUS AMYLOIDOSIS

This occurs histopathologically as an epiphenomenon within skin tumors such as basal cell carcinoma, Bowen's disease, trichoepithelioma, pilomatricoma, sweat gland tumors, etc. It also occurs in seborrheic keratosis, porokeratosis, intradermal melanocytic nevi, and dermatofibroma. It is also reported to occur following PUVA therapy.

Primary Systemic Amyloidosis (Lubarsh–Pick Disease)

This form of amyloidosis is usually associated with underlying plasma cell dyscrasias or multiple myeloma. AL amyloid is deposited in the skin as well as other internal organs such as the kidneys, heart, gastrointestinal tract, peripheral nerves, and tongue.

Clinical Features

The presenting symptoms are nonspecific. Fatigue, syncope, weight loss, dyspnea, and paresthesia occur in such patients.

Cutaneous findings include spontaneous petechiae, purpura, and ecchymoses. They appear over the eyelids, neck, axillae, and anogenital regions, usually following minor trauma. It is also known as "pinch purpura." The periorbital purpura is very characteristic, and known as "raccoon eyes sign." It is precipitated by coughing, Valsalva maneuver or post-proctoscopy. Waxy, translucent, purpuric papules, nodules, and plaques are seen on the face **(Fig. 2)**, neck, scalp, and anogenital areas. Smooth and erythematous waxy infiltration of amyloid occurs over the palms, soles, and fingertips. Diffuse cutaneous infiltration can give rise to a sclerodermoid appearance. The scalp skin can be thrown into folds resembling cutis verticis gyrata. Hemorrhagic blisters, nail dystrophy and cutis laxa have also been described.

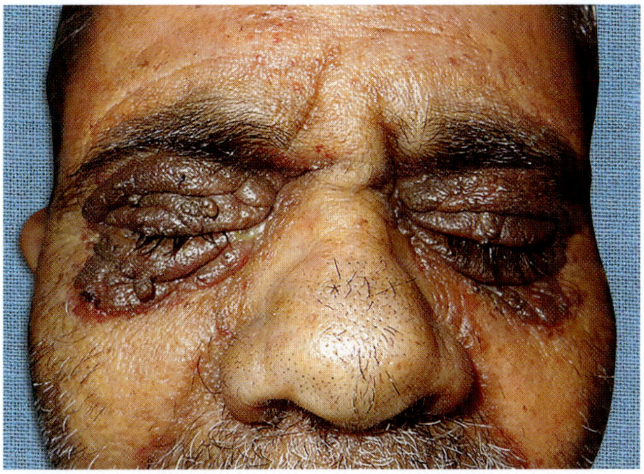

Fig. 2: Primary systemic amyloidosis.

Amyloid deposits appear as soft rubbery hemorrhagic swelling in the oral mucosa. The tongue is uniformly enlarged and firm, and may have hemorrhagic papules, plaques, or bullae on its surface. Xerostomia may be present if the salivary glands are affected.

Systemic symptoms depend on the organs which are involved. Renal involvement can lead to proteinuria and pedal edema. Cardiac involvement can cause dyspnea, arrhythmias, elevated jugular venous pressure, and bilateral pedal edema. Hepatomegaly and splenomegaly can occur. Nervous system involvement leads to sensory and autonomic neuropathy and carpal tunnel syndrome.

Pathology

Amyloid deposits can be demonstrated in rectal and mucosal biopsies in 80–90% of patients. In the skin, the amyloid deposits are present in the dermis and subcutaneous fat. It is also found around the sweat glands and blood vessel walls.

Differential Diagnosis

The differential diagnosis of waxy papules includes xanthelasma, necrobiotic xanthogranuloma, papular mucinosis, nodular amyloidosis, adnexal tumors, and lipoid proteinosis. The nodules need to be differentiated from cysts, lipomas, nevus lipomatosis, and lymphomas. Causes of purpura and sclerodermoid skin also need to be investigated and ruled out.

Management

The treatment of primary systemic amyloidosis is similar to that of multiple myeloma. High-dose melphalan followed by autologous peripheral blood stem cell transplantation is the treatment of choice in younger patients. In older

TABLE 3: Causes of secondary systemic amyloidosis.

Chronic infections	*Chronic inflammatory diseases*
• Tuberculosis • Lepromatous leprosy • Hidradenitis suppurativa • Chronic skin infections in drug addicts	• Rheumatoid arthritis • Ankylosing spondylitis • Scleroderma • Dermatomyositis • Systemic lupus erythematosus • Generalized psoriasis • Chronic pustular psoriasis • Epidermolysis bullosa acquisita • X-linked anhidrotic ectodermal dysplasia • Recurrent venous ulcers • Chronic burns

patients or those with cardiac involvement, lenalidomide and bortezomib are used alone or in combination with systemic corticosteroids, colchicine, or melphalan. Supportive therapy is given according to the organs involved and their manifestations.

Secondary Systemic Amyloidosis

It is also known as reactive systemic amyloidosis, this occurs as a complication of chronic infections and chronic inflammatory diseases **(Table 3)**. It is characterized by deposition of amyloid A protein. The precursor is an acute phase protein which is synthesized by the liver. The kidneys, liver, spleen, and adrenals are usually affected. There is usually no skin involvement. Treatment is by treating the underlying cause.

KEY POINTS

- Amyloidosis is a heterogeneous group of diseases in which amyloid accumulates within various tissues and organs. It is broadly classified as systemic and localized amyloidosis.
- Systemic amyloidosis is generalized and several organ systems are involved. In the localized form of amyloidosis, single organs (such as the skin) are involved. Macular, lichen, nodular, biphasic, and dyschromic amyloidosis are types of localized primary cutaneous amyloidosis.
- The mechanism by which amyloid gets deposited in tissues is unknown. Genetic predisposition, friction, Epstein–Barr virus infection, and environmental factors are proposed as etiological factors of primary cutaneous amyloidosis. The amyloid material is possibly derived from keratinocytes.
- The amyloid deposits are restricted to the upper papillary dermis. It may expand the papillae and displace the elongated rete ridges laterally. The overlying epidermis shows irregular acanthosis and hyperkeratosis. Congo stain gives amyloid an orange-red color, which is doubly refractive and apple-green when examined in polarized light.
- Secondary cutaneous amyloidosis occurs within skin tumors such as basal cell carcinoma, Bowen's disease, trichoepithelioma, pilomatricoma, sweat gland tumors, etc.
- Primary systemic amyloidosis is usually associated with underlying plasma cell dyscrasias or multiple myeloma. AL amyloid is deposited in the skin as well as other internal organs such as the kidneys, heart, gastrointestinal tract, peripheral nerves, and tongue.
- The cutaneous findings of primary systemic amyloidosis include spontaneous petechiae, purpura, and ecchymoses. They appear over the eyelids, neck, axillae, and anogenital regions.
- Secondary systemic amyloidosis occurs as a complication of chronic infections and chronic inflammatory diseases.
- High-potency topical corticosteroids, salicylic acid, topical DMSO, topical calcineurin inhibitor, topical PUVA therapy, and UVB phototherapy have been tried for cutaneous amyloidosis. Dermabrasion helps to reduce the papules of lichen amyloidosis. Fractional, Q-switched, and pulsed dye lasers have been tried with variable success.
- High-dose melphalan followed by autologous peripheral blood stem cell transplantation is the treatment of choice in primary systemic amyloidosis. In older patients or those with cardiac involvement, lenalidomide and bortezomib are used alone or in combination with systemic corticosteroids, colchicine, or melphalan.

SUGGESTED READING

1. Breathnach SM. Amyloid and amyloidosis. J Am Acad Dermatol. 1988;18:1-16.
2. Castanedo-Cazares JP, Lepe V, Moncada B. Lichen amyloidosis improved by 0.1% topical tacrolimus. Dermatology. 2002; 205(4):420-1.
3. Jiang Y, Kong Q, Hui Y, Sang H. Atrophic nodular cutaneous amyloidosis. An Bras Dermatol. 2018;93(1):111-3.
4. Kyle RA, Gertz MA. Primary systemic amyloidosis: clinical and laboratory features in 474 cases. Semin Hematol. 1995;32:45-59.
5. Weidner T, Illing T, Elsner P. Primary localized cutaneous amyloidosis: a systematic treatment review. Am J Clin Dermatol. 2017;18(5):629-542.
6. Wong CK. Mucocutaneous manifestations in systemic amyloidosis. Clin Dermatol. 1990;8(2):7-12.

EXAMINATION QUESTIONS

1. What is the pathogenesis of cutaneous amyloidosis?
2. What are the histopathological features of cutaneous amyloidosis?
3. What are the systemic associations of amyloidosis?
4. What are the cutaneous manifestations of primary systemic amyloidosis?

69 CHAPTER Other Metabolic Disorders

Remya Raj R, Satyaki Ganguly

ALKAPTONURIA

Alkaptonuria is a rare autosomal recessive disorder characterized by dark urine in children, musculoskeletal system involvement in the form of arthritis, and ochronosis later in life.

Nomenclature

Alkaptonuria is also known as black urine disease or black bone disease. Ochronosis is used to explain the bluish-gray appearance in gross examination and yellowish discoloration in microscopic examination caused by the deposition of homogentisic acid in connective tissues. The condition is commonly caused by alkaptonuria but can also occur from topical administration of hydroquinone.

History

An ochronotic Egyptian mummy Harwa (1500 BC) probably had alkaptonuria. In 1908, Sir Archibald Garrod described alkaptonuria and proposed that it results from a deficiency of an enzyme that normally splits the aromatic ring of homogentisic acid. He also coined the term "inborn error of metabolism" and alkaptonuria was the first designated inherited metabolic disease.[1]

Epidemiology

Frequency 1 in 250,000.

Pathogenesis

Alkaptonuria is due to the deficiency of homogentisate 1, 2-dioxygenase resulting in accumulation of homogentisic acid which is an intermediate metabolite of phenylalanine and tyrosine metabolism. Homogentisic acid is further oxidized to benzoquinone acetate, which polymerizes to melanin-like polymers, and gets deposited in fibrous tissue and cartilage resulting ochronosis. As homogentisic acid has affinity to alkalis, it was named as alkapton and the condition was named as alkaptonuria. The alkaptonuria gene has been mapped to chromosome 3q13.33.[2]

Clinical Features

- Alkaptonuria is a classical triad of dark-colored urine, ochronosis, and ochronotic arthropathy.
- The first symptom of alkaptonuria is darkening of urine on standing due to oxidation of homogentisic acid. Scleral pigmentation or Osler's sign starts in the third decade. Skin pigmentation starts in the fourth decade from the ear cartilage followed by forehead, cheeks, axilla, genitalia, palms, and soles. Brown staining of the nails is also seen.
- The arthropathy also starts around the fourth decade involving the weight-bearing joints such as knees, intervertebral joints and shoulders, with narrowing of joint spaces, and disk calcifications.
- Pigment deposits can also be seen in the respiratory and gastrointestinal mucosa, dura mater, and tympanic membrane. There can be cardiovascular involvement after 50 years. High urinary homogentisic acid excretion can result in prostatic and renal calculi.[2]

Histopathology: Skin biopsy from palms and soles without special stains revealed the deposition of brownish-yellow (ochre) pigment in the mid-dermis and degeneration of collagen bundles.[3]

Approach and Management

History

History of urine turning black on standing or black discoloration of diapers in pediatric age group, pigmentation of ears, and joint pains in adults.

Examination

- Grayish-black pigmentation of the pinna, photoexposed areas, genitalia, palms, and soles
- Grayish black scleral pigmentation
- Pain in knee, back, and shoulders

Dermoscopy: Dermoscopy showed bluish-green pigmentation in the dermis.[3]

Laboratory Workup

Definitive diagnosis is by quantification of homogentisic acid in urine using gas-liquid chromatography.

- *Urine examination:*
    - Blackish discoloration of urine upon standing for 1 hour
    - Immediate brownish-black discoloration after adding sodium hydroxide solution
    - Benedict's test—reducing substance in spite of normal blood sugar levels
- X-ray and MRI of the affected joints

Differential Diagnosis

- Exogenous ochronosis due to topical application of hydroquinone can be differentiated by the involvement of pinna, sclera, and concomitant arthropathy.
- Other causes of arthropathy have to be differentiated by early onset, severity along with presence of pigmentary changes, and black urine.

Treatment

Dietary restriction of phenylalanine and tyrosine can reduce the excretion of homogentisic acid and prevent further progression of arthropathy.[4] Vitamin C 500 mg twice daily inhibits the polymerization of homogentisic acid. Nitisinone, which inhibits 4-hydroxyphenylpyruvate dioxygenase and decreases formation of homogentisic acid significantly, reduces the excretion of homogentisic acid by inhibiting the homogentisic acid synthesizing enzyme 4-hydroxyphenylpyruvate dioxygenase.[2,4] Physiotherapy has been tried, but timely spinal surgery and arthroplasty are recommended as mainstay for treatment for spondyloarthropathy.

Key Points

- It is caused by deficiency of homogentisate 1, 2-dioxygenase.
- Autosomal recessive disorder
- Triad of dark-colored urine, ochronosis, and ochronotic arthropathy
- Urine turning black on standing or black discoloration of diapers is the first clue.
- Nitisinone decreases formation of homogentisic acid.

PHENYLKETONURIA

Phenylketonuria is an autosomal recessive disorder caused by deficiency of phenylalanine hydroxylase manifesting with pigmentary dilution, mental retardation, growth retardation, and mousy odor in the urine.

History and Nomenclature

In 1934, Dr Asbjørn Følling described "oligophrenia phenylpyrouvica" in two severely mentally retarded children. It was later renamed as phenylketonuria.[5]

Incidence

It varies according to the ethnicity, lowest (<1 in 100,000) in Japan and Finland to highest in Turkey (1 in 2,600).[6]

Pathogenesis

Phenylalanine hydroxylase enzyme converts phenylalanine to tyrosine and tetrahydrobiopterin acts as a cofactor for the enzyme. Phenylketonuria develops due to deficiencies in phenylalanine hydroxylase or dihydrobiopterin reductase, the enzyme involved in the synthesis of tetrahydrobiopterin.[7]

Clinical Features

- Commonly detected in newborn screening
- Reduced pigmentation of hair, skin, and iris
- Unscreened patients present with vomiting, psychomotor retardation, behavior problems, peculiar gait, hypertonicity, and seizures in early childhood
- Atopic dermatitis-like features
- Photosensitivity
- Scleroderma-like induration of the extremities
- Eight subtypes have been described.

Approach and Management

History and Examination

- Decreased pigmentation of skin and eyes
- Dermatitis
- Neurological features

Laboratory Workup[6]

- Definitive diagnosis is by detection of elevated serum phenylalanine concentration and by tandem mass spectrometry.
- The diagnosis is supported by presence of normal or low serum tyrosine levels and urinary ferric chloride test.
- It should be confirmed by molecular genetic testing.
- Newborn screening is advised.[7]
- Prenatal diagnosis is by chorionic villus sampling, amniocentesis, and DNA sampling.

Differential Diagnosis

- *Albinism*: Absence of neurological features
- *Chédiak-Higashi syndrome*: Presence of recurrent pyogenic infections
- *Hermansky-Pudlak syndrome*: Presence of bleeding disorder
- *Atopic dermatitis*: Absence of neurological features
- *Scleroderma*: Absence of neurological features

Treatment[6-8]

- Phenylalanine restricted diet helps in avoiding permanent brain damage.
- Tetrahydrobiopterin 4 chaperone treatment in phenylketonuria patients with tetrahydrobiopterin deficiency. Tetrahydrobiopterin, a cofactor for phenylalanine hydroxylase enzyme, can stabilize the defective enzyme, increasing the activity of the enzyme.
- *Large neutral amino acid therapy*: Competes with phenylalanine for amino acid transporters to cross the blood–brain barrier, thereby decreasing the concentration of phenylalanine in the brain.
- Enzyme replacement therapy
- Gene therapy

Key Points

- Autosomal recessive disorder caused by deficiency of phenylalanine hydroxylase.
- Pigmentary dilution, mental retardation, growth retardation, and mousy odor in the urine.
- Ataxia is the most common neurological feature.
- Elevated serum phenylalanine concentration demonstrated by tandem mass spectrometry.
- Phenylalanine-restricted diet prevents permanent brain damage.

HARTNUP DISEASE

Hartnup disease is an autosomal recessive disorder of gastrointestinal and renal neutral amino acid transport resulting in pellagra-like appearance and neurological features.

History and Nomenclature

Named after the Hartnup family where it was described in two siblings in 1956.[9]

Epidemiology

Incidence in newborn screening is 1:25,000, but clinical presentation is rarer.[9]

Pathogenesis

Mutations in the *SLC6A19* gene located in the short arm of chromosome 5 cause it.[9] This gene encodes a neutral amino acid transporter expressed in the intestine and kidneys. Therefore, mutation in this gene results in malabsorption of tryptophan, a neutral amino acid, resulting in decreased synthesis of niacin, giving rise to the picture-like pellagra. The tryptophan in the intestinal lumen gets converted to indole compounds, which after absorption, further gets converted to 3-hydroxyindole or indicant, resulting in indicanuria.[10,11]

Clinical Features

- Presentation between 3 and 9 years of age.
- Well-demarcated dry scaly plaques on sun-exposed areas such as face, dorsum of hands, arms, and feet.
- Sun exposure causes erythema and blistering resolving with desquamation and depigmentation.
- Most common neurological feature is cerebellar ataxia.
- Diarrhea could be present.
- The biochemical disorder is always present, but the clinical manifestations are variable, even asymptomatic cases have been recognized through screening.

Approach and Management

History

- History of photosensitive scaly rash
- Dietary history ruling out possibility of pellagra
- Neurological features

Examination

- Erythema and blistering on face and extremities
- Well-demarcated scaly plaques on the dorsum of hands and feet.

Laboratory Workup

Definitive diagnosis is by urine chromatography which shows presence of neutral amino acids including tryptophan in the urine. The urine analysis also shows indicanuria along with presence of kynurenine and serotonin. Calculation of the Hartnup amino acids/other amino acids (HAA/OAA) ratio can help in differentiating Hartnup disease from other aminoacidurias.[11]

Differential Diagnosis

- *Pellagra*: Ruled out by dietary history and presence of neutral amino acids in the urine.
- *Lupus erythematosus*: Absence of joint pains and other systemic involvement clinically along with antinuclear antibody (ANA) and urine analysis are the differentiating features.
- *Seborrheic dermatitis*: Facial lesions and scaling may appear similar, but the presence of lesions on extremities rules out seborrhoeic dermatitis.
- *Acrodermatitis enteropathica*: Some of the patients of Hartnup disease present with a similar picture, but with a normal serum zinc level and fail to improve with zinc supplementation.
- *Carcinoid syndrome*: The lesions are persistent in Hartnup disease rather than episodic flushing attacks, as in carcinoid syndrome.

Treatment

50–300 mg of oral nicotinamide daily.

Key Points

- Autosomal recessive disorder of gastrointestinal and renal neutral amino acid transport
- Malabsorption of tryptophan, a neutral amino acid, resulting in decreased synthesis of niacin
- Pellagroid appearance
- Ataxia most common neurological feature
- Presence of neutral amino acids in the urine
- Rapid improvement with nicotinamide supplementation

MAPLE SYRUP URINE DISEASE

Maple syrup urine disease (MSUD) is an autosomal recessive disorder affecting branched-chain amino acids (BCAAs) in which neonates present with metabolic crisis and neurological symptoms.

Nomenclature

Maple syrup urine disease is also known as branched-chain ketoacid (BCKA) dehydrogenase deficiency or branched-chain ketoaciduria. The name is derived from the distinctive sweet odor of urine and cerumen similar to that of maple syrup in affected babies at the time of crisis.

Epidemiology

Frequency 1 in 185,000.[12]

Pathogenesis

Maple syrup urine disease is caused by decreased activity of branched-chain α-ketoacid dehydrogenase (BCKAD) complex, the second enzymatic step in the degradative pathway of BCAAs. BCKAD has four subunits and is essential in the metabolism of leucine, isoleucine, and valine. When there is a mutation in any of the genes coding for the enzyme complex, the amino acids and their toxic metabolic by-products get accumulated in plasma, resulting in symptoms.[13] 4,5-dimethyl-3-hydroxy-2[5H]-furanone (sotolone), which is also found in maple syrup and fenugreek, is the compound responsible for the characteristic odor of MSUD.

Clinical Features

- In classic MSUD, neonates will have a maple syrup odor in cerumen by 12 hours after birth.
- By 12–24 hours, there will be a rise in the plasma concentrations of BCAAs leucine, isoleucine, valine, and alloisoleucine, as well as a generalized disturbance of plasma amino acid concentration ratios.
- By the age of 2–3 days, neonate will have ketonuria, irritability, and poor feeding.
- In 4–5 days, the encephalopathy will worsen resulting in lethargy, intermittent apnea, opisthotonus, and stereotyped movements such as "fencing" and "bicycling."
- By the age 7–10 days, affected neonate might fall into coma and central respiratory failure.
- Other common clinical features include anemia, anorexia, acrodermatitis, alopecia, osteoporosis, and esophageal candidiasis.[14]
- Those with partial BCKAD enzyme deficiency will have intermediate MSUD and can have manifestations intermittently.

Approach and Management

History

- History of sweet odor of urine
- Neurological symptoms

Examination

- Maple syrup odor in cerumen
- Irritability and poor feeding
- Focal dystonia
- Opisthotonus
- Respiratory failure

Laboratory Workup

- Elevated BCAAs in plasma
- Elevated plasma alloisoleucine
- Elevated BCKAs in urine
- Positive urine dinitrophenylhydrazine (DNPH) test
- Ketonuria
- For screening of newborns, whole blood concentration ratios of leucine and isoleucine to alanine and phenylalanine is done using tandem mass spectrometry.[15]

Differential Diagnosis

- Conditions which can present with encephalopathy in neonates such as birth asphyxia, hypoglycemia, meningitis, encephalitis, kernicterus, and status epilepticus.
- Other inborn errors of metabolism which can have similar presentation such as urea cycle disorders, glycine encephalopathy, β-ketothiolase deficiency, and propionic or methylmalonic academia.

Treatment

Management of MSUD consists of dietary leucine restriction and BCAA-free formula feeds, along with judicious supplementation of isoleucine and valine. Metabolic decompensation has to be corrected by treating the precipitating stress. Hemofiltration can be tried to remove BCAAs from the extracellular compartment. In case patient develops brain edema, management in an intensive care setting is necessary. Liver transplantation is an effective step in the management of MSUD. Genetic counseling and tests for prenatal diagnosis also constitute an essential part in the management.

Key Points

- It is caused by the decreased activity of branched-chain α-ketoacid dehydrogenase complex.
- Autosomal recessive disorder
- Characteristic maple syrup odor of urine and cerumen
- It may present with metabolic crisis or neurologic symptoms.
- Formula feeds devoid of BCAAs form the mainstay of management.

FABRY DISEASE

Fabry disease is a rare X-linked recessive disorder of glycosphingolipid catabolism characterized by the presence of multiple angiokeratomas on skin with renal and ocular symptoms.

History and Nomenclature

Fabry disease, also known as Anderson Fabry disease or angiokeratoma corporis diffusum universale was independently described by Anderson and Fabry in 1898.

The term "angiokeratoma" is derived from the Greek words for "'vessel," "horn," and "tumor."

Epidemiology

Frequency 1 in 40,000–60,000 males.[16]

Pathogenesis

Fabry disease is an X-linked lysosomal storage disorder caused by the deficiency of the lysosomal enzyme, α-galactosidase A resulting from mutations in the α-galactosidase A gene at *Xq22.1*. This results in progressive deposition of uncleaved neutral glycosphingolipids, predominantly, α-galactosyl-lactosyl ceramide, otherwise known as globotriaosylceramide (Gb3) or trihexosylceramide, within the lysosomes of endothelium and pericytes of blood vessels, eyes, kidneys, lungs, heart, intestine, and nervous system leading to characteristic clinical features in the patients.

Clinical Features

- Symptoms usually start in early childhood with acral paresthesia.
- Females present with symptoms around one decade later than males and have less severe organ damage.
- Multiple angiokeratomas presenting as clustered symmetrical erythematous papules over lower trunk, genitals, and thighs in "swimming suit" pattern.
- Renal manifestations include proteinuria, RBC, and epithelial cell casts in urine in the initial stages followed by uremia and renal failure eventually.
- Ocular manifestations include whorl-like corneal opacities, aneurysmal dilation of conjunctival veins, granular, spoke-like deposits in the posterior lens known as Fabry cataract, and tortuous retinal vessels.
- Additional features include hypohidrosis, gastrointestinal manifestations, bone pain, tinnitus, and hearing loss.[17]
- Death may occur in 3rd to 4th decade of life due to renal failure, cardiovascular event, or stroke.

Approach and Management

History

- History of burning sensation in hands and feet with grouped dark-red papules over trunk in children or young adults
- Clouding of vision and azotemia symptoms in older age group

Examination

- Multiple angiokeratomas over trunk and thighs in "bathing trunk" distribution
- Telangiectasias predominantly over sun-exposed sites
- "Pseudoacromegalic" facies
- Mucosal involvement of oral cavity and conjunctiva may occur.
- Finger nails may show "turtle back" configuration.
- Vasomotor changes such as bluish discoloration or flushing of hands are suggestive of Raynaud's phenomenon
- Hypohidrotic lax skin
- Lymphedema
- Corneal opacities, deposits in anterior capsule and posterior lens, and tortuous retinal vessels in ophthalmological examination
- Features suggestive of worsening renal function

Dermoscopy: Dermoscopy of angiokeratoma papules shows sharply demarcated round, dark, and red lacunae (corresponding to dilated vessels with and without thrombosis respectively) with whitish veil (corresponding to acanthosis).[18]

Laboratory Workup

Histopathology: Skin biopsy from angiokeratoma lesions show acanthotic epidermis with superficial ectatic capillaries in upper dermis lined by normal-appearing endothelial cells. The epidermis often appears to be encircling the dilated vascular space in papillary dermis.

Periodic acid–Schiff (PAS) positive diastase-resistant deposits may be seen in endothelial cells and pericytes of capillaries. Characteristic, electron dense, lamellated intracytoplasmic vacuolar inclusions (zebra bodies) are typically seen on electron microscopy.

- Renal function test
- Urine microscopy to detect casts, protein
- Polarization microscopy of the urinary sediment demonstrates birefringent lipid globules known as "mulberry cells" with characteristic "maltese cross" configuration.
- Renal biopsy
- Leukocyte α-Gal A enzyme assay
- Urinary ceramide trihexoside levels
- Molecular genetic analysis of the *GLA* gene mutation is the most accurate method of diagnosis in females.
- Demonstration of low α-galactosidase A activity in chorionic villus sampling helps in prenatal diagnosis.

Differential Diagnosis

- Localized angiokeratomas such as solitary papular type, Fordyce-type occurring on scrotum or vulva, Mibelli type occurring over bony prominences of the hands and feet, and angiokeratoma circumscriptum neviforme, which is a congenital zosteriform verrucous lesion of the lower legs.
- Other lysosomal storage diseases which can present with angiokeratomas including GM1 gangliosidosis, mannosidosis, sialidosis, fucosidosis, aspartylglucosaminuria, galactosialidosis, and Kanzaki disease.

Treatment

- Treatment is predominantly symptomatic.
- Angiokeratomas can be treated using 1064-nm long pulsed Nd:YAG lasers or intense-pulsed light (IPL) systems.

- Carbamazepine or gabapentin may help in managing episodes of neuropathic pain.
- Antiplatelet drugs such as aspirin or clopidogrel may be advised to prevent recurrent ischemic strokes.
- Warfarin may be help in preventing cardioembolic stroke.
- Renal replacement therapy including kidney transplantation
- Enzyme replacement therapy with agalsidase-α (Replagal) or agalsidase-β (Fabrazyme) helps in reversing substrate storage in lysozyme thus normalizing renal, cerebral, and cardiovascular function.[19]

Key Points

- It is caused by deficiency of the lysosomal enzyme α-galactosidase A
- X-linked inheritance
- Angiokeratomas distributed in swimming-suit pattern over trunk and thighs
- Ocular and renal manifestations are predominant.
- Enzyme replacement therapy forms the mainstay of management.

REFERENCES

1. Phornphutkul C, Introne WJ, Perry MB, Bernardini I, Murphey MD, Fitzpatrick DL, et al. Natural history of alkaptonuria. N Engl J Med. 2002;347:2111-21.
2. Tharini GK, Ravindran V, Hema N, Prabhavathy D, Parveen B. Alkaptonuria. Indian J Dermatol. 2011;56:194-6.
3. Chandrakala C, Tharini GK, Ananthi M, Subha R. A case of alkaptonuria with degenerative collagenous plaques and foot drop. Indian J Dermatol. 2016;61:678-80.
4. Thapa M, Bhatia M, Maurya VK. Alkaptonuria. Med J Armed Forces India. 2018;74:394-6.
5. Følling I. The discovery of phenylketonuria. Acta Paediatr Suppl. 1994;407:4-10.
6. Sumaily KM, Mujamammi AH. Phenylketonuria: a new look at an old topic, advances in laboratory diagnosis, and therapeutic strategies. Int J Health Sci (Qassim). 2017;11:63-70.
7. van Wegberg AMJ, MacDonald A, Ahring K, Bélanger-Quintana A, Blau N, Bosch AM, et al. The Complete European Guidelines on Phenylketonuria: Diagnosis and Treatment. Orphanet J Rare Dis. 2017;12:162.
8. Al Hafid N, Christodoulou J. Phenylketonuria: a review of current and future treatments. Transl Pediatr. 2015;4:304-17.
9. Ciecierega T, Dweikat I, Awar M, Shahrour M, Libdeh BA, Sultan M. Severe persistent unremitting dermatitis, chronic diarrhea and hypoalbuminemia in a child: Hartnup disease in setting of celiac disease. BMC Pediatr. 2014;14:311.
10. Patel AB, Prabhu AS. Hartnup disease. Indian J Dermatol. 2008;53:31-2.
11. Haijes HA, Prinsen HCMT, de Sain-van der Velden MGM, Verhoeven-Duif NM, van Hasselt PM, Jans JJM. Accurate discrimination of Hartnup disorder from other aminoacidurias using a diagnostic ratio. Mol Genet Metab Rep. 2019;22:100551.
12. Liu Y, Chu X, Liu R, Sun Y, Kong Q, Li Q. Paroxysmal spasticity of lower extremities as the initial symptom in two siblings with maple syrup urine disease. Mol Med Rep. 2019;19:4872-80.
13. Blackburn PR, Gass JM, Vairo FPE, Farnham KM, Atwal HK, Macklin S, et al. Maple syrup urine disease: mechanisms and management. Appl Clin Genet. 2017;10:57-66.
14. Morton DH, Strauss KA, Robinson DL, Puffenberger EG, Kelley RI. Diagnosis and treatment of maple syrup urine disease: a study of 36 patients. Pediatrics. 2002;109:999-1008.
15. Imperlini E, Santorelli L, Orrù S, Scolamiero E, Ruoppolo M, Caterino M. Mass spectrometry-based metabolomic and proteomic strategies in organic acidemias. Biomed Res Int. 2016;2016:9210408.
16. Mehta A, Ricci R, Widmer U, Dehout F, Garcia de Lorenzo A, Kampmann C, et al. Fabry disease defined: baseline clinical manifestations of 366 patients in the Fabry Outcome Survey. Eur J Clin Invest. 2004;34:236-42.
17. Hsu TC, Yang CC, Ling CC, Lee CN. Hypohidrosis as a clue to the early diagnosis of fabry disease and prevention of late complications. Dermatol Sin. 2019;37:235-6.
18. Cuestas D, Perafan A, Forero Y, Bonilla J, Velandia A, Gutierrez A, et al. Angiokeratomas, not everything is Fabry disease. Int J Dermatol. 2019;58:713-21.
19. Sanchez-Niño MD, Ortiz A. Enzyme Replacement Therapy for Fabry Disease. J Inborn Errors Metab. Screen. 2016;4:1-7.

EXAMINATION QUESTIONS

Write short note on the following:

1. Hartnup disease
2. Fabry disease

70 CHAPTER

Nutritional Disorders of Skin

Anup Kumar Tiwary, Piyush Kumar

INTRODUCTION

Nutrition provides energy and is essential for life. It plays an important role in building and maintaining body organs, and in various metabolic processes. Deficiency or excess of nutrition poses both short-term and long-term challenges to health and recognition of signs of nutritional deficiency (or excess) allows timely correction of these deficiencies. Skin often bears the brunt of various nutritional deficiency (and excess), and provides necessary clinical clues for early diagnosis and subsequent therapeutic correction. Understanding dermatoses related to nutritional deficiency and excess requires knowledge of different nutrients (outlined in **Flowchart 1**). This chapter discusses cutaneous and some specific systemic manifestations of common macro- and micronutrients and their management. Recommended dietary allowances and dietary sources are enlisted in **Tables 1 and 2**, respectively.

DEFICIENCY DISORDERS

PROTEIN-ENERGY MALNUTRITION IN CHILDREN AND ADULTS

Introduction

The term "*protein-energy malnutrition*" (PEM) denotes variegated clinical conditions ranging from mild impairment of physical growth in children to *kwashiorkor* (characterized by the presence of edema) *and nutritional marasmus* (characterized by severe wasting).[1] The view that kwashiorkor is the result of protein deficiency and nutritional marasmus the result of energy deficiency is an oversimplification. The current view is that most PEM is not a deficiency of one specific nutrient or protein but the result of inadequate intake or poor utilization of food and energy. Of note, both these clinical types of PEM constitute only the small tip of the iceberg accounting for less than 5% in developing countries whereas up to 70% of children (<5 years of age) have mild or moderate PEM. The common causes of PEM in children are listed in **Box 1**.

Adult kwashiorkor and marasmus do exist with much lesser incidence but similar spectrum of presentations except growth and development aspects for obvious reasons. Chief causes of PEM in adults are inadequate food intake, infections, malabsorption, malignancy, and eating disorders.[1]

Pathophysiology of PEM

To understand the pathophysiology, conceptually, marasmus is considered as adapted state and kwashiorkor is considered as nonadapted state.

In a child consuming much less food/energy than needed, insulin production is decreased and increased secretion of catabolic hormones lead to hepatic gluconeogenesis and breakdown of fat and muscles. In untreated conditions, marked wasting ensues which can lead to death. Such cascade of metabolic events is characteristic of marasmus. Clinical features of kwashiorkor supervene when relatively more carbohydrates are ingested at the expense of protein and fat intake. It leads to reduced protein synthesis, hypoproteinemia and edema.[2] Concomitant infections can cause increased nitrogen loss and aggravate the protein deficiency and water retention.

Flowchart 1: Various nutrients.

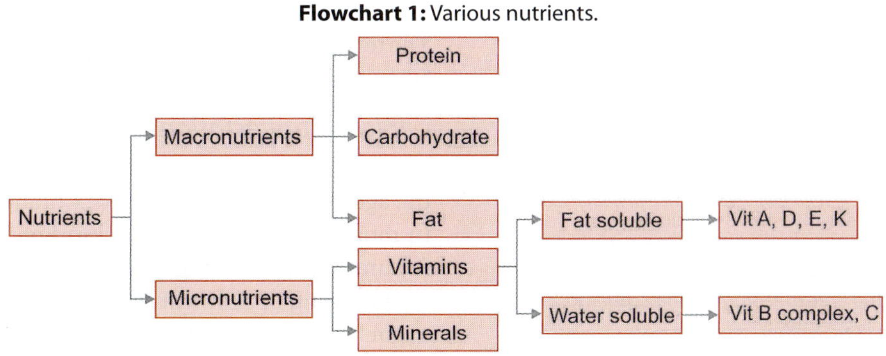

TABLE 1: Recommended dietary allowance (RDA) of common macro- and micronutrients.

Nutrients	*Recommended dietary allowance*
Proteins	0.8–1.0 g/day/kg of body weight
Essential fatty acids (EFA)	At least 10% of total daily calories should come from polyunsaturated fat and 2–4% of calories from EFA *α-linolenic acid (ω-3 fatty acid):* Adult male: 1.6 g/day Adult female: 1.1 g/day <14 years: 0.5–1.2 g/day *Linoleic acid (ω-6 fatty acid):* Adult male: 12–16 g/day Adult female: 10–12 g/day <14 years: 4–10 g/day
Vitamin A	*Infants and children:* 300–500 µg retinol equivalents (µg RE) *Adults:* 600–900 µg RE *Pregnancy:* 75–770 µg RE *Lactation:* 1,200–1,300 µg RE
Vitamin B_2	*Infants:* 0.3–0.4 mg/day *Children (1–3 years):* 0.5 mg/day *Children and adolescents (4–18 years):* 0.6–0.9 mg/day *Adults:* 1.3 mg/day (male) and 1.0 mg/day (female) *Pregnancy:* 1.4 mg/day *Breastfeeding:* 1.6 mg/day
Vitamin B_3	*Infant:* 8 mg/day *Adult:* 16 mg/day (male), 14 mg/day (female) *Pregnancy:* 18 mg/day *Lactation:* 17 mg/day
Vitamin B_{12}	*0–12 months:* 0.4–0.5 µg/day *1–3 years:* 0.9 µg/day *9–13 years:* 1.8 µg/day *14 plus onward:* 2.4 µg/day *Pregnant women:* 2.4 µg/day *Lactating mother:* 2.8 µg/day
Vitamin C	*Children:* 40–50 mg/day *Adults:* 60–100 mg/day
Vitamin D	(1 µg = 40 IU) *<18 years:* 200 IU *19–50 years:* 400 IU *51–65 years:* 600 IU *>65 years:* 800 IU *Pregnancy and lactation:* 200 IU
Biotin	*Infants:* 5 mg/day *1–6 years:* 8–12 mg/day *7–18 years:* 20–25 mg/day *>19 years:* 30 mg/day
Iron	*Infants:* 11 mg *Children:* 7–10 mg *14–18 years:* 11 mg (male) and 15 mg (female) *>18 years of age:* 8 mg (male) and 18 mg (female) *Pregnant women:* 27 mg *Lactating women:* 9 mg
Zinc	*Adults:* 8–11 mg/day *Children <8 years:* 2–5 mg/day
Copper	0.9 mg/day for adults
Selenium	*Children <3 years of age:* 15–20 µg/day *Children 3–13 years of age:* 20–40 µg/day *Adolescents and adults:* 55 µg/day *Pregnant and breastfeeding mothers:* 60 and 70 µg/day, respectively

TABLE 2: Food sources of nutrients.

Nutrients	*Food sources*
Proteins	Cereals, nuts, meat, eggs, fish, milk, dairy products
Essential fatty acids	Fish, nuts and seeds, flaxseed oil, soybean oil
Vitamin A	• *Plant sources:* Contain β-carotene or retinal in dark green leafy vegetables, carrot, papaya, mango, tomato, apricot • *Animal sources:* Contain retinyl esters, e.g., egg yolk, liver, fish, dairy products
Vitamin B_2	Milk and other dairy products, almonds, whole grain, mushrooms, soybeans, eggs, broccoli, spinach, liver
Vitamin B_3	Liver, lean pork, salmon poultry, red meat, dairy products, green leafy vegetable, beans, nuts
Vitamin B_{12}	Fish, red meat, milk, and milk products
Vitamin C	Citrus fruits and vegetables such as potatoes, tomatoes, berries, green vegetables
Vitamin D	Plant sources—vitamin D_2 Animal sources, e.g. liver, eggs, cod-liver oil—vitamin D_3
Biotin	Soy flour, milk, hazelnuts, peanuts, mushroom, egg yolk, liver
Iron	Green leafy vegetables, grains, dried fruits and beans, nuts, fish, red meats, and poultry
Zinc	Meat, fish, shellfish, eggs, dairy products, and legumes
Copper	Whole grains, legumes, potato, nuts, shellfish, beef, and pork liver
Selenium	Sea foods, cereals, red meat, chicken, fish, egg yolks, and kidney

BOX 1: Etiology of PEM in infants and children.[2]

- Prematurity or low birth weight
- No or inadequate breastfeeding
- Faulty weaning practices
- Inappropriate use of infant formula in place of breastfeeding for very young infants
- Low energy staple diets (protein and fat content also low)
- Inadequate availability of food
- Inadequate food intake or absorption due to infections or infestations

Clinical Features in Infants and Children

The clinical hallmark of kwashiorkor is acral pitting edema, and the predominating feature of nutritional marasmus is severe underweight. Children who have both edema and severe underweight are diagnosed as marasmic kwashiorkor.[2] A comparison has been summarized in **Table 3**.

Kwashiorkor (Wet PEM)

The term "kwashiorkor" is derived from the Ghanese term for "the one who is deposed."[1]

Clinical Manifestations

The symptoms of kwashiorkor usually first develop between the age of 6 months and 5 years. Cutaneous changes are seen in most of the cases of kwashiorkor, initially affecting the flexural skin. Following findings can be observed:

- Fissuring of skin with desquamation suggesting cracked or "*crazy pavement*."[2]

TABLE 3: Comparative clinical features of kwashiorkor and marasmus.

Features	*Kwashiorkor*	*Marasmus*
Age group	6 months to 5 years	Below 1 year
Predominant etiology	Protein deficiency >Energy deficiency	Energy deficiency
Dermatosis, flaky-paint	Flaky-paint dermatosis, crazy pavement dermatitis	Wrinkled, dry skin
Hair changes	Common, "Flag sign" and "salt and pepper" appearances	Less common
Subcutaneous fat	Reduced	Extreme loss
Pitting edema	Present on extremities and face	Absent
Face	May be edematous, moon face	Drawn in, monkey-like
Growth retardation	Present (–2 SD)	Present (–3 SD)
Wasting	Present but not severe	Severe
Appetite	Poor	Usually good
Mental changes	Very common (irritability, apathy)	Uncommon
Anemia	Severe (sometimes)	Present, less severe
Fatty infiltration of liver and hepatomegaly	Present	Usually absent
Fasting plasma Insulin level	Elevated	Decreased
Response to treatment	Relatively faster	Slower

- Hyperpigmentation along with dermatitis (on extensor surfaces of the arms and legs) sometimes resembles the old sunbaked, blistered paint has given rise to the term *"flaky-paint/enamel paint dermatosis."*[1]
- Skin is atrophic and depigmented beneath the flaky-paint areas.
- Angular cheilitis, vulvovaginitis and xerophthalmia may also occur due to accompanying micronutrient deficiencies.
- *Hair changes:* Hair becomes thinner, lusterless, dull and brittle with reddish tint. In severe cases, hair may appear greyish-white as *"salt and pepper"* appearance. Due to intermittent periods of improved nutrition, alternating light and dark colored bands (*"flag sign" or "signabandera")* within the hair shaft are seen. Increased lanugo hair may also be observed.[1]
- *Edema:* Pitting edema first develop on lower legs then involve hands and face giving the appearance of moon face.
- Other findings include *fatty infiltration of the liver (due to* decreased synthesis of lipoproteins), and mental changes (Irritability, apathy and poor appetite).[1]
- *Growth retardation:* Shorter height and weight than normal (usually 60–80% of standard or below 2 standard deviation).

BOX 2: Laboratory investigations for protein-energy malnutrition.[1,2]

- Serum albumin (<2.5 g/dL in severe cases) and electrolytes level
- Serum transferrin and retinol binding protein levels—usually low
- Fasting plasma insulin level—elevated in kwashiorkor and low in marasmus
- Serum level of soluble CD14—indicates low body mass index and muscle atrophy
- Urinary excretion of creatinine and hydroxyproline—low
- Urinalysis, peripheral blood smear and stool test—to detect infections and infestations
- Mantoux testing for tuberculosis
- Chest radiography—to rule out bacterial pneumonia, tuberculosis
- Cutaneous histopathology—hyperkeratosis, attenuation of the granular layer, increased basal layer pigmentation, decreased dermal collagen fibers and crowding of elastic fibers, atrophy of the hair appendages *(spares eccrine glands)*

Marasmus

Derived from the Greek word *marasmos* meaning wasting.[2]

Clinical Manifestations

Marasmus typically affects infants under 1 year of age. Skin appears thin, dry, and wrinkled skin (especially over thighs and buttocks). Angular cheilitis and pressure ulcers over bony prominences may also be present:

- *Hair and nail changes:* Thinner and brittle hair with poor growth and alopecia is marked. Nails may have longitudinal ridges and beau's lines with decreased growth rate.
- *Stunting and wasting:* Very low weight (below 60% or -3 SD of the standard) with extreme wasting of muscles with pot belly and monkey facies are hallmark in severe cases.[1] Perianal fat loss can lead to rectal prolapse and abdominal muscle hypotonia may result in abdominal distension.
- Children with marasmus are usually alert and less irritable. Anemia, diarrhea, decreased resting body temperature, and bradycardia may also be noted.

Laboratory Investigations

Laboratory tests **(Box 2)** are only to assess the seriousness of the condition and to differentiate between kwashiorkor and marasmus.

Management of PEM

- Patients with severe PEM often require hospitalization due to the concurrent risks of hypoglycemia, hypothermia, dehydration, and sepsis.[2]
- Individuals who are not awake and responsive may require intravenous hyperalimentation during the initial stages of therapy; care must be taken to avoid excessively rapid rehydration due to the risks of congestive heart failure.
- Oral refeeding is generally preferred using oral rehydration salts containing a mixture of essential electrolytes at least until diarrhea subsides or fortified formulas as soon as these can be tolerated.[2]
- Response to treatment is likely to be slower with marasmus than with kwashiorkor.

ESSENTIAL FATTY ACID DEFICIENCY

Introduction, Dietary Sources and Biological Functions of Essential Fatty Acids

Essential fatty acids (EFA) are polyunsaturated fatty acids (18–22 carbons) that cannot be synthesized as humans lack the enzymes required. There are two such EFAs: linoleic acid (ω-6 fatty acid) found in vegetable oils; and α-linolenic acid (ω-3 fatty acid) present in fish oil and flaxseed.[1] Apart from being an energy source, EFAs serve many functions such as formation of epidermal barrier to control transepidermal water loss (TEWL), insulation for temperature regulation, intestinal absorption of fat-soluble vitamins and chemical signaling in order to regulate inflammation, gene expression and protein translation.

Clinical Manifestations

Patients with EFA deficiency initially present with xerotic scaly skin with or without erythema.[1] It can lead further to erosions, particularly in intertriginous areas. Delayed wound healing, purpura due to weak capillary walls, brittle nails, and nonscarring alopecia with canities may also occur.

Systemic manifestations include growth retardation in child, fatty liver infiltration, increased susceptibility to infection due to impaired immunity response, anemia, thrombocytopenia, and neurological dysfunctions such as paresthesia, pain and inability to walk and cloudy vision.

Laboratory Diagnosis

Clinical signs of EFA deficiency can be supported by some laboratory parameters such as elevation in serum triene (mead acid or eicosatrienoic acid) : tetraene (arachidonic acid) ratio (>0.2).[1]

Management

Essential fatty acids supplementation can be done orally or parenterally. Topical application of vegetable oils (sunflower, soybean and safflower) can improve the xerotic scaly skin only.[1] The weekly administration of injectable lipid emulsion (ILE) is advocated for patients on parenteral nutrition.

VITAMIN DEFICIENCIES

Vitamin A (Retinol)

Vitamin A is a fat soluble, cyclic polyene alcohol "retinol" which can be converted into two other biologically important metabolites: retinal and retinoic acid.[2] Plant derived foods contain β-carotene or retinal and animal foods have retinol or retinyl esters (preformed vitamin A). Of note, enterocytes can absorb any form of vitamin A except retinyl ester (has to be hydrolyzed into retinol) and to get released into the circulation from enterocyte, it again needs to be esterified into retinyl ester form. Thus, retinyl ester form goes to liver, get stored there and released into the blood circulation when required. Before being released from liver, ester form is again converted into retinol and gets bound to retinol binding protein (RBP). Thus, the storage form of vitamin A is retinyl ester and circulating form is retinol. Vitamin A is essential for the reproductive system, bone formation, vision (photoreceptor "rhodopsin" generation) and epithelial growth and differentiation.[2] Zinc can increase the plasma retinol level by alcohol dehydrogenase (zinc dependent)-mediated conversion of retinol to retinyl ester. Zinc also increases the hepatic synthesis of retinol binding protein.

Vitamin A Deficiency

Risk factors include inadequate intake, conditions causing fat malabsorption (pancreatic or biliary tract disease, celiac disease, Crohn's disease, Shwachman–Diamond syndrome, cystic fibrosis, cholestatic liver disease, chronic intestinal parasitic infection, and gastric bypass surgery), protein, and zinc deficiency lead to low plasma RBP.

Clinical Features

Common cutaneous changes are due to abnormal keratinization leading to xerosis, scaling and fissuring. *Phrynoderma* (toad-like skin) is a classical cutaneous presentation of vitamin A deficiency, usually in children but may also be seen in other deficiencies such as of vitamin B-complex, vitamins C, E, as well as essential fatty acid deficiency and PEM. These appear as dark-brown, hyperkeratotic follicular papules with central spiny projection **(Fig. 1)**.[2] The classical sites are extensor surfaces of the extremities (elbows, knees), posterolateral aspect of upper arms, anterolateral thighs and buttock. Later on, abdomen, shoulders, face, neck and back may also get involved.[1] Mucosal changes includes squamous metaplasia of oral and nasal mucosa resulting in xerostomia, hyposmia, and hypogeusia. Salivary glands and other mucosal linings may also be affected (laryngeal, bronchial, and vaginal mucosa).

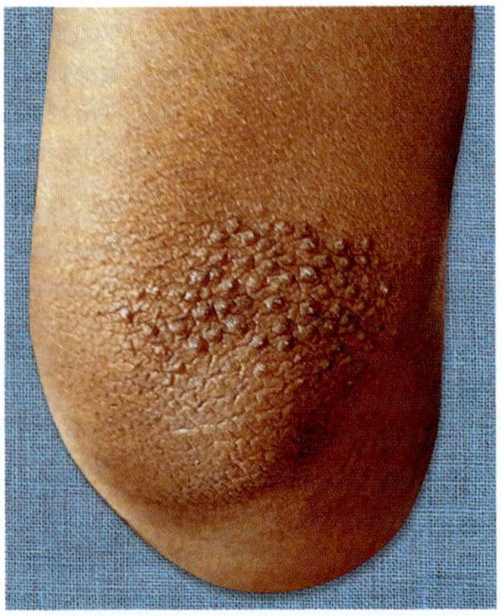

Fig. 1: Multiple hyperkeratotic conical papules on elbow in phrynoderma.

Ocular manifestations can be various types of ocular involvement, collectively called as "Xerophthalmia," depending upon the severity but night blindness is the earliest to manifest.[2] It has been classified into eight categories given in **Table 4**.

Other nonspecific effects: Lowered immunity, increased risk of secondary infections such as measles and growth retardation are seen more frequently in vitamin A deficient children.

Laboratory Diagnosis

Although laboratory tests are rarely employed to detect vitamin A deficiency, following findings favor the deficiency of vitamin A:

- *Decreased serum retinol level* <20 μg/dL (N = 30–50 μg/dL).
- *Decreased plasma levels of RBP* <30 mg/dL (normal is 30–40 mg/dL).
- *Positive retinylglucuronidehydrolysis (RAG) test:*
  - It can detect marginal vitamin A deficiency without clinical signs or symptoms.
  - Presence of retinoic acid at 4 hours after giving oral RAG indicates vitamin deficiency.
- *Positive conjunctival impression cytology* (conjunctival cells are stained and examined microscopically to detect squamous metaplasia).

Treatment

- Treatment for children 1 year of age or over should consist of 110 mg of retinylpalmitate or 66 mg of retinyl acetate (200,000 IU of vitamin A) orally or preferably 33 mg (100,000 IU) of water-miscible vitamin A (retinylpalmitate) by intramuscular injection (half dose for infants).
- The oral dose should be repeated on the second day and again on discharge from hospital or 7 days after the first dose.
- Vitamin A in oil should not be used for injection.
- Severe corneal involvement should be treated as emergencies to prevent blindness.

Vitamin B_2

Introduction

Riboflavin is water soluble and heat stable vitamin and is required for energy production, functioning of many enzymes, and normal fatty acid and amino acid synthesis.

TABLE 4: Classification of xerophthalmia.

Ocular signs	*Classification*
Night blindness	XN
Conjunctival xerosis	X1A
Bitot's spots	X1B
Corneal xerosis	X2
Corneal ulceration/keratomalacia < 1/3 corneal surface	X3A
Corneal ulceration/keratomalacia ≤ 1/3 corneal surface	X3B
Corneal scar	XS
Xerophthalmia fundus	XF

Physiological Roles

The derivatives of riboflavin, riboflavin 5' phosphate [flavin mononucleotide (FMN)] and riboflavin 5' adenosine diphosphate [flavin adenine dinucleotide (FAD)],[2] act as coenzymes for energy-producing respiratory pathways, and carbohydrate, amino acid, and fat metabolism. It is also needed for the functioning of enzyme lysyl oxidase that is required to initiate the cross-linking of newly formed collagen. Impaired maturity and or defective cross linking of collagen resulting from ariboflavinosis is thought to be responsible for the skin lesions. In cornea, riboflavin molecule breaks down, releasing 2,3-butanedione which binds with stromal proteins and help in final maturation.

Clinical Manifestations

Its deficiency is called as ariboflavinosis which is seen after 3–5 months of inadequate diet. The most striking features are pallor and angular stomatitis (perleche).[2] Cheilosis with erythema, xerosis and vertical fissuring of lips are also common.[2] Glossitis with smooth magenta red tongue with atrophic and red enlarged fungiform papillae are seen.

Oro-oculo-genital syndrome: It consists of seborrheic dermatitis such as rash affecting the nasolabial folds alaenasi, nasal bridge, nasolabial dyssebacia, forehead, cheeks, postauricular region, eyelids, scrotum, and vulva are involved.[2]

Extracutaneous manifestation: These are red and itchy eyes, night blindness, cataract, migraine, peripheral neuropathy, anemia secondary to interference with iron absorption, fatigue, malignancy (esophageal and cervical dysplasia).

Investigations

Increased erythrocytes glutathione reductase activity of more than 1.2 IU/L indicates riboflavin deficiency. Urinary excretion of less than 30 mg of riboflavin per gram of creatinine is associated with clinical signs.

Treatment

It consists of riboflavin replenishment **(Box 3)**, with care taken not to overlook coexisting B-complex deficiencies.

Vitamin B_3

Introduction

Vitamin B_3 (Niacin) is a water soluble vitamin and plays an important role in oxidation reduction reaction, biosynthesis of lipid (e.g., ceramide) and maintenance of epidermal barrier function by decreasing the transepidermal water loss. Vitamin B_3 refers to both molecules, nicotinic acid and niacinamide.[3]

BOX 3: Dosage for riboflavin for deficiency treatment.

- *Age <3 years:* Not established
- *Age 3–12 years:* 3–10 mg PO divided daily
- *Age >12 years and adults:* 6–30 mg PO divided daily for replenishment when deficiency is suspected

Physiological and Biochemical Role

In human, dietary niacin is absorbed from stomach and intestine. Most tissues takes up both the forms of vitamin to synthesize nicotinamide adenine dinucleotide (NAD) and nicotinamide adenine dinucleotide phosphate (NADP), key molecules which donate or accept hydrogen ions in oxidation-reduction reactions.[3] Thus these molecules play an important role in glycolysis, protein and amino acid metabolism, pyruvate metabolism, pentose biosynthesis, high-energy phosphate bond generation, glycerol metabolism, and fatty acid metabolism. In addition to its synthesis from dietary niacin, NAD can also be obtained from dietary amino acid tryptophan via kynurenine pathway. The conversion of niacin from tryptophan requires vitamin B_6, riboflavin, and heme (iron) as cofactor.

Clinical Features of Niacin Deficiency

The deficiency of vitamin B_3 (and/or its precursor tryptophan) results in pellagra, which presents with the classical triad of (photosensitive) dermatitis, diarrhea, and dementia. Severe and untreated cases may die of disease.[3] It is associated classically with a diet overtly composed of corn, millet, or sorghum. Other causes of niacin deficiency are Hartnup's disease (tryptophan converted to serotonin), chronic alcoholism, cirrhosis, carcinoid tumor, malabsorption, and drugs (isoniazid, pyrazinamide, azathioprine, 5-fluorouracil, and anticonvulsants).

The characteristic mucocutaneous finding of disease is photosensitive eruption. It occurs symmetrically on face, neck (*Casal's necklace*),[3] upper chest, and on extensors of arms and feet (usually does not extend proximal to malleoli) **(Fig. 2)**. Initially, the lesions starts as erythema on photo-exposed skin, progressing later to hyperpigmented with scab and crust (shellac like appearance). Prolonged and recurrent phototoxic events lead to dry, smooth paper thin glassy skin with a parchment like consistency. In severe cases eruption can be vesicular or bullous (wet pellagra). Other associated findings include painful fissure on palms and soles, cheilitis, glossitis, vaginitis with ulceration.[3]

Systemic involvement does occur. Gastrointestinal involvement results in weakness, abdominal pain, diarrhea, anorexia, esophagitis. Peripheral and central nervous system involvement (peripheral neuropathy, dysesthesia, disorientation, depression, attacks of dizziness, hallucinations, dementia, and psychosis) too is known.[3]

Diagnosis

Diagnosis is primarily done on clinical grounds. Low serum niacin, tryptophan, NAD, and NADP levels are noted in niacin deficiency and confirm the diagnosis of pellagra. Other supportive findings are low urinary excretion of N-methylnicotinamide and its pyridine derivative (N-methyl-2-pyridone, 5-carboxamide).

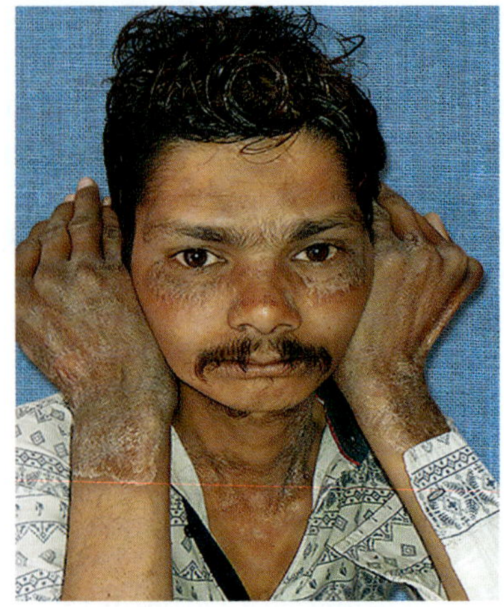

Fig. 2: Pellagra with symmetric erythematous scaly plaques on face, neck and dorsa of the hands.
Courtesy: Dr Hiral Shah, Baroda Medical College, Vadodara, Gujarat, India.

Treatment

Nicotinamide is preferred over nicotinic acid as it does not precipitate the flushing, itching, and burning observed after the ingestion of large doses of niacin. For adults, the daily recommended dose is 300 mg of nicotinamide in divided doses, and treatment should continue for 3–4 weeks. Glossitis and other oral features as well as diarrhea subside in a few days. The dementia and dermatitis usually improve significantly within the first week of therapy.

Vitamin B_{12}

Introduction

Vitamin B_{12}, also known as cyanocobalamin, is a water soluble vitamin and is essential for normal functioning of brain and nervous system as it is required for synthesis of myelin. Also, it plays a key role in formation of red blood cell. It is absorbed through the distal ileum after binding to the gastric intrinsic factor in an acidic pH. Deficiency is caused by gastrointestinal abnormalities-such as deficiency of intrinsic factor, achlorhydria, ileal disease, and malabsorption syndromes.[4] It is primarily found in animal products, so strict vegetarians are more prone to develop vitamin B_{12} deficiency.

Biochemical and Physiological Roles

The active form of vitamin B_{12}, methylcobalamin acts as cofactor for methionine and tetrahydrofolate synthesis. Tetrahydrofolate is required for DNA synthesis. The derivative of methionine is required for polyamine synthesis and transmethylation reactions. These reactions are needed for myelin maintenance and synthesis.

Clinical Features

Vitamin B_{12} is stored in body in large amount and symptoms of deficiency appear usually after 3–6 years of gastrointestinal abnormalities. Glossitis, hyperpigmentation and canities are the main dermatological finding. Glossitis with fissures of the tongue and angular stomatitis are early signs even prior to development of anemia.[4] Diffuse or patchy hyperpigmentation over any part of the body; though mainly on exposed part is seen **(Figs. 3 and 4)**. Hyperpigmentation involving flexural area, palm, sole, nail, and oral cavity resembling Addison's disease is noted **(Fig. 5)**.[4] Hyperpigmentation is thought to occur because of increased tyrosinase activity, and defect in melanin transport between melanocytes and keratinocytes. In contrast to skin, premature graying of hair is noted.

Extracutaneous findings include megaloblastic anemia, and neuropathy.[4] Long-standing cases develop signs of peripheral nervous system and spinal cord involvement. Neuropsychiatric manifestations, such as recent memory loss, depression, hypomania, paranoid psychosis with auditory or visual hallucinations (megaloblastic madness), violent behavior, personality changes, blunted affect, and emotional liability too are observed in some cases.

Laboratory Investigations

- *Peripheral blood picture:* Macrocytic anemia and hypersegmented neutrophils are seen.
- *Serum cobalamin level:* Less than 200 pg/mL is suggestive.

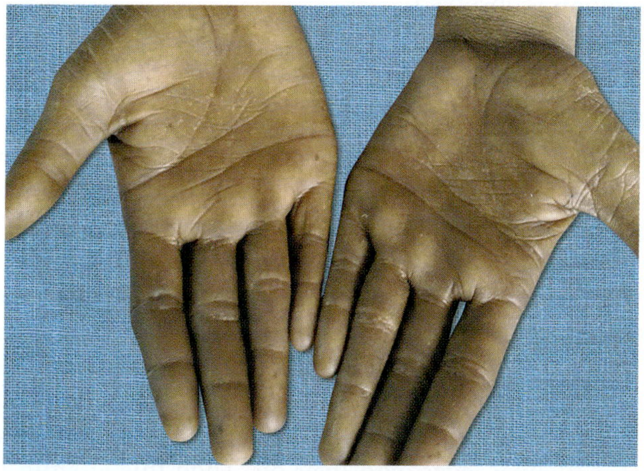

Fig. 3: Palmar hyperpigmentation in vitamin B_{12} deficiency.

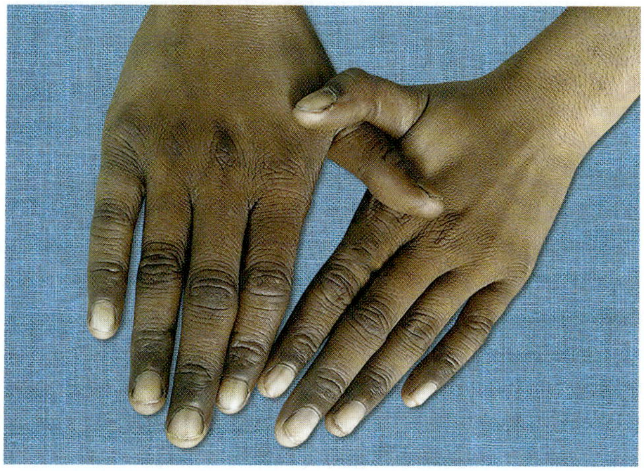

Fig. 4: Hyperpigmented dorsa of hands in vitamin B_{12} deficiency.

- *Antibodies detection*: Detect antibodies to intrinsic factor.
- *Methylmalonic acid (MMA) test:* MMA level higher in vitamin B_{12} deficiency.
- *Schilling test:* Less than 10% of the radiolabeled vitamin B_{12} in urine is suggestive.

Treatment and Prognosis

Parenteral replacement with intramuscular injection of vitamin B_{12}, 1 mg/week given for 1 month, followed by 1 mg per month given. It results in improvement of the pigmentary changes in the skin, nail, mucous membrane, and hair. Oral supplementation can be done in patients with pernicious anemia, in higher doses-1–2 mg/day. Neurological defect may not improve with vitamin B_{12} replacement.

Vitamin C (Ascorbic Acid)

Introduction

Vitamin C, also known as ascorbic acid, is an important antioxidant and protects DNA, protein, and vessel walls from damage caused by free radicals. Another important role of vitamin C is seen in formation of triple-helix formation of collagen. It is obtained from citrus fruits and vegetables as human are unable to synthesize.

Physiological Roles

The most important role of vitamin C is observed in formation of collagen. Impaired collagen synthesis seen in vitamin C deficiency accounts for typical changes seen in scurvy, notably hemorrhagic manifestations (defective collagen in blood vessels), bleeding gum (defective dentition), poor wound healing, and bone changes. Another important function of vitamin C is antioxidant activity, as described earlier. In addition, it enhances absorption of iron in intestine (distal part of small bowel) and is required for conversion of folic acid to biologically active form folinic acid, and thus affects hematopoiesis. Additionally, it acts as a cofactor in the metabolism of tyrosine and cholesterol and the synthesis of

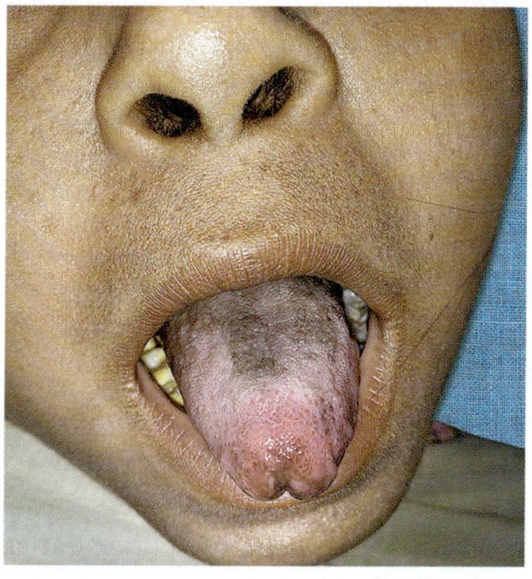

Fig. 5: Tongue in vitamin B_{12} deficiency showing hyperpigmentation and smooth surface due to atrophic papillae.

carnitine, neurotransmitters (e.g., norepinephrine), peptide hormones, corticosteroids, and aldosterone.

Clinical Features of Vitamin C Deficiency

Collagen rich tissues such as skin, cartilage, dentine, osteoid, and capillary blood vessels are primarily affected and are responsible for typical clinical findings. Poor wound healing, defective bone growth (in children) and dentition (resulting in bleeding gums) and hemorrhagic manifestations (including bleeding into hair follicles) are hallmark of scurvy. The bony changes are seen in children and occur at the junction between diaphysis and growth cartilage. There is failure of new bone matrix formation. Calcification of the growth cartilage at the end of the long bones continues, leading to the thickening of the growth plate. Bone resorption continues at normal rate, resulting in brittle bones and microscopic fractures. Periosteum becomes loosened, and classic subperiosteal hemorrhage at the ends of the long bones is noted. Bleeding into the joints may occur causing extremely painful hemarthroses. In advanced cases, clinically noticeable beading may be present at the costochondral junctions of the ribs, known as scorbutic rosary (i.e., sternum sinks inward). This needs to be distinguished from rickety rosary which is knobby and nodular.

Classical cutaneous findings include perifollicular hyperkeratotic papules, perifollicular hemorrhages, purpura, and ecchymoses are seen most commonly on the legs and buttocks. The central hairs are twisted like corkscrews, and are often fragmented. Poor wound healing and breakdown of old scars may be noted. Gums appear bluish-purple and have spongy feel. Loosening of teeth and mucosal petechiae may be seen.

Other notable extracutaneous findings include anemia, hypotension (in late stages), ocular disease (subconjunctival hemorrhage, bleeding within the optic nerve sheath, fundoscopic changes like flame-shaped hemorrhages, and cotton-wool spots), anorexia, and gastrointestinal mucosal bleeding.

Infantile scurvy (Barlow's disease): The hallmark clinical manifestation is extreme pain and tenderness of the arms and the legs. The baby is irritable and tends to remain in a characteristic pseudo-paralytic posture (due to subperiosteal pain) with semiflexion of the hips and the knees (*"pithed frog or frog leg posture"*).

Diagnostic Methods

Clinical diagnosis can be made with many pathognomonic clinical findings. These are four "H"—hemorrhagic signs, hyperkeratosis, hematologic abnormalities, and hypochondriasis. Capillary fragility can be checked by inflating a blood pressure cuff and looking for petechiae on the forearm. Plasma level is not the accurate indicator of body vitamin C store. The level of vitamin C in leukocytes more accurately correlates to tissue stores and can be measured by high-pressure liquid chromatographic method. Urinary ascorbic acid level estimation after a load of 1 g of ascorbic acid in water is helpful.

Radiology plays an important role in identifying bone changes. The common findings include subperiosteal elevation, fractures and dislocation, alveolar bone reabsorption and ground-glass appearance of cortex. Radiological signs described in scurvy include *white line of Frankel* (zone of provisional calcification becomes dense and widened), *Pelkan spurs* (metaphyseal spurs), Scurvy line or *Trummerfeld zone* (transverse band of radiolucency in the metaphysis), *Wimberger ring* (a ring of increased density surrounding the epiphysis), and *corner sign of Park* (triangular zone of rarefaction in metaphysis).

Replacement Therapy

Adults are treated with oral ascorbic acid at 100 mg 3–5 times a day until a total of 4 g is reached, and then they should decrease intake to 100 mg daily. Parenteral doses are necessary in those with gastrointestinal malabsorption. The recommended adult dose is 200 mg IV daily for not more than 7 days. Infants and children are usually treated with vitamin C 100–300 mg daily until full recovery of clinical signs and symptoms is observed.

Vitamin D

Source and Synthesis of Vitamin D_3

Vitamin D is a group of seco-steroid which, before being biologically active, has two primary forms: plant derived ergocalciferol or vitamin D_2 (plant derived); and vitamin D_3 or cholecalciferol which is mostly synthesized in the stratum spinosum and stratum basale layer of skin from 7-dehydrocholesterol (provitamin D_3) by the UV-B component of sunlight (290–320 nm) as previtamin D_3 form, followed by a temperature-dependent conversion into vitamin D_3. Vitamin D_3 can also be obtained from animal source of diet, e.g., liver, eggs, cod-liver oil. Then this vitamin D_3 (cholecalciferol) is released into the circulation, enters the liver and get hydroxylated to form 25-hydroxyvitamin D_3. Further hydroxylation takes place in the kidney to form the biologically active 1,25-dihydroxyvitamin D_3 (calcitriol).

Biological Roles

Vitamin D, acting like a hormone, primarily regulates the blood levels of calcium and phosphorus in order to maintain several vital functions in our body such as mineralization of bone, contraction of muscles, nerve conduction and immunomodulations. Certain specific cells such as keratinocytes, osteoclasts and enterocytes tend to differentiate under the action of vitamin D, thereby increasing the gastrointestinal absorption of dietary calcium and phosphate, bone resorption, and reabsorption of calcium and phosphate by renal tubules.

Causes of Vitamin D Deficiency

Vitamin D deficiency is usually affected by local cultural practices and circumstances. Chief causes are inadequate sunlight exposure, particularly in densely populated cities and in temperate countries, low intake of plant derived foods, fat malabsorption (due to gastrointestinal surgery, celiac disease and pancreatico-biliary disease), chronic renal failure and regular use of sunscreens. High-risk groups such as infants, adolescents, elderly people, and pregnant and lactating women.

Clinical Features

The most common clinical manifestations of vitamin D deficiency are rickets (in children) and osteomalacia (in adults). Rickets is softening of bones due to defective mineralization of cartilage in the epiphyseal growth plate, leading to several types of skeletal deformities in children. Osteomalacia is characterized by decreased mineralization of newly formed osteoid at sites of bone turnover in adults. In both types, patients usually complain of gastrointestinal upset, muscle weakness, hypotonia, carpopedal spasm, tetany, diffuse bone and joint pain (pelvic, lumbar and legs) and increased risk of fractures but some features are typical of rickets owing to the poor cartilaginous development in child. These are epiphyseal widening, fraying and widening of the metaphysis, rachitic rosary (at costochondral junctions of the anterior ribs), craniotabes, frontal bossing, lateral bowing of legs, widening of the wrists, scoliosis, fractures, and enamel hypoplasia in untreated cases.

Since, the therapeutic approach is a little different for different types of rickets and cutaneous changes are seen in a particular type of rickets, a brief discussion about rickets is worth.

Its most common type is true vitamin D deficient type. There are two other hereditary (autosomal recessive)types of rickets due to genetic mutation (gene loci on 12q13) causing functional deficiency of vitamin D, hence known as pseudo-deficiency rickets or vitamin D dependent rickets type I (VDDR-I) and type II (VDDR-II). VDDR-I is due to the deficiency of renal 25-hydroxyvitamin D-1 alpha-hydroxylase enzyme and VDDR-II is caused by mutation in the vitamin D receptor leading to end organ resistance to physiologic level of 1,25-dihydroxyvitamin D_3. There is another rare type, due to decreased intraluminal bile salts leading to poor absorption of vitamin D, called as "*hepatic rickets*."

There are some peculiar cutaneous manifestations of VDDR-II which resembles the syndrome of "generalized atrichia with papules and milia." Such patients lose all the hairs 1–3 months after birth except eyebrows and eyelashes and present with small papules and milia on the face and scalp. This is seen in about 50% of patients with VDDR-II.

Other systemic changes include increased systolic blood pressure, raised fasting plasma glucose, hyperinsulinemia, dilated cardiomyopathy and increased risk of *Mycobacterium tuberculosis* infection.

Diagnosis

Vitamin D deficiency results in hypocalcemia, hypophosphatasia, decreased serum levels of 25-hydroxyvitamin D and alkaline phosphatase. Radiological examination is necessary to see the bony changes of rickets which may be osteopenia, widening of the epiphyseal plate and metaphysis and growth plate deformities such as cupping, fraying, formation of cortical spurs, rachitic rosary, fractures.

Treatment

Patients with clinical and laboratory evidence of vitamin D deficiency must be treated with oral 1,25-dihydroxyvitamin D_3 (200 µg daily or 60,000 IU weekly) for 6–8 weeks followed by 800 IU daily along with calcium. Calcium supplementation is particularly needed to treat VDDR-II.

Biotin (Synonyms: Vitamin H, Vitamin B_7)

Introduction and Biologic Roles

Biotin is a water-soluble, heterocyclic, sulfur-containing, monocarboxylic acid and essential coenzyme of four carboxylase enzymes: pyruvate carboxylase, methyl crotonyl-CoA carboxylase, propionyl-CoA carboxylase, and acetyl-CoA carboxylase. It is essential in the metabolism of all macromolecules; carbohydrates, fatty acids, amino acids, and nucleotides.

Biotin Absorption and Avidin

Dietary biotin is usually a protein-bound complex "biocytin" (biotin with lysine) which needs to be acted upon by pancreatic biotinidase to get released and absorbed via enterocytes. A protein found in egg whites, called "avidin" binds free biotin in the gut and prevent the biotin absorption.[4]

Causes of Biotin Deficiency

Increased consumption of raw egg-white (containing avidin which binds biotin and makes it poorly absorbable), short bowel syndrome, parenteral nutrition without biotin supplementation, drugs (valproate, carbamazepine, phenytoin), long-term use of antibiotics (eradicate gut flora).

Clinical Features

Although uncommon, but biotin deficiency can develop due to inadequate dietary intake or impaired intestinal absorption because of the above mentioned factors. Patients can be of any age groups (but usually adults). Clinical presentation simulates the picture of zinc deficiency and essential fatty acid deficiency. It starts with seborrheic dermatitis like erythematous scaling around the nose, eyes, mouth and perianal region followed by crusting.[5] Glossitis, conjunctivitis, alopecia, and neurological alterations (irritability, lethargy, paresthesias and hypotonia) may also occur in untreated cases.[4]

There are two examples of inborn error of biotin metabolism (autosomal recessive) which result in the functional deficiency of biotin despite of adequate dietary intake.[4] These are:

1. *Holocarboxylase synthetase deficiency (neonatal onset):* It is a fatal condition resulting from failure of incorporation of biotin to several carboxylase enzymes. Neonate presents with erythematous scaly scalp dermatitis extending to eyebrows, eyelashes and multiple periorificial areas.[4] It can also cause total alopecia. Neurological findings include feeding and breathing difficulty, recurrent vomiting, severe metabolic acidosis, hypotonia and hypertonia, ataxia, seizures, and developmental delay.
2. *Biotinidase deficiency (infantile onset):* Deficiency of biotinidase, due to *BTD* gene mutation, leads to decreased biotin absorption resulting in low serum level of biotin. Onset is typically after 3 months of age. The clinical presentations are overlapping with acrodermatitis enteropathica and holocarboxylase synthetase deficiency.

Laboratory Investigations

Biochemical indicators are useful to rule out inborn error of biotin metabolism in child patients. Low urinary levels of biotin, increased urinary excretion of 3-hydroxyisovalerate (reflecting the activity of b-methyl-crotonyl-CoA carboxylase) and 3-methylcrotonylglycine, lactic academia and hyperammonemia favor the diagnosis of holocarboxylase synthetase deficiency. Serum biotinidase level is usually <30% of normal value in case of biotinidase deficiency.

Treatment and Prognosis

The recommended daily value increases from 100 to 200 μg in adults. Dietary deficiency should be treated with daily oral supplementation of biotin, 30 μg in neonates and 150 μg in adults until symptoms resolve. This dose is higher in metabolic types, being 10–40 mg biotin per day. Neurological alterations may not reverse with treatment.

MINERAL DEFICIENCIES

Zinc Deficiency

Introduction

Zinc is the second-most abundant trace element in the body (after iron). Most of the zinc in the body is intracellular; only around 0.1% of total zinc is found in plasma, bound to albumin and α-2 macroglobulin. It is present in all tissues and body fluids but predominantly located in skeletal muscle and bone. Total body pool of zinc in a healthy adult has been estimated to be around 2–3 g.

Physiological Role

Zinc is an integral component of more than 300 enzymes including carbonic anhydrase, alkaline phosphatase, glutamate dehydrogenase, lactate dehydrogenase, alcohol dehydrogenase, carboxypeptidase, DNA polymerase, protein chain elongation factor, and copper (Cu)–Zn superoxide dismutase. Collectively, these enzymes are needed for metabolism of carbohydrate, fat, and protein and clearance of reactive oxygen species. Other than this catalytic role, zinc has structural and regulatory roles as well. No wonder, zinc is essential for the normal functioning of anabolic processes, such as growth, tissue maintenance, and wound healing.

Absorption and Excretion

Zinc is absorbed in the small intestine by a carrier-mediated mechanism and absorption is enhanced by citric acid and inhibited by iron, copper, calcium, fiber, and phytates. There are two families of zinc transporters which have opposing roles- ZnT transporters reduce intracellular zinc while ZIP transporters increase intracellular zinc concentration.[6] Zinc absorbed in gut is either transported to the liver through the portal system or bound to metallothionein intracellularly in enterocytes. Some of metallothionein bound fraction is reabsorbed and undergoes enterohepatic circulation; rest is lost during shedding of enterocytes. Zinc is excreted in bile and urine; skin and hair loss account for additional physiologic loss of zinc.

Clinical Features

Zinc deficiency may be hereditary or acquired. Acquired zinc deficiency is seen in pregnancy, lactation, extensive cutaneous burns, generalized exfoliative dermatoses, parenteral nutrition, intestinal malabsorption syndromes, cystic fibrosis, alcoholism, HIV infection, malignancy, uremia, and chronic renal disease (especially nephrotic syndrome).

The clinical features in both hereditary and acquired types are similar; however, manifestations are milder in acquired forms. Hereditary type, called acrodermatitis enteropathica (AE), presents with perioral erosive dermatitis and perleche, that progresses to involve the face, acral parts, and diaper area **(Figs. 6A to C)**.[6] Alopecia and extracutaneous features like diarrhea and photosensitivity may accompany the skin lesions. The skin lesions in acquired forms develop over a few days and are typically periorificial in location. The lesions are eczematous scaly plaques and may develop into vesicles, bullae, or pustules. The underlying skin has a "scald like" erythematous appearance.[6] Skin lesions in milder acquired forms are less dramatic and lack features of inflammation. They usually present with psoriasiform plaques, annular plaques with brown black crusts at advancing margins and scaling at the center, crusted plaques, or pigmented lichenoid lesions on areas subject to repeated pressure and trauma, such as elbows, knees, knuckles, malleolar regions of the ankles, and the sacral area. Long standing cases exhibit frequent infections, delayed wound healing, growth retardation, anorexia, anemia, photophobia, hypogonadism, delayed puberty, and altered mental status.

Diagnosis

The determination of a low plasma zinc level is diagnostic. Hypoalbuminea, hemolyzed samples, and contamination may give erroneous values for zinc. Also, cases of AE with

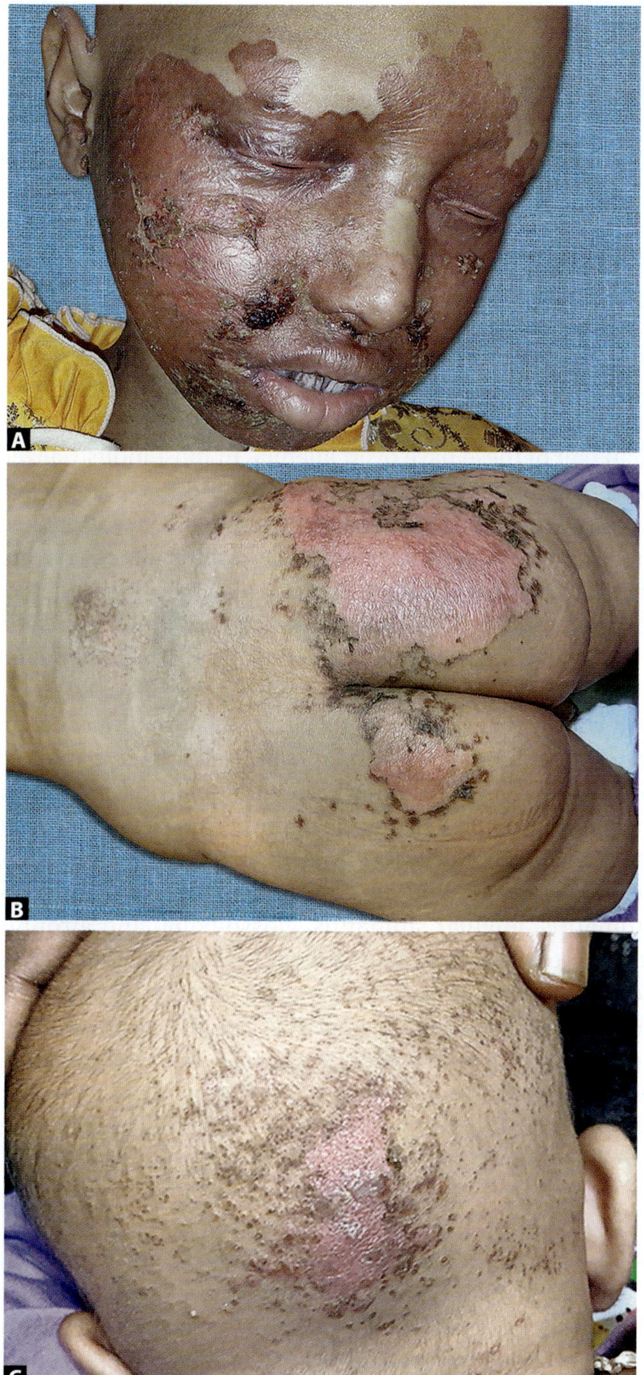

Figs. 6A to C: (A) Scald-like erythematous facial lesions in acrodermatitis enteropathica; (B) Scald-like erythema and scaling on the gluteal region in acrodermatitis enteropathica; (C) Involvement of pressure bearing area of the scalp in acrodermatitis enteropathica.

normal serum zinc levels are known. Zinc-dependent enzyme, serum alkaline phosphatase estimation may serve as surrogate marker of hypozincemia.

Histopathologic Features

The diagnostic pathological finding is necrolysis, cytoplasmic pallor, vacuolization, ballooning degeneration, and subsequent confluent necrosis of keratinocytes in the upper part of the epidermis.[6] Chronic lesions may lack features of necrolysis and mimic psoriasis. Clinical suspicion and treatment response to zinc supplementation are the keys to diagnosis.

Prognosis and Treatment

The condition may be fatal in the absence of zinc therapy. Zinc supplementation with a dose of 1–2 mg/kg results in rapid improvement. Diarrhea responds within 24 hours and skin lesions usually heal in 1–2 weeks without sequelae. Patients with severe features of zinc deficiency may require long-term treatment with zinc. Overzealous treatment should be avoided because zinc supplementation can lower blood copper levels and large accidental overdoses may cause multisystem organ failure. In addition, predisposing factors should be identified and must be taken care of.

Copper Deficiency

Introduction and Biological Functions of Copper

Being a cofactor of many enzymes such as tyrosinase, lysyl oxidase, cytochrome oxidase, and superoxide dismutase, copper plays an important role in melanogenesis, heme synthesis, collagen cross-linking, free radical detoxifications, and maintaining the integrity of the myelin sheath of nerve fibers. Ninety percent of plasma copper is bound to ceruloplasmin (a serum ferroxidase, helps in hepatobiliary excretion of copper) and the rest is bound to albumin (transport protein), competing for the zinc explaining the interaction between these two elements in plasma.

Etiological Factors

Apart from the compromised nutritional states, other conditions can also precipitate its deficiency such as excessive intake of antacids, zinc, iron, or vitamin C (decreases absorption), celiac disease, cystic fibrosis, gastric bypass surgery, and short bowel syndrome.

Clinical Manifestations

Patients usually presents with anemia, neutropenia, and hypopigmentation of skin and hairs. Chronic cases may develop osteoporosis, fractures, symmetrical sensorimotor neuropathies in extremities, and optic neuropathies.

There are two well-known systemic disorders related to copper metabolism:

Menkes kinky hair disease and Wilson's disease: It was first described by John Menkes in 1962 as an X-linked neuro-degeneration syndrome caused by mutation in "*ATP7A* or *MNK gene*" (codes copper-transporting *P*-type ATPase) on Xq13.3-q21.[2] It leads to decreased intestinal absorption of copper and presents with characteristic tricho-osteo-cutaneous changes. Its incidence is less than 10 cases per million.

The disease become clinically apparent classically at 2–3 months of age with the development of characteristic "*cherubic facial appearance*" comprising of depressed nasal bridge, ptosis, and reduced facial movements. The other presenting signs are delayed developmental milestones, failure to thrive, truncal hypotonia with poor head control, seizures, inability to visual fixation and hyperactive deep tendon reflexes.[2]

Hair becomes sparse, lusterless, and depigmented hair with *steel wool appearance* (especially on scalp and eyebrows). Other structural changes are pilitorti, monilethrix and trichorrhexisnodosa.[2] Cutaneous findings include follicular hyperkeratosis and soft, inelastic, depigmented skin especially at the nape of the neck, axillae, and trunk.

Bony changes occur in the form of osteoporosis, diaphyseal periosteal reaction, widening of metaphysic and lateral spur formations in long bones, skull, ribs, and vertebrae.

Laboratory Investigations

In all cases of copper deficiency disorders, serum copper level is usually <70 μg/dL (normal range is 70–140 μg/dL). Other features include microcytic anemia, and neutropenia (earliest and most sensitive prognostic measure).

Management

Copper supplementation is done to correct the deficiency in acquired cases but there is no effective treatment for Menkes disease till date. Medical therapy for Wilson's disease are chelating agents such as penicillamine, trientine or zinc. Surgical modalities include transjugular intrahepatic shunting and orthotopic liver transplantation.

Iron Deficiency

Introduction and Biological Roles

Iron is an essentially present in hemoglobin, myoglobin and many enzymes such as cytochrome P450, catalase, xanthine oxidase, aldehyde oxidase, succinic dehydrogenase, and monoamine oxidase. It serves several vital functions in the body including heme synthesis for oxygenation of tissues and muscles, synthesis of collagen, steroid hormones and bile acids, detoxification and signal controlling of some neurotransmitters, such as the dopamine and serotonin systems in the brain. Dietary iron has two main forms: (1)heme (ferrous form) and (2) nonheme (ferric). Plants and iron-fortified foods contain nonheme iron only, whereas meat, seafood, and poultry contain both heme and nonheme iron.

Dietary Absorption

Iron is absorbed by duodenal enterocytes in ferrous states only, hence acidic medium facilitates its absorption by reducing ferric iron to ferrous form. This is why heme iron is better absorbed (20–25%) than nonheme iron (5–10%) and ascorbic acid enhances its absorption while calcium and phytates inhibits. It also explains why iron tablets should be taken in empty stomach.

Etiology

Decreased dietary intake, malabsorptive states such as coeliac sprue, Crohn's disease, gastrectomy, increased demand (as in infancy, adolescence or pregnancy) or from chronic blood loss (menstrual, hookworm infestation, bleeding peptic ulcers, etc.) may result in iron deficiency. The high-risk groups are weaning infants, children, adolescents, and women of childbearing age, especially pregnant women.

Clinical Features

Iron deficiency is the most prevalent important nutritional problem of humans. It threatens over 60% of women and children in most nonindustrialized countries, and more than half of these have overt anemia. In most industrialized countries in North America, Europe and Asia, 12–18% of women are anemic. Functionally, iron deficiency is defined as declining of iron stores combined with signs of an iron-deficient erythropoiesis.

General symptoms of iron deficiency are nonspecific generalized pruritus, fatigue and anorexia. Growth retardation and increased susceptibility to infections are seen in infants and young children. Iron deficiency has profound effect on mucous membranes, hair, and nails. Nails become thinned out and flattened, brittle with longitudinal ridges. Chronic cases may develop spoon-shaped concavity known as "koilonychias" (mostly involving index and third fingernails). Hair looks lusterless, brittle, dry with split hair ends. Aphthous stomatitis, angular stomatitis, glossodynia, and atrophic filiform papillae of tongue are mucosal changes. Impaired collagen synthesis causes blue sclera. Along with the above signs of iron deficiency anemia (IDA), predominantly middle aged women may develop dysphagia due to esophageal web formation (having risk of malignant transformation to postcricoid carcinoma), called as "*Plummer-Vinson syndrome*" or "*Patterson-Brown-Kelly syndrome*."

Laboratory Diagnosis

Hemoglobin and hematocrit tests are the most commonly used measures to screen patients for iron deficiency, even though they are neither sensitive nor specific. Hemoglobin concentrations lower than 13 g/dL in men and 12 g/dL in women (11 g/dL in pregnant women) indicate the presence of anemia. Typically, iron deficiency states show microcytic hypochromic picture on peripheral blood film, having low hematocrit value, low serum values of iron (<30 μg/dL), ferritin (<15 μg/L) and transferring saturation (<10%), elevated TIBC (>360 μg/dL), increased RDW index, raised red cell zinc protoporphyrin level (>100 μg/dL).

Prevention

Iron deficiency can be prevented by following three strategies: (1) oral iron supplementation to high-risk groups such as pregnant women and preschool children; (2) iron fortification of certain foods, such as flour; and (3) food and nutrition education to improve the bioavailability of the dietary iron.

Treatment

The management approach depends upon the underlying cause and severity of the anemia. Most of the cases of iron deficiency anemia are pregnant women, growing children and adolescents having inadequate iron intake. Such groups also respond to oral ferrous salts (sulfate, fumarate, gluconate or ascorbate salts). Usually, up to 300 mg of ferrous sulphate (elemental iron is 60 mg) is given twice daily in empty stomach as food may inhibit its absorption. In other group of patients with severe anemia due to continuing blood loss and/or cardiovascular instability, parenteral therapy (intravenous iron dextran) and blood transfusion should be preferred.

Of note, as per CDC recommendations, all pregnant women with IDA should be treated with 60–120 mg/day of oral iron. To add, breastfed infants who were born preterm or with a low birthweight should receive 2–4 mg/kg/day of iron drops (to a maximum of 15 mg/day) from ages 1–12 months. Treatment for IDA in children should be with 3 mg/kg/day of iron drops given between meals.

KEY POINTS

- PEM is not a deficiency of any specific nutrient or protein but the result of poor intake or utilization of food.
- Flaky paint dermatosis and flag sign are the characteristic features of kwashiorkor.
- Storage form of vitamin A is retinyl ester and circulatory form is retinol.
- Zn increases plasma retinol level by alcohol dehydrogenase-mediated conversion of retinol to retinyl ester which is absorbed into the circulation.
- Zn deficiency results in increased Cu absorption and hence, hypercupremia and a copper: zinc ratio > 1.5 have been suggested as markers of hypozincemia.
- Vitamin A may antagonize the vitamin D-mediated intracellular signaling pathways affecting calcium metabolism resulting in skeletal changes.
- Neutropenia is the earliest and most sensitive hematologic measure of copper deficiency.
- Vitamin A in oil should never be injected (can cause lipogranuloma).
- Vitamin D_3 is mostly synthesized in the stratum spinosum and stratum basale layer.
- Glossitis with smooth magenta-red tongue with atrophic and red enlarged fungiform papillae are striking features of ariboflavinosis.
- Casal's necklace refers to the classic dermatitis on neck seen in pellagra.
- Perifollicular hemorrhages and cork screw hairs are hallmark of vitamin C deficiency.
- Avidin protein found in egg whites binds free biotin in the gut and prevent the biotin absorption.
- Functional deficiency of biotin metabolism can result due to the deficiency of: Holocarboxylase synthetase (neonatal onset) and Biotinidase (infantile onset).
- *Triene:* Tetraene in serum >0.2 indicates essential fatty acid deficiency.
- Menkes kinky hair disease is an X-linked neurodegeneration syndrome caused by mutation in "*ATP7A* or *MNK* gene" on Xq13.3-q21.
- Steel wool appearance of hair of scalp and eyebrows is a characteristic feature of copper deficiency.
- Koilonychia due to iron deficiency is more marked on thumb and index finger.
- Plummer vinson syndrome consists of IDA, mucocutaneous signs of IDA such as glossitis, cheilitis, and esophageal webs causing dysphagia.
- Cherubic facial appearance of Menkes disease consists of depressed nasal bridge, ptosis, and reduced facial movements.
- Iron tablets should ideally be taken in empty stomach because iron is better absorbed in ferrous states.

REFERENCES

1. Lee LW, Yan AC. Skin manifestations of nutritional deficiency disease in children: modern day contexts. Int J Dermatol. 2012; 51(12):1407-18.
2. Orozco-Covarrubias L, Durán McKinster C. Skin manifestations of nutritional disorders. In: Irvine AD, Hoeger PH, Yan AC (Eds). Harper's Textbook of Pediatric Dermatology, 3rd edition. NJ: Wiley-Blackwell; 2011. pp. 65.1-65.10.
3. Mac Donald A, Forsyth A. Nutritional deficiencies and the skin. Clin Exp Dermatol. 2005;30(4):388-90.
4. Heath ML, Sidbury R. Cutaneous manifestations of nutritional deficiency. Curr Opin Pediatr. 2006;18:417-22.
5. Haight RR, Norman RA. The cutaneous manifestations of nutritional deficiencies. In: Norman RA (Ed). Diagnosis of Aging Skin Diseases, 1st edition. London: Springer; 2008. pp. 193-203.
6. Kumar P, Lal NR, Mondal AK, Mondal A, Gharami RC, Maiti A. Zinc and skin: a brief summary. Dermatol Online J. 2012;18(3):1.

EXAMINATION QUESTIONS

1. What are the cutaneous manifestations of vitamin A deficiency?
2. Discuss the management of vitamin B_{12} deficiency.
3. Explain acrodermatitis enteropathica.
4. Write a short note on pellagra.
5. Explain diet in dermatology.

8 SECTION | Hair, Nail, Mucosa, Adnexa and Connective Tissue

71 CHAPTER Acne and Other Acneform Diseases

Souvik Sardar

INTRODUCTION[1,2]

Acne is a chronic inflammatory disease of the sebaceous follicles due to its obstruction. Sebaceous follicle is a type of pilosebaceous unit having a sebaceous gland and a rudimentary hair. It can affect any age group. Early diagnosis and treatment is necessary as the disease and its related temporary and permanent complications can have a deep psychosocial impact on the patient's quality-of-life.

HISTORY[3]

The term *acne* was coined by, Aëtius Amidenus, a physician of Emperor Justinian, in the 6th century AD.

EPIDEMIOLOGY[4]

Acne is one of the most common skin diseases in the world affecting the adolescents and young adults in majority (85% prevalence in 12–24 years of age). Most commonly, it starts at puberty and spontaneously remits by 30 years. Individuals may have acne eruption till 5th or 6th decade and are termed as persistent acne.

PATHOGENESIS[1,5-16]

There is an interplay of multiple factors in the pathogenesis of acne **(Table 1)**.

CLASSIFICATION[16,17]

Based on morphology, acne has been classified as described in **Table 2**.

Box 1 represents different types of comedones.

Grading of acne has been described in **Table 3**.

TABLE 1: Factors in the pathogenesis of acne.

Four main factors			
Seborrhea and change in quality of sebum	*Altered infundibular keratinization*	*Overcolonization of Propionibacterium acnes*	*Inflammation at the sebaceous follicle*
In puberty ↑ DHEAS and DHT (conversion from testosterone) ↓ ↑ Size and numbers of lobules Decrease in linoleic acid	Retention hyperkeratosis of the infrainfundibular epithelium ↓ Keratinous plug formed in the pilar canal (Microcomedone)	Proliferation of aerobic *P. acne* ↓ Releases lecithinase, lipase, and proteinase ↓ Rupture of comedones and inflammation (Papule and pustule)	• Activation of both innate and adaptive immunity • Increased TLR-2, 4 expressions • Release of IL-1, 2, 8, 12, TNF-α leading to influx of CD-4 T cells, neutrophils which in turn degranulates • All these further causes rupture of comedones and spread of inflammation (Nodule formation and scarring)
Other factors			
• *Genetic:* Number, size, and activity of sebaceous glands are inherited • *Hormones:* Androgens and progestins • *Environmental:* – Hot and humid – Exposure to oils and halogenated chemicals • *Stress:* Release of substance-P contributing towards seborrhea • *Diet:* – Milk and milk products – High glycemic foods – Sugary products • *Cosmetics:* Comedogenic ones • *Drugs*			

(DHEAS: dehydroepiandrosterone sulfate; DHT: dihydrotestosterone; IL: interleukin; TLR: toll-like receptor; TNF-α: tumor necrosis factor alpha)

TABLE 2: Classification of acne (based on morphology).

Noninflammatory acne	*Inflammatory acne*
• *Open comedones (blackheads)* ***(Fig. 1)***: Nonerythematous papules with dilated follicular opening turning black due to lipid oxidation and melanin deposition. Contains inspissated keratin • *Closed comedones (Whiteheads)* ***(Fig. 2)***: Skin colored papules with no visible opening. Better appreciated by palpation or stretching of skin	• Erythematous papules • Pustules • Nodules • Cysts (not a true cyst)—may coalesce to form inflamed plaques, abscess, and sinus tracts

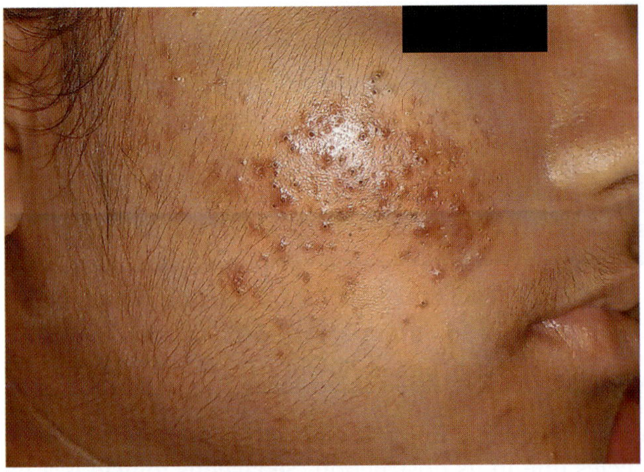

Fig. 1: Open comedones (blackheads) with few papules—Indian Acne Alliance (IAA) grade I. *Courtesy*: Souvik Sardar.

BOX 1: Types of comedones.[7]

- Open comedones
- Closed comedones
- Missed comedones—seen only after stretching of skin
- Submarine comedones—ill-defined closed comedone
- Grouped comedones
- Macrocomedones
- Sandpaper comedones
- Nevoid comedones
- Drug-induced comedones

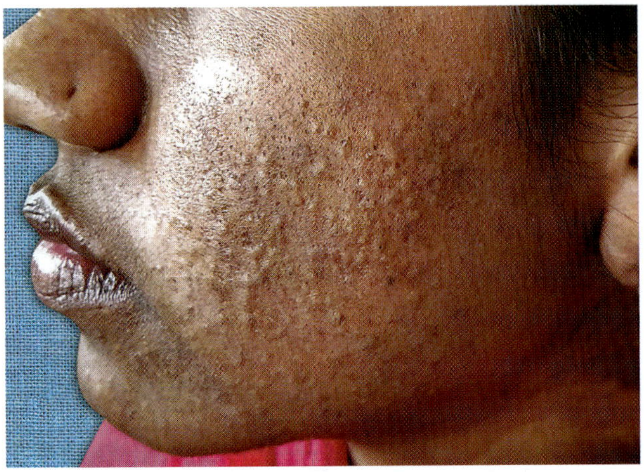

Fig. 2: Multiple closed comedones, few open comedones (IAA grade I). Ice-pick scars can also be seen. *Courtesy:* Souvik Sardar.

TABLE 3: Grading of acne.[18]

Mild (grade I) ***(Figs. 1 and 2)***: Predominantly comedones	Comedones <30 Papules <10 No scarring
Moderate (grade II) ***(Fig. 3)***: Predominantly papules	Comedones any number Papules >10 Nodules <3 Scarring ±
Severe (grade III) ***(Fig. 4)***: Many nodules	Comedones and papules any number Nodules/cysts >3 Scarring +

CLINICAL FEATURES[16,17,19]

- Present with comedones, papules, pustules, nodules, abscess, draining sinuses, and scars.
- Lesions can occur in the seborrheic zones most frequently in the face followed by back, chest, and shoulder.
- Primary lesion is a microcomedone.
- Acne vulgaris means the common acne (Latin word *Vulgaris* means common) starting in puberty.

Neonatal Acne

- *Onset*: 2–3 weeks of birth.
- *Morphology*: Papules and pustules. No comedones.
- *Cause*: Excess androgenic activity with *Malassezia* spp. infection.

Infantile Acne

- *Onset*: 3–6 months of birth.
- *Morphology*: Typical comedones, papules, pustules, and rarely nodules.

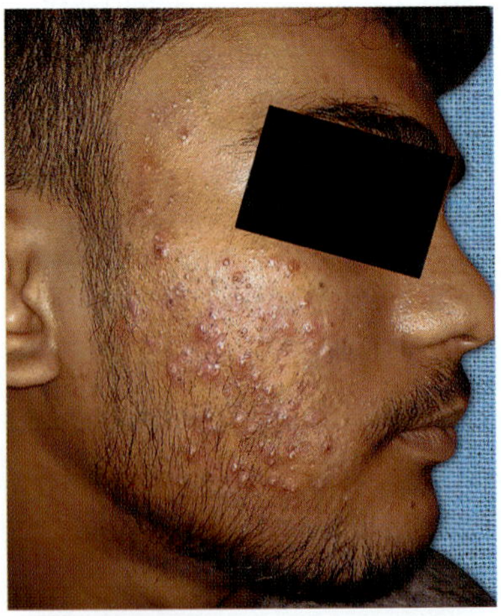

Fig. 3: Multiple papules and pustules [Indian Acne Alliance (IAA) grade II). *Courtesy:* Souvik Sardar.

- *Cause*: Infantile gonadal testosterone and adrenal dehydroepiandrosterone sulfate (DHEAS).

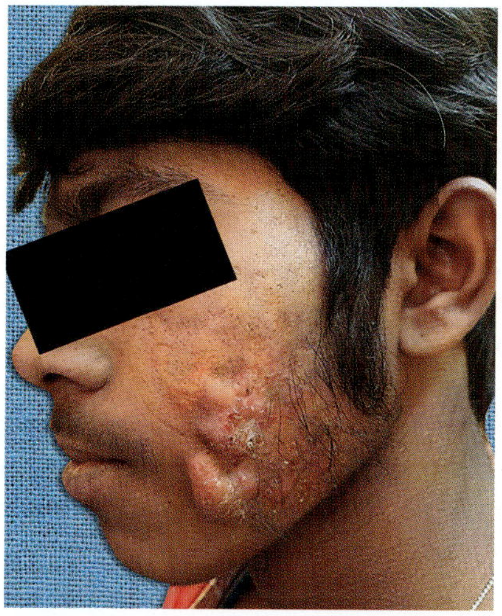

Fig. 4: Nodular acne with multiple abscesses [Indian Acne Alliance (IAA) grade III].
Courtesy: Dr Uttam Kumar Lenka, Kolkata, West Bengal, India.

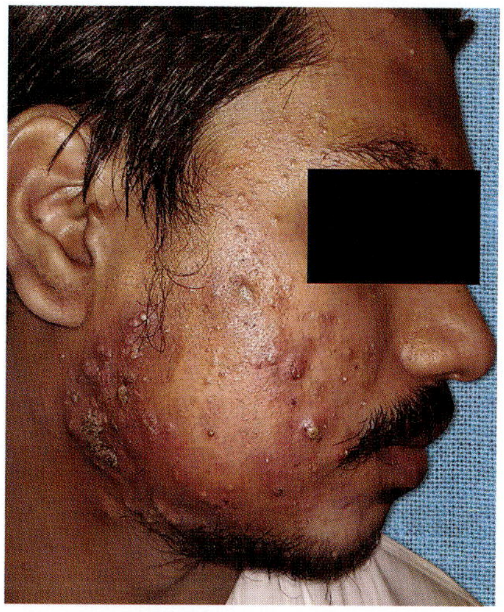

Fig. 5: Acne conglobata.
Courtesy: Souvik Sardar.

Mid-Childhood Acne

- *Onset*: 1–7 years of age.
- Acne is generally uncommon in this age. Need to be investigated for underlying hormonal imbalances, adrenal gland tumor, and congenital adrenal hyperplasia.

Preadolescent Acne

Onset: 7–12 years of age.

Postadolescent Acne

Two varieties: Persistent acne (continuation of acne from adolescence to adult life) or late onset acne (occurring after 25 years of age, mostly in females with endocrinological or metabolic abnormalities or stress).

Perimenopausal Acne

- *Onset*: Just before and within 2 years of menopause.
- *Cause*: Imbalance caused by lack of estrogen from ovary and continuous androgen from adrenal glands.
- Rarely, androgen-secreting tumors may be found if postmenopausal acne is associated with signs of virilism and hirsutism.

Acne Conglobata (Fig. 5)

- *Onset*: Adolescence and early adulthood.
- May have positive family history.[20]
- *Morphology*: Multiple comedones, papules/pustules join to form inflamed tender nodules, mostly in the back. Polyporous comedones are characteristic **(Fig. 6)**. Abscess may be found.
- Follicular occlusion triad [acne conglobata, dissecting folliculitis of scalp, hidradenitis suppurativa (HS)] and tetrad (triad with pilonidal sinus).

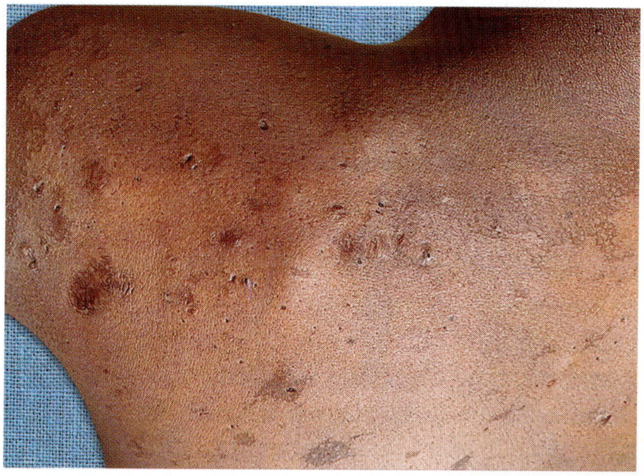

Fig. 6: Polyporous comedones with scarring in acne conglobata.
Courtesy: Dr Uttam Kumar Lenka, Kolkata, West Bengal, India.

- *Complication*: Irregular scars (atrophic/hypertrophic) due to high inflammation.

Acne Fulminans

- Acne conglobata patients having systemic features of fever, myalgia, arthralgia, erythema nodosum, and focal bony erosions in sternum and clavicle.
- Suppurative abscess and ulcers are commonly found.
- May be associated with anabolic steroid use and late-onset congenital adrenal hyperplasia.
- High chance of scarring.

Solid Facial Edema

- *Onset*: Adolescence or early adulthood.
- *Morphology*: Hard nonpitting edema involving the midface. May have prior papulopustular acne lesions.
- *Treatment*: Oral isotretinoin.

Hormonal Acne

- Mostly in adult females.
- *Site*: Lower face, chin, and jawline involvement are characteristic.
- *Associated with:* Polycystic ovarian disease (PCOD) (as in **Fig. 7**); ovarian/adrenal tumors, congenital adrenal hyperplasia; hyperandrogenism, insulin resistance, and acanthosis nigricans (HAIR-AN) syndrome; and seborrhea, acne, hirsutism, alopecia (SAHA) syndrome.
- *Other features*: Hirsutism, obesity, seborrhea, acanthosis nigricans, androgenetic alopecia, premenstrual flares, menstrual irregularities, and clitoromegaly.
- Hormonal workup is necessary (described below).

Acne Excorée

- Due to habit of pricking and excoriating the acne lesions.
- Common in young women.
- *Associated with*: Obsessive-compulsive disorder (OCD), body dysmorphic disorders, depression, and anxiety. Hence, antidepressants may be helpful in treatment.

Acne Tropicalis

- Common in extreme hot and humid weather.
- Mostly among furnace workers and military personnel.
- Change of environment resolves the problem to great extent.

Acne Associated with Syndromes

- *Apert syndrome*: Craniosynostoses with syndactyly of hands and feet.
- Synovitis, acne, pustulosis, hyperostosis, osteitis (SAPHO) syndrome.
- *PAPA syndrome*—sterile *p*yogenic *a*rthritis, *p*yoderma gangrenosum and *a*cne conglobata.
- *PAPASH syndrome*—sterile *p*yogenic *a*rthritis, *p*yoderma gangrenosum, *a*cne conglobata and *s*uppurative *h*idradenitis.
- *PASH syndrome*—*p*yoderma gangrenosum, *a*cne conglobata, and *s*uppurative *h*idradenitis.

ACNEIFORM ERUPTIONS (FIG. 8)[16,17]

Follicular papulopustular eruptions similar in appearance to acne but does not involve all four factors in pathogenesis:

- *Acne mechanica*: Repeated friction and mechanical trauma causing obstruction of the sebaceous follicles. For example, rubbing due to violin over lateral neck and crutches in armpits.
- *Acne aestivalis*: Due to exposure to ultraviolet (UV) light (natural or artificial).
- *Acne venenata*: Epicutaneous contact with topical irritants and comedogenic ingredients causing pilosebaceous canal obstruction. It is of three types:
  1. *Acne cosmetica*: Certain ingredients such as lanolin and cocoa butter in cosmetics.
  2. *Pomade acne*: Due to hair products.
  3. *Occupational acne*: Cutting oil acne (most common), petroleum oil acne, and oil/tar/pitch acne.
- *Chloracne*:
  - *Cause*: Percutaneous absorption, inhalation, or ingestion of halogenated aromatic hydrocarbons, polychlorinated naphthalenes, etc.
  - *Site*: Causes noninflamed comedo-like lesions in the malar and retroauricular areas as well as axilla, neck, back, and scrotum.
- *Drug-induced acneiform eruptions:*[1,21] Certain drugs can cause acne-like lesions. A list of drugs has been given in **Table 4**.

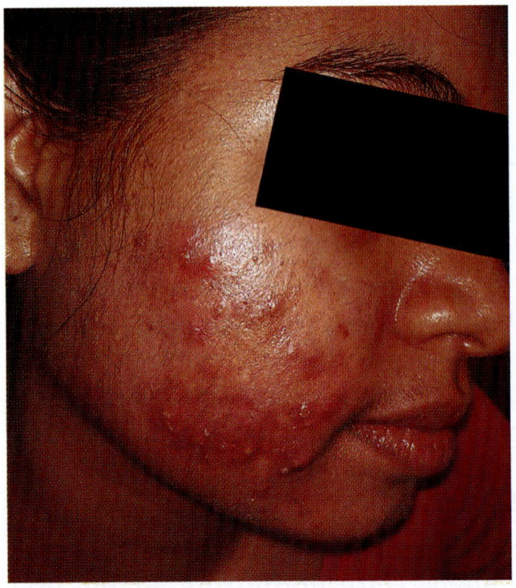

Fig. 7: IAA grade III acne with polycystic ovarian disease (PCOD). Note the involvement of lower face.
Courtesy: Souvik Sardar.

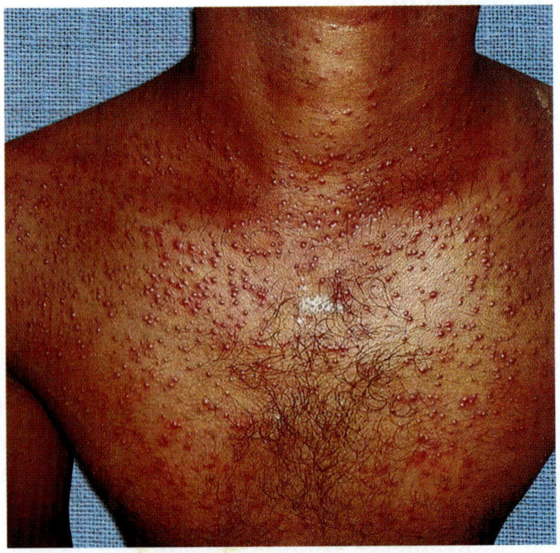

Fig. 8: Widespread acneiform eruptions after oral corticosteroid therapy.
Courtesy: Dr Uttam Kumar Lenka, Kolkata, West Bengal, India.

Differences between Acne and Acneiform Eruptions

Vide **Table 5**.

COMPLICATIONS[2,22,23]

Inflammation is the single most important factor determining the burden of complications. Both degree and depth of inflammation plays an important role. In addition to the clinical complications, acne can cause severe impact as far as the psychosocial aspect is concerned:

- *Epidermal damage*: Erythema and postinflammatory hyperpigmentation.
- Dermal damage produces scars (vide **Table 6**).

DIFFERENTIAL DIAGNOSES

- Rosacea
- Milia
- Sebaceous hyperplasia
- Demodecidosis
- Pityrosporum folliculitis
- Gram-negative folliculitis
- Staphylococcal folliculitis
- Eosinophilic folliculitis
- Pseudofolliculitis barbae
- Facial idiopathic granulomas with regressive evolution (FIGURE) [also called lupus miliaris disseminatus faciei (LMDF)]
- Trichoepithelioma
- Osteoma cutis
- Angiofibroma (tuberous sclerosis)
- Syringoma
- Molluscum contagiosum
- Steatocystoma multiplex
- Perioral dermatitis
- Verruca plana
- Hidradenitis suppurativa

TABLE 4: Drugs causing acneiform eruptions.

Common drugs	*Uncommon drugs*
• Isoniazid • Corticosteroids • Phenytoin • eGFR inhibitors • Anabolic steroids • Progestin • Lithium	• Phenobarbital • Azathioprine • Cyclosporine • Propylthiouracil • Vitamin B_6 and B_{12} • TNF inhibitors

(eGFR: estimated glomerular filtration rate; TNF: tumor necrosis factor)

TABLE 5: Differences between acne and acneiform eruptions.

Acne	*Acneiform eruptions*
• Typical polymorphic eruptions including comedones, papules, pustules, nodules, and abscess • May form scar • Gradual onset in the pubertal age group • *Cause:* Multifactorial including follicular keratinization, seborrhea, bacterial overgrowth, and inflammation • Involve seborrheic zones	• Monomorphic papules or pustules • Less chance of scarring • Abrupt onset in any age group • Drugs, topical irritants, and certain foods • Any area may be involved

TABLE 6: Complications due to dermal damage.

Atrophic	*Hypertrophic*
• Rolling scar • Boxcar scar **(Fig. 9)** • Ice pick scar **(Fig. 9)**	• Hypertrophic scars • Keloid • Papular scars of nose and chin[24] • *Perifollicular elastolysis:*[25] Soft atrophic scars in the shoulder/upper back

APPROACH TO A PATIENT WITH ACNE

- *History*: A detail history is necessary regarding:
  - *Age*: Early (neonatal/infantile), adolescent, and adult onset.
  - *Onset*: Sudden (drug and hormonal) and gradual (majority cases).
  - *Family history*: Acne conglobata or fulminans can have positive parental history.
  - *Drugs, supplements, and diet*: Can cause acneiform eruptions or aggravation of existing acne.
  - *Menstrual history*: Any irregularities (less than nine cycles indicates oligomenorrhea).
  - *Occupation*: Exposure to industrial gases, oils, and petroleum products.
  - Agents used for routine skin care including cosmetic use.

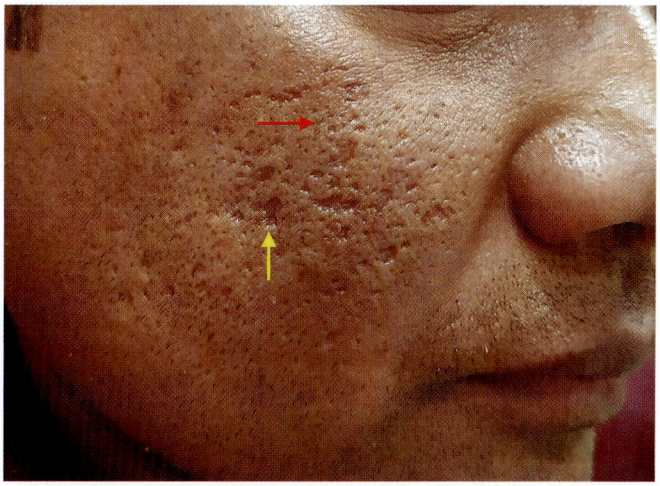

Fig. 9: Boxcar scars (yellow arrow) and ice pick scars (red arrow).
Courtesy: Souvik Sardar.

- *Examination*:
  - Skin type
  - Morphology and severity
  - Distribution
  - Presence of features of hyperandrogenism or hormonal imbalances
  - Dermoscopy—to rule out acne differentials like demodecidosis where mite can be seen.

INVESTIGATIONS[16,17]

Vide **Table 7** for investigations.

TREATMENT[8,16,17,26-29]

General advices **(Box 2)** and specific management of acne **(Table 8)** have been discussed below.

TABLE 7: Investigations in acne patients.

Related to disease	*Related to treatment*
• *Hormonal investigations:* Testosterone (free and total), DHEAS, 17-OH progesterone, prolactin, LH, FSH, SHBG, TSH, and FBS/PPBS • USG lower abdomen/trans-vaginal—to check adrenals and ovaries • Microbiological examination to rule out gram-negative folliculitis	• Routine investigations before isotretinoin prescription—LFT, UPT, and lipid profile • K^+ level (for spironolactone)

(DHEAS: dehydroepiandrosterone sulfate; FBS: fasting blood sugar; FSH: follicle-stimulating hormone; LFT: liver function test; LH: luteinizing hormone; 17-OH: 17-hydroxyprogesterone; PPBS: postprandial blood sugar; TSH: thyroid-stimulating hormone; SHBG: sex hormone binding globulin; UPT: urine pregnancy test; USG: ultrasonography)

KEY POINTS

- Follicular obstruction, bacterial overcolonization, altered sebum quality, and inflammations contribute to the pathogenesis of globally one of the most common skin diseases.
- Microcomedone is the primary lesion. Papules, pustules, nodules, abscess, and cysts may also be found.
- Acne conglobata and fulminans are severe forms causing inevitable scarring.
- PCOD is a common association with acne in females.
- Hormonal workup is very important in females with lower face, adult-onset acne, not responding to conventional regime.
- Acneiform eruptions are monomorphic.
- Anabolic steroids, isoniazid, phenytoin, and corticosteroids are common offenders for drug-induced acneiform eruptions.
- Occupational exposure to hydrocarbons and coal tar derivatives can cause noninflamed comedones.
- Acne sequelae include irregular scars and pigmentation.
- Combination of topical retinoid and benzoyl peroxide (BPO) is first-line therapy in mild-to-moderate cases.

BOX 2: General advices for acne patients.

- Proper counseling is of utmost importance
- Avoid using comedogenic moisturizer, OTC products, heavy makeup, and scrubbers/facials
- *Diet:* Avoid milk and milk products, foods with high caloric value, and gym supplements/whey protein
- Do not prick or squeeze
- Take proper sun protection
- Avoid stress
- Weight reduction (mostly in PCOD and hormonal acne patients)

(PCOD: polycystic ovarian disease; OTC: over-the-counter)

TABLE 8: Specific management of acne.

Topical drugs	*Role in acne treatment*	*Remarks*
Retinoids—adapalene, tretinoin, and tazarotene	Comedolytic, anti-comedogenic and anti-inflammatory action	• Chance of retinoid dermatitis and photosensitivity • Can be combined with topical antibiotics or BPO (first line in mild and moderate) • Tazarotene is pregnancy category X, rest two are category C
Benzoyl peroxide (BPO)	• Antibacterial action by free radical release • Reduces antibiotic resistance	• Combined with topical retinoids or topical antibiotics • Pregnancy category C
Topical antibiotics—clindamycin and erythromycin	Reduces *P. acne* infection	• Prolonged use and monotherapy can cause antibiotic resistance • Combined with topical niacinamide, retinoids, or BPO • Pregnancy category B
Azelaic acid	• Reduces PIH • Mildly antibacterial, anti-inflammatory, and comedolytic	• Good for sensitive skin • Pregnancy category B
Topical dapsone (5%)	Anti-inflammatory action	• Can be combined with topical retinoids • Pregnancy category C
Salicylic acid—0.5–2%	Comedolytic and anticomedogenic	Pregnancy category C

Contd...

Contd...

Topical drugs	*Role in acne treatment*	*Remarks*
	Systemic drugs	
• Oral antibiotics • Erythromycin, clindamycin, and azithromycin • Doxycycline, minocycline, and lymecycline • Amoxycillin and cephalexin • Trimethoprim—sulfamethoxazole	• Reduces *P. acne* infection • Antimetalloproteinase activity reduces inflammation	• Tetracyclines avoid in pregnancy and children ≤ 8 years • Should not be used beyond 2–3 months continuously or as monotherapy • Doxycycline—1.7–2.4 mg/kg • Minocycline—1 mg/kg
Oral isotretinoin	Works in all four stages of pathogenesis	• Dose—0.5–1 mg/kg/day • Low dose 0.25–0.4 mg/kg is also given • Preferred in severe nodular acne or treatment resistant moderate acne or those producing considerable scarring or psychological stress
Hormonal therapy: • Combined OCP • Spironolactone • Flutamide • Low dose corticosteroids	• Reduces androgen release, sex hormone binding globulin, and free testosterone • Spironolactone blocks androgen receptor • Reduces 5-α reductase activity	Used in female acne—airway hormonal imbalance, not responding to conventional treatment, clinical signs of hyperandrogenism with normal biochemical profile
Metformin	Reduces IGF-1 and hence sebum production	Used in patients with hyperandrogenism
Oral corticosteroids	• Low dose intake in adrenal hyperandrogenism • Reduce inflammation (hence reduced chance of scarring) • Reduce isotretinoin flare	Dose—0.5–1 mg/kg/day short course with gradual tapering
	Procedural treatment	
Comedone extraction	For open and closed comedones	
Intralesional triamcinolone acetonide	• For severe nodular acne, abscess, hypertrophic, or keloidal scars • Dose—10 mg/mL to be diluted with normal saline to 2.5 mg/mL. 0.1 mL is given at each site	
Phenolisation of abscess wall	In recurrent abscess	
Chemical peeling: Salicylic acid, mandelic acid, retinol, glycolic acid, black vinegar containing peel and TCA	• Reduce active acne • Reduce PIH • TCA CROSS done in ice pick scars	
Acne scar: • Subcision • Scar excision, punch floatation/grafting/ excision • Microneedling RF, dermaroller, dermaplaning • Dermabrasion/microdermabrasion • IPL • Ablative, nonablative, and fractional laser • Autologous fat transfer and fillers	 • For rolling scars • Mostly in boxcar scars • Rolling scars mostly • Except in ice pick and deep boxcar scar • Active acne and scar erythema • For all types of scars • For depressed scars	

(CROSS: chemical reconstruction of skin scars; IGF-1: insulin-like growth factor 1; IPL: intense pulsed light; OCP: oral contraceptive pill; PIH: postinflammatory hyperpigmentation; RF: radiofrequency; TCA: trichloroacetic acid)

- BPO can reduce the chance of antibiotic resistance.
- Oral isotretinoin is an excellent modality of treatment in severe and treatment-resistant moderate acne.
- Short course oral corticosteroid may be added in severe cases to reduce inflammation and isotretinoin induced flares.
- Treatment of scars is multipronged where combination of both energy and nonenergy-based modalities are necessary.

REFERENCES

1. Degitz K, Placzek M, Borelli C, Plewig G. Pathophysiology of acne. J Dtsch Dermatol Ges. 2007;5:316-23.
2. Tan JK. Psychological impact of acne vulgaris: evaluating the evidence. Skin Ther Lett. 2004;9:1-3.
3. Goolamali SK, Andison AC. The origin and use of the word 'acne'. Br J Dermatol. 1977;96:291-4.
4. White GM. Recent findings in the epidemiologic evidence, classification, and subtypes of acne vulgaris. J Am Acad Dermatol. 1998;39:S34-7.

5. Gollnick H, Cunliffe W, Berson D, Dreno B, Finlay A, Leyden JJ, et al. Management of acne: a report from a global alliance to improve outcomes in acne. J Am Acad Dermatol. 2003;49:S1-38.
6. Paugam C, Corvec S, Saint-Jean M, Le Moigne M, Khammari A, Boisrobert A, et al. Propionibacterium acnes phylotypes and acne severity: an observational prospective study. J Eur Acad Dermatol Venereol. 2017;31:e398-9.
7. Cunliffe WJ, Holland DB, Clark SM, Stables GI. Comedogenesis: some new aetiological, clinical and therapeutic strategies. Br J Dermatol. 2000;142:1084-91.
8. Thiboutot D, Gollnick H, Bettoli V, Dréno B, Kang S, Leyden JJ, et al. New insights into the management of acne: an update from the Global Alliance to Improve Outcomes in Acne group. J Am Acad Dermatol. 2009;60:S1-S50.
9. Auffret N. What's new concerning the pathophysiology of acne? Ann Dermatol Venereol. 2003;130:101-6.
10. Jeremy AH, Holland DB, Roberts SG, Thomson KF, Cunliffe WJ. Inflammatory events are involved in acne lesion initiation. J Invest Dermatol. 2003;121:20-7.
11. Webster GF. The pathophysiology of acne. Cutis. 2005;76 (Suppl 2):4-7.
12. Herane MI, Ando I. Acne in infancy and acne genetics. Dermatology. 2003;206:24-8.
13. Singh R, Reddy B, Singh G. Acne cornea or oil-acne simulating Pityriasis rubra pilaris. Indian J Dermatol Venereol Leprol. 1976;42:7-9.
14. Zouboulis CC, Böhm M. Neuroendocrine regulation of sebocytes: a pathogenetic link between stress and acne. Exp Dermatol. 2004;13:31-5.
15. Adebamowo CA, Spiegelman D, Danby FW, Frazier AL, Willett WC, Holmes MD. High school dietary dairy intake and teenage acne. J Am Acad Dermatol. 2005;52:207-14.
16. Danby FW. Acne: causes and practical management, 1st edition. West Sussex: Wiley-Blackwell; 2015.
17. Plewig G, Kligman A. Acne and rosacea, 3rd edition. New York: Springer; 2000.
18. Kubba R, Bajaj AK, Thappa DM, Sharma R, Vedamurthy M, Dhar S, et al. Acne in India: guidelines for management—IAA consensus document. Indian J Dermatol Venereol Leprol. 2009;75(Suppl 1):1-62.
19. Gollnick HP, Bettoli V, Lambert J, Araviiskaia E, Binic I, Dessinioti C, et al. A consensus-based practical and daily guide for the treatment of acne patients. J Eur Acad Dermatol Venereol. 2016;30(9):1480-90.
20. Ghodsi SZ, Orawa H, Zouboulis CC. Prevalence, severity, and severity risk factors of acne in high school pupils: a community-based study. J Invest Dermatol. 2009;129:2136-41.
21. Williams C, Layton AM. Persistent acne in women: implications for the patient and for therapy. Am J Clin Dermatol. 2006;7:281-90.
22. Jacob CI, Dover JS, Kaminer MS. Acne scarring: a classification system and review of treatment options. J Am Acad Dermatol. 2001;45:109-17.
23. Fife D. Evaluation of acne scars: how to assess them and what to tell the patient. Dermatol Clin. 2016;34:207-13.
24. Ali FR, Kirk M, Madan V. Papular acne scars of the nose and chin: an under-recognised variant of acne scarring. J Cutan Aesthet Surg. 2016;9:241-43.
25. Wilson BB, Dent CH, Cooper PH. Papular acne scars. A common cutaneous finding. Arch Dermatol. 1990;126:797-800.
26. Zaenglein AL, Pathy AL, Schlosser BJ, Alikhan A, Baldwin HE, Berson DS, et al. Guidelines of care for the management of acne vulgaris. J Am Acad Dermatol. 2016;74:945-73.e33.
27. Layton AM, Cunliffe WJ. Guidelines for optimal use of isotretinoin in acne. J Am Acad Dermatol. 1992;27:S2-7.
28. Gollnick H, Abanmi AA, Al-Enezi M, Al Hammadi A, Galadari I, Kibbi A-G, et al. Management of acne in the Middle East. J Eur Acad Dermatol Venereol. 2017;31(Suppl 7):4-35.
29. Del Rosso JQ, Kircik L, Gallagher CJ. Comparative efficacy and tolerability of dapsone 5% gel in adult versus adolescent females with acne vulgaris. J Clin Aesthet Dermatol. 2015;8:31-7.

EXAMINATION QUESTIONS

1. Explain the etiopathogenesis of acne.
2. How will you approach to a female with late onset acne?
3. Write short note on acne conglobata.
4. Write short note on acne fulminans.
5. Discuss newer management options in acne.
6. Discuss management of hormonal acne.

72 CHAPTER Rosacea and Related Diseases

Indrashis Podder, Anupam Das

INTRODUCTION

Rosacea is a relatively common chronic inflammatory acneiform disorder arising from the facial pilosebaceous units. It can present with myriad clinical features ranging from persistent facial erythema to papules, pustules, and nodules, primarily affecting the facial convexities. In addition, occasional vascular changes, hypertrophic changes, or ocular involvement has been reported.

EPIDEMIOLOGY[1]

This disorder commonly affects fair-skinned people (Fitzpatrick skin types I, II, or III), peak incidence reported between 30 and 50 years. There is a predilection for female gender; however, men are more prone to develop severe disease and rhinophyma. It is less frequent in darker skin tones (Fitzpatrick skin types V or VI).

PATHOGENESIS[1,2]

The exact pathogenesis is unclear. Several possible etiopathogenic factors have been proposed such as genetic predisposition (increased expression of *HLA-DRA* and *BTNL2*), altered innate immunity [elevated levels of cathelicidin, kallikrein 5, LL-37, and altered toll-like receptor 2 (TLR2) expression], defective skin barrier function (increased transepidermal water loss and dry skin), ultraviolet radiation exposure [ultraviolet A (UVA)-induced collagen denaturation, ultraviolet B (UVB)-induced activation of fibroblast, vascular endothelial growth factor, and increased reactive oxygen species generation], microorganisms (*Demodex folliculorum* and *Helicobacter pylori*), and neurological dysfunction [significantly lower heat pain threshold due to increased activation of transient receptor potential vanilloid (TRPV) 1–4 and an transient receptor potential ankyrin receptor 1 (TRPA1)].

All these factors engage in a complex interaction to promote and regulate leukocyte chemotaxis, angiogenesis, and create a local inflammatory milieu—the hallmarks of rosacea pathogenesis.

CLINICAL FEATURES AND DIAGNOSIS[1]

A classical history is episodic/transient redness (flushing) of the face in response to hot liquids, spicy foods, alcohol, and/or sun and heat exposure. Coexistence of acne may be noted frequently.

However, in the absence of any specific diagnostic tests for this condition till date, the National Rosacea Society Expert Committee laid down the primary and secondary clinical features of rosacea in 2004.

Presence of at least one primary feature with or without secondary features is required for diagnosis.

The classification of clinical features is given in **Table 1**.

Clinical Subtypes

There are four subtypes of this disease and their further variants depending on the primary and secondary features:

1. *Erythematotelangiectatic rosacea (ETR)*: Persistent erythema and telangiectasia
2. *Papulopustular rosacea (PPR)*: Predominantly papules and pustules.
3. *Phymatous rosacea*: Nodular, thickened skin with patulous follicles, and predominantly affecting the nose bulb. Marked sebaceous hyperplasia and lymphedema can cause facial disfigurement. Following types of phymas have been reported:
   - Rhinophyma (enlarged nose)
   - Metophyma (enlarged cushion like swelling of forehead)
   - Blepharophyma—swollen eyelids
   - Otophyma—cauliflower-like swelling of earlobes
   - Gnathophyma—swollen and thickened chin
4. *Ocular rosacea*: Red eyes, dry, and gritty sensation may lead to burning and stinging. May result in blepharitis, conjunctivitis, and episcleritis.

TABLE 1: Primary and secondary clinical features of rosacea.

Primary features	*Secondary features*
• Flushing (transient erythema) • Nontransient erythema • Papules and pustules • Telangiectasia	• Burning or stinging • Plaques • Dry appearance • Edema • Ocular manifestations • Peripheral location • Phymatous changes

Staging (Plewig and Kligman Classification) and Severity

Plewig and Kligman have proposed a staging system for this disease and graded its severity:

- *Rosacea diathesis*: Episodic erythema and transient flushing
- *Stage I*: Persistent erythema and telangiectasia, characteristic flushy "red face". It can be graded as mild, moderate, or severe depending on degree of flushing and erythema.
- *Stage II*: Stage I plus tiny papules and papulopustules (2–3 mm). No comedones.
  - *Mild:* Few papules/pustules (<5)
  - *Moderate:* 5–10 papules/pustules
  - *Severe:* >10 papules/pustules
- *Stage III*: Stage II plus dusky red papules and nodules. Marked sebaceous hyperplasia and lymphedema can occur in chronic cases resulting in different phymas and facial disfigurement. This stage indicates severe disease.

NB: Sequential progression of stages may not occur, disease may start with stage II or III, and frequent overlap is seen.

Site: Classically, bilateral, symmetric involvement of the face is noted with predilection for malar areas. Nasolabial folds are involved [differentiating it from malar rash of systemic lupus erythematosus (SLE)]. This disease is often associated with seborrheic dermatitis.

Diagnosis

As mentioned before, rosacea is a clinical diagnosis having diagnostic criteria (mentioned above). However, occasionally diagnostic modalities may be needed to confirm the diagnosis and rule out differentials.

Dermoscopy: It is noninvasive diagnostic modality. Dermoscopic signs of rosacea include linear or arborizing vessels in a polygonal network, dark red background, scattered white scales, follicular plug, Demodex tails, and Demodex follicular openings.

Skin biopsy: Not recommended routinely. Findings include nonspecific perivascular and periappendageal lymphohistiocytic infiltrate, dilated capillaries, and occasional "tuberculoid" granulomas without caseation. May be useful in detecting *Demodex mites* (≥5 mite/cm^2 is considered pathogenic).

Skin scraping: May reveal *Demodex folliculorum* infestation.

Bacterial culture: May be utilized to rule out *Staphylococcus aureus* infection.

DIFFERENTIAL DIAGNOSES

Some important differential diagnoses, categorized according to clinical presentation, have been presented in **Table 2**.

TREATMENT[1,3]

The treatment can be broadly categorized as follows:

- General measures for prevention
- Specific measures:
  - Topical
  - Systemic
  - Physical and light based

General Measures

These measures are necessary for all patients to avoid triggering factors and minimize relapse. Proper patient counseling is of paramount importance to avoid specific triggering factors such as strong winds, temperature variations, sun exposure, exercise, spicy foods, alcohol, physical, and/or emotional stress. Several photoprotection measures are recommended such as covered clothing, shade-seeking behavior, umbrellas and shades, and broad-spectrum sunscreens (having sun protection factor of at least 30+). Both UVA and UVB radiation are implicated in its pathogenesis by stimulating free radical generation. Other general measures include use of facial cleansers (to remove excess sebum) and facial moisturizers (to avoid dryness of facial skin).

Specific Measures

Topical

Topical treatment of rosacea has been presented in **Table 3**.

TABLE 2: Differential diagnoses of rosacea and their identifying features.

Clinical presentation	*Differential diagnoses*
Facial papules/pustules	• Acne (presence of comedones) • *Staphylococcus aureus* folliculitis, gram-negative folliculitis, demodicidosis (ruled out by microbiologic investigations) • Perioral dermatitis (restricted to perioral region, thin clear area between involved area and upper lip)
Facial flushing/erythema	• Seborrheic dermatitis—involvement of scalp, seborrheic areas, malar area not classically involved • Prolonged use to topical corticosteroids—history of topical steroid abuse • SLE—nasolabial fold not involved • Dermatomyositis—typical periorbital swelling and redness (heliotrope sign)

(SLE: systemic lupus erythematosus)

TABLE 3: Topical treatment of rosacea.

US FDA approved	*Off-label drugs*
• Azelaic acid • Metronidazole • Sodium sulfacetamide • α-adrenergic agonist (brimonidine)	• Retinoids • Calcineurin inhibitors • Macrolides • Benzoyl peroxide • Permethrin • Ivermectin • Clindamycin

(US FDA: United States Food and Drug Administration)

The commonly used topical agents are briefly discussed below:

- *Azelaic acid (15% and 20% gel/cream):*
  - United States Food and Drug Administration (US FDA) approved topical agent, recently, been recommended as the first-line treatment for mild to moderate inflammatory or PPR by the ROSacea COnsensus (ROSCO) panel of experts.
  - *Mode of action (MoA)*: Reducing the levels of kallikrein 5 and cathelicidin (inflammatory cytokines) aggravating rosacea.
  - Once at night use, may be safely used for 6 months continuously.
  - *Adverse drug reaction (ADR)*: Burning and stinging sensation.
- *Metronidazole (0.75% and 1% gel/cream):*
  - Reduces the rate of ultraviolet-induced reactive oxygen species generation and also inactivates the existing reactive oxygen species.
  - Recommended use—twice daily
  - It increases the remission free period following treatment.
  - *ADR*: Burning and stinging
- *Topical α-adrenergic agonist (Brimonidine)*:
  - Recently approved by the US FDA for the treatment of rosacea-associated persistent erythema.
  - *MoA*: Perilesional vasoconstriction, thus reducing erythema.
  - *Dose*: Brimonidine tartrate (0.5%) gel; once-daily usage.
  - *ADR*: Usually well tolerated, but associated with rebound erythema on discontinuation.
- *Topical ivermectin (1% cream):*
  - Not yet approved by US FDA, but extensively studied in rosacea with encouraging results.
  - MoA:
    - Acts against the *Demodex* mites, a key pathogenic factor.
    - Also reduces inflammation by checking neutrophilic migration and phagocytosis, downregulating inflammatory cytokines such as interleukin-1β (IL-1β) and tumor necrosis factor-alpha (TNF-α) and upregulating the anti-inflammatory cytokine IL-10.
  - *Dose:* 1% cream; once-daily usage is recommended.
  - *ADR:* Sporadic reports of mild dryness, burning, and stinging sensation, all are transient.

TABLE 4: Systemic treatment of rosacea.

Systemic anti-rosacea medications	
US FDA approved	*Off-label usage*
Tetracyclines	• β-adrenergic receptor antagonists • Isotretinoin • Oral ivermectin

(US FDA: United States Food and Drug Administration)

Systemic Agents

Systemic treatment of rosacea has been presented in **Table 4**.

Some important systemic medications are briefly discussed below:

- *Tetracyclines:*
  - Only US FDA approved systemic medication for rosacea.
  - Second-generation tetracyclines such as doxycycline and minocycline are preferred, because of their better safety profile.
  - *MoA*: They act in papulopustular/inflammatory rosacea by downregulating proinflammatory cytokines such as kallikrein 5 and cathelicidin resulting in decreased neutrophil chemotaxis, reduced generation of toxic reactive oxygen species, and inhibition of nitric oxide-mediated vasodilatation.
  - *Dose*: Subantimicrobial doses of doxycycline (40 mg/day) and minocycline (45 mg/day) have proven effectiveness.
  - Contraindicated in pregnant or lactating women and children less than 12 years.
- *Isotretinoin:*
  - May be used off-label in severe cases (pyoderma faciale) not responding to topical therapies and systemic tetracyclines.
  - *MoA*: Downregulation of monocytic TLR2 expression.
  - *Dose*: A lower dosage (10 mg/day) has been found to be effective with minimal adverse effects.
  - *ADR*: Dry lips and xerosis (tolerable and transient), and mild-to-moderate elevation of serum triglyceride levels may occur in some. Absolutely contraindicated during pregnancy and lactation (category X).
- *Oral ivermectin*:
  - Sporadic case reports have indicated oral ivermectin (200 μg/kg) along with topical medications for eradication of *Demodex mites.*

Physical and Light-based Therapies

- Physical and light-based modalities may be attempted for certain manifestations such as telangiectasias, persistent facial erythema, and phymas (especially rhinophymas), not responding to conventional therapy.

- *Pulsed dye laser and intense pulsed light rays*: Telangiectasia and persistent erythema by targeting dilated blood vessels.
- *CO_2 laser/surgery*: Removal of excess tissues in phymas.
- *ADR*: Purpura, bruising and overheating, and postinflammatory hyperpigmentation are the occasional adverse effects.

DISEASE COURSE AND PROGNOSIS

This disease usually has a prolonged course with frequent recurrences. Rarely, disease may disappear spontaneously after few years, but usually lifetime prevalence is noted.

COMPLICATIONS

Although, this condition is not lethal, it is a morbid condition significantly impairing the patient's quality of life by inducing stigma and anxiety. Recently, systemic associations have been reported such as inflammatory bowel disease (Crohn's disease or ulcerative colitis), dementia, Alzheimer's disease, and Parkinson's disease.

KEY POINTS

- Rosacea can present with persistent facial erythema to papules, pustules, and nodules, primarily affecting the facial convexities.
- A classical history is episodic/transient redness (flushing) of the face in response to hot liquids, spicy foods, alcohol, and/or sun and heat exposure.
- Major clinical subtypes are erythemotelangiectatic, papulopustular, phymatous, and ocular rosacea.
- Patients should be counseled to avoid triggering factors such as strong winds, temperature variations, sun exposure, exercise, spicy foods, alcohol, physical, and/or emotional stress.
- It has a prolonged course with frequent recurrences.

REFERENCES

1. Sarkar R, Podder I, Jagadeesan S. Rosacea in skin of color: a comprehensive review. Indian J Dermatol Venereol Leprol. 2020;86:611-21.
2. Ahn CS, Huang WW. Rosacea pathogenesis. Dermatol Clin. 2018;36:81-6.
3. Dursun R, Daye M, Durmaz K. Acne and rosacea: What's new for treatment? Dermatol Ther. 2019;32:e13020.

EXAMINATION QUESTIONS

1. Describe the pathogenesis, clinical features, and management of rosacea.
2. Discuss the clinical differentials of different types of rosacea.
3. Explain management of rosacea.

73 CHAPTER Disorders of Eccrine and Apocrine Glands

Aarti Sarda, Varsha Vaidyanathan, Abhishek De

INTRODUCTION

Human sweat glands are of two types: (1) Eccrine; and (2) Apocrine. Eccrine and apocrine glands differ in their origin, structure, size, distribution, mode of secretion, and functions. Eccrine sweat glands are present all over the body excluding certain sites such as the lips, nailbed, external ear canal, clitoris, and labia minora. These glands are present since birth but become completely functional only at about 2 years of age. Apocrine glands on the other hand enlarge and become functional only at the time of puberty and are distributed in specific areas such as the axilla, periumbilical and perianal areas, labia minora, prepuce, and the areolae of the breasts (Montgomery's tubercles). Moll's glands on the eyelid, mammary glands, and the ceruminous glands of the ear canal are all believed to be modified apocrine glands.

Structurally, the eccrine and apocrine glands are roughly similar with the presence of a coiled secretory portion in the lower dermis or subcutaneous fat and a double-layered ductal portion. Apocrine glands are larger than eccrine glands and have only a straight duct which opens into the follicular infundibulum or on to the surface. The eccrine duct has a straight dermal portion and a coiled epidermal segment (acrosyringium) which opens onto the skin surface.

The main function of the eccrine glands is sweat production via which excess heat is dissipated from the body. It also serves to excrete substances from the body as well as moisten the palms leading to a better grip. Although the exact function of apocrine glands is not known, it is believed to play a role in human behavioral and sexual interactions via release of pheromones.

Disorders of sweat glands are common and can be due to an alteration in the quantity and quality of sweat production, blockage of their ducts, or benign and malignant neoplasms of the glands.

In this chapter, we will focus on the disorders of eccrine and apocrine sweat glands **(Table 1)**.

TABLE 1: Disorders of eccrine and apocrine sweat glands.

Disorders of sweat glands	
Eccrine glands	*Apocrine glands*
Hyperhidrosis	Bromhidrosis
Hypohidrosis and anhidrosis	Chromhidrosis
Miliaria	Fox–Fordyce disease
Periporitis	Hidradenitis suppurativa
Granulosa rubra nasi	
Neutrophilic eccrine hidradenitis	

DISORDERS OF ECCRINE GLANDS[1,2]

Hyperhidrosis[3,4]

Hyperhidrosis is defined as sweat secretion in excess of the amount required for normal body thermoregulation. This excessive sweating is pathological and occurs in low temperature and low stress settings as opposed to physiological sweating. It can be divided into two types: (1) Primary and (2) Secondary.

Primary hyperhidrosis is idiopathic and the diagnostic criteria require the presence of at least four of the following factors for a duration of 6 months or more.

- Involvement of eccrine dense areas such as palms, soles, and axilla
- Bilateral and symmetrical
- No episodes at night
- Episodes occurring at least once a week
- Onset at <25 years of age
- Positive family history
- Impaired daily activities

Secondary hyperhidrosis is due to an underlying disease or disorder which secondarily affects the sweat glands.

Depending upon the areas affected, hyperhidrosis can be classified as:

- *Generalized*: Here the hyperhidrosis involves the entire body. Some of the causes are listed here and must be looked for in patients but many times the cause is elusive.
    - Endocrinal disease—diabetes mellitus, hyperthyroidism, and hyperpituitarism
    - Neurological disease—Parkinson's disease, spinal injury, and peripheral neuropathies
    - Infections—febrile episodes in tuberculosis, malaria, etc.
    - Drugs—propranolol, pilocarpine, and tricyclic antidepressants
    - Lymphomas and other solid organ malignancies
    - Menopause, obesity, and pregnancy.

- *Focal:* Here, only certain areas of the body have excessive sweating. There is significant mental and emotional distress due to the symptoms. Most of the cases of hyperhidrosis presenting to the dermatologist tend to be of the focal variant.
  - *Palmoplantar*: There is excessive sweating of the palms and soles and occurs in young adults. It may be continuous or phasic which may be triggered by emotional stimuli. It may be so severe as to cause sweat to drip onto the floor. The hands and feet tend to be cold and acrocyanotic. It may be associated with palmoplantar keratoderma. There is a predisposition to pompholyx, allergic sensitization to footwear, fungal infections, and pitted keratolysis due to maceration of the hands and feet.
  - *Axillary*: Similar to palmoplantar hyperhidrosis, it may be continuous or phasic. There is excessive sweating from the axilla but it tends to not have a foul odor since it is due to overactivity of the eccrine glands and not the apocrine. In some cases, the condition may spontaneously resolve itself in the late twenties.
  - *Craniofacial*: The excessive sweating is localized to the face and scalp, and it is seen in middle-aged people. It may be triggered by heat, exercise, or spicy food. It tends to be persistent.
- *Localized*: Here, a circumscribed area of the skin shows hyperhidrosis. It may be due to neurological conditions affecting the sympathetic supply of the sweat gland. It may be compensatory due to loss of activity in adjacent glands due to diabetes, neurological conditions, or after sympathectomy. It may even be due to sweat gland nevi.
- *Cold-induced*: In this condition, paradoxically, there is hyperhidrosis on cold exposure and anhidrosis/hypohidrosis due to heat. Other features may be associated like a high-arched palate, kyphoscoliosis, and neuropathy.
- *Gustatory*: Sweating in response to spicy food is physiological in many persons, and it is bilateral and symmetrical but gustatory hyperhidrosis may be pathological in conditions involving the autonomic nervous system. The most common cause is trauma to the sympathetic nerves on the head and neck resulting in misalignment during regeneration. Here, the sweating is generally unilateral and involves specific areas such as preauricular or submental.

For example, in Frey's syndrome, trauma or surgery in the parotid areas causes damage to the auriculotemporal nerves which while regenerating synapse in such a way that chewing which normally causes parotid secretion, instead causes localized sweating over the skin overlying the parotid gland. The parasympathetic fibers meant to stimulate the secretomotor function of the parotid gland join instead with the sympathetic fibers innervating the overlying sweat glands and blood vessels.[5] Damage to the chorda tympani nerve during surgery around submandibular gland causes sweating on the submental area while eating. This is known as chorda tympani syndrome. In a similar manner, injury to the vagus nerve during cervical sympathectomy causes gustatory sweating localized to the upper arm. It may also be seen in diabetes or after herpes zoster.

Management of Hyperhidrosis

- Trigger avoidance—such as spicy food, alcohol, and highly-charged emotional provocations.
- Clothing—avoid tight clothing and synthetic fabrics, frequent change of socks, and use of talcum powder.
- Topical antiperspirants—for focal cases, 6.25–40% aluminum chloride hexahydrate can be applied to dry skin once at night and left on for 6–8 hours. They form precipitates that block the sweat ducts and reduce perspiration.
- Oral anticholinergics—used in generalized hyperhidrosis and treatment-resistant cases. Glycopyrrolate is commonly used at a dose of 1–2 mg bd. Oxybutynin can be started at 2.5 mg OD going up to 15 mg OD. Side effects such as dry mouth, blurred vision, drowsiness, and urinary retention may prove troublesome for the patients. It is not approved by the Food and Drug Administration (FDA).
- Iontophoresis—primarily for palmoplantar hyperhidrosis. It uses galvanic current transmission through undamaged skin immersed in water. Interference with electrochemical gradient of sweat secretion and blockade of sympathetic transmission is thought to be the mechanism of action. Multiple sessions are required.
- Botulinum toxin A—injection of BTX into the dermal-subcutaneous junction prevents the cholinergic transmission to eccrine sweat glands. It is immensely useful in axillary and palmoplantar hyperhidrosis. It is FDA approved and requires 1–2 sessions per year for maintenance.
- Sweat reduction devices—such as microwave thermolysis, ultrasound therapy, and fractional microneedle radiofrequency.
- Surgery—this is the last resort when all other treatments have failed. Local techniques include excision, curettage, and liposuction. In severe cases, sympathectomy may be performed.

Anhidrosis/Hypohidrosis

Decreased sweat production (hypohidrosis) or absent sweat production (anhidrosis) may occur due to neurological causes (organic brain lesions, spinal cord lesions, tabes dorsalis, syringomyelia, Ross syndrome, peripheral neuropathies, diabetes, leprosy, etc.) or conditions causing atrophy or obstruction of the sweat gland and duct such as miliaria, psoriasis, eczema, burns, scleroderma. It is also seen in congenitally absent or reduced sweat glands as in anhidrotic ectodermal dysplasia or congenital sensory neuropathy type IV. Since the body's temperature control mechanism is dysregulated due to impaired sweat production, symptoms include fatigue, drowsiness, and fever.

Localized hypohidrosis can be due to various causes, leprosy being an important one.

Miliaria

Miliaria occurs in hot and humid conditions when there is an obstruction to the eccrine sweat ducts leading to the leakage of eccrine sweat into the epidermis. Depending upon the level at which the obstruction occurs, the different types may present as follows:

- *Miliaria crystallina*: It is also known as sudamina, here, the obstruction is at the level of the stratum corneum. Consequently, the leaked sweat pools superficially in the form of clear, thin-walled noninflammatory vesicles 1–2 mm in size. They are asymptomatic and develop on the trunk in crops after a febrile episode. After rupturing, these vesicles desquamate with thin branny scales.
- *Miliaria rubra*: The obstruction of the sweat duct is at the deeper epidermal level. There is keratinization of the sweat ducts associated with leakage of sweat. Clinically, there is appearance of multiple erythematous papules on the trunk, flexures, and areas of friction by clothing or jewelry. These papules are intensely itchy and have a pricking sensation, hence the condition is also known as prickly heat.
- *Miliaria profunda*: Following repeated attacks of miliaria rubra, there may be rupture of the eccrine duct at or below the dermoepidermal junction leading to formation of 1–3 mm sized pale, firm, and asymptomatic papules on the trunk.

Miliaria causes severe discomfort but after a few months of acclimatization to the heat and humidity, the intensity decreases. Miliaria may be complicated by superadded bacterial infection leading to the formation of pustules (miliaria pustulosa). Permanent damage to the sweat ducts may cause disturbance of temperature regulation.

Treatment is by avoidance of sweating via cool baths, use of fans, and air coolers. Avoidance of restrictive clothing also helps. Calamine lotion combined with emollients reduces the discomfort. Vitamin C orally has been found to be helpful.[6]

Periporitis[7,8]

Periporitis is a condition wherein there are multiple sweat gland abscesses. This may be a primary pyoderma of the eccrine sweat glands or it may occur as a secondary complication of miliaria. It is seen in infants and young children mostly over the face. *Staphylococcus aureus* is the usual culprit. This condition is common in summers, especially in hot countries.

Clinically, the hallmark is single or multiple dome-shaped, erythematous papules without a tendency to point. When untreated, there is development of pus in the center and a breakdown of the lesion. Diagnosis is mostly clinical and the child is treated with oral and topical antibiotics. Measures must be taken to keep the child in a cool environment to prevent a recurrence.

Granulosa Rubra Nasi

This is a rare condition involving hyperhidrosis of the nose and surrounding skin. Symptoms start in childhood and generally resolve at the time of puberty. Sometime sit may persist into adulthood. Initially, there is only excess visible sweating on the tip of the nose. Over time other skin changes such as redness, telangiectasias, papules, vesicles develop over the nose, cheeks, and lips. This condition does not require any treatment but if the patient insists, botulinum toxin A injection can be considered.

Neutrophilic Eccrine Hidradenitis[1,9]

As the name suggests, this is an acute inflammation of the eccrine sweat glands. On biopsy, there is degeneration of the eccrine sweat glands along with a dense neutrophilic infiltration, and hence this condition is considered to be part of the neutrophilic dermatoses. Following types are seen:

- Chemotherapy-induced—this usually presents around 8–10 days after administration of chemotherapy drugs such as cytarabine, daunorubicin, and vincristine, with tender red papules and plaques on the face and extremities. It usually resolves within 2 weeks of the stopping the chemotherapy but tends to recur with further courses.
- Infectious—mostly occurs due to *Serratia,* staphylococci, and streptococci infections in immunocompromised patients. Common underlying conditions are hematological malignancies and solid-organ cancers.
- Palmoplantar—this is a self-resolving condition mainly seen in otherwise well children with no underlying disease. They present with tender plaques and nodules on soles more often than on palms.
- Associated with HIV infection
- Associated with Behçet's disease

In most of the cases, there is spontaneous resolution without scarring within a few days to weeks. In some patients, dapsone, colchicine, and systemic steroids have been used to manage the condition and also prevent a recurrence.

DISORDERS OF APOCRINE GLANDS

As the apocrine glands do not become completely functional until puberty, the disorders of these glands only start to manifest after that age.

Bromhidrosis[4]

Apocrine secretions are generally odorless but in the moist areas of the axilla, there is a proliferation of microorganisms such as *Staphylococcus, Micrococcus,* corynebacteria, and propionibacteria which act upon these secretions to release volatile fatty acids and thioalcohols which have an offensive odor. This excessive and offensive odor is known as bromhidrosis (Greek: bromos—stench, hidros—sweat). Poor hygiene can further exacerbate the condition. The patient may be aware of the malodor himself or may be made conscious by friends and family. Management is by general measures such as curbing dietary garlic, frequent baths, use of local antibacterial substances (clindamycin, erythromycin), antiperspirants, deodorants, and fragrances. Reduction of eccrine sweating may reduce the malodor by making the area less conducive for the growth of microorganisms. Hence, botulinum toxin injection and local surgeries may be considered in severe and resistant cases.

Chromhidrosis

This condition involves the secretion of apocrine sweat which may be colored blue, yellow, or green. This occurs due to the release of lipofuscin which lends its color to the apocrine sweat. It occurs at the time of puberty and may naturally fade away in old age. It may be exacerbated by exercise and emotional provocation. The most common site affected is the axilla. Others include the face and nipples. Sometimes, even the breast milk may have a green or blue tinge. Treatment options include topical capsaicin especially for the face and nipples, and botulinum toxin injections in the axillary areas.

Apocrine Miliaria (Fox–Fordyce Disease)[10]

Similar to the eccrine gland miliaria, apocrine miliaria is caused by obstruction of the apocrine duct at the follicular infundibulum. It is a rare condition with a female preponderance. It is seen soon after puberty in areas with apocrine abundance such as the axilla, nipples, and anogenital areas. Recently, there has been an increased incidence secondary to laser hair reduction procedures.[11,12] They present as skin-colored, dome-shaped, and uniform follicular papules which are intensely itchy. This condition tends to persist until old age when the apocrine glands senesce. Pregnancy may offer an interim relief in some cases.

Treatment is not very satisfactory. They involve use of topical or intralesional steroids, topical clindamycin, adapalene, and tacrolimus. Ultraviolet radiation and oral retinoids may be helpful. There has been some interest in use of fractional CO_2 lasers and pulsed-dye lasers to treat this condition.[13,14]

Hidradenitis Suppurativa (Acne Inversa/Apocrinitis)

This is a chronic and relapsing disorder characterized by suppurative follicular papules, pustules, and nodules in the apocrine areas such as genitocrural areas and axilla. It often becomes indolent due to subcutaneous extension with induration, scarring, and sinus formation.

It is commonly seen in young females, usually after the onset of puberty. Obstruction of the apocrine gland follicle obstructs the outflow of the apocrine gland in addition to that of the sebaceous gland, and is believed to be the initiating event in hidradenitis. Genetic factors play a role. Smoking, obesity, and hormonal factors may contribute. *Staphylococcus* and streptococci are frequently isolated from the lesions and bacterial infection seems to be important in the extension of the disease and probably in the destructive scarring.

The disease is characterized by multiple papules, nodules, and pustules. The nodules coalesce to form abscesses which rupture to form sinus tracts and have a recurrent discharge. Comedones, often polyporous, are usually present on or next to the affected skin **(Fig. 1)**.[15-17]

The axillae and the perineal region (including genital, pubic, inguinal and perianal areas, buttocks, and upper thighs) are therefore the main sites, the more severe disease usually occurring in the latter. Hidradenitis suppurativa can be associated with acne conglobata, dissecting cellulitis of the scalp and pilonidal sinus, together forming the follicular occlusion triad. Differential diagnosis includes scrofuloderma, actinomycosis, granuloma inguinale, and lymphogranuloma venereum.

The condition is difficult to treat. Improvement in local hygiene including weight reduction in the obese and the use of antiseptic–detergent agents for washing is advised. Acute episodes and relapses should be treated as bacterial infections. The anti-inflammatory effects of systemic corticosteroids may be useful in acute exacerbations. Treatment modalities include isotretinoin, antibiotics and immunosuppressives, and biologics such as adalimumab. Surgery should be considered in refractory cases. Relatively minor techniques include deroofing or exteriorization of sinus tract, curettage and electrocoagulation of sinus tracts, CO_2 laser excision, and simple excision of troublesome areas with direct closure or grafting **(Fig. 1)**.

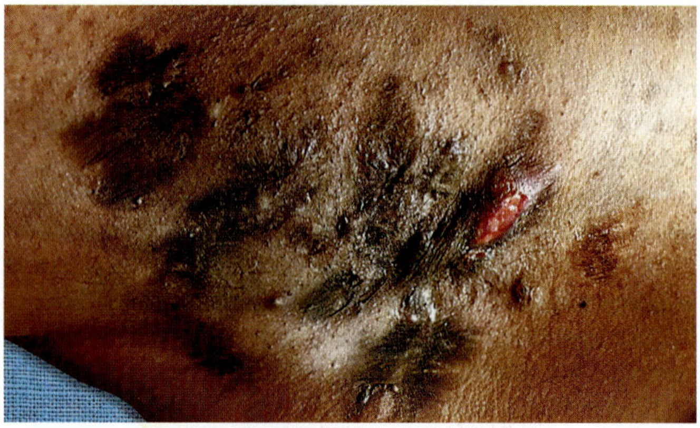

Fig. 1: Hidradenitis suppurativa.
Courtesy: Dr Koushik Lahiri.

CONCLUSION

Disorders of eccrine and apocrine sweat glands, while not life-threatening, have a considerable effect on the quality of life of the patients and as such all efforts must be made to manage and treat the conditions to the patients' satisfaction and comfort.

KEY POINTS

- Primary hyperhidrosis is mainly seen in children, emotional stress precipitates excessive sweating of the palms and soles. Secondary hyperhidrosis can be due to neurological cause, endocrine disorder, drugs, or malignancy.
- Hypohidrosis can be due to congenital ectodermal dysplasias, sensory neuropathy, neurological causes, and drugs.
- Hidradenitis suppurativa is a chronic disorder usually seen in young adult females. It is characterized by suppurative scarring follicular papules, pustules, and nodules in the apocrine areas and the formation of multiple sinuses, double comedones, and cribriform and bridging scars.

REFERENCES

1. Coulson IH, Wilson NJE. Disorders of the Sweat Glands. In: Griffiths C, Barker J, Blelker T, Chalmers R, Creamer D (Eds). Rook's Textbook of Dermatology, 9th edition. UK: Wiley-Blackwell Publication; 2016. pp. 94.1-18.
2. Babu KKR. Disorders of sweat glands. In: Valia RG, Valia AR, (Eds). IADVL Textbook of Dermatology, 3rd edition. Mumbai: Bhalani Publishing House; 2008. pp. 799-828.
3. Nawrocki S, Cha J. The etiology, diagnosis, and management of hyperhidrosis: a comprehensive review—therapeutic options. J Am Acad Dermatol. 2019;81(3):669-80.
4. Semkova K, Gergovska M, Kazandjieva J, Tsankov N. Hyperhidrosis, bromhidrosis, and chromhidrosis: Fold (intertriginous) dermatoses. Clin Dermatol. 2015;33(4): 483-91.
5. Sato K, Wang KH, Saga K, Sato KT. Biology of sweat glands and their disorders. II. Disorders of sweat gland functions. J Am Acad Dermatol. 1989;20:713-26.
6. Hindson TC, Worsley DE. The effects of administration of ascorbic acid in experimentally induced miliaria and hypohidrosis in volunteers. Br J Dermatol. 1969;81(3):226-7.
7. Maibach HI, Kligman AM. Multiple sweat gland abscesses. JAMA. 1960;174:140-2.
8. Dhar S. Infections and Infestations. In: Dhar S (Ed). Color Atlas and Synopsis of Pediatric Dermatology, 3rd edition. Jaypee Brothers Medical Publishers; 2019. p. 86.
9. Bachmeyer C, Aractingi S. Neutrophilic eccrine hidradenitis. Clin Dermatol. 2000;18(3):319-30.
10. Yost J, Robinson M, Meehan SA. Fox-Fordyce disease. Dermatol Online J. 2012;18(12):28.
11. Sammour R, Nasser S, Debahy N, El Habr C. Fox-Fordyce Disease: An under-diagnosed adverse event of laser hair removal? J Eur Acad Dermatol Venereol. 2016;30(9):1578-82.
12. Bernad I, Gil P, Lera JM, Giménez de Azcárate A, Irarrazaval I, Idoate MÁ. Fox-Fordyce disease as a secondary effect of laser hair removal. J Cosmet Laser Ther. 2014;16(3):141-3.
13. Ahmed Al-Qarqaz F, Al-Shannag R. Fox-Fordyce disease treatment with fractional CO_2 laser. Int J Dermatol. 2013;52(12): 1571-2.
14. Fordyce disease with pulsed dye laser. Photodermatol Photoimmunol Photomed. 2016;32(5-6):311-3.
15. Fitzsimmons JS, Guilbert PR, Fitzsimmons EM. Evidence of genetic factors in hidradenitis suppurativa. Br J Dermatol. 1985;113:1-8.
16. Highet AS, Warren RE, Weeks AJ. Bacteriology and antibiotic treatment of perineal suppurative hidradenitis. Arch Dermatol. 1988;124:1047-51.
17. Bell BA, Ellis H. Hydradenitis suppurativa. JR Soc Med. 1978; 71:511-5.

EXAMINATION QUESTIONS

1. Classify sweat gland disorders.
2. Enumerate the causes of hyperhidrosis and their management.
3. Write short note on hidradenitis suppurativa.
4. How will you approach to a case of hyperhidrosis?

74 CHAPTER Alopecias

Bela J Shah

INTRODUCTION

Hair loss is increasingly becoming a common reason to visit a medical professional especially a dermatologist. The causes of hair loss are varied hence the diagnosis and treatment become challenging at times.

Trichoscopy and biopsy are invaluable tools in the hands of a trained dermatologist. Treatment should be directed at addressing the cause, wherever possible.

HAIR

Hair is a protein filament that grows from follicles found in the dermis, the innermost layer of the skin. It is a unique appendageal organ of the skin associated with a heightened cosmetic importance and minimal phylogenetic significance.

Structure of Hair (Figs. 1 and 2)

Longitudinal section of hair: It is made of three parts:

1. *Hair shaft*: The part of hair visible above the skin.
2. *Hair follicle*: The part of hair embedded in skin.
3. *Hair bulb*: The deeper distended part of the follicle.

Structure of the Hair Follicle[1]

- *Upper segment*:
  - Infundibulum
  - Isthmus
- *Lower segment*:
  - Bulb
  - Stem

Bulb: A follicular papilla is located at the center of the bulb which contains follicular germinative keratinocytes that divide every 24–48 hours to form inner six layers of the hair follicle. Melanocytes are found interspersed between them.

Upper bulb comprises cells that undergo complete keratinization to form hard anucleated keratin. This area is called Adamson's fringe.

Stem: Extends from the Adamson's fringe up to the insertion of arrector pilorum (bulge).

Isthmus: Narrow part of follicle between the attachment of arrector pilorum and opening of the sebaceous duct.

Infundibulum: Funnel-shaped connection of follicular canal with the surface epidermis.

Structure of the Hair Shaft

From inner to outer layers:

Medulla: It may be absent or interrupted at times. It consists of few layers of rounded cells containing glycogen vacuoles that turn into air-filled cavities as the hair grows out.

Cortex: It forms the bulk of the hair shaft. It consists of numerous layers of elongated flattened cells packed together.

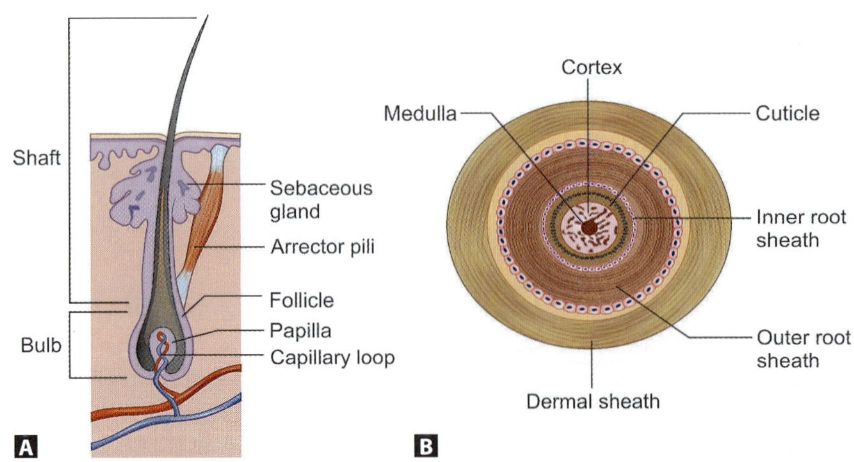

Figs. 1A and B: (A) Structure of hair follicle; (B) Transverse section of structure of hair shaft.

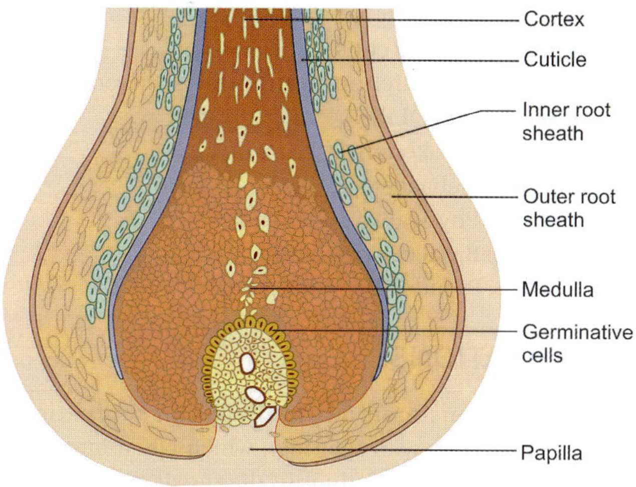

Fig. 2: Longitudinal section of structure of hair shaft.

TABLE 1: Functions of hair.

Vital functions (lost during evolution except on scalp and eyelashes)	*Accessory functions*
Protection against cold and sunlight	Cosmesis
Mechanical protection	Screen nasal passage
Disseminate apocrine odor	Tactile sense
Camouflage	Minimize intertriginous friction

Flowchart 1: Classification of alopecia.

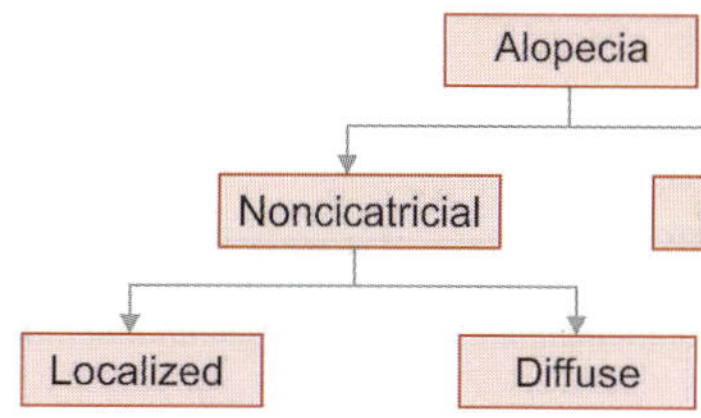

Cuticle: It consists of 5–10 layers of flattened cells arranged in roof tile pattern.

Inner root sheath (IRS): Molds the emerging hair shaft. It disintegrates and disappears at the isthmus:
- Cuticle of IRS
- *Huxley's layer*: It has 4–6 layers of elongated cells
- *Henle's layer*: It has two layers of thick cells. It is the first layer to get keratinized.

Outer root sheath: It is continuous with the surface epidermis through which its terminal part, the acrotrichium, passes.

Perifollicular fibrous sheath: It is a thin layer of connective tissue that envelopes the hair follicle throughout its length.

Types of Hair

Hair is classified into three main types:
1. *Lanugo hair (wool like)*: Fine and soft hair of fetus which is shed in utero.
2. *Vellus hair*: Fine, short, nonmedullated, and nonpigmented hair present on most part of body.
3. *Terminal hair*: Long, coarse, medullated, and pigmented hair present on scalp, eyebrows, eyelashes, pubis, axilla, beard, and moustache. A normal scalp averages seven terminal hairs per vellus hair.

Hair Cycle and Growth

Hair passes through following stages of growth and shedding:
1. *Growth phase/anagen*: Has pigmented angulated bulb. Duration is 2–7 years.
2. *Involution phase/catagen*: Duration is 2–3 weeks.
3. *Resting phase/telogen*: Hair shows depigmented club-shaped bulb. Duration is 2–3 months.

- *Shedding phase/teloptosis*: Club hair is eventually shed by active process called exogen.
- *Kenogen/lag phase*: Hair follicle remains empty.

Average rate of growth of hair in different parts of body:[1]
- *Scalp hair*: 0.45 mm/day
- *Beard hair*: 0.35 mm/day
- *Extremities*: 0.25 mm/day.

Functions of Hair (Table 1)

Hair has no vital function in humans, yet it is esthetic and psychological functions are extremely important, as any clinical dermatologist can readily attest to it from daily practice. It can be distressing to have excess or lack of hair.

ALOPECIA

Alopecia or baldness refers to a loss of hair from part of the head or body. Typically, at least the head is involved. The severity of hair loss can vary from a small area to the entire body.

Classification of Alopecia

Classification of alopecia is shown in **Flowchart 1**.

Noncicatricial Alopecia

Type of loss of hair without the presence of scarring: In this type of alopecias, follicles appear preserved on clinical and histological examination, although they can sometimes be difficult to appreciate when miniaturized. The three most common forms of nonscarring alopecias are androgenetic alopecia (AGA), telogen effluvium, and alopecia areata (AA).

Localized type of noncicatricial alopecia:
- Alopecia areata
- Trichotillomania
- Pressure alopecia
- Loose anagen syndrome
- Hair shaft disorders.

Generalized type of noncicatricial alopecia:

- *Congenital and hereditary alopecias*:
  - Congenital universal atrichia
  - Hereditary vitamin D resistant rickets
  - Ectodermal dysplasia
  - Trichorhinophalangeal syndrome.
- *Alopecia due to hair cycle defects:*
  - Telogen hair loss
  - Anagen hair loss
  - Short anagen syndrome.
- *Alopecia due to hair shaft defects:*
  - Hair fractures
  - Hair nodes
  - Hair narrowings
  - Hair twists and curls
  - Hair bands
  - Unruly hairs.
- *Others:*
  - Alopecia totalis (AT)
  - Alopecia universalis (AU).

Cicatricial Type of Hair Loss

Permanent loss of hair is due to destruction of hair follicles.

Its causes are:

- *Congenital*: Aplasia cutis
- *Inflammatory*: Lichen planopilaris, discoid lupus erythematosus (DLE)
- *Infective*: Favus, kerion
- *Nevi*: Nevus sebaceous
- *Traumatic*: Physical and chemical
- *Neoplastic*: Basal cell carcinoma
- *Idiopathic*: Pseudopelade of Brocq.

INVESTIGATIONS

There are various methods available for evaluation of patients presenting with hair loss, which when interpreted with caution, provide valuable diagnosis and facilitate management of the patient.

Detailed history covering this questionnaire includes duration of hair loss, patient's nutritional status, occupation, any concomitant medical or surgical illness in order to exclude conditions such as telogen effluvium. To evaluate hair loss, multiple tools are used, as shown in **Table 2**.

The trichoscopic findings of alopecia are described in **Flowchart 2**.

TABLE 2: Evaluation of hair loss.

Test	*Description*
Trichoscopy[2]	Done by handheld dermatoscope. Rapid and high-resolution examination of scalp to measure hair growth parameters such as hair diameter, hair length, and to assess signs of inflammation
Videodermoscopy	Permits rapid and high-resolution photographs with several magnifications which can be captured and stored. It also helps to identify ideal site to take biopsies
Wood's lamp examination	Uses wavelength 320–450 nm, peak 365 nm. Used mainly for tinea capitis. Fluorescence results due to pteridine
Daily hair counts	• Helps to assess hair bulb and hair shaft • Helps to distinguish telogen effluvium from anagen effluvium and active diffuse alopecia areata
Hair pull test	• Traction test or Sabouraud's sign • More than 10% hairs if pulled out means positive pull test, indicates active hair shedding
Hair pluck test	• It is done mainly to assess percentage of scalp hairs in different phase of hair cycle and thus helps to identify the hair cycle-related growth disorders • Normally 80–88% of hairs are in anagen, 10–20% in telogen, and 1–2% in catagen
Unit area trichogram	• It refers to the proportion of the various types of hairs counted after epilating all hairs in small marked out area (300 mm^2) • Anagen, catagen, and telogen hairs seen and helps to calculate ratio of anagen to telogen hairs • It helps to know hair density and hair diameter
Wash test	• It helps to differentiate telogen effluvium from female-pattern hair loss • Patients who have at least 10% telogen vellus hairs can be classified as having androgenetic alopecia
Hair weight estimation	Used mainly in clinical trials. Target area hairs are clipped and after a fixed period of time they are collected and subsequently weighed
Trichometry	• Trichometry refers to the measurement of hair diameter as an objective way of assessing patients with alopecia • Dermoscopy and laser beam diffraction can be used for trichometry
Trichotillometry	The mean force required for epilation can be measured by a trichotillometer. The normal epilation force of >36 g reduces to less than 19 g in Kwashiorkor. Easy pluckability of hair is observed in malnutrition and loose anagen hair syndrome
Laboratory investigations	Mainly includes hemoglobin (Hb), serum, serum vitamin B_{12}, and serum TSH (thyroid-stimulating hormone) level to rule out the most common causes of hair loss. Other investigations include hormonal profile in female patients of hair loss showing signs of virilization

Contd...

Contd...

Test	*Description*
Global photography	• A stereotactic positioning device is used • Photographs help to see the difference pre- and post-treatment. Most widely used in clinical practice
Phototrichogram	• It is a noninvasive procedure • It helps in evaluation of scalp at regular interval • It helps in evaluation of hair density, hair thickness, hair length, and linear growth rate
Polarizing light microscopy	• It is the light in which all the rays vibrate in one plane • It is a good tool for diagnosis in hair shaft disorders *Example*: "Tiger tail" appearance (alternate light and dark bands) in trichothiodystrophy
Electron microscopy of hair	• It provides better resolution but is expensive and is used rarely for diagnosis of alopecia • It gives a resolution of about 2 nm *Example*: Loose anagen hair syndrome in which cuticle shows rippled appearance
Confocal microscopy of hair	• Based on principle that the object and its image are having same focus, so that image resolution is increased many time • It helps in understanding morphogenesis of hair and diagnosing conditions such as trichothiodystrophy of hairs
Scalp biopsy	• It is indicated in cases of cicatricial alopecia and undiagnosed cases of noncicatricial alopecia • It helps in assessing stage of hair cycle and for confirmatory diagnosis of cicatricial alopecias • *Cicatricial alopecia*: The punch should be taken from areas of inflammation; two types of sections: (1) Vertical and (2) horizontal (preferred in cicatricial alopecia) • *Noncicatricial alopecia*: A punch in the center of the lesion is appropriate
X-ray diffraction	It is used for ultrastructural studies of normal hair and effects of pollution and hair dye

Flowchart 2: The trichoscopic findings of alopecia.

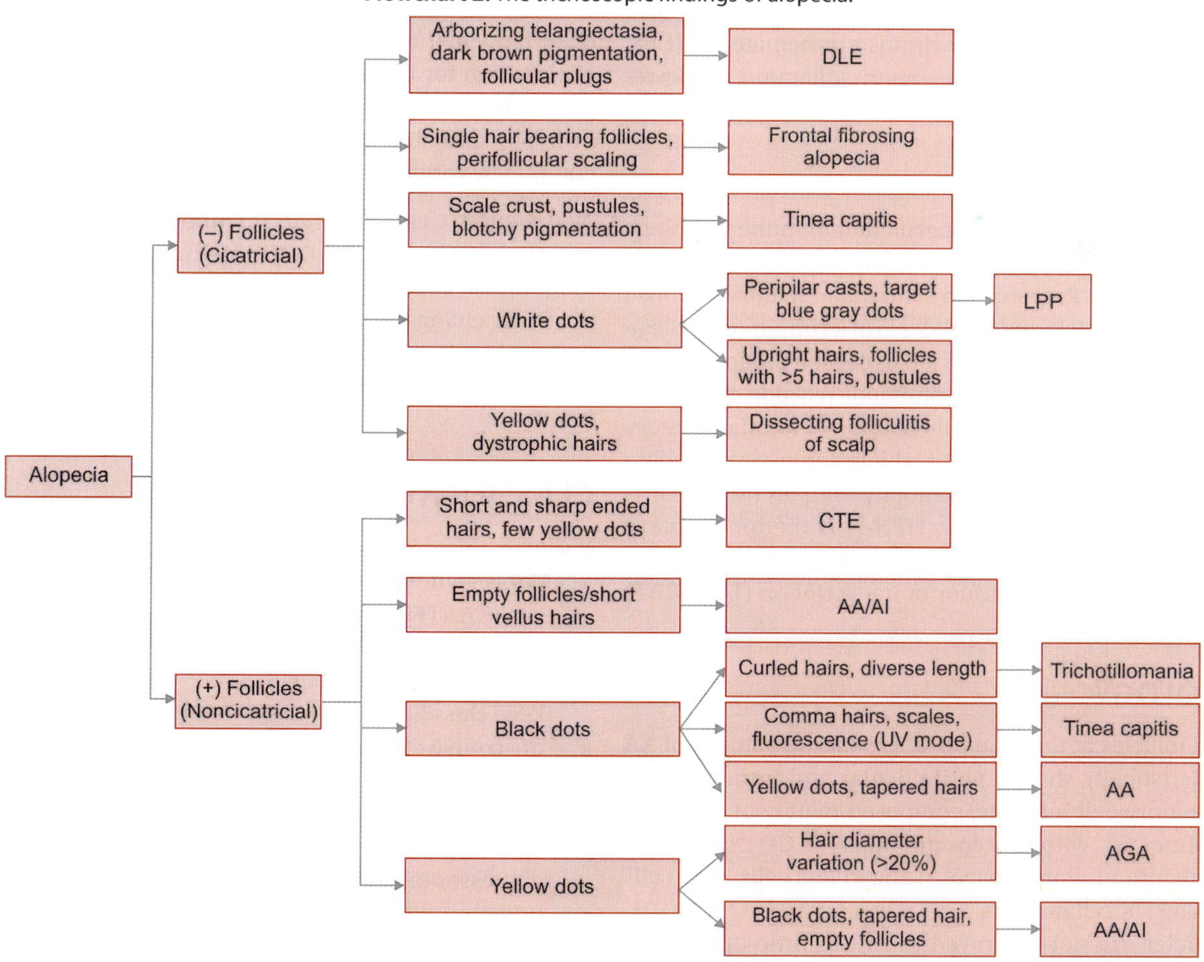

(AA: alopecia areata; AI: alopecia incognito; CTE: chronic telogen effluvium; DLE: discoid lupus erythematosus; LPP: lichen planopilaris; UV: ultraviolet)

ALOPECIA AREATA

INTRODUCTION

Alopecia areata (AA) is a common, chronic, and inflammatory disease that causes reversible nonscarring hair loss. Celsus is credited with describing patterns of hair loss using the Greek word *alopekia*, meaning fox mange. Sauvages coined the term "alopecia areata" in 1763. Among the many factors involved in the pathogenesis of AA, the most important is the T-cell-mediated autoimmune mechanism occurring in genetically predisposed individuals. Environmental factors may be responsible for triggering the disease.

EPIDEMIOLOGY

The average lifetime risk of developing AA is estimated to be 1.7%. The frequency of AA is the same in both sexes. It occurs across all ethnic groups mostly before the age of 40 years, with the peak age of onset between the second and fourth decades.

ASSOCIATED DISEASES

Alopecia areata is associated with several autoimmune diseases including thyroiditis, lupus erythematosus (LE), vitiligo, psoriasis, type 1 diabetes, atopy, inflammatory bowel disease, and autoimmune polyendocrinopathy type 1.

PATHOGENESIS

The etiology of AA is an organ-specific autoimmune pathology to which both genetic predisposition and environmental factors contribute. Perpetuation of the inflammatory response within the hair follicle and breakdown of its immune privilege in genetically predisposed individuals cause a predominantly CD8-driven, Th1-type T-cell autoimmune reaction against the hair follicles that results in acute hair loss. Proinflammatory signals, including substance P and interferon-γ, upregulate expression of major histocompatibility complex (MHC) class Ia inside the hair. Interferon-γ (IFN-γ) is the most potent inducer of ectopic MHC class I expression.[3] Janus kinase-signal transducer and activator of transcription (JAK-STAT) pathway is involved.

PATHOLOGY

Anagen follicles at the margins of expanding patches of AA characteristically show a perifollicular and intrafollicular inflammatory cell infiltrate, composed mainly of activated T-lymphocytes, with a preponderance of CD4 cells, and an admixture of macrophages, Langerhans cells, and cells expressing NK cell markers.

Follicles are not destroyed in AA, as little or none of the inflammatory infiltrate is seen around the isthmus of the hair follicle, the site of hair follicle stem cells. Follicles are smaller than normal and anagen follicles do not develop beyond the anagen III–IV stage.

Genetics

The lifetime risk of AA in the children of a proband is approximately 6%. The strongest allelic associations are with:

- *HLA DQB1*0301*
- *HLA DRB1*1104*

CLINICAL FEATURES

Alopecia areata usually presents as well-defined patches of hair loss on the scalp but any hair-bearing skin can be involved. Typically, the surface of patches is smooth and of normal skin color without any secondary changes such as scaling and follicular changes. The eyebrows and eyelashes are lost in many cases of AA and may be the only sites affected. Characteristic "exclamatory mark hairs" are seen either within or at the border of the patches. These are short hairs with proximal tapering, close to scalp and distal thickening and widening. The diagnosis is mostly clinical. The pigmented hairs are predominantly affected and white hairs are spared. This may result in a dramatic change in hair color if the alopecia progresses rapidly, and is probably the explanation for historical accounts of people "going white overnight." During the regrowth phase, hairs may be non- or hypopigmented but hair pigmentation usually recovers completely within few months.

Nail changes: Classically, fine, multiple, small, and superficial stippled pits regularly distributed along transverse and longitudinal lines are most commonly seen.

Other changes include geometric punctate leukonychia (multiple white spots in a grill pattern), trachyonychia (sandpaper nails), Beau's lines, onychomadesis, and red lunulae.

CLASSIFICATION

Based on the extent of hair loss, it is classified as:

- Alopecia universalis (AU) **(Fig. 3)**
- Patchy AA **(Fig. 4)**
- Alopecia totalis (AT)
- Alopecia subtotalis **(Fig. 5)**.

Ikeda classification is based on the associated conditions and the course of the disease:

- *Common type*: It is most commonly seen and affecting adults aged 20–40 years and AT develops in 5–15% of cases.
- *Atopic type*: It begins early in life and mostly (30–75%) progresses to AT.
- *Autoimmune type*: It is seen in middle-aged groups and is associated with autoimmune diseases, and progresses to AT in 10–50%.

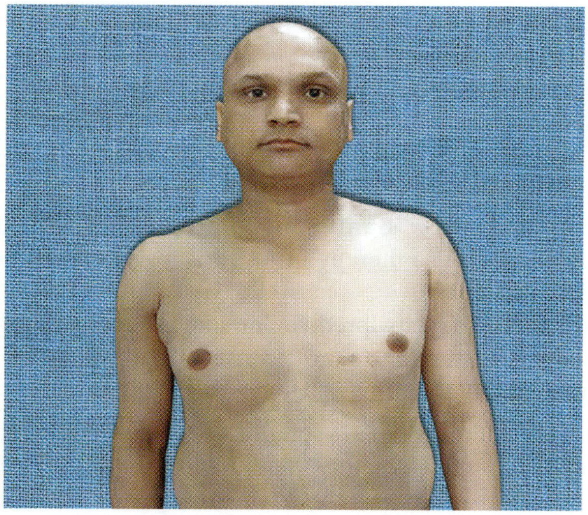

Fig. 3: Alopecia universalis.

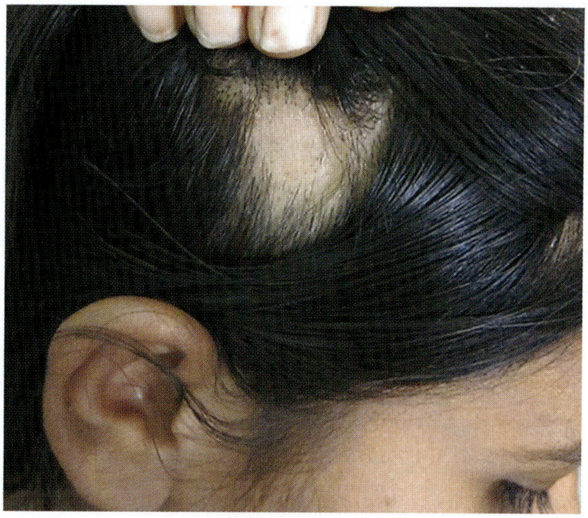

Fig. 4: Patchy alopecia areata.

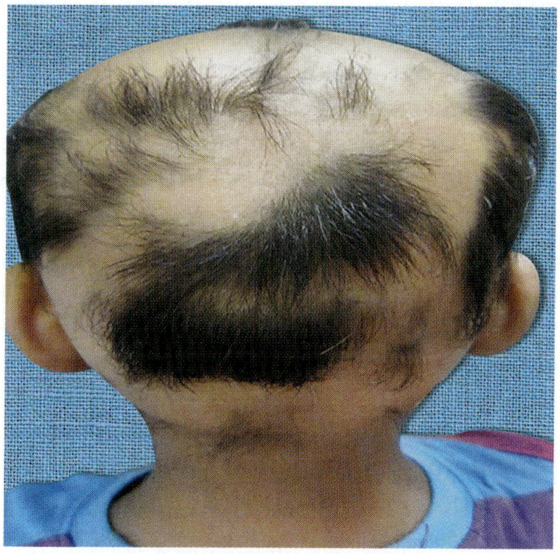

Fig. 5: Alopecia subtotalis.

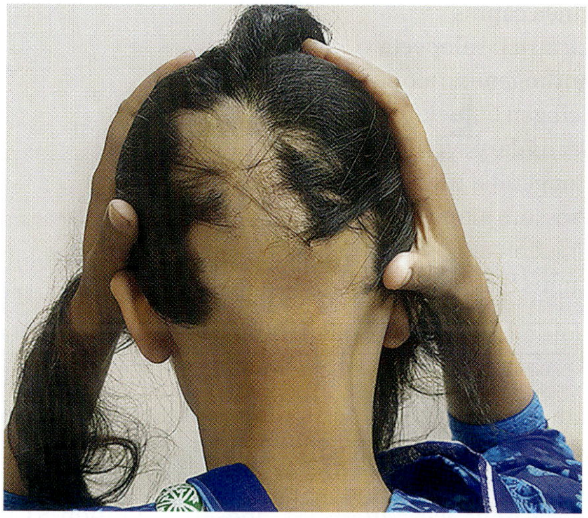

Fig. 6: Ophiasis.
Courtesy: Dr Abhijit Saha.

- *Prehypertensive type*: It is seen in young adults whose parents are hypertensive and progress rapidly to AT in 40% of cases.

Based on the pattern of hair loss, alopecia areata is classified into:

- *Reticular*: Small distinct patches may merge and form larger patches.
- *Ophiasis*: Band-like AA along the posterior occipital and temporal margins **(Fig. 6)**.
- *Sisaipho*: Ophiasis inversus presents with alopecia involving the frontal, temporal, and parietal scalp but spares hair along the scalp periphery, mimicking AGA.
- *Diffuse*: Extends over whole scalp but usually does not affect all hairs. A highly positive pull test will help to differentiate it from other causes.
- *Perinevoid type*: Unusual and rare form with patches around a nevus.

Scoring system in alopecia areata: Severity of alopecia tool (SALT) score is useful to find out the quantitative assessment of scalp hair loss. In SALT score, the entire scalp in divided into four parts based on the surface area: (1) Vertex (top) (40%—0.4); (2) posterior (24%—0.24); (3) right side (18%—0.18); and (4) left side of scalp (18%—0.18). Percentage of hair loss in each area is determined independently and is multiplied by the percentage of scalp covered in that area of the scalp, and summing the products of each area gives the SALT score. SALT score is easily reproducible and validated. However, it does not include hair pigmentation, body hair, and nail involvement.

DIAGNOSIS

The diagnosis of AA is mainly clinical and investigations are usually not needed in majority of the cases. The presence of exclamatory mark hairs at the border and the hair pull test with six or more hairs from the periphery suggests that the patch may be active and progressive.

Shuster described coudability hairs (a kink in the normal looking hairs, at a distance of 5–10 mm above the surface, when the hair was bent inward) in patchy AA.

Characteristic dermoscopic features of AA are yellow dots, black dots, broken hairs, tapering hairs (exclamation marks), cadaverized hairs, and short regrowing vellus hairs. Long-standing cases may reveal empty follicles.

A scalp biopsy may be rarely required, helpful for diffuse AA subtype, and early scarring alopecia. Peribulbar and intrabulbar lymphocytic inflammatory infiltrate resembling "swarm of bees" is characteristic acute phase of AA on histopathology.

DIFFERENTIAL DIAGNOSIS

- Trichotillomania
- Tinea capitis
- Cicatricial alopecia
- Androgenetic alopecia
- Telogen effluvium
- Secondary syphilis
- Congenital triangular alopecia
- Pressure alopecia
- Traction alopecia
- Lupus hair

COURSE AND PROGNOSIS

Spontaneous regrowth occurs in up to 80% of patients of limited AA within 1 year. Poor prognostic factors include younger age of onset, family history, history of atopy, pattern (ophiasis, reticular pattern, AT, and AU), duration >1 year, and presence of nail disease and other autoimmune diseases.

MANAGEMENT

Alopecia areata is mainly a cosmetic concern, causing more emotional problems, especially in children and women. In limited patchy alopecia, a potent topical steroid (e.g., clobetasol), is the first-line management. It is recommended to use 1 cm beyond the involved area. Treatment should be continued for at least 3 months.

Intralesional steroids are also an effective treatment in patchy AA. A depot steroid (hydrocortisone acetate 25 mg/mL or triamcinolone acetonide 5–10 mg/mL) is administered by a 0.5-inch long 30-gauge needle into deep dermis or upper subcutaneous tissue at multiple sites, 1 cm apart and 0.1 mL into each site, once in 4–6 weeks. Local atrophy is a common side effect which recovers within a few months.

In extensive and rapidly progressive AA, long-term 12–16 weeks daily or pulse treatment with oral corticosteroids produces regrowth of hair.

Mini Pulse Corticosteroid Therapy

Oral betamethasone has been given in a dose of 10 mg once weekly. 5 mg of betamethasone is split in two equal doses on two consecutive days in a week.

Prednisolone Pulse Therapy

Few studies show significant improvement with oral prednisolone pulse therapy in AA. It is given 200 mg once weekly.[4]

1,000 mg IV methylprednisolone or 100 mg of dexamethasone pulse therapy on three consecutive days at 1 month intervals for AT and universalis can also be given.

Minoxidil: Minoxidil in 5% solution stimulates proliferation at the base of the bulb and differentiation above the dermal papilla and leads to hair regrowth. Young patients respond better than older patients.

Contact sensitizers: Contact immunotherapy is a well-documented treatment for AA. The patient is sensitized to a potent allergen and the same allergen is then applied to the scalp, usually at weekly intervals, in a concentration sufficient to induce a mild contact dermatitis. The contact allergens commonly used include dinitrochlorobenzene (DNCB), squaric acid dibutylester (SADBE), and diphenylcyclopropenone (DPCP).

Anthralin: Anthralin being an irritant and is effective because of its immunosuppressive and anti-inflammatory properties by generating free radicals. It is used as 0.5–1% cream with short contact therapy. It is applied daily for 20–30 minutes, for 2–3 weeks, gradually increasing contact time daily by 5 minutes up to 1 hour or till erythema and/or pruritus develops and maintained the same time of contact for 3–6 months. It was found to be effective in patchy AA in children <10 years.

Phototherapy: Psoralen and ultraviolet A (PUVA) therapy in combination with oral steroids has been found effective in recalcitrant AT and AU. Mild erythema, burning and increased risk for melanoma are some of the side effects observed with PUVA. Narrowband ultraviolet B (NBUVB) phototherapy has been found ineffective in AA.

Cyclosporine: Oral cyclosporine, 2.5–6 mg/kg/day for 2–12 months in age groups of 12–40 years having various patterns of AA and in treatment resistant patients, is a beneficial treatment option for severe AA.

Cases with poor prognosis-like AT require wigs.

TRICHOTILLOMANIA (FIG. 7)

INTRODUCTION

Trichotillomania is a behavioral disorder characterized by compulsive hair pulling. The term "trichotillomania" is derived from the Greek *thrix*, hair; *tillein*, pulling out; and *mania*, madness. It is seen more commonly in females than in males (7:1) and in children more than adults.

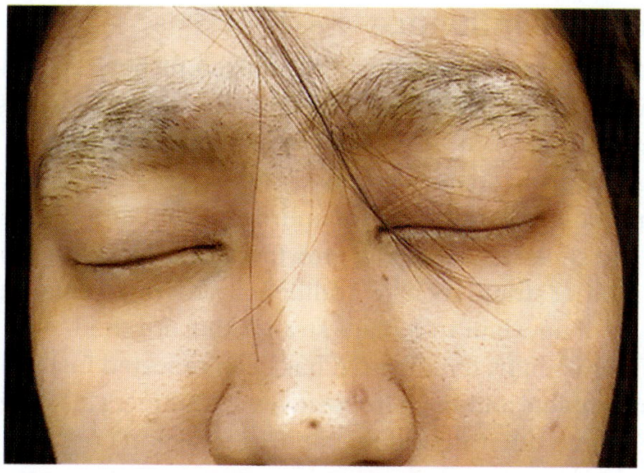

Fig. 7: Trichotillomania.
Courtesy: Dr Aarti Sarda.

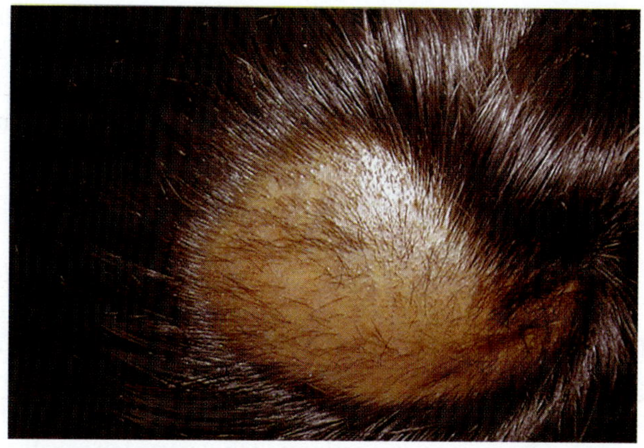

Fig. 8: Irregular, asymmetric patchy alopecia on the scalp.

DSM-IV CRITERIA FOR TRICHOTILLOMANIA

- Recurrent pulling out of one's hair resulting in noticeable hair loss.
- An increasing sense of tension immediately before pulling out the hair or when attempting to resist the behavior.
- Pleasure, gratification, or relief when pulling out the hair.
- The disturbance is not better accounted for by another mental disorder and is not due to a general medical condition (e.g., a dermatological condition).
- The disturbance causes clinically significant distress or impairment in social, occupational, or other important areas of functioning.

Many patients with chronic disease do not meet all the criteria.

CLINICAL FEATURES

Individuals with trichotillomania usually pluck scalp hair most frequently from one frontoparietal area, resulting in irregular and asymmetrical patchy or full alopecia of the scalp **(Fig. 8)**. Patients may also pluck from other hair-bearing regions such as the eyebrows, eyelashes, face, extremities, or pubic region. The patches of hair loss are often in a bizarre or angular pattern, having twisted or broken hair, of variable lengths at various distances from the clinically normal scalp. In young children, the hair-pulling tic develops gradually and unconsciously:

- Broken hair shafts of variable length with longitudinal splitting/fraying
- Coiled and fractured hairs (sometimes resemble a question mark hair)
- Less common findings—yellow dots, short vellus hair, perifollicular erythema, pigmentation, and hemorrhages
- These are histopathological (HP) findings.

Scalp biopsy may be required where dermoscopy is doubtful. Scalp histology will vary according to the severity and duration of the hair plucking. Most consistent feature is the presence of numerous empty canals. Some follicles are severely damaged; there are clefts in the hair matrix, the follicular epithelium is separated from the connective tissue sheath, and there are intraepithelial and perifollicular hemorrhages and intrafollicular pigment casts.

DIFFERENTIAL DIAGNOSIS

The differential diagnosis includes tinea capitis, AA, and monilethrix, which can be excluded by history, physical examination, trichoscopy, KOH examination, fungal culture, and scalp biopsy.

MANAGEMENT

No specific treatment approach has been established as effective. Counseling, hypnosis, behavioral modification therapy, insight-oriented psychotherapy, and pharmacologic therapy, such as clomipramine or selective serotonin-reuptake inhibitors (SSRIs), have all been tried. The habit tic in young children is often self-limiting, but help from a pediatric psychologist can be helpful.

ANDROGENETIC ALOPECIA

(Androgenic Alopecia, Male/Female Pattern Hair Loss/ Patterned or Premature Baldness)

INTRODUCTION

Androgenetic alopecia is one of the most common forms of hair loss in both men and women. Hair loss begins above both temples. Hair also thins at the crown often progressing to partial or complete baldness. The pattern of hair loss in women differs from male-pattern baldness. In women, the hair becomes thinner all over the head, and the hairline does not recede. In women, it rarely leads to total baldness.

Associated diseases: Androgenetic alopecia in men has been associated with several other medical conditions including coronary heart disease and prostate enlargement. Additionally, prostate cancer, disorders of insulin resistance, and hypertension have been related to AGA. In women, this form of hair loss is associated with an increased risk of polycystic ovary syndrome (PCOS). In women, it is found to be associated with hyperaldosteronism, hyperandrogenism, and hypertension.

EPIDEMIOLOGY

The incidence of AGA is generally considered to be greater in males than females, although according to some, this difference in incidence may be a reflection of different expression in males and females. AGA can affect all races, but the prevalence rates vary. Prevalence is considered to be highest in Caucasians. It is estimated that prevalence rates in Caucasian populations is around 30% for men in their 30s, 40% for men in their 40s, and 50% for men in their 50s. In the Indian context, a population-based study of 1,005 subjects showed a 58% prevalence of AGA in males aged 30–50 years. In women, hair loss is most likely after menopause.[5]

Frequency

Androgenetic alopecia is an extremely common disorder that affects roughly 50% of men and perhaps as many women older than 40 years. 13% of premenopausal women reportedly have some evidence of AGA. However, its incidence increases greatly in women following menopause, it may affect 75% of women older than 65 years.

Race

The incidence and the severity of AGA tend to be the highest in white men, second highest in Asians and African Americans, and lowest in Native Americans and Eskimos.

Age

Almost all patients with AGA have an onset prior to age of 40 years, although many of the patients show evidence of the disorder by age of 30 or even by 20 years or even before.

PATHOGENESIS

Genetics

Androgenetic alopecia is postulated to be a dominantly inherited disorder with variable penetrance and expression. However, it may be of polygenic inheritance. This condition tends to cluster in families. Numerous studies have identified two major genetic risk loci. These are the X-chromosomal AR/EDA2R locus and the PAX1/FOXA2 locus on chromosome 20. The *AR* gene provides instructions for making a protein called an androgen receptor. Androgen receptors allow the body to respond appropriately to dihydrotestosterone and other androgens.

In a recent genome-wide association study, *HDAC9* is found to be the third AGA susceptibility gene. In a study, 3q26 site on the X chromosome was found be strongly linked to AGA.[6]

Hormonal Influence

Androgens particularly dihydrotestosterone have key role in pathogenesis of this form of hair loss. Androgen is necessary for progression of AGA, as it is not found in males. The progression of AGA is stopped if postpubertal males are castrated. Increased levels of androgens in hair follicles can lead to a shorter cycle of hair growth and the growth of shorter and thinner strands of hair. Additionally, there is a delay in the growth of new hair to replace strands that are shed.

Interestingly, female AGA has been reported in a patient with complete androgen insensitivity syndrome. This suggests that factors other than direct androgen action contribute to patterned hair loss and systemic or external factors may play a role in AGA.

Hair Follicle Miniaturization (Fig. 9)

Normally on the top of scalp, there are androgen sensitive follicles while on the sides and back of the scalp—androgen independent follicles. In genetically predisposed individual (under influence of androgens) terminal hair follicles are transformed into indeterminate and finally into miniaturized vellus hairs. Follicular miniaturization leaves behind stellae as dermal remnant of full-sized follicle which is a small cluster of elastic fibers in the neck of dermal papilla.

Role of Prostaglandin E2

Garza et al. found elevated levels of prostaglandin D2 synthase at mRNA and protein levels and low levels of prostaglandin E2 (PGE2) in bald scalp. They also showed that both prostaglandin D2 and its nonenzymatic metabolite, 15-deoxy-D12,14-prostaglandin J2, inhibit hair growth in both mouse and human hair follicles.

Hair Cycle Dynamics

There is reduction in anagen and prolongation of telogen phase that corresponds to period of excessive hair shedding, that is responsible for "eraser-like areas" especially in female pattern hair loss (FPHL) **(Table 3)**. Length of each hair shaft is reduced. Terminal : vellus hair ratio is also reduced.

Grading

- *Ludwig scale*: Three-point scale grading of FPHL with diffuse thinning of the crown region with preservation of the frontal hairline **(Fig. 12)**.
- *Sinclair scale*: Five-point scale for grading of FPHL with diffuse thinning of the crown region with preservation of the frontal hairline **(Fig. 13)**:
  - *Grade 1* Is normal. This pattern is found in all girls prior to puberty but in only 45% of women 80 years or over.
  - *Grade 2* Shows a widening of the central part.
  - *Grade 3* Shows a widening of the central part and thinning of the hair on either side of the central part.

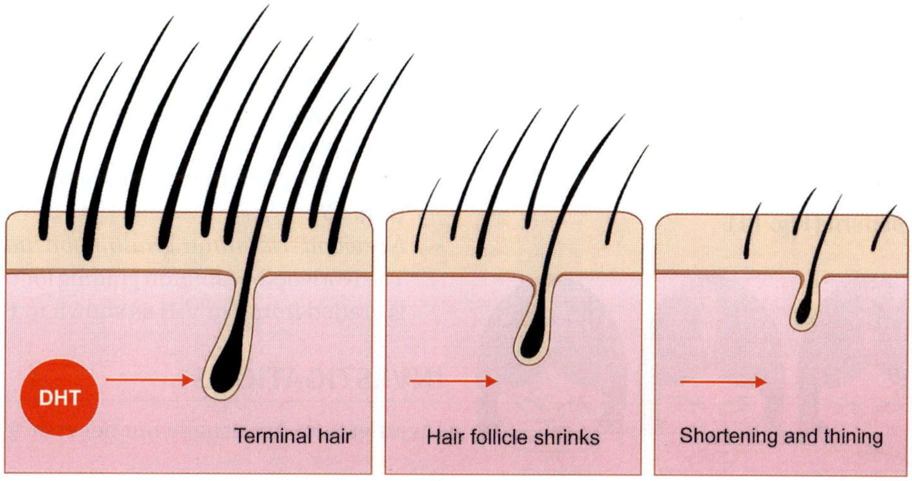

Fig. 9: Hair follicle miniaturization.

TABLE 3: Description of female and male pattern baldness.

Female pattern baldness	*Male pattern baldness*
Alopecia in women; baldness—female; hair loss in women; androgenetic alopecia in women; hereditary balding or thinning in women	Alopecia in men; baldness—male; hair loss in men; androgenetic alopecia
Most common type of hair loss in women	Most common type of hair loss in men
Peak age of onset—third to fourth decade	Peak age of onset—bimodal third and fifth decade
History of first-degree relative with AGA—common	History of first-degree relative with AGA—less common
Causes: • Aging • Changes in the levels of androgens (male hormones). For example, after reaching menopause, many women find that the hair on their head is thinner, while the hair on their face is coarser	*Causes*: • Male pattern baldness is related to genes and male sex hormones. It usually follows a pattern of receding hairline and hair thinning on the crown
Symptoms: • Hair thins mainly on the top and crown of the scalp. It usually starts with a widening of central parting **(Fig. 10)** • The front hairline remains unaffected except for normal recession, which happens to everyone as time passes • The hair loss rarely progresses to total or near total baldness, as it may be seen in men	*Symptoms*: • The typical pattern of male baldness begins at the hairline • The hairline gradually moves backward (recedes) and forms an "M" shape • Eventually the hair becomes finer, shorter, and thinner, and creates a U-shaped (or horseshoe) pattern of hair around the sides of the head • Areas of complete baldness—present **(Fig. 11)**
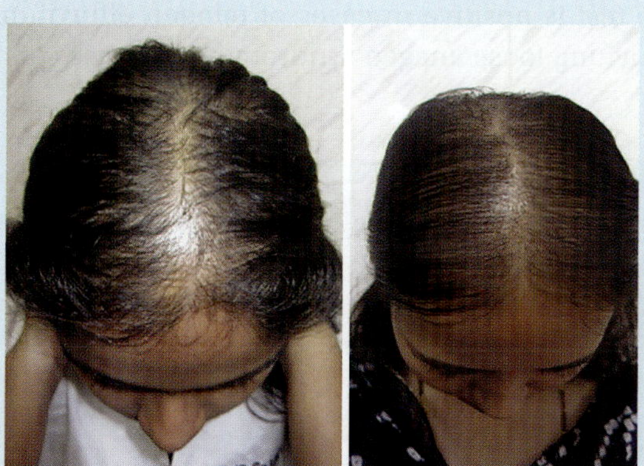 **Fig. 10:** Widening of central partition in FPHL.	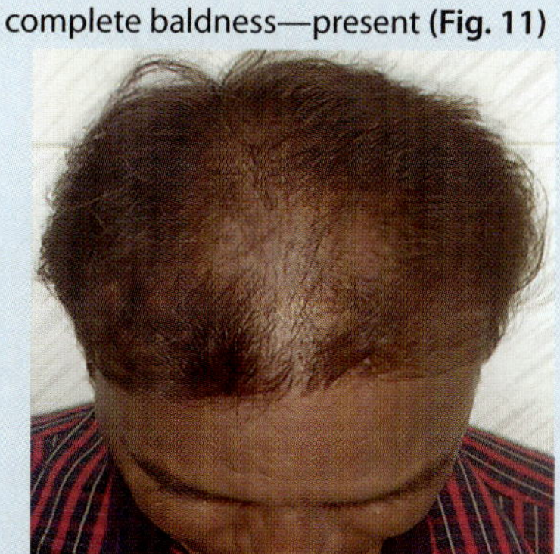 **Fig. 11:** U-shaped pattern of hair loss with areas of complete baldness.
Grading of FPHL: • Ludwig scale • Sinclair scale • Olsen scale • BASP	*Grading*: Norwood–Hamilton grading for male pattern baldness

(AGA: androgenetic alopecia; BSAP: basic and specific; FPHL: female pattern hair loss)

Grade 4 Reveals the emergence of a diffuse hair loss over the top of the scalp.

Grade 5 Indicates advanced hair loss.

- *Olsen scale*: Olsen proposed a classification similar to Ludwig classification but incorporated the accentuation of frontovertical alopecia, which has a triangular or "Christmas tree" pattern **(Fig. 14)**.

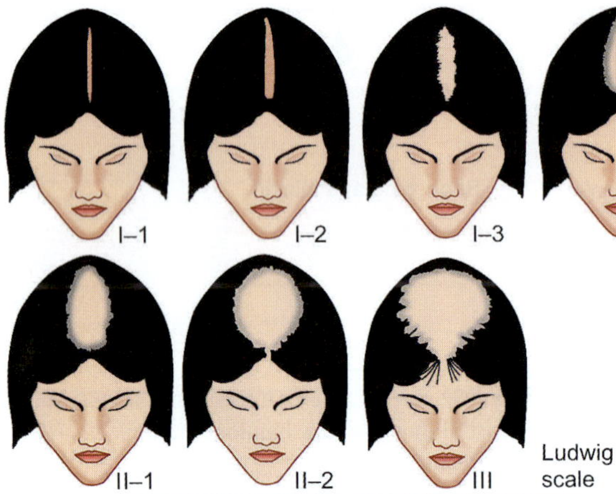

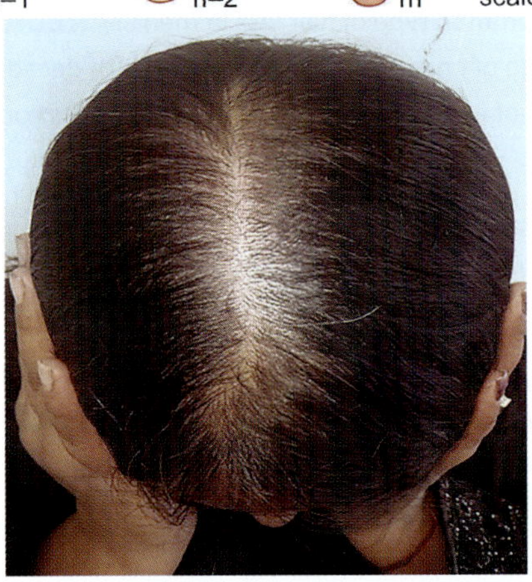

Fig. 12: A 34-year-old female with female pattern hair loss (FPHL) (Ludwig scale—stage I–2).

- *Basic and specific (BASP)*: The BASP classification was designed by Lee et al. This included four basic types and two specific types. The basic type represents the shape of the anterior hairline and the specific type represents the density of hair on the frontal and vertex area. The final type is the combination of the basic and the specific type **(Fig. 15)**.
- *Norwood–Hamilton grading for male pattern baldness:* The Norwood–Hamilton grading for male pattern baldness is graded from I to VIII as shown in **Figure 16**.

INVESTIGATIONS

Investigations are usually not necessary in men with AGA.

Blood Investigations

- *Complete blood count*:
  - Serum ferritin
  - Thyroid function test
  - Fasting lipid profile
  - Fasting glucose.

If there are signs of virilization (such as infertility, hoarseness, clitoromegaly, and increased muscle mass) or hirsutism: Serum testosterone can be done.

Dehydroepiandrosterone sulfate (morning sample on days 1–5 of cycle; make sure the patient is not on oral contraceptive pill):

- 17-hydroxyprogesterone for congenital adrenal hyperplasia
- Androstenedione
- Ovarian ultrasound to rule out polycystic ovarian syndrome
- Adrenal imaging

Pull Test

The test is positive in cases of telogen effluvium, anagen effluvium, loose anagen syndrome, early cases of patterned

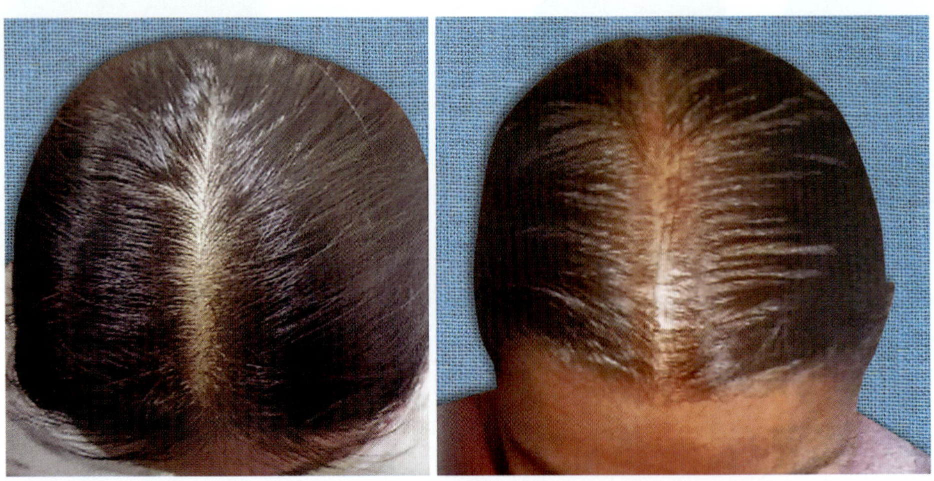

Fig. 13: Females with grade I and III—according to Sinclair scale.

alopecia, and at the advancing edge of AA. In cases of acute telogen effluvium, the pull test is positive over the entire scalp whereas in cases of AGA, it could usually be positive over the area of thinning. But negative tests do not exclude the diagnosis.

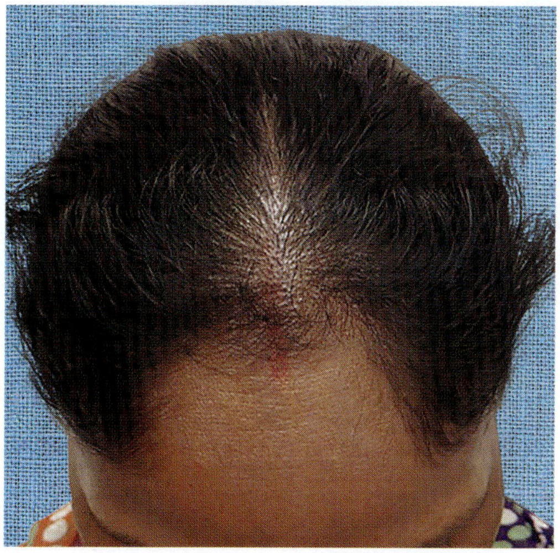

Fig. 14: A 42-year-old female with frontovertical accentuation of female pattern hair loss (FPHL).

Trichoscopy

Trichoscopy of AGA shows anisotrichosis and white dots as shown in **Figure 17**.

Anisotrichosis: Hair diameter diversity >20% vellus hairs.

Peripilar sign: Brown halo, roughly 1 mm in diameter, at the follicular ostium around the emergent hair shaft in early FPHL.

White peripilar signs of larger diameter may be a sign of atrophy which can be present in long-standing FPHL.

Focal atrichia is seen as pencil-erased areas of hair loss in advanced FPHL.

White dots: white spots with diameter ranging from 0.2 to 0.3 mm are distributed uniformly between the follicular ostia and not around the follicular ostia and may be seen in long-standing cases of AGA, represent hypertrophied sebaceous glands. What do they signify?

Yellow dots correspond to dilated follicular infundibulum filled with sebum and keratinous matter.

Histopathology

In evolving-pattern alopecia, the diameter of hair shafts varies. Fibrous tract remnants (so-called streamers) can be

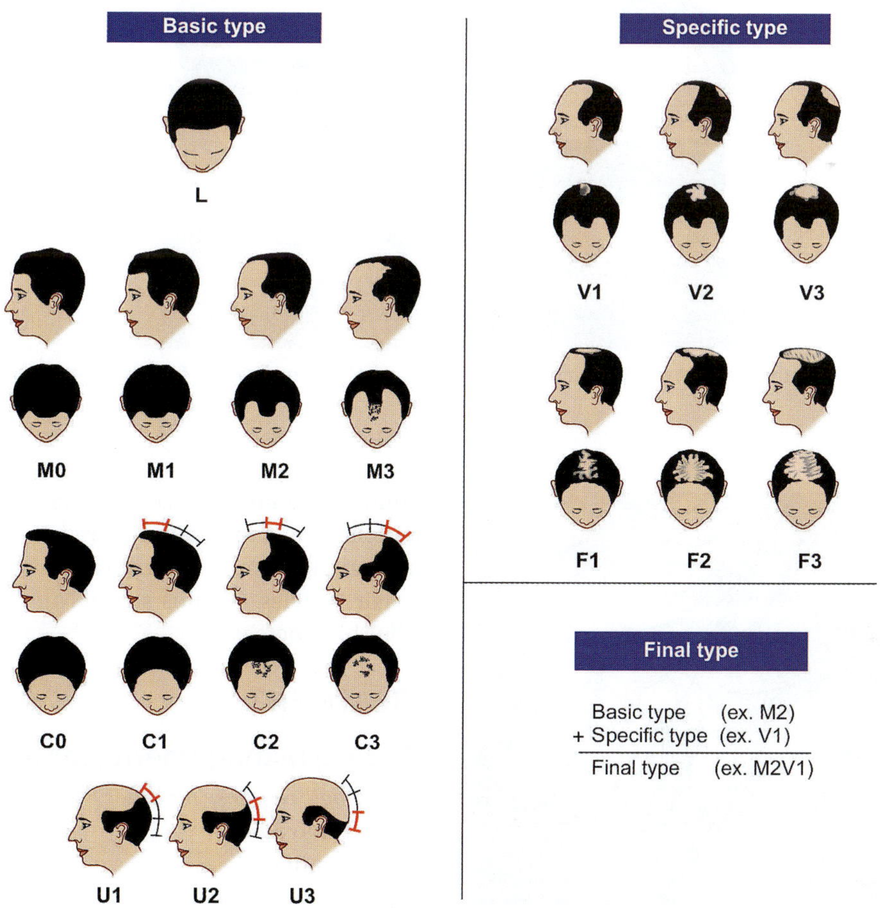

Fig. 15: Basic and specific grading of female pattern hair loss.

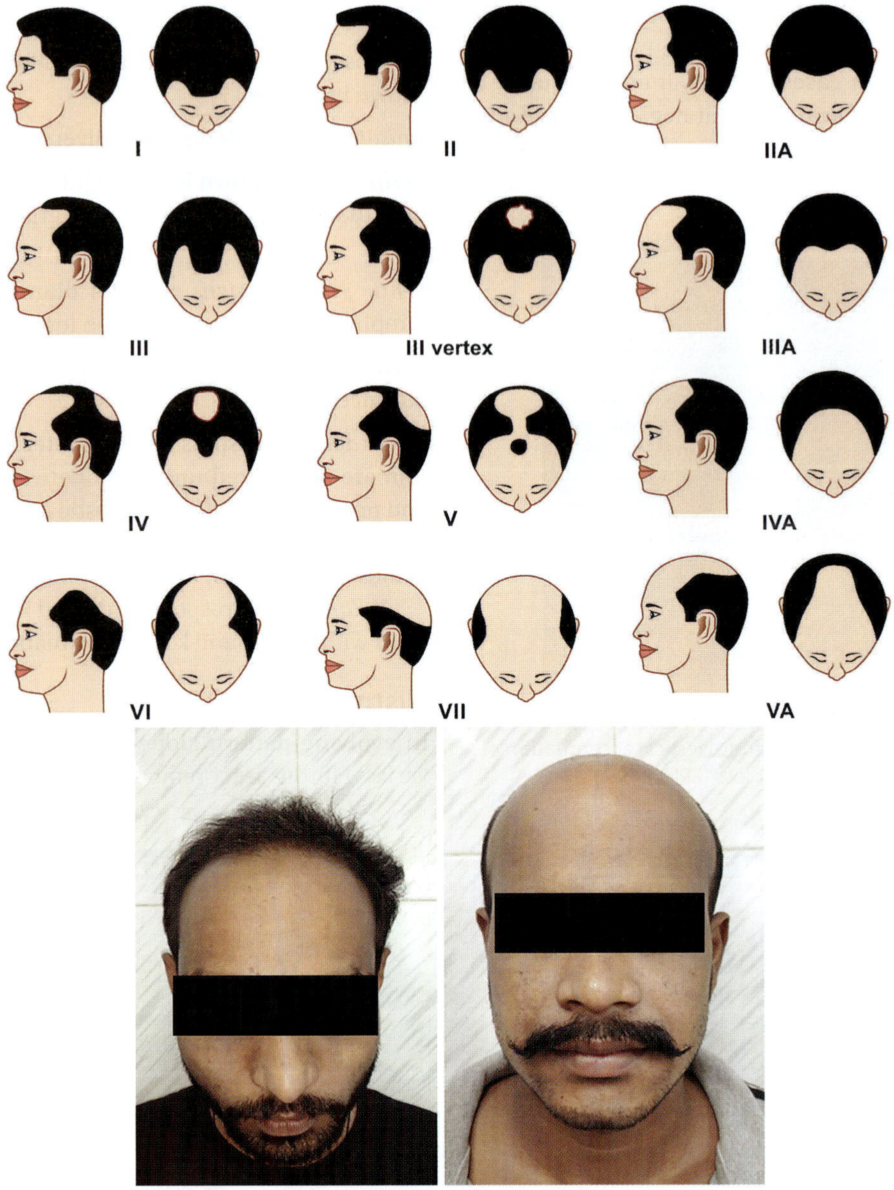

Fig. 16: Males with grade IIIA and V—according to Norwood–Hamilton grading for male pattern baldness.

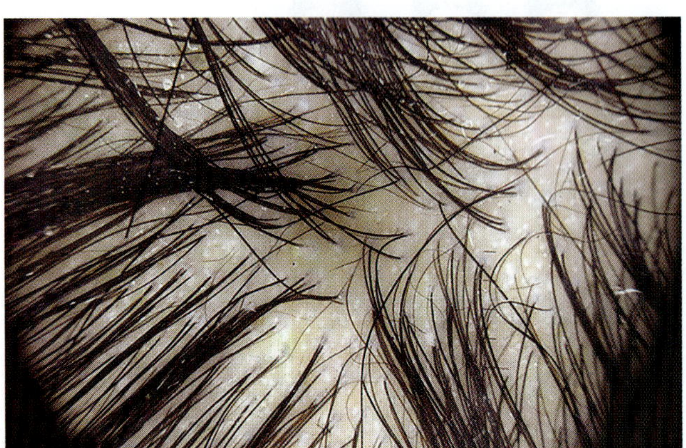

Fig. 17: Trichoscopy showing anisotrichosis and white dots.

found below miniaturized follicles. At times, a superficial, perifollicular, and inflammatory infiltrate is noted. A mildly increased telogen-to-anagen ratio is often observed. Number of hair follicles remains same. Number and percentage of vellus hair increase.

TREATMENT

Medical Management (Tables 4 and 5)

- *Biologic response modifier*:
  - Minoxidil
  - Peptides
- *Hormone modifier*:
  - Finasteride (5-a-reductase inhibitor), dutasteride

TABLE 4: Medical management of AGA.

Topicals	*Minoxidil*	*Aminexil*	*Tretinoin*
Mechanism of action	• Converted to minoxidil sulfate (active form) which opens ATP-sensitive potassium channels in cell membranes, leading to a vasodilatory effect • Lengthen the duration of the anagen phase, and it may increase the blood supply to the follicle • Increased expression of (VEGF) mRNA in the dermal papillae • Activation of cytoprotective prostaglandin synthase-1, an enzyme that stimulates hair growth • Increased expression of hepatocyte growth factor (HGF) m-RNA which is another hair growth promoter	An antifibrotic agent that inhibits collagen formation around hair follicle and maintains follicle survival resulting in increase in hair density and growth by preventing perifollicular fibrosis	Prolongs anagen phase and increases percutaneous absorption of minoxidil three-fold if used in combination with minoxidil
Formulation and strength	Lotion, gel The drug is marketed as a 2% or a 5% solution, with the 5% solution being somewhat more effective (available off label in higher concentrations)		• 58% with tretinoin 0.025% alone • 66% with tretinoin 0.025% combined with 0.5% minoxidil
Side effects	*Local*: Aggravation of seborrheic dermatitis, psoriasis, allergic contact dermatitis, irritation, and pain *Systemic*: Hypertrichosis, headache, and hypotension		
Remarks	Patients who respond best to this drug are those who have a recent onset of androgenetic alopecia and small areas of hair loss		
Hormone response modifiers	*Finasteride*	*Dutasteride*	*Antiandrogens*
	5-α-reductase type 2 inhibitor	Dual 5-α-reductase inhibitor, i.e., inhibits both type 1 and type 2 5-α-reductase isoenzymes	Antiandrogens such as cyproterone acetate, spironolactone, flutamide, and finasteride are more effective in females with hyperandrogenism
Mechanism of action	Prevents the conversion of testosterone to its more potent form DHT within hair follicles **(Fig. 18)** 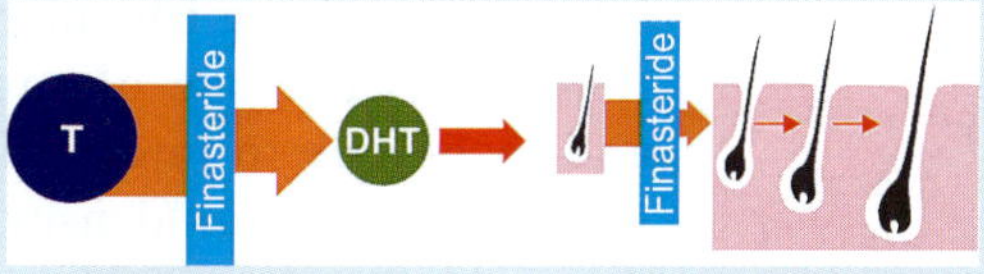 **Fig. 18:** Mechanism of action of finasteride.	Reversing the miniaturization process that occurs in AGA may be useful in treating hirsutism, acne, and other hormone-related disorders	
Dosage	1 mg/day	0.5 mg daily	*Cyproterone acetate*: 50–100 mg daily taken on days 5–14 of the menstrual cycle supplemented by 50 µg ethinylestradiol on days 5–25 *Spironolactone*: 100–200 mg over a period of 6 months in patients of FPHL *Flutamide*: 250 mg/day when given for at least a year *Drospirenone*: 3 mg/day +30 µg of ethinylestradiol during a 21-day cycle
Side effects	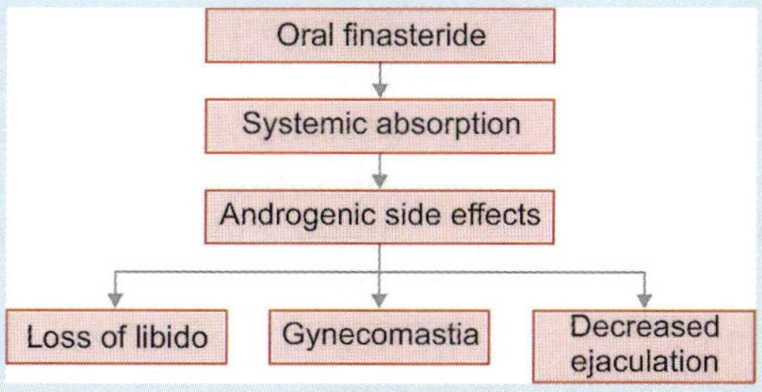	• Erectile dysfunction • Decreased libido • Ejaculation disorder • Gynecomastia	• Feminization of a male fetus is a serious concern with its use in females of the childbearing age • Spironolactone causes metrorrhagia and hence should be administered with oral contraceptives

(AGA: androgenetic alopecia; ATP: adenosine triphosphate; DHT: dihydrotestosterone; FPHL: female pattern hair loss; mRNA: messenger ribonucleic acid; VEGF: vascular endothelial growth factor)

TABLE 5: Other medical modalities.

Prostaglandin F2α analogs	*Latanoprost* and *bimatoprost*	• Topical latanoprost 0.1%—increase in the number, length, and thickness of eyelashes (alopecia areata) • Stimulate hair follicle activity, treating hair loss
Capixyl: Biochanin A+ Acetyl tetrapeptide-3		*Biochanin A*: Effective inhibitor of 5-α-reductase type 1 and 2 *Acetyl tetrapeptide-3*: Direct effect on hair follicle, increases size of hair follicle for better anchoring and vitality
Caffeine		• Higher transfollicular penetration rate • Prevent progression and induce hair regrowth in androgenetic alopecia
Plant extracts	• Allium cepa root extract, Kerarice • Baicapil • Serenoa repens	*Serena repens* extract—inhibits both types of 5-α-reductase and, when taken orally, has been shown to increase growth in androgenetic alopecia patients
Procapil	Procapil combines vitaminated matrikine with apigenin and oleanolic acid	Anti-hair loss complex that targets: • 5-α-reductase • Inadequate blood perfusion • Failing anchorage of the hair in the dermal papilla

  - Spironolactone
  - Cyproterone acetate
- *Prostaglandin analogs*: Prostaglandin F2α analogs *latanoprost* and *bimatoprost.*

Only two drugs currently have US Food and Drug Administration (FDA)-approved indications for treatment of androgenetic alopecia: minoxidil and finasteride.

OTHER MEDICAL MODALITIES (TABLE 5)

Low-level laser light: Low-level laser light therapy, in particular a red light hairbrush-like device, has been marketed as an over-the-counter technique for hair growth:

- *Microneedling*:
  - Release of platelet-derived growth factor (PDGF)
  - Epidermal growth factors are increased
  - Activation of stem cells in hair bulge area.

  Microneedling involves the use of a microneedle-tipped instrument, most commonly a dermaroller or a dermapen, which has recently been shown to enhance expression of hair-related genes and stimulation of hair in mice by Jeong et al. and Kim et al.
- *Platelet-rich plasma (PRP)*:
  - Growth factors present in PRP induce follicular stem cells to shift from a dormant state to an active state that starts the process of hair production.
  - Vascular endothelial growth factor 8 (VEGF-8) and PDGF-4 found in PRP are known to facilitate angiogenesis around the hair follicle.

Platelet-rich plasma contains high concentrations of over 20 growth factors such as PDGF, transforming growth factor, VEGF, epidermal growth factor, fibroblast growth factor, connective tissue growth factor, and insulin-like growth factor 1 (IGF-1) that are actively secreted from the α-granules of platelets and are thought to stimulate hair regrowth. These essential proteins regulate cell migration, attachment, proliferation, and differentiation and promote extracellular matrix accumulation. Activated autologous PRP has also been noted to activate the proliferation of dermal papilla cells by upregulating fibroblast growth factor-7 and β-catenin, in addition to extracellular signal-related kinase and Akt signaling.

- *Surgical hair restoration*:
  - Hair transplantation **(Table 6)**
  - *Scalp micropigmentation*: Micro hair pigmentation, also named tricopigmentation, or cosmetic hair follicle replication is a nonsurgical treatment which uses the latest technology to create the effect of a full head of hair. Unlike classic tattoo, no permanent ink is used during iricopigmentation treatments. It involves the use of specialized equipment and technique to inject pigment into the scalp. A tricopigmentation "density" treatment is ideal for those with first signs of thinning hairs. By treating the skin we can take away or reduce the contrast between skin color and hair color, thus resulting in an optical illusion of more density.

    Indications in AGA:
    - In cases of low Norwood scale or in cases where thinning of the follicles is in general, observed in order to achieve the effect of density in the suffering areas
    - In cases of high Norwood scales, usually combined with a hair transplant
    - In cases of achieving the desired density where:
      - There is a very poor or exhausted donor area
      - The extraction of the follicles has exceeded 50% of the donor area. In that case the micropigmentation can be applied to both donor and recipient area
      - The patient uses prosthetic hair piece and wants to get rid of it.
  - Scalp flaps
  - Scalp reduction

TABLE 6: Differences between follicular unit transplant (FUT) and follicular unit extraction (FUE).

Follicular unit transplant by strip harvesting	*Follicular unit extraction*
Strip excision of donor skin and suturing done	Extraction of individual units one by one through small punch holes; each alternate hair unit is removed. No suturing
Healing: Single linear scar (1–3 mm wide)—over 1–2 weeks	*Healing*: Multiple tiny scars in between hairs—over 2–3 days
Donor hairs not trimmed; suture completely hidden	Donor hairs trimmed
Quicker • 4–5 hours for 2, 000 grafts • Transection rate 1–2%	*Slower* • 8–10–12 hours for 2,000 grafts • Transection rate 2–5%
More precise (microscopic dissection)	Less precise as units are pulled blindly
Large sessions, up to 3,000 grafts possible	Large sessions difficult
More comfortable *Position*: Sleeping face up	More uncomfortable *Position*: Head-down position for several hours
Operation site over donor hidden	Operation site over donor shaven and hence visible

- *Other treatment options:*
  - Wigs
  - Hair pieces
  - Cosmetic camouflage
  - Hair weaving.

PROGNOSIS

The prognosis of AGA is unknown. Some patients progress to the point where they lose almost all of the hair on the scalp. Others have a patterned or nonpatterned thinning but retain a considerable number of scalp hairs. Women with AGA usually show thinning of the crown rather than developing truly bald areas. Along with affecting the patient psychologically, AGA is significant in that and it allows ultraviolet light to reach the scalp and, thus, increases the amount of actinic damage. In addition, males with AGA may have an increased incidence of myocardial infarction.

A study by Sanke et al. indicated that early AGA (i.e., prior to 30 years of age) in males is the phenotypic equivalent of PCOS and that these males may be at risk of developing complications found in association with PCOS such as obesity, metabolic syndrome, insulin resistance, cardiovascular disease, and infertility.

DIFFUSE ALOPECIA

INTRODUCTION

Diffuse hair shedding can be quite distressing and can affect both sexes at any age. Any factor that interrupts the normal hair cycle can trigger diffuse hair loss including a wide variety of physiologic or emotional stress, endocrine imbalance, nutritional deficiencies, etc. Finding the cause, or trigger, of the hair loss requires a thorough history and examination and this will enable appropriate treatment. Patient education is the key in the management of diffuse hair loss.

The most common type of diffuse shedding is telogen effluvium. Other common causes of diffuse hair loss include early AGA, anagen hair loss, and diffuse type of AA. The rare causes of diffuse hair loss include loose anagen hair syndrome, congenital atrichia, congenital hypotrichosis, and hair shaft abnormalities (hair breakage, unruly hairs).

TELOGEN EFFLUVIUM

Telogen effluvium is defined as increased shedding of telogen club hairs because of premature termination of the anagen phase of the hair cycle. Establishing a cause requires a thorough history to identify known triggers, investigations to exclude endocrine, nutritional or autoimmune etiologies and, in persistent cases, histology to look for early changes of AGA. Normal telogen shedding should be about 70 hairs per day.

Pathogenesis

Five functional types of telogen effluvium, as described by Headington, based on different phases of the follicular cycle are the following:

- Immediate anagen release is a short onset effluvium where follicles leave anagen and enter telogen prematurely, resulting in increased hair shedding at the end of telogen, about 2–3 months later. It is common after a physiological stress such as severe illness and with drug induced hair loss.
- Delayed anagen release is the cause of postpartum hair loss.
- Short anagen syndrome is caused by shortening of the duration of anagen.
- Immediate telogen release is caused by premature exogen. This could also be associated with a shortening of telogen duration. The follicles may remain empty for weeks before the initiation of anagen. This empty telogen follicle, called kenogen, has a prolonged duration in AGA. Drugs such as minoxidil can also precipitate exogen, which causes the temporary increase in hair shedding commonly noticed 4–6 weeks after minoxidil therapy.

- Delayed telogen release occurs after prolonged telogen followed by transition to anagen. It may occur seasonally in some humans.

Acute Telogen Effluvium

- Acute onset scalp hair loss occurring 2–3 months after a triggering event such as high fever, sudden starvation, surgical trauma, or hemorrhage.
- Procedures done on the hair for cosmetic purpose such as smoothening, straightening, pumming, spa therapy, and ironing can also lead to diffuse hair loss of various degrees.
- In about one-third patients of acute telogen effluvium, no trigger is identified.
- The functional mechanism of hair loss is immediate anagen release. The patient may notice an increase in hair on the pillow, or when brushing, or in the shower drain.
- The daily loss ranges from under 100 to over 1,000 hairs, which results in diffuse reduction in hair density if it continues at higher rates.
- Spontaneous complete regrowth is expected to occur within 3–6 months unless the trigger is repeated. Telogen gravidarum is the telogen hair shedding seen 2–3 months after childbirth (an example of delayed anagen release). Most cases resolve but a small proportion of women may experience persistent episodic diffuse or localized shedding.

Investigations

- The hair pull test is usually strongly positive for telogen hairs at the vertex and the scalp margins, with normal club hairs, in acute telogen effluvium, but a negative hair pull test does not exclude the diagnosis.
- The trichogram analysis usually shows >25% of telogen hairs in acute telogen effluvium.
- Histological examination fails to show any abnormality apart from an increase in the proportion of telogen follicles.
- Expectant management and observation is advisable when an obvious explanation exists for acute telogen effluvium.

Chronic Telogen Effluvium

- Chronic diffuse telogen hair loss is defined as telogen hair shedding lasting for longer than 6 months.
- It is due to an idiopathic change in hair cycle dynamics [primary chronic telogen effluvium (CTE)] or secondary to a variety of causes including FPHL.
- Various causes of chronic diffuse telogen hair loss include thyroid disorders (both hyperthyroidism as well as hypothyroidism including drug-induced hypothyroidism), acrodermatitis enteropathica, acquired zinc deficiency (due to long-standing parenteral nutrition), profound iron deficiency anemia, and malnutrition.
- The shedding in the early stages of FPHL can be diffuse and episodic, mimicking a telogen effluvium, but this shedding tends to be chronic and relapsing, and recovery is generally incomplete. Crash dieting with severe protein-calorie restriction, chronic starvation, hypoproteinemia of metabolic/dietary origin, pancreatic disease (including other forms of malabsorption), essential fatty acid deficiencies (seen in prolonged parenteral nutrition and hypervitaminosis A), liver disorders, chronic renal failure, advanced malignancies, secondary syphilis, systemic lupus erythematosus (SLE), and dermatomyositis may all cause telogen hair loss.

Primary Chronic Telogen Effluvium

- Primary CTE affects middle-aged women (30–50 years) and is an idiopathic and sometimes self-limiting condition distinct from chronic diffuse telogen effluvium secondary to organic causes.
- Sudden onset of increased hair shedding lasting for at least 6 months.
- Absence of visible widening of the central parting line, and scalp biopsy fails to reveal any miniaturization of hair follicles.
- CTE differs from the acute form due to its prolonged fluctuating course and less frequent occurrence.
- In most cases, no trigger can be identified.
- CTE is believed to be related to a reduction in the variation of anagen duration without any reduction in the mean duration of the anagen phase of the hair cycle.

Investigations

- The diagnosis of CTE is reached by excluding other causes of diffuse telogen hair loss by taking a thorough history, including a detailed drug and dietary history.
- The routine investigations include a complete blood count and thyroid function tests. Serum zinc levels, antinuclear antibody (ANA) titer, syphilis serology, and other investigations of nutritional status should be performed if clinically suspected.
- The hair pull test is commonly positive over the vertex and occipital scalp but a negative hair pull test on any one day does not exclude the diagnosis of CTE.
- Scalp dermoscopy fails to reveal miniaturized hair fibers and compound hair follicles with 2–3 fibers exiting from each pore is usually seen.

The diagnosis of CTE is usually suspected from the history and examination, but some cases may require scalp biopsy for differentiating it from early AGA.

Management: While the hair continues to shed, it is replaced, and this condition does not lead to baldness. Antiandrogens have little effect but minoxidil can reduce hair shedding in CTE.

Drug-induced Telogen Effluvium

- Usually starts 6–12 weeks after starting treatment and is progressive while the drug is continued.

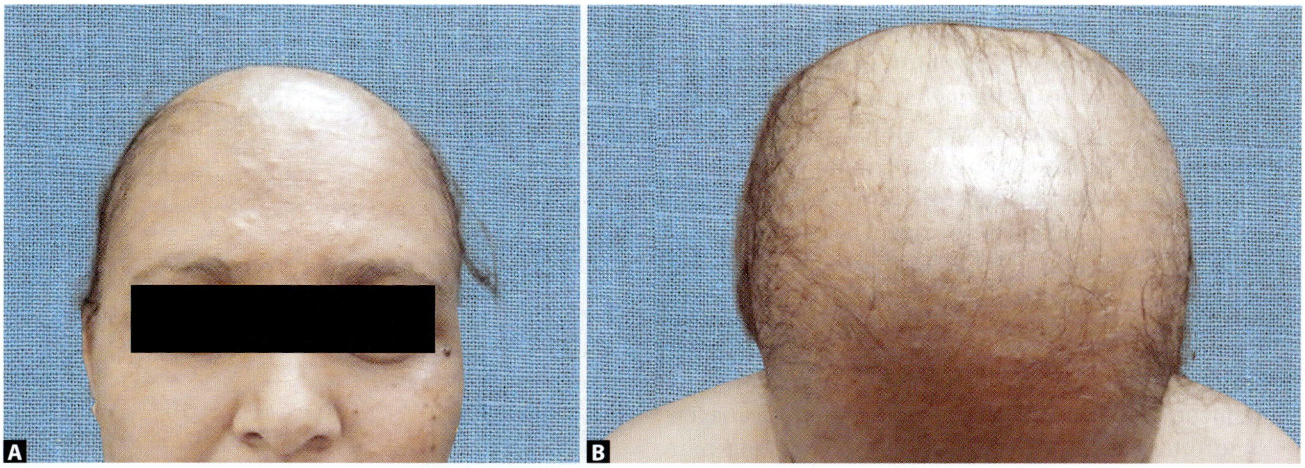

Figs. 19A and B: Anagen effluvium after cisplatin therapy.

- Most commonly caused by immediate anagen release.
- The diagnosis is made by identifying and correlating the chronology of drug exposure and the onset of the hair loss, and excluding other causes of alopecia.
- A suspected drug needs to be stopped for at least 3 months and regrowth following discontinuation with recurrence on re-exposure supports the diagnosis.
- A dose-related diffuse telogen hair loss is common with acitretin,[8] but less common with isotretinoin. Minoxidil causes telogen shedding for a short duration by immediate telogen release. Other drugs known to cause telogen effluvium are oral contraceptive pills, androgens, β-blockers, angiotensin-converting enzyme inhibitors, anticonvulsants, antithyroid drugs, antidepressants, and the anticoagulants heparin and warfarin. Withdrawal of the trigger will lead to arrest of hair shedding within 3 months but a full recovery in hair density may take 6 months.
- Unrecognized coincidental AGA is a possibility if there is persistent shedding after 3 months, or incomplete recovery after 6 months.

ANAGEN HAIR LOSS

As a result of interruption of the anagen hair cycle, anagen hair loss presents as abrupt anagen hair shedding with a severe diffuse scalp alopecia. Anagen effluvium is usually of short-onset compared with telogen effluvium, occurring within days to weeks of the insult. The hair-pull test is positive for dystrophic anagen hairs with tapered ends. If the insult ceases, hair growth restarts within weeks.

Antimitotic chemotherapeutic agents induce arrest of the anagen phase, presenting a toxic insult to the rapidly dividing hair matrix. Hair loss usually begins within 1–2 weeks of chemotherapy and is most noticeable by 1–2 months. The scalp hair is usually most affected, but all body hair can be affected. Chemotherapeutic agents commonly implicated in causing hair loss include cisplatin, carboplatin, cyclophosphamide, docetaxel, paclitaxel, fluorouracil, epirubicin, gemcitabine, vincristine, etc. **(Figs. 19A and B)**.

Other triggers of anagen hair loss include AA, radiation, heavy-metal poisoning, and boric acid poisoning.

OTHER CAUSES

In "congenital atrichia with papules," patients are born with hairs but shortly thereafter lose hair (including the eyebrows and eyelashes), which are never replaced again. Elbows and knees show development of papular lesions histopathologically consistent with milia. Scalp biopsy reveals malformed and reduced hairs and absence of any inflammation. Severe congenital hypotrichosis is very commonly associated with other defects. In most of these conditions, the hair is abnormal in quantity as well as quality. Alopecia is one of the striking features of a host of ectodermal dysplastic syndromes.

Hair in Human Immunodeficiency Virus Disease

Human immunodeficiency virus (HIV) disease, symptomatic as well as asymptomatic, shows several hair abnormalities [acquired immunodeficiency syndrome (AIDS) trichopathy]. The hairs are thin, sparse, and lighter in color. Individuals with curly hair loose their curls with the hair growing straighter. Premature graying and faster progression of pattern alopecia may occur in the HIV infected. Various medications given for HIV (zidovudine, lamivudine, indinavir, cidofovir, and fluconazole) may cause alopecia.

Scanning electron microscopy showed various hair shaft disorders such as longitudinal ridging, trichoschisis, indentation, variation in irregularly altered shaft diameter and twisting as well as irregular surface of the hair shaft. The presence of prominent apoptotic keratinocytes in the upper external root sheath just below the junction of the sebaceous duct and follicular canal is believed to be a characteristic feature of hair in the HIV infected.

Short Anagen Syndrome

Short anagen syndrome is seen at birth or early childhood as diffuse thinning of scalp hairs that "never grow." Most of the hairs are of the telogen type without any hair shaft abnormalities in the trichogram. Anagen duration is usually markedly reduced and scalp biopsy shows fewer hair follicles and absence of inflammation or scarring. The condition may improve spontaneously by puberty. Topical minoxidil can be tried as it prolongs anagen.

Loose Anagen Hair Syndrome

It is an uncommon cause of anagen hair loss, loose anagen hair syndrome presents as easily pluckable anagen hair without pain or breakage in young children (girls more commonly than boys) and may occur in families. The hair grows only up to a short length, is sparse but covers the scalp adequately and rarely requires cutting, leading to complaints that they "do not grow."

Light microscopy reveals anagen hair without an inner or outer root sheath. Scanning electron microscopy shows a rippled or "floppy sock" appearance of the cuticle and shafts which may be triangular, grooved or with ridges. A biopsy demonstrates that the hair cuticle is not attached with the IRS. The follicles are seen to be triangular/rhomboid on horizontal sectioning. The condition improves spontaneously over the years, particularly during adolescence, and at times even recurs.

Early stage trichogram reveals numerous tapering "pencil point" hair shafts (dystrophic anagen hairs). In the late stages, only telogen hairs can be pulled out because of complete loss of anagen hairs and hence, whenever telogen hairs constitute about 100% of hairs sampled, the diagnosis should be anagen effluvium rather than telogen effluvium.

HAIR SHAFT DISORDERS

Hair shaft disorders are classified according to fragility.

Hair shaft disorders associated with increased fragility are:
- Monilethrix
- Pili torti
- Netherton syndrome
- Trichorrhexis nodosa
- Trichothiodystrophy.

Hair shaft disorders not associated with increased fragility:
- Pili annulati
- Woolly hair
- Uncombable hair syndrome
- Loose anagen hair syndrome
- Trichostasis spinulosa
- Pili multigemini
- Trichoptilosis
- Bubble hair.

TABLE 7: Classification based on morphology of defect.

Fractures: • Trichoclasis • Trichoschisis • Trichorrhexis nodosa	*Narrowings*: • Monilethrix • Pohl–Pinkus mark • Tapered hair • Exclamation mark
Nodes: • Pseudomonilethrix • Trichorrhexis invaginata • Trichorrhexis nodosa • Trichonodosis • Nits, piedra, hair casts • Trichomycosis axillaris	*Twists and curls*: • Pili torti • Woolly hair • Circle hair • Corkscrew hair • Trichomalacia
Bands: • Pili annulati • Trichothiodystrophy	*Splits*: • Trichoptilosis • Pili bifurcate
Shaft nondefects: Loose anagen hair syndrome	

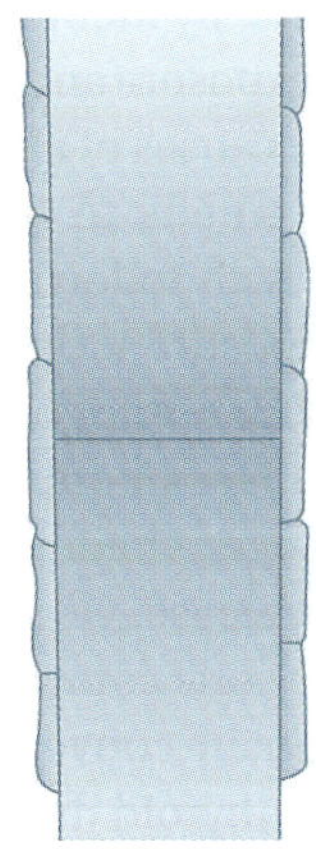

Fig. 20: Trichoclasis.

Classification based on morphology of defect is given in **Table 7**.

TRICHOCLASIS

It is a common greenstick fracture of the shaft occurring due to weathering and cosmetic trauma. Cuticle partly remains in continuity with the fracture **(Fig. 20)**.

TRICHOPTILOSIS (SPLIT HAIR)

Mechanical and chemical trauma in the form of curling irons, other heat treatment, and chemical procedure causes longitudinal fracture of hair shaft toward the tip or may occur within the hair shaft sparing the tip.

MONILETHRIX (BEADED HAIR, SPINDLE HAIR) (FIGS. 21A AND B)

Introduction

Radcliffe and Crocker suggested the term monilethrix, which is a rare condition of the hair.

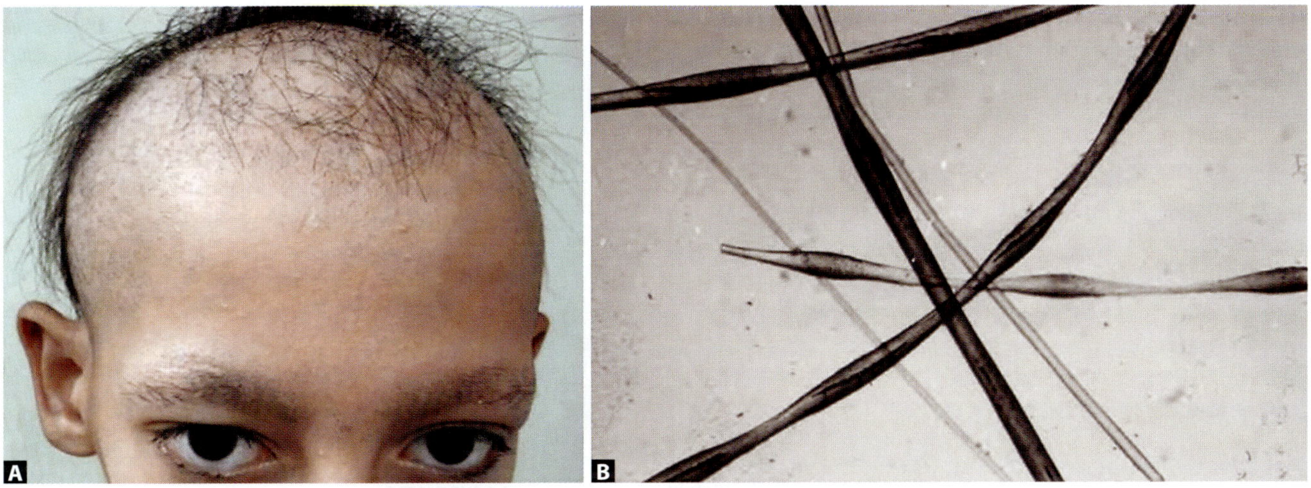

Figs. 21A and B: Monilethrix: (A) Clinical picture; (B) DPXmount.

Pathophysiology

True monilethrix must be distinguished from pseudomonilethrix. It is an artifact produced by tweezers or compressing overlapping hairs between two glass slides. Elliptical nodes 0.7–1 mm apart are separated by narrower internodes, resembling the body and neck of a skittle. The widths of the nodes and the distances between them vary between the hairs of an individual and between members of the same family. The hair shaft is beaded and breaks easily.

Histology

The follicle shows wide and narrow zones corresponding to the nodes and internodes. Node formation may be related to the diurnal rate of hair growth. Intermittent administration of an antimitotic agent can give rise to zones of constriction alternating with zones of normal diameter.

Recent reports suggest defective cortical cell keratinization as the mechanism for the hair constrictions and breakage.

Clinical Features

Typically, patient presents with sparse and short hairs. Age of onset, severity, and expression within a family and course of the disease may show variations. Hair loss or broken hair is accompanied by follicular keratoses most commonly on the nape and occiput. In some cases, the eyebrows, eyelashes, pubic and axillary hair, and general body hair may be affected. Spontaneous improvement or complete recovery has occurred, even during pregnancy or it may persist with little change throughout life. Trichoscopy?

On trichoscopy, beaded hair shaft with regularly spaced nodes and internodes ("regularly bended ribbon" sign) are seen.

PILI TORTI (TWISTED HAIR)

INTRODUCTION

Hairs are flattened and at irregular intervals completely rotated through 180° around their long axis. Three to five twists occur before the shaft normalizes. True pili torti of Menkes syndrome and the isolated expression of the abnormality in an otherwise unaffected person demonstrate the same distinct twisting. Scanning electron microscopy suggests that not all twisted hairs are pili torti. Occasional twists of varying angles should not be taken to this distinctive anomaly. Screening with dermoscopy and microscopy will help in sampling.

Menkes syndrome, Bjornstad syndrome with sensorineural deafness and Crandall syndrome are all associated with pili torti. It can also be found in some scarring alopecia **(Figs. 22A and B)**.

CLINICAL FEATURES

The hair may be normal at birth and change in the first few months. Affected hairs are brittle and may break off at a length of 5 cm or less, or grow longer in areas of the scalp which are less subjected to trauma and friction. There may be only short, coarse stubble hair over the whole scalp or there may be circumscribed baldness, or sometimes irregularly patchy or occipital hair loss present.

TRICHORRHEXIS NODOSA (FIG. 23)

Introduction

"Tricho" means hair, "rrhexis" means breakage, "nodosa" means knots or bulges. If the degree or frequency of the injury is sufficient, it can be induced in normal hair. The cuticular cells become disrupted, allowing the cortical cells to splay out to form nodes. It may be congenital or acquired.

Trichorrhexis nodosa is a feature of the rare metabolic defect argininosuccinic aciduria where there is a deficiency of the enzyme argininosuccinase, and it is associated with mental retardation, dry, brittle and lusterless hairs and may show trichorrhexis nodosa, but it does not occur in all patients. Trichorrhexis nodosa can be seen in biotinidase deficiency and trichohepatoenteric syndrome. It may occur in certain

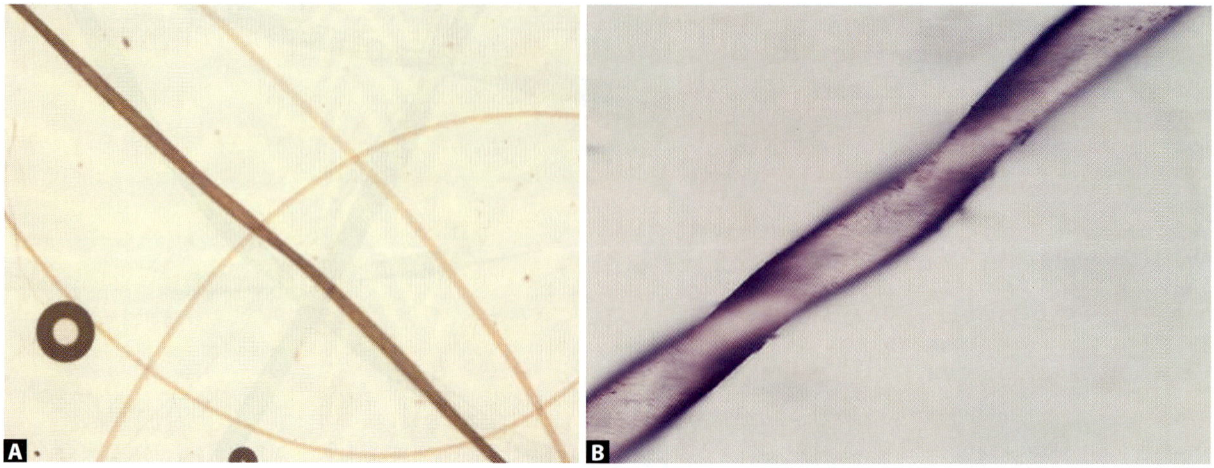

Figs. 22A and B: Pili torti in Menkes kinky hair syndrome.

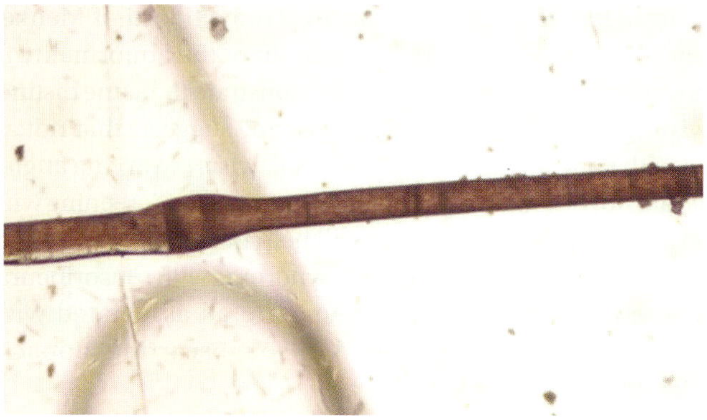

Fig. 23: Trichorrhexis nodosa.

families as an apparently isolated defect of the hair node formation and fracture is induced by minimal trauma and develop during the early months of life.

The cumulative effect of shampooing, brushing, sea bathing, and sunlight has led to damage the cuticular cells and node formation in acquired form of trichorrhexis nodosa. Trichorrhexis nodosa is an extreme form of weathering.

Trichoscopy shows brush-like hair fractures and fraying at nodes.

LOCALIZED AUTOSOMAL RECESSIVE HYPOTRICHOSIS

Introduction

Extensive hair loss occurs due to brittle hairs which fracture readily. Hair microscopy shows either trichorrhexis nodosa or monolethrix-like breading. It is due to mutation in gene *dsg4*.

Pathophysiology

At the nodes, the cuticle bulges and is split by longitudinal fissures. If fracture occurs transversely through a node (trichoclasis), the end of the hair resembles a small paintbrush.

Clinical Features

In trichorrhexis nodosa complicating a congenital defect of the hair shaft, the hair breaks so easily that large or small portions of the scalp show only broken stumps and alopecia may be gross. However, the common situation is where trauma plays a major part, there are three principal clinical presentations:

1. Distal trichorrhexis nodosa occurs in all races, incidental, and only a few whitish nodules are seen near the ends of scattered hairs. If many hairs are affected, the patient may complain that the hair is dry, dull, or brittle. The longer the hair, the more likely it is to occur.
2. Proximal trichorrhexis nodosa is a generalized variant seen in Afro-Caribbean women. The scalp hair is universally short and brittle and demonstrates severe weathering on light microscopic examination.
3. The third clinical form was well described by Sabouraud but it appears now to be rare. In a localized area of scalp, moustache or beard, some hairs are broken and others show from one to five or six nodules.

Investigations

The congenital forms must be differentiated from other shaft defects. The distal acquired form may simulate dandruff or even pediculosis. In all cases, diagnosis depends on careful microscopy:

- Bamboo hair/trichorrhexis invaginata
- Kindly rewrite with emphasis on trichorrhexis invaginata where Netherton syndrome could be a part.

Bamboo hair or trichorrhexis invaginata is due to abnormal keratinization. The hair shaft cortex is structurally weak at specific points along its length. Harder adjacent segments of the hair shaft impact into these softer portions creating a ball and socket appearance. The hair shaft may break with minimal trauma. It is suggested that the weakness in the hair cortical region arises from the incomplete sulfhydryl conversion into sulfide bridges in the cortical region.[7] Trichorrhexis invaginata is a classical feature of Netherton syndrome. The cause is a mutation in the *SPINK5* gene.

Netherton syndrome is a rare autosomal recessive genodermatoses characterized by congenital ichthyosiform erythroderma, atopic diathesis, and hair shaft abnormality. The patient may present primarily either with cutaneous changes or complaining of sparse and fragile hair. Generalized scaling and erythema are present from birth or early infancy, but the degree, extent, and persistence of the erythema are very variable. The hair is short, dry, lusterless, and brittle, and the eyebrows and lashes are sparse or absent. In many, it has the characteristics of atopic eczema accompanied by an elevated immunoglobulin E (IgE).

Light microscopy is the best tool for detecting features of Netherton syndrome in hair. Alternatively, finding a single trichorrhexis invaginata node in a single hair is a conclusive positive. Electron microscopy will only allow assessment of small lengths of a small number of hairs. Detail of the surface features is enhanced using partially crossed polarizing filters. Where diagnosis is difficult, sampling eyebrows hairs may provide confirmation. Make trichoscopic description more lucid with simpler term.

By trichoscopy, it is possible to visualize hairs that invaginate in several spots and nodular structures along its axis, typical of bamboo hair as well as golf-tee hair.

Management

There is no specific treatment for the hair dystrophy other than avoidance of physical and chemical trauma.

TRICHOTHIODYSTROPHY (FIG. 24)

Introduction

The term trichothiodystrophy (TTD) was coined to describe brittle hair with abnormally low sulfur content (tricho—hair, thio—sulfur, dys—faulty, and trophe—nourishment). TTD can be classified according to the constellation of features that accompany the hair changes. It is one of a group of nucleotide excision repair disorders that have overlapping characteristics and etiology.

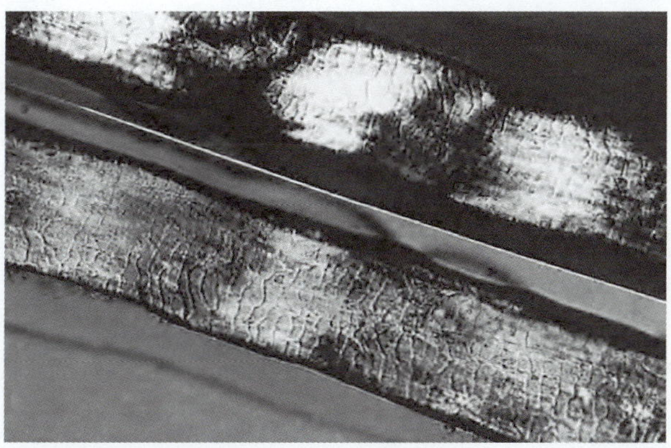

Fig. 24: Trichothiodystrophy showing alternating bright and dark zones under a polarizing microscope.

Pathophysiology

Sulfur amino acid reduction is commensurate with clinical abnormality in the hair of those with associated autism. With trauma, it may fracture with a clean transverse break (trichoschisis) or may form nodes resembling trichorrhexis nodosa. The hairs are flattened and can be twisted into various shapes—rather like a ribbon or shoelace. Transmission electron microscopy demonstrates a decrease in high sulfur protein staining in the hair shaft and a reduction of this protein in the exo-cuticular part of the cuticle cells.

Clinical Features

There is a wide range of phenotypic characteristics, depending on the variant of TTD. The hair is sparse, short and brittle, but the degree of alopecia varies considerably.

Classification of trichothiodystrophy:

A—isolated hair defect
B—A + nail dystrophy
C—B + mental retardation
D—C + growth retardation
E—D + decreased fertility
F—E + ichthyosis
G—F + photosensitivity (similar to xeroderma pigmentosum type D)
H—G + neutropenia

Diagnosis

Microscopic diagnosis of trichothiodystrophy requires that all hair should exhibit tiger-tail banding along with hair shaft abnormalities such as irregular contour, trichoschisis, and trichorrhexis nodosa-like defects. Cysteine in the hair can be quantified by sodium azide-dependent oxidation to cysteic acid.

PILI ANNULATI (RINGED HAIR)

Introduction

This abnormality is characterized by hair showing alternate light and dark bands along its length. The condition is inherited as an autosomal dominant disorder, the genetic defect maps to chromosome 12q.

Pathophysiology

With the light microscope, the abnormal dark bands alternating with normal light bands are reversed. The bright appearance of the abnormal bands in reflected light is caused by air spaces in the cortex. Detection of the cortical defect is made easier with microscopy. Dermoscopy is not as reliable because the perception is based largely on light transmission through the hair and not reflection.

Clinical Features

Pili annulati is normally diagnosed as a coincidental finding or as part of a pursuance of the unusual, but quite attractive and spangled appearance. Fragility is occasionally a presenting feature and more prone to weathering.

Prognosis

The prognosis is good in the sense that the severity of the defect does not increase with age.

WOOLLY HAIR

Woolly hair is more or less tightly coiled hair occurring over all or part of the scalp. In those of African origin, woolly hair is the normal. In non-African individuals, it may be generalized or localized. The generalized forms are autosomal dominant. Hair microscopy in all the woolly hair disorders reveals nonspecific features. This usually arises in association with grooves, partial twists, irregularity of bore, and sometimes features of trauma.

Woolly Hair Nevus

Woolly hair nevus presents with a circumscribed patch of hair showing altered color and texture. The hair may be fine in infancy, becoming coarser with age, especially at puberty. It is commonly associated with melanocytic or epidermal nevi elsewhere on the skin. Associated ocular and auditory defects, digital abnormalities and precocious puberty have been reported.

Acquired Woolly Hair

It occurs most commonly in the context of patterned hair loss (acquired progressive kinking of hair). It may also be caused by drugs such as valproate, retinoids, and antiretroviral agents protease inhibitors.

UNCOMBABLE HAIR SYNDROME: SPUN-GLASS HAIR, CHEVEUX INCOIFFABLES, PILI TRIANGULI ET CANALICULI

Introduction

It is a distinctive hair shaft defect first described by Dupre and Bonafe, mode of inheritance is probably autosomal dominant.

Pathophysiology

Light microscopy reveals the triangular cross-section and longitudinal grooving. Twisting can also be present and contributes to stiffness to a minor degree. Scanning electron microscopy of selected hairs can be helpful. The pili canaliculi are present in all cases, followed by pili trianguli and pili torti.

Clinical Features

The condition first becomes obvious from 3 months to 12 years of age. The hair is normal in quantity and length, but the wild and disorderly appearance totally resists all efforts to control it with a brush or comb. The hair is often a silvery blonde color. It is associated with increased fragility. The eyebrows and eyelashes are normal.

Histological examination shows premature keratinization of the IRS layers of Huxley and Henle. Trichograms show 98–100% anagen hairs. Keratin K6 is an IRS keratin proposed as a protein that might control manifestations of the disorder.

Management involves advice on gentle hair grooming and reassurance that the defect usually resolves spontaneously with age. Oral biotin therapy has been suggested.

HAIR CASTS (PERIPILAR KERATIN CASTS, PSEUDONITS) (FIG. 25)

Hair casts (HCs) are thin, elongated 2–8 mm long, firm, whitish cylindrical concretions which ensheath the hair shaft and can be easily dislodged. They are of two different types: (1) peripilar (idiopathic) and (2) parakeratotic (secondary) keratin cast. The secondary form is more common and often coexists with pathological conditions involving scalp scaling such as in psoriasis, tractional alopecia, pityriasis amiantacea, seborrheic dermatitis, or scalp infections such as tinea capitis, folliculitis decalvans or hair shaft defects. Due to its clinical resemblance to pediculosis capitis, the entity is also known as pseudonits.

Hair casts of both parakeratotic and peripilar keratin casts results due to the failure of disintegration of root sheath which gets pulled out of hair follicle and surrounds the shaft leading to its persistence during hair growth.

Macroscopical and microscopical examination together will differentiate HCs from the other possibilities such as white piedra—due to trichosporon cutaneum/beigelii—a yeast-like fungus which surrounds the hair-shaft and may eventually invade the cortex causing severance, trichorrhexis nodosa, pediculus capitis, seborrheic dermatitis, trichomycosis nodosa. Hair cast in tractional alopecia denotes ongoing traction and the disease is likely to progress.

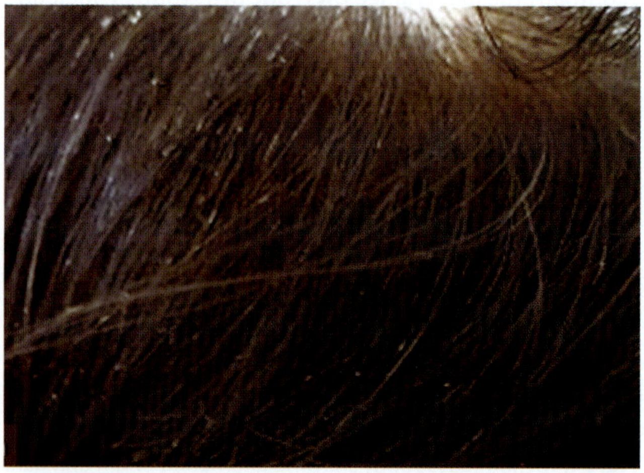

Fig. 25: Hair casts—whitish concretions along hair shaft.

Treatment involves soaking the HCs in acetic acid and combing them off the shaft at the distal end.

TRICHOSTASIS SPINULOSA

Felix Franke first described this condition and termed it "Pinselhaar" meaning "paint brush hair." It is a common condition which sometimes goes unnoticed.

Trichostasis spinulosa affects the skin of the nose of adults, and is often confused with blackheads. Lesions may also occur on the scalp, chest, back, and elsewhere. It can affect both men and women and usually occurs in older adults. Trichostasis spinulosa lesions appear as numerous tiny open pores filled with multiple tiny short hairs. Each follicular plug may contain between 5 and 25 hairs and is usually >1 mm in size.

There are two variants:

1. *Classical variant*: Solitary or very few asymptomatic comedone-like papules over nose.
2. Another variant is typified by multiple, pruritic, and follicular papules, predominantly distributed over the trunk and arms of young persons.

Diagnosis is made by microscopic examination.

It should be differentiated from keratosis pilaris, chloracne, eruptive vellus hair cyst, Darier's disease, ichthyosis follicularis, pityrosporum folliculitis, and keratotic follicular papules of scurvy.

Treatment: Topical retinoic acid and pulsed diode laser.

BUBBLE HAIR

Bubble hair is an acquired hair shaft deformity characterized by bubble-like areas in the hair shaft seen with light microscopy and corresponding cavitary defects with scanning electron microscopy. It occurs due to thermal injury caused by hair dryers, heating tongs, or hot curls. Hair appears dry and wiry, with patchy loss of hair due to excessive fragility. It may be associated with other acquired hair shaft defects such as trichorrhexis nodosa and trichoptilosis. On cross-section, these hairs reveal either a single large cavity or a reticulated "swiss cheese-like loss of cells."

PILI BIFURCATI (FIG. 26)

The shaft bifurcates into two halves and is covered by its own cuticle, the parts may rejoin distally. In contrast to this, in trichoptilosis, the split hairs do not have complete cuticular cover around them.

PILI MULTIGEMINI

Between the two and eight matrices and papillae hair with separate IRS are formed in the same follicular canal. The jawline is the most common site and there may be nodular inflammatory lesions.

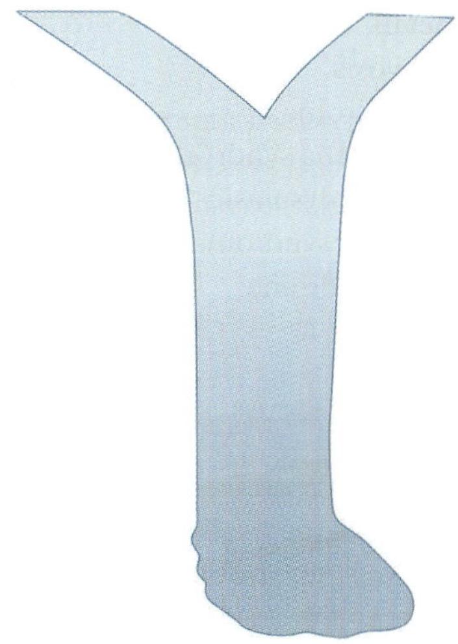

Fig. 26: Pili bifurcati.

CICATRICIAL ALOPECIA

Cicatricial alopecia, also known as scarring alopecia, can result from many causes and are permanent alopecias because of irreversible loss of hair follicles.

INTRODUCTION

One of the earliest descriptions of cicatricial alopecia was given by Brocq in 1885 (pseudopelade of Brocq), in which destruction of follicles leads to permanent patchy baldness and is not accompanied by any clinically evident inflammatory pathology. Quinquaud described folliculitis decalvans, a form of scarring alopecia in which pustular folliculitis of the advancing margin was a conspicuous feature.

Cicatricial alopecias are classified as primary or secondary:

- *Primary cicatricial alopecia*: The hair follicle is the target of a destructive inflammatory process.
- *Secondary cicatricial alopecia*: Destruction of the hair follicle is secondary to a non-follicle-directed process or external injury, such as severe infections, burns, radiation, or tumors.

CLASSIFICATION OF CICATRICIAL ALOPECIA

Developmental/Hereditary

- Aplasia cutis
- Focal dermal hypoplasia
- Dystrophic epidermolysis bullosa
- Incontinentia pigmenti
- Conradi syndrome
- Keratosis pilaris atrophicans faciei
- Keratosis follicularis spinulosa
- Folliculitis decalvans
- Darier's disease
- Porokeratosis of Mibelli

- Epidermal nevus
- Lamellar ichthyosis
- Marie-Unna syndrome
- Follicular hamartoma syndrome
- Polyostotic fibrous dysplasia
- Hallermann-Streiff syndrome
- Rapp-Hodgkin syndrome

Traumatic

- Mechanical injury
- Thermal injury
- Electrical burns
- Persistent traction alopecia
- Persistent trichotillomania
- Factitious injury

Neoplastic

- Basal cell carcinoma
- Squamous cell carcinoma
- Syringolymphoid hyperplasia
- Cutaneous angiosarcoma
- Lymphomas
- Metastasis

Follicular Inflammation with Pustules

- Tinea capitis
- Bacterial folliculitis
- Folliculitis decalvans
- Dissecting cellulitis of scalp
- Acne keloidalis nuchae
- Tufted folliculitis
- Hidradenitis suppurativa

Follicular Inflammation without Pustules

- Pseudopelade of Brocq
- Follicular lichen planus
- Graham-Little-Piccardi-Lasseur syndrome
- Discoid lupus erythematosus
- Lichen sclerosus et atrophicus
- Follicular mucinosis

Dermal Inflammation Leading to Secondary Follicular Damage

- Cicatricial pemphigoid
- Pyoderma gangrenosum
- Morphea
- Facial hemiatrophy
- Dermatomyositis
- Necrobiosis lipoidica
- Sarcoidosis
- Temporal arteritis
- Ecthyma and deep secondary pyodermas
- Syphilis
- Tuberculosis
- Leishmaniasis
- Myiasis
- Herpes zoster

The North American Hair Research Society (NAHRS) classified primary cicatricial alopecia based on the inflammatory infiltrate around hair follicle as follows:

Lymphocytic

- Chronic cutaneous lupus erythematosus
- *Lichen planopilaris*: Classic lichen planopilaris (LPP), frontal fibrosing alopecia (FFA), and Graham-Little-Piccardi syndrome
- Classic pseudopelade of Brocq
- Central centrifugal cicatricial alopecia
- Alopecia mucinosa
- Keratosis follicularis spinulosa decalvans

Neutrophilic

- Folliculitis decalvans
- Dissecting cellulitis/folliculitis of scalp (perifolliculitis abscedens et suffodiens)

Mixed

- Acne keloidalis nuchae
- Acne necrotica
- Eruptive pustular dermatosis

Nonspecific (End stage)

CAUSES

All types of cicatricial alopecias involve inflammation directed at stem cell niche in the outer root sheath at the level of insertion of the arrector pili muscle (the bulge) which destroys any potential for hair regrowth. Histologically, the follicles ultimately disappear or are replaced by fibrous stelae. Patients may complain of itching, burning, soreness, scaling, or discharge. Primary cicatricial alopecia tends to run a chronic and progressive course and ultimately leads to disfigurement.

EPIDEMIOLOGY

Cicatricial alopecia is not rare. It represents approximately 7% of patients seen in specialist hair loss clinics.

Age, Sex and Ethnicity

Most cases of LPP are seen in women aged 30-50 years. Discoid lupus erythematosus occurs twice as commonly in women than men. Frontal fibrosing alopecia occurs almost exclusively in postmenopausal women. Folliculitis decalvans occurs equally in men and women from the age of 30 years. Dissecting cellulitis is most common in men in their twenties.

Associated Diseases

Scalp lichen planus and discoid lupus of the scalp will have cutaneous disease elsewhere either at presentation or during follow-up. Linear morphea may be associated with facial hemiatrophy. Follicular mucinosis may be associated with cutaneous T-cell lymphoma. Scalp metastases may be solitary or associated with widespread metastatic disease. Dissecting cellulitis may be associated with the follicular occlusion tetrad. Keratosis pilaris spinulosa decalvans may be associated with keratosis pilaris elsewhere on the body.

INVESTIGATIONS

After the preliminary diagnosis of cicatricial alopecia, examination of scalp is needed to find cause of the hair loss such as folliculitis, follicular plugging, or broken hairs. Dermoscopy reveals a loss of follicular ostia. Hairs, even if grossly normal in appearance, should be extracted from the edge of the bald area for microscopy and culture in folliculitis decalvans. In most cases, a diagnostic biopsy is indicated. The site for biopsy must be carefully selected: early lesions are likely to yield more information. Several punch biopsies are preferable to a single elliptical biopsy. In this way, different stages of the disease process can be investigated. Ideally, at least one 4 mm biopsy should be taken from a clinically active area, prepared for horizontal section and stained with hematoxylin and eosin.

MANAGEMENT

A number of treatments are used empirically. The aim of treatment is to reduce symptoms and to slow or stop the progression of hair loss. Early treatment is the key to minimize the extent of permanent alopecia. Surgical correction with a combination of scalp reduction and hair transplantation is generally recommended for secondary cicatricial alopecia. Camouflage powders and sprays as well as wigs are useful.

Conditions presenting with cicatricial alopecia are discussed here.

Follicular Lichen Planus

Lichen planus is an idiopathic inflammatory disease that may affect the skin, hair, and nails. When it affects hair, cicatricial alopecia occurs.

Three varieties are:

1. Classical lichen planopilaris
2. Frontal fibrosing alopecia
3. Graham-Little-Piccardi-Lasseur syndrome (GLPLS)

Classical Lichen Planopilaris

This is the most common form of follicular lichen planus and typically presents with progressive scarring alopecia of the scalp. This occurs in middle age and preferentially affects females. Involvement of areas other than the scalp is seen in 17–28% of patients at presentation and in 50% during the course of the disease.

Pathophysiology: Karnik et al. investigated the molecular basis for LPP using microarray analysis and identified a decreased expression of genes required for lipid metabolism and peroxisome biogenesis. The expression of peroxisome proliferator-activated receptor-γ (PPAR-γ), a transcription factor that regulates these processes, was found to be significantly decreased in LPP. Immunohistochemical analysis of biopsies from LPP showed a progressive loss of peroxisomes, proinflammatory lipid accumulation, and infiltration of inflammatory cells preceding the destruction of the pilosebaceous unit.

Pathology: Epidermal changes include fibrillar changes in the basal cells that lead to the formation of colloid bodies. Macrophages containing pigment may be seen in the dermis. Fibrin and immunoglobulin M (IgM) may be detected in the upper dermis and various components of complement in the basement membrane zone in immunofluorescence (IF). In classical lesion, horny and granular layers are thickened and there is irregular acanthosis. Flattening of the rete pegs gives rise to a saw-tooth configuration. There is liquefaction degeneration of the basal cells. Close-up against the epidermis is a dense infiltrate of lymphocytes and some histiocytes. When the process involves hair follicles, the infiltrate extends around them and the hairs are replaced by keratin plugs. The follicles may ultimately be totally destroyed.

Clinical features: It initially starts as violaceous follicular scaly papular lesion which spreads peripherally and eventually these papules are replaced by follicular plugs and scarring. The plugs are shed from the scarred area, which remains white, smooth, and atrophic. A well-developed lesion is a patch of smooth, skin-colored, scarring alopecia with or without follicular plugging at the periphery, and tufts of unaffected hairs within it. Hyperkeratotic papules are seen in peripherally extending lesion. Hair pull test will be positive at the margins. Symptoms of itching, burning, pain, and tenderness are often present. Disease activity is maximum at periphery which differentiates it from DLE and alopecia mucinosa.

On trichoscopy, perifollicular inflammation leading to formation of tubular scales called peripilar casts, is seen usually at the periphery of the patch. Also seen are target "blue-gray dots" which reflect perifollicular pigment incontinence. Chronic cases show white dots which are the fibrous tracts that replace the scarred follicles. The spared interfollicular skin shows the honeycomb pigment pattern and some spared follicles bearing terminal hairs. Pulled hairs reveal anagen roots with preserved hair sheaths.

Sites of predilection for LPP other than the scalp include the axillae, inguinal folds, sacrum, and limb flexures. It manifests as grouped or disseminated follicular, flat, elevated, or hemispherical erythematous papules or punctate keratoses.

Treatment: A short course of systemic corticosteroid may be desirable initially to stabilize the disease. Intralesional corticosteroids are helpful when active inflammatory changes are still present. Potent topical steroids such as clobetasol propionate ointment or shampoo once daily usually relieves associated symptoms such as itch or pain, and may slightly inhibit the process. Cyclosporine is very effective for cutaneous lichen planus. Retinoids (acitretin, isotretinoin), chloroquine, griseofulvin, and thalidomide can be used. Specific PPAR-γ targeted therapy with agents such as pioglitazone is disappointing till now.

Frontal Fibrosing Alopecia

Introduction: This is a clinical variant of LPP, with similar histologic features.

Clinical features: It has been associated with the postmenopausal state. Clinically, it is identified by progressive symmetric band-like alopecia with recession of frontal hair line. In contrast to AGA, the recession is in straight line. Recession of posterior hair line is also seen. There is loss of follicular ostia. Margin toward hair line is serrated. There is perifollicular erythema and hyperkeratotic papules at margin. Eyebrow, eyelash, and axilla are also involved. The natural history of FFA is one of slow progression over many years. Recession of the hairline eventually stops in most cases but this cannot be predicted.

The trichoscopy findings in FFA include absence of follicular openings, follicular hyperkeratosis, perifollicular scaling, and perifollicular erythema.[8] Broken hair shafts and pili torti can be seen occasionally too. Perifollicular erythema is a characteristic feature of FFA, but not always evident on trichoscopy for being an evolutive sign that is followed by interfollicular erythema.[8]

Differential diagnosis includes keratosis follicularis spinulosa decalvans, traction alopecia, and ophiasis.

Treatment includes topical minoxidil and topical as well as systemic steroids. Systemic retinoids, hydroxychloroquine, and griseofulvin have been tried with a variable response. Finasteride 2.5 mg/day was found to arrest the progression of disease in women.

Graham–Little–Piccardi–Lasseur Syndrome

In 1915, Graham–Little reported the case of a woman aged 55 years who had suffered for 10 years from slowly progressive cicatricial alopecia and for 5 months from groups of horny papules.

Pathophysiology: In the scalp, the mouths of affected follicles are filled by horny plugs. The underlying follicle is progressively destroyed and eventually an atrophic epidermis covers sclerotic dermis. In the axillae and pubic region, the follicles are likewise destroyed, although the skin does not appear clinically to be atrophic.

Middle-aged or elderly women are the commonly affected. It is a rare lichenoid dermatosis defined by the triad of multifocal cicatricial alopecia of the scalp; noncicatricial alopecia of the axilla and groin; and a follicular lichen planus eruption on the body, scalp, or both.

In most patients, the earliest change has been patchy cicatricial alopecia of the scalp.

The keratosis pilaris is referred to in early case reports as lichen spinulosus. In most cases, they have developed aggressively and have been grouped into plaques, often on the trunk, or the trunk and limbs, but occasionally involving the eyebrows and the sides of the face.

Management: No treatment is universally effective. A short course of oral prednisolone is used to stabilize rapidly progressive disease. Cyclosporine can also be used.

KERATOSIS PILARIS ATROPHICANS

It is characterized by keratotic follicular papules that are followed by permanent follicular loss. Three well-known types are included:

1. Keratosis pilaris atrophicans facei
2. Keratosis follicularis spinulosa decalvans
3. Atrophoderma vermiculata

Biopsy shows follicular plugging and a perifollicular lymphocytic infiltrate in early phase, while later lesions show follicular destruction.

Topical emollients, keratolytics, tretinoin, and steroids have been tried. Systemic retinoids can be used, keeping in mind the side effects.

CENTRAL CENTRIFUGAL CICATRICIAL ALOPECIA (FOLLICULAR DEGENERATION SYNDROME, HOT COMB ALOPECIA)

It is a scarring alopecia that mainly affects women of African descent. Thermal trauma induced by a hot comb used for hair straightening can lead to hair damage and hence was termed "hot comb alopecia." More women with scarring alopecia had a history of hair weaving and long duration of chemical relaxer usage. Now it is thought to be due to premature degeneration of the IRS and hence, it has been called follicular degeneration syndrome. There is developing evidence that the etiology of central centrifugal cicatricial alopecia (CCCA) may be multifactorial. The current name CCCA reflects the clinical appearance of the condition.

Clinical Features

It presents usually in the third or later decades, average age of onset at 38 years, as a patch of diminished density of hair on the posterior vertex of the scalp that continues to widen irregularly but bilaterally while leaving behind few short and brittle hairs. There may be clinical evidence of inflammation at the advancing margin. It follows a pattern similar to FPHL. Additionally, pustules and crusting may be found in patients with superimposed folliculitis decalvans.

The trichoscopy shows perihilar white halos, loss of follicular openings, disrupted pigmented network, irregularly distributed pinpoint white dots, and individual broken hair follicles.

Differential diagnosis: Female pattern hair loss, AA, LPP, or telogen effluvium.

Treatment

It involves avoiding hair styles that require heat treatment or produce traction and avoiding relaxers. For folliculitis decalvans, topical corticosteroids, and oral tetracyclines can be used. Hair transplantation can be useful in patients with advanced disease. Olsen postulated an overlap between this condition and FPHL with fibrosis and advocated the use of topical minoxidil.

FOLLICULITIS DECALVANS (QUINQUAUD'S DISEASE)

Folliculitis decalvans (FD) is a rare neutrophilic inflammation of the scalp leading to progressive cicatricial alopecia. This entity was first described by Quinquaud. It is also known as tufted folliculitis.

Various terminologies such as lupoid sycosis (Brocq 1888), ulerythema sycosiforme (Unna 1889), and epilating folliculitis of the glabrous skin (Arnozan 1892 and Dubreuilh 1894) essentially imply the same process. Similar lesions involving the hairy regions of the lower limbs are termed as folliculitis depilans and folliculitis cruris et atrophicans. It is believed that all these entities are variants of a single syndrome.

Tufted folliculitis occurs when the infundibular epithelium of damaged follicles heals with the formation of a large, common infundibulum. Tufted folliculitis is not specific for folliculitis decalvans. It can occur in different cicatrical alopecia by the afore-mentioned mechanism. Up to 30 hairs may emerge through a common dilated pore. Tufted folliculitis with multiple hairs emerging from a single follicular ostium gives "dolly hair" appearance.

It typically starts as crops of pinhead-sized follicular pustules which is followed by round or oval patches of scarring hair loss. The disease may remain limited to a few small patches or may progress over time causing extensive hair loss.

Although the scalp is the most common affected region, any body site such as the beard, axillae, groins, and pubes may be involved. *Staphylococcus aureus* is frequently demonstrable in these lesions.

Pathophysiology

Histology reveals follicular abscesses, with a dense perifollicular polymorphonuclear infiltrate, and scattered eosinophils and plasma cells in the upper portion of the follicle with partial or complete epithelial disruption. In mature lesions, foreign-body granulomatous inflammation around hair shaft bits within the dermis may be seen. Eventually all that remains of the follicle is extensive fibrosis.

Investigations

As fungal kerion may mimic folliculitis decalvans, hairs should be plucked for fungal culture and a periodic acid–Schiff (PAS) stain should be performed on the scalp biopsy. The purulent discharge from lesions should be cultured and tested for antibiotic sensitivity in all cases.

On trichoscopy, it is characterized by presence of multiple upright hairs (>5) emerging from a single ostium, corresponding to the classic clinical picture. Follicular scaling is seen representing follicular inflammation. In addition, follicular pustules are seen at the active border. Twisted capillary loops may be seen in the interfollicular region. The inactive scarred areas are seen as pinkish-white patches with absent follicular openings.

Treatment

- Oral antibiotics during initial stage can halt the inflammation and prevent scarring. Cotrimoxazole has given good results. Clindamycin (300 mg bid), ciprofloxacin, or clarithromycin should be given along with high dose. Rifampicin (300 mg bid) for 10 weeks.
- Rifampicin not only cures the infection but also eliminates the *S. aureus* carrier state.
- Topical antibacterials such as mupirocin 1%, fusidic acid 1%, or erythromycin 2% bid can be used.
- In some severe forms, addition of an oral corticosteroid may be necessary.
- Oral isotretinoin can result in long-term remissions in some patients.
- Methyl aminolevulinate photodynamic therapy is reported to result in clinical improvement.

CHRONIC CUTANEOUS LUPUS ERYTHEMATOSUS

Lupus erythematosus is an autoimmune, connective tissue disease characterized by the presence of circulating nonorgan-specific autoantibodies to cell nuclear antigens.

Three different forms are described: (1) Systemic lupus erythematosus (SLE), (2) Subacute cutaneous lupus erythematosus (SCLE), and (3) Chronic cutaneous lupus erythematosus (CCLE). However, only CCLE regularly produces cicatricial alopecia. CCLE in most of the cases does not present with systemic involvement but it might be a presentation of SLE.

Scalp lesion in cutaneous LE is a marker of chronicity of disease.

Pathophysiology

There is hyperkeratosis with follicular plugging, a perivascular and periadnexal lymphoid infiltrate. Focal basal layer vacuolar degeneration is seen. Colloid body formation, pigmentary incontinence, papillary dermal edema, thickening of the basement membrane zone and exocytosis of lymphocytes into the epidermis, and follicular epithelium are seen.

Scarring occurs only in CCLE and manifests as homogenized collagen fibers running parallel to the surface, a loss of appendages and lone arrector pili muscles.

In contrast to lichen planus, hypergranulosis, saw- toothed rete ridges, perifollicular fibrosis, and clefts are absent in lupus. There is linear staining of deposits of complement (C3), IgM and IgG on the basement membrane in >80% of cases of LE, but not in lichen planus. Also direct immunofluorescence (DIF) is positive in lupus.

Clinical Features

Scarring alopecia occurs in 20% of men and 50% of women affected with CCLE. It starts as erythematous scaly patches that may go unnoticed until the hairs are lost. The IRS, which molds the hair shaft, gets twisted and deformed due to follicular fibrosis, and hence, gives rise to curly hairs in nonalopecic plaques of scalp DLE. Erythematous plaques covered with adherent scales that show "carpet tacks" on the undersurface are visible at this stage. It is followed by atrophic, depigmented scars with telangiectases in the center and hyperpigmentation at the periphery **(Fig. 27)**.

Investigations

Antinuclear antibody is positive in approximately 35% of patients with CCLE. Anti-Ro antibodies are found in 10%.

Trichoscopy of the affected skin shows atrophy with complete loss of follicular openings. Arborizing telangiectasia is seen over the patch. Prominent hyperkeratotic follicular plugging is seen at the periphery of the plaque. Dark brown to blue-gray pigment pattern is seen in DLE affecting the interfollicular area unlike in LPP where it is concentrated around the follicles.

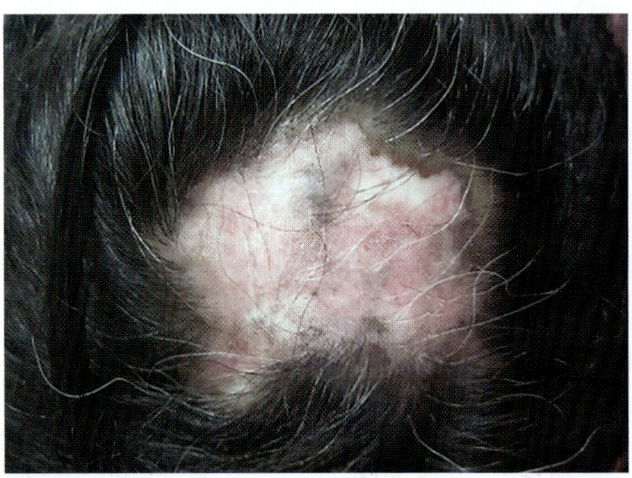

Fig. 27: Scarring alopecia in discoid lupus erythematosus lesion.

Treatment

Photoprotection with a hat or a broad-spectrum sunscreen can be used. Topical potent steroids or intralesional steroids are the drug of choice for limited disease. Many topical agents, viz., tacrolimus (0.1%), tazarotene (0.05%), imiquimod (5%), and intralesional IFN-α2 have been used with variable results.

In cases with rapid progression, antimalarials, oral prednisolone, and isotretinoin can be used. Antimalarials form the mainstay of treatment in chronic cases refractory to topical steroids. Hydroxychloroquine in a regimen of 200–400 mg/day produces a remission within 3 months in the majority and the dosage can then be tapered gradually. Scarring is permanent, but early treatment may produce a surprising amount of regrowth.

Other modalities tried are dapsone, clofazimine, methotrexate, azathioprine, mycophenolate mofetil, systemic IFN-α2 and monoclonal anti-CD4 antibodies.

CICATRICIAL PEMPHIGOID

Recurrent bullae finally lead to scarring alopecia. In Brunsting–Perry variant, the scalp and face may be involved in the absence of mucosal lesions.

PSEUDOPELADE OF BROCQ

Pelade is the French term for alopecia areata. While some believe pseudopelade is a unique entity, most now believe that it is an end stage or clinical variant of various forms of cicatricial alopecia.

The following two types of pseudopelade of Brocq are recognized:

1. *Primary idiophathic pseudopelade:* Pathophysiology unknown.
2. *Secondary psuedopelade:* It occurs as end stage or burnt out stage of other cicatricial disorders such as follicular lichen planus, morphea, DLE, etc.

Pathophysiology

Early lesions may have a light lymphocytic infiltrate around the upper two-thirds of the hair follicle. This infiltrate invades sebaceous glands and eventually destroys the entire pilosebaceous unit. Single hairs may survive within a patch for many years.

Later patches are smooth, soft and slightly depressed, and histology reveals thin atrophic epidermis overlying a sclerotic dermis containing fibrotic streams extending into the subcutis. There are no inflammatory changes at this stage. These fibrotic streams are follicular "ghosts." Arrector pili muscles may be seen inserting into these fibrous remnants of hair follicles.

With an acid-alcohol orcein stain, elastic fibers are seen around the lower part of the follicle, whereas in all the other scarring alopecias, the scar tissue consists of collagen devoid of elastin.

Clinical Features

It is a very uncommon type of alopecia mainly affecting females between ages 30 and 50 years. Lesions are distributed randomly. The alopecia is asymptomatic and is often discovered by chance. It classically presents as porcelain white hypopigmented and slightly depressed atrophic plaque. Lesions often are shaped irregularly, as opposed to the round or oval patches usually seen in AA. Irregular and confluent patches form "foot print in snow" appearance.

The course is extremely variable. Most often there is slow development over many years of small, round patches of alopecia that ultimately converge to produce larger irregular areas of hair loss.

Braun-Falco (1986) proposed clinical and histological criteria for making the diagnosis.

Clinical Criteria

- Irregular and confluent patches of hair loss
- Moderate atrophy (late stage)
- Mild redness around hair follicles (early stage)
- Female predominance (3:1)
- Long course of >2 years
- Slow progression
- Spontaneous termination possible.

Histological Criteria

- No marked inflammation
- No widespread scarring
- No significant plugging of hair follicles
- No sebaceous (oil) glands
- Normal epidermis
- Fibrotic streamers in dermis.

Immunohistochemistry

Negative: Disease progression eventually ends spontaneously. Topical corticosteroids, intralesional triamcinolone acetonide (10 mg/mL), prednisone, oral mini pulse, hydroxychloroquine, isotretinoin, and mycophenolate mofetil are some of the options with almost nil results. Autologous hair transplantation and scalp reduction surgery can be done in stable alopecia.

LIPEDEMATOUS SCALP

Lipedematous scalp is a rare entity characterized by an increased thickness of subcutaneous tissue in the scalp giving soft spongy appearance of the surface and occasionally causes pruritus and pain in the affected area. The scalp is soft, spongy, or thick in the forehead area (apex) and in the back (occiput) of the head. Symptoms include diffuse pain, abnormal sensations (paresthesia), headache, burning, thickening of the scalp with localized or generalized sensitivity of the scalp or itching.

The cause is unknown, but there may be mechanical factors, such as the prolonged wearing of tight headwear and hormonal factors. Lipedematous scalp may be associated with diseases such as diabetes mellitus, renal failure, loose joints and skin, Sjögren's syndrome, hyperlipidemia, and ovarian cysts. There is no definitive treatment to stop the progression of the disease.

TRACTION ALOPECIA

Hairstyles that impose sustained pulling on the hair roots lead to traction alopecia. It can be associated with headache and relieved when the hair is loosened. Fringe sign? Trichoscopy?

Hair loss is usually seen along the marginal hairline (frontal, temporal, or occipital) with decreased retained follicular markings and the presence of a "fringe" of finer, or miniaturized hairs. The characteristic finding is the retention of hair follicles of lesser diameter along the frontal and/or temporal hairline. This sign is called the "fringe sign," and it correlates with the presence of vellus hairs seen in the histology.[9]

Trichoscopy reveals the presence of hair casts (HC) (typical of traction alopecia). In patients with a patchy and marginal type of alopecia secondary to traction, a reduction in the density of hair follicles, the absence of follicular openings, and the presence of a large number of freely mobile HCs at the periphery of the patch are seen. In the patient with a diffuse type of alopecia secondary to traction, trichoscopy reveals a normal density of hair with numerous HCs. The HCs due to traction alopecia are nonadherent, white or brown in color, cylindrical in shape, and tend to encircle the proximal hair shaft.[10]

It may be reversible during early stages. The patient or parents need to be educated to adopt hairstyles that do not pull the hair tight. Where there is inflammation, mild steroids can be helpful.

KEY POINTS

- Alopecia refers to hair loss which can be localized, partial or complete involving scalp, eyebrows, moustache, beard, or body hair, and is broadly classified into cicatricial and noncicatricial.
- Basic approach is to have a thorough history and clinical examination.
- Trichoscopy is a great and handy tool to evaluate these cases. Laboratory investigations also aid in many cases.
- Scalp biopsy and DIF may also be indicated in cases of cicatricial alopecia.
- Noncicatricial alopecia (nonscarring alopecia) is further classified into localized and diffuse. Treatment is aimed at the underlying cause.
- Alopecia areata has an autoimmune pathology and genetic predisposition.

- Androgenetic alopecia is one of the most common causes of hair loss and can present with male or female pattern baldness.
- Diffuse hair shedding can have wide variety of triggers and the most common type is telogen effluvium.
- Trichotillomania is a behavioral disorder with compulsive hair pulling resulting in alopecia.
- Hair shaft disorders are broadly classified into two main types: (1) those associated with increased fragility and (2) those not associated with increased fragility.
- Cicatricial alopecias (scarring alopecia) are classified as primary or secondary and also classified on the basis of inflammatory infiltrate histologically.
- Various causes of cicatricial alopecia include lichen planus, CCLE, FFA, CCCA, folliculitis decalvans, pseudopelade of Brocq, lipedematous scalp, etc.
- Aim of treatment in cicatricial alopecia is to reduce symptoms and to arrest the disease process. Early treatment is required to minimize the extent of hair loss and surgical correction may also be indicated.

REFERENCES

1. Dawber RPR, Ebling FJG, Wojnarowska FT. Disorders of hair. In: Champion RH, Burton JL, Ebling FJG (Eds). Textbook of Dermatology, 5th edition. Oxford: Blackwell Scientific; 1991. pp. 2533-638.
2. Jain N, Doshi B, Khopkar U. Trichoscopy in alopecias: diagnosis simplified. Int J Trichology. 2013;5:170-8.
3. McElwee KJ, Gilhar A, Tobin DJ, Ramot Y, Sundberg JP, Nakamura M, et al. What causes alopecia areata? Exp Dermatol. 2013;22(9):609-26.
4. Efentaki P, Altenburg A, Haerting J, Zouboulis CC. Medium-dose prednisolone pulse therapy in alopecia areata. Dermatoendocrinol. 2009;1(6):310-3.
5. Shankar DK, Chakravarthi M, Shilpakar R. Male androgenetic alopecia: population-based study in 1,005 subjects. Int J Trichology. 2009;1:131-3.
6. Brockshmidt FF, Heilmann S, Ellis JA, Eigelshoven S, Hanneken S, Herold C, et al. Susceptibility variants on chromosome 7p21.1 suggest *HDAC9* as a new candidate gene for male-pattern baldness. Br J Dermatol. 2011;165(6):1293-302.
7. Duquia RP, Almeida HL Jr, Souza PRM, Vettorato G. Netherton's syndrome with a 20-year follow-up. An Bras Dermatol. 2006; 81:559-62.
8. Toledo-Pastrana T, Hernández MJ, Camacho Martínez FM. Perifollicular erythema as a trichoscopy sign of progression in frontal fibrosing alopecia. Int J Trichology. 2013;5:151-3.
9. Pulickal JK, Kaliyadan (2020). Traction Alopecia. In: StatPearls [Internet]. Available from: https://www.ncbi.nlm.nih.gov/books/NBK470434/ [Last accessed January 2021].
10. Polat M. Evaluation of clinical signs and early and late trichoscopy findings in traction alopecia patients with Fitzpatrick skin type II and III: a single-center, clinical study. Int J Dermatol. 2017;56(8):850-5.

EXAMINATION QUESTIONS

1. Explain DD of a 35-year-old female with non-scarring alopecia.
2. Describe the pathogenesis and management of alopecia areata. What are the newer management modalities of alopecia areata?
3. Explain trichoscopy in non-scarring alopecia.
4. Explain trichoscopy in alopecia areata.
5. Write a short note on hair shaft disorders.

75 CHAPTER

Hirsutism and Hypertrichosis

Rajetha Damisetty

INTRODUCTION

Hair in human beings is considered largely vestigial; yet abnormalities of hair, both its loss from the scalp and its presence anywhere on the body in excess are fraught with emotional distress. The onslaught of images of smooth faces and hair-less bodies on social media has made even normal body hair relatively unacceptable. It is prudent to expect those with excess hair due to either hypertrichosis or hirsutism to be more anguished than ever. The onus on the dermatologist to make an etiologic diagnosis of excess hair and to manage it effectively is also particular high in today's world.

HYPERTRICHOSIS VERSUS HIRSUTISM

Hypertrichosis is defined as the presence of excess hair growth anywhere on the body irrespective of the gender.[1] Excess hair is in comparison with what is considered normal for individuals of the same age, race, and sex. Hirsutism is the presence of increased number of terminal hairs in a male pattern in a female. It is important to distinguish hypertrichosis from hirsutism as endocrine evaluation is usually warranted in the latter.[2] The latter is a marker of androgen excess, either in the circulation or at the level of the receptor and the hair follicle.

HYPERTRICHOSIS: CLASSIFICATION

Hypertrichosis may be classified based on:

- Age of onset (congenital or acquired)
- Extent of distribution (generalized or circumscribed)
- Type of excess hair (lanugo, vellus, or terminal)
- Site involved
- Isolated or associated with other anomalies

Congenital hypertrichosis is rare and may be an isolated condition of the skin or a component feature of other disorders **(Flowchart 1)**. Acquired hypertrichosis is far more frequent.

Acquired Hypertrichosis

It may be generalized or localized **(Figs. 1 and 2)**.

- Drug induced
- Metabolic disorders (porphyrias, mucopolysaccharidoses such as Hurler, Hunter, and Sanfilippo syndrome)

Flowchart 1: Classification of congenital hypertrichosis.

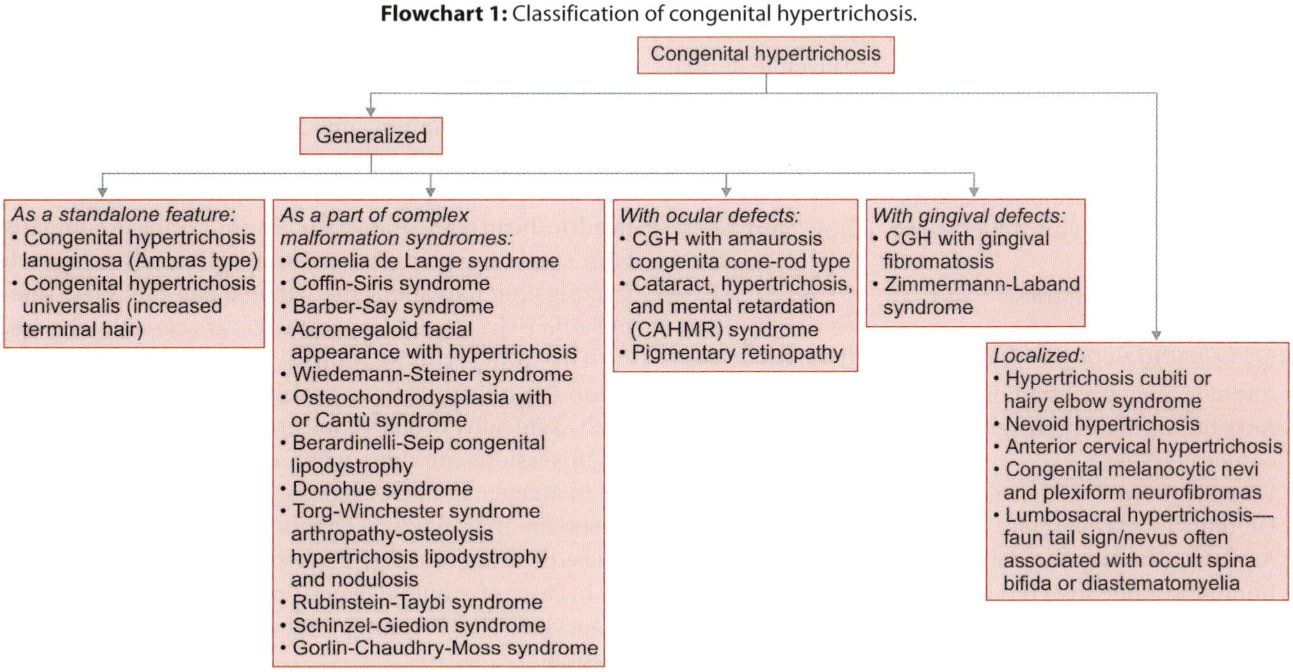

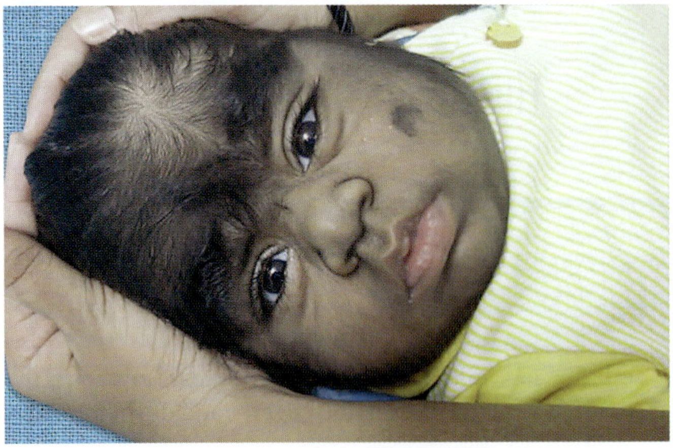

Fig. 1: Congenital generalized hypertrichosis.

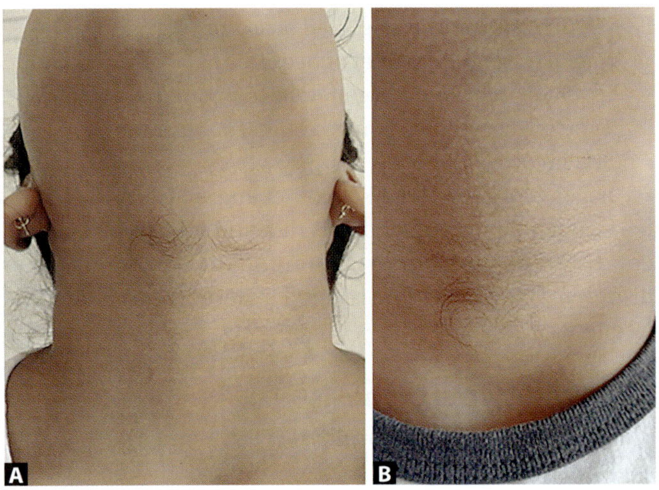

Figs. 2A and B: Anterior cervical hypertrichosis in nonidentical twins.

- Endocrine disorders (juvenile hypothyroidism and acromegaly)
- Cutaneous autoinflammatory diseases (juvenile dermatomyositis)
- Infectious diseases [advanced human immunodeficiency virus (HIV) infection, varicella scars]
- Malnutrition and anorexia nervosa
- Paraneoplastic syndromes (lung, colon, and breast carcinomas)
- Traumatic brain injuries

Drugs Causing Acquired Generalized Hypertrichosis

- Antibiotics such as streptomycin
- Anti-inflammatory drugs such as benoxaprofen and corticosteroids
- Vasodilators (diazoxide, minoxidil, and prostaglandin E1)
- Diuretics (acetazolamide)
- Anticonvulsants (phenytoin)
- Immunosuppressives (cyclosporine and mycophenolate mofetil)
- Psoralens (methoxypsoralen and trimethylpsoralen)
- Antiseptic agents (hexachlorobenzene)
- Chelators (penicillamine)
- Interferon-alpha
- Fenoterol
- Epidermal growth factor receptor (EGFR) inhibitors (cetuximab, panitumumab, erlotinib, and gefitinib)

Topical Formulations Causing Hypertrichosis

- Topical corticosteroids
- Sclerotherapy
- Tacrolimus
- Bimatoprost and latanoprost

It is important to carefully evaluate all patients with hypertrichosis and reach a precise diagnosis which may unearth systemic concerns. All of them should be offered a solution for the cosmetic problem which may weigh heavily on the mind.

MANAGEMENT OF HYPERTRICHOSIS

Temporary methods of hair removal such as shaving and waxing are frequently resorted to by those with hypertrichosis. Permanent laser hair reduction (LHR) has revolutionized the management of unwanted hair and should be offered to all patients with hypertrichosis.[3] Many of them are discriminated against and distressed emotionally. Neodymium-doped yttrium aluminum garnet (Nd:YAG) (1,064 nm) and diode (800 or 810 nm) lasers are the most popular; alexandrite (755 nm) laser has been gaining acceptance for the past few years, especially after In-motion technology has become widely available and understood. Intense pulse lights (IPLs) have lost favor, particularly the inexpensive ones with narrow pulse widths **(Fig. 3)**.

Combination of wavelengths has become trendy with double wavelengths (755 nm and 810 nm Reveal Vega, 755 and 1,064 nm Lumenis Splendor X, Lutronic Clarity and Candela), triple wavelengths (755, 810, and 1,064 nm in Alma Soprano Platinum and Titanium and 810, 940, 1,060 nm in Cocoon's) primelase and quadruple wavelengths (755 nm, 810 nm, 940 nm, and 1,064 nm Milesman Compact blend). Large scale head-to-head comparative studies are lacking in comparison with single wavelengths. 755 nm has an advantage while treating finer hair and lighter colored hair but is less safe for melanin rich skin unless parameters are carefully chosen.

The number of sessions would depend on the skin color, the hair thickness, and the device and parameters used. Typically, 6–8 sessions are required. Efficacy is high when sessions are done when maximum number of hairs are in anagen, at intervals of 2–3 months. Unlike those with hirsutism, maintenance sessions are not usually required unless the drug causing hirsutism needs to be continued.

In cases of acquired hypertrichosis, the root cause should be tackled. The offending drug should be withdrawn when possible.

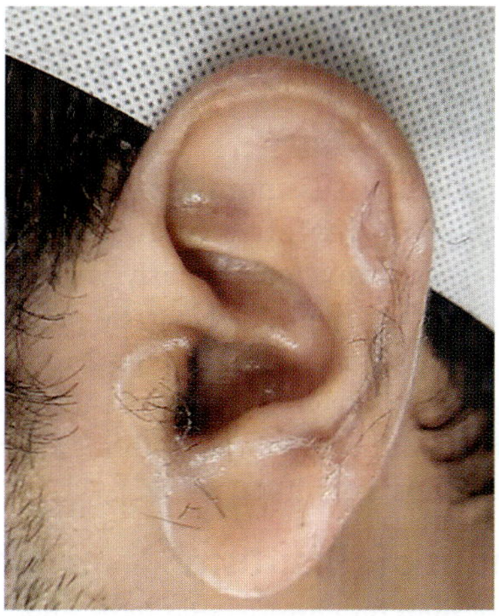

Fig. 3: Y-chromosome linked pinna hypertrichosis after marking for laser hair reduction (LHR).

BOX 1: Etiology of hirsutism.

- *PCOS*: 70–90% of hirsutism approximately
- *Idiopathic*: 5–17%
- *Nonclassic congenital adrenal hyperplasia (NCCAH)*: 1–8%
- *Pituitary or other endocrine abnormalities (present as secondary PCOS)*:
  - Hyperprolactinemia
  - Cushing's syndrome
  - Severe hypothyroidism
  - GH abnormalities
- Ovarian/adrenal tumors
- Ovarian hyperthecosis (a severe variant of PCOS with a tumor-like presentation)
- *Drugs*: Androgens, corticosteroids, progestins, estrogen antagonists (clomiphene and tamoxifen), danazol, phenytoin, and D-penicillamine
- *Drugs causing hyperprolactinemia:* Metoclopramide and phenothiazines

(GH: growth hormone; PCOS: polycystic ovarian syndrome)

HIRSUTISM

Defining Hirsutism

Hirsutism is defined as excess terminal hair in a woman in a male pattern.[2,3] Typically affected areas are the lower face, upper neck, chest, and lower abdomen. A change in the form and rate of hair growth is an important determinant in making the diagnosis of hirsutism, particularly in the early days. It affects approximately 5–15% of premenopausal women across the world.

Normal amount of hair for women is heavily dependent on ethnicity with some races being naturally more hairy. Terminal hair on either the chin or the lower abdomen (score ≥ 2) was close to 100% sensitive and 27% specific at predicting total body hirsutism.[4] Semiquantitative definition of a score exceeding 8 in modified Ferriman-Gallwey (mFG) scoring is popular but the cutoff is not sacrosanct. A score of 5 and 7 has been found to be relevant in Guangdong province, China[5] and in Filipino[6] women, respectively.

Hirsutism has to be distinguished from hypertrichosis which may be localized or generalized but without confirming to a male pattern.

Grading of Hirsutism

The mFG score takes into account hair growth in nine androgen-sensitive body areas—(1) the upper lip, (2) chin, (3) chest, (4) upper and (5) lower back, (6) upper and (7) lower abdomen, (8) upper arm, and (9) thigh. A score of 0 implies the absence of terminal hair growth, and a score of 4 represents extensive growth.

Etiology of Hirsutism

Polycystic ovarian syndrome (PCOS) is the most common cause of hirsutism. Idiopathic hirsutism accounts for 5–17% of all hirsutism.[7] The other important cause is nonclassic congenital adrenal hyperplasia (NCCAH/LOCAH), an autosomal recessive condition with a deficiency of 21-hydroxylase, constituting 1–8%. All the other etiologies account for <1–2%. They are enlisted in **Box 1**. Most Indian studies have underestimated the presence of PCOS in hirsute patients as transabdominal ultrasonography has a low sensitivity for identifying polycystic ovarian morphology.[8]

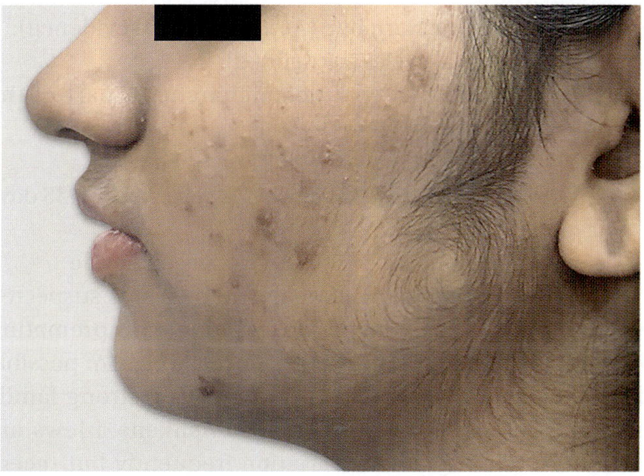

Fig. 4: A 14-year-old girl with acne excoriée, extensive truncal acne, axillary acanthosis nigricans, and irregular cycles 3 years after menarche with nonclassic congenital adrenal hyperplasia (NCCAH).

Etiologic Diagnosis of Hirsutism

Hirsutism may be termed a morphologic diagnosis or a symptom; a specific etiological diagnosis is essential in order to exclude potentially fatal conditions such as androgen-secreting tumors or the lifelong consequences of some disorders associated with hirsutism such as PCOS and NCCAH **(Fig. 4)**.

Polycystic ovarian syndrome is suspected in the setting of slowly progressing hirsutism of moderate to severe degree. Onset of hirsutism is usually in adolescence. Signs of insulin resistance (IR) (acanthosis nigricans and acrochordons) may be seen, even in the absence of excess body mass index (BMI).

Polycystic ovarian syndrome is usually diagnosed using the Rotterdam criteria[9] when two out of the following criteria are present.

1. Clinical (acne or hirsutism) and/or biochemical hyperandrogenemia (measured elevated androgen levels)
2. Menstrual irregularity
3. Polycystic ovarian morphology on transvaginal ultrasonography

It is a diagnosis that can be made only after excluding other specific disorders, such as nonclassic adrenal 21-hydroxylase deficiency, anterior pituitary disorders including Cushing syndrome, hyperprolactinemia, growth hormone (GH) abnormalities, severe hypothyroidism, and androgen-producing tumors. In patients with irregular menstrual cycles and hyperandrogenism, an ovarian ultrasound is not necessary for PCOS diagnosis, if there is no evidence of grossly excess thyroid-stimulating hormone (TSH), prolactin (laboratory evidence), and elevated GH and adrenocorticotropic hormone (ACTH) (clinical evidence). Irregular menstrual cycles are defined[10] as:

- Normal in the first year postmenarche as part of the pubertal transition
- *>1 to <3 years post menarche*: <21 or >45 days
- *>3 years postmenarche to perimenopause*: <21 or >35 days or <8 cycles per year
- >1 year postmenarche > 90 days for any one cycle

Nonclassic congenital adrenal hyperplasia is suspected when hirsutism has an early onset along with premature adrenarche. These girls are usually normal weight or possibly underweight, lack features of IR and have a strong family history.[7] Certain ethnicities such as Ashkenazi Jews are purported to have genetic variation frequently but recent studies have shown that the prevalence of these mutations has been overestimated. Since most patients with NCCAH carry one allele with a severe mutation for CYP21A2, there is a risk for having offspring with classic CAH. Premarital counseling is warranted once this diagnosis is made.

Idiopathic hirsutism underlies roughly 50% of mild hirsutism and 5–17% of all hirsutism.[7] Many patients diagnosed with idiopathic hirsutism may have subtle or overt PCOS which is missed due to the insensitivity of the diagnostic modalities used. A common scenario is when transabdominal ultrasonography is used in unmarried women, particularly those who are obese, the abdominal fat prevents the delineation of polycystic ovaries and a misdiagnosis of idiopathic hirsutism is made. In such situations, assay of anti-Müllerian hormone (AMH) may be of value.

Tumoral hirsutism should be considered when hirsutism is rapidly progressive and severe. Signs of virilization such as clitoromegaly change in voice and body habitus to a male phenotype with loss of breast mass and broadening of shoulders should make the clinician perform a keen search for a functional ovarian or adrenal tumor. Total testosterone is usually elevated beyond 150–200 ng/dL in such situations. Ovarian hyperthecosis, a severe variant of PCOS can closely mimic androgen secreting tumors.

Workup for Hirsutism

A thorough clinical assessment[11] including history taking for menstrual and obstetric history and evidence of hormonal dysregulation, particularly with respect to GH, ACTH, and hyperinsulinemia have to be performed prior to advising laboratory assessment. **Boxes 2 to 6** elaborate the laboratory investigations that need to be undertaken.

Flowchart 2 summarizes an algorithmic approach to reach an etiologic diagnosis of hirsutism.

Management of Hirsutism

Some patients may be comfortable with physical modes of removal such as shaving, threading, or waxing the unwanted hair. For many others, permanent or at least long-term reduction of cosmetically unacceptable hair is the aim

BOX 2: First-line investigations for hirsutism.

- Serum prolactin
- Thyroid-stimulating hormone (TSH)
- Serum total testosterone in the early follicular phase
- Ultrasonography of the pelvis in the early follicular phase, ideally using a high resolution transvaginal probe
- 17-hydroxyprogesterone in case of peripubertal onset

BOX 3: First-line investigations best done under endocrinologist's supervision.

- Insulin-like growth factor 1 (IGF-1) assay—in cases of associated acromegaly only
- Overnight dexamethasone suppression test—in the presence of Cushingoid features only

BOX 4: Second-line investigations.

- DHEAS—when tumoral origin is suspected but total testosterone is not grossly elevated
- Free androgen index
- Oral glucose tolerance test
- Fasting serum insulin and HOMA-IR

(DHEAS: dehydroepiandrosterone sulfate; HOMA-IR: homeostasis model assessment-insulin resistance)

BOX 5: Investigations that are frequently performed but do not add value.

- Free testosterone
- LH:FSH ratio
- Dihydrotestosterone
- Androstenedione
- Sex hormone binding globulin (SHBG)

(FSH: follicle-stimulating hormone; LH: luteinizing hormone)

BOX 6: Investigations done to facilitate pharmacologic therapy or to screen for metabolic abnormalities.

- Lipid profile
- Serum creatinine
- Serum electrolytes

Flowchart 2: Algorithmic approach to determine the etiology of hirsutism.

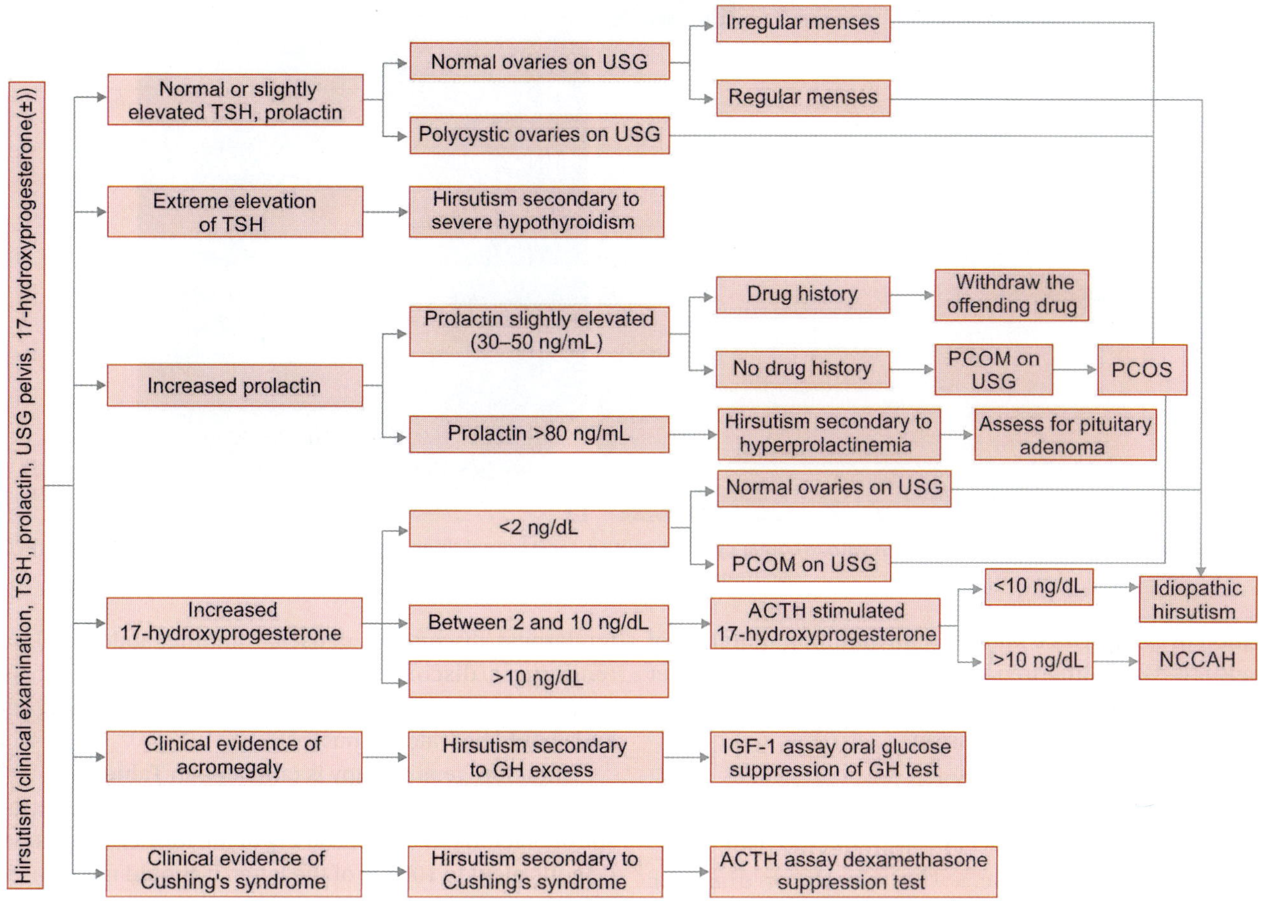

(ACTH: adrenocorticotropic hormone; GH: growth hormone; IGF-1: insulin-like growth factor 1; PCOM: polycystic ovary morphology; TSH: thyroid-stimulating hormone; USG: ultrasonography)

of management.[3] Optimal outcomes would be possible only if light or laser-based treatments and suppression of androgens are done simultaneously. This caveat holds good irrespective of the etiology of hirsutism and is applicable for idiopathic hirsutism too where peripheral androgen blockade is essential; antiandrogens need to be used concomitantly with combined oral contraceptive (COC) pills in women in the reproductive age to avoid irregular menses and possible feminization of the male fetus.

Polycystic Ovarian Syndrome Management

Lifestyle changes[11] including optimal diet, exercise, sleep, and stress management are integral to managing PCOS and need to be continued for life. Weight loss, more precisely "fat loss" helps in reducing both insulin and testosterone excess and reduces hirsutism. Ideal BMI of 23 should be the target but even 5% loss in weight can result in significant improvements.

Pharmacologic Treatment of PCOS ***(Figs. 5A and B)***

Most effective medical therapy of hirsutism associated with PCOS is combination therapy using COC pills and antiandrogens, with the addition of insulin in the presence of significant IR. Androgen suppression by the estrogenic component of COCs is the first-line therapy for PCOS. A minimum dose of 30 µg of ethinylestradiol (EE) is needed to exert this effect. Antiandrogenic progesterones such as drospirenone (Yasmin, Dronis 30, Crisanta, etc., with 3 mg drospirenone and 30 µg EE) or cyproterone acetate (Diane 35, Krimson 35, Ginette 35, etc., with 2 mg cyproterone acetate and 35 µg EE) are ideal. The former has a less unfavorable effect on metabolic parameters while the latter is slightly more effective.

The feared side effect is venous thromboembolism (VTE). The risk is doubled from 4–5/10,000 women years in reproductive age non-COC users to 8–9/10,000 women years in reproductive age COC users. Drospirenone containing COCs may be associated with a higher risk of VTE than COCs containing the progestin levonorgestrel or some other progestins. The relative risk ranged from no increase to a threefold increase. Risk is maximal during the first 6 months of therapy, gradually settles after that period and increases after restarting COCs.

The World Health Organization (WHO) list of absolute and relative contraindications should be used as a checklist before

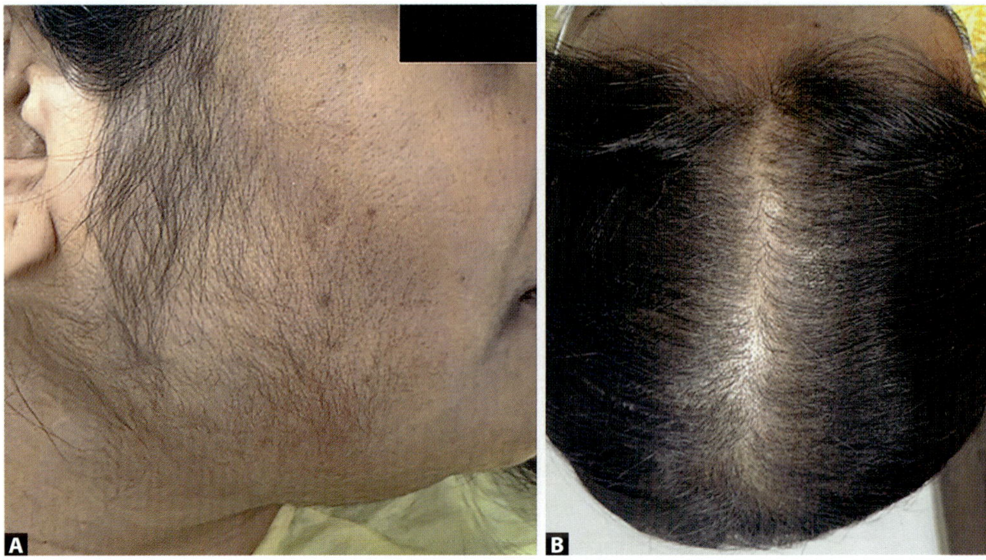

Figs. 5A and B: A 28-year-old obese women with irregular cycles, hirsutism, and frontal thinning with polycystic ovary morphology (PCOM) on transvaginal ultrasonography.

initiation of COCs. Once initiated, the minimum duration of therapy is 6–12 months, frequently up to 18 months or longer for patients with hirsutism to allow 6–8 sessions of LHR during the period of androgen suppression.

Absolute contraindications to COCs:

- <6 weeks postpartum
- Smoker over the age of 35 (>15 cigarettes per day)
- Hypertension (systolic > 160 mm Hg or diastolic >100 mm Hg)
- Current or past history of VTE
- Ischemic heart disease
- History of cerebrovascular accident
- Complicated valvular heart disease (pulmonary hypertension, atrial fibrillation, and history of subacute bacterial endocarditis)
- Migraine headache with focal neurological symptoms
- Breast cancer (current)
- Diabetes with retinopathy/nephropathy/neuropathy
- Severe cirrhosis
- Liver tumor (adenoma or hepatoma)

Relative contraindications to COCs:

- Smoker over the age of 35 (<15 cigarettes per day)
- Adequately controlled hypertension
- Hypertension (systolic 140–159 mm Hg or diastolic 90–99 mm Hg)
- Migraine headache over the age of 35
- Currently symptomatic gallbladder disease
- Mild cirrhosis
- History of combined oral contraceptive pill (OCP)-related cholestasis
- Users of medications that may interfere with OCP metabolism.

The most frequent adverse reactions (≥2%) are premenstrual syndrome, headache/migraine, breast pain/tenderness/discomfort, nausea/vomiting, abdominal pain/tenderness/discomfort, and mood changes. Depressive symptoms are more common in adolescents and young adults and should be watched out for.

Antiandrogens therapy is tabulated in **Table 1**.

Flutamide is potent antiandrogen deemed superior to spironolactone by some; 250 mg of the former was shown to be equivalent to 100 mg of the latter. It should not be used in hirsute women as idiosyncratic hepatotoxicity can occur and can lead to even fatal consequences.

Cyproterone acetate as a stand-alone drug (25–100 mg/day) is a steroidal antiandrogen; it is not available in India except as a COC.

Insulin Sensitizers

Metformin is the drug of choice for significant IR, manifests as moderate to severe acanthosis nigricans, elevated homeostasis model assessment-insulin resistance (HOMA-IR) (≤2.5) or both. It is used in doses of 1,000-2,500 mg/day for at least 3–6 months, till IR is well controlled. Caution is needed in the presence of renal or hepatic impairment. Lactic acidosis is a dreaded side effect while bloating, flatulence, and diarrhea are common but usually settle with continued usage, especially if doses are reduced.

Myo-inositol 2 g and N-acetylcysteine 600 mg were found to have effects equivalent to metformin 500 mg and are better tolerated and accepted by patients but the cost is significantly higher. Insulin sensitizers do not play any role in hirsutism except in the presence of IR. Hence, they should not be used in idiopathic hirsutism or in hirsutism due to other etiologies.

Box 7 summarizes the pharmacologic treatment of moderate to severe hirsutism. Only physical (laser) modalities may suffice for mild hirsutism. However, the dermatologist

TABLE 1: Antiandrogens used in hirsutism management.

Antiandrogen	*Description*	*Dosage*	*Contraindications*	*Adverse events*	*Monitoring*	*Comments*
Spironolactone	Potassium sparing diuretic that blocks androgen receptors	100 mg once a day to 200 mg in two divided doses	Renal failure and hyperkalemia	Frequent micturition, postural hypotension, and breast tenderness	Serum sodium and potassium for dosages higher than 100 mg/day or in women older than 45 years of age	Should be used in combination with COCs in reproductive age women. Potassium rich foods need to be restricted
Bicalutamide	Nonsteroidal antiandrogen similar to flutamide	50 mg Q24H	Severe hepatic impairment	• Elevated liver enzymes • Extremely rare interstitial pneumonitis	Hepatic trans-aminases and GGT	Pregnancy category X drug; has to be used in combination with COCs in reproductive age women
Finasteride	Competitive inhibitor of type II 5α-reductase	5 mg	Possibility of conceiving	Usually well tolerated	None	Mild antiandrogenic effect, inferior to above two drugs. May be used independent of COCs if pregnancy can be reliably avoided

(COC: combined oral contraceptive; GGT: gamma-glutamyltransferase)

BOX 7: Pharmacologic treatment for moderate to severe hirsutism.

- *PCOS:*
  - *COC:* First-line treatment
  - Antiandrogens (usually spironolactone): For moderate and severe hirsutism from the outset and for mild hirsutism that responds poorly
  - Metformin or other insulin sensitizers, if IR is present
- *Idiopathic hirsutism*: Antiandrogens (usually spironolactone) + COC
- *Nonclassic congenital adrenal hyperplasia*: Oral corticosteroids
- *Pituitary or other endocrine abnormalities*:
  - Hyperprolactinemia—cabergoline
  - Cushing's syndrome—treat the cause
  - Severe hypothyroidism—supplement thyroxine
  - GH abnormalities
- Tumors—surgery
- Ovarian hyperthecosis—similar to PCOS; GnRH agonists may be needed
- Drugs—stop the offending agent
- Post-menopausal hirsutism—spironolactone monotherapy ± metformin for IR; finasteride 5 mg is an option if electrolytes cannot be monitored

(COC: combined oral contraceptive; GH: growth hormone; GnRH: gonadotropin-releasing hormone; PCOS: polycystic ovarian syndrome)

should assess response to LHR and be ready to institute pharmacologic therapy in case of poor response.

Procedural Management of Hirsutism

This has been described in the hypertrichosis section in detail. LHR for hirsute women typically needs numerous sessions; the typical number ranges from 6 to 8 sessions for women in their 40s to 10–12 sessions or more for adolescent girls. A finite number can be predicted only if effective androgen suppression is done while LHR is being performed, usually for a minimum period of 12–18 months continuously. Maintenance sessions may be needed for few stray coarse hair every 4–6 months in some patients. Excellent results are possible when right laser parameters are used in conjunction with appropriate pharmacologic therapy **(Figs. 6 and 7)**.

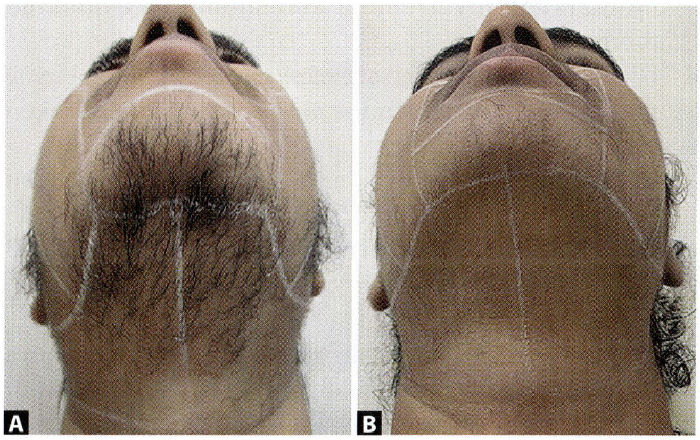

Figs. 6A and B: A 20-year-old women with PCOS and NIDDM 3 months after third session of diode LHR, used in combination with Yasmin, spironolactone, sitagliptin, metformin, and lifestyle measures. Her weight reduced from 99 kg to 81.9 kg (BMI 39.6 till 32.8) during this period.
(BMI: body mass index; LHR: laser hair reduction; NIDDM: noninsulin-dependent diabetes mellitus; PCOS: polycystic ovarian syndrome)

Eflornithine hydrochloride is a topical agent that can delay hair growth temporarily.[3] It has to be used twice a day consistently for optimal effects. It is expensive has potential to cause irritation. It is best used a stop gap method when LHR or other physical methods cannot be used. Combination with LHR leads to good results temporarily but poor results in the long term as it reduces anagen hair which is when LHR is most effective.

For older women with white hair, electrolysis is an option. Punch excision using punches <1 mm has also been done without scarring.

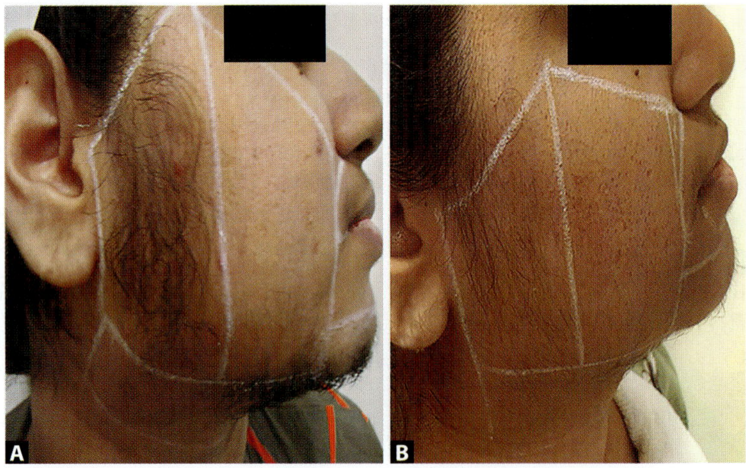

Figs. 7A and B: Same patient as in **Figures 6A and B**. In motion 755 nm LHR was used for finer hair on the cheeks.

KEY MESSAGES

- Hypertrichosis, whether congenital or acquired, localized or generalized, can be a clue to a systemic disease or multisystem involvement and should be evaluated thoroughly.
- Hirsutism is a presence of excess terminal hair in a male pattern in a woman and is always a sign of androgen excess.
- Androgen excess may be at the level of the androgen receptor as in idiopathic hirsutism or in the circulation in most other conditions that cause hirsutism. Except in mild cases, where treatment is not sought, thorough evaluation is mandatory.
- Polycystic ovarian syndrome is the most common cause of hirsutism. It usually presents with normal or slightly high testosterone levels. If testosterone level is grossly elevated, androgen secreting tumors of the ovary or the adrenal or ovarian hyperthecosis should be considered.
- Careful clinical evaluation for anterior pituitary hormone excess along with assays of prolactin and TSH are usually sufficient to confirm a diagnosis of PCOS in the presence of irregular menstrual cycles.
- Assessment of numerous hormones such as dehydroepiandrosterone sulfate (DHEAS), luteinizing hormone (LH), follicle-stimulating hormone (FSH), and free testosterone comes at a huge cost and does not add value.
- Rotterdam criteria should be used for the diagnosis of PCOS. Transabdominal ultrasonography is unreliable to assess polycystic ovarian morphology particularly in obese women. Where possible, high resolution or 3D ultrasound probes should be used, especially in unmarried girls where transvaginal sonogram cannot be done.
- Polycystic ovarian syndrome is a syndrome with health and fertility implications and should be managed in a holistic manner, ideally in collaboration with a sensible endocrinologist. Lifestyle measures including weight and body fat control should be given utmost importance and should be continued for life, well after hirsutism is treated.
- All hirsute women and all patients with hypertrichosis should be given the option of physical methods of depilation and permanent options such as laser hair reduction.
- Almost all patients with moderate to severe hirsutism need pharmacologic therapy alongside laser hair reduction to achieve optimal outcomes.
- Spironolactone along with COCs is the first-line therapy for most patients of hirsutism, be it secondary to PCOS or idiopathic hirsutism. All other etiologies are ideally managed by an endocrinologist.
- A good laser hair reduction machine with a long wavelength (810 nm diode or 1,064 nm Nd:YAG), alone or in combination, with a moderate to long pulse width and cooling apparatus will yield satisfactory results provided the right fluence and pulse width are chosen and simultaneous androgen suppression instituted.

REFERENCES

1. Pavone P, Praticò AD, Falsaperla R, Ruggieri M, Zollino M, Corsello G, et al. Congenital generalized hypertrichosis: the skin as a clue to complex malformation syndromes. Ital J Pediatr. 2015;41:55-63.
2. Azziz R. The evaluation and management of hirsutism. Obstet Gynecol. 2003;101:995-1007.
3. Messenger AG, Sinclair RD, Farrant P, de Berker DAR. Disorders of hair. In: Griffiths C, Barker J, Bleiker T, Chalmers R, Creamer D (Eds). Rook's Textbook of Dermatology, 9th edition, Vol 4. West Sussex: Wiley Blackwell; 2016.pp. 64-8.
4. Knochenhauer ES, Hines G, Conway-Myers BA, Azziz R. Examination of the chin or lower abdomen only for the prediction of hirsutism. Fertil Steril. 2000:74:980-3.
5. Zhao XM, Ni RM, Huang J, Huang LL, Du SM, Ma MJ, et al. Study on the facial and body terminal hair growth in women in Guangdong by using modified Ferriman-Gallwey scoring system. Zhonghua Fu Chan Ke Za Zhi. 2013;48(6):427-31.

6. Ilagan MKCC, Paz-Pacheco E, Totesora DZ, Clemente-Chua LR, Jalique JRK. The Modified Ferriman-Gallwey Score and Hirsutism among Filipino Women. Endocrinol Metab (Seoul). 2019;34(4):374-81.
7. Unluhizarci K, Kaltsas G, Kelestimur F. Non polycystic ovary syndrome-related endocrine disorders associated with hirsutism. Eur J Clin Invest. 2012;42(1):86-94.
8. Chhabra S, Gautam RK, Kulshreshtha B, Prasad A, Sharma N. Hirsutism: A clinico-investigative study. Int J Trichology. 2012;4:246-50.
9. Rotterdam ESHRE/ASRM Sponsored PCOS Consensus Workshop Group. Revised 2003 consensus on diagnostic criteria and long-term health risks related to polycystic ovary syndrome (PCOS). Hum Reprod. 2004;19:41-7.
10. Teede HJ, Misso ML, Costello MF, Dokras A, Laven J, Moran L, et al. Recommendations from the international evidence-based guideline for the assessment and management of polycystic ovary syndrome. Fertil Steril. 2018;110(3):364-79.
11. Martin KA, Anderson RR, Chang RJ, Ehrmann DA, Lobo RA, Murad MH, et al. Evaluation and Treatment of Hirsutism in Premenopausal Women: An Endocrine Society Clinical Practice Guideline. J Clin Endocrinol Metab. 2018;103(4):1233-57.

EXAMINATION QUESTIONS

1. How will you approach to a case of hirsutism?
2. Discuss the management of hirsutism.

76 CHAPTER Nail Disorders

Chander Grover, Shikha Bansal

INTRODUCTION

The nail subserves important functions in humans like protection of phalanges and fingertips; enhancement of fine touch; execution of fine digital movements; amelioration of itching; and contribution toward a better aesthetic appearance. The main function however is to produce a protective nail plate (NP) over the dorsal surface of each digit.

ANATOMY AND PHYSIOLOGY OF THE NAIL UNIT

The human nail comprises of six components: Nail matrix; nail plate; cuticular system; nailbed mesenchyme and phalangeal bone; anchoring ligaments; and nailfolds **(Table 1) (Figs. 1 and 2)**.[1] It has a rich blood supply derived from digital arteries, which form a cruciate anastomosis.

The average rate of growth of fingernails is 0.1 mm/day or 3 mm/month (1.8–4.5 mm/month) while for toenails, it is half to one-third (12–18 months to fully regenerate). Structurally, nails have a higher content of hard keratins (responsible for strength) as well as phospholipids (responsible for flexibility of the NP).[2] The high sulfur content in keratin is responsible for their rugged physical qualities. The normal water content is 10–30% and is directly related to the relative humidity.

ETIOLOGY OF NAIL DISORDERS

Nail disorders lead to unpleasant social stigma, significant functional compromise, or act as reservoir of infection with potential of spread. These can be broadly classified as summarized in **Box 1**.

INFECTIOUS NAIL DISORDERS

Onychomycosis

Onychomycosis is fungal infection of the nail unit caused by yeasts, molds, or dermatophytes. Toenails are more commonly involved than finger nails; predisposing factors being excessive perspiration, tight-fitting footwear, preexisting nail disorders, trauma, diabetes mellitus, immunosuppression, and poor peripheral circulation.

TABLE 1: Components of the nail unit.

Component of nail unit	*Anatomical description*	*Clinical changes produced*
Nail matrix	The germinative epithelium of the nail unit. The major part of NP arises from matrix	Beau's lines, pitting, longitudinal ridging, trachyonychia, true leukonychia
Nail plate	Keratinized structure formed due to maturation and keratinization of the nail matrix epithelium The visible, hard, transparent structure comprising the majority of nail unit	Brittle nails, pachyonychia (thickening), pincer nail, koilonychia
Nailbed	Modified epithelium placed between the isthmus and distal margin of lunula Does not have granular layer and melanocytes	Onycholysis, subungual hyperkeratosis, apparent leukonychia, splinter hemorrhages
Nail folds	Hold the NP in place. There are two lateral nail folds, and one each of proximal and distal nail fold	Acute and chronic paronychia, changes in nail fold capillary patterns
Eponychium (cuticle)	Thin strip of cornified epithelium. It arises from the proximal nail fold and adheres to the superficial surface of the proximal NP	Breach in cuticle can lead to paronychia
Hyponychium	Keratotic barrier at the physiological point of separation of the NP from the distal nail fold	Pterygium inversum unguis
Lunula	Visible part of the nail matrix. It demarcates the junction between matrix and nailbed	Absent lunula, blue lunula, red lunula
Onychodermal band / Isthmus	Thin transverse white band. It indicates the most distal part of the firm attachment of NP to nailbed	Trauma, exposure to irritants can lead to disruption of isthmus causing onycholysis

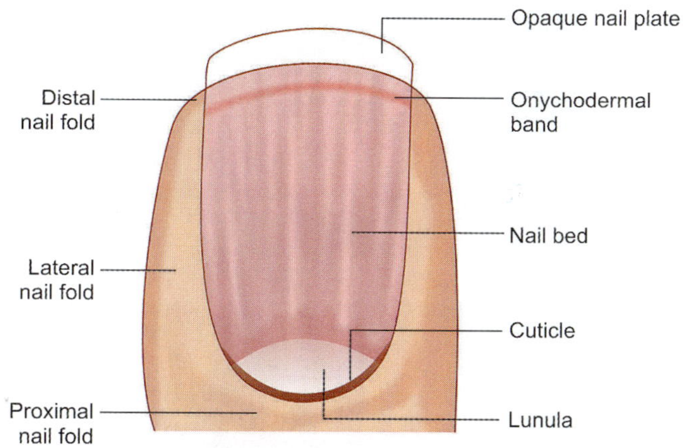

Fig. 1: The surface landmarks of nail unit.

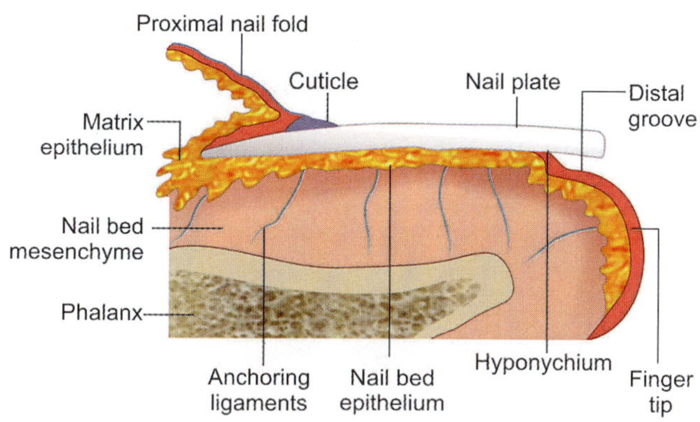

Fig. 2: Sagittal section of nail unit.

Majority of cases are caused by anthropophilic dermatophytes, especially *Trichophyton rubrum*, followed by *Trichophyton mentagrophytes var. interdigitale*. Nondermatophytes molds, such as *Scopulariopsis vicaulis* and *Aspergillus* spp., can be involved in onychomycosis as primary pathogens, contaminants, or secondary pathogens.[3]

Clinical Types

These include:

- *Distal and lateral subungual onychomycosis (DLSO)*: It is the most common clinical type, caused mostly by *Trichophyton rubrum*. It is primarily a nailbed infection, initially showing a yellowish or blackish discoloration of lateral or distal NP **(Fig. 3)** with subsequent hyperkeratosis, crumbling, or disintegration of NP. Severe cases may show yellow spikes, representing concentrated foci of fungal elements (Dermatophytoma) **(Fig. 4)**.[2] One hand, two feet dermatophytosis may demonstrate concomitant onychomycosis.
- *Proximal subungual onychomycosis (PSO)*: There is whitish discoloration under proximal part of the NP due to invasion under proximal nail fold **(Fig. 5)**. It is commonly caused by *Trichophyton rubrum* and *Trichophyton megninii*. It can be an indicator of HIV infection.

BOX 1: Causes of abnormal nails.

- Infectious nail disorders:
  - Onychomycosis
  - Parasitic infections
  - Viral infections
  - Bacterial infections
  - HIV-associated nail changes
- Nail manifestations of dermatological disorders:
  - Nail psoriasis
  - Nail lichen planus
  - Eczematous nail changes
  - Darier's disease
  - Alopecia areata
  - Bullous disorders
  - Erythema multiforme/TEN
- Abnormalities of nail pigmentation:
  - Leukonychia
  - Melanonychia
  - Pigmentation of lunula
- Nail in systemic diseases
- Drug-induced nail changes
- Nail tumors:
  - Benign tumors
  - Malignant tumors
- Traumatic nail disorders:
  - Acute trauma
  - Chronic repetitive trauma
- Pediatric nail disorders:
  - Physiological changes
  - Congenital malformations
  - Thickened nails in children
  - Blistering disorders
  - Inflammatory disorders
  - Trachyonychia
- Nail disorders in elderly:
  - Age-associated nail changes
  - Physical nail abnormalities
  - Disorders of nail

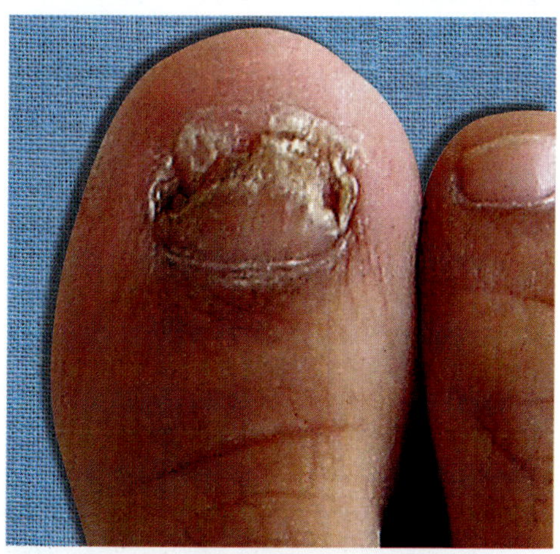

Fig. 3: Involvement of lateral and distal part of toe nail suggestive of DLSO (distal and lateral subungual onychomycosis).

- *Superficial white onychomycosis (SWO)*: It presents as a chalky white discoloration of the NP **(Fig. 6),** also known as "leukonychia trichophytica." The underlying nailbed is completely normal. Common causes include *Trichophyton mentagrophytes, Cephalosporium, acremonium,*

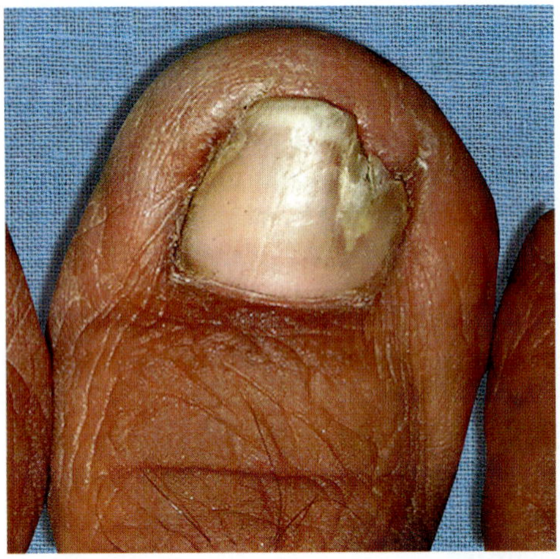

Fig. 4: Dermatophytoma seen as a prominent, thick localized involvement of distal nail plate (NP).

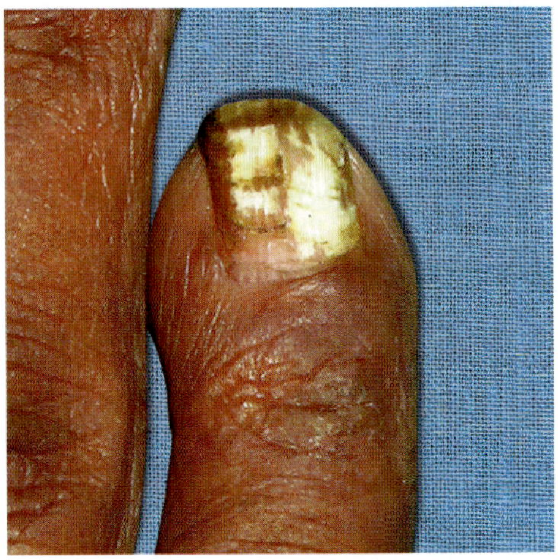

Fig. 5: Proximal subungual onychomycosis (PSO).

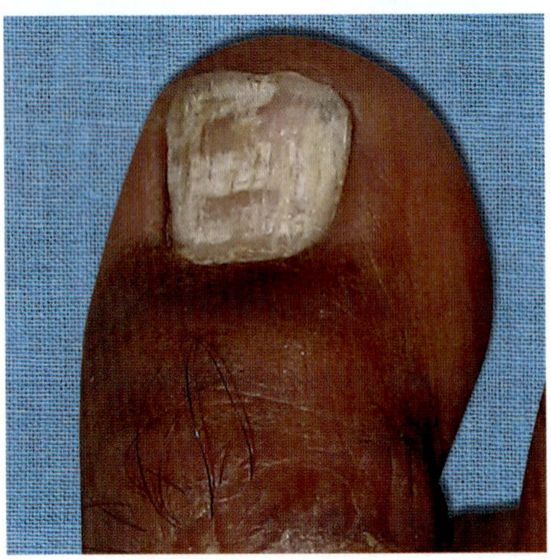

Fig. 6: Superficial white onychomycosis (SWO) caused by dermatophytes.

Aspergillus, and *Fusarium oxysporum.* This is the only form that can be treated with topical medications because of the superficial nature of infection.

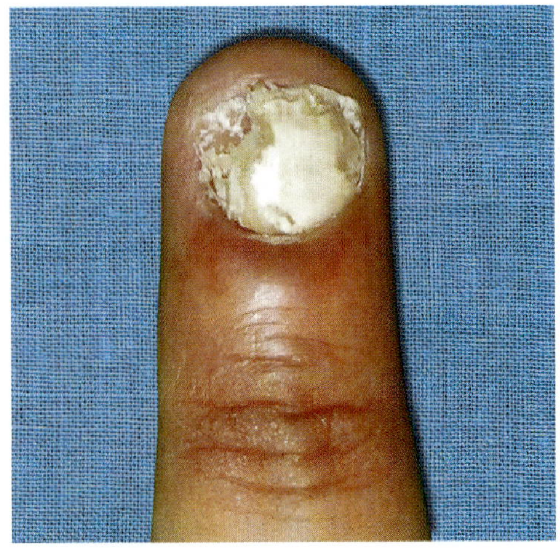

Fig. 7: Endonyx onychomycosis.

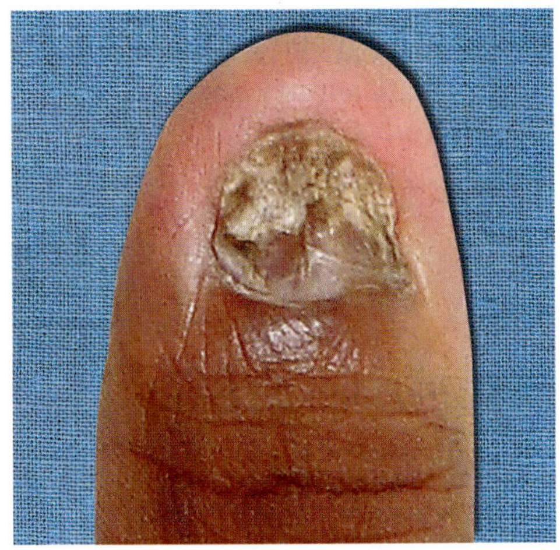

Fig. 8: Total dystrophic onychomycosis (TDO) involving up to the matrix area.

- *Endonyx onychomycosis (EOM):* The NP is primarily involved with the fungus growing between the NP lamellae **(Fig. 7)**. It is mainly caused by *T. sudanenses.* Clinically, EOM is seen as a diffuse milky-white discoloration of the affected nail, with an absence of nailbed hyperkeratosis or onycholysis.
- *Total dystrophic onychomycosis (TDOM):* There is a total destruction of the nail apparatus involving the whole thickness of NP, nailbed and matrix **(Fig. 8)**. The plate becomes thick, dystrophic and crumbles down. TDO may be primary (e.g., in cases with chronic mucocutaneous candidiasis) or secondary to any of the four previous forms.

Diagnosis

A definitive laboratory diagnosis of onychomycosis is important to institute adequate and appropriate treatment. The specimen is obtained from the most affected part of the NP, but should also include subungual debris as much as possible. Samples obtained by drilling give much higher yield than simple clippings. The commonly used tests include:

- *Direct microscopy*: Nail clippings are dissolved in 10% KOH (potassium hydroxide) and examined to assess for fungal elements. The process can be hastened by the use of Dimethyl sulfoxide (DMSO). Dyes such as Chlorazol black E, Parker's blue-black ink, Congo red; methylene blue, etc. improve the sensitivity. Fluorescent microscopy is also a useful technique.
- *Fungal culture*: It provides an identification of the species to enable proper treatment. It is also useful in microscopy negative cases. Culture should simultaneously be obtained on media with and without cycloheximide, so as to identify the presence of saprophytic species.
- *Dermatoscopy*: Onychomycosis shows a jagged proximal edge of onycholytic area; "spikes" within onycholytic areas **(Fig. 9)**; white-yellow longitudinal striae within the onycholyzed NP and parallel bands of varying colors ("Aurora Borealis" pattern). Specific patterns like dendritic pattern (endonyx) and grid pattern (SWO) have been described in literature. Other features include blackish dots and globules, matte homogenous color of detached NP and dryness and scaling of adjacent skin.[4]
- *Histopathology*: It has proved more sensitive than either KOH or culture. It also helps document actual invasion of NP by fungal elements.

Treatment

Many patients are not symptomatic and may not seek treatment. Even then, patients with comorbidities such as diabetes or peripheral neuropathy are at a higher risk of complications like cellulitis related to onychomycosis. Treatment is based on the following general principles: [1]

- Systemic antifungals are the mainstay of therapy.
- Topical antifungals or surgical approaches have only an adjuvant role.

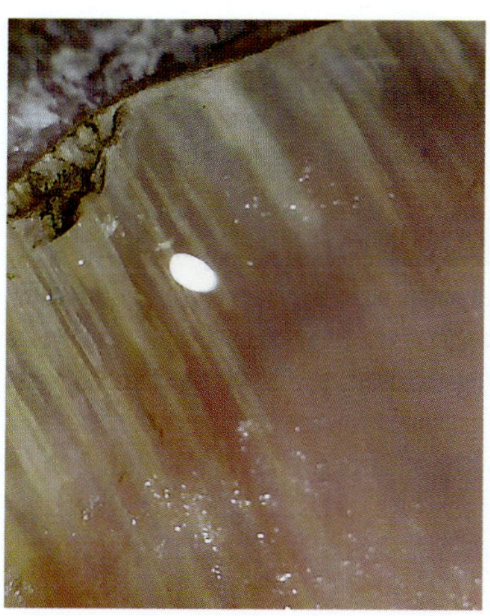

Fig. 9: Dermoscopy of a case of onychomycosis showing "jagged" proximal edge of onycholysis (DinoLite AM7915MZT 50×).

- Due consideration should be given to the likely causative organism.
- Patient specific factors are important while deciding the agent or treatment regime to be followed.

Oral antifungal drugs:

- *Terbinafine* (allylamine) is the only fungicidal drug. It is not effective against some species of *Candida* and molds. The drug is retained in the NP for a long period of time (30 and 36 weeks respectively for 6- and 12-week therapy). The treatment is given for 6 weeks for finger nail disease and for 12 weeks for toe nail disease. The *treatment regime* followed is 250 mg tablet, once a day (>40 kg), 125 mg tablet, once a day (20–40 kg), and 62.5 mg tablet, once a day (<20 kg).
- *Itraconazole* (azole) has a broad spectrum of activity against dermatophytes, Candida and saprophytes. It persists in the NP for 6–9 months. There is a potential for drug interactions and hepatotoxicity. *Treatment regimens* could be *continuous* (200 mg daily, for 6 weeks in finger nail disease and 12 weeks in toe nail disease) or *pulse regime* (200 mg twice a day in adults for 1 week/month, with 2 and 3 pulses being given for finger and toe nail respectively; 5 mg/kg/day in children for 1 week/month).
- *Fluconazole* (azole) has a broad spectrum of activity and is considered safe for comedication. The *pulse regime* incorporates a dose of 150 mg once a week, which can be increased to 300–450 mg for nonresponders for 6–9 months. The dose in children is 6 mg/kg/week for 3–4 month for finger nail and 5–7 month for toe nail. It can be detected in NP for 6 month after discontinuation of therapy.
- *Griseofulvin* is probably the least effective drug covering only dermatophytes. It needs to be administered in daily doses till growth of normal nail (6–9 months for fingernail and 12–18 months for toenail). It is given as 10–15 mg/kg/day in divided doses.

Absorption of itraconazole and griseofulvin are affected by food. Griseofulvin has better absorption when taken with fatty food. Itraconazole capsule after meal or empty stomach with cola beverage and suspension in empty stomach.

Topical therapies:

- *Indications*:
    - Primary therapy in mild infections
    - Palliative in those unable to take oral antifungals
    - Prophylactic agent.
- *Agents used*:
    - 8% ciclopirox nail lacquer
    - Amorolfine lacquer
    - 40% urea gel 10% efinaconazole solution
    - 5% tavaborole[5]
    - 5% luliconazole solution

Special considerations:

- *Children*: An assessment should be done for simultaneous tinea capitis, pedis, etc. Fluconazole or terbinafine are the preferred agents.
- *Elderly*: An assessment should be made for possible drug interactions. The most convenient dosage schedules should be used.
- *Nondermatophyte molds*: Successful treatment is difficult to achieve. Nail avulsion and topical therapies are important adjuncts. Systemic antifungals may be totally ineffective. Better response is seen with itraconazole.
- *Candida onychomycosis*: Oral azoles are the treatment of choice. Topical therapies have useful adjunctive role. Associated paronychia or onycholysis also needs to be treated effectively.

Viral Infections

- *Verrucae* can involve subungual or periungual location **(Fig. 10)**. Periungual warts involving perionychial area are common in nail biters. Treatment of subungual or periungual warts can be frustrating. Although, most warts remit spontaneously, proper attention to extensions under the nail are imperative to completely eradicate the infection. Dermatoscopy of small periungual lesions which clinically appear as scaly papules can show dilated and thrombosed vessels.[4] Treatment options available include intralesional bleomycin, keratolytics, cryosurgery, imiquimod, laser therapy, interferons, and immunotherapy.
- *Herpetic whitlow* is an intensely painful infection with HSV-1 or 2 (Herpes Simplex Virus); involving one or more finger, typically affecting terminal phalanx. Local tenderness, erythema, pain, vesiculation, erosion and ulceration may be seen; gradually healing over 2–3 weeks It is seen in medical and dental personnel; nail biters; finger-suckers and patients with herpes labialis or gingivostomatitis. Following universal precautions can prevent infections in healthcare workers. It can also be due to autoinoculation from genital herpes. Periodic recurrences may occur. Confirmation of diagnosis can be done with Tzanck smear, culture or rapid immunofluorescence techniques.
- *Treatment* is needed as condition is highly contagious as well as painful. Hand elevation, analgesics, and immobilization of extremity if required. Oral acyclovir or valaciclovir are the drugs of choice. Severe or recurrent cases may require therapy with famciclovir or foscarnet.

Bacterial Infections (Paronychia)

Paronychia is inflammation of the nailfolds. Although, it may be infectious or noninfectious in origin; bacterial causes are commonly implicated. Noninfectious causes include contact dermatitis, dyshidrotic eczema, fixed drug eruption, etc.

Clinical Types

- *Acute paronychia* is generally associated with a history of trauma. Erythema, tenderness or visible collection of pus is present. Generally, only one nail is involved **(Fig. 11)**. If several nails are involved, one should consider chronic dermatitis, dermatoses, or drug induced causes.
- *Chronic paronychia* is a very recalcitrant inflammatory disorder affecting nailfolds. It is defined as inflammation lasting >6 weeks, involving one or more of the three nailfolds (proximal or lateral). The patient presents with redness, tenderness and swelling around nails, fluid under the skin, and thick, discolored and deformed nail. There is induration and rounding off of the paronychium, recurring episodes of inflammation, and drainage and lost cuticle **(Fig. 12)**. NP thickening, ridging, onychomadesis, transverse striations, and pitting can be present due to inflammation of nail matrix. Greenish discoloration suggests *Pseudomonas* colonization. Chronic paronychia

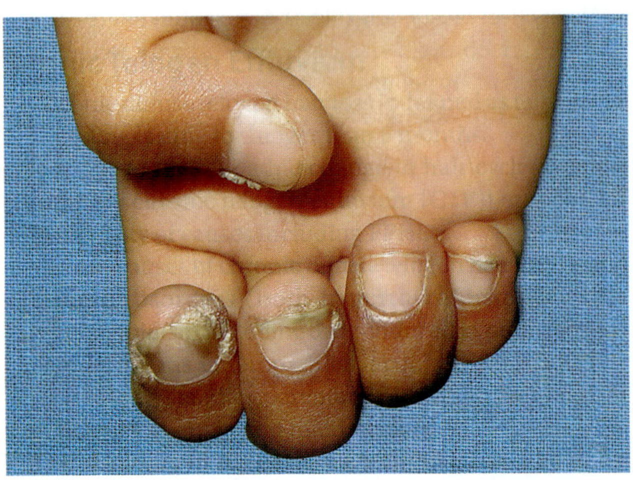

Fig. 10: Subungual and periungual wart with extensive destruction of the NP.

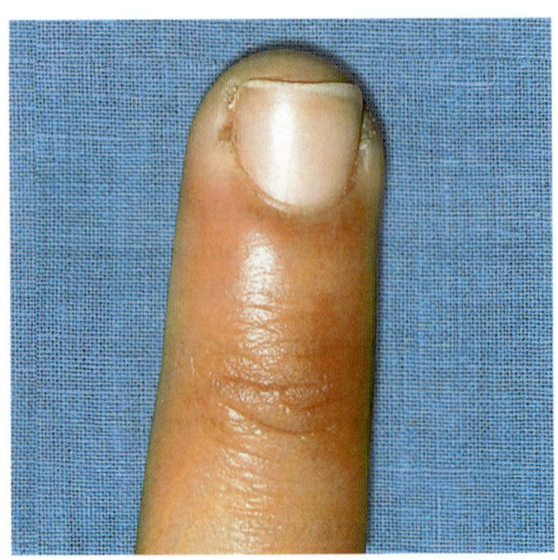

Fig. 11: Acute paronychia of showing extensive inflammation and collection of pus pocket in the nailfold.

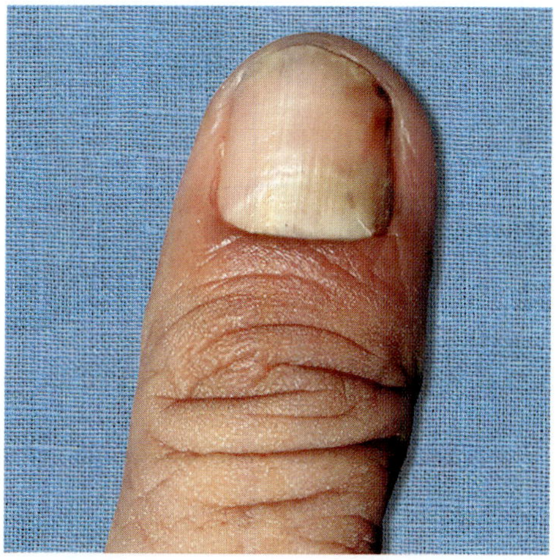

Fig. 12: Chronic paronychia showing disruption of cuticle, swelling and inflammation of proximal nail fold. Note yellowish discoloration underneath the proximal part of NP suggestive of pus formation.

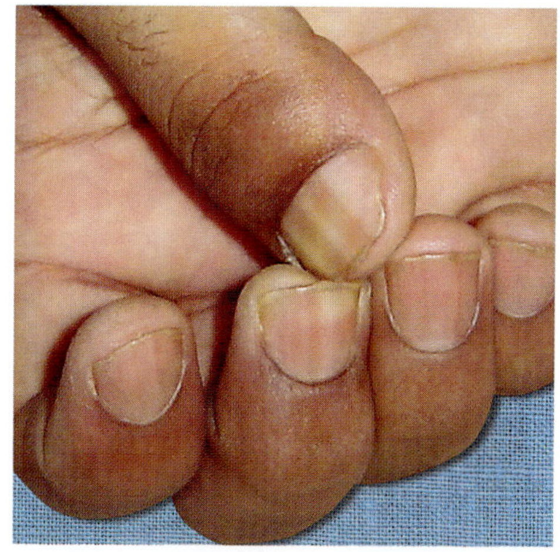

Fig. 13: New onset melanonychia in a patient with HIV/AIDS on antiretroviral therapy.

commonly afflicts house and office cleaners, laundry workers, food handlers, cooks, dishwashers, bartenders, chefs, nurses, swimmers, diabetics, and patients on HIV-ART. The role of *Candida* is probably minor; it may be a form of hand dermatitis. An eczematous condition with a multifactorial etiology could be responsible.

Treatment

- Acute paronychia requires antibacterial, analgesics, soothing soaks and drainage of pus, if required.
- For chronic paronychia, treatment principles include:
  - Determination and elimination/minimization of the cause
  - Strict avoidance of excessive moisture/contact irritants
  - No physical trauma to the cuticle
  - Treatment of secondary infection with yeast or bacteria
  - Mid or high potency steroids used topically for several weeks
  - Topical tacrolimus can also be used
  - Surgical treatment needed for cases with extensive fibrosis and thickening of the proximal nailfold; aim being to excise the fibrosed tissue and expose the inflamed germinal matrix to permit unrestricted drainage.[6]

HIV-associated Nail Changes

Nail changes are present in 47.7% of HIV patients as compared to 34% of normal controls. Although several of these changes increase the index of suspicion for HIV infection, there are no pathognomonic changes:

- Onychomycosis is seen in 6.3% HIV patients. PSO is very characteristic, even though the incidence is low.[7] Mycotic keratoderma, and SWO (in fingernails without toe nail involvement) should raise the suspicion of HIV. Candida may produce a hypertrophic nailbed infection and is the major fungus affecting pediatric patients. Others such as *Pityrosporu movale* and *Alternaria* have also been implicated in onychomycosis in AIDS patients.
- Viral infections seen are relapsing herpetic whitlow and severe HPV infection.
- Crusted scabies, with massive subungual colonization can be seen.
- Neoplasms such as squamous cell carcinoma, metastatic lesions and sarcoma may appear in the nail region, apart from nail unit lymphoma. Almost 100% of AIDS patients with Kaposi's sarcoma have onychomycosis.
- Inflammatory diseases involving nail produce similar manifestations, though there is an increased risk of secondary infection and delayed healing. Psoriasis may show a granulomatous, proliferative response in nails of HIV positive.
- There is an increased incidence of erythematous crescents, slower nail growth, yellowing of nails and Beau's lines.
- Therapy with azathioprine produces dark brown discoloration or blue nails **(Fig. 13)**. Paronychia and pyogenic granuloma of great toe have been reported with indinavir.[8]

NAIL MANIFESTATIONS OF DERMATOLOGICAL DISORDERS

The nail is involved in many dermatological diseases. Although, the pattern of involvement may not be pathognomonic of a particular disorder; mostly a combination of different findings point toward a diagnosis.

Nail Psoriasis

About 10–50% of psoriasis patients have nail involvement. In 1–5%, psoriatic nail disease may be seen without concomitant

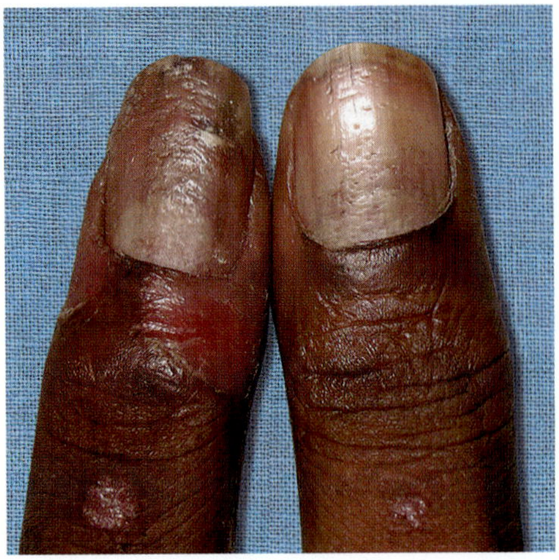

Fig. 14: Multiple, irregular pits in a patient with nail psoriasis.

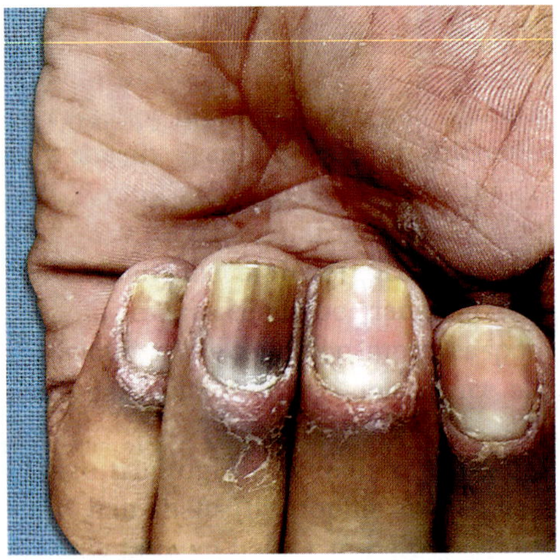

Fig. 15: Distal onycholysis with subungual hyperkeratosis involving multiple nails in a patient with psoriasis. Note the characteristic erythematous border.

or overt cutaneous disease. Up to 53–86% patients with psoriatic arthritis are known to have nail manifestations.

Clinical findings of nail psoriasis depend on the anatomical location of the affected part of nail unit. In order of reducing frequency, psoriatic nail changes include pitting (irregular, deep, randomly arranged) **(Fig. 14)**, onycholysis, subungual hyperkeratosis **(Fig. 15)**, NP discoloration, uneven surface, splinter hemorrhages,[9] and acute or chronic paronychia. Presence of *salmon patch* or oil spots suggests psoriatic disease **(Fig. 16)**. The most common nail finding is *pitting* in fingernails and *subungual hyperkeratosis* in toenails. According to the anatomical location of the psoriatic pathology, the various nail changes are as outlined in **Table 2**.

Severity of nail psoriasis is evaluated by *Nail Psoriasis Severity Index (NAPSI)* which assesses extent of nailbed and nail matrix involvement **(Fig. 16)**. Each nail is divided into four quadrants, each of which is assessed for the presence of matrix disease (pitting, leukonychia, red spots in lunula,

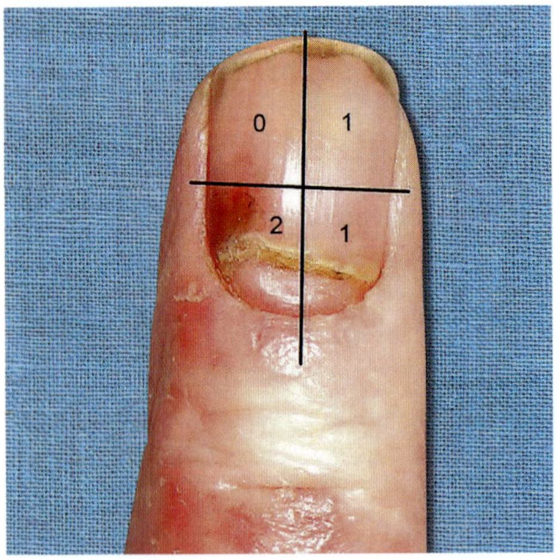

Fig. 16: "Salmon patch" seen in the nailbed. Calculation of NAPSI. Nail is divided into 4 imaginary quadrants and presence of NP and nailbed changes is graded in each of them to calculate the total score.

TABLE 2: Nail changes in psoriasis.

Clinical manifestations	*Anatomical part of the nail affected*
Pitting, longitudinal striations	Proximal matrix
Focal, subtotal or total leukonychia	Intermediate matrix
Focal onycholysis, thinned out NP, erythema of the lunula	Distal matrix
"Oil drop" sign or "salmon patch," splinter hemorrhages	Nailbed
Subungual hyperkeratosis, onycholysis	Hyponychium

NP crumbling) or bed diseases (oil-drop discoloration, onycholysis, hyperkeratosis, and splinter hemorrhages).

Special morphological types of nail psoriasis include:

- *Acro pustulosis* is destructive pustulation of the nail unit, generally presenting as a part of pustular psoriasis. Sterile pustules in the nailbed and the matrix lift the NP. Erythema and discomfort of the digits is associated.
- *Acrodermatitis continua of Hallopeau* is a form of localized pustular psoriasis, beginning in the periungual location, affecting a single digit mostly and following a relapsing course **(Fig. 17)**. Long-standing cases may show an atrophic thinning of distal digit and resorption of distal phalanx.

Psoriatic nail disease needs to be differentiated from other cause of dystrophic nails including onychomycosis which may be ruled out by direct microscopic examination of KOH preparation or culture. However, histopathological examination is much more informative. Dermatoscopy findings vary depending on the part of the nail unit affected. The NP characteristics include pitting in the form of irregularly sized and shaped depressions which may be surrounded by whitish halo **(Fig. 18)**. Characteristic nailbed features include onycholysis surrounded by an erythematous border **(Fig. 19)**;

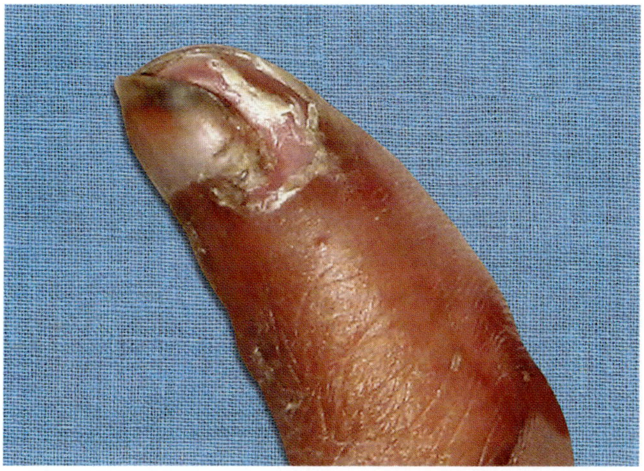

Fig. 17: Acrodermatitis continua of Hallopeau with acral involvement of thumb.

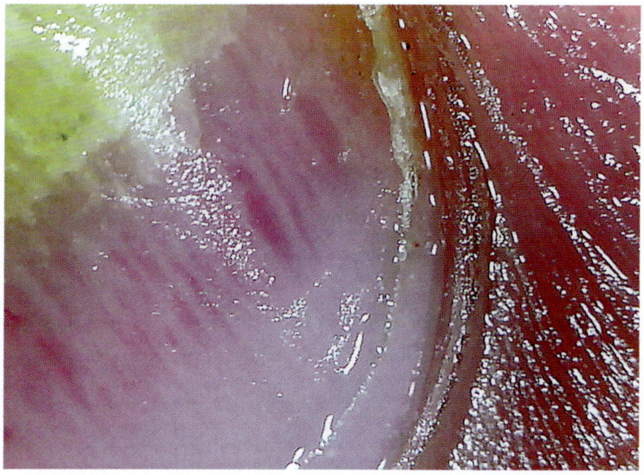

Fig. 19: Dermoscopic image showing erythematous border of onycholysis with reddish globules surrounded by whitish halo (DinoLite AM7915MZT 30×).

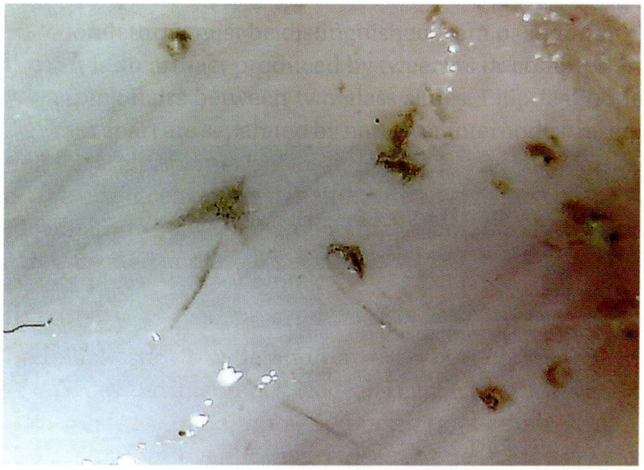

Fig. 18: Dermoscopy showing characteristics pits of nail psoriasis (DinoLite AM7915MZT 50×).

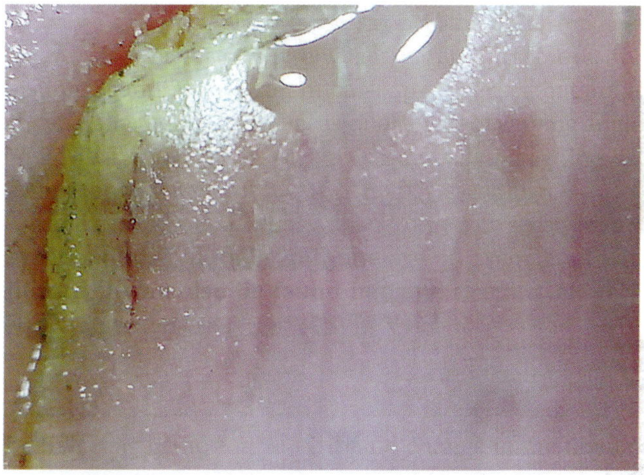

Fig. 20: Dermoscopic image showing multiple splinter hemorrhages and salmon patch (DinoLite AM7915MZT 50×).

salmon patch; pustular lesions and splinter hemorrhages **(Fig. 20)**. The erythematous border of onycholysis shows globose, dilated blood vessels surrounded by a prominent halo **(Fig. 19)**. Salmon patches are irregular in size and shape and variable in color (red to orange) **(Fig. 20)**. The hyponychium and proximal nailfold show characteristic vascular pattern of psoriasis (irregularly distributed, dilated and tortuous capillaries). In pustular psoriasis, nailbed may show small pustules, scaling, hemorrhages, and dilated vessels.

Treatment depends on clinical presentation and patient considerations. Most patients have mild nail disease without joint involvement and topical therapy, e.g., calcipotriol, steroids, tazarotene, etc. only may be needed; however, for severe nail disease, a major impact on quality-of-life, moderate-to-severe skin disease or psoriatic arthritis, systemic therapy is warranted. Patient specific considerations are important for choice of therapy. Recommended general measures include avoidance of microtrauma (to prevent Koebnerization).[1] Commonly used agents are outlined in **Table 3**.

Nail Lichen Planus

Nail LP may be seen alone without any cutaneous or mucous membrane changes. Varied nail manifestations include onychorrhexis, onychoschizia, nail pigmentation, pterygium, and onychomadesis. Early treatment during active inflammatory stage can help prevent pterygium formation and irreversible loss.

Onychorrhexis (longitudinal ridging and splitting) is the hallmark of nail LP **(Fig. 21)**, occurring due to focal matrix involvement resulting in patchy *thinning*. Extensive involvement of matrix may cause scarring resulting in *pterygium or anonychia* **(Fig. 22)**. LP of nailbed results in a *bluish discoloration,* or *onycholysis* **(Fig. 23)**. *Trachyonychia* **(Fig. 24)** and *Idiopathic atrophy of NP* are less common variants usually seen in children.

Diagnosis of nail LP is difficult in cases where nail involvement occurs in isolation; Histopathological examination is useful in such cases to avoid permanent sequelae.

TABLE 3: Treatment options for nail psoriasis.

Therapeutic agent	*Indication for use*	*Expected side-effects*
Topical calcipotriol	Nailbed hyperkeratosis, pustular psoriasis limited to one or two nails	Secondary to systemic absorption of the drug
Topical tazarotene	Nailbed hyperkeratosis	Irritant potential
Topical steroids	Nailbed features	Long-term skin and even bone atrophy
Intralesional steroids	Nail matrix injections for features of matrix disease especially thickened nails	Pain, PNF atrophy and hypopigmentation, subungual hematoma
Intralesional steroids	Nailbed injections for nailbed disease especially subungual hyperkeratosis	Pain, nailbed atrophy, subungual hematoma, pigmentary changes
Systemic retinoids	Severe nail matrix and nailbed psoriasis	Brittleness, paronychia, pyogenic granulomas
Combination (Acitretin and Calcipotriol)	Severe pustular psoriasis of nails	
Systemic MTX	Effective but recommended only in cases with cutaneous involvement	
Systemic cyclosporin	Effective but recommended only in cases with cutaneous involvement	
PUVA (Psoralen and UVA therapy)	Not effective, may even worsen nail signs	Pigmentary changes, melanonychia striata
Biologics (Infliximab, Alefacept, Etanercept)	Effective in nail psoriasis	

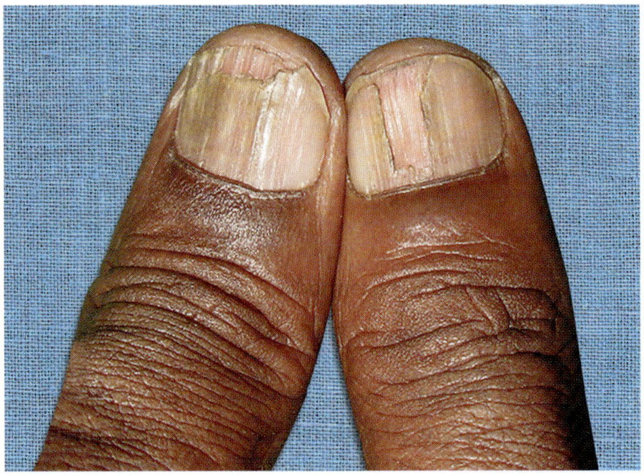

Fig. 21: Onychorrhexis in a case with nail lichen planus.

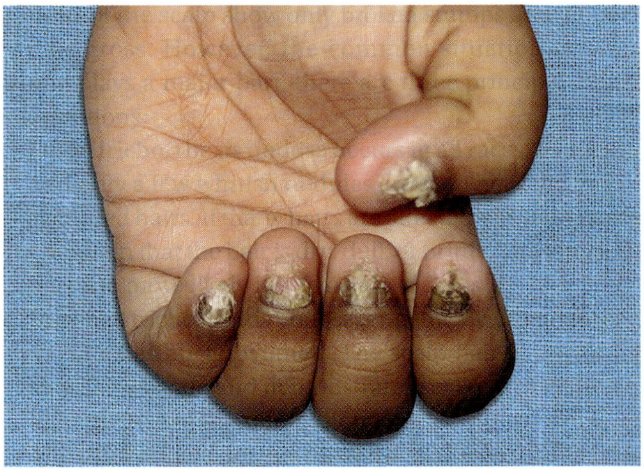

Fig. 23: Distal onycholysis with subungual hyperkeratosis in a patient with nail lichen planus. Note the prominent melanonychia.

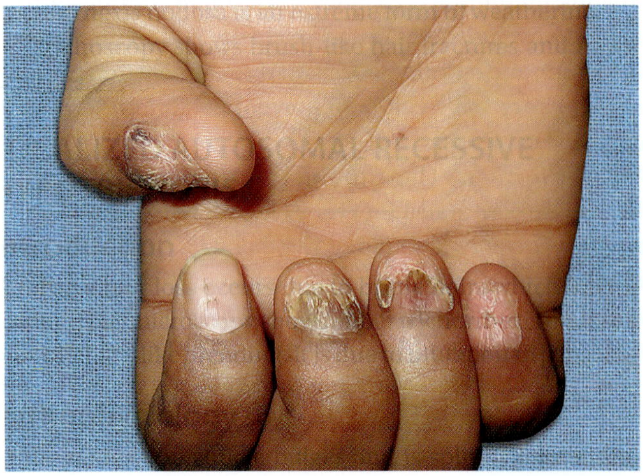

Fig. 22: Pterygium formation in multiple nails in a case of nail lichen planus.

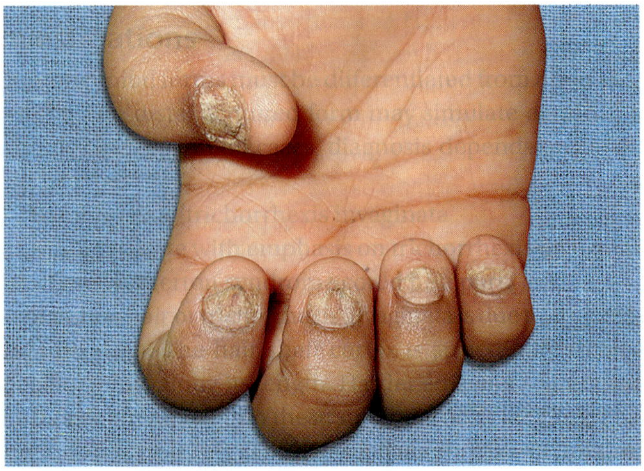

Fig. 24: Trachyonychia in a child with nail lichen planus.

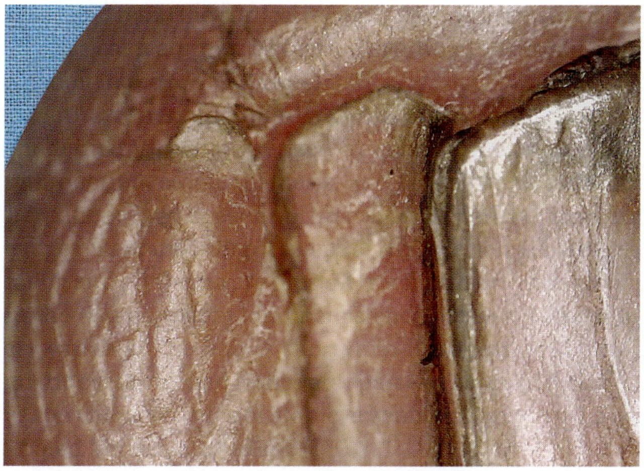

Fig. 25: Dermoscopic images of NP showing prominent onychorrhexis (DinoLite AM7915MZT 50×).

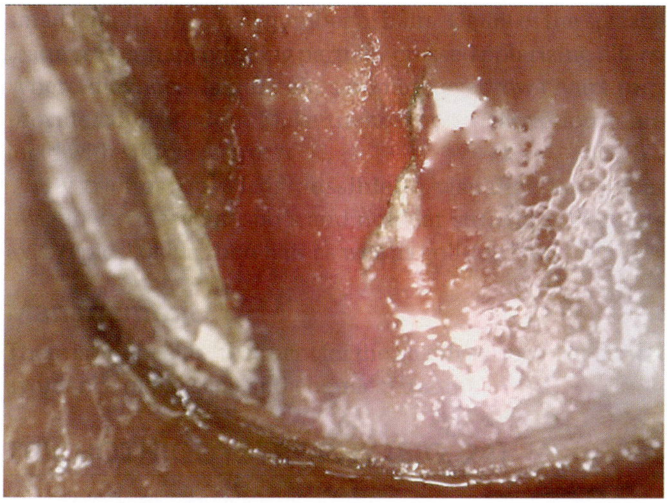

Fig. 26: Dermoscopic image showing distinct chromonychia involving the nailbed (DinoLite AM7915MZT 50×).

Dermatoscopy of nail can help decide whether or not to initiate aggressive therapy. The onychoscopic abnormalities are of nail matrix, bed, and paronychial origin. Nail matrix features seen are onychorrhexis, trachyonychia, pitting and pterygium **(Fig. 25)**. Nailbed features highlighted are chromonychia, and onycholysis and subungual hyperkeratosis **(Fig. 26)**.[4]

Treatment is necessary because of the most dreaded complication of permanent anonychia and pterygium. Steroids either systemic or intramatricial can produce near total regression of early changes. Intramatricial steroids (triamcinolone 2.5–5 mg/mL) injected in the proximal nailfold at 4 weekly intervals are helpful. Systemic steroids may be needed with multiple nail involvement. Triamcinolone acetonide (0.5 mg/kg monthly for 4–6 months), can be given. Etanercept and alitretinoin have also been found useful.

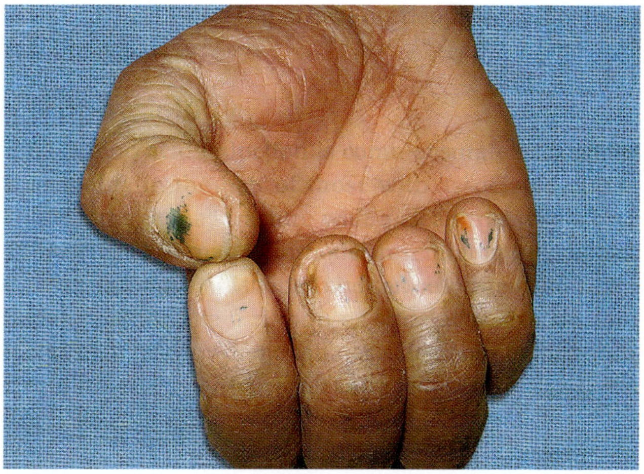

Fig. 27: Prominent eczematous nail changes in housewives' dermatitis, seen as paronychial inflammation, roughness, and lateral discoloration of nails.

Eczematous Nail Changes

Nail involvement due to paronychial or matrix inflammation may occur in isolation or as part of eczema elsewhere. Although nail involvement can occur in all forms of eczematous dermatitis, most commonly it seen with atopic dermatitis or contact allergic dermatitis of hands. Mostly, a combination of atopy and exogenous irritant or allergic reaction is common. Cyanoacrylates used in prosthetic nails can induce local as well as distant allergic reactions with NP showing roughening, thickening, transverse ridging, coarse pitting, or onycholysis.

Nail matrix disturbances manifest as thickening, pitting, transverse ridges and furrows; while bed disease presents as subungual hyperkeratosis, splinter hemorrhages, onycholysis, and pain. Acute or chronic paronychial inflammation, polished appearance, koilonychias on prolonged contact with certain oils, and acute onycholysis may also occur **(Fig. 27)**.

Keratosis Follicularis (Darier's Disease)

About 95–99% of patients with Darier's disease show characteristic nail changes like longitudinal white streaks, fragile, thickened or longitudinally splintered NP with distal, V-shaped nicks. Alternating longitudinal, red and white bands are also characteristic (sandwich appearance). There is no effective treatment for these nail changes.

Alopecia Areata

Nail abnormalities due to nail matrix inflammation are common (10–66% of patients) and usually not severe. *Fine pitting* affects up to 34% patients, is uniform and shallow and presents in regular rows (glen-plaid configuration) **(Fig. 28)**. Others alterations include *trachyonychia*, punctate leukonychia, mottled lunula, and onychomadesis. Nail involvement tends to regress spontaneously with time and also improves with systemic steroids. It may precede,

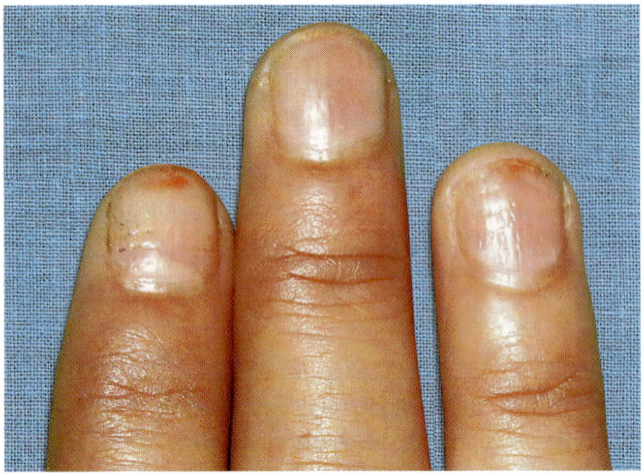

Fig. 28: Regular pitting in a case with alopecia areata.

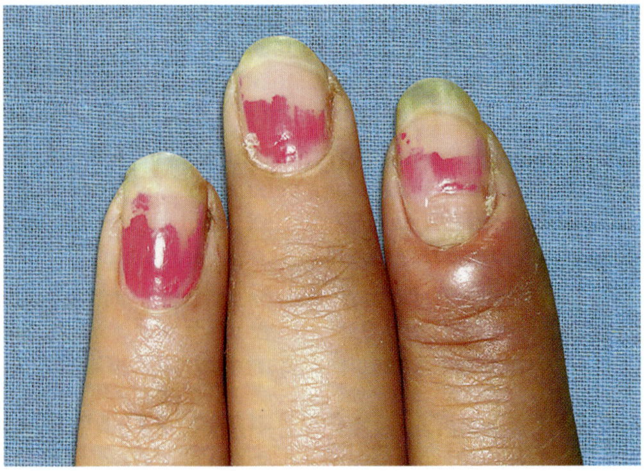

Fig. 29: Pemphigus vulgaris with periungual involvement seen as inflammation of nail fold with secondary nail changes in the form of Beau's lines.

coincide with or follow hair loss and represents a poor prognostic marker.

Bullous Disorders

Paronychia and onychomadesis are nail manifestations of autoimmune bullous disorders. Nail involvement is mainly a contiguous affliction, with secondary changes in the form of onychomadesis, pterygium, chronic paronychia, Beau's lines, pigmentary changes, or super infection **(Fig. 29)**:

- In *pemphigus vulgaris,* nail abnormalities can even precede skin findings. Nail lesions often relapse just before disease exacerbation/recurrence. Severe nail changes are often associated with extensive and severe disease.
- Nail scarring and pterygium are rare complications of *bullous pemphigoid*.
- Nail loss has been occasionally reported in *epidermolysis bullosa acquisita*.

ABNORMALITIES OF NAIL PIGMENTATION

Many disorders present with only an alteration in nail color as the primary or secondary manifestation of the disease.

Pigmented Nails

Abnormal nail pigmentation can be due to varied mechanisms like increased matrix melanogenesis, imperfect keratinization, infection, by-products of metabolism, ischemia, genetic abnormalities, or lack of nutrients. The pigmentation may be present in the NP or nailbed.

While evaluating any case of nail pigmentation, one needs to identify the anatomical unit involved in the pigmentary process. Nail discoloration following the shape of lunula is likely to be a result of internal factors; whereas, that corresponding to shape of proximal nailfold is likely to be external in origin.

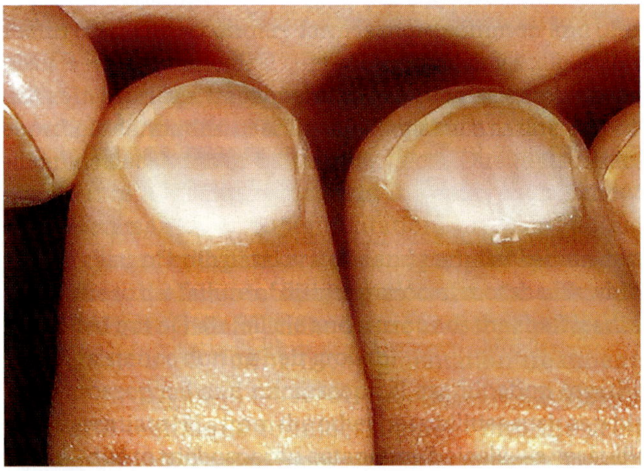

Fig. 30: Half and half nails with prominent distal brown discoloration.

Some named entities responsible for nail pigmentation include:

- *Brown arcs* seen distally, due to melanin deposition in the NP (with chronic renal failure).
- *Bissell's lines* seen as longitudinal brown lines in adrenal insufficiency.
- *Erythematous Crescents* seen as distal red bands due to vascular alterations in various systemic illnesses.
- *Expedition nails* seen as transverse white bands, probably due to protein deficiency.
- *Half and half nails* seen as proximal white or normal nail, with a distal brown color occupying 20–60% of nail **(Fig. 30)**. These are seen in chronic renal failure.
- *Terry's nails* (apparent leukonychia) seen as ground glass opacification of nearly entire nail, obliteration of lunula, and a narrow band of normal, pink nailbed at the distal border. These are characteristically described in cirrhosis. The nail is white proximally and normal distally.

- *Neapolitan nails* seen in elderly as bands of white, brown and red, from the proximal to the distal end.
- *Muehrcke's paired white bands* seen as pair of two white lines with an intervening area of normal pink color. These lines run parallel to the lunula and are described in patients with hypoalbuminemia.

Leukonychia

It is whitish discoloration of nails which may be congenital or acquired. Generally, the texture of nails is normal and there are no associated abnormalities of skin or its appendages. Two different mechanisms cause leukonychia:

1. *True leukonychia* (majority cases) is because of an aberration of dorsal nail matrix maturation resulting in dyskeratinization and parakeratotic foci or airspaces, imparting a whitish color to the ventral NP. It may occur in a variety of patterns:
   - *Total leukonychia* is a rare, inherited form in which all the nails are milky or porcelain white **(Fig. 31)**.
   - *Subtotal leukonychia* is a white proximal two-thirds of the nail. It is attributed to a delay in keratin maturation **(Fig. 32)**.
   - *Punctate leukonychia* consists of 1–3 mm diameter spots, attributed to a minor matrix trauma or alopecia areata **(Fig. 33)**.
   - *Longitudinal leukonychia* occurs due to parakeratotic focus in matrix, e.g., Darier's disease.
   - *Striate leukonychia* consists of horizontal bands as in cases of psoriasis and trauma **(Fig. 32)**.
2. *Apparent leukonychia* is due to vascular changes in the nailbed, with a normal overlying plate. It may occur in various patterns as described previously.

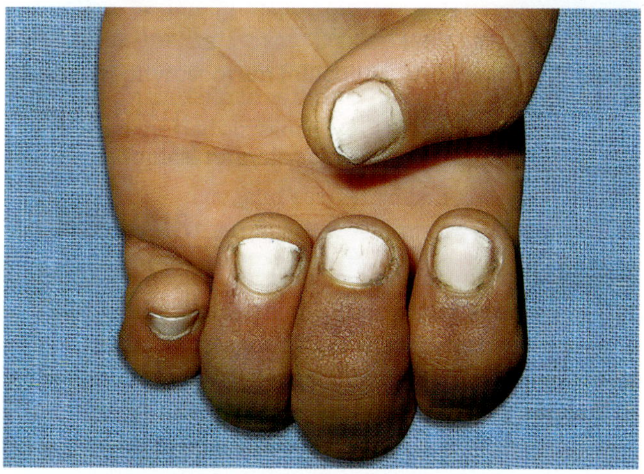

Fig. 31: Hereditary total leukonychia.

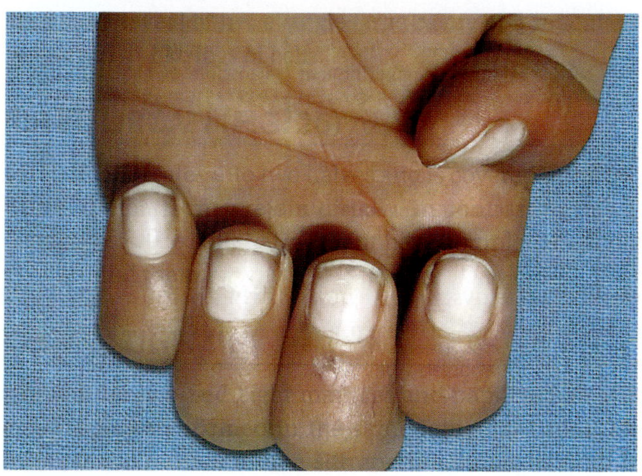

Fig. 32: Subtotal leukonychia: Striate pattern seen in between.

Leukonychia may also be classified *etiologically* as *congenital* or *acquired*. Factors responsible for *acquired leukonychia* include:

- Trauma induced matrix injury causing dyskeratinization or airspaces.
- Drugs or ingestants including antimony, carbon monoxide, formaldehyde, arsenic, lead, sulfonamides, etc.
- Systemic insults such as renal transplantation, anemia, cirrhosis, chronic renal failure, gout, hypoalbuminemia, pellagra, leprosy, pneumonia, malaria, syphilis, tuberculosis, etc.
- Dermatological disorders such as acrokeratosis verruciformis, alopecia areata, Darier's disease, dyshidrosis, SWO, herpes zoster, etc.

Melanonychia

Melanonychia is a normal finding in heavily pigmented races seen as *longitudinal pigmented bands (LPB)* in multiple nails. However, in white races, its presence may be an important pointer towards melanoma. Multiple causes (mostly benign) are implicated including physiologic bands, systemic disorders, trauma, inflammatory disorders, fungal infections, drugs, benign melanocyte hyperplasia, etc. Chronic inflammatory conditions such as onychomycosis, paronychia, psoriasis, lichen planus, amyloidosis, and chronic radio dermatitis may also lead to melanocyte activation and light-brown bands.

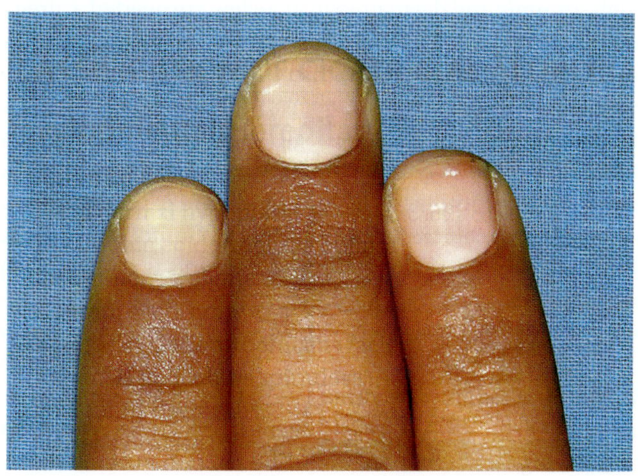

Fig. 33: Punctate leukonychia.

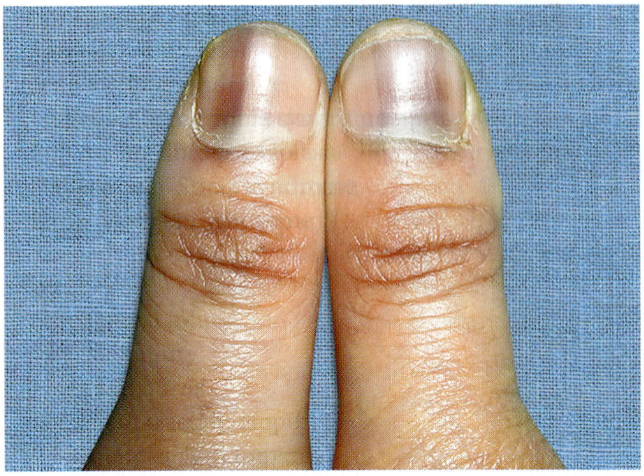

Fig. 34: Longitudinal melanonychia involving multiple nails with faint brown to black bands.

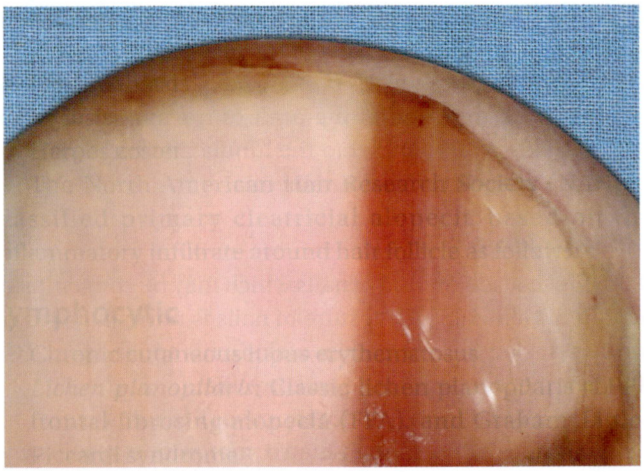

Fig. 36: Dermoscopic image showing brownish band with regular lines involving the thumb nail; suggestive of melanocyte activation (DinoLite AM7915MZT 20×).

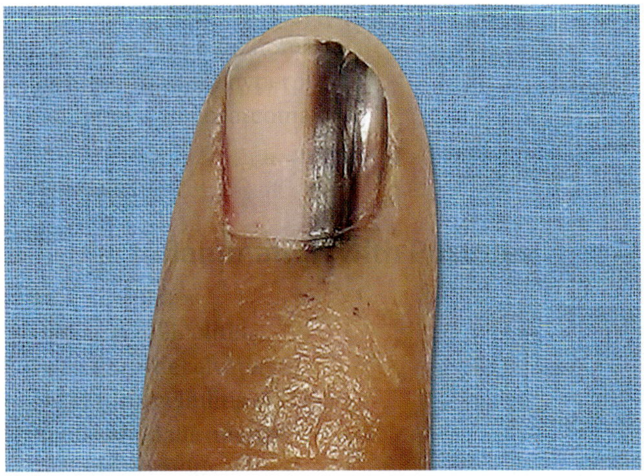

Fig. 35: Longitudinal melanonychia: Thick black band involving the thumb nail. Probably due to a nail matrix nevus.

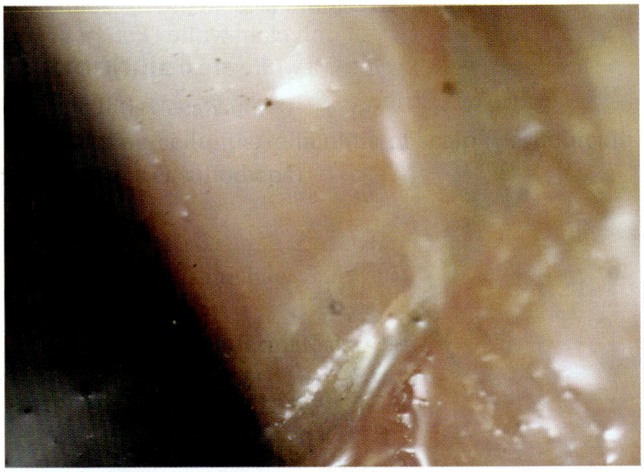

Fig. 37: Dermoscopic image showing dark black band with regular lines and peripheral pigment granules; suggestive of melanocyte proliferation (DinoLite AM7915MZT 20×).

Etiologically, LPB's can arise due to melanocyte activation **(Fig. 34)** or melanocyte proliferation **(Fig. 35)**. Multiple bands are usually non-neoplastic. A complete drug history and thorough systemic and dermatological review are needed. Clinical features differentiating these two causes have been reviewed by Baran. Onychoscopy can also help differentiate to some extent. Bands caused by *melanocyte activation* are benign and need not be evaluated pathologically **(Fig. 36)**. *Melanocyte proliferation* shows granular inclusions (<0.1 mm) within the bands. Benign proliferations produce regular patterned and spaced, brown-black parallel bands with uniform color and thickness **(Fig. 37)**. Malignant proliferation is suggested by irregular patterned, varying colored, irregular spaced, bands with varying thickness and evidence of crossing over of lines. LPB with onset in a single digit, during 6th decade of life, developing abruptly, becoming darker or wider suddenly, or occurring in the thumb, index finger or great toe are suggestive of a subungual melanoma (SM). The band may demonstrate blurred, rather than sharp lateral borders and may be accompanied by nail dystrophy. Findings which raise the suspicion of nail melanoma are summarized in **Box 2**.

BOX 2: Indicators/high-risk factors for nail unit melanoma.

- A personal or family history of melanoma
- New vertical brown-black nail pigmentation specially in fair-skinned
- Involvement of a "high-risk" digits (thumb, index finger, great toe)
- Changes in the band such as darkening, widening, and bleeding
- A bandwidth greater than 6 mm
- A band that is wider proximally than distally
- Nonuniform color of the line
- Indistinct lateral borders
- Associated with pigmentation of the nailfold (the Hutchinson sign, representing subungual melanoma) NP dystrophy, bleeding, or ulceration

ABCDE rule is a sensitive, and specific clinical tool for screening SM *in situ*. ABCDE rule includes several clinical features of melanoma. The features include—asymmetry, border irregularity, color variation, diameter >6 mm, and a new or changing lesion).

Various causative factors for LPB include:
- Benign racial pigmentation is the most common cause.
- Dermatological disorders like lichen planus, Bowen's disease, Peutz Jegher's syndrome, porphyria, etc.
- Drugs including antimalarials, doxorubicin, minocycline, azidothymidine (AZT), phenytoin, psoralens, sulfonamides, methotrexate, etc.
- Fungal agents such as *Acrotherium niger, Alternaria tenuis, Trichophyton soudanenses, Fusarium* spp., *Hendersonula toruloidea.*
- Nonfungal infections such as AIDS, secondary syphilis, *Proteus mirabilis,* and verruca vulgaris.
- Systemic factors leading to increased production of MSH (melanocyte stimulating hormone) include adrenal insufficiency (Cushing's syndrome), hypopituitarism, hemosiderosis, hyperbilirubinemia, hyperthyroidism, or irradiation.
- Local factors such as carpal tunnel syndrome, local radiotherapy, exostosis, foreign body, naevi, tumors, or onychophagia.
- Systemic conditions such as malnutrition, vitamin B_{12} deficiency, postinflammatory hyperpigmentation, pregnancy, etc.
- Frictional melanonychia due to the use of tight footwear.
- A substantial number of cases remain idiopathic.

Pigmentation of the Lunula

The lunula may also show pigmentary abnormalities in various conditions, e.g.:
- *Blue lunula* seen in cases of argyria, bacterial paronychia or with AZT therapy;
- *Punctate red spots* over lunula are seen in alopecia areata, psoriasis, dermatomyositis or twenty-nail dystrophy;
- *Yellow lunula* can be seen with tetracycline therapy, etc.

NAIL IN SYSTEMIC DISEASES

Generally, there is involvement of multiple nails. Assessment is better done in fingernails. A large number of reaction patterns have been seen to be associated with systemic disorders:
- *Splinter hemorrhages* arising in multiple nails, especially in the proximal part, are more likely to be due to a systemic cause like bacterial endocarditis, Trichinosis, anemia, cirrhosis, diabetes, antiphospholipid syndrome, septicemia, SLE, hypertension, Buerger's disease, Raynaud's disease, drug reactions, onychomycosis, HIV, irradiation, etc. Most commonly due to trauma, longitudinal arrangement is due to orientation of nailbed capillaries.
- *Beau's lines* **(Fig. 38)**: These are transverse grooves in the NP arising due to temporary suppression of matrix as a result of acute or chronic stress or systemic illness. Precipitating events may be local trauma, paronychia, chemotherapeutic agents cytotoxic to the nail matrix, or abrupt onset of systemic disease. Involvement of multiple nails at the same level arise suspicion regarding systemic cause. The width of the transverse groove corresponds to the duration of the disease that has affected the matrix. The distal limit of the furrow, if abrupt, indicates a sudden attack of disease; if sloping, a more protracted onset.

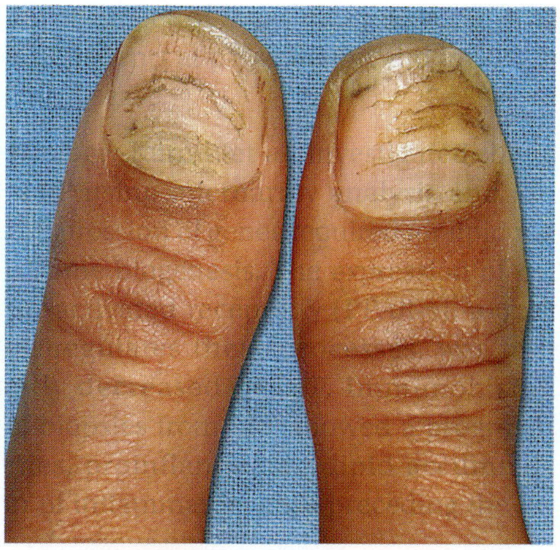

Fig. 38: Multiple Beau's lines.

- *Onycholysis* may be seen with anemia, bronchiectasis, SLE, pellagra, vitamin C deficiency, etc. even though it is less commonly associated with systemic disorders. *Plummer's nail* is a special type of onycholysis seen with thyroid disorders, usually starting in the 4th or 5th finger. Other causes may include pregnancy, impetigo herpetiformis, hereditary onycholysis, photo-onycholysis, or occupational causes.
- *Transverse white bands* may be in the form of *Mee's lines* (tend to be single) or *Muehrcke's paired white bands.* This should be distinguished from traumatic white lines.
- *Longitudinal erythronychia* may be localized (involving one nail) or polydactylous (involving more than one nail). The localized form is usually due to a neoplastic process, whereas involvement of many nails indicates underlying regional or systemic disease.
- *Erythematous crescents* are abnormally prominent erythematous bands at the distal portion of nail vascular bed occurring in chronic medical illnesses like renal failure.
- *Clubbing* is focal bulbous enlargement of the terminal segments of fingers and/or toes due to proliferation of connective tissue between nail matrix and the distal phalanx **(Fig. 39)**. A number of causes have been proposed including hereditary, idiopathic or acquired clubbing (most common). Acquired causes could be pulmonary (80%), cardiovascular (10–15%), hepatic, gastrointestinal, renal or occupational disease. Unilateral or unidigital clubbing is due to vascular abnormality confined to an extremity.

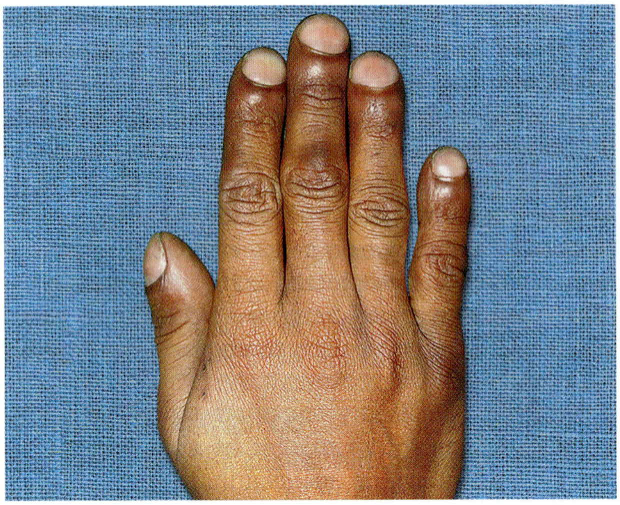

Fig. 39: Clubbing involving multiple nails.

- *Koilonychia* (spoon-shaped nails) is an abnormality of nail curvature wherein a drop of water placed on nail surface will not roll off. It can be hereditary or idiopathic, but again acquired causes are the most common. The most common causes are trauma, psoriasis, alopecia areata, onychomycosis, and digital ischemia (Raynaud's disease). Anemia is classically related with koilonychia and iron deficiency is the most common systemic association. Occupational koilonychia is a common cause of koilonychia seen in car mechanics, cabinet makers, mushroom growers, glass workers, chimney sweeps, rickshaw pullers, coil winders, and pin threaders. Koilonychia is physiological in some children, seen in 2nd to 4th toe in children aged between 1 and 4 years and disappear spontaneously.

DRUG-INDUCED NAIL CHANGES

Drugs may cause nail alterations in growth rate or pigmentation. Rarely, there may be shedding or permanent deformity of the nails **(Table 4)**. Commonly implicated drugs are:

- *Antibiotics*: Tetracyclines produce yellowish coloration and phototoxic reaction. Chloramphenicol may also cause phototoxicity. Cephaloridine and cloxacillin may result in onychomadesis.
- *Cancer chemotherapeutic agents:* They can lead to reduced nail growth (Beau's lines, onychomadesis), or increased pigmentation like cyclophosphamide, doxorubicin, methotrexate, 5-flourouracil **(Fig. 40)**. They can also cause true and apparent leukonychia.
- *Heavy metals*: Lead and arsenic may produce transverse white bands. Silver produces a blue lunula.
- *Antimalarials*: They commonly produce various kinds of pigmentation.
- *Others*: Carbamazepine, phenytoin, practolol, retinoids, etc., may also lead to nail changes.
- *Paronychia, pyogenic granuloma*

TABLE 4: Drug-induced nail changes.

Nail unit component affected	*Nail change*	*Drug responsible*
Nail matrix	Beaus lines	Chemotherapeutic agents-Docetaxel, cisplatin, fluorouracil, taxane, retinoids
	NP thinning	Chemotherapeutic agents, retinoids, antivirals
	True leukonychia	Chemotherapeutic agents—Doxorubicin, cyclophosphamide
Nailbed	Onycholysis	Taxanes, immunosuppressive drugs
	Photo-onycholysis	Tetracyclines, PUVA
Nail fold damage	Acute paronychia	Taxanes, retinoids, gemcitabine
	Pyogenic granuloma	Retinoids, EGFR inhibitors
NP	Nail pigmentation	Antineoplastic agents, e.g., doxorubicin, bleomycin, cyclophosphamide

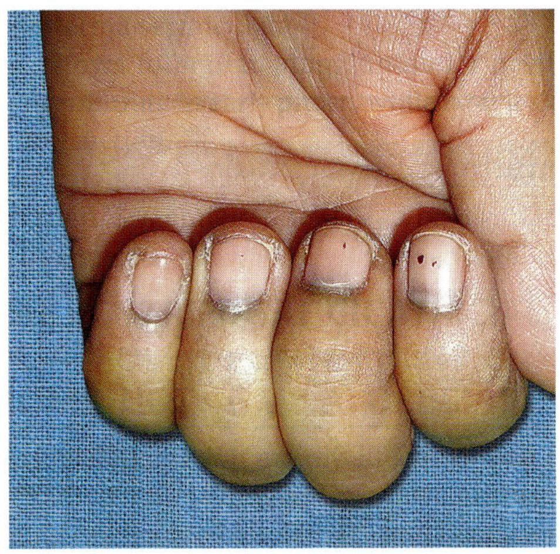

Fig. 40: Proximal nail discoloration in a patient on chemotherapeutic drugs.

NAIL TUMORS

A large number of nail tumors have been described, arising from different parts of the nail unit, except the NP. The diagnosis is generally delayed due to altered morphology. Investigational tools include onychoscopy, X-ray examination, MRI, and histopathology.

Benign Tumors

- *Wart* is the most common tumor involving the nail unit. It has been dealt with above.
- *Mucous cyst (*peri or subungual) is the second most common ungual tumor. It is a pseudocyst produced by localized, degenerative tissue reaction, containing a clear viscous fluid.

- *Pyogenic granulomas* are the third most common tumor, representing a reactive vascular overgrowth. They generally present along the lateral nailfold, as reddish-black, friable mass bleeding easily on touch **(Fig. 41)**. Tissue specimens should always be obtained before therapeutic destruction to rule out melanoma.
- *Glomus tumors* are hamartomatous growths due to hyperplastic neuromyoarterial glomus body. They are usually solitary, presenting with sharply localized pain and discoloration visible through the nail plate **(Fig. 42)**. Pain may be relieved by warmth or by tourniquet application (Hildreth test). The tumor may be localized with an X-ray (50% cases), ultrasonography (not very useful in subungual location), or an MRI (diagnostic test of choice). Onychoscopy may show discrete linear vascular structures. A more useful role is intraoperative (after nail plate removal), which can help localize the lesion, delineate surgical margins, thus ensuring complete removal and minimizing recurrences.[4] Excision is the treatment of choice.
- *Onychomatricoma* is a unique subungual tumor arising from the nail matrix. It is filamentous matrix tumor characterized by the triad of xanthonychia, longitudinal ridging with transverse over curvature and splinter hemorrhages.
- A number of fibromatous tumors have been described in the nail region. *Acquired digital fibrokeratoma* (garlic clove fibroma) is a benign, asymptomatic lesion with a hyperkeratotic tip and narrow base **(Fig. 43)**. It commonly arises from the periungual, especially near the matrix.
- Periungual fibromas (*Koenen's tumors*) are rare, benign fibrous tumors occurring around the nail plate **(Fig. 44)**. They are generally present at puberty and are associated with tuberous sclerosis. The tumor usually develops from under the proximal or lateral nailfold and rests on the nail plate.
- Four types of *bone tumors* may involve the nail unit. *Exostosis* (most common) is a slow growing tumor, mainly found on the great toe. Radiology shows a trabeculated bony growth with an expanded distal portion covered with

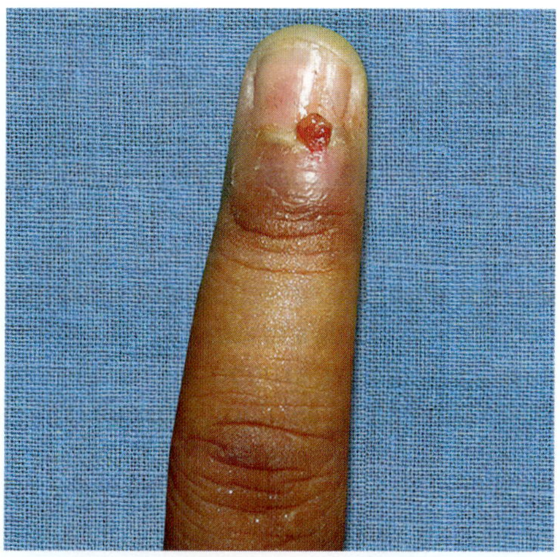

Fig. 41: Pyogenic granuloma involving the proximal nailfold area.

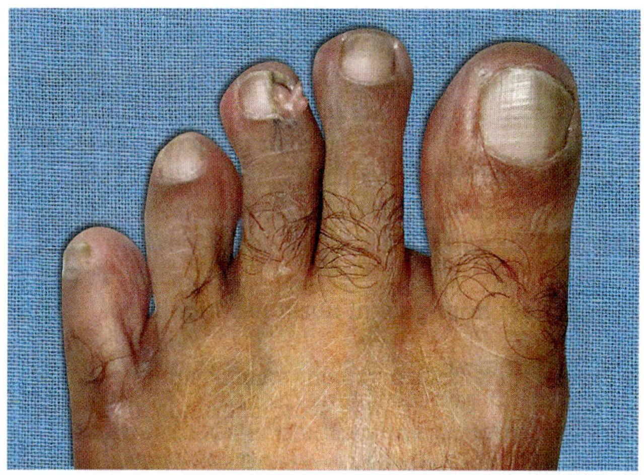

Fig. 43: Acquired digital fibrokeratoma.

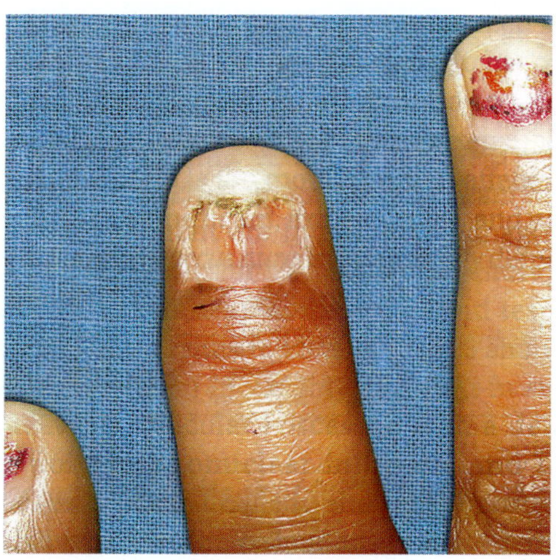

Fig. 42: Glomus tumor with severe pain and secondary nail dystrophy.

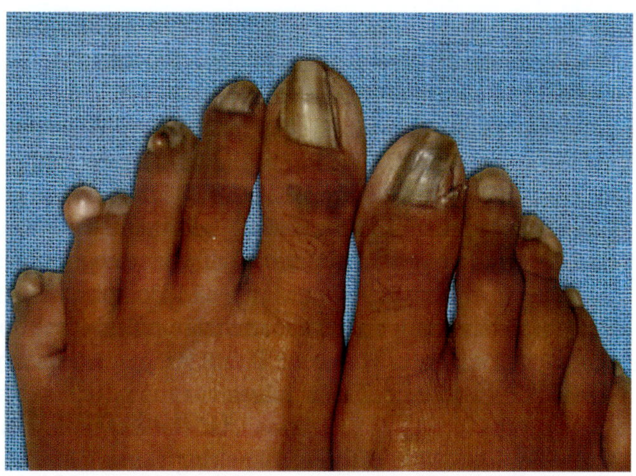

Fig. 44: Multiple Koenen's tumors in a patient with tuberous sclerosis.

radiolucent fibrocartilage. *Osteochondroma* manifests as benign, painful neoplasm loosely attached to the bone with islands of hyaline cartilage. *Enchondroma* is a cartilage tumor presenting as a painful solitary tumor of distal phalanx with clubbing, paronychia, nail thickening, discoloration, ridging, and elevation of nail. It is a rapidly growing tumor with X-ray showing a loculated radiolucent cyst with flecks of calcification. *Osteoid osteoma* presents as enlargement of entire digital tip with thickening of nail, clubbing and increased local sweating. The pain is nagging, characteristically relieved with NSAIDs.

- *Benign melanocytic nevus* can lead to longitudinal pigmented bands. The characteristic features have been discussed above.

Malignant Tumors

- *Squamous cell carcinoma* is the most common malignant tumor of nail unit. It commonly involves thumb; metastasis is infrequent and late. Histopathologically, atypical cells are seen extending into the dermis. Clinical presentation includes erythema and onycholysis initially and later on ulceration can occur.
- *Carcinoma cuniculatum* or *verrucous carcinoma* is known for its local aggressive behavior, but has a low potential for metastasis. It presents as a warty growth with discharge of foul-smelling yellowish material. Histologically, both exophytic and endophytic growth patterns are seen. There is an invaginated proliferation of well-differentiated keratinocytes with central crypts containing keratinous debris.
- *Basal cell carcinoma* is extremely rare in the subungual location, primarily because of relative sun protection in this region.
- *Subungual melanoma* typically presents as a darkened longitudinal band; may present as diffuse pigmentation also. It is frequently misdiagnosed with delay in appropriate treatment. About 20% of the melanomas may be amelanotic; hence, index of suspicion should be kept high for an inflammatory process which fails to resolve completely. A biopsy of suspicious changes, particularly if there are progressive changes in color or size, should be done. Dermoscopy can add valuable information and help decide regarding the need for biopsy. Clinical forms seen are lentigo maligna, superficial spreading, nodular or acral lentiginous melanoma (most common). Histopathology has a confirmatory role. The prognosis is guarded, depending on the level of invasion, and duration.
- *Metastatic carcinomas* of the nail unit are very rare. They may mimic acute or chronic infections such as cellulitis, paronychia, whitlow or osteomyelitis. The most common primary source for fingernails is lung tumors and for toenails are genitourinary tumors.

TRAUMATIC NAIL DISORDERS

These are very common due to the acral location of the nail unit. Both acute severe trauma, and chronic repetitive trauma can produce characteristic nail changes.

Clinical Features

- *Acute trauma* may manifest with a spectrum of changes ranging from simple subungual hematoma to complete nail avulsion **(Fig. 45)**. A classification system has been proposed to facilitate the management of traumatic nail lesions **(Table 5)**.

  Dermatoscopy shows subungual hematomas as well-delineated globular structure with color variation (black, purple, red to brown) **(Fig. 46)**. Recent hematoma tends be deeply located, reddish purple with irregular margins; whereas older hematomas are more superficial, roundish and deep red. Delayed subungual hematomas need to be differentiated from a subungual melanomas; dermoscopy is again useful in this regard. A small punch biopsy of NP can also differentiate clotted blood vs melanoma.

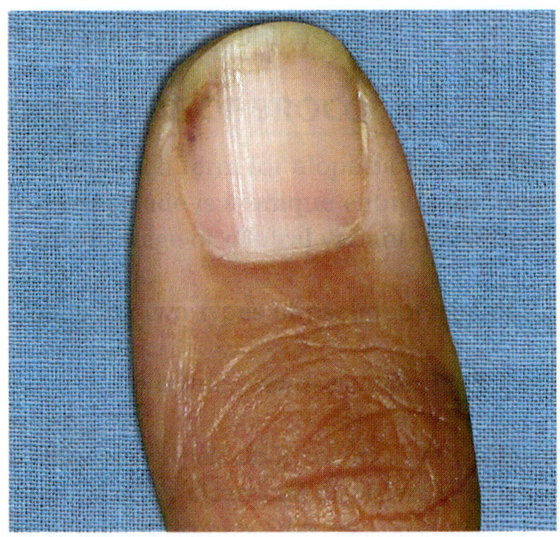

Fig. 45: Distal resolving subungual hematoma.

TABLE 5: Management of acute nail injuries.

Type	*Effect*	*Therapy*
I	Small hematoma associated with a small break in the nailbed	Fenestration of nail over the hematoma
II	Large hematoma with significant nailbed injury	Remove nail to identify site and nature of subungual damage
III	Large hematoma, NP displaced	X-ray may reveal fracture of terminal phalanx, with laceration of nailbed
IV	Severe crush injury	Nail avulsion to reveal matrix for careful reconstruction of lacerations
V	Amputation of tip of digit, may include parts of the matrix	If tip can be retrieved, it should be used as a graft

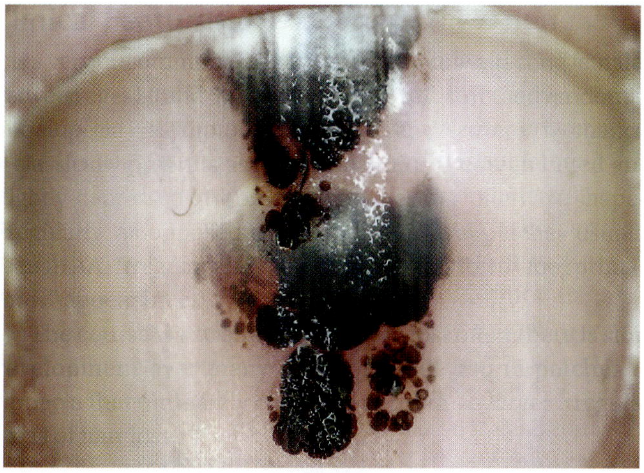

Fig. 46: Dermoscopic image of subungual hematoma (DinoLite AM7515MZT 35×).

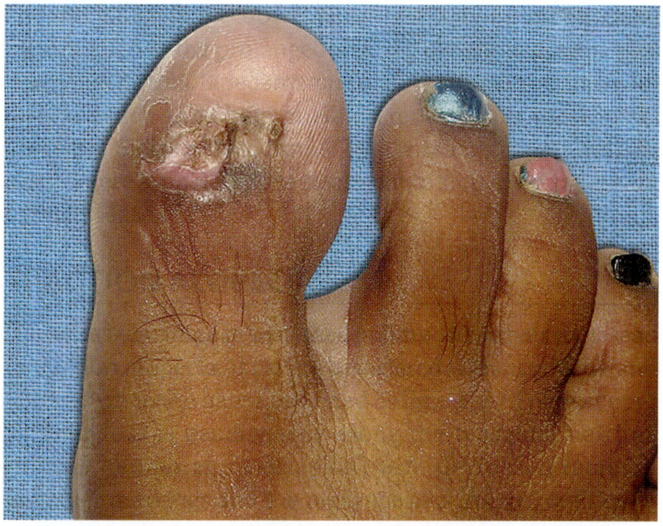

Fig. 47: Post-traumatic nail loss with pterygium formation.

It must be remembered that acute injuries may also sometimes lead to chronic deformities like split nail deformity or post traumatic pterygium **(Fig. 47)**. Management of these is very difficult.

- *Chronic repetitive trauma* can lead to variety of manifestations including *chronic paronychia*:
  - *Habit-tic deformity* (washboard nails) is due to a conscious or inadvertent, self-induced habit of causing chronic repetitive trauma to the proximal nailfold. It is common on thumbnails where the individual is in the habit of constantly rubbing the central portion of PNF. Central transverse Beau's lines, not covering the entire width of the NP are characteristically seen **(Fig. 48)**. The cuticle is usually distorted.
  - *Median canaliform dystrophy of Heller* manifests as inverted fir tree like split or canal in the nail plate. It may extend from the cuticle to free edge of the nail plate; however, cuticle is preserved (c.f. Habit-tic deformity). It is reported with repetitive trauma, as familial transmission, or with oral retinoid therapy.
  - *Nail biting (onychophagia)* presents as short nails, exposed nailbed, ragged free edge or surface abnormalities **(Fig. 49)**. Most of the cases are not associated with any psychological abnormality. Severe cases may show subungual hemorrhage, strips of nail loss, residual spurs, or disappearing nail.
  - *Onychotillomania* is defined as self-induced trauma to the nail unit, either by picking or pulling at the nails. It may lead to severe irreversible nail dystrophy, melanonychia, or infections. Nails are rough, with irregular nailfolds. Secondary complications such as warts, pterygium, secondary infection, chronic paronychia, or osteomyelitis may occur.
  - *Hang nails* are characterized by hard pieces of epidermis breaking away from the lateral and proximal nailfolds **(Fig. 49)**. This occurs due to nail biting or minor injuries.

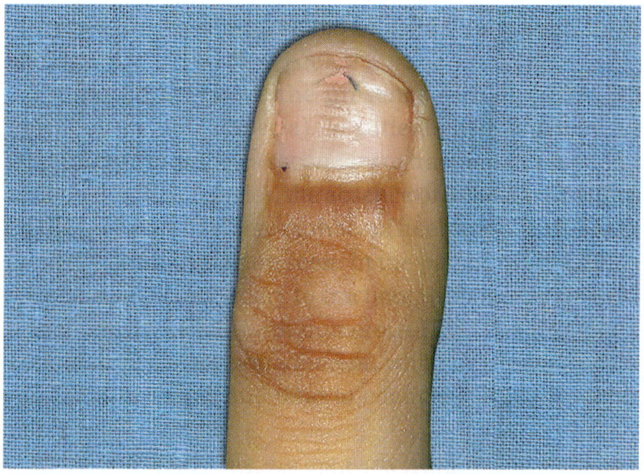

Fig. 48: Habit-tic deformity of the thumb nail with multiple, central Beau's lines placed closely.

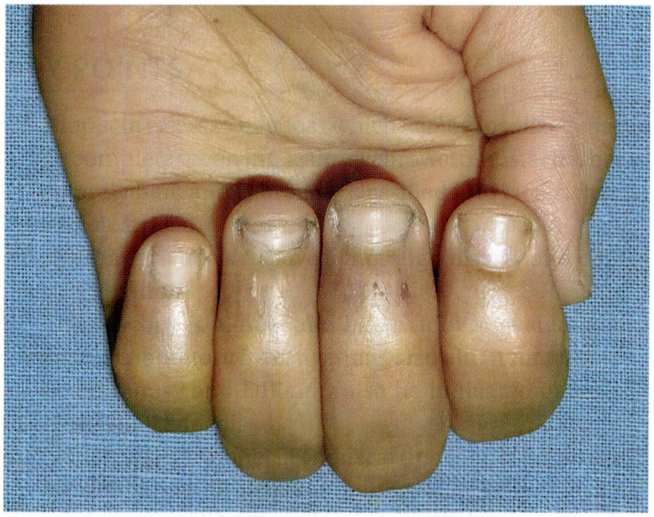

Fig. 49: Onychophagia with distinctly shortened nails, disruption of onychodermal band and changes in surrounding skin. Hang nails seen as the dry, exfoliating proximal nail fold with linear erosions.

PEDIATRIC NAIL DISORDERS

Altered appearance of nails in children may have a profound psychosocial impact due to ridicule from the peer group.

Physiological Changes

- At birth, the nail plate is thin and transparent; barely extending beyond the hyponychium.
- Temporary koilonychia may be seen, especially on great toenails.
- Superficial longitudinal ridges in *herring-bone pattern* may persist in infancy and normalizes gradually. It reflects a gradual change in the maturation of the matrix.
- *Onychoschizia* (<5 years of age), prominent onychodermal band, *Beau's lines* (present by 2 months of age in 92% of infants), *onychomadesis* (due to intrauterine asphyxia), or *paronychia* (due to finger sucking) may also occur.
- Assessment of gestational age of newborn can be done by observing the length and texture of nails. Nails of preterm (and some term infants) fall shorter than the distal digital pulp (*pseudo-ingrown toenail*) whereas, the nails of a post-term or large for gestational age infants, extend well beyond the hyponychium.

Congenital Malformations

- *Congenital malalignment of the great toenails* is seen with laterally deviated nail plate (rarely medially) with respect to the longitudinal axis of phalanx. Transverse ridging may occur because of intermittent trauma to the matrix. If not corrected early, it may result in paronychia, ingrown nails (most common cause of ingrowing toe nail in children and adolescent) or onychomadesis.
- *Congenital anonychia* may be inherited or may occur sporadically. It may be associated with underlying defects of the digit such as ectrodactyly, bizarre flexural pigmentation, coarse spare hair, etc.
- Rare abnormalities include *polyonychia* (without polydactyly), *onychoheterotopia* (true ectopic nails), etc.
- Nail abnormalities may be associated with specific skeletal dysplasias such as racket nails, acro-osteolysis, Apert's syndrome, cleidocranial dysostosis, nail-patella syndrome, etc.
- Chromosomal disorders associated with nail deformity include Down syndrome (macronychia, clubbing); Trisomy 18 (hypoplasia of 5th finger); or Turner syndrome (narrow, hyper convex, deep set nails).
- Teratogenic effects of drugs including phenytoin (hypoplastic nails with longitudinal pigmented bands) or alcohol (anonychia of the 5th digit) may induce nail changes.
- Ectodermal dysplasias show nail changes and in the Freire-Maia Taxonomic System, nails belong to subclass 3. Nail plate may be small, brittle, and discolored or even thickened in some cases.

Thickened Nails in Children

Thickened nails in children may be a result of:

- *Pachyonychia congenita*, an autosomal dominant genodermatosis with variable penetrance and expressivity, is characterized by subungual hyperkeratosis, keratosis palmaris et plantaris and leukokeratosis of oral mucosa. The nails are generally normal at birth, but within 2–8 weeks, the classical changes begin to develop in the form of smooth but hard nail plate with massive subungual hyperkeratosis.
- *Onychauxis* (brittle, thickened nails with a distorted rough surface) may be a manifestation of chronic mucocutaneous candidiasis. There is massive thickening of nails caused by *Candida albicans*, along with widespread involvement of skin and oral mucosa. There is paronychia, subungual hyperkeratosis, onycholysis and bulbous digital tips. It can also be seen in immunosuppressed states (primary or secondary); atopic erythroderma, alopecia totalis, vitiligo, or recurrent infections.
- Localized nail hypertrophy is generally a manifestation of dermatophytosis, psoriasis or benign nail tumors (e.g., neurofibromas, exostosis).

Blistering Disorders

- Intrauterine finger sucking may lead to blisters involving distal digital pulp. In such a case, bacterial or herpetic infection needs to be ruled out.
- *Epidermolysis bullosa* may produce sub or periungual bullae along with nail deformities in the form of anonychia, dystrophy, onychogryphosis or onychomadesis **(Fig. 50)**.
- Older children may manifest herpetic whitlow or blistering distal dactylitis which is a nontender, localized, bacterial infection of the distal volar pad of fat, due to group A β-hemolytic streptococci. The blister may spread dorsally to the nailfolds, leading to paronychia or latent onychomadesis.

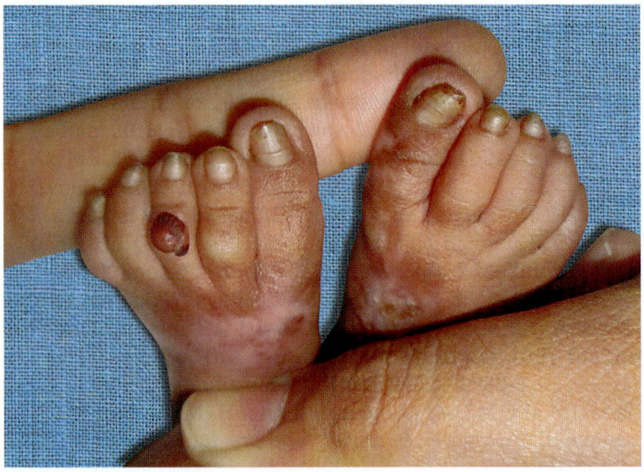

Fig. 50: Epidermolysis bullosa with characteristic nail changes.

Inflammatory Disorders

Apart from many inflammatory diseases like erythema multiforme, Kawasaki's disease or childhood atopic dermatitis, which may affect the nails; distinct entities include:

- *Parakeratosis pustulosa*: A benign, inflammatory condition predominantly seen in girls less than 5 years of age. There is a well demarcated, bright red, swollen, nontender distal phalanx with few periungual pustules. It may go off spontaneously or can get converted into psoriasis in future.
- *Paronychia* is common in children and is generally associated with finger sucking. Systemic disorders such as mucocutaneous candidiasis, acrodermatitis enteropathica may also present with these lesions.
- *Onychophagia*, seen in up to 50% of children, is a common pediatric problem. It leads to traumatic nail abnormalities, apart from increasing the spread of warts and infectious agents.
- Nail dystrophy with a linear skin disorder can be seen with ILVEN (inflammatory verrucous epidermal naevus), incontinentia pigmenti, lichen nitidus, lichen planus, linear porokeratosis, or lichen striatus.

Twenty-nail Dystrophy/Trachyonychia

Twenty-nail dystrophy (TND) is a term popularized by Hazelrigg et al in their initial report of children with acquired trachyonychia of all 20 nails.[10] *Trachyonychia or sand-blasted nails* refers to nails with closely spaced *longitudinal striations, onychorrhexis, onychoschizia*, distal chipping and a dull, opalescent appearance giving them a rough appearance **(Fig. 51)**. This term describes a *reaction pattern* rather than a specific disease. The onset is insidious, either simultaneously in all nails or in individual nails, gradually over many months. According to some reports, the appearance of the nail plate may vary from rough, lusterless, sand papered appearance to a shiny appearance (variant) with numerous, small, superficial pits **(Fig. 52)**.

Most commonly, twenty-nail-dystrophy is seen as an isolated nail abnormality (spongiotic trachyonychia); however, many associations have been attributed including lichen planus, alopecia areata, eczematous changes, IgA deficiency, ichthyosis vulgaris, primary biliary cirrhosis, pemphigus, vitiligo, etc. Most of these cases resolve spontaneously over several years.

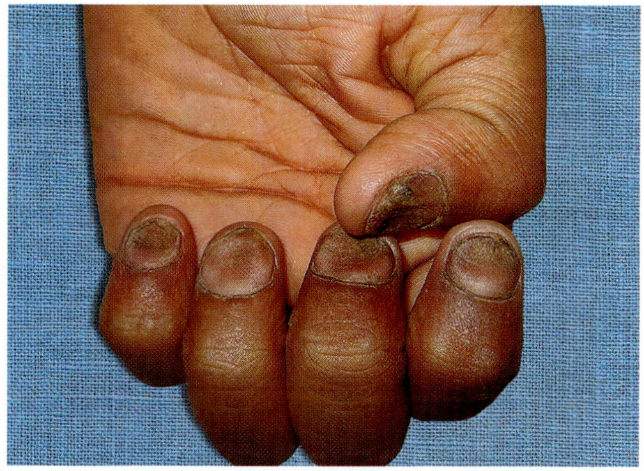

Fig. 51: Twenty-nail dystrophy: Trachyonychia with rough appearance of nails.

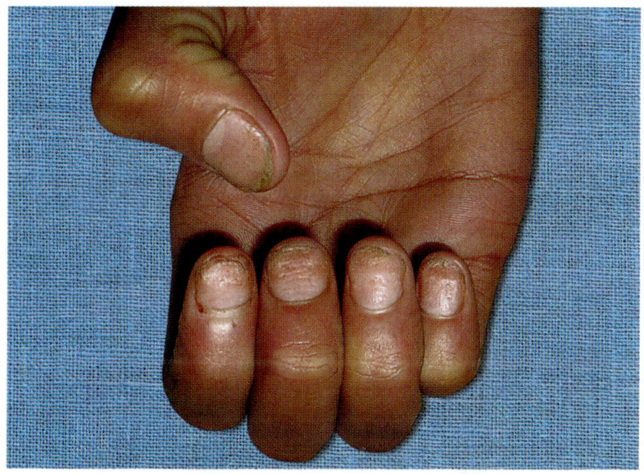

Fig. 52: Shiny trachyonychia.

NAIL DISORDERS IN ELDERLY

These include age-related changes; disorders due to concurrent dermatological and systemic diseases; or secondary to tumors of nail or surrounding structures.

Age-associated Nail Changes

- Linear nail growth is decreased.
- Nails become dull and opaque with color varying from yellow to gray.
- Smaller lunula with Neapolitan nails may be seen.
- Generally, transverse curvature of nail increases and longitudinal decreases.
- An increased friability and onychorrhexis may be seen (up to 85% of subjects >50 years). The thickness may increase, decrease or remain the same.

Physical Nail Abnormalities

- *Onychauxis* is localized hypertrophy of nail plate **(Fig. 53)**. Many cases can be attributed to onychomycosis; even though, idiopathic cases exist. These would need periodic partial or total debridement of nail plate.
- *Onychoclavus* is subungual corn; it may occur because of anatomical abnormality or mechanical changes. It is a painful process typically occurring under the great toenail.
- *Onychocryptosis* is ingrown nail due to penetration of the lateral nailfold by the nail plate. It may be due to over-curvature of nail plate, or hypertrophy of lateral nailfold. It presents as inflamed, tender, granulation tissue **(Fig. 54)**. It can be a devastating problem in the elderly with

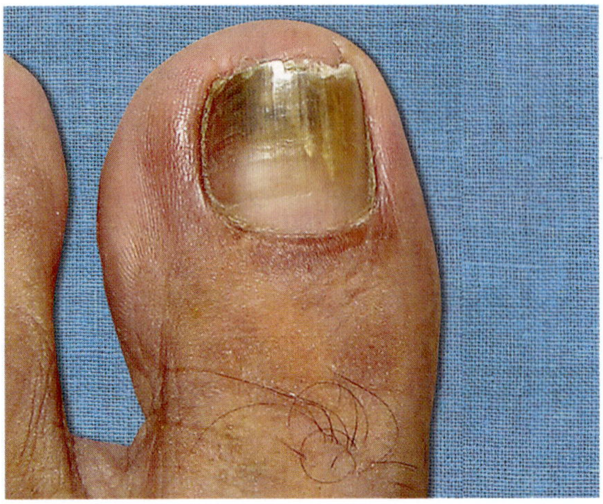

Fig. 53: Onychauxis with focal thickening and discoloration of distal nail plate.

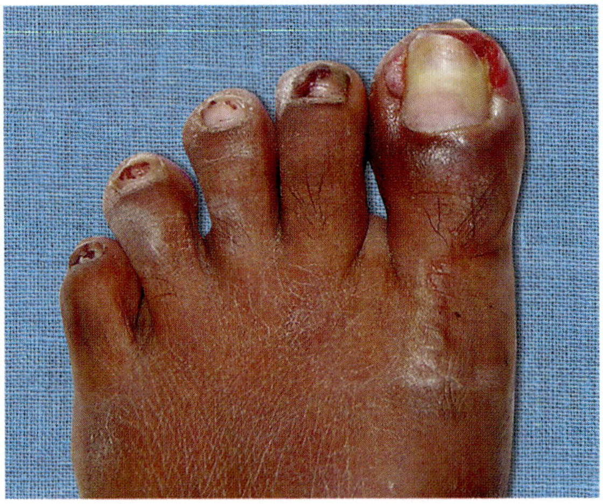

Fig. 54: Onychocryptosis or ingrown toenail.

neuropathy. An extreme ingrown is known as *Pincer nail* (trumpet shaped, embedding both the lateral nailfolds) **(Fig. 55)**. Lateral Nail matrix phenolization is required for advanced cases.

- *Onychogryphosis* is an enlarged nail plate with exaggerated curvature, commonly seen in elderly, involving the toenails. Primary onychogryphosis occurs due to self-neglect or an inability to perform adequate foot care. Secondary factors including nail trauma, nailbed hypertrophy or biomechanical abnormalities. Thickened, opaque nail plate is prone to trauma and further infection.
- *Onychophosis* is the presence of localized or diffuse hyperkeratotic tissue on the nailfolds or subungually. It is common in elderly, involving the 1st and 5th toes. Predisposing factors include repeated minor trauma, nailfold hypertrophy, onychocryptosis, xerosis, etc.

Disorders of Nail

Nail disorders in elderly age group are quite common, however, data regarding their exact prevalence are lacking:

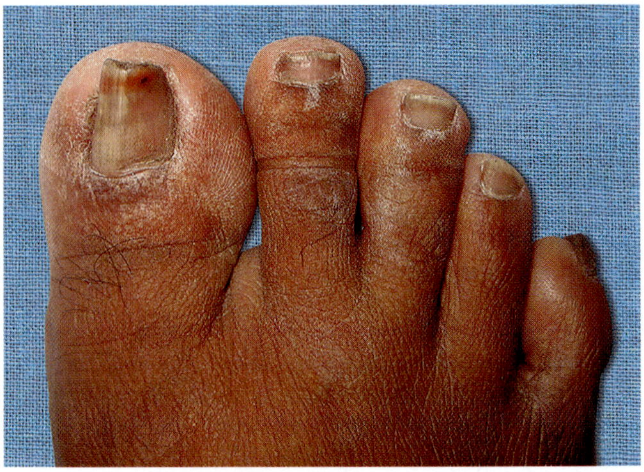

Fig. 55: Pincer nail deformity.

- *Brittle nails* are seen in 20–35% of elderly.
- Elderly are especially prone to nail abnormalities due to faulty pedal biomechanics. Bony abnormalities in elderly (hammer toes, hallux rigidus, hallux valgus, etc.) can lead to nail abnormalities including *onychauxis, onychoclavus, onychophosis, subungual exostosis,* etc. Shoe-induced biomechanical abnormalities are also seen due to foot and shoe incompatibility.
- Rarely, onychotillomania or onychophagia may be seen.
- Large number of infections may involve the nail unit in elderly. *Onychomycosis* is more common in the elderly and saprophytic molds are most common organisms involved. In elderly, only topical therapy may be recommended at times. Paronychia and onycholysis are also common.

KEY POINTS

- Nail abnormalities constitute a significant number of patients attending the dermatology departments. These disorders significantly affect the quality-of-life and functionality of the patients and that is why they deserve special attention.
- Nail has a unique structure and different reaction patterns as compared to the rest of the skin and appendages.
- It is useful to know the appearance of nail in health and disease states to be able to recognize and treat these conditions effectively.
- Infectious conditions comprise of only 50% of nail dystrophies. Other causes deserve special mention and care, including the physiological and pathologic causes of abnormal nails.

REFERENCES

1. Scher RK, Daniel CR. Nails: Therapy, Diagnosis and Surgery, 3rd edition. Philadelphia: Elsevier Saunders; 2005.
2. Lawry M, Rich P. The nail apparatus: a guide for basic and clinical science. Curr Probl Dermatol. 1999;11:161-208.

3. Nouripour-Sisakht S, Mirhendi S, Shidfar H, Ahmadi MR, Rezaei-Matehkolaei B, Geramishoar A, et al. Aspergillus species as emerging causative agents of onychomycosis. J Mycol Med. 2015;25:101-7.
4. Grover C, Jakhar D. Onychoscopy: a practical guide. Indian J Dermatol Venereol Leprol. 2017;83:536-49.
5. Gupta AK, Hall S, Zane LT, Lipner SR, Rich P. Evaluation of the efficacy and safety of tavaborole topical solution, 5%, in the treatment of onychomycosis of the toenail in adults: a pooled analysis of an 8-week, post-study follow-up from two randomized phase 3 studies. J Dermatolog Treat. 2017;30:1-5.
6. Pabari A, Iyer S, Khoo CT. Swiss roll technique for treatment of paronychia. Tech Hand Up Extrem Surg. 2011;15:75-7.
7. Kore SD, Kanwar AJ, Vinay K, Wanchu A. Pattern of mucocutaneous manifestations in human immunodeficiency virus-positive patients in North India. Indian J Sex Transm Dis. 2013;34:19-24.
8. Bouscarat F, Douchard C, Bouhour D. Paronychia and pyogenic granuloma of great toes in patients treated with Indinavir. N Engl J Med. 1998;338:1776-7.
9. Dawber RPR, Baran R, de Berker D. Disorders of nails. In: Burns T, Breathnach S, Cox N, Griffiths C (Eds). Rook's Textbook of Dermatology, 6th edition. New Jersy: Blackwell Science; 1998. pp. 2815-68.
10. Hazelrigg DE, Duncan WC, Jarratt M. Twenty-nail dystrophy of childhood. Arch Dermatol. 1977;113:73-5.

EXAMINATION QUESTIONS

1. Discuss the components of nail unit. Discuss in brief the clinical importance of each component. Draw a diagram of blood supply of nail unit.
2. Discuss the principles of dermatoscopy and role of onychoscopy in dermatology.
3. Discuss nail changes in five different dermatological disorders.
4. Describe nail changes and their pathogenesis in:
   (a) Lichen planus.
   (b) Psoriasis.

Write short notes on the following:

5. Onychomycosis.
6. Topical antifungals in onychomycosis.
7. Trachyonychia/twenty-nail dystrophy.
8. Nail manifestations of internal disease.
9. Nailfold capillaroscopy.
10. Nail psoriasis.
11. Nail LP.

77 CHAPTER

Dermal Hypertrophies

Somenath Sarkar

INTRODUCTION

Dermal hypertrophies are benign or malignant fibroblastic and myofibroblastic disorders. The benign hypertrophies are more common than the malignant hypertrophies. Some of them develop in childhood, but it is not rare among adults. They have characteristic clinical and histological features. Histopathology is the key for proper diagnosis and treatment. Fibroblast on histology looks like spindle-shaped cell with a tapered nucleus, while myofibroblast looks like spindle-shaped cell with a cigar-shaped nucleus. On immunohistochemistry, fibroblast is positive with vimentin and CD4, while myofibroblast is positive with vimentin, muscle-specific actin (MSA), and smooth muscle actin (SMA).

CLASSIFICATION

Benign Dermal Hypertrophy

- *Both adult and children*:
  - Hypertrophic scar
  - Keloid
  - Acrochordon
  - Dermatofibroma
- *In children*:
  - *Solitary lesion*:
    - Infantile digital fibromatosis
    - Myofibrosis
    - Calcifying aponeurotic fibroma
    - Plantar fibromatosis
    - Infantile fibromatosis
    - Fibrous hamartoma of infancy
    - Fibromatosis colli
    - Cranial fasciitis
  - *Multiple lesions*:
    - Juvenile hyaline fibromatosis
  - *Aggressive lesion*:
    - Infantile fibromatosis
    - Infantile myofibromatosis
- *In adults*:
  - *Solitary lesion*:
    - Acquired digital fibrokeratoma
    - Dupuytren's contracture
    - Dermatomyofibroma
    - Pleomorphic fibroma
    - Collagenous fibroma
    - Myofibroma
    - Solitary fibrous tumor
  - *Multiple lesions*:
    - Fibromatosis (palmoplantar, penile, knuckle pads)
    - Pachydermodactyly
  - *Reactive lesions:*
    - Nodular fasciitis
    - Elastofibroma dorsi
  - *Aggressive lesion*:
    - Desmoid tumor
  - *Clinically distinctive hypertrophies*:
    - Cutis verticis gyrata (CVG)
    - Pachydermoperiostitis
    - Cerebriform fibrous proliferation

Malignant Dermal Hypertrophy

- Dermatofibrosarcoma protuberans (DFSP)
- Atypical fibroxanthoma
- Giant cell fibroblastoma
- Malignant fibrous histiocytoma (MFH)
- Epithelioid sarcoma (ES)

Hypertrophic Scar and Keloid

- Hypertrophic scar and keloid are two forms of abnormal wound healing characterized by increased uncontrolled collagen synthesis and deposition at the site of injury. Both of them have higher predilection to develop in dark-skinned races and in Asians (16%).[1] Keloid can occur at any age commonly between 10 and 30 years.
- Both of them favor the line of increased skin tension, such as shoulder, sternum, mandible, and arm. But keloid can appear in a site where there is minimal tension such as ear lobe and any site of injury. Keloid appears as pruritic, pink to hyperpigmented, smooth-surfaced plaque with claw-like well-circumscribed borders.
- The basic difference between keloid and hypertrophic scar is that keloid extends beyond the original wound with claw-like extension but hypertrophic scar remains confined to the wound margin. Hypertrophic scar is asymptomatic keloid is pruritic, hypertrophic scar regress spontaneously and keloid never regresses spontaneously but recurs after treatment. In hypertrophic scar, both the number of fibroblast and density of collagen bundles

TABLE 1: Key features of hypertrophic scar and keloid.

	Hypertrophic scar	*Keloid*
History of injury	Yes	Not always
Onset	Immediate	May be delayed
Extension beyond the wound margin	No	Yes
Symptom	Usually absent	May be pruritic
Clinical profile	Raised	Raised
Erythema	Prominent	Varies
Number of fibroblast	Increased	Increased
Density of collagen	Increased	Increased
Orientation of collagen bundle	Parallel to skin surface	Haphazard
Myofibroblast	Present	Absent
Spontaneous resolution	Sometimes, may be gradual	Rare
Response to treatment	Good	Poor

TABLE 2: Vancouver scar scale.

Parameter	*Interpretation*	*Score*
Vascularity	Normal Pink Red Purple	0 1 2 3
Pigmentation	Normal Hypopigmented Hyperpigmented	0 1 2
Pliability	Normal Supple Yielding Firm Ropes Contracture	0 1 2 3 4 5
Height	Flat <2 mm 2–5 mm >5 mm	0 1 2 3
	Total score	*13*

are increased and collagen bundles are parallel to skin surface but keloid has thick bundle of collagen oriented in haphazard array with increased number of fibroblast. Key clinical features, similarities, and differences are elaborated in **Table 1**.

- Assessment of scar can be done by its extent, volume, maximum dimensions, and thickness. A subjective scale known as Vancouver scar scale is available for overall assessment of the quality of scar **(Table 2)**.[2] In the first decade of 21st century, both patients and observer scar assessment scale have been developed and found to be reliable.[3] Noninvasive techniques such as observation of scar color, blood flow, hardness, and elasticity; imaging techniques such as high-frequency ultrasound, laser Doppler perfusion, and magnetic resonance imaging (MRI); dedicated scar photography can be employed to evaluate the scar objectively.[4]
- Treatment of both of entity is challenging to clinicians. Intralesional triamcinolone injection is the mainstay of therapy. To avoid recurrence steroid injection combined with cryotherapy, 5-fluorouracil (5-FU).[5] Other injectables with varying success rate are injection bleomycin and interferons. Topical self-adherent silicone gel sheet pressure garments, retinoids, and tacrolimus are other modalities of treatment. For larger lesion debulking followed by intralesional steroid and interferon injection can be done.

Skin Tag

- Skin tag or acrochordon is the most common entity that effect both male and female and incidence increase with age. Predisposing factors are family history, obesity, and diabetes mellitus. In Birt–Hogg–Dubé syndrome acrochordon associated with fibrofolliculoma and trichodiscoma.[6]
- Clinically, it is asymptomatic soft skin color or hyperpigmented single or multiple, pedunculated papule over eyelid, neck, axilla, groin, trunk, and upper thigh. It may be painful if pedicle gets strangulated or irritated.
- Treatment is solely cosmetic issue but surgical excision, electrocauterization, or radiofrequency ablation may be considered when get twisted, irritated, or causing cosmetic concern.

Dermatofibroma

- Dermatofibroma is the second most common fibrohistiocytic tumor after skin tag. Dermatofibroma commonly appear in women at their 20s and 30s over lower extremities than men. Precise dermatofibroma etiology is unknown.
- Common triggering factors are trauma and arthropod bite. Multiple eruptive dermatofibroma is seen in patients with autoimmune disease (e.g., lupus erythematosus), immunosuppression [human immunodeficiency virus (HIV)], and atopic dermatitis.[7]
- Dermatofibromas are characterized by dermal proliferation of spindle-shaped fibroblast and myofibroblast arranged in short interlacing fascicles. An increased number of small blood vessels and presence of mitotic figures on histology indicates that it may be due to some reactive or neoplastic process.
- Clinically, it is solitary or multiple, firm, shiny or keratotic, tan to pink or hyperpigmented, dome-shaped papule or nodule measuring 0.5 mm to 1 cm in diameter. On palpation, lesion is indurated, mobile but fixed to the subcutaneous tissue and on lateral pressure tumor moves downward with dimple-like depression on overlying skin ("dimple sign" or "button holing"). Common clinical differentials of dermatofibroma are elaborated in **Table 3**.

TABLE 3: Common clinical differentials of dermatofibroma.

Benign lesion	*Malignant lesion*
• Cyst • Hypertrophic scar • Neurofibroma • Tophus • Schwannoma • Erythema elevatum diutinum	• Basal cell carcinoma • Dermatofibrosarcoma protuberans • Nodular melanoma • Giant cell tumor of the skin

- Histologically, overlying epidermis is hyperplastic with hyperpigmented basal layer ("dirty fingernail sign") and elongation of rete ridges, which is separated by a clear zone (grenz zone) from the tumor in the dermis. Dermis has short interlacing fascicles of plump of spindle-shaped cells (fibroblasts and myofibroblasts) without atypia, arranged in a characteristic storiform pattern.[8] Blood vessels, foamy histiocytes, and multinucleated giant cells containing lipid or hemosiderin are frequently present. Large number of capillaries along with associated sclerosis may present, such lesion may termed as "sclerosing hemangioma." Prominent lipid accumulation may be seen in lipidized ("ankle type") dermatofibroma. Few dermatofibroma may be poorly cellular, with spindle-shaped cells extending between the collagen bundles. The major histologic variants and histological differentials of dermatofibroma are elaborated in **Boxes 1 and 2**, respectively.
- Deeper variant is usually seen in young adults on trunk and extremities measuring 1–2 cm and clinically difficult to differentiate from dermatofibrosarcoma protuberans (DFSP), lipoma, and cyst. Histologically, infiltrative storiform pattern of occupying the entire dermis, extension to subcutis in vertical and radial pattern, increased cellularity, and fascial plane showing no defined border with normal tissue favors the diagnosis of DFSP. In contrast, dermatofibroma is usually confined to dermis. Positive immunohistochemical staining with vimentin, factor XIIIa, stromelysin, CD68 and α-SMA, and negative staining with CD34 supports the diagnosis of dermatofibroma. In atypical, the cell variant seen in the middle-aged adult lesion is >2 cm and invade superficial subcutis. Histology shows pleomorphic plump spindle or polyhedral cells with large hyperchromatic, irregular, or bizarre nuclei in a context of classical dermatofibroma. Individual cell may be mono- or multinucleated with abundant cytoplasmic vacuoles and hemosiderin deposit. Atypical mitotic figures are present with local recurrence and distant metastases.
- Tumor remains either static or regression over time leaving behind hyperpigmentation. Symptomatic tumor needs fusiform excision up to superficial subcutis to prevent recurrence. In deeper variant excision up to deep subcutis is required as it recurs more frequently.

BOX 1: Histologic variants of dermatofibroma.

- Extension in the subcutaneous tissue (deep dermatofibroma)
- With atypical cells (monster cells)
- Atrophic
- Palisading
- Aneurysmal
- Ossifying
- Clear cell
- With osteoclast-like cell
- With granular cells
- Cellular
- Xanthomatous
- Myxoid

BOX 2: Histological differentials of dermatofibroma.

- Keloid
- Scar
- Dermatomyofibroma
- Dermatofibrosarcoma protuberans (DFSP)
- Nodular Kaposi sarcoma

Infantile Digital Fibromatosis

- Infantile digital fibromatosis is a benign fibroblastic tumor present as solitary, smooth, flesh-colored, dome-shaped asymptomatic nodule on the dorsolateral aspect of fingers and toes.
- It primarily affects infant but has been present since birth in one-third of cases. It affects the third to fifth digits, rarely second, and saves the thumb and hallux. It can also occur at extradigital sites such as arm, breast, thigh, and tongue.
- Histopathology of the tumor shows poorly circumscribed proliferation of spindle-shaped myofibroblast arranged in interlacing bundle in collagenous stroma in dermis. Pathognomonic feature is the presence of eosinophilic perinuclear intracytoplasmic inclusion body stains red with Masson trichrome stain and purple with phosphotungstic acid hematoxylin. These inclusions are actin filament arranged in whorled pattern and immunoreact with SMA and vimentin.
- Differential diagnosis is infantile myofibromatosis and congenital infantile fibrosarcoma.
- Clinically, it has a benign course but may cause functional impairment such that surgical intervention may be required. Recurrence rate is very high (up to 60%) after wide local excision.[9] Therefore, 5-FU and triamcinolone are also given after excision for better result.

Fibromatosis Colli

- It is self-limiting to present rapidly growing tumor in the first week of life. It includes less than one-third of sternocleidomastoid muscle as a neck lump with or without torticolis and rarely bilateral. The etiology is uncertain, birth trauma suggested as possible cause. It should be differentiated from other cause of torticolis in infants. Common clinical differentials include branchial cyst, thyroglossal cyst, cystic hemangioma, tubercular lymphadenitis, neuroblastoma, rhabdomyosarcoma, lymphoma, etc. Ultrasonography is the preferred imaging modality that confirms the diagnosis in most of the cases. Computed tomography and MRI are used where there is doubt on sonography.

- Fine-needle aspiration cytology (FNAC) reveals benign plump spindle fibroblast. Histologically, there is benign proliferation of fibroblasts.
- It usually resolves within first year of life, only physiotherapy is needed surgical tenotomy can be done in refractory cases. Botulinum toxin may be used if there are ongoing symptoms despite physiotherapy.

Calcifying Aponeurotic Fibroma

- Calcifying aponeurotic fibroma is a very rare benign slow growing fibrous tumor. This tumor is more common in boys than girls and peak incidence is seen in between 8 and 14 years of age.
- It is clinically characterized by asymptomatic solitary, firm, subcutaneous nodule on the hand, and feet and close to aponeurosis such as neck, forearm, popliteal fossa, lower back, and thigh. Uncommon sites involved are knee and elbow.[10]
- Histology shows tumor composed of sheets of spindled epithelioid fibroblast cell in collagenous stroma. There is characteristic island of central calcification with chondroid and osseous metaplasia surrounded by palisading fibroblast with occasional multinucleated giant cells. X-ray showing calcific stippling within the tumor. MRI should be done to determine the extent of calcification for treatment purpose.
- Treatment of the tumor is surgical excision but recurrence rate is 50% and is higher in patients younger than 3 years of age.

Fibrous Hamartoma of Infancy

- Fibrous hamartoma of infancy is a rare childhood benign tumor. About one-fourth cases are congenital and 91% cases occur during the first year of life with a male-female ratio of 3:1/2:1. This tumor appears as a painless, solitary, rapidly growing skin or flesh-colored ill-defined subcutaneous nodule or plaque over the axilla, shoulder, upper arm, upper trunk, groin, and external genitalia. These lesions often include hypertrichosis, alteration of color, eccrine gland hyperplasia, etc.[11] Multiple lesions occur rarely. These lesions have alteration of skin color, pinkish hue, hypertrichosis, eccrine gland hyperplasia, and fixity to underlying structure.
- Histology of the tumor has three features: (1) proliferation of spindle-shaped myofibroblast oriented in broad fascicle in a collagenous stroma; (2) nest of aggregates of small round plump, spindle-shaped immature mesenchymal cell in myxoid matrix; and (3) mature adipocytes.
- Treatment of choice is complete local excision.

Infantile Myofibromatosis

- It is the most common childhood fibromatosis occurs below 2 years of age with 50% of patients having disease since birth.[12] Solitary or multiple firm to rubbery skin colored to purple dermal or subcutaneous nodules located in the head, neck, trunk, and internal organs including gastrointestinal tract, kidney, heart, lung, muscle, and lytic bone metaphyseal lesions. Females have higher chance of visceral involvement.
- It is of three types: (1) solitary (prognostically good), (2) multicentric, (3) generalized (prognostically poor) due to visceral involvement and mortality rate is 75%.
- Histopathology demonstrates circumscribed nodule of plump spindle myofibroblast arranged in fascicles within a collagenous stroma and stag pattern of dilated branching blood vessels. Myofibroblasts are positively stained with actin and vimentin.
- Solitary lesion resolves spontaneously. Extensive surgical excision, chemotherapy, and radiotherapy are recommended for multicentric and generalized disease.

Hyaline Fibromatosis Syndrome

- It includes infantile juvenile hyaline fibromatosis and systemic hyalinosis. Both diseases are autosomal recessive genodermatosis due to mutation of capillary morphogenesis protein-2 gene. Few authorities believe both the entities belonged to same spectrum of disease. They only differ with regards of severity and organ involvement.
- Both entities affect both sexes equally and present from 4 months to 2 years of age. Initially, the lesion started as firm, pearly, subcutaneous papules over the lips, ear, nose, and chin (perinasal and perioral areas); firm nodule and tumor over the scalp, head, neck, and trunk; verrucous perianal nodule and reddish-blue to brown plaque on extensor surface of joint. Hyaline material deposited in internal organ and skin leading to gingival hypertrophy, periodontal disease, caries, recurrent infection, persistent diarrhea, and multiorgan failure. Joint contracture, osteolysis and muscle weakness may cause severe debilitation.
- Histology shows spindled myofibroblast in hyalinized and chondroid stroma. Osteoclast-like giant cells present in the perivascular area and the presence of calcosphorules are diagnostic.
- There is no appropriate treatment available to date. Physiotherapy can stop the progression of the disease.[13]

Infantile Fibromatosis

- Infantile fibromatosis is a highly aggressive, rapidly growing nodule on the trunk. This tumor regressing spontaneously.
- It has three histological patterns: (1) immature mesenchymal pattern, (2) collagenous pattern, and (3) desmoids pattern.
- This tumor is locally infiltrative but rarely metastasized.

Adult Onset Fibromatosis

- Dupuytren's contracture or palmar fibromatosis is a fibroproliferative disorder of the palmar fascia. It has commonly seen in Caucasians and rarely in dark-skinned people. It affects middle aged to older males than females.
- Triggering factors include North European ancestry, family history, old age, male sex, seizures, alcohol-induced liver disease, smoking, trauma, and diabetes mellitus.
- It is clinically characterized by fixed flexion joint deformity or contracture along the ulnar distribution of palmar fascia. It most commonly begin as a nodule over 4th and 5th metacarpal head gradually converts a cord-like structure, contracture, deformity, joint immobility, nerve injury, and development of reflex sympathetic dystrophy.
- Fasciotomy is the mainstay of therapy followed by splinting and range of movement exercise. Recently, injection collagenase (*Clostridium histolyticum*) can be given within each cord of contracture having a success rate of 45–56% and is also approved by the FDA.[14] The recurrence rate is very high with more deformity and less common with good surgical correction and postoperative rehabilitation.

Peyronie's Disease

- Peyronie's disease is fibrosis of tunica albuginea that surrounded corpus cavernosa and placed in between corpus spongiosum and corpora cavernosum. This condition is more common with increasing age.
- Risk factors are genetic predisposition, penile trauma, systemic vascular disease, smoking, and alcoholism. About 4% have Dupuytren's contracture. This disease causes pain, hardening, erectile dysfunction, indentation, and loss of penis girth. This condition is associated with painful sexual intercourse.
- Ultrasound provides a definitive diagnosis.
- Spontaneous regression over many years has been observed in one-third of cases. Collagenase injection, vitamin E supplementation, and pentoxifylline, may be given. Surgical procedures such as corporeal placation and Nesbit operation may be performed with good results.[15]

Dupuytren's Contracture (Palmar Fibromatosis)

- Flexion contracture of the affected digits, mostly in ulnar distribution, predominantly affecting the ring finger. Ledderhose disease is the plantar counterpart of Dupuytren's contracture. It includes plantar fascia that causes fibrosis over medial sole of the foot.
- Fibrogenic cytokines such as TGF-β and TGF-β_2 are thought to be involved in the pathogenesis, causing increased proliferation of fibroblast and differentiation toward myofibroblast.
- Proliferations of myofibroblasts are key histological findings, but when cord develops myofibroblast disappear.
- Common differentials are ganglion cyst, soft tissue sarcoma, callus, tenosynovitis, giant cell tumor of the tendon sheath, etc.
- Surgical therapy with fasciotomy, releasing the joint contracture is the mainstay of therapy. Injectable collagenase may be used to relieve the contracture.

Knuckle Pad

- It is benign asymptomatic circumscribed, smooth, firm, skin-colored hyperkeratotic fibrous growth over dorsal aspect of metacarpophalyngeal, and interphalangeal joint.
- It can be idiopathic, genetic or acquired (repetitive trauma). It may be associated with palmar plantar and penile fibromatosis. Rarely, it can be associated with Bart–Pumphrey syndrome, having knuckle pad leukonychia and hearing loss.[16]
- It should differentiate from false knuckle pad and synovitis.
- Treatment is not necessary in most of the cases. Intralesional triamcinolone and 5-FU may reduce the size of the lesion.

Nodular Fasciitis

- It is a benign self-limiting reactive fibroproliferative disorder that mainly affects young adult without any sex and racial predilection. It presents as rapidly growing tender subcutaneous nodules, usually occurring in the upper extremity, trunk, head, neck, and lower extremity in descending order of frequency.
- Common clinical differentials include proliferative fasciitis, proliferative myositis, fibromyxoid sarcoma, inflammatory myofibroblastic tumor, myxoma, myofibroma, myositis ossificans, desmoid fibromatosis, etc.
- Histopathology demonstrates poorly demarcated nodule of spindle fibroblast, ganglion cell-like fibroblast, and myofibroblast in an edematous, myxoid, and highly vascular stroma imparting a parental appearance. Common histological mimickers are pleomorphic adenoma and spindle cell sarcoma. Abundance of plasmacytoid cells and presence of cytokeratin and S100 on immunohistochemistry favors the diagnosis of pleomorphic adenoma. Frequent cellular pleomorphism, presence of atypical mitotic figure and coarse granular chromatin points the diagnosis of spindle cell sarcoma.
- On immunohistochemistry, nodular fasciitis is reactive with SMA, MSA, vimentin, and CD68.
- The condition is usually self-limiting. Surgical excision is the treatment of choice. Recurrence is rare.[17]

Elastofibroma Dorsi

- It is benign fibroproliferative tumor appearing in periscapular region of middle-aged woman. It may occur over the head, neck, abdominal, and thoracic cavity following a microtrauma.

- It presents as a poorly circumscribed, mobile, firm, and bilateral asymptomatic mass. Histopathology shows eosinophilic, partly fragmented elastic fiber combined with swollen collagen bundle, fibroblast, and mature fat cell.
- MRI is the best noninvasive technique to detect the tumor.
- Surgical excision is recommended when it causes functional disability, compression symptoms, or pain.

Pachydermodactyly

- It is a rare digital fibromatosis of adolescent boy. It presents as symmetrical, painless, well-circumscribed soft tissue swelling on the lateral side of proximal interphalangeal joint of 2nd to 4th finger sparing the thumb. Mechanical trauma may be the predisposing factor.

Acquired Digital Fibrokeratoma

- It presents, as a solitary skin, a pink colored, mildly keratotic, exophytic papulonodule with a collarette of elevated skin.
- It occurs after a trauma in middle-aged adult. It should be distinguished from verruca, periungual fibroma, cutaneous horn, and supernumerary digit.
- Histopathology shows orthokeratosis, variable epidermal hyperplasia along with collagen bundle, perpendicular to the epidermis, and decreased elastic fibers.[18]
- Treatment of choice is simple excision, electrosection, or radiofrequency ablation.

Dermatomyofibroma

- It presents as well-defined, skin-colored to red-brown plaque with smooth surface, commonly seen in young women, mostly in shoulder, axilla, upper arm, and neck.
- It should be differentiated with dermatofibroma, granuloma annulare, pseudolymphoma, fibrosed cyst, and DFSP.
- Histopathology shows well-defined myofibroblastic growth in the reticular dermis and upper subcutis.
- Simple excision cures the condition. Recurrence is rare when marginally or incompletely removed.[8]

Pleomorphic Fibroma

- It is slow growing asymptomatic dome-shaped or polypoid skin-colored papule seen mainly in adult women on extremities, nose, forehead, retroauricular region, etc.
- It should be differentiated from neurofibroma, fibrokeratoma, fibroepithelial polyp, etc.
- Histology shows well-defined dermal lesion with thick, haphazardly arranged collagen bundle with low cellularity. Cells are spindle-shaped fibroblast, myofibroblast, and irregular-shaped multinucleated cell.
- Complete surgical excision is the treatment of choice.

Collagenous Fibroma

- It is a solitary, asymptomatic, mobile, and slow-growing adult male fibrous tumor that occurs mainly in the arm, shoulder, neck, upper back, and abdominal wall. It usually occurs in the 5th to 6th decade of life.
- Pathologically, it is located in subcutis and is only superficial to the skeletal muscle.
- Surgery is the preferred treatment option with no confirmed recurrence of tumor.

Solitary Fibrous Tumor

- It is a rare soft tissue tumor of mesenchymal origin, typically arising in the plural cavity, but can involve the skin, presents as firm painless nodule in the head and neck region and extremities.
- Histologically, it is characterized by bland spindle cells with variable amount of fibrous element with a completely hyalinized collagenous stroma in the dermis. It is reactive with vimentin.
- Treatment is simple surgical excision. The recurrence is rare.

Desmoid Tumor

- They are highly aggressive but benign musculoaponeurotic fibromatosis characterized by deep seated infiltrative mass with high recurrence rate.
- It is of two types: (1) intra-abdominal and (2) extra-abdominal. The intra-abdominal variant is usually present after pregnancy on abdominal wall or surgical scar. Extra-abdominal variant located in neck, shoulder, chest wall, and pelvic girdle. About 10–15% cases of intra-abdominal variant is associated with familial adenomatous polyposis and Gardner syndrome.
- It rarely transforms into sarcoma and lack of ability to metastasis. Histopathology demonstrates poorly circumscribed proliferation of mature fibroblast in collagenous stroma.
- Surgical excision is the treatment of choice for extra-abdominal variety.[19] Recurrence rate is very high (25–65%).

Cutis Verticis Gyrata

- It is a symmetric cerebriform fold on the scalp. These folds are aligned from crown to vertex in an anteroposterior manner. It is usually seen in puberty. It is soft on palpation. The density of hair is less on the folds but not on the furrows.
- It has two variants: (1) essential (isolated) and (2) non-essential, and associated with neurological and ophthalmic disorder. Primary disease is commonly seen in male, but secondary disease can occur at any age with equal sex ratio.
- Secondary one is asymptomatic and associated with acromegaly, pseudomegaly, myxedema, insulin resistance,

Turner syndrome, Noonan syndrome, fragile X syndrome, Klinefelter syndrome, hereditary neuralgic amyotrophy, tuberous sclerosis, hyper IgE syndrome, Graves' disease, and paraneoplastic due to metastatic carcinoma **(Table 4)**.
- It requires no treatment but excision can be tried.[20]

Pachydermoperiostosis

- It is a rare syndrome presenting with pachydermia (thickening of skin), periostitis or thickening of long bones and clubbing due to altered proteoglycan synthesis. Other associated clinical features include coarse facial features, CVG, floppy eyelid, palmoplantar hyperhidrosis, periostitis and acro-osteolysis.
- It is a self-limiting condition, though arthralgia is debilitating but improves with oral tamoxifen therapy.

Dermatofibrosarcoma Protuberans

- Dermatofibrosarcoma protuberans is a rare locally aggressive mesenchymal neoplasm that usually occurs in the third and fourth decade of life. The normal clinical appearance is firm, indurated plaque often skin colored with exophytic nodules. Ulceration occurs rarely. It can present as nonprotuberant atrophic lesions resembling sclerosing basal cell carcinoma, morphea, anetoderma, etc. The most common site is trunk, followed by lower limbs and head and neck region.
- Differential diagnosis includes keloid, dermatofibroma, nodular melanoma, morphea, lichen sclerosus, fibrous histiocytoma, etc. **(Table 5)**.
- On histology, DFSP shows poorly circumscribed proliferation of slender or plump spindle cells with pleomorphism arranged in a storiform pattern.[21] Proliferation is commonly infiltrated by subcutaneous fat isolating adipocytes to form lucencies, called honeycomb or Swiss-cheese appearance. Less than 5% of DFSPs contain melanin-producing cells with schwannian differentiation, and termed as Bednar tumor.
- Immunohistochemical staining with CD34 helps distinguish between DFSP and dermatofibroma, which positively stains with factor XIIIa.
- This tumor has a tendency to local invasion and recurrence. In rare cases, recurrent tumor with fibrosarcomatous area has metastasized to lung.[22]
- Surgical removal with 1–3 cm clear margin is the gold standard of therapy. Mohs microsurgery is preferred surgical approach of many practitioners. Adjuvant radiotherapy may help to reduce local recurrence. Imatinib mesylate, which targets PDGF receptor, has been tested as a medical therapy in inoperable or recurrent DFSPs with partial response.[23] Recently, FDA approved imatinib for unresectable, recurrent and/or metastatic DFSP in adults at a dose of 800 mg daily.

Atypical Fibroxanthoma

- Atypical fibroxanthoma (AFX) is a relatively common, fast growing neoplasm of intermediate potential; occurs mainly over sun-exposed areas in elderly people with no sexual predilection.
- AFX presents as asymptomatic, fast-growing, solitary papulonodular lesion often resembling necrotic pyogenic granuloma, squamous cell carcinoma, and basal cell carcinoma.[24] Treatment is mostly surgical.

Giant Cell Fibroblastoma

- It is a rare neoplasm thought to be juvenile variant of DFSP that occurs most frequently in the trunk, thigh, or inguinal region. It usually appears during early childhood, with a strong male preponderance.[25]
- Clinical presentation is the same as DFSP. On histology, this tumor has dense connective tissue with lack of fibroblast and sometimes wreath-like giant cells. Treatment is same as DFSP.

Malignant Fibrous Histiocytoma

- Pleomorphic sarcoma and myxofibrosarcoma are two dermatologically significant MFH entities. They present as the most commonly occurring subcutaneous mass on limbs. About 10–15% of cases of lesion occur in the head and neck region. Typically present as a solid, rapidly growing skin colored subcutaneous nodule.
- Common histology pattern is the storiform spindle cell pattern. Immunohistochemistry with broad antibody panel excludes metastatic carcinoma.
- About 50% of patients with pleomorphic sarcoma have distant metastasis. Recurrence is high (30–50%). Complete surgical excision is the gold standard of therapy. Surgical excision with radiotherapy increases the control of recurrence.

TABLE 4: Diseases associated with cutis verticis gyrata.

Primary	*Secondary*
• Mental retardation • Seizure disorder • Cataract • Optic atrophy	• Myxedema • Acromegaly • Turner syndrome • Noonan syndrome • Fragile X syndrome • Klinefelter syndrome • Grave's disease • Tuberous sclerosis • Metastatic carcinoma

TABLE 5: Common clinical and histological differentials of DFSP.

Clinical	*Histological*
• Keloid • Hypertrophic scar • Large dermatofibroma • Dermatomyofibroma • Morphea	• Dermatofibroma • Dermatomyofibroma • Neurofibroma • Fibrosarcoma • Malignant peripheral nerve sheath tumor

Epithelioid Sarcoma

- It is an extremely rare aggressive sarcoma that occurs most frequently in the hand and fingers of young males. ES usually presents as firm dermal subcutaneous nodule with ulceration with occasional ulcer and sinus formation.
- Histology shows that majority of the lesions originating from fascia, tendon, and subcutaneous tissues are only 25% of those resulting from dermis. Histology shows epithelioid cell admixed with spindle cells and a collagenous and myxoid stroma.
- Radical excision is the treatment of choice. Conservative surgery with adjuvant radiotherapy can be done.[26] There is a very high recurrence (up to 50%).

KEY POINTS

- Hypertrophic scars are confined to the margin of the wound, while keloid extends beyond the margin of the wound.
- Hypertrophic scars have good response to therapy, whereas keloid has a bad response to therapy.
- Fibrous and fibrohistiocytic proliferation of the skin can be reactive or neoplastic.
- Immunohistochemical staining with CD34 and factor XIIIa (dermal dendrocytes), CD68 (for histiocytes), MSA (for myofibroblast), and vimentin (mesenchymal component) are helpful in assessing these conditions.
- Hyaline fibromatosis and systemic hyalinosis are autosomal recessive, presents with papulonodular lesion in the head and neck area. Systemic hyalinosis may include internal organs.
- Cutis verticis gyrata is characterized by fold in the scalp. Primary type has an onset at puberty and predominantly affects males.
- Dermatofibroma is a fibrohistiocytic tumor characterized by the proliferation of spindle-shaped fibroblasts and myofibroblasts in the storiform pattern. Surgical excision is the best choice for treatment.
- Acquired digital fibrokeratoma presents exophytic papules or nodules with collarette of elevated skin. Excision is the therapy of choice.
- Palmar fibromatosis (Dupuytren's contracture) is characterized by flexion contracture of digits, predominantly affecting the ring finger. Surgical therapy and collagenase injection are the mainstays of therapy.
- Skin tags are causing cosmetic concern. Electrocauterization, radiofrequency ablation, and surgical excision may be used for this purpose.
- Infantile digital fibromatosis predominantly affects 3rd or 4th digits. Wide local excision in the treatment of choice, but recurrence is normal.
- Fibromatosis colli is a self-healing tumor that develops in the infants in first week of life in the lower third of sternocleidomastoid.
- Peyronie's disease is caused by the fibrosis of tunica albuginea, causing painful erection. Collagenase injection, oral vitamin E, and pentoxifylline are the treatment options.
- Knuckle pads are benign and may be inherited or caused by repetitive trauma.
- Nodular fasciitis presents with rapidly growing subcutaneous swelling in the upper torso of the body. It is reactive with SMA, vimentin, and CD68.
- Desmoid tumor is benign musculoaponeurotic fibromatosis with high recurrence rate. Surgical excision is the main treatment option.
- DFSP is a locally aggressive mesenchymal tumor. It is CD38 positive. The gold standard therapy is a surgical excision with a broad clear margin. Imatinib mesylate can be used as medical treatment.

REFERENCES

1. Robles DT, Berg D. Abnormal wound healing: keliods. Clin Dermatol. 2007;25:26-32.
2. Sullivan T, Smith J, Kermode J, McIver E, Courtemanche DJ. Rating of burn scar. J Burn Care Rehabil. 1990;11:256-60.
3. van de Kar AL, Corion LU, Smeulders MJ, Draaijers LJ, van der Horst CM, van Zuijlen PP. Reliable and feasible evaluation of linear scars by the patient and Observer Scar Assessment Scale. Plast Reconstr Surg. 2005;116:514-22.
4. Oliveira GV, Chinkes D, Mitchel C, Oliveras G, Hawkins HK, Herndon DN. Objective assessment of burn scar vascularity, erythema, pliability, thickness, and planimetry. Dermatol Surg. 2005;31:48-58.
5. Darougheh A, Asilian A, Shariati F. Intralesional triamcinolone alone or in combination with 5-fluorouracil for the treatment of keloid and hypertrophic scars. Clin Exp Dermatol. 2009;34: 219-23.
6. De Ia Torre C, Ocampo C, Dovel IG, Osada A, Cruces MJ. Acrochordons are not a component of the Birt-Hogg-Dubé syndrome: dose this syndrome exists? Case reports and review of the literature. Am J Dermatopathol. 1999;21:369-74.
7. Yazici AC, Baz K, Ikizoglu G, Koca A, Kokturk A, Apa DD. Familial eruptive dermatofibroma in atopic dermatitis. J Eur Acad Dermatol Venereol. 2006;20(1):90-2.
8. Mentzel T, Kutzner H. Dermatomyofibroma: clinicopathologic and immunohistochemical analysis of 56 cases and reappraisal of a rare and distinct cutaneous neoplasm. Am J Dermatopathol. 2009;31: 44-9.
9. Dabney KW, MacEwen GD, Davis NE. Recurring digital fibrous tumor of childhood: case report with long-term follow-up and review of the literature. J Pediatr Orthop. 1986;6:612-7.
10. Fetsch JF, Miettinen M. Calcifying aponeurotic fibroma: a clinicopathologic study of 22 cases arising in uncommon sites. Hum Pathol. 1998;29(12):1504-10.
11. Yoon TY, Kim JW. Fibrous hamartoma of infancy manifesting as multiple nodules with hypertrichosis. J Dermatol. 2006;33:427-9.
12. Wiswell TE, Davis J, Cunningham BE, Solenberger R, Thomas PJ. Infantile myofibromatosis: the most common fibrous tumor of infancy. J Pediatr Surg. 1988;23:315-8.
13. Thomas JE, Moossavi M, Mehregan DR, McFalda WL, Mahon MJ. Juvenile hyaline fibromatosis: a case report and review of the literature. Int J Dermatol. 2004;43:785-9.

14. Desai SS, Hentz VR. The treatment of Dupuytren disease. J Hand Surg Am. 2011;36(5):936-42.
15. Ralph DJ, Minhas S. The management of Peyronie's disease. BJU Int. 2004;93:208-15.
16. Gönül M, Gül Ü, Hizli P, Hizli Ö. A family of Bart-Pumphrey syndrome. Indian J Dermatol Venereol Leprol. 2012;78(2):178-81.
17. Bernstein KE, Lattes R. Nodular (pseudosarcomatous) fasciitis, a nonrecurrent lesion: clinicopathologic study of 134 cases. Cancer. 1982;49:1668-78.
18. Kint A, Baran R, De Keyser H. Acquired (digital) fibrokeratoma. J Am Acad Dermatol. 1985;12:816-21.
19. Devata S, Chugh R. Desmoid tumors: a comprehensive review of the evolving biology, unpredictable behavior, and myriad of management options. Hematol Oncol Clin North Am. 2013;27(5):989-1005.
20. Zhao L, Fang F, Xu J, Wang Y, Qian G, Lin J, et al. Giant primary cutis verticis gyrata successfully treated with surgical excision and tissue expansion. Dermatol Surg. 2006;32:753-5.
21. Terrier-Lacombe MJ, Guillou L, Maire G, Terrier P, Vince DR, de Saint Aubain Somerhausen N, et al. Dermatofibrosarcoma protuberans, giant cell fibroblastoma, and hybrid lesions in children: clinicopathologic comparative analysis of 28 cases with molecular data—a study of the French Federation of Cancer Centers Sarcoma Group. Am J Surg Pathol. 2003;27: 27-39.
22. Mentzel T, Beham A, Katenkamp D, Dei Tos AP, Flatcher CD. Fibrosarcomatous ("high-grade") dermatofibrosarcoma protuberans: clinicopathologic and immunohistochemical study of a series of 41 cases with emphasis on prognostic significance. Am J Surg Pathol. 1998;22:576-87.
23. Rutkowski P, Van Glabbeke M, Rankin CJ, Ruka W, Rubin BP, Debiec-Rychter M, et al. Imatinib mesylate in advanced dermatofibrosarcoma protuberans: pooled analysis of two phase II clinical trials. J Clin Oncol. 2010;28:1772-9.
24. Fretzin DF, Helwig EB. Atypical fibroxanthoma of the skin: a clinicopathological study of 140 cases. Cancer. 1973;31: 1541-52.
25. Jha P, Moosavi C, Fanburg-Smith JC. Giant cell fibroblastoma: an update and addition of 86 new cases from the Armed Forces Institute of Pathology, in honor of Dr. Franz M. Enzinger. Ann Diagn Pathol. 2007;11:81-8.
26. Callister MD, Ballo MT, Pisters PW, Patel SR, Feig BW, Pollock RE, et al. Epithelioid sarcoma: results of conservative surgery and radiotherapy. Int J Radiat Oncol Biol Phys. 2001;51:384-91.

EXAMINATION QUESTIONS

1. Explain keloid.
2. Discuss pathogenesis and newer treatment options for keloid.
3. Write a short note on dermatofibroma.
4. What are the types and HPE of dermatofibroma?
5. Explain DFSP.

78 CHAPTER

Cutaneous Atrophy

Nishant Choudhary

INTRODUCTION

Cutaneous atrophy refers to clinical changes due to decrease in dermal connective tissue. Changes seen are:

- Loss of elasticity
- Thinning
- Telangiectasia and prominent veins
- Dry and soft skin
- Loss of hair follicles

Cutaneous atrophy can be broadly classified as:

- Generalized cutaneous atrophy
- Localized cutaneous atrophy

GENERALIZED CUTANEOUS ATROPHY

Aging and Wrinkles

Wrinkles are furrows or creases in the skin surface. Three morphological types of wrinkles are:

1. *Crinkles*:
   - Fine wrinkles in aging skin.
   - Disappear when skin is stretched.
   - Can be seen even in sun protected areas.
2. *Glyphic wrinkles*:
   - Wrinkles due to accentuation of normal skin markings.
   - Caused by sun light-induced elastotic degeneration.
3. *Linear furrows*: Grooves (straight or curved) seen on the face of elderly people. For example, crow's feet and frown lines.

Treatment of Wrinkles

- Topical retinoid
- Dermabrasion
- Botulinum toxin
- Fillers
- Chemical peels
- CO_2 laser
- Surgical corrections

Histology

- Thinning of epidermis
- Deposition of abnormal elastic tissue in papillary dermis
- Decrease in chondroitin sulfate

Glucocorticosteroids-induced Atrophy

- Both oral and topical steroids can lead to atrophy.
- It can present as thinning, striae or localized atrophy.[1]
- Steroids cause atrophy by decreasing activity of enzymes involved in collagen production, decreased fibroblast activity, and vasoconstriction involving superficial vascular network leading to ischemia.
- More the potency more the chances

Histology

- Thinning of epidermis
- Flattening of rete ridges
- Thinning of dermis

Treatment

- Topical retinoids
- Oral and topical vitamin C
- CO_2 laser

Idiopathic Mid-dermal Elastolysis

- Widespread fine wrinkling often seen in young females due to postinflammatory elastolysis in mid-dermis
- Ultraviolet (UV) radiation, insect bite, and borreliosis are suspected triggers
- No definite treatment

Atrophic Skin with Rheumatoid Disease

- Seen in patients of rheumatoid arthritis over 60 years of age
- Skin on dorsum of hands and forearm become loose, thin, inelastic, and transparent skin. Underlying veins become more clear

Striae (*Synonyms:* Stretch Marks, Striae Atrophicans, and Striae Distensae)

- Linear scars in areas of dermal damage due to stretching of skin **(Fig. 1)**.
- It is supposed to be due to damage to connective tissue structure commonly due to:
  - Sudden growth in adolescence
  - Drugs—steroids and indinavir[2]
  - Over abdomen and breasts in pregnancy
  - Cushing's disease

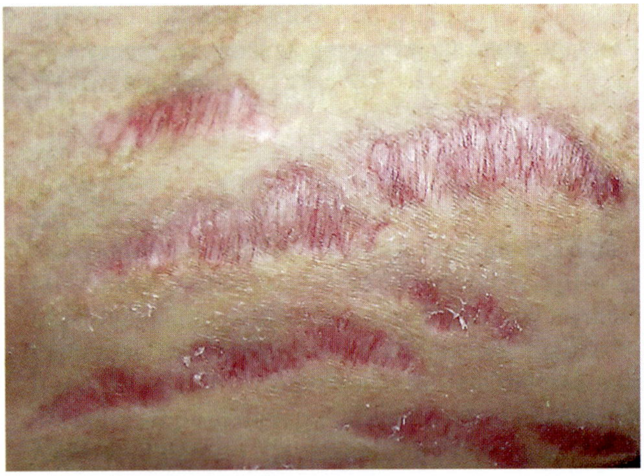

Fig. 1: Striae.

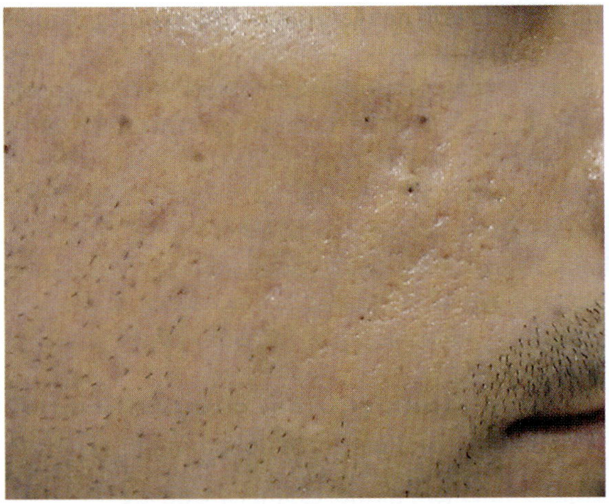

Fig. 2: Atrophic scars following acne.

Histopathology

- Thinning of epidermis
- Dermal collagen bundles arranged parallel to surface

Treatment

- Reassurance
- Topical retinoids
- Lasers—pulsed dye, neodymium-doped yttrium aluminum garnet (Nd:YAG), and CO_2 lasers

LOCALIZED CUTANEOUS ATROPHY

Atrophoderma

Follicular Atrophoderma

- Dimple-like defects at follicular orifice present since birth or early life. Commonly seen at dorsa of hands and feet.
- May occur as isolated defect or in association with genetic defects such as Conradi syndrome, Bazex syndrome, palmoplantar hyperhidrosis, and hyperkeratosis palmoplantaris.

Vermiculate Atrophoderma

- Honeycomb or reticulate atrophy around horny follicular plugs commonly seen over cheeks in symmetrical and crowded fashion.
- Also seen over upper lips, forehead, and ears.
- Associated with congenital heart defects, Down syndrome, and neurofibromatosis.
- It can occur as part of keratosis pilaris syndrome.

Atrophoderma of Pasini and Pierini

- Occur as single or multiple lesions of varying size (2 cm or larger) slightly depressed than surrounding normal skin.
- Most commonly seen over back. Also seen over chest and abdomen and sometimes proximal part of limbs.

Linear Atrophoderma of Moulin

Presents as unilateral and hyperpigmented atrophic bands following the line of Blaschko.[3]

Atrophic Scars

Usually seen following connective tissue destruction either due to trauma or inflammatory reaction **(Fig. 2)**.

Stellate and Pseudoscars

- Pseudoscars are white irregular atrophic scars usually seen in elderly people.
- Common on light-exposed area like forearm.
- Occur after mild trauma and associated with senile purpura.
- Brown pseudoscars are seen commonly over shin in diabetics.

Anetoderma (*Synonym:* Macular Atrophy)

Uncommon condition due to loss of dermal elastic tissue resulting in localized area of lax skin. Herniation or outpouching may be seen.

Primary Anetoderma

- Exact cause is unknown.
- Occurs in crops and may remain unchanged while new lesions may continue to develop. Etiology can be:
  - Familial
  - Antiphospholipid syndrome
  - Human immunodeficiency virus/acquired immunodeficiency syndrome (HIV/AIDS)
  - Complement activation

Secondary Anetoderma

Lesion appears at the site of primary lesion. It is seen following acne, syphilis, leprosy, discoid lupus erythematosus (DLE), dermatofibroma, xanthogranuloma, and tuberculosis.

Acrodermatitis Chronica Atrophicans (*Synonym:* Late Phase Lyme Borreliosis)

- It is a late-stage skin manifestation of chronic Borrelia infection (Lyme disease).
- There is persistent inflammation of the skin of extremities with atrophy.
- Lesions increase in centrifugal pattern for some time (months to years) then atrophy occurs leaving hairless, tissue paper like, or poikilodermatous skin.
- Caused by *Borrelia burgdorferi sensu lato*
- Amoxicillin, doxycycline, ceftriaxone, and cefotaxime have been useful in treatment.

Local Panatrophy

- It is atrophy of skin accompanied by loss (partial/total) of subcutaneous fat.
- It is sometimes associated with impaired growth or atrophy of underlying muscles and bone.

Panatrophy of Grower

- Well-defined areas of atrophy irregular in size, shape, and distribution without any sclerotic changes. Commonly involves back, buttock, thighs, and upper arm
- Females are affected more.

Sclerotic Panatrophy

Atrophy follows morphea, sometimes can occur in its absence. Usually affects limbs of a child, progress for some time then stops. Mostly lesions are solitary.

Parry–Romberg Syndrome (*Synonym:* Facial Hemiatrophy)

- It is progressive unilateral dysplasia of superficial facial tissue which can sometimes involve underlying muscle, bone, and cartilage. Rarely bilateral.
- It is associated with neurological signs such as trigeminal neuralgia, migraine, Horner's syndrome, syringomyelia, epilepsy, muscle spasms, heterochromia of iris, and ipsilateral cerebral atrophy. "En coup de sabre" morphea may be associated with some degree of facial hemiatrophy.
- Plastic surgery is useful in correcting the defects.

Poikiloderma

Poikiloderma refers to skin changes described by atrophy, telangiectasia, and macular or reticulate pigmentation.

Acquired Poikiloderma

Poikiloderma can occur following:

- Ionizing radiation
- Heat or cold exposure
- Dermatomyositis
- Systemic lupus erythematosus (SLE)
- Mycosis fungoides
- Rarely systemic sclerosis

Poikiloderma of Civatte commonly affects side of neck due to reaction because of photosensitizing chemicals in cosmetics. Females are affected more.

Congenital Poikiloderma

- *Rothmund–Thomson syndrome*: Autosomal recessive disorder. Patient has poikiloderma, congenital skeletal abnormality, juvenile cataract, short stature, premature aging, and increased risk of malignant disease.
- *Dyskeratosis congenita*: Bone marrow failure with reticulated skin hyperpigmentation, nail dystrophy, and oral leukoplakia
- *Mendes da costa syndrome*: Erythrokeratodermia variabilis
- *Hereditary sclerosing poikiloderma of Weary:*
  - Autosomal dominant
  - Generalized poikiloderma in childhood
  - Sclerosis of palms and soles
  - Linear hyperkeratotic bands on flexure
- *Hereditary acrokeratotic poikiloderma of Weary:*
  - Autosomal dominant
  - Generalized poikiloderma in childhood
  - Persistent keratotic papules on hands, feet knees, and elbow
- *Kindler syndrome*: Autosomal recessive disorder with congenital acral skin blistering, photosensitivity, progressive poikiloderma, and diffuse cutaneous atrophy.[4] Kindlin-1 expression is defective.
- *Diffuse and macular atrophic dermatosis*: Generalized poikiloderma since birth giving appearance of premature aging.
- *Degos–Touraine syndrome*: Incontinentia pigmenti with poikiloderma of sun-exposed areas.

KEY POINTS

- Cutaneous atrophy classified as: Generalized and local cutaneous atrophy.
- Wrinkles are a form of generalized cutaneous atrophy associated with the aging process and exacerbated by sun exposure. Treatment ranges from botolinium toxoid injections to surgical intervention. Preventive measures include photoprotection.
- Glucocorticoid-induced local atrophy is part of topical steroid damaged/dependent facies, with a spectrum encompassing erythema, monomorphic acne, steroid atrophy, steroid rosacea, telangiectasia, perioral dermatitis, striae, and severe addiction to the TC.
- Poikiloderma constitutes a triad of atrophy, telangiectasia, and macular or reticulate pigmentation.

REFERENCES

1. Coondoo A. Topical steroid misuse: The Indian Scenario. Indian J Dermatol. 2014;59:451-5.
2. Darvay A, Acland K, Lynn W, Russell-Jones R. Striae formation in two HIV-positive persons receiving protease inhibitors. J Am Acad Dermatol. 1999;41(3 Pt 1):467-9.
3. Moulin G, Hill MP, Guillaud V, Barrut D, Chevallier J, Thomas L. Acquired atrophic pigmented band-like lesions following Blaschko's lines. Ann Dermatol Venereol. 1992;119:729-36.
4. Kinder T. Congenital poikiloderma with traumatic bulla formation and progressive cutaneous atrophy. Br J Dermatol. 1954;66:104-11.

EXAMINATION QUESTION

1. What is poikiloderma? Name various syndromes associated with it.

79 CHAPTER Panniculitis

Abhijit Saha

INTRODUCTION

Panniculitis refers to inflammation of subcutaneous fat and infiltration with inflammatory cells. There are enumerable causes of panniculitis with overlapping clinical and histopathological features, therefore pose considerable amount of diagnostic challenge both to dermatologists and pathologists. Clinical similarities are stated as erythematous, painful, tender subcutaneous nodule and plaque which may ulcerate and drain in some cases. Histopathological differences are also subtle because there are only limited ways how subcutaneous tissue responds to different insults. Stage of the disease and specimen of adequate depth are further points of consideration.

Classification of panniculitis is exhaustive and beyond the scope of this chapter. Readers are requested to consult any standard dermatology textbook.

ERYTHEMA NODOSUM

- Erythema nodosum (EN) is the most common form of panniculitis in both adult and children.
- It commonly manifests at third decade of life.
- Women are usual victims.
- *Etiology:* Delayed type of hypersensitivity reaction to plethora of stimuli. Several intermediate steps have been described like reactive oxygen species production,[1] expression of adhesion molecules,[2] and release of pro-inflammatory cytokines.[3]
  - Idiopathic (one-third to half of the cases)
  - Streptococcal pharyngitis
  - Nonstreptococcal upper respiratory tract infection
  - *Gastroenteritis: Yersinia, Campylobacter, Salmonella*
  - Tuberculosis
  - *Mycoplasma* or *Chlamydia pneumonia*
  - Histoplasmosis, coccidiomycosis
  - Sarcoidosis
  - Ulcerative colitis, Crohn's disease
  - Malignancy
  - *Drugs:* Sulfonamide, oral contraceptive pills, penicillins, iodide, bromide, granulocyte-colony stimulating factor
- *Findings pointing toward systemic causes of EN:*
  - Preceding upper respiratory tract infection
  - Diarrhea
  - Synovitis
  - Abnormal chest X-ray
  - Elevated antistreptolysin O and/or anti-DNase B titer
  - Positive tuberculin test or interferon-gamma release assay
- *Clinical features:*
  - Symmetrically distributed bilateral erythematous, tender subcutaneous nodules distributed over anterior lower leg
  - Ulceration is not a feature of EN
  - Bruise-like discoloration occurs before subsidence
  - Lesions subside within 2–6 weeks without any sequela
  - Recurrence may occur in cases associated with sarcoidosis or Crohn's disease
  - Systemic symptoms which do not point toward systemic cause: Fever, malaise, arthritis, and arthralgia.[4]
  - *Variants:* Subacute nodular migratory panniculitis, chronic erythema nodosum, erythema nodosum migrans
  - One-third cases of EN may recur.
- *Histopathology:*
  - Septal panniculitis without vasculitis
  - Infiltrate initially is neutrophilic; gradually changes to mixed infiltrate with lymphocytes, giant cells, and granulation tissue
  - Miescher granuloma is characteristic but not pathognomonic;[4,5] composed of macrophages at septa or septolobular junction surrounding neutrophils or cleft-like septa. Older lesion of Miescher granuloma main contains epitheloid or multinucleated giant cells.
  - *Late stage:* Fibrosis of septa and spillage of infiltrate into lobules causing diagnostic difficulties.
- *Investigations:*
  - Complete blood count
  - C-reactive protein
  - Erythrocyte sedimentation rate
  - Liver function test
  - Throat swab culture
  - Antistreptolysine O titer

- Tuberculin skin test
- Chest X-ray
- Inflammatory bowel disease panel
- Stool culture for *Yersinia, Campylobacter, Salmonella*
- Skin biopsy in doubtful cases

- *Treatment:*
  - *Supportive:* Bed rest, nonsteroidal anti-inflammatory drug
  - Discontinuation of culprit drug
  - Treatment of underlying infection
  - Saturated solution of potassium iodide
  - Systemic steroid
  - Colchicine
  - Dapsone
  - Thalidomide
  - Infliximab

ERYTHEMA INDURATUM

- Historically, this entity erythema induratum was considered as tuberculid and the term nodular vasculitis referred to the cases which are of nontuberculous origin.
- Erythema induratum is actually type four hypersensitivity response to several organism (nocardia, hepatitis C) or drug (propylthiouracil) among which tuberculosis is considered as strongest association.[6,7]
- Young or middle-aged adult women are common victims.
- *Clinical features:*
  - Lesions are erythematous, tender nodules, and plaques with predilection for posterior lower leg.
  - Lesions have tendency to ulcerate and heal with postinflammatory hyperpigmentation or atrophic scarring.[6,8]
  - Course is relapsing.
- *Histopathology:*
  - Lobular or mixed panniculitis with vasculitis in more than 90% cases.
  - Initially, infiltrate is predominantly neutrophilic followed by mixture of neutrophils, lymphocytes, macrophages, and multinucleated giant cells.
  - Vasculitis may be lymphocytic or neutrophilic or granulomatous
  - Coagulative or caseous necrosis presents in half of the cases.
- *Treatment:*
  - Supportive
  - *Tuberculous origin:* Antituberculous drugs
  - *Nontuberculous origin:* Systemic steroid, potassium iodide, tetracycline, mycophenolate mofetil.

TRAUMATIC PANNICULITIS

- It is due to trauma of varied etiology which may be accidental or iatrogenic, accidental, or purposeful.
- It can occur due to:
  - Cold injury (cold panniculitis)
  - Excessive heat
  - Blunt trauma
  - Electrical injury
  - Injection of substances due to cosmetic (silicon) or other purpose (drugs such as vitamin K, morphine, pentazocine, vaccine, meperidine)
  - Megavolt radiation
- *Clinical features:*
  - *Cold panniculitis:*
    - More common in infant and children
    - Infant and children are more susceptible than adult because higher percentage of saturated fat and higher melting point of the same. Therefore slight drop in temperature leads to crystallization of fat.[9,10]
    - Lesions are erythematous, ill-defined, indurated plaque, or nodule
    - Lesions usually appear 24–72 hours after cold exposure
    - Cheek is the most common site to be involved
    - Lesions heal within few weeks with post-inflammatory hyperpigmentation but without any scarring.
    - *Variants:*
      - Popsicle panniculitis due to sucking ice lollies
      - Application of ice pack on cheek due to supraventricular tachycardia
      - Due to generalized cold exposure
      - Scrotal cold panniculitis due to swimming in cold water
      - Equestrian panniculitis on superior-lateral aspect of thigh due to cold exposure through tight fitting clothes of women horse rider.
  - In injection-induced panniculitis causative agent could be suspected from distribution of lesions.[11,12]
    - *Panniculitis due to vitamin K injection (Texier disease):* Sclerotic lesion with lilac border on thigh and buttock.
    - *Lesions are distributed in easily accessible areas with bizarre pattern:* Factitious panniculitis due to injection of noxious substances such as mineral oil, milk, feces by patients with psychological conflicts.
    - *Self-injection of insulin:* Thigh or lower abdomen
    - *Drug injected by nurse:* Deltoid or buttock.

These subcutaneous nodules undergo liquefaction, ulceration, and discharge of thick oily fluid or pus and heal with depressed scar.

  - Sclerosing lipogranuloma is a special entity due to injection of oil into the male genitalia by the patient himself. It may occur due to topical application of vitamin E or accidental firing of grease gun.
  - Lesions due to blunt trauma look-like ecchymoses and favor arm, hand, and shin area.

- Panniculitis due to excessive heat or electrical injury is associated with ulceration and eschar formation
- *Histopathology:* Histopathology varies depending upon cause:
  - In cold panniculitis, it is predominantly septal/lobular panniculitis composed of mainly lymphocytes and histiocytes. It is often associated with perivascular infiltrate of lymphocytes around the deep vascular plexus near the dermis and subcutis junction.
  - *Panniculitis due to injection:* Initially, there is acute inflammation with fat necrosis, hemorrhage, and neutrophilic infiltration. Gradually, infiltrate is replaced by lymphocytes, macrophages with associated fibrosis sets in. Polarized foreign material might be seen with polarized light.
  - Injection of oil (sclerosing lipogranuloma) produces formation of many pockets of fatty material throughout dermis and subcutis surrounded by intense fibrosis with macrophages in between. During routine histopathological processing extraction of fats give rise to "Swiss cheese appearance"
- *Treatment:*
  - Removal of triggers
  - Topical or intralesional steroid
  - Surgical debridement

INFECTION-INDUCED PANNICULITIS

- Variety of organisms, viz., bacteria, fungus, and virus has been implicated in the causation of panniculitis.
- Pathogens involved are:
  - *Bacteria: Staphylococcus aureus, Pseudomonas aeruginosa*
  - *Fungus: Candida* spp., *Aspergillus* spp., *Fusarium* spp., *Microsporum* spp., *Histoplasma capsulatum, Cryptococcus neoformans*
  - *Mycobacteria: M. tuberculosis, M. avium-intracellulare, M. ulcerans*
  - *Coxiella burnetii*
  - *Borrelia burgdorferi*
- *Pathogens reach subcutis through following routes:*
  - Direct inoculation
  - Extension from underlying infection
  - Hematogenous spread
  - Transfascial from enteric source
  - *Persorption of Candida:* Through intact epithelium from gut to subcutis.
- Immunosuppressed patients (diabetes mellitus, organ transplant, hematological malignancy, AIDS, connective tissue disorder) are usual victims[13,14] but it is not a rule. Immunocompetent individuals can get infection.[15]
- Clinically, patient presents with local swelling and erythema which ulcerate and drain. Lower extremity is the common site of involvement.
- *Differentials:* All the panniculitis with nodule formation and ulceration-like pancreatic panniculitis, alpha-1 antitrypsin deficiency panniculitis, and traumatic panniculitis.
- *Histopathology:* Though classically described as lobular panniculitis without vasculitis, many a times presents as mixed lobular-septal panniculitis. Additional features are neutrophilic infiltration, necrosis, hemorrhage, and vascular proliferation.
- Organism can be identified with special stain or tissue culture of biopsy specimen.
- *Treatment:* Antibiotics, surgical debridement.

LUPUS PANNICULITIS

- It is a form of cutaneous lupus erythematosus
- It can be an isolated finding or may progress to discoid lupus erythematosus (DLE) in at least one-third cases and systemic lupus erythematosus (SLE) in 10–15% cases.[16] Though DLE or SLE can occur simultaneously or before the occurrence lupus panniculitis. Patients who develop SLE usually have milder systemic manifestation.
- Commonly occur in women and adults.
- *Clinical features:*
  - Lesions are inflamed tender plaque or nodule which heal with lipoatrophy
  - Lesions have predilection for face, upper extremities and trunk
  - Rarity of involvement of distal extremities is important diagnostic clue
  - There might be no epidermal changes or might be associated with DLE-like changes such as scales, follicular plugging, telangiectasia, atrophy, and scarring
  - Overlying skin may be tethered to the underlying lesion causing surface depression
  - Lupus panniculitis has a chronic relapsing course and subsides with lipoatrophy.
- *Histopathology:*
  - Lobular panniculitis with predominantly lymphocytic infiltrate
  - Lymphoid follicle
  - Hyaline necrosis
  - Mucin deposition
  - Calcification
  - Epidermal or dermal features of DLE may or may not present (seen in 1/2 to 2/3rds cases).[17]
  - *Direct immunofluorescence:* Linear deposition of IgM and C_3 at dermoepidermal junction in 50% cases.
  - *Major histopathological differential:* Subcutaneous panniculitis-like T-cell lymphoma.[18,19] Sometimes, it is difficult to distinguish between two entities based on histopathology ground having features of both the entities.

- *Treatment:*
    - Systemic/topical steroid
    - Hydroxychloroquine
    - Immunosuppressive drugs
    - Photo protection

PANCREATIC PANNICULITIS

- Seen in pancreatic disorders such as acute pancreatitis, chronic pancreatitis, pancreatic carcinoma, traumatic pancreatitis, and pseudocyst pancreas.
- Pancreatic enzymes such as lipase, trypsin, amylase, phosphorylase are responsible to liquefactive fat necrosis and inflammation. Trypsin and amylase increase vessel wall permeability and allow lipase to hydrolyze neutral fat to free fatty acid glycerol which incites inflammation.
- Commonly seen in adults.
- Panniculitis precedes the onset of pancreatic disorders and act as sign of internal disease.
- Patients usually present with erythematous tender nodule mainly over distal lower extremities. They may become fluctuant and ulcerative followed by draining of oily greasy material.
- When panniculitis involves visceral fat-like omentum, preperitoneal fat and periarticular fat additional features would be fever, arthritis,[20] abdominal pain, ascites, and pleural effusion.[21]
- *Histopathology:*
    - Mainly lobular or mixed lobular/septal panniculitis
    - Liquefactive necrosis of fat cells leads to formation of "ghost cells" with loss of nucleus and thick shadowy wall
    - Saponification of fat by calcium results in dystrophic calcification; deposition of homogeneous or granular basophilic material[22]
- *Treatment:* Treatment of the underlying pancreatic disorders

ALPHA-1 ANTITRYPSIN DEFICIENCY PANNICULITIS

- Alpha-1 antitrypsin deficiency is a rare cause of panniculitis
- Usual manifestations of this entity are cirrhosis, hepatitis, pancreatitis, emphysema, urticaria, angioedema, vasculitis, membranoproliferative glomerulonephritis.
- Alpha-1 antitrypsin is a serine protease inhibitor which inactivates several proteolytic enzymes[23] such as collagenase, pancreatic and neutrophilic elastase, trypsin, and chymotrypsin. Alpha-1 antitrypsin is also involved inhibition of activation of lymphocyte and macrophages and activation of complement cascade acting upon different enzymes. Deficiency is most severe in patients who are homozygous for the Z allele of *SERPINA1* gene. In these patients aberrant alpha-1 antitrypsin accumulates in the liver and small amount which is released into the circulation form inactive polymer. This polymer is chemotactic for neutrophils. Unchecked activities of proteolytic enzymes and complement activation also contribute to the pathogenesis.[24]
- *Clinical features:*
    - Painful tender subcutaneous nodule or plaque with predilection for lower extremities (buttock, thigh) through any body part may be involved.
    - Lesions can ulcerate with discharge of oily substance and heal with atrophic scarring.
    - Course is chronic relapsing.
- *Histopathology:*
    - In early-stage, neutrophils are recruited between collagen bundle of reticular dermis then spread through septa to lobules. Then there is liquefactive necrosis of fat lobules and separation of the same from adjacent septa.
    - Adjacent skip areas of normal fat to the necrosed area are a characteristic finding.[25]
    - Lymphocytic vasculitis is noted in area of heavy neutrophilic infiltration or necrosis.
- *Treatment:*
    - Steroids, immunosuppressive drugs, colchicine, tetracyclines are not that much effective
    - Dapsone is one effective drug
    - Most effective therapy is alpha-1 antitrypsin intravenous infusion
    - Other effective therapies are plasma exchange, liver transplantation.

SUBCUTANEOUS PANNICULITIS-LIKE T-CELL LYMPHOMA

- Malignant proliferation of T-cells in the subcutaneous fat mimicking panniculitis
- Diagnosis is challenging and based upon constellation of clinical, histopathological, immunohistochemistry, and molecular finding.
- According to the World Health Organization (WHO)/European Organization for Research and Treatment of Cancer (EORTC) classification of cutaneous lymphoma this entity includes the cases only with alpha/beta T-cell receptor phenotype.
- Epstein–Barr virus may play role in pathogenesis.
- *Clinical features:*
    - Erythematous plaque or nodule distributed mainly over trunk and extremities which may ulcerate
    - There may be associated fever, malaise
    - Less frequently associated with hemophagocytic syndrome than gamma/delta phenotype
    - Development of hemophagocytic syndrome is associated with poor prognosis.

- *Histopathology:*
  - Lobular infiltration of lymphocytes
  - Cytological atypia
  - Riming of adipocytes with malignant cells
  - *Immunohistochemistry:* CD3+, CD8+, CD56–
  - *T-cell receptor gene rearrangement:* Monoclonal proliferation
- *Treatment:*
  - Systemic corticosteroid
  - Chemotherapy such as cyclophosphamide, vincristine, doxorubicin
  - Radiotherapy

CYTOPHAGIC HISTIOCYTIC PANNICULITIS

- The term "cytophagic histiocytic panniculitis" (CHP) denotes to clinically panniculitis presented as subcutaneous plaque or nodule which on histopathological examination shows benign appearing histiocytes engulfing different cells such as erythrocytes, lymphocytes.
- Many patients with CHP have lymphoma[26] mainly primary cutaneous gamma/delta T-cell lymphoma or Epstein–Barr virus associated NK/T-cell lymphoma nasal type. CHP and lymphoma are considered to fall into the same spectrum of disease.
- Commonly occurs in adults
- Lesions are distributed over trunk and extremities.
- Patients usually have chronic relapsing course.
- A subset of patients may have fatal hemophagocytic syndrome where macrophages phagocytose cells of hematopoietic system throughout liver, spleen, and lymph node. Clinically, these patients present with cytopenia, elevated liver enzymes, lymphadenopathy, hepatosplenomegaly, and coagulopathy.
- *Histopathology:* Fat lobules are infiltrated with benign histocytes engulfing erythrocytes, nuclear debris, platelets appearing as bean bag.[27]
- *Treatment:*
  - Systemic steroids
  - Chemotherapy
  - Peripheral stem cell transplantation

SUBCUTANEOUS FAT NECROSIS

Please go through the topic in chapter 32 written by same author.

KEY POINTS

- Panniculitis denotes inflammation of subcutaneous fat.
- Erythema nodosum is the most common form of panniculitis for both adults and children.
- Erythema nodosum can be differentiated clinically from erythema induratum by absence of ulceration and involvement of anterior lower leg.
- Infant and children are more susceptible than adult to cold panniculitis because higher percentage of saturated fat and higher melting point of the same.
- Distribution of lesions in case of injection-induced panniculitis point toward possible inciting agents.
- Infection-induced panniculitis usually occurs in immunosuppressed patients (diabetes mellitus, organ transplant, hematological malignancy, AIDS, connective tissue disorder).
- *Panniculitis with nodule formation and ulceration:* Pancreatic panniculitis, alpha-1 antitrypsin deficiency panniculitis, traumatic panniculitis, infection-induced panniculitis, and subcutaneous panniculitis-like T-cell lymphoma.
- Lupus panniculitis tends to involve face and upper extremities and may progress to discoid lupus erythematosus (DLE) in at least one-third cases and systemic lupus erythematosus (SLE) in 10–15% cases.
- When pancreatic panniculitis involves visceral fat such as omentum, preperitoneal fat, and periarticular fat additional features would be fever, arthritis, abdominal pain, ascites, and pleural effusion.
- Panniculitis is a rare manifestation of alpha-1 antitrypsin deficiency and presents with ulcerative subcutaneous nodule over thigh or buttock.
- Subcutaneous T-cell like lymphoma is a close histopathological differential with lupus panniculitis. Suspicion arises when there are cellular atypia and peripheral riming of adipocytes with malignant cells.

REFERENCES

1. Kunz M, Beutel S, Brocker E. Leucocyte activation in erythema nodosum. Clin Exp Dermatol. 1999;24:396-401.
2. Senturk T, Aydintug O, Kuzu I, Düzgün N, Tokgöz G, Gürler A, et al. Adhesion molecule expression in erythema nodosum-like lesions in Behçet's disease: a histopathological and immunohistochemical study. Rheumatol Int. 1998;18:51-7.
3. Nicol MP, Kampmann B, Lawrence P, Wood K, Pienaar S, Pienaar D, et al. Enhanced anti-mycobacterial immunity in children with erythema nodosum and a positive tuberculin skin test. J Invest Dermatol. 2007;127:2152-7.
4. White WL, Hitchcock MG. Diagnosis: erythema nodosum or not? Semin Cutan Med Surg. 1999;18:47-55.
5. Kim B, LeBoit PE. Histopathologic features of erythema nodosum-like lesions in Behçet's disease: a comparison with erythema nodosum focusing on the role of vasculitis. Am J Dermatopathol. 2000;22:379-90.
6. Mascaro JM Jr, Baselga E. Erythema induratum of Bazin. Dermatol Clin. 2008;26:439-45.
7. Baselga E, Margall N, Barnadas MA, Coll P, de Moragas JM. Detection of *Mycobacterium tuberculosis* DNA in lobular granulomatous panniculitis (erythema induratum—nodular vasculitis). Arch Dermatol. 1997;133:457-62.
8. Cho KH, Lee DY, Kim CW. Erythema induratum of Bazin. Int J Dermatol. 1996;35:802-8.
9. Quesada-Cortes A, Campos-Munoz L, Diaz-Diaz RM, Casado-Jimenez M. Cold panniculitis. Dermatol Clin. 2008; 26:485-9.

10. Rajkumar SV, Laude TA, Russo RM, Gururaj VJ. Popsicle panniculitis of the cheeks: a diagnostic entity caused by sucking on cold objects. Clin Pediatr (Phila). 1976;15:619-21.
11. Sanmartin O, Requena C, Requena L. Factitial panniculitis. Dermatol Clin. 2008; 26:519-27.
12. Pang BK, Munro V, Kossard S. Pseudoscleroderma secondary to phytomenadione (vitamin K1) injections: Texier's disease. Australas J Dermatol. 1996;37:44-7.
13. Oecker AH. Infection-induced panniculitis. J Cutan Pathol. 1989;16:183-93.
14. Maioriello RP, Merwin CF. North American blastomycosis presenting as an acute panniculitis and arthritis. Arch Dermatol. 1970;102:92-6.
15. Pao W, Duncan KO, Bolognia JL, Carroll CB, Hotez PJ, Bessen DE. Numerous eruptive lesions of panniculitis associated with group A *Streptococcus* bacteremia in an immunocompetent child. Clin Infect Dis. 1998;27:430-3.
16. Ng PP, Tan SH, Tan T. Lupus erythematosus panniculitis: a clinicopathologic study. Int J Dermatol. 2002;41:488-90.
17. Riccieri V, Sili Scavalli A, Spadaro A, Taccarim E, Zoppini A. Lupus erythematosus panniculitis: an immunohistochemical study. Clin Rheumatol. 1994;13:641-4.
18. Willemze R, Jansen PM, Cerroni L, Berti E, Santucci M, Assaf C, et al. Subcutaneous panniculitis-like T-cell lymphoma: definition, classification, and prognostic factors: an EORTC Cutaneous Lymphoma Group Study of 83 cases. Blood. 2008; 111:838-45.
19. Fraga J, Garcia-Diez A. Lupus erythematosus panniculitis. Dermatol Clin. 2008;26:453-63.
20. Dahl PR, Su WP, Cullimore KC, Dicken CH. Pancreatic panniculitis. J Am Acad Dermatol. 1995;33:413-17.
21. Heykarts B, Anseeuw M, Degreef H. Panniculitis caused by acinous pancreatic carcinoma. Dermatology. 1999;198:182-3.
22. Garcia-Romero D, Vanaclocha F. Pancreatic panniculitis. Dermatol Clin. 2008;26:465-70.
23. Valverde R, Rosales B, Ortiz-de Frutos FJ, Rodriguez-Peralto JL, Ortiz-Romero PL. Alpha-1-antitrypsin deficiency panniculitis. Dermatol Clin. 2008; 26:447-51.
24. Irvine C, Neild V, Stephens C, Black M. Alpha-1-antitrypsin deficiency panniculitis. JR Soc Med. 1990;83:743-4.
25. Su WP, Smith KC, Pittelkow MR, Winkelmann RK. Alpha-1 antitrypsin deficiency panniculitis: a histopathologic and immunopathologic study of four cases. Am J Dermatopathol. 1987;9:483-90.
26. Wick MR, Patterson JW. Cytophagic histiocytic panniculitis: a critical reappraisal. Arch Dermatol. 2000;136:922-4.
27. Gallardo F, Pujol RM. Subcutaneous panniculitic-like T-cell lymphoma and other primary cutaneous lymphomas with prominent subcutaneous tissue involvement. Dermatol Clin. 2008; 26:529-40.

EXAMINATION QUESTIONS

1. Give example of predominantly septal panniculitis without vasculitis.

Write short notes on the following:

2. Lupus panniculitis
3. Erythema induratum
4. SPTCL
5. Erythema nodosum
6. Panniculitis:
   (a) Classification
   (b) Clinical features and diagnosis
   (c) Management

80 CHAPTER

Lipodystrophies

Chinmay Kar

INTRODUCTION

Lipodystrophies are a heterogeneous group of disorders characterized by selective loss of adipose tissue (lipoatrophy). Lipodystrophy and lipoatrophy may use interchangeably. Some defines lipodystrophy as an abnormality of fat that is usually associated with atrophy and/or infrequently hypertrophy of adipose tissue. The lipodystrophy may be congenital or acquired, generalized or partial or localized, autosomal recessive or dominant. Patients are usually complicated with various metabolic abnormalities such as insulin-resistant diabetes mellitus, hypertriglyceridemia, acanthosis nigricans, hepatic steatosis, etc.

EPIDEMIOLOGY

The genetic lipodystrophies are rare syndromes. Due to recent advancement of genetic studies and other sophisticated investigations, the diagnosis is becoming earlier age group and more in number than previous era. The estimated prevalence of genetic lipodystrophies may be less than 1 in one million population.[1] Congenital generalized lipodystrophy has been reported in approximately 500 patients and most common familial partial lipodystrophy of Dunnigan variety was also found in 500 patients.

Incidence of acquired variant is much more than congenital due to antiretroviral therapy containing mainly Protease inhibitors of HIV patients. But acquired generalized variant has been reported only about 100 patients[2] and acquired partial lipodystrophy was found in 250–300 patients.[3]

CLASSIFICATION

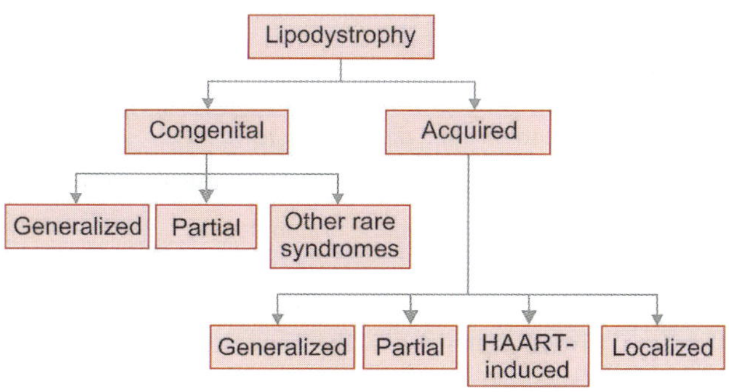

Congenital generalized lipodystrophy (CGL)		
Types	*Mode of inheritance*	*Gene involved*
CGL type 1	Autosomal recessive	*AGPAT2*
CGL type 2	Autosomal recessive	*BSCL2*
CGL type 3	Autosomal recessive	*CAV1*
CGL type 4	Autosomal recessive	*PTRF*

Familial partial lipodystrophy (FPLD)		
Types	*Mode of inheritance*	*Gene involved*
FPLD type 1	Not known	Unknown
FPLD type 2	Autosomal dominant	Lamin A/C *(LMNA)*.
FPLD type 3	Autosomal dominant	*PPARG*
FPLD type 4	Autosomal dominant	*PLIN1*
FPLD type 5	Autosomal recessive	*CIDEC*
FPLD type 6	Autosomal recessive	*LIPE*

Extremely rare genetic syndromes	
Types	*Gene involved*
Mandibuloacral dysplasia (MAD) type A	*LMNA*
MAD type B	*ZMPSTE24*
JMP/CANDLE	*PSMB8*
SHORT syndrome	*PIK3R1*
MDP syndrome	*POLD1*
Neonatal progeroid syndrome, type A	*FBN1*
Neonatal progeroid syndrome, type B	*CAV1*
Atypical progeroid syndrome	*LMNA*
Hutchinson-Gilford progeria	*LMNA*

Etiology of acquired generalized variant can be autoimmune, panniculitis associated or idiopathic. Whereas partial variant may be autoimmune, membranoproliferative glomerulonephritis associated or idiopathic. Localized form may be due to drug induced, panniculitis associated, pressure induced, idiopathic or centrifugal type. Highly active antiretroviral therapy (HAART)-induced lipodystrophy is mostly due to protease inhibitors. But nucleoside reverse transcriptase inhibitor (NRTI) especially stavudine and zidovudine-induced lipodystrophy may also be seen.

Clinical Features

Congenital Lipodystrophies[4]

Types	*Subtypes*	*Main clinical features*
Congenital generalized lipodystrophy (Berardinelli–Seip syndrome) characterized by near total absence of the body fat starting at birth or shortly after, with generalized muscularity and metabolic abnormalities such as diabetes mellitus, hypertriglyceridemia, acanthosis nigricans, hepatomegaly	CGL1	Loss of metabolically active fat with sparing of mechanically functioning fat. There are lytic bone lesions.
	CGL2	• Both metabolically active and mechanical adipose tissues are lost • Cardiomyopathy, cirrhosis, mental retardation
	CGL3	Absent metabolically active adipose tissue and preserved mechanical and bone marrow adipose tissue. Short stature, vitamin D resistance, hypocalcemia, hypomagnesemia
	CGL4	Absent metabolically active adipose tissue. Preserved mechanical and bone marrow adipose tissue. Myopathy, skeletal abnormalities, pyloric stenosis and gastrointestinal motility problems, cardiac arrhythmias
Familial partial lipodystrophy is characterized by loss of fat from the limbs, metabolic abnormalities	FPLD type 1 (Kobberling syndrome)	Loss of subcutaneous fat from the limbs, although they usually have truncal obesity. Palpable "ledge" formation between the normal and lipodystrophic areas.
	FPLD type 2 (Dunnigan syndrome)	Increased muscularity and loss of fat in the limbs, excess fat accumulation in the face and neck
	FPLD type 3	Loss of subcutaneous fat from the limbs, specifically distally
	FPLD type 4	Loss of subcutaneous fat from the limbs. Histologically, there is small adipocytes, macrophage infiltration and fibrosis of adipose tissue
	FPLD type 5	Loss of subcutaneous fat from the limbs, small, multilocular lipid droplets in adipocytes
	FPLD type 6	Increased visceral fat, dyslipidemia, hepatosteatosis, insulin resistance, and diabetes, some may present with muscular dystrophy and elevated serum creatine phosphokinase
Rare genetic lipodystrophy syndromes	MAD type A	Mandibular and clavicular hypoplasia, acro-osteolysis. Partial lipodystrophy affecting the extremities and trunk
	MAD type B	• Mandibular and clavicular hypoplasia, acro-osteolysis • More generalized loss of fat, premature renal failure, progeroid features
	JMP/CANDLE	Joint contractures, muscle atrophy, microcytic anemia and panniculitis-induced lipodystrophy (JMP) including chronic atypical neutrophilic dermatosis with lipodystrophy and elevated temperature (CANDLE)
	SHORT syndrome	Short stature, hyperextensibility of joints or hernia, ocular depression, Rieger anomaly, teething delay (SHORT)
	MDP syndrome	Mandibular hypoplasia, deafness, and progeroid features
	Neonatal progeroid syndrome, type A	• Generalized loss of body fat and muscle mass, and progeroid appearance at birth • Marfanoid habitus
	Neonatal progeroid syndrome, type B	Generalized loss of body fat and muscle mass, and progeroid appearance at birth
	Atypical progeroid syndrome	Partial or generalized loss of subcutaneous fat, progeroid features
	Hutchinson-Gilford progeria	Generalized loss of subcutaneous fat, progeroid features

Acquired Lipodystrophies

Acquired generalized lipodystrophy (Lawrence syndrome) is suspected when there is near total absence of the body fat commonly develops during childhood or adolescence, and metabolic abnormalities such as hepatic steatosis, fibrosis, diabetes and hypertriglyceridemia	Autoimmune	AGL follows an autoimmune disease like JDM
	Panniculitis-associated	Tender subcutaneous nodules that herald the onset of AGL
	Idiopathic	No history of autoimmune disease or panniculitis

Contd...

Contd...

Acquired partial lipodystrophy (Barraquer–Simons syndrome) starts with loss of subcutaneous fat from face, neck and upper extremities, and progresses to the trunk	Autoimmune	Coinciding autoimmune disorders; dermatomyositis/polymyositis and SLE are most commonly associated disorders
Lower limbs are typically spared, some patients have excess fat over the gluteal region, thighs and calves. Usually, there is no metabolic complication. Female: Male is 4:1	Membranoproliferative glomerulonephritis-associated	Low serum complement 3, glomerulonephritis, hematuria, urinary casts, proteinuria, nephritic syndrome, renal failure
	Idiopathic	No history of autoimmune disease or MPGN
Highly active antiretroviral therapy-induced lipodystrophy in HIV-infected patients	Protease inhibitor (PI) induced	It starts from face, trunk and extremities. But some patients develop buffalo hump, double chin and intra-abdominal fat gain. Diabetes, hyperlipidemia and coronary heart disease may occur. Usually starts after 2–4 years of HAART initiation
	NRTI-induced	Same as PI induced but incidence is low
Localized lipodystrophy occurs in locally affected areas[5]	Drug-induced	Insulin therapy, steroids and antibiotics injections cause local production of TNF-α that differentiates adipocytes. Other probable mechanisms include presence of lipases, repeated trauma and/or autoimmune processes. More common in patients with high titers of anti-insulin antibodies. May have deposition of IgA and C3 locally. Sometimes responds to local corticosteroids
	Pressure-induced	Fat atrophy localized to the area exposed to repeated pressure. Trauma and decreased perfusion caused by repeated pressure to the same area over a long period of time. This tends to improve when the pressure is avoided
	Panniculitis-associated	Initial development of panniculitis followed by localized fat loss when these lesions heal. It is usually associated with ANA, dsDNA or autoimmune disease like SLE
	Centrifugal (lipodystrophia centrifugalis abdominalis infantalis)	More common in Asians. Fat loss spreads in a centrifugal pattern from abdomen and groin area, and is associated with peripheral panniculitis. It begins in infancy, stops spreading between the ages of 3 and 8 and then in most cases, resolves by itself. Etiology is unknown
	Idiopathic	Localized form without any detectable cause

Investigations

Investigations should be carried out for suspected cases. These are:

- *Blood sugar level* with glycosylated hemoglobin—high.
- *Free insulin level*—increased due to insulin resistance.
- *Lipid profile*—hypertriglyceridemia with low HDL cholesterol (resistant to treatment).
- *Liver function test*—increased bilirubin and transaminase level.
- *Serum leptin level*—low but not diagnostic. This measurement is helpful in replacement treatment of lipodystrophy by human recombinant leptin (metreleptin). In generalized lipodystrophy, serum leptin and adiponectin levels are very low.
- *Serum C3 estimation*—low in acquired partial lipodystrophy
- *Imaging study*—digital X-ray, dual energy X-ray absorptiometry (DEXA) scan (for lytic bone lesions and osteoporosis), whole-body magnetic resonance imaging (MRI), and computed tomography (CT) scan.[6]
- Genetic testing

Differential Diagnosis

Generalized lipodystrophy	*Partial lipodystrophy*
• Uncontrolled diabetes mellitus • HIV-associated wasting • Anorexia nervosa, cachexia and starvation • Chronic infections • Adrenocortical insufficiency • Thyrotoxicosis	• Cushing's syndrome • Truncal obesity • Multiple symmetric lipomatosis • Progeroid syndromes • Acromegaly/gigantism

Approach to Diagnosis

Lipodystrophy is difficult to diagnose because of its rare incidence and lack of experience. Diagnosis can be done by history, general appearance, physical examinations, and appropriate investigations.

- *History:*
    - Congenital or acquired (though specific diagnosis of congenital form is usually made during childhood or even adulthood when they start developing metabolic abnormalities).
    - Parental consanguinity and the mode of inheritance for congenital lipodystrophy[7]

- Disproportionate hyperphagia (inability to stop eating, waking up to eat, fighting for food)
- *Body distribution of adipose tissue:* Generalized or partial loss of fatty tissue
- *Physical examination:*
  - Muscle hypertrophy and prominent veins (phlebomegaly)
  - Cushingoid appearance or progeroid appearance or pseudo-acromegaloid appearance
  - Acanthosis nigricans (associated with insulin resistance)
  - Renal dysfunction, proteinuria
  - Reproductive dysfunction (reduced fertility, hyperandrogenism, oligomenorrhea, hirsutism and/or polycystic ovaries)
  - Occasionally musculoskeletal abnormalities, cardiomyopathy, low intelligence.
- *Metabolic abnormalities:*[8]
  - Relatively early onset of insulin-resistant diabetes which is severe in some patients with requirement for high doses of insulin, e.g., requiring ≥200 U/day, ≥2 U/kg/day, or early development of complications.
  - Dyslipidemia which is characterized by elevated triglycerides and low HDL cholesterol. Hypertriglyceridemia can be very severe (≥500 mg/dL) and is unresponsive to treatment with associated history of acute pancreatitis.
  - Hepatomegaly and/or elevated transaminases in the absence of a known cause of liver disease (e.g., viral hepatitis). Hepatic steatosis (radiologic evidence), hepatomegaly, non-alcoholic steatohepatitis (NASH), cirrhosis.

Treatment

Treatment of lipodystrophies is challenging. Main target of treatment is to treat the complications along with cosmetic surgery. The loss of adipose tissue can be reverted back by cosmetic surgeries such as autologous adipose tissue transplant or implantation of hyaluronic acid, silicone, polyacrylamide gels, calcium hydroxylapatite as dermal fillers or muscle grafting. Excess fat can be removed by surgical excision or liposuction.

Common complications such as diabetes mellitus, hypertriglyceridemia, hepatic steatosis, lytic bone lesions, cardiomyopathy can be treated accordingly. Subcutaneous metreleptin replacement therapy improves blood sugar, lipids in markedly hypoleptinemic patients with generalized lipodystrophies. Metreleptin may be useful in FPL patients with severe metabolic derangements or low leptin level.[9] Withdrawal of offending drug(s) is the treatment of drug-induced cases.

KEY POINTS

- Lipodystrophies are a heterogeneous group of disorders characterized by selective loss of adipose tissue.
- Two main types—Genetic and acquired.
- According to involvement, genetic lipodystrophies can be generalized or partial. Generalized variety is always autosomal recessive. Partial type may be autosomal dominant or recessive.
- Acquired lipodystrophies may be generalized, partial, localized or HAART induced. They can be autoimmune, panniculitis-associated, drug-induced or idiopathic.
- Generalized and partial variants are always associated with metabolic abnormalities, mostly diabetes mellitus, hyperlipidemia, hepatic steatosis, and their complications.
- Abnormal lipoatrophy with or without abnormal deposition of fat associated with diabetes mellitus, lipid abnormality, acanthosis nigricans, hepatic problems can be a clue for investigating the case of lipodystrophy.
- Cosmetic surgery with treatment of metabolic abnormalities is the treatment of choice.
- Subcutaneous metreleptin replacement is also used in metabolic abnormalities.

REFERENCES

1. Kang S, Amagai M, Bruckner AL, Enk AH, Margolis DJ, McMichael AJ, et al. Fitzpatrick's Dermatology, 9th edition. New York: McGraw-Hill education; 2019. pp. 1295-307.
2. Misra A, Garg A. Clinical features and metabolic derangements in acquired generalized lipodystrophy: case reports and review of the literature. Medicine. 2003;82:129-46.
3. Misra A, Peethambaram A, Garg A. Clinical features and metabolic and autoimmune derangements in acquired partial lipodystrophy: report of 35 cases and review of literature. Medicine. 2004;83:18-34.
4. Hussaina I, Garg A. Lipodystrophy syndromes. Dermatol Clin. 2008;26(4):569-78.
5. Garg A. Lipodystrophies. Am J Med. 2000;108(2):143-52.
6. Handelsman Y, Oral EA, Bloomgarden ZT, Brown RJ, Chan JL, Daniel Einhorn D, et al. The clinical approach to the detection of lipodystrophy: an AACE consensus statement. Endocr Pract. 2013;19:107-16.
7. Garg A. Clinical review: Lipodystrophies: genetic and acquired body fat disorders. J Clin Endocrinol Metab. 2011;96:3313-25.
8. Akinci B, Sahinoz M, Oral E. Lipodystrophy syndromes: presentation and treatment. In: Feingold KR, Anawalt B, Boyce A (Eds). South Dartmouth (MA): MDText.com, Inc.; 2000.
9. Diker-Cohen T, Cochran E, Gorden P, Brown RJ. Partial and generalised lipodystrophy: comparison of baseline characteristics and response to metreleptin. J Clin Endocrinol Metab. 2015;100:1802-10.

EXAMINATION QUESTION

1. Write short notes on lipodystrophies/lipodystrophies syndromes.

81 CHAPTER Disorders of Oral Cavity and Mucosa

Ankur Talwar, Kshama Talwar

INTRODUCTION

Dermatologic diseases are characterized by numerous primary diseases that affect the skin but may also involve the mucosa of the body, including the oral mucosa. Currently, dermatologic diseases constitute an area of great scientific and odontological interest, considering that oral lesions can precede cutaneous lesions for long periods of time, being, sometimes, the only signs of the disease.

CLASSIFICATION

The various disorders of the oral cavity can be classified according to the anatomical area involved **(Table 1)**.

DISORDERS OF LIPS

Fordyce Spots

- Variant of sebaceous glands (the glands that normally produce sebum and are usually found within hair follicles).
- Present as slightly elevated yellowish or white papules on the vermilion border of the lips **(Fig. 1)**.

TABLE 1: Classification of disorders of oral cavity.

Lips	• Exfoliative cheilitis • Actinic cheilitis • Angular cheilitis • Granulomatous cheilitis • Glandular cheilitis • Plasma cell cheilitis • Eczematous cheilitis • Fordyce spots
Tongue	• Oral hairy leukoplakia • Black hairy tongue • Geographic tongue • Fissured tongue/scrotal tongue • Median rhomboid glossitis • Strawberry tongue • Glossitis
Buccal mucosa	• Oral submucous fibrosis • Leukoplakia • Candidiasis/moniliasis • Recurrent aphthous stomatitis (RAS) • Oral lichen planus (OLP) • Oral pemphigus/pemphigoid
Gums/ periodontium	• Chronic gingivitis • Desquamative gingivitis • Gingival fibromatosis

- They may also be seen on the glans or shaft of the penis, or the vulva of the female, the inside of the cheeks.
- They are easier to see when the skin is stretched.
- Can occur as a solitary lesion or more frequently in crops.
- These are generally harmless and do not require any treatment.
- In case of cosmetic concern, electrosurgery or CO_2 laser have been used successfully to remove the spots.

Exfoliative Cheilitis

- Also known as factitial cheilitis.
- Presents as continuous peeling of the vermilion part of the lips.
- It may affect just one lip, usually the lower. When both lips are involved, the lower lip is usually more affected than the upper.
- There may be fissuring, peeling, crusting, or hemorrhagic crusting over the lips **(Fig. 2)**.
- The peeling appears to be cyclical and proceeds at different rates in different sites.
- May be representative of obsessive-compulsive tendency to pick or chap the lips.
- Diagnosis of exclusion and there is no specific diagnostic test for it.
- Typically resistant to treatment. Treatment of an associated mood or anxiety disorder must. Factitial cheilitis should be considered as an underlying cause of exfoliative cheilitis, especially in the presence of concomitant psychiatric disorders.

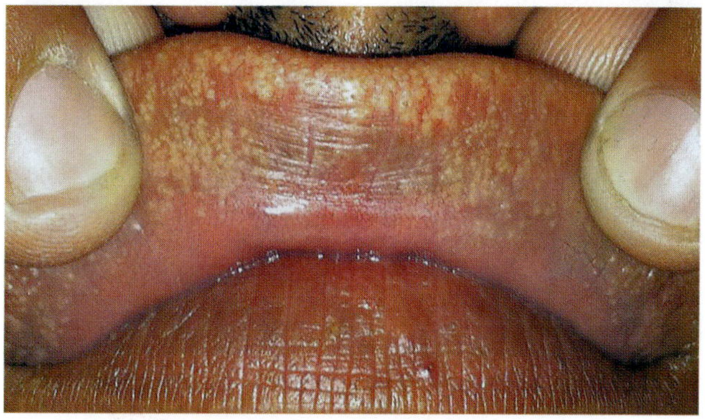

Fig. 1: Fordyce's spots.

- Successful use of keratolytic lip balms, sunscreen, topical steroids, systemic steroids, antibiotics, calcipotriol, and cryotherapy have been described.

Actinic Cheilitis

- Due to chronic sun exposure.
- Adults with fair skin who live in tropical areas, especially outdoor workers.
- Ninety percent of cases involve the lower lip. Three times more common in males than in females.
- Presents as swelling, redness, scaly plaques, fissuring, focal ulceration and crusting, and loss of the demarcation between the vermilion border of lower lip and surrounding skin (earliest change to occur, rest follows) **(Fig. 3)**.
- *Premalignant condition*: It has a predisposition towards progression to squamous cell carcinoma hence a biopsy is warranted in long standing cases.
- *Treatment*: Limit sun exposure; apply sunscreen-containing lip balm frequently.

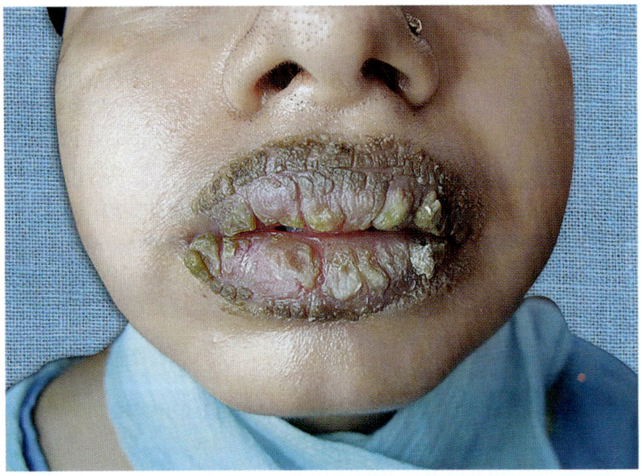

Fig. 2: Exfoliative cheilitis.

- Topical therapies include topical retinoids, 5-fluorouracil cream, imiquimod cream, photodynamic therapy, cryo, and laser ablation.

Angular Cheilitis

- Affects the corners of the mouth or oral commissures.
- Also called angular stomatitis, cheilosis, and perleche (perlèche).
- Painful cracks/fissures at the corners of the mouth.
- May be accompanied by redness, bleeding, and crusting.
- May progress to impetigo or candidal skin infection.
- Treatment may include lip balm or thick emollient ointment, topical antibiotic, topical antifungal cream, and topical steroid ointment.

Granulomatous Cheilitis

- Also known as Miescher cheilitis.
- May represent a spectrum of Crohn's disease, sarcoidosis, and orofacial granulomatosis.
- Recurrent chronic (long lasting) swelling and enlargement of one or both lips.
- The enlarged lip appears cracked and fissured, with reddish brown discoloration and scaling **(Fig. 4)**.
- The fissured lip becomes painful and eventually acquires the consistency of firm rubber.
- Enlargement of regional lymph nodes in 50% of cases.
- Fissured or plicated tongue in 20–40% of cases.
- *Miescher–Melkersson–Rosenthal syndrome* is the term used when the cheilitis occurs as part of a symptomatic triad including facial palsy and plicated (fissured) tongue.
- Histologically characterized by granulomatous infiltrate consisting of epithelioid cells and multinucleate giant cells, without caseous necrosis, associated with some degree of lymphedema and fibrosis.[1]
- *Treatment*: Intralesional corticosteroids, high-dose clofazimine, and doxycycline/tetracycline.

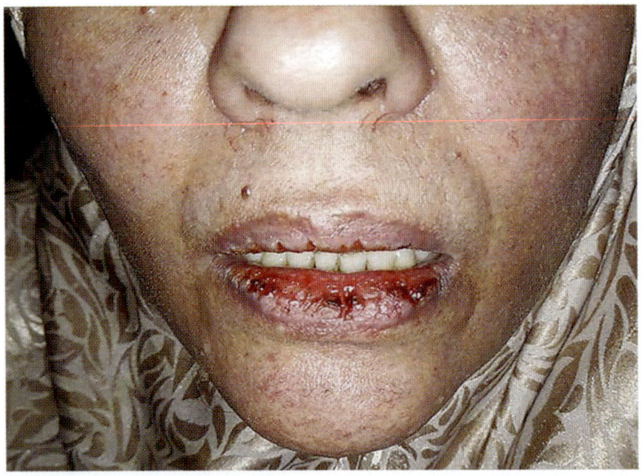

Fig. 3: Actinic cheilitis.

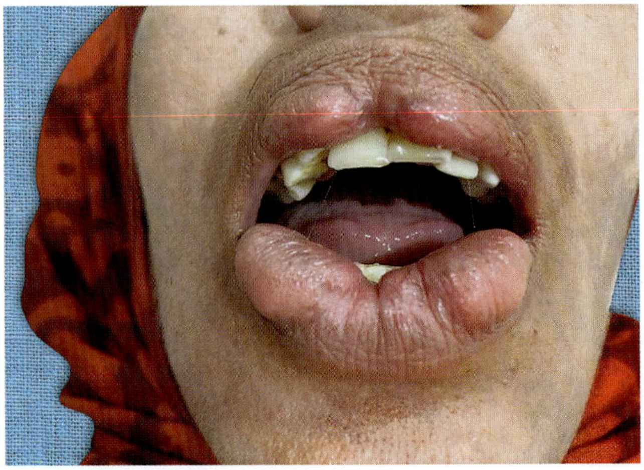

Fig. 4: Granulomatous cheilitis.

DISORDERS OF TONGUE

Oral Hairy Leukoplakia

- Corrugated white lesion seen on ventral and lateral surfaces of tongue
- Commonly associated with human immunodeficiency virus (HIV)
- Epstein-Barr virus (EBV)—causative agent
- Lesions are shaggy and frayed **(Fig. 5)**
- Plaque like and often bilateral
- Microscopy—reveals viral nuclear inclusions with a rim of chromatin
- No treatment is required usually unless patient is bothered by unsightly appearance.
- Resolves with zidovudine, acyclovir, and ganciclovir
- Topically application of podophyllin resin and tretinoin
- Oral hairy leukoplakia (OHL) is highly predictive of acquired immunodeficiency syndrome (AIDS) development.[2]

Black Hairy Tongue/Lingua Villosa/ Lingua Nigra

- Seen in smokers and persons with poor oral hygiene
- Increased coffee and tea drinking—predisposing factors
- Use of broad-spectrum antibiotics, radiation therapy may also be causative
- Defective desquamation of filiform papillae
- Accumulation of excess keratin on filiform papillae of the dorsal part of tongue
- Dark color results from trapping of debris and bacteria
- No treatment is required
- Gentle tongue scrapping and removal of etiology
- Surgical removal of papillae—laser and electrodesiccation

Geographic Tongue

- Benign migratory glossitis—psoriasiform inflammation in dorsal part of tongue.
- Often patients have a family history of geographic tongue or fissured tongue.
- Characterized by irregularly-shaped, red, map-like, smooth, and swollen patches surrounded by white lines **(Fig. 6)**.
- Occurs more often in patients who have psoriasis, especially pustular psoriasis.[3]
- Also known as wandering rash of tongue.
- This condition may occur suddenly and persist for months or longer.
- No treatment is necessary. Usually it resolves over time without treatment.

Fissured Tongue/Scrotal Tongue/ Lingua Plicata

- Characterized by grooves that vary in depth
- Seen on dorsal and lateral aspects of tongue
- Seen in Melkersson-Rosenthal syndrome and Down syndrome in association with geographic tongue and normal individual
- Debris can be trapped in the fissure.
- Depth of fissure varies about 6 mm
- No treatment is required.

Median Rhomboid Glossitis

- Also known as central papillary atrophy of tongue—susceptibility for candidiasis.
- Presents as rhomboid-shaped, well-defined, and erythematous plaque in the central tongue due to localized atrophy of the filiform papillae. Presents at posterior midline of dorsum of tongue.
- Soft palate erythema at the area of contact with the underlying tongue—kissing lesion.
- No treatment is necessary.
- Antifungal therapy—reduces clinical erythema and inflammation in *Candida* infection.

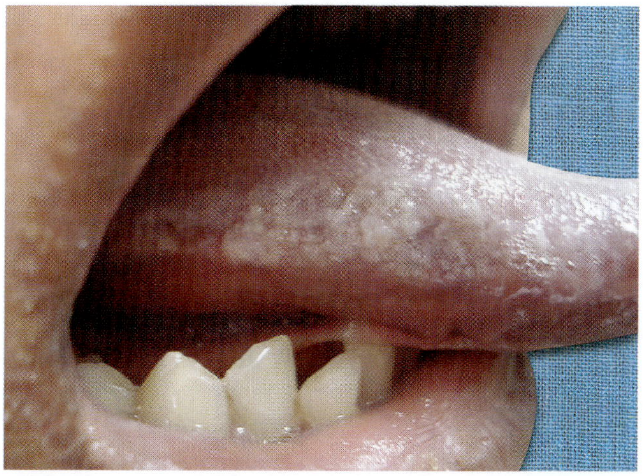

Fig. 5: Oral hairy leukoplakia.

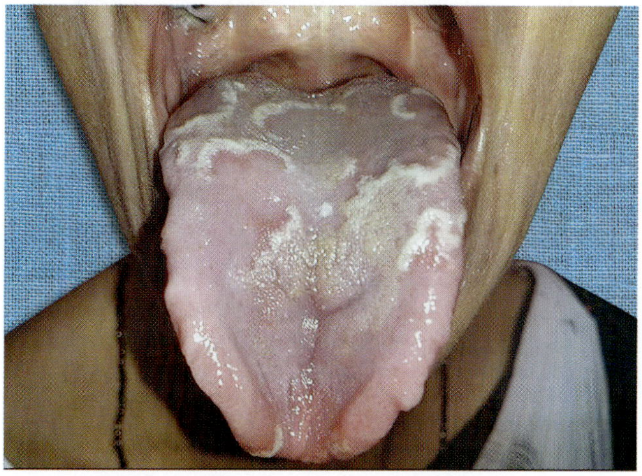

Fig. 6: Geographic tongue.

Strawberry Tongue

- In this, the tongue takes the distinctive red color of a strawberry.
- This is characterized by enlargement of the fungiform papillae.
- Thus, along with the reddening of the tongue, it is dotted with raised papillae giving it the look of a strawberry **(Fig. 7)**.
- Generally reflects a systemic disease rather than oral disorder.
- May be seen with scarlet fever, Kawasaki disease, and toxic shock syndrome.

Glossitis

- Due to dietary deficiency of folate or vitamin B_{12} and/or niacin.
- Common in alcoholics and in patients with Crohn's disease.
- Loss of the tiny, finger-like projection on the tongue—the papillae leading to an abnormally smoothed tongue.
- A dark red discoloration of the tongue may be seen.

DISORDERS OF BUCCAL MUCOSA

Oral Submucous Fibrosis

- Chronic insidious painless process characterized as dense white patch in oral cavity and pharynx due to juxta-epithelial deposition of fibrous tissue
- Typical to Indian subcontinent/genetic or racial
- Premalignant (40% may progress to oral cancers)
- Age 20–50 years, female > male
- *Etiology*: Paan/tobacco/supari (prolonged betel nut chewing), cigarette/bidi smoking + alcohol, spicy food, nutritional deficiency—iron, vitamins A, B, and zinc
- Stage I—stomatitis—ulcers, soreness, and burning sensation in mouth, intolerance to chillies/spicy food

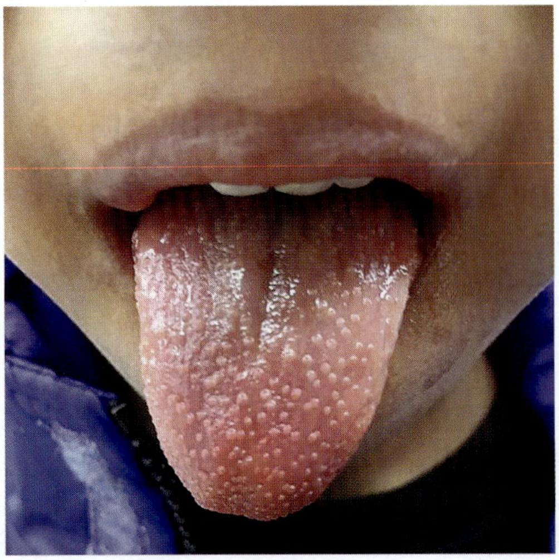

Fig. 7: Strawberry tongue.

- Stage II—fibrosis—white fibrotic bands over soft palate, pillars, and buccal mucosa
- Stage III—sequelae—marked trismus, ankyloglossia, poor orodental hygiene, leukoplakia, dysphagia, and speech deficit
- *Treatment*: Local injection steroids—injection steroid (dexamethasone 4 mg) + injection hylase (1,500 units)
- Good orodental hygiene, vitamins, zinc, and antioxidants
- *Surgical*: Incision/sectioning of fibrous bands and grafting

Leukoplakia

- Clinical white patch that cannot be characterized clinically and pathologically as any other disease and which cannot be rubbed off.
- *Causes*: Tobacco smoking/chewing (betel nut), alcohol, spices, dental sepsis/ill-fitting dentures, chronic candidal infection/viral/SMF, vitamin deficiency/Plummer–Vinson syndrome.
- Male > female, age 30–40 years.
- White, gray, or yellowish surface with well-defined margins—most common site—buccal mucosa and oral commissure.
- There are four types of leukoplakia which are discussed in **Table 2**.
- About 1–20% chance of malignancy and 20% chance of recurrence.
- Lesions on ventral and lateral borders of the tongue, soft palate, floor of the mouth, and oropharynx are considered high risk for malignant transformation.
- Lesions showing moderate-to-severe dysplasia, surgical excision, or laser surgery should be considered as treatment of choice.
- Cryotherapy ablation and carbon dioxide laser ablation are helpful.[4]

Candidiasis/Moniliasis

- In immunocompromised individuals, destruction of other organisms in oral cavity leads to overgrowth of *Candida* and it becomes pathogenic.
- Risk factors—immunosuppression (drug, HIV, and diabetes), xerostomia overuse of antibiotics/steroids,

TABLE 2: Types of leukoplakia.

Clinical type	*Clinical features*
Homogeneous thin leukoplakia	• Most common type • Usually asymptomatic, white uniform patch **(Fig. 8)**
Nodular speckled leukoplakia	Nodular growths overlying the homogeneous white plaque
Erosive/erythroleukoplakia	• Highly malignant • White patches have erosions and interspaced with red patches
Proliferative/verrucous type	• High recurrence • Seen in women

postchemotherapy, malignancy, elderly/newborns/pregnancy, and cytotoxic drugs.

- Gram stain—fungal hyphae; potassium hydroxide (KOH) examination—branching hyphae.
- **Table 3** depicts types, age group, clinical features, and treatment of candidiasis/moniliasis.

Recurrent Aphthous Stomatitis

- Most common nontraumatic form of oral ulcer involving oral cavity and oropharynx
- Ulcers are superficial and shallow in mobile or nonkeratinized epithelium areas—lips, tongue, and buccal mucosa
- Very painful
- Most common site—lower vestibule; does not involve hard palate and gingiva
- Generally seen in women aged 10–30 years

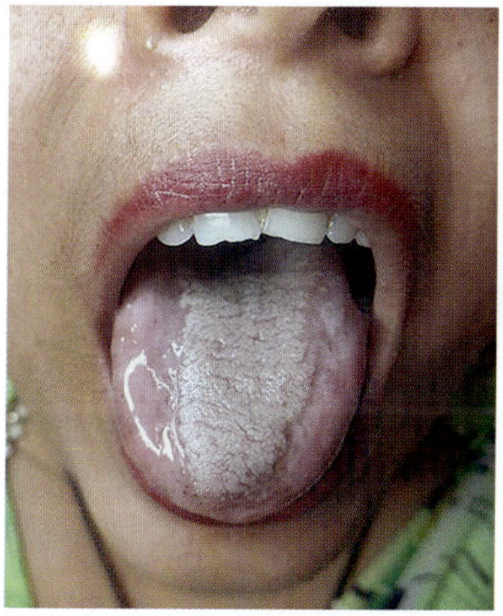

Fig. 8: Homogeneous thin leukoplakia.

- *Causes*: Local physical trauma, psychological/stress, drug-induced—nonsteroidal anti-inflammatory drug (NSAID), food allergy—nuts, spices, vitamin deficiency—B_{12}, folic acid, and habitual constipation
- Clinical types and features are presented in **Table 4**.
- *Treatment*: Avoid spicy food, vitamin supplements, and topical steroids
- Topic lignocaine gel, oral steroids, and intralesional steroids for large ulcers
- Cauterization of base of ulcer with 10% silver nitrate and trichloroacetic acid
- Tablet tetracycline 250 mg dissolved in 50 mL of water five times a day, rinse it, and then swallow it.

Oral Lichen Planus

- Word lichen planus derived from the Greek word leichen meaning tree moss and the Latin word planus meaning flat.
- Oral lichen planus affects 50% of patients with cutaneous lichen planus but may occur without skin lesions elsewhere.
- *Causes*: Contact allergens in dental restorative materials, viral infection—particularly hepatitis C, drugs—this is called oral lichenoid drug reaction. It is most often due to gold therapy.
- Clinical types and features of oral lichen planus are depicted in **Table 5**.
- *Grinspan's syndrome*[5] is the association of oral lichen planus (OLP) with diabetes and hypertension.
- Graham Little syndrome and vulvo-vagino-gingival syndrome are other syndromes associated with OLP, in which there is mucosal involvement of gingival and genital region, usually of erosive type.

TABLE 3: Types, age group, clinical features, and treatment of candidiasis/moniliasis.

Type	*Age group*	*Clinical features*	*Treatment*
Acute pseudomembranous candidiasis (thrush)	Infants/children/immunocompromised	• White gray patch on oral mucosa and tongue • Associated with inflammation of surrounding mucosa	• Topical application of nystatin/clotrimazole • 1% gentian violet application • Systemic antifungals—fluconazole (100–150 mg daily for 10 days), ketoconazole, and itraconazole • Intravenous amphotericin B
Chronic hypertrophic candidiasis/candidial leukoplakia	Usually presents in elderly and immunosuppressed individuals	• Dense chalky plaque more thicker which cannot be wiped off • Most common site—anterior buccal mucosa • High incidence of malignancy	• Surgery—excision • Long-term antifungal treatment—nystatin and amphotericin B
Acute erythematous candidiasis		Painful over hard palate	
Chronic erythematous candidiasis		Asymptomatic	
Angular candidiasis		Involves angle of mouth extends to skin	
Median rhomboid glossitis		On dorsum of tongue in front of foramen cecum, asymptomatic, and needs no treatment	

TABLE 4: Clinical types and features of recurrent aphthous stomatitis.

Clinical type	*Clinical features*
Minor aphthous ulcers (85%)	• Small and multiple 2–5 mm ulcers with central necrotic area surrounded by red halo **(Fig. 9)** • Last for 7–10 days, heals without scar
Major aphthous ulcers (10%)	• Single ulcer >2–4 cm, posterior part of oral cavity, and very painful • Take 3–6 weeks to heal, heals with scar **(Fig. 10)**
Herpetiform aphthous ulcers (5%)	• Multiple tiny ulcers occur close together and coalesce to form large ulcer • Take 7–10 days, heal without scar

- OLP is considered a premalignant condition. Reported transformation rates vary from 0.5 to 2% over a period of 5 years.
- *Histology*: "Saw-tooth" rete pegs, liquefaction necrosis of basal layer—Max-Joseph spaces, civatte (hyaline or cytoid) bodies, and juxta-epithelial band of inflammatory cells
- *Treatment*: Steroids—topical steroids/intralesional steroids/oral steroids
- Topical tacrolimus—0.1%, causes irritation, and burning sensation
- Topical retinoids—tretinoin 0.1%—rapid elimination but with relapse

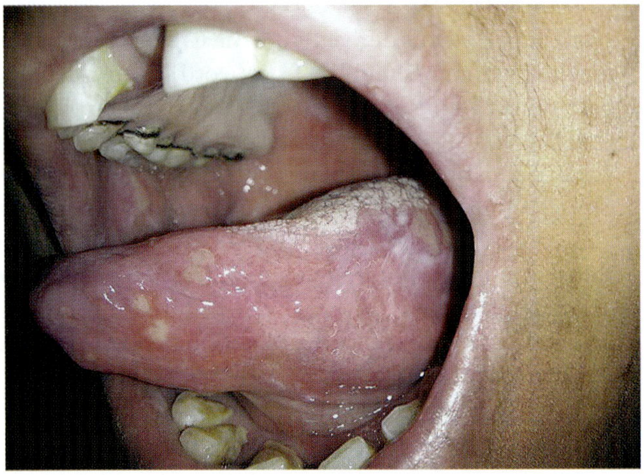

Fig. 9: Minor aphthous ulcers.

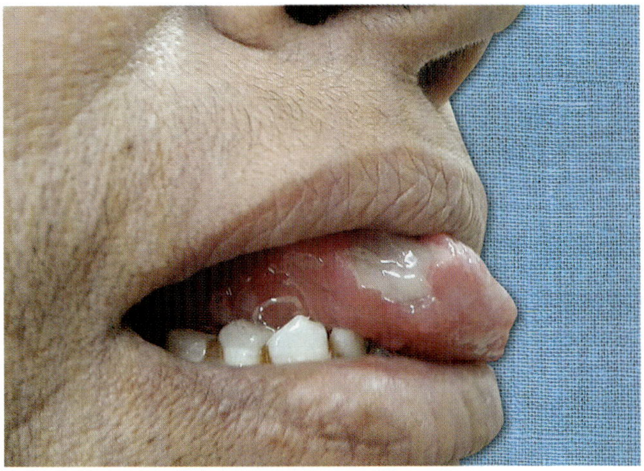

Fig. 10: Major aphthous ulcers.

TABLE 5: Clinical types and features of oral lichen planus (OLP).

Clinical type	*Clinical features*
Reticular lichen planus	• Symmetrical white lace-like pattern on buccal mucosa • May affect tongue or gums • They are usually bilaterally seen • Characteristic pattern of interlacing white lines (Wickham striae) **(Fig. 11)** • Usually asymptomatic. May ulcerate
Papular OLP	• Characterized by small white papules • Merge with reticular striae as part of the natural course
Plaque type OLP	• Homogenous well-demarcated white plaque, often, but not always surrounded by striae • Clinically may be very similar to homogenous leukoplakia
Atrophic type	• Characterized by a homogeneous red area • Smooth, poorly defined erythematous areas with or without peripheral striae • Usually associated with desquamative gingivitis
Erosive OLP	• Atrophic areas with central ulceration • Periphery of the atrophic regions is bordered by fine, white radiating striae • Pain, burning sensation, bleeding, and desquamative gingivitis • Ulcer may be covered by pseudomembrane
Bullous type	• Rare form characterized by large vesicles or bullae • Usually have peripheral radiating striae • Lesions rupture immediately leaving painful ulcers
Ulcerative type OLP	• Most disabling form of oral lichen planus • Fibrin-coated ulcers surrounded by an erythematous zone frequently displaying radiating white striae

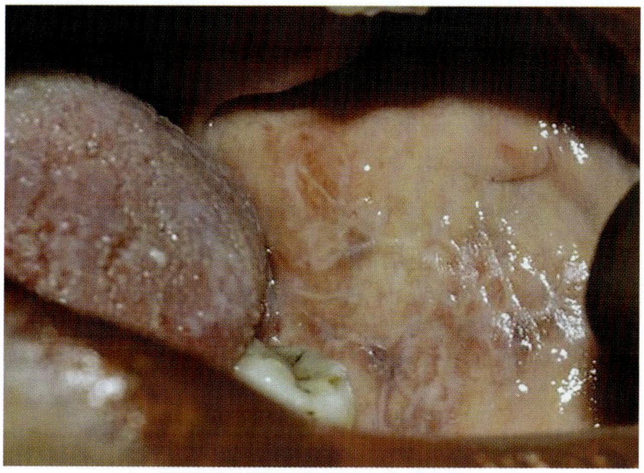

Fig. 11: Reticular lichen planus.

- Cyclosporin—for more sever variants like erosive or ulcerative OLP, solution can be used as oral swish and spit method.

CONCLUSION

Examination and knowledge of the oral mucosa forms a vital part of complete dermatological examination. Many diseases may start in the oral cavity and oral lesions may precede the cutaneous lesions by months to years. There are also common conditions that are unique to the oral mucosa; hence, a dermatologist should have a thorough understanding of the oral cavity.

KEY POINTS

- Exfoliative cheilitis presents as fissuring, peeling, crusting, or hemorrhagic crusting and may be representative of underlying factitial or obsessive-compulsive behavior.
- Actinic cheilitis usually presents in outdoor workers, fair-skinned individuals on the lower lip, and is considered as a premalignant condition with possible progression to squamous cell carcinoma.
- Cheilitis granulomatosis may be associated with various systemic conditions (sarcoidosis, Crohn's disease, and tuberculosis) and is characterized by firm and rubber-like consistency of lips.
- Leukoplakia presenting on ventral and lateral borders of the tongue, soft palate, floor of the mouth, and oropharynx are considered high risk for malignant transformation and surgical excision or laser surgery should be considered.
- Recurrent aphthous stomatitis is characterized by shallow, superficial ulcers over nonkeratinized epithelium areas such as lips, tongue, buccal mucosa, and is classified into minor (size 2–5 mm) and major (>2–4 cm) depending on the size of the ulcers.
- Oral lichen planus affects 50% of patients with cutaneous lichen planus, but may occur in isolation. There are seven variants described according to the morphology.

REFERENCES

1. Grave B, McCullough M, Wiesenfeld D. Orofacial granulomatosis—a 20-year review. Oral Dis. 2009;15(1):46-51.
2. Chapple IL, Hamburger J. The significance of oral health in HIV disease. Sex Transm Infect. 2000;76(4):236-43.
3. Tarakji B, Umair A, Babaker Z, Azzeghaiby SN, Gazal G, Sarraj F. Relation between psoriasis and geographic tongue. J Clin Diagn Res. 2014;8(11):ZE06.
4. Lin HP, Chen HM, Cheng SJ, Yu CH, Chiang CP. Cryogun cryotherapy for oral leukoplakia. Head Neck. 2012;34(9):1306-11.
5. Lamey PJ, Gibson J, Barclay SC, Miller S. Grinspan's syndrome: a drug-induced phenomenon?. Oral Surg Oral Med Oral Pathol. 1990;70(2):184-5.

EXAMINATION QUESTIONS

1. What are the different types of oral candidiasis?
2. Write a short note on leukoplakia.
3. What are various types and management of oral lichen planus (OLP)?

Postgraduate Dermatology

The photographs on the cover of the textbook depict images as under:

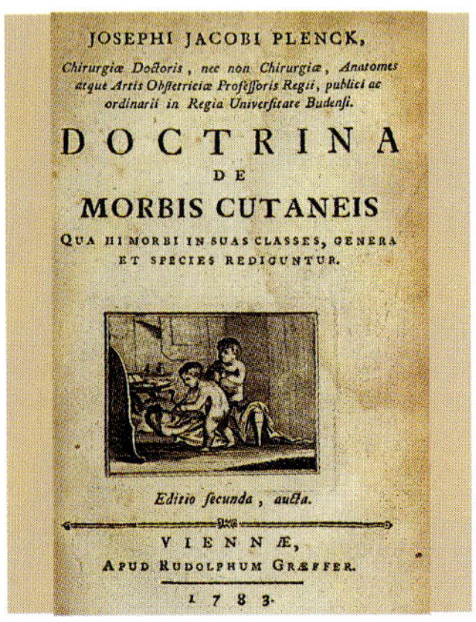

This image from the second edition of (1783) of *Doctrina De Morbis Cutaneis* of Joseph Jacob Plenck (1735–1807), a Viennese Military Surgeon and polymath. Plenck was the first to introduce a method of classifying skin diseases in 1776. This profoundly influenced Robert Willan (1757–1812), the Father of English Dermatology to introduce the modern classification. The first four orders namely Papulae, Squamae, Exanthemata and Bullae published as a book entitled *On Cutaneous Diseases* Vol. I in 1808.

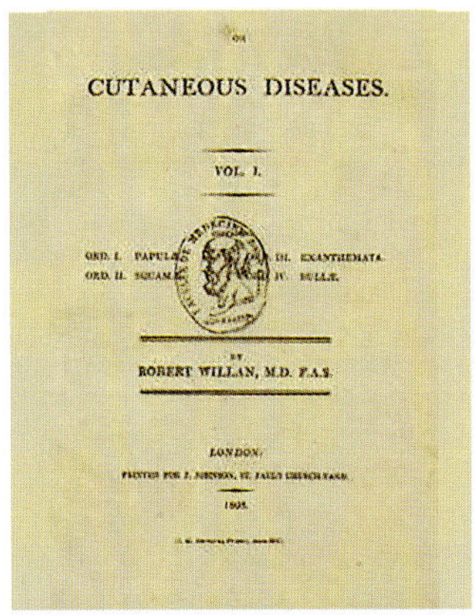

A water color from Willan's book depicting the various orders. Willan was also the first physician to give clear clinical description of psoriasis, another milestone in the history of psoriasis.

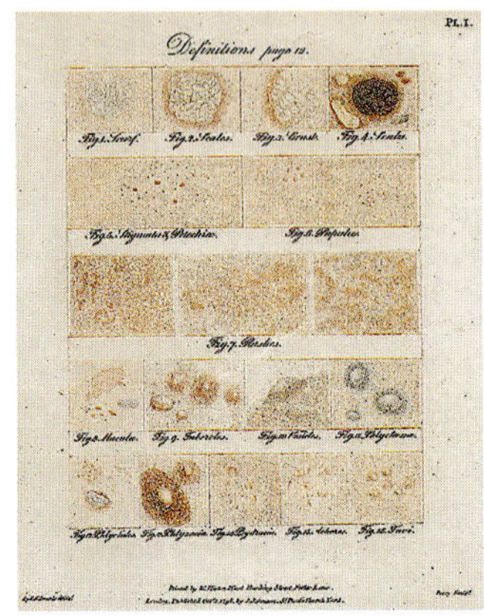

A collage of four landmark images which formed the most important milestones in the history of modern dermatology.

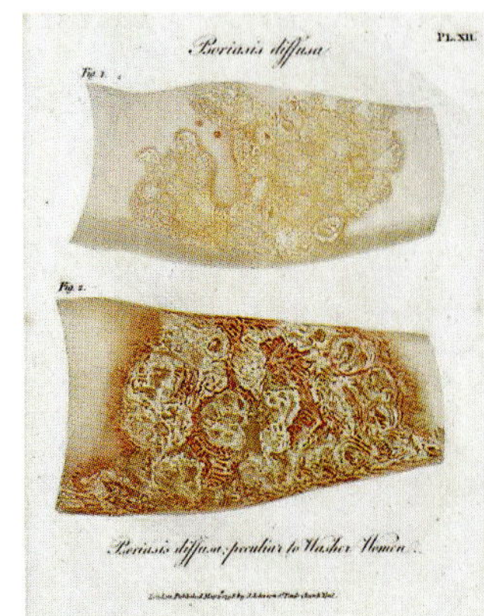

A water color entitled *Psoriasis diffusa,* taken from Willan's aforesaid treatise.

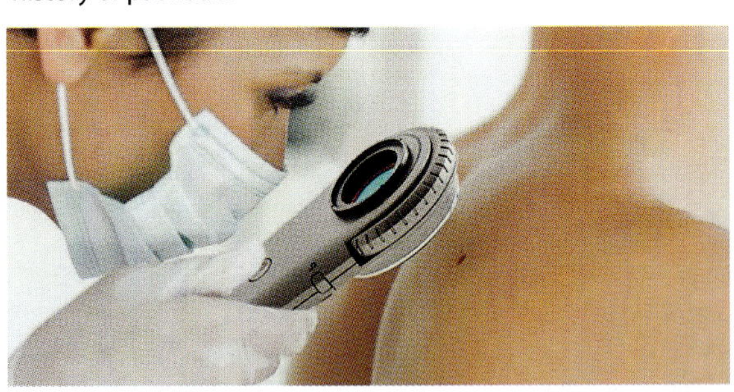

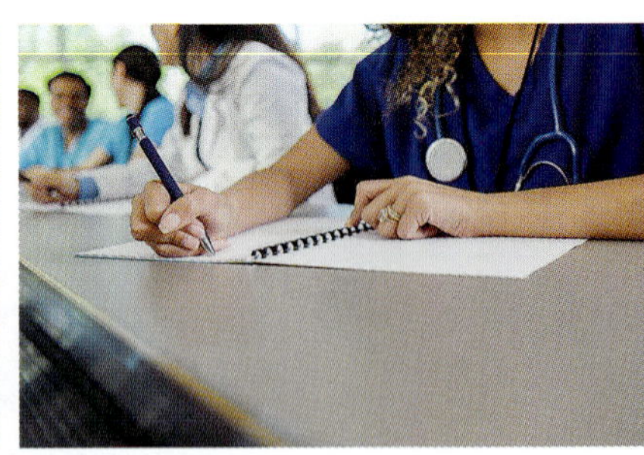

Postgraduate Dermatology

Volume 2

Editors

Koushik Lahiri

MBBS DVD (CAL) FIAD FFAADV FRCP (Glasgow) FRCP (Edin) FRCP (London)
Professor and Distinguished Academician (AHERF)
Senior Consultant Dermatologist
Apollo Multispecialty Hospitals Limited
Honorary Medical Director
Wizderm Speciality Skin and Hair Clinic
Kolkata, West Bengal, India
Vice President, International Society of Dermatology (2017–2021)
President, Association of Cutaneous Surgeons (I) (2013–2015)
Chairperson, ACSI Academy of Dermatosurgery (2017–2019)
Editor, Indian Journal of Dermatology (2012–2017)

Abhishek De

MD FAGE MRCP-SCE (Dermatology)
Associate Professor
Calcutta National Medical College
Kolkata, West Bengal, India
Associate Editor, Indian Journal of Dermatology
Associate Editor, Indian Journal of Skin Allergy
Honorary Secretary, Skin Allergy Research Society of India
Assistant Editor, Journal of Cutaneous and Aesthetic Surgery (JCAS)

Assistant Editors

Aarti Sarda

MD FAGE MRCP-SCE (Dermatology)
Consultant Dermatologist
Department of Dermatology
Wizderm Speciality Skin and Hair Clinic
Kolkata, West Bengal, India

Anupam Das MD

Assistant Professor
Department of Dermatology
KPC Medical College and Hospital
Kolkata, West Bengal, India

Abhijit Saha MD

Consultant Dermatologist
Institute of Child Health
Kolkata, West Bengal, India

Surajit Gorai

MD (Gold Medalist) DNB MNAMS (Dermatology)
Associate Professor (AHERF)
Consultant Dermatologist
Apollo Gleneagles Hospital
Kolkata, West Bengal, India

Barnali Chowdhury MD

Consultant Dermatologist
Rabindranath Tagore International
Institute of Cardiac Sciences
Kolkata, West Bengal, India

Foreword

S Premalatha

JAYPEE

JAYPEE BROTHERS MEDICAL PUBLISHERS

The Health Sciences Publisher

New Delhi | London

Jaypee Brothers Medical Publishers (P) Ltd

Headquarters
EMCA House
23/23-B, Ansari Road, Daryaganj
New Delhi 110 002, India
Landline: +91-11-23272143, +91-11-23272703
+91-11-23282021, +91-11-23245672
E-mail: jaypee@jaypeebrothers.com

Corporate Office
4838/24, Ansari Road, Daryaganj
New Delhi 110 002, India
Phone: +91-11-43574357
Fax: +91-11-43574314
E-mail: jaypee@jaypeebrothers.com

Overseas Office
J.P. Medical Ltd
83 Victoria Street, London
SW1H 0HW (UK)
Phone: +44 20 3170 8910
E-mail: info@jpmedpub.com

EU GPSR Authorised Representative
Logos Europe, 9 rue Nicolas Poussin
17000, La Rochelle, France
Phone: +33 (0) 6 67 93 73 78
E-mail: contact@logoseurope.eu

Website: www.jaypeebrothers.com
Website: www.jaypeedigital.com

Inquiries for bulk sales may be solicited at: jaypee@jaypeebrothers.com

Postgraduate Dermatology (Volumes 1 and 2)

First Edition: **2022**

Reprint: **2026**

ISBN: 978-93-5270-463-7

Printed at: Samrat Offset Pvt. Ltd.

Contents

VOLUME 1

SECTION 1 OVERVIEW OF BASICS IN DERMATOLOGY

SECTION 2 PRURITUS, URTICARIA, ALLERGY, AND ECZEMAS

SECTION 6 PAPULOSQUAMOUS DISEASES

SECTION 7 SKIN AND SYSTEMIC DISEASE

SECTION 8 HAIR, NAIL, MUCOSA, ADNEXA AND CONNECTIVE TISSUE

VOLUME 2

SECTION 9 VASCULAR DISEASES

SECTION 10 NEOPLASTIC SKIN DISEASES

SECTION 11 PIGMENTARY AND MISCELLANEOUS SKIN DISORDERS

SECTION 12 LEPROSY

SECTION 13 SEXUALLY TRANSMITTED DISEASE

9 SECTION | Vascular Diseases

82 CHAPTER Raynaud's Phenomenon

Nidhi Choudhary

INTRODUCTION

Raynaud's phenomenon is an episodic and reversible vasospasm of peripheral arteries (usually digital) characterized clinically by a triphasic color change of pallor followed by cyanosis and/or redness.

It is usually associated with pain and sometimes with paresthesia.

The episode is precipitated by cold and emotional stress.

Such type of color change is because of: pallor due to ischemia, cyanosis due to deoxygenation, and erythema due to reperfusion.[1]

HISTORY

First described by Maurice Raynaud, a French physician.[2]

In his thesis, he described several patients who developed discoloration of their fingers on cold exposure.

INCIDENCE

- It affects 3–5% of population.[3]
- Females are four times more commonly affected than males.

CLASSIFICATION

Primary Raynaud's phenomenon: Idiopathic or classic.

Secondary Raynaud's phenomenon: Secondary to some underlying disease or cause.[4]

CAUSES OF SECONDARY RAYNAUD'S PHENOMENON[5]

Causes of secondary Raynaud's phenomenon are given in **Table 1**.

TABLE 1: Causes of secondary Raynaud's phenomenon.

Connective tissue diseases	Systemic sclerosis, MCTD, SLE, Sjögren's syndrome
Drugs and toxins	Beta-blockers, ergot derivatives, vinyl polychloride, cyclosporine, bleomycin, vinca alkaloids, cisplatin, and carboplatin
Endocrine diseases	Hypothyroidism
Vascular diseases	Vasculitis, thromboembolic diseases
Hematological diseases	Cryoglobulinemia, cryofibrinogenemia Cold agglutinin disease Myeloproliferative disorders such as essential thrombocythemia and polycythemia, etc.
Occupational	Vibration injury, cold injury
Obstructive cause	Thoracic outlet syndrome, atherosclerosis, Takayasu arteritis, Buerger disease, crutch pressure
Neurological diseases	Carpal tunnel syndrome, pheochromocytoma, carcinoid syndrome, reflex sympathetic dystrophy, migraine

(MCTD: mixed connective tissue disease; SLE: systemic lupus erythematosus)
Source: Fitzpatrick's Dermatology in General Medicine 7th edition, vol 2, p. 1647.

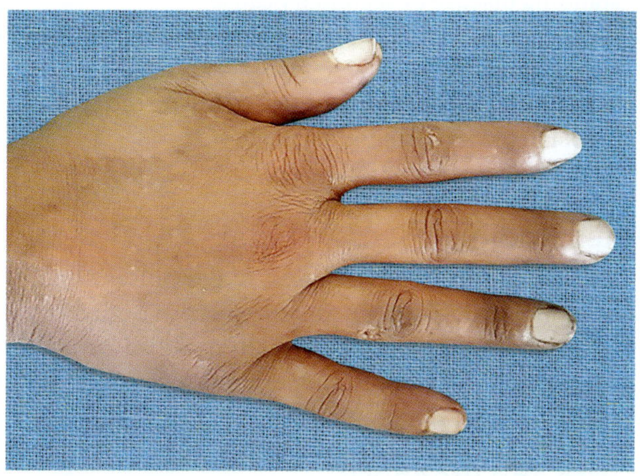

Fig. 1: *Raynaud's phenomenon:* Ischemic phase of attack.

CLINICAL FEATURES

History

- Patients complain of episodic attacks of well-demarcated, white **(Fig. 1)**, or blue digits induced by exposure to cold or emotional stress **(Fig. 2)**.
- The classic triphasic color change is rarely described by the patient; most describe only pallor or cyanosis along with numbing of digits.
- A throbbing pain may occur which is more common in secondary Raynaud's phenomenon.

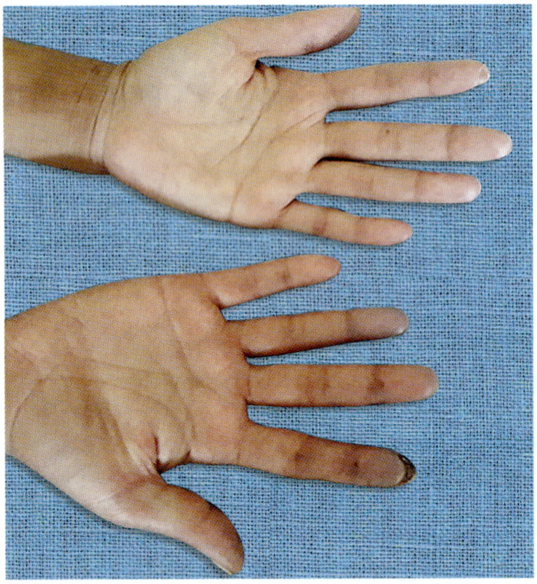

Fig. 2: *Raynaud's phenomenon:* Bluish discoloration of digits.

- Apart from finger and toes, sometimes earlobes, nose tip, and nipples may be involved.
- History should be taken to rule out connective tissue diseases (CTDs) (arthritis, dysphagia, dyspnea, photosensitivity, skin rash, muscle weakness, etc.), drug intake, and occupational exposure to vibration.

Cutaneous Finding

- There is well-demarcated blanching or cyanosis of the digit.
- The digits distal to line of ischemia are cold while proximal digits are warm.
- Associated findings like sclerodactyly point toward long-standing disease or secondary cause.
- Trophic or ischemic changes may occur in prolonged or severe attacks.
- Sclerodactyly, painful ulcers, and pitted scars are associated with systemic sclerosis.
- Gangrene may occur rarely.

Other Findings

- To rule out obstructive causes, major pulses should be examined along with BP measurement in both arms.
- Adson maneuver—a diminished radial pulse with exaggerated neck and shoulder movement point toward thoracic outlet syndrome.

Course and Prognosis

- Spontaneous remission may occur in primary Raynaud's phenomenon.
- This is not seen with secondary Raynaud's phenomenon.
- Pregnancy has been shown to improve Raynaud's phenomenon since there is an improvement in peripheral blood flow and oxygenation.

BOX 1: Diagnostic criteria for primary Raynaud's phenomenon.

By Allen and Brown[7] and Le Roy and Medsger,[8]
- Presence of Raynaud's phenomena for 2 years or more
- Normal vascular examination with symmetric peripheral pulses and normal nailfold capillary microscopy
- Bilateral involvement of extremities
- Vasospastic attacks precipitated by exposure to cold or emotional stimuli
- Negative or low titer ANA
- Absence of gangrene, or if present, limited to the skin of fingertips
- No evidence of an underlying disease, drug, or occupational exposure responsible for attacks
- Normal ESR

(ANA: antinuclear antibody; ESR: erythrocyte sedimentation rate)
Source: Fitzpatrick's Dermatology in General Medicine, 7th edition, Vol 2, p. 1647.

- Since Raynaud's phenomenon may be the initial manifestation, all patients should be evaluated to rule out an underlying cause. About 10% of patients may eventually go on to develop the disease later.[6]

DIAGNOSTIC CRITERIA FOR PRIMARY RAYNAUD'S PHENOMENON

Diagnostic criteria for primary Raynaud's phenomenon are given in **Box 1**.

DIFFERENCE BETWEEN PRIMARY AND SECONDARY RAYNAUD'S PHENOMENON

Difference between primary and secondary Raynaud's phenomenon is given in **Table 2**.

INVESTIGATIONS

- CBC with ESR
- Urine routine
- Antinuclear antibody (ANA)
- Antibodies against specific antigens (in patients with abnormal ANA or when history or clinical features are suggestive of CTD)
- Chest X-ray (for interstitial lung disease or cervical rib)
- Nailfold capillary microscopy (to distinguish between primary and secondary Raynaud's phenomenon)
- Doppler ultrasound if vascular/obstructive cause is suspected.
- Special investigations are required only if there are suggestive history and physical findings.

Nailfold Capillary Microscopy

- Capillaroscopy is the most reliable method to distinguish between primary and secondary Raynaud's phenomenon through identification of an early pattern of systemic sclerosis.[9]
- Nailfolds are examined as this area is easily accessible and here axis of capillaries lies parallel to skin surface.

- The morphological changes are evaluated under following parameters:
  - Loop density and findings are described ahead.
  - Capillary length variability
  - *Architectural derangement*: Tortuous, meandering, giant, and bushy capillaries
  - Irregular distribution of capillary array and extravasations into perivascular tissue.

Normal Capillaroscopic Pattern[10]

- The capillaries have homogeneous size, shape, and color.
- Arranged transversely across the cuticle in hairpin loop pattern.
- The normal capillary density ranges from 7 to 12 capillaries, averaging 9 capillaries/mm.
- Some morphological variations, such as crossed or meandering loops may be present.
- Some capillary dilation and small areas of microbleeding associated with daily microtrauma may be present.

Scleroderma Pattern

Maricq et al.[11] described the scleroderma pattern characterized by:

- Presence of dilated capillaries (ectasia and/or megacapillaries)
- Loss of capillary loops (capillary drop-out)
- Microbleeding and neoangiogenesis (branched capillaries)

TABLE 2: Differences between primary and secondary Raynaud's phenomenon.

	Primary Raynaud's phenomenon	*Secondary Raynaud's phenomenon*
Sex ratio	F:M—20:1	F:M—4:1
Precipitants	Cold, emotional Stress	Cold
Etiology	Idiopathic	Secondary to some underlying disease
Median age of onset	14 years	Above 30 years
Pain	Less severe	Severe throbbing pain may be present
Involvement	Bilateral involvement of extremities	May be unilateral/ bilateral
Associated features	No evidence of an underlying disease	Features suggestive of a CTD, drug intake, occupational exposure may be present
Ischemic changes	Severe ulceration and gangrene usually absent	Ulcer, gangrenous changes, digital scars may occur
Antinuclear antibody	Negative or low titer ANA positive	ANA positive in 90–95%
Frequency of attacks	Usually <5 per day	5–10+ per day
Nailfold capillaroscopy	Normal	Abnormal in >95% cases

(ANA: antinuclear antibody; CTD: connective tissue disease)
Source: Bolognia Dermatology, 4th edition.

DIFFERENTIAL DIAGNOSIS

Chilblain: Erythematous papules/nodule, edema, and burning sensation on cold exposure. In severe cases, ulcers or bullae may develop. Lesions leave a residual hyperpigmentation on healing.

Acrocyanosis: On cold exposure, the hands and feet acquire a bluish color which becomes purplish or red on rewarming, the pallor phase is absent. The extremities become cold, clammy, and swollen.

TREATMENT

General Measures

Behavioral modifications—Minimize exposure to cold:

- Wearing layered clothes to maintain core temperature
- Limiting time spent outdoors in winter
- Wearing insulated gloves
- Hand warming
- Cessation of smoking
- Stop offending drug
- Avoid caffeine
- Counseling and stress management.

Drug Therapy

Drug therapy is given in **Table 3**.

Newer therapies for Raynaud's phenomena are given in **Table 4**.

TABLE 3: Drug therapy.

Mild attacks	General measures such as protection from cold and cessation of smoking are sufficient.
Frequent or severe attacks	Calcium-channel blockers (nifedipine 10–20 mg tid to qid, diltiazem 60 mg tid or qid), antiadrenergic drugs (prazosin), angiotensin-receptor blockers (losartan), and topical nitroglycerin
Acute severe ischemia	IV PGE1 or prostacyclin, low molecular weight heparin, digital sympathectomy, microvascular surgery
Digital ulcers	Antiseptic soaks, topical antibiotics, dressing, CCB, PGE1
Digital gangrene	Antibiotics, analgesics, surgical debridement, amputation

(CCB: clinical cardiopulmonary bypass; IV: intravenous; PGE1: prostaglandin E1)
Source: Fitzpatrick's Dermatology in General Medicine, 7th edition, Vol 2, p. 1647.

TABLE 4: Newer therapies for Raynaud's phenomena.[12]

Drug class	*Route of administration*	*Effect*
Endothelin antagonist (bosentan)	Oral	Reduced number of new ulcers
Phosphodiesterase type 5 inhibitor (sildenafil, tadalafil)	Oral	Reduced duration, frequency, and severity of attacks; improved ulcer healing
SSRI (fluoxetine)	Oral	Reduced attack frequency and severity
Selective serotonin 5HT2 antagonist (sarpogrelate)	Oral	Reduced attack frequency and severity
Antioxidants (N-acetylcysteine)	IV	Reduced frequency and severity of attacks and improved ulcer healing
Botulinum toxin-A	Interdigital injection	Decreased pain, numbness, attack frequency, improved blood flow, and ulcer healing
Statins (atorvastatin)	Oral	Reduction in number of ulcers

(SSRI: selective serotonin reuptake inhibitor)

KEY POINTS

- Episodic, reversible, and triphasic color change in response to cold or emotional stress.
- Classified into primary and secondary types.
- Secondary is most commonly associated with connective tissue diseases particularly systemic sclerosis.
- A proper history and clinical examination should be done to rule out CTD.
- Nailfold capillary microscopy is a good tool to distinguish between the two types.

REFERENCES

1. Cooke JP, Marshall JM. Mechanisms of Raynaud's disease. Vasc Med. 2005;10(4):293-307.
2. Kaiser H. Maurice Raynaud (1834-1881) and the syndrome named after him. Z Rheumatol. 2011;70(7):620-4.
3. Pope JE. The diagnosis and treatment of Raynaud's phenomenon: a practical approach. Drugs. 2007;67:517-25.
4. Block JA, Sequeira W. Raynaud's phenomenon. Lancet. 2001;357:2042-8.
5. Wigley FM. Raynaud's phenomenon. N Engl J Med. 2002; 347:1001-8.
6. Goundry B, Bell L, Langtree M, Moorthy A. Diagnosis and management of Raynaud's phenomenon. BMJ. 2012; 344:e289.
7. Allen EV, Brown GE. Raynaud's disease: a critical review of minimal requisites for diagnosis. Am J Med Sci. 1932;183: 187-200.
8. LeRoy EC, Medsger TA Jr. Raynaud's phenomenon: a proposal for classification. Clin Exp Rheumatol. 1992;10:485-8.
9. De Angelis R, Grassi W, Cutolo M. A growing need for capillaroscopy in rheumatology. Arthritis Rheum. 2009;61: 405-10.
10. Souza E, Kayser C. Nailfold capillaroscopy: relevance to the practice of rheumatology. Rev Bras Reumatol. 2015;55(3): 264-71.
11. Maricq HR. Comparison of quantitative and semiquantitative estimates of nailfold capillary abnormalities in scleroderma spectrum disorders. Microvasc Res. 1986;32(2):271-6.
12. Levien TL. Advances in the treatment of Raynaud's phenomenon. Vasc Health Risk Manag. 2010;6:167-77.

EXAMINATION QUESTION

1. What are the differences between primary and secondary Raynaud's phenomena?
2. What are the common causes of secondary Raynaud's phenomena?
3. How would you approach and manage a case of Raynaud's phenomena?

83 CHAPTER Purpura

Kingshuk Chatterjee

INTRODUCTION

Purpura is a group of disorders characterized by discoloration of skin and/or mucous membrane due to extravasation of red blood cells. Any mechanism that disturbs the integrity of vasculature and its support will lead to purpura. The various causes range from minor alterations to serious fatal abnormalities.

PATHOGENIC FACTORS

- Vascular damage
- Defective connective tissue support to the vasculature
- Reduction in number/abnormal function of platelets
- Deficiency/abnormal consumption of coagulation factors

CLINICAL SIGNS

Purpura is a sign and not a disease per se, described by the following signs:

- *Petechiae*: Pinhead sized, round macules evolving from bright red to brown in color. Classically, they appear in crops over dependent areas of body and indicate defective platelets
- *Vibices (singular: vibex)*: Linear streaks of hemorrhage on skin
- *Ecchymoses (bruise)*: Bluish patch formed by deep extensive hemorrhage, which gradually becomes yellow and fade away
- *Hematoma*: Large pool of extravasated blood in a dead space, leading to a fluctuant swelling
- *Palpable purpura*: Bright red hemorrhagic papules, indicative of underlying vascular inflammation. These lesions are nonblanchable.

COMMON CAUSES OF PURPURA

- *Platelet disorders*:
    - Platelet function abnormalities
    - Thrombocytosis
    - Thrombocytopenia
- *Coagulation disorders*:
    - Inherited (hemophilia, Von Willebrand disease)
    - *Acquired*:
        - Disseminated intravascular coagulation (DIC)
        - Purpura fulminans
        - Drugs (e.g., anticoagulants)
        - Metabolic (liver disease, vitamin K deficiency)
- *Vascular disorders*:
    - *Inflammatory*:
        - Leukocytoclastic vasculitis
        - Capillaritis [e.g., pigmented purpuric dermatoses (PPD)]
    - *Direct vascular damage*:
        - Infections
        - Toxins and drugs (e.g., aspirin, barbiturates)
    - Raised intravascular pressure (e.g., coughing, vomiting, tourniquets)
    - Defective vasculature support (e.g., steroid-induced purpura, senile purpura, scurvy)
    - Vascular abnormality (e.g., tufted angioma, acro-angiodermatitis)
- *Microvascular occlusion*:
    - Embolic (e.g., cholesterol, septic)
    - Cryoproteins (e.g., cryoglobulinemia, cryofibrinogenemia)
    - Infective (e.g., ecthyma gangrenosum, disseminated strongyloidiasis)
    - Platelet plugs [e.g., thrombotic thrombocytopenic purpura (TTP), myeloproliferative disorders]
- *Miscellaneous*:
    - Physical and artifactual purpura
    - Contact purpura
    - Purpura in nonpurpuric dermatoses (lichen sclerosus, lichen nitidus, erythema multiforme)
    - Painful bruising syndrome
    - Paroxysmal finger hematoma[1]

EVALUATION IN A CASE OF PURPURA

It is prudent to determine whether the purpura is associated with an underlying systemic abnormality, warranting urgent attention with detailed laboratory investigations or an innocuous condition, to be managed by counseling and reassurance.

HISTORY

- Onset and distribution of rash
- Associated mucocutaneous symptoms
- Bleeding from other sites including orifices
- Constitutional and systemic symptoms
- Drug history

CLINICAL EXAMINATION

- Number of rash
- Size
- Distribution
- Palpability
- Associated features (e.g., pustule, nodule, necrosis, ulceration)
- Systemic associations

LABORATORY INVESTIGATIONS

- *Routine hemogram*: To detect hematological abnormalities
- *Platelet count and platelet function tests*: Most important investigation to assess a case of nonpalpable purpura
- Bleeding time
- Coagulation profile
- Capillary resistance test
- Occult blood test
- Histopathology in case of palpable purpura

Purpura due to platelet disorders: An essential component of the hemostatic mechanism is presence of adequate number of circulating and functional platelets. Either reduction in number or loss of function leads to purpura.

CLASSIFICATION

Thrombocytopenia

- *Reduced production*:
  - Bone marrow disease (aplasia, neoplasia, replacement, others)
  - Metabolic (uremia, alcoholism)
  - Infection
  - Drugs
- *Reduced survival*:
  - Autoantibody mediated—idiopathic thrombocytopenic purpura, systemic lupus erythematosus (SLE), antiphospholipid antibody (APLA)
  - Alloantibody mediated—post-transfusion, neonatal
  - Infection
  - Drugs
- *Excessive consumption*:
  - Thrombotic thrombocytopenic purpura
  - Disseminated intravascular coagulation
  - Hemolytic uremic syndrome

Abnormal Platelet Function

- *Inherited*: Von Willebrand disease, Glanzmann's disease, storage pool disease
- Drugs
- *Others*: Uremia, dysproteinemia, myeloproliferative disorders

Thrombocytosis

- Essential thrombocythemia
- Myeloproliferative diseases
- *Others*: Blood loss, postsplenectomy, sarcoidosis, malignancy[2]

Immune Thrombocytopenic Purpura (*Synonym:* Idiopathic Thrombocytopenic Purpura)

- Manifested by mucocutaneous bleeding due to reduced platelet count
- If duration is <6 months, it is termed acute and chronic in case duration is >6 months.[3]
- Surface glycoproteins of platelets act as autoantigens leading to platelet loss through attachment with Fc receptors on macrophages, mainly in the spleen.
- The childhood-onset immune thrombocytopenic purpura (ITP) is acute in onset; sudden onset of petechiae or purpura after a bout of infection and spontaneous remission are seen.
- The adult-onset ITP is chronic in nature; more common in women; associated with other autoimmune disorders and infection; crops of mucocutaneous petechiae, epistaxis, gum bleeding, and menorrhagia are commonly seen; splenomegaly is rare.
- The diagnosis is generally one of exclusion and blood count and smear are usually within normal limits.
- Prednisolone 1–1.5 mg/kg/day is the treatment of choice. Persistent low platelet count < 5,000/mm^3 may require intravenous immunoglobulin (IVIG) infusion.[4,5]
- Platelet infusions are needed to tackle severe bleeding. Patients requiring heavy dose of steroids to maintain a platelet count >30,000/mm^3 may be recommended splenectomy within 3–6 months.
- Chronic refractory cases may require immunosuppressives, e.g., azathioprine, cyclosporine, cyclophosphamide, anti-D IgG (immunoglobulin G) and rituximab (anti-CD20 monoclonal antibody).[6,7]

Thrombotic Thrombocytopenic Purpura

- Widespread thrombotic microangiopathy leads to a conundrum of fever, thrombocytopenic purpura, hemolytic anemia, renal dysfunction, and neurological manifestations.

- Genetic form of the disease is due to deficiency of a protease (ADAMST13). The acquired form may result from drugs (ticlopidine, cyclosporine) and connective tissue disorders (SLE, Sjögren's syndrome, and scleroderma).
- Infusion of platelet-poor-fresh frozen plasma or cryo-precipitate-poor plasma can prevent episodes of familial TTP in children.
- Plasma exchange is recommended for the older children and adults with acquired TTP. Glucocorticoid therapy or splenectomy can interfere with antibody production.[8]

Disseminated Intravascular Coagulation

- It is a complex disorder of consumption of coagulation factors and platelets with generation of intravascular fibrin, leading to systemic thrombosis and hemorrhage.
- It is generally precipitated by many factors including obstetric complications, bacterial sepsis, malignancy, snakebite, and excessive tissue damage.
- Notable systemic features include fever, hypotension, respiratory distress, circulatory failure, hematemesis, epistaxis, hematuria, uterine bleeding, and renal failure.
- Variable dermatological manifestations include widespread purpura, hemorrhagic bullae, acral hemorrhagic necrosis, purpura fulminans, acral cyanosis, localized infarction, gangrene, and deep hematoma.
- In addition to the clinical condition, suggestive of DIC, thrombocytopenia, prolonged prothrombin time and activated partial thromboplastin time with presence of fibrin degradation product and D-dimer can lead to the diagnosis.
- Treatment of the underlying cause is the mainstay of treatment. Intensive therapy, replacement of blood constituents and anticoagulants are supportive measures.[9,10]

Purpura Fulminans

- Abnormal coagulation and microvascular occlusion lead to acute severe hemorrhagic necrosis of the skin.
- Usually after an infectious episode, children are affected with this potentially lethal condition.
- Sudden appearance of ecchymotic lesions of retiform or stellate pattern appears on trunk, extremities, buttocks, and pressure points. Hemorrhagic bullae and necrosis on skin are common. Febrile illness, internal hemorrhage, and shock may cause mortality.
- Homozygous deficiency of protein C or less commonly protein S lead to the disease in neonatal period.
- In childhood, the postinfectious disease is usually common, characterized by widespread necrosis and sepsis. Meningococcal meningitis, group A streptococcal infection, staphylococcal, and pseudomonal infections are the usual perpetrators. Purpura fulminans in a case of SLE should arouse the suspicion of APLA.
- Cutaneous necrosis without inflammation and vascular occlusion with platelet fibrin thrombi is the histological hallmark of the disease.
- Treatment is mainly supportive with antibiotics for underlying disease and replacement with fresh frozen plasma. If facilities are available, protein C and anti-thrombin therapy may be instituted. Acral necrosis may require amputation.[1]

Pigmented purpuric dermatoses: They consist of a group of disorders, characterized by extravasation of red blood cells from the superficial dermal capillaries, causing hemosiderin deposition resulting in pigmented purpuric lesions, most commonly over lower extremities of young adults but also in children sometimes. The extravasation has been attributed to increased capillary fragility due to an interplay of cell-mediated hypersensitivity reaction, disturbed humoral immunity, and vascular abnormality. Venous stasis is associated in many cases. Contact with textile dyes and drugs, e.g., nonsteroidal anti-inflammatory drugs (NSAIDs), diuretics and glipizide may give rise to PPD.

CLINICAL TYPES

- *Schamberg's disease (progressive pigmented purpuric dermatosis)*:
  - Most common type of PPD; may be familial.
  - Punctate purpuric macules are seen, particularly around ankle and pretibial region.
  - Confluence of lesions may produce larger brownish macules; they are rarely pruritic.[11]
- *Majocchi's disease (purpura annularis telangiectodes)*:
  - Punctate purpuric macules are associated with annular telangiectatic patches.
  - Symmetrically distributed on lower legs with proximal spread.
  - Central clearing and peripheral spreading may lead to ring like or concentric patterns.
- *Pigmented purpuric lichenoid dermatosis of Gougerot and Blum*: Plaques are formed by coalescence of lichenoid papules on lower legs.
- *Eczematid-like purpura of Ducas and Kapetanakis*: It is a variant of Schamberg's disease with scaly, eczematous pigmented purpuric macules.
- *Lichen aureus*:
  - Grouped, rusty, golden, or violaceous papules on lower limb
  - Sometimes involvement of trunk, upper limb, and segmental distribution have been noted.[12]
- *Granulomatous PPD*: It is a rare variant, characterized by a granulomatous picture on histology.[13]

HISTOPATHOLOGICAL FEATURES

- Upper dermal capillaries show lymphocytic vasculitis.
- Upper dermis shows a perivascular or lichenoid mononuclear infiltrate.

- Lymphocytic spongiosis and exocytosis is typically seen in the eczematid-like purpura.
- Extravasation of RBC and presence of hemosiderin, either in free form or inside macrophage is the constant features in all variants.[14]

MANAGEMENT

- They do not show satisfactory response to treatment.
- Reassurance, limb elevation, and supporting hosiery are helpful.
- Topical corticosteroids might offer symptomatic relief in terms of pruritus and pigmentation.
- Pentoxifylline, psoralen plus ultraviolet A (PUVA), ascorbic acid, griseofulvin, and cyclosporine have been claimed as beneficial in some reports.

Drugs and Toxin-mediated Purpura

- Drugs may lead to thrombocytopenia, either by bone marrow toxicity or by platelet destruction.
- Common drugs leading to thrombocytopenic purpura include sulfonamides, thiazides, gold, cytotoxic agents, NSAIDs, heparin, aspirin, carbimazole, carbamazepine, phenytoin, hydralazine, cephalosporins, rifampicin, and isoniazid.
- Drugs causing purpura by vascular damage include, aspirin, allopurinol, barbiturates, furosemide, isoniazid (INH), and quinidine.
- Topical EMLA cream may damage the capillaries directly on site of application, to cause purpura.
- Alcohol, snake venom, and various food additives can also cause purpura.

Purpura from Raised Intravascular Pressure

- Bouts of cough and vomiting may cause crops of purpura over face and neck.
- Gravity and venous stasis are important factors for localized purpura on lower limbs in elderly.
- Prolonged standing and sitting with legs lowered may produce purpura on legs (orthostatic purpura).

Purpura from Diminished Vascular Support

- Aging and solar damage leads to diminished connective tissue support leading to senile or actinic purpura.
- Corticosteroids in any form (topical, systemic, or endogenous over secretion) lead to purpuric spots.
- Abnormal collagen synthesis in vitamin C deficient patients lead to perifollicular purpura in scurvy.
- Disorders of connective tissues, e.g. Ehlers–Danlos syndrome or pseudoxanthoma elasticum (PXE) may produce purpura like lesions.

Painful Bruising Syndrome (Gardner–Diamond Syndrome, Psychogenic Purpura, Autoerythrocyte Sensitization Syndrome)

- Characterized by recurrent crops of tender, extremely painful ecchymotic spots over limbs and other parts, frequently after trauma in emotionally disturbed young females.
- Occasional presence of systemic symptoms, e.g., headache, joint pain, and gastrointestinal upsets.
- Autoimmune mechanisms and increased cutaneous fibrinolytic activities have been implicated as pathogenic factors.
- Histopathology shows extravasation of RBCs, perivascular inflammatory infiltrate without vasculitis.
- Neuropsychiatric therapy has only proven beneficial in this condition.

Physical and Artifactual Purpura

- Ecchymoses occur commonly from physical trauma, indicating child abuse and domestic violence.
- Bizarre pattern of purpura and ecchymoses indicate self-inflicted trauma and cultural remedial maneuvers.
- Punctate black hemorrhagic macules on heels (talon noir) are produced by sheering stress of various sports.[1]

KEY POINTS

- Purpura is an umbrella term to encompass a variety of disorders affecting vasculature.
- Direct damage to the blood vessel or their wall, platelet dysfunction and defective coagulation are the major underlying factors leading to development of purpura.
- Thrombocytopenia due to various causes leads to purpura in a majority of cases.
- Pigmented purpuric dermatoses is a unique group of disorders affecting superficial dermal capillaries.
- Identification of the underlying cause is most important for the management of purpura.

REFERENCES

1. Bandyopadhyay D. Purpura, Vasculitis, and neutrophilic dermatoses. In: Sacchidanand S, Oberai C, Inamadar AC (Eds). IADVL Textbook of Dermatology, 4th edition. Mumbai: Bhalani Publishing House; 2016.
2. Cox NH, Piette WW. Purpura and microvascular occlusions. In: Burns T, Breathnach S, Cox N, Griffiths C (Eds). Rook's Textbook of Dermatology, 7th edition. Oxford: Blackwell Science; 2004.
3. Cines DB, Blanchette VS. Immune thrombocytopenic purpura. N Engl J Med. 2002;346:995-1008.
4. George JN, el Harake MA, Aster RH. Thrombocytopenia due to enhanced platelet destruction by immunologic mechanisms. In: Beutler E, Lichtmann MA, Coller BA, Kipps TJ (Eds).

Williams' Hematology, 5th edition. New York: McGraw-Hill; 1995. pp. 1315-55.
5. Kumar P, Clarke M (Eds). Clinical Medicine, 6th edition. Edinburgh: Elsevier Saunders; 2005.
6. McMillan R. Therapy for adults with refractory chronic immune thrombocytopenic purpura. Ann Intern Med. 1997;126:307-14.
7. Carcao MD, Zipursky A, Butchart S, Leaker M, Blanchette VS. Short course oral prednisone therapy in children presenting with acute immune thrombocytopenic purpura (immune thrombocytopenic purpura). Acta Paediatr Suppl. 1998;424:71-4.
8. Moake J. Thrombotic microangiopathies. N Engl J Med. 2002; 347:589-600.
9. Levi M, Ten Cate H. Disseminated intravascular coagulation. N Engl J Med. 1999;341:586-92.
10. Levi MM, Schmaier AH, Nagalla S. (2020). Disseminated intravascular coagulation (DIC). e-Medicine. https://emedicine.medscape.com/article/199627-overview [Last accessed February, 2021].
11. Kanwar AJ, Thami GP. Familial Schamberg's disease. Dermatology. 1999;198:175-6.
12. Mishra D, Maheshwari V. Segmental lichen aureus in a child. Int J Dermatol. 1991;30:654-5.
13. Wong WR, Kuo TT, Chen MJ, et al. Granulomatous variant of chronic pigmented purpuric dermatosis: report of two cases. Br J Dermatol. 2001;145:162-4.
14. Weedon D. Skin Pathology, 2nd edition. Edinburgh: Churchill Livingstone; 2002.

EXAMINATION QUESTIONS

1. Define purpura? How do you classify purpura clinically? Enumerate the causes of purpura.
2. Write in brief about pigmented purpuric dermatosis.
3. How do you investigate a case of purpura?

84 CHAPTER

Leg Ulcer

Falguni Nag

INTRODUCTION

Leg ulcers represent a break of the skin, sometimes extending through the dermis or deeper structure. A chronic leg ulcer (CLU) is defined as one lasting for 6 weeks or more.[1] Prevalence of ulcers was reported to be 0.1–1%,[2] and 3–5% in the population over 65 years of age.[3]

Incidence of ulceration is rising as a result of the aging population[4] and increased risk factors for atherosclerotic occlusion such as smoking, obesity, and diabetes, etc.[5,6] It is more common in female.[1] Although most leg ulcers are caused by venous insufficiency (45–60%), arterial insufficiency (10–20%), diabetes (15–25%), and combinations of these are also well-known etiological factors (10–15%).[5,6] Less frequent causes are infection, vasculitis, and malignancy **(Table 1)**.

VENOUS ULCER

Overall incidence of venous ulcer is 0.2%. It is an age-related disease, mainly affecting older women.[1] Lipodermatosclerosis (LPDS) may be associated with venous ulcer which precedes ulceration.

Pathogenesis

Hippocrates was the first to note the association between varicose veins and ulceration.

Venous ulceration is caused by increased pressure in the venous system. The main cause of venous hypertension is insufficiency of the valves in the deep venous system and the lower perforating veins. Intact valves but absent muscle contraction may also cause edema and ulceration, a condition known as dependency syndrome. Valve insufficiency is usually acquired as in post-thrombotic syndrome or rarely congenital.[3]

Clinical Features

Venous insufficiency presents with lower leg edema, varicose eczema, LPDS, hyperpigmentation, hyperkeratosis,

TABLE 1: Causes[3] of leg ulceration.

Venous	• Venous insufficiency and dependency • Valve incompetence (post-thrombotic, congenital)
Arterial	Peripheral arterial disease (arteriosclerosis) • Arterial thrombosis • Embolism • Hypertension (Martorell ulcer) • Mixed (venous ulcer with peripheral arterial disease) • Thromboangiitis obliterans (Buerger disease) • Raynaud phenomenon, scleroderma • Physical or chemical injury, burn wounds • Pressure (decubitus), pressure by shoes, compression bandages
Infectious diseases	Erysipelas, ecthyma, ulcerating pyoderma, gas gangrene *(Clostridium)*, ecthyma gangrenosum *(Pseudomonas)*, toe-web infection, atypical mycobacteria, eumycetoma/mycetoma, osteomyelitis, tropical ulcer
Neuropathic diseases	Diabetes, leprosy, alcohol neuropathy, tabes dorsalis, syringomyelia, spina bifida, paraplegia, paresis, multiple sclerosis, poliomyelitis
Vasculitis	• Small vessel-leukocytoclastic vasculitis, microscopic polyangiitis, Wegener's granulomatosis, Churg–Strauss disease, Henoch-Schönlein purpura, essential cryoglobulinemic vasculitis, erythema induratum (Bazin), livedo reticularis, livedo vasculitis • Polyarteritis nodosa
Hematological	Sickle cell anemia, polycythemia, leukemia, myeloma, lupus anticoagulant, anticardiolipin (antiphospholipid syndrome) antithrombin III deficiency, protein C or S deficiency
Metabolic diseases	Diabetes mellitus, calcinosis cutis, homocystinuria
Others	Basal cell carcinoma, squamous cell carcinoma, malignant melanoma, metastasis, Marjolin ulcer, pyoderma gangrenosum, pemphigoid and other bullous diseases, systemic lupus erythematosus, scleroderma, trench foot, lymphedema, perniosis (chilblains), rheumatoid arthritis

and atrophie blanche preceding ulceration.[7] The ulcer is characteristically situated on the medial aspect of the lower leg, the "gaiter" region and usually do not develop initially below the level of the malleoli or in the foot unless complicated by livedoid vasculitis or arterial disease.[1]

Ankle-brachial pressure index (ABPI) ≤ 0.9 is defined as peripheral arterial disease (PAD).[1] Clinically diagnosed venous ulcer patient may have associated PAD and the ulcer may be called as mixed ulcer due to venous and arterial pathology.

Treatment

The mainstay of treatment and mode of prevention is the control of edema by avoiding prolonged leg dependency and adequate compression therapy.[6] Elastic compression stocking is more effective in daily practice than standard compression therapy with bandages.[1]

Dressing with warm tap water or sterile saline is usually sufficient.[1] Wound debridement by removal of slough, eschar is important.

Systemic antibiotics are used only when there is clear evidence of infection.

Skin grafting is indicated when the ulcers are large in size, of a prolonged duration and refractory to conservative treatment.

Surgical intervention for incompetent communicating/perforator veins in the setting of normal deep venous system is only helpful to reduce the recurrence of ulcer.[1]

ARTERIAL ULCERATION

Arterial ulceration or ischemic ulceration is due to a reduced arterial blood supply to the lower limb that causes tissue hypoxia and tissue damage. Atherosclerosis is responsible for >90% of all arterial disease in the Western world. It affects 5% of men over the age of 50 years, of which 10% may develop critical limb ischemia.[1] Other causes include diabetes, thromboangiitis, and vasculitis, some of which may predispose to the atheroma formation. Thrombotic and atheroembolic episodes lead to tissue damage and ulcer formation.[8] Modifiable risk factors for peripheral vascular disease include smoking, hyperlipidemia, hypertension, diabetes, and obesity. There may be history of angina, myocardial infarction, and stroke[8] Most common presenting features are intermittent claudication, ischemic ulceration, and skin infarction.[1] Arterial ulceration typically occurs over the tip of toes, heels, and bony prominences of the foot. The ulcer appears "punched out," with well-demarcated edges and a pale, nongranulating, often necrotic base. The surrounding skin may be cool to touch, hairless, thin, shiny, and with thickened toenails. There may be a decreased or absent pulse in the dorsalis pedis and posterior tibial arteries.[8]

Presence of palpable peripheral pulse does not rule out the PADs **(Fig. 1)**.

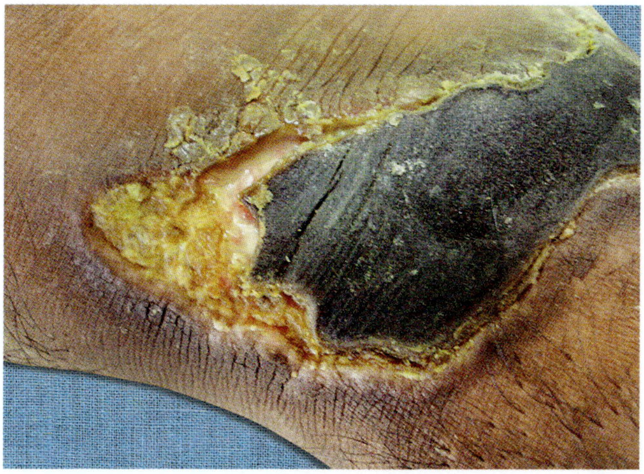

Fig. 1: Arterial ulcer.

Management

Cessation of smoking, control of diabetes, hypertension, hyperlipidemia, and treatment of infection are essential component of management. Reconstructive surgery for diffuse disease or angioplasty for localized stenosis, is the most common surgical intervention for ulcer healing. Operative indications for chronic ischemia include non-healing ulceration, gangrene, rest pain, and progression of claudication.[8]

In patients with critical limb ischemia, when revascularization therapy is not possible conservative treatment with analgesics, vasodilators, and/or anticoagulants may be used.

THROMBOANGIITIS OBLITERANS

Thromboangiitis obliterans (TAO) or Buerger's disease is an episodic inflammatory and thrombo-occlusive vascular disease of unknown origin. Distal vessels and nerves within the neurovascular bundles are involved in the legs and occasionally in arms. Male gender and genetic background, cigarette smoking, infectious agents; and environmental factors such as chronic anxiety and mental stress as a consequence of low socioeconomic status are the main predisposing factor.[9]

The diagnosis of TAO is difficult due to the lack of specific clinical, radiological, histopathological features, and a lack of diagnostic criteria. Claudication in the arch of the foot is an early sign and even specific to TAO.[10] The traditional diagnosis of Buerger's disease is based on five criteria (history of smoking, onset before the age of 50 years, infrapopliteal arterial occlusive disease, phlebitis migrans, and absence of atherosclerotic risk factors other than smoking). Angiographic usually shows "corkscrew or "tree roots" pattern **(Fig. 2)**.

Treatment

The aim of treatment is to stop smoking to prevent ulceration and to hasten the period of ulcer healing, without major

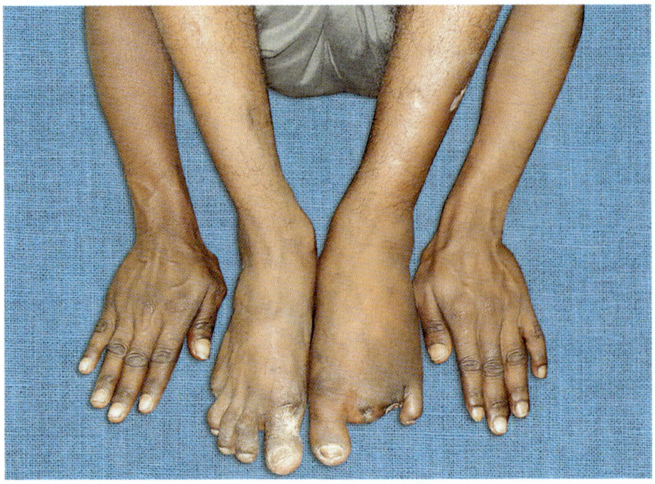

Fig. 2: Buerger ulcer.

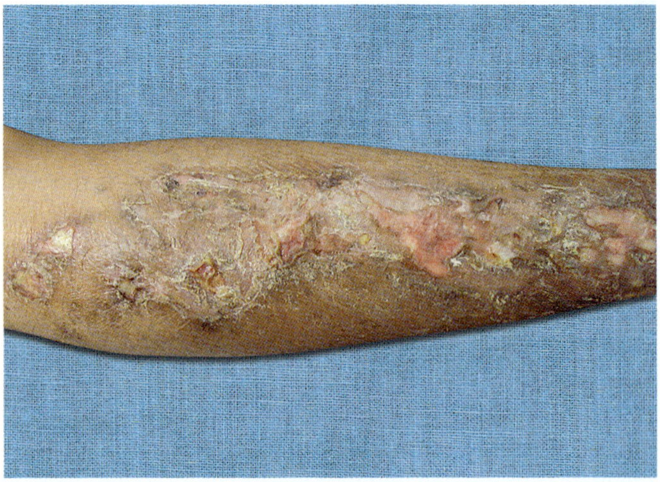

Fig. 3: Traumatic ulcer.

amputation, as ulceration and gangrene in TAO are limited to the most distal part of the limbs. Surgical or chemical sympathectomy sometime needed in nonresponsive cases.

DIABETIC FOOT ULCER

Diabetic patients may develop foot ulcer. Distal sensorimotor and autonomic neuropathy along with arterial insufficiency and decreased ability to fight infection predisposes to ulcer formation.

In the neuropathic type, ulcers commonly develop on the plantar surface of the foot, toes, and in neuroischemic type around the edges of the foot, including tips of the toes and the back of the heel, and are associated with trauma or from unsuitable shoes.[1]

The main principles of treatment are relief of any pressure at the wound site, surgical debridement, control of infection, and strict control of glucose levels. Pressure relief may be accomplished by total contact casting.

TRAUMATIC ULCER

Ulceration due to trauma, in the absence of proper management, may present with chronic non-healing leg ulcer **(Fig. 3)**.

TROPHIC ULCER DUE TO LEPROSY

Trophic ulcer due to leprosy mostly located on the plantar region of the foot, primarily on weight bearing areas, metatarsal head area, the fifth metatarsal bone and calcaneus area **(Fig. 4)**.

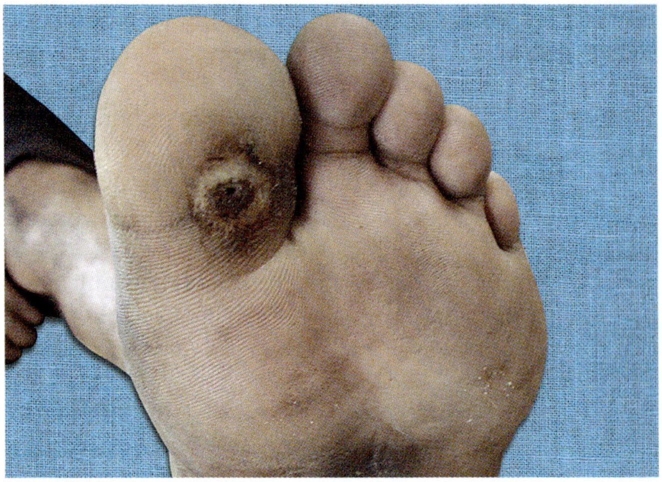

Fig. 4: Trophic ulcer.

MYCETOMA

Mycetoma mainly affects the feet and lower extremities, present worldwide, and endemic in tropical and subtropical regions. Inoculation commonly follows minor trauma, more among the barefoot-walking populations, and common among adult males. The infection is caused by fungus (eumycetoma) or a bacterium (actinomycetoma) and generally remains localized, causing cutaneous and subcutaneous tissue swelling, nodule formation, and drainage through sinus tracts. Actinomycetomas are responsive to antibiotics, but eumycetomas require surgical excision along with antifungals.

UNCOMMON CAUSES OF ULCERATION

Vasculitis

Cutaneous vasculitis may present as purpura, or skin infarction leading to ulceration. Cutaneous ulceration is usually caused by small- to medium-vessel vasculitis.

Martorell Ulcer

It is seen in patients with prolonged, severe hypertension. The ulceration is secondary to tissue ischemia caused by increased vascular resistance. The ulcers are usually located at the lower limb, above the ankle region, contain black necrosis, and are extremely painful with normal distal arterial pulsations. Management consists of treatment of hypertension.

Pyoderma Gangrenosum

It is primarily clinical diagnosis of exclusion but may be associated with specific features on histology. The patient often has a history of a painful sterile pustule or nodule with surrounding erythema, which eventually ruptures and ulcerates. The ulcer has a characteristic erythematous or violaceous overhanging edge.[3] The wound bed is often purulent and may extend to muscle. Pyoderma gangrenosum is associated with underlying active or quiescent systemic disease; these include inflammatory bowel disease, seronegative rheumatoid arthritis, and lymphoproliferative diseases.

APPROACH TO DIAGNOSIS OF A CASE OF CHRONIC LEG ULCER

History

How did ulcer start? (trauma, pressure, etc.), duration, recurrence, previous treatments history (medical or surgery), history of prolonged standing or sitting.

Risk Factors

- Varicose vein, prior venous ulceration, past surgery, deep vein thrombosis (DVT), obesity, congestive cardiac failure, and traumatic injury are important for venous ulcer.
- Peripheral, vascular disease, angina, ischemic heart disease, acute myocardial infarction, diabetes mellitus, hypertension, dyslipidemia, hyper-homocystenemia, antiphospholipid antibody, and smoking are important for ischemic ulcer.
- Leprosy and diabetic neuropathy are important for trophic ulcer.

Nature of Pain

- Patient with venous ulcer feels more pain, aching or heaviness in leg, when the leg is in dependent position.
- Patient with ischemic ulcer feels more pain in the leg raised position.
- Intermittent claudication, rest pain and night pain may be associated with ischemic ulcer.
- Numbness, tingling more in favor of diabetic ulcer.

Examination

Sign

- Pigmentation (brown staining), varicose eczema, contact dermatitis, itching over vein, atrophie blanche, ankle flare, edema, indurations (hard feeling in skin), LPDS, ulcer over malleolus, ulcer within Gaiter area associated with venous ulcer.
- Dusky skin color on foot, cold foot, loss of hair on leg/atrophic, shiny skin shin, muscle wasting, ulcer on toe or lateral malleolus, gangrene on toe or foot leg blanche when leg raised, thickened toe nails, absent or diminished pulse more in favor of ischemic ulcer.
- Trophic changes, fissure, callus, warm temperature, ulcer over ball of great toe or heel, decreased sensitivity to touch more in favor of diabetic ulcer or ulcer due to leprosy.

Ulcer Description

- Site of ulcer (medial malleoli/lateral malleoli/digital/planter/other)
- Measurement depth (superficial/dermal/deep dermal/tendon exposed/bone exposed)
- Appearance of ulcer bed (black/yellow/red/pink/green)
- Type of tissue in ulcer bed (necrotic/sloughy/granulating/epithelializing/infected)
- Edges of ulcer (shallow/rolled out/punched out)
- Sign of infection (redness/inflamed/purulent)

Condition of Surrounding Skin

- Venous dermatitis (erythematic/scaling/crusting) and hemosiderosis (brown staining)
- Lipodermatosclerosis, edema (pitting/nonpitting), scaring from previous ulcer, cellulitis
- Shiny/taut/thin dry skin, pallor, hair loss
- Atrophy of subcutaneous tissue
- Temperature (decreased/cold)
- Necrosis/eschar/gangrene

Limb Examination

- Peripheral edema
- Peripheral pulses
- Nerve examination (thick/tender)
- Ankle-brachial pressure index.

Laboratories

- Routine blood examination
- Consideration of skin biopsy
- Doppler study
- *Others investigations*:
    - Investigation for hyperviscosity syndrome: Serum homocysteine assay, anticardiolipin antibody, antiphospholipid antibody, lupus anticoagulant, antithrombin III function
    - Rheumatoid arthritis (RA) factor
    - Antinuclear antibody (ANA)
    - X-ray (to exclude osteomyelitis).

KEY POINTS

- Chronic ulceration of the lower leg including the foot is a common condition, causing pain, social discomfort, and morbidity.

- The diagnosis is mostly clinical aided with thorough clinical examination of the ulcer along with detailed history.
- *ABPI* and *Doppler study* are helpful to distinguish any arterial compromise not only in ischemic ulcer but also in long-standing venous ulcer.

REFERENCES

1. Mortimer PS, Burnand KG, Neumann HAM. Diseases of the Veins and Arteries: Leg ulcers. In: Burns T, Breathnach S, Cox N, Griffiths C (Editors). Rook's Textbook of Dermatology, 8th edition. West Sussex: Wiley-Blackwell; 2010;p 47.1-47.58.
2. Graham ID, Harrison MB,Nelson EA, Lorimer K, Fisher A. Prevalence of lower-limb ulceration: a systematic review of prevalence studies. Adv Skin Wound Care. 2003;16:305-16.
3. Mekkes JR, Loots MA, Van Der Wal AC, Bos JD. Causes, investigation and treatment of leg ulceration. Br J Dermatol. 2003;148:388-401.
4. Margolis DJ, Bilker W, Santanna J, Baumgarten M. Venous leg ulcer: incidence and prevalence in the elderly. J Am Acad Dermatol. 2002;46: 381-6.
5. Liedberg E, Persson BM. Increased incidence of lower limb amputation for arterial occlusive disease. Acta Orthop Scand. 1983;54:230-4.
6. Bello YM, Phillips TJ. Management of venous ulcers. J Cutan Med Surg. 1998;3:6-12.
7. Valencia IC, Falabella A, Kirsner RS, Eaglstein WH. Chronic venous insufficiency and venous leg ulceration. J Am Acad Dermatol. 2001;44:401-21.
8. Grey JE, Harding KG, Enoch S. Venous and arterial leg ulcers. BMJ. 2006;332:347-50.
9. Fazeli B, Rezaee SA. A review on thromboangiitis obliterans pathophysiology: thrombosis and angiitis, which is to blame? Vascular. 2011;19:141-53.
10. Fiessinger JN. Thromboangiitis obliterans or Buerger's disease: challenges for the rheumatologist. Rheumatology. 2007;46:192-9.

EXAMINATION QUESTION

1. How will you approach to diagnose and manage a case of chronic leg ulcer?

85 CHAPTER

Vasculitis

Snehal Siddhesh Kalantri, Aarti Sarda

INTRODUCTION

Vasculitis can be defined as inflammation of vessel walls with reactive damage of mural structures. This leads to loss of vessel integrity, which may lead to bleeding and thrombosis resulting in downstream ischemia (particularly with end arteries) and necrosis. The vasculitides are often serious and sometimes fatal diseases that require prompt recognition, complete evaluation of organs at risk, and therapy. The only clue may be in form of dermatologic manifestation. Patients with skin vasculitis are at risk for vasculitis involving other organs. This chapter will focus mainly on cutaneous manifestations of various vasculitis.

ETIOPATHOGENESIS

Cutaneous vasculitis occurs due to inflammatory processes that occur in and damage small- or medium-sized blood vessels in the skin. Small blood vessels are capillaries, postcapillary venules, and nonmuscular arterioles in the superficial and mid-dermis (<50 μm). Medium-sized vessels consist of 50–150 μm vessels with muscular walls in the deep dermis and subcutis.[1] A wide variety of disorders can lead to the development of cutaneous vasculitis. It is estimated that infections, medications, connective tissue diseases, and malignancy account for 23%, 20%, 12%, and 4% of cases of cutaneous vasculitis, respectively.[2] In contrast, the primary systemic vasculitides (granulomatosis with polyangiitis, polyarteritis nodosa, microscopic polyangiitis, and eosinophilic granulomatosis with polyangiitis) are less common causes of cutaneous vasculitis, less than 4% of cases of vasculitis. Recent classification of vasculitis is given in **Box 1**.[3]

BOX 1: Classification of vasculitis according to Chapel Hill Consensus Conference on Nomenclature of Vasculitis 2012.

Large vessel vasculitis:
- Takayasu arteritis
- Giant cell arteritis

Medium vessel vasculitis:
- Polyarteritis nodosa
- Kawasaki disease

Small vessel vasculitis:
- *ANCA associated:*
  - Microscopic polyangiitis
  - Wegener's granulomatosis
  - Churg–Strauss disease
- *Immune complex mediated:*
  - Anti-glomerular basement membrane (Anti-GBM) disease
  - Cryoglobulinemic vasculitis
  - IGA vasculitis (Henoch–Schönlein)
  - Hypocomplementemic urticarial vasculitis

Variable vessel vasculitis:
- Behçet's syndrome
- Cogan's syndrome

Single organ vasculitis:
- Cutaneous leukocytoclastic vasculitis
- Cutaneous arteritis
- Primary CNS vasculitis
- Isolated aortitis
- Others

Vasculitis with systemic disease:
- Lupus vasculitis
- Rheumatoid vasculitis
- Sarcoid vasculitis
- Others

Vasculitis with probable etiology:
- Hepatitis C-associated cryoglobulinemic vasculitis
- Hepatitis B-associated vasculitis
- Syphilis-associated aortitis
- Drug-associated immune complex-mediated vasculitis
- Drug-associated ANCA positive vasculitis
- Cancer-associated vasculitis
- Others

(ANCA: antineutrophil cytoplasmic antibody; CNS: central nervous system; IgA: immunoglobulin A)

COMMON CUTANEOUS FEATURES OF VASCULITIS

Due to Involvement of Small Vessel

- *Petechiae*: Petechiae are nonblanchable and nonpalpable pinpoint macules (less than a few millimeters in diameter) that result from capillary inflammation and red blood cell extravasation.
- *Palpable purpura*: These are raised, nonblanchable (on diascopy) caused due to leakage of blood from vasculature into interstitium.
- *Hemorrhagic bullae*: Involvement of small vessels throughout the dermis can result in necrosis of overlying tissue and extravasation of red blood cells and thus hemorrhagic bullae.

- *Urticarial plaques*: Lesions of urticarial vasculitis usually persist for more than 24 hours, and frequently are associated with a burning sensation or pain rather than pruritus. Lesions may contain purpuric areas and can resolve with hyperpigmentation.
- Superficial ulcers

Due to Involvement of Medium Size Vessels

Subcutaneous Nodules

These are formed due to intense inflammation of medium-sized vessels. Deep ulceration or digital necrosis occurs due to reduced skin perfusion.

Livedo Reticularis

It presents as a localized or widespread patchy, reticulated, and vascular network with a red-blue or violaceous hue. It occurs due to reduced blood flow. It can in conditions other than vasculitis, such as vasculopathy due to vasospasm, hypercoagulable states, thrombosis, increased blood viscosity, or embolic phenomena.

Livedo Racemosa

It presents with a more abrupt and broken vascular pattern than livedo reticularis. It is strongly associated with Sneddon's syndrome, a nonvasculitic disorder characterized by livedoid skin lesions and cerebrovascular accidents, but may also occur in vasculitis and other disorders.[4]

DISTRIBUTION OF LESIONS

Distribution is most commonly symmetrical and on the lower legs, dependent areas, or on areas of constrictive clothing due to increased hydrostatic pressure in these sites.

SYMPTOMS

The skin lesions are often asymptomatic, but may be associated with pruritus, burning sensations, or pain.

Course

Course is variable; some patients experience a single, limited episode of vasculitis (mostly vasculitis secondary to medications or infection), while other have relapsing or course.

Duration of Symptoms

It ranges from several days to decades.

DIFFERENTIAL DIAGNOSIS OF CUTANEOUS VASCULITIS[5]

- Pigmented purpuric dermatoses
- Macular purpura due to chronic sun exposure, glucocorticoid therapy, trauma, or anticoagulants
- Inflammatory disorders on the lower extremities or other dependent sites (e.g., stasis dermatitis)
- Arthropod bites

LESS COMMON DIFFERENTIALS

- Scurvy (perifollicular hemorrhage)
- Platelet deficiencies or dysfunction (petechiae or macular purpura)
- Hypercoagulable and thrombotic disorders (noninflammatory retiform purpura)
- Cholesterol emboli (noninflammatory retiform purpura, digital gangrene, and livedo reticularis)
- Septic emboli (petechiae on the distal extremities and noninflammatory retiform purpura)
- Systemic amyloidosis (periorbital and pinch purpura)
- Strongyloidiasis (periumbilical purpura)
- Purpura fulminans
- Livedoid vasculopathy

APPROACH TO A CASE OF CUTANEOUS VASCULITIS

Clinical Assessment

History to Rule Out Cause

- Drug intake
- Symptoms of infections particularly upper respiratory tract
- Symptoms and risk factors for hepatitis

History to Rule Out Systemic Involvement

- Fatigue, chills, and night sweats
- Myalgias or arthralgias
- Tea-colored urine or gross hematuria
- Abdominal pain or melena
- Chest pain
- Dyspnea, cough, or hemoptysis
- New-onset or worsening asthma
- Peripheral neuropathy

INVESTIGATIONS

Biopsy

Biopsies should be performed in all patients with lesions suggestive of vasculitis to confirm diagnosis and to differentiate between different forms.

Histopathologic Diagnostic Criteria

Small vessels require two out of three of the following criteria for a definitive diagnosis of vasculitis:[2]

- Angiocentric and/or angioinvasive inflammatory infiltrates

- Disruption and/or destruction of vessel walls by the inflammatory infiltrate
- Fibrinoid necrosis

Medium-sized vessels require both the criteria to confirm vasculitis:
- Inflammatory infiltrate infiltrating the muscular vessel wall
- Fibrinoid necrosis

Other histopathologic findings that suggest but are not diagnostic for vasculitis are extravasated erythrocytes, nuclear debris (leukocytoclasia), necrosis of eccrine glands, endothelial cell damage swelling or necrosis, cutaneous ulceration, infarction, or necrosis.

Findings that suggest particular forms of vasculitis:
- Granulomas in Wegener's granulomatosis or Churg-Strauss syndrome
- Interface dermatitis in vasculitis associated with connective tissue disorders

Timing of Biopsy

Lesions that are between 24 and 48 hours old are best to demonstrate findings of vasculitis.

Site

Biopsies from most of the lesions should be taken from within the lesion while biopsies of livedo racemosa should be taken from within the center of an erythematous ring.[1] Biopsies of ulcers should be taken from the edge.

Type

Punch biopsies 4 mm in diameter are sufficient for petechial lesions, palpable purpura, or urticarial lesions. Nodules, ulcers, or livedo racemosa require large punch biopsies (8–10 mm) or excisional wedge biopsies.

Direct Immunofluorescence Studies

It should always be performed when facilities are available. Direct immunofluorescence (DIF) is particularly important for the diagnosis of immunoglobulin A vasculitis (Henoch-Schönlein purpura).

Direct immunofluorescence is also of value for immune complex-mediated vasculitides from pauci-immune vasculitis.

Obtaining the Specimen

Ideally, DIF should be performed on a lesion that is less than 24 hours old. Specimens from vasculitic lesions should be taken from within the lesions. Specimens can be placed in Michel's transport medium or normal saline or can be flash-frozen with liquid nitrogen; it should not be put in formalin. Tissue placed in saline must be processed within 24 hours.

ADDITIONAL STUDIES

Initial Studies

- Complete blood count with differential and platelets
- Liver function tests
- Blood urea nitrogen (BUN)/creatinine
- Urinalysis with microscopy

Secondary Studies

When the etiology is unclear, the following testing can be done:
- Hepatitis B and C serologies
- Serum complement levels (CH50, C3, and C4)
- Antinuclear antibody (ANA) and anti-double stranded deoxyribonucleic acid (dsDNA), anti-Ro, anti-La, anti-RNP, and anti-Smith antibodies
- Rheumatoid factor
- Serum cryoglobulins
- Antineutrophil cytoplasmic antibodies (ANCAs)
- Serum and urine protein electrophoresis and immunofixation
- Human immunodeficiency virus (HIV) antibody

In patients with pulmonary symptoms, chest radiographs should be done. High-resolution computed tomography (HRCT) can be done for further evaluation.

Evaluation for Malignancy

It should be done in suspected cases with no known cause for vasculitis and signs and symptoms suggestive of malignancy.

Evaluation for Vasculitis due to Levamisole-contaminated Cocaine

Antineutrophil cytoplasmic antibodies [perinuclear ANCA (pANCA) or both pANCA and cytoplasmic ANCA (cANCA)], antiphospholipid antibodies, and leukopenia or neutropenia are frequently detected in patients with vasculitis or vasculopathy due to levamisole-contaminated cocaine. Urine toxicology testing for cocaine and testing for levamisole in serum or urine can be done.[6]

MANAGEMENT

Management depends on diagnosis of type of vasculitis, presence of systemic involvement, and disease severity. Underlying infection should be treated. Triggering drugs should be stopped. Underlying malignancy or rheumatological disease is to be treated. Systemic involvement needs a multidisciplinary approach. Treatment of individual disease is mentioned in respective tables.

Features of different vasculitis with cutaneous features are discussed in **Tables 1 to 3**.

TABLE 1: Medium vessel vasculitis with cutaneous findings.

	PAN	*cPAN*	*NV*	*Kawasaki*
Synonym	Kussmaul-Maier disease, necrotizing arteritis		Erythema induratum	Mucocutaneous lymph node syndrome, infantile polyarteritis
Vessel size	Medium	Medium	Medium	Medium
Triggering factors associated	Hepatitis B	Hepatitis B	Tuberculosis	Unidentified infection
Cutaneous findings	• Nodules • Ulcers • Livedo racemosa • Infarcts	• Nodules • Ulcers • Livedo racemosa • Infarcts	• Nodules • Ulcers • Lower extremity edema	• Redness and edema of palms and soles • Perianal desquamation • Dry-cracked lips • Strawberry tongue
Systemic features and involvement	• Weight loss • Myalgia • Fatigue • Neuropathy • Hypertension • Decrease renal perfusion	• Weight loss, myalgia • Fatigue • Neuropathy	Tuberculosis features	• Unresponsive fever • Cervical lymphadenopathy • Conjunctivitis • Reactivation of BCG scar • Coronary artery disease in 30% cases
Important laboratory studies	Negative ANCA	Negative ANCA	• Chest X-ray • Mantoux	• Diagnosis is clinical • ECG for cardiac involvement
DIF	Negative	Negative	Negative	Negative
Treatment	• NSAIDs • Systemic steroids, antivirals, if hepatitis present • Methotrexate *Second line:* • Cyclophosphamide • Plasma exchange *Third line:* • Rituximab	• NSAIDs • Systemic steroids	ATT	*First line:* • IVIgG (2 g/kg) and aspirin *Second line:* • High-dose steroids

(ANCA: antineutrophil cytoplasmic antibody; ATT: antitubercular therapy; BCG: bacillus Calmette-Guérin; cPAN: cutaneous polyarteritis nodosa; DIF: direct immunofluorescence; ECG: electrocardiogram; IVIgG: intravenous immunoglobulin G; NSAIDs: nonsteroidal anti-inflammatory drugs; NV: nodular vasculitis; PAN: polyarteritis nodosa)

TABLE 2: Small vessel vasculitis.

	WG	*CSS*	*MPA*	*CV*
Synonym	Granulomatosis with polyangiitis	• Eosinophilic granulomatosis with polyangiitis • Allergic granulomatous angitis	Microscopic polyangiitis	Type 2 and type 3 cryoglobulinemia
Vessel size	Medium and small	Medium and small	Medium and small	Medium and small
Possible triggering factors	*Staphylococcus aureus*, farming, and occupational solvents	Not known	Farming	• Hepatitis C • Sjögren syndrome • B-cell lymphomas
Cutaneous findings	• Nodules • Ulcers • Infarcts • Livedo racemosa • Palpable purpura • Saddle nose deformity • Strawberry gums	• Nodules • Ulcers • Infarcts • Livedo racemosa • Palpable purpura	• Nodules • Ulcers • Infarcts • Livedo racemosa • Palpable purpura	• Nodules • Ulcers • Infarcts • Livedo racemosa • Palpable purpura
Systemic features and involvement	• Weight loss, myalgia • Fatigue • Neuropathy • Glomerulonephritis • Necrotizing granulomatous	*Three phases:* 1. Allergies and asthma and nasal polyps 2. Peripheral blood eosinophilia 3. Vasculitis weight loss, myalgia	• Weight loss, myalgia • Fatigue • Neuropathy • Alveolar hemorrhage • Glomerulonephritis	• Weight loss, myalgia • Fatigue • Neuropathy • Membranoproliferative glomerulonephritis

Contd...

Contd...

	WG	*CSS*	*MPA*	*CV*
	• Inflammation of respiratory tract	• Fatigue • Neuropathy • Allergies asthma • Heart and GI involvement (especially if pANCA –) • Glomerulonephritis and neuropathy (especially if pANCA +)		
Important laboratory studies	• cANCA positive • Positive PR3 • *HP:* Leukocytoclastic vasculitis and granulomas	• pANCA + • MPO + • Eosinophilia • *HP:* – Eosinophilic infiltrates, extravascular granulomas – Vasculitis of both arteries and veins	• pANCA + • MPO + • No eosinophilia • *HP:* – Segmental vascular necrosis – Leukocytoclastic vasculitis – No granulomas	• Hepatitis C + • Cryoglobulins+ • *HP:* Pandermal leukocytoclastic vasculitis
DIF	Negative	Negative	Negative	Positive IgM
Treatment	*First line:* • Cyclophosphamide • Methotrexate with steroids, • Plasmapheresis in patients with renal crisis *Second line:* • Rituximab *Third line:* • IVIgG	• Localized disease • Oral steroids • Systemic disease • Pulsed cyclophosphamide • Refractory cases rituximab	• Oral and IV steroids • Cyclophosphamide • Rituximab	• If hepatitis C positive • Antiviral • If negative • Steroids and immunosuppressants

(ANCA: antineutrophil cytoplasmic antibody; cANCA: cytoplasmic ANCA; CSS: Churg-Strauss syndrome; CV: cryoglobulinemic vasculitis; DIF: direct immunofluorescence; HP: hypertrophic pachymeningitis; IgM: immunoglobulin M; IV: intravenous; MPA: microscopic polyangiitis; MPO: myeloperoxidase; pANCA: perinuclear ANCA; RV: rheumatoid arthritis; WG: Wegener's granulomatosis)

TABLE 3: Small vessel vasculitis continued.

	HSP	*UV*	*CSSV*	*EED*
Synonym	• IgA vasculitis • Anaphylactoid purpura • Hemorrhagic vasculitis	McDuffie syndrome	• Hypersensitivity vasculitis • Cutaneous leukocytoclastic vasculitis	Burys disease
Vessel	Small	Small	Small	Small
Triggering factor	*Streptococcus*	May be SLE Pyogenic infections	Infections, drugs, malignancy Exercise	Infections Connective tissue disorders
Cutaneous features	• Urticaria • Papules • Purpura • Petechiae	• Urticaria • Papules • Purpura • Petechiae	• Urticaria • Papules • Purpura • Petechiae	• Symmetrical red violaceous papules and nodules on dorsum of hands and feet • Scaring
Systemic features	• Arthritis • Abdominal pain • Renal involvement	• Fatigue • Fever • Angioedema • Arthralgia • Abdominal pain • Raynaud's phenomenon • Uveitis • Obstructive lung disease	No systemic involvement	None
Laboratory studies	• Urine analysis for renal involvement • *HP:* Leukocytoclastic vasculitis	• Low compliment levels • *HP:* Leukocytoclastic vasculitis	• To rule out triggering factors • *HP:* Leukocytoclastic vasculitis	• ANCA positive in some cases • *HP:* – Leukocytoclastic vasculitis in initial stage – Late stages—fibrosis and macrophages

Contd...

Contd...

	HSP	*UV*	*CSSV*	*EED*
DIF	Perivascular IgA	IgG, C3, and fibrin can be seen along the DEJ	IgG, IgM, C3, IgA	IgG, IgA, and fibrin
Treatment	• Supportive care • Systemic steroids • Other immunosuppressants	*First line:* • Systemic steroids *Second line:* • Dapsone • Hydroxychloroquine *Third line:* • MMF • Cyclophosphamide	*First line:* • Oral steroids *Second line:* • Colchicine • Dapsone *Third line:* • Azathioprine • Methotrexate • Cyclosporine • Cyclophosphamide	*First line:* • Dapsone *Second line:* • Niacinamide • Topical or intralesional steroids *Third line:* • Immunosuppressants

(ANCA: antineutrophil cytoplasmic antibody; CSVV: cutaneous small vessel vasculitis; DEJ: dermoepidermal junction; DIF: direct immunofluorescence; EED: erythema elevatum diutinum; HP: hypertrophic pachymeningitis; HSP: Henoch-Schönlein purpura; Ig: immunoglobulin; MMF: mycophenolate mofetil; SLE: systemic lupus erythematosus; UV: urticarial vasculitis)

KEY POINTS

- Infections and medications are the most common etiologies of cutaneous small vessel vasculitis.
- Careful history and physical examination is to be done to identify the type of vasculitis and systemic involvement.
- Biopsies of lesions of cutaneous vasculitis should be taken from a lesion that is 24–48 hours old.
- Histopathologic features of vasculitis include fibrinoid necrosis and an inflammatory infiltrate invading or damaging the vessel wall.
- DIF offers valuable clues for diagnosis, and should be performed when possible.
- Appropriate initial laboratory studies for patients with cutaneous vasculitis include a complete blood count, liver function tests, blood urea nitrogen and creatinine, and urinalysis with microscopy. Additional tests are performed if the cause of vasculitis is unclear or if systemic involvement is suspected.
- Treatment of vasculitis depends on type of vasculitis and extent of systemic involvement.

REFERENCES

1. Carlson JA. The histological assessment of cutaneous vasculitis. Histopathology. 2010;56:3-23.
2. Carlson JA, Ng BT, Chen KR. Cutaneous vasculitis update: diagnostic criteria, classification, epidemiology, etiology, pathogenesis, evaluation and prognosis. Am J Dermatopathol. 2005;27:504-28.
3. Jennette JC, Falk RJ, Bacon PA, Basu N, Cid MC, Ferrario F, et al. 2012 revised International Chapel Hill Consensus Conference Nomenclature of Vasculitides. Arthritis Rheum. 2013;65: 1-11.
4. Dhadly M, Dean SM, Eberhardt RT. Cutaneous changes in peripheral vascular arterial disease. In: Wolff K, Goldsmith LA, Katz SI (Eds). Fitzpatrick's Dermatology in General Medicine, 7th edition. New York: McGraw Hill; 2008. p. 1667.
5. Piette W. Purpura: mechanisms and differential diagnosis. In: Bolognia JL, Jorizzo JL, Rapini RP (Eds). Dermatology, 2nd edition. Spain: Elsevier; 2008. p. 321.
6. Gross RL, Brucker J, Bahce-Altuntas A, Abadi MA, Lipoff J, Kotlyar D, et al. A novel cutaneous vasculitis syndrome induced by levamisole-contaminated cocaine. Clin Rheumatol. 2011;30:1385-92.

EXAMINATION QUESTIONS

1. Classify vasculitis. How do you differentiate it from vasculopathy? Describe approach to a case of vasculitis.
2. Describe ANCA-associated vasculitis.
3. Write a short note on Kawasaki disease.
4. Discuss Henoch-Schönlein purpura. How will you approach a case with palpable purpura?
5. Write a short note on urticarial vasculitis.
6. Describe the HPE of vasculitis.

86 CHAPTER

Diseases of Arteries Veins and Lymphatics

Kinnor Das, Surajit Gorai

INTRODUCTION

The main functions of cutaneous circulation are nutrition and thermoregulation. Pathology of vascular system can have myriad of presentations. Alteration in cutaneous vasculature can be caused by underlying systemic disorder(s) as well.

THROMBOANGIITIS OBLITERANS[1-4]

Thromboangiitis obliterans is a nonatherosclerotic segmental inflammatory disease of medium sized and small vessels.

They are classified as a type of vasculitis.

Etiology

- Smoking → thrombosis → oxygen and nutrients deficiency to tissue
- Presence of antibodies to endothelial cell
- Diminished response to acetylcholine
- Chronic arsenic poisoning and long-term cannabis smoking

Clinical Features

- Unilateral painful and purple discoloration of the fingers or toes (blue toe syndrome)
- Pain is aggravated at night, after exercise, and with reduction in surrounding temperature
- With time ulceration and gangrene occurs
- On examination, the peripheral pulses are lost or feeble.
- Other associated features include:
    - Venous thrombosis (recurrent)
    - Impaired blood supply to internal organs.

Diagnostic Criteria

- Smoking or tobacco use
- Onset at <45–50 years
- Infrapopliteal, segmental arterial occlusions with sparing of the proximal vasculature
- Frequent arterial involvement in the distal upper extremities (reflected by Raynaud phenomenon or digital ulcers)
- Superficial phlebitis
- Exclusion of other conditions like diabetes, arteriosclerosis, true arteritis, proximal emboli, and hypercoagulable states.

Investigations

- *Histopathology:* Intraluminal thrombosis with microabscess. A mixed infiltrate of leukocytes and giant cells can be visualized in all layers of the vessel wall. Internal elastic lamina is typically spared.
- *Arteriogram:* Normal proximal vessels. Numerous occlusions and narrowing seen in distal vessels. New corkscrew collaterals develop to maintain blood supply.
- Tests to rule other pathology should be performed.

Treatment

- Smoking termination
- The extremities should be kept warm and protected from injuries
- Intravenous (IV) iloprost
- Sympathectomy
- Debridement if required

MARTORELL'S HYPERTENSIVE LEG ULCER[5,6]

- A Martorell ulcer is an extremely painful leg ulcer that develops in due to longstanding uncontrolled high blood pressure.
- *Other names:* Martorell's hypertensive leg ulcer/arteriosclerotic ulcer of Martorell/Martorell hypertensive ischemic leg ulcer.
- *Associated disease:* Diabetes mellitus
- Female > Male
- *Age:* 50s and 60s

Clinical Features

- Painful red blister → blue → ulcer develops.
- *Location:* Outer aspect of the lower leg (above the ankle)
- Ulcer characteristics may include:
    - Pain out of proportion to appearance of the ulcer
    - Shape is irregular
    - Usually solitary (if multiple then symmetrical)
    - *Edge:* Inflamed
    - There may be sudden enlargement of ulcer due to tissue necrosis.
    - Satellite ulcer may be present.
    - Deeper tissues may be exposed.
- Rest pain/intermittent claudication → absent

Investigations

Skin biopsy to rule out other causes of leg ulcer.

Treatment

- Blood pressure control is primary.
- *Ulcer care:*
  - Surgical debridement
  - Compression therapy
  - Vacuum-assisted closure
  - Skin grafting
  - Antibiotics (for secondary skin infections)
- Pain relief

Preventative Measures

- Complete termination of smoking habit
- Compression stockings
- Protection from physical trauma

ERYTHROMELALGIA[7,8]

Erythromelalgia is of two types:

1. Primary erythromelalgia
2. Secondary erythromelalgia.

Primary erythromelalgia + family history = Weir-Mitchell disease.

For primary erythromelalgia, Male:Female ratio = 1:2.5 while M:F ratio in secondary erythromelalgia is 3:2.

Etiology

- Primary erythromelalgia → *SCN9A* mutation
- Secondary erythromelalgia
  Associated with:
  - Myeloproliferative disorders. Erythromelalgia appears before the myeloproliferative disorder in around 85% patients
  - Paraneoplastic diseases
  - Autoimmune neuropathies
  - Diabetes
  - Rheumatological
  - Infectious diseases
- For primary erythromelalgia, there is no age bar. Secondary erythromelalgia occurs mostly after 4th decade.
  - Extremities most commonly involved (atypical variants can involve other parts of the body)
  - Secondary erythromelalgia is usually bilateral.

Clinical Features

- Erythromelalgia is typified by intense burning pain, erythema, and elevated temperature of skin of extremities.
- The symptoms are amplified on warming of extremities and reduced on cooling and on raising limb upward.
- The symptoms may be continuous or intermittent.

Complications

- Ulceration
- Necrosis
- Gangrene
- Secondary infection of wounds

Investigations

- Investigation for underlying causes
- Diagnosis based on clinical picture

Treatment

Generally cases of primary erythromelalgia are refractory.

Secondary erythromelalgia → Underlying cause to be treated

- Cooling
- Topical capsaicin cream
- *Oral medications:*
  - Aspirin—relieves symptoms of erythromelalgia related to thrombocytosis
  - Sodium channel blockers—mexiletine (in patients with *V872G* mutation)
  - Calcium antagonists (nifedipine, diltiazem)
  - Prostaglandin (misoprostol)
  - IV nitroprusside/lignocaine/prostaglandin
  - SSRI (venlafaxine, sertraline, fluoxetine, paroxetine)
  - TCS (amitriptyline, imipramine)
  - Anticonvulsants (gabapentin, carbamazepine)
  - NAV1.7 channel modulator → PF-05089771
  - NAV1.7 channel blockers → TV-45070
- *Surgical intervention:* Sympathectomy

CALCIPHYLAXIS[9,10]

Calciphylaxis is typified by necrosis of the skin and fatty tissue.

Also known as: Calcific uremic arteriolopathy/calcific vasculopathy.

Etiology

It generally associated with end-stage kidney disease (secondary hyperthyroidism).

Other conditions associated:

- Obesity
- Diabetes
- Caucasians
- Females
- Hypoalbuminemia
- Warfarin

Clinical Features

- Calciphylaxis mostly occurs on the fatty areas of lower limb.

- Initially starts as retiform purpura → bleeding → Stellate purple lesions with black areas in the center → supply (dry gangrene).
- Severe pain is present.

Outcome

- Deep ulceration with a chronic course
- Secondary infection
- Sepsis
- Death

Investigations

- *Skin biopsy:*
  - Ca^{++} deposited within blood vessels in the subcutaneous tissue
  - Perieccrine calcium deposition may be present.
  - There may also be panniculitis.
- X-rays → vascular calcification
- Bone scintigraphy → enhanced radiotracer uptake in indurated plaques affected by calciphylaxis (but these findings are absent in ulcers as a result of diminished blood flow at sites of tissue necrosis).

Treatment

- If warfarin is the cause, anticoagulant to be replaced.
- Normalize the calcium and phosphate product levels
  - Calcium and phosphate restricted diet
  - Dialysis using lower dialysate calcium concentration
- Parathyroidectomy
- Cinacalcet
- Thorough wound management is essential.

Other Drugs

- Etidronate
- Matrix metalloproteinases inhibitors → such as doxycycline

Mortality in patients with calciphylaxis associated with chronic renal disease → 60–80%. Death as a result of infection.

DISEASES OF VEINS

Livedo Vasculitis[11]

It is a chronic vascular disorder characterized by persistent painful ulceration of chiefly but not exclusively lower leg.

Livedo vasculitis alias "livedoid vasculopathy"/"livedoid vasculitis"/"livedo reticularis with summer ulceration."

Associated Condition(s)

- Antiphospholipid antibodies (APLAs)
- Protein C deficiency
- Factor V mutation (Leiden)
- Arteriosclerosis
- Homocysteinemia
- Hyperlipoproteinemia

8% patients → Prothrombin *G20210A* gene mutation has been found.

Clinical Features

Bilateral and mostly involves lower extremities:

- Small, tender, irregular ulcers
- Painless, irregular atrophie blanche
- Livedo reticularis
- Raynaud phenomenon
- Occasional acrocyanosis.

Histopathology

- Hyalinization
- Thick blood vessel walls
- Deposition of fibrin
- Vascular occlusion
- Mild inflammation

Deposition of fibrinogen C3 IgM can be found in most of the cases.

Investigations

- Complete blood count
- Coagulation studies
- Antinuclear antibody (ANA)
- Lupus coagulant and anticardiolipin antibodies
- Levels of homocysteine

Transcutaneous oximetry → reduced oxygen flow

Differential Diagnosis

- Venous or arterial insufficiency
- Rheumatoid arthritis
- Systemic lupus erythematosus (SLE)
- Systemic sclerosis
- Small vessel vasculitis
- Cutaneous polyarteritis nodosa (PAN)
- Malignant atrophic papulosis

Treatment

- Protect the area injuries
- Antibiotics for infection
- Leg elevation, compression therapy, bed rest, and occlusive wound dressings may aid healing.
- Stop smoking, if relevant, as smoking reduces peripheral blood flow.
- *Drugs:*
  - Pentoxifylline
  - Antiplatelet agents like aspirin
  - Fibrinolytic agents such as danazol, tissue plasminogen activator
  - Anticoagulant agents such as heparin or warfarin
  - Vasodilators such as nifedipine
  - Folic acid, vitamin B_{12}, and vitamin B_6 which act as cofactors of homocysteine metabolism.

LIVEDO RETICULARIS AND LIVEDO RACEMOSA[12]

Livedo Reticularis

Livedo reticularis (LR) is a benign and primary disorder typified by is symmetric, reversible, and uniform livid conical discoloration.

Livedo reticularis may be classified into four types:
1. Physiological
2. Primary
3. Idiopathic
4. Amantadine-induced

Physiologic LR is also called as cutis marmorata. It is mainly seen in young females and occurs commonly on the lower limbs on exposure to cold and resolves slowly on rewarming.

In primary LR, skin color changes are unrelated to ambient temperature.

Idiopathic LR is persisting. The diagnosis is made by exclusion. It seldom denotes the early stage of antiphospholipid syndrome (APS) or Sneddon's syndrome.

Livedo Racemosa

Although livedo racemosa (LRC) is a secondary and pathologic disorder. There is clinically livid conical discoloration which is symmetric, irreversible, and in a "broken" like pattern.

It is more generalized and noninfiltrated as compared to LR. LRC found on the limbs, trunk, and buttocks. LRC is classically seen in Sneddon's syndrome. Other disorders associated with LRC include livedoid vasculopathy, APS, SLE, essential thrombocythemia, thromboangiitis obliterans, polycythemia vera, and polyarteritis nodosa.

SUPERFICIAL THROMBOPHLEBITIS

Superficial thrombophlebitis is an inflammation of a superficial vein(s) as a result of blood clot just below the skin. Risk factors for superficial thrombophlebitis:
- Past history of superficial phlebitis, deep vein thrombosis (DVT), and/or pulmonary embolism
- Varicose veins
- Intravenous injection or infusion
- Existing clotting disorders
- Pregnancy
- Hormone therapy
- Vasculitis
- Smoking
- Cancer
- Long-term immobility

Clinical Features

- Swelling, erythema, and tenderness
- There may be bluish discoloration
- Due to the clot the vein may feel hard or rope like.

Management

Mild cases resolve within a month.

For severe cases:
- Raise the leg and apply warm compresses
- Elastic support
- Analgesics
- Low-molecular-weight heparin (LMWH)
- Puncture and evacuation if needed
- Surgical excision

VENOUS ULCERS[13,14]

Venous ulcers are those ulcers which occur as a result of improper functioning of venous valves.

Pathogenesis

- Venous hypertension
- Fibrin cuff theory
- Inflammatory cuff theory
- Cytokine dysregulation

Clinical Features

- Moderate pain → improves on limb elevation (in arterial ulcers pain worsen with limb elevation)
- Irregular and sloping edges
- Associated edema, as a result of increased hydrostatic pressure, which leads to "atrophie blanche"
- "Atrophie blanche" → localized loss of skin pigmentation as a result of death of red blood cells (RBCs) and scarring
- Lipodermatosclerosis → hardening of the skin → "inverted champagne bottle" appearance of leg
- Associated superficial varicose veins or "ankle flare" may be present.

Treatment

- Dressing
- *Debridement:*
  - Sharp
  - Wet to dry
  - Autolytic
  - Enzymatic (chemical)
  - Maggot debridement
- Topical
- Systemic
- Compression
- Surgery
- *Other supportive measures:*
  - Leg elevation
  - Calf muscle exercise
  - Nutritional supplement
  - Electrical stimulation therapy
  - Hyperbaric oxygen

Flowchart 1: Treatment of venous ulcers.

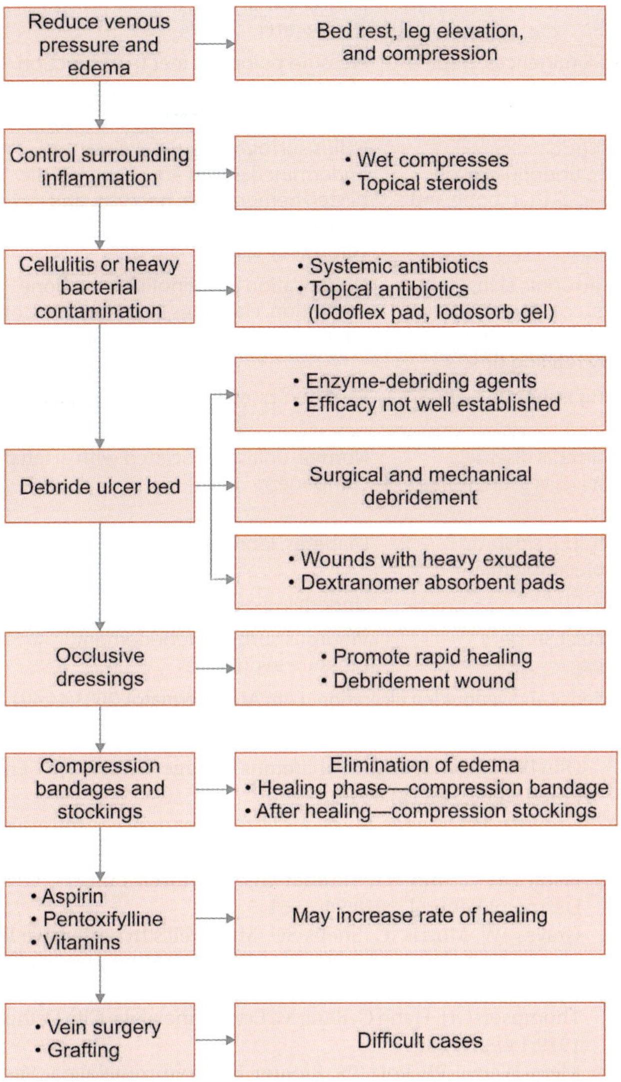

Source: Clinical Dermatology: A Color Guide to Diagnosis and Therapy by Thomas P Habif.

- Vacuum-assisted closure
- Sclerotherapy using hypertonic saline, sodium tetradecyl sulphate, polidocanol
- Manual lymph drainage

Poor Prognostic Factors

- Duration >1 year
- Larger wounds
- Fibrin in >50% of wound surface
- ABPI < 0.8
- History of venous stripping or ligation

LYMPHEDEMA

Lymphedema is localized swelling of a part of the body which occurs as a result of abnormal accumulation of lymph.

Localized Lymphedema

- Scar lymphedema
- Solid facial edema
- Large firm skin tags
- Genital swelling in Crohn disease

Diffuse Lymphedema

There are two types of diffuse lymphedema: (1) Primary lymphedema and (2) Secondary lymphedema.

Primary Lymphedema

- Primary lymphedema is as known as Milroy disease.
- Usually due to underdevelopment of lymphatic system
- About 70–80% of cases are female.
- Age of onset is variable.

Secondary Lymphedema

- Occurs due to some other primary disorders
- Chronic venous disease
- Postsurgery
- Radiotherapy
- Trauma, or infection
- Reduced mobility

Clinical Features

- Swelling
- Tightness and heaviness
- Altered sensation
- Joint discomfort
- Occasional tenderness
- Changes in temperature
- Reduced range of movement

In advanced stages, skin becomes thick with folds and bulges. Dry warty lesions appear on the lower limbs called elephantiasis nostras verruciformis or lymphatic papillomatosis.

Complications

- Impetigo and cellulitis
- Chronic inflammation and fibrosis (scarring)
- Skin cancer → angiosarcoma (Stewart–Treves syndrome), basal cell carcinoma, squamous cell carcinoma, and sebaceous carcinoma. Tumors are often multiple.
- Viral warts
- Elephantiasis nostras verruciformis may be due to human papillomavirus activation.

Management

The main target of treatment is to reduce the swelling.

Mild-to-moderate swelling → Complex physical (lymphatic/lymphedema) therapy (CPT/CLT)

- Skin care
- Simple lymphatic drainage

TABLE 1: Differences between main three types of ulcer.

	Venous	*Arterial*	*Neuropathic*
Ulcer location	Medial malleolus; trauma or infection may localize ulcers laterally or more proximally	Distal, over bony prominences; trauma may localize ulcers proximally	Pressure points on feet (e.g., junction of great toe and plantar surface, metatarsal head, heel)
Ulcer appearance	Shallow, irregular borders; base may be initially fibrinous, but later develops granulation tissue	Round or punched-out, well-demarcated border, fibrinous yellow base or true necrotic eschar; bone and tendon exposure may be seen	Callus surrounding the wound and undermined edges are characteristic; blister, hemorrhage, necrosis, and exposure of underlying structures are commonly seen
Physical examination	Varicose veins, leg edema, atrophie blanche, dermatitis, lipodermatosclerosis, pigmentary changes, purpura	Loss of hair, shiny, atrophic skin, dystrophic toenails, cold feet, femoral bruit, absent or decreased pulses, prolonged capillary refilling time	No sensation to monofilament; bone resorption, claw toes, flat foot, Charcot joints
Frequent symptoms	Pain, odor, and copious drainage from the wound; pruritus	Claudication, resting ischemic pain	Foot numbness, burning, paresthesias
Ankle–brachial pressure index (ABI)	>0.9	ABI < 0.7 suggests arterial disease; calcification of vessels gives falsely high Doppler readings	Normal, unless associated with arterial component
Risk factors	Deep venous thrombosis, significant leg injury, obesity	Diabetes, hypertension, cigarette smoking, hypercholesterolemia	Diabetes, leprosy, frostbite
Complications	Allergic contact dermatitis, cellulitis	Gangrene	Underlying osteomyelitis
Treatment pearl	Compression therapy, leg elevation	Pentoxifylline, vascular surgery assessment if ABI < 5	Vigorous surgical debridement, pressure avoidance

Source: Valencia IC, Falabella A, Kirsner RS, Eaglstein WH. Chronic venous insufficiency and venous leg ulceration. J Am Acad Dermatol. 2001;44:401.[15]

- Compression bandaging
- Exercise and movement

For severe swelling, additional treatments include:

- Manual lymphatic drainage
- Multilayer lymphedema bandaging
- Drug therapy (under trial)
- Surgery

KEY POINTS

- Thromboangiitis obliterans mostly happens due to smoking related vasoconstriction of distal arteries.
- Calciphylaxis may indicate underlying life-threatening conditions.
- Livedoid vasculopathy leads to stellate-shaped ulcers on the skin as it involve arterioles or venioles.
- Lymphedema can be localized or diffuse. Secondary diffuse edema may be due to obstruction, infection or radiation mostly.

REFERENCES

1. Abdullah A, Hayden A, Gabana CA, Appleton BE. A challenging case of thromboangiitis obliterans. Br Columbia Med J. 2016;58(3):126-9.
2. Klein-Weigel PF, Richter JG. Thromboangiitis obliterans (Buerger's disease). Vasa. 2014;43(5):337-46.
3. Olin JW. Thromboangiitis obliterans (Buerger's disease). N Engl J Med. 2000;343(12):864-9.
4. Gregory P, Creager Mark A. Thromboangiitis obliterans. Circulation. 2010;121(16):1858-61.
5. Fistal EY, Vatutin NT, Taradin GG. Martorell's ulcers. Vestn Dermatol Venerol. 2018;94(3):51-5.
6. Graves JW, Morris JC, Sheps SG. Martorell's hypertensive leg ulcer: case report and concise review of the literature. J Hum Hypertens. 2001;15(4):279-83.
7. Thompson GH, Hahn G, Rang M. Erythromelalgia. Clin Orthop. 1979;144:249-54.
8. Klein-Weigel PF, Volz TS, Richter JG. Erythromelalgia. Vasa. 2018;47(2):91-7.
9. Nigwekar SU, Thadhani R, Brandenburg VM. Calciphylaxis. N Engl J Med. 2018;378(18):1704-14.
10. Nigwekar SU, Kroshinsky D, Nazarian RM, Goverman J, Malhotra R, Jackson VA, et al. Calciphylaxis: risk factors, diagnosis, and treatment. Am J Kidney Dis. 2015;66(1):133-46.
11. DermNet. (2006). Livedoid vasculopathy. [online] Available from https://dermnetnz.org/topics/livedoid-vasculopathy/. [Last accessed May, 2021].
12. Sajjan VV, Lunge S, Swamy MB, Pandit AM. Livedo reticularis: a review of the literature. Indian Dermatol Online J. 2015; 6(5):315.
13. Etufugh CN, Phillips TJ. Venous ulcers. Clin Dermatol. 2007;25(1):121-30.
14. Collins LG, Seraj S. Diagnosis and treatment of venous ulcers. Am Fam Phys. 2010;81(8):989-96.
15. Valencia IC, Falabella A, Kirsner RS, Eaglstein WH. Chronic venous insufficiency and venous leg ulceration. J Am Acad Dermatol. 2001;44(3):401-24.

EXAMINATION QUESTIONS

1. Classify different types of leg ulcers.
2. Discuss the management of venous ulcers.
3. Write a short note on livedo reticularis.

87 CHAPTER

Neutrophilic Dermatoses

Varsha Vaidyanathan, Aarti Sarda, Abhishek De

INTRODUCTION

Neutrophils are inflammatory cells which accumulate and get activated at sites of infection or injury. They release contents from their cytoplasmic granules which kill the microorganisms after phagocytosis. Sometimes these neutrophils get activated without any discernable source of infection and they end up damaging the normal tissue. Dermatologically they manifest as neutrophilic dermatoses which are comprised of a spectrum of different diseases all linked by a similar histopathological picture of diffuse sterile neutrophilic infiltrate. As the pathogenic mechanism is similar, they share a common treatment approach as well.

They are classified[1] as shown in **Table 1**.

Most dermatologists only consider the nonvasculitis-associated dermal dermatoses as true neutrophilic dermatoses. Of these, Sweet syndrome, pyoderma gangrenosum, and Behçet's disease are of particular importance and hence will be discussed in greater detail in this chapter.

SWEET SYNDROME[1-3]

Sweet syndrome, also known as acute febrile neutrophilic dermatosis, is the prototypic neutrophilic dermatosis and is characterized by the appearance of tender, nonpruritic, erythematous papules, and plaques over the head, neck, shoulders, and upper extremities with associated fever, leukocytosis, and neutrophilic infiltrate on histopathology.

Sweet syndrome has a worldwide distribution with no predilection for race or ethnicity. There is a female preponderance and most cases occur between the ages of 30 and 60.

The exact etiology of Sweet syndrome is unknown but several conditions have been found in association and it is possible that these may trigger the neutrophilic activation seen in Sweet syndrome. Some of these conditions are as follows:

- *Infections:* Upper respiratory tract infections, gastrointestinal infections
- *Malignancies:* Hematological malignancies such as leukemias, lymphomas, aplastic anemia, myelodysplasias, solid organ malignancies involving breast, prostate, genitourinary
- *Inflammatory bowel disease:* Ulcerative colitis, Crohn's disease
- *Immunological conditions:* Collagen vascular disorders like lupus erythematosus, Sjögren's syndrome
- *Medications:* Colony-stimulating factors, imatinib mesylate, propylthiouracil, oral contraceptives
- *Other neutrophilic dermatosis:* Pyoderma gangrenosum, neutrophilic eccrine hidradenitis, Behçet's disease
- *Other diseases:* Sarcoidosis, rheumatoid arthritis
- Pregnancy.

Pathogenesis

An external or internal trigger causes changes in cell signaling and cytokine production resulting in increased neutrophil production and migration into the skin. Cytokines like IL-1, IL-3, IL-6, IL-8, and granulocyte colony-stimulating factor (GCSF) are found to be elevated but it is as yet unclear how much of a role they play in the pathogenesis of Sweet syndrome specifically as they are elevated in nearly all inflammations regardless of cause. One hypothesis is that a person may fail

TABLE 1: Classification of neutrophilic dermatoses.

Neutrophilic dermatoses		
Epidermal	*Dermal*	
	With associated vasculitis	*Without associated vasculitis*
• Pustular psoriasis • Acute generalized epidermal pustulosis • Reiter's disease • Immunoglobulin A (IgA) pemphigus • Infantile acropustulosis • Transient neonatal pustulosis	• Leukocytoclastic vasculitis • Erythema elevatum diutinum • Medium-sized vessel vasculitis	• Sweet syndrome • Pyoderma gangrenosum • Behçet's disease (small vessel vasculitis may be present) • Bowel-associated dermatosis-arthritis syndrome • Still's disease • Erythema marginatum • Neutrophilic eccrine hidradenitis • Dermatitis herpetiformis • Linear IgA bullous disorder • Periodic fever syndrome

to respond rapidly and effectively to an infection leading to a larger stimulus for neutrophilic activation and migration the second time around and subsequently leads to the development of Sweet syndrome. There may be a genetic predisposition.

Classification

Largely, Sweet syndrome can be classified as:

- *Classical type:* Generally have a fever and history of infection. Upper respiratory tract infection (URTI) precedes the appearance of skin lesions by 2–3 weeks.
- *Malignancy associated:* With associated hematological malignancy, generally they are already diagnosed prior to appearance of Sweet syndrome. However, solid-organ malignancies tend to be detected within a year of development of Sweet syndrome.
- *Drug-induced*—they are further divided into:
  - Granulocyte colony-stimulating factor (GCSF)-induced (which is more common)
  - Secondary to other drugs such as propylthiouracil, oral contraceptive pills (OCPs), imatinib, antiepileptics, nonsteroidal anti-inflammatory drugs (NSAIDs).

Clinical Features

Tender, erythematous papules, plaques and nodules distributed over the head, neck, trunk and upper extremities is the classical presentation. They appear acutely along with constitutional symptoms of fever, malaise, myalgia and arthralgia. Asymmetric, nonerosive, sterile arthritis affecting knees and wrists may occur. The plaques are well-defined with sharp, irregular borders. Due to intense dermal edema, the plaques develop a shiny, transparent appearance and almost look-like vesicles and are hence known as pseudovesicles. True vesicles and pustules with subsequent crusting and scarring may also be seen. Extracutaneous involvement of the central nervous system (CNS), respiratory system, and eyes has been noted.

Variants

- *Neutrophilic dermatosis of the dorsal hands:* Lesions clinically and histopathologically similar to typical Sweet syndrome appear on the dorsal hands. Hemorrhagic papules and bullae may dominate. In almost half of the cases, lesions are present at other sites as well. There is some amount of overlap with pyoderma gangrenosum (PG) and some authors consider it to be a variant of PG.
- *Subcutaneous variant[4]:* Erythema nodosum-like tender nodules appear on the legs. Histopathologically they resemble Sweet syndrome lesions and there may be an associated malignancy.
- *Histiocytoid variant[5]:* Clinically, they may resemble typical or subcutaneous variant of Sweet syndrome but histopathologically there is a dense infiltrate of histiocytoid cells which are immature myeloid cells and precursors of neutrophils. It can be associated with malignancies and drugs.

Differential Diagnosis

- Infections like erysipelas, cellulitis, tuberculosis
- Other neutrophilic dermatoses such as pyoderma gangrenosum, Behçet's disease
- Erythema nodosum, erythema multiforme
- Vasculitis like erythema elevatum diutinum, polyarteritis nodosa, urticarial vasculitis, granuloma faciale.

Investigations

- Skin biopsy
- Complete blood counts, C-reactive protein (CRP), erythrocyte sedimentation rate (ESR), liver, and renal function tests
- Suspected malignancies should be investigated according to guidelines. If no apparent cause, then full clinical examination including lymph nodes, breast, genitals, mouth, and prostate should be carried out.

Histopathology

There is a dense, diffuse neutrophilic infiltrate in the dermis which may extend into the subcutaneous tissue creating a septal or lobular panniculitis. There may also be some eosinophils and lymphocytes but the overall picture is dominated by neutrophils. There is intense dermal edema. Leukocytoclasis and vasculitis may or may not be seen. If present, leukocytoclasis occurs with endothelial swelling but without fibrinoid necrosis. Epidermal changes are insignificant but may occasionally show subcorneal pustules and intraepidermal vesiculation. Three histological variants—histiocytoid, lymphocytic and eosinophilic—have been described.

Diagnostic Criteria

In order to be diagnosed, patients must satisfy two major and two minor criteria out of those mentioned here:

Major Criteria

- Acute onset of typical lesions
- Dense neutrophilic dermal infiltrate on biopsy

Minor Criteria

- Temperature >38°C
- Preceding respiratory or gastrointestinal infection, associated malignancy, drug exposure, or pregnancy
- Excellent response to systemic steroids
- Abnormal lab values. Any 3 out of 4 (ESR > 20, WBCs > 8,000, neutrophils >70%, raised CRP)

Treatment

- Mild cases may resolve with topical corticosteroids alone. In most other cases, systemic treatment in the form of prednisolone (0.5–1 mg/kg for 4–6 weeks) is required. Prolonged low dose for 2–3 months more may be required in some patients. If there is no response even after 3 months, then a steroid-sparing agent is added.

- Any one of dapsone (50–100 mg/day), potassium iodide (300 mg tid) or colchicine (0.5 mg tid) may be prescribed as a steroid-sparing second-line agent.
- Other drugs may be considered such as indomethacin, cyclosporine, clofazimine, interferon alpha.
- Tumor necrosis factor (TNF) inhibitors have been used in the treatment of recalcitrant Sweet syndrome but may also be a cause of drug-induced Sweet syndrome.

Prognosis

Even without treatment, the disease resolves spontaneously within 3 months without scarring. There is rapid response to systemic corticosteroids. About one-third of the cases recur after resolution.

PYODERMA GANGRENOSUM[1,2,6]

Introduction

Pyoderma gangrenosum is a rare, chronic, recurrent neutrophilic dermatosis presenting with nonhealing ulcers and is generally associated with an underlying systemic condition. There are four main variants. As the histopathological picture is not the same across all its variants, clinicohistopathological correlation must be relied on to make an accurate diagnosis. The term pyoderma gangrenosum is a misnomer as there is no infectious etiology as was initially supposed by the names Brunsting, Goeckerman and O'Leary.

Pyoderma gangrenosum is present all over the world. Although it can affect any age, there is preponderance in women between the ages of 20 and 50. In half of the patients, the condition arises idiopathically. In the other half there is an underlying systemic or autoimmune disorder. These include inflammatory bowel disease (IBD) like ulcerative colitis and Crohn disease, hematogenous malignancies, solid organ malignancies, and rheumatoid arthritis.

Pathogenesis

Due to the association with autoimmune conditions, an underlying defect in cell-mediated immunity and neutrophil function has been suspected to play a causative role. In particular, enhanced activity of the IL-1 pathway is considered to be involved similar to that seen in autoimmune conditions. There is an overexpression of IL-1, IL-1-beta, IL-1 receptor, IL-8, and TNF-alpha in lesional skin. Support for this proposed pathogenesis comes from the effectiveness of canakinumab (anti-IL-1-beta antibody) in suppressing the condition. Corticosteroids may also be acting via their ability to reduce IL-1 formation.

Clinical Features

The classical presentation of PG is the ulcerative type. The lesions begin as solitary or multiple painful papules, pustules or nodules with surrounding red or violaceous color. Then these break down to form an ulcer which may be shallow or deep enough to expose the underlying muscles and tendons. The ulcer has a purulent base and an irregular, violaceous border extending centrifugally. Generally, the ulcers expand rapidly. When healing occurs, there is re-epithelialization from the margins with the eventual formation of an atrophic cribriform scar. PG demonstrates the phenomenon of pathergy wherein a penetrating trauma gives rise to new lesions. This is seen in around 25% of the cases.

The main features of the four important variants are given in **Table 2**.

TABLE 2: Features of pyoderma gangrenosum variants.

	Classical ulcerative	*Vesiculobullous*	*Pustular*	*Superficial granulomatous/ vegetative*
Associations	Idiopathic or IBD	Hematogenous malignancies such as AML, CML, myelodysplasias	Most commonly associated with IBD	• Usually not associated with underlying disorders. • May be related to Wegener's granulomatosis
Site	Frequently appear on pretibial region of legs but can occur anywhere	Face and upper extremities especially back of hands	Trunk and extensor surfaces of limbs	Trunk, areas of trauma
Clinical appearance	Classical lesion of PG, i.e., deep or shallow ulcer with irregular violaceous undermined border	Rapid appearance of superficial, hemorrhagic vesicles and bullae which ulcerate then heal with scarring	Discrete tender pustules surrounded by a halo of erythema	Begin as a single superficial ulcer with elevated and verrucous borders
Histopathology	Central necrosis, ulceration of epidermis and dermis with intense neutrophilic infiltrate. Suppuration and abscess formation at dermo-epidermal junction	Neutrophilic infiltrate with intraepidermal vesiculation	Perifollicular neutrophilic infiltrate with subcorneal pustule formation	Granulomatous response with peripheral palisading histiocytes and giant cells

(AML: acute myeloid leukemia; CML: chronic myeloid leukemia; IBD: inflammatory bowel disease; PG: pyoderma gangrenosum)

Aside from these major subtypes, there are some others such as:

- *Parastomal PG:* Lesions are similar to that of ulcerative PG and are present at the site of stoma. They appear as a response to pathergy caused by trauma of stoma devices and fecal irritation. They are commonly associated with ileostomy done for IBD. Factors such as obesity, female gender, and associated autoimmune conditions increase the chances of developing parastomal PG.
- *Pyostomatitis vegetans:* Chronic, verrucous plaques studded with pustules occur on the lips and buccal mucosa. May be associated with other variants of PG and with IBD.
- *Neutrophilic dermatosis of the dorsal hands:* As mentioned earlier, this may be associated with both Sweet syndrome and PG.
- *Extracutaneous PG:* PG can involve other sites such as the lungs, brain, muscles, bones, heart, and gastrointestinal (GI) tract in the form of aseptic abscesses **(Fig. 1)**.

Differential Diagnosis

Pyoderma gangrenosum is a disease of exclusion and the following conditions have to be ruled out:

- Arterial and venous ulcers
- Vasculitis
- External trauma causing wounds
- Atypical mycobacterial infection
- Squamous cell carcinoma, mycosis fungoides
- Fungal infections such as sporotrichosis, mucormycosis, blastomycosis, histoplasmosis.

Diagnostic Criteria for Ulcerative Variant of Pyoderma Gangrenosum

Major (Must be Met)

- Rapidly progressive painful cutaneous ulcer with undermined, irregular, violaceous borders
- Other causes of cutaneous ulcers excluded.

Minor (Any two)

- History of pathergy or cribriform scarring evident
- Associated systemic diseases such as IBD, hematological malignancies, etc.
- Histopathology suggestive of PG
- Rapid response to systemic corticosteroids.

Investigations

- Thorough clinical examination including lymph nodes
- Skin biopsy—not essential for diagnosis but helps to rule out other causes
- Tissue/swab for bacterial, fungal and atypical mycobacterial organisms
- Complete blood count, peripheral smear, bone marrow examination if indicated
- Liver and renal function tests

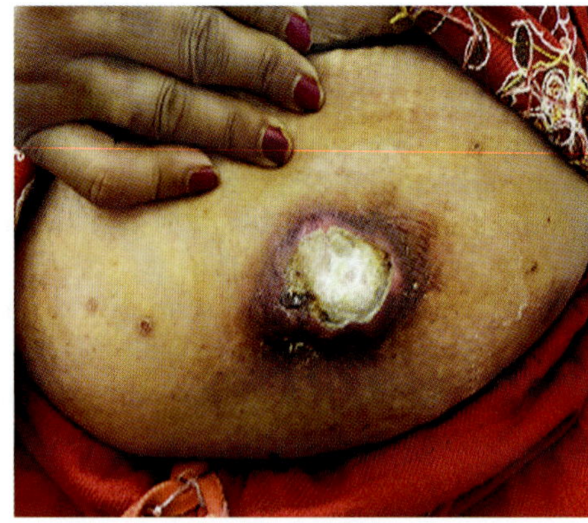

Fig. 1: Pyoderma gangenosum.

- Stool for occult blood
- Chest X-ray, urinalysis
- Test for malignancies as the clinical situation indicates

Treatment

- General measure for ulcers on legs like daily dressing, keeping the ulcer clean and moist, compression stockings, weight reduction
- For small lesions, topical or intralesional corticosteroids
- For severe and recalcitrant PG, systemic treatment is started. Options include oral prednisolone (0.5–1 g/kg), cyclosporine (5 mg/kg), pulse therapy with 3 consecutive days of 1 g methylprednisolone, dapsone (50–100 mg/day). Other immunosuppressants such as methotrexate, azathioprine, mycophenolate mofetil, cyclophosphamide.
- Biologicals such as infliximab, anakinra, ustekinumab, adalimumab, etanercept
- Other modalities that have been tried include hyperbaric oxygen, topical nicotine.
- Skin grafting should not be done in the early inflammatory phase because of the phenomenon of pathergy but later when the disease process has been controlled with immunosuppressants there can be a role for skin grafting.
- Recently, there have been reports of improvement with injection of platelet-rich plasma[7] around the ulcer and application of autologous platelet-rich fibrin.[8]

Prognosis

Pyoderma gangrenosum follows a chronic course and takes months to years to resolve. Even after resolution, there is recurrence in more than half the cases. Long-term preventative and maintenance strategies are required.

BEHÇET'S DISEASE[2,9,10]

Introduction

Behçet's disease, also known as Adamantiades-Behçet disease, is a neutrophilic dermatosis with multisystemic manifestations such as recurrent oral and genital ulcerations, ocular abnormalities, and cutaneous lesions. It is named after

Benediktos Adamantiades, a Greek ophthalmologist who reported it in 1931 and Hulusi Behçet who reported a similar constellation of findings in 1937.

Epidemiology

Behçet's disease has a worldwide prevalence and is endemic in east and central Asia and the Mediterranean countries, i.e., along the ancient Silk Route. The highest prevalence is in Turkey (80/100,000) in contrast to the US (0.12/100,000). In the Mediterranean and Middle East countries, it is more common and more severe in men, whereas in Japan and Korea, the reverse is true. The peak incidence is in the twenties and thirties.

Pathogenesis

The HLA-B51 allele is an important risk factor for those living along the Silk Route as it is present in over 80% of the patients here. Earlier theories hypothesized that an infectious agent (HSV, hepatitis C virus, *Streptococcus*) triggered an immune response in genetically susceptible individuals leading to Behçet's disease, but these theories have not been substantiated. Overall, the etiology remains largely unknown although other factors like environmental pollution, clotting factors, drugs have been studied.

Whatever the trigger may be, the neutrophils in Behçet's disease get activated and produce increased amounts of superoxides and lysosomal enzymes which ultimately result in mucocutaneous lesions. Elevated levels of TNF-alpha, IL-1-beta, and IL-8 may activate the neutrophils and encourage the interactions between neutrophils and endothelial cells.

Clinical Features

The lesions in Behçet's disease may start with one system and then involve the others or may be multisystemic from the start. Lesions may present acutely or slowly over a period of months to years.

Mucocutaneous Lesions

Aphthous stomatitis is present in almost 70% of the patients. Oral ulcers begin as multiple red papules which go on to form a painful 1–3 cm sized sharply defined ulcers with a yellowish base and surrounding red halo. These ulcers usually heal without scarring. In contrast, the anogenital lesions are larger, have a more irregular base, are more painful, and heal with scarring. The usual sites are the penis and scrotum in men, and the vulval folds in women. They can also be seen in the vagina, urethra, perineum, inguinal, and perineal areas.

Primary cutaneous lesions manifest as vesiculopustules, pustules, and purpuric papules on the face and limbs. Despite the papulopustular lesions not being folliculocentric, they have been described as acneiform. Erythema nodosum-like lesions appear on the legs and buttocks. The phenomenon of pathergy is seen as in PG. Lesions similar to those in PG and Sweet syndrome may be present.

Extracutaneous/Systemic Lesions

- Ocular manifestations are more severe in men and include posterior uveitis (which may lead to blindness), anterior uveitis, hypopyon, cataract, glaucoma, retinal detachment, and optic nerve atrophy.
- Joint involvement is seen in about half of the patients. A nonerosive, sterile, asymmetrical, seronegative oligoarthritis is characteristic. A migratory monoarthritis may be present. Knees, wrists, and ankles are commonly affected.
- Abdominal pain and hemorrhage may be seen, similar to that in IBD. Ulcerations resembling anogenital aphthae may develop in the small intestine.
- Neurological signs and symptoms appear late in the disease process and are associated with a poor prognosis. Cranial nerve palsies, meningoencephalitis, benign intracranial hypertension, brainstem lesions may be seen in approximately 10% of patients. Headache, gait disturbances, seizures, hemiplegia, depression, psychosis are all part of the manifestations.
- Vascular involvement manifest as venous thrombosis, arterial thrombosis, and aneurysms. Patients with pulmonary artery aneurysms present with coughing and hemoptysis. Myocarditis, endocarditis, and valvular involvements are all signs of cardiac involvement.
- Renal involvement presents with glomerulonephritis.

Histopathology

Early lesions show dense neutrophilic infiltrate along with endothelial swelling, RBC extravasation, and leukocytoclasia. Leukocytoclastic vasculitis with fibrinoid necrosis may be present. Aneurysms involving the larger arteries may be seen.

Diagnostic Criteria

There are many sets of criteria which can be applied for Behçet's disease. The most commonly used one is the Revised International Criteria for Behçet's Disease. Here, each feature is ascribed points and a diagnosis of Behçet's disease is reached if the sum of the points is at least 4.

Clinical Feature	Points
Recurrent oral lesions	2
Recurrent oral ulcers	2
Recurrent genital ulcers	2
Recurrent skin lesions	1
CNS manifestations	1
Vascular lesions	1
Positive pathergy test	1

Investigations

- *Pathergy test:* 0.1 mL normal saline is injected intradermally using a 20G needle at a 45° angle either on the volar aspect of the forearm or on the inner aspect of the lips. After 48 hours, a reading is done. The appearance of a papule more than 2 mm in size or a pustule indicates a positive pathergy test.

However, it is not pathognomonic of Behçet's disease as it is also seen in PG, Crohn disease, and rheumatoid arthritis.
- Evidence of arthritis can be found on X-rays.
- In general, there are no diagnostic tests as such. Diagnosis depends on fulfilling the criteria as discussed earlier.

Treatment

Depends upon extent, severity, and systems involved.
- *Mucocutaneous lesions:* For oral ulcers, topically 1% silver nitrate, 5% hydrogen peroxide, chlorhexidine mouthwashes, tetracycline mouthwashes, triamcinolone paste, lidocaine before meals, and cyclosporine 500 mg solution as mouthwash. Oral agents include colchicine 1–2 mg/day, 5–60 mg/day prednisolone depending on severity, dapsone 100 mg, azathioprine 2.5 mg/kg/day.
- *Ocular lesions:* Topically steroids, mydriatics, and cycloplegics. Systemic steroids, azathioprine, cyclosporine, anti-TNF alpha agents
- *Joint involvement:* NSAIDs, colchicine, azathioprine, sulfasalazine, steroids, methotrexate
- *Vascular involvement:* Systemic steroids are the mainstay of the treatment. Other agents include azathioprine, methotrexate, cyclosporine, anticoagulation, anti-TNF alpha agents and surgical modalities in certain cases.
- *CNS involvement:* Similar to that of vascular management
- *GI involvement:* Steroids, sulfasalazine, anti-TNF agents.

Prognosis

Behçet's disease has a variable and unpredictable clinical course. Markers of severe disease include male sex, HLA-B51 positivity, and early systemic involvement. Aggressive treatment is required to prevent complications like blindness. Spontaneous remissions have been noted. The mucocutaneous lesions tend to recur and remit chronically.

CONCLUSION

Neutrophilic dermatoses lead to significant morbidity and poor quality of life for the patient. It is incumbent on the treating dermatologist to be up-to-date with the current research so as to be able to accurately and quickly diagnose the patients and offer effective treatment modalities.

KEY POINTS

- Neutrophilic dermatoses are a heterogeneous group of diseases linked by a common histological picture of dense neutrophilic infiltrate.
- Sweet syndrome presents with tender, erythematous papules, and plaques in the head and neck area associated with constitutional signs and symptoms.
- Sweet syndrome may be classical, malignancy-associated, or drug-induced. It tends to remit spontaneously even without treatment but there is rapid response to corticosteroids.
- PG classically presents with nonhealing ulcers on the legs. Other variants include vesiculobullous, pustular, and vegetative. Vesiculobullous type is associated with hematological malignancies and the pustular type with IBD.
- PG follows a chronic course.
- Behçet's disease has recurrent oral and genital ulcers, ocular lesions, and erythema nodosum-like and acneiform lesions. There is a multisystem involvement.
- Pathergy is seen in PG and Behçet's disease.
- Treatment approach is similar for the neutrophilic dermatoses and involves immunosuppression using various drugs.

REFERENCES

1. Davis MDP, Moschela SL. Neutrophilic dermatoses. In: Bolognia JL, Schaffer JV, Cerroni L (Eds). Dermatology, 4th edition. Amsterdam, Netherlands: Elsevier Publication; 2018. pp. 453-71.
2. Ormerod AD, Hampton PJ. Neutrophilic dermatoses. In: Griffiths C, Barker J, Blelker T, Chalmers R, Creamer D (Eds). Rook's Textbook of Dermatology, 9th edition. New Jersey, USA: Wiley-Blackwell Publication; 2016. pp. 49.1-17.
3. Cohen PR. Sweet's syndrome--a comprehensive review of an acute febrile neutrophilic dermatosis. Orphanet J Rare Dis. 2007;2:34.
4. Guhl G, García-Díez A. Subcutaneous sweet syndrome. Dermatol Clin. 2008;26(4):541-51.
5. Wark KJ, Crawshaw H. Histiocytoid Sweet syndrome. Med J Aust. 2019;211(9):400-400.e1.
6. Alavi A, French LE, Davis MD, Brassard A, Kirsner RS. Pyoderma gangrenosum: an update on pathophysiology, diagnosis and treatment. Am J Clin Dermatol. 2017;18(3):355-72.
7. Alvarez-Lopez MA, Burón-Alvarez I, Villegas-Fernández C. Refractory pyoderma gangrenosum treated with platelet-rich plasma. J Eur Acad Dermatol Venereol. 2016;30(8):1423-4.
8. Fortunato L, Barone S, Bennardo F, Giudice A. Management of facial pyoderma gangrenosum using platelet-rich fibrin: a technical report. J Oral Maxillofac Surg. 2018;76(7):1460-3.
9. Nelson CA, Stephen S, Ashchyan HJ, James WD, Micheletti RG, Rosenbach M. Neutrophilic dermatoses: pathogenesis, Sweet syndrome, neutrophilic eccrine hidradenitis, and Behçet disease. J Am Acad Dermatol. 2018;79(6):987-1006.
10. Bulur I, Onder M. Behçet disease: new aspects. Clin Dermatol. 2017;35(5):421-34.

EXAMINATION QUESTIONS

Write short notes on the following:
1. Neutrophil dermatoses
2. Sweet syndrome
3. Pyoderma gangrenosum
4. Behçet's disease

10 SECTION Neoplastic Skin Diseases

88 CHAPTER Benign Acanthomas of Skin

Shouvik Ghosh, Anupam Das

INTRODUCTION

Benign acanthomas are a group of benign skin neoplasms, composed of epidermal keratinocytes and located in the prickle cell layer of the epidermis. They may be simulated by lesions which are not benign (actinic keratosis) or not an epidermal lesion (dermatofibroma). Examples of benign acanthomas arising out of normal (epidermoid) keratinization process are seborrheic keratosis and related conditions [viz. dermatosis papulosa nigra (DPN)]

There are also acanthomas which show aberrant keratinization process such as:

- *Epidermolytic acanthoma* with epidermolytic hyperkeratosis
- *Warty dyskeratoma* with dyskeratosis
- *Acantholytic acanthoma* with acantholysis
- *Lichen planus-like keratosis* with lichenoid hyperplasia
- *Clear cell acanthoma* with absence of keratinization.

Acanthomas are benign tumors of epidermal keratinocytes. The proliferating cells may show normal epidermoid keratinization or a wide range of aberrant keratinization. Keratoacanthomas are not usually considered in this category, although there is no logical reason for their exclusion. The following acanthomas are discussed here:

- Seborrheic keratosis
- Dermatosis papulosa nigra
- Stucco keratosis (Keratoelastoidosis verrucosa)
- Acantholytic acanthoma
- Epidermolytic acanthoma
- Warty dyskeratoma
- Melanoacanthoma
- Clear cell acanthoma
- Clear cell papulosis
- Large cell acanthoma
- Lichen planus-like keratosis
- Keratoacanthoma.

SEBORRHEIC KERATOSIS

Seborrheic keratoses (senile warts, basal cell papillomas) are common, often multiple, benign tumors seen commonly among older individuals. They may occur on any part of the body except the palms and soles, although there is a predilection for face, chest, interscapular region, and waistline. Extremities are also affected. Occasionally solitary, seborrheic keratoses more commonly present as multiple, tan/light brown to black, sharply demarcated lesions. Seborrheic keratosis typically evolves from a macule and may progress to become papular or verrucous. They appear "stuck on" the skin, as if they can be removed with the flick of a fingernail. Most lesions are not more than a centimeter or so in diameter, but larger variants, sometimes even pedunculated, have been reported. Lesions may become inflamed due to rupture of the small pseudocysts they contain, or from trauma or rarely from infection with microorganisms such as *Staphylococcus aureus*. Although usually asymptomatic, traumatized or inflamed lesions may become tender, pruritic, erythematous, crusted and, rarely, pustular. The development of a basal cell or squamous cell carcinoma or a keratoacanthoma in a seborrheic keratosis is a rare event. More common is the juxtaposition or "collision" of these lesions. Rarely, a malignant melanoma may develop in a seborrheic keratosis.[1]

Histopathologically, most seborrheic keratoses show acanthosis, varying degree papillomatosis, and hyperkeratosis. They are composed of basaloid cells with a varying admixture of squamoid cells. Keratin-filled invaginations and small cysts (horn cysts) are a characteristic feature. Nests of squamous cells (squamous eddies) may be present, particularly in the irritated type.

At least nine distinct histological patterns have been recognized: acanthotic (solid), reticulated (adenoid), hyperkeratotic (papillomatous), clonal, irritated, inflamed, desmoplastic, adamantinoid, and with pseudorosettes. Overlapping features are not uncommon.

Acanthotic type is the most common histologic type and composed of broad columns or sheets of basaloid cells with horn cysts.

Reticulated (adenoid) type has interlacing thin strands of basaloid cells, often pigmented, enclosing small horn cysts.

Hyperkeratotic type is exophytic, with varying degrees of hyperkeratosis, papillomatosis, and acanthosis. Basaloid and squamous cells, both are present.

Clonal seborrheic keratosis have intraepidermal nests of basaloid cells resembling the Borst–Jadassohn phenomenon.

Irritated variant, there is a heavy inflammatory cell infiltrate often lichenoid in nature within the upper dermis. Apoptotic cells are present in the base of the lesion and in areas of squamous differentiation. The term *lichenoid* seborrheic keratosis is a preferable term to irritated seborrheic keratosis. Kamino bodies are rarely found in this type. Sometimes there is a heavy inflammatory cell infiltrate without lichenoid qualities, rarely neutrophils are abundant in the infiltrate. This may be regarded as a true *inflammatory* variant, although often lesions with features overlapping with those of the irritated type are found.

Desmoplastic variant, there are irregular squamous nests and cords of cells extending into a desmoplastic stroma. The trapped cells may mimic a squamous cell carcinoma.

Adamantinoid type is a variant with intercellular mucin and small basaloid keratinocytes with spindled cytoplasm.

Variant with pseudorosettes, basaloid cells are radially arranged around central, small empty spaces. The lesion is acanthotic with occasional horn cysts.

Treatment of asymptomatic seborrheic keratoses is largely performed for cosmetic reasons. Symptomatic lesions are usually removed by destruction, curettage or shave excision. The most common method of destruction is cryotherapy. Other methods include laser vaporization (pulsed CO_2, erbium:YAG) or electrodesiccation.

Leser–Trélat Sign

The sign of Leser–Trélat is a rare cutaneous-marker of internal malignancy (in particular gastric or colonic adenocarcinoma, breast carcinoma, and lymphoma). It is characterized by sudden appearance of numerous seborrheic keratosis, may be associated with an internal cancer. The seborrheic keratoses may precede, follow, or develop concurrently with the onset of symptoms of the cancer. Involution of the seborrheic keratoses has followed treatment of the cancer. They lesions are often pruritic. Malignant acanthosis nigricans, tripe palms other cutaneous paraneoplastic features may appear at the same time or shortly after. Rarely, in other conditions such as inflammatory dermatoses, erythrodermic conditions and pregnancy an abrupt appearance or increase in the number and size of SK lesions has also been reported.

DERMATOSIS PAPULOSA NIGRA

Although considered by some as a variant of seborrheic keratosis, DPN is a clinically distinctive entity, found almost exclusively in black adults, with a female preponderance. A familial predisposition is often present. There are multiple small, sessile to filiform, hyperpigmented papules, with a predilection for the malar eminences and forehead. The neck and upper part of the trunk may also be involved. An eruptive form has been reported in association with an adenocarcinoma of the colon. DPN is characterized by acanthosis, papillomatosis, and hyperkeratosis in a pattern quite similar to the acanthotic type of seborrheic keratosis. Horn pseudocysts, however, are not a common feature. Electrodesiccation is the treatment of choice.

STUCCO KERATOSIS (KERATOELASTOIDOSIS VERRUCOSA)

Typically, it occurs as multiple 1–5 mm grayish-white "stuck on" warty popular lesions over lower extremities of elderly adults. They are usually distributed symmetrically below the knee, especially on the dorsal and lateral aspects of the foot and ankle. Occasionally, they may also be noted on the thighs and the forearms. Characteristically, the central keratotic part of the lesions can be scratched off, without any bleeding leaving a colarette of dry, fine scales. Histologically, orthokeratotic hyperkeratosis is seen interdigitating in a church-spire pattern with an acanthotic stratum malpighii, fusion of rete ridges, and, in many cases, solar elastosis. The microscopic pattern is indistinguishable from hyperkeratotic seborrheic keratoses and some authorities believe stucco keratosis is a variant of seborrheic keratosis. Ammonium lactate solution may be tried to improve the appearance of the lesions.

ACANTHOLYTIC ACANTHOMA

Acantholytic acanthoma is a solitary tumor with a predilection for the trunk in adults. It usually presents as an asymptomatic, solitary keratotic papule or nodule. Sometimes, there may be multiple lesions in the genital area. Histologically, there is acantholysis with or without dyskeratosis in a hyperplastic epidermis with an overall flat architecture.[2]

EPIDERMOLYTIC ACANTHOMA

Epidermolytic acanthoma may appear any time during adulthood. No particular race or gender predilection is seen. Two varieties are there—an isolated form and a disseminated form. Both the forms present as pigmented keratotic papules that may resemble verrucae or seborrheic keratosis. Lesions are generally 1 cm or less in diameter. Isolated epidermolytic acanthoma may appear on any part of the body. Lesions are discrete but they may occur in clusters and still be considered to represent the isolated variant. The disseminated form has a predilection for the trunk, especially the back; it has also been reported in the genital region. Lesions are usually asymptomatic, but they may be pruritic. The histologic pattern of epidermolytic hyperkeratosis consists of four components:

1. Clear spaces surrounding nuclei in the stratum spinosum and stratum granulosum.
2. Indistinct cellular boundaries consisting of reticulated, lightly staining material

3. Markedly thickened granular zone containing a large number of, irregularly shaped, basophilic keratohyaline-like bodies
4. Compact hyperkeratosis

The basal layer is normal. Epidermolytic acanthoma generally demonstrates more papillomatosis than is typically seen in other conditions with the histologic pattern of epidermolytic hyperkeratosis. There is often a slight superficial perivascular lymphocytic infiltrate in the dermis. Treatment is not required as the lesions are benign. Destruction, shave excision, or linear excision may be tried.

WARTY DYSKERATOMA

Warty dyskeratomas are rare, usually solitary, rarely multiple, verrucous, often crusted, skin-colored to brown papulonodular lesions with a predilection for the head and neck area in middle-aged and elderly individuals. A central keratotic plug is there within the lesion. Warty dyskeratomas typically range in size from several millimeters to 2 cm in diameter. Most warty dyskeratomas are asymptomatic, though some may rarely complain of itching or burning. Histologically there is a central cup-like invagination filled with cornified debris. The epithelium lining of the invagination contains suprabasilar clefting, with numerous acantholytic and dyskeratotic cells within the cleft.[3]

MELANOACANTHOMA

Melanoacanthoma, first described by Bloch, is a rare benign pigmented cutaneous lesion which is composed of both melanocytes and keratinocytes. The lesion is a slowly growing, usually solitary, tumor of the head and neck, or trunk and seen in older men. Clinically, a melanoacanthoma resembles a pigmented seborrheic keratosis or a melanoma, and may be growing up to 3 cm or more in diameter. Melanoacanthoma arising from mucous membranes has been reported.[4]

Histologically, it is a benign epidermal neoplasm composed of both heavily pigmented dendritic melanocytes containing mature melanosomes and keratinocytes essentially devoid of melanin.

CLEAR CELL ACANTHOMA

Clear cell acanthoma presents as a firm, brown-red, dome-shaped nodule or papule or plaque most commonly in the lower part of the legs of middle-aged and elderly individuals. Other sites can also be involved. Generally lesions are almost asymptomatic. A scaly collarette is common. Sometimes they are crusted or slightly eroded and a serous exudate may be present on the surface. There is often prominent vascularity that occasionally simulates a pyogenic granuloma, although the erythema can be blanched with application of pressure. Although usually solitary, multiple tumors have been described and a few patients with multiple clear cell acanthomas have also had varicose veins and/or ichthyosis in association. They range in size from 0.3 to 2 cm in diameter, although rarely larger lesions have been described. Growth is slow and the tumor may persist over a period over 2–10 years. Spontaneous involution has been reported.

Histological examination shows a well-demarcated area of psoriasiform epidermal hyperplasia in which the keratinocytes have pale-staining cytoplasm. The granular layer is diminished. PAS stains the pale cytoplasm of the keratinocytes red. The material that stains with PAS is diastase-sensitive, confirming it is glycogen. Electron microscopy also demonstrates abundant glycogen within the cytoplasm. Epidermal rete ridges are elongated. There are intermittent broad and slender rete ridges, and a tendency for the acanthosis to be more prominent centrally. There may be fusion of the acanthotic downgrowths. Other epidermal changes include mild spongiosis, exocytosis of neutrophils which may form tiny intraepidermal microabscesses, and thinning of the suprapapillary plates. The epidermal surface shows parakeratotic scale and sometimes focal pustulation.

Clear cell acanthomas may be treated with excision, shave excision, cryotherapy, and curettage and electrofulguration.[5]

CLEAR CELL PAPULOSIS

Clear cell papulosis is an extremely rare condition characterized by multiple asymptomatic white macules and papules on the face, anterior chest, abdomen, or lumbar region. Lesions may be arranged along the "milk lines." There is a predisposition for Asian children. The lesions measure 2–10 mm in size.

The epidermis is mildly acanthotic with a slightly disorganized arrangement of the epidermal cells. There are numerous number of clear cells scattered mainly among the basal cells with a few cells in the stratum spinosum also. The cells are larger than the adjacent keratinocytes and have cytoplasmic vacuolization. The clear cells are variably stained by the periodic acid Schiff (PAS), mucicarmine, Alcian blue, and colloidal iron methods. There is no known treatment.

LARGE CELL ACANTHOMA

Large cell acanthoma characteristically presents as an asymptomatic, solitary, sharply demarcated, scaly, lightly pigmented papule or plaque approximately 3–10 mm in diameter, on the sun-exposed skin of elderly individuals. Face and neck are mainly involved. It may be also found on the upper or lower extremities and the trunk. Large cell acanthoma is thought to comprise sunlight-induced clones of abnormal cells, without a tendency to malignancy. However some investigators have proposed bowenoid transformation.

Histologically, there is epidermal thickening with uniform large keratinocytes with abundant cytoplasm and enlarged nuclei. Other features include orthokeratosis, a prominent granular layer, mild papillomatosis, epidermal rete ridge elongation, or basal layer hyperpigmentation. Mild cytologic atypia may be appreciated. Shave or simple excision as well as destruction is treatment options.[6]

LICHEN PLANUS-LIKE KERATOSIS

Lichen planus-like keratosis (benign lichenoid keratosis, solitary lichenoid keratosis) almost invariably occurs as a solitary, pink to red brown acanthoma on sun-exposed skin (most commonly on upper chest and forearm) of middle-aged or older individuals (35–65 years). Women are diagnosed more frequently than men. Clinical differential diagnosis includes BCC, basal cell carcinoma, actinic keratosis, seborrheic keratosis, Bowen's disease, and nevus. Histologically, lichen planus-like keratosis features hyperkeratosis and hypergranulosis, occasional local parakeratosis (unlike typical lichen planus), and irregular acanthosis. The dermoepidermal junction is partially obscured by a lichenoid infiltrate composed mainly of lymphocytes with scattered histiocytes. Eosinophils and plasma cells are sometimes present. All other features of interface dermatitis like basal vacuolar degeneration, melanin incontinence, and colloid bodies are seen. Cellular atypia and anaplasia are not seen, but mild dysplasia is observed sometimes. No treatment is required. Lesions may be removed by excision, curettage and electrofulguration or cryotherapy, etc.[7]

KERATOACANTHOMA

Keratoacanthoma, a biologically benign acanthoma with clinical and histologic features that make it a distinctive entity, often displays remarkable cellular atypia, and so traditionally discussed together with SCC. It has rarely been emphasized that some keratoacanthomas do not show dysplastic changes and may be histologically indistinguishable from other benign acanthomas.

Keratoacanthomas are usually considered to be a well-differentiated SCC, but sometimes are considered to be benign, especially when lesions spontaneously regress or occur as multiple lesions in one of those syndromes mentioned here. Typically, a rapidly enlarging papule evolving into a sharply circumscribed crateriform nodule with a keratotic core persisting for 2–3 months and then may resolve slowly over 4–6 months, leaving a depressed scar. Most lesions occur on the head or sun-exposed areas of the extremities, with or without symptoms of pain, or tenderness. There are several distinct clinical presentations, including solitary, multiple, grouped, giant, subungual, intraoral, multiple spontaneously regressing (Ferguson–Smith), multiple nonregressing, generalized eruptive (Grzybowski), keratoacanthoma centrifugum marginatum. By far the most common presentation is the solitary keratoacanthoma.

Keratoacanthoma typically has a volcano architecture. The tumor is comprised of well-differentiated keratinocytes with a brightly eosinophilic glassy cytoplasm surrounding a core filled with cornified material. An inflammatory infiltrate of lymphocytes, and often eosinophils, is usually present. Small intratumoral abscesses of neutrophils are common. Elastic fibers are often seen within the epithelium at the base of the lesion. As the lesion regresses, the dome-shaped architecture flattens and fibrosis develops at the base of the lesion.[8]

KEY POINTS

- Benign acanthomas are a group of benign skin neoplasms, composed of epidermal keratinocytes, and located in the prickle cell layer of the epidermis.
- Some of the clinically relevant disorders include seborrheic keratosis, dermatosis papulosa nigra, stucco keratosis, and keratoacanthoma.

REFERENCES

1. Greco MJ, Bhutta BS. Seborrheic keratosis. In: StatPearls. Treasure Island (FL): StatPearls Publishing; 2021.
2. Brownstein MH. Acantholytic acanthoma. J Am Acad Dermatol. 1988;19(5 Pt 1):783-6.
3. Rambhia KD, Makhecha MB. A case of warty dyskeratoma on an unusual location. Indian Dermatol Online J. 2019;10:343-5.
4. Vasani RJ, Khatu SS. Melanoacanthoma: uncommon presentation of an uncommon condition. Indian Dermatol Online J. 2013;4:119-21.
5. Benedetto CJ, Athalye L. Clear cell acanthoma. In: StatPearls. Treasure Island (FL): StatPearls Publishing; 2020.
6. Patsatsi A, Lazaridou E, Fotiadou C, Kyriakou A, Sotiriadis D. Large cell acanthoma: a debate throughout the decades. Dermatol Pract Concept. 2014;4(1):43-5.
7. Prieto VG, Casal M, McNutt NS. Lichen planus-like keratosis. A clinical and histological reexamination. Am J Surg Pathol. 1993;17(3):259-63.
8. Zito PM, Scharf R. Keratoacanthoma. In: StatPearls. Treasure Island (FL): StatPearls Publishing; 2020.

EXAMINATION QUESTIONS

Write short notes on the following:

1. Keratoacanthoma.
2. Warty dyskeratoma.
3. Lichen planus-like keratosis.

89 CHAPTER Premalignant Conditions of Skin

Souvik Sardar

INTRODUCTION[1,2]

The term premalignant refers to a group of diseases with the tendency to transform into invasive carcinoma. Histologically, these diseases feature dysplastic changes restricted to the epidermis and hence also called carcinoma in situ.

The new term advocated by World Health Organization (WHO) for such oral lesions is *"potentially malignant disorders"* which means that some, but not all of the lesions can progress to frank malignancy. The common premalignant lesions are given in **Table 1**.

ORAL

Leukoplakia and Erythroplakia

Definition[2]

- *Leukoplakia:* A predominantly white plaque of questionable risk having excluded (other) known diseases or disorders that carry no increased risk for cancer (WHO definition).
- *Erythroplakia:* A fiery red that cannot be characterized clinically or pathologically as any other definable disease (WHO definition).

Epidemiology

Common in males of 40–60 years age group.

Risk Factors

- Tobacco
- Smoking. Reverse smoking is an important factor for erythroplakia (palatal lesions in reverse smoking)
- Alcohol
- Betel
- Human papillomavirus (HPV) infection.

Clinical Features

- Leukoplakia has two variants:
  - *Homogeneous*: Uniform white plaque mostly in cheek mucosa.
  - *Nonhomogeneous*:
    - Speckled type—erythematous eroded patches in between white patches (erythroleukoplakia). More in soft palate, floor of mouth, and ventrolateral tongue areas
    - Verrucous—corrugated surface
    - Nodular—small polyp-like outgrowths
  - Proliferative verrucous leukoplakia (PVL) is a distinct entity having multifocal involvement.
- Erythroplakia presents as flat or slightly elevated sharply defined red plaque.
- The lesions cannot be rubbed off and are mostly asymptomatic.

Prognosis

The chances for malignant transformation are:[11]

- *Homogeneous leukoplakia:* 1–7%
- *Speckled leukoplakia:* 18–47%
- *Verrucous leukoplakia:* 4–15%
- Nonsmokers, lesions in floor of mouth, and erythroplakia are more prone for malignant transformation.

TABLE 1: Common premalignant lesions of skin and mucosa.

Oral	*Genital*	*Cutaneous*	*Diseases not potentially malignant but reported with malignancy later*
• Leukoplakia and erythroplakia • Actinic cheilitis • Oral submucosal fibrosis • Palatal lesions in reverse smokers	• Erythroplasia of Queyrat • Bowenoid papulosis • Bowen's disease of penis • Penile horn • Squamous intraepithelial neoplasia and squamous hyperplasia • Pseudoepitheliomatous keratotic and micaceous balanitis	• Bowen's disease • Actinic keratosis • Atypical/dysplastic nevus[3] • Lentigo maligna[4] • Radiation keratosis • Arsenic keratosis • *Psoralen and ultraviolet A* (PUVA) keratosis • Thermal keratosis • Scar carcinoma • Chemical keratosis • Epidermodysplasia verruciformis	• Disseminated superficial actinic keratosis[5]/linear[6]/giant[7] • Vulvar lichen sclerosus[8] • Oral nonreticular lichen planus[9] and hypertrophic lichen planus[10]

Histology

- *Leukoplakia*: Hyperkeratosis. Epithelial dysplasia may vary from none to mild-moderate-severe grades.
- *Erythroplakia*: Severe epithelial dysplasia.

Differential Diagnosis[2]

Common diseases presenting as white lesions in oral mucosa are:

- Leukoedema
- Morsicatio buccarum
- White sponge nevus
- Acute pseudomembranous candidiasis
- Oral lichen planus (LP) (plaque type)
- Lichenoid reaction
- Frictional keratosis
- Chemical burn
- Smoker's palate
- Hairy leukoplakia
- Discoid lupus erythematosus (DLE)

Erythroplakia

- Oral candidiasis (erythematous)
- Oral LP (erythematous)
- DLE
- Oral pemphigus vulgaris
- Desquamative gingivitis
- Chronic mechanical trauma
- Hemangioma
- Kaposi sarcoma

Management

- Cessation of predisposing factors
- If no or mild dysplasia—periodic checkup may be done depending on the areas involved.
- If moderate-to-severe dysplasia—excision is the best.
- Other modalities—cryotherapy, photodynamic therapy, CO_2 ablative laser therapy, 5-fluorouracil (5-FU), and 5% imiquimod

Actinic Cheilitis

Introduction

Premalignant disease of the lip due to chronic ultraviolet (UV) exposure

Epidemiology[12]

Common in fair-skinned males in fourth to eighth decade of life

Risk Factors[12]

- Cumulative UV radiation is the single most predisposing factor
- Tobacco
- Smoking
- Immunosuppression

Clinical Features

- Initial lesion is red and edematous which later becomes dry and scaly with gradual thickening.
- Commonly affects the lower lip vermillion border. Demarcation of the vermillion and skin is lost.
- Ulceration, bleeding, and nodularity indicates malignant transformation.[13]

Histology

Hyperkeratosis, acanthosis, or epidermal atrophy and plasma cell infiltration may be noted. Degree of epithelial dysplasia may vary in a single lesion. Hence, multiple samples may be necessary.

Differential Diagnosis[14]

- Lichen planus
- DLE
- Cheilitis glandularis
- Granulomatous cheilitis
- Plasma cell cheilitis
- Squamous cell carcinoma (SCC).

Management[14]

Refer **Table 2**.

Prognosis[12]

Malignant transformation is higher than actinic keratosis (AK).

Oral Submucosal Fibrosis[2,15]

It is defined as thickening and fibrosis of the oral mucosa including oropharynx and upper esophagus, which clinically presents with burning sensation. Chewing betel nut and slaked lime are predisposing factors. Chance of malignant transformation is 7.6%.

GENITAL

Bowenoid Papulosis

Introduction

The term is specifically used for SCC in situ appearing in the background of oncogenic HPV infection in the genitalia.

Cause

Infection by oncogenic HPV (16, 18, 39, and 51).

TABLE 2: Management of actinic cheilitis.

General	*Specific*
• Sun protection measures • Avoidance of smoking	• Topical: 5-fluorouracil (5-FU), tretinoin, and 5% imiquimod • Cryotherapy • CO_2 laser ablation • Photodynamic therapy • Vermilionectomy

Clinical Features

- Multiple small flat reddish or brownish papules in the genitalia with tendency to coalesce.
- *Site*—glans and shaft of penis, vulva, and perineum.
- *Age*—young sexually active population

Histology

Widespread intraepidermal keratinocytic atypia giving rise to "windblown appearance".

Differential Diagnosis

- Genital wart
- Bowen's disease (BD)
- Intraepithelial neoplasia
- Lichen planus

Treatment

5-fluorouracil, 5% imiquimod, electrodessication, cryotherapy, and excision

Prognosis

- 1–2.6% chance of transformation into SCC[16]
- Female patients and sexual partners of male patients have chance for cervical neoplasia.

Erythroplasia of Queyrat

Introduction

Bowen's disease of the nonkeratinized part of penis is called erythroplasia of Queyrat whereas BD involving the keratinized surface is separately diagnosed as Bowen' disease of penis.

Clinical Features[17]

Well defined, erythematous shiny plaque on the glans penis or coronal sulcus or inner side of prepuce in uncircumcised male.

Histology

Dysplasia restricted to the epidermis occasionally with plasma cells in the dermis.

Dermoscopy

Diffuse or clustered arrangement of glomerular vessels.

Prognosis

- 30% cases may progress to invasive SCC.[18]
- Malignant transformation in BD of penis is 10%.[19]

Differential Diagnosis

- Zoon's balanitis
- Ulcerative lichen planus
- Pemphigus vulgaris
- Fixed drug eruption (FDE)
- Psoriasis

Treatment

- *Topical*: 5-FU and 5% imiquimod
- *Procedural*: Excision, cryotherapy, electrodessication, and photodynamic therapy

Prevention

Circumcision and smoking abstinence

Squamous Intraepithelial Neoplasia[16]

Introduction

Dysplastic changes restricted to epithelium of anogenital area with intact basement membrane are called *intraepithelial neoplasia.*

Types

- *Vulvar intraepithelial neoplasia (VIN):* Further divided into differentiated and undifferentiated type.
- *Penile intraepithelial neoplasia (PeIN)*: Includes erythroplasia of Queyrat and BD of penis.
- *Anal intraepithelial neoplasia (AIN) and perianal intraepithelial neoplasia (PaIN)*: Divided into low and high grade.

Predisposing Factors

- HPV infection
- Smoking
- Human immunodeficiency virus (HIV)
- Uncircumcised male
- Immunosuppression
- Anal intercourse
- Genital lichen sclerosus.

Clinical Features

- *VIN*: Shiny erythematous plaque, seborrheic keratosis-like lesions, or warty growth. Background lesions of lichen sclerosus can be seen in differentiated type. Pruritus, dysuria, and pain may be present.
- Pruritus ani may be found in AIN.

Differential Diagnosis

- *VIN*: Lichen planus, condyloma accuminatum, and lichen sclerosus
- *AIN*: SCC and genital warts.

Prognosis

- *PaIN*: 5% chance of malignant transformation
- *VIN*: 10% of undifferentiated type progress to invasive SCC whereas chance is more for differentiated.

Treatment

Five percent imiquimod, 5-FU, electrosurgery, Mohs micrographic surgery, and wide local excision.

Prevention

Human papillomavirus vaccine can reduce the chance of intraepithelial neoplasia in younger females.

Pseudoepitheliomatous Keratotic and Micaceous Balanitis[20]

Introduction

Very rare penile proliferative condition with thick scales

Clinical Features

- Asymptomatic hyperkeratotic hard plaque with thick adherent micaceous scale.
- Perimeatal hyperkeratosis causing multi-farcated urinary streams, a condition described as "watering can penis".
- Most commonly affects uncircumcised elderly individuals.

Histopathology

- Pseudoepitheliomatous hyperplasia
- Mild lower epidermal dysplasia

Treatment

- *Topical*: 5-FU and podophyllin resin
- *Procedural*: Cryotherapy, radiation, and excision

Prognosis

Progression to invasive SCC may occur but rate is unknown.

Penile Horn[21]

- Arises over pseudoepitheliomatous keratotic and micaceous balanitis (PKMB), verrucous carcinoma, and squamous carcinoma.
- Adequate excision is the treatment of choice.

CUTANEOUS

Bowen's Disease[22]

Introduction

The carcinoma in situ of the skin, mucosa, and nails is called BD. This was first described in 1912.

Epidemiology

Male preponderance. Mostly in older individuals

Risk Factors

- UV exposure
- Arsenicosis
- HPV infection
- Immunosuppression
- Actinic keratosis

Clinical Features

- Well-defined, solitary, mostly asymptomatic erythematous plaque with hyperkeratotic or scaly or crusted surface.
- *Site*: Sun-exposed areas such as head and neck.
- In chronic arsenicosis, the disease is multifocal mostly involving the sun-protected areas.
- *Morphological variants*:
  - Pigmented
  - Intertriginous
  - Periungual
  - Subungual.

Histology

- Hyperkeratosis and diffuse confluent parakeratosis with full thickness epidermal atypia.
- Hyperchromatic, dysplastic, and pleomorphic atypical keratinocytes with loss of polarity are found giving rise to "windblown" appearance. Some keratinocytes may be vacuolated.
- Basement membrane is intact.
- Inflammatory infiltrate in upper dermis.
- *Histological variants:* Psoriasiform, atrophic, acantholytic, epidermolytic, and pagetoid.
- If basement membrane is damaged then there is chance of regional metastasis or even visceral.[23]

Dermoscopy

Glomerular vessels (characteristic) and dotted vessels with superficial scales

Clinical Differential Diagnosis

- *Hyperkeratotic*: Psoriasis, superficial basal cell carcinoma (BCC), nummular dermatitis, AK, seborrheic keratosis, and DLE
- *Pigmented*: Melanoma
- *Intertriginous*: Inverse psoriasis, seborrheic dermatitis, and intertrigo
- *Subungual/periungual*: Onychomycosis and periungual wart
- *Genital*: Zoon's balanitis and FDE

Histological Differential Diagnosis

- Paget's disease
- Bowenoid AK
- Pagetoid melanoma in situ
- Bowenoid papulosis

Treatment

- *Topical*: 5-FU and 5% imiquimod
- *Surgical or destructive*: Excision, Mohs micrographic surgery, cryotherapy, and electrosurgery
- *Ablative*: Radiation, laser ablation, and photodynamic therapy

Prognosis

- 3–5% extragenital cases may develop invasive SCC.[19]
- SCC over BD has predilection for metastasis.
- Recurrence may be noted in small percentage due to subclinical lateral spread and narrow margin of excision.

Actinic Keratosis

Introduction

Also known as solar keratosis as it is related to chronic UV ray exposure.

Risk Factors[24]

- Chronic UV ray exposure
- Elderly
- Fitzpatrick type 1 skin
- Male
- Immunosuppression
- Albinism.

Clinical Features

- *Site*: Sun-exposed areas such as bald scalp, face, ears, dorsum of hands, and lips (actinic cheilitis).
- *Morphology*: Multiple scaly erythematous or skin colored, flat or slightly elevated rough or verrucous plaques.
- Mostly asymptomatic. May have burning, bleeding, crusting, or overlying cutaneous horn.
- Associated findings of chronic sun damage.
- *Clinical grades*: More easily felt than seen (grade 1), moderately thick (grade 2), and severely thickened (grade 3).[25]
- *Clinical variants*: Hypertrophic, atrophic, lichenoid, pigmented, and actinic cheilitis.
- Subclinical lesions may be there in vicinity of clinically evident lesions—a phenomenon called *field cancerization*.
- *Clinical clues to malignant transformation*: Induration, inflammation, pain, ulceration, rapid increase in size, and resistant to treatment.

Histopathology

- *Flag sign*: Alternate orthokeratosis (uninvolved basophilic corneum in acrosyringeal or acrotrichial ostia) and focal parakeratosis (eosinophilic corneum in involved area).
- Atypical keratinocytes involving mostly the lower layers of epidermis varying with clinical gradings.
- Hyperchromatic nuclei with loss of polarity.
- Elastosis in upper dermis due to actinic damage.
- *Histological variants*: Hypertrophic, atrophic, pigmented, acantholytic, and bowenoid.

Differential Diagnosis

- Seborrheic keratosis
- Lentigo maligna
- Bowen's disease
- Superficial BCC
- Squamous cell carcinoma.

Dermoscopy

- Strawberry pattern with interfollicular vessels and rosettes (facial nonpigmented type)
- Can have surface scales
- Hyperpigmented follicular openings with broken brownish pseudonetwork (facial pigmented type).

Treatment

Refer **Table 3**.

- *Chemoprevention*:
  - Oral retinoids
  - Oral nicotinamide
  - 5% imiquimod cream

Prognosis

Can progress to invasive SCC (1–10% chance per lesion in 10 years).[26]

Radiation Keratosis[27]

Ionizing radiation may cause hyperkeratotic lesions developing into SCC.

Arsenic-induced Squamous Cell Carcinoma In Situ[28]

Introduction

Prolonged exposure to arsenic in inorganic form leads to keratoses and can cause cutaneous precancerous lesions like multifocal BD and cancerous lesions such as multifocal SCC or BCC.

Clinical Features

- Keratotic punctate papules over the palms and soles.
- An erythematous halo or thickening can be an early sign of transformation to carcinoma in situ.
- Multifocal Bowen's disease, mostly in sun-protected area is characteristic.

TABLE 3: Management of actinic keratosis.

General	*Specific*
• Sun protection measures	• 1% or 5% 5-fluorouracil (5-FU)—twice daily × 2–4 weeks • 5% imiquimod—thrice weekly × 4 weeks • Cryotherapy • Electrodessication • Ablative lasers • Photodynamic therapy • Excision removal

Histology

Hyperkeratosis, parakeratosis, and acanthosis along with atypical keratinocytes.

Prognosis

Rate of progression to malignancy is unknown. SCC arising from this is more aggressive.

Treatment

- *Topical*: Tretinoin and 5-FU
- *Procedural*: Ablative laser, cryotherapy, and excision

Psoralen and Ultraviolet A Keratosis[29]

Prolonged exposure can cause keratinocytic atypia leading to SCC.

Thermal Keratosis

- Chronic exposure to infrared radiation or heat from sources such as log burning stoves, locomotive engines, heating pads, and kangri (in Kashmiris).
- *Clinical feature*: Hyperkeratotic papule or plaque in erythema ab igne lesions.[30]

Scar Carcinoma

- SCC may develop on chronic burn scars, chronic ulcers, osteomyelitic scar, etc., and are highly metastasizing.
- Malignant transformation is 2% for burn scars.[31]

Chemical Keratosis[32]

Occupational exposure to tar, pitch, and coal combined with UV exposure can lead to cancerous lesions.

Epidermodysplasia Verruciformis

- Actinic keratosis, BD, and SCC can develop on exposed wart-like lesions of epidermodysplasia verruciformis (EDV).
- Rate of malignant transformation is quite high, 30–70%.[33]

KEY POINTS

- Premalignant conditions are those which can transform into invasive carcinoma later.
- Leukoplakia is a diagnosis of exclusion.
- Erythroplakia is less common, but have high chance of malignancy.
- Actinic cheilitis is a mucosal variant of AK with higher malignant transformation than AK.
- Cumulative UV exposure is the single most important risk factor for the disease involving the lower lip.
- Bowenoid papulosis is an SCC in situ with background coinfection by oncogenic HPV.
- It affects the sexually active youngs with rare malignant transformation.
- Erythroplasia of Queyrat has high chance of malignancy and it presents as solitary erythematous shiny plaques on glans penis of older uncircumscribed individuals.
- Intraepithelial neoplasia is restricted to carcinoma in situ involving the anogenital areas namely, vulval, penile, anal, and perianal type.
- Undifferentiated vulval type in young females is prognostically better than differentiated type of elderly.
- PKMB is a rare disease with thick adherent scales on the glans.
- Cutaneous horn, particularly penile ones, is commonly associated with underlying premalignant or malignant conditions.
- Bowen's disease is common in sun-exposed skin and is mostly unifocal.
- There is loss of polarity of the nuclei with widespread dysplasia—"windblown appearance".
- SCC over BD tends to be more aggressive than other SCCs.
- AK is more common in Caucasians.
- Subclinical lesions in the vicinity of clinical lesions can cause recurrence of AK—field cancerization.
- Rate of transformation to SCC is very low in AK.
- Chronic arsenicosis can cause BD, SCC, BCC, and internal malignancies also.
- Bowen's disease in arsenicosis patient is multicentric and involves sun-protected areas and arsenical keratotic lesions of palms and soles.
- EDV patients are highly prone to develop malignancy in later stage, which can be slowed down by systemic retinoids, sun protection measures, and regular follow-ups.

REFERENCES

1. Fonseca E. Tumores epiteliales. In: Ferrándiz C (Ed). Dermatología clínica, 4th edition. Barcelona: Elsevier; 2014.
2. Warnakulasuriya S, Johnson NW, van der Waal I. Nomenclature and classification of potentially malignant disorders of the oral mucosa. J Oral Pathol Med. 2007;36(10):575-80.
3. Ko JS, Matharoo-Ball B, Billings SD, Thomson BJ, Tang JY, Sarin KY, et al. Diagnostic distinction of malignant melanoma and benign nevi by a gene expression signature and correlation to clinical outcomes. Cancer Epidemiol Biomarkers Prev. 2017;26(7):1107-13.
4. Stevenson O, Ahmed I. Lentigo maligna: prognosis and treatment options. Am J Clin Dermatol. 2005;6(3):151-64.
5. Shrum JR, Cooper PH, Greer KE, Landes HB. Squamous cell carcinoma in disseminated superficial actinic porokeratosis. J Am Acad Dermatol. 1982;6:58-62.
6. Murase J, Gilliam AC. Disseminated superficial actinic porokeratosis co-existing with linear and verrucous porokeratosis in an elderly woman: update on the genetics and clinical expression of porokeratosis. J Am Acad Dermatol. 2010;63:886-91.
7. Sawai T, Hayakawa H, Danno K, Miyauchi H, Uehara M. Squamous cell carcinoma arising from giant porokeratosis: a case with extensive metastasis and hypercalcemia. J Am Acad Dermatol. 1996;34:507-9.

8. Heymann WR. Lichen sclerosus. J Am Acad Dermatol. 2007;56:683-4.
9. Braun KA, Massa L. Oral lichen planus with malignant transformation to invasive squamous cell carcinoma. Cutis. 2015; 96(3):E12-4.
10. Singh SK, Saikia UN, Ajith C, Kumar B. Squamous cell carcinoma arising from hypertrophic lichen planus. J Eur Acad Dermatol Venereol. 2006;20(6):745-6.
11. Mortazavi H, Baharvand M, Mehdipour M. Oral potentially malignant disorders: an overview of more than 20 entities. J Dent Res Dent Clin Dent Prospects. 2014;8:6-14.
12. Jadotte YT, Schwartz RA. Solar cheilosis: an ominous precursor: part I. Diagnostic insights. J Am Acad Dermatol. 2012;66:173-84.
13. MacFarlane GE, Terezhalmy GT. Actinic cheilitis. Diagnosis, prevention, and treatment. US Navy Med. 1982;73:22-4.
14. Jadotte YT, Schwartz RA. Solar cheilosis: an ominous precursor part II. Therapeutic perspectives. J Am Acad Dermatol. 2012;66(2):187-200.
15. Passi D, Bhanot P, Kacker D, Chahal D, Atri M, Panwar Y. Oral submucous fibrosis: newer proposed classification with critical updates in pathogenesis and management strategies. Natl J Maxillofac Surg. 2017;8(2):89-94.
16. Heppt MV, Schlager G, Berking C. Epithelial precancerous lesions. In: Kang S, Amagai M, Bruckner AL, Enk AH, Margolis DJ, McMichael AJ, Orringer JS (Eds). Fitzpatrick's Dermatology, 9th edition. New York: McGraw-Hill; 2019.
17. Goette DK. Erythroplasia of Queyrat. Arch Dermatol. 1974; 110:271-3.
18. Mikhail GR. Cancers, precancers, and pseudocancers on the male genitalia. A review of clinical appearances, histopathology, and management. J Dermatol Surg Oncol. 1980;6:1027-35.
19. Kao GF. Carcinoma arising in Bowen's disease. Arch Dermatol. 1986;122:1124-6.
20. Adya KA, Palit A, Inamadar AC. Pseudoepitheliomatous keratotic and micaceous balanitis. Indian J Sex Transm Dis AIDS. 2013;34(2):123-5.
21. Yu RC, Pryce DW, Macfarlane AW, Stewart TW. A histopathological study of 643 cutaneous horns. Br J Dermatol. 1991;124: 449-52.
22. Bowen JT. Precancerous dermatosis. J Cutan Dis. 1912;30: 241-55.
23. Graham JH, Helwig EB. Bowen's disease and its relationship to systemic cancer. Arch Dermatol. 1959;80:133-59.
24. Flohil SC, van der Leest RJ, Dowlatshahi EA, Hofman A, de Vries E, Nijsten T. Prevalence of actinic keratosis and its risk factors in the general population: the Rotterdam Study. J Invest Dermatol. 2013;133(8):1971-8.
25. Olsen EA, Abernethy ML, Kulp-Shorten C, Callen JP, Glazer SD, Huntley A, et al. A double-blind, vehicle-controlled study evaluating masoprocol cream in the treatment of actinic keratoses on the head and neck. J Am Acad Dermatol. 1991;24(5 Pt 1):738-43.
26. Glogau RG. The risk of progression to invasive disease. J Am Acad Dermatol. 2000;42(1 Pt 2):23-4.
27. Edwards MJ, Hirsch RM, Broadwater JR, Netscher DT, Ames FC. Squamous cell carcinoma arising in previously burned or irradiated skin. Arch Surg. 1989;124:115-7.
28. Neubauer O. Arsenical cancer: a review. Br J Cancer. 1947;1: 192-251.
29. Stern RS, Laird N, Melski J, Parrish JA, Fitzpatrick TB, Bleich HL. Cutaneous squamous cell carcinoma in patients treated with PUVA. N Engl J Med. 1984;310:1156-61.
30. Arrington JH III, Lockman DS. Thermal keratoses and squamous cell carcinoma in situ associated with erythema ab igne. Arch Dermatol. 1979;115:1226-8.
31. Stromberg BV, Keiter JE, Wray RC, Weeks PM. Scar carci-noma: prognosis and treatment. South Med J. 1977;70(7): 821-22.
32. O'Donovan WJ. Cancer of the skin due to occupation: tar carcinoma. Arch Dermatol Syphilol. 1928;19:595-606.
33. Lowy DR, Androphy EJ. Warts. In: Freedberg IM, Eisen AZ, Wolff K (Ed). Fitzpatrick's Dermatology in General Medicine, 6th edition. New York: McGraw Hill; 2003. pp. 2119-31.

EXAMINATION QUESTIONS

1. Discuss the differential diagnosis of leukoplakia and erythroplakia.
2. Discuss the histologic and dermoscopic findings of Bowen's disease.
3. Name the premalignant and malignant lesions of skin associated with arsenic exposure.

Write short notes on the following:

4. Premalignant lesions in skin
5. Verrucous carcinoma

90 CHAPTER

Squamous Cell Carcinoma and Basal Cell Carcinoma

Barnali Chowdhury, Koushik Lahiri

SQUAMOUS CELL CARCINOMA

INTRODUCTION

Squamous cell carcinoma (SCC) is also known as Bowen's disease (BD). It is more commonly seen in older individual but can also be seen in younger individual with significant sun exposure. BD may arise from a pre-existing actinic keratoses or it may arise *de novo*. Erythematous scaly patch or slightly elevated plaque is the classical lesion of SCC which typically arise in the sun-exposed areas such as head and neck, extremities, and trunk in the descending order **(Fig. 1)**.[1]

RISK FACTORS[2]

- Fair skin
- Light-colored hair and blue, green, or gray eyes
- Long-term exposure to UV radiation
- Living in sunny regions or at a high altitude
- History of multiple severe sunburns, especially if they occurred early in life
- History of being exposed to chemicals such as arsenic

Bowenoid papulosis: This term is used when histopathological changes of SCC in situ are found within general warts.[1]

INVASIVE CUTANEOUS SCC[3]

Invasive cutaneous SCC is most commonly found in bald scalp, face, neck, dorsal hands, and shins and usually arises within a background of damaged skin. The color of the lesion usually varies from erythematous to skin color. SSC are usually papulonodular but it can be plaque-like, papillomatous, or exophytic. Natural history of these lesions varies from slowly enlarging to rapidly growing with significant tenderness and even associated with pain **(Fig. 2)**.

STAGING[3]

TNM Staging (Table 1)

Primary tumor (T):

- TX: Primary tumor cannot be assessed.
- T0: No evidence of primary tumor
- Tis: Carcinoma in situ
- T1: Tumor $\leq$2 cm in greatest dimension with <2 high-risk features
- T2: Tumor > 2 cm in greatest dimension or tumor any size with $\geq$2 high-risk features
- T3: Tumor with invasion of maxilla, orbit, or temporal bone
- T4: Tumor with invasion of skeleton (axial or appendicular) or peridural invasion of skull base

Regional lymph nodes (N):

- NX: Regional lymph nodes cannot be assessed.
- N0: No regional lymph-node metastasis
- N1: Metastasis in a single ipsilateral lymph node, $\leq$3 cm in greatest dimension
- N2: Metastasis in a single ipsilateral lymph node; >3 cm but <6 cm in greatest dimension (2a); or in multiple ipsilateral

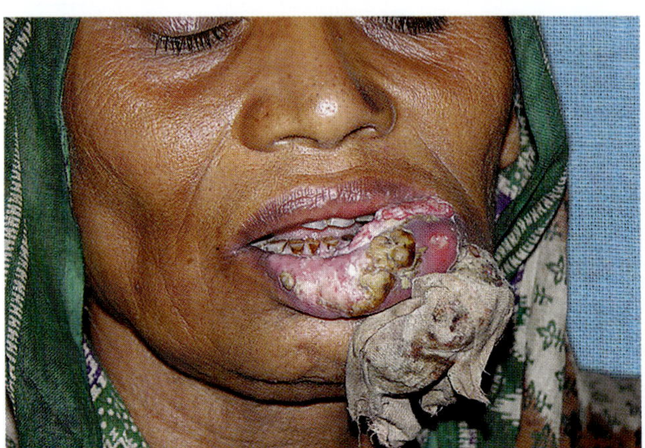

Fig. 1: Extensive hyperkeratosis and leukoplakia of the lower vermillion lip.

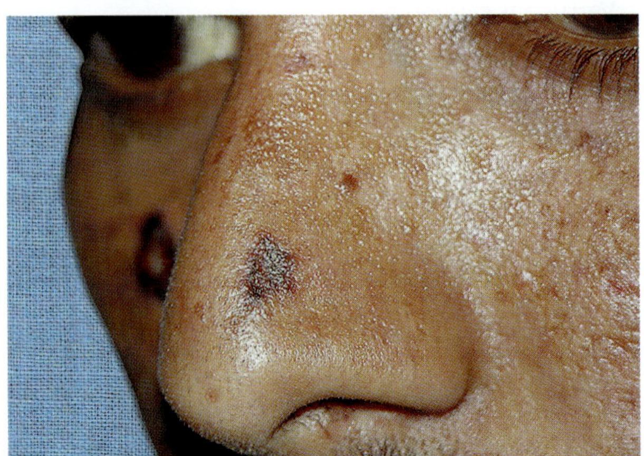

Fig. 2: Small hyperkeratotic lesion over the nose.

TABLE 1: TNM staging.

Stage	*T*	*N*	*M*
0	Tis	N0	M0
I	T1	N0	M0
II	T2	N0	M0
III	T3	N0	M0
	T1	N1	M0
	T2	N1	M0
	T3	N1	M0
IV	T1	N2	M0
	T2	N2	M0
	T3	N2	M0
	T Any	N3	M0
	T4	N Any	M0
	T Any	N Any	M1

Source: Adopted from the American Joint Committee on Cancer, 2010.

lymph nodes; none >6 cm in greatest dimension (2b); or in bilateral or contralateral lymph nodes, none >6 cm in greatest dimension (2c)

- N3: Metastasis in a lymph node, >6 cm in greatest dimension

Distant metastasis (M):

- M0: No distant metastasis
- M1: Distant metastasis

KERATOACANTHOMA

It was first described in 1889 by Jonathan Hutchinson. Other terminologies for keratoacanthoma (KA) are molluscum sebaceum, molluscum pseudocarcinomatosum, self-healing primary SCC, and keratocarcinoma. It is a variant of SCC with several distinct clinical presentations include solitary multiple rapidly growing crateriform nodules. The fully developed lesion is volcano shaped with buttresses of normal epidermis. Within the volcano is abundant hyaline keratin, which has a glassy appearance **(Fig. 3)**.

Keratoacanthomas can be difficult to distinguish histologically from conventional SCCs. This has prompted some to consider KAs and SCCs to be the same. Clinically, they are differentiated by their history of rapid growth and their volcano shape, yet histologically there are too many features that overlap with SCC to allow reliable separation **(Fig. 4)**.

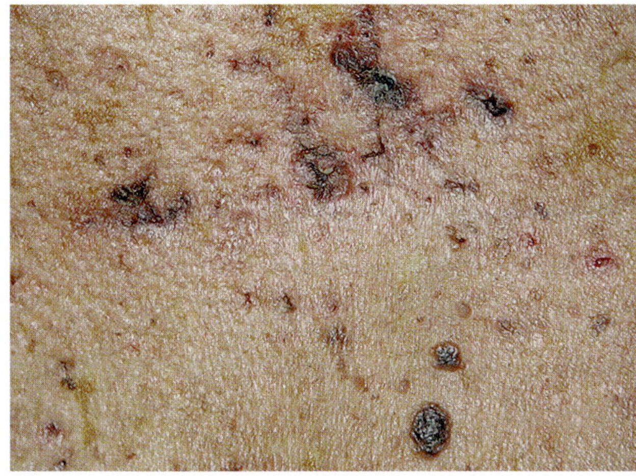

Fig. 3: Multiple superficial SCC along with hypertrophic AKs. (AK: actinic keratosis; SCC: squamous cell carcinoma)

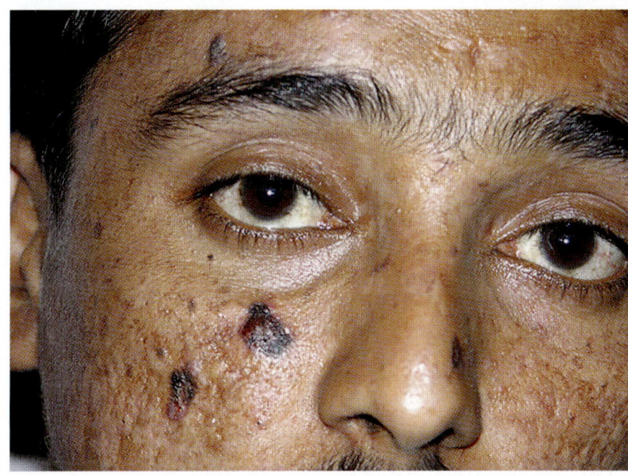

Fig. 4: Large keratotic nodules over the infraorbital area.

VERRUCOUS CARCINOMA

It is a low-grade variant of SCC with little potential for distant metastases. The term “verrucous carcinoma” was first used by Ackerman in 1948 to describe a carcinoma of the oral cavity. It is a rare and well-differentiated variant of SCC. It is usually seen in middle-aged and older adults. In addition to occurring in the oral cavity, genital area, and the plantar surface, verrucous carcinoma may occur anywhere on the skin **(Figs. 5 and 6)**.

Low-grade malignancy with three major subtypes:

1. Epithelioma cuniculatum
2. Giant condyloma acuminatum
3. Oral florid papillomatosis

PATHOGENESIS

Human papillomavirus (HPV) infection, chronic irritation, and chemicals have been implicated in the pathogenesis. Diagnosis is usually challenging due to bland histologic features. Deep incisional biopsy is recommended to differentiate among three subtypes.[4,5]

Dermoscopic images:[6]

- Linear irregular vessels
- Elongated vessels with hairpin
- Dotted vessels or combination of both

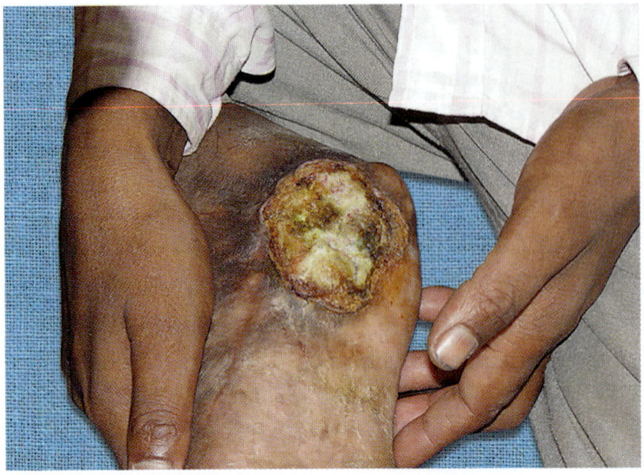

Fig. 5: Verrucous and ulcerated lesion.

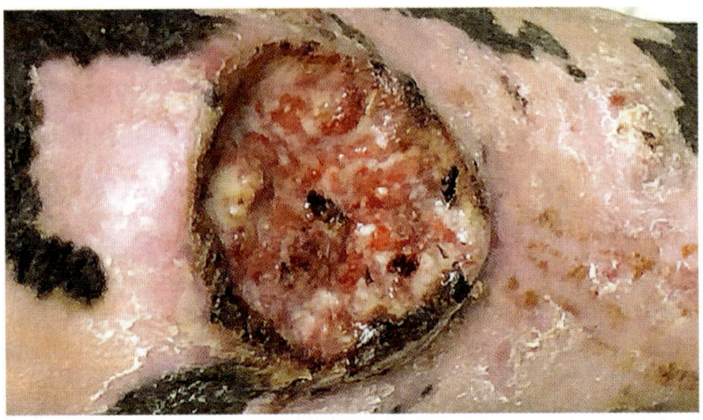

Fig. 6: Squamous cell carcinoma.
Courtesy: Dr Koushik Lahiri.

- Vessels are surrounded by whitish halo
- Ulcerated and hemorrhagic crust appear as red brown black-colored surface blotches

Histopathological examination (HPE):[5] Following are the HPE characteristics of different SCC.

SCC in situ:
- Full-thickness atypia of epidermis over a broad zone
- Nuclear pleomorphism and apoptosis and mitosis
- Epidermis shows acanthosis.
- A number of different histopathologic variants are seen.

Invasive SCC:
- Well differentiated
- Intercellular bridges often apparent along with keratin pearls and apoptotic cells
- Nucleoli may be prominent.
- The degree of nuclear atypia and cellular differentiation vary within and among tumors.

Keratoacanthoma:
- Typically has a "volcano-like" architecture.
- Well-differentiated keratinocytes
- Minimal cytologic atypia
- Diagnosis of invasive KA-like SCC should be considered in the presence of hyperchromatic nuclei or abnormal mitoses.

Verrucous carcinoma
- Well-differentiated and distinct clinic pathologic variant of SCC with warty appearance
- Minimal cytologic atypia
- Pushing border as opposed to an infiltrative invasive edge
- Major distinguishing features are the massiveness, depth of the lesion, and pronounced irregular architecture

SIMULATORS OF SCC

- Irritated seborrheic keratosis
- Verruca vulgaris
- Warty dyskeratoma
- Inverted follicular keratosis
- Prurigo nodularis
- Hypertrophic lichenplanus
- Hypertrophic lupus erythematous

DIFFERENTIAL DIAGNOSIS

- *Actinic keratosis:* Smaller lesion compared to usual SCC
- *Superficial basal cell carcinoma:* More translucent quality with slight elevation of the leading edge
- *Psoriasis:* Difficult to differentiate especially in presence of concomitant psoriatic papules
- Chronic eczema

TREATMENT OF SCC[7]

Squamous cell carcinomais highly curable if found early. Different modalities of treatments are available for SCC. It depends on the size, location, aggressiveness of the tumor, and person's immune status. Very small, localized tumor can be treated by less invasive methods such as curettage and electrodessication, laser therapy, cryosurgery, and photodynamic therapy. For the larger tumor surgical excision, Mohs surgery and radiotherapy are recommended. Chemotherapy and immunotherapy are used for the lesion which has spread beyond the skin.

Treatment of Localized Tumor[7]

- *Curettage and electrodessication (C and E):* C and E applied for the very small and superficial low-risk lesions including SCC in situ. It involves removing the lesion with a scraping instrument and then searing the base of the lesion with an electric needle.
- *Cryosurgery*: This treatment involves destroying the lesion with liquid nitrogen. It is often used to treat small tumor with clear and smooth border. This treatment is usually done when other surgical options are not possible.

- *Photodynamic therapy*: In this treatment, photosensitizers are used to make the tissue more susceptible to phototherapy. Again, this modality is useful for only superficial lesion. Examples of photosensitizers include aminolevulinic acid (ALA), Silicon Phthalocyanine Pc4, m-tetrahydroxyphenylchlorin (mTHPC), and mono-L-aspartyl chlorin e6 (NPe6).
- *Excision*: Standard surgical excision with clear margins is effective for superficial small lesions. In case of SCC of <2 cm diameter, 4-mm margins are adequate, whereas high-risk SCC requires 6-mm margins with size >2 cm, poor differentiation, invasion to fat and location in the high-risk areas.
- *Mohs micrographic surgery (MMS):* Mohs surgery is especially useful for SCC with high-risk characteristics such as >2 cm, recurrent tumor after excision, poorly defined edges, and in cancers with certain areas such as face and genital areas. MMS results in better histologic verification of complete removal by allowing maximum preservation of the surrounding tissue.
- *Radiation therapy (RT)*: RT is preferred treatment option in patients for whom surgery is contraindicated or as an adjuvant therapy following treatment of advanced and high-risk SCC. RT is associated with higher recurrence than surgery. It is preferred in patients with advanced age (>60 years) and unwilling to undergo surgery. RT is associated with poor cosmetic outcome.
- *Medical treatment:* Imiquimod and fluorouracil creams are used locally. Imiquimod is an immune response modifier. It is best used for superficial lesions <2 cm diameter and to be applied 3–5 times each week for 6–16 weeks. Fluorouracil cream is a topical cytotoxic agent and used to treat small superficial basal cellcarcinomas. It is usually applied twice daily for 6–12 weeks. It has high recurrence rates.
- *Immunotherapy:*[8] The US Food and Drug Administration (FDA) has approved one immunotherapy medication for the treatment of advanced SCC of the skin. It is called *cemiplimab-rwlc*. Studies have shown significant shrinkage of tumor by >50% and its effect persists for >6 months. *Cemiplimab-rwlc* is given by an intravenous (IV) infusion, once every 3 weeks. Pembrolizumab is another immunotherapy currently under investigation to treat advanced SCC of the skin.[9]

Prophylaxis[10]

Retinoids have been suggested for prophylaxis against skin cancer development. Acitretin is preferred over isotretinoin for the prophylaxis in solid organ transplant recipient due to its better side-effect profile. Triglyceride level and liver function should be monitored during therapy. Other agent used for the prevention in transplant recipients includes low-dose oral capecitabine.

KEY POINTS

- SCC commonly known as Bowen's disease.
- Risk factors associated with SCC are fair skin, prolong exposure to UV radiation, chemical exposure.
- TNM staging important for prognosis and treatment.
- SCC is curable if found early.
- Mohs surgery and radiotherapy are recommended for large tumor.

BASAL CELL CARCINOMA

INTRODUCTION

Basal cell carcinoma (BCC) is also known as basal cell epithelioma or rodent ulcer. It is the most common cancer in the human beings and usually arises from the sun-damaged skin involving commonly exposed area such as head and neck, and occasionally over the trunk and extremities **(Fig. 7)**. BCC is a slow-growing tumor with rare occurrence of metastases. It can be managed with local therapy such as excision. BCC usually appears as pink-colored pearly papules with overlying ulceration or telangiectatic vessels **(Figs. 8 to 10)**.[11]

ETIOLOGY/RISK FACTORS[11]

- *Age and sex:* Commonly found in the elderly males
- Patients with history of other skin cancers such as SCC or melanoma
- Damage of the skin following prolonged sun exposure
- Patients with fair skin types are more likely to develop compared to dark-skinned individual
- Presence of other skin diseases such as cutaneous lupus, sebaceous nevus or thermal injury to the skin
- Inherited syndromes such as Gorlin syndrome, Bazex-Dupré-Christol syndrome, Rombo syndrome, Oley syndrome, and xeroderma pigmentosum

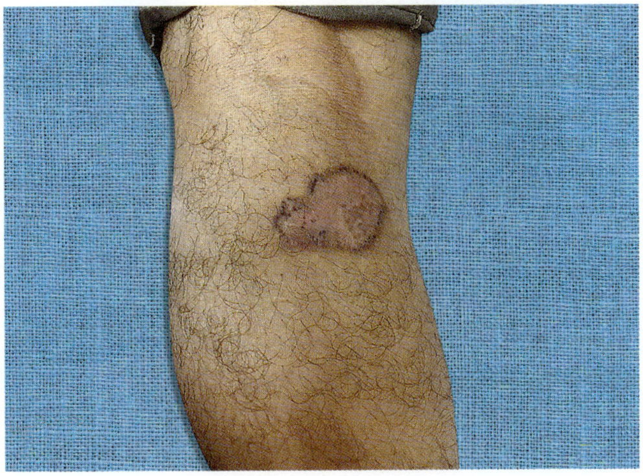

Fig. 7: Basal cell carcinoma.
Courtesy: Dr Aarti Sarda.

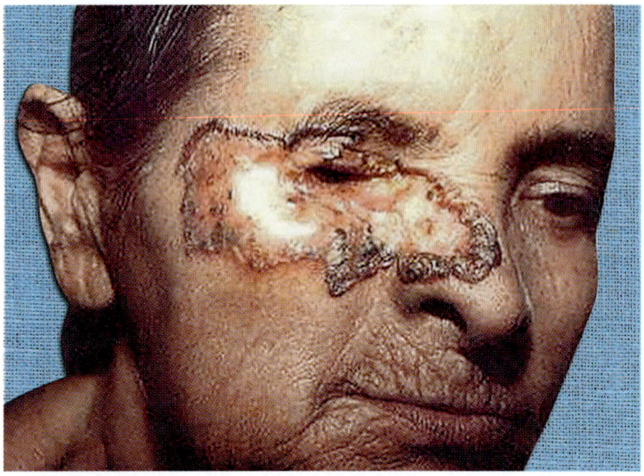

Fig. 8: Nodulo-ulcerative tumor of the periorbital region with rolled border.

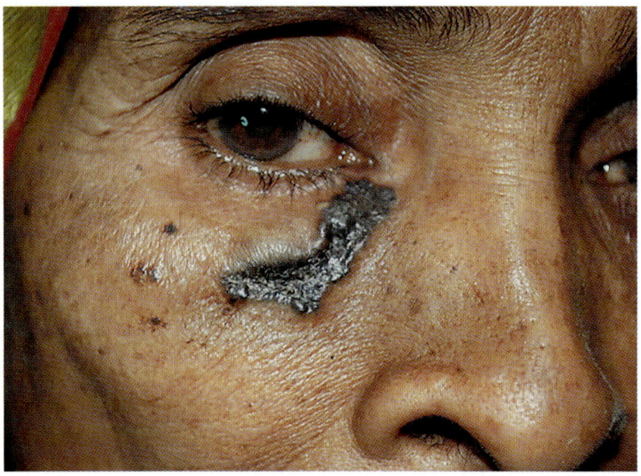

Fig. 9: Ulcerative lesion with rolled border at preorbital area.

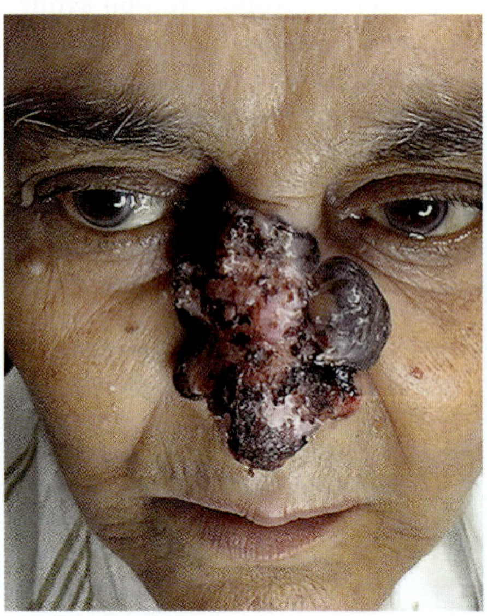

Fig. 10: Noduloulcerative basal cell carcinoma.
Courtesy: Dr Koushik Lahiri.

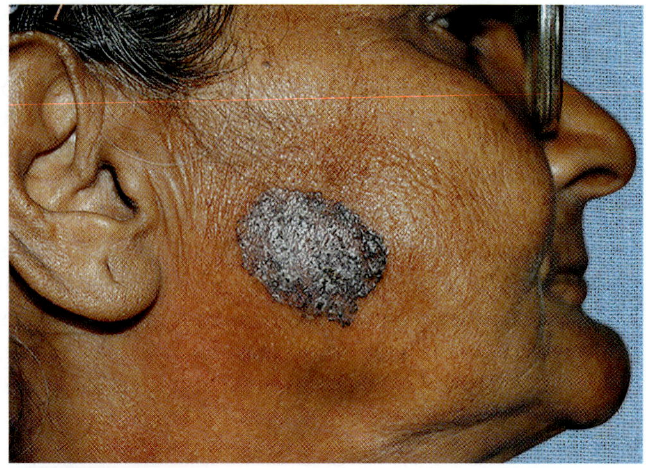

Fig. 11: Rounded lesion over the face with admixture of scale and hemorrhagic crusts.

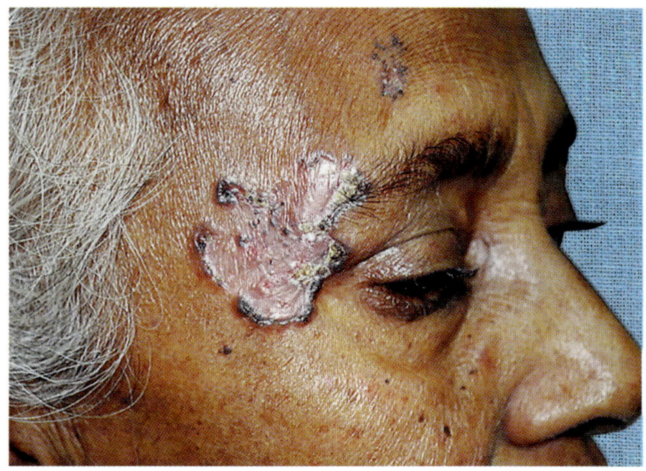

Fig. 12: Hypopigmented firm plaque-like lesion with translucent rolled border.
Courtesy: Dr Koushik Lahiri.

- Other risk factors such as ionizing radiation, arsenic exposure, and immunosuppression

CLINICAL FEATURES[11,12]

Basal cell carcinoma usually appears as a painless swelling or nodule. Later, it turns to an open ulcer with a hard edge. In >90% of cases, BCCs develop on the face. It can develop at any part of body exposed to sun—the face, ears, neck, back, chest, arms, and legs. Most commonly BCC remains confined to the skin and does not spread to other organs, but it can invade surrounding tissue leading to disfigurement of the skin **(Figs. 11 and 12)**.

The main characteristics are:

- Slowly growing plaque or nodule **(Fig. 13)**
- Skin colored, pink or pigmented
- Varies in size from a few millimetres to several centimeters in diameter
- Spontaneous bleeding or ulceration **(Fig. 14)**

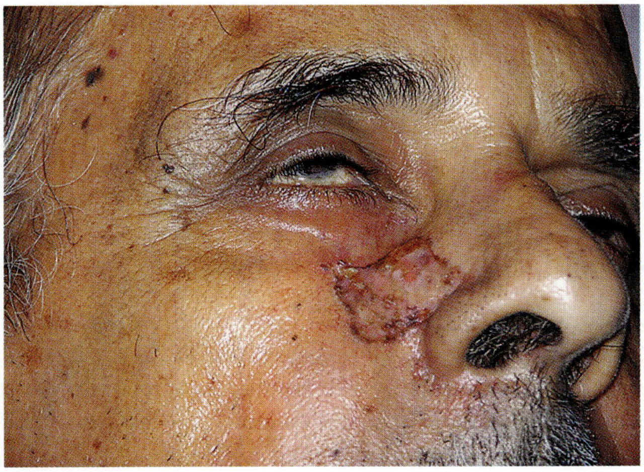

Fig. 13: Hypopigmented rounded lesion with scale and crusts.

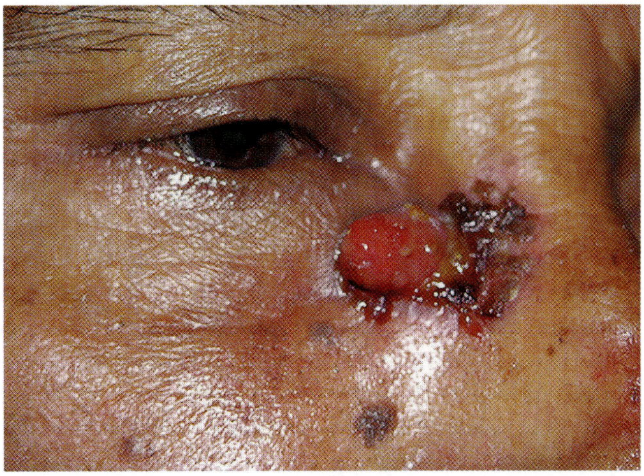

Fig. 14: Oval ulcerated lesion with hemorrhagic crusts and rolled border.

PATHOPHYSIOLOGY[13]

The cause of BCC is multifactorial. Following are the two important pathogenesis have been described.[12]

1. *Genetic factors*:[14] Association with the following genetic mutations were found in the development of BCC.
   - Mutationsin the patched (PTCH1) tumor suppressor gene, part of hedgehog signaling pathway in 70% of patients with sporadic BCC.
   - Mutation in the *P53* genes
   - Mutations in smoothened (*SMO*) gene and at CDNK2A loci
2. *Sun exposure and ultraviolet radiation*: Chronic sun exposure leads to development in the BCC by following pathways:
   - *UV damage:* Direct DNA damage by UV radiation and indirect DNA damage through reactive oxygen species (ROS) and immune suppression.[15]
   - Direct damage of the DNA and RNA by UVB with mutations involving C/T or CC/TT transition.[15]

TYPES OF BCC

Histologically, BCC has been classified into multiple variants. Four most common variants will be discussed in detail.

- *Nodular BCC:* Typically seen as a small pearly nodule with smooth surface and rolled out edges. It is commonly found over the face. Occasionally, central depression or umbilication noted over the nodules. Another variant of nodular form is cystic type which is soft in consistency filled with jelly-like content. On microscopic examination, nodular BCC composed of central island cells with peripheral palisading. Micronodular, microcystic, and infiltrative types are potentially aggressive type of nodular BCC and known as nodulocystic carcinoma.
  1. *Superficial BCC:* It is most commonly seen in young adults and found over the trunk and shoulders. On macroscopic examination, irregular plaques-like scaly lesion with translucent rolled border noted.
  2. *Morphoeic BCC:* It has typical appearance of white waxy scar-like lesion and commonly found over the face. Occasion borders of this lesion are not clearly demarcated with extension of the lesion deep into the skin is noted in this type of BCC. Even infiltration of cutaneous nerves is also seen. This is the least common and aggressive form of BCC.
  3. *Basosquamous carcinoma:* This is another aggressive variant of BCC with mixed pattern. Infiltrative pattern of growth noted with local invasion to lymph nodes and nerves. This tumor has got very high chance of local recurrence after treatment.
  4. *Infundibulocystic variant:* In this variant, localized small tumor usually found over the face. Multiple cystic infundibular structure filled with keratin and sometimes melanin found within the tumor.

DIAGNOSIS[12,16]

Diagnosis of BCC is most often done clinically by typical appearance of slow-growing lesion, and excision biopsy is done for confirmation and for histopathological characterization. Sometimes typical small superficial lesions on trunk or extremities are clinically diagnosed and treated without doing biopsy.

TREATMENT OF PRIMARY BCC[12,13]

The treatment for a BCC depends on its type, size, and location, the number to be treated, patient factors, and the preference or expertise of the doctor. Most BCCs are treated surgically.

- *Excision biopsy:* It is typically recommended for the treatment of nodular, infiltrative, and morpheic BCCs.

At least 3–5 mm surrounding normal skin margins are needed to remove during excision. Adequate skin clearance has to be confirmed with pathological examination. In case of inadequate excision, further treatment with surgery or radiotherapy is recommended to prevent the recurrence of lesion.

- *Mohs micrographically controlled excision:* In this type of excision, tumor is carefully examined under the microscope to confirm the adequacy of the excision. Excised tissue is marked to examine under microscope and in case of incomplete excision, further layers of tissues are removed to clear the tumor. With the expert hand, excellent result can be obtained with this procedure. This procedure is usually applied for the lesion in the face around eyes, lips, and nose. It is suitable for ill-defined, morpheic, infiltrative, and recurrent subtypes.
- *Superficial skin surgery:* It is a quick and easy technique which includes shave, curettage, and electrocautery. A small bandage is usually applied over the area without doing suture. Wound is healed by secondary intention and this procedure is used for the small well-defined lesions over trunk and limbs.
- *Cryotherapy:* In this procedure, liquid nitrogen is used to destroy the lesion by freezing the area. It is used for the superficial small lesion over the trunk and limbs. As this procedure leaves permanent scar over the treatment area, this is avoided for the lesions over the head and neck.
- *Photodynamic therapy:* In this two-stage procedure, first photosensitizers such as aminolevulinic acid lotion and methyl aminolevulinate cream are used over the lesion and then lights are used to destroy the cancer cells and precancerous tissue. Photosensitizers are activated at the specific wavelength of the lights. This procedure is applied for the lesion with low risk and superficial location. Cosmetic outcome is usually excellent with this procedure.
- *Imiquimod cream:* It is used for local therapy as a cream. It exerts its antitumor activity by binding with toll-like receptor 7 and 8 of the macrophages, monocytes, and dendritic cells and directly through activation of apoptosis. It is mainly used to treat very small superficial BCC. It is applied for at least 6–12 weeks and has high recurrence rate.
- *Fluorouracil cream:* It is a topical cytotoxic agent which inhibits thymidylate synthase activity thereby impairs deoxyribonucleic acid (DNA) synthesis. It is also used to treat very small superficial BCC and applied for at least 6–12 weeks.
- *Radiotherapy:* Most of the BCC can be treated with local therapy as mentioned above. In rare cases where there are positive margins reported in histopathology or in a large tumor, radiotherapy is applied as an adjunct therapy for cure.

Treatment for Advanced or Metastatic BCC

Locally advanced primary, recurrent, or metastatic BCC requires combined therapy including surgery and radiotherapy. Experimental therapies under investigations include vismodegib and sonidegib. Mechanism of actions of these agents are hedgehog signaling pathway inhibition.

PROGNOSIS[17]

Most small BCCs can be cured by treatment. About 50% of them are prone to develop second lesion, so regular skin examination preferably by a dermatologist is recommended. People with history BCC are also prone to develop other types of skin cancers such as melanoma.

PREVENTION[18]

- The most important way is to avoid sunburn.
- Adequate sun protection, especially among with high risks of developing BCC. These categories include individual with fair skin and with family history of BCC.
- Avoid going out under the sun without adequate cover of the exposed areas.
- Use of high protection factors—SPF 50+ sunscreen
- Avoid use of sun beds or solaria.
- *Chemoprophylaxis:* Oral nicotinamide (vitamin B_3)—500 mg twice a day to reduce the severity and number of the lesions.

KEY POINTS

- Basal cell carcinoma is the most common types of skin cancer.
- BCC is commonly found in fair-skinned individual after prolonged sun exposure.
- There are four main clinical variants of BCC. These are nodular, superficial spreading, sclerosing, and pigmented BCCs.
- BCC is a slow-growing tumor and rarely spread in other organs.
- Diagnosis is established with histology.
- Most BCC lesions are treated surgically with excision or Mohs micrographic surgery with excellent prognosis.
- Prevention is best done by avoiding sun exposure.

REFERENCES

1. Anadolu-Brasie R, Patel AR. Squamous cell carcinoma of the skin." In: Nouri K. Skin Cancer. China: McGraw Hill Medical; 2008. pp. 86-114.
2. Riddel C, Rashid R, Thomas V. Ungual and periungual human papillomavirus associated squamous cell carcinoma: a review. J Am Acad Dermatol. 2011; 64(6):1147-53.
3. Que SKT, Zwald F, Schmults CD. Cutaneous squamous cell carcinoma: Incidence, risk factors, diagnosis, and staging. J Am Acad Dermatol. 2018;78(2):237-47.

4. Nadhan KS, Chung CL, Buchanan EM, Shaver C, Shipman S, et al. Risk factors for keratinocyte carcinoma skin cancer in nonwhite individuals: a retrospective, analysis. J Am Acad Dermatol. 2019;81(2):373-8.
5. Omland SH, Ahlstrom MG, Gerstoft J, Pedersen G, Mohey R, Pedersen C, et al. Risk of skin cancer in patients with HIV: a Danish nationwide cohort study. J Am Acad Dermatol. 2018;79(4):689-95.
6. Weber P, Tschandl P, Sinz C, Kittler H. Dermatoscopy of neoplastic skin lesions: recent advances, updates, and revisions. Curr Treat Options Oncol. 2018;19(11):56.
7. Que SKT, Zwald FO, Schmults CD. Cutaneous squamous cell carcinoma: management of advanced and high-stage tumors. J Am Acad Dermatol. 2018;78(2):249-61.
8. US Food and Drug Administration. (2018). FDA approves cemiplimab-rwlc for metastatic or locally advanced cutaneous squamous cell carcinoma. [online] Available from: https://www.fda.gov/drugs/drug-approvals-and-databases/fda-approves-cemiplimab-rwlc-metastatic-or-locally-advanced-cutaneous-squamous-cell-carcinoma. [Last accessed April, 2021].
9. Vaidya P, Mehta A, Ragab O, Lin S, In GK. Concurrent radiation therapy with programmed cell death protein 1 inhibition leads to a complete response in advanced cutaneous squamous cell carcinoma. JAAD Case Rep. 2019;5(9):763-6.
10. Ribero S, Stucci LS, Daniels GA, Borradori Luca. Drug therapy of advanced cutaneous squamous cell carcinoma: is there any evidence? Curr Opin Oncol. 2017;29(2):129-35.
11. Cameron MC, Lee E,Hibler BP, Barker CA, Mori S, Cordova M, et al. Basal cell carcinoma: epidemiology, pathophysiology, clinical, and histological subtypes, and disease associations. J Am Acad Dermatol. 2019;80(2):303-17.
12. Invited Reviewers; Kim JYS, Kozlow JH, Mittal B, Moyer J, Olencki T, Rodgers P. Guidelines of care for the management of basal cell carcinoma. J Am Acad Dermatol. 2018;78:540-59.
13. Bichakjian CK, Olencki T, Aasi SZ, Alam M, Andersen JS, Berg Daniel, Bowen GM. Basal cell skin cancer, Version 1.2016, NCCN Clinical Practice Guidelines in Oncology. J Natl Compr Canc Netw. 2016;14(5):574-97.
14. Xie P, Lefrançois P. Efficacy, safety, and comparison of sonic hedgehog inhibitors in basal cell carcinomas: a systematic review and meta-analysis. J Am Acad Dermatol. 2018;79:1089-100.
15. Ferrucci LM, Cartmel B, Molinaro AM, Leffell DJ, Bale AE, Mayne ST. Indoor tanning and risk of early-onset basal cell carcinoma. J Am Acad Dermatol. 2012;67:552-62.
16. Weber P, Tschandl P, Sinz C, Kittler H. Dermatoscopy of neoplastic skin lesions: recent advances, updates, and revisions. Curr Treat Options Oncol. 2018;19(11):56.
17. Drucker AM, Adam GP, Rofeberg V, Gazula A, Smith B, Moustafa F, et al. Treatments of primary basal cell carcinoma of the skin: a systematic review and network meta-analysis. Ann Intern Med. 2018;169(7):456-66.
18. Hughley BB, Schmalbach CE. Cutaneous head and neck malignancies in the elderly. Clin Geriatr Med. 2018;34(2):245-58.

EXAMINATION QUESTIONS

1. Explain the types and HPE of basal cell carcinoma.
2. Discuss Mohs micrographically controlled excision.

91 CHAPTER Vascular Tumor and Malformations

Surajit Gorai, Adhyatm Bhandari, Kinnor Das

ARTERIOVENOUS MALFORMATION[1,2]

An arteriovenous malformation refers to communication between an artery and a vein. The affected skin feels warmer than the surrounding skin. It may be possible to feel a "thrill" due to the high flow of blood through the arteriovenous malformation. The doctor listening with a stethoscope may hear a rumble or "bruit".

Arteriovenous Fistula[3]

An arteriovenous fistula is an abnormal connection or passageway between an artery and a vein. It may be congenital, surgically created for hemodialysis treatments, or acquired due to pathologic process, such as trauma or erosion of an arterial aneurysm.

Salmon Patch[4,5]

- Also known as stork bites or angel kisses
- These are extremely common anomalies. Histologically there is dilatation of the subpapillary capillaries.
- Clinically, the lesions take the form of irregular, dull pinkish red, macular areas often featuring fine, linear telangiectasia.
- The nape of the neck and occiput are by far the most commonly affected areas. But face and rest of the scalp are often affected.
- Sacral lesions are of significance because of the association with spinal dysraphism.
- They subside with age.

Port-Wine Stain Nevus Flammeus[5]

It is a vascular malformation of developmental origin characterized pathologically by *ectasia of superficial dermal capillaries* and clinically by persistent macular erythema. The vascular ectasia *gradually involves the deeper dermal vessels.* The endothelium is of normal appearance. It is suggested that it results from a *developmental weakness* of the supporting structures of the vessel wall or from diminished neural influence on the vascular tone.

- They are *almost always present at birth.*
- They vary in color from a *fairly pale pink to deep red or purple* and in size from a few mm to many cm in diameter.
- The *face* is the most frequently affected site.
- It is *most often unilateral* with sharp midline demarcation.
- They *may be associated with areas of nevus anemicus.*
- Associated *eye and brain abnormalities* occur.
- A *variety of venous and lymphatic abnormalities* may be associated with port-wine stains, particularly when these occur on the limbs and trunk.
- Granuloma telangiectaticum is a frequent complication of port-wine stain. Other angiomatous lesions can occur in the vicinity of port-wine stain.
- Occasionally, the development of *basal cell and/or squamous cell carcinoma* has been reported.
- On the face, the general rule is for the port-wine stain to darken very slowly and gradually become raised and thickened sometimes taking a cobblestone appearance, paradoxically, on the limbs and trunk, port-wine stains will often fade somewhat over the years.
- *Ocular problems* associated with facial port-wine stain:
  - Dilated conjunctival vessels
  - Abnormal plexus of episcleral vessels
  - Tortuous retinal vessels
  - Glaucoma
  - Choroidal angioma
  - Orbital vascular malformation causing proptosis.

Syndromes Associated with Port-Wine Stains[6]

- *Sturge-Weber syndrome (Encephalofacial angiomatosis):*[7]
  - Facial port-wine stain in the distribution of the first branch of trigeminal nerve.
  - *Homolateral leptomeningeal angiomatosis:* This leads to convulsions of grand mal type, behavioral problems, subnormal intelligence, contralateral hemiparesis, and EEG abnormalities. Characteristic S-shaped intracranial calcifications are found in the leptomeninges within the first few months of life on CT scan and on X-rays after the age of 2 years.
  - *Ocular involvement* occurs in 40% of patients in the form of ipsilateral glaucoma, buphthalmos, congestion, strabismus, and loss of vision.
- *Klippel-Trenaunay syndrome:*[8]
  - This is a syndrome characterized by a *triad of port-wine stain, varicose veins and bony and soft-tissue hypertrophy of an extremity.*

Vascular anomalies classification.[1]

Vascular malformations		*Vascular tumors*
High flow • Arteriovenous malformation (AVM) • Arteriovenous fistula	Both high-flow malformations can be classified into: • Sporadic • Associated with hereditary hemorrhagic telangiectasia (HHT) • In capillary malformation, AV syndrome	**Benign** • *Infantile hemangioma (IH)*: – Diffuse neonatal hemangiomatosis – Multifocal IH (with/without systemic involvement) – Hepatic hemangioma • *Congenital hemangioma (CH):* – Rapidly involuting CH – Non-involuting CH – Partially involuting CH • Tufted angioma • Spindle cell hemangioma • Epithelioid hemangioma • Pyogenic granuloma
Low flow • *Capillary malformations:* – Salmon patch – Port-wine stain – Hereditary hemorrhagic telangiectasia (HHT) – Reticulate vascular nevus • *Venous malformations (VM):* – Common VM – Familial VM – Blue rubber bleb nevus – Glomangioma – Zosteriform nevus malformation		
Combined (AVMs): • AVMs of major vessels • AVM associated with other anomalies		**Locally aggressive** • Kaposiform hemangioendothelioma • Retiform hemangioendothelioma • Composite hemangioendothelioma • Kaposi sarcoma • Dabska tumor
		Malignant • Angiosarcoma • Epithelioid hemangioendothelioma

- Deeper vessels are usually absent or hypoplastic.
- *Problems* which may arise are *compensatory scoliosis, cutaneous ulcerations, edema and stasis from varicosities*. Thrombophlebitis of the varicosities occasionally occurs.
- Diagnosed by Doppler flowmetry, venous occlusion plethysmography, MRI, and plain radiographs.
- *Treatment:* A difference of more than 1 cm in leg length should be treated with sole raise of healthy foot + elastic support stockings + varicotomy if the deeper veins are patent. Extreme overgrowth (more than 2 cm) of an affected limb may be corrected by orthopedic procedures such as epiphysiodesis and tibial osteotomy.

- *Parkes-Weber syndrome:*[9] In this syndrome, AV fistulae are seen with features of Klippel-Trenaunay syndrome.

Hereditary Hemorrhagic Telangiectasia[10,11]

- Hereditary hemorrhagic telangiectasia (HHT) is also known as Osler-Rendu-Weber syndrome. It is a rare autosomal dominant disorder that affects blood vessels throughout the body and is characterized by a tendency for bleeding (haemorrhage, American spelling "hemorrhage"), in particular recurrent epistaxis (nosebleeds); and skin telangiectasia (skin lesions resulting from dilation of blood vessels).
- The diagnostic criteria for HHT are:
  - Spontaneous recurrent nosebleeds
  - Multiple telangiectases on skin and mucous membranes
  - Involvement of internal organs
  - An affected parent, sibling or child
- The two major types of HHT are HHT1 and HHT2. They are caused by mutations in the endoglin (ENG) and activin receptor-like kinase type 1 *(ACVLR1)* genes found on chromosome 9 and 12, respectively.
- *Treatment:*
  - Nosebleeds—laser coagulation therapy/septal dermoplasty
  - Telangiectases—cautery or dye laser surgery
  - GI bleeding—iron replacement therapy. For advanced cases, blood transfusion and/or endoscopic treatments

Reticulate vascular nevi are closely related to port-wine stains. The main difference is that reticulate naevi usually spontaneously improve by fading with time.[12]

VENOUS MALFORMATIONS[13]

- Venous malformation is the most common type of congenital vascular malformation (CVM) with an incidence of 1–2 in 10,000 and a prevalence of 1%.
- Although present at birth, they are not always clinically evident until later in life and tend to grow

in concert with the child and without spontaneous regression.

- VMs are composed of ectatic venous channels found usually in the head, neck, limbs, and trunk and are thought to be sporadic in most cases, though familial inheritance patterns exist.
- VMs can be challenging to diagnose and are often confused with hemangioma.

Positive and negative clinical findings and characteristics of venous malformations

Positive	• Bluish/purple superficial appearance • Occasionally palpable phleboliths and spontaneous thrombi • Soft and compressible mass • Swelling • Pain • Well-defined or diffuse and infiltrative • Can involve superficial or deep structures • May enlarge during Valsalva maneuver, puberty or pregnancy
Negative	• Hyperemia • Pulsatility • Palpable local thrill
Characteristics	• Occur in childhood or early adulthood • Can occur anywhere in the body, but are predominantly located in the head and neck (40% of cases), trunk (20%), and extremities (40%) • Lesions are categorized as: (i) Microcystic small diameter locules; (ii) macrocystic (large, more translucent subcutaneous masses in the neck, pelvis or axilla); (iii) mixed • VMs are postcapillary, by definition, and represent enlarged and engorged structures. These may demonstrate abnormal and sparse smooth muscle cells within the thin vessel wall, absent or insufficient valves, chaotic vascular branching, and are nonfunctional hemodynamically

Indications of Treatment

- Bleeding from below skin to intramuscular or retroperitoneal hematoma, hematuria, rectal bleeding, hematemesis, hemoptysis, or intracerebral or intraspinal bleeding
- Lesions are in close proximity to important structures or obstruct inflow and outflow of important structures
- Lesions are in life-threatening areas or in areas with high probabilities of complications
- Lesions cause excessively adverse hemodynamic effects.
- Disabling pain
- Functional impairment
- Excessive cosmetic implications
- Recurrent thrombosis

Treatment modalities available:

- Surgery
- Sclerotherapy
- Laser therapy

Blue Rubber Bleb Nevus Syndrome[14]

The blue rubber bleb nevus syndrome or Bean syndrome is a rare form of venous malformation in which there are skin and gastrointestinal tract lesions. There is frequently a family history, with autosomal dominant inheritance, i.e., the tendency to the syndrome is passed on to half of one's children.

The skin lesions present as compressible blue or purple rubbery nodules with a wrinkled surface. There may be a single lesion or hundreds of lesions occurring all over the body. Lesions in the GI tract (mouth to rectum) may bleed and cause anemia or rarely, sudden death. The nodules remain unchanged for life.

Surgical excision, sclerotherapy, and/or laser therapy may be indicated. However in most cases, no treatment is required.

Glomangioma[15]

Glomuvenous malformation is also known as glomangioma, or glomangiomatosis. These differ from standard venous malformations by being multiple, slightly raised, blue, or bluish-purple in appearance. There are characteristic features of this lesion on skin biopsy (histology). Glomuvenous malformations may be inherited as an autosomal dominant trait, which means half the children of an affected person will have a tendency to develop these lesions to a variable extent. They are due to a specific mutation in the *glomulin gene.*

Glomuvenous malformations should be distinguished from solitary glomus tumors, which usually occur under or beside a nail in an adult, and are not inherited. They are small, but exquisitely tender blue or purple nodules with a fibrous rim. An X-ray may show underlying erosion of the bone. Solitary glomus tumors are due to a proliferation of glomus cells; the diagnosis is confirmed by skin biopsy.

Zosteriform Venous Malformations[16]

Venous malformations with a dermatomal distribution is called as "zosteriform venous malformations", while the terms "zosteriform cavernous hemangiomas" and "unilateral dermatomal cavernous hemangiomatosis" were previously used to describe the lesions.

Zosteriform venous malformations was first reported in 1977 by Steinway and Fretzin.

They have a distinct distribution pattern limited to unilateral single or multiple adjacent dermatomes, further characterized by the absence of visceral lesions or enchondromas, and a negative family history.

Although there are no established treatments for this disease, possible therapeutic options include compression garments, aspirin, sclerotherapy, and surgical removal.

Vascular Malformation Associated with Other Anomalies[1]

- *Klippel-Trenaunay syndrome:* CM + VM +/- LM + limb overgrowth
- *Parkes Weber syndrome:* CM + AVF + limb overgrowth
- *Servelle-Martorell syndrome:* Limb VM + bone undergrowth
- *Sturge-Weber syndrome:* Facial + leptomeningeal CM + eye anomalies ± bone and/or soft tissue overgrowth
- Lim CM + congenital non-progressive limb hypertrophy
- *Muffucci syndrome:* VM ± spindle-cell hemangioma + enchondroma
- *Macrocephaly:* CM (M-CM/MCAP)
- *Microcephaly:* CM (MICCAP)
- *CLOVES syndrome:* CM, VM and/or LM + asymmetrical somatic overgrowth
- *Proteus syndrome:* CM, VM and/or LM + asymmetrical somatic overgrowth
- *Bannayan-Riley-Ruvalcaba syndrome:* AVM + VM + macrocephaly, lipomatous overgrowth

Infantile Hemangioma[17-19]

- Benign vascular neoplasms
- Most common neoplasms of infancy
- *Incidence:* 1–3%
- Female:Male = 3:1
- Usually sporadic
- Enlarge by rapid cellular proliferation of endothelial cells

Risk Factors

- *Low birth weight:* Most significant risk factor (40% risk increase for every 500 g decrease in birth weight)
- Preterm infants
- Advanced maternal age (older than 30 years of age), pre-eclampsia, placenta previa, and other placental anomalies
- Female child more prone to complicated infantile hemangiomas (IH)
- Use of in vitro fertilization
- Mothers with autoimmune diseases such as inflammatory bowel disease, RA, psoriasis

Stages of Infantile Hemangiomas

Stage	*Clinical features*
Nascent (at birth)	Subtle findings such as blanched erythematous macule, telangiectatic patch, cluster of bright red papules, or bluish area
Proliferating phase (first few weeks of life)	Rapid proliferation during 3–6 months of life, then growth rate slows down and the hemangioma attains maximum size by 9–12 months
Involution phase (12–18 months)	• Begins from the center of lesion • Bright cherry red color changes into dull red purple color and subsequently into grey white • Accompanied by flattening of surface and breaking up of superficial plaque into smaller islands
Involuted phase	• Residual pallor, telangiectasia, atrophic skin or altered skin texture seen. Redundant fibrofatty tissue seen in hemangiomas with dermal component • If no signs of regression by 5–6 years. Complete regression is unlikely

Histopathology

- *Early growth phase:* Well-defined, solid, nonencapsulated masses composed of proliferating plump endothelial cells and pericytes characterize proliferating hemangiomas.
- *Late proliferative phase:* Capillary-sized lumina are present
- *Phase of involution:* Apoptosis, hemangioma becomes more organized, a lobular appearance develops with islands of fibrous and fatty tissue between the lobules, vascular channels decrease, may assume a cavernous appearance.
- Mast cells are evident at all phases.

Immunohistochemistry: Positive for GLUT-1 (characteristic of placental microcirculation), factor VIII, CD31, and von Willebrand factor, FcγRII, merosin, and Lewis Y-antigen.

Clinical Features

Evolution of hemangioma of infancy

Macular area of hyperemia or grouped punctate telangiectasia
↓
Group of small, closely packed angiomas develop within the area and enlarge/coalesce
↓
Circumscribed oval/round, soft, dome-shaped red/purple plaque called as strawberry nevus
Based on location, IH may be superficial, deep, and mixed

Superficial Infantile Hemangiomas (Capillary/Strawberry)

- Usually appears in first 4 weeks of life
- May present as precursor lesions at the time of birth.
- Involves superficial dermis
- Vivid, scarlet red color, sharply circumscribed dome shaped papules and plaques
- Rubbery consistency
- Blanches partially on pressure
- *M/C site:*
  - Head and neck (60%)

- Trunk (25%)
- Extremities (15%)
- 80% of cases have single lesion.

Size ranges from <1–25 cm or more; attains maximum size usually by 3–6 months.

There is frequently a deep element to superficial hemangioma in larger lesions (termed as mixed infantile type). Superficial element usually emerges from center of swelling.

Deep Infantile Hemangioma

- Involves reticular dermis and subcutis
- Soft, warm, round bluish masses beneath normal skin–often feel like *bag of worms*
- Compressible to half the original size
- Often become larger/darker when the child screams or cries

Mixed Infantile Hemangioma

Mixed IH (25–35%) has superficial and deep components giving poached egg appearance due to well-defined superficial portion overlying a less well-defined deeper portion.

Segmental Hemangiomas

Segmental hemangiomas are generally plaque-like in presentation, demonstrate a geographic distribution over a specific cutaneous region and are more likely to be associated with complications, require more aggressive therapy, and have a poorer overall outcome.

Distribution pattern:

- Focal (77%)—solitary, discrete, circular, or plaque-like lesion
- Segmental (18%)—plaques in an anatomic or developmental distribution commonly associated with local complications or structural anomalies and continued growth beyond 6 and occasionally 9 months of age (3%)
- Multifocal (3%)—several discrete localized lesions distributed over more than one anatomic site
- Indeterminate—the lesions are not definitively focal or segmental.

Investigations for hemangioma:

- Doppler ultrasonography
- MRI for suspected anatomical associations such as PHACE syndrome, SACRAL, LUMBAR and PELVIS syndromes
- Laryngoscopy to investigate stridor with or without beard lesions
- For visceral involvement—thyroid and liver function tests, ultrasound of abdomen, MRI or ultrasound of the head, or echocardiogram
- Skin biopsy shows uniform vessel morphology with an outer layer of pericytes and inner lining of endothelial cells containing typical microtubular Weibel-Palade bodies
- Immunohistochemical staining for GLUT1 confirms a diagnosis of IH, although GLUT1 is also positive in angiosarcoma, epithelioid endothelioma, angiokeratoma, and verrucous hemangioma. Staining is negative in congenital hemangioma and other vascular malformations.

Indications for intervention:

- Function-threatening hemangiomas (ocular, auricular, nasal tip, and genitalia)
- Life-threatening hemangiomas (impending respiratory distress)
- Disfiguring hemangiomas (large facial hemangiomas)
- Ulceration
- Associated systemic involvement (>5 IH lesions)

Components for nonactive intervention:

- Assure and educate the parents on the natural course of IH, its heterogeneity, and need for follow-ups
- Advocate regular follow-ups—serial photographs, hemispheric measurements need to be recorded to assess the course of the lesions
- Apply bland emollients over the lesion to keep it soft and trim the patient's nails regularly
- Address emotional and psychosocial issues arising from cosmetic appearance and social reaction
- Alert—identify existing or impending sequelae which can necessitate intervention

Treatment options:

- Oral propranolol is the preferred low-risk nonsurgical approach.
- Topical timolol—for lesions less than 2 cm^2.
- Laser-pulsed dye or Nd:YAG lasers can be used as adjuvant or monotherapy for ulcerated and residual lesions, such as telangiectases, after the proliferative period.
- Surgical excision with primary closure can be useful; for example, an ulcerated scalp lesion that can cause bleeding, scarring, and alopecia.
- Plastic surgery—for lesions with a risk of slow involution and scarring such as the tip of nose, lip, and parotid.
- Embolization and sclerotherapy (less commonly used).

Propranolol—Mechanism of action, indications, dosage, and routes of administration:

Mechanism of action	• Vasoconstriction • Decreases VEGF and β fibroblasts GF genes • Apoptosis of capillary endothelial cells • Blocks G-protein coupled receptor kinase Leu41 • Reduces MP-9 • Effect on mesenchymal stem cells
Dosage	2 mg/kg/day (oral)

Contd...

Contd...

Indications	• First line in nonresolving IH • Failure/contraindications to other treatment modalities • IH located in sites inaccessible to surgery and/or parents unwilling for surgery • Compromised airway, visual axis, or other vital structures • Severe cosmetic embarrassment • Complicated IH • Intolerance to other therapies, i.e., deranged liver function tests
Routes of administration	Oral, intralesional, and topical

(IH: infantile hemangioma; VEGF: vascular endothelial growth factor; GF: growth factor)

An Algorithm to Manage Infantile Hemangioma with Oral Propranolol

Step 1
- Identify indication
- Assess contraindications—bronchial asthma, heart failure, sinus bradycardia, hypoglycemia, hypotension, heart block, and known propranolol allergy
- Evaluate cardiopulmonary status (ECG, CXR, and echocardiogram), timed sugars

Step 2
- Administering propranolol
- Two regimens currently in practice:
  - 0.33 mg/kg/dose given Q 8 h for 1 week—double the dose to 0.67 mg/kg/dose to get the recommended 2 mg/kg/day dose
  - 1 mg/kg/day Q 8 h—increase to 2 mg/kg/day after 1 week

Note: Each dose prepared by pharmacist in small packets—dissolve in rose syrup/honey

Step 3
- Watch for complications:
  - Hypoglycemia (can be as late as 6 months after initiating therapy)
  - Hypotension
  - Bradycardia (<60), hypotension (<50/30)
  - Sleep disruption
  - Acrocyanosis
  - Diarrhea
- Safety instructions for patients:
  - Administer during daytime hours only
  - Frequent feeds
  - If refusing feeds—skip the dose
  - Exact dose, at least 6 hours apart
  - If missed/if child spurts out the dose—wait until next dose
  - If sick/not feeding—stop propranolol—pediatric consult

Step 4
- Monitor:
  - BP, timed sugars, pulse rate 1–3 hours after initial dose—after every dose hike—after every 2–3 months
  - Weight—for dose revision
  - Response:
    - Serial photographs
    - Color and texture (softer and lighter in 48 hours)
    - Growth (stops within 24 hours to 2 weeks, complete resolution by 4 months)
  - Special circumstances

Contd...

Contd...

  - Ulcerated hemangiomas:
    - Propranolol as an adjuvant to local barrier creams/oral antibiotics/POL/topical morphine 0.1% in hydrogeljbe-caplermin
    - Average healing time is 4.3 weeks
  - PHACES: Lowest dosage, slow dose titration, 3 times/day dosing, close neurological follow-up

(ECG: electrocardiogram; CXR: chest X-ray; PDL: pulsed dye laser; BP: blood pressure)

Complications

Local complications	Ulceration (common complication, seen in 5–13%), hemorrhage, infection, and necrosis
According to location	
Periorbital and retrobulbar	Visual axis obscured, astigmatism, amblyopia, and optic nerve compression
Auricular	External auditory canal obstruction, otitis externa, and hearing impairment
Nasal tip and large facial hemangiomas	Permanent scarring (e.g., Cyrano nose) and disfigurement
Mandibular/beard area distribution	Airway obstruction
Perioral	Feeding difficulties, ulceration, and disfigurement
Subglottic	Strider and respiratory failure
Perineal	Ulceration
Multiple hemangiomas	Visceral involvement (liver and GIT)
Large hemangiomas	High-output cardiac failure
Associated anomalies	
PHACES syndrome	Posterior fossa malformations, hemangiomas (plaque such as segmental facial hemangiomas), arterial anomalies, cardiac defects, eye abnormalities, sternal clefts, and supraumbilical raphe
PELVIS syndrome	• Perineal hemangiomas and external genitalia malformations • Lipomyelomeningocele, vesicorenal abnormalities, imperforate anus, and skin tags
SACRAL syndrome	Spinal dysraphism, anogenital anomalies, cutaneous anomalies, renal and urological anomalies, associated angioma of lumbosacral localization

(PHACES: posterior fossa malformations-hemangiomas-arterial anomalies-cardiac defects-eye abnormalities-sternal cleft and supraumbilical raphe syndrome; GIT: gastrointestinal tract)

Vascular malformations	*Hemangiomas*
Result from errors of vascular morphogenesis, present since birth	Benign neoplasms, result from proliferation of endothelial cells, usually appear after birth

Contd...

Contd...

Vascular malformations	*Hemangiomas*
M:F = 1:1	F>M [3 : 1], premature infant <1,500 g, infant who had chorionic villous sampling
Enlarge proportional to child's growth, noninvoluting	1st proliferate f/b involution
Have a persistent color hue	Bright red color—deepens during 1st year
On palpation—soft and easily compressible	Firm/rubbery consistency
Frequent association with malformation syndromes, e.g., Sturge–Weber, phakomatosis pigmentovascularis, Klippel–Trenaunay syndrome, etc.	PHACES syndrome, spinal dysraphism

Congenital Hemangioma[20,21]

- Type of hemangioma that is *fully developed at birth.*
- Detected by USG from the 12th week of gestation.
- Clinically, the feature that distinguishes them is their lack of a proliferative phase and their tendency to involute very rapidly with the whole process generally being complete within the first year.
- Based on their progression, they can be classified into:
  - Rapidly involuting congenital hemangioma
  - Noninvoluting congenital hemangioma
  - Partially involuting congenital hemangioma

Infantile hemangioma	*Congenital hemangioma*
Present at birth and potentially diagnosable during fetal development via ultrasound	Visible between 2 weeks and 4 months of age
Growth is complete at birth, or it may grow proportionately as your child grows	Grows rapidly for about 6–12 months (average is around 8 months)
Occurs equally in males and females	Occurs in five females for every male
Less common than infantile hemangiomas, but not rare	Common (4–5% incidence in newborns)
Rapid or no involution (shrinking)	Slow shrinking that takes months or years

Tufted Angioma[22]

- Vascular tumors typified by tightly packed capillaries ("tufts") in discrete lobules
- They usually present before 5 years of age
- Presents as brown, red or purple areas of skin, and are firm and tender
- *HPE:* Canon ball appearance seen
- Spontaneous regression is unusual.

Spindle Cell Hemangioma[23]

- It is an rare vascular tumor → presents as subcutaneous or deep dermal nodule
- Usually present over the extremities
- Usually <2 cm in size
- It is benign in nature
- *Treatment options:*
  - Surgery
  - Systemic steroids
  - Cryotherapy
  - Laser and radiation therapy
  - Cytotoxic drugs
  - Selective embolization
- Recombinant interleukin-2

Epithelioid Hemangioma[24,25]

- Called as angiolymphoid hyperplasia by some authors
- It is characterized by a benign although locally aggressive behavior, composed by proliferated small-caliber blood vessels lined by plump endothelial cells with an epithelioid morphology.
- Eosinophils are often rich in the lesion.
- Treatment options:
  - Intralesional steroids (ILS)
  - Cryotherapy
  - Laser cauterization
  - Irradiation

Pyogenic Granuloma[26,27]

- It is also called *lobular capillary hemangioma.*
- It is one of the most common vascular tumors of infants and children and can also occur in adults, particularly in pregnant women.
- Solitary, red, rapidly growing papule or nodule, often with a subtle collarette of scale
- *Typical locations:* Cheek or forehead, but virtually any body site including the mucous membranes may be affected.
- Erosion can occur with subsequent profuse bleeding (Band-Aid disease)
- Rare association with vascular anomalies including arteriovenous malformations and congenital hemangioma
- PG does not typically involute spontaneously.
- Even after definitive treatment, recurrence and even satellite lesions surrounding the original PG
- Simple curettage with electrocautery is usually curative.
- Other options include excision, laser surgery (carbon dioxide or pulsed-dye laser), and cryotherapy
- Imiquimod and timolol—topical options.

Kaposiform Hemangioendothelioma[28]

- Kaposiform hemangioendothelioma (KHE) is a rare vascular endothelial tumor.
- Mostly occurs in infancy and early childhood.
- The sites of predilection:
  - Skin
  - Deep regions (retroperitoneum)

- Clinical feature
- Blue-red lesion, ill-defined borders
- Looks like Kaposi sarcoma
- It is associated with lymphatic vessel proliferation and Kasabach–Merritt phenomenon (KMP)
- Resection is the treatment of first choice
- *Treatment of KHE:* Systemic corticosteroids ± vincristine, vincristine, propranolol, aspirin, rapamycin
- Treatment of KHE + Kasabach–Merritt syndrome = systemic corticosteroids and vincristine

Retiform Hemangioendothelioma[29]

- Retiform hemangioendothelioma (RH) is a rare vascular neoplasm (<50 cases reported till now) which presents clinically as a slow growing asymptomatic solitary nodule or plaque either on extremities or trunk in 2nd-4th decade of life.
- Slow indolent course with very high local recurrence and metastasizes rarely
- *HPE:* Elongated, arborizing blood vessels lined by monomorphic bland endothelial cells with prominent apical nuclei and scanty cytoplasm resembling *"match stick" or hobnail appearance.*
- Treatment of choice—Moh's micrographic surgery
- Adjuvant radiotherapy for:
  - Large tumor size
  - Local recurrence
  - Lymph node metastasis

Composite Hemangioendothelioma[30]

- Composite hemangioendothelioma (HE), defined by the World Health Organization (WHO) as "a locally aggressive, rarely metastasizing neoplasm with vascular differentiation, containing an admixture of histologically benign, intermediate, and malignant components."
- It is an extremely rare entity with a handful of cases reported till.
- Composite HE should be treated with wide excision and patients should be carefully followed for several years after diagnosis as it recurs in approximately 50% of cases, sometimes aggressively, but only rarely metastasizes.

Kaposi Sarcoma[31,32]

- Vascular tumor which is locally aggressive
- *Clinical features:* Progressive, enlarging red to violaceous skin lesions
  - *Patch stage:* Red or purple macules or patches
  - *Plaque stage:* Thickened red, purple or brown plaques
  - *Tumor stage:* Nodule formation

All four clinical subtypes of Kaposi may show these stages and multiple different stages may be present simultaneously.

- *Types of Kaposi sarcoma:*
  - *Classic/sporadic:*
    - Elderly men > women
    - Lower extremity skin lesions
    - Central equatorial Africa, Mediterranean, and Eastern European
    - May be associated with secondary malignancy
    - Clinically indolent course
  - *Endemic/African:*
    - Lower extremity skin lesions
    - Children and young to middle-aged adults
    - Not related to HIV
    - Sub-Saharan Africa
    - May be aggressive if lymph nodes involved
  - *Iatrogenic:*
    - Predominantly transplant associated
    - Skin, visceral, and mucosa involvement
  - *AIDS associated:*
    - Patients infected with HIV1
    - Predilection for certain risk groups
    - Risk for homosexual men greater than hemophiliac
    - Affinity for skin but may be disseminated
    - Most aggressive of all Kaposi subtypes
- *Treatment:*
  - No definitive cure but variety of possible treatments for
  - Removal of immunosuppressive agents in iatrogenic variant
  - Highly active antiretroviral therapy (HAART) for AIDS associated variant
  - Other options include surgical excision (of symptomatic lesions only; wide local excision usually not indicated), radiation, systemic chemotherapy, topical drugs, cryoablation therapy.

Dabska Tumor[33]

- Dąbska tumor is extremely rare, low-grade angiosarcoma
- Found in children
- HPE anastomosing vascular channels with intravascular papillary outpouchings projecting, sometimes in a glomerulus like pattern, into a lumen lined by atypical columnar endothelial cells.
- *Treatment of choice:* Wide local excision

Angiosarcoma[34,35]

Angiosarcoma is an uncommon and aggressive malignant tumor (cancer) that arises from endothelial cells, which normally line the walls of blood or lymphatic vessels.

Cutaneous angiosarcoma is the most common form of angiosarcoma not associated with chronic lymphoedema. The disease is primarily located on the head and neck of elderly persons and is also known as Wilson–Jones angiosarcoma, senile angiosarcoma, or malignant angioendothelioma.

- Clinical features of this form of angiosarcoma are lesions that most commonly appear on the scalp or upper forehead.
- In the early stages of disease, lesions may be singular or multifocal, slow spreading patches of livid or dusky red color, somewhat like an ill-defined bruise.

- Lesions may develop into elevated nodules or plaques that may bleed and ulcerate.
- Lesions grow rapidly and spread, making margins difficult to define.
- Treatment of angiosarcoma is dependent on the location of the angiosarcoma and the extent of the tumor. Treatment includes chemotherapy, surgery, radiotherapy, or a combination of these treatment modalities.

Epithelioid Hemangioendothelioma[36]

Epithelioid hemangioendothelioma occurs equally in both sexes and at any age, although it is rarely seen in childhood. This tumor presents as poorly defined painful, subcutaneous mass, either superficial or deeper of variable size. Lung, liver, and bone may also be primary sites. Approximately half of EHEs are associated with blood vessels. As such, venous occlusion with resultant edema or thrombophlebitis can occur. EHE metastasizes and produces multifocal lesions in around a third of cases with a 15% direct-cause overall lifetime mortality rate.

Treatment: Wide local excision.

Kasabach–Merritt syndrome[37]

It is a combination of:

- A rapidly growing vascular tumor
- Thrombocytopenia (low platelets)
- Microangiopathic hemolytic anemia (destruction of red blood cells)
- Consumptive coagulopathy (impaired clotting)

KEY POINTS

- Arteriovenous malformation may be surgically created for hemodialysis.
- Vascular malformations are mostly low flow capillary malformations such as salmon patch, port-wine stain, etc.
- Vascular tumor may be locally aggressive Kaposiform hemangioendothelioma or Kaposi sarcoma; or it might be invasive angiosarcoma.
- Infantile hemangiomas are most common vascular tumor that present since infancy.
- Infantile hemangioma involutes by its own in most of the cases thus needs no treatment.
- Deep variant of it needs evaluation.
- Lasers, sclerotherapy or surgical modalities are needed to treat these disorders.

REFERENCES

1. Wassef M, Blei F, Adams D, Alomari A, Baselga E, Berenstein A, et al. Vascular anomalies classification: recommendations from the International Society for the Study of Vascular Anomalies. Pediatrics. 2015;136(1):e203-14.
2. Larralde M, Gonzalez V, Marietti R, Nussembaum D, Peirano M, Schroh R. Pseudo-Kaposi sarcoma with arteriovenous malformation. Pediatr Dermatol. 2001;18(4):325-7.
3. Jayroe H, Foley K. Arteriovenous Fistula. In: StatPearls [Internet]. Treasure Island (FL): StatPearls Publishing; 2021. Available from: http://www.ncbi.nlm.nih.gov/books/NBK559213.
4. Leung AKC, Telmesani AMA. Salmon patches in caucasian children. Pediatr Dermatol. 1989;6(3):185-7.
5. McLaughlin MR, O'Connor NR, Ham P. Newborn Skin: Part II. Birthmarks. Am Fam Physician. 2008;77(1):56-60.
6. Garzon MC, Huang JT, Enjolras O, Frieden IJ. Vascular malformations: Part II: Associated syndromes. J Am Acad Dermatol. 2007;56(4):541-64.
7. Thomas-Sohl KA, Vaslow DF, Maria BL. Sturge-Weber syndrome: A review. Pediatr Neurol. 2004 May 1;30(5):303-10.
8. Berry SA, Peterson C, Mize W, Bloom K, Zachary C, Blasco P, et al. Klippel-Trenaunay syndrome. Am J Med Genet. 1998;79(4):319-26.
9. Banzic I, Brankovic M, Maksimović Ž, Davidović L, Marković M, Rančić Z. Parkes Weber syndrome—Diagnostic and management paradigms: a systematic review. Phlebology. 2017;32(6):371-83.
10. McDonald J, Bayrak-Toydemir P, Pyeritz RE. Hereditary hemorrhagic telangiectasia: an overview of diagnosis, management, and pathogenesis. Genet Med. 2011;13(7):607-16.
11. Guttmacher AE, Marchuk DA, White RI. Hereditary hemorrhagic telangiectasia. N Engl J Med. 1995;333(14):918-24.
12. Ngan V. Capillary vascular malformation [Internet]. DermNet NZ. 2003. Available from: https://dermnetnz.org/topics/capillary-vascular-malformation/.
13. Behravesh S, Yakes W, Gupta N, Naidu S, Chong BW, Khademhosseini A, et al. Venous malformations: clinical diagnosis and treatment. Cardiovasc Diagn Ther. 2016;6(6):557-69.
14. Oranje AP. Blue Rubber Bleb Nevus Syndrome. Pediatr Dermatol. 1986;3(4):304-10.
15. Boon LM, Mulliken JB, Enjolras O, Vikkula M. Glomuvenous Malformation (glomangioma) and venous malformation: distinct clinicopathologic and genetic entities. Arch Dermatol. 2004;140(8):971-6.
16. Noda S, Asano Y, Sugie R, Mizuno K, Adachi M. Zosteriform venous malformations with an atypical presentation. Acta Derm Venereol. 2011;91(3):369-71.
17. Mendiratta V, Jabeen M. Infantile hemangioma: an update. Indian J Dermatol Venereol Leprol. 2010;76(5):469.
18. Holland KE, Drolet BA. Infantile Hemangioma. Pediatr Clin. 2010;57(5):1069-83.
19. Darrow DH, Greene AK, Mancini AJ, Nopper AJ, the Section on Dermatology S on O-H and NS. Diagnosis and Management of Infantile Hemangioma. Pediatrics. 2015;136(4):e1060-104.
20. Mulliken JB, Enjolras O. Congenital hemangiomas and infantile hemangioma: missing links. J Am Acad Dermatol. 2004;50(6):875-82.
21. Liang MG, Frieden IJ. Infantile and congenital hemangiomas. Semin Pediatr Surg. 2014;23(4):162-7.
22. Okada E, Tamura A, Ishikawa O, Miyachi Y. Tufted angioma (angioblastoma): case report and review of 41 cases in the Japanese literature. Clin Exp Dermatol. 2000;25(8):627-30.
23. Tomasini C, Aloi F, Soro E, Elia V. Spindle cell hemangioma. Dermatology. 1999;199(3):274-6.
24. Sw W, Kg I, Dh D, De S, Fm E. Epithelioid hemangioendothelioma and related lesions. Semin Diagn Pathol. 1986;3(4):259-87.

25. Kalil RK. Epithelioid hemangioma. In: Santini-Araujo E, Kalil RK, Bertoni F, Park Y-K (Eds). Tumors and Tumor-like Lesions of Bone: For Surgical Pathologists, Orthopedic Surgeons and Radiologists [Internet]. London: Springer; 2015. pp. 479-85. Available from: https://doi.org/10.1007/978-1-4471-6578-1_33
26. Lin RL, Janniger CK. Pyogenic granuloma. CUTIS-N Y-. 2004;74:229-36.
27. Patrice SJ, Wiss K, Mulliken JB. Pyogenic granuloma (lobular capillary hemangioma): a clinicopathologic study of 178 cases. Pediatr Dermatol. 1991;8(4):267-76.
28. Fernández Y, Bernabeu-Wittel M, García-Morillo JS. Kaposiform hemangioendothelioma. Eur J Intern Med. 2009;20(2):106-13.
29. Tan D, Kraybill W, Cheney RT, Khoury T. Retiform hemangioendothelioma: a case report and review of the literature. J Cutan Pathol. 2005;32(9):634-7.
30. Fletcher CD, Unni KK, Mertens F. Pathology and genetics of tumours of soft tissue and bone. Vol. 4. Iarc; 2002.
31. Cesarman E, Damania B, Krown SE, Martin J, Bower M, Whitby D. Kaposi sarcoma. Nat Rev Dis Primer. 2019;5(1):1-21.
32. Radu O, Pantanowitz L. Kaposi sarcoma. Arch Pathol Lab Med. 2013;137(2):289-94.
33. Schwartz RA, Dabski C, Dąbska M. The Dąbska tumor: a thirty-year retrospect. Dermatology. 2000;201(1):1-5.
34. Spiker AM, Mangla A, Ramsey ML. Angiosarcoma. In: StatPearls [Internet]. Treasure Island (FL): StatPearls Publishing; 2021. Available from: http://www.ncbi.nlm.nih.gov/books/NBK441983/.
35. Mendenhall WM, Mendenhall CM, Werning JW, Reith JD, Mendenhall NP. Cutaneous angiosarcoma. Am J Clin Oncol. 2006;29(5):524-8.
36. Sardaro A, Bardoscia L, Petruzzelli MF, Portaluri M. Epithelioid hemangioendothelioma: an overview and update on a rare vascular tumor. Oncol Rev. 2014;8(2):259. Available from: https://www.ncbi.nlm.nih.gov/pmc/articles/PMC4419652/.
37. Singh S, Bhari N, Jassi R. Kasabach-Merritt phenomenon. Indian J Paediatr Dermatol. 2019;20(4):295.

EXAMINATION QUESTIONS

1. What are the differences between vascular malformation and hemangioma?
2. Discuss the management of infantile hemangioma.
3. Classify vascular tumors and vascular malformations.
4. Discuss propranolol for infantile hemangioma.
5. Write syndromes associated with hemangioma.
6. Write a short note on PHACES syndrome.

92 CHAPTER

Malignant Melanoma

Arijit Coondoo

INTRODUCTION

Malignant melanoma is a neoplasm of melanocytes which mutate and divide uncontrollably. Benign growth of melanocytes results in benign melanocytic nevi, ephelides, and lentigines. Malignant growth of melanocytes causes melanoma. Melanomas may appear de novo or develop from a precursor lesion such as benign melanocytic nevus, dysplastic nevus, atypical lentiginous junctional nevus, cellular blue nevus, solar lentigo, and lentiginous junctional nevus.[1] The ABCDE criteria (*Asymmetry; Border irregularity; Color variegation; Diameter increasing; Evolving*) have been formulated as warning signs that a mole is changing in nature from benign to malignant. Additionally, a criterion "F" (*funny looking*) incorporating the "Ugly duckling sign" referring to the one among many mole that looks different and sticks out from the rest has been proposed.[2]

Melanomas can develop anywhere on the skin, but are more common on the chest, back, face, head, and neck in men and the arms and legs in women. Though most melanomas are induced by solar radiation some may also occur in areas of the unexposed areas such as the palms, soles, and perineum. Nondermatological sites include the eyes, mucosa, gastrointestinal tract, genitourinary tract, and leptomeninges. Though both black and white skin contain an equal number of melanocytes, the amount of melanin produced by black skin is much more than in white skin. Hence the damage due to UV radiation is much less in dark brown or black skin than in white skin. Hence, the disease is relatively less common in people with darker skin.[1]

ETIOPATHOGENESIS

Melanomagenesis is the sequence of events whereby normal melanocytes are converted to melanoma cells. It is a complex process of interaction between ultraviolet radiation (UVR) and genetic factors.

Solar ultraviolet radiation (UVR) comprising of UVC (200–290 nm), UVB (290–320 nm), and UVA (320–400 nm) is the major environmental risk factor for melanoma. UVB is considered to be the most carcinogenic of the three. UVR induces melanoma through different mechanisms, including induction of melanocyte cell division, suppression of the immune system of the skin, and production of free radicals. UVR also causes DNA damage, forming products such as cyclobutane pyrimidine dimers (CPD) and 6-4-pyrimidone photoproducts (6-4PP) which cause oxidative DNA damage leading to DNA mutations which contribute to melanoma formation.[3]

The increased risk of melanoma due to sun exposure also depends on sun exposure patterns and timing. Intense and intermittent sun exposure (as in sunburn cases) is associated with a higher risk compared to a chronic continuous pattern of sun exposure.[5] For example, those who work in airplanes have an increased risk of melanoma due to greater exposure to UV.[4] Artificial light and intense sun exposure on the beach or tanning in tanning beds may also increase the risk of development of melanoma.[5]

Genetic predisposition leading to development of melanoma include family history, fair skin, blue eyes and freckles (as seen in Fitzpatrick types I and II), presence of more than 100 typical nevi, or atypical nevi and xeroderma pigmentosum. Inherited genes which have been implicated in the development of melanoma are *CDKN2A (p16), CDK4, RB1, CDKN2A (p19),* MDm, *PTEN/MMAC1, ras.TYR, TYRP1,* and *ASIP*. *CDKN2A (p16)* located on band 9p21, and its mutation plays an important role in melanomas. Mutations may occur in genes such as *BRAF, EGF, Fas, PTEN* which are not inherited but are acquired due to environmental factors such as exposure to solar UV rays of the sunlight can increase the risk of melanoma.[6]

Melanoma is an immunogenic tumor. It secretes factors affecting the immunologic characteristics of the tumor microenvironment, including TGF, IL10 indolamine 2,3-dioxygenase and other factors which affect the immunological characteristics of the tumor environment. Immunosuppression, as observed in organ transplant recipients, lymphoma patients and HIV patients may induce melanoma. A strong intrinsic immune response and extrinsic response due to immunotherapy (interferon a-2b and IL-2) can result in a better prognosis.[7]

Recent studies have shown that patients with Parkinson disease have increased risk of preexisting melanoma, similarly patients with melanoma have a similar risk of developing Parkinson's disease.[8]

The risk factors for development of melanoma are enumerated in **Table 1**.[9]

TABLE 1: Risk factors for development of melanoma.

Level of risk	*Factor*
High	• Changing mole • Dysplastic nevi in familial melanoma • More than 50 nevi, 2 mm or greater in diameter
Moderate	• One family member with melanoma • Previous history of melanoma • Sporadic dysplastic nevi • Congenital nevus
Slight	• Immunosuppression • Sun sensitivity • History of acute, blistering sunburns • Freckling

TABLE 2: 2018 WHO classification of melanomas.

Melanomas arising in sun-exposed skin	• *Low cumulative solar damage (CSD)*: Superficial spreading melanoma • *High CSD*: Lentigo maligna melanoma • *High CSD*: Desmoplastic melanoma
Melanomas arising at sun-shielded sites or without known association with UV exposure	• Spitz melanoma • Acral melanoma • Mucosal melanoma • Melanoma arising in congenital nevus • Melanoma arising in blue nevus • Uveal melanoma

2018 WHO CLASSIFICATION[10]

According to this classification melanomas can be divided into those caused by sun exposure and those that are not. Melanomas caused by sun exposure were further sub-divided by the histopathologic degree of CSD of the surrounding skin and degree of associated solar elastosis, into low and high CSD **(Table 2)**.

HISTOPATHOLOGICAL CLASSIFICATION[11]

There are two growth phases of melanomas: radial and vertical.

In the radial growth phase, melanoma cells are confined to the epidermis, and start as flat patches. They grow slowly, but may, at any time, become thickened or become nodular by progressing to a vertical growth phase where they enter the dermis and later metastasize **(Table 3)**.

TABLE 3: Histopathological classification.

Tumor confined to epidermis (*in situ*)	• Superficial spreading melanoma • Lentigo maligna melanoma • Acral lentiginous melanoma
Tumors which invade dermis rapidly	• Nodular melanoma • Spitzoid melanoma • Mucosal melanoma • Desmoplastic melanoma • Spindle-shaped melanoma
Tumors which spread to other tissues (metastatic)	

Superficial Spreading Melanoma

It accounts for 70% of all cutaneous malignant melanomas. They usually arise from stable pigmented dysplastic nevi which may ulcerate, enlarge, or change color. They usually occur at sites of intermittent sun exposure especially the head, neck, and trunk of males and the lower extremities of females but may occur anywhere on the body. Characteristically SSMs exhibit the ABCDE characteristics of the changing mole. The surface is smooth at first but become dry or warty later on. There may be skin colored skip areas or white scars caused by regression.[12]

Lentigo Maligna and Lentigo Maligna Melanoma

Lentigo maligna (LM) is type of melanoma in situ characterized by atypical melanocyte proliferation within the basal epidermis. It occurs in the elderly, especially women on the sun exposed skin of the face or neck, especially the nose and cheek, growing slowly in diameter over 5 to 20 years. It has a smooth surface, variable pigmentation, and an irregular shape.[13] In a few cases (less than 5%), it invades the dermis and deeper tissues, and transforms into lentigo maligna melanoma (LMM) (Hutchinson's melanotic freckle). The risk of development of invasive melanoma is greater in larger lesions usually with diameter above 4 cm. Transformation to LMM should be suspected when there is itching or stinging; ulceration or bleeding, increased number of colors or a thickening of a part of the lesion.[14]

Desmoplastic Melanoma

Desmoplastic melanoma (DM) is a rare form of invasive melanoma often involves nerve fibers (neurotropic melanoma). It sometimes arises under a LM. It appears as a flat or raised papule, plaque or nodule, 6 cm or more in size, with a smooth or irregular surface, and borders and a firm consistency. There are various shades of pigmentation —usually skin-colored or pink, but may also be gray, brown, blue or black.[15]

Spitzoid Melanoma

Spitzoid melanoma (SM) is a malignant melanoma that is clinically, histologically, and cytologically very similar to the benign Spitzoid nevus. Spitzoid melanoma looks very much like the benign Spitz nevus. SM may arise de novo or from within a Spitz nevus.

In contrast to Spitzoid nevus SM has a larger size (10 mm or more in diameter); lacks symmetry, is poorly circumscribed, may ulcerate or penetrate deeply into the dermis. It is often round in shape, has uniform color and usually does not follow the ABCDE criteria.[16]

Acral Lentiginous Melanoma

Acral lentiginous melanoma (ALM), a rare type of melanoma found usually in Africans and Asians occurs mainly on the palms, soles, and nail beds. Subungual melanomas may resemble subungual hematomas. It can develop within an existing melanocytic nevus or arise *de novo*. In the initial *in situ* phase, which persists for months or years it appears as a slow growing flat patch of discolored skin. The malignant cells remain confined to the epidermis. When ALM becomes invasive the melanoma cells cross the basement membrane and enter the dermis to become a rapidly growing nodular melanoma proliferating deeply in the skin.[17]

Nodular Melanoma

Nodular melanoma (NM) is characterized by vertical growth of melanoma cells after a short-lived or absent radial growth. It comprises about 10–15% of all melanomas. It may arise *de novo* or within a different type of existing melanoma. It appears as a dome-shaped, symmetrical, brown or black, rapidly growing nodule with a smooth, crusted or warty surface. There may be ulceration or bleeding.[18]

Mucosal Melanoma

Mucosal melanoma is a rare type of melanoma that occurs on mucosal surfaces of nasal cavity, paranasal sinuses, oral cavity, gastrointestinal tract, anus, respiratory tract, genitourinary tract, vulva, and vagina.[19]

Amelanotic Melanoma

Amelanotic melanoma is a melanoma which is devoid of pigment. It accounts for 1–8% of all melanomas. Any subtype of melanoma can be amelanotic. It may be skin colored, red, pink, or erythematous. The borders may be well-defined or indistinct. It may occur in young children and in chronic photodamaged skin of elderly.[20]

DIAGNOSIS

Laboratory studies, imaging studies, surgical procedures for histopathology and dermoscopy are important tools for the diagnosis of the primary tumor and metastasis.

Laboratory Studies

The following laboratory studies are needed: Complete blood count and complete chemistry panel (including liver function tests and lactate dehydrogenase).

Imaging

Chest X-ray, CT scan of chest and/or abdomen, MRI of brain, ultrasonography for lymph node involvement and positron emission tomography/computed tomography scanning (PET/CT) is done to seek other sites of metastasis.

Surgical procedures performed for diagnosis are complete excisional biopsy of a suggestive lesion and sentinel lymph node biopsy (SLNB).[21]

Immunohistochemistry is used for diagnosis of difficult cases. There are two types of biomarkers for melanoma used for diagnosis and prognosis: Melanocytic markers and proliferative markers. Melanocytic markers such as Melan-A, MART-1. HMB-45, Gp100, S100 protein, micropthlamia transcription factor (MITF), tyrosinase and SOX10 are used to determine if a lesion is melanocytic in origin. Proliferation makers such as Ki-67 and PHH3 are used to evaluate cell cycle activity in a lesion.[22]

Histopathology

Complete excision of the suspicious lesion with a 2 mm lateral margin and including the full thickness of skin with a little subcutaneous fat is recommended. A punch or shave biopsy is done only when complete excision is difficult (e.g., a lesion on face).

Histologically, melanomas are asymmetrical, poorly circumscribed lesions which exhibit architectural disturbance and prominent cytological atypia. Specific features include pagetoid involvement of the epidermis, nests of melanocytes which have variable size and shape (may be confluent and lack maturation), melanocytes inside lymphovascular spaces, atypical and mitoses and increased apoptosis. Ulceration is an indicator of prognosis. Mitotic figures are commonly seen. Melanoma cells are of two major types: epithelioid and spindle cells. Epithelioid cells seen commonly in superficial spreading melanoma are large and round with abundant eosinophilic cytoplasm and prominent vesicular nuclei with large nucleoli. Spindle cells are found in spindle cell melanoma, a rare subtype of melanoma composed of spindled neoplastic cells arranged in sheets and fascicles.[23]

The biopsy report should include a macroscopic description of the lesion and a microscopic description. In case of invasive melanoma the Breslow thickness to the nearest 0.1 mm, and Clark level of invasion should be reported. The Breslow level of thickness is measured in millimeters from the top of the granular layer (or base of ulceration) to the deepest point of tumor. It is important for prognosis because the chance of metastasis increases with increasing thickness.

The Clark level indicates the anatomical level of invasion **(Table 4)**.

Dermoscopy

Dermoscopy helps in the diagnosis of melanoma in clinically suspicious lesions. Various diagnostic criteria such as the 7-point checklist, the Menzies method, the ABCD rule, the CASH algorithm, and the TAA method of sequential questioning have been developed for the early detection of

TABLE 4: Clarke level of invasion.

Clarke level	*Level of invasion*
1	Epidermis (*in situ* melanoma)
2	Papillary dermis
3	Papillary/Reticulate dermal interface
4	Reticular dermis
5	Subcutis

BOX 1: 1-point checklist.

Diagnostic criteria

Major criteria (2 points each):
- Atypical pigment network
- Blue-white veil
- Atypical vascular pattern

Minor criteria (1 point each):
- Irregular streaks
- Irregular pigmentation
- Irregular dots/globules
- Regression structures

TABLE 5: Staging of melanoma and treatment.

Stage	*Features*	*Treatment*
Stage 0 (in situ)	Tumor present in epidermis only	Excision, imiquimod, Moh's surgery, radiation therapy
Stage I A/B	Tumor 2 mm thick. No spread to lymph nodes. Ulcer +/–	Excision with or without lymph node management
Stage II A, B, C	Tumor thickness 4 mm or more. May or may not spread to lymph nodes. Ulcer +/–	Excision, with or without lymph node management
Stage III A, B, C, D	Melanoma has spread to 2 or more lymph nodes and nearby lymphatics. Original tumor is more than 4 mm and ulcerated or may not be visible at all	Excision, lymph node dissection. Removal of nearby lymph vessels if involved

melanoma. The 7-point checklist **(Box 1)** has three major criteria (allotted 2 points each) and 4 minor criteria (allotted 1 point each). A total of 3 or more should raise the suspicion of melanoma.[24]

TREATMENT

The main treatment for early stage melanoma is widespread local excision with sentinel lymph node biopsy or regional lymph node dissection if indicated. Medical management is reserved for adjuvant therapy in patients with advanced melanoma. Adjuvant therapy for resectable stage III melanoma includes the following agents—interferon alpha, pegylated interferon, immunotherapy with ipilimumab; nivolumab, pembrolizumab **(Table 5)**.[25]

The extent of the surgery depends on the thickness of the melanoma and its spread. This is indicated by staging of the melanoma **(Table 4)**.[26]

Nonsurgical therapy for unresectable stage III, stage IV, and recurrent melanom are immunotherapy, chemotherapy, palliative local therapy, signal-transduction inhibitors, and intralesional therapy.

KEY POINTS

- Benign growth of melanocytes results in benign melanocytic nevi, ephelides, and lentigines. Malignant growth of melanocytes causes melanoma.
- The ABCDE criteria (Asymmetry; Border irregularity; Color variegation; Diameter increasing; Evolving) have been formulated as warning signs that a mole is changing in nature from benign to malignant.
- Melanoma genesis is a complex process of interaction between ultraviolet radiation (UVR) and genetic factors.
- Melanomas can be divided into those caused by sun exposure and those that are not. Those caused by sun exposure were further subdivided by the histopathologic degree of cumulative solar damage (CSD) of the surrounding skin and degree of associated solar elastosis, into low and high CSD.
- Histopathologically melanomas are classified into those in the radial growth phase (spreading in the epidermis) and those in the vertical growth phase (entering the dermis).
- The most common type of melanoma is superficial spreading melanoma (SSM) which accounts for 70% of all melanomas.
- Laboratory studies, imaging studies, surgical procedures for histopathology, and dermoscopy are important tools for the diagnosis of the primary tumor and metastasis.
- Histologically, melanomas are asymmetrical, poorly circumscribed lesions which exhibit architectural disturbance and prominent cytological atypia.
- The 7-point dermaoscopy checklist has 3 major criteria (allotted 2 points each) and 4 minor criteria (allotted 1 point each). A total of 3 or more should raise the suspicion of melanoma.
- The main treatment for early stage melanoma is widespread local excision with sentinel lymph node biopsy or regional lymph node dissection if indicated.

REFERENCES

1. Longo C, Pellacani G. Melanoma. Dermatol Clin. 2016;34(4):411-9.
2. Daniel Jensen J, Elewski BE. The ABCDEF rule: combining the "ABCDE Rule" and the "Ugly Duckling Sign" in an effort to improve patient self-screening examinations. J Clin Aesthet Dermatol. 2015;8(2):15.

3. Sun X, Zhang N, Yin C, Zhu B, Li X. Ultraviolet radiation and melanoma genesis: from mechanism to immunotherapy. Front Oncol. 2020;10:951.
4. Sanlorenzo M, Wehner MR, Linos E, Kornak J, Kainz W, Posch C, et al. The risk of melanoma in airline pilots and cabin crew: a meta-analysis. JAMA Dermatol. 2015;151(1): 51-8.
5. Miller AJ, Mihm MC Jr. Melanoma. N Engl J Med. 2006;355(1): 51-65.
6. Ribero S, Glass D, Bataille V. Genetic epidemiology of melanoma Eur J Dermatol. 2016;26(4):335-9.
7. Kubica AW, Brewer JD. Melanoma in immunosuppressed patients. Mayo Clin Proc. 2012;87(10):991-1003.
8. Bose A, Byrne Á, Rinzel J. Parkinson's disease and melanoma: co-occurrence and mechanisms. PLoS Comput Biol. 2019; 15(5):e1006450.
9. Rastrelli M, Tropea S, Rossi CR, Alaibac M. Melanoma: epidemiology, risk factors, pathogenesis, diagnosis and classification. In Vivo. 2014;28(6):1005-11.
10. Elder DB, Bastion BC, Cree IA, Massi D, Scolyer RA. The 2018 World Health Organization classification of cutaneous, mucosal, and uveal melanoma: detailed analysis of 9 distinct subtypes defined by their evolutionary pathway. Arch Pathol Lab Med. 2020;144(4):500-22.
11. Barnhill RL, Mihm MC Jr. The histopathology of cutaneous malignant melanoma. Semin Diagn Pathol. 1993;10(1): 47-75.
12. Singh P, Kim HJ, Schwartz RA. Superficial spreading melanoma: an analysis of 97702 cases using the SEER database. Melanoma Res. 2016;26(4):395-400.
13. Robinson M, Primiero C, Guitera P, Hong A, Scolyer RA, Stretch JR, et al. Evidence-based clinical practice guidelines for the management of patients with lentigo maligna. Dermatology. 2020;236(2):111-6.
14. Situm M, Bolanca Z, Buljan M. Lentigo maligna melanoma: the review. Coll Antropol. 2010;34:299-301.
15. Shi P, Xu Z, Lei X, Yibulayin F, Wushou A. Desmoplastic melanoma: demographic and clinicopathological features and disease-specific prognostic factors. Oncol Lett. 2019;17(6): 5619-27.
16. Kamino H. Spitzoid melanoma. Clin Dermatol. 2009;27(6): 545-55.
17. Goydos JS, Shoen SL. Acral lentiginous melanoma. Cancer Treat Res. 2016;167:321-9.
18. Kalkhoran S, Milne O, Zalaudek I. Historical, clinical, and dermoscopic characteristics of thin nodular melanoma. Arch Dermatol. 2010;146(3):311-8.
19. Tyrrell H, Payne M. Combating mucosal melanoma: recent advances and future perspectives. Melanoma Manag. 2018;5(3): MMT11.
20. Bono A, Maurichi A, Moglia D, Camerini T, Tragni G, Lualdi M, et al. Clinical and dermatoscopic diagnosis of early amelanotic melanoma. Melanoma Res. 2001;11:491-4.
21. Markovic SN, Erickson LA, Rao RD, Weenig RH, Pockaj BA, Bardia A, et al. Malignant melanoma in the 21st century, Part 1: epidemiology, risk factors, screening, prevention, and diagnosis. Mayo Clin Proc. 2007;82(3):364-80.
22. Davis LE, Shalin SC, Tackett AJ. Current state of melanoma: diagnosis and treatment. Cancer Biol Ther. 2019;20(11): 1366-79.
23. Fllosa A, Fllosa G. Melanoma diagnosis: the importance of histopathological report. Dermatopathology (Basel). 2018;5(1): 41-3.
24. Holmes GA, Vassantachart JM, Limone BA, Zumwalt M, Hirokane J, Jacob SE. Using dermoscopy to identify melanoma and improve diagnostic discrimination. Fed Pract. 2018; 35(Suppl 4):S39-45.
25. National Cancer Institute (USA.gov). Melanoma Treatment (PDQ®)–Health Professional Version. [online] Available from: https://www.cancer.gov/types/skin/hp/melanoma-treatment-pdq#link/_25_toc. [Last accessed March, 2021].
26. Grishenwald JE, Scolyer RA, Hess KR, Sondak VK, Long GV, Ross MI, et al. Melanoma staging: evidence-based changes in the American Joint Committee on Cancer eighth edition cancer staging manual. CA Cancer J Clin. 2017;67:472-92.

EXAMINATION QUESTIONS

1. Explain acral lentigious melanoma.
2. What are the types of melanoma? What are the dermoscopic features necessary for diagnosis of melanomas?
3. Describe newer treatment agents for melanoma.

93 CHAPTER Primary Cutaneous Lymphomas

Arijit Coondoo

INTRODUCTION

Primary cutaneous lymphomas (CL) are a group of non-Hodgkin's lymphomas caused by malignant proliferation of lymphocytes. They primarily involve the skin without involvement of lymph nodes, bone marrow or viscera at the time of diagnosis. These lymphoproliferative neoplasms originate from various types of lymphocytes. Around 65% of them are cutaneous T-cell lymphomas (CTCL), 25% are cutaneous B-cell lymphomas (CBCL) and 10% originate from natural killer (NK) cells [(CD4+/CD56) + hematodermic neoplasm (blastic NK-cell lymphoma)].[1]

CUTANEOUS T-CELL LYMPHOMAS

The term cutaneous T-cell lymphoma was coined in 1979 at an international workshop sponsored by the National Cancer Institute (NCI). In 2005 CTCL was classified by WHO-EORTC (World Health Organization-European Organization of Research and Treatment of Cancer) into mainly two subtypes—those with indolent clinical behavior and those with aggressive behavior. An updated version of the WHO-EORTC incorporating some changes in nomenclature was published in 2018 **(Table 1)**.[2]

TABLE 1: WHO-EORTC classification (2018).

CTCLs with indolent clinical behavior	• Mycosis fungoides • Mycosis fungoides variants and subtypes • Primary cutaneous CD30+ lymphoproliferative disorder (primary cutaneous anaplastic large cell lymphoma, lymphomatoid papulosis) • Subcutaneous panniculitis-like T-cell lymphoma • Primary cutaneous CD4+ small/medium T-cell lymphoproliferative disorder (provisional)
CTCLs with aggressive clinical behavior	• Sézary syndrome • Adult T-cell leukemia/lymphoma • Extranodal NK/T-cell lymphoma, nasal type • Primary cutaneous acral CD8+ T-cell lymphoma (provisional) • Primary cutaneous CD8+ aggressive epidermotropic cytotoxic T-cell lymphoma (provisional) • Primary cutaneous gamma/delta-positive T-cell lymphoma

(CTCL: cutaneous T-cell lymphomas; WHO-EPRTC: World Health Organization-European Organization of Research and Treatment of Cancer)

While mycosis fungoides (MF) accounts for approximately 60% of CTCL cases and 50% of all primary cutaneous lymphomas, its leukemic variant, Sezary's syndrome (SS) represents around 5% of CTCL cases. Primary cutaneous CD30+ lymphoproliferative disorders including primary cutaneous anaplastic large lymphoma and lymphomatoid papulosis accounts for 25% of all cases other subtypes are very rare.[3]

Etiopathogenesis

The etiology of CTCL has still not been fully elucidated. Previously it was thought to be mainly due to infection with Human T-cell leukemia virus type 1, Epstein–Barr virus, *Staphylococcus aureus* or other infective agents. However, recent studies do not support this hypothesis. Environmental factors (such as environmental and occupational exposure to carcinogens), antigen-driven T-cell lymphoproliferation, dyscrasia following medication use and genetic factors, such as HLA class II alleles have been reported as predisposing factors. The genomic panorama of CTCL shows a high level of heterogenicity. Mutations have been found in 17 genes including genes involved in T-cell activation and apoptosis, chromatin remodeling, NF-κB signaling, and DNA damage response.[4] Copy number variations, fusion 4 proteins, and somatic mutations in diverse cellular and signaling pathways might contribute to the pathogenesis of the disease. Aberrations are seen in chromosome 10 have been demonstrated. Ectopic expression of cancer testis genes in the CTCLs inhibiting apoptosis inducing resistance to various therapeutic modalities, and contributes to oncogenesis by targeting tumor suppressor genes such as *p53* and *p21* has also been seen.[5] In most CTCLs, the neoplastic T-cells express cutaneous lymphocyte antigens (CLA) indicating that these are the neoplastic types of normal skin-homing T-cells. T-cells have a strong affinity for the epidermis resulting in epidermotropism as well as the formation of Pautrier microabscesses. Cytotoxic CD8+ T-cells, which play an important role in anti-tumor immunity are found in the infiltrate along with the T-helper cells. In the early stages, the skin infiltrates have a higher CD8+/CD4 ratio. The higher percentage of CD8+ cells indicate a better prognosis.[6]

MYCOSIS FUNGOIDES (ALIBERT-BAZIN SYNDROME, GRANULOMA FUNGOIDES)

Mycosis fungoides is historical name for a type of CTCL.[7] It is a misnomer because it has no relation to any fungal infection. The disease progresses through various stages, usually sequentially or arising de novo in any of these stages **(Table 2)**.[8] The clinical phases of the disease are:

Premycotic phase: Classic MF may be preceded by a nonspecific inflammatory process. At this stage, it may appear similar to nonspecific chronic dermatitis, atopic dermatitis or large-plaque parapsoriasis. Some authors regard large plaque parapsoriasis as the patch stage which may later progress to early plaque-stage of MF.

Patch phase is characterized by oval or annular dry patches on nonexposed skin. They may disappear spontaneously, retain the same size for years or enlarge gradually. The skin may be thin or atrophic, and may or may not itch. At this stage the lesions may be similar in appearance to eczema, psoriasis, or parapsoriasis.

Plaque phase is characterized by thickened, well-defined, erythematous to violaceous, pruritic patches (resembling psoriasis) with lymphadenopathy. If lesions involve up to 10% of body surface area (BSA) are classified as stage IA. Those occupying more than 10% BSA are classified as stage IB. In many cases the disease remains static at these stages for many years without progression to later stages.

Tumor phase may develop from plaques. They may be accompanied by lymphadenopathy (Stage IIA) or may be without lymphadenopathy (Stage IIB). There are erythematous to violet colored nodules which may ulcerate. They are usually present on the face (resembling leonine facies), axillae, anticubital fossae, and groins. There is an increase in the malignant behavior of the tumor cells and the disease may spread to other organs or transform into a large cell lymphoma. They may rarely occur without preceding patches or plaques (*D'emblee mycosis fungoides*).

Erythrodermic phase (Stage III) is characterized by widespread erythema and scaling covering 90% of body surface with islands of normal skin, sparing body folds (deck chair or folded luggage sign). The lesions are severely pruritic. Alopecia, palmoplantar hyperkeratosis and nail dystrophy may be present.

MYCOSIS FUNGOIDES VARIANTS

MF may present as numerous clinical and histological variants which are enumerated in **Table 3**.[9,10]

Diagnosis

In addition to the history and clinical features the histomorphologic and cytomorphologic findings help in the diagnosis of MF. In addition to demonstration of a dominant T-cell clone in skin biopsy specimens by a molecular assay [i.e., Southern blot, polymerase chain reaction (PCR)] also helps to distinguish MF from other lichenoid dermatosis. Genetic testing may also be helpful.[11]

Histopathology

The histopathological features diagnostic of MF are enumerated in **Box 1**.[12] The histopathology varies according to the stage.[12]

Patch stage: Superficial lichenoid infiltrate of lymphocytes and histiocytes with exocytosis (atypical cells infiltrating the epidermis without significant spongiosis). It may mimic eczema or lichenoid dermatoses. Epidermotropism may not be clearly evident.

Plaque stage: Epidermotropism is more evident. Pautrier microabscess present. Dermal infiltrate is denser.

TABLE 2: Staging of mycosis fungoides (MF).

Stage	*Cutaneous lesions*	*Red skin*	*Lymph nodes*	*Sezary cell in blood*	*Metastasis*
IA	Patches, papules, plaques on >10% BSA	Nil	Normal	Low	Nil
IB	Patches, papules, plaques on <10% BSA	Nil	Normal	Low	Nil
IIA	Patches, papules plaques on any amount of BSA	Nil	Abnormal but not cancerous	Low	Nil
IIB	Patches, papules, plaques and single or multiple tumors 1 cm or larger	Nil	Abnormal but not cancerous	Low	Nil
III	Patches, papules, plaques or tumors covering any amount of BSA	80% or more of BSA	Abnormal but not cancerous	Low	Nil
IVAI	Patches, papules, plaques or tumors covering any amount of BSA	80% or more of BSA	Abnormal but not cancerous	High	Nil
IVAII	Patches, papules, plaques or tumors covering any amount of BSA	80% or more of BSA	Very abnormal/ cancerous	High	Nil
IVB	Patches, papules, plaques or tumors. Any amount of BSA	80% or more of BSA		High	To other organs, e.g., liver/spleen

(BSA: body surface area)

TABLE 3: Variants of mycosis fungoides.

Variants	*Features*
Folliculotropic mycosis fungoides (MF)	Alopecia, follicular cyst, comedones, follicular mucinosis, infiltrated plaques and papules
Pagetoid reticulosis	Solitary psoriasiform or hyperkeratotic patch or plaque localized to extremities
Hypopigmented MF	Well-demarcated, hypopigmented or white pruritic patches
Hyperpigmented MF	Diffuse macular hyperpigmentation resembling erythema dyschromicum perstans
Pustular MF	Pustular lesions limited to palms
Bullous MF	Tense or ruptured bullae with an erythematous base arising on normal skin or within the MF patches or plaques on the trunk and extremities
Unilesional MF	Single lesion of typical MF
Syringotropic MF	Involvement of the eccrine gland or duct. Red to skin-colored papules, red to brown patches, or red scaly plaques with hair loss. No mucinous degeneration
Poikilodermic MF (Poikiloderma vasculare atrophicans)	Poikilodermatous lesions arising in normal cases of MF
Granulomatous slack skin syndrome	Pendulous, more-or-less infiltrated folds of skin in intertriginous areas, especially the axillae and groin. May give rise to Hodgkin's disease
Others Hyperkeratotic Vegetating Purpura-like Urticarial Papular Psoriasiform Photosensitive	

BOX 1: Histological features diagnostic of mycosis fungoides (MF).

- Band-like infiltrate in upper dermis comprising of lymphocytes and other inflammatory cells, with no Grenz zone
- Epidermotropism of mononuclear cells
- Small amount of spongiosis in the epidermis
- Hyperchromatic and convoluted or cerebriform nuclei of lymphocytes

Tumor stage: The dermal infiltrate is denser. There may be no exocytosis of lymphocytes. Transformation to large cells may occur.

Two prominent histological features of MF are:

1. *Epidermotropism*: Characteristic infiltrates of malignant T-cell usually colonize the basal cell layer, mostly at the tips of rete ridges.
2. *Pautrier microabscesses* clear halo surrounding an intraepidermal mononuclear cell singly or in clumps. Its presence is suggestive but not diagnostic of MF.

SEZARY SYNDROME

Sezary syndrome (SS) is a CTCL where there is a combination of leukemia with erythroderma. Following a nonspecific dermatitis (as in MF) the skin becomes itchy, thickened or edematous, dry, scaly, and bright red (red man syndrome) with lymphadenopathy. It is characterized by the presence of neoplastic T-cells (Sézary cells) in the skin, lymph nodes, and peripheral blood. The patient may have palmar and/or plantar hyperkeratosis, nail dystrophy, alopecia, and ectropion along with hepatosplenomegaly.

The prognosis is poor. Median survival varies between 2 and 4 years. Mortality is usually due to opportunistic infections due to immunosuppression.[13]

Histopathological Features

- Epidermotropism
- Atypical lymphocytes infiltrating dermis
- Lymphocytes with a single cerebriform nucleus
- Pautrier microabscesses, or intraepidermal aggregates of atypical cells
- Immunohistochemistry stains positive for CD3+ and CD4+ cell.

Diagnostic Criteria

Presence of one or more of the following criteria is necessary for diagnosis:

- *Absolute Sézary cell count:* 1,000 cells/μL or more
- Immunophenotypic abnormalities (expanded CD4+ T-cell population resulting in a CD4/CD8 ratio of more than 10; loss of any or all of the T-cell antigens CD2, CD3, CD4, and CD5; or loss of both CD4 and CD5)
- A T-cell clone in the peripheral blood by molecular or cytogenetic methods.[13]

PRIMARY CUTANEOUS CD30+ LYMPHOPROLIFERATIVE DISORDERS

It accounts for 30% of all CTCL cases. It includes the following:

- *Primary cutaneous anaplastic large cell lymphoma*: Solitary or multiple nodules and tumors which may or may not be ulcerated. They are usually localized. Lymph nodes may be involved. Spontaneous regression may occur either partially or completely. Hence, the prognosis is good.[14]
- *Lymphomatoid papulosis*: Recurrent papulonodular or papulonecrotic lesions are seen on the trunk and limbs. Spontaneous regression may occur after 3–12 weeks. The disease is chronic. Healed lesions may leave behind scars.[15]

SUBCUTANEOUS PANNICULITIS-LIKE T-CELL LYMPHOMA

A rare type of CTCL characterized by solitary or multiple plaques and nodules principally involving the leg but may be generalized. Rarely, scalp alopecia may be present. Ulceration is rare. Systemic symptoms such as fever, fatigue, and weight loss may occur. Dissemination to extracutaneous sites is unusual.[16]

ADULT T-CELL LEUKEMIA/LYMPHOMA

It is characterized by cutaneous lesions (tumors, papules, and plaques) in 50% cases along with leukemia, lymphadenopathy, hypercalcemia, and organ involvement. The cutaneous lesions are mostly tumors generalized papules (22%), or plaques (19%). The cutaneous lesions may be similar to those of MF.[17]

TREATMENT OF MYCOSIS FUNGOIDES AND SEZARY'S SYNDROME

Topical therapies alone are generally used in stage I patients while a combination of topical and systemic therapies or systemic therapies alone are used for the later stages or for refractory Stage I cases. The drugs used for treatment of MF and SS are enumerated in **Table 4**.[18,19]

Localized MF is also treated by radiotherapy, intralesional steroids, or surgical excision, allogenic stem cell transplantation, unrelated cord blood transfusion, and multiagent chemotherapy.[20]

CUTANEOUS B-CELL LYMPHOMAS

They are malignant proliferation of B-lymphocytes. Different types of lymphoma occur due to different types of mutations occurring at different points in the development of B-cells.[21]

TABLE 4: Drugs used for treatment of mycosis fungoides/Sezary syndrome (MF/SS).

Topical	*Systemic*
Emollients	Retinoids
Antipruritics	Immunomodulators (e.g., recombinant IFN-α2b)
Corticosteroids	Monoclonal antibody antineoplastics (e.g., alemtuzumab)
Retinoids (Alitretinoin, Tazarotene Bexarotene)	Fusion toxins
Nitrogen mustard	Antineoplastics (chlorambucil, vorinostat, methotrexate, etoposide, romidepsin, denileukin diftitox, carmustine, mechlorethamine)
Imiquimod	Corticosteroids (e.g., prednisone, prednisolone)
UVB phototherapy	Gemcitabine
PUVA	Histone deacetylase inhibitors
Total body electron beam radiation	Extracorporeal photopheresis

WHO/EORTC Classification of CBCL

- *Primary cutaneous marginal zone B-cell lymphoma [mucosa-associated lymphoid tissue (MALT) type]*: Manifests as reddish, solitary or multiple, indolent lymphoma on the upper torso and upper extremities and sometimes on the head and neck.

  Histology: Nodular or diffuse infiltrates of marginal zone B-cells, lymphocytes, lymphoplasmacytoid cells, plasma cells mixed with reactive T-cells, and centroblast or immunoblast-like cells in the dermis. Treatment is by chemotherapy with CHOP (cyclophosphamide, doxorubicin, vincristine, and prednisone).
- *Primary cutaneous follicle center lymphoma*: Indolent lymphoma of follicle characterized by nodules and tumors with a firm consistency mainly on the head and neck.

  Histology: Proliferation of centrocytes and centroblasts in a follicular and/or diffuse growth pattern in the dermis and subcutaneous tissue. Treatment is by radiotherapy or surgery.
- *Cutaneous diffuse large B-cell lymphoma (DLBCL)*: It is classified as: (1) DLBCL (leg type); (2) DLBCL (other). Aggressive type of CBCL manifesting as a solitary nodule or multiple tumors restricted to one anatomic area. They exhibit a tendency for extracutaneous spread to regional lymph nodes and other sites.

  Histology: Diffuse dermal proliferation of centroblasts and immunoblasts with large round nuclei with open chromatin, prominent nucleoli, and identifiable mitotic figure. Sparse T-cells found in perivascular areas. Treated by chemotherapy with R-CHOP (Rituximab + CHOP).
- *Intravascular large B-cell lymphoma*: It involves the skin secondarily. It includes: (1) Mantle cell lymphoma; (2) Lymphomatoid granulomatosis; (3) Chronic lymphocytic leukemia; (4) Burkitt lymphoma.[22]

PRIMARY CUTANEOUS NK/T-CELL LYMPHOMA

This rare Epstein-Barr virus (EBV)-associated neoplasm develops usually in nonlymph node sites. Around 80% of cases are the nasal type and occur on and inside the nasal cavity up to the upper respiratory and upper digestive tract. They are referred to as nasal NK/T-cell lymphomas. Around 20% of these lymphomas are found non-nasal sites, including the skin, muscle, testis, salivary glands, and gastrointestinal tract. They are referred to as non-nasal NK/T-cell lymphomas. These lymphoma can rarely metastasize and infiltrations may occur on the skin, liver, spleen, skin, lymph nodes, and bone marrow. Involvement of the peripheral blood may occur in aggressive NK-cell leukemia/lymphoma.[23]

KEY POINTS

- Primary cutaneous lymphomas are malignant proliferation originating from T-cell lymphocytes, B-cell lymphocytes, and NK cell lymphocytes which involve the skin without involvement of internal organs.

- Cutaneous T-cells lymphomas are divided into those with indolent behavior (mainly mycosis fungoides) and those with aggressive behavior (mainly Sezary syndrome).
- Apart from infectious factors various environmental factors and genomic factors play a role in the pathogenesis of cutaneous T-cell lymphomas (CTCL).
- Clinically mycosis fungoides passes through the premycotic phase, patch phase, plaque phase, tumor phase, and erythrodermic phase before metastasizing to various internal organs.
- Tumors may rarely occur without preceding patches or plaques (*D'emblee mycosis fungoides*).
- Mycosis fungoides (MF) may present as numerous clinical and histological variants.
- In addition to the history and clinical features, the histomorphologic and cytomorphologic findings help in the diagnosis of MF.
- Two histopathological characteristics of CTCL are epidermotropism and Pautrier microabscess.
- Sezary syndrome is a CTCL where there is a combination of leukemia with erythroderma.
- Topical therapies alone are generally used in stage I patients of CTCL while a combination of topical and systemic therapies or systemic therapies alone are used for the later stages or for refractory stage I cases.

REFERENCES

1. Kempf W, Zimmermann AK, Mitteldorf C. Cutaneous lymphomas: an update 2019. Hematol Oncol. 2019;37 (Suppl 1):43-7.
2. Willemze R, Cerroni L, Kempf W, Berti E, Facchetti F, Swerdlow SH, et al. The 2018 update of the WHO-EORTC classification for primary cutaneous lymphomas. Blood. 2019;133(16):1703-14.
3. Bobrowicz M, Fassnacht C, Ignatova D, Chang YT, Dimitriou F, Guenova E. Pathogenesis and therapy of primary cutaneous T-cell lymphoma: Collegium Internationale Allergologicum (CIA) update 2020. Int Arch Allergy Immunol. 2020;181(10): 733-45.
4. Choi J, Goh G, Walradt T. Genomic landscape of cutaneous T-cell lymphoma. Nat Genet. 2015;47(9):1011-9.
5. Phyo ZH, Shanbhag S, Rozati S. Update on biology of cutaneous T-cell lymphoma. Front Oncol. 2020;10:765.
6. Larocca CA, LeBoeuf NR. An overview of cutaneous T-cell lymphomas. Hematol Oncol Clin North Am. 2019;33(4): 669-86.
7. Cerroni L. Mycosis fungoides: clinical and histopathologic features, differential diagnosis, and treatment. Semin Cutan Med Surg. 2018;37(1):2-10.
8. Olsen E, Vonderheid E, Pimpinelli N, Willemze R, Kim Y, Knobler R, et al. Revisions to the staging and classification of mycosis fungoides and Sezary syndrome: a proposal of the International Society for Cutaneous Lymphomas (ISCL) and the cutaneous lymphoma task force of the European Organization of Research and Treatment of Cancer (EORTC). Blood. 2007;110(6):1713-22.
9. Willemze R. Mycosis fungoides variants: clinicopathologic features, differential diagnosis and treatment. J Dtsch Dermatol Ges. 2018;16(5):543-57.
10. Muñoz-González H, Molina-Ruiz AM, Requena L. Clinicopathologic variants of mycosis fungoides. Actas Dermosifiliogr. 2017;108(3):192-208.
11. Panda S. Mycosis fungoides: current trends in diagnosis and management. Indian J Dermatol. 2007;52:5-20.
12. Smoller BR, Santucci M, Wood GS, Whittaker SJ. Histopathology and genetics of cutaneous T-cell lymphoma. Hematol Oncol Clin North Am. 2003;17(6):1277-31.
13. Larocca C, Kupper T. Mycosis fungoides and Sézary syndrome: an update. Hematol Oncol Clin North Am. 2019;33(1):103-20.
14. Brown RA, Fernandez-Pol S, Kim JJ. Primary cutaneous anaplastic large cell lymphoma. Cutan Pathol. 2017;44(6):570-7.
15. Sica A, Vitiello P, Sorriento A, Ronchi A, Calogero A, Sagnelli C, et al. Lymphomatoid papulosis. Minerva Med. 2020;111(2): 166-72.
16. Baxi KD, Rathod SP, Chaudhary RG, Jagati A. Subcutaneous panniculitis-like T-cell lymphoma. Indian J Dermatol Venereol Leprol. 2020;86(5):606.
17. Chen YP, Wu ZJ, Liu W, Wang JC, Zhu WF, Chen FF, et al. Clinicopathological characteristics of adult T-cell leukemia/ lymphoma. Zhonghua Bing Li Xue Za Zhi. 2019;48(1):11-6.
18. Photiou L, van der Weyden C, McCormack C, Prince HM. Systemic treatment options for advanced-stage mycosis fungoides and Sézary syndrome. Curr Oncol Rep. 2018;20(4):3.
19. Lovgren ML, Scarisbrick JJ. Update on skin directed therapies in mycosis fungoides. Chin Clin Oncol. 2019;8(1):7.
20. Valipour A, Jäger M, Wu P, Schmitt J, Bunch C, Weberschock T. Interventions for mycosis fungoides. Cochrane Database Syst Rev. 2020;7(7):CD008946.
21. Selva RL, Violetti SA, Delfino C, Grandi V, Cicchelli S, Tomasini C, et al. A literature revision in primary cutaneous B-cell lymphoma. Indian J Dermatol. 2017;62:156-67.
22. Wilcox RA. Cutaneous B-cell lymphomas: 2019 update on diagnosis, risk stratification, and management. Am J Hematol. 2018;93(11):1427-30.
23. Tse E, Kwong YL. The diagnosis and management of NK/T-cell lymphomas. J Hematol Oncol. 2017;10:85.

EXAMINATION QUESTIONS

1. Define and classify primary cutaneous lymphomas.
2. Explain approach to a case of CTCL.
3. Discuss the HPE of various stages of mycosis fungoides.
4. Name the systemic therapies used for treatment of CTCL.

94 CHAPTER Mastocytosis

Abhijit Saha

INTRODUCTION

Mastocytosis is a heterogeneous group of disorder characterized by growth and accumulation of mast cell in the skin and/or other organs like bone marrow, liver, spleen, etc.[1] These clonal mast cells originate from bone marrow. Mastocytosis can be considered as spectrum of clinical disorder where clinical presentations vary widely from childhood to adult onset disease. Childhood onset mastocytosis present solely with cutaneous involvement whereas adult mastocytosis may or may not have cutaneous involvement. Prognostically more than 50% of childhood mastocytosis resolves spontaneously by adolescence. Adult mastocytosis persists for life.

EPIDEMIOLOGY

Mastocytosis may occur at any age with no sex predilection. But more than half of the cases present between birth and 2 years of age.[2] Adult mastocytosis usually develops during third or fourth decade of life. Familial cases have been reported.

PATHOGENESIS

- Mast cells originate from pluripotent stem cells in bone marrow and possess CD34 and CD117 (KIT). They come in the peripheral blood as agranular monocyte like cells. They acquire granules after getting into tissue. For growth, maturation, differentiation and survival of mast cell KIT (tyrosine kinase receptor) need to be activated. Activation of KIT receptor occurs only upon binding with KIT ligand stem cell factor (SCF). SCF is expressed by variety of cells like fibroblasts, endothelial cells, and keratinocytes. Similarly KIT is not a monopoly of mast cells.
- Four different type of hypothesis has been postulated for causation of mastocytosis:
  1. Alteration of structure and activity of KIT
  2. Alteration of SCF (in tissue or blood)
  3. Chromosomal abnormality
  4. Increased survival of BCL-X and BCL-2 protein preventing apoptosis
- Out of these four mechanism alteration of KIT is most widely accepted, activating mutation per say. Somatic activating mutation of KIT at codon 816 is the most common described. This leads to replacement of aspartic amino acid (D) with valine (V, D816V). Ultimate outcome is ligand independent constitutive activation of KIT receptor.[3] This mutation has been found in most of the adults and forty percent of children. Profound diversity of clinical presentation and lack of KIT mutation in some patients and families point toward additional factors might have significant contribution in disease causation.
- Certain other somatic mutations such as TET2, JAK2, CBL has been demonstrated in different forms of systemic mastocytosis associated with poorer prognosis.[4]

CLASSIFICATION

- Mastocytosis can be classified as cutaneous and systemic mastocytosis and localized extracutaneous mast cell proliferation by World Health Organization (WHO).[5]
- Cutaneous mastocytosis (CM) are of three type: Mastocytoma, maculopapular mastocytosis (urticaria pigmentosa), and diffuse cutaneous mastocytosis.
- All these three forms of mastocytosis may undergo bullae formation.
- Childhood-onset mastocytosis comprises a greater portion of cutaneous mastocytosis.
- Only less than 10–15% of childhood mastocytosis continue in the adulthood.
- Only indolent systemic mastocytosis (ISM) and smoldering systemic mastocytosis (SSM) are of dermatological significance because they may present with cutaneous lesions.
- Cutaneous mastocytosis is diagnosed on the basis of clinical and histopathological finding in absence of criteria required to establish systemic mastocytosis.
- Criteria to diagnose systemic mastocytosis are also established by WHO beyond the scope of this book. Diagnostic criteria for systemic mastocytosis will be available in any standard textbook.

CLINICAL FEATURES

- Patients may present with wide variety of symptoms due to functional effect of mast cell mediators **(Box 1)** in response to various triggers **(Table 1)**.

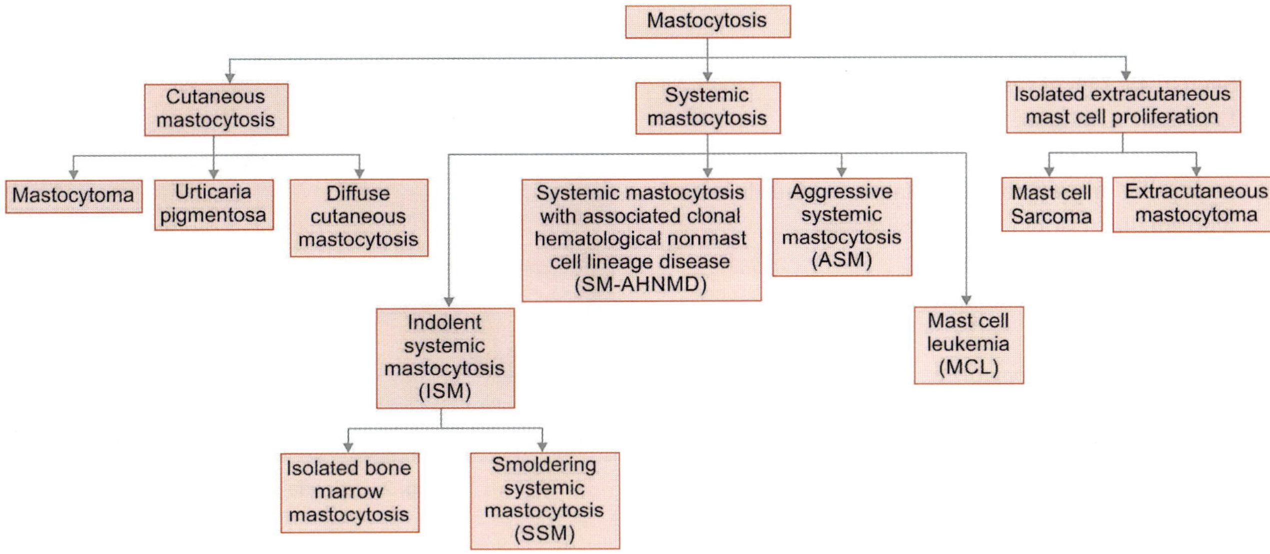

BOX 1: Mast cell mediators.

- Histamine
- Heparin
- Tryptase/chymase
- Prostaglandin D2
- Leukotriene
- Platelet activating factor
- Tumor necrosis factor-α
- Interleukin (IL)-4, IL-5, IL-6

TABLE 1: Triggers for mast cell mediators.

Physical triggers	Friction, stress, sun light, exercise, heat, cold, hot bath
Drugs	Alcohol, aspirin, NSAIDs, anticholinergic drug, opiates, morphine, amphotericin B, polymyxin B, radiocontrast material containing iodine, quinine, thiamine
Anesthetics	Procaine, tetracaine, D-tubocurarine, scopolamine, gallamine
Food	Lobster, egg white, citrus food, chocolate
Others	Snake venom, hymenoptera venom, jellyfish sting

- Common symptoms are pruritus, urticaria, flushing, abdominal pain, diarrhea, dizziness, and syncope.
- Certain symptoms such as bone pain, epigastric pain, and cognitive impairment point toward extracutaneous disease.

Cutaneous Mastocytosis

Children frequently present with cutaneous mastocytosis. Children have excellent prognosis with 50–70% of patients show spontaneous resolution by adolescence. Involvement of other system (extracutaneous) is almost invariably absent in children.

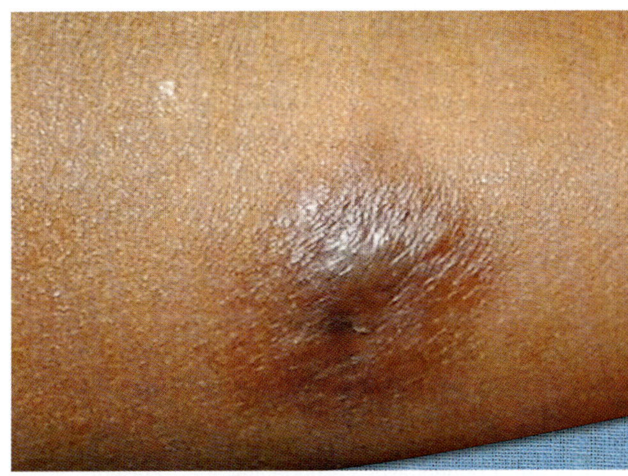

Fig. 1: Mastocytoma with central blistering.
Courtesy: Dr Sandipan Dhar.

Darier's sign could be demonstrated by stroking or rubbing of any skin lesion leading to formation of urticaria-like wheal (blister occasionally) due to release of mast cell mediators. It may occur spontaneously. It is positive in 90% of cases and depends upon lesional mast cell density. Darier sign can easily be seen in pediatric patients up to 2 years of age and difficult to appreciate in adult mastocytosis with skin lesion.

Cutaneous mastocytosis include three different presentation: solitary mastocytoma, maculopapular cutaneous mastocytosis (urticaria pigmentosa), and diffuse cutaneous mastocytosis.

- *Solitary mastocytoma* ***(Fig. 1)***:
  - Congenital or appear within first 2 years of life
  - Seen in 15–50% of cases
  - Solitary or less than/up to three lesions
  - Tan to brown nodule or plaque over distal extremity or neck or trunk
  - Surface resemble pitted skin of orange (peau d'orange)
  - Blister may occur.

- *Maculopapular mastocytosis* ***(Fig. 2)****:*
  - Congenital or appear within first year of life
  - Seen in 45–75% of cases
  - Less than 10 to more than 100 lesions
  - Lesions are either monomorphic(tan to brown macule or papule) or polymorphic (plaque or nodule mixed with smaller lesions)
  - Mainly distributed over trunk
  - Face and acral areas are usually spared
  - Blister may occur.
- *Diffuse cutaneous mastocytosis:*
  - Seen in less than 5–10% cases
  - Presents during first few months of life
  - Generalized involvement of skin
  - Two type of presentation; one is generalized, thickened, hyperpigmented and leathery appearance. Another is extensive blistering and excoriation[6] resembling erythroderma
  - Highest risk of systemic disease
- *Adult patients may present with following presentations:*
  - Reddish-brown macule and papule
  - Tan to red brown papulonodule or nodule
  - Telangiectasia macularis eruptive perstans (TMEP)

Features	*Mastocytoma*	*Maculopapular cutaneous mastocytosis (CM)*	*Diffuse CM*
Percentage of involvement	Seen in 15–50% of cases of CM	Seen in 45–75% of cases of CM	Seen in less than 5–10% cases of CM
Age of onset	Congenital or appear within first two year of life	Congenital or appear within first year of life	Presents during first few months of life
Number of lesion	Solitary or less than/up to three lesion	Less than 10 to more than 100 lesion	Generalized
Morphology	Tan to brown nodule or plaque	Lesions are either monomorphic (tan to brown macule or papule) or polymorphic (plaque or nodule mixed with smaller lesions)	Two type of presentation; one is generalized, thickened, hyperpigmented and leathery appearance. Another is extensive blistering and excoriation[6] resembling erythroderma
Distribution	Over distal extremity or neck or trunk	Trunk sparing acral area and face	Generalized
Blister	Yes	Yes	Yes
Systemic symptoms	Rare, may occur	May occur	Common

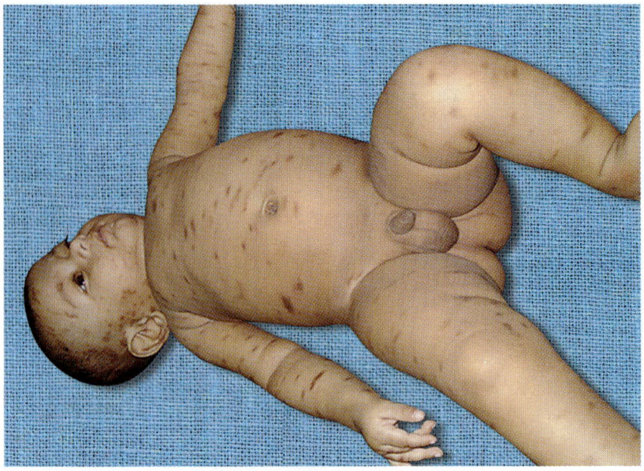

Fig. 2: Urticaria pigmentosa.
Courtesy: Dr Sandipan Dhar.

Systemic Mastocytosis

- More common in adults, children are rarely affected.
- At least two organ system need to be involved.
- Cutaneous involvement may occur with some form of systemic mastocytosis.
- Bone and gastrointestinal system are most commonly affected.
- Patients with skeletal involvement presents with bone pain.
- Bony lesions vary from radiolucent, radiopaque to mixture of both.
- Nausea, vomiting, diarrhea, abdominal pain are most common gastrointestinal symptoms.
- Patients are at risk to develop gastrointestinal hemorrhage secondary to gastritis or peptic ulcer.
- Liver and spleen involvement are usually asymptomatic
- Alteration of hepatic function is less frequent.
- Lymph node is rarely involved unless very advanced case.

Differential Diagnosis

Mastocytoma	• Juvenile xanthogranuloma • Pseudolymphoma • Arthropod bite • Spitz/melanocytic nevus • Café-au-lait macule
Urticaria pigmentosa (UP)	• Acute urticaria • Multiple lentigines • Juvenile xanthogranuloma • Histiocytosis • Bullous impetigo • Herpes simplex infection • Early lesion of incontinentia pigmenti • Chronic bullous disease of childhood • Bullous pemphigoid (Bullous impetigo to Bullous pemphigoid: in UP with Blisters **(Fig. 3)**)
Diffuse cutaneous mastocytosis	• Toxic epidermal necrolysis • Epidermolysis bullosa • Staphylococcal scalded skin syndrome[7] • Leukemic infiltration

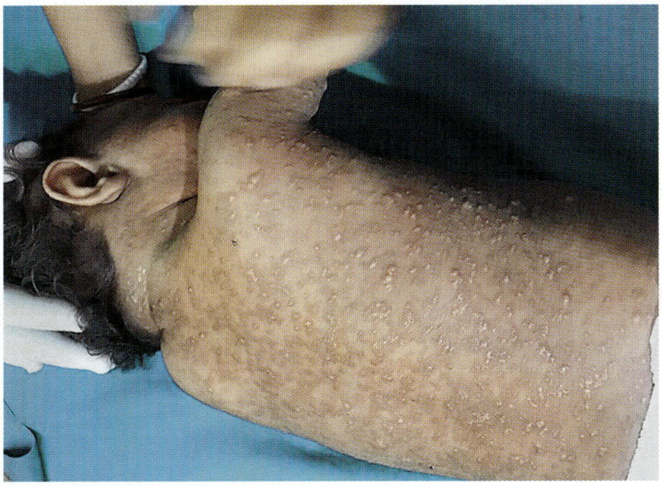

Fig. 3: Bullous mastocytosis.
Courtesy: Dr Sandipan Dhar.

Diagnosis

- Cutaneous mastocytosis can be easily diagnosed by clinical features, Darier's sign and demonstration of mast cell in dermis in biopsy specimen.
- Several special stains such as Giemsa, Toludine blue, KIT or tryptase antibody help in proper identification of mast cell in the infiltrate.
- Bone marrow or gastrointestinal biopsy is indicated in suspected cases of systemic mastocytosis.
- Indirect evidence of systemic involvement are high serum tryptase level and high urinary N-methylhistamine level.

Treatment

- Aim of the treatment is symptomatic control.
- Avoidance of potential triggers such as friction, heat, medications, etc.
- Counseling of the parents regarding natural course, prognosis, and available treatment options.[8]
- Children with mastocytosis are at increased risk of anaphylaxis therefore epinephrine autoinjector should be kept ready.
- Topical therapy includes topical steroid under occlusion and topical pimecrolimus for mastocytoma.
- Second generation H1 receptor antagonists (cetirizine, levocetrizine, loratadine, desloratadine, fexofenadine) are the initial treatment of choice.[9]
- For severe symptomatic cases first generation H1 receptor antagonists (hydroxyzine, cyproheptadine) can be used.
- Short course of systemic steroid may be required in severe symptomatic cases.
- Other treatment modalities which can be used are:
  - Cromolyn sodium
  - Ketotifen
  - Psoralen plus ultraviolet light A (PUVA) therapy
  - Narrow band ultraviolet light B (NBUVB) therapy
  - Cyclosporine
  - Tyrosine kinase inhibitor (imatinib, dasatinib, nilotinib)
  - Interferon alfa-2b

Prognosis

Overall prognosis of childhood cutaneous mastocytosis is very good in comparison with adults. Around 50–70% cases of childhood cutaneous mastocytosis undergo resolution by adolescence where adult cutaneous mastocytosis persists for life. Complete resolution is rare.[10] A good number of patients show marked reduction in the number of symptomatic lesions. Less than 10–15% cases go into adulthood.

KEY POINTS

- Mastocytosis is a spectrum of clinical disorder of bone marrow origin where mast cell accumulates in skin and/or other organ.
- Activating mutation of *KIT* gene of codon 816 (D816V) leads to constitutive, ligand-independent activation of the said receptor.
- About 55% cases appear between birth to 2 years of age.
- Urticaria pigmentosa is the commonest form of childhood mastocytosis characterized by tan to yellow-brown macule, papule, plaque or nodule distributed mainly over trunk.
- Adult mastocytosis is less commonly associated with cutaneous involvement.
- Treatment is mainly symptomatic control with oral antihistamine and other systemic agents, avoidance of triggers, and patient education.
- Prognosis of childhood-onset mastocytosis is excellent where adult mastocytosis persists for life.

REFERENCES

1. Horny HP, Sotlar K, Valent P, Hartmann K. Mastocytosis. Dtsch Arztebl Int. 2008;105:686-92.
2. Hartmann K, Henz BM. Mastocytosis: recent advances in defining the disease. Br J Dermatol. 2001;144:682-95.
3. Bodermer C, Hermine O, Palmerini F, Yang Y, Grandpeix-Guyodo C, Leventhal PS, et al. Pediatric mastocytosis is a clonal disease associated with D816V and other activating c-KIT mutation. J Invest Dermatol. 2010;130:804-15.
4. Schwaab J, Schnittger S, Sotlar K, Walz C, Fabarius A, Pfirrmann M, et al. Comprehensive mutational profiling in advanced systemic mastocytosis. Blood. 2013;122:2460-6.
5. Horny H, Akin C, Metcalfe DD, Escribano L, Bennett JM, Valent P, et al. Mastocytosis (mast cell disease). In: Swerdlow SH, Campo E, Harris NL, Jaffe ES, Pileri SA, Stein H, et al. (Eds). World Health Organization (WHO) Classification of Tumors.

Pathology and Genetics. Tumors of Hematopoietic and Lymphoid Tissues. Lyon, France: IARC Press; 2008. pp. 54-63.
6. Heide R. Clinical Aspects of Pediatric and Adult Onset Mastocytosis of the Skin. Rotterdam: Erasmus University Rotterdam; 2008.
7. Ghosh A, Choudhury J, Dhar S. An infant with bullous mastocytosis: a rare form of bullous disorder. Indian J Paediatr Dermatol. 2017;18:122-4.
8. Srinivas SM, Dhar S, Parikh D. Mastocytosis in children. Indian J Paediatr Dermatol. 2015;16:57-63.
9. Metcalfe DD. The treatment of mastocytosis: an overview. J Invest Dermatol. 1991;96:55S-6S.
10. Middelkamp Hup MA, Heide R, Tank B, Mulder PGH, Oranje AP. Comparison of mastocytosis with onset in children and adults. J Eur Acad Dermatol Venereol. 2002;16:115-20.

EXAMINATION QUESTION

1. Classify mastocytosis. How do you treat a case of cutaneous mastocytosis?

95 CHAPTER

Other Neoplasm of Skin

Varsha Vaidyanathan, Aarti Sarda, Abhishek De

INTRODUCTION

Cutaneous neoplasms or tumors are autonomous proliferations of cutaneous cells and they may be malignant or benign. This chapter will address neoplasms other than the commonly known ones such as basal cell carcinoma, squamous cell carcinoma, melanomas, and premalignant conditions. There are various neoplasms and many of them are more likely to be diagnosed histologically than clinically.

For ease of understanding, these neoplasms will be classified as follows depending upon the structure of origin:

- *Appendageal tumors:*
    - Tumors with eccrine/apocrine differentiation
    - Tumors with sebaceous differentiation
    - Tumors with follicular differentiation
- Fibrous and fibrohistiocytic tumors
- Skeletal muscle tumors
- Smooth muscle tumors
- Tumors of subcutaneous tissue
- Neural tumors

Within each group, a few key neoplasms will be dealt with in more detail.

APPENDAGEAL TUMORS[1-3]

These are tumors arising from the skin appendages, i.e., eccrine gland, apocrine gland, pilosebaceous apparatus (hair follicle and adjoining sebaceous gland). As the pilosebaceous apparatus is more densely concentrated in the face and scalp, the tumors arising from these structures are more likely to be found in these areas.

Tumors with Eccrine/Apocrine Differentiation

Hidrocystoma

It is a tumor formed by cystic dilatation of eccrine or apocrine ducts. Eccrine hidrocystoma is more commonly seen in middle-aged women while apocrine hidrocystomas have no such predilections. It is usually solitary but can be multiple and presents as a well-defined, smooth, and dome-shaped nodule containing serous fluid. The color varies from skin-colored to blue-black. It is asymptomatic and slowly increases in size to about 1 cm. The most common site is the face, especially around the eyelids. Apocrine hidrocystomas may also occur in the penis, vulva, and axilla. Eccrine hidrocystomas are affected by the temperature with the size increasing in summer and flattening in winters.

Histology shows a cystic lesion in the dermis double-lined by columnar cells and myoepithelial cells and show either eccrine or apocrine differentiation.

Treatment is by surgical excision, electrodessication, CO_2 laser, or pulsed dye laser. Topical atropine and scopolamine have also been used.

Poroma

Most poromas are eccrine in origin and arise from the acrosyringium, i.e., the intraepidermal part of the eccrine duct. Some poromas may however be apocrine in nature. It is usually seen in adults. They are most commonly found on the palms and soles; however, other sites such as head and neck may also be affected. These lesions are solitary, dome-shaped, moist red nodules around 1 cm in size, and may be mistaken for pyogenic granulomas.

Histologically, there is a distinct margin between normal epidermis and adjacent cuboidal cells with broad columns reaching down into the dermis. The tumor cells are basaloid, cuboidal, and have a clear cytoplasm.

The tumor is benign. In few cases, it may go on to develop into a porocarcinoma.

Treatment is by surgical excision.

Syringoma

These tumors arise from sweat ducts. They are relatively common in women. They appear in adolescence and increase during adulthood. They present as multiple tiny skin-colored cystic lesions although some may be flat. Most commonly they appear on the face, around the eyes, and on the upper cheeks. They can also appear on the neck, chest, and buttocks. They tend to be bilaterally symmetrical.

Histologically, multiple convoluted and cystic ducts lined by a double layer of cells and containing an amorphous material are found in the upper dermis. They characteristically show a tadpole or comma appearance wherein a tail-like strand of cells juts from the duct into the surrounding stroma.

Syringomas are treated with electrofulguration, CO_2 lasers or enucleation with a hypodermic needle. However, they may recur.

Hidradenoma

This is a relatively rare tumor which may arise from either eccrine or apocrine sweat glands. It is more commonly seen in adult females. Hidradenoma tends to be solitary and is seen on the head, neck, chest, and limbs. They present as firm dermal nodules up to 3 cm in size with a thickened or ulcerated surface. There may be a history of serous discharge. The ulcerated nodules may be mistaken for basal cell carcinoma.

On histology, circumscribed masses with two types of cells—clear cells containing glycogen and elongated darker cells, are seen in the dermis. Interspersed within these masses, double-layered ducts and clefts are present. The tumor mass may be connected to the epidermis.

Surgical excision is curative.

Cylindroma

This is a relatively rare tumor of sweat gland origin seen usually in women. They present as multiple, well-demarcated, smooth, and pink nodules on the scalp. Uncommonly they may be seen on the face, neck, or chest. Some may be pedunculated. They grow slowly and although most are small, some cylindromas may grow up to 5 cm or more. Large ones give rise to the appearance of so-called "turban tumors".

On histology, a characteristic jigsaw puzzle appearance is noted. There are multiple tumor lobules surrounded by a lining of hyaline basement membrane material and they are closely placed next to each other simulating puzzle pieces. Cells in the lobules are of two types—small peripheral cells and larger cells with pale cytoplasm towards the center.

Surgical excision is the treatment of choice. Wide excision and graft replacement may be required if the lesions are extensive.

Syringocystadenoma Papilliferum

This tumor is apocrine in origin. Although they may present at birth or early childhood, mostly they are seen in adults. Clinically, there are multiple pink or red papules arranged in a linear pattern on the head and neck or more rarely the vulva, scrotum, breast, or external ear. They may arise *de novo* or from a preexisting nevus sebaceous. The papules may become warty, crusted, or ulcerated.

On biopsy, papillary projections are seen on the epidermal surface of the tumor mass along with cystic invaginations which show a double layer of columnar cells with an apocrine secretion pattern.

Treatment is by surgical excision.

Extramammary Paget's Disease

Primary disease (75%) is an in situ carcinoma arising from the intraepidermal duct of the apocrine glands. Secondary disease (25%) occurs due to upward spread onto the skin of an underlying adenocarcinoma. These two are indistinguishable on biopsy.

It is usually seen in women in their 50s or older. Clinically, it presents on apocrine-rich areas such as vulva, anogenital region, and axilla as a pruritic, well-defined, erythematous plaque with rounded raised margins. The surface may be scaly with crusting, weeping, and erosions. Later there may be lichenification. Leukoplakia and hyperpigmentation may also develop. It resembles an eczema, but there is no response to steroids which may be the first clue to alert diagnosticians to its true nature.

Biopsy shows large oval cells with abundant pale cytoplasm and large nuclei and nucleoli present singly or in groups in the epidermis.

An underlying adenocarcinoma must be looked for and if found must be treated appropriately. Complete excision of the lesion of extramammary Paget's disease must be carried out. Mohs surgery may be of use. The lesions may recur postsurgery. Photodynamic therapy, topical imiquimod, and radiotherapy have been used as adjunct management or as primary treatment in very elderly patients who cannot undergo surgery.

Paget's Disease of the Nipple

This is an intraepidermal adenocarcinoma strongly associated with an underlying carcinoma of the breast. It is almost always seen in women in their 50s and 60s. It presents initially with a moist and crusted itchy eczematous area on the nipple and surrounding areola. The lesion is sharply marginated with a slightly raised surface. Over a period of time, the lesion increases in size and discomfort with itching, burning, and serosanguinous discharge. A lump may be palpable in the breast.

Histopathologically, it is similar to extramammary Paget's disease.

Patients should be investigated for presence and extent of underlying breast carcinoma, which should be appropriately managed. Surgery should include the whole nipple-areola complex.

Tumors with Sebaceous Differentiation

Sebaceous Adenoma

This is a relatively rare benign tumor composed of undifferentiated sebaceous cells and is more commonly seen in the elderly population. The lesion is a solitary rounded, sessile, or pedunculated skin-colored or yellowish papule less than 1 cm in size usually seen on the scalp or face, especially the eyelid. Multiple lesions are seen in association with Muir–Torre syndrome.

On histology, well-demarcated sebaceous lobules are seen in the dermis. Most of the cells are mature sebocytes except for a peripheral row of small basaloid cells. There are cystic spaces lined by eosinophilic matter and they contain sebaceous material.

Management is by surgical excision.

Sebaceous Carcinoma

This is a rare malignant tumor of sebaceous origin usually seen in middle-aged and elderly males. It is slow-growing and presents as a solitary, yellowish-orange, firm lesion on the face and scalp, especially around the eyelids where it may be mistaken for a chalazion. It is generally a nonaggressive tumor, but it may sometimes show a rather invasive nature.

Biopsy shows multiple sebaceous lobules of varying shapes and sizes. The cells range from mature sebocytes to undifferentiated basaloid cells. Nuclear atypia, mitosis, and necrosis may be seen.

These lesions need a complete surgical excision. Mohs surgery is of particular utility here.

Tumors with Follicular Differentiation

Trichoblastoma

Trichoepitheliomas, which were earlier considered a separate entity, also now fall under this same group. These arise from the follicular germ cells. Usually they are small solitary papules appearing on the head and neck. In Brooke–Spiegler syndrome and Brooke–Fordyce disease, they may be multiple waxy papules on the nasolabial folds. It is generally benign but may transform into a malignancy.

Histopathologically, they occur in nodular, retiform, cribriform, columnar, and racemiform patterns. Multiple lobular aggregates of basophilic basaloid cells with invaginating stroma are present in the dermis. There is follicular differentiation.

Management is by complete surgical excision.

Pilomatricoma

This is a benign tumor arising from the hair matrix and is the most common hair follicle tumor. Most of the patients are children. It presents as a solitary, firm to hard, and lobular dermal nodule less than 3 cm in size on the head and neck. The surface is generally smooth but may ulcerate.

Biopsy shows well-demarcated islands of cells surrounded by fibrous capsule in the dermis. In these islands, basophilic nucleated basaloid cells are present in the periphery whereas enucleated ghost cells are seen in the center.

Treatment is by complete surgical excision.

FIBROUS AND FIBROHISTIOCYTIC TUMORS[4,5]

As the name suggests, these are soft tissue tumors of fibroblastic and fibrohistiocytic origin. They tend to present as a nonspecific nodule on the body.

Dermatofibroma

Also known as a fibrous histiocytoma, this is a benign dermal tumor composed of cells resembling histiocytes, fibroblasts, and myofibroblasts. The exact etiology is as yet unknown. They occur in young to middle-aged adults. It is commonly seen on lower limbs and presents as a firm, slightly scaly, and yellowish-brown papule. Fitzpatrick sign or dimple sign is frequently positive wherein lateral pressure on the lesion causes a depression due to epidermal tethering. Usually the lesions are solitary but may be multiple or eruptive, which may be familial or associated with immunosuppression or autoimmune diseases. The clinicopathological variants of dermatofibroma include the cellular, aneurysmal, pseudosarcomatous (atypical), epithelioid, and atrophic types. Unlike cellular and aneurysmal variants, the ordinary dermatofibroma almost never recurs after excision. Some may transform and behave in an aggressive fashion.

On biopsy, there is epidermal hyperplasia mimicking lichen simplex chronicus or squamous papilloma. In the dermis, there is an aggregation of cells resembling histiocytes and fibroblasts along with mononuclear inflammatory cells. At the periphery, hyalinized collagen bundles are seen. The tumor tends to blend into the surrounding normal tissue.

Ordinary dermatofibromas are usually merely a cosmetic nuisance. Merely a cosmetic nuisance and can be surgically excised if the patient so desires. However, in the case of atypical, aneurysmal and cellular types, it is better to definitively excise them since they tend to recur and there is a chance of malignant transformation.

Acquired Digital Fibrokeratoma

This is a benign tumor seen on the periungual area of fingers and toes in adults possibly as a reaction to trauma and presents as a solitary skin-colored, dome-shaped, or conical lesion with a collarette of raised skin at the base. The surface may be slightly verrucous. Multiple tumors may be seen in tuberous sclerosis.

These are diagnosed clinically and do not usually require a biopsy which shows thick collagen bundles, thin elastic fibers, increased vascularity, and fibroblasts.

Treatment is by simple excision.

Dermatofibrosarcoma Protuberans

This is a locally invasive tumor with fibroblastic differentiation. It usually presents during the third to fifth decades of life. In about 50% cases, it is situated on the flexural aspect of the trunk. It can also occur on proximal parts of the limbs and scalp. There is a tendency to develop on scars and sites of previous trauma. It tends to be slow growing and starts out as a well-defined plaque with irregular contours, which eventually becomes a firm reddish blue dermal nodule occasionally with an ulcerated surface.

On histopathology, a multinodular mass composed of uniform slender spindle-shaped cells is seen in the dermis and subcutis. The tumor cells infiltrate deeper and laterally into normal dermis to form spokes of a wheel—known as "storiform" pattern. The subcutis is also infiltrated in a lace-like fashion—"honeycomb" pattern.

Management is by wide local excision with a margin of 2–4 cm. Mohs micrographic surgery can reduce the chances of recurrences which otherwise are quite high.

Soft Fibroma (Skin Tag)

Also known as acrochordons, they present as multiple pedunculated or filiform skin-colored soft papules in the neck, axilla, and groin. Histologically, they show hyperkeratosis, acanthosis, and papillomatosis. The filiform variant shows an underlying fibrovascular stalk.

Treatment is by electrocautery, chemical cauterization, or simple excision.

SKELETAL MUSCLE TUMORS

These are tumors arising from the skeletal muscles. They very rarely appear on the skin primarily. Rhabdomyosarcomas may involve the skin by direct extension from deeper tissues. Other tumors include rhabdomyoma and rhabdomyosarcomatous congenital hamartoma.

SMOOTH MUSCLE TUMORS

Leiomyoma

This is a benign tumor derived from smooth muscles. Depending upon the origin of the smooth muscle, they are classified as pilar leiomyoma (from arrector pili muscle), angioleiomyoma (from the vascular media), or genital leiomyoma (from smooth muscle of scrotum, labia majora, or nipple). Of these, the pilar type is the most common while the genital type is the rarest. They can appear at any age except for angioleiomyoma which is more frequently found in middle-aged females.

Pilar leiomyoma presents as solitary or multiple pink to red firm nodules less than 1.5 cm in size on the extremities, trunk, or head and neck. Multiple small nodules may coalesce to form a larger nodule. These nodules are very painful, especially when triggered by cold temperature or emotional disturbance.

Angioleiomyoma presents as a solitary skin-colored deep dermal or subcutaneous nodule on the extremities. It may be up to 4 cm in size and is frequently painful which can be exacerbated by temperature changes, menstruation, and pregnancy.

Genital leiomyoma presents most frequently on the scrotum as a solitary dermal nodule. Incidence of pain is less frequent as compared to the other types.

Histologically, interwoven bundles of eosinophilic spindle-shaped cells with long and thin nuclei are found in the dermis. These cells are positive for actin and desmin confirming their muscular origin.

Gabapentin and calcium channel blockers may temporarily ease the pain. Definitive therapy is surgical excision.

Smooth Muscle Hamartoma

This rare tumor represents a hamartomatous proliferation of smooth muscles within the dermis. It is usually congenital with a slight male preponderance. It appears on the trunk and extremities as a hyperpigmented and hypertrichotic patch or plaque. Pseudo-Darier sign[6] (rubbing or stroking of the lesion produces transient induration, piloerection, and redness of the skin) may be present. Histologically and clinically it resembles a Becker's nevus and it may be considered to be part of the same spectrum.

On biopsy, variably arranged bundles of smooth muscles are seen in the dermis. Follicles may be seen prominently.

It is a benign condition and does not require treatment except for cosmetic reasons in which case a complete excision is performed.

TUMORS OF SUBCUTANEOUS TISSUE

Lipoma

This is a benign tumor composed of mature adipose tissue. They are common in adults, especially in the obese. They present as solitary or multiple asymptomatic, slow-growing, soft, lobular, subcutaneous nodules of varying size with overlying normal epidermis commonly on the trunk, limbs, and neck. Multiple painful lipomas are seen in adiposis dolorosa (Dercum's disease).

On biopsy, these are well-encapsulated tumors containing lobules of normal mature fat cells divided by fibrous septae. Fat necrosis may be seen.

A lipoma can be managed with simple excision. Injection lipolysis by injection of phosphatidyl choline/sodium deoxycholate in the lipoma has been tried with variable success.[7]

NEURAL TUMORS

Neurofibroma

It is a relatively common tumor composed of all the neural elements such as Schwann cells, fibroblasts, endothelial cells, and axons. It may be common/cutaneous (extraneural) or plexiform (intraneural). The common neurofibroma is a soft, skin-colored small nodule with buttonhole sign positive (on pressure with a fingertip they can be pushed back into the dermis). Multiple such neurofibromas are found all over the body in neurofibromatosis type I. Plexiform neurofibromas involve the entire nerve along with its branches and they are pathognomonic of neurofibromatosis I. They are large and pedunculated skin-colored to hyperpigmented swellings with a squishy "bag of worms" feel on palpation. There is also a diffuse type of neurofibroma which presents as poorly defined plaques in children and adolescents.

Histologically, the tumor is unencapsulated and contains spindle-shaped cells with wavy nuclei in collagenous stroma along with multiple mast cells. In plexiform neurofibromas, nerve trunks of varied sizes are scattered in the tumor mass.

Common neurofibromas can be easily excised; however, this may be hard to do when the lesions are extensive as in neurofibromatosis I. Surgical excision of plexiform neurofibromas is quite difficult as they are extensive and there is a risk of intratumor hemorrhage.

Schwannoma (Neurilemmoma)

This benign tumor originates from nerve sheaths and is composed of Schwann cells. It is a relatively rare tumor and may be seen in women in their 40s and 50s. Mostly it is seen arising from the acoustic nerve in the setting of neurofibromatosis type II. Rarely, it may be seen in the elbow, wrist, knee, or head and neck in association with the main regional nerves where it presents as a firm or cystic, yellowish-grey round nodule less than 5 cm in size.

Histologically, the tumor is circumscribed and encapsulated in the subcutaneous tissue along the course of the nerve. The tumor cells are spindle-shaped with elongated basophilic nuclei and are arranged in interwoven bands. In the Antoni A pattern, the nuclei are arranged in a palisading pattern at the periphery with intervening eosinophilic substance and this is called a Verocay body. In the Antoni B pattern, there is no palisading. Thin spindle-shaped cells are present in a clear matrix along with wavy collagen bundles.

Management of cutaneous schwannomas is by simple excision.

CONCLUSION

Many of these neoplasms present with nondescript features clinically and hence may be overlooked by both the patient and the doctor. However, some of them may be a clue to an underlying disorder or even have a malignant potential. So it is always a good practice to keep a weather eye out for these lesions, biopsy them to determine their exact nature, and then treat them accordingly.

KEY POINTS

- Appendageal tumors are those arising from the skin appendages, i.e., eccrine glands, apocrine glands and pilosebaceous unit.
- Most of the benign tumors of eccrine and apocrine origin are present on the head and neck except for poroma which is usually seen on the palms and soles.
- On histopthology, cylindromas have a typical 'jigsaw puzzle' appearance. Syringomas show a 'tadpole' or 'comma' appearance.
- Long-standing eczematous lesions in middle-aged women in apocrine-rich areas which do not respond to topical steroids must be investigated for Paget's disease of the nipple and extramammary Paget's disease.
- Multiple sebaceous adenomas are seen in Muir–Torre syndrome.
- Fitzpatrick sign or dimpling sign (lateral pressure on the lesion producing a depression due to epidermal tethering) is elicited in dermaofibromas.
- Leiomyomas are extremely painful nodules especially when triggered by cold are of three types depending upon origin—pilar leiomyomas, angioleiomyomas and genital leiomyomas.
- Smooth muscle hamartomas show pseudo-Darier sign wherein rubbing of the lesion produces transient induration, redness and piloerection.
- Lipomas are generally asymptomatic but multiple painful lipomas are found in adiposis dolorosa (Dercum's disease).

REFERENCES

1. Khandpur S, Ramam M. Skin tumors. In: Valia RG, Valia AR (Eds). IADVL Textbook of Dermatology, 3rd edition. Mumbai: Bhalani Publishing House; 2008. pp. 1475-529.
2. Calonje E. Tumours of skin appendages. In: Griffiths C, Barker J, Blelker T, Chalmers R, Creamer D (Eds). Rook's Textbook of Dermatology, 9th edition. New Jersey, United States: Wiley-Blackwell; 2016. pp. 138.1-44.
3. Storm CA, Seykora JT. Cutaneous adnexal neoplasms. Am J Clin Pathol. 2002;118(Suppl):S33-49.
4. Luzar B, Calonje E. Cutaneous fibrohistiocytic tumours: an update. Histopathology. 2010;56(1):148-65.
5. Calonje E. Soft-tissue tumours and tumour-like conditions. In: Griffiths C, Barker J, Blelker T, Chalmers R, Creamer D (Eds). Rook's Textbook of Dermatology, 9th edition. New Jersey, United States: Wiley-Blackwell; 2016. pp. 137.1-66.
6. Bilgiç Ö, Tunçez Akyürek F, Altınyazar HC. Pseudo darier sign: a distinctive finding for congenital smooth muscle hamartoma. J Pediatr. 2016;169:318.
7. Amber KT, Ovadia S, Camacho I. Injection therapy for the management of superficial subcutaneous lipomas. J Clin Aesthet Dermatol. 2014;7(6):46-8.

EXAMINATION QUESTION

1. Write a short note on dermatofibroma.

CHAPTER 96

Histiocytosis and Xanthomas

Deblina Bhunia, Ravi Ranjan

HISTIOCYTOSIS

INTRODUCTION

Histiocytoses comprise a group of proliferative disorders characterized by abnormal accumulation and behavior of cells of the mononuclear phagocytic system which consists of dendritic cells, monocytes, and macrophages. These disorders include a wide variety of conditions that can affect both children and adults, ranging from benign skin lesions to life-threatening systemic disorders.[1]

CLASSIFICATION

The initial classification of histiocytosis in 1987 by the Histiocyte Society, classified these diseases into three categories: (1) Langerhans cell related, (2) non-Langerhans cell related, and (3) malignant. In the most recent classification proposed by Emile et al., the histiocytic disorders are grouped into five categories based on clinical, genetic, and immunohistologic features: (1) Langerhans-related (L); (2) cutaneous and mucocutaneous (C); (3) Rosai-Dorfman disease (R); (4) malignant (M); and (5) hemophagocytic lymphohistiocytosis (H) **(Table 1)**.[2]

According to this recent proposed classification,[2] Langerhans cell histiocytosis (LCH) and Erdheim-Chester disease (ECD) are thought to be the part of same group (L-related group) as nearly 20% of cases of ECD have associated LCH lesions, along with same genetic mutations in majority and some similar clinical complications.

Indeterminate cell histiocytosis also has some clinical and histological overlap with LCH, suggesting a shared primary component in disease pathogenesis.

TABLE 1: Histiocytoses classification: A brief overview.[2]

Group	Family	Disorders
L group (Langerhans related)		• Langerhans cell histiocytosis (LCH) • Erdheim-Chester disease (ECD) • Mixed (LCH/ECD) • Indeterminate cell histiocytosis
C group (non-LCH with skin and mucosal involvement)	Xanthogranuloma (XG) family*	• Juvenile XG • Adult XG • Solitary reticulohistiocytoma • Benign cephalic histiocytosis • Generalized eruptive histiocytosis • Progressive nodular histiocytosis • Xanthoma disseminatum
	Non-XG family	• Necrobiotic XG • Multicentric reticulohistiocytosis, • Cutaneous Rosai-Dorfman disease
R group		Rosai-Dorfman and related diseases
M group		Malignant histiocytoses
H group		Hemophagocytic lymphohistiocytosis

*Phenotype of dermal dendritic cells; positive for factor XIIIa, CD68, CD163, etc., negative for S100 and CD1a.

DESCRIPTIONS OF INDIVIDUAL HISTIOCYTOSIS

Langerhans Cell Histiocytosis

Langerhans cell histiocytosis was initially divided into eosinophilic granuloma, Hand-Schüller-Christian disease, and Abt-Letterer-Siwe disease, depending on the sites and severity. Later, these diseases were found to be manifestations of a single entity and were unified under the term histiocytosis X. This designation was changed to LCH as Langerhans cell represented the primary cell involved in the pathophysiology.

- Characterized by proliferation and accumulation of CD1a+ Langerhans cells in various tissues.
- Children are more commonly affected than adults.
- Age of onset is important factor influencing the disease course.
- May begin with any pattern and evolve or relapse to another.
- Most cases of LCH demonstrate clonality and telomere shortening. BRAF V600E mutations have been detected in a majority.

Childhood Langerhans Cell Histiocytosis[3]

- Boys are more commonly affected.
- Bony lesions are present in almost two-thirds of cases and skin disease in one-third.

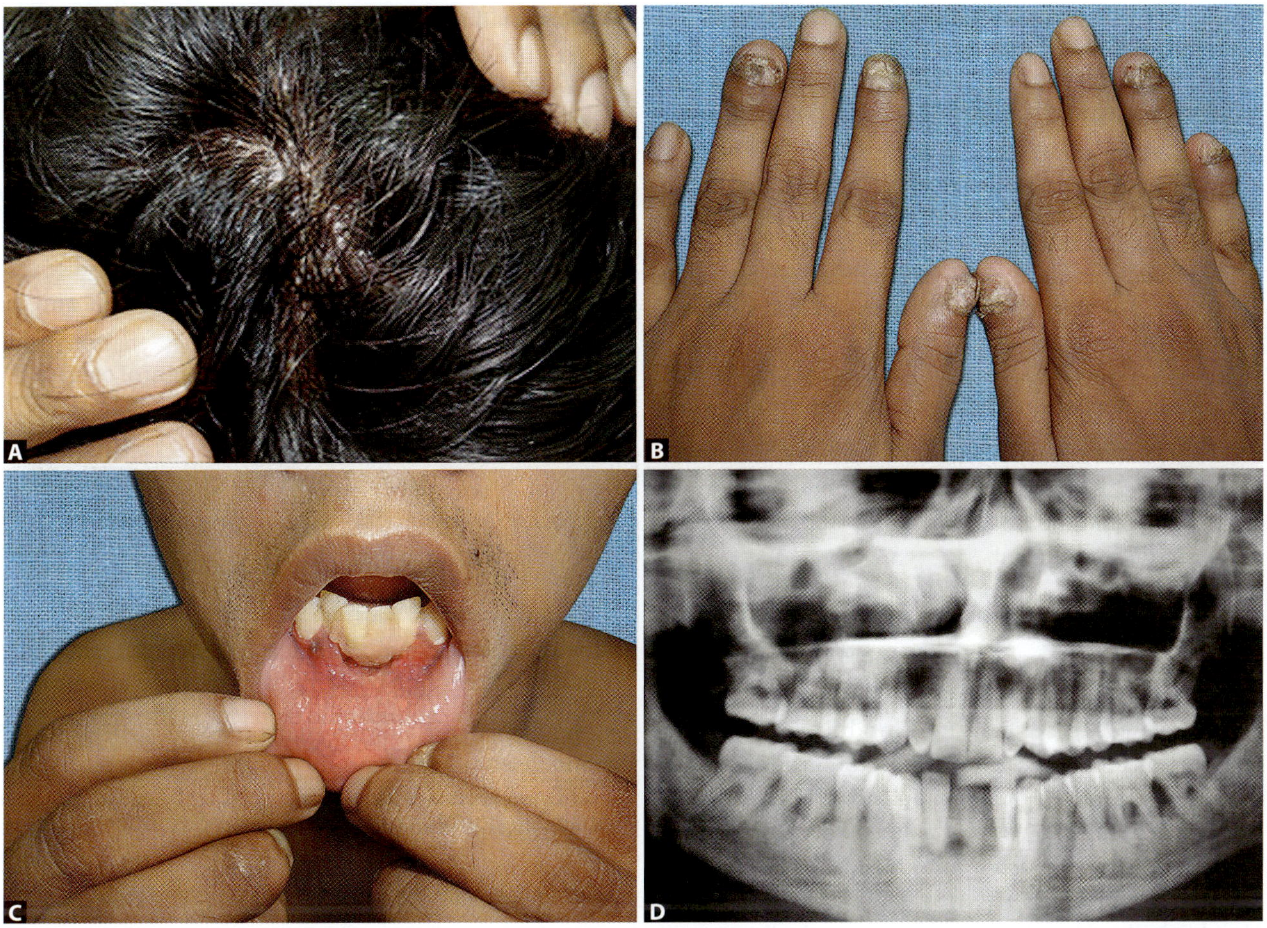

Figs. 1A to D: Langerhans cell histiocytosis in an adult patient with (A) crusted lesions on scalp; (B) Nail involvement; (C) Gingival lesion; (D) Destruction of alveolar bone (radiography).

- The prognosis for children <1 year is worse due to multisystem (MS) involvement.

Adult Langerhans Cell Histiocytosis[3]

- Common age of presentation: 20–35 years.
- Multisystem disease in up to two-thirds cases.
- Bones are the most common organ involved, followed by skin and mucosa.
- Diabetes insipidus occurs in 20% of patients, and other endocrine abnormalities can result from hypothalamic-pituitary involvement.

Clinical Features[3,4] ***(Figs. 1 and 2)***

- The LCH is subdivided into: single system (SS) and MS disease.
- SS-LCH can be unifocal or multifocal.
- MS-LCH is divided into "low-risk" and "high-risk" disease. High risk of mortality is associated with involvement of the hematopoietic system, liver, and spleen.
- Single system bone LCH is the most common form. Skull vault is frequent site; followed by long and flat bones. It usually occurs in older children and young adults.
- *Skin* is the second most commonly involved organ.

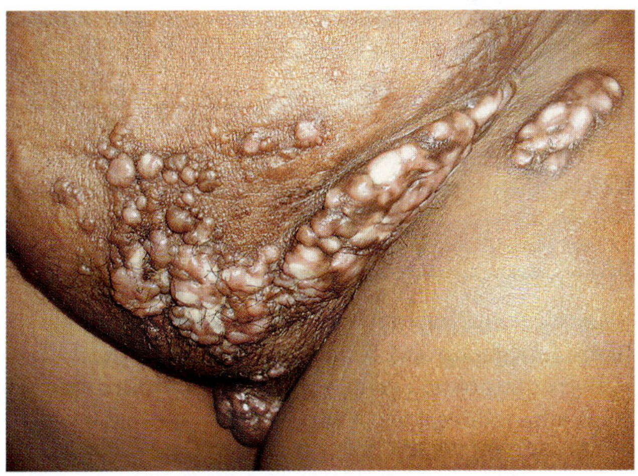

Fig. 2: Papulonodular lesions with ulceration in the groin of a woman with Langerhans cell histiocytosis.

- Lesions are variable; macules, papules, plaques, vesicles, pustules, bullae, and ulcerations can be seen.
- *Characteristic lesion in children*: Papulosquamous lesions with greasy scales, affecting the scalp, flexors, and midline of trunk resembling seborrhoeic dermatitis; often associated with *hemorrhage and petechial component*.

- *Nail changes* can occur, mostly in MS disease, as nail dystrophy, nail plate loss, nail bed purpura, and paronychia.
- Painful *oral ulceration* (mostly buccal mucosal), alveolar bone lesion leading to periodontitis, gingival involvement, and tooth detachment can occur. Cervical adenopathy and bilateral parotid swelling may be seen.
- Painful and ulcerative lesions restricted to genitalia seen rarely.
- Bone marrow involvement may cause cytopenias.
- The liver may be involved either by direct infiltration or due to obstruction by enlarged nodes in porta hepatis; both can lead to biliary cirrhosis.
- Pulmonary disease with diffuse micronodular infiltrates and cysts are commonly seen in adults (mostly smokers). Pneumothorax can occur.

Variants[4]

- *Congenital or neonatal onset SS-LCH [congenital self-healing reticulohistiocytosis (CSHRH) or Hashimoto-Pritzker disease]*: Solitary/multinodular lesions over any part of the body, usually 0.2–2.5 cm in diameter; red, brown, pink, or dusky papules, nodules, or rarely hemorrhagic bullae with/without ulceration. Lesions commonly regress over few months.
- *Skin LCH as part of low-risk MS disease, formerly known as Hand-Schüller-Christian syndrome*: Chronic disease with lytic bone lesions, diabetes insipidus, exophthalmos, and skin lesions. Age of onset is usually 2–6 years. Cutaneous manifestations are variable; oral mucosa may be involved.
- *Skin involvement as part of disseminated disease, previously known as Letterer-Siwe disease*: The most extensive and severe form, occurs in <15% of pediatric cases; commonly seen <2 years of age. Multiple organs including bones, lungs, liver, spleen, central nervous system (CNS), and bone marrow are involved.

Histopathology

- Dense dermal infiltrate of Langerhans cells, with abundant, amphophilic cytoplasm and eccentric round/kidney bean-shaped nucleus; can be superficial, folliculocentric, or deep and diffuse.
- Frequent exocytosis of the abnormal cells.
- Mixed dermal infiltrate of neutrophils, eosinophils, lymphocytes, and plasma cells.
- The Langerhans cells are positive for S100, CD1a, and langerin (CD207).

Other Investigations

- Complete blood count
- Electrolytes, urea, and creatinine
- Liver function tests
- Coagulation studies
- Erythrocyte sedimentation rate (ESR) and C-reactive protein (CRP)
- Chest X-ray
- Abdominal ultrasound
- Skeletal survey

Tests Indicated in Some Patients

- Magnetic resonance imaging of the brain and water deprivation test
- High-resolution computed tomography of chest
- Lung function tests
- Lung biopsy
- Liver biopsy
- Bone marrow biopsy
- Full hormone screening

Management[5]

- Approach depends on the extent and severity of disease and patient's age.
- Children with SS-LCH may not require aggressive treatment.
- *Unifocal bone lesions*: Curettage or intralesional steroid injection.
- *Skin only disease*: Topical steroids, tacrolimus, nitrogen mustard, or phototherapy.
- *Recalcitrant/MS disease with organ dysfunction*:
    - Children—prednisolone with vinblastine.
    - Adults—first line is etoposide, maintenance with azathioprine.
    - In patients unresponsive to conventional therapy, 2-chlorodeoxyadenosine may be effective.
    - *Other drugs*: Methotrexate, thalidomide, interferon-α, 6-mercaptopurine, cytosine arabinoside, cyclosporine, etc.
    - In severe cases—bone marrow transplantation.
    - Vemurafenib and other BRAF inhibitors can be tried.

Erdheim-Chester Disease[2,4]

- *Erdheim-Chester disease* is primarily a visceral disorder with cutaneous lesions.
- May begin at any age; common group is 40–70 years.
- Male predominance.
- *The characteristic feature*: Sclerosis of the metaphyseal and diaphyseal regions of long bones (mostly bilateral and symmetric). Bone pain may be the presenting feature.
- *Cutaneous lesions*: Diverse; periorbital xanthelasma-like lesions are common. Xanthoma-like or red-brown papular lesions involving the extremities or trunk can be seen.

- *Other systemic*:
  - Diabetes insipidus
  - Pulmonary, cardiovascular, and CNS involvement can occur.
- Overlap with LCH reported in some cases.

Histopathology

- Infiltration with foamy histiocytes with small nucleus; occasional Touton giant cells
- Fibrosis present in most cases
- Histiocytes are positive for CD68 and CD163 and negative for CD1a. Few are positive for S100.

Prognosis

Often fatal, usually from pulmonary fibrosis and cardiac failure. Mortality rate is 60%.

Treatment

- Surgical debulking, radiotherapy, high-dose systemic steroid, cyclosporine, interferon-α and vinca alkaloids, anthracyclines, and cyclophosphamide can be tried.
- Vemurafenib in patients with BRAF V600E mutation.

Indeterminate Cell Histiocytosis[2,3]

- Rare histiocytosis composed of dendritic cells staining variably with Langerhans cell markers (S100 and CD1a), negative for langerin (CD207) and lacks Birbeck granules.
- Skin lesions can resemble other forms of histiocytosis.
- Single/multiple, asymptomatic, papules, plaques, or nodules of 3–10 cm, over trunk and extremities.
- Mucosal involvement is rare.
- Visceral involvement and hematologic malignancies accompanied in some.
- Phototherapy, pravastatin, thalidomide, and methotrexate can be tried.

Juvenile Xanthogranuloma[2-4,6-8]

- Most common non-LCH.
- Appears within first year of life in majority.
- Male predominance.

Cutaneous

- Solitary (more common) or multiple lesions
- Well-demarcated, firm, rubbery, round to oval dermal papules/nodules
- Early lesions are pink to red brown, later become yellowish
- *Distribution*: Head and neck, followed by upper trunk and upper extremities
- *Three types of lesions*:
  1. Small nodular (2–5 mm)
  2. Large nodular (5–20 mm)
  3. Giant xanthogranuloma (>20 mm)
- Usually *regress within 3–6 years*
- Subcutaneous lesion commonly appears in infancy, often in <3 months.
- Oral juvenile xanthogranuloma (JXG) may develop as solitary lesion on tongue, lip, or palate.

Extracutaneous Involvement

- Ocular involvement in 0.3–0.4% cases with multiple JXGs; iris is the most common location.
- Uncommonly involves lung, liver, testis, CNS, kidney, spleen, retroperitoneum, etc.
- Juvenile myelomonocytic leukemia (JMML) and neurofibromatosis (type 1) have been reported in JXG.

Dermoscopy

"Setting sun" appearance, an orange yellow background, and subtle erythematous border with branched and linear vessels running from the edge to the center.

Histopathology

- *Early lesions*: Mononuclear cells with less vacuolated abundant amphophilic cytoplasm.
- *Mature lesions*: Foam cells, Touton, and foreign body giant cells
- Histiocytes are positive for factor XIIIa, CD68, CD163, vimentin, fascin, and MS-1; negative for CD1a, and S100 **(Table 2)**.

Treatment

- Usually not required
- Excision of persistent lesions

TABLE 2: Antigenic markers of the non-Langerhans-related cutaneous histiocytoses.[3,7]

Histiocytic disorder	*S100 protein*	*CD1A*	*CD68*	*Factor XIIIA*
Juvenile xanthogranuloma	–(+)	-	+	+
Solitary reticulohistiocytoma	–	–	+	+
Benign cephalic histiocytosis	–	–	+	+
Generalized eruptive histiocytosis	–	–	+	+
Progressive nodular histiocytosis	–	–	+	+
Xanthoma disseminatum	–	–	+	+
Papular xanthoma*	–	–	+	+/–
Necrobiotic xanthogranuloma	–	–	+	–
Multicentric reticulohistiocytosis	–	–	+	–(+)
Rosai-Dorfman disease	+	–	+	–(+)

Note: The bracket denotes rare occurrence.
*Papular xanthoma is not mentioned in the recent classification.

- Combination of surgery, chemotherapy, radiotherapy, or immunotherapy may be required in visceral involvement.

In *adult xanthogranuloma*, lesions usually occur in late 20s to early 30s. Lesion is frequently *solitary and persistent*.[2]

Solitary reticulohistiocytoma (SRH): Asymptomatic, commonly solitary papules/nodules of <1 cm in diameter seen over any part of body including mucosa with features like xanthogranuloma in which oncocytic macrophages and ground-glass giant cells dominate. This entity was previously considered as a part of reticulohistiocytosis group, but clinical and immunohistochemistry findings differ in solitary and multicentric form.[2,4,7,8]

Benign Cephalic Histiocytosis[3]

- Onset: 2 months to 3 years
- Starts from head, then cheeks, forehead, eyelids, and ears; may spread to neck and trunk.
- Multiple (often 5–20 in number) reddish-yellow papules, 2–4 mm in size; may coalesce to from reticular pattern.
- *Resolves by 2–8 years*, with hyperpigmentation. Some cases may evolve into JXG.
- No systemic or mucosal involvement.

Histopathology

Diffuse dermal infiltration of monomorphous macrophages.

Generalized Eruptive Histiocytosis[3]

Clinical Features

- Multiple papules, involving the trunk and proximal extremities, and sparing flexors.
- Mucosal involvement is rare.
- No visceral involvement.
- New lesions appear in crops, over several years.
- *Spontaneous involution* with hyperpigmentation.
- *In children*: May appear after bacterial/viral infection.
- *In adults*: May be associated with malignancy, e.g., leukemia/lymphoma.

Histopathology

- Dermal infiltration of monomorphous and vacuolated macrophages.

Treatment

- Usually not required.
- Psoralen-ultraviolet A (PUVA) therapy or isotretinoin may be considered in adults.

Progressive Nodular Histiocytosis[2,3]

- Common age group: 40–60 years.
- *Two types of lesions*:
    - Superficial small xanthomatous papules up to 5 mm in diameter; distributed all over body, sparing the flexors.
    - Larger deep lesions up to 5 cm in diameter, associated with pain, ulceration, and disfigurement.
- Smaller papules may evolve to larger lesions.
- On the face, lesions may coalesce. Leonine facies and ectropion can be seen.
- Conjunctival, oral, or laryngeal lesions may occur.
- *Regress rarely* after many years.

Xanthoma Disseminatum[3,7]

Clinical Feature

- Insidious onset.
- Onset before 25 years in >60% cases.
- Asymptomatic yellow, red, and brown papules symmetrically distributed on face, trunk, and extremities.
- Characteristically involves *eyelid and flexors* (axilla, inguinal, antecubital, and popliteal fossa).
- May heal with atrophy.
- Mucosal involvement in 40–60% cases, may lead to following complications:
    - Oropharynx—dysphagia.
    - Larynx—dysphonia and airway obstruction.
    - Conjunctiva and cornea—blindness.
- Central nervous system and bone involvements can occur.
- Diabetes insipidus in around 40% patients; may present with triads of cutaneous lesions, mucosal lesions, and diabetes insipidus.
- Rare association with monoclonal gammopathy.
- Hyperlipidemia reported in few cases.

Prognosis

About one-third cases persistent or progressive; complete or partial resolution in others.

Histopathology

- *Early lesion*: Scalloped macrophages in dermis
- *Later*: Foam cell and Touton giant cell.

Treatment

- Surgery, radiotherapy, cryosurgery, laser therapy, and medications such as 2-chlorodeoxyadenosine (2-CdA), cyclophosphamide, and cyclosporine have been tried.

Papular Xanthoma[3,9]

- Rare non-LCH.
- May appear in early childhood or after adolescent.
- Male predominance.
- Solitary or multiple small, yellowish papules, or nodules of 1–10 mm.
- Multiple lesions are generalized, but *do not favor flexors*.
- In adults, mucosal involvement may occur.
- Usually no systemic involvement or hyperlipidemia.

Necrobiotic Xanthogranuloma[3,7,10]

Clinical Features

- Average age of onset—the sixth decade.
- *Cutaneous*: Yellowish papules, nodules, or plaques involving the face (*periorbital areas—common*), trunk, and extremities; sometimes with *telangiectasias, atrophy, ulceration,* and *scarring.*
- *Ophthalmic*: Orbital masses, ectropion, ptosis, conjunctival lesions, keratitis, scleritis, uveitis, etc., in approximately 50% patients.
- Immunoglobulin G (IgG) monoclonal gammopathy accompany in majority (>70% cases).
- Plasma cell dyscrasia, cryoglobulinemia, and/or lymphoproliferative disorder may be present.
- *Others*: Hepatosplenomegaly, cardiovascular and respiratory involvement, leukopenia, anemia, hypocomplementemia, etc.

Histopathology

- *Palisading xanthogranuloma* in mid dermis extending into panniculus.
- Histiocytes foam cells, lymphoid follicles, plasma cells, and giant cells with zones of *necrobiosis.*
- *Cholesterol clefts* in areas of "necrobiosis".
- Touton giant cells and foreign body giant cells.

Treatment

Management options include low-dose chlorambucil, melphalan, or cyclophosphamide (with/without steroids), radiotherapy, plasmapheresis, CO_2 laser, etc.

Multicentric Reticulohistiocytosis[3,7,11]

- Usually begins at around 50 years.
- Female predominance.
- *Primary manifestations*: Skin lesions and arthritis.
- In 40% patients—joint disease occurs first; in 30%—skin lesions first appear; rest—both simultaneous.
- *Skin lesions*:
    - Multiple firm skin colored, yellowish, pink or red-brown papules and nodules, 2–10 mm in size.
    - *Distribution*: Mostly *acral and symmetrical.*
    - *Favored sites*: The head, hands, fingers, ears, and articular regions of the limbs.
    - Lesions often arranged around nail folds, giving a "*coral bead*" appearance; sometimes associated with nail dystrophy.
    - Facial lesions can lead to "leonine facies".
- Mucosa involved in one-third; oral (lips, tongue—common), nasopharynx, larynx, and sclera.
- One-third patients can have hypercholesterolemia and xanthelasma.
- *Bone involvement*:
    - Inflammatory, symmetrical, destructive polyarthritis, predominantly involving small joints (distal interphalangeal most common) of hands and wrist, with absorption and telescopic shortening of phalanges (opera-glass fingers).
- *Associated diseases*: Malignancies (e.g., breast, gastrointestinal and genitourinary tract, leukemia, lymphoma, etc.), autoimmune diseases (e.g., thyroiditis, Sjögren syndrome, etc.), tuberculosis, and others.

Histopathology

- Mononuclear and multinuclear macrophages in the dermis with abundant smooth/slightly granular, eosinophilic "ground-glass" cytoplasm.
- Epidermis may be thinned, with a grenz zone.
- Mixed dermal infiltration.

Management

- Screening for associated diseases.
- Systemic steroid, methotrexate, tumor necrosis factor (TNF)-alpha inhibitor, tocilizumab, and others.

Rosai-Dorfman Disease[4,7,12]

- *Synonym*: Sinus histiocytosis with massive lymphadenopathy (SHML)
- Children and young adults commonly affected.
- Characterized by *massive, painless, and bilateral cervical lymphadenopathy*; may be associated with fever, anemia, neutrophilia, elevated ESR/CRP, and polyclonal hypergammaglobulinemia. Other nodal involvement can occur.
- Over 40% of patients with Rosai-Dorfman disease (RDD) have at least one extranodal site involved: skin, soft tissues, respiratory tract, bone, genitourinary system, CNS, etc.
- *Cutaneous involvement*:
    - Seen in approximately 10% patients with systemic form or present rarely as skin only disease.
    - In cutaneous RDD, there is female predominance; mostly seen in adults.
    - Lesions are often multiple; nonspecific red-brown or xanthomatous macules, papules, nodules, or plaques.
    - May affect any site; *eyelids and malar region common.*
- Clinical course—unpredictable, with episodes of exacerbation and remission.

Histopathology

- Florid, mixed inflammatory infiltrate, very large cells with abundant water-clear cytoplasm.
- Emperipolesis—presence of intact lymphocytes (and plasma cells) in the histiocytes.

Treatment

- Necessary in vital organ involvement or significant nodal enlargement

- Debulking surgery
- Radiotherapy and medications such as systemic steroid, thalidomide, 2-chlorodeoxyadenosine, imatinib, clofarabine, and rituximab have been tried.

Malignant Histiocytosis[2,4]

Classification of Malignant Histiocytosis

- *Primary malignant histiocytosis (MH)*:
  - Skin
  - Lymph nodes
  - Digestive system
  - Central nervous system
  - Other or disseminated
- *Secondary MH to*:
  - Follicular lymphoma
  - Lymphocytic leukemia/lymphoma
  - Hairy cell leukemia
  - Acute lymphoblastic leukemia
  - Histiocytosis (LCH, RDD, and others)
  - Another hematologic neoplasia

Subtypes

- Langerhans cell sarcoma
- Histiocytic sarcoma
- Interdigitating dendritic cell sarcoma
- Indeterminate cell sarcoma

Clinical Features

- Mostly seen in adults.
- *Skin lesions*: Variable and nonspecific, solitary or multiple papules, nodules or erythematous plaques, sometimes with ulceration.
- *Other systems*: Lymph nodes, gastrointestinal, respiratory, genitourinary, bone marrow, etc.; variable in different subtypes.

Histopathology

In *rapidly progressive lesion* with histiocytic cells, *prominent mitotic activity* with atypical mitoses and *cellular atypia* are important diagnostic features.

Hemophagocytic Lymphohistiocytosis[2,4]

Types

- Primary [Mendelian inherited conditions leading to hemophagocytic lymphohistiocytosis (HLH)]
- *Secondary*: Associated with infection, malignancy, chemotherapy, defined rheumatologic conditions [macrophage activation syndrome (MAS)-HLH], transplant, iatrogenic immune-suppression or activation, etc.

Clinical Features

- *Age*: Familial—before 1 year, secondary—adults.
- Prolonged high fever, hepatosplenomegaly, lymphadenopathy, neurological symptoms (e.g., seizure), etc.
- *Skin lesions*: Transient, nonspecific, maculopapular rash, often in time of high fever.

Investigations

- *Histopathology*: Hemophagocytosis (histiocytes with active phagocytosis of erythrocytes, leukocytes, or platelets) in spleen, bone marrow, and lymph node.
- *Skin biopsy*: Often nonspecific.
- *Others*: Cytopenia, elevated ferritin level, hypertriglyceridemia, hypofibrinogenemia, hyponatremia, elevated soluble CD25, decreased natural killer cell activity, etc.

Treatment

Stem cell transplant, systemic steroid, chemotherapy, biologicals, etc.

XANTHOMA (TABLE 3; FIGS. 3 AND 4)[3,7,13]

Xanthomas are macules, papules, nodules, or plaques with characteristic yellow to orange hue and they usually develop as a result of lipid deposition in the dermis, within macrophages (primarily) and extracellular tissue.

TABLE 3: Clinical features and diseases associated with different types of xanthomas.

Type	*Cutaneous lesions*	*Distribution of lesions*	*Associated disorders*
Tuberous xanthoma	Flat/elevated and rounded, grouped, yellowish/orange nodules; may coalesce	Over the joints, especially elbows and knees; may occur over face, knuckles, toe joints, axillary and inguinal folds, and buttocks	Familial dysbetalipoproteinemia (Fredrickson type III) and familial hypercholesterolemia (Frederickson type II) *Secondary:* Primary biliary cirrhosis, monoclonal gammopathy, multiple myeloma, leukemia, etc.
Tendinous xanthoma	Skin colored papules or nodules, 5–25 mm in diameter	Extensor tendons on backs of hands, dorsa of feet and Achilles tendons.	Familial hypercholesterolemia (Frederickson type II), familial dysbetalipoproteinemia (Frederickson type III), cerebrotendinous xanthomatosis, phytosterolemia *Secondary:* Cholestasis, hypothyroidism, etc.

Contd...

Contd...

Type		*Cutaneous lesions*	*Distribution of lesions*	*Associated disorders*
Eruptive xanthoma		Small, yellowish orange to reddish brown papules; appear in crops, sometimes with inflammatory halo Pruritus or tenderness may be present	All over body; commonly—buttocks, extensor surfaces of arms and thighs, knees, inguinal and axillary folds, and oral mucosa	Hypertriglyceridemia associated with familial lipoprotein lipase deficiency, Apo C-II deficiency (Frederickson type I), Apo A-I and Apo A-I/C-III deficiency, familial hypertriglyceridemia (Frederickson type IV), Frederickson type V hyperlipidemia *Secondary:* Obesity, diabetes mellitus, alcohol, medications like retinoids, etc.
Plane xanthoma	Xanthelasma palpebrarum	Soft, yellowish orange oblong plaques	Eyelids, near inner canthus.	• Familial hypercholesterolemia (Frederickson type II) • Familial dysbetalipoproteinemia (Frederickson type III)
	Palmar xanthoma	• Irregular yellowish plaques • Striated xanthoma as yellowish streaks	• The palms and flexural surfaces of fingers • Striated xanthoma-palmar and plantar creases	Familial dysbetalipoproteinemia, homozygous Apo A-I deficiency
	Other plane xanthomas	Flat macules/slightly elevated plaques with yellowish-orange color	Neck, trunk, shoulders, axillae, inner surface of thighs, antecubital and popliteal spaces	Familial hypercholesterolemia *Secondary:* Cholestasis due to primary biliary cirrhosis, biliary atresia, monoclonal gammopathy in normolipidemic
Verruciform xanthoma		Persistent, solitary, reddish, or light orange verrucous lesion	Oral mucosa, anogenital, periorificial region, lower extremities	Recessive dystrophic epidermolysis bullosa, lymphedema, graft versus host disease, CHILD syndrome, epidermal nevi, etc.
Xanthoma disseminatum		Asymptomatic yellow, red, brown papules	All over body; especially on eyelids and flexors, mucous membrane involved	• Diabetes insipidus, monoclonal gammopathy • Hyperlipidemia uncommon
Papular xanthoma		Solitary/multiple small, yellowish papules/nodules of 1–10 mm diameter	Generalized; do not favor flexors, mucosal involvement in adults	Usually not associated with hyperlipidemia or systemic disease

(CHILD: congenital hemidysplasia with ichthyosiform nevus and limb defects)

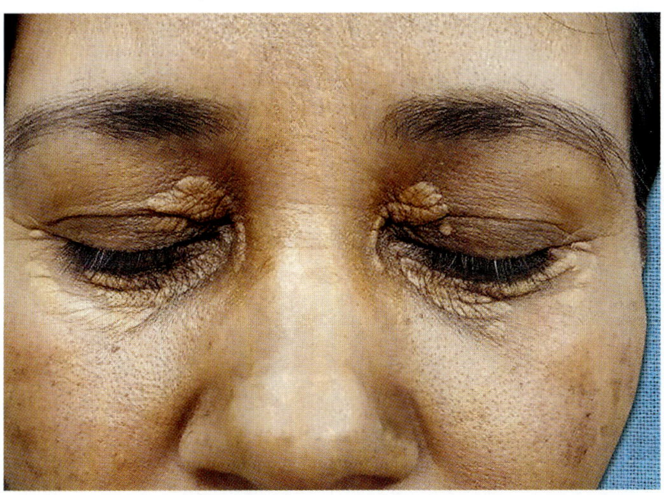

Fig. 3: Xanthelasma palpebrarum over the upper and lower eyelid in a middle-aged woman.

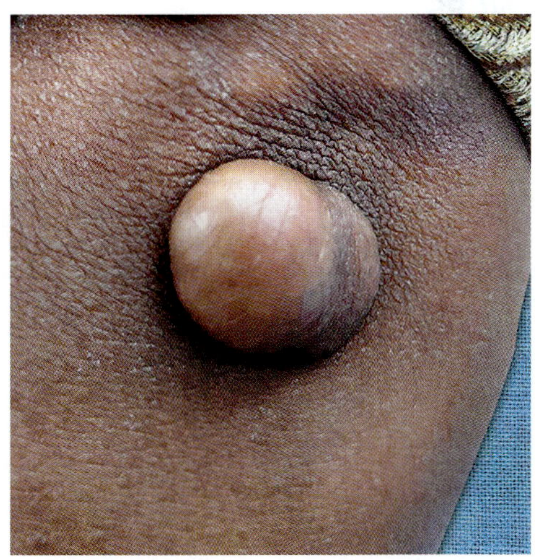

Fig. 4: Tuberous xanthoma over elbow of a woman.

Xanthomas commonly develop in association with primary or secondary disorders of lipid metabolism, except some normolipidemic variants.

Most of the cutaneous xanthomas usually appear in adulthood, with the exception of those related to homozygous familial hypercholesterolemia or secondary to diseases which occur in childhood.

The morphology and distribution of lesions sometimes aid in diagnosis of different types of lipid disorders or paraproteinemia.

KEY POINTS

- Histiocytoses encompass a group of proliferative disorders of the mononuclear phagocytic system which consists of dendritic cells, monocytes, and macrophages; presentations range from benign skin lesions to life-threatening systemic disorders.
- In the most recent classification, the histiocytic disorders are grouped into five categories: (1) Langerhans-related (L); (2) cutaneous and mucocutaneous (C); (3) Rosai-Dorfman disease (R); (4) malignant (M); and (5) hemophagocytic lymphohistiocytosis (H).
- Langerhans cell histiocytosis is characterized by proliferation and accumulation of CD1a+ Langerhans cells; can be subdivided into SS and MS disease. Most characteristic skin lesions are papulosquamous lesions resembling seborrheic dermatitis; often associated with purpura.
- Juvenile xanthogranuloma is the most common non-LCH.
- Xanthoma disseminatum and multicentric reticulohistiocytosis are cutaneous histiocytoses which usually have major systemic involvements. Necrobiotic xanthogranuloma can also be associated with paraproteinemia and other systemic disorders.
- Diagnosis of histiocytosis is based mostly on careful clinical examination, histopathology, and immunohistochemistry.
- Xanthomas commonly develop in association with disorders of lipid metabolism, except some normolipidemic variants such as verruciform xanthoma, papular xanthoma, and xanthoma disseminatum.

REFERENCES

1. Filipovich A, McClain K, Grom A. Histiocytic Disorders: Recent Insights into Pathophysiology and Practical Guidelines. Biol Blood Marrow Transplant. 2010;16:S82-9.
2. Emile JF, Abla O, Fraitag S, Horne A, Haroche J, Donadieu J, et al. Revised classification of histiocytoses and neoplasms of the macrophage-dendritic cell lineages. Blood. 2016;127:2672-81.
3. James WD, Elston DM, Treat JR, Rosenbach MA, Neuhaus IM. Andrews' Diseases of the Skin: Clinical Dermatology, 13th edition. Philadelphia, PA: Elsevier; 2020.
4. Tran TH, Pope E, Weitzman S. Cutaneous histiocytoses. In: Griffiths CEM, Barker J, Bleiker T, Chalmers R, Creamer D (Eds). Rook's Textbook of Dermatology, 9th edition. Oxford: Wiley-Blackwell; 2016. pp. 136.1-29.
5. Borysiewicz C, Chu AC. Langerhans cell histiocytosis. In: Lebwohl MG, Heymann WR, Berth-Jones J, Coulson IH (Eds). Treatment of Skin Diseases, 5th edition. Philadelphia, USA: Elsevier; 2018. pp. 1385-400.
6. Oliviera TE, Tarlè RG, Mesquita LAF. Dermoscopy in the diagnosis of juvenile xanthogranuloma. An Bras Dermatol. 2018;93:138-49.
7. Bolognia JL, Schaffer JV, Cerroni L. Dermatology, 4th edition. China: Elsevier; 2018.
8. Zelger B, Cerio R, Soyer HP, Misch K, Orchard G, Wilson-Jones E. Reticulohistiocytoma and multicentric reticulohistiocytosis. Histopathologic and immunophenotypic distinct entities. Am J Dermatopathol. 1994;16:577-84.
9. Jadhav S, Choudhary N, Ahar R, Ghosh A, Singha J, Saha A. Papular xanthoma in a child: Report of a rare entity. Indian J Paediatr Dermatol. 2015;16:78-80.
10. Wood AJ, Wagner MV, Abbott JJ, Gibson LE. Necrobiotic xanthogranuloma: a review of 17 cases with emphasis on clinical and pathologic correlation. Arch Dermatol. 2009;145:279-84.
11. Sinha A, Dhungana S, De D, Prakash M, Sharma SK, Das A. Multicentric reticulohistiocytosis: A clinicoradiological review. Indian J Rheumatol. 2018;13:195-201.
12. Foucault E, Rossi J, Dorfman R. Sinus histiocytosis with massive lymphadenopathy (Rosai-Dorfman disease): review of the entity. Semin Diagn Pathol. 1990;7:19-73.
13. Schaefer EJ, Santos RD. Xanthomatoses and lipoprotein disorders. In: Goldsmith LA, Katz SI, Gilchrest BA, Paller AS, Leffell Dj, Wolff K (Eds). Fitzpatrick's Dermatology in General Medicine, 8th edition. New York: McGraw-Hill; 2012. pp. 1600-12.

EXAMINATION QUESTIONS

1. Describe clinical features, investigations and management of childhood Langerhans cell histiocytosis.

Write short notes on the following:

2. Juvenile xanthogranuloma.
3. Necrobiotic xanthogranuloma.
4. Multicentric reticulohistiocytosis.
5. LCH.
6. Describe clinical features and association of different types of Xanthomas.

11 SECTION

Pigmentary and Miscellaneous Skin Disorders

97 CHAPTER Disorders of Hyperpigmentation

Barnali Chowdhury, Koushik Lahiri

INTRODUCTION

Hyperpigmentation of the skin is a common dermatological disorder and commonly encountered in the skin of color, which is generally categorized as Fitzpatrick skin types IV-VI. This type of skin is characterized by higher melanin content compared to white skin and higher eumelanin to pheomelanin ratio.[1] Hyperpigmentation occurs due to accumulation of the excessive melanin in the skin. It has significant psychological impact. There are various causes of hyperpigmentation of which melasma and hyperpigmentation due to inflammation and drugs are the common causative factors. In this chapter we will discuss in detail about the common etiologies and other differentials will be discussed in brief.

Differential diagnosis of hyperpigmentation:[2]

- Melasma
- Postinflammatory hyperpigmentation (PIH)
- Drug-induced hyperpigmentation
- Macular amyloidosis
- Acanthosis nigricans
- Exogenous ochronosis
- Riehl melanosis
- Dermatosis papulosa nigra (DPN)
- Nevus of Ota
- Hori nevi
- Ephelides
- Lentigines
- Lichen planus pigmentosus (LPP) **(Fig. 1)**
- Erythema dyschromicum perstans (EDP)
- Actinic lichen planus (ALP)
- Pigmentary demarcation lines (PDL)
- Linear and whorled nevoid hypermelanosis (LWNH)
- Incontinentia pigmenti

MELASMA

Melasma is one of the most common disorders of acquired hyperpigmentation in patients with skin of color. It is most commonly found over the face and in predominantly affect Fitzpatrick skin types III and IV **(Table 1)**. Melasma mostly seen in female. The reported prevalence of melasma and other facial hypermelanosis ranges from 8.8% among Latino females in the Southern United States to as high as 40% in Southeast Asian populations. Some individual with melasma reports deterioration in summer. Person with seborrheic melanosis often enjoys clearance of lesion in summer.[3]

Factors associated with development of melasma includes pregnancy, use of oral contraceptive pills, and prolonged sun exposure. The high incidence of melasma among family members suggests a genetic component. Instead of increase in the melanocytes it has been proposed that pathogenesis include mainly presence of more biologically active melanocytes producing excessive melanin. It appears as dark brown patches with indistinct border present over the malar, mandibular, and centrofacial area. The centrofacial pattern of melasma is the most common. It is classified as epidermal, dermal, and mixed types depending on the presence of the melanin.[4]

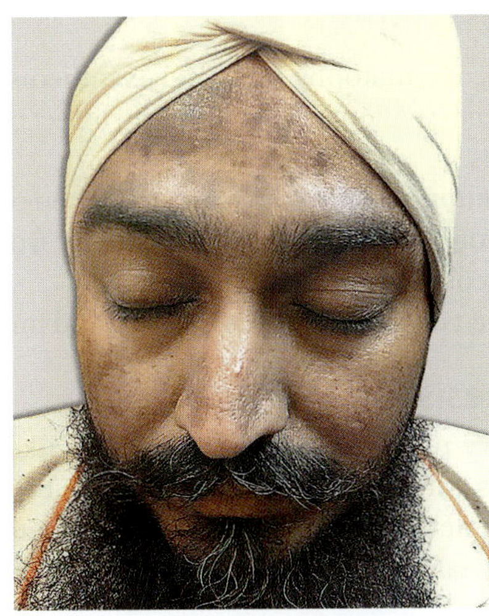

Fig. 1: Lichen planopigmentosus.
Courtesy: Dr Aarti Sarda.

TABLE 1: Types and features of melasma.[5]

Types of melasma	*Clinical features*
Epidermal	• Well-defined border • Dark brown color • Appears more obvious under black light • Responds well to treatment
Dermal	• Ill-defined border • Light brown color • Unchanged under black light • Responds poorly to treatment
Mixed	• Combination of light and brown patches • Partial improvement with treatment

Clinical features of different types are mentioned in the following table. Other pigmentary disorders such as PIH, solar lentigines, acanthosis nigricans, exogenous ochronosis, LPP, and EDP should be kept in the mind while diagnosing melasma. While a Wood lamp examination was previously thought to accurately predict epidermal versus dermal pigment deposition, recent studies have shown that dermal melanin deposition is common and may be underrecognized. First line of treatment primarily includes sun protection with broad-spectrum sunscreen and other topical agents to reduce pigment production. Chemical peels can be used as second line therapy in patients not responding to first line treatment. Laser and light therapy can be used in refractory cases. For women who note the onset of melasma after beginning a course of an oral contraceptive, the medication should be stopped if possible.

POSTINFLAMMATORY HYPERPIGMENTATION

It is an acquired hypermelanosis commonly seen in Fitzpatrick skin types IV to VI, but it can affect all skin types. Pigmentary changes are seen in greater frequency in African Americans, Hispanics/Latinos, Asians, and Native Americans.[6]

Etiology

- *Infections*: Dermatophytosis, viral exanthems
- *Inflammatory*: Allergic reactions from insect bites, contact dermatitis
- *Papulosquamous diseases*: Psoriasis, lichen planus
- Medication induced or hypersensitivity from irritants, burns or cosmetic procedure
- After acne vulgaris, atopic dermatitis, and impetigo.

Pathogenesis

Inflammatory process released mediators like cytokines, chemokines and prostanoids, which in turn increase melanocytic activity leading to increase production and transfer of melanin to surrounding keratinocytes.

Clinical Features

Usually appear as macule or patches at the site of previous inflammatory process. It may appear as tam brown or dark brown if it is localized to epidermis otherwise blue gray appearance if it involves dermis.

Management[7]

Treatment of the underlying inflammatory condition; broad spectrum sunscreen with SPF 50+ can be used as a depigmenting agent in the sun-exposed areas. It is important to note that the users of sunscreen are prone to develop vitamin D deficiency particularly among the dark-skinned individuals. Adequate intake of vitamin D (at least 1,000 mg daily) either through diet or supplement should be encouraged.

Topical Depigmenting Agents[8]

Hydroquinone (HQ) remain as the mainstay of medical therapy in the treatment of PIH. It acts by blocking the conversion of dihydroxyphenylalanine (DOPA) to melanin due to inhibition of the enzyme tyrosinase. HQ can be used as monotherapy or in combination with other topical agents. These agents should be continued for at least 8–12 weeks although studies have shown significant reduction in melatonin activity after 4 weeks of therapy. Other depigmenting agents include azelaic acid, kojic acid, cysteamine cream, vitamin C cream, retinoids, and corticosteroids. These agents help in lightening the lesion if it is caused by epidermal hyper melanosis. Success rate varies but it can be used in combination with other agents. Retinoids are structural analogue of vitamin A and act by modulating cell proliferation and differentiation and apoptosis induction. Tropical tretinoin can be used in the concentration between 0.01 and 0.1% and it can be used as cream or gel formulations. In a 40-week randomized double controlled trial in the skin of color patients it was found to be effective however almost half of them developed tretinoin dermatitis.

Surgical Therapy

It includes chemical peels, laser treatment, and intense pulse light therapies (IPL). Superficial chemical peels can be done with glycolic acid, salicylic acid and trichloroacetic acid (TCA) with good result. Most chemical peels are well tolerated with side effects include erythema, burning sensation, PIH, superficial desquamation, and vesiculation. Photoprotection should be continued after the procedure to prevent or avoid worsening PIH.

DRUG-INDUCED FACIAL PIGMENTATION

Patchy dyspigmentation is commonly enhanced by sun exposure and thus tends to occur in sun-distributed areas on the face, neck, V of the chest, upper back, and distal upper extremities. Specific drugs such as amiodarone, daunorubicin, gold, methotrexate, psoralens, and 5-fluorouracil induce hyperpigmented changes in this topographic distribution. Generalized dyspigmentation, in contrast, usually appears uniform and along the entire length of the body. Changes such as these are commonly seen with minocycline use and can resemble those incited by other metabolic or endocrinologic diseases such as Addison disease or hypothyroidism, anti-psychotics (chlorpromazine and related phenothiazines). Bluish-gray pigmentation, especially in sun-exposed areas. Pigmentation is cumulative and some areas may develop a purplish tint.[9]

- *Phenytoin/anticonvulsants:*
    - 10% of patients develop pigmentation of the face and neck resembling chloasma (clearly defined, roughly symmetrical dark brown patches)
    - Fades after a few months when drug has been stopped

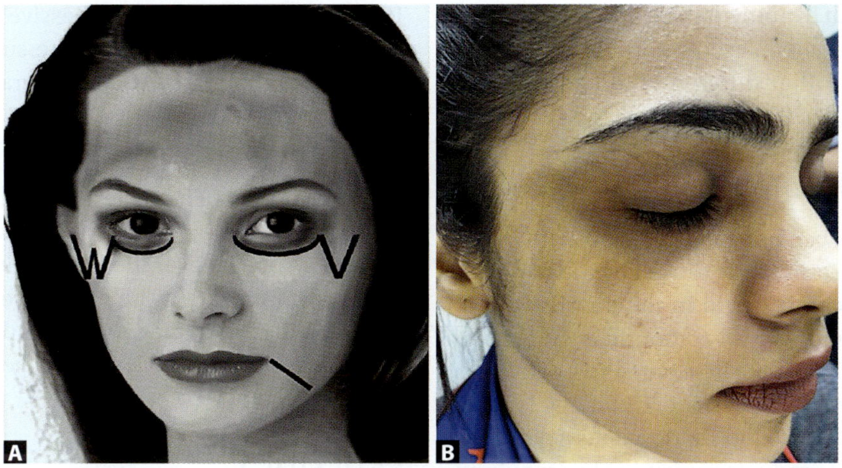

Figs. 2A and B: Pigmentary demarcation lines over the face. Some of these margins or some parts often appeared as sharp and clearly distinct. For example, the inferomedial margins of the zygomatic patches were found to be often very sharp and distinct. Interestingly, this was observed to conform to what has been previously mentioned as pigmentary demarcation line type F (PDL-F). It was also described that PDL-F extended as periorbital pigmentation. We have also observed that the lateral margins of the perioral pigmentation roughly follow the nasolabial fold in the upper part and the mentolabial fold in the lower part. Possibly, parts of this margin represent what has been previously mentioned as PDL-H pattern.

- *Antimalarials:* About 25% of patients receiving chloroquine or hydroxychloroquine for several years develop bluish-gray pigmentation on face, neck and sometimes lower legs and forearms. Continuous long-term use may lead to blue-black patches, especially in sun-exposed areas.
- *NSAIDs:*
  - Often associated with fixed drug eruptions (drugs that cause a single or few sharply demarcated erythematous lesions) which resolve promptly but leave a local brown pigmentation
  - May occur on the face, lips
- *Others:*
  - Busulfan, cyclophosphamide, bleomycin and adriamycin have all produced hyperpigmentation to some degree
  - Amiodarone can cause blue-gray pigmentation in sun-exposed areas.

Pigmentary demarcation lines on face are shown in **Figures 2A and B**.[10]

MACULAR AMYLOIDOSIS

Amyloidosis can be primary and secondary depending on the origin of the amyloid protein. It is an insoluble protein deposited in the organs and cause dysfunction of the organs. Amyloid deposition in the skin called cutaneous amyloidosis. In this condition amyloid or amyloid-like protein deposited in the dermis.[11]

The different types of amyloidosis are given in **Table 2**.

Features of macular amyloidosis:

- Flat of dusky brown color spots seen over the skin
- Occasionally spots are coalesced to form patches

TABLE 2: Types of amyloidosis.

Types	
Primary amyloidosis	• Occasionally associated with multiple myeloma • AL amyloid • Skin involvement occurs in 30–40% patients • Localized primary cutaneous amyloidosis can be of the following four types: 1. Lichen amyloidosis 2. Macular amyloidosis 3. Nodular amyloidosis 4. Amyloidosis cutis dyschromica
Secondary amyloidosis	• Associated with chronic inflammatory conditions such as rheumatoid arthritis known as AA amyloidosis • Sin involvement is rare

- Can be moderately or severely itchy
- Usually located over the upper parts of the body like shoulder arm or upper chest
- Women are more commonly involved than man
- Facial acanthosis nigricans (FAN)

ACANTHOSIS NIGRICANS

Acanthosis nigricans (AN) is clinically manifested as dark, velvety, and thickened skin, symmetrically distributed over the neck, axillae, and other flexural regions of the body. Rarely it can be found over the face. It is commonly associated with metabolic syndrome. Strong association has been found in patients with obesity, diabetes mellitus, and insulin resistance. Rarely it can be seen as a congenital disorder. Other clinical conditions associated with AN include Addison's disease, hormonal therapy like growth hormone, oral contraceptive use, and in patients with hypothyroidism. It can also be seen as a manifestation of paraneoplastic syndrome.[12]

Salient features of other differential diagnosis of the hyperpigmentary disorder.

EXOGENOUS OCHRONOSIS

It typically presents as banana-shaped lesion with yellow-brown deposits in the dermis. It is caused by the deposition of polymerized homogentisic acid in the dermis which is similarly found in patients with alkaptonuria or endogenous ochronosis.[2] Unlike alkaptonuria, exogenous ochronosis does not exhibit systemic manifestation. Etiology is mostly attributed to the use of skin products and patients typically give history of application of products containing hydroquinone, phenol, mercury, and picric acid. Differential diagnosis of this disorder includes PIH, pigmented contact dermatitis, and melasma. It can be managed by dermabrasion, chemical peel using glycolic acid, and by laser therapy but the result is not always satisfactory.

RIEHL MELANOSIS

It is also known as pigmented contact dermatitis of face. Typically present as a brownish gray color diffuse hyperpigmentation over the sites of application of cosmetics. Erythema and pruritus preceded by the lesion. A photopatch testing or a closed patch testing to standard series, cosmetic series fragrance series usually help us in the diagnosis. Treatment includes complete avoidance of the suspected allergens or chemicals and by application of sun protection cream and skin lightening agents. Chemical peel can be used in patients with lesions not responding to the above therapy.[2]

DERMATOSIS PAPULOSA NIGRA

It is primarily diagnosed in the patients with African descent. Although it can be found in other races. These are tiny (1–5 mm), pigmented papules seen over the face, predominantly over forehead, and malar prominence.[13] Most often these lesions do not cause any symptoms but rarely they can be pruritic. DPN should be differentiated from seborrheic keratoses, melanocytic nevi, lentigines, and verrucae. These lesions are treated with curettage, cryotherapy, electrodessication, and laser destruction.[14]

NEVUS OF OTA

It usually seen in the skin of colors especially in the Asians and black people. The lesions appear in the newborn and most often presenting at birth. These are distinct tiny macules of varying size with appearance of blue-gray confluence surrounding the eyes. Size varies from few centimeters to unilateral extensive facial involvement. Distribution along the area innervated by trigeminal nerve has been observed. Pathophysiology includes excessive melanocyte deposition in the tissues. These lesions are successfully treated with Q-switched ruby, Nd:YAG laser therapy or cryotherapy.[15]

HORI NEVI

It is an acquired bilateral lesion predominantly found in the Asian populations primarily Chinese or Japanese women. It usually appears over the zygomatic area with blue-gray or gray-brown macules. The eye and oral mucosa are usually spared. Differential diagnosis includes melasma, lentigines, or ephelides. Treatment is similar like naevus of Ota with laser and cryotherapy.

EPHELIDES

These are commonly known as freckles. Appears as small light brown well demarcated lesions over the exposed area so the skin because of the formation of the more than usual pigment formation by the melanocytes. It typically appears in the summer and fade in the winter months. Treatments include sun protection, cryotherapy, and laser therapy.[16]

LENTIGINES

Appearance of the lesions are almost similar like ephelides, but it does not fade in the winter months. More commonly seen in white skin but can happen in Asians. Solar lentigines are tan to dark brown colored well-circumscribed round macules or patches of 2–3 cm in diameters; usually caused by sun exposure, after tanning, phototherapy or radiation. Inherited pattern lentigines are associated with familial syndrome like mutation I the Ras-MAP kinase, mTOR signaling, and PTEN pathways. Treatment includes sun protection, skin lightening agents, laser, and cryotherapy.[16]

LICHEN PLANUS PIGMENTOSUS

It is a variants of lichen planus most commonly seen in middle aged adults with Fitzpatrick skin type III-V. It typically present as irregularly shaped or oval shaped gray-brown macule or patches over the sun exposed areas. Rarely lips are involved with patchy dark pigmentation. UV radiation appears to have pathogenic role in the development of LPP considering its distribution in the sun exposed areas. The differential diagnosis includes melasma, lichenoid drug eruption, EDP, and PIH. Treatment includes topical steroids, immunomodulators, and skin lightening agents. Successful treatment with topical tacrolimus for 12–16 weeks has been reported.

ERYTHEMA DYSCHROMICUM PERSTANS

It is characterized by asymptomatic, well demarcated irregular patches on the face, neck, and trunk with gray or blue in color.[17]

EDP is more commonly seen in Latin Americans without any specific gender predilection. It has been hypothesized that a cell-mediated reaction to the ingested medications or allergens, exposure to pesticides, and toxins, leading to development of an inflammatory phase with rim of erythema over the sun exposed areas. Probable association with the HLA-DR4 allele and development of EDP in Mexican patients has been postulated. Differential diagnosis includes lichenoid drug eruption, leprosy, and pinta and other forms of PIH. Treatment includes topical corticosteroids, immunomodulators like tacrolimus, antibiotics, antimalarial, isoniazid, chemical peels and laser therapy.[13]

ACTINIC LICHEN PLANUS

It is rare variant of lichen planus mainly reported from Middle Eastern countries. These lesions are erythematous brownish scaly lesion with annular configuration, typically found in young adults and children. Typically found over the sun exposed areas like forehead, face, upper extremities, and neck. Lesions should be differentiated from lichenoid drug eruptions and polymorphous drug eruption. Treatment includes topical or intralesional corticosteroids and acitretin along with sun protective measures. Antimalarials such as hydroxychloroquine and immunomodulators such as cyclosporine have been found to be effective in the treatment.[18]

PIGMENTARY DEMARCATION LINES

These are lines of demarcation between dorsal and ventral surface most commonly seen in darkly pigmented skin. It is physiologic pattern of human pigments, most commonly seen in anterolateral and posteromedial thigh. It does not require specific treatment, usually resolve on its own.

LINEAR AND WHORLED NEVOID HYPERMELANOSIS

Linear and whorled nevoid hypermelanosis is a genetically heterogenous mosaic skin condition characterized by a clone of skin cells with increased pigment production. Clinical features of LWNH include swirls and streaks of brown pigmentation seen in early first year of life. Occasionally pigmentary mosaicism is seen. Involvement of other systems include neurologic, musculoskeletal or cardiac has been reported. There is no proven effective therapy for this condition. Use of camouflage cosmetic may be helpful in this condition.

INCONTINENTIA PIGMENTI

It is a rare genetic disorder with X-linked dominant inheritance. It is a multisystem disorder involves skin, eye, teeth, and central nervous system. Skin lesion depends on the stage of the disease. It is seen due to mutation in the *IKBKG* or *NEMO* gene.

- *Stage 1*: Vesicular
- *Stage 2*: Verrucous
- *Stage 3*: Hyperpigmented
- *Stage 4*: Atrophic or hypopigmented.

KEY POINTS

- Hyperpigmentation is a commonly encounter disorder seen in the outpatient clinic. Treatment is sometime challenging.
- Several methods can be used depending on the etiology of the disorder and also depending on the availability of expertise.
- A proper understanding of this disorder is necessary to decide exact treatment option.

REFERENCES

1. Sharma VK, Sahni K, Wadhwani AR. Photodermatoses in pigmented skin. Photochem Photobiol Sci. 2013;12(1):65-77.
2. Vashi NA, Kundu RV. Facial hyperpigmentation: causes and treatment. Br J Dermatol. 2013;169(Suppl 3):41-56.
3. Khanna N, Rasool S. Facial melanoses: Indian perspective. Indian J Dermatol Venereol Leprol. 2011;77(5):552-63.
4. Sheth VM, Pandya AG. Melasma: a comprehensive update: part I. J Am Acad Dermatol. 2011;65(4):689-97.
5. Sheth VM, Pandya AG. Melasma: a comprehensive update: part II. J Am Acad Dermatol. 2011;65(4):699-714.
6. Shenoy A, Madan R. Post-inflammatory hyperpigmentation: a review of treatment strategies. J Drugs Dermatol. 2020;19(8):763-8.
7. Lee YJ, Shin HJ, Noh TK, Choi KH, Chang SE. Treatment of melasma and post-inflammatory hyperpigmentation by a picosecond 755-nm Alexandrite laser in Asian patients. Ann Dermatol. 2017;29(6):779-81.
8. Bae YC, Rettig S, Weiss E, Bernstein L, Geronemus R. Treatment of post-inflammatory hyperpigmentation in patients with darker skin types using a low energy 1,927 nm non-ablative fractional laser: a retrospective photographic review analysis. Lasers Surg Med. 2020;52(1):7-12.
9. Gimenez Garcia RM, Carrasco Molina S. Drug-induced hyperpigmentation: review and case series. J Am Board Fam Med. 2019;32(4):628-38.
10. Malakar S, Dhar S. Pigmentary demarcation lines over the face. Dermatology. 2000;200(1):85-6.
11. Kanchanapoomi M, Rosenstein R, Shvartsbeyn M, Meehan SA, Dolly N, Femia A. Primary diffuse macular amyloidosis. Dermatol Online J. 2015;21(12).
12. Das A, Datta D, Kassir M, Wollina U, Galadari H, Lotti T, et al. Acanthosis nigricans: a review. J Cosmet Dermatol. 2020; 19(8):1857-65.
13. Mahajan VK, Chauhan PS, Mehta KS, Sharma AL. Erythema dyschromicum perstans: response to topical tacrolimus. Indian J Dermatol. 2015;60(5):525.
14. Xiao A, Muse ME, Ettefagh L. Dermatosis papulosa nigra. Treasure Island (FL): StatPearls; 2020.
15. Vishnevskia-Dai V, Moroz I, Davidy T, Zloto K, Birger Y, Fabian ID, et al. Naevus of Ota: clinical characteristics and proposal

for a new ocular classification and grading system. Br J Ophthalmol. 2021;105(1):42-7.

16. Praetorius C, Sturm RA, Steingrimsson E. Sun-induced freckling: ephelides and solar lentigines. Pigment Cell Melanoma Res. 2014;27(3):339-50.
17. Leung AKC, Lam JM. Erythema dyschromicum perstans in an 8-year-old Indian child. Case Rep Dermatol Med. 2018;2018: 2143089.
18. Bouassida S, Boudaya S, Turki H, Gueriani H, Zahaf A. Actinic lichen planus: 32 cases. Ann Dermatol Venereol. 1998;125 (6-7):408-13.

EXAMINATION QUESTIONS

Write short note on following:

1. Melasma.
2. Reticulate pigmentary disorders.
3. Dyskeratosis congenita.

98 CHAPTER

Albinism and Genetic Disorders of Pigmentation

Belliappa P Raju, Umashankar Nagaraju

INTRODUCTION

Pigmentation has long fascinated the human race, with developmental melanocyte abnormalities reported by ancient Greeks, Romans, and Egyptians.[1] The melanins responsible for mammalian pigmentation include reddish-hued pheomelanin and brown/black-colored eumelanin, and these melanins are produced by melanocytes through a process known as melanogenesis. Melanocytes develop from the neural crest (NC), a multipotent vertebrate cell population. The wide variation in basal human skin color and tanning response results from differences in amount and/or cellular distribution of melanin rather than differing melanocyte numbers. Human pigmentation disorders can be classified by phenotype, including hypo- or hyperpigmentation, congenital or acquired presentation, effects on melanocyte number (hypo- or hyperplasia), or effects on melanocyte function. Here we discuss about the genetic pigmentation disorders.

CLASSIFICATION

Genetic disorders of pigmentation can be classified into hypopigmentation and hyperpigmentation disorders.

Hypopigmentation Disorders

- *Hypopigmentation from altered melanocyte function*:
  - Oculocutaneous albinism (OCA)
  - Hermansky–Pudlak syndrome
  - Chediak–Higashi syndrome
  - Griscelli syndrome
  - Cross-McKusick-Breen syndrome
  - Oculocutaneous albinoidism.
- *Hypopigmentation from melanocyte hypoplasia*:
  - Piebaldism
  - *Neurocutaneous disorders*:
    - Waardenburg syndrome (WS)
    - Tietze syndrome
    - Fisch's syndrome
    - Woolf syndrome
    - Ziprowski-Margolis syndrome
    - Tuberous sclerosis
    - Hypomelanosis of Ito
    - Ataxia-telangiectasia.
  - *Inborn metabolic error-related disorders*:
    - Menkes kinky hair syndrome
    - Phenylketonuria
    - Histidinemia
    - Homocystinuria.
- *Developmental anomaly*:
  - Nevus depigmentosus
  - Nevus anemicus.

Albinism

Albinism is an inherited hypopigmentation disorder where defective melanin production causes severe reduction to complete absence of all skin, hair, and eye pigmentation. When the eyes are also affected, it is called OCA; when only the eyes are involved, it is called ocular albinism. Ocular phenotypes may include nystagmus, reduced visual acuity, and misrouting of optic nerves. While OCA is autosomal recessive in nature, ocular albinism is a rare sex-linked recessive condition.[2] These conditions are associated with either failure of synthesis of tyrosinase or defect in tyrosinase activity. OCA patients are generally called "albinos." Oculocutaneous albinism is the most frequent form of diffuse hypopigmentation worldwide with a prevalence estimated around 1/20,000. The prevalence of the various OCA subtypes varies considerably from one continent to another, but OCA1 is the most frequent form worldwide.

The various OCA forms are classified based upon their associated genetic mutations **(Table 1)**.

Differential diagnosis: Diagnoses to be considered in the case of ocular and cutaneous hypopigmentation include histidinemia, homocystinuria, phenylketonuria, Hermansky–Pudlak, and Chediak–Higashi syndromes, as well as Cross and Tietze syndromes.

Complications and comorbidities: Incidence of skin cancer which appears early and may lead to death is increased in patients with OCA, especially squamous cell carcinoma. Melanoma is far less common.

Disease course and prognosis: Lifespan is normal, and medical problems are generally not increased compared to general population. Development and intelligence are normal. They have a normal fertility.

TABLE 1: Classification and salient features of different types of oculocutaneous albinism (OCA).

Types	*OCA1*	*OCA2*	*OCA3*	*OCA4*	*Hermansky–Pudlak syndrome (HPS)*[3]	*Chediak–Higashi syndrome*[3]
Synonyms	1. *OCA1A:* Tyrosinase-negative type OCA (TNA) 2. *OCA1B*: Yellow mutant type OCA (YMA), Amish albinism	Tyrosinase-positive type OCA (TPA)	Brown OCA and red OCA			
Inheritance	Autosomal recessive	Autosomal recessive	Autosomal recessive	Autosomal recessive	Autosomal recessive	Autosomal recessive
Genetic defect	Mutations in tyrosine gene	Mutations of the *P* gene on chromosome 15	Mutations in the *TYRP1* gene	Defect in the membrane-associated transporter protein (MATP) gene	Causative gene (HPS) is on chromosome 10q23	Causative gene (CHS1) is on chromosome 1q43
Clinical features	• Absent skin and hair pigmentation, no ability to tan (0CA1A) • Partial albinism, hair darkens with age (OCA1B)	Prevalent in black people, blond to red-brown hair with age, ephelides	Rufous albinism in black people	Similar to OCA1, more common in Japan	Decreased pigmentation in eyes, hair and skin, easy bruisability and bleeding tendency, lung interstitial fibrosis, granulomatous colitis	Partial albinism (blond hair, fair skin) accompanied by immunodeficiency (pyogenic infections, hemophagocytic syndrome) and cerebellar syndrome

Management: Management consists of avoidance of sun exposure, adoption of sun protection measures, clinical examinations at least once a year or two for early detection and appropriate treatment of premalignant and malignant lesions, and ophthalmologic consultations. Genetic counseling can help affected individuals assess their chances of transmitting the disorder to their progeny.

Griscelli Syndrome

Synonym: Griscelli-Pruniéras syndrome.

Inheritance: Autosomal recessive.

Types and genetics: Type 1 results from mutations in *MYO5A*, encoding myosin 5a. Type 2 results from mutations in *RAB27A* gene. Type 3 is caused by mutations in *MLPH* encoding melanophilin or by a specific genetic defect in *MYO5A*. Genetic alterations result in defective transport of melanosomes and consequently abnormal accumulation of melanosomes in melanocytes.[4]

Clinical features:

Type 1: Silvery gray hair and fair skin, neurological defects.

Type 2: Silvery gray hair and fair skin, immunological defects (hemophagocytic lymphohistiocytosis).

Type 3: Silvery gray hair and fair skin.

Differential diagnosis: Chédiak–Higashi and Elejalde syndromes. Elejalde syndrome is inherited in an autosomal recessive fashion and is characterized by pigment dilution, silvery gray hair and neurological defects.

Management: Bone marrow transplantation.

Cross-McKusick-Breen Syndrome

Synonyms: Oculocerebral syndrome with hypopigmentation/Cross syndrome/Kramer syndrome.

History: Initially described in an inbred Amish family.

Inheritance: Autosomal recessive.

Clinical features: Generalized hypopigmentation, white/silvery hair, severe mental retardation with spastic tetraplegia, and athetosis. Ocular anomalies (microphthalmos, small opaque cornea, and coarse nystagmus).

Oculocutaneous Albinoidism

Inheritance: Autosomal dominant.

Clinical features: Mildly expressed form of tyrosinase-positive oculocutaneous albinism (ty-pos OCA). Skin looks white but slightly tanned and the hair is white to yellow or reddish. Ocular involvement such as nystagmus and markedly decreased visual acuity is rare with variable degree of photophobia and blue iris. Diffuse punctate pattern of pigmentation is present in the retina and iris. Hair bulb incubation test shows DOPA positivity.

Piebaldism

Inheritance: Autosomal dominant.

Genetics: Heterozygous mutations in *KIT*, encoding c-KIT, a membranal tyrosine kinase receptor responsible for triggering cell proliferation and migration. It results in impaired migration of melanocytes to the skin in the hypopigmented patches. Heterozygous mutation in the gene encoding the zinc finger transcription factor *SNAI2* can also result in piebaldism.[5]

Epidemiology: The incidence is estimated at <1 in 20,000. Both sexes are affected equally.

Clinical features: Typical and common feature is a white forelock, often associated with a V-shaped area of leukoderma on the mid-forehead. Depigmented patches on ventral or lateral trunk and mid-extremities with hands and feet spared. Small spots of hyperpigmentation arise subsequently within the hypopigmented lesions or even on the background of normal skin. Piebaldism with deafness but without other features of WS indicates *Woolf syndrome*.

Differential diagnosis: Vitiligo, Vogt-Koyanagi syndrome, Alezzandrini syndrome, Woolf syndrome, and WS.

Management: Sun protection, epidermal cell or skin grafting.

Neurocutaneous Disorders

Waardenburg syndrome

Waardenburg syndrome is a genetic disorder characterized by piebaldism and sensorineural deafness with an estimated incidence of 1 in 20,000–40,000 **(Table 2)**.

Management: Early detection and management of the hearing defect for mental development.

Tietze syndrome

History: Reported in a six-generation pedigree by Tietze in 1963.

Inheritance: Autosomal dominant, mutation in *MITF* gene such as WS2.[7]

Clinical features: Rare condition characterized by a generalized form of piebaldism (somewhat like albinism) with loss of pigment in hair, total deaf-mutism, hypoplastic eyebrows, but with normal eye color.

Fisch's syndrome: It presents with early graying of hair, partial heterochromia, and deafness. It is distinguished from WS by the absence of lateral displacement of the inner canthi.[8]

Ziprkowski-Margolis syndrome

Synonyms: Woolf syndrome/albinism-deafness syndrome.

Inheritance: X-linked recessive, Xq26.3-q27.1.

Clinical features: Congenital deafness and partial albinism with a piebald pattern.

Hypomelanotic macules of tuberous sclerosis

Inheritance: Autosomal dominant.

Clinical features: Ash-leaf macules—hypopigmented multiple, irregularly scattered, lance-ovate-shaped macules. Neurocutaneous disorder characterized by the classical triad of epilepsy, low intelligence, and adenoma sebaceum.

Hypomelanosis of Ito

Synonym: Incontinentia pigmenti achromians of Ito.

History: Neuroectodermal disorder described by Ito in 1952.

Inheritance: Autosomal dominant, cutaneous mosaicism.

Incidence: Between 1/10,000 and 1/8,500, females more affected.

Etiopathogenesis: Decreased number of melanocytes with fewer melanosomes.

Clinical features: May appear years after birth and tend to fade in later life. Unusual unilateral or bilateral cutaneous macular hypopigmented whorls, streaks, and patches, corresponding to the lines of Blaschko. Extracutaneous findings include neurological (mental retardation and epilepsy), ophthalmological (ptosis, symblepharon, nystagmus, strabismus, cataracts, myopia, and corneal opacity), and skeletal defects (short stature, scoliosis, syndactyly, polydactyly, brachydactyly, and asymmetry of limbs).[9]

TABLE 2: Types and features of Waardenburg syndrome.[6]

Disease name	*Inheritance*	*Genes*	*Clinical features*
WS1	AD	*PAX3*	White forelock, hypopigmented patches, dystopia canthorum, iris heterochromia, deafness, synophris, and mild facial dysmorphism (broad nose root)
WS2	AD	*MITF/SLUG*	Same as WS1, but no facial dysmorphism
WS3	AD	*PAX3*	Same as WS1 with musculoskeletal anomalies (syndactyly, carpal bone fusion)
WS4	AR	*EDN3/EDNRB/ SOX10*	Shah-Waardenburg syndrome (SWS) phenotype accompanied by Hirschsprung disease, neurological symptoms if caused by *SOX10* mutation

(AD: autosomal dominant; AR: autosomal recessive)

TABLE 3: Inborn metabolic error-related disorders.

Disease	*Inheritance*	*Biochemical profile*	*Cutaneous findings*	*Other features*
Phenylketonuria	Autosomal recessive	Hyperphenylalaninemia, phenylpyruvic, and phenylacetic oligophrenia	Hypomelanization of skin, hair, and eyes	Mental retardation
Menkes kinky hair syndrome	X-linked recessive	Defect in copper metabolism	• Found only in females (probably lethal in males) • Sparse depigmented kinky hair, generalized hypopigmentation, and seborrheic dermatitis-like lesions	Growth retardation, developmental delay of CNS including cerebellar degeneration, and usually early death in infancy
Histidinemia	Autosomal recessive	Elevated blood and urinary histidine levels and defective histidase activity in liver and skin	Deficient eye and skin color, fair, or reddish hair	Mental retardation and speech difficulties
Homocystinuria	Autosomal recessive	Elevated plasma and urinary levels of methionine and homocysteine	Generalized lack of melanin in the skin and hair	Mental retardation, seizure, myopia, posterior dislocation of lens, osteoporosis, pes cavus, genu valgum, and Marfanoid features. Thromboembolic events leading to hypertension, anemia, and cardiomegaly

(CNS: central nervous system)

Differential diagnosis: Nevus depigmentosus and incontinentia pigmenti.

Ataxia-telangiectasia
Inheritance: Autosomal recessive.

Clinical features: Depigmented tiny circumscribed macules in about one-third on the extremities and trunk. Neurocutaneous disorder characterized by cerebellar ataxia, choreoathetosis, oculocutaneous telangiectasia, bronchiectasis with recurrent pulmonary infections, and premature graying of hair.

Inborn Metabolic Error-related Disorders (*Table 3*)

Nevus Depigmentosus

Synonym: Achromic nevus.

History: First reported by Lesser in 1884.

Etiopathogenesis: Developmental defect of melanocytes with aggregation of melanosomes and defect in transfer to the keratinocytes.

Clinical features: Asymptomatic depigmented macule of varying sizes present at birth or early onset in life which is stable in size and distribution throughout life with regular/serrated borders. These are common on trunk, neck, face, and proximal extremities, which do not cross the midline. Different types are focal, segmental, whorled, and generalized.[10]

Differential diagnosis: Vitiligo and hypomelanosis of Ito.

Treatment: Counseling, suction blister grafting, and epidermal cell suspension for cosmetic reasons.

Nevus Anemicus

It is benign, localized, developmental anomaly, usually present since birth, and manifested by a hypopigmented macule with a well-defined serrated margin. On diascopy, it merges with the surrounding colored skin. Wood's lamp examination reduces the hypopigmentation.

KEY POINTS

- Human pigmentation disorders can be classified by phenotype, including hypo- or hyperpigmentation, congenital or acquired presentation, effects on melanocyte number (hypo- or hyperplasia), or effects on melanocyte function.
- Albinism is an inherited hypopigmentation disorder where defective melanin production causes severe reduction to complete absence of all skin, hair, and eye pigmentation.
- Piebaldism is an autosomal dominant condition with depigmented skin, white forelock, scattered islets of hyperpigmented macules within the depigmented patches.
- Waardenburg syndrome is a genetic disorder characterized by piebaldism and sensorineural deafness.
- Hypomelanosis of Ito presents with unusual unilateral or bilateral cutaneous macular hypopigmented whorls, streaks, and patches, corresponding to the lines of Blaschko.
- Ataxia-telangiectasia presents with depigmented tiny circumscribed macules on the extremities and trunk along with cerebellar ataxia, choreoathetosis, oculocutaneous

telangiectasia, bronchiectasis with recurrent pulmonary infections, and premature graying of hair.

- Nevus depigmentosus presents as depigmented macule of varying sizes present at birth or early onset in life which is stable in size and distribution throughout life with regular/ serrated borders.
- Nevus anemicus presents as a developmental anomaly, manifested by a hypopigmented macule with a well-defined serrated margin. On diascopy, it merges with the surrounding colored skin.

REFERENCES

1. Thomas I, Kihiczak GG, Fox MD, Janniger CK, Schwartz RA. Piebaldism: an update. Int J Dermatol. 2004;43:716-9.
2. Shah BH, Desai BA. Genealogical aspects of albinism. Indian J Dermatol Venereol. 1967;33:260-3.
3. Huizing M, Helip-Wooley A, Westbroek W, Gunay-Aygun M, Gahl WA. Disorders of lysosome-related organelle biogenesis: clinical and molecular genetics. Annu Rev Genomics Hum Genet. 2008;9:359-86.
4. Baxter LL, Pavan WJ. The etiology and molecular genetics of human pigmentation disorders. Wiley Interdiscip Rev Dev Biol. 2013;2:379-92.
5. Richards KA, Fukai K, Oiso N, Paller AS. A novel KIT mutation results in piebaldism with progressive depigmentation. J Am Acad Dermatol. 2001;44:288-92.
6. Pingault V, Ente D, Dastot-Le Moal F, Goossens M, Marlin S, Bondurand N. Review and update of mutations causing Waardenburg syndrome. Hum Mutat. 2010;31:391-406.
7. Izumi K, Kohta T, Kimura Y, Ishida S, Takahashi T, Ishiko A, et al. Tietz syndrome: unique phenotype specific to mutations of MITF nuclear localization signal. Clin Genet. 2008;74:93-5.
8. Fisch L. Deafness as part of hereditary syndrome. J Laryngol Otol. 1959;73:355-82.
9. Pavithran K. Incontinentia pigmenti achromians. Indian J Dermatol Venereol Leprol. 1984;50:223-4.
10. Dhar S, Kanwar AJ, Kaur S. Nevus depigmentosus in India: experience with 50 patients. Pediatr Dermatol. 1993;10:299-300.

EXAMINATION QUESTIONS

1. Classify genetic disorders of pigmentation. Write a short note on piebaldism.
2. Write a short note on hypopigmentary disorders in dermatology and its approach.

99 CHAPTER Vitiligo

Abhijit Saha, Maitreyee Sengupta

INTRODUCTION

Vitiligo is an acquired, idiopathic disorder of localized depigmentation resulting from progressive loss of melanocytes.[1] It is characterized by sharply demarcated depigmented macules and patches. It is one of the most common forms of acquired melanocytopenic hypomelanosis.

EPIDEMIOLOGY

- Vitiligo has a worldwide prevalence of 0.5–1% of the general population.[1]
- It can affect any age from birth to senescence but onset is most common between 20 and 30 years of age.
- Vitiligo affects all races and both sexes equally.

Pathogenesis and Pathophysiology

Vitiligo is a multifactorial disorder. Both genetic and nongenetic theories have been proposed for its causation. Immunohistochemical studies have shown a lack of DOPA-positive identifiable melanocytes in the epidermis of vitiligo skin. The KIT receptor, a protein expressed early in melanocyte differentiation, is undetectable in vitiligo skin, suggesting that putative melanocyte precursors are no longer present. Considering the various theories suggested for the causation of vitiligo, the same may not apply for all cases:

- *Autoimmune destruction of melanocytes:* This is the leading theory regarding vitiligo causation. Dysfunction of humoral immunity is supported by the association of vitiligo with autoimmune endocrinopathies such as hypo- and hyperthyroidism, pernicious anemia, Addison's disease, or polyglandular insufficiencies.[2] Antibodies have been detected against several melanocyte antigens such as tyrosinase and tyrosinase-related proteins 1 and 2 (TYRP1 and TYRP2) in the sera of vitiligo patients. CD8+T-cells have been found in perilesional epidermis as well as blood of vitiligo patients. Several components of the innate immune system have been found to be associated with vitiligo, e.g., NLRP-1, XBP-1, HSP-70.
- *Intrinsic defect in the structure and function of melanocytes:* An abnormality in the structure and/or function of the rough endoplasmic reticulum may play a role in the pathogenesis of vitiligo. Vitiligo melanocytes have increased sensitivity to oxidative stress (UVB), resulting in early cell death.
- *Defective free radical defenses:* With Wood's lamp illumination, the clinically white skin of vitiligo has a characteristic yellow/green or bluish fluorescence. This fluorescence is due to the accumulation of two different oxidized pteridines: 6-biopterin (bluish fluorescence) and 7-biopterin (yellow/green fluorescence).
- *Reduced melanocyte survival and dysregulation of melanocyte apoptosis:* A deficiency of the stem cell factor/KIT/MITF/Bcl-2 survival pathway within melanocytes might be responsible for their passive death.[2,3]
- Destruction of melanocytes by autocytotoxic metabolites, originating from the transepidermal melanocytorrhagy due to defective adhesion
- Membrane lipid alterations in melanocytes
- Deficiency of unidentified melanocyte growth factors
- Destruction of melanocytes by neurochemical substances
- Viral infection [e.g., cytomegalovirus (CMV)]
- *Genetic factors:* A genetic factor is undoubtedly involved in vitiligo.[3] Approximately 30% of patients have a positive family history and vitiligo has been reported in monozygotic twins. The inheritance of vitiligo cannot be explained by simple Mendelian genetics. Rather, it is characterized by incomplete penetrance, multiple susceptibility loci, and genetic heterogeneity. Several genomic susceptibility loci have been identified for vitiligo, most of which encode for components of the immune system, while a few for the enzyme tyrosinase.
- *Convergence theory:* All the above hypotheses are not mutually exclusive, a "convergence" theory has been proposed in which genetic factors, stress, accumulation of toxic compounds, infection, autoimmunity, altered cellular environment, and impaired melanocyte migration, and proliferation all contribute to the phenomenon of vitiligo.

Clinical Features

- The most common form of vitiligo is a totally amelanotic macule surrounded by normal skin. The lesions are usually symmetrically distributed, except for the segmental type where it is unilateral.
- The macules usually have a convex outline, increase irregularly in size, and fuse with neighboring lesions to form complex patterns.

- The most commonly involved sites are areas of repeated friction, chronic pressure or trauma, like the hips, dorsa of the hands/fingers, feet, elbows, knees, and ankles. Vitiligo is also frequently localized to areas that are normally hyperpigmented, such as face, axillae, nipples, umbilicus, sacrum, inguinal, and anogenital regions.
- Hair within the lesions may be normally pigmented, but may also become depigmented-leukotrichia. Vitiligo of the scalp usually presents as a localized patch of white or gray hair (poliosis). Spontaneous repigmentation of depigmented hair in vitiligo does not occur.
- Vitiligo macules are mostly asymptomatic, but few may complain of pruritus. Lesions in exposed areas are particularly prone to sunburn and it may be the presenting complaint.
- *Koebner's phenomenon:* Vitiligo may develop in sites of specific trauma, such as cut, burn, or abrasion.[4] It has also been reported to develop on striae.[5] This is more common in progressive vitiligo.

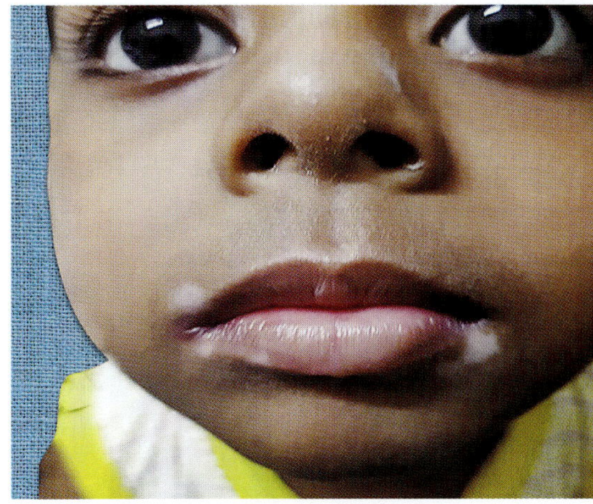

Fig. 1: Focal vitiligo
Courtesy: Dr Abhijit Saha.

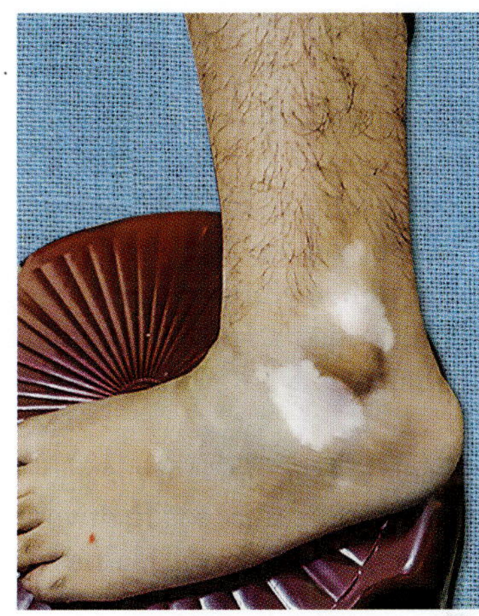

Fig. 2: Focal vitiligo
Courtesy: Dr Abhijit Saha.

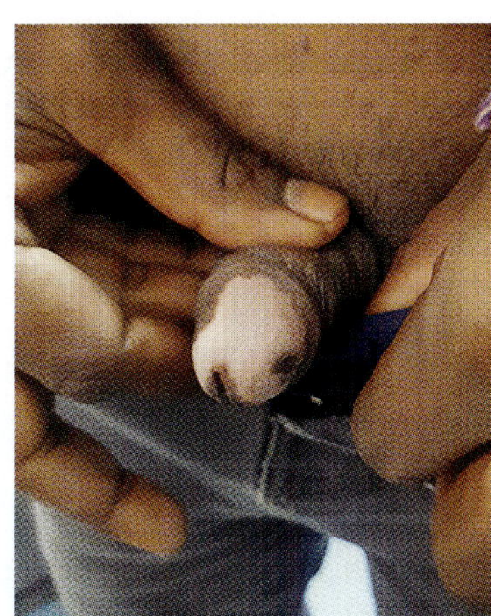

Fig. 3: Mucosal vitiligo
Courtesy: Dr Abhijit Saha.

CLINICAL CLASSIFICATION OF VITILIGO

Vitiligo has been traditionally classified into two groups: (1) Localized, which does not cross the midline, and (2) generalized, which involves bilaterally.[6]

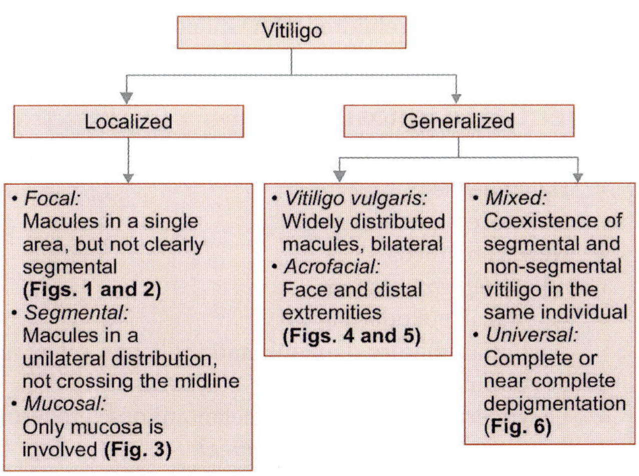

Clinical Variants

- *Trichrome vitiligo:* Lesions show an intermediate hypopigmented zone of varying width between the normal and totally depigmented skin.
- *Quadrichrome vitiligo:* Reflects the presence of a fourth color (dark brown) at sites of perifollicular repigmentation.
- *Hypochromic vitiligo/vitiligo minor:* This is a form of vitiligo seen in dark-skinned individuals where there is a partial defect in pigmentation leading to hypopigmented rather than depigmented lesions.
- *Halo nevi-associated leukoderma:* Discrete amelanotic macules develop at sites distant from the halo naevi. This phenomenon differs from classical vitiligo in that the depigmented macules are often more limited and not as clearly demarcated from normal skin as in vitiligo and often do not progress.
- *Vitiligo ponctue:* Small confetti-like amelanotic macules occurring on normal skin or on a hyperpigmented macule.

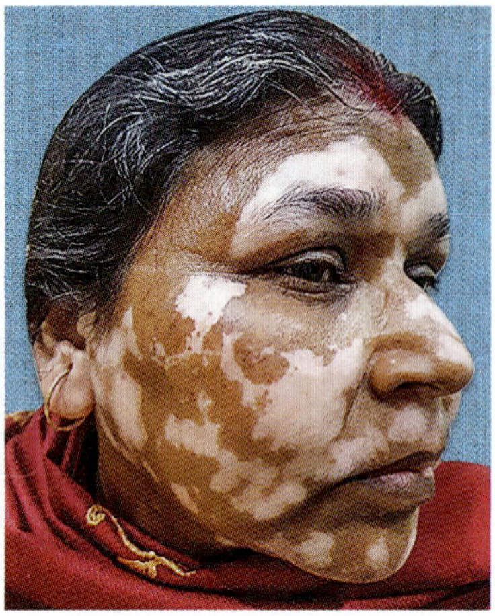

Fig. 4: Acro facial vitiligo
Courtesy: Dr Abhijit Saha.

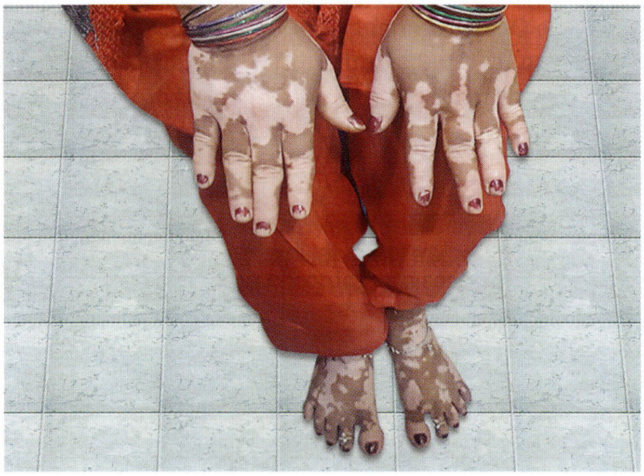

Fig. 5: Acro facial vitiligo
Courtesy: Dr Abhijit Saha.

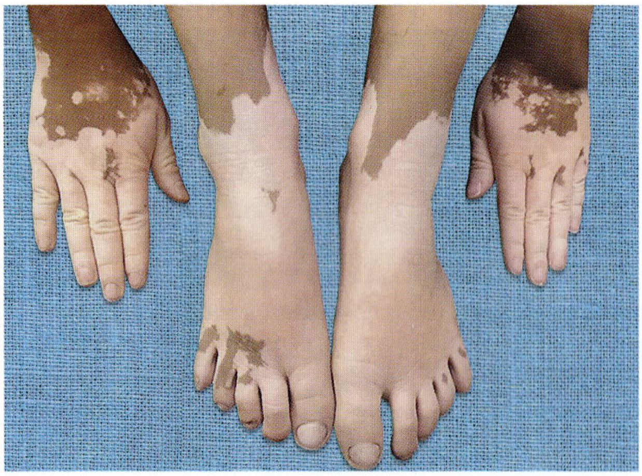

Fig. 6: Acral vitiligo.
Courtesy: Dr Aarti Sarda.

- *Blue vitiligo:* Vitiligo macules occurring in areas already affected by postinflammatory hyperpigmentation.
- Uncommonly, vitiligo macules may have a hyperpigmented margin or even a raised inflammatory border with erythema.

DISORDERS ASSOCIATED WITH VITILIGO[7]

- Thyroid diseases (hyperthyroidism and hypothyroidism, i.e., Graves' disease, Hashimoto's thyroiditis)
- Pernicious anemia
- Addison's disease
- Diabetes
- Hypoparathyroidism
- Myasthenia gravis
- Alopecia areata
- Morphea and lichen sclerosus
- Halo naevus
- Malignant melanoma
- Uveitis including Vogt-Koyanagi-Harada syndrome and Alezzandrini syndrome.

Course of the Disease

- The onset of vitiligo is insidious. Most frequently, vitiligo is gradually progressive, sometimes extending rapidly over a period of several months and then remaining quiescent for many years.[8]
- Sun-induced or spontaneous repigmentation may occur, but complete and stable repigmentation is rare.
- In children, segmental vitiligo is far more common than in adults, although vitiligo vulgaris is still the most common form. The incidence of associated endocrinopathies is significantly less in children with vitiligo but they have an increased incidence of autoantibody production.

Differential Diagnosis

- *Single circular lesion:*
  - Halo naevus
  - Nevus depigmentosus
  - Nevus anemicus
- *Complete depigmentation:*
  - Chemical leukoderma
  - Postinflammatory depigmentation, lichen sclerosus et atrophicus
  - Leukoderma associated with melanoma or scleroderma
- *Early lesions or partial loss of pigment:*
  - Postinflammatory hypopigmentation
  - Pityriasis versicolor and other cutaneous infections like leprosy
  - Progressive macular hypomelanosis
  - Inherited hypomelanosis in piebaldism, tuberous sclerosis, and Waardenburg syndrome.

Treatment

- The diagnosis of vitiligo is clinical. Supportive evidence includes family history, Koebner's phenomenon, leukotrichia, and fluorescence on Wood's lamp examination.
- The aims of treatment in vitiligo are halting the depigmenting process and stabilization of lesions, and repigmentation of the affected areas.

- *Narrowband-UVB:* The treatment of choice in generalized vitiligo is narrowband UVB (NB-UVB).[9] The starting doses vary from 100 to 250 mJ/cm^2, with increments of 10–20% at each subsequent exposure until satisfactory erythema is achieved within the lesions. Treatments are administered two to three times per week. The advantages of NB-UVB over PUVA therapy include shorter treatment times, no drug costs or gastrointestinal side effects, reduced phototoxic reactions, and no need for post-treatment photoprotection; NB-UVB can be used safely in children, pregnant or lactating women, and in individuals with hepatic or kidney dysfunction.
- *Psoralen plus phototherapy:* Psoralen photochemotherapy involves the use of psoralens combined with UVA light. The psoralens most commonly used are 8-methoxypsoralen (8-MOP) and 4, 5', 8-trimethylpsoralen (TMP). Psoralens can be applied either topically (topical PUVA) or orally (oral PUVA), followed by exposure to either artificial UV light or natural sunlight (PUVASOL). 8-MOP is administered at a dose of 0.4–0.6 mg/kg two to four times a week. This dose is gradually increased until minimal asymptomatic erythema of the involved skin occurs. Topical psoralen formulations have a high risk of phototoxicity (blistering, koebnerization). Low concentrations (≤0.1%) should be used and, approximately 20–30 minutes after applying the topical preparation (cream or ointment), the patient should be exposed to UVA. When sunlight is the source of UVA, it is known as PUVASOL. The response rate of PUVA is variable, and complete repigmentation is achieved in only a few, while cosmetically acceptable improvement is obtained in a majority of patients. The total number of PUVA treatments required is between 50 and 300.
- *Other phototherapies:* Khellin plus UVA (KUVA) and phenylalanine plus UVA have also been tried for the treatment of vitiligo but not recommended due to doubtful efficacy and hepatic toxicity.
- *Corticosteroids:* Topical corticosteroids are useful for small localized areas, but intralesional corticosteroids should be avoided. To minimize cutaneous atrophy, treatment should be discontinued if there is no visible improvement after 2 months. Systemic corticosteroids (high-dose pulsed therapy, mini-pulsed regimen, or low-dose daily oral dose) have been claimed to rapidly arrest spreading vitiligo and induce repigmentation. Combination therapy using a topical corticosteroid and UVA irradiation has been shown to be more effective than either the topical corticosteroid or UVA alone.
- *Topical immunosuppressants:* Topical application of 0.1% tacrolimus ointment has resulted in repigmentation of vitiligo, also in children. The best results were obtained when it was combined with sun exposure. Topical tacrolimus can also be used in conjunction with the 308 nm excimer laser and topical corticosteroids. Topical pimecrolimus has also been used.
- *Surgical therapies:* For vitiligo patients who fail to respond to medical therapy, autologous transplantation can be performed. The general selection criteria for autologous transplantation are stable vitiligo (for at least 6 months), unsatisfactory response to medical therapy, absence of Koebner phenomena, positive minigrafting test, no tendency for scar or keloid formation, and age above 12 years.
  - Mini punch grafting is the simplest method.[10] Small punch grafts (1–2 mm) from uninvolved skin are implanted within achromic areas. A cobblestone effect, variegated appearance of the grafts, sinking pits and infection are potential side effects. When combined with phototherapy, it has been shown to be more effective than mini punch grafting alone.[11]
  - Suction blister epidermal grafting has also been used. The advantages are absence of scarring and possibility of reusing the donor site.
  - Thin split skin grafting has been used with success in experienced hands.
  - *Melanocyte transfer:* Grafting of cultured autologous melanocytes is an expensive technique that requires specialized laboratory expertise but gives excellent results. Grafting of non-cultured epidermal cell suspensions that include melanocytes has also been advocated. Grafting of follicular melanocytes to repigment vitiligo leukotrichia has also been performed successfully.
  - Microneedling or transverse needling of small localized lesions in combination with topical 5-fluorouracil cream is a newer modality of treatment.
- *Micropigmentation:* Permanent dermal micropigmentation, i.e., tattooing with a non-allergenic iron oxide pigment, can be used to camouflage recalcitrant areas of vitiligo where repigmentation rates are poor, e.g., the lips, nipples, and distal fingers.
- *Laser and microphototherapy:* Lasers are not widely used for vitiligo treatment but the 308 nm excimer laser with wavelength equivalent to NB-UVB has been used with some success for localized lesions. Focused microphototherapy with UVB light where only the depigmented skin is irradiated, through a dark pad with 2 mm holes, has also been tried.
- *Depigmentation:* Patients with widespread disease and only a few areas of normally pigmented skin can be treated with depigmenting agents to give a uniform color. The most commonly used agent is 20% monobenzyl ether of hydroquinone (MBEH), applied once to twice daily to the affected areas for 9–12 months or longer. It is a potent irritant/allergen and skin test should be performed over a small area before wider use. Side effects include contact dermatitis, exogenous ochronosis and leukomelanoderma en confetti. Depigmentation requires lifelong strict photoprotection (sunscreens, clothing, umbrellas). Other

agents for skin bleaching include laser therapy (e.g., Q-switched alexandrite 755 nm, Q-switched ruby 694 nm) and cryotherapy.

- *Psychological support:* The impact of this disorder on quality of life is very severe in many patients. Patients should be counseled regarding the nature of the disease process and current therapies available. They should be reassured that something beneficial can always be done.
- *Others:* Camouflage creams and treatments form an important part of the management as they provide immediate benefit in covering up recalcitrant vitiligo particularly in cosmetically-sensitive areas. Certain other therapies such as pseudocatalase with NB-UVB and systemic antioxidants have been used with inconsistent results.

KEY POINTS

- Vitiligo is a multifactorial, acquired depigmenting disorder.
- Various theories have been proposed in vitiligo causation such as autoimmunity, melanocyte defects, genetic factors, and damage by toxic free radicals.
- Vitiligo lesions are characterized by amelanotic macules with convex borders that are sharply demarcated from normal skin. Leukotrichia and poliosis may be seen.
- Sunburns may occur over the lesions and Koebner's phenomenon may be seen.
- Vitiligo may be associated with other autoimmune disorders particularly endocrinopathies.
- Topical corticosteroids and photo-therapy (NB-UVB and PUVA) form the mainstay of therapy. Recalcitrant lesions may require surgical grafting.
- Psychological support and counseling, along with camouflage techniques, form an important part of the management.

REFERENCES

1. Nordlund JJ, Boissy RE, Hearing VJ, King RA, Oetting WS, Ortonne JP. The Pigmentary System: Physiology and Pathophysiology, 2nd edition. Maldon, MA: Blackwell; 2006.
2. Richmond JM, Frisoli ML, Harris JE. Innate immune mechanisms in vitiligo: danger from within. Curr Opin Immunol. 2013;25:676-82.
3. Passeron T, Ortonne JP. Physiopathology and genetics of vitiligo. J Autoimmun. 2005;25(Suppl):63-8.
4. van Geel N, Speeckaert R, Taieb A, Picardo M, Böhm M, Gawkrodger DJ, et al. Koebner's phenomenon in vitiligo: European position paper. Pigment Cell Melanoma Res. 2011; 24:564-73.
5. Lahiri K, Sengupta SR. Vitiligo developing on striae: an isomorphic phenomenon. Ind J Dermatol. 1996;41(2):70-1.
6. Ezzedine K, Lim HW, Suzuki T, Katayama I, Hamzavi I, Lan CCE, et al. Revised classification/nomenclature of vitiligo and related issues: The Vitiligo Global Issues Consensus Conference. Pigment Cell Melanoma Res. 2012;25:E1-13.
7. Spritz RA. The genetics of generalized vitiligo and associated autoimmune diseases. Pigment Cell Res. 2007;20:271-8.
8. Lahiri K, Malakar S. The concept of stability of vitiligo: A reappraisal. Indian J Dermatol. 2012;57:83-9.
9. Scherschun L, Kim JJ, Lim HW. Narrow-band ultraviolet B is a useful and well-tolerated treatment for vitiligo. J Am Acad Dermatol. 2001;44:999-1003.
10. Lahiri K. Evolution and evaluation of autologous mini punch grafting in vitiligo. Indian J Dermatol. 2009:54(2): 159-67.
11. Lahiri K, Malakar S, Sarma N, Banerjee U. Inducing repigmentation by regrafting and phototherapy (311 nm) in punch grafting failure cases of lip vitiligo: a pilot study. Indian J Dermatol Venereol Leprol. 2004;70:156-8.

EXAMINATION QUESTIONS

1. Describe etiopathogenesis of vitiligo.
2. Describe clinical features and associations of vitiligo.
3. Discuss role of phototherapy in the management of vitiligo.
4. Discuss role of surgical techniques in the management of vitiligo.
5. What are recent advances in the management of vitiligo?
6. Describe dermoscopy in vitiligo.
7. Enlist various severity scores in dermatology, assessment of psychosocial impact in vitiligo, and counseling in vitiligo.

100 CHAPTER Other Hypopigmented Disorders

Ivoreen Darung, Maitreyee Sengupta, Abhijit Saha

INTRODUCTION

Pigmentary disorder is a common phenomenon we encounter in our daily clinical practice. They can be hypopigmented, depigmented, or hyperpigmented. In this chapter, we will restrict ourselves with hypo/depigmented disorders only. Classification of this group is cumbersome and exhaustive. A proper classification is extremely needed for holistic approach as far as diagnosis, management, and prognosis are concerned.

Understanding each disorder and their underlying pathology is important to diagnose underlying systemic disorders.[1,2]

UNDERSTANDING PATHOPHYSIOLOGY

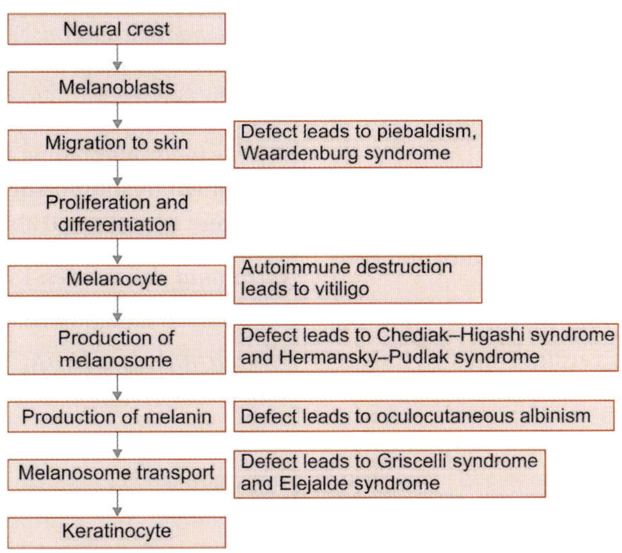

TYPES OF HYPOPIGMENTATION

1. Diffuse
2. Localized

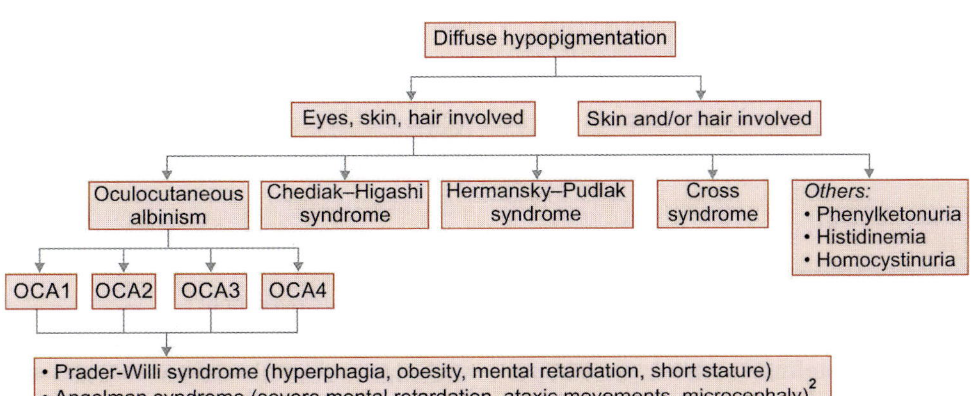

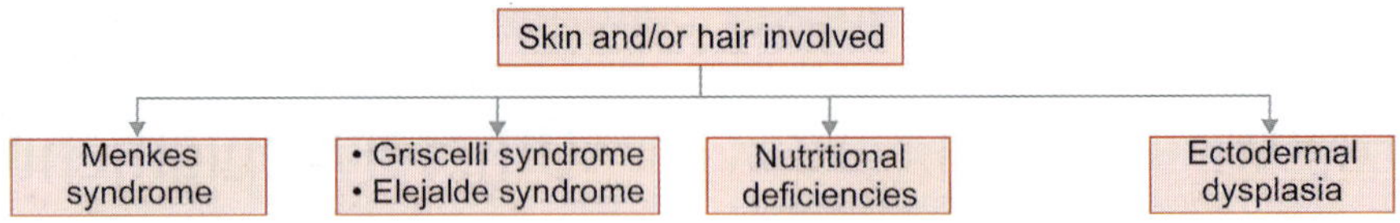

Oculocutaneous albinism:
- Predominantly autosomal recessive disorder
- *Types*: OCA1, OCA2, OCA3, OCA4
- *On examination*: Pigmentary dilution of skin, hair, eyes
- *Ocular findings*: Translucent iris, photophobia, reduced visual acuity, strabismus and nystagmus (due to misrouting of optic fibers)
- *Histopathology*: Normal number of melanocytes but reduced melanin
- *Management*: Symptomatic, photoprotection
- *Complications*: Cutaneous photocarcinogenesis (esp. squamous cell carcinoma).[2]

Chediak–Higashi syndrome:
- Autosomal recessive disorder
- Cutaneous and ocular findings similar to oculocutaneous albinism
- *Systemic associations*: Severe immune deficiency, bleeding diathesis.

Hermansky–Pudlak syndrome:
- Autosomal recessive
- Cutaneous and ocular findings similar to oculocutaneous albinism
- *Systemic associations*: Bleeding diathesis, immune deficiency, pulmonary fibrosis, cardiomyopathy, inflammatory bowel disease, renal disease.[3]

Cross syndrome:
- Pigmentary dilution of skin, silvery hair, ocular anomalies
- *Systemic associations*: Psychomotor impairment, progressive neurologic manifestations.[2]

Menkes syndrome:
- X-linked disorder
- Due to inappropriate copper storage
- Pigment dilution of skin and hair
- Progressive deterioration of central nervous system
- Death by 3 years of age.

Griscelli syndrome:
- Autosomal recessive disorder
- *Cutaneous*: Pigmentary dilution of skin, silvery hair
- *Systemic association*: Neurologic abnormalities, immunologic impairment
- *Light microscopy of hair shaft*: Pigment clumping.[3]

Elejalde syndrome:
- Pigmentary dilution of skin, silvery hair
- Severe neurological abnormalities.[4]

Nutritional deficiencies: Kwashiorkor, selenium, and copper deficiency

Ectodermal dysplasia: EEC syndrome (Ectrodactyly-ectodermal dysplasia-cleft lip/palate).[2]

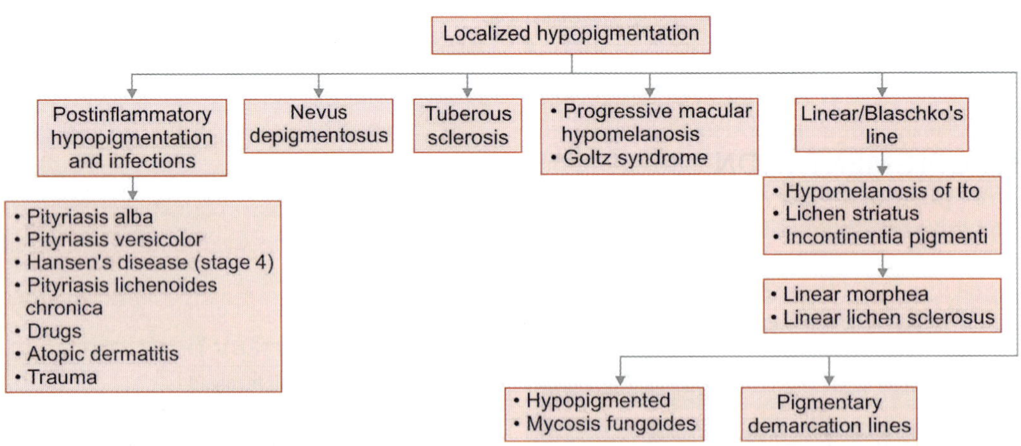

Postinflammatory Hypopigmentation (Fig. 1)

Pityriasis alba:
- Solitary or multiple ill-defined, round, oval hypopigmented patch with slightly scaly surface
- Commonly over face
- History of atopy
- Decreased number of melanocytes and melanosomes
- Decreased size of melanosomes.[2]

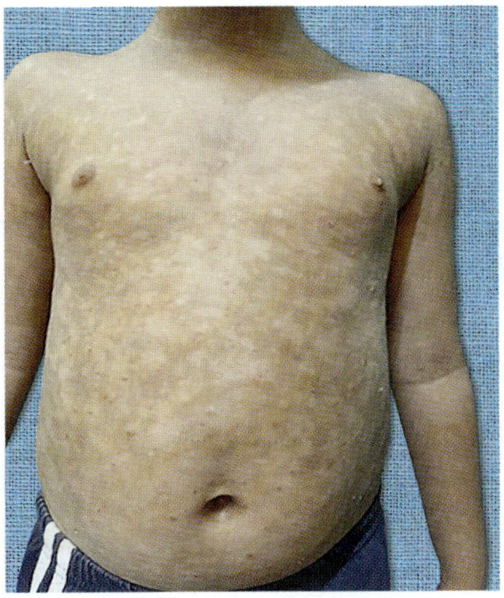

Fig. 1: Postinflammatory hypopigmentation in pityriasis lichenoides chronica.
Courtesy: Dr Abhijit Saha.

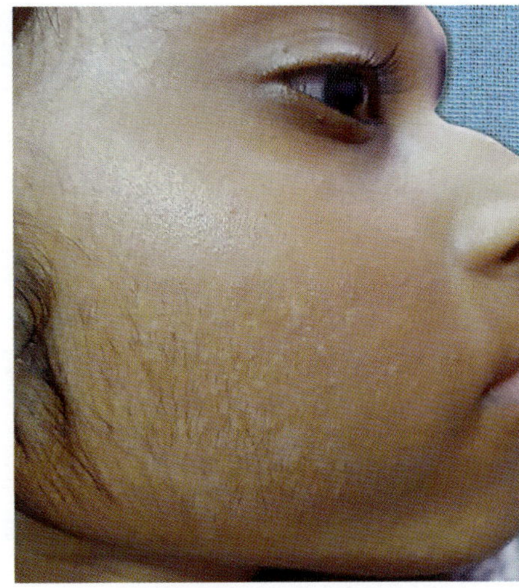

Fig. 2: Pityriasis versicolor.
Courtesy: Dr Abhijit Saha.

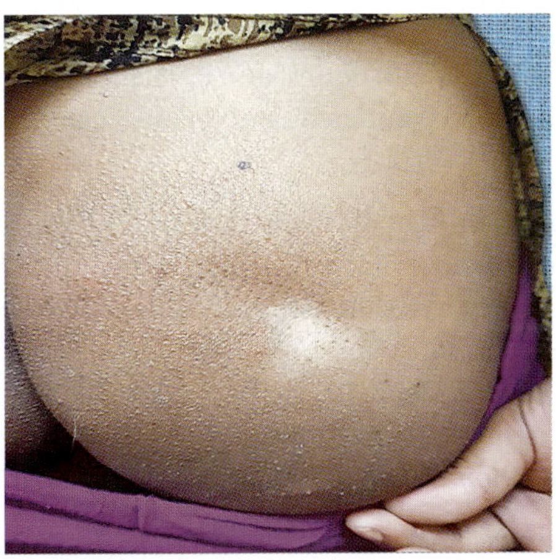

Fig. 3: Steroid-induced hypopigmentation and atrophy.
Courtesy: Dr Abhijit Saha.

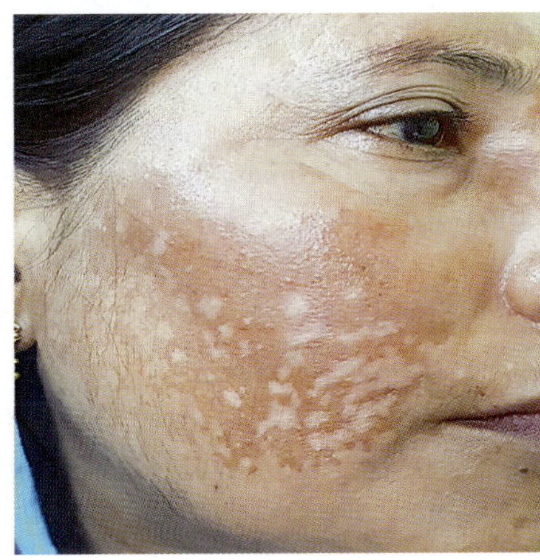

Fig. 4: Hydroquinone-induced hypopigmentation.
Courtesy: Dr Abhijit Saha.

Pityriasis versicolor **(Fig. 2)**:
- Superficial dermatophytosis
- Caused by *Malassezia* spp. (*M. globosa, M. restricta, M. sympodialis, M. furfur, M. obtusa*)
- Discrete perifollicular hypopigmented, scaly, coalescing macules over seborrheic areas
- *Woods lamp*: Yellow-green fluorescence
- *KOH*: "Spaghetti and meatballs."[5]

Hansen's disease:
- *Indeterminate leprosy*: Hypopigmented patch with ill-defined border and smooth surface, sensation ±, nerve thickening ±, AFB ±
  Majority resolve spontaneously after few months.
- *Tuberculoid leprosy*: Well-demarcated anesthetic hypopigmented xerotic patch, thickened nerve present
- *Borderline tuberculoid leprosy*: Well-demarcated, anesthetic hypopigmented, xerotic patch with irregular borders, presence of pseudopodia and marginal breakdown, satellite lesions, thickened nerve present.[6]

Drugs: Topical/intralesional corticosteroids **(Fig. 3)**, hydroquinone **(Fig. 4)**, arsenic, mercury, chloroquine, imatinib mesylate, etc.

Nevus depigmentosus:
- Misnomer
- Lesions are hypopigmented rather than depigmented
- Asymptomatic well-demarcated patch with irregular and serrated border.[2]

Progressive macular hypomelanosis:
- Onset in early adolescence
- Asymptomatic discrete and coalescing round/oval, nonscaly, ill-defined hypopigmented macules distributed over seborrheic areas.[7]

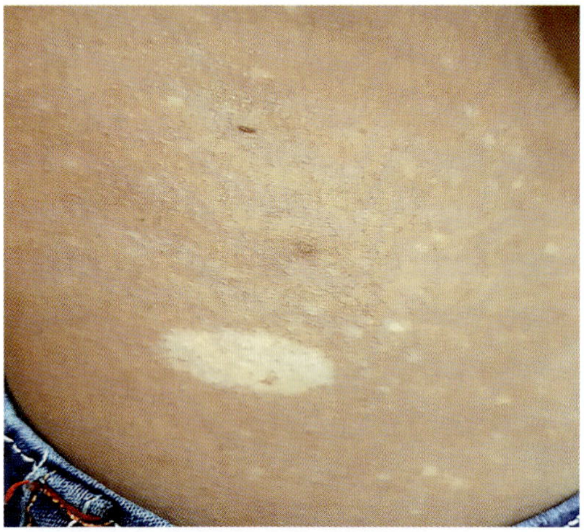

Fig. 5: Ash-leaf macule.
Courtesy: Dr Abhijit Saha.

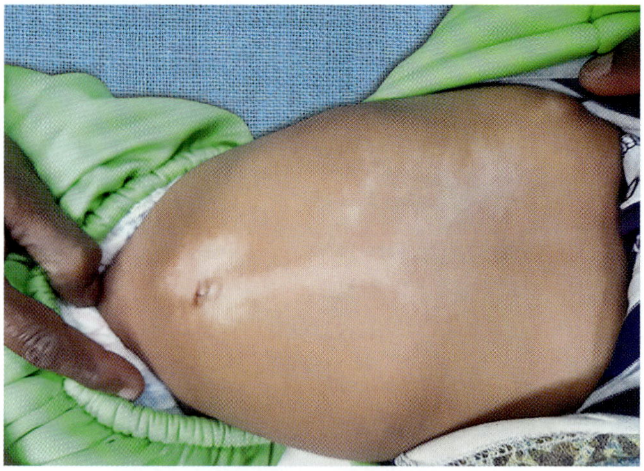

Fig. 6: Pigmentary mosaicism.
Courtesy: Dr Abhijit Saha.

Ash-leaf macules in tuberous sclerosis ***(Fig. 5)***:
- Early cutaneous sign of tuberous sclerosis
- Three or more "Ash leaf" macules greater than 5 mm size is diagnostic
- *Other findings*: Angiofibromas, shagreen patch, Koenen tumors, gingival fibromas
- Systemic involvement.[5]

Hypomelanosis of Ito ***(Fig. 6)***:
- Also known as pigmentary mosaicism[1]
- Hypopigmentation follows lines of Blaschko
- *Associations*: Skin, hair, nail, dental, ocular, central nervous system (CNS), musculoskeletal anomalies.

Lichen striatus:
- Pruritic or asymptomatic, discrete erythematous and slightly scaly papules with hypopigmented macules along the lines of Blaschko down the extremities or around the trunk
- Nail involvement (can occur if the lesion extends down the digit) nail plate thinning, longitudinal ridging, splitting, nail bed hyperkeratosis
- *Histopathology*: Lichenoid interface dermatitis, spongiosis, deep dermal lymphoid periappendageal infiltrate (around eccrine sweat glands and ducts).[5]

Incontinentia pigmenti:
- X-linked dominant disorder
- *Onset*: First few weeks after birth
- *Clinical features*: Whorled pigmentation over the trunk
- Consists of four stages:

Vesicular phase → verrucous phase → hyperpigmented phase → hypopigmented phase (usually seen in adult women)
- *Associations*: Teeth, bones, and CNS anomalies
- Encephalopathy and neonatal seizures can occur.[6]

Linear morphea:
- May follow lines of Blaschko
- *Clinical features*: Linear, smooth, indurated, slightly depressed, ivory-white or hyperpigmented lesions
- *Associated syndromes*:
  - En coup de sabre
  - Parry Romberg syndrome
- *Complications*: Joint contractures and frozen joints.[6]

Goltz syndrome:
- *PORCN* gene mutation
- X-linked dominant disorder
- *Clinical features*: Asymmetric linear and reticulated atrophy along Blaschko's lines, progressive hyperpigmented freckling within the hypopigmented patches, telangiectasias.
- *Associated findings*: Periorificial papillomas, lipomas,
- *Systemic*: Skeletal defects, ocular, dental abnormalities.[8]

Pigmentary demarcation lines: *Type E*: Hypopigmented macules and patches oriented obliquely, bilaterally symmetric over chest (mid-third of the clavicle to periareolar skin).[2,5]

Hypopigmented mycosis fungoides:
- Early stage mycosis fungoides
- *Clinical features*: Pruritic/asymptomatic hypopigmented patches over trunk and limbs
- *Histopathology*: Typical features of mycosis fungoides.[2]

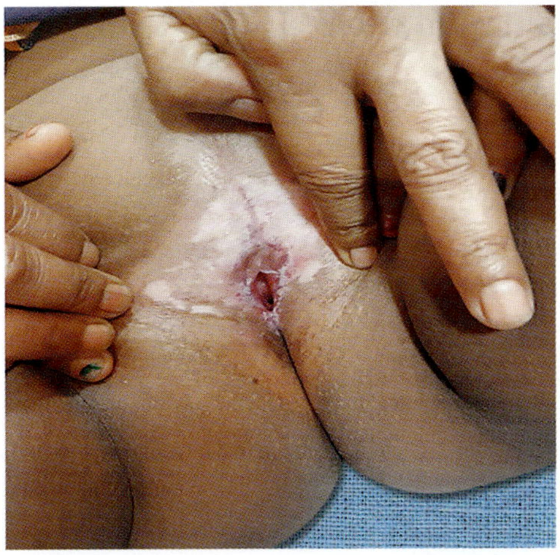

Fig. 7: Genital lichen sclerosus et atrophicus.
Courtesy: Dr Abhijit Saha.

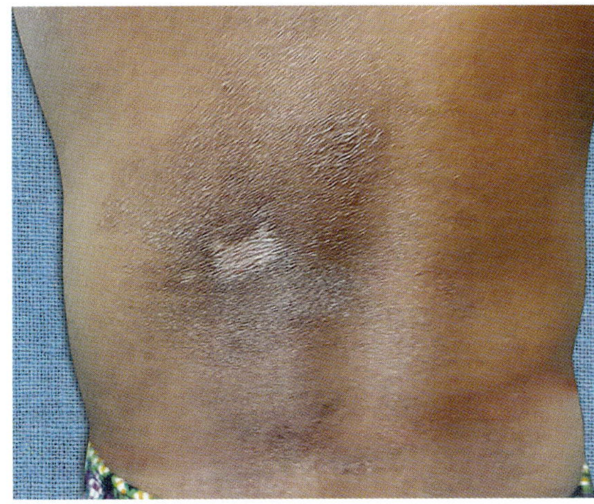

Fig. 8: Extragenital lichen sclerosus et atrophicus.
Courtesy: Dr Abhijit Saha.

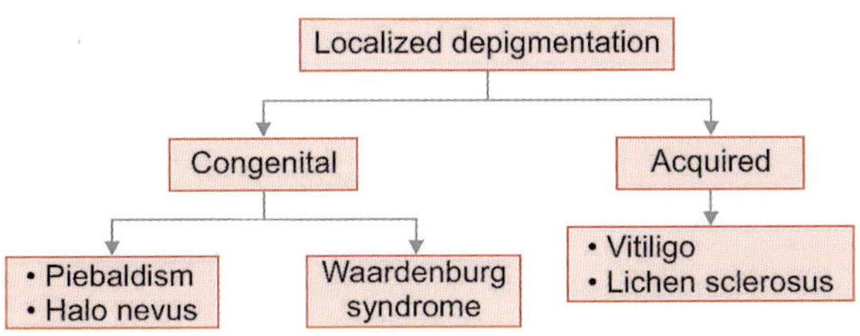

Piebaldism:

- Autosomal dominant
- Characterized by white forelock and patchy absence of skin pigment
- *Onset*: Since birth
- Well-demarcated, static, depigmented patch with irregular margins consisting of hyperpigmented and normally pigmented macules over the surface
- Distribution over anterior/posterior trunk/mid upper arm to wrist/mid-thigh to mid-calf/shins
- *Histopathology*: Absence of melanocytes in the depigmented patches[6]
- *Associations*: Hirschsprung's disease, neurofibromatosis type 1.[9]

Waardenburg syndrome:

- Autosomal dominant/recessive
- *Cutaneous findings*: White forelock and patchy depigmentation of skin
- *Systemic findings*: Congenital deafness, partial/total heterochromia iridis, synophrys, broad nasal root, dystopia canthorum
- Subtypes:
  Type 1—classic form
  Type 2—absence of dystopia canthorum
  Type 3—associated with limb abnormalities
  Type 4—associated with Hirschsprung's disease.[2]

Lichen sclerosus ***(Figs. 7 and 8)***:

- *Bimodal age distribution in females*: Prepubertal and postmenopausal
- Solitary or multiple depigmented atrophic papules and plaques with flat surface, associated with fissuring, erosions, purpura, telangiectasias and bullae
- Genital lesions are pruritic.[5]

Halo nevus:

- Asymptomatic
- Characterized by a melanocytic nevus surrounded by a round/oval hypopigmented annulus.
- Four stages of evolution:
  1. Appearance of halo
     ↓
  2. Loss of pigment in the central nevus
     ↓
  3. Disappearance of nevus
     ↓
  4. Disappearance of halo
- Halo phenomenon can be seen in blue nevi, neurofibromas, congenital melanocytic nevi, and melanoma[1]
- *Myerson's nevus*: Eczematous change around a nevus.[6]

Differential Diagnosis of Linear Hypopigmentation/Depigmentation

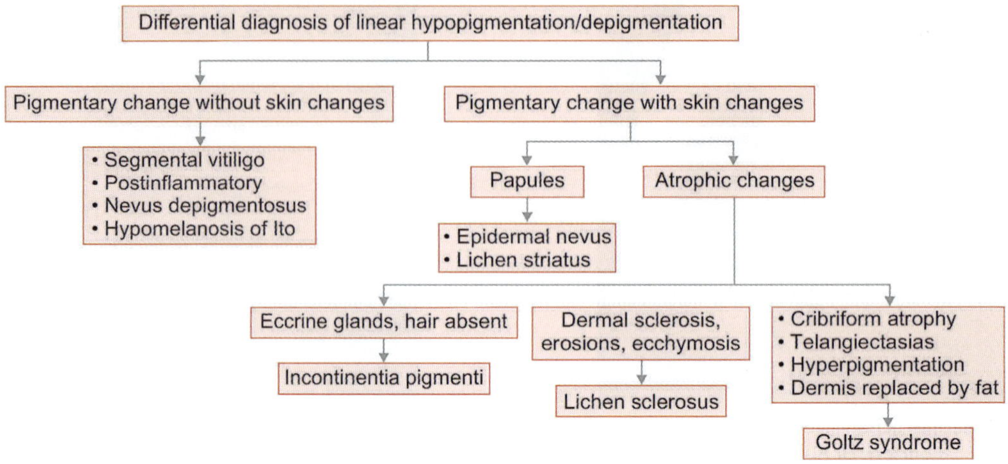

- Differential diagnosis of scalp poliosis (focal depigmentation of hair)

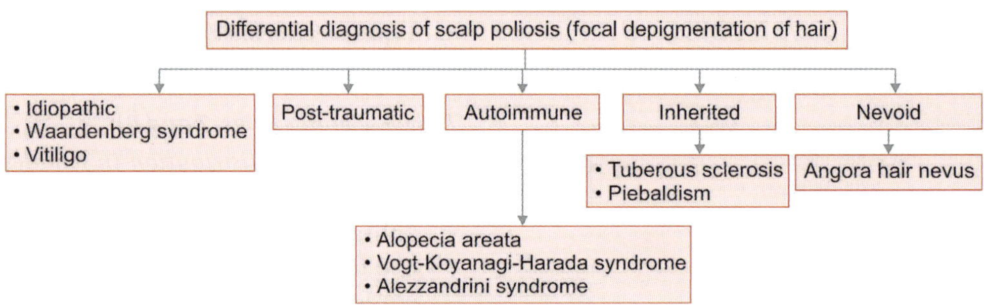

Causes of Hypopigmentation/Depigmentation of Scalp Hair

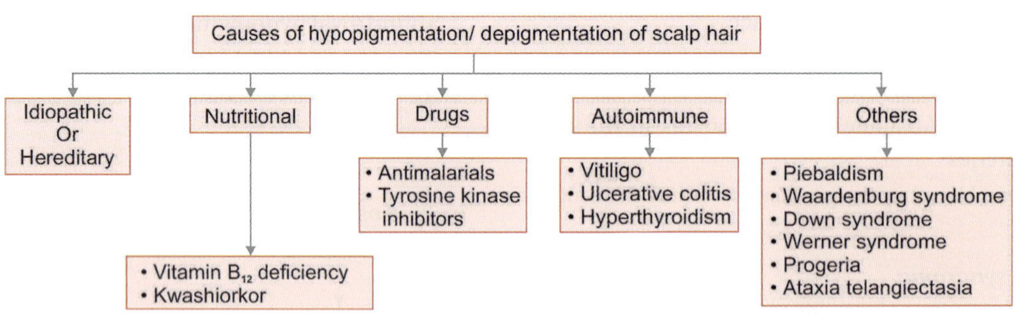

KEY POINTS

- Not all clinically hypopigmented lesions have an underlying pigmentary disorder, e.g., nevus anemicus, Bier's spots, Woronoff's ring.
- Nevus anemicus is caused due to hypersensitivity to catecholamines. Characterized by well-defined irregular shaped macule/patch present since birth. Margin blanches on diascopy.
- Bier's spots are caused due to underlying vascular anomaly. Characterized by multiple hypopigmented macules with erythematous intervening skin which blanches upon pressure, distributed over limbs.[3]
- Woronoff's ring is a hypopigmented halo around psoriatic plaque, caused due to vasoconstriction.
- Anemia and cutaneous edema can also cause skin lightening.
- *Disorders associated with silvery hair*: Chediak–Higashi syndrome, Griscelli syndrome, Elejalde syndrome.

REFERENCES

1. Giam YC. Approach to pigmented skin disorders in children. Hong Kong J. Dermatol. Venereol. 2018:26;113-21.
2. Bolognia JL, Jorizzo JL, Schaffer JV, Callen JP, Cerroni L, Heymann WR, et al (Eds). Dermatology, 3rd edition. Elsevier Saunders; 2012.
3. Van Geel N, Speeckaert M, Chevolet I, De Schepper S, Lapeere H, Boone B, et al. Hypomelanoses in children. J Cutan Aesthet Surg. 2013;6:65-72.
4. Tey HL. A practical classification of childhood hypopigmentation disorders. Acta Derm Venerol. 2010;90:6-11.
5. James WD, Elston DM, Treat JR, Rosenbach MA, Neuhaus IM. Andrew's Diseases of the Skin Clinical Dermatology, 13th edition. Elsevier Inc. 2020.
6. Kumar B, Dogra S. IAL Textbook of Leprosy, 2nd edition. New Delhi: Jaypee Brothers Medical Publishers. 2016;15:239-42.
7. Desai SR, Owen JL. Progressive macular hypomelanosis: An update. Pigment Int. 2014;1:52-5.
8. Ghosh SK, Dutta A, Sarkar S, Nag SS, Biswas SK, Mandal P. Focal dermal hypoplasia (Goltz syndrome): A cross-sectional study from Eastern India. Indian J Dermatol. 2017;62:498-504.
9. Agarwal S, Ojha A. Piebaldism: A brief report and review of literature. Indian Dermatol Online J. 2012:3;144-7.

EXAMINATION QUESTIONS

1. Discuss differential diagnosis of linear hypopigmented disorders.
2. Write a short note on mosaicism.

101 CHAPTER

Cutaneous Drug Reactions

Yogesh S Marfatia, Ruchi Shah, Reema R Baxi

INTRODUCTION

Adverse drug reactions (ADRs) [World Health Organization (WHO)] are described as "response to a medicine in humans or animals which is noxious and unintended and which occurs at any dosage and can also result from an overdose, misuse, or abuse of a medicine."[1]

INCIDENCE

Incidence of cutaneous drug reactions in hospitalized patients range from 1 to 3%, 2% of which are life-threatening severe cutaneous adverse drug reactions (SCADRs).

Increasing incidence of ADRs can be attributed to longer survival rates, improved treatment options and outcomes, polypharmacy, increased frequency, and duration of drug exposure.[2]

MECHANISM OF CUTANEOUS DRUG REACTIONS[1]

Drugs cause cutaneous adverse reactions by different mechanisms as highlighted in **Flowchart 1**.

Various factors that affect cutaneous adverse drug reaction (CADR) are shown in **Figure 1**.

Flowchart 1: Mechanism of cutaneous drug reactions.

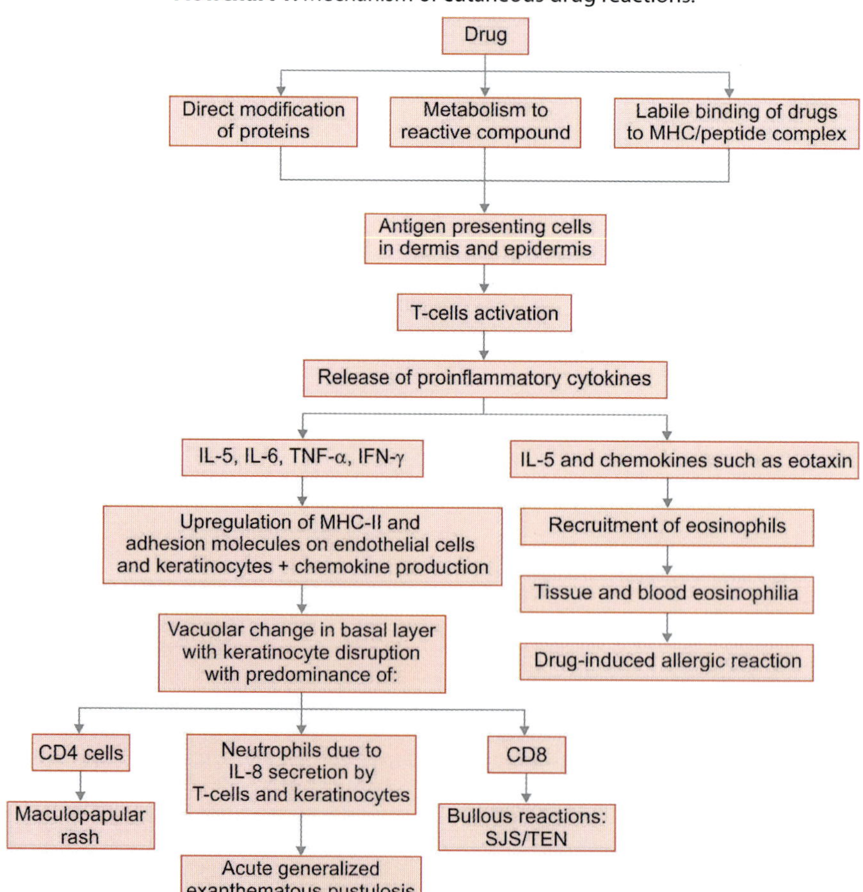

(IFN-γ: interferon gamma; IL-5: interleukin-5; MHC: major histocompatibility complex; SJS/TEN: Stevens–Johnson syndrome/toxic epidermal necrolysis; TNF-α: tumor necrosis factor alpha)

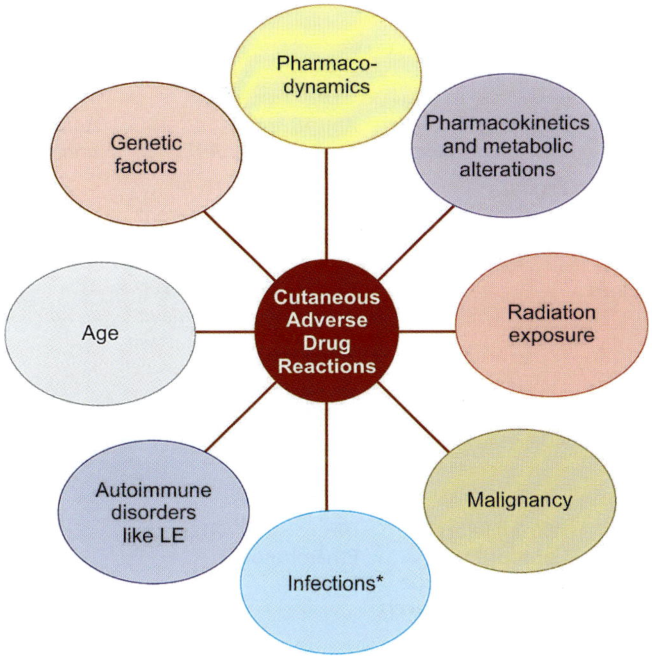

Fig. 1: Factors affecting cutaneous adverse drug reaction (CADR). *Infections such as HIV, EBV, HHV-6 and 7 [drug reaction with eosinophilia and systemic symptoms (DRESS)], CMV [acute generalized exanthematous pustulosis (AGEP)], *Mycoplasma* [Stevens–Johnson syndrome/toxic epidermal necrolysis (SJS/TEN)].[3]
(LE: lupus erythematosus)

PHARMACOGENOMICS

Pharmacogenomics is the discipline of pharmacology with a special focus on the application of genomic technologies to drug discovery and further characterization of older drugs. Prior human leukocyte antigen (HLA) screening of susceptible population can help in preventing potential severe cutaneous adverse reactions (SCARs) **(Table 1)**.

TABLE 1: HLA screening for SCADRs.

Drug	*HLA*	*SCADR*	*Population at risk*[4]
Abacavir	HLA-B*57:01	DHS	All
Carba-mazepine	HLA-B*15:02 HLA-A*31:01	SJS/TEN DRESS	Chinese Chinese, Japanese, Korean, Caucasian
Allopurinol	HLA-B*58:01	DRESS and SJS/TEN	Chinese, Japanese, Korean, Thai, European
Dapsone	HLA-B*1301	DHS/SJS/TEN/DRESS	Chinese, Thai

(DHS: drug hypersensitivity syndrome; DRESS: drug reaction with eosinophilia and systemic symptoms; HLA: human leukocyte antigen; SCADR: severe cutaneous adverse drug reaction; SJS: Stevens–Johnson syndrome; TEN: toxic epidermal necrolysis)

BENIGN CUTANEOUS ADVERSE DRUG REACTIONS[5]

The following are the benign cutaneous ADR that are commonly encountered due to drugs:

Drug-induced Exanthems

Exanthems are the most common benign CADR and have been reported in about 2% of hospitalized patients.

Mechanism: Type IV hypersensitivity.

Clinical Features

- *Symptoms*: Pruritic maculopapular rash.
- *Morphology*: Scarlatiniform, morbilliform, rubelliform, or large macules.
- *Distribution*: Symmetrical involvement of trunk and extremities, intertriginous areas might be involved but face and pressure areas are usually spared. Rash starts from trunk and then involves the face.
- *Course*: The first eruption occurs after a sensitization phase of 5–7 days and usually fades with desquamation.

Allopurinol can cause morbilliform rash. Other drugs causing maculopapular rashes have been summarized in **Table 2**. Try to provide mnemonics of most important drugs (PCAP: *P*enicillin, *C*ephalosporin, *A*spirin, *P*henytoin).

Differential Diagnosis

Viral exanthems can be differentiated by:

- Presence of accompanying fever and sore throat
- May be associated with enanthems
- Viral exanthems start from face and acral sites and progress to involve the trunk.

Management

- Stoppage of offending drug
- Emollient application
- Antihistamines and medium potency topical corticosteroids in pruritic cases.

Symmetrical Drug-related Intertriginous Flexural Exanthem (Drug-induced Baboon Syndrome)

- It is a bilaterally symmetrical eruption involving thighs, groin, gluteal region, and other intertriginous areas such as axillae, knees, elbows, and neck without the presence of systemic signs and symptoms.
- Penicillins and cephalosporins are the most common drugs causing such eruptions.

Drug-induced Pruritus

- It is commonly seen with opioids (morphine, codeine) antimalarials (chloroquine, mepacrine), statins, paclitaxel, and hydroxyethyl starch.
- Opioids and chloroquine cause mast cell degranulation leading to pruritus.
- Cessation of drug causes relieves the pruritus.

TABLE 2: Common drugs causing cutaneous ADR.[1]

Cutaneous ADR	Class of drugs						
	Antibiotics and antifungals	*NSAIDs*	*Anticonvulsant and drugs acting on CNS*	*Antihypertensive and antiarrhythmic*	*Anti-TB and antileprosy*	*ART*	*Antimalarials*
Exanthem	*Penicillins (Pn):** Ampicillin, amoxicillin-morbilliform rash *Cephalosporin (CS):** Cephalexin, cefaclor, cefuroxime, cefotaxime, ceftriaxone *Macrolides:** Azithromycin, roxithromycin *Vancomycin:* Red man syndrome *Sulfonamides:** Cotrimoxazole	*Aspirin:* Scarlatiniform eruptions *Diclofenac* *Indomethacin*	*Phenytoin:* Carbamazepine, valproate Barbiturates Phenothiazines	Digitalis	INH[1] Dapsone	NVP[2], Efavirenz Abacavir TDF[3] Ritonavir Indinavir Tipranavir	–
Urticaria	*Penicillins:*CS—* Cephalexin, cefaclor, ceftriaxone, cefixime, cefoperazone *Macrolides:** Erythromycin *Tetracyclines** *Sulfonamides* *Fluoroquinolones* *Antifungals:* Fluconazole, ketoconazole, griseofulvin*	Aspirin* Ibuprofen* Naproxen* Piroxicam Phenylbutazone Paracetamol	Amitriptyline Paroxetine Fluoxetine	*ACE Inhibitors** Captopril Angioedema due to bradykinin levels	INH Ethambutol	Abacavir	–
Lichenoid eruptions	Minocycline Terbinafine (drug-induced LE)	Diclofenac	Lithium, phenothiazines	*ACE inhibitors:* Captopril-eczematous lesions *Beta blockers:* Atenolol *Thiazides* *Procainamide,* Quinidine, diltiazem, hydralazine, *Statins,* *Methyldopa* *LE-like lesions*	–	–	CHQ[4]
Fixed drug eruptions	*Tetracyclines:* Doxycycline *Aminoglycosides:* Streptomycin *Fluoroquinolones:* Ciprofloxacin *Cotrimoxazole* *Metronidazole* *Penicillins* *Itraconazole* *Amphotericin (gray syndrome)*	Aspirin, phenylbutazone, diclofenac, naproxen (bullous eruptions)	Phenytoin, phenobarbitone Barbiturates, codeine	Quinidine	Dapsone, rare with INH	Rare	Rare
Acneiform eruptions	Rare	Rare	Phenytoin, carbamazepine Lithium	Rare	INH, rifampicin	Rare	Rare
Photosensitivity	*Tetracyclines:* Doxycycline, minocycline *Macrolides:* Azithromycin *Fluoroquinolones:* Sparfloxacin, ciprofloxacin, *Sulfonamides:* Cotrimoxazole *Griseofulvin*	Naproxen	Imipramine	Thiazide diuretics Quinidine	Clofazimine		CHQ

Contd...

Contd...

Cutaneous ADR	Class of drugs						
	Antibiotics and antifungals	NSAIDs	Anticonvulsant and drugs acting on CNS	Antihypertensive and anti-arrhythmic	Anti TB and antileprosy	ART	Antimalarials
Pigmentary changes	*Tetracyclines:* Doxycycline, minocycline	–	Mephenytoin	–	Clofazimine-mahogany brown pigmentation	Zidovudine	Mepacrine (acquired ochronosis)
Pellagroid changes	–	–	Phenytoin Phenobarbital	–	INH	–	–
Ichthyotic changes	–			Pravastatin Nicotinic acid	INH Clofazimine	–	–
Erythema nodosum	*Penicillins Sulfonamides*	Ibuprofen	–	–	–	–	–
Pityriasis rosea-like lesions	*Metronidazole Terbinafine*	Ibuprofen, naproxen	Clozapine, lamotrigine, nortriptyline	ACE inhibitors	–	–	–

*Drugs strongly associated
(ACE: angiotensin-converting enzyme; CNS: central nervous system; CHQ: chloroquine; INH: isoniazid; LE: lupus erythematosus; NSAIDs: nonsteroidal anti-inflammatory drugs; NVP: nevirapine; TDF: tenofovir)
Mnemonic: AAAAAAN (A–Antibiotics and Antifungals, A—Anticonvulsants, A—Antihypertensives, A—Anti-TB and Anti-leprosy drugs, A–ART, A–Antimalarials, N—NSAIDs)

Drug-induced Urticaria and Angioedema

Urticaria is the second most common CADR after maculopapular exanthem.

Mechanism and Pathophysiology

- Aspirin causes idiopathic urticaria by nonallergic mechanism and the reaction is dose dependent.
- Release of mediators from mast cells either directly (radiocontrast media, local anesthetics, and dextran) or indirectly by cross-linking of immunoglobulin E (IgE) on mast cell after repeated exposure to drug.
- Angiotensin-converting enzyme (ACE) inhibitors also inhibit bradykininase thereby leading to increased levels of bradykinin which is responsible for angioedema.

Clinical Features

- Urticaria and angioedema arise within 24–36 hours and occur when the drug is first ingested. ACE inhibitors may take much longer time.
- Withdrawal of the drug leads to improvement in 24–48 hours.

Common drugs causing urticarial and angioedema have been summarized in ***Table 2****:*

- Biologics, anesthetic agents, neuromuscular blockers, and analgesics have been reported to cause anaphylaxis.
- Serum sickness like illness can be caused by penicillins and cephalosporins (such as cefaclor).

Management

Oral antihistamines and oral corticosteroids can be given. Selective cyclooxygenase-2 (COX-2) inhibitors can be given in NSAID sensitive patients.

Lichenoid Eruptions[6]

Lichenoid drug reactions may be clinically seen as lesions of lichen planus or lupus erythematosus and are characterized by band-like lymphocytic infiltrate the dermoepidermal junction.

Mechanism and Pathophysiology

- Offending drug binds to major histocompatibility complex on keratinocytes and Langerhans cells and T-cells are directed against this complex.
- HLA-DR4 and HLADQB1 have been linked with drug-induced lupus erythematosus (LE) such as hydralazine and minocycline.

Clinical Features

- Resembles classical lichen planus (LP)/LE and it is difficult to differentiate clinically.
- Apoptotic keratinocytes are more commonly seen with drug-induced LP/LE and the number of plasma cells and eosinophils is also higher as compared to classical LE/LP.

Gold, mercury amalgam, and penicillamine have been reported to cause lichenoid eruptions. Other common drugs causing lichenoid eruptions have been listed in **Table 2**.

Common drugs causing LE-like lesions have been listed in **Table 2**.

Management

Potent to superpotent topical corticosteroids such as clobetasol propionate 0.05% ointment/cream can be used.

Fixed Drug Eruptions

Fixed duration eruption (FDE) is a cutaneous ADR characterized by well-defined lesions occurring at the same sites each time the causative drug is given.

Mechanism and Pathophysiology

- FDE is a type of delayed type hypersensitivity.
- Tissue resident memory T cells (T_{RM}) are memory T cells that reside in the tissue and are responsible for FDE.
- Exposure of the drug everytime leads to reactivation of these TRM and release of interferon gamma (IFN-γ) leading to drug eruptions occurring at the same site.

Clinical Features

- *Morphology*: Sharply defined round to oval erythematous plaque which evolves to become dusky and violaceous. Extensive FDE may sometimes present as bullous lesions—generalized bullous FDE (GBFDE).
- *Distribution*: Lips, genitals, palms, and soles.
- *Variants of FDE: Pigmented and nonpigmented FDE, generalized FDE, linear FDE, wandering FDE, bullous FDE, urticarial FDE, eczematous and psoriasiform FDE, erythema dyschromicum perstans-like eruption.*
- Common drugs causing FDE have been listed in **Table 1**. Other drugs causing FDE are:
  - Carbocysteine—over face
  - Methimazole—over trunk and extremities
  - Pseudoephedrine.

Differential Diagnosis (Fig. 2)

Generalized bullous FDE must be differentiated from toxic epidermal necrolysis (TEN) by:

- Prior history of similar episodes
- Sparing of mucosal areas
- Absence of multiple purpuric/target lesions and presence of intervening normal skin.

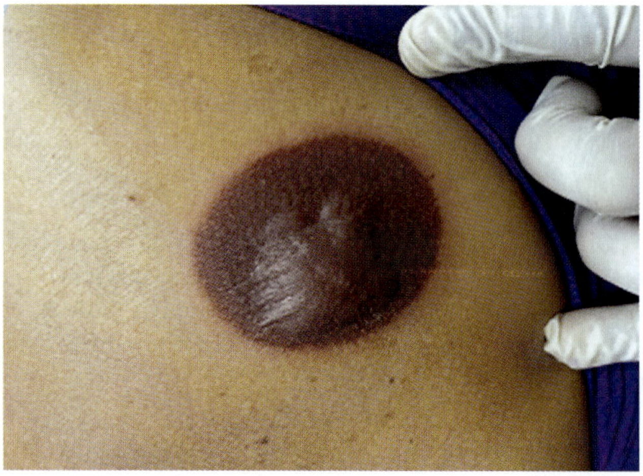

Fig. 2: Bullous fixed drug reaction.
Courtesy: Dr Subhra Sankar Sahoo.

Management

- Medium potency topical corticosteroids and systemic corticosteroids must be given in multiple lesions.
- GBDFE needs hospitalization and intensive care.

Drug-induced Acneiform Eruptions

These are characterized by:

- A medical history for drug intake
- Sudden onset of eruptions
- Absence of triggering factors
- An unusual age of onset.

Clinical Features

Morphology: Monomorphic papules and pustules.

Distribution: Arms, lower back and genitalia (beyond the seborrheic areas).

Common drugs causing acneiform eruptions are:

- *Corticosteroids*: Oral and topical
- *Anabolic steroids*: Danazol/stanazol
- Lithium
- Vitamin B_{12}, Vitamin B_6
- Cyclosporine
- *Epidermal growth factor receptor inhibitors*: Cetuximab.

Other commonly used drugs causing acneiform eruptions have been listed in **Table 1**.

MANAGEMENT

2.5/5% benzoyl peroxide gel for 2–3 weeks.

Drug-induced Erythema Nodosum

Erythema nodosum is a cutaneous reactive septal panniculitis which is a type IV hypersensitivity to various antigens, like medications.

Clinical Features

- *Symptoms*: Fever might be present
- *Morphology*: Symmetrical, erythematous, and tender subcutaneous nodules, or plaques
- *Distribution*: Anterior aspects of limbs
- *Course*: Self-limiting and resolves within 2–4 weeks after withdrawal of the offending drug.

Common drugs causing erythema nodosum are oral contraceptives and hormonal replacement therapy.

Other drugs causing erythema nodosum have been listed in **Table 1**.

Management: Self-limiting. NSAIDs may be given.

Severe Cutaneous Adverse Drug Reactions[7]

Heterogeneous group of delayed hypersensitivity reactions to drugs **(Table 3)**.

MNEMONICS are mentioned in **Table 3**.

TABLE 3: Drugs causing SCARs.

SCADRs	*Common drugs implicated*		
	Antibiotics	*Anticonvulsants*	*Others*
Acute generalized exanthematous pustulosis (AGEP)	• Ciprofloxacin • *PAIDS:* Penicillin/phenytoin, amoxycillin, allopurinol, azithromycin, isoniazid, doxycycline, and diclofenac, streptomycin and sulfonamides	• Phenytoin • Carbamazepine	• Chloroquine • HCQ • Diltiazem • Nifedipine • Diclofenac • Furosemide • Allopurinol • Acetaminophen
Drug reaction with eosinophilia and systemic symptoms (DRESS)	• Vancomycin • Amoxycillin • Piperacillin-tazobactam • Minocycline • Sulfasalazine • Dapsone (DDS) • Sulfadiazine	• Phenytoin • Carbamazepine • Lamotrigine	• Allopurinol • Omeprazole • Furosemide • Ibuprofen
Drug-induced generalized exfoliative dermatitis	• Penicillins • Cotrimoxazole • Cephalosporins • Vancomycin • ATT • ART	• Phenytoin • Carbamazepine • Phenobarbital	• Allopurinol • Acitretin • NSAIDs • Omeprazole/lansoprazole • CCBs • Lithium • Imatinib, INF-α
Stevens–Johnson syndrome/ toxic epidermal necrolysis (SJS/ TEN)	• Sulfamethoxazole and other sulfa antibiotics • Sulfasalazine • Nevirapine • Rifampicin • Isoniazid • Tetracycline	• *CLAPS:* Carbamazepine, lamotrigine, allopurinol, AKT (isoniazid), ART (nevirapine), allopurinol, phenytoin/ phenobarbital, sulfonamides	• Allopurinol • Oxicam NSAIDs • Salicylates

(ART: antiretroviral therapy; ATT: antitubercular therapy; CCBs: calcium channel blockers; DDS: diaminodiphenyl sulfone; HCQ: hydroxychloroquine; IFN-α: interferon α; NSAIDs: nonsteroidal anti-inflammatory drugs; SCADRs: severe cutaneous adverse drug reactions; SCARs: severe cutaneous adverse reactions)

Acute Generalized Exanthematous Pustulosis (Exanthemic Pustular Psoriasis, Pustular Drug Reaction, Toxic Pustuloderma)

- *Clinical features*: Appearance of hundreds of sterile nonfollicular pustules on edematous erythematous base at flexural sites such as neck, axillae, inframammary, and inguinal folds, typically 2–5 days after ingestion of culprit drug **(Table 3)**.
- Fever>38°C.
- *Effector mechanism*: Activation and proliferation of specific CD4 and CD8 T cells, perforin and granzyme B, and Fas ligand mechanisms to induce apoptosis.
- *Histopathology*: Spongiosis, epidermal pustule formation, and leukocytoclastic dermal infiltrate.
- *Laboratory findings*: Leukocytosis, typically neutrophilia $>7 \times 10^9$/L and eosinophilia.
- Hypocalcemia.
- *Management*:
  - Intravenous (IV) fluid and careful hemodynamic monitoring
  - Oral corticosteroids
  - Emollients.

Drug Reaction with Eosinophilia and Systemic Symptoms/Drug Hypersensitivity Syndrome

- Idiosyncratic drug reaction characterized by widespread exanthematous eruption with facial edema with eosinophilia, lymphadenopathy (>2 cm), fever and systemic involvement usually 2–6 weeks after administration of culprit drugs **(Table 3)**.
- *Cutaneous findings*: Urticated papular exanthem (widespread papules and plaques with cutaneous edema), morbilliform eruption, erythroderma, erythema multiforme (EM)-like lesions.
- *Hematological findings*: Eosinophilia (most common), leukocytosis, lymphopenia/lymphocytosis, thrombocytosis/thrombocytopenia, pancytopenia, and atypical lymphocytes on peripheral smear.
- *Effector mechanism*: T-cell-mediated perforin-granzyme B as well as Fas-/FasL-dependent cell death.
- *Systemic involvement*:
  - *Liver*: Hepatocellular and obstructive patterns of hepatitis
  - Mild to transient hepatitis with alanine aminotransferase (ALT) < 250 IU/L to fulminant hepatic failure requiring liver transplantation

- *Renal*: Interstitial nephritis. Hematuria, proteinuria and urinary eosinophils
- *Cardiac*: Pericarditis, myocarditis—manifesting as chest pain, dyspnea, tachycardia, hypotension, and signs of pleural/pericardial effusion. Elevated cardiac enzymes
- Acute necrotizing eosinophilic myocarditis (ANEM)
- *Pulmonary*: Pleural effusion, pleuritis, and acute interstitial pneumonia
- *Central nervous system (CNS)*: Seizures, cranial nerve (CN) palsies, limbic encephalitis, and human herpesvirus 6 (HHV-6) may be demonstrated by polymerase chain reaction (PCR) in cerebrospinal fluid (CSF)
- *Gastrointestinal*: Eosinophilic esophagitis, ulcerative colitis with or without eosinophilia
- Hypo-/hyperthyroidism in convalescent phase.

- *Complications and sequelae*:
  - Fulminant liver failure, late-onset interstitial nephritis, persistent interstitial pneumonitis, and myocarditis
  - Autoimmune phenomena such as LE and autoimmune thyroid disease. Presence of antinuclear antibodies (ANAs), anti-thyroglobulin antibody, and anti-TPO (thyroid peroxidase)
- *Management*:
  - Intravenous fluids, thermoregulation
  - Catheterization to facilitate fluid balance management
  - Supplemental oxygen
  - *First-line treatment*: Oral corticosteroids 1–3 mg/kg/day
  - *Second-line treatment*: Cyclosporine, intravenous immunoglobulin (IVIg)
  - *Third-line treatment*:
    - Plasmapheresis and extracorporeal membrane oxygenation (ECMO)
    - Rituximab
    - Valganciclovir (virus reactivation theory)
    - *Severe liver failure*: N-acetylcystine.

Drug-induced Generalized Exfoliative Dermatitis

- Drug-induced erythema, pruritus, and scaling effecting more than 90% BSA **(*see* Table 3)**.
- *Pathophysiology*: Increased epidermal turnover, decreased transit time an increased mitotic activity.
- Associated constitutional symptoms such as malaise, hypothermia, or fever as well as signs of lymphadenopathy, cardiomegaly, and high output cardiac failure.
- *Management*: Identification and withdrawal of offending drug and initiation of systemic corticosteroids.

Stevens–Johnson Syndrome/Toxic Epidermal Necrolysis (Figs. 3 and 4)[2]

- Severe mucocutaneous drug eruption characterized by blistering and epidermal sloughing typically 7–10 days after administration of culprit drug **(*see* Table 3)**.
- *Mortality rates*: 1–5% in Stevens–Johnson syndrome (SJS), 10–15% in transitional SJS/TEN, and 30–40% in TEN.[1]
- *Effector mechanism*: CD8+ cytotoxic T lymphocyte-mediated Fas-FasL and granulysin-mediated apoptosis.
- *Clinical presentation*: Malaise, fever, upper respiratory tract symptoms → atypical targets or purpuric macules on face, upper torso, and proximal limbs which gradually progress → confluence of erythematous lesions → blistering (positive Nikolsky sign—detachable epidermis).
- *Body surface area (BSA) involvement*: <10%: SJS, >30%: TEN, 10–30%: SJS/TEN overlap.
- *Sequelae*:
  - *Mucocutaneous*: Acute skin failure, mucosal stricture and stenosis, loss of nails, and hypopigmentation
  - *Ocular*: Synechia, xerophthalmia, symblepharon, corneal ulcers, panophthalmitis, and blindness
  - *Pulmonary*: Pulmonary edema, bacterial pneumonitis, and atelectasis
  - *Gastrointestinal*: Mucosal erosions and bloody diarrhea
  - *Renal*: Hematuria and proteinuria.

SCORTEN

SCORTEN (Severity-of-Illness Score for Toxic Epidermal Necrolysis) is a simple assessment tool to decide severity and predict mortality in cases having TEN. The parameters versus their score are discussed in **Table 4**. Score versus predicted mortality is discussed in **Table 5**.

- *Investigations at presentation*:
  - Complete blood count (CBC)
  - Urea and electrolytes
  - Amylase
  - Bicarbonate
  - Glucose
  - Liver function test (LFT), liver function test (RFT)
  - Erythrocyte sedimentation rate (ESR), C-reactive protein (CRP)
  - Coagulation studies
  - Mycoplasma serology
  - ANA and extractable antigen
  - Complement
  - Indirect immunofluorescence.

TABLE 4: SCORTEN parameters and their score.

Risk factor	*Points*
Age > 40 years	1
Presence of malignancy	1
Heart rate > 120 beats/min	1
Epidermal detachment >10% body surface area (BSA)	1
Serum urea > 10 mmol/L	1
Serum glucose > 14 mmol/L	1
Bicarbonate < 20 mmol/L	1

TABLE 5: SCORTEN versus predicted mortality rate.

Score	*Predicted mortality rate*
0–1	3%
2	12%
3	35%
4	58%
≥5	90%

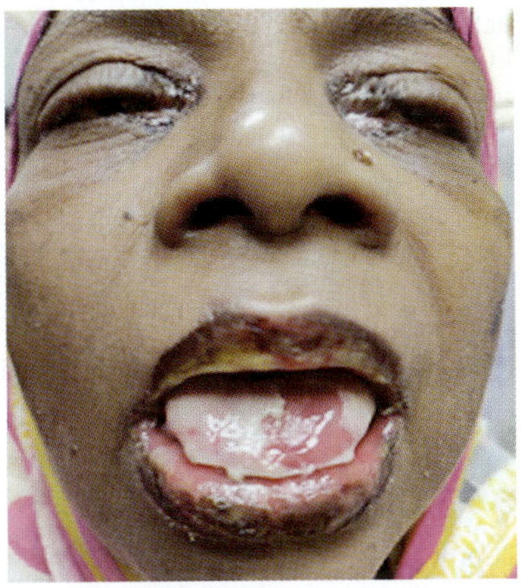

Fig. 3: Stevens–Johnson syndrome.
Courtesy: Dr Subhra Sankar Sahoo.

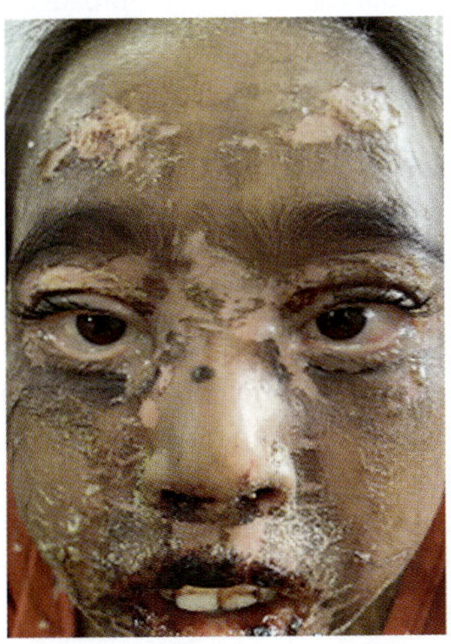

Fig. 4: Toxic epidermal necrolysis.
Courtesy: Dr Subhra Sankar Sahoo.

- *Management*:
  - Withdrawal of culprit drug
  - ICU admission
  - *Intensive care including:*
    - Thermoregulation at around 30–32°C to reduce calorie losses through skin and resultant shivering
    - *Fluid replacement*: Calculated according to Parkland's formula:

  Fluid requirement for first 24 hours = 4 mL/kg body weight × percentage of BSA involved.
  3/4th of the calculated requirement is given in first 8 hours and the rest in remaining 16 hours.
  Ringer lactate is the fluid of choice.
  Thereafter, fluid replacement = Urine output + 500 mL:
  - *Nutritional regimen*: Enteral preferred over parenteral
  - *Analgesia*: Morphine, ketamine, or gamma aminobutyric acid (GABA)
  - Preventing/treating infection
  - Topical therapy/dressing to minimize heat and fluid loss as well as prevent infections
  - Systemic corticosteroid (0.5–1 mg/kg prednisolone for 10 days or 500 mg IV methylprednisolone for 3 days) can be started within first 72 hours of onset to reduce mortality and morbidity. However, it should be rapidly tapered after 3–5 days.

  Long-term steroid administration can hamper wound healing, mask underlying sepsis or can lead to gastrointestinal bleeding. It increases hospital stay and mortality:
  - Cyclosporine (3–4 mg/kg/day) for up to 2 weeks followed by weaning for 2 weeks. It inhibits T-lymphocytes, macrophages as well as keratinocytes involved in TEN and also has antiapoptotic properties. Encouraging results reported if instituted early and for uncomplicated, limited disease.
  - Intravenous immunoglobulin (0.5–1 g/kg/day for 3–4 consecutive days) within 2–3 days of onset of symptoms. Role is debatable.

Adverse Drug Reactions in Special Situations

Cutaneous ADR due to Radiotherapy and Chemotherapy[8,9]

Radiotherapy consists of irradiating the affected area with high energy ionizing radiation in order to destroy the tumor cells.

Clinical features:
- *Acute radiation dermatitis*: Within 90 days of exposure; erythema and edema → moist desquamation → necrosis and ulceration
- *Chronic radiation dermatitis*: 15 days to 10 years; hypopigmented and atrophic skin
- Postirradiation morphea
- Vitiligo.

Management:
- Emollients (in mild cases)
- *Topical antiseptics*: Silver sulfadiazine
- Moderate potency steroids.

Chemotherapy-induced ADR

Radiation recall:
- Drug-induced inflammatory eruption confined to area that was previously irradiated in radiation recall.
- It usually occurs on an average of 8 days after irradiation.
- Commonly due to actinomycin D, doxorubicin, and etoposide.

  Other ADR have been summarized in **Table 6**.

  Drugs causing/aggravating bullous diseases, psoriasis,

TABLE 6: Chemotherapy associated cutaneous adverse drug reaction (ADR).[8]

Cutaneous ADR	*Pathophysiology*	*Clinical features*	*Offending drugs*	*Management*
Toxic erythema of chemotherapy: 1. Palmoplantar dysesthesia 2. Intertriginous eruption 3. Neutrophilic eccrine hidradenitis	Direct toxicity via excretion through eccrine ducts → palms and soles involved	Pain, burning, pruritus with papulovesicular lesion over palms and soles	Cytarabine Doxorubicin 5-fluorouracil	Symptomatic, spontaneous resolution
Papulopustular eruption	Growth arrest of keratinocytes → inflammation	Follicular pustules and papules over trunk	Epidermal growth factor inhibitors (EGFRs) (cetuximab, panitumumab), tyrosine kinase inhibitors (erlotinib)	Topical hydrocortisone 1%, oral doxycycline 100 mg BD
Alopecia (anagen effluvium)	Cytostatic effect on hair follicles in anagen	Diffuse alopecia, reversible and dose dependent	Paclitaxel Doxorubicin Cyclophosphamide	Scalp cooling → vasoconstriction → slower uptake of drug, minoxidil 2% lotion
Nail changes	Direct toxicity to nail plate	Onycholysis, onychomadesis, Beau's lines, leukonychia, melanonychia, pyogenic granuloma	EGFR inhibitor	Topical corticosteroids, doxycycline
Hyperpigmentation	Direct toxic effect on melanocytes Pigmentary effect of the deposited drug	Flagellate hyperpigmentation — multiple macular linear streaks, generalized	Bleomycin Busulfan Fluorouracil	–
Photosensitivity	Phototoxic, photoallergic and UV recall	Erythema and burning over anterior chest	5-fluorouracil Methotrexate Dactinomycin	Broad-spectrum sunscreens, topical corticosteroids

TABLE 7: ADR due to newer drugs/biologicals.[10]

Biological drug	*Common cutaneous adverse effects*
Rituximab	• Infusion-related reaction such as rash, pruritus, or urticaria, angioedema • Severe mucocutaneous reactions in the form of SJS, lichenoid dermatitis, vesiculobullous dermatitis, and paraneoplastic pemphigus • Rash, exfoliation, vasculitis
Infliximab	• Cutaneous vasculitis • Drug rash • *Others:* Erythema nodosum, Sweet's syndrome, bullous eruption, necrotizing fasciitis, cutaneous ulcerations, atopic dermatitis, nevi
Etanercept	• Injection site bleeding, bruising • Cutaneous vasculitis • Lupus-like syndrome • EM and TEN
Adalimumab	• *Injection site reaction:* Erythema, edema, itching • Infectious skin complications such as cellulitis, erysipelas, herpes zoster
Secukinumab	• Candidial infection • Oral herpes, tinea pedis, otitis externa • Urticaria
Omalizumab	• Pruritus, dermatitis • Injection site reactions • Anaphylaxis

(ADR: adverse drug reaction; EM: erythema multiforme; TEN: toxic epidermal necrolysis)

connective tissue diseases are mentioned in **Table 8**. Salient points to differentiate drug induced versus idiopathic aggravations are mentioned in **Table 9**.

Diagnosis of Drug Reactions

Definite drug reaction can be considered when:

- Temporal relationship can be established with drug levels in body fluids
- Recognized response to suspected drug
- Improved with drug withdrawal
- Reappearance of reaction on re-exposure.

Approach to a Patient with Drug Reaction

Take detailed history of suspected drug—date of administration, formulation, and dosage along with date of onset of lesions →

History of previous medications and drug reactions → any associated medical/surgical illnesses→ drug provocation challenge (administration of test dose of the suspected drug after recovery for confirmation).

Test dosing is to be avoided in cases of SCADRs and anaphylactic reactions.

Causality assessment is mainly done through:

- Clinical, i.e., Naranjo scale
- In vivo and Ex vivo tests.

TABLE 8: Drugs aggravating chronic skin diseases.

Disease	*Drugs*
Psoriasis	*Drugs with well-known causal association:* • Beta blockers • Lithium • Synthetic antimalarials • NSAIDs • Tetracyclines • *Antimalarial:* Chloroquine *Drugs with considerable but insufficient data:* • ACE inhibitors • Interferons • Antifungals *Emerging reports of new drugs:* • TNF-α blockers • VEGF inhibitors • Anti-PD 1 drugs • Other biologics *Others*
Bullous disorders	*Pemphigus:* • *Thiol drugs:* Penicillamine, captopril, and tiopronine • *Phenol drugs:* Aspirin, heroin, rifampin, and levodopa • *Nonthiol and nonphenol drugs:* NSAIDs, and calcium-channel blockers *Bullous pemphigoid:* Diuretics (furosemide), ACE inhibitors (captopril), and antibiotics, NSAIDs; ibuprofen, phenacetin, penicillamine, etanercept *Epidermolysis bullosa acquisita:* Penicillins, cephalosporins, diclofenac, captopril, and glibenclamide
Autoimmune diseases	*Systemic sclerosis:* Bleomycin, paclitaxel, pentazocine, cocaine, appetite suppressants, and D-penicillamine *Systemic lupus erythematosus:* Sulfadiazine, hydralazine, procainamide, isoniazid, methyldopa, quinidine, minocycline, chlorpromazine

(ACE: angiotensin-converting enzyme; NSAIDs: nonsteroidal anti-inflammatory drugs; TNF-α: tumor necrosis factor alpha; VEGF: vascular endothelial growth factor)

Drug Skin Tests

It is useful for CADRs in which immediate or delayed hypersensitivity is involved. It can be performed within 6 months after the reaction.

Test includes:

- Intradermal testing using a sterile diluted solution of suspected drug with a control performed with 0.9% normal saline.
- *Skin window technique*: Surface application of suspected drug over abraded skin.
- Passive transfer tests.
- Patch testing.
- Prick test.

Other in vivo tests:

- Detection of reaginic antibody
- Basophil degranulation test
- Release of histamine from sensitized tissues and leukocytes
- RAST (radioallergosorbent test for specific IgE antibodies)
- Leukocyte migration test
- Hemagglutination test.

Ex vivo tests: Lymphocyte transformation tests.

TABLE 9: Drug induced versus idiopathic aggravation in chronic skin diseases.

Condition	*Drug induced*	*Idiopathic*
Psoriasis[11]	Exacerbation of preexisting psoriasis → remission following treatment discontinuation is seen in case of drug-induced psoriasis; while certain drugs can aggravate psoriasis and on discontinuation remission is not seen Drug can also induce new lesions over uninvolved skin or can induce psoriasis de novo in a case not having personal/past history of psoriasis	No history of drug ingestion
Bullous disorders:		
• *Pemphigus*[12]	Pemphigus foliaceous	Oral and skin lesions
• *Bullous pemphigoid*[13,14]	Mostly skin lesions Younger patients Rare relapse Induced forms of BP are usually transient, often localized and generally disappear after discontinuation of the drug	Elderly patients
• *Epidermolysis bullosa acquisita*[15]	Vancomycin	
Autoimmune diseases:		
• *SLE*[16]	More common in males	No gender predisposition
• *Systemic sclerosis*	Clinical features less severe	More severe clinical features

(SLE: systemic lupus erythematosus)

Prevention of Cutaneous Adverse Drug Reaction

- *Identification of offending drug and refraining from consumption of the drug responsible for CADR*: Education of the patient plays an important role in the prevention of ADR. This can be done by providing lists of drugs which have been responsible for CADR to patients **(Tables 2, 3, 7, 10 and 11)**.
- *Pharmacovigilance:*[19] Pharmacovigilance is the science of collecting, monitoring, researching, assessing, and evaluating information from healthcare providers and patients on the adverse effects of medications, biological

TABLE 10: Drugs causing hair changes.[17]

Hair changes	*Drugs*
Hair loss	
Telogen effluvium	• Heparin and its derivatives • Isoniazid • Indinavir • Beta blockers (propranolol and metoprolol), ACE inhibitors (captopril) • Antidepressants such as fluoxetine, lithium, levodopa • Systemic retinoids, tacrolimus • MMF • Metformin, glibenclamide • Antithyroid drugs • Terbinafine
Anagen effluvium	• Antineoplastic agents and immunosuppressives • Levodopa • Colchicine
Hypertrichosis	• Beta blockers (atenolol), CCBs (nifedipine, verapamil) • Cyclosporine, methotrexate, corticosteroids • Minoxidil • Psoralens • Retinoids • Streptomycin, ethambutol • Indomethacin, TCAs (imipramine), vincristine, zidovudine
Hair discoloration	
Darkening	• Indinavir, zidovudine • Levodopa/carbidopa • Minoxidil • Verapamil • Acitretin
Lightening/ graying	• Benzoyl peroxide • Cyclosporine • Hydroquinone • Valproic acid • Inhaled corticosteroids • IFN-α, Imatinib
Color changes	• Selenium sulfide (yellow) • Anthralin (yellow)

(ACE: angiotensin-converting enzyme; CCBs: calcium channel blockers; MMF: mycophenolate mofetil; IFN-α: interferon α; TCAs: tricyclic antidepressants)

TABLE 11: Drugs causing nail changes.[18]

Nail changes	*Drugs*
Nail discoloration	
Melanonychia	• Cyclophosphamide, methotrexate, 5-FU imatinib • Hydroxyurea • Psoralen • Zidovudine (black), lamivudine (longitudinal brown/black bands) • Phenothiazines, clofazimine • Chloroquine (blue-black) • Lithium (golden) • Heparin (transverse red lines), carotene (yellow) ketoconazole (longitudinal pigmented bands), lead (hyperpigmentation), silver (slate blue)
Photo-onycholysis	• Tetracyclines, fluoroquinolones • Sulfonamides • NSAIDs • Griseofulvin • Thiazides • Chlorpromazine • Captopril • OCPs • Quinine • Paroxetine • Psoralens
Onychomadesis	• Azithromycin • Sulfonamides • Lead
Pitting	• Fluorine, mepacrine
Nail pterygium	• Nifedipine
Onychocryptosis	• Isotretinoin • Protease inhibitors • Terbinafine
Increased rate of nail growth	• Fluconazole, itraconazole • L-dopa • OCPs • Retinoids
Decreased rate of nail growth	• Cyclophosphamide, azathioprine, cyclosporine, methotrexate • Retinoids • Heparin

(NSAIDs: nonsteroidal anti-inflammatory drugs; OCPs: oral contraceptive pills)

products, herbalism, and traditional medicines with a view to identify new information about hazards associated with medicines and preventing harm to the patient.

Adverse Event Reporting System

- It is a computerized database which has been designed for FDA's post-marketing surveillance programs for all FDA approved drugs.
- MedWatch is the FDA safety information and adverse event reporting program.

National Pharmacovigilance Program of India

Identified 179 ADRs Monitoring Centers (AMCs) across the country which report to the National Coordination Center (NCC) with the help of softwares developed for international networking such as VigiFlow and WHO-Uppsala Monitoring Centre (UMC).

Currently, the contribution of India to the WHO global Individual Case Safety Reports (ICSRs) database is 3%.

GENERAL MANAGEMENT

- Suspected drug causing lesions to be confirmed. Avoid the offending drugs and other cross reactive medications.
- *Relevant investigations*: Basic laboratory testing—CBC/absolute EC/LFT/RFT.

Specific tests before starting drug: Glucose 6-phosphate dehydrogenase (G6PD) (dapsone)/thiopurine methyltransferase (TPMT) (azathioprine)/HLA testing (as mentioned in **Table 1**):

- *Treatment*:
  - Topical treatment
  - Topical corticosteroids/emollient
  - *Oral*: Antihistamines and oral corticosteroids (0.5–1 mg/kg/day of prednisone).
- *Hospitalization indicated when*:
  - *Cutaneous*: Skin surface > 60%, erythema confluence, facial edema, skin pain, palpable purpura, skin necrosis, bullae or epidermal detachment, positive Nikolsky sign, mucosal erosions, urticaria and/or tongue edema.
  - *General*: High fever, lymphadenopathy, arthralgia, or arthritis, expiratory dyspnea, hypotension.
  - *Biological*: Eosinophilia >1,000/mm^3, lymphocytosis with atypical lymphocytes, and liver function abnormalities.

KEY POINTS

- Awareness about potential ADRs of commonly prescribed drugs is essential.
- Most of the benign ADRs are self-limiting and need supportive treatment.
- Severe cutaneous adverse reactions are associated with high degree of morbidity, mortality, complications, and sequelae. Prompt identification and earliest possible withdrawal of the drug is the essence.
- Systemic corticosteroids are helpful in DRESS and AGEP.
- Early institution and fast tapering of systemic steroids can be considered in SJS/TEN in resource limited setup but it must be avoided for longer duration.
- There are encouraging reports on benefit of cyclosporine when instituted early and in uncomplicated cases.
- Biologics, anticancer drugs, and radiotherapy are being now increasingly used and awareness about their ADRs is essential.
- Association between HLA genotype and ADR is established for some drugs. HLA testing in susceptible population prior to institution of those drugs is an important preventive measure.
- Patient must be given a comprehensive list of drugs to be avoided. Even first-degree relatives of the patient must be advised to avoid drugs causing SCARs.
- It is a moral and ethical responsibility of every treating doctor to take part in National Pharmacovigilance Program of India (PvPi).

REFERENCES

1. Pujara SB, Shah BJ. Drug reactions. In: Sacchidanand S, Oberai C, Inamadar AC (Eds). IADVL Textbook of Dermatology, 4th edition. India: Bhalani Publishers; 2015. pp. 2344-95.
2. Hoetzenecker W, Nägeli M, Mehra ET, Jensen AN, Saulite I, Schmid-Grendelmeier P, et al. Adverse cutaneous drug eruptions: current understanding. Semin Immunopathol. 2016;38(1):75-86.
3. Adler NR, Aung AK, Ergen EN, Trubiano J, Goh MSY, Phillips EJ. Recent advances in the understanding of severe cutaneous adverse reactions. Br J Dermatol. 2017;177(5):1234-47.
4. Yip VL, Marson AG, Jorgensen AL, Pirmohamed M, Alfirevic A. HLA genotype and carbamazepine-induced cutaneous adverse drug reactions: a systematic review. Clin Pharmacol Ther. 2012;92:757-65.
5. Arden-Jones MR, Lee HY. Benign cutaneous adverse reactions to drugs. In: Griffiths C, Barker J, Bleiker TO, Chalmers R, Creamer D (Eds). Rook's Textbook of Dermatology, 9th edition. Oxford: Wiley Blackwell; 2016. pp. 118.1-118.17.
6. Halevy S, Shai A. Lichenoid drug eruptions. J Am Acad Dermatol. 1993;29(2 Pt 1):249-55.
7. Walsh S, Lee HY, Creamer D. Severe cutaneous adverse reactions to drugs. In: Griffiths C, Barker J, Bleiker TO, Chalmers R, Creamer D (Eds). Rook's Textbook of Dermatology, 9th edition. Oxford: Wiley Blackwell; 2016. pp. 119.1-119.23.
8. Fearfield L, Natkunarajah J. Cutaneous side effects of chemotherapy and radiotherapy. In: Griffiths C, Barker J, Bleiker TO, Chalmers R, Creamer D (Eds). Rook's Textbook of Dermatology, 9th edition. Oxford: Wiley Blackwell; 2016. pp. 120.1-120.14.
9. Hymes SR, Strom EA, Fife C. Radiation dermatitis: clinical presentation, pathophysiology, and treatment 2006. J Am Acad Dermatol. 2006;54:28-46.
10. Dogra S, Daroach M. Adverse effects of biologics: feared or real? In: Neema S, Chatterjee M (Eds). Handbook of Biologics and Biosimilars in Dermatology, 1st edition. New Delhi: Jaypee Brothers Medical Publishers; 2018. pp. 206-18.
11. Balak DM, Hajdarbegovic E. Drug-induced psoriasis: clinical perspectives. Psoriasis (Auckl). 2017;7:87-94.
12. Pile HD, Yarrarapu SNS, Crane JS. Drug Induced Pemphigus. Treasure Island (FL): StatPearls Publishing; 2020.
13. Kanahara SM, Agrawal A. Drug-induced bullous pemphigoid. J Gen Intern Med. 2016;31(11):1393-4.
14. Rawson K, Vinod S, Sreenivasan B, Roy G. Drug-induced bullous pemphigoid: a case report with review. J Indian Acad Oral Med Radiol. 2018;30(4):427-31.
15. Delbaldo C, Chen M, Friedli A, Prins C, Desmeules J, Saurat JH, et al. Drug-induced epidermolysis bullosa acquisita with antibodies to type VII collagen. J Am Acad Dermatol. 2002;46(5):S161-4.
16. Niklas K, Niklas AA, Majewski D, Puszczewicz M. Rheumatic diseases induced by drugs and environmental factors: the state-of-the-art - part one. Reumatologia. 2016;54(3):122-7.
17. Feroze Kaliyadan, Ashique KT. Cutaneous adverse drug reactions and hair. In: Gupta LK, Martin AM (Eds). IADVL's Textbook of Cutaneous Adverse Drug Reactions: A Comprehensive Guide, 1st edition. India: Bhalani Publishers; 2018. pp. 187-95.
18. Kaul S, Singhal A. Nail changes due to drugs. In: Gupta LK, Martin AM (Eds). IADVL's Textbook of Cutaneous Adverse Drug Reactions: A Comprehensive Guide, 1st edition. India: Bhalani Publishers; 2018. pp. 209-20.
19. Kalaiselvan V, Thota P, Singh GN. Pharmacovigilance Programme of India: recent developments and future perspectives. Indian J Pharmacol. 2016;48(6):624-8.

EXAMINATION QUESTIONS

1. Explain immune-mediated adverse drug reactions.
2. Discuss the pathophysiology of DRESS.
3. How will you approach to diagnosis and management of DRESS.
4. What are the pathophysiology and HPE features of DRESS.
5. Describe and discuss mechanism, pathophysiology, and clinical features of drug-induced urticarial and angioedema.
6. Explain drug-induced lichenoid eruptions and drug-induced acneiform eruptions.
7. Discuss the management of Stevens–Johnson syndrome and toxic epidermal necrolysis.
8. What are the advances in etiopathogenesis of SJS/TEN?
9. Write a short note on AGEP.

102 CHAPTER Topical Steroid Damaged Skin

Arijit Coondoo, Koushik Lahiri

INTRODUCTION

An important landmark in the history of treatment of dermatological disorders was achieved in 1952 when compound F, the first topical corticosteroid (TC), was introduced for the treatment of inflammatory disorders of the skin. For the dermatologists, TC became the ultimate healer bringing welcome relief to a large number of patients. Taking advantage of this euphoria, a number of modifications were made in the hydrocortisone molecule and TCs of higher potencies were introduced in the next few decades by the pharmaceutical companies. Whereas such molecules of various potency made the therapy of inflammatory disorders more effective they were also overused, misused, and abused indiscriminately resulting in severe local and systemic side effects as well as psychological dependence on the drug.[1] The face is the most common and most severely affected site of such abuse resulting in a phenomenon which has been labeled as "topical steroid dependent facies" (TSDF).[2] However, the face is not the only site affected in this manner—damage can affect any part of the skin particularly the folds such as groin and axilla resulting in topical steroid-damaged skin.[3]

HISTORY

As mentioned earlier, it was Sulzberger and Witten who introduced the first TC in 1952. After a decade of judicious and injudicious use in a wide range of cutaneous disorders the first reports of side effects of TC gradually started appearing in the world literature since 1963.[4] TC addiction was first reported in 1973 and the entity was fully described by Kligman and Frosch in 1979.[5] Further reports of TC addiction on the face were published under various names such as dermatitis rosaeciformis steroidica, red skin syndrome, and steroid-induced rosacea-like dermatitis.[2] In 2006, the first report of misuse of TC on face in India was published.[6] Subsequently, the entity of damage due to TC application on face and the resultant dependence on the drug was labeled as "topical steroid-dependent/damaged face" (acronym TSDF) by Lahiri in March 2008 and defined as an entity by Lahiri and Coondoo in 2016.[2] A multicentric pan-Indian study was conducted at 12 centers by the Indian Association of Dermatologists, Venereologists and Leprologists (IADVL) from April through July 2008 and the results were published in 2011.[7] Further reports of TC misuse and damage led to the publication of a symposium on this topic in the Indian Journal of Dermatology in 2014.[1] To tackle this growing menace IADVL formed the IADVL Taskforce against Topical Steroid Abuse (ITATSA) in 2014.

ETHICAL USE OF TOPICAL CORTICOSTEROID

Due to their anti-inflammatory, immunosuppressive, antiproliferative, antipruritic melanopenic, and atrophogenic effect on the skin, TCs are useful in inflammatory, immunologic, and hyperproliferative disorders **(Table 1)**.[7] Based on their vasoconstrictive effect on the skin, TCs are classified according to their potency into seven classes (USA classification). Judicious use of TC is dependent on the potency of the TC, site of application, indication, age of the patient and amount, duration, and frequency of usage **(Box 1)**. TCs of lower potencies (preferably class VI or class VII) should be applied on the thin skin of the face and folds and in the extremes of age (children and elderly) when the skin is thinner than in adults. TCs of higher potencies should not be used beyond a

TABLE 1: Principal indications of topical corticosteroids.

Eczematous disorders	• Atopic dermatitis • Contact dermatitis • Seborrheic dermatitis
Papulosquamous disorders	• Psoriasis • Lichen planus • Erythroderma
Bullous disorders	• Pemphigus • Pemphigoid
Connective tissue disorders	• Discoid lupus erythematosus • Morphea
Pigmentary disorders	• Vitiligo • Melasma (Kligman's formula)
Neutrophilic diseases	• Sweet's syndrome • Behçet's syndrome
Cutaneous malignancies	• Lymphocytoma cutis • Cutaneous T-cell leukemia • Lymphomatoid papulosis
Miscellaneous	• Alopecia areata • Papular urticaria • Lichen sclerosus et atrophicus

BOX 1: Factors of ethical use of topical corticosteroids (TC).

- *Indication*: Should be used only in proper indication; avoid in contraindicated diseases
- *Site of application*: Avoid TC of higher potency on soft sites such as face and folds
- *Potency of TC*: Should be kept in mind while prescribing
- *Age of the patient*: TC of lower potency to be applied in children and geriatric patients
- *Duration of application*: TC of higher potency should not be applied for >2 weeks

certain period (preferably 2 weeks) due to their atrophogenic potential. In such cases, once daily application along with proper amount based on finger-tip unit (FTU) is recommended. Combination of TC with other drugs such as antibiotics, antifungals, hydroquinone retinoids, etc. should be avoided or used judiciously (keeping in mind the modalities of use).[8]

PRECIPITATING FACTORS

A number of precipitating factors have contributed to the phenomenal increase in the incidence of damage to the skin due to TC. An apathetic bureaucracy, pharmaceutical companies producing unethical TC, marketing executives of such companies promoting TCs and combinations to nondermatologists including quacks, salesmen at chemists selling TCs randomly to the gullible public, dermatologists writing incomplete prescriptions, and prescription repeating by patients are the major factors which contribute to this massive misuse of TC in India leading to almost an epidemic of TC damaged skin.[1] Pharmaceutical companies unethically market two, three, four, and five drug combinations for financial benefits. One such combination of TC with other drugs—the so-called "modified Kligman's formula" containing mometasone—deserves special mention because of its widespread use as a "fairness cream."[7] This craze is aggravated the biased attitude toward fair skin which is continuously being fanned by the promotion of fairness creams by celebrities. Most TCs are available as over-the-counter (OTC) products at nominal price. Patients also apply TCs on nonsteroid responsive diseases as well as dermatoses like dermatophytosis on the recommendation of relatives, friends, and neighbors. During the past few years, incidence of dermatophytosis has risen to epic proportions resulting in an increasing tendency among patients to apply 2 or 3 drug combinations containing antifungals and steroids on the lesions on the advice of laymen and chemists. Misuse of TC on fungal lesions lead to both antifungal resistance as well as spread to unusual sites such as the face.[10]

ETIOLOGY

Topical steroid-damaged skin is an adaptive state that occurs due to repeated administration of TC. Hence, it is a form of drug dependence caused by chronic misuse, overuse, and abuse of the drug. Dependence on the drug is not only psychological but also physical. Withdrawal of the drug results in a flare of symptoms known as rebound phenomenon. This causing immense physical distress to the patient. Unable to bear the discomfort, the patient resumes applying the TC. Further attempts to withdraw the drug are resisted.[11] The addiction to TC occurs when it is overused in the proper indication but either without prescription or unsupervised (e.g., eczemas) or misused for the wrong indication (e.g., acne vulgaris). Addiction to TC may occur after short-term use of TCs of higher potency or prolonged use of TCs of any potency. Dependence may also occur when the TC of higher potency are applied in children and geriatric patients on the face and folds.[2,11] Withdrawal of TC becomes more difficult with higher potencies of TC used. Vasoconstriction plays an important role in the action of TC. When the TC is withdrawn, it results in withdrawal of the vasoconstrictive effect of TC. The fixed vasodilatation, which ensues causes, occurs as an important part of rebound phenomenon seen after withdrawal of the drug. It has been postulated that the chronic vasoconstriction, which occurs after repeated application of TC, is caused by inhibition of nitrous oxide (NO). The endothelial NO is released when the TC is withdrawn. This causes erythema due to dilatation of blood vessels. The erythema is further enhanced dermal atrophy and resultant lack of support to the blood vessels. It has been further postulated that chronic immunosuppression caused by the prolonged application of TC causes overgrowth of microorganisms which act as superantigen. This immunosuppressive effect is removed when the TC is withdrawn resulting in a superantigen-induced inflammatory reaction which is clinically manifested as inflammatory lesions (papules and pustules).[12]

CLINICAL FEATURES

Topical corticosteroid should always be applied on diseased skin for the proper indication and avoided in diseases where they are contraindicated **(Table 2)**. As mentioned earlier, topical steroid-damaged skin may be caused by overuse of TC on diseased skin for the proper indication or misuse of TC for the wrong indication (dermatophytosis, acne, etc.) or on normal skin (as fairness cream). Continuous use of the TC causes an initial improvement of symptoms such as pruritus followed by an aggravation of symptoms. The disease for which the TC has been initially applied becomes gradually resistant to the drug with aggravation of symptoms and signs and appearance of newer lesions. Such lesions, which appear as a result of TC misuse and overuse together constitute the features of topical steroid-damaged skin **(Table 3)**. This phenomenon is seen particularly on skin of face and folds as also on lesions of existing diseases such as bacterial and fungal infections (dermatophytoses, candidiasis, and pityriasis versicolor) where the TC has been misused. On the face erythematous papules and pustules **(Fig. 1)**,

TABLE 2: Contraindications of topical corticosteroids.

Absolute	*Relative*
Hypersensitivity to the drug	Infections (bacterial, fungal, viral)
Hypersensitivity to the vehicle	Infestation by parasites
Ulcers	

TABLE 3: Features of topical steroid-damaged skin.

Cutaneous features	*Other effects*
Atrophy and striae	Status cosmeticus
Acneiform eruptions	Chronic actinic dermatitis
Hypopigmentation	Photosensitivity
Hyperpigmentation	Rebound phenomenon on withdrawal of TC
Hypertrichosis	Tachyphylaxis
Erythema	
Telangiectasia	
Infections occurring due to TC application	
Aggravation of fungal (including Tinea incognito), bacterial, and viral infections	
Perioral dermatitis	
Allergic contact dermatitis	

(TC: topical corticosteroid)

acneiform eruptions **(Fig. 2)**, bacterial infections **(Fig. 3)**, fungal infections **(Fig. 4)**, telangiectasia **(Fig. 5)**, hypertrichosis **(Fig. 6)**, dryness, hypo- and hyperpigmentation, eyelid dermatitis, allergic contact dermatitis **(Fig. 7)**, perioral dermatitis **(Fig. 8)**, and photosensitivity may be observed after TC misuse. When the TC is withdrawn, the patient may develop intense itching, dryness, and intense erythema (red face syndrome) for 2 weeks. This is followed by desquamation of the skin. The flare and erythema resolves after a couple of weeks but reappears again after 2 weeks with decrease intensity. This cycle of flare and resolution continues for some time but with decreasing intensity and increasing intermission till complete cure. The rebound phenomenon may also occur in areas beyond the original site or even at distant sites. Symptoms similar to status cosmeticus or chronic actinic dermatitis may also be seen.[3] At other sites, the patients may exhibit acneiform eruptions **(Fig. 9)**, atrophy and striae **(Figs. 10 to 12)**, tinea incognito **(Figs. 13 and 14)**, hypopigmentation **(Fig. 15)**, purpura, ulcerations, and stellate pseudoscars. Application of TC on lesions of dermatophytosis may result in development of tinea incognito. Tachyphylaxis may occur after chronic use particularly in cases of psoriasis.[3]

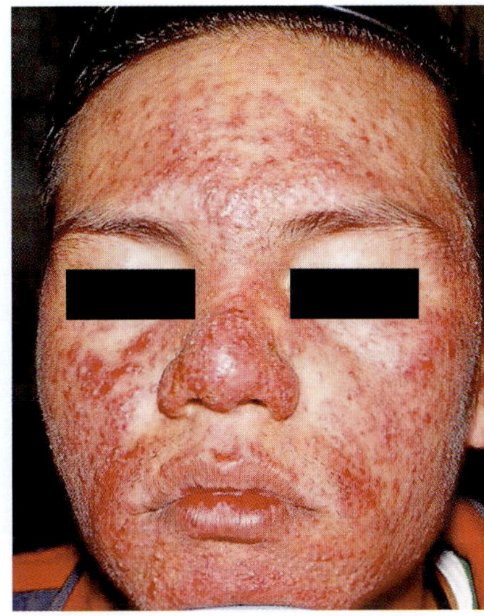

Fig. 1: *Erythema:* The hallmark of topical steroid dependent/damaged face (TSDF).

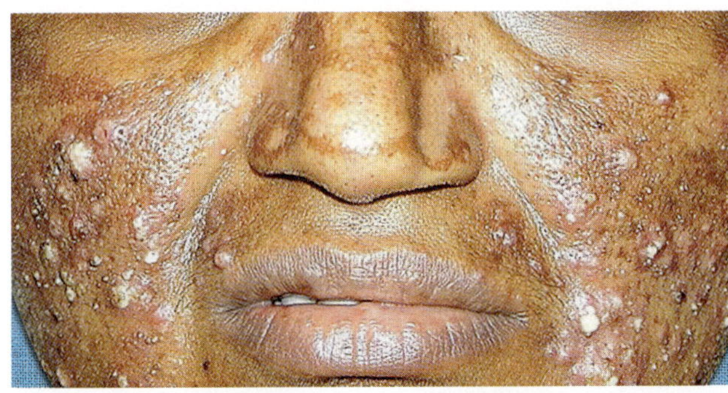

Fig. 2: Acneiform eruption.

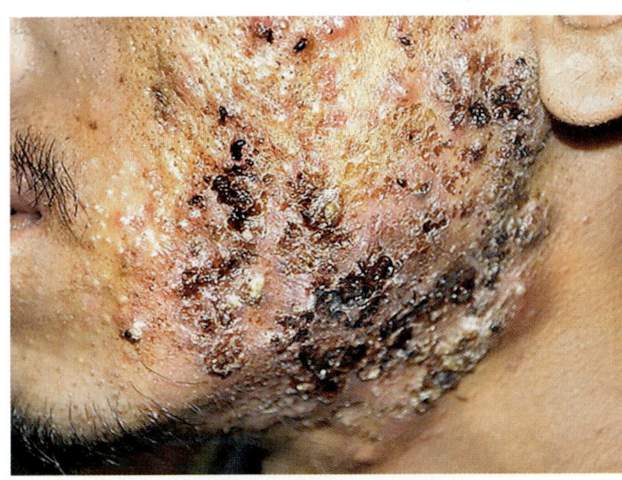

Fig. 3: Severe bacterial infection.

MANAGEMENT

Management of topical steroid-damaged skin poses a challenge to the dermatologist. Controlling the rebound phenomenon and reversal of the damages caused by the TC involves a good amount of counseling as well as therapy.

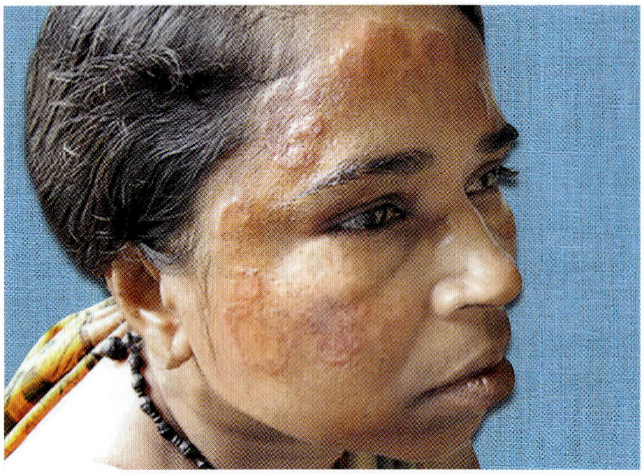

Fig. 4: Tinea incognito on face.

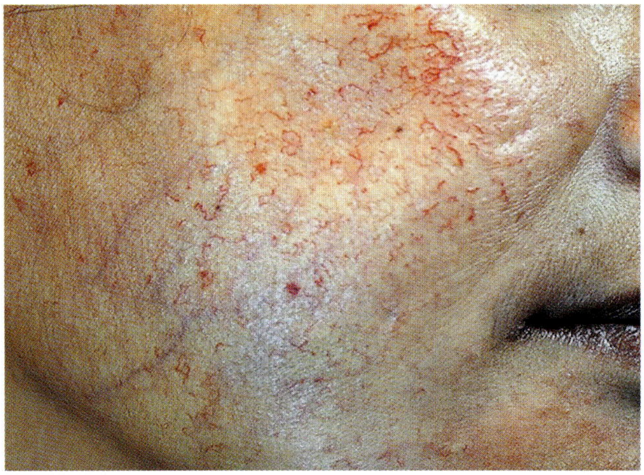

Fig. 5: Telangiectasia.

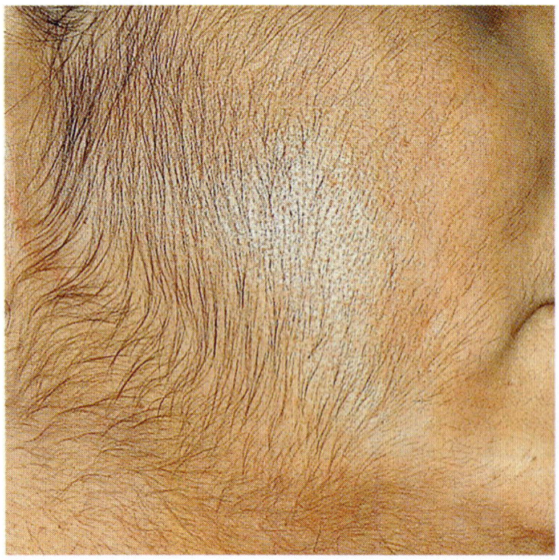

Fig. 6: Hypertrichosis.

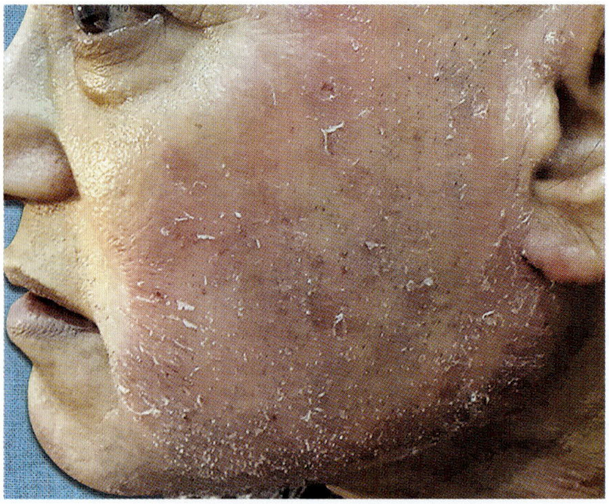

Fig. 7: Allergic contact dermatitis.

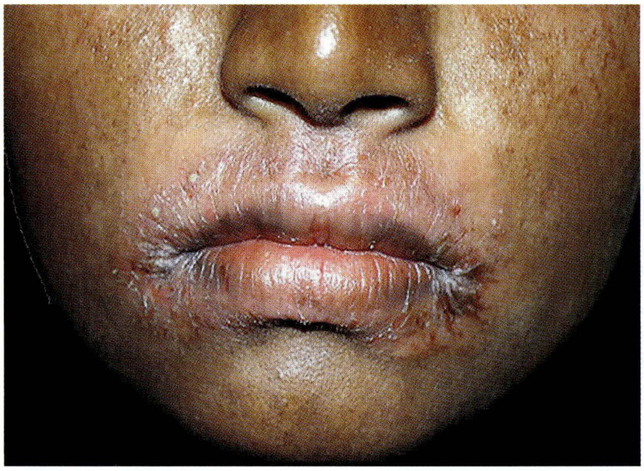

Fig. 8: Perioral dermatitis.

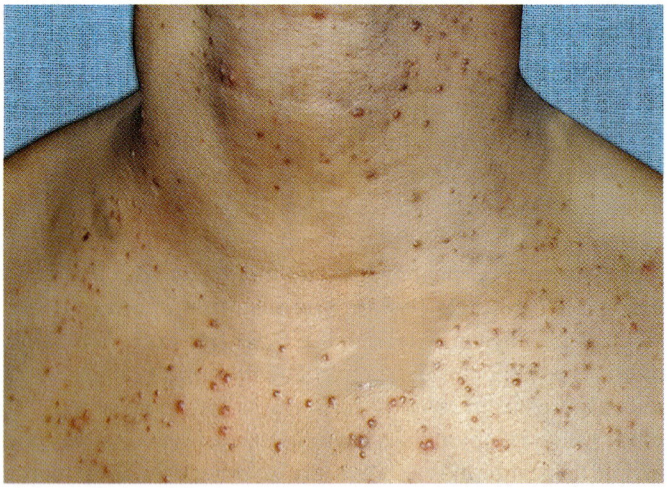

Fig. 9: Monomorphic acne on chest.

The recovery period is quite harassing and painful. Hence, these patients need intense psychological support. They should be advised to use TCs only as per the prescription of a dermatologist never on the advice of nonprofessionals, friends, relatives, and particularly the salespersons at chemist's counters. Repeating prescription and use of the TC beyond the prescription period must be strictly prohibited. During flares the patient should not use any soap, emollients

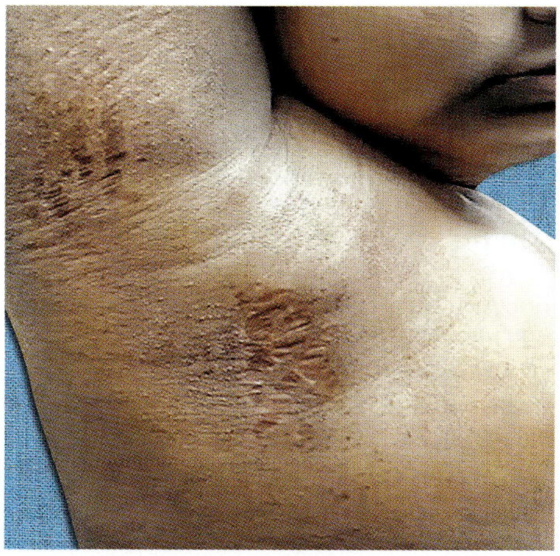

Fig. 10: Atrophy of skin due to application of potent topical steroid on soft skin of axilla in a child.

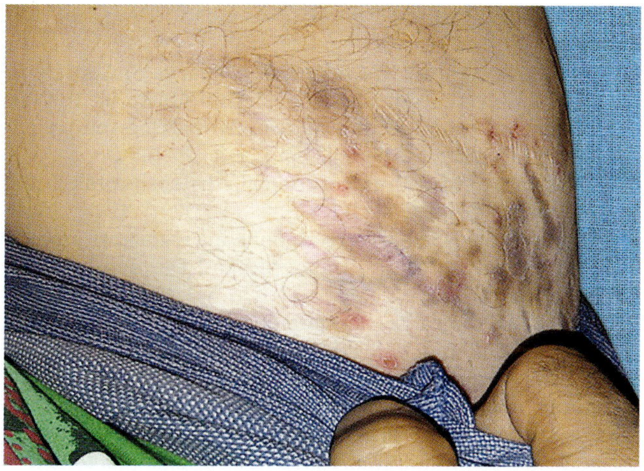

Fig. 11: Striae on thigh.

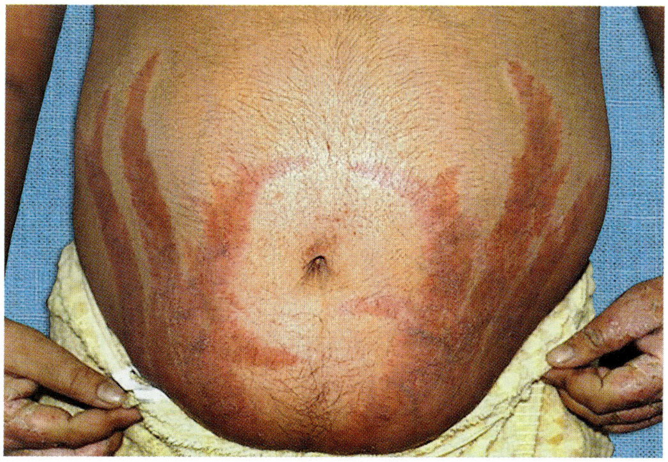

Fig. 12: Topical steriod induced striae.

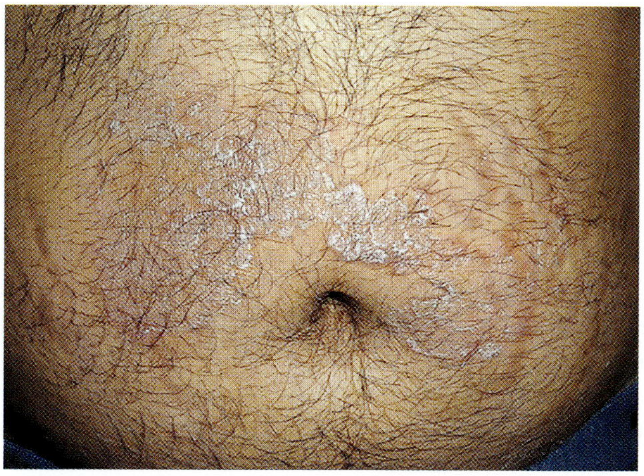

Fig. 13: Tinea incognito on abdomen.

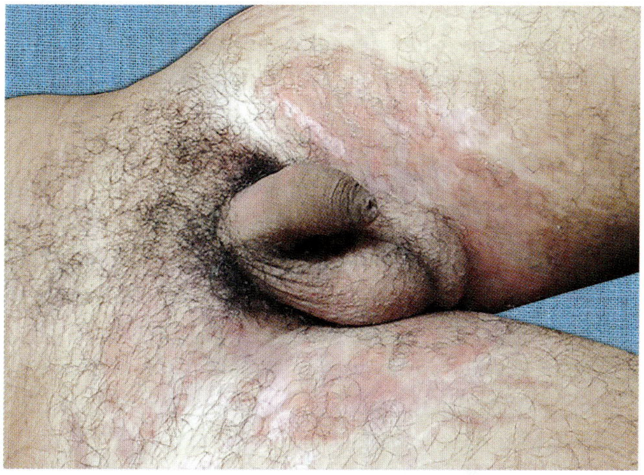

Fig. 14: Tinea incognito with erythema on groin.

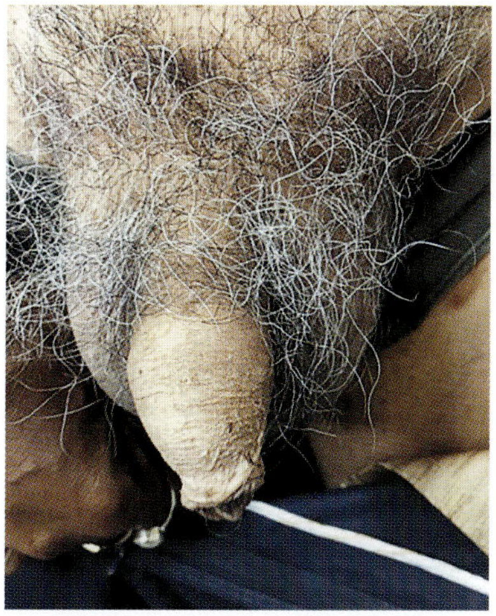

Fig. 15: Hypopigmentation on genitalia.

containing glycolic acid, lactic acid, etc. or cosmetics on the face which must be washed with lukewarm water only.[12] Counseling about the bad effects of overuse and misuse of TC as well as prior advice to the patient about the rebound phenomenon that may occur on stoppage of the drug forms an important part of management.[3] The method of withdrawal of TC is controversial and remains a matter of debate. Gradual withdrawal of TC to minimize the discomfiture caused by the rebound phenomenon is advocated by some authorities. However, other clinicians prefer complete stoppage of TC immediately after the treatment is started.[12] Some workers advocate replacement of the TC with calcineurin inhibitors.[2] However, some patients complain of a burning sensation on application of calcineurin inhibitors on the steroid-damaged skin.[12] Other drugs such as metronidazole, doxycycline, and minocycline have also been tried.[2] Ancillary drugs that have been recommended by various workers are oral antihistaminics to control the intense itching associated with the rebound phenomenon, bland emollients for the dryness, repeated ice compresses for the burning sensation, and Burrow's solution for the weeping lesions.[2]

KEY POINTS

- The first TC was introduced in 1952 by Sulzberger and Witten for the treatment of inflammatory disorders of the skin.
- During the next few decades, modifications were made in the steroid molecule and TCs of higher potencies were introduced.
- Based on their potency, TCs are classified into seven different classes.
- Ethical use of TCs involves an understanding of their potency, mode of application, and awareness of side effects.
- Topical corticosteroids are misused, overused, and abused due to a number of factors.
- The face is the most common site of misuse of TCs.
- Misuse of TCs on the face can result in a number of serious physical and psychological side effects.
- These side effects have been collectively named topical steroid dependent/damaged face (TSDF) by Lahiri and Coondoo.
- To combat the menace of topical steroid misuse, DVL has formed a taskforce named IADVL Task Force Against Topical Steroid Abuse (ITATSA).
- Management of TSDF is difficult and involves both physical measures and psychological counseling.

REFERENCES

1. Coondoo A. Topical corticosteroid misuse: the Indian scenario. Indian J Dermatol. 2014;59:451-5.
2. Lahiri K, Coondoo A. Topical steroid damaged/dependent face (TSDF): an entity of cutaneous pharmacodependence. Indian J Dermatol. 2016;61:265-72.
3. Abraham A, Roga G. Topical steroid-damaged skin. Indian J Dermatol. 2014;59:456-9.
4. Epstein NN, Epstein WL, Epstein JH. Atrophic striae in patients with inguinal intertrigo. Arch Dermatol. 1963;87:450-7.
5. Kligman AM, Frosch PJ. Steroid addiction. Int J Dermatol. 1979;18(1):23-31.
6. Rathi S. Abuse of topical steroid as cosmetic cream: a social background of steroid dermatitis. Indian J Dermatol. 2006; 51:154-5.
7. Saraswat A, Lahiri K, Chatterjee M, Barua S, Coondoo A, Mittal A, et al. Topical corticosteroid abuse on the face: a prospective, multicentre study of dermatology outpatients. Indian J Dermatol Venereol Leprol. 2011;77:160-6.
8. Saraswat A. Ethical use of topical corticosteroids. Indian J Dermatol. 2014;59:469-72.
9. Verma SB. Sales, status, prescriptions and regulatory problems with topical steroids in India. Indian J Dermatol Venereol Leprol. 2014;80:201-3.
10. Verma SB. Topical corticosteroid misuse in India is harmful and out of control. BMJ. 2015;351:h6079.
11. Ghosh A, Sengupta S, Coondoo A, Jana A. Topical corticosteroid addiction and phobia. Indian J Dermatol. 2014;59:465-8.
12. Rapaport MJ, Rapaport V. The red skin syndromes: corticosteroid addiction and withdrawal. Expert Rev Dermatol. 2006;1:547-61.
13. Coondoo A, Phiske M, Verma S, Lahiri K. Side-effects of topical steroids. A long overdue revisit. Indian Dermatol Online J. 2014;5:416-25.

EXAMINATION QUESTION

1. Discuss the approach and management of topical steroid-damaged skin.

103 CHAPTER

Erythema Multiforme, Stevens–Johnson Syndrome, and Toxic Epidermal Necrolysis

Reena Rai, Janani Adityan

INTRODUCTION

Erythema multiforme (EM), Stevens–Johnson syndrome (SJS), and toxic epidermal necrolysis (TEN) are cutaneous reactions characterized by mucocutaneous involvement. Although they have clinical similarity, EM is recently considered as a different variant.

ERYTHEMA MULTIFORME

Introduction

It is an acute, recurrent, and self-limiting cutaneous disorder characterized by abrupt onset of symmetrical red papules which evolve into characteristic target-like lesions **(Fig. 1)**. It is usually precipitated by infection.

History

- Ferdinand Von Hebra, an Australian dermatologist first described EM in 1860.
- The disease he described was mild and accompanied with onset of hundreds of papules.
- From his daily observation, he found that papules evolved into lesions with concentric zones of color change henceforth he named the lesions as target lesions.
- Bernard Thomas later divided into EM major (EMM) (severe mucosal necrosis with EM-like cutaneous) and EM minor (EMm) (Von Hebra's disease).

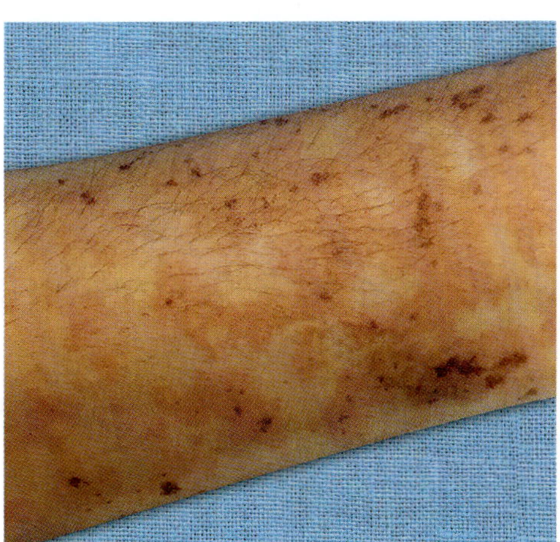

Fig. 1: Targetoid lesions in an erythema multiforme patient.

Epidemiology

- Young adults
- Recurrent in at least 10% in EMM and 30% in EMm
- Male preponderance.

Etiology

The etiology of erythema multiforme is enlisted in **Table 1**.

Immunological Basis

The immunological basis of erythema multiforme is shown in **Flowchart 1**.

Clinical Features

- Erythema multiforme is common in young adults but can occur at any age.
- Resolves around 2–3 weeks.

Erythema Multiforme Minor/ Papular/Simplex Form

About 80% present with minor form.

Distribution: Most common areas to be involved are palms, trunk, mucosal membranes such as oral and genital. They spread in a centripetal manner **(Fig. 2)**.

TABLE 1: Etiology of erythema multiforme (EM).

Viral	• Herpes simplex • Adenovirus • Cytomegalovirus • Hepatitis B • HIV • Infectious mononucleosis • Mumps • Varicella	• Variola • Polio • Orf
Bacterial	• Rickettsiae • *Mycoplasma pneumoniae*	
Fungal	• Histoplasmosis	
Drug reactions	• Vaccinations	
Miscellaneous	• Contact reactions • Malignancy • Polyarteritis nodosa • Polymorphic light eruption (PLE) • Granulomatosis with polyangiitis • Lupus erythematosus	Sarcoidosis

Flowchart 1: Immunological basis of erythema multiforme.

Associations with HLA B62, HLA B35, and HLA DR53 have been observed with recurrent cases
↓
Mononuclear cells infected with herpes simplex
↓
Activates SP1 and IFN δ—mediated by viral polymerase
↓
Initiates an inflammatory cascade
↓
Recruitment of HSV-specific CD4 T-cells produce INF-α
↓
Increased expression of IFN-α leads to increased sequestration of leukocytes, monocytes, and natural killer cells and recruitment of autoreactive T-cells
↓
Perforin positive cells mediate apoptotic cell death in EM and SJS

(EM: erythema multiforme; HLA: human leukocyte antigen; HSV: herpes simplex virus; IFN: interferon; SJS: Stevens–Johnson syndrome)

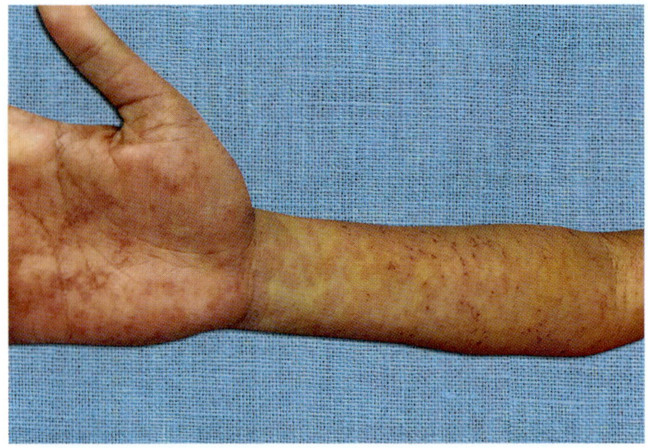

Fig. 2: Targetoid lesions in erythema multiforme (EM).

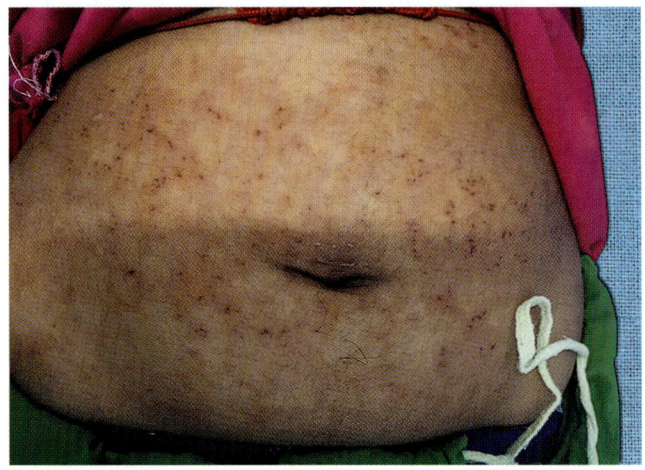

Fig. 3: Targetoid lesions in abdomen.

Morphology:

- Macular, papular, or urticarial lesions can occur with classic "iris" or target lesions **(Figs. 1 and 3)**
- Target lesions have three characteristic zones:
  1. Central area of dusky erythema or purpura
  2. Middle paler zone of edema
  3. Outer ring of erythema with well-defined edge
- Atypical target lesions show only two zones
- Erosions/bullae over mucous membrane can be present
- Photoaggravation
- Koebner phenomenon.

Localized Vesiculobullous Form

Larger lesions have a central bulla and marginal ring of vesicles (*herpes iris of Bateman*).

Erythema Multiforme Major

- More extensive mucosal membrane involvement with extensive target lesions.
- Sudden in onset.
- Prodromal systemic symptoms occur 1–13 days before eruption.

Mucous Membrane Lesions

- 70% oral cavity involvement.
- Mucosal lesions appear in lips, gingivae, ventral side of the tongue while the hard palate is spared.
- Bilateral conjunctivitis and pain in eyes.
- Nasal, urethral, and anal involvement can be seen.
- *Fuchs syndrome:* Ectodermis pluriorificialis is a rare occurrence characterized by severe involvement of 2–3 mucosal sites with absence of skin lesions. It has a relapsing course and is associated with herpes simplex virus (HSV).
- *Rowell syndrome*: Lupus erythematosus with EM-like lesions with immunological finding of speckled antinuclear antibodies, anti-LA or anti-RO antibodies, and positive test for rheumatoid factor.

Natural Course

- Lesions appear with 24 hours and remain for 7 days or longer.
- Each episode lasts for 2 weeks and heals without sequelae.

Pathology

- *Epidermis*: Keratinocyte necrosis with exocytosis of lymphocytes
- Interface dermatitis
- *In dermis*: Mild perivascular inflammatory cell infiltrate
- Immunofluorescence—nonspecific

Differential Diagnosis

- Stevens–Johnson syndrome
- Urticaria

- *Vasculitis*: Kawasaki disease
- Fixed drug eruption
- Paraneoplastic pemphigus

Complications

- Transient discoloration
- *Persistent EM or continuous EM*: Prolonged and overlapping attack of EM

Treatment

- Limited or localized lesions can be treated symptomatically.
- In severe cases, systemic steroids of 0.5–1 mg/kg/day for 3–5 days can be given.
- Antiviral therapy for herpes simplex triggered EM.
- Long-term prophylactic dose of oral acyclovir 10 mg/kg/day in divided doses for at least 6 months can be given for recurrent cases.
- Other drugs such as thalidomide, dapsone, azathioprine, mycophenolatemofetil and cyclosporine can be given in recurrent EM resistant to prophylactic antiviral therapy.

Key Points

- Erythema multiforme is a self-limiting, recurrent disease with target lesions in acrofacial distribution.
- Infections such as HSV and drugs are frequent cause.
- Subtypes EM major—skin lesions with mucosal involvement; EM minor—skin lesions without mucosal involvement.
- *Histopathology:* Keratinocyte necrosis, lymphocyte exocytosis with interface dermatitis.
- Prophylactic antiviral therapy for prevention of recurrences.

STEVENS–JOHNSON SYNDROME AND TOXIC EPIDERMAL NECROLYSIS

Introduction

TEN also known as "Lyell's syndrome" is a rare, acute, life-threatening condition with severe mucosal erosions and skin detachment **(Figs. 4 and 5)**. This is usually caused by intake of drugs **(Table 2)**. TEN is a most extensive form whereas SJS is milder variant.

History

- In 1956, Alan Lyell observed eruption of skin resembling scalding both objectively and subjectively in a group of four patients, he called it "toxic epidermal necrolysis."
- In 1922, US physicians, Stevens and Johnson, observed an acute form of mucocutaneous disease in two young males.
- The characteristic of SJS was extensive mucosal necrosis along with severe purulent conjunctivitis and stomatitis.

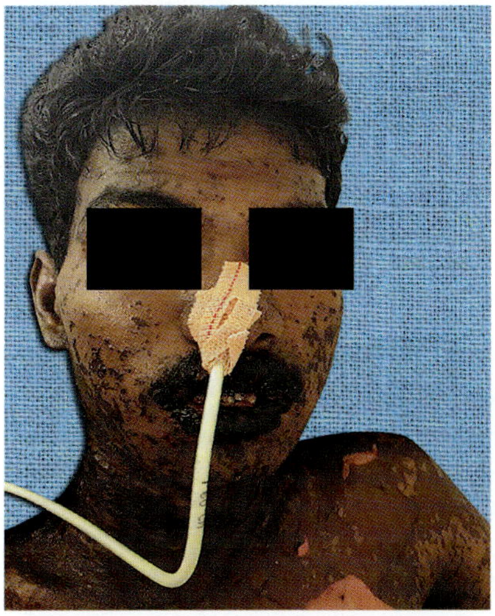

Fig. 4: Hemorrhagic crusted lips in a toxic epidermal necrolysis (TEN).

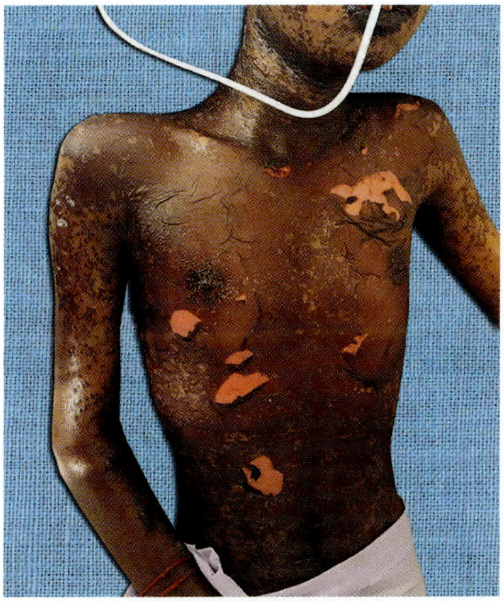

Fig. 5: Epidermal detachment in toxic epidermal necrolysis (TEN).

TABLE 2: Common drugs precipitating SJS/TEN.

Allopurinol	Lamotrigine
Aminopenicillins	Piroxicam
Nevirapine	Sulfadoxine/sulfadiazine
Barbiturates	Sulfasalazine
Phenytoin	Trimethoprim/sulfamethoxazole
Carbamazepine	Thioacetazone

(SJS/TEN: Stevens–Johnson syndrome toxic epidermal necrolysis)

Nomenclature

- The word toxic refers to the toxemia which is caused by the circulation of toxins. The toxin is responsible for epidermal necrosis and its constitutional symptoms.
- By combining the key clinical feature "epidermolysis" with histological feature "necrosis"—Lyell has termed it "necrolysis."

Classification

Patient can be classified into three groups depending on the extent of skin detachment:

1. <10% of body surface area (BSA)—SJS.
2. 10–30% of BSA—SJS–TEN.
3. >30% of BSA—TEN.

Risk Factors

- Immunosuppression as in HIV, lymphoma, diabetes, etc.
- Slow acetylators
- Administration of concomitant of radiotherapy and anticonvulsants
- *HLA-B* 1502*: Asian and East Indians exposed to carbamazepine
- *HLA-B* 5801*: Han Chinese exposed to allopurinol
- *HLA-A* 3101*: European exposed to carbamazepine

Pathogenesis: Revise New Concepts Fitzpatrick Latest Edition, Bolognia Recent Edition, CD8 T-Cell, IL-15, See Pathogenesis

- The evidence of specific drug-related human leukocyte antigen (HLA) alleles highlights genetic susceptibility as a major risk factor.
- The drug metabolites have reduced capacity to detoxify. These metabolites react with host tissue and initiate an immune response—antigen and antibody reaction.
- The antigen antibody complexes is formed by three different concepts.
  1. *Hapten/Prohapten concept:* Drug binds with a cellular peptide covalently.
  2. *p-i concept:* Drug directly interacts with a specific MHC class 1 molecule or T-cell receptor non- covalently.
  3. *Altered peptide concept:* Drug interacts with MHC 1 directly presenting an altered self.
- These drugs initiate apoptosis of epidermal keratinocytes causing denudation and skin blistering by the following ways:
  i. Upregulation of Fas ligands on the keratinocytes induced by the medication leads to death receptor mediated apoptotic activity.

     Apoptotic pathway:

     Fas ligands area member of tumor necrosis family of cytokines

     ↓

     Fas ligands bind to Fas death receptors which are specific cell surface receptors

     ↓

     Receptors detect the intracellular death signals there by inducing cellular destruction by apoptosis

  ii. These drugs mainly interact with major histocompatibility complex (MHC) class 1 and also drug-specific CD8 cytotoxic T cells which accumulate within the epidermal blisters. The CD8 cells in turn secrete high concentration of granzyme B and perforin, which leads to death of keratinocytes.
  iii. Activation of CD8 T-cells, natural killer, and natural killer T-cells and nitric oxide play a major role in keratinocyte apoptosis.
  iv. Drugs activate the monocytes to secrete annexin A1. They bind to formyl peptide receptor 1 (FPR1) to induce necroptosis of keratinocytes.
  v. Recently, circulating levels of IL-15 have shown to be associated with severity and mortality rate of SJS/TEN.

Clinical Features

- The period of latency between initiation of the vulnerable drug and onset of features of SJS/TEN is 7–21 days. It is reduced with re-exposure.
- Fever, malaise, and upper respiratory tract infections usually precedes.
- Initially, atypical skin lesions appear on trunk then slowly creeping to the neck, face, and extremities. Lesions are erythematous, dusky red, or purpuric macules which coalesce together on a later stage **(Figs. 5 and 6)**.
- Erosions of buccal, ocular, and genital mucosa along with erythema are seen in >90% of the patient presenting with SJS/TEN.
- Distal extremities are generally spared whereas palms and soles have target lesions.
- The skin lesions are erythematous and tender and necrotic **(Fig. 7)**.
- Pseudo-Nikolsky sign due to epidermal necrolysis

Eye Involvement

- Visual impairment is caused by sudden inflammation of mucosal surface of eye and eyelids.
- Chemosis, conjunctivitis, pseudomembrane formation, corneal, and conjunctival epithelial defects are some of the other eye signs seen in SJS/TEN.

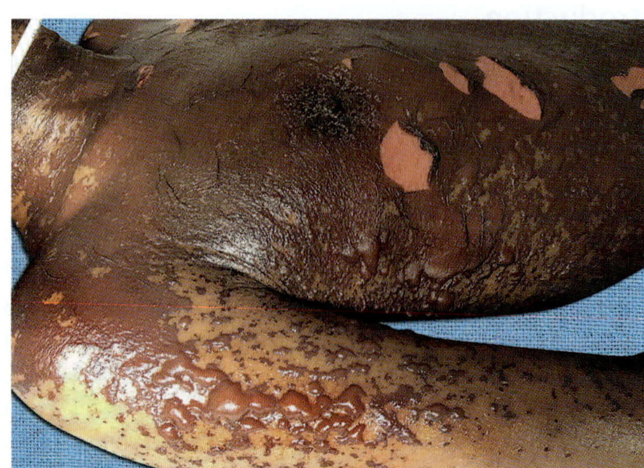

Fig. 6: Bullous lesions in toxic epidermal necrolysis (TEN).

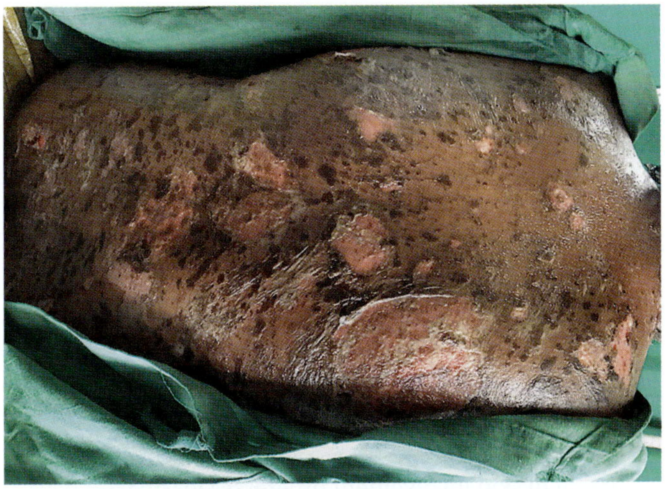

Fig. 7: Epidermal necrosis with erosions in toxic epidermal necrolysis (TEN).

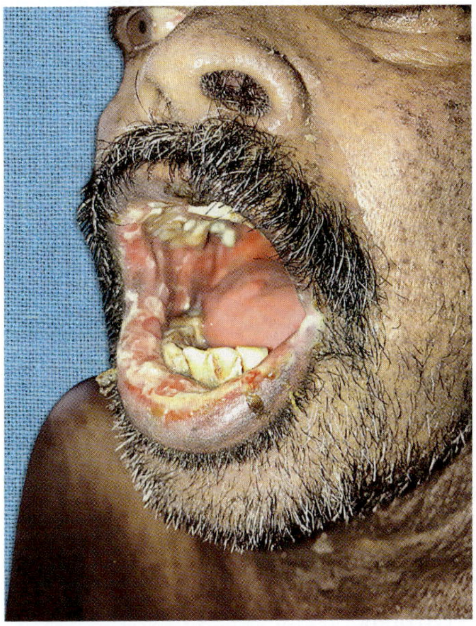

Fig. 8: Oral erosions in a toxic epidermal necrolysis (TEN).

Oral Involvement

- Blistering and ulcerations along with painful mucosal erythema **(Fig. 8)**
- Adherent hemorrhagic crusts are seen in the lips **(Figs. 4 and 9)**.

Urogenital Involvement

Pain and urinary retention

Pulmonary Involvement

- Dyspnea and hemoptysis
- Hyperventilation and bronchial hypersecretion

Gastrointestinal Involvement

Diarrhea and esophagitis

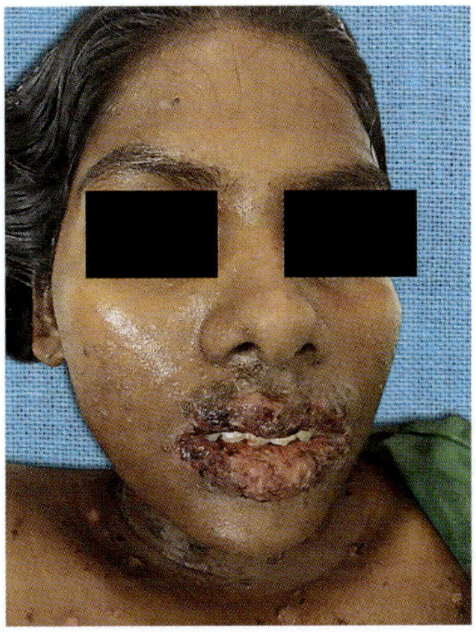

Fig. 9: Eye and oral involvement in Stevens–Johnson syndrome (SJS).

Histopathology

- *In early lesions:* Epidermal spongiosis and exocytosis with moderate perivascular mononuclear cell infiltration in papillary dermis. Satellites cell necrosis with opposition of mononuclear cells to necrotic keratinocytes.
- *In established lesions*: Necrosis of the whole epidermis with perivascular infiltrate composed of lymphocytes and subepidermal split.
- *Direct immunofluorescence (DIF)*: Negative

Differential Diagnosis

- *Erythema multiforme*: Typical target lesions, mostly related to herpes Infection
- *Staphylococcal scalded skin syndrome (SSSS)*: High incidence in children. It can occur in immunocompromised adults and those with renal failure. It spares palms and soles. It is induced by *Staphylococcus* toxin. Histologically, it is subcorneal.
- *Acute generalized exanthematous pustulosis (AGEP)*: Large area of erythema studded with multiple, small, and nonfollicular pustules. Histopathology—dense neutrophilic infiltrate and no epidermal necrolysis.
- *Generalized fixed drug eruptions*: Lesions develop after exposure to a drug with dusky violaceous plaques and fades leaving residual postinflammatory pigmentation. New lesions occur at the site of previous lesions.
- *Paraneoplastic pemphigus*: Severe mucosal erosions.
- *Drug-induced linear IgA bullous dermatosis*: Vancomycin can cause TEN. DIF is positive.
- *Erythema of chemotherapy*: It occurs after exposure to chemotherapeutic agent. Symmetrical involvement of lesions in folds. Biopsy shows enlarged atypical keratinocytes with less necrosis.

- DRESS—drug reaction with eosinophilia and systemic symptoms. Widespread erythema with facial edema, peripheral eosinophilia. Biopsy shows dense inflammatory infiltrate with eosinophils. Necrosis is usually absent.

Complications

Acute

- Septicemia caused by *Pseudomonas* and *Staphylococcus aureus*.
- Hypothermia due to deranged thermoregulatory control.
- Transcutaneous fluid losses due to reduced intake and oral lesions which are extremely painful.
- *Epidermal detachment of 50% body surface area*: Acute kidney injury due to fluid depletion and end-organ hypoperfusion. Water losses accounts for 2–3 L/day.
- Leukopenia and anemia
- Hepatic failure
- Hyperglycemia and hypoalbuminemia
- *Epithelial necrolysis in bronchi*: Airway obstruction by sloughed epithelium and bronchial erosions

Chronic

- Postinflammatory dyspigmentation
- Eruptive melanocytic nevi commonly found in children
- Onychomadesis—shedding of nails due to arrest of nail matrix
- Telogen effluvium
- Pruritus, abnormal photosensitivity, and abnormal sweating.

Ocular Complications

- Corneal and conjunctival ulceration with or without scarring, dry eyes, distichiasis, entropion, and trichiasis
- Introital adhesions—destruction of conjunctival goblet cells
- Scarring of the conjunctival fornix obstructs the ductal opening of the lacrimal glands causing dryness
- Symblepharon and ankyloblepharon
- Ectropion and entropion
- Permanent blindness and visual impairment.

Oral Complications

Scarring of the oral mucosa causes gingival synechiae which leads to food trapping and limitation of oral mobility.

Pulmonary Involvement

Bronchiolitis obliterans: Airway epithelial injury followed by scarring and regeneration which leads to severe obstruction and dyspnea.

Gastrointestinal

- Esophageal stricture
- Diarrhea due to intestinal ulceration
- *Cholestasis and histological loss of interlobular bile duct*: Vanishing bile duct syndrome.

Urogenital

- *Vaginal and introital adhesion*: Dyspareunia
- *Vaginal adenosis*: Replacement of noncornified vaginal epithelium with metaplastic epithelium of endocervical differentiation.

Psychological

Post-traumatic stress disorder

Disease Course and Prognosis: Mortality Rate?

- Extent of skin involvement progresses for first 5–7 days.
- Re-epithelialization takes 2–3 weeks once the triggering agent is removed.
- *Prognosis:* SCORTEN prognostic scoring system **(Table 3)**.
- *Approach to a patient with TEN/SJS*: Mortality rate varies from 5 to 12% for SJS to 30% for TEN.
- *Mortality:* SCORTEN mortality scoring **(Table 4)**.

Investigations

- Complete blood count, erythrocyte sedimentation rate (ESR)
- Urea, electrolytes
- Amylase
- Bicarbonate
- Glucose

TABLE 3: Prognostic scoring system—SCORTEN.

Factors	*Points*
Age > 40 years	1
Heart rate >120 bpm	1
Cancer/hematological malignancy	1
Body surface area (BSA) on day 1 >10%	1
Serum urea (>10 mmol/L) >28 mg/dL	1
Serum bicarbonate (<20 mmol/L)	1
Serum glucose level (>14 mmol/L)	1

Note: SCORTEN scoring system is used to access the patients with TEN.

TABLE 4: SCORTEN mortality scoring.

Score	*Mortality rate*
0–1	3.2
2	12.1
3	35.8
4	58.3
≥5	90

- Liver function text (LFT), C-reactive protein (CRP)
- Antinuclear antibody (ANA), extractable nuclear antigens (ENA)
- Complement
- Indirect immunofluorescence
- Biopsy, DIF
- Chest X-ray
- Blood culture
- Urine culture
- Pus culture.

Treatment for SJS/TEN

- Stop the offending drug
- Correct electrolyte and fluid balance
- Thermoregulation
- Topical antibiotic can be used on open wound
- Dressing on denuded area reduces fluid to protein loss, limits colonization of bacteria
- Vaseline dressings are recommended for exposed areas.

Local Therapy

Eyes:

- Ocular lubricant should be administered every 2 hours.
- Break down of conjunctival adhesions and inflammatory debris should be removed.
- Topical antibiotic is recommended for corneal ulcer.
- Topical steroids if used reduce ocular surface damage.
- Extensive loss of ocular surface—amniotic membrane transplantation.

Mouth:

- Application of lubricants frequently to the lips
- Clean mouth with warm saline
- Use an antiseptic mouthwash twice or thrice a day
- Topical steroids in the form of mouthwash (Betnesol 0.5 mg in 10 mL water).

Urogenital:

- Application of emollients
- Topical steroids and antibiotics for noneroded surfaces
- To prevent urethral strictures catheterization can be done.

Fluid replacement:

- *Parklands formula*: 4 mL × TBSA (%) × body weight (kg)
- 50% given in first 8 hours
- 50% given in next 16 hours

Nutrition

- Early catabolic phase—20–25 kcals/kg/day
- Anabolic phase—20–30 kcals/kg/day

Other support

- Analgesics for pain
- Proton pump inhibitors for gastric protection
- Blood sugars should be monitored regularly
- If infection is present treat with antibiotics

Specific Treatment

Corticosteroids

- The use of corticosteroids is controversial.
- It should be given only when the patient presents within 48–72 hours.
- Early administration of steroids may reduce the inflammation. However, it increases the risk of impaired re-epithelialization and risk of sepsis.
- *Dose*: Steroids equivalent to prednisolone 0.5–1 mg/kg daily for short period and taper.

Cyclosporine:

- Immunosuppressant which works by inhibition of CD8 cytotoxic mechanism and it has antiapoptotic effect by inhibition of Fas ligand, nuclear factor κB and tumor necrosis factor-α (TNF-α).
- *Dose*: 3–5 mg/kg/day in divided doses for 10 days then tapered.

Intravenous immunoglobulin:

- High dose of normal immunoglobulin inhibits Fas—Fas ligand apoptosis and interaction through anti-Fas activity.
- *IVIG dose*: 0.5–1 g/kg/day for 3–4 consecutive days.

Plasmapheresis or hemodialysis: Plasmapheresis helps in removal of offending drugs, its metabolites, and inflammatory mediators such as cytokines.

Anti-TNF agents:

- Thalidomide
- Etanercept
- Infliximab

Prevention

- Patients should avoid re-exposure of the drug.
- First-degree relatives should be notified and warned about the risk of reaction to same drugs.

Key Points

- *TEN/SJS:* Acute, fatal mucocutaneous disease
- Usually occurs 7–21 days after initiation of drug.
- Most common causative agents are drugs. Prognosis is determined by SCORTEN scoring system.
- *SJS:* <10% of body surface area; SJS overlap TEN—10–30% of body surface; TEN > 30% of body surface area.
- *Histopathology:* Satellite cell necrosis with sparse perivascular infiltrate.
- *Treatment:* Discontinuation of causative drug with symptomatic management.

REFERENCES

1. Rook A, Barker J, Bleiker T, Chalmers R, Creamer D, Griffiths C. Rook's Textbook of Dermatology. Chichester, West Sussex (UK): Wiley Blackwell; 2016.
2. Bolognia JL, Schaffer JV, Cerroni L. Dermatology. Philadelphia: Elsevier; 2017.

3. Rai R, Srinivas CR. Suprapharmacologic doses of intravenous dexamethasone followed by cyclosporine in the treatment of toxic epidermal necrolysis. Indian J Dermatol Venereol Leprol. 2008;74(3):263-5.
4. Fitzpatrick T, Freedberg I. Fitzpatrick's Dermatology in General Medicine. New York: McGraw-Hill, Medical Publishing Division; 2003.
5. Elder DE. Lever's Histopathology of the Skin. Philadelphia, PA: Wolters Kluwer; 2015.
6. Gupta LK, Martin AM, Agarwal N, D'Souza P, Das S, Kumar R, et al. Guidelines for the management of Stevens–Johnson syndrome/toxic epidermal necrolysis: an Indian perspective. Indian J Dermatol Venereol Leprol. 2016;82(6):603-25.
7. Wolverton SE. Comprehensive Dermatologic Drug Therapy, 3rd edition. Edinburgh (UA): Saunders; 2013.
8. James W, Elston D, Treat J, Rosenbach M, Neuhaus I. Andrews' Diseases of the Skin: Clinical Dermatology. Philadelphia: Elsevier; 2019.

EXAMINATION QUESTIONS

1. Describe the HPE of erythema multiforme.
2. Discuss the etiopathogenesis of toxic epidermal necrolysis (TEN).
3. Explain the management of TEN.
4. Write a short note on Rowell's syndrome.

104 CHAPTER

Graft-versus-host Disease

Prerna Raj, Aarti Sarda, Abhishek De

INTRODUCTION

Graft-versus-host disease (GVHD) is a multisystem multiorgan failure disease due to transfer of foreign donor hematopoietic stem cells into a host recipient via an allogeneic hematopoietic stem-cell transplant (HSCT).[1] GVHD may also occur following transfusion of nonirradiated blood products in maternal to fetal transmission or in the setting of solid organ transplantation.

Based on the type and time of presentation, GVHD can be classified into:

- Acute GVHD (aGVHD), which occurs within the first 100 days of transplantation, with the triad of dermatitis, enteritis, and hepatitis.
- Chronic GVHD (cGVHD), which develops after 100 days and consist of an autoimmune syndrome involving the skin and multiple organs.

HISTORY

The first successful allogeneic bone marrow transplant was performed in 1968. Subsequent advances in histocompatibility antigen testing increased the safety while establishment of bone marrow donor registries made HSCT accessible to large number of patients. Most recently, use of umbilical cord blood and reduced intensity conditioning regimens has led to further increase in number of transplants. However, use of mismatched unrelated donor (MUD) transplants carries a greater likelihood of mismatch of minor human leukocyte antigen (HLA) loci.

EPIDEMIOLOGY

Currently, 25,000 allogeneic HSCTs are performed worldwide each year. The most important predictor of GVHD remains HLA compatibility between donor and recipient. Approximately, 40% of HLA-identical HSCT recipients and 60–70% of HLA mismatched HSCT recipients will develop GVHD.

Cord blood transplant is associated with a decreased incidence of GVHD, but higher rates of nonengraftment. Also, because number of stem cells in cord blood is limited, two cord blood units are often required for successful engraftment in an adult recipient.

BOX 1: Risk factors associated with development of graft-versus-host disease.

- *Donor:*
  - HLA incompatibility with recipient
  - Unrelated to recipient
  - Female with male recipient
- *Recipient:* Age (older > middle-aged > pediatric)
- *Stem-cell source:*
  - Peripheral blood > bone marrow > cord blood
  - T-cell replete graft
- *Other:* Myeloablative-conditioning regimen

(HLA: human leukocyte antigen)

Peripheral blood has clearly emerged as a stem cell source at many transplant centers.[2] In peripheral blood HSCTs, the donor is treated with a colony-stimulating factor (e.g., filgrastim) which mobilizes the donor stem cells from the marrow into circulation. Cells are then collected via apheresis and infused into the recipient.

Removal of donor T-cells (T-cell depletion) prior to transplantation through ex vivo graft manipulation, or in vivo treatment of the recipient (e.g., antithymocyte globulin and alemtuzumab) significantly decreases the risk of GVHD.

Box 1 presents risk factors associated with development of GVHD.

PATHOGENESIS

The pathogenesis of aGVHD can be summarized in a three-step process **(Flowchart 1)**:[3]

I. HSCT conditioning and consequent damage to host tissues leading to activation of host antigen-presenting cells (APC).
II. Donor T-cells proliferate in response to contact with activated APC.
III. Destruction of target tissues (skin, liver, and gastrointestinal tract) occurs via cytotoxic T-lymphocytes, natural killer cells, and soluble factors [tumor necrosis factor-α (TNF-α), interferon-γ (INF-γ), interleukin-1 (IL-1), and nitric oxide (NO)]

In contrast, a clear understanding of cGVHD is still lacking. Alloreactive T-cells are again thought to play a central role. B-cells appear to prime the T-cells to minor histocompatibility antigens and levels of B-cell activating factor of the TNF family (BAFF), correlate with cGVHD. Multiple autoantibodies are often present, including antinuclear, anti-dsDNA (anti-double-stranded deoxyribonucleic acid) and anti-smooth muscle antibodies. Early-onset cGVHD (3–9 months) is associated with IFN-γ, increased regulatory T-cells, and a T-cell cytokine response (IL-2Rα).

Late-onset cGVHD (>9 months) is characterized by B-cell activation via soluble BAFF, induction of toll-like receptor 9 (TLR 9), and autoantibody formation.

CLINICAL FEATURES

Acute GVHD presents in the skin as morbilliform exanthem with increased predilection for acral areas. Pruritus is variable and a follicular pattern is observed. There may be a hemorrhagic appearance due to thrombocytopenia. The gastrointestinal tract (nausea, voluminous diarrhea, and abdominal pain) and liver (transaminitis, cholestasis, and bilirubin elevation) are two other primary organ systems affected. The most severe variant of aGVHD presents with generalized involvement of bullae formation leading to skin sloughing resembling toxic epidermal necrolysis and has poor prognosis. Clinical staging and histological grading of acute GVHD has been presented in **Table 1**.

Chronic GVHD may manifest in nearly any organ system, skin and mucosal involvement being most common. Other sites of involvement include the eyes (keratoconjunctivitis sicca, blepharitis, and corneal erosion), salivary gland (sicca syndrome), esophagus (strictures and webs), liver, pancreas (exocrine insufficiency), and lungs (bronchiolitis obliterans).

The most characteristic manifestation of epidermal cGVHD involvement is reticulate pink to violet papules and plaques with overlying scale, which resembles lichen planus. Lesions involve dorsal aspect of hands, feet, forearms, and trunk which may become widespread. In addition, psoriasiform plaques, keratosis pilaris-like follicular erythema, subacute cutaneous lupus erythematosus (LE)-like eruption, or poikiloderma may develop.

Similar to "lichenoid", there is a "sclerodermoid" pattern of involvement.[4] It includes superficial lichen sclerosus such as shiny, wrinkled, and gray-white plaques on upper back, localized or widespread morphea-like[5] involvement frequently at sites of injury or friction like waistband, and subsequent rippling of skin with joint contractures resembling eosinophilic fasciitis. Long-standing fibrosis may result in skin ulceration particularly of legs and proliferation of benign angiomatous nodules.

Flowchart 1: Mechanism of development of GVHD.

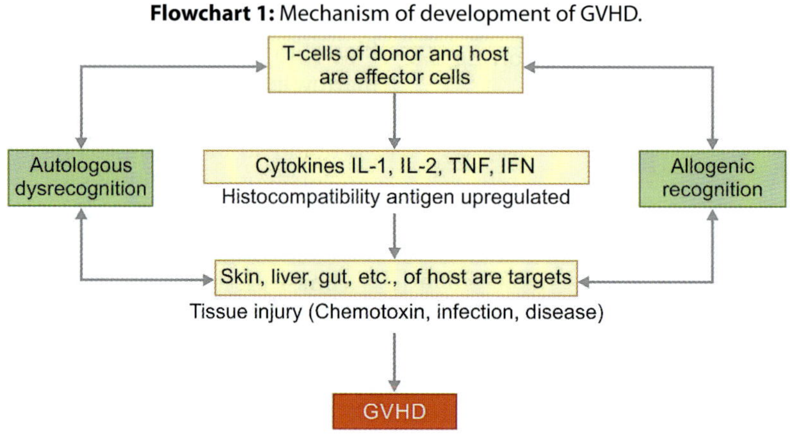

(GVHD: graft-versus-host disease; IFN: interferon; IL: interleukin; TNF: tumor necrosis factor)

TABLE 1: Clinical staging and histological grading of acute GVHD.

Stage	*Skin*	*Liver (bilirubin)*	*Gut*	*Grade*	*Histologic*
1	Erythematous macules and papules, <25% BSA	2 to <3 mg/dL	Diarrhea, 500–1,000 mL/day, persistent nausea	I	Focal vacuolar change of basal keratinocytes
2	Erythematous macules and papules, 25–50% BSA	3–6 mg/dL	Diarrhea, 1,000–1,500 mL/day	II	Grade I plus necrotic keratinocytes in epidermis and a dermal lymphocyte infiltrate
3	Erythematous macules and papules (>50% BSA) to generalized erythroderma	6–15 mg/dL	Diarrhea, >1,500 mL/day	III	Grade II plus fusion of basilar vacuoles to form clefts and microvesicles
4	Generalized erythroderma with bulla formation	>15 mg/dL	Severe abdominal pain with or without ileus	IV	Grade III plus large areas of separation of epidermis from dermis

(BSA: body surface area; GVHD: graft-versus-host disease)

BOX 2: Mucocutaneous manifestations of chronic GVHD.

Skin
- Alopecia
- Angiomatous papules
- Bullae
- Eczema
- Edema
- Erythema
- Hypo-/hyperpigmentation
- Ichthyosis-like
- Keratosis pilaris-like
- Lichen planus-like
- Lichen sclerosus-like
- Morbilliform
- Morphea-like
- Poikiloderma
- Scleroderma-like
- Sweat impairment
- Ulceration

Nails
- Brittleness
- Longitudinal ridging/splitting
- Onycholysis
- Pterygium unguis (dorsal)

Subcutaneous tissue
- Fasciitis[6,7]
- Panniculitis

Oral mucosa
- Erythema
- Gingivitis
- Keratotic plaques
- Lichen planus-like
- Mucocele
- Mucosal atrophy
- Mucositis
- Pseudomembranes
- Restriction of oral opening from sclerosis
- Ulceration
- Xerostomia

Genital mucosa
- Lichen planus-like
- Vaginal scarring/stenosis[8]
- Vulvar erosions/fissures

(HLA: human leukocyte antigen)

Mucocutaneous manifestations of chronic GVHD are given in **Box 2**.

DIFFERENTIAL DIAGNOSIS

The primary differential diagnosis of aGVHD is a viral or drug exanthem and engraftment syndrome.[9] Engraftment syndrome is a nonspecific erythematous skin eruption, fever, and pulmonary edema at the time of neutrophilic engraftment. When there is palmoplantar involvement, toxic erythema of chemotherapy is possible.

Differentials of cGVHD is broader, includes lichenoid drug eruptions, autoimmune connective tissue diseases (lupus, dermatomyositis, morphea, systemic sclerosis, and papulosquamous disorders), transient acantholytic dermatosis, and voriconazole-associated photosensitivity.

TREATMENT

Acute GVHD

- With limited cutaneous involvement, may be managed with topical corticosteroids.[10]
- First-line therapy consists oral prednisolone or intravenous (IV) methylprednisolone (1 mg/kg twice daily).
- Systemic calcineurin inhibitor (tacrolimus/cyclosporine).
- Other immunosuppressants such as mycophenolate mofetil and TNF-α inhibitors (e.g., etanercept and infliximab).

Chronic GVHD

- It is a major therapeutic challenge.
- Localized—topical corticosteroids and topical calcineurin inhibitors.
- Psoralen ultraviolet A (PUVA) and narrow band ultraviolet B (NBUVB) shows some benefits.
- Oral steroids in addition with hydroxychloroquine, mycophenolate mofetil, imatinib mesylate,[11] rituximab,[12] acitretin, and basiliximab.
- Extracorporeal photophoresis may be tried.
- With ocular symptoms, special contact lenses can prove helpful.
- Long term, sun protection needs to be emphasized.
- Patients should be educated regarding skin cancer risk in the setting of immunosuppression thus undergo regular surveillance.

KEY POINTS

- Multiorgan disorder that most commonly results from the transfer of donor hematopoietic stem cells into a recipient via an allogeneic HSCT.
- Despite advances in HSCT procedures and post-transplant immunosuppressive therapy, more than half of HSCT recipients develop chronic GVHD, which remains a major cause of morbidity and mortality.
- Divided into acute and chronic based on clinical features and histopathology.
- Acute is treated with topical CS/systemic CS, systemic calcinurin inhibitor, other immunosuppressants such as MMF, TNF-α inhibitor.
- Chronic is treated with topical/systemic CS, calcinurin inhibitors, phototherapy, imatinib, acitretin, rituximab, sun protection and prolonged immunosuppression.

REFERENCES

1. Ferrara JLM, Levine JE, Reddy P, Holler E. Graft-versus-host disease. Lancet. 2009;373:1550-61.
2. Pidala J, Anasetti C, Kharfan-Dabaja MA, Cutler C, Sheldon A, Djulbegovic B. Decision analysis of peripheral blood versus bone marrow hematopoietic stem cells for allogeneic hematopoietic cell transplantation. Biol Blood Marrow Transplant. 2009;15(11):1415-21.

3. Schultz K. Pathophysiology of Chronic Graft-versus-host disease: Interdisciplinary Management. Cambridge, United Kingdom: Cambridge University Press; 2009.
4. Chosidow O, Bagot M, Vernant JP, Roujeau JC, Cordonnier C, Kuentz M, et al. Sclerodermatous chronic graft-versus-host disease. Analysis of seven cases. J Am Acad Dermatol. 1992; 26(1):49-55.
5. Patel AR, Pavletic SZ, Turner ML, Cowen EW. The isomorphic response in morphealike chronic graft-vs-host disease. Arch Dermatol. 2008;144;1229-31.
6. Schaffer JV, McNiff JM, Seropian S, Cooper DL, Bolognia JL. Lichen sclerosus and eosinophilic fasciitis as manifestations of chronic graft-versus-host disease. Expanding the sclerodermoid spectrum. J Am Acad Dermatol. 2005;53:591-601.
7. Filipovich AH, Weisdorf D, Pavletic S, Socie G, Wingard JR, Lee SJ, et al. National Institutes of Health consensus development project on criteria for clinical trials in chronic graft-versus-host disease: I. Diagnosis and staging working group report. Biol Blood Marrow Transplant. 2005;11;945-56.
8. Zantomio D, Grigg AP, MacGregor L, Panek-Hudson Y, Szer J, Ayton R. Female genital tract graft-versus-host disease: Incidence, risk factors and recommendations for management. Bone Marrow Transplant. 2006;38:567-72.
9. Nishio N, Yagasaki H, Takahashi Y, Hama A, Muramatsu H, Tanaka M, et al. Engraftment syndrome following allogeneic hematopoietic stem cell transplantation in children. Pediatr Transplant. 2009;13:831-7.
10. Martin PJ, Schoch G, Fisher L, Byers V, Anasetti C, Appelbaum FR, et al. A retrospective analysis of therapy for acute graft-versus-host disease: initial treatment. Blood. 1990;76: 1464-72.
11. Olivieri A, Locatelli F, Zecca M, Sanna A, Cimminiello M, Raimondi R, et al. Imatinib for refractory chronic graft-versus-host disease with fibrotic features. Blood. 2009;114: 709-18.
12. Cutler C, Miklods D, Kim HT, Treister N, Woo SB, Bienfang D, et al. Rituximab for steroid-refractory chronic graft-versus-host disease. Blood. 2006;108:756-62.

EXAMINATION QUESTION

1. Describe the pathogenesis, clinical features and management of Graft-versus-host disease.

105 CHAPTER Skin Sign of Abuse

Shailvi Banka Biyani, Surajit Gorai

INTRODUCTION

Abuse is defined as any act which harms the other person physically, mentally, and emotionally. It is a major health problem, affecting all socioeconomic classes, races, gender, age. There are four major types of abuse: (1) Physical abuse, (2) sexual abuse, (3) emotional abuse, and (4) neglect.

Cutaneous injury is the most common and recognizable form of abuse hence dermatologist play a major role in diagnosis.[1]

EPIDEMIOLOGY

Children and elderly are most commonly affected. Children's protective services (CPS) have reported a steady increase in cases of alleged abuse or neglect since the 1960s.

Measurement of child abuse is inherently difficult, as cases reported represent the tip of the iceberg.[2] Parents are the main culprits in 90% of the time.[3]

In sexual abuse, females outnumber males (F:M = 2.5:1) and risk is more in preadolescent group.

Emotional abuse or neglect may precede or accompany other forms of abuse and is the most common form of abuse.[4]

Children who are abused also suffer from anemia, gastrointestinal tract infections, vitamin deficiencies, respiratory tract infections, skin diseases, and malnutrition.[5]

Elder abuse is on the rise and those above 80 years are more susceptible.

RISK FACTORS

Age, child disability, teenage pregnancy, unwanted pregnancy, prematurity, developmental disorders, chronic illness, substance abuse, poverty, improper parenting, dangerous neighborhoods, and poor recreational facilities.[6]

CUTANEOUS SIGNS OF PHYSICAL ABUSE

1. *Abrasions, bruises and lacerations:*
   - Most common physical sign is bruising[7]
   - Rare in <6 months of age as they are immobile
   - *Sites involved*: Knees, anterior tibia, upper arms, medial and posterior thighs, hands, trunk, cheeks, ears, neck, genitalia, and buttocks
   - Pattern bruising is a strong indicator.[8]

   Differential diagnosis: Mongolian spots, lichen sclerosus, bleeding disorders, hypersensitivity vasculitis, infections, chilblains, connective tissue disorders, erythema nodosum, phytophotodermatitis, neuroblastoma, purpura fulminans.
2. *Burns*: Scalds (most common), pattern burns, flame burns, cigarette burns, and electrical/chemical burns

   Scalds:
   - Immersion burns (tide marks)[9]—stocking and glove distribution, zebra stripes, donut hole sparing[10]
   - Splash/spill burns

   Differential diagnosis: Fixed drug eruption, cellulitis, sunburn, toxic epidermal necrolysis, contact dermatitis, phytophotodermatitis, staphylococcal scalded skin syndrome, dermatitis herpetiformis, epidermolysis bullosa, bullous impetigo.
3. *Bite marks*: Adult bite marks can be differentiated from those of a child by findings of maxillary intercanine distance >3 cm and the tooth pattern.[6] Swab should be taken for all bite marks for DNA testing.
4. *Oral trauma*: Bruising, abrasions on lip, petechiae on palate, ageusia, halitosis.
5. *Traumatic alopecia*: *Differential diagnosis*: Tinea capitis, trichotillomania, loose anagen syndrome, alopecia areata.

   Cultural practices: Cupping, coining, spooning, moxibustion, caida de mollera and salting.[6]

CUTANEOUS SIGNS OF SEXUAL ABUSE

Sexual abuse is defined by the *American Academy of Pediatrics* as the engaging of a child in sexual activities that the child cannot comprehend, for which the child is developmentally unprepared, and cannot give informed consent and violate the social taboos of society.[11]

Types: Genital penetration, inappropriate touching, fondling, sexual kissing, exhibitionism, voyeurism, involvement of a child in sexual talks, showing or using in pornographic pictures.

Signs and symptoms: Symptoms are nonspecific such as abdominal pain, encopresis, enuresis, phobias, sleep disturbances, or delayed milestones.[12] History is the gold standard of diagnosis. There are often no physical signs.[6]

Differential diagnosis: Lichen sclerosus et atrophicus, anogenital warts, seborrheic dermatitis, atopic dermatitis, lichen planus, psoriasis, Crohn's disease, hemangiomas, perianal streptococcal dermatitis, vulvovaginitis, Behηet's disease, foreign bodies, labial adhesions, urethral caruncle, Crohn's disease, hemolytic uremic syndrome, and neurogenic anus.

CUTANEOUS SIGNS OF EMOTIONAL ABUSE AND NEGLECT

Emotional abuse is defined as mistreating one emotionally in the form of verbal abuse, disparagement, criticism, threat, or ridicule.[4] Neglect can be described as the inability to fulfil the basic needs of the dependent such as clothing, health, safety or education.[4]

Signs and symptoms: Subcutaneous wasting, severe dermatitis, ichthyosis, hypovitaminosis, poor hygiene, scabies, pediculosis, and trichotillomania.

Munchausen syndrome by proxy: An emotional abuse in which adults fake their own symptoms in their own children.

CUTANEOUS SIGNS OF DRUG ABUSE

Illicit drug use may be suspected or diagnosed on the basis of cutaneous finding. Intravenous drug users frequently have definite skin manifestation.[13] Drug abuse may indirectly contribute to various systemic complications **(Tables 1 and 2)**.

TABLE 1: Cutaneous signs of drug abuse.

Skin tracks	*Drugs given by IV route*	*Lymphedema*
Skin popping scars	Drugs given by SC or dermal route	Lymphedema
Ulcerations	• IV propoxyphene • IV cocaine • SC barbiturates • SC, IM pentazocine	Circumferential pigmented bands (IV administration)
Palmar and digital hyperkeratosis	Smoking/crack cocaine	Madarosis, linear and circular black plaques in hands
Pseudoaneurysm	Drugs given by arterial route	• Purpura • Diminished pulses
Delusions of parasitosis	Cocaine, methamphetamine	
Papulopustular acneiform eruption	MDMA (ecstasy)	
Acne vulgaris	• Methamphet-amine • Marijuana • Anabolic steroids	• Male and female pattern alopecia • Gynecomastia • Hirsutism • Coarse skin • Testicular atrophy
Nasal verrucae	Snorting of cocaine or heroin	• Nasal irritation • Septal perforation

(IM: intramuscular; IV: intravenous; MDMA: methylenedioxy-methamphetamine; SC: subcutaneous)
Source: Adapted from Bolognia, Section 13, Chapter 18, p. 1514.

TABLE 2: Infectious complications of drug abuse.

Bacterial	*Fungal*	*Viral*
• Abscesses and cellulitis • Necrotizing fasciitis • Pyomyositis • Septic thrombophlebitis • Septic arthritis • Osteomyelitis • Endocarditis	• Candidiasis • Aspergillosis • Zygomycosis	• Hepatitis • HIV

Source: Adapted from Bolognia, Section 13, Chapter 18, p. 1515.

ELDER ABUSE

Abuse in >65 years of age and >80 years is more susceptible. The US National Academy of Sciences has defined[14] elder abuse as:

- Intentional actions that cause harm or create a serious risk of harm (whether or not harm is intended) to a vulnerable elder by a caregiver or other person who stands in a trust relationship to the elder, or
- Failure by a caregiver to satisfy the elder's basic needs or to protect the elder from harm.

Types:[12]

- Neglect—55%
- Physical abuse—15%
- Financial and material abuse—12%
- Emotional or psychological abuse—8%
- Sexual abuse—1%
- Unspecified forms of abuse—9%

Risk factors: Shared living arrangement, social isolation, mental illness, and alcohol.

CONCLUSION

Abuse requires a multidisciplinary approach. Legal authorities must be approached wherever abuse is suspected.

KEY POINTS

- Abuse is any maltreatment done to a person against his/her consent.
- Physical, sexual, emotional, and neglect are the four important types of abuse.
- Dermatologist are an important bridge in diagnosis as the cutaneous signs are the earliest to appear.
- Children and elder are the most affected age group although no age is bar.
- Sexually transmitted disease in <3 years, hymenal rupture, abrasions and lacerations of genitalia, bites or suction marks on genitalia or inner thighs are suggestive of child abuse.

REFERENCES

1. Heymann WR. Cutaneous signs of child abuse. J Am Acad Dermatol. 2005;53:138-9.
2. Dubowitz H, Bennett S. Physical abuse and neglect of children. Lancet. 2007;369:1891-9.
3. US Department of Health and Human Services, Administration on Children, Youth and Families. Child Maltreatment 2007. Washington, DC: US Government Printing Office; 2009.
4. Larcher V. Physical and sexual abuse. In: Harper J, Oranje A, Prose N (Eds). Textbook of Pediatric Dermatology, 2nd edition. Oxford: Blackwell Publication; 2006. pp. 1850-66.
5. Banerjee SR, Bharati P, Vasulu TS, Chakrabarty S, Banerjee P. Whole time domestic child labor in metropolitan city of Kolkata. Indian Pediatr. 2008;45:579-82.
6. Swerdlin A, Berkowitz C, Craft N. Cutaneous signs of child abuse. J Am Acad Dermatol. 2007;57:371-92.
7. Chadwick DL. The diagnosis of inflicted injury in infants and young children. Pediatr Ann. 1992;21:477-83.
8. Kos L, Shwayder T. Cutaneous manifestations of child abuse. Pediatr Dermatol. 2006;23:311-20.
9. Yeoh C, Nixon JW, Dickson W, Kemp A, Sibert JR. Patterns of scald injuries. Arch Dis Child. 1994;71:156-8.
10. Stratman E, Melski J. Scald abuse. Arch Dermatol. 2002; 138:318-20.
11. Johnson CF. Abuse and neglect of children. In: Kliegman RM, Behrman RE, Jenson HB, Stanton BF (Eds). Nelson's Textbook of Pediatrics, 18th edition. Philadelphia: Saunders-Elsevier; 2007. pp. 171-84.
12. Finkelhor D. Current information on the scope and nature of child sexual abuse. Future Child. 1994;4:31-53.
13. Del Giudice P. Cutaneous complications of intravenous drug abuse. Br J Dermatol. 2004;150:1-10.
14. Abbey L. Elder abuse and neglect: when home is not safe. Clin Geriatr Med. 2009;25:47.

EXAMINATION QUESTION

1. What are the types of abuse? Write a short note on cutaneous signs of physical abuse.

106 CHAPTER Sports Dermatology

Priyankar Misra

INTRODUCTION

Sports dermatology is a very interesting and new branch of dermatology focusing mainly on dermatoses which are commonly seen in athletes and sportsmen. The skin of an athlete is subjected to repetitive and prolonged mechanical, physical, and environmental stressors, which can damage the skin along with increased susceptibility to infections in body contact sports such as boxing and wrestling.

The commonly encountered cutaneous conditions by a dermatologist are being classified into:

- Mechanical or traumatic
- Inflammatory
- Exacerbation pre-existing conditions
- Conditions seen in aquatic sports

MECHANICAL/TRAUMATIC CONDITIONS

Friction Blisters

- These blisters are commonly seen due to multiple and severe frictional forces that a competitive athlete is exposed to. When the severity and repetition of these forces is more blisters are formed faster in comparison to forces which are prolonged and of lower intensity.
- Poor fitting shoe, heat, and moisture are some factors that lead to the formation of blisters.[1,2]
- The chronologies of clinical signs are as follows: Erythema → pallor → vesicles or bullae. This is generally associated with pain and burning sensation. The commonly affected sites are the bony prominences which bear the brunt of forces such as the tips of the toes, heel, and balls of the feet.
- Taking adequate preventive measure is the key to maintaining a long and injury free sporting career. In this case, preventive measure are:
  - Using highly absorbent socks or multiple layers of socks of differing materials.
  - Using drying powders or other antiperspirant agents such as topical or oral anticholinergics, 20% aluminum chloride applied topically. In resistant cases, iontophoresis and botulinum toxin injection can be used.
  - Application of petroleum jelly post workout leads to proper moisturization and skin barrier function.
- *Treatment of a friction blister:*
  - A 11-blade can be used for sterile drainage of the site but blister roof should be intact to serve as a natural dressing, which relieves the discomfort and protects the site from superinfection.
- If the blister roof gets detached, then it should be treated as an open wound with appropriate antiseptic dressing and topical antibiotics, if required. Rarely, it requires oral antibiotic if there is secondary infection.
- Secondary infection is a complication that can lead to osteomyelitis, cellulitis, and sepsis if proper care is not taken.

Corns and Callosity

- The skin in the areas of repetitive friction becomes thickened, which is nothing but a protective reaction mainly seen over bony prominences.[3] They generally develop as a result of uneven and repetitive friction, which may arise from footwear, gait abnormality, or high level of activity.
- Corns are often misdiagnosed as calluses, which are clinically similar in appearance.[4] Most corns are dry, firm, and painful on vertical pressure with a shiny surface. On removal of the upper layers, translucent central core may be visible which is small (1–2 mm) and translucent.[5] Calluses are generally painless and do not have this central core, which is characteristically seen in corns.
- Warts are another entity which looks similar, but they lack the dermatoglyphics on the skin and they are painful on lateral pressure from the sides. They show pinpoint bleeding when paring is done.
- *Treatment:*[6]
  - *Surgical*: Paring or surgical debridement.
  - *Medical*: Topical retinoids, warm water soaks, topical cantharides, and intralesional steroids. If there is pain and inflammation associated then that has to be addressed as well.
  - Pressure offloading should be done by using specialized shoe with a soft sole to prevent recurrence following treatment.

Knuckle Pads and Athletes Nodule

- Knuckle pads are callosities that develop only over the knuckles in specific professional occupations or hobby sports. It is very commonly seen among boxers.
- They are benign firm, smooth, skin-colored papules, nodules, or plaques which are asymptomatic. Most common site of occurrence is on the dorsal aspect of the proximal interphalangeal joint of the fingers.
- Athlete's nodules are small, asymptomatic, skin-colored nodules on the dorsum of the feet, knees, or knuckles as a result of recurrent friction, pressure, and trauma. The term "athlete's nodule" is a general term referring to a hyperplastic and reactive dermatosis in various athletes. These are common in surfers, boxers, and football and hockey players and are accompanied by thickening of the overlying epidermis. Boxers typically develop athlete's nodules on the knuckles although have the susceptibility for lesions to develop on the feet or toes.[6] Surfers knots are benign, acquired subcutaneous nodules which are typically seen in tibial tuberosities, dorsum of the feet, and the chest which occur due to repetitive low-grade friction of bony prominences with the paddle board. Most cases improve by cessation of surfing.[7]
- Microscopic examination of athlete's nodule shows an increase collection of collagen bundles in the reticular dermis.[6]
- None of the treatment measures are very satisfactory be it medical or surgical. Taking proper protection so as to reduce the repetitive trauma is the most effective way of preventing formation of knuckle pad or athlete's nodule. Local injections of corticosteroids at the site may reduce the size of the lesions. Similarly keratolytics, such as salicylic acid or urea, reduce the lesion size and soften the lesion. If there is functional difficulty, then surgical intervention may be tried out although there is chance of recurrence and scar formation.[6]

Piezogenic Papules (Cutaneous Hernia) (Fig. 1)

- Multiple, skin- or yellow-colored, small, nontender papules found in weight-bearing areas of the feet mainly over the medial or lateral aspect are known as piezogenic papules. Prolonged standing and exercise leads to subdermal fat herniation as a result of excess pressure that accumulates.[8]
- Lower limb is mostly affected in long distance runners whereas similar lesions are around the hand in boxers because of constant vigorous pressure over wrist or palm.[9,10]
- Several treatment modalities have been tried with varying degrees of success such as injectable corticosteroids, electroacupuncture, compression, and padding inserted into the athlete's shoe. Injectable fillers can also be tried in severe cases.

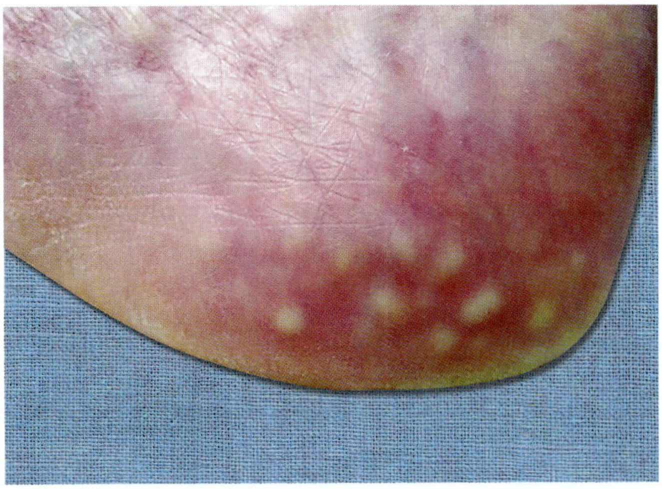

Fig. 1: Piezogenic papules. Asymptomatic, compressible, and skin-colored to yellow papules of the posterior heel as a result of increased heel pressure from sporting activities.[6]

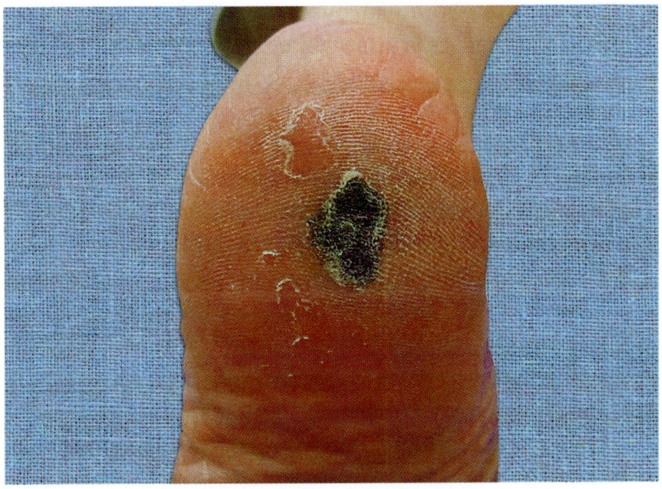

Fig. 2: Talon noir. Asymptomatic, trauma-induced, and dark plaque of the heel that occurs predominantly in young adult athletes and clinically resembles malignant melanoma.[6]

Black Heel (Talon Noir or Calcaneal Petechiae) and Black Palm (Tache Noir) (Fig. 2)

- Black heel is a localized hyperpigmentation or darkening seen on the pressure points mainly on the posterolateral aspect of the heel. They are asymptomatic and self-limiting in nature. It is almost exclusively seen in young adults engaged in active sports, which involve frequent abrupt starts and stops such as basketball, tennis, and lacrosse as these are sports associated with frequent quick starts and stops. However, it can be seen in any sports associated with abrupt impact with the hard ground.
- Similar looking lesion on palm, especially on the thenar eminence, is called black palm (tache noir) which is seen in gymnasts, weightlifters, and in other such sports where an athlete need to put immense pressure on their hands.

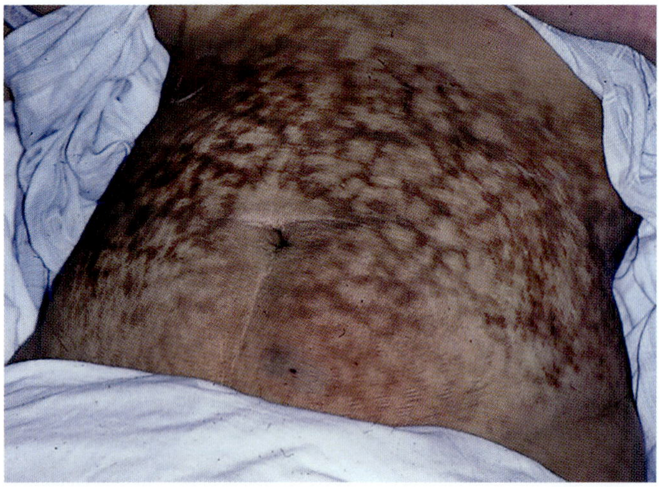

Fig. 3: Erythema ab igne. Reticulated and hyperpigmented patches over the trunk secondary to exposure of an external heating source (a heating pad).[6]

- *Runner's rump* is a cutaneous condition characterized by a small ecchymoses in upper gluteal cleft caused by constant friction with each stride when running.
- It is caused by hemorrhage of superficial blood vessels within stratum corneum, which are minimal surrounding protective fatty tissue.[11]
- They are harmless, self-limiting, and resolves on their own within a few weeks from time of onset and should not hamper an athlete from taking part in any sporting event. In severe cases, pairing can be done to relieve the pain.

Erythema Ab Igne (Fig. 3)

- This is a skin condition which develops as a result of chronic heat exposure in athletes from heating pads, hot water bottles, sauna and steams rooms, and heated recliners that are used for joint or muscle aches. Clinically, it presents as persistent, reticulate or lacy-like, telangiectatic, and erythematous patches that may become hypo- or hyperpigmented in areas exposed to extreme localized heat.[12]
- Complication includes malignant transformation which can be squamous cell carcinoma (SCC), Merkel cell carcinoma, and cutaneous marginal zone lymphoma.
- Due to this malignant potential, it is important to readily diagnose lesions, discontinue offending heat exposure, follow the lesion over time, and biopsy suspicious lesions.
- Generally, treatment is aimed at avoidance of heat exposure. In chronic cases when there is hyperpigmentation, topical lightening agents and/or laser therapy can be tried out.

Tennis Toes

- It is a condition where there is pooling of blood under the toenails, i.e., subungual hematoma, and it is generally painful involving mostly the great toe.
- It is commonly seen in tennis players or runners following repeated injury to the toenail, which results from using ill-fitting shoes.
- If the shoe size is too small, the toe gets crammed up in the toe box of the shoe and the built up of pressure leads to subungual bleed. Whereas, if the shoe size is too large, the feet can slide back and forth forcing the toe against the front of the shoe leading to the same painful condition.
- Prevention consists of wearing shoes of proper size and keeping the nail short so that it does not grow beyond the end of toe.
- Treatment is usually not required as it heals on its own but if it is very painful, drainage might be required. Subungual hematomas are treated by either releasing the pressure conservatively, by drilling a hole through the nail into the hematoma (trephining) within 48 hours of injury,[13] or by removing the entire nail. Trephining is generally accomplished by using a heated instrument[14] to pass through the nail into the blood clot.

Turf Toe

- It refers to an injury of any soft-tissue structure in the plantar complex around the metatarsophalangeal (MTP) joint which may be lead to injury from mild sprain to even dislocation of the MTP joint.
- It commonly affects the great toe MTP joint which may present as pain, swelling, bruising around the joint, and movement restriction.
- Initial management includes rest, ice application, compression bandage, and elevation. Following this in severe cases further investigation using X-ray and magnetic resonance imaging (MRI) may be required to further determine the line of treatment.

INFLAMMATORY CONDITIONS

Contact Dermatitis

- It is a type of inflammatory reaction of the skin that resulting from direct contact with an offending agent. Athletes are repeatedly exposed to allergic chemicals along with represent a unique population of patients who are frequently exposed to various allergens and chemicals on top of repeated exposure to trauma, heat, and moisture that can precipitate the dermatitis.
- Allergic contact dermatitis (ACD) affects those who have a past history of sensitization to the particular substance and represent a delayed-type hypersensitivity reaction. The reaction shows a lag period ranging from hours to days from contact to development of the clinical manifestation. It is seen in athletes from sports equipment, such as shoes or gloves, goggles, swim caps, knee, and shin pads, athletic tapes, antibiotics and anti-inflammatory creams and sprays.

- Direct injury to the skin results in irritant contact dermatitis (ICD) immediately within seconds to minute after exposure and without involving the immune system pathway. ICD is seen due to contact from clothing, hockey sticks, basketballs, pool water, rafts and boards, coral, and seaweed.
- Clinically, they look similar to contact dermatitis seen elsewhere, but the area of distribution varies depending on the source of the contact allergen. The causative allergen can be determined by patch testing.
- *Treatment*:
  - *Topical corticosteroid*: Depending on the severity and site, mid-potent to high-potent steroid is given. Topical antibiotic can be added depending on the presence of secondary bacterial infection.
  - *Topical calcineurin inhibitors*: They are generally given as maintenance after stopping topical steroids or can be tried out for mild reactions.
  - *Systemic corticosteroids*: In severe cases, systemic corticosteroids are given. Oral antibiotics are given, if there is associated secondary infection.
- Prevention of direct skin contact is the primary preventive strategy. Emollients can be given to improve the skin barrier function to prevent such occurrence in future.[6]

Sunburn and Sun-related Conditions

- Athletes are chronically exposed to intense sunlight. This might lead to acute sunburn that presents with pain, irritation, and erythema over the affected area. Over a period of time, they are at a high risk of developing premalignant lesions such as actinic keratosis and others which may progress to cancer such as melanoma, SCC, and basal cell carcinoma. Cosmetic skin changes such as freckles, solar lentigines, and wrinkles are common.
- *Prevention*: The following measures to be regularly taken up in order to prevent development of sun-induced skin changes:
  - Waterproof broad-spectrum [ultraviolet A (UVA) and ultraviolet B (UVB)] sunscreen with sun protection factor (SPF) at least 30 should be applied 30 minutes prior to sun exposure and repeated every 2 hours as per guidelines of American Academy of Dermatology.
  - *Sun protective clothing*: UV protection factor (UPF) determines the amount of UV radiation that can be blocked by a particular fabric of clothing. The higher the UPF, the better is the protection provided by the clothing to UV light. For athletes, it is advisable that they wear clothing with UPF greater than 40.
  - A fern extract named *Polypodium leucotomos* (PL) has shown full body sun protection and has anti-aging benefits. The recommended dose is 240 mg capsule taken orally once daily 2–3 hours prior to sun exposure.[14]

EXACERBATION OF PRE-EXISTING CONDITIONS

Acne Mechanica (Sports-induced Acne)

- Acne mechanica (AM) resembles acne vulgaris and presents as papulopustular eruptions mainly over forehead, jawline, chin, or shoulders. It mainly develops over areas which are occluded by heavy protective equipment and clothing. Predisposition factors include heat, friction, pressure, and occlusion.
- The common sporting events associated with this condition are those that use body or head gear, such as hockey, lacrosse, and football.[15]
- Treatment is not as straightforward as a case of typical acne vulgaris. Prevention is the most important strategy of management. They should be advised to wear such as wearing moisture-absorbing clothing beneath any sport equipment and regular thorough cleansing of the skin after any extreme physical activity. For medical management, topical or systemic antibiotics, topical and systemic retinoids, and topical benzoyl peroxide can be used just like acne vulgaris.

Physical Intertrigo

- Inflammation of skin folds that is induced by mechanical factors is called physical intertrigo. Mechanical factors include skin-to-skin rubbing and friction which gets aggravated by moisture, heat, and infection. Constant rubbing of opposing surfaces lead to itching and irritation which leads to inflammation and erythema followed by erosion, maceration, and fissuring which makes the area very tender and painful. This condition gets often complicated by colonization with bacterial, viral, or fungal elements.
- The sites commonly affected are the intertriginous areas **(Fig. 4)** such as groin, axillae, webspaces of fingers, and toes and inframammary and abdominal folds.

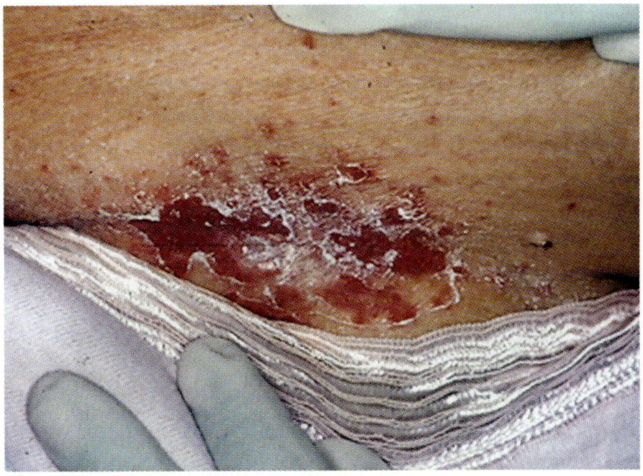

Fig. 4: Intertrigo.[6]

TABLE 1: Conditions seen in aquatic sports.[16]

Condition	*Etiopathology*	*Clinical features*	*Treatment*
Swimmer's xerosis	Loss of protective sebum and long jacuzzi baths	Dry, scaly, and itchy skin mainly over extremities	Moisturizing Syndet soap, oil-based moisturizer applied immediately after pat-drying, topical steroid (severe)
Bikini bottom (deep bacterial folliculitis)	*Streptococcus, Staphylococcus aureus*	Firm, tender, and deep-seated nodules over the inferior gluteal creases	Systemic antibiotics therapy with skin flora coverage like cephalexin or co-amoxiclav
Hot-tub folliculitis	*Pseudomonas aeruginosa*	Follicular erythematous papules and pustules (self-limiting)	Acetic acid 5% compresses, antihistaminic, oral ciprofloxacin therapy
Jellyfish sting reaction	Jellyfish also known as man-of-war stings, in salt-water swimmers	Linearly-oriented urticarial lesion immediately following stinging	Tentacles removed with tweezers, acetic acid soaks, and topical steroids
Swimming pool granuloma or fish tank granuloma	*Mycobacterium marinum*, an atypical *Mycobacterium* found in fresh or salt water	Asymptomatic indurated red to hyperpigmented papules or nodules on the knees, elbows, or dorsal surface of the hands and feet, may ulcerate	Rifampicin (600 mg), ethambutol (1.2 g) daily for 3–4 months continued 4–6 weeks following resolution
Seabather's eruption	Larvae of *Edwardsiella lineata* and *Linuche unguiculata* (thimble jellyfish)	Stinging sensation followed by an intensely pruritic vesiculopapular or urticarial eruption on areas covered by the swimming suit where the larvae get trapped	Cold packs, oral antihistamine therapy, and mid-potency topical corticosteroid therapy
Swimmer's itch or cercarial dermatitis	Allergic reaction to freshwater schistosome (flatworm) larva	Itchy, transient erythematous maculopapular eruption over areas of contact	Self-limiting, supportive with cold packs, and oral antihistaminics

- Jogger's or runner's nipple is a specific condition seen due to friction from the cloth of a loose shirt or a poorly fitting bra can rub against the sensitive nipple skin, causing chafing, cracks, and even bleeding. Nipple fissures caused by friction may also occur in surfers and bodyboarders due to the board and seawater rubbing against the nipples while paddling.
- *Preventive strategy*:
  - The skin folds have to be kept cool and dry by wearing light, nonocclusive, and absorbent clothing. Wool and synthetic fabrics should be avoided.
  - Topical antifungal medications are helpful, especially if used with a low-dosage topical corticosteroid or topical calcineurin inhibitor for a short duration as these medications help to decrease inflammation and associated pruritus.[6]

CONDITIONS SEEN IN AQUATIC SPORTS[16]

Conditions seen in aquatic sports along with their clinical features and treatment are given in **Table 1**.

CONCLUSION

Sports dermatology is an emerging subspecialty in the field of dermatology which aims at identifying common and unique sports-related conditions. Athletes are different from others since their heightened and repetitive physical activities along with environmental stressors place them at a higher risk to some dermatological conditions. Failure to identify these conditions early may lead to complications later that can reduce the performance level and even curtail vital years of sporting life for the athlete. So it is important for a dermatologist to be familiar with these conditions and identify them early and provide adequate treatment.

KEY POINTS

- Athlete's nodules are small, asymptomatic, skin-colored nodules on the dorsum of the feet, knees, or knuckles as a result of recurrent friction, pressure, and trauma.
- Black heel is a localized hyperpigmentation or darkening seen on the pressure points.
- Tennis toes is due to subungal hemorrhage seen in runners or tennis players.
- Sportsmen involved in aquatic sports are predisposed to certain dermatological conditions such as swimmer's itch, swimming pool granuloma, etc. due to exposure to aquatic flora and fauna.

REFERENCES

1. Helm TN, Bergfeld WF. Sports dermatology. Clin Dermatol. 1998;16:159-65.
2. Freiman A, Barankin B, Elpern DJ. Sports dermatology part 1: common dermatoses. CMAJ. 2004;171:851-3.

3. Singh D, Bentley G, Trevino SG. Callosities, corns, and calluses. BMJ. 1996;312:1403-6.
4. Houston SD, Knox JM. Skin problems related to sports and recreational activities. Cutis. 1977;19:487-91.
5. Richards RN. Calluses, corns, and shoes. Semin Dermatol. 1991; 10:112-4.
6. Emer J, Sivek R, Marciniak B. Sports dermatology: Part 1 traumatic or mechanical injuries, inflammatory conditions, and exacerbations of pre-existing conditions. J Clin Aesthet Dermatol. 2015;8(4):31-43.
7. Payton L. Multiple bumps seen on the heels. Piezogenic pedal papules. JAAPA. 2007;20:15.
8. Zaidi Z, Jafri N, Noori B, Thawerani H. Piezogenic papules: a study of 100 cases. J Pak Med Assoc. 1995;45:93-4.
9. Cox NH, Broome G. Piezogenic palmar papules: a novel physical sign of palmar lipoma. Br J Dermatol. 2008;159:757-8.
10. Ayres S Jr, Mihan R. Calcaneal petechiae. Arch Dermatol. 1972;106:262.
11. Dissemond J, Grabbe S. Erythema ab igne. Intern Med J. 2008; 38:675.
12. Chan CC, Chiu HC. Images in clinical medicine: erythema ab igne. N Engl J Med. 2007;356(9):e8.
13. Farhadian JA, Tlougan BE, Adams BB, Leventhal JS, Sanchez MR. Skin conditions of baseball, cricket, and Softball players. Sports Med. 2013;43:575-89.
14. Choudhry SZ, Bhatia N, Ceilley R, Hougeir F, Lieberman R, Hamzavi I, et al. Role of oral *Polypodium leucotomos* extract in dermatologic diseases: a review of the literature. J Drugs Dermatol. 2014;13:148-53.
15. Farber GA, Burks JW, Hegre AM, Brown GR. Football acne: an acneiform eruption. Cutis. 1977;20:356-60.
16. Freiman A, Barankin B, Elpern DJ. Sports dermatology part 2: swimming and other aquatic sports. CMAJ. 2004;171(11):1339-41.

EXAMINATION QUESTIONS

1. Write a short note on erythema ab agne.
2. Describe the dermatolgical conditions commonly seen in sportsmen involved in aquatic sports.
3. Write a short note on talon noir.

107 CHAPTER

Teledermatology

Dipayan Sengupta, Surajit Gorai

WHAT IS TELEDERMATOLOGY?

Teledermatology is a concept in which individual patient-related information is transmitted electronically to a different physical location ("tele" means distant, such as telephone) for the purpose of better management of that patient. We can define it as: *Teledermatology (TD) is a subspecialty of dermatology that uses the information and communications technologies to diagnose, monitor, treat, prevent, research, and educate over a distance.*[1]

TYPES

Teledermatology and as a whole the concept of remote care has traditionally been classified into various types. However, we need to understand that no such classification is absolute and in reality, all or some of the models work together to optimize the care process. Below we are mentioning some of the ways it can be classified:

- *Based on between whom the communication is made:*
    - *Primary or patient-assisted or direct teledermatology*: When there is direct communication between the patient and the provider (dermatologist).
    - *Secondary teledermatology*: The patient visits a nondermatologist doctor (in-person), who in turn communicate with a dermatologist for better management. Also mentioned as assisted teledermatology.
    - *Tertiary teledermatology*: It means communication between multiple dermatologists for better management of some patient.[2]

Primary teledermatology can be used and preferred by educated patients who can use smartphones and have some amount of digital literacy as often they need to capture photographs as per instruction and often need to do online payment. On the other hand, secondary dermatology is most preferred in rural areas where digital literacy is yet to penetrate. Tertiary dermatology is most preferred among dermatologists usually for getting a second opinion from their peers usually through a digital platform such as WhatsApp or Facebook group.

- *Based on the mode of communication:*
    - *Synchronous teledermatology*: The patient and the provider must be connected at the same time. It is possible via phone, WhatsApp, video call, or real time chat.
    - *Asynchronous teledermatology:* Here usually photos/audio clips or other documents are sent to the dermatologist who can give an opinion on a later time.[3]

Synchronous technology is currently more preferred as without real-time communication, medical history is often incomplete.

However, nowadays a hybrid approach is also preferred where some information is sent beforehand (including images) and later a real-time communication is scheduled. The initial information is collected by an assistant, or a digital form or even by a virtual assistant (the later is often powered by cutting-edge technologies such as machine learning).

ADVANTAGES

- According to most studies, diagnostic accuracy is not much inferior to in-person settings.
- Waiting time, efforts, travel expenses, need for a physical space, manpower are saved for both dermatologists and patients as both of them can do it from their home.
- Secondary teledermatology can provide better treatment even to remote areas, where no specialized dermatologist is physically available.
- Tertiary teledermatology may lead to better patient management.
- Data are usually stored virtually. So less use of paper that is also environment friendly.
- As prescription is typed in phone or laptop, ambiguity in prescription writing is totally eliminated.
- A detail advice can be given for some diseases such as atopic dermatitis and it can be saved for future.
- We can provide the service even in difficult situations such as in prison, air, sea or mobile ambulance, warfront, etc. Also a resource-poor country can have best dermatology care from other countries.
- Prescriptions and reports are easily saved and used in next visits.[4,5]

DISADVANTAGES AND CHALLENGES

There are certain core challenges in teledermatology which must be properly dealt with before it becomes mainstream.

- Time consuming so less attractive for many dermatologists.

- Physical examination is not possible. So chance of inaccurate diagnosis.
- Dependent on third party software or applications as there are legal issues about medical data protection and storage, to be known by the patient or difficulty in reaching the patient, to have payment for consultation.
- Insurance companies do not cover teledermatology.
- Patient satisfaction is low. Real-time teleconsultation dependent on good internet connection from both side, good quality of phone camera and skill.[6,7]

INDIAN SCENARIO

During the onset of COVID-19 pandemic in India; in collaboration with NITI Aayog, Ministry of Health and Family Welfare of India, took a visionary step to make telemedicine legal in India and published a detail guideline on 25th March, 2020. Till date this is regarded as standard telemedicine guideline for us. While readers are encouraged to read the full telemedicine guideline from the official website (https://www.mohfw.gov.in/pdf/Telemedicine.pdf), we are mentioning some important points here.

- A Registered Medical Practitioner is entitled to provide telemedicine consultation to patients from any part of India.
- All currently registered medical practitioners need to complete a mandatory online course within 3 years of notification of these guidelines to provide consultation via telemedicine.
- Any medium including phone call/WhatsApp/chat platforms are allowed. Which one is appropriate in a particular case is up to the judgement of the doctor.
- It is up to the judgement of the doctor whether telemedicine is appropriate in a particular case.
- It cannot be anonymous. Both doctor and patient must know each other's identity in detail. If in doubt, proof (such as age proof) can be asked for.
- Every doctor shall display the registration number accorded to him/her by the State Medical Council/National Medical Commission, on prescriptions, website, electronic communication (WhatsApp, Email, etc.) and receipts, etc., given to his/her patients.
- If the patient initiates the consultation, then the consent is implicit. Official consent is required only if the doctor initiates the consultation.
- The doctor shall maintain all patient records including case history, investigation reports, images, etc. as appropriate.
- Follow-up consultation means for the same problem within 6 months. No new symptoms develop and the doctor can properly recall the context.
- The doctor may prescribe medicines via telemedicine only when he/she is satisfied that he/she has gathered adequate and relevant information about the patient's medical condition and prescribed medicines are in the best interest of the patient.
- *Medications that can be prescribed:*
  - *List O*: OTC medicines. No restrictions.
  - *List A*: It can be given in both first contact and follow-up but only after video consult, includes antifungal medicines for tinea and topical skin medicines.
  - *List B*: It can be given in follow-up only (in addition to ongoing medicines in that case)
  - *Prohibited list*: It cannot be given via teleconsultation, e.g., Medicines listed in Schedule X of Drug and Cosmetic Act and Rules or any Narcotic and Psychotropic substance listed in the Narcotic Drugs and Psychotropic Substances Act, 1985.
- Standard of care and nature of prescription is not different in case of online consultation. E-prescription or photo of written prescription both is allowed.
- In case the doctor is transmitting the prescription directly to a pharmacy, he/she must ensure explicit consent of the patient that entitles him/her to get the medicines dispensed from any pharmacy of his/her choice.
- An authorized caregiver can take the consultation on behalf of the patient.
- Patient's privacy and confidentiality must be maintained. Doctors are not permitted to solicit patients for telemedicine through any advertisements or inducements.
- At any stage of the consultation, the patient and doctor, both can refuse to continue and end the consultation there.
- Telemedicine consultations should be treated the same way as in-person consultations from a fee perspective. Doctors may charge an appropriate fee for the telemedicine consultation provided. A receipt should be given.
- Technology platforms shall conduct their due diligence before listing any doctor on its online portal. Platform must provide the name, qualification and registration number, contact details of every RMP listed on the platform.[8]

TELEDERMATOLOGY TECHNOLOGIES

- *Mobile phones and computers*: By far, the most common gadget used in India for teleconsultation. Though poor quality of video or image hampers exact diagnosis yet it is being used due to ease of use. In dermatology, minimum resolution of image is considered 1024 × 768 pixels, better to have 1280 × 1024. Mobile or computer of these quality gradually becoming available and affordable.[9]
- *Still picture-based instruments*: Conventionally, cameras are point and shoot and can be used for this purpose. Single lens reflex (SLRs) are having better quality in terms of exposure control and manual settings but more expensive. In comparison to video consultation, still picture-based images are of high quality and better to use to delineate the minute lesional details. As good resolution can be achieved with mobile cameras, nowadays they gradually replacing point and shoot cameras.[10]

- *Advanced videoconferencing unit*: Modern videoconferencing unit, a fixed setup in tertiary care hospital, and its peripheral center; being used for proper telemedicine consultation these days. It is usually done with a high-resolution camera mounted on top of a computer that can be used for radiology, dermatology, and even for eye examination. From patient's side, it is assisted by a general practitioner most of the time.[11]
- *Information display and archiving system*: Ideally in advanced setup large monitor more than 19 inch, high-resolution display of 1760 × 2140 pixels or greater should be used. Computers should be capable of handling large image or video files. Medical images and other medical documents (EHR, Electronic Health Record) are stored personally by dermatologist, in mobile and it should be archived to any computer/drive time to time. Hard disk, CD, or any compliant online storage medium can be used for storage and archive. In US, EHR should be HIPAA (Health Insurance Portability and Accountability Act)[11,12] compliant while in India similar kind of act is DISHA (Digital Information Security in Healthcare Act).[13]

FUTURE SCOPE AND DIRECTION

There are chances of huge advancement in the field as more and more sophisticated technologies are coming to address all the challenges and regulatory authorities are gradually lifting the legal obstacles especially after the COVID-19 pandemic. The authors believe that we are gradually moving toward an O2O (offline to online) landscape where there will be no strict distinction between traditional and teledermatology. For example, a patient's first visit may be in-clinic and later visits are online or vice versa. As it is a growing subject, rules and regulation are yet to be crystallized all over the globe. Timely update on the same is necessary.

Teledermatology have great potential to provide and revolutionize dermatology services in wide geographical range in cost-effective way. It can assist primary care physician to deliver better care to patients, to those who are bedbound and unable to go to a distance.[14] However, before its widespread application, its reliability, accuracy and safety to be determined in scientific way. Medical data protection and prevent them from being misused will be a huge problem in a country like India. In future, it will be an integrated part of our healthcare system.

KEY POINTS

- Post COVID teledermatology or telemedicine is a well-known entity.
- It can assisted teledermatology by another doctor from patient's side.
- It can significantly reduce time, cost and effort involve in physical consultation.
- Can serve a distant community with exact diagnosis by an expert sitting distantly.
- Till now clinical examination is not possible making it less desirable to most physicians.
- In India, it is legal since 25th March, 2020 within detail rules and regulations

REFERENCES

1. Pasquali P, Sonthalia S, Moreno-Ramirez D, Sharma P, Agrawal M, Gupta S, et al. Teledermatology and its current perspective. Indian Dermatol Online J. 2020;11:12.
2. van der Heijden JP, de Keizer NF, Witkamp L, Spuls PI. Evaluation of a tertiary teledermatology service between peripheral and academic dermatologists in the Netherlands. Telemed e-Health. 2014;20:332-7.
3. Lee JJ, English JC. Teledermatology: a review and update. Am J Clin Dermatol. 2018;19:253-60.
4. Coates SJ, Kvedar J, Granstein RD. Teledermatology: from historical perspective to emerging techniques of the modern era: part I: history, rationale, and current practice. J Am Acad Dermatol. 2015;72:563-74.
5. Moreno-Ramirez D, Ferrandiz L, Ruiz-de-Casas A, Nieto-Garcia A, Moreno-Alvarez P, Galdeano R, et al. Economic evaluation of a store-and-forward teledermatology system for skin cancer patients. J Telemed Telecare. 2009;15:40-5.
6. Whited JD. Teledermatology research review. Int J Dermatol. 2006;45:220-9.
7. Eber EL, Janda M, Arzberger E, Hofmann-Wellenhof R. Survey on the status of teledermatology in Austria. JDDG: Journal der Deutschen Dermatologischen Gesellschaft. 2019;17:25-31.
8. Ministry of Health and Family Welfare of India (2020). Telemedicine Guideline. [online] Available from: https://www.mohfw.gov.in/pdf/Telemedicine.pdf [Last accessed February, 2021].
9. Ratner D, Thomas CO, Bickers D. The uses of digital photography in dermatology. J Am Acad Dermatol. 1999;41:749-56.
10. Loane MA, Corbett R, Bloomer SE, Eedy DJ, Gore HE, Mathews C, et al. Diagnostic accuracy and clinical management by real-time teledermatology. Results from the Northern Ireland arms of the UK Multicentre Teledermatology Trial. J Telemed Telecare. 1998;4:95-100.
11. Loane MA, Gore HE, Corbett R, Steele K, Mathews C, Bloomer SE, et al. Effect of camera performance on diagnostic accuracy: preliminary results from the Northern Ireland arms of the UK Multicentre Teledermatology Trial. J Telemed Telecare. 1997;3:83-8.
12. HHS (2003). Summary of the HIPAA privacy rule. Office for Civil Rights. [online] Availble from: https://www.hhs.gov/hipaa/for-professionals/privacy/laws-regulations/index.html [Last accessed February, 2021].
13. Shrivastava S, Srikanth TK. e-Governance for healthcare service delivery in India: challenges and opportunities in security and privacy. In: Proceedings of the 13th International Conference on Theory and Practice of Electronic Governance; 2020. pp. 180-3.
14. Kaliyadan F. Teledermatology in India: practical implications. Indian J Med Sci. 2008;62:208.

EXAMINATION QUESTIONS

Write a short note on following:

1. Teledermatology
2. Artificial intelligence in dermatology

12 SECTION

Leprosy

108 CHAPTER History and Introduction to Leprosy

Abhishek De, Aarti Sarda, Sachi Gupta

INTRODUCTION

- Leprosy is one of the oldest diseases in the world.
- In the ancient texts about the disease there is no clear and precise description of its clinical practice, leading to confusion of its exact origin.
- The confusion starts with a linguistic issue.
- The Hebrew word, "tsara'ath," translated "leprosy" in the authorized version of the Old Testament, is a generic and nonscientific term that refers to any disease produce scaly lesions on the skin
- It is not clear at what point of time the word referred to the disease leprosy
- Before the third century BC, there are no specific written records describing leprosy as a specific human disease in the western world.

HISTORICAL ASPECTS OF LEPROSY

History of World Leprosy[1]

- The word leprosy comes from ancient Greek Λέπρα [léprā], "a disease that makes the skin scaly"
- Leprosy probably originated in East Africa or the Near East and traveled with humans along their migration routes, including those of trade in goods and slaves.
- The four strains of *M. leprae* are based in specific geographic regions. Strain 1 occurs predominantly in East Africa, Asia, and the Pacific region; strain 2 in Ethiopia, Malawi, Nepal/North India, and New Caledonia; strain 3 in Europe, North Africa, and the America; and strain 4 in West Africa and the Caribbean.
- There are two possibilities of mode of spread of leprosy in Europe. One, it might have been brought in by the men of Alexander from India, or it might have been introduced by the Persian during their invasion of Europe.
- Leprosy was first described in China by Chao Yuanfang in Etiology of Diseases in 610 BC
- In the third century BC in Greece, Straton, a disciple of the physician Erasistratos (c. 300–250 BC), accurately leprosy, which was called elephantiasis.
- The word "graecorum" was added later to differentiate it from elephantiasis arabum (known as bancroftian filariasis)
- Leprosy was reliably described only by Alexandria-trained physicians, who distinguished it well from other diseases.
- The first hospital for lepers was founded early in the fourth century in Rome, during the reign of Constantine.
- Numerous leprosaria, or leper hospitals, were founded in the Middle Ages; Matthew Paris, a Benedictine monk, estimated that in the early thirteenth century, there were 19,000 across Europe.
- Vilhelm Møller-Christensen, was a Danish medical historian and paleopathologist who pioneered and developed the subject of leprosy osteoarchaeology. Møller-Christensen excavated a place near Naestved, Zealand which was the place of old St George's Hospital, and examined bone changes in the skeleton excavated and performed comparisons with modern-day leprosy patients.
- Gerhard Henrik Armauer Hansen discovered the pathogenic leprosy bacillus in 1873. His discovery was published in Norsk Magazin for Laegevidenskaben in 1874. Hansen's finding was opposed principally by his father-in-law, Daniel Cornelius Danielssen, who considered it a hereditary disease.
- Many scientists rejected Hansen's theory initially because he was unable to satisfy the Koch's postulates, which required that the microorganisms be isolated and inoculated into another animal, causing the disease. Desperate to prove he was right, Hansen inoculated the leprous material into a woman's eye, which caused great moral damage to his career.
- Dr Charles Shepherd of the Center for Disease Control in 1959 discovered the multiplication of the bacillus in the mouse footpad.
- Dr Waldemar Kirchheimer of Carville and Dr Eleanor Storrs of the Southern Gulf Research Institute in 1968 demonstrated that the nine-banded armadillo is susceptible to developing disseminated Hansen's disease after inoculation with leprosy bacillus.

History of Leprosy in India[2]

- India may be the point of origin of leprosy with skeletal evidence of the disease dating to 2000 BC.
- Leprosy in India was mentioned in the Vedic writing in 1450 BC.

- In Susruta Samhita of 600 BC, there was reasonable account of clinical feature and management of leprosy
- In the 15th century, an Indian physician named Gopal Krishna produced a comprehensive work on the Materia Medica of India in which he described "galita kushtari rasa" which was used for the treatment of leprosy. It was a combination of mercury, sulfur, iron, copper, and vegetable oils.
- Dutch built the first asylum for the lepers in Cochin in 1728.
- In 1859, Mout, a British surgeon of Indian Medical Service, introduced chaulmoogra oil as therapy for leprosy.
- In colonial India, the government enacted the Lepers Act, 1898.

History of Chemotherapy of Leprosy[3]

- Sun Si-Mao (581–682 AD) was a famous traditional medical doctor from the Tang Dynasty in China who personally treated more than 600 people with leprosy. His writings, Qian Jin Yao Fang and Qian Jin Yi Fang, contain 8 dissertations and 20 recipes on leprosy, as well as commentary on principles for the treatment of leprosy.
- A common premodern treatment of leprosy was chaulmoogra oil. The oil has long been used in India as an Ayurvedic medicine for the treatment of leprosy and various skin conditions. It has also been used in China and Burma. It was introduced to the West by Frederic John Mouat, a professor at Bengal Medical College. He tried the oil as an oral and topical agent in two cases of leprosy and reported significant improvements in an 1854 paper.
- In 1894, Chaulmoogra was used as an injection in Egypt (Feeny).
- Promin was synthesized in 1940 by Feldman of Parke-Davis and company. Until the introduction of treatment with promin in the 1940s, there was no effective treatment for leprosy.
- Between 1940 and 1947, Guy Henry Faget, MD, Director, National Leprosarium, United States Marine Hospital, Carville, USA, pioneers of sulfone drug therapy. Dr Faget and his staff demonstrated the efficacy of sulfone drugs, including Promin, Diasone, and Promizole in the treatment of Hansen's disease, which gives new hope to sufferers. Promin was introduced as a specific treatment for leprosy in 1943.
- Although the parent sulphone, Diamino Diphenyl Sulphone – (DDS) or Dapsone was available before Promin it was not used due to its toxicity in the doses of 1 to 2 gm daily which was generally applicable in the case of sulphonamides. Dapsone was first used for leprosy in 1941.
- Dapsone was introduced later in pharmacologic doses in the 1940s by Cochrane and Muir in India, Lowe and Davey in Nigeria, and Souza Lima in Brazil.
- Clofazimine was first used by Browne and Hogerzeill in the treatment of leprosy
- A forerunner of rifampicin, rifamycin SV, was introduced by Opromolla in Brazil in 1963. Shepard et al. also confirmed the rapid bactericidal activity of Rifampicin. Pattyn et al. were the first to use the drug in intermittent doses in leprosy and found it to be bactericidal.
- Ethionamide/Prothionamide which could be used interchangeably has been used to a limited extent in leprosy following favorable results by Floch et al.
- Seventies saw a number of efforts on improving chemotherapy of leprosy including among others the regimen used in Malta by Freerksen, also known as the Borstel regimen. This involved a combination of Rifampicin, Isoniazid, Prothionamide, and Dapsone.
- In 1965, Thalidomide was introduced by Sheskin for the treatment of lepra reaction.
- In 1964, Pettit and Ress first reported Dapsone resistance.
- In 1981, A WHO Study Group recommended multi drug (MDT) regimens—a combination of rifampicin, clofazimine and dapsone—for the treatment of leprosy patients.

Clinical Approach to a Patient of Leprosy

The diagnosis of leprosy is usually made on clinical examination but preferably should be supplemented by microbiological examination.

Cardinal Signs of Leprosy

1. *Anesthetic patches or anesthesia:* This may be a suggestive skin lesion(s) (hypopigmented or erythematous) with sensory impairment or loss, or else there may be just an area of sensory deficit, more often in the distribution of a nerve trunk or limited to the distal parts of extremities.
2. Thickened peripheral nerves or cutaneous nerves
3. *Acid-fast bacilli:* Finding of acid-fast bacilli (*M. leprae*) on slit skin smears or biopsy specimen is diagnostic of leprosy.[4]

History

- *Chief complaints:* Primary skin lesions, appearance of redness/swelling/pain/ulceration in skin lesions, history of impaired or loss of sensation, history of shooting pain in limbs, history of deformity, history of difficulty in walking or chappals falling off feet, history of inability to close eye, history of ulcer over hand or feet.
- Onset, duration, progress of the disease.
- Details of history, including the name, age, sex, education, occupation, place of birth, visit/stay in hyperendemic or endemic areas for leprosy, and presenting complaints, should be recorded
- Rule out other complaints
- *Precipitating factors for reactions:*
  - History of cough/cold/fever/dysuria/loose motions.
  - History of mental stress/exertion/surgery/vaccinations/drug intake.

- In females, history of pregnancy/postpartum period/menstruation
- *History of nerve involvement:*
  - History of tingling/numbness/shooting pains in upper/lower limbs
  - History of developing numb areas in R/L arm/forearm/leg/face, etc.
- *History of sensory system involvement:* History of impairment or loss of sensation to touch of sudden gradual onset noticed by the patient over the medial or lateral side of hand/feet/soles or any other part of the body.
- *History of motor system involvement:*
  - History of difficulty in buttoning shirts/grasping pen, keys, etc.
  - History of inability to straighten fingers, inability to extend wrist.
  - History of difficulty in walking where the patient has to walk by raising the foot high off the ground as compared to the opposite foot
  - History of chappals/sandals falling off feet
  - History of inability to close R/L eye
- *History of trophic changes:* History of developing blisters/ulcers/corns/cracks/resorption, i.e., shortening of fingers or toes/nail changes.
- *History of eye involvement:* History of pain/redness/watering/photophobia/diminished vision of sudden/gradual onset.
- *History of involvement of breast and genitalia:*
  - History of enlargement of breast (especially in case of LL Hansen in males),
  - History of pain, swelling of testicles.
- *Treatment history:*
  - History of taking any red/brown/white capsules/tablets every month from the hospital
  - History of taking any treatment for reactions
  - History of improvement/no improvement following treatment.
- *Past history:* Diabetes mellitus/hypertension/ischemic heart disease/tuberculosis.
- *Family history:*
  - History of leprosy in family
  - History of diabetes mellitus /hypertension/ischemic heart disease/tuberculosis in family
- *Personal history:* Bowel/bladder habits, addictions, etc.
- *Examination:*
  - Clinical examination should be conducted preferably in daylight and privacy should be ensured.
  - The patient should be seated comfortably and the physician's attitude should be sympathetic and devoid of stigma for the disease.
- *General examination:*
  - If the patient is conscious and co-operative
  - Built
  - Pallor/cyanosis/clubbing/icterus
  - Pulse, BP, jugular venous pressure
  - Lymphadenopathy
  - Edema of hands, feet, face.
- *Cutaneous examination:*
  - *Areas of involvement:* Unilateral/bilateral/symmetrical/asymmetrical involvement of face/trunk/extremities/buttocks with/without involvement of palms/soles/genitals, etc.
  - *Morphology of lesions:*
    - Macule/plaque
    - Papules/nodules
    - Diffuse infiltration of face
    - Nodular infiltration of ears
    - Ulcers/sinuses
    - Ichthyosis
  - Description of lesion
  - Number of lesion
  - *Color of lesion:* Hypopigmented/erythematous/coppery red, etc.
  - *Shape:* Oval/round/bizarre/geographic/annular, etc.
  - Size of lesion
  - *Margins of lesion:* Well defined/ill-defined, regular/irregular, raised/flat.
  - *Presence of Satellite lesions:* An independent lesion close to the big lesion (within <1 cm of parent lesion) (seen in borderline spectrum).
  - *Surface of lesion:*
    - Dry/rough – Tuberculoid spectrum
    - Smooth/shiny– BB, BL, LL
    - Scaly/non scaly
    - If the surface shows any ulceration
  - *Sensations:* Temperature/pain/light touch, impaired/lost more at center or periphery of lesion or uniformly all over the lesion.
  - *Loss of hair:* Sparsity/total loss over the lesion
  - *Loss of sweating:* Dryness.
  - Consistency/induration
  - Warmth over the lesion
  - *Tenderness:* Tenderness over lesion is seen in reactional states.
  - *Local cutaneous nerves:* Run the thumb around the lesion and feel for thickened nerves. They are often enlarged in tuberculoid lesions.
- *Examination of nerves:*
  - Number of nerves involved
  - peripheral/ central
  - Unilateral/bilateral
  - Symmetrical/asymmetrical
- Examination of peripheral nerves (REDRAW)
- *Nerves examined* ***(Fig. 1 and Box 1):***
  - *Cutaneous nerve:*
    - Face and neck (supraorbital, infraorbital, zygomatic, greater auricular, supratrochlear, supraclavicular).

- Forearm (medial, lateral and posterior cutaneous nerves of forearm, radial cutaneous nerve, ulnar cutaneous nerve).
- Thigh (medial, intermediate, lateral and posterior cutaneous nerves of thigh).
- Leg and foot (infrapatellar, sural, superficial, peroneal, and anterior tibial).

- *Peripheral nerve trunks:*
  - *Upper limb:* Radial, ulnar, median
  - *Lower limb:* Lateral popliteal and posterior tibial
  - Mention whether nerves are thickened/soft/firm/tender/nontender.

- While examining a nerve the following points should be noted:
  - Tenderness and paresthesia on palpation. Tenderness is detected by watching the patient's face while exerting slight pressure; if the nerve is tender the patient winces.
  - The nerve's consistency, whether soft or firm.
  - Rarely, if there is a swelling, whether it is fusiform, rounded with fluctuation, or nodular.
- Examination for sensory loss
- Testing should be done for temperature, pain, light touch.
- *Semmes-Weinstein monofilament testing:*
  - Nylon monofilaments are easier to use and those bending at a force of 200 mg, 2 g, and 10 g are recommended.

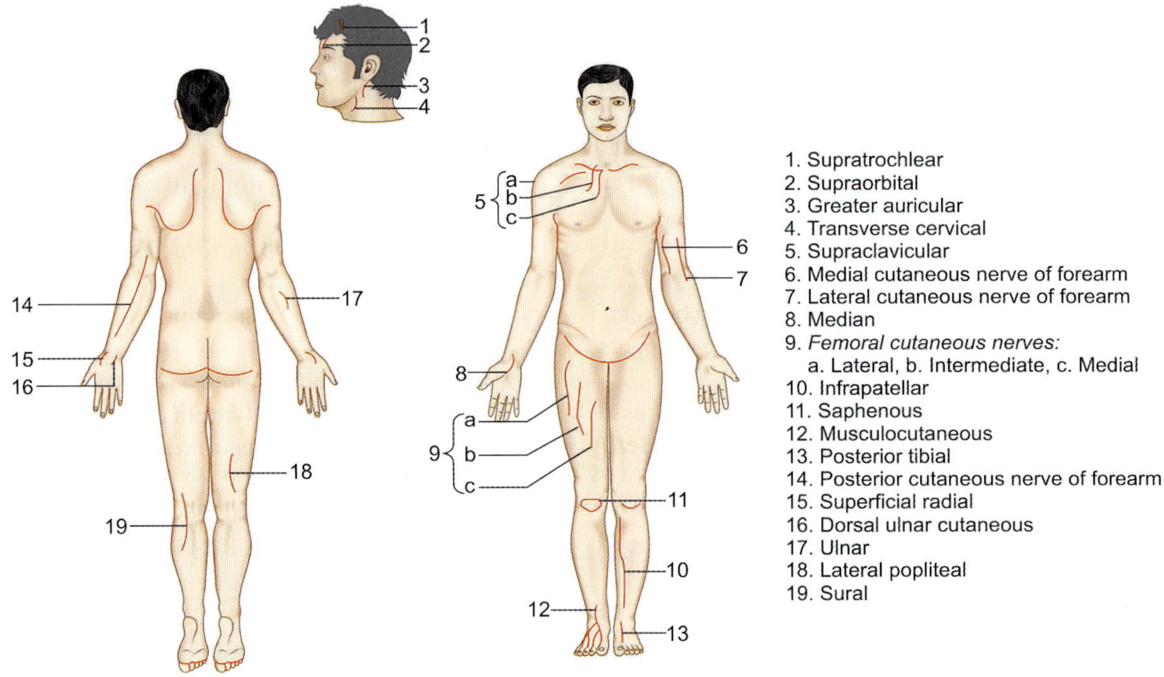

Fig. 1: Diagrammatic representation of sites of commonly thickened nerves.

BOX 1: Clinical examination of the important cutaneous nerves.

- The ulnar nerve, above the bend of the elbow. The nerve is best felt with the elbow joint slightly flexed. With the point of the patient's elbow resting on the examiner's palm, the examiner hooks two fingers around the elbow to palpate the nerve in the ulnar groove and traces it proximally where it is usually enlarged.
- The lateral popliteal or common peroneal nerve is felt behind the knee over the head of the fibula with the knee slightly flexed and is traced as it winds around the neck of the fibula.
- The posterior tibial nerve is felt below and behind the medial malleolus midway between the heel and the medial malleolus.
- The median nerve is felt on the anterior aspect of the wrist between the palmaris tendon and the tendon of the flexor digitorum superficialis. It is best palpated with the fist clenched and the wrist in flexion.
- The radial nerve is felt in the radial groove in the arm behind the insertion of the deltoid muscle.
- The supraorbital and supratrochlear nerves are felt by rolling them against the frontal bone above the orbit.
- The greater auricular nerve is seen or felt over the sternomastoid muscle with the head turned to the opposite side.
- The transverse cervical nerve is felt as it emerges from below the sternomastoid muscle across the middle of the neck.
- Branches of the supraclavicular nerve, if enlarged, can be seen crossing the clavicle.
- The medial cutaneous nerve of the forearm is seen and felt coursing on the medial side of the forearm from the bend of the elbow. The lateral and posterior cutaneous nerves are less commonly enlarged.
- The superficial radial and ulnar cutaneous nerves are examined on the lateral and medial sides, respectively, of the dorsum of the hand with the fist clenched.
- The medial, intermediate, and lateral femoral cutaneous nerves are looked for in the front of the thigh with the knee flexed.
- The infrapatellar branch of the saphenous nerve is felt by rolling it against the bone on the medial side below the patella.
- The sural nerve is felt at the junction of the upper two-thirds and lower one-third of the leg and lower down as it winds around the lateral malleolus, lateral to the tendo-Achilles.
- The superficial peroneal (or musculocutaneous) is palpated in front of the ankle on the dorsum of the foot between the tendons of the extensor hallucis longus and extensor digitorum longus.

- The length of the filament should be 38 mm.
- The normal sensory threshold for the hands is 200 mg and that of the feet, 2 g. If 2 g and 10 g are not felt over the hands and the feet, respectively, there is a loss of protective sensations.

- *Moving 2 point discrimination test:*
  - This is most sensitive test for sensory loss for all sites but for the feet.
  - There is good correlation among Moving 2 point discrimination test and Semmes-Weinstein monofilament testing and pinprick test.
  - The only limitation of Moving 2 point discrimination test is that it is difficult to explain to the patient.
- *Pinprick test:*
  - Paper pins cleaned with spirit or alcohol before use
  - A paper pin should be pressed sufficiently to produce pain but not to draw blood and should be discarded after single use.
  - Testing with a paper pin is subjective
- *Testing thermal sensation:*
  - It is important, as in early lesions it may be the only sensation impaired.
  - It is traditionally carried out by applying test tubes containing cold water and tepid water (40–50°C).
- *Examination of motor system:*
  - *Hands should be examined for:*
    - *Deformity:* Clawing of fingers/ape thumb/splaying of fingers/wrist drop.
    - *Muscle bulk:* Wasting of thenar, hypothenar eminences and guttering of interosseous spaces.
    - *Tone:* Hypotonia (thenar, hypothenar muscles).
    - Power.
  - *WHO disability grading:*
    - *Hands and feet:*
      - *Grade 0:* No anesthesia, no visible deformity or damage
      - *Grade 1:* Anesthesia present, but no visible deformity or damage
      - *Grade 2:* Visible deformity or damage present
    - *Eyes:*
      - *Grade 0:* No eye problem due to leprosy; no evidence of visual loss
      - *Grade 1:* Eye problems due to leprosy present, but vision not severely affected as a result (vision: 6/60 or better; can count fingers at 6 meters).
      - *Grade 2:* Severe visual impairment (vision worse than 6/60; inability to count fingers at 6 meters); also includes lagophthalmos, iridocyclitis, and corneal opacities.
  - *Feet should be examined for:*
    - *Gait:* Normal/high stepping gait
    - *Deformity:* Foot drop, claw toes
    - *Muscle bulk:* Wasting of tibialis anterior/posterior, guttering of interosseous spaces.
    - *Tone:* Hypotonia
    - Power
  - *Examination of the facial muscles:*
    - Light and tight eye closure (orbicularis oculi)
    - Lid gap
  - *Reflexes:* In leprosy, deep tendon reflexes are normal.
- *Trophic changes:* Blisters/ulcers/scars/callosities/fissures/nail changes/resorption of fingers or toes.
- *Systemic examination:*
  - Abdominal, respiratory system, cardiovascular and central nervous system.
  - *Eyes:* Eyebrows or eyelashes madarosis, lagophthalmos
  - *Nose:* deformity (depression of tip or bridge of nose, columellar retraction, clover leaf deformity).
  - *Breast:* Gynecomastia
  - *Genitalia:* Testicular swelling/tenderness

KEY POINTS

- Gerhard Henrik Armauer Hansen discovered the pathogenic leprosy bacillus in 1873.
- Promin was introduced as the first specific treatment for leprosy in 1943.
- Dapsone was introduced in the 1940s by Cochrane and Muir in India, Lowe and Davey in Nigeria, and Souza Lima in Brazil.
- Clofazimine was first used by Browne and Hogerzeill in the treatment of leprosy.
- Three cardinal signs of leprosy are anesthetic patches or anesthesia, thickened peripheral nerves and finding of acid-fast bacilli (*M. leprae*) on slit-skin smears or biopsy specimen.

REFERENCES

1. Couto Dal Secco RG, França K, Castillo D, AlHarbi M, Lotti T, Fioranelli M, et al. A synopsis of the history of Hansen's disease. Wien Med Wochenschr. 2017;167(Suppl 1):27-30.
2. Bhattacharya SN, Sehgal VN. Leprosy in India. Clin Dermatol. 1999;17(2):159-70.
3. Noordeen SK. History of chemotherapy of leprosy. Clin Dermatol. 2016;34(1):32-6.
4. Sirumban P, Kumar A, Durai V, Neelan PN. Diagnostic value of cardinal signs/symptoms in paucibacillary leprosy. Indian J Lepr. 1988;60(2):207-14.

EXAMINATION QUESTIONS

1. Write a brief note on the history of leprosy.
2. How will you approach to a suspected case of leprosy?

Ultrastructure and Microbiology of *Mycobacterium Leprae*

109 CHAPTER

Arnab Dutta, Abhishek De, Aarti Sarda

INTRODUCTION

Taxonomy:

- Order—Actinomycetales
- Family—Mycobacteriaceae[1]

Gerhard Armauer Hansen, a Norwegian physician, discovered *Mycobacterium leprae* in 1873. There are at least four strains of *M. leprae* known to cause human infection, such as TN (India), Thai-53 (Thailand), NHDP-63 (United States), and Br4923 (Brazil). Comparative genomics show remarkable conservation (99.99%) of genome among the four strains. In 2008, a second species, *Mycobacterium lepromatosis,* also found to be causing diffuse lepromatous leprosy. This species has more than 9% difference in genomic analysis from that of *M. leprae*. Till now, *M. lepromatosis* had been described from Brazil, Mexico, Canada, Myanmar, and Singapore. Evolutionally, *M. Leprae* had undergone reductive evolution, which made them an obligatory intracellular bacillus unlike other free-living *Mycobacterium*.[2]

ULTRASTRUCTURE[2]

Lepra bacilli ultrastructure was given by Draper[3] **(Figs. 1A and B)**.

The ultrastructural components of *M. leprae* can be summated in **Table 1**.[4]

IMPORTANCE OF RECOGNIZING BACTERIAL STRUCTURE

- Knowledge of structures recognized by antigen-presenting cell (APC)/T-cells help in vaccination, immunomodulation.
- Newer drugs that can interfere with the synthesis of cellular constituents and devising drugs with better penetration.
- Specific components that will help in confirming that cultivated bacillus is *M. leprae*.
- Ensure phagocytosis of cells.[5]

MICROBIOLOGY OF *MYCOBACTERIUM LEPRAE*

Mycobacterium leprae is an obligate intracellular parasite. It is a rod-shaped bacterium, measuring 1–8 microns in length and 0.3 microns in diameter, with parallel sides and rounded ends. *M. leprae* lives in Schwann cells, chondrocytes of cartilage, melanocyte, endothelial cell, muscle cell, and macrophages. It is acid fast (weaker than *Mycobacterium tuberculosis*) and alcohol fast. Acid fastness is pyridine extractable. *M. leprae* is weakly gram positive.

It divides by binary fission. It is a noncultivable bacillus but capable of limited multiplication following mouse footpad inoculation. Macrophages occur in very large clumps—globi

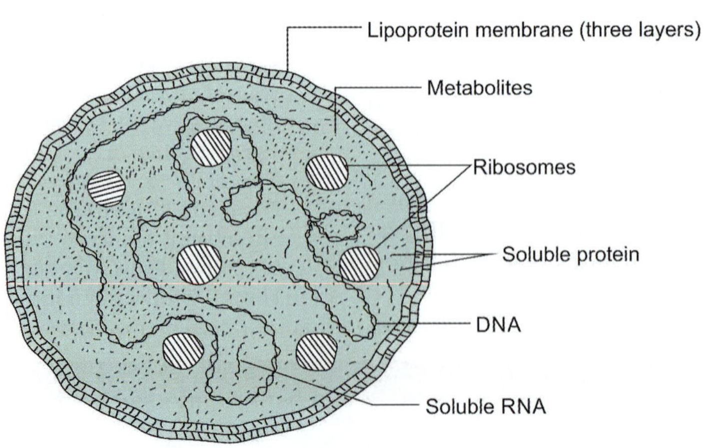

Fig. 1A

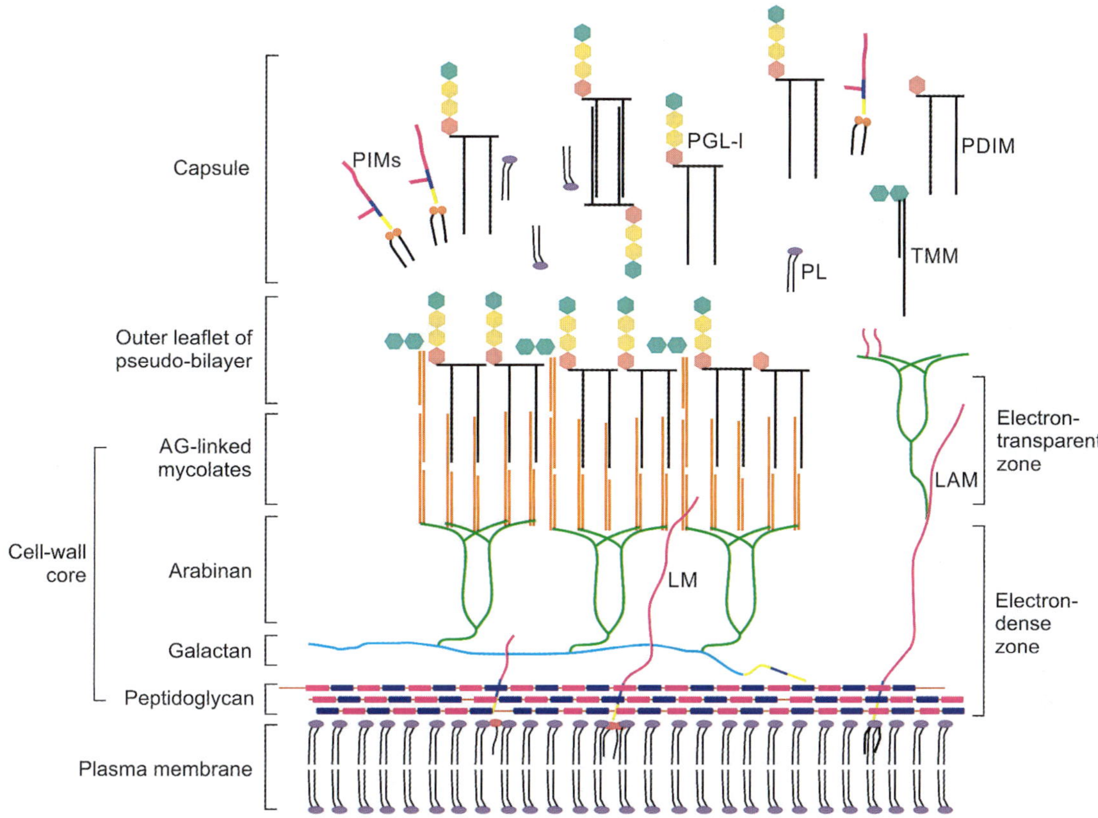

Fig. 1B

Figs. 1A and B: Schematic diagram of ultrastructure of the *Mycobacterium leprae*.
(AG: arabinogalactan; DNA: deoxyribonucleic acid; LAM: lipoarabinomannan; LM: lipomannan; PDIM: phthiocerol dimycocerosate; PGL-1: phenolic glycolipid-1; PIMs: phosphatidylinositol mannosides; PL: phospholipid; RNA: ribonucleic acid; TMM: trehalose monomycolate)

TABLE 1: Ultrastructural components of *Mycobacterium leprae*.

Components	*Description*	*Functions and applied*
Outer capsule	• Suggested by Hanks • Electron transparent zone of foamy vesicular material • Composed of two lipids—phthiocerol dimycocerosate, passive protective role and phenolic glycolipid—active role, 3-methylated sugar molecules attached through a phenol molecule to fat	• Antigenic specificity to *M. leprae* • Form the foam of Virchow cell • The terminal trisaccharide of phenolic glycolipid-1 (PGL-1) which is a surface exposed *M. leprae*-specific antigen, was shown to bind to laminin-2, indicating that PGL-1 also plays a part in the invasion of *M. leprae* into Schwann cells. • *Techniques to demonstrate:* – TLC – HPLC – Mass spectrometry – Freeze etching – ELISA
Cell wall	• 20 nm thick • Outer layer—electron transparent, lipopolysaccharides composed of arabinogalactan esterified with long chain mycolic acid • Inner layer—electron dense, repeated disaccharide units cross-linked with short peptides	• Maintain shape of cell • Protection
Cell membrane	Consists of polar lipids, proteins, and enzymes	• Controls transport in and out of the cell • Surface protein antigens • Candidates for selective toxicity of drugs
Cytoplasm	• Electron dense • Contain DNA, mesosomes, storage granules, and ribosomes • DNA composition—55% GC rather than 65–70%	Maintain cell rigidity

(DNA: deoxyribonucleic acid; ELISA: enzyme-linked immunosorbent assay; HPLC: high-performance liquid chromatography; GC: guanine-cytosine; TLC: thin-layer chromatography) or smaller clumps/parallel array resembling "bundle of cigars". It has a generation time of about 12–14 days.

In practice, in a stained smear, *M. leprae* shows highly polymorphic morphology. Few are brightly and uniformly stained with parallel sides, rounded ends, and length being five times the breadth, such bacteria are called "solid bacteria". Mostly *M. leprae* in smear appears irregularly stained and fragmented or granular.[6,7]

RESISTANCE

- Viable for 9–16 days in warm and human environment
- In moist soil for 46 days
- Direct sunlight for 2 hours
- Ultraviolet for 30 minutes

VIABILITY ASSAYS

- *Molecular viability assay*: Reverse transcriptase (RT) polymerase chain reaction (PCR) of 16S ribosomal ribonucleic acid (rRNA)
- Mouse foot pad inoculation
- *Morphological index*: This is calculated by counting the numbers of solid-staining acid-fast rods. Only the solid-staining bacilli are viable. It is not unusual for solid-staining *M. leprae* to reappear for short periods in patients being successfully treated with drugs.
- *Fluorescent vital dyes*: Fluorescein diacetate and ethidium bromide, rhodamine-123, and propidium iodide
- *Metabolic profiling*: Mass spectrometry to measure Na^+/K^+ ratio, adenosine triphosphate (ATP) content, and phenolic glycolipid-1 (PGL-1) synthesis
- Radiorespirometry

KEY POINTS

- *Mycobacterium leprae* is an obligate intracellular parasite.
- It is a weakly gram positive, weakly acid fast, and alcohol fast noncultivable bacillus with parallel sides and rounded ends.
- Main structural components of *M. leprae* are from outside inwards—outer capsule, cell wall, cell membrane, and cytoplasm.
- PGL-1 of outer capsule provides antigenic specificity to *M. leprae*.
- Cell membrane of *M. leprae* consists of polar lipids, proteins, and enzymes.
- Knowledge of structural components recognized by APC/T-cells help in vaccination and immunomodulation.

REFERENCES

1. Kumar B, Kar H. Bacteriology of leprosy. In: Kumar B (Ed). IAL Textbook of Leprosy, 2nd edition. New Delhi: Jaypee Brothers Medical Publishers; 2015. pp. 90-4.
2. Chatterjee BR. Mycobacterium leprae and the bacteriology of leprosy. In: Chatterjee BR (Ed). Leprosy: Etiobiology of Manifestations, Treatment and Control. Calcutta: Statesman Commercial Press; 1993. pp. 42-80.
3. Draper P. Cell walls of *Mycobacterium leprae*. Int J Lepr Other Mycobact Dis. 1976;44:95-8.
4. Draper P, Kandler O, Darbre A. Peptidoglycan and arabinogalactan of *Mycobacterium leprae*. J Gen Microbiol. 1987;133:1187-94.
5. Young DB. Detection of mycobacterial lipids in skin biopsies from leprosy patients. Int J Lepr Other Mycobact Dis. 1981; 49:198-204.
6. Cole ST, Eiglmeier K, Parkhill J, James KD, Thomson NR, Wheeler PR, et al. Massive gene decay in the leprosy bacillus. Nature. 2001;409:1007-11.
7. Vissa V, Brennan PJ. The genome of *Mycobacterium leprae*: a minimal mycobacterial gene set. Genome Biol. 2001;2:1-7.

EXAMINATION QUESTIONS

1. Draw a neat labeled diagram of *Mycobacterium leprae*.
2. Write a short note on ultrastructure and microbiology of *M. leprae*.

110 CHAPTER Immunology of Leprosy

Adrija Datta, Nilay Kanti Das

INTRODUCTION

Disease occurs due to interaction between host, agent, and environment and the immune response of the host towards the pathogen determines the clinicopathological expression. Leprosy constitutes the ideal example of immunologically-mediated infectious disease where immune response towards intracellular bacteria guides disease expression. In 1966, Ridley and Jopling suggested classifying leprosy in two stable forms [tuberculoid (TT) and lepromatous leprosy (LL)] and the three intermediate forms lying in between the two poles based primarily on immunological and histological criteria. This chapter will highlight on how the immune response of host determines the host susceptibility for infection, the spectrum of manifestations, and also the response to therapy.

Mycobacterium leprae, an acid-fast bacillus with a slow generation time is an intracellular organism that resides primarily within macrophages and dendritic cells. It also affects the peripheral nervous system by infecting the Schwann cells. Capsular lipid phenolic glycolipid-1 (PGL-1) and lipoarabinomannan (LAM) in the mycobacterial cell membrane play important roles in immune response. The pathogen has to encounter the innate immune system first, which identify certain pathogenic structures called pathogen-associated molecular patterns and activate pathways to eliminate the organism. The adaptive immunity is activated when specific epitopes are presented to the T lymphocyte by antigen-presenting cell. However, there is considerable overlap between the two, indicating interdependence of the two systems for successful control of infection.

IMMUNOPATHOGENESIS

Transmission of Leprosy

With the exception of armadillos, humans are the only known hosts of lepra bacilli and contacts of patients with multibacillary LL are at high risk of contracting the disease. Lepra bacilli may remain viable in nasal discharge for up to 48 hours. Multiple studies have considered the upper respiratory airway via nasal droplets to be the main mode of entry of leprosy. In vitro studies have demonstrated attachment of mycobacterial adhesion molecules histone-like protein and heparin-binding hemagglutinin to nasal epithelial cells thus promoting survival of bacteria in the upper airway tract. Bacilli reach their target sites most probably by hematogenous spread.[1]

Mycobacterium leprae can enter the host cell in different ways. Receptors to complement fragments CR1, CR3, and CR4 help in phagocytosis, where PGL-1 is specifically recognized by complement 3.[2] Interaction with macrophage scavenger receptors CD163 and CD209 also promotes bacillary entry into macrophages.[3]

FATE OF INFECTION

About 90–95% individuals do not develop any disease following infection with *M. leprae*. Following subclinical infection, patients may present with one to few ill-defined hypopigmented lesions with weak or no cell-mediated immunity with mild dermal and perineural inflammation on histology—a stage called indeterminate leprosy, which may be the initial feature in 20–80% of patients. Majority (about three-fourths) regress spontaneusly, while few may remain indeterminate for a prolonged time. Others proceed to the more definite form of leprosy and may present in any sperctrum **(Flowchart 1)**.[4]

Flowchart 1: Fate of Infection in case of *Mycobacterium leprae*.

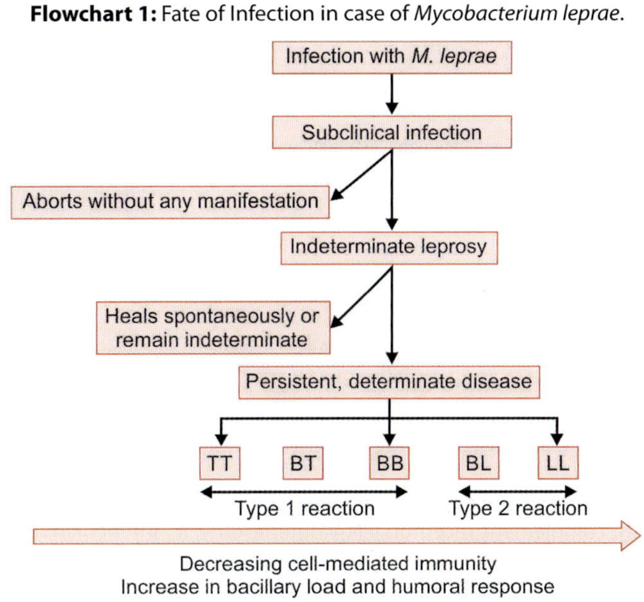

INNATE IMMUNITY

Innate immunity comprises the first line of defense against any external agent. In the pathogenesis of an intracellular parasite, pattern recognition receptors identify antigenic components, which lead to phagocytosis and subsequent activation of intracellular pathways leading to antigen presentation **(Fig. 1)**. Multiple toll-like receptors (TLRs) as well as nucleotide-binding oligomerization domain 2 (NOD2) of NOD-like receptor (NLR) family are involved in pathogenesis of leprosy. Several mycobacterial cell wall components such as lipomannan, LAM, and 19-kDa lipoprotein act as agonists to TLR1/TLR2 heterodimers, whereas phosphatidylinositol dimannoside can activate TLR2 homodimers. Activation of TLR1 and 2 initiate differentiation of macrophages and dendritic cells leading to secretion of proinflammatory cytokines interleukin 12 (IL-12) and tumor necrosis factor (TNF) which regulates and maintains a T helper type 1 (Th1) protective response. TLR1 and TLR2 are thus expressed abundantly in paucibacillary TT lesions. *M. leprae* can inhibit TNF-α-mediated inflammatory response through interaction with TLR4. Human NOD2 receptor is capable of dendritic cell differentiation via an IL-32-mediated pathway. Activation of NOD2 is mediated by mycobacterial muramyl dipeptide and is associated with autophagy and antigen presentation.[5] Activation of TLR2 and interferon gamma (IFN-γ) receptor stimulates the vitamin D-dependent pathway to produce antimicrobial peptides cathelicidin and human beta-defensin which are recruited in autophagolysosomes for intracellular killing of *M. leprae*.[6]

Recent years have revealed importance of autophagy in induction of dichotomy of leprosy. Autophagic protein Beclin 1 is expressed in TT lesions while antiapoptotic B-cell lymphoma-2 (BCL2) protein that inhibits autophagy has been found in lepromatous lesions. Similarly, apoptosis is related to containment of infection in TT pole, with antiapoptotic molecules propagating infection in multibacillary patients.[1]

Clinical Implications

Polymorphisms in genes for TLRs, NOD2, and autophagic proteins are associated with susceptibility to leprosy **(Table 1)**.

MACROPHAGES IN LEPROSY

Macrophages play a crucial role in the pathogenesis of leprosy. Traditionally they have been classified as M1 or inflammatory macrophages and M2 or healing macrophages, with different expression of surface molecules. Though this specificity cannot coexist once they reach specific tissues, still the concept of this duality of macrophages helps in our lucid understanding of the polar expression of leprosy **(Table 2)**. IFN-γ and bacterial lipopolysaccharide induce M1 phenotype with production of inflammatory cytokines and enzymes like induced nitric oxide synthase which generate free radicals for killing of *M. leprae*. Protein Jagged 1 also regulates polarization of monocytes into M1 macrophages by IFN-γ stimulated endothelial cells. On the other hand, unstimulated endothelial cells differentiate monocytes into M2 macrophages.[7] They may also be induced by IL-4, IL-10, and IL-13 or immune complexes. Anti-inflammatory cytokines, growth factors

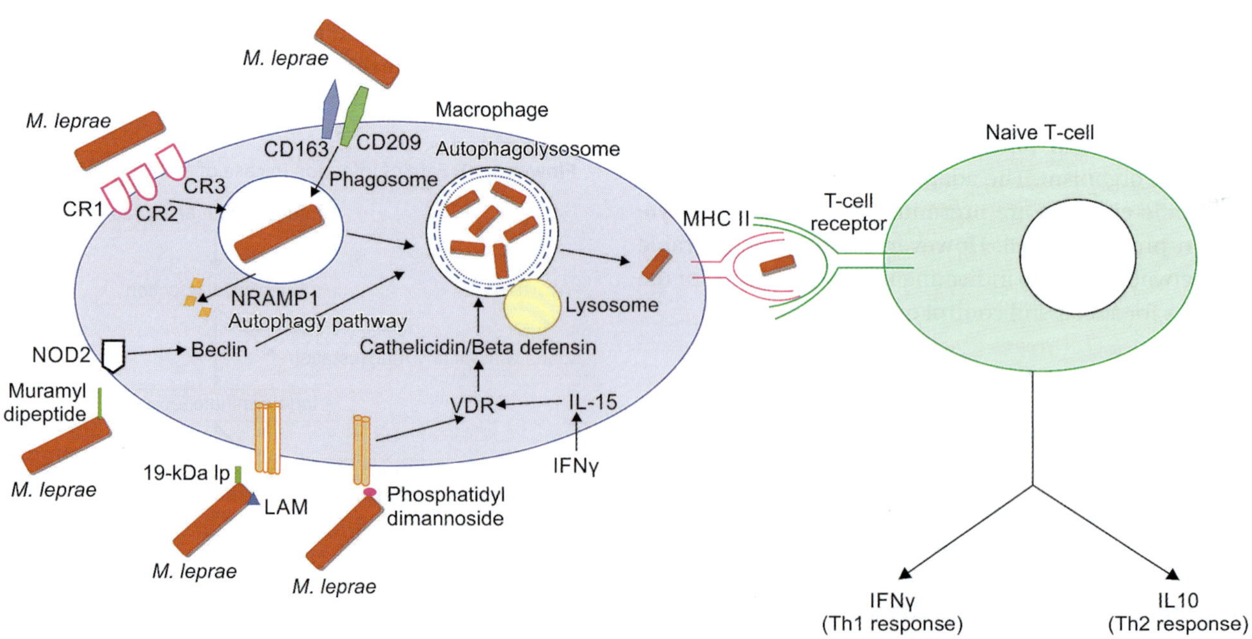

Fig. 1: Interaction of *Mycobacterium leprae* with innate immunity and subsequent antigen presentation.
(CR: complement receptor; IFN-γ: Interferon γ; IL: interleukin; LAM: lipoarabinomannan; Lp: lipoprotein; MHC: major histocompatibility complex; NOD2: nucleotide-binding oligomerization domain 2; NRAMP: natural resistance-associated macrophage protein; TCR: T-cell receptor; Th2: T helper type 2; TLR: toll-like receptor)

TABLE 1: Genetic polymorphisms that affect leprosy susceptibility.

Genes implicated in leprosy	*Role of genetic variant*
• MHC genes • Innate immune receptors—TLR1, TLR2, TLR4, NOD2, MRC1, and *VDR* • Cytokines—*TNF, IL-10, IL-6, and IFN-γ* • Transport molecules—SLCA11/NRAMP1 • PARK2, PACRG, and LTA • Transporters associated with peptide loading 1 and 2 (TAP1 and TAP2) • MHC class I chain-related gene A (MICA)	• SNPs of HLA-DRB1/DQA1 susceptible • TLR1—602S allele protective (India); 248S/SS allele susceptible but protective for ENL (Bangladesh) • TLR2—N199N susceptible to reversal reaction • TNF-308A inconsistent association • *IL-10* promoter region SNP in paucibacillary leprosy • *IL-6* polymorphism susceptible to ENL • Modulates leprosy susceptibility • PARK2—multiple SNPs susceptible (India, Brazil, and Vietnam); LTA+80 SNP susceptible in young individuals (Vietnam and India) • TAP1 A637G variant susceptible (India) • Protective against multibacillary in Brazil and China; susceptible in India

(ENL: erythema nodosum leprosum; IFN-γ: interferon gamma; IL: interleukin; MHC: major histocompatibility complex; MRC1: mannose receptor 1; NOD2: nucleotide-binding oligomerization domain 2; NRAMP1: natural resistance-associated macrophage protein 1; SNP: single-nucleotide polymorphism; TLR: toll-like receptor; VDR: vitamin D receptor)

TABLE 2: Immunological features of polar forms of leprosy.

Typical tuberculoid leprosy	*Lepromatous leprosy*
Strong cell-mediated immunity—Th1 response	Weak cell-mediated immunity—Th2 response, with increased humoral response
Proinflammatory cytokines—IL-2, IFN-γ, TNF-α, and IL-12	Anti-inflammatory cytokines—IL-4, IL-5, and IL-10
Granuloma: Well-differentiated macrophages and epithelioid cell	*Granuloma:* Poorly organized granuloma with microvacuolated macrophages (foamy macrophages)
Diffuse infiltrate of CD4+ cells, with CD8+ cells in periphery (CD4:CD8 = 2:1)	CD4+ and CD8+ cells distributed throughout granuloma (CD4:CD8 = 1:2)
Lepromin test—positive	Lepromin test—negative

(IL: interleukin; IFN-γ: interferon γ; Th1: T helper type 1; Th2: T helper type 2; TNF-α: tumor necrosis factor α)

like transforming growth factor β (TGF-β), fibroblast growth factor (FGF), and enzymes like arginase produced by M2 macrophages cause immunosuppression and promote healing and fibrosis. Expression of costimulatory molecules such as CD68 and CD163 on cell surface aids bacillary entry into these cells. Leukocyte immunoglobulin-like receptor subfamily A member 2 (LILRA2) expressed by lepromatous macrophages inhibits IL-12 release. The sustained IL-10 release augments uptake of *M. leprae* and oxidized phospholipids which in turn has an inhibitory effect on inflammatory meditators. This amplified phagocytosis continues without induction of antimicrobial program. Concomitant uptake of hemoglobin-haptoglobin complex CD163 provides iron for survival of bacteria.[7]

Clinical Implications

Cytokines like IFN-γ, TNF-α, and IL-2 in a proinflammatory framework limits proliferation of *M. leprae* giving rise to localized paucibacillary TT lesions. Enhanced phagocytosis without killing ensures unrestricted bacillary growth and is associated with the widespread multibacillary form of leprosy, with intracellular lipid droplets providing a foamy appearance of macrophages on histology.

ROLE OF KERATINOCYTES

Apart from dendritic cells, keratinocytes are critical in mounting an epidermal immune response against *M. leprae*. They express mannose-binding receptors, TLRs, and intercellular adhesion molecule-1 (ICAM-1) with a capacity to secrete cytokines and antimicrobial peptides mediating a strong cellular response, as observed in TT leprosy and reversal reactions. Human beta defensins (HBD2 and HBD3) are expressed by keratinocytes in response to *M. leprae* antigens and are stimulated by TNF-α, thereby maintaining a Th1 cytokine milieu. Cytokines and chemokines secreted by keratinocytes are responsible for skin homing of dendritic cells, T-cells, and neutrophils. HLA-DR+ keratinocytes may also function as antigen-presenting cells.[1,2]

ADAPTIVE IMMUNITY

Acquired immunity or adaptive immunity is a highly specific form of immunity that has a "memory" against previously exposed antigen and involves T and B lymphocytes and their diverse receptors. Cell-mediated immunity provides protection against intracellular organisms like mycobacteria whereas humoral immunity acts mostly against extracellular organisms.

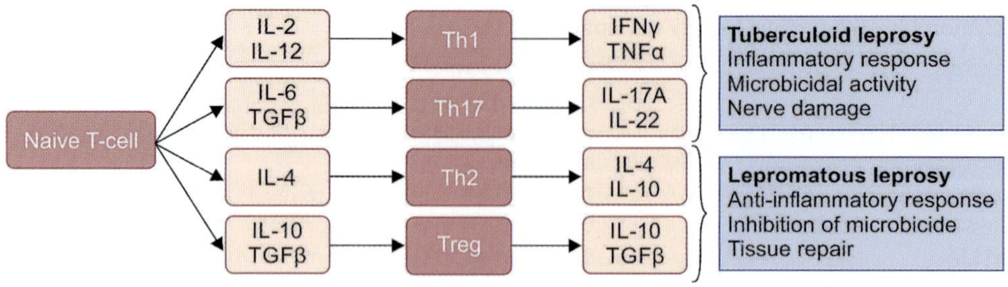

Fig. 2: T-cell responses in leprosy.
(IFN-γ: interferon γ; IL: interleukin; TGF-β: transforming growth factor β; Th: T helper; Treg: regulatory T-cell)

CELL-MEDIATED IMMUNITY

In leprosy, T-cells are activated when antigenic peptides expressed by class II major histocompatibility complex (MHC) molecule on antigen presenting cell interact with T-cell receptor, leading to induction of helper T-cell response (Th1 or Th2). The type of T-cell response is governed by the local cytokine and chemokine subset, which directs whether the infection will be contained or permitted **(Fig. 2)**.

T Helper Type 1 Response

Proinflammatory cytokines IL-2, TNF-α, IFN-γ, lymphotoxin-α, IL-12, and IL-15 comprise the Th1 cytokines. Secretion of IL-12 potentiated by IFN-γ differentiates the naive CD4+ T- cell to Th1 lymphocyte, which further induces macrophages and dendritic cells to produce IL-12, IL-15, and IL-18. These interleukins amplify the Th1 inflammatory response through proliferation of CD4+ T-cells and enhanced T-cell-mediated IFN-γ secretion. Th1 cytokines are responsible for increased antigen presentation, recruitment of inflammatory cells, proliferation of lymphocytes, differentiation of macrophages, and induction of antimicrobial pathways (IL-5-induced vitamin D-dependent pathway).[8]

T Helper Type 2 Response

T helper type 2 cytokines are responsible for activation of B cells and antibody production along with inhibition of Th1 inflammatory responses. In leprosy, Th2 response is initiated against *M. leprae* in presence of IL-10 and TGF-β, with production of IL-4, IL-5, and IL-13. Th2 cytokine profile is responsible for immunosuppression seen in LL, along with antibody production, inhibition of TNF, and activation of regulatory T-cells. Immune complex formation additionally contributes to anti-inflammatory effect.[9]

The borderline spectrum of leprosy represents a zone of immunological instability, with decreasing T-cell response from TT to lepromatous pole and increasing bacillary load. The resulting granuloma is also mixed type. This instability is responsible for the acute inflammatory episodes or reactions causing inflammation in both skin lesions and affected nerves, making the patient prone to sudden loss of nerve function or impairment and deformities.

Clinical Implication

Tuberculoid leprosy presents as single to few hypopigmented hypoesthetic/anesthetic lesions consistent with the Th1 response of resistance to *M. leprae* infection. An anti-inflammatory Th2 response with well-developed but ineffective humoral immunity correlates with small infiltrated lepromatous lesions in a widespread and symmetrical distribution.

T Helper Type 17 Response

Naive T-cells are transformed into Th17 cells when subjected to IL-6, IL-22, and TGF-β to elicit an inflammatory response in leprosy through cytokines IL-17A, IL-17F, and IL-23 acting on epithelial cells. Stimulated epithelial cells engage and activate inflammatory cells through IL-6, IL-1β, and chemokines. Additionally antimicrobial peptides like defensins are produced, justifying higher levels of Th17 cytokines in paucibacillary leprosy and TT leprosy as compared to LL patients. In both type 1 and type 2 reactions, Th17 cytokines incite a surge in inflammatory cytokines and chemokines to mobilize inflammatory cells and activate endothelial cells. IL-26 is a recently illustrated Th17 cytokine with a presumable role in autophagy, with higher expression in TT and reversal reactions.[10]

Regulatory T-cells (Treg)

Suppressor T-cells function to prevent autoimmunity and limit chronic inflammation. In leprosy suppressor functions are orchestrated by forkhead box P3 (FOXP3) inducible T-cells bearing CD4+CD25+FOXP3+ phenotype. They are capable of suppressing inflammatory responses by Th1, Th17, and Th9 cells through direct contact or through suppressive cytokines IL-10 and TGFβ. Borderline leprosy (BL)/LL patients exhibit a higher proportion of Treg cells than patients in the TT spectrum. Sadu et al. demonstrated a negative correlation between Th17 cells and regulatory T-cells in LL.[2,10]

T Helper Type 9 and T Helper Type 22 Responses

Newer subsets of T helper are steadily gaining importance. Th9 cells are generated on stimulation with IL-4 and TGF-β and through production of IL-9 generate a proinflammatory response. Th22 cells, differentiated in response to IL-6 and TNF-α, secrete FGF-β, IL-22, and IL-13 influencing phagolysosome maturation and reparative responses in LL.[11]

HUMORAL IMMUNITY AND IMMUNOLOGIC UNRESPONSIVENESS

Lepromatous leprosy is characterized by a polyclonal B-cell response of immunoglobulin M (IgM), IgG, and IgA classes, with a T-cell anergy specific for *M. leprae*. Stimulation of B cells by IL-4 and IL-5 leads to formation of antibodies against multiple *M. leprae* antigens, without any effective protective response to the intracellular pathogen. In 90–95% patients of lepromatous patients, antibodies against PGL-1 and its glycoconjugates are found, the titers of which decline on administration of therapy. Various theories have been proposed for the immunologic unresponsiveness: (1) direct inhibition of T-cells or macrophages by *M. leprae*, probably PGL-1 mediated, (2) inhibition of T-cell responses by soluble factors secreted from *M. leprae* stimulated macrophages, and (3) negative regulation by FOXP3+ regulatory T-cells.[2]

IMMUNE-MEDIATED NERVE DAMAGE IN LEPROSY

Peripheral neuropathy is a distinctive feature of leprosy. Perineural and intraneural inflammation and destruction are responsible for loss of sensory and motor functions resulting in the most disabling consequences of leprosy. Schwann cell is the primary cell to be affected and nonmyelinating Schwann cells are predominantly affected. Following initial bacillemia, the lepra bacilli reach Schwann cell via blood vessels of perineurium into the endoneurium. Mannose capped LAM and PGL-1 as well as surface antigen laminin-binding protein 21 (LBP21) facilitate entry of *M. leprae* into the Schwann cell by binding to laminin-2 in basal lamina of Schwann cells and α-dystroglycan. Infected Schwann cells may get reprogrammed to stem-cell like phenotype under the influence of *M. leprae* thereby ensuring bacillary survival and enhancing spread of infection. Schwann cells have been shown to express TLR2 and also TNF and TNF receptors, which are known to induce demyelination, apoptosis, and subsequently nerve damage. *M. leprae* sensitizes Schwann cell to TNF-mediated demyelination. LAM triggers axonal injury through complement activation and deposition of membrane attack complex (MAC) along axons in lepromatous patients. Infected Schwann cells have been shown to express adhesion molecules [ICAM-1, neural cell adhesion molecule (NCAM), and N-cadherin) and MHC class II molecules, followed by antigen presentation to CD4+ T-cells. In TT lesions and reversal reactions, nerve damage is arbitrated through proinflammatory cytokines. Immunostaining of skin biopsy specimen has revealed inverse correlation between IL-17 and nerve growth factor and its receptor (NGF/NGFR), with excess IL-17 in TT form, contributing to the Th1 inflammatory response in nerve damage.[12]

Nonimmune-mediated neuronal damage occurs either by direct contact with bacteria and activation of ErbB2 kinase pathway or production of nitric oxide and its metabolites.

REACTIONAL STATES

Leprosy reactions are immunologically-mediated acute inflammatory episodes occurring usually in the unstable borderline spectrum of the disease, with mycobacterial antigens acting as the potential triggers for the T-cell response. These episodes may occur any time before, during, or after multidrug therapy. They cause severe nerve function impairment and if not promptly treated paves way for significant morbidity. Two types of leprosy reactions are usually described—type 1 reactions or reversal reactions in the borderline types and type 2 reaction or erythema nodosum leprosum (ENL), occurring in borderline lepromatous and LL. Lucio's phenomenon with necrotic lesions occurs in diffuse non-nodular LL.

Type 1 Reaction or Reversal Reaction

It is a delayed type hypersensitivity reaction, noted in the unstable borderline spectrum of leprosy usually after initiation of multidrug therapy. Both innate and adaptive immunity are involved in the pathogenesis of type 1 reactions. Increased antigen presentation by macrophages and Schwann cells to the T-cells leads to increase in cell-mediated immunity and lesional infiltration of CD4+ cells is observed with secretion of proinflammatory cytokines IFN-γ, TNF-α, IL-2, IL-12, IL-1β, IL-6, IL-8, and generation of free radical producing inducible nitric oxide synthase. Vitamin D-dependent antimicrobial pathway is also initiated. IFN-γ levels are higher than that in type 2 reactions. Endothelial cells express marked increase in adhesion molecules. Immunoregulatory molecules IL-10 and TGFβ have also been demonstrated in type 1 reactions. Recent research points a single-nucleotide polymorphism (SNP) in TLR2 as protective factor for reversal reactions and increased serum levels of IFN-γ-induced chemokine CXCL10/IP10 and IL-6 as potential markers for type 1 reactions.[11,13]

Clinical Implication

Type 1 reaction presents with edema and erythema of preexisting skin lesions, with or without pain and tender swollen nerve, resulting in sudden loss of function of the affected nerve. Neuritis is more common and severe than in type 2 reactions.

Type 2 Reaction or Erythema Nodosum Leprosum

It is a type 3 hypersensitivity reaction mediated by immune complexes in multibacillary leprosy with a high antibody load, with a simultaneous T-cell response to mycobacterial antigens. It is characterized by infiltration of CD4 cells, in excess of CD8 cells, and subsequent influx of neutrophils. Increase in IL-2 receptors is indicative of increasing cellular immunity. Cytokine profile is similar to type 1 reaction, but higher levels of IL-4, IL-5, IL-6, IL-10, and TNF are observed in type 2 reactions. TNF and IFN-γ levels correlate with the severity of type 2 reactions. Despite this heightened T-cell response, delayed hypersensitivity does not develop in such patients and there is persistence of lepromin negativity. Platelet-derived growth factor-BB (PDGF-BB), an angiogenic growth factor may function as a marker for type 2 reaction.[13,14] Leprosy patients with IL-6 polymorphism are at greater risk of developing these types of inflammatory episodes.

Clinical Implication

Type 2 reaction manifests as crops of tender erythematous papules and nodules, with fever, malaise, joint pain, and other constitutional symptoms.

IMMUNOGENETICS

It is well established that host factors are paramount to the expression of clinical features of leprosy. Genetic polymorphisms in the immune system determine susceptibility or resistance to leprosy or predilection towards a certain pole in disease spectrum. Multitude of studies on many a genes in different populations across the world has given rise to considerable heterogeneity.

The *MHC* genes or human leukocyte antigens (HLAs) are the most polymorphic genes in the human genome and thus are implicated heavily in genetic association with leprosy. HLA-A*11, B*40, and Cw7 have been noted in Indian population with increased susceptibility to ENL with A11. HLA-A*11 and HLA-B*38 have been observed in leprosy patients from Brazil as well. HLA-DR2 polymorphisms have consistently been associated with leprosy, with predominance of TT leprosy in Indian population. Polymorphisms in HLA-DRB1/DQA1 (rs1071630 and rs9270650) are consistent with leprosy per se.

Low incidence of leprosy occurs with 602S allele of *TLR1*, found among white Europeans, whereas 1805G allele offered protection from reversal reaction in a large case control study in Nepalese population. C597T polymorphism in *TLR2* was significantly associated with protection from type 1 lepra reaction. Multiple *NOD2* variants have rendered susceptibility to leprosy in Chinese, Vietnamese, and Nepalese population, with few SNPs offering protection to reversal reaction (rs2287195 and rs8043770). Mutation in murine *NRAMP1* resulted in defective innate immunity, but human polymorphisms have been inconsistently associated with leprosy susceptibility. Polymorphisms in *LTA*, the gene for T-cell cytokine lymphotoxin-α, have been implicated in susceptibility to leprosy in younger population of endemic countries like India. *TAP1* variant A637G has been reported to increase susceptibility to leprosy in Indian population.[15] TNF-308A variant provided heterogenous results in populations across the globe. SNP in the promoter region of IL-10 influences leprosy susceptibility in Brazilian, Malawi, and Indian populations, preferentially the paucibacillary form of leprosy. *IL-6* polymorphisms [(GG) and (GG+CG) rs2069840] confer protection to type 2 lepra reactions in Brazilian population, but most *IL-6* polymorphisms increase risk of developing ENL.

CONCLUSION

The host immune response is an important facet for understanding the disease pathology and also its clinical manifestations. Understanding the fact that leprosy manifestations are not influenced by the geographical locations and neither on the strain differences; the pivotal role lies on the host immunology. Both the innate and adaptive immunity plays their respective roles in leprosy pathogenesis and the understanding the immunology help us to learn more about the risk factors for the susceptibility and clinical outcome. Immunology is an evolving subject with more and more information pouring in every day. Essentially, all the above informations are like the pieces of the jigsaw puzzle and we are far from completing the entire picture. So we look forward for more information to help us with the understanding of the immunology of leprosy.

KEY POINTS

- Receptors of innate immunity like TLR1/2, TLR4, TLR6, NOD-like receptors, Scavenger receptors and vitamin D receptors interact with lepra bacilli and create Th1/Th2 cytokine milieu.
- Macrophages play an important role - M1 macrohages in TT spectrum: Antimicrobial; M2 macrophages in LL spectrum: Phagocytic.
- Th1 response pattern seen in tuberculoid spectrum involves IFN-γ and TNF-α-induced inflammation, lymphocyte proliferation and induction of antimicrobial pathway whereas Th2 response pattern seen in lepromatous spectrum involves IL-4, IL-10 and TGF-β-mediated suppression of imflammation, production of antibodies and induction of regulatory T-cells.
- Th17 cells are seen in tuberculoid pole and have strong proinflammatory function.
- Schwann cells facilitate adhesion and entry of lepra bacilli and cause nerve damage directly as well as indirectly through membrane attack complex.
- Type 1 reaction is a delayed type hypersensitivity with increase in TNF-α and IFN-γ whereas Type 2 reaction is an immune-complex reaction with increased levels of IFN-γ and IL-17.

REFERENCES

1. Pinheiro RO, Schmitz V, Silva BJA, Dias AA, de Souza BJ, de Mattos Barbosa MG, et al. Innate immune responses in leprosy. Front Immunol. 2018;9:518.
2. Nath I, Saini C, Valluri VL. Immunology of leprosy and diagnostic challenges. Clin Dermatol. 2015;33:90-8.
3. Jin S, Ahn KJ, An KS. Importance of the immune response to Mycobacterium leprae in the skin. Biomed Dermatol. 2018;2:1.
4. Harboe M. Overview of host-parasite relations. In: Hastings RC (Ed). Leprosy, 2nd edition. United Kingdom: Churchill Livingstone; 1994. p. 87-112.
5. Misch EA, Berrington WR, Vary JC Jr, Hawn TR. Leprosy and the human genome. Microbiol Mol Biol Rev. 2010;74:589-620.
6. Modlin RL. The innate immune response in leprosy. Curr Opin Immunol. 2010;22:48-54.
7. da Silva Prata RB, de Mattos Barbosa MG, de Andrade Silva BJ, da Paixão de Oliveira JA, Bittencourt TL, Pinheiro RO. Macrophages in the pathogenesis of leprosy. In: Bhat KB (Ed). Macrophage Activation - Biology and Disease. [Online] IntechOpen 2019 Sep 26. Available from: https://www.intechopen.com/books/macrophage-activation-biology-and-disease/macrophages-in-the-pathogenesis-of-leprosy.
8. Weiss DI, Do TH, de Andrade Silva BJ, Teles RMB, Andrade PR, Ochoa MT, et al. Adaptive immune response in leprosy. In: Scollard D, Gillis T (Eds). International Textbook of Leprosy.
9. Scollard DM, Adams LB, Gillis TP, Krahenbuhl JL, Truman RW, Williams DL. The continuing challenges of leprosy. Clin Microbiol Rev. 2006;19:338-81.
10. Sadhu S, Mitra DK. Emerging concepts of adaptive immunity in leprosy. Front Immunol. 2018;9:604.
11. de Sousa JR, Sotto MN, Simoes Quaresma JA. Leprosy as a complex infection: breakdown of the Th1 and Th2 immune paradigm in the immunopathogenesis of the disease. Front Immunol. 2017;8:1635.
12. Ebenezer GJ, Polydefkis M, Scollard D. Mechanisms of nerve injury in Leprosy. In: Scollard D, Gillis T (Eds). International Textbook of Leprosy.
13. Fonseca AB, Simon MD, Cazzaniga RA, de Moura TR, de Almeida RP, Duthie MS, et al. The influence of innate and adaptative immune responses on the differential clinical outcomes of leprosy. Infect Dis Poverty. 2017;6:5.
14. Moubasher AD, Kamel NA, Zedan H, Raheem DD. Cytokines in leprosy, I. Serum cytokine profile in leprosy. Int J Dermatol. 1998;37:733-40.
15. Shinde V, Marcinek P, Rani DS, Sunder SR, Arun S, Jain S, et al. Genetic evidence of *TAP1* gene variant as a susceptibility factor in Indian leprosy patients. Hum Immunol. 2013;74:803-7.

EXAMINATION QUESTIONS

1. Discuss the role of macrophages in pathogenesis of leprosy.
2. Discuss Th1/Th2 paradigm in immunopathogenesis of leprosy.
3. What is the role of innate immunity in leprosy?
4. Write briefly on immune-mediated nerve damage in leprosy.
5. Discuss immunopathogenesis of leprosy reactions.
6. Briefly describe immunology of leprosy.

111 CHAPTER Classification through Ages

Fenil Patel

INTRODUCTION[1,2]

Leprosy is a chronic granulomatous disorder caused by *Mycobacterium leprae*. Various clinical manifestations of leprosy depend on host immune response. If the host immunity is strong enough to kill *M. leprae,* person has no disease. If host immunity is poor, person can develop various clinical manifestation of leprosy according to host immune resistance against *M. leprae*. Leprosy can involve nerves, skin, or both. Due to wide range or spectrum of clinical presentation, disease course, prognosis, and complication, it is absolute necessity to classify it. Though, till now different classification was given for leprosy, none cater all the requirement of field leprosy worker, clinician, and researcher. Recently World Health Organization (WHO) classification is used for treatment purpose and Ridley–Jopling classification is used for academic and research purpose.

CRITERIA FOR CLASSIFICATION[1]

Bacteriological Criteria

In this criterion, bacterial index (BI) is measured. There are two methods of BI measurement:

1. Slit-skin smear technique (used by field leprosy workers where facility of histopathology is not available, widely used technique).
2. Skin biopsy (used where the facility of histopathology in laboratory is available).

Immunological Criteria

In this criterion, cell-mediated immunity (CMI) against leprosy bacilli is measured. Lepromin test is performed for measuring host CMI. Lepromin test positive has good immune response and negative has poor immune response against *M. leprae*.

Histopathological Criteria

This criterion is widely used for research purpose. Different lesions have their own unique histopathological findings; disease can be classified definitely in various classes according to these findings.

Clinical Criteria

This criterion depends on various clinical features of the disease. It is the easiest way to classify the disease. Recently classification based on clinical criteria is widely used for treatment purpose.

In *Sushruta Samhita*, three forms of the disease were described. The disease without skin lesions but sensory changes and deformities was described under the "*Vat Rakta*" or "*Vat Shonita*". The disease with skin lesions was described under two categories of "*Aruna Kustha*": in one, prominent symptoms were sensory involvement and in other ulceration.[2]

Pre-Manila Classifications[2]

Danielssen and Boeck (1848)

- Nodular
- Anesthetic

Hansen and Looft (1895)

- Tuberosa
- Maculoanesthetic

Neisser (1903)

- Lepra tuberosa
- Lepra cutanae
- Lepra nervorum

The Manila Classification (1931)[3]

In Manila, Philippines the Leonard Wood Memorial organized a round table meet. In this meet, first attempt was made for international classification of leprosy.

Leprosy was divided into three types:

1. Cutaneous
2. Neural
3. Mixed

Administrative Classification of Cases

Mycobacterium leprae can be disseminated through skin, mucous membrane, or excretion of the infected host.

- *Open cases*: Cases from which dissemination is possible.
- *Closed cases*: Cases from which dissemination is not possible.

The Cairo Classification (1938)[2,4]

The International Leprosy Congress, Cairo coined the classification.

Classified in:

- Lepromatous (L)
- Neural
  - Anesthetic (Na)
  - Simple macular (Ns)
  - Tuberculoid (Nt)—"major" and "minor" forms

This classification has two defects:

1. For neural lesions separate class is given in this classification but in lepromatous patients, nerve lesions are also present. So it is ambiguous to classify neural lesion under separate class.
2. Some patients have features of both the classes; there is no intermediate class in this classification. So we cannot classify this kind of patient particularly.

The Pan-American Classification (1946)[5]

The second Pan-American Leprosy Congress, Rio de Janeiro coined a South American classification. This classification was based on histopathology.

This classification has three types:

1. Lepromatous (L)
2. Tuberculoid (T)
3. Uncharacteristic or unidentified (I)

Defect

The only defect of this classification is where to classify the pure neural leprosy. Pure neural leprosy is classified in all three types based on histopathological findings.

The Havana Classification (1948)[6]

The Fifth International Leprosy Congress, Havana coined this classification. It is the variant of the Pan-American classification. The term "uncharacteristic" was changed to "indeterminate".

This classification has three types:

1. Lepromatous
2. Tuberculoid
3. Indeterminate

This classification has same defect like the Pan-American classification, where to classify pure neural cases.

The Madrid Classification (1953)[7]

The technical committee of the International Leprosy Congress, Madrid described The Madrid Classification **(Box 1)**.

Two changes were made in Pan-American classification and Havana classification:

1. "Uncharacteristic" was changed to "indeterminate".
2. New group "borderline" added as per WHO Expert Committee recommendation, 1952.

BOX 1: The Madrid classification.

Lepromatous type (L):
- Macular
- Diffuse
- Infiltrated
- Nodular
- Neuritic, pure (?)

Tuberculoid type (T):
- Macular (Tm)
- Minor tuberculoid (micropapuloid) (Tt)
- Major tuberculoid (plaques and annular lesions) (TT)
- Neuritic, pure (Tn)

Indeterminate group (I):
- Macular (Im)
- Neuritic, pure (In)

Borderline (dimorphous) group (B):
- Infiltrated
- (Others ?)

BOX 2: The Indian classification.

- Lepromatous (L)
- Tuberculoid (T)
- Maculoanesthetic (MA)
- Borderline (B)
- Polyneuritic (P)
- Indeterminate (I)

Definitions

- "Type" connotes clinically and biologically stereotyped features, characterized by marked stability and mutual incompatibility.
- "Group" connotes less distinctive or positive characteristics, less stability, and less certainty with respect to evolution.
- "Variety" connotes a subdivision of a type or group.

Defect

Pure neuritic type is classified in lepromatous type, tuberculoid type, and indeterminate group, but it is not kept under borderline group where it is most commonly seen.

The Indian Classification (1955)[8]

The Indian classification was given by Indian association of leprologists **(Box 2)**. It is almost similar to the Madrid classification.

According to Madrid classification, it was difficult to classify primary neuritic cases (pure neuritic-only nerve involvement) from secondary neuritic cases (nerve involvement is secondary to skin lesion). Solution of this difficulty was given in Indian classification. Secondary neuritic case is classified according to type of skin lesions and symbol (n) is added after it. This symbol indicated that the sensory changes are secondary to skin involvement.

The Revised Indian Classification (1981)[2]

This classification was adopted at general meeting of the Indian Association of Leprologists in Agra. There was only one difference from the original Indian classification, "maculoanesthetic" type was removed and placing it as a variety of tuberculoid type. So there are only five classes in compare to original Indian classification in which there were six classes.

Classification Suggested by Job and Chacko[2]

Job and Chacko include the maculoanesthetic or macular tuberculoid under the borderline tuberculoid (BT) type and separate type for primary neuritic lesions **(Box 3)**. They also divided the borderline group into two separate types:

1. Borderline tuberculoid
2. Borderline lepromatous

Compare to revised Indian classification, maculoanesthetic was kept under the BT type instead of tuberculoid type.

The Ridley–Jopling Immunological Classification[9]

This classification is mainly used for research purposes **(Box 4)**.

Ridley and Jopling defined all above groups on clinical, bacteriological, immunological, and histological findings. Due to difference in CMI of host to *M. leprae*, leprosy is classified in various groups. Tuberculoid case and lepromatous case are seen at either end of the spectrum depending on CMI. In between this, two wide spectrums are divided in various subgroups. These various subgroups are nothing but the borderline cases. These borderline cases are divided into three subgroups:

1. Near the tuberculoid end (BT)
2. In between tuberculoid and lepromatous end (BB)
3. Near the lepromatous end (BL)

These cases show the upgrading or downgrading due to change in the host immune status. So, borderline cases are the unstable form of the leprosy.

BOX 3: The Job and Chacko classification.

- Lepromatous leprosy (L)
- Tuberculoid leprosy (T)
- Borderline tuberculoid leprosy (BT)
- Borderline lepromatous leprosy (BL)
- Indeterminate leprosy (I)
- Polyneuritic leprosy (P or N)

BOX 4: The Ridley–Jopling immunological classification.

- Tuberculoid leprosy (TT)
- Borderline tuberculoid leprosy (BT)
- Mid-borderline leprosy (BB)
- Borderline lepromatous leprosy (BL)
- Lepromatous leprosy (LL)

In Ridley–Jopling classification, pure neuritic cases and indeterminate skin lesions are not kept under any spectrum.

WHO Classification (1982)[10]

This classification is based on the BI.

- Paucibacillary leprosy: BI <2+
- Multibacillary leprosy: BI ≥2+

WHO Classification (1988)[11]

Paucibacillary leprosy: All smear negative cases belonging to:

- Indeterminate (I), tuberculoid (TI), and borderline tuberculoid (BT) cases as classified under Ridley–Jopling classification
- Indeterminate (I) and tuberculoid (T) cases under Madrid classification

Multibacillary leprosy: This includes all:

- Mid-borderline (BB), borderline lepromatous (BL), and lepromatous (LL) under Ridley–Jopling classification
- Borderline (B) and lepromatous (L) cases under Madrid classification
- Any other smear positive case

WHO Classification (1998)[12]

Based on number of lesions:

- Single lesion paucibacillary leprosy (SLPB)
- Paucibacillary leprosy (two to five skin lesions)
- Multibacillary leprosy (six or more skin lesions and all smear positive cases)

WHO Classification (2017)[13]

Paucibacillary leprosy: One to five skin lesions without demonstrated presence of bacilli in a slit-skin smear.

Multibacillary leprosy: More than five skin lesions; or with nerve involvement (pure neuritis or any number of skin lesions and neuritis); with demonstrated presence of bacilli in a slit-skin smear irrespectively from the number of skin lesions.

Classification of Leprosy under National Leprosy Eradication Programme[14]

The classification of leprosy under National Leprosy Eradication Programme is given in **Table 1**.

TABLE 1: Classification of leprosy under National Leprosy Eradication Programme.

Characteristics	*Paucibacillary (PB)*	*Multibacillary (MB)*
Skin lesions	One to five lesions	Six and above
Peripheral nerve	No nerve or only one nerve involvement	More than one nerve involvement
Skin smear	Negative at all sites	Positive at any site

KEY POINTS

- Four criteria for leprosy classification are bacteriological criteria, immunological criteria, histopathological criteria, and clinical criteria.
- Recently WHO classification is used for treatment purpose. Leprosy is classified as paucibacillary or multibacillary. According to this, multidrug therapy (MDT) is given to the patients.
- For academic and research purpose Ridley–Jopling classification is widely used.

REFERENCES

1. Kumar B, Kumar H. IAL Textbook of Leprosy, 2nd edition. New Delhi: Jaypee Brothers Medical Publishers (P) Ltd.; 2017.
2. Hastings RC. Leprosy (Medicine in the Tropics). London, United Kingdom: Churchill Livingstone; 1985.
3. Leonard Wood Memorial for the Eradication of Leprosy. Conference. Report of the Leonard Wood Memorial Conference on Leprosy. Manila, Philippine Island: Bureau of Printing; 1931.
4. The Cairo Congress number. Int J Lepr. 1938;6(3):371-76.
5. Leprosy News and Notes. Int J Lepr. 1947;15(1):91-123.
6. Wade HW. Classification at Havana. Int J Lepr. 1948;16(3): 383-6.
7. Sixth International Congress of Leprosy. Int J Lepr. 1953; 21(4):484-557.
8. Current literature. Int J Lepr. 1956;24(2):220-43.
9. Ridley DS, Jopling WH. Classification of leprosy according to immunity a five group system. Int J Lepr. 1966;34(3): 255-73.
10. WHO study group. Chemotherapy of leprosy for control programmes. World Health Organ Tech Rep Ser. 1982;675: 1-33.
11. WHO Expert Committee on Leprosy, Sixth Report. World Health Organ Tech Rep Ser. 1988;768:1-51.
12. WHO. WHO Expert Committee on Leprosy, Seventh Report. Geneva: World Health Organization; 1998.
13. WHO. Guidelines for the diagnosis, treatment and prevention of leprosy. New Delhi: World Health Organization, Regional Office for South-East Asia; 2017.
14. National Leprosy Eradication Programme (2019). Training Manual for Medical Officers. [online] Available from: https://cltri.gov.in/MO%20Training%20Manual.pdf [Last accessed January, 2021].

EXAMINATION QUESTIONS

1. Describe the criteria for leprosy classification and write notes on the WHO classification.
2. Explain the classification of leprosy.
3. Name various classifications of leprosy and write notes on Ridley-Jopling immunological classification.

112 CHAPTER

Animal Models in Leprosy

Varsha Vaidyanathan, Aarti Sarda, Abhishek De

INTRODUCTION

The bacterial etiology of leprosy was demonstrated in 1873 by Armauer Hansen. However, researchers had long been stymied by their inability to cultivate *Mycobacterium leprae* outside of the human host. Various animals and birds were tried as viable hosts but ultimately proved to be unsuccessful due to the prolonged growth cycle of *M. leprae* as well as its need for cooler temperatures. Finally in the 1960s, Charles Shepard managed to successfully cultivate *M. leprae* in the footpad of mice.[1] Rees, in 1966 first obtained disseminated infection in an immature mice previously treated with thymectomy and whole body irradiation. Few years later, Kirchheimer and Storrs succeeded in establishing the nine-banded armadillo as a model for the study of leprosy.[2] Since then, other animals like rhesus monkey, sooty mangabey and African green monkey have been used to grow lepra bacilli.

Flowchart 1 gives an overview of the animal models used in leprosy.

As the mouse footpad and the nine-banded armadillo are still the gold standard animal models in leprosy, in this chapter, we will take an in-depth look at these models.

MURINE MODELS

The mouse (*Mus Musculus*) is a small, inexpensive, prolific breeder with a short gestation period. This makes it ideal for various experiments in medical research.

Mice can be infected experimentally in the following ways:

- Footpad infection—this area is cooler than the rest of the mouse body with an average temperature of 20–25°C, and hence is ideal for the growth of *M. leprae*.

There are two footpad infection protocols:

1. Shepard's mouse footpad (MFP) assay—$<10^4$ viable bacilli are inoculated. The mice thus infected are monitored for 18 months. Bacterial growth and tissue granulomas can be studied.
2. Based on lepromin tests, $>10^6$ leprae bacilli are inoculated. Here, long-term effects can be evaluated.

- Ear infection—like the footpad, the ear pinna too is cooler than the rest of the body. Unlike in the footpad, growth of lepra bacilli here is rapid.
- Intraneural infection—unlike in humans, mouse Schwann cells are not readily infected by *M. leprae*. This can be overcome by direct injection of bacilli in the nerve.[3] However, the survival and growth of the bacilli is compromised in this method. This route may have some utility in the investigation of nerve damage in leprosy.

Types of Mice/Rat Used

- *Immunocompetent mice:* MFP is sensitive in detecting small number of bacilli, infection produced in consistent, however yield is less (10^6 *M. leprae*). BALB/C, CBA, CFW mouse lines provide higher plateau level. Inoculation is done by subcutaneous injection in the footpad with not more than 5,000–10,000 AFB in a volume of 0.03 mL. AFB reaches detectable level in 90–120 days. In 150–180 days count grows to 10^6. For the next 1 year level remains constant. Some strains with better growth are called "Fast" strains and others "Slow" strains. Fast strains achieve higher and faster plateau level. Growth of *M. leprae* is limited in immunocompetent mice and histopathological changes are also minimal. Nerves are usually not infected.

Flowchart 1: Overview of animal models in leprosy.

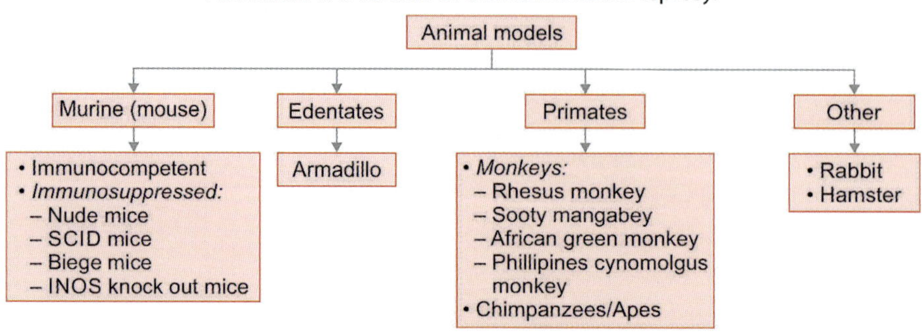

(SCID: severe combined immunodeficiency)

- *Immunocompetent rats:* Lewis strain of rat commonly used.
- *Immunosuppressed mice:* Growth of *M. leprae* ceases at 10^6 because of T-cell immune response. Several models involving T-cell deprivation have therefore been used, all involve thymus deficiency.
    - *Thymectomized and irradiated mice:* These are unable to mount an immune response. Thymectomy is done in normal adult mice followed by irradiation. Growth of *M. leprae* is slow but continuous and at the end of 2 years, average is 10^7 to 10^8.
    - *Nude mice:* Nude mice is a congenitally athymic mice used as experimental leprosy model. These are mice with "nu" mutation and are hairless and have rudimentary thymus. The "nu" genes are inherited as autosomal recessive. They are susceptible to *M. leprae* and also other infections. They are best maintained in insulators at germ-free conditions. Following injection of *M. leprae*, at first there is a localized swelling, then generalized disease occurs within 18 weeks involving all organs except CNS. Accumulation in liver and spleen is limited. Bacterial count may become 10^{10} to 10^{11}.
    - *Severe combined immunodeficiency (SCID) mice:* These mice are deficient in T and B cell immunity. 10^6 *M. leprae* are inoculated in footpad which become 10^9 in 8 months.
    - *Beige mice:* They have an almost entirely defective immune system. There is deficiency of both macrophage and NK cells. The lepra bacilli here multiply and most of the normal tissue is replaced by heavily infected foamy macrophages.
    - *ALY mice (Alymphoplasia mice):* There is absence of lymph nodes and Payer patches. These mice are deficient in T and B cell immunity, highly susceptible to infection by *M. leprae*.
    - *INOS knock out mice:* Inducible nitric oxide synthetase knocks out mice. These are genetically incapable of producing NOS which is responsible for producing reactive nitric oxide intermediates, which is a major antimicrobial mechanism of activated macrophages.
- *Genetically modified mice:* Here, genes specific to different parts in the pathway of the immune system are knocked out. The mice thus infected with *M. leprae* have broadened our understanding of the role of the immune system in the disease process of leprosy.

Uses of the Mouse Model

- *Drug testing:*[4] MFP assay is the gold standard for evaluating the efficacy of drugs in leprosy. There are three different methods for this as discussed in **Table 1**.
- To detect drug resistance/experimental chemotherapy MFP assay can also be used to detect drug resistance. Drugs such as rifampicin, ofloxacin and dapsone can be evaluated using alternative methods but for clofazimine, MFP assay is the chief method of ascertaining resistance.
- *Evaluation of vaccines:* Vaccinated mice are inoculated with a low dose challenge. Bacilli are then counted after 6 months. Both the mouse footpad and ear pinna have been used.
- *Diagnosis:* MFP tests are being used in studies to develop standardized protocols for immunodiagnosis of leprosy, studying mechanism of reversal reaction.

Limitations of the Mouse Model

- At the end of the day, mice are immunologically different from humans so not all the data can be extrapolated
- The mouse model is not ideal for the study of nerve disease.

ARMADILLO MODEL (AMERICAN ANTEATER)

The armadillo is a natural host of *M. leprae*. They are found only in America. There are 21 different species but the ones of interest in leprosy research are the nine-banded armadillo (*Dasypus novemcinctus*) and to a lesser extent the seven-banded armadillo (*Dasypus septumcinctus*), six-banded armadillo (*Euphractus sexcinctus*) and hairy armadillo.

Since leprosy in armadillo closely reflects the natural course and progression in humans and also due to the heavy

TABLE 1: Different methods of drug testing using the mouse model.

Continuous method	*Proportional bactericidal method*	*Kinetic method*
<10^4 bacilli inoculated in immunocompetent mice	Groups of immunocompetent mice are inoculated with serial 10-fold dilutions starting from 10^4/footpad	<10^4 bacilli inoculated in immunocompetent mice
Daily administration of drugs started on the same day as inoculation and continued till the animals are humanely killed	Drug administration is started on the same day as inoculation. Length of treatment is variable	Drug administration is started 60 days after inoculation
Drug activity is measured by comparison of inhibition of multiplication in treated mice and placebo mice	Bacilli in the footpad are counted 12 months post-treatment to calculate the "proportion" of bacilli that survived	Drug efficacy is measured by time lag between treated and placebo mice in reaching 10^6 bacilli
Cannot differentiate between bactericidal and bacteriostatic activity of drugs	• Used to determine efficacy of a drug or treatment regimen • Cannot detect a drug's bacteriostatic activity	• In bactericidal drugs, growth will not resume after stopping treatment • In bacteriostatic drugs, growth will resume with a measurable growth delay
Simple and straightforward method	Can be tedious	Can be tedious

bacillary load they carry, the long life span (~12 years) and lower body temperature (32–35°C), the armadillo has become an ideal model for leprosy research.

Most armadillos are susceptible to infection with leprosy and can be infected via various routes—intradermal, intravenous, and via respiratory droplets. They exhibit the full spectrum of leprosy including tuberculoid, lepromatous, and borderline types. Most infections are lepromatous. Outwardly few signs are present as the armadillo skin is covered with a tough armor plate.[5] Plantar ulceration is commonly seen in the late stages of the disease and it mimics those seen in humans.

Uses of the Armadillo Model

- *Evaluation of nerve disease:* Like humans and unlike mice, armadillos are capable of developing extensive neurological disease. Since their nerves are easily accessible, they can be biopsied for further studies. Histopathologically, there is a characteristic interstitial neuritis with presence of bacilli in perineurium, epineurium, and endoneurium. Armadillo nerve segments can be used for gene expression profiling and compared to that of normal nerves. Nerve conduction studies can also be performed to study the effect of leprosy on the nerves and to evaluate the disease progress over time.
- *Evaluation of myopathies:* As seen in humans, armadillo foot muscles can be paralyzed due to nerve injury secondary to leprosy. These muscles can be evaluated by antibody-labeling and nuclear labeling. The skeletal muscle features resemble the impairment seen in human leprosy patients suggesting that the armadillo model can be used to evaluate myopathies related to leprosy.
- *Diagnosis of leprosy:* An IgM response can be detected in infected armadillos and these antibodies persist over the course of the disease with the titers correlating well with the bacillary load. The antigens used include the *M. leprae* specific PGL-1 antigen and the LID-1 antigen.
- To study drug resistant-strains and persisters.

Limitations of the Armadillo Model

- Armadillos are not available easily and must be caught from the wild.
- Armadillos are found only in America.
- As compared to mice, management and upkeep of armadillos in a laboratory setting is more difficult.
- Armadillos do not breed well in captivity.

CONCLUSION

Mouse and armadillo models effectively provide a large number of viable *M. leprae* bacilli for experimental and research purposes. This has enhanced our understanding of the disease process and is a useful tool in reliably testing for drug efficacy, resistance and for vaccine research.

KEY POINTS

- *M. leprae* cannot be grown in culture. A host is required. Animals used include mouse, nine-banded armadillo, rhesus monkey, sooty mangabey, and African green monkey.
- Mice can be infected through the footpad, ear pinna, or direct intraneural injection.
- The mouse model is used for evaluations of drugs, resistance, and vaccines.
- Mouse model is unsuitable for research on nerve disease.
- Leprosy in armadillo closely reflects the disease in humans and also shows a similar nerve involvement and hence is useful for nerve studies.

REFERENCES

1. Shepard CC. The experimental disease that follows the injection of human leprosy bacilli into foot-pads of mice. J Exp Med. 1960;112(3):445-54.
2. Kirchheimer WF, Storrs EE. Attempts to establish the armadillo (*Dasypus novemcinctus* Linn.) as a model for the study of leprosy. Report of lepromatoid leprosy in an experimentally infected armadillo. Int J Lepr Other Mycobact Dis. 1971;39(3):693-702.
3. Shetty VP. Animal model to study the mechanism of nerve damage in leprosy: a preliminary report. Int J Lepr Other Mycobact Dis. 1993;61(1):70-5.
4. Adams LB, Pena MT, Sharma R, Lahiri R, Truman RW. Experimental leprosy: contributions of animal models to leprosy research. In: Kumar B, Kar HK (Eds). IAL Textbook of Leprosy, 2nd edition. New Delhi, India: Jaypee Brothers Medical Publishers; 2017. pp. 186-204.
5. Truman R. Armadillos as a source of infection for leprosy. South Med J. 2008;101(6):581-2.

EXAMINATION QUESTION

1. Discuss animal models in leprosy.

113 CHAPTER

Histopathology of Leprosy

Bhabani STP Singh, Swetalina Pradhan

INTRODUCTION

Mycobacterium leprae (M. leprae) is an obligate intracellular bacterium with an affinity towards the Schwann cells of the neurons. It is also found in the macrophages, melanocytes, and chondrocytes. The slow division time and the obligate intracellular habitat of the bacillus make the infection chronic. Tissue reaction to *M. leprae* is a granuloma surrounding the infected site to prevent further spread of the infection. The host cell-mediated immunity determines the degree of granulomatous response to the organism and thereby ascertains the clinical and histopathological manifestation of the disease.

A clinical diagnosis of leprosy is mostly made by the help of three cardinal signs of the disease. These were primarily devised for the healthcare providers in the field. Accepting a diagnosis of leprosy based on these criteria has some inherent fallacies. A biopsy and histopathologic study of the specimen serves as useful tool in confirming the diagnosis in cases of ambiguity in the cardinal signs. The diagnosis and classification of a leprosy patient should be based on a detailed clinicopathologic correlation. Clinical and morphological diagnoses of early lesions remain challenging, and the histopathologic study of the cases should always be interpreted in correlation with clinical findings.[1]

REQUIREMENT OF SKIN BIOPSY

Histopathology in a patient of leprosy serves various crucial purposes, such as:

- Diagnostic confirmation in case of inadequacy or ambiguity of cardinal signs of the disease.
- Classify the disease into a particular spectrum.
- Assess the response to chemotherapy and thereby suspect resistance to therapy, if any.
- Distinguish reactions and relapse from the disease.
- To measure the bacterial load and disease activity in the patient by use of special stains.
- Academic purpose of teaching and research in the pathological aspect of the disease.

TECHNIQUE OF A SKIN BIOPSY

Accuracy of the information about the disease obtained from the skin biopsy depends upon factors such as timing of the biopsy during lesional evolution, site of the biopsy, and adequacy of the tissue sample. Usually a disposable punch of 5 mm including the full thickness of the dermis along with the subcutaneous tissue is ideal for the histopathologic study. An incisional biopsy of 1.5 cm long and 0.5 cm wide is preferred by some authors. However, the later requires minor surgical expertise. A punch biopsy is easier to perform and causes a smaller postoperative wound which heals faster. Proper site selection of biopsy is important. The most active and representative site of the disease should be considered for biopsy:[2]

- *Small hypopigmented patch:* Center of the lesion.
- *Annular patch:* Active edge of the lesion.
- *Different morphological lesions:* Multiple site biopsies.
- *Suspected type 1 reaction:* Most edematous and infiltrated area.
- *Suspected type 2 reaction:* Deep biopsy including subcutaneous fat.

Diagnostic Confirmation and Classification of the Disease

Indeterminate Leprosy

This is an evolutionary stage of the disease, characterized by hypopigmented patch with a doubtful loss of sensory loss. Nearly 70% of the lesions heal spontaneously without any progression. Skin biopsy shows an occasional acid-fast bacillus (AFB) in the noninflamed nerve, erector pilorum, or subepidermal zone. As lesions evolve, neural inflammation begins evidenced by lymphocyte and nonspecific histiocytic infiltration in the perineurium or nerve parenchyma. Schwann cell proliferation is also seen **(Fig. 1)**.

Tuberculoid Leprosy

The classic most feature of tuberculoid leprosy (TT) leprosy is compact well-organized granuloma composed of epithelioid cells surrounded by a mantle of lymphocytes. The tuberculoid granuloma usually effaces the epidermis obliterating the subepidermal space. Langhans giant cells are seen. The nerves

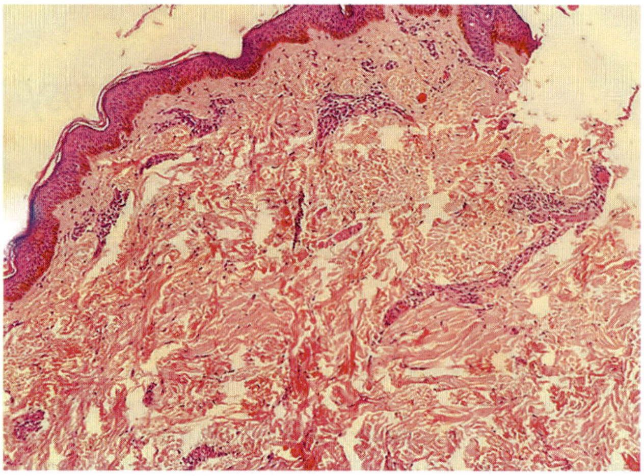

Fig. 1: Perineural lymphocyte and nonspecific histiocytic infiltration in indeterminate leprosy (H&E ×100).

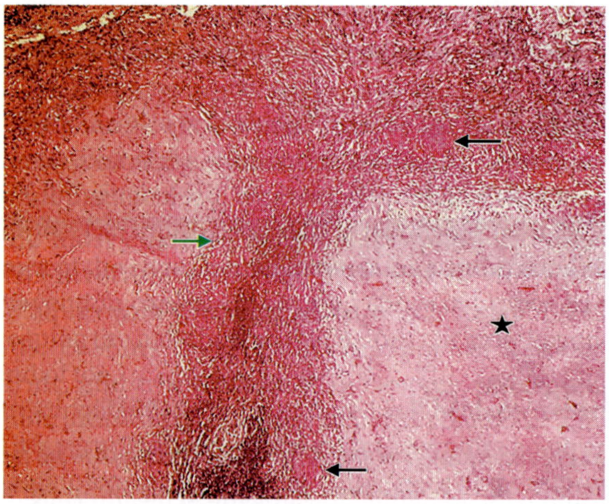

Fig. 2: Caseation necrosis in nerve centre along with epithelioid cells and few giant cells. Black arrows—foreign body giant cells; Green arrow—neural elements; Black asterix—caseation necrosis (H&E ×100).

are replaced by the infiltrating epithelioid cells, making the nerve unidentifiable. Caseation limited to the nerves can be seen **(Fig. 2)**.[2] The sections mostly are negative for AFB.

Borderline Tuberculoid Leprosy

There is epithelioid cell granuloma in a branching pattern, following the neurovascular bundle. The number of lymphocytes is lesser than that of TT. Infiltration of the nerve is typically seen with few AFB [bacterial index (BI) 0–2]. Periеccrine and periappendageal (erector pili) can be seen. A clear subepidermal is always found **(Fig. 3)**.

Borderline Borderline Leprosy

There are no compact granuloma formations seen. Both epithelioid cells and macrophages almost found in equal numbers. Lymphocytes are scanty. AFB may be frequent (BI 2–4). This stage of leprosy is unstable and has few clinical as well as histopathological features of type 1 reaction.[2] Subepidermal clear zone is always seen. Nerve is usually intact with laminated perineurium which resembles a cut onion appearance in cross-section. Multinucleate giant cells are not seen.

Borderline Lepromatous Leprosy

Macrophage granuloma is seen with early foamy changes in few of the cells. A few epithelioid cells may be seen. There is a clear subepidermal zone. The nerves may show laminated appearance secondary to perineal proliferation similar to cut onion appearance. This laminated appearance is due to the end neural repair mechanism following injury to epineurium, as the nerve is not completely destroyed here as in TT and borderline tuberculoid (BT) leprosy. Plenty of bacilli are found either singly or in clumps within macrophages (BI 3–5) **(Fig. 4)**.

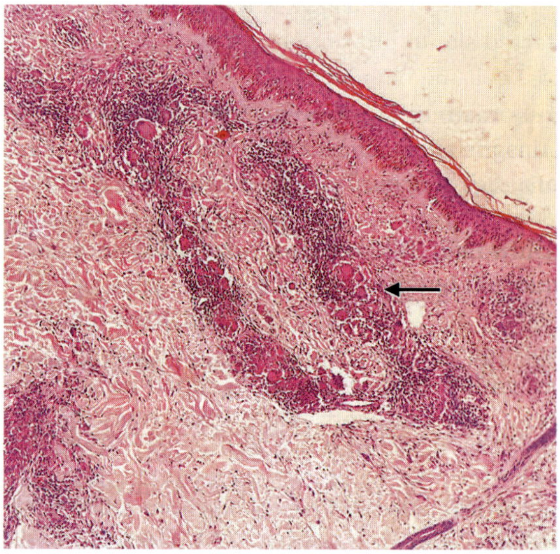

Fig. 3: Oblong granuloma following neurovascular bundle with numerous giant cells (indicated by black arrow) in borderline tuberculoid leprosy (H&E ×100).

Lepromatous Leprosy

The epidermis is thinned out with loss of rete ridges. There is a clear subepidermal grenz zone. There are macrophage granulomas with a lot of foamy histiocytes. Lymphocytes are rarely present. The foamy macrophages contain plenty of AFB (BI 4–6). These solid bacilli are stacked-like cigars and are called globi. The nerves are infiltrated with abundant of AFB, but their architecture is well-preserved **(Fig. 5)**. Presence of lymphocytes forming clusters along with macrophage granulomas differentiates subpolar lepromatous leprosy (LL) from polar LL, where lymphocytes are sparse.

Histoid Leprosy

The epidermis is atrophied due to the expansile nature of the histoid leproma. The surrounding tissue is compressed giving

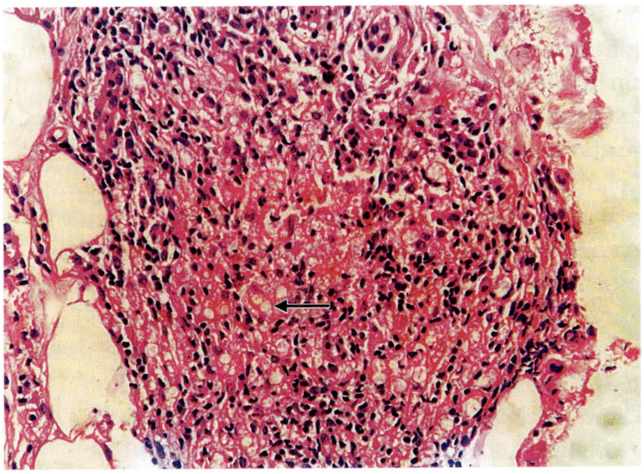

Fig. 4: Macrophage granuloma with foamy changes (indicated by black arrow) and numerous lymphocytes and few epithelioid cells in borderline lepromatous leprosy (H&E ×400).

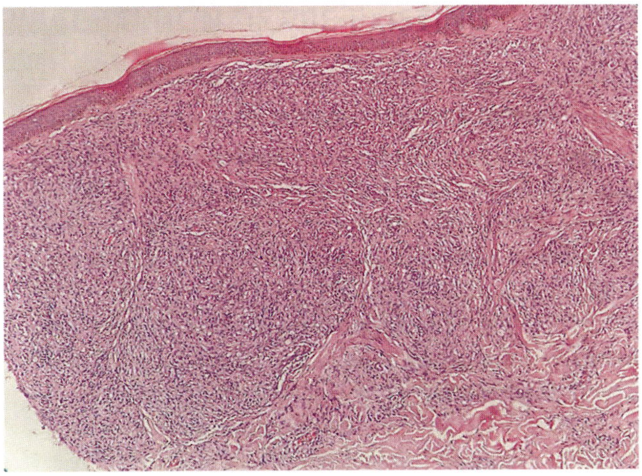

Fig. 6: Collection of spindle-shaped histiocytes in whorls in histoid leprosy (H&E ×100).

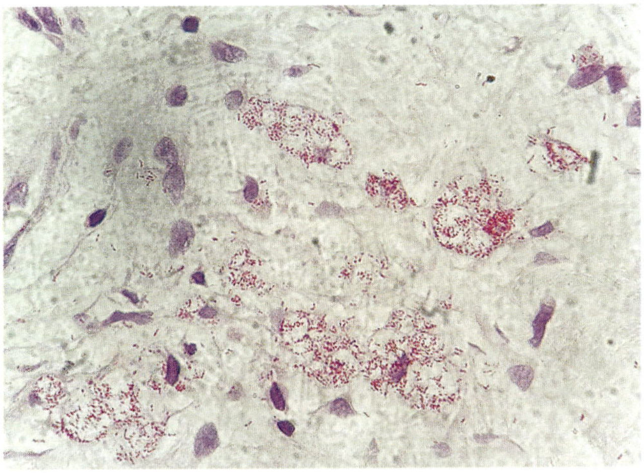

Fig. 5: Staining with acid-fast bacillus (AFB).

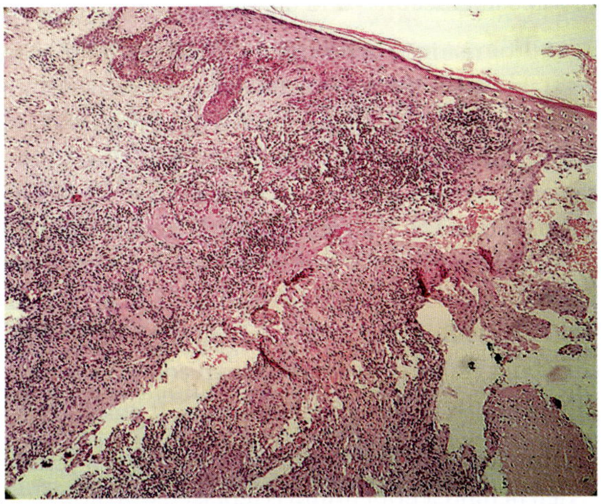

Fig. 7: Disorganized granuloma with increased infiltration of lymphocytes and increased giant cells in type 1 reaction (H&E ×100).

the appearance of a pseudocapsule. This is mostly seen in case of active disease. There is a collection of spindle-shaped histiocytes in whorls and bands interlacing with each other **(Fig. 6)**. A feature typical to this morphological form of leprosy is the histoid habitus of the lepra bacilli. They are arranged in bundles parallel to the long axis of the histiocyte. The bacilli are uniform staining and are longer than the bacilli seen in other types of leprosy. The histoid leproma could be seen in the dermis or the subcutis or both. Histopathological variants of histoid leprosy are described to be pure fusocellular, fusocellular with epithelioid component, and fusocellular with vacuolated cells.[3]

Distinguish Reactions and Relapse from the Disease

Type 1 Reaction

Type 1 reaction usually occurs in borderline leprosy mainly in BT, borderline borderline (BB), and at times in borderline lepromatous (BL) leprosy. It is a delayed type hypersensitivity reaction characterized by increased infiltration of lymphocytes, macrophages, and neutrophils. There is increased edema in the superficial dermis and in the granuloma as well making it disorganized. More number of foreign body giant cells appear. Langhans giant cells also become larger and increased in number **(Fig. 7)**.[4] In case of severe reaction, there is erosion of the epidermis with necrosis.[5]

Type 2 Reaction

It is an immune complex type of hypersensitivity reaction. This reaction occurs in cases with high bacillary load, i.e., in BL and LL leprosy. The granulomas are infiltrated with neutrophils, which are accepted as the most reliable sign of skin lesion typical of type 2 reaction **(Fig. 8)**. Immune complexes are deposited in the walls of venules and arterioles causing vasculitis. Vasculitis may cause full necrosis of the epidermis and erosion. Vasculitis is though not universally

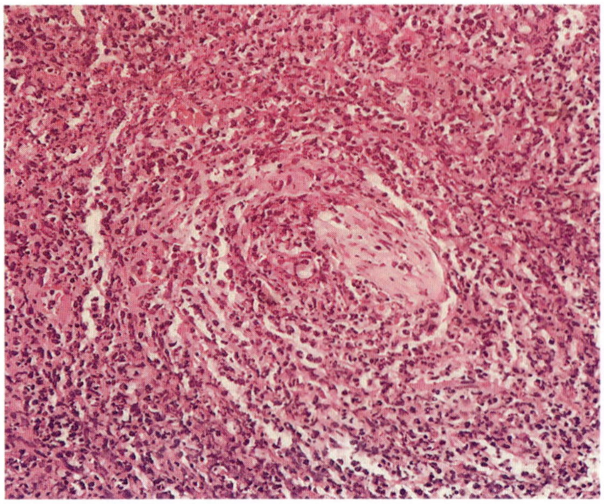

Fig. 8: Granuloma infiltrated with neutrophils with leukocytoclasia in type 2 reaction (H&E ×400).

seen.[6] Vascular lumen may be occluded in deeper dermis and subcutis causing necrosis and ulceration of overlying skin.

Relapse: A 2 log rise in BI is indicative of a relapse. Reappearance of solid staining bacilli in a previously treated case of leprosy indicates relapse. Preexisting granuloma tends to become irregular at the edge and extend spurs to extend between the dermal fascicles during relapse.[7] On the contrary, the granuloma becomes disorganized with increase in number of giant cells in case of reaction.

Assess the Response to Chemotherapy (Resolving Disease) and Relapse

Multibacillary Leprosy

The granuloma gradually diminishes in size without any fibrosis left behind. Perineurium is replaced with fibrous tissue and nerve parenchyma is left hyalinized. With treatment, macrophages become increasing foamy, reflecting the fragmentation and granularity of the AFB. Foamy macrophages along with periadnexal lymphocytes are found in the tissue sections even years after smear negativity.[8]

Paucibacillary Leprosy

There is intraneural and perineural fibrosis with treatment. There is reduction in the size of the granuloma without any fibrosis of the adnexal tissue.

Type 1 reaction: Edema gets reduced and granuloma becomes organized.

Type 2 reaction: Neutrophils become sparse and monocytes become the predominant cells with subsidence of type 2 reaction.

Bacterial Load and Disease Activity

There are a number of indices which can be obtained from the histopathologic slide. Granuloma fraction is defined as the fraction of the dermis in a section occupied by a granuloma as observed under a (×4) low power objective. This index is expressed as a fraction and reflects the extent of skin involvement. Granuloma fraction is mathematically the area of granuloma per unit area of dermis. The accuracy of the granuloma index measurement can be increased by use of planimetry.[9]

Bacillary index is the measure of bacterial load in the tissue section. It is graded using an oil immersion objective as:

- *0:* No bacilli found in 100 microscopic fields
- *1+:* 1–10 bacilli in 100 microscopic fields
- *2+:* 1–10 bacilli in 10 microscopic fields
- *3+:* 1–10 in one microscopic field
- *4+:* 10–100 in one microscopic field
- *5+:* 100–1,000 bacilli in one microscopic field
- *6+:* Over 1,000 bacilli and globi in one microscopic field.

The final bacillary index is the calculated as the mean value of all the sites.

CONCLUSION

Histopathology of leprosy is an important tool for diagnosis of clinically doubtful cases, assign the disease to a spectrum, and monitor the disease regression.

KEY POINTS

- Histopathology of leprosy is required for confirmation of diagnosis, spectral classification, distinguishing reactional states, and assessing the response to treatment.
- The most active and representative site of the disease should be considered for biopsy.
- Epithelioid granuloma eroding into the epidermis with destruction of the nerves is classically seen in TT leprosy.
- There is less compact epithelioid granuloma in BT leprosy with more giant cells as compared to TT leprosy.
- Admixture of epithelioid cells and macrophages are seen in mid borderline leprosy.
- BL and LL leprosy have macrophage granuloma with high bacillary index and a cut onion appearance of nerves.
- Spindle shaped histiocytes arranged in whorls and bands compressing the surrounding tissue are seen in histoid Hansen's disease.
- Type 1 reaction is characterized by disorganized granuloma with influx of lymphocytes and increase in giant cells.
- Increased infiltration of neutrophils is the hallmark of type 2 reaction.

REFERENCES

1. Semwal S, Joshi D, Goel G, Asati D, Kapoor N. Clinico-histological correlation in Hansen's disease: three-year experience at a newly established tertiary care center in central India. Indian J Dermatol. 2018;63:465-8.
2. Singh A, Weng X, Nath I. Skin biopsy in leprosy. In: Khopkar U (Ed). Skin Biopsy—Perspectives. Rijeka, Croatia: InTech; 2011. pp. 73-86.

3. Gupta SK. Histoid leprosy: review of the literature. Int J Dermatol. 2015;54(11):1283-8.
4. Lockwood DN, Lucas SB, Desikan KV, Ebenezer G, Suneetha S, Nicholls P. The histological diagnosis of leprosy type 1 reactions: identification of key variables and an analysis of the process of histological diagnosis. J Clin Pathol. 2008;61:595-600.
5. Tripathy T, Panda M, Kar BR Thakur TK, Singh BSTP. Facial Lazarine Leprosy in Post-elimination Era: A Case Report. Indian J Lepr. 2018;90:313-8.
6. Adhe V, Dongre A, Khopkar U. A retrospective analysis of histopathology of 64 cases of lepra reactions. Indian J Dermatol. 2012;57:114-7.
7. Ridley DS. Reactions. In: Ridley DS (Ed). Pathogenesis of Leprosy and Related Diseases. UK: Butterworth and Co-publishers Ltd.; 1988. pp. 118-34.
8. Job CK. Histopathological features of relapsed leprosy. Indian J Lepr. 1995;67:69-80.
9. Cree IA, McDougall AC, Coghill G, Beck JS. Quantitation of the granuloma fraction in leprosy skin biopsies by planimetry. Int J Lepr Other Mycobact Dis. 1985;53:582-6.

EXAMINATION QUESTIONS

1. What is the HPE of leprosy?
2. What is the HPE of leprosy reactions?

114 CHAPTER

Clinical Features of Leprosy

Surajit Gorai, Kinnor Das

INTRODUCTION

The clinical features of leprosy depend on the immune status of an individual. With downgrading cell-mediated immunity (CMI), bacillary load increases and clinical features shifts from tuberculoid pole to lepromatous one. **Figure 1** explains it.

Clinical features of leprosy were classified in many ways such as Indian classification, WHO classification, Ridley Jopling classification, etc. No classification is all inclusive. For our understanding purpose we will discuss Ridley Jopling one as it is widely accepted and based on:[1,2]

- Clinical
- Bacteriological
- Immunological
- Histopathological

The clinical features will be classified according to the Ridley Jopling classification and those types of Hansen's which are not included in the Ridley Jopling classification is discussed later.

How to describe the type of Hansen's?[3]

- Number of lesion(s)
- Distribution and symmetry
- Definition and clarity of lesion
- Anesthesia
- Surface of lesion
- Peripheral nerve involvement
- Mucosal and/or systemic involvement
- Number of *Mycobacterium leprae* in skin smears
- Lepromin test
- *Histopathology (HPE):*
  - *Strong host immunity:*
    - Larger lesion
    - Strong immunity → try to restrict bacilli → well-defined lesions
    - Asymmetrical
  - *Weak host immunity:*
    - Smaller lesion
    - Poor defined lesion
    - Symmetrical

TUBERCULOID LEPROSY[3-5]

- Single or few (up to 3)
- Asymmetrical
- Large, dry erythematous/hypopigmented patches with well-defined margins

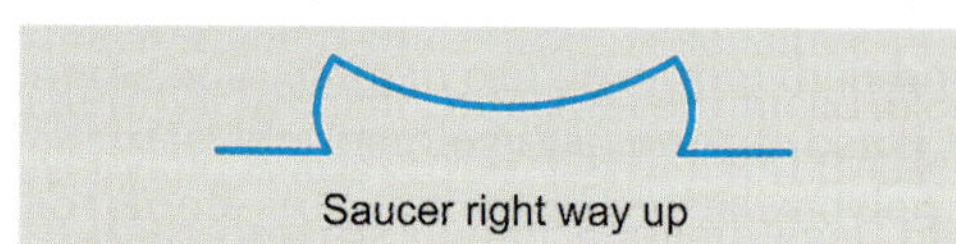

- *Anesthesia:* Present
- *Sweating:* Lost, loss of hair present
- *Nerves:* Thickened, presence of feeding nerves, nerve abscesses
- No systemic involvement
- *Skin smears:* Negative
- *Lepromin test:* Strongly positive

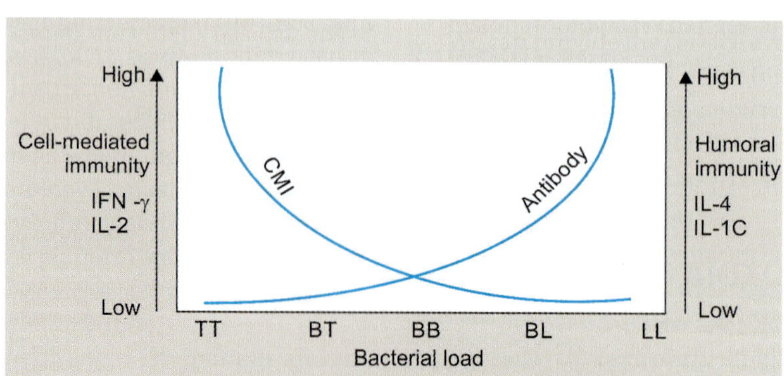

Fig. 1: CMI and antibody response in leprosy.
(BT: borderline tuberculoid; BB: mid-borderline leprosy; BL: borderline lepromatous leprosy; LL: lepromatous leprosy; TT: tuberculoid leprosy; CMI: cell-mediated immunity)

- *HPE:* Foci of lymphocytes, epithelioid cells and giant cells invading papillary zone and sometimes eroding epidermis. Cutaneous nerves, if not destroyed, are greatly swollen by epithelioid cell granuloma; they may caseate.
- *Course:* Polar tuberculoid leprosy (TT) stable and subpolar TT may downgrade.

Borderline Leprosy[3–5]

- Common type of leprosy
- Subdivided into borderline tuberculoid (BT), mid-borderline leprosy (BB), and borderline lepromatous leprosy (BL)
- *Course:* Unstable with variable prognosis, may progress to subpolar lepromatous leprosy (LL) leprosy
- Most prone to reactions

BORDERLINE TUBERCULOID

- Few (up to 10)
- Asymmetric
- Large, hypopigmented or skin-colored macules plaques with ill-defined margins with presence of satellite lesion near the advancing margin of patch (*Tap sign* can be elicited: Deep tenderness upon tapping over lesions which are overlying bone in tuberculoid leprosy)[6]

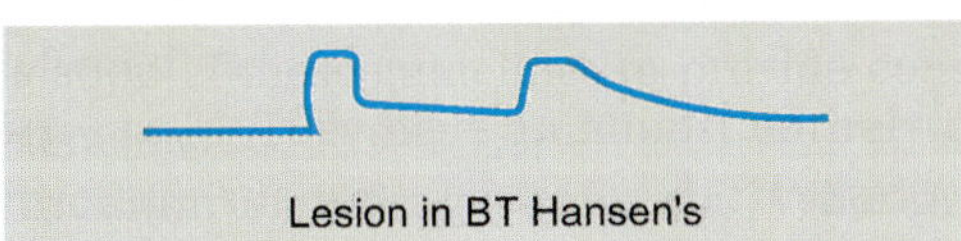

- *Anesthesia*: Marked
- *Surface*: Dry with hair loss
- *Nerve involvement*: Irregular and asymmetrical
- No systemic involvement
- *Skin smears*: Negative
- *Lepromin test*: Weakly positive
- *HPE*: BT there is a tuberculoid reaction more diffuse than in TT.

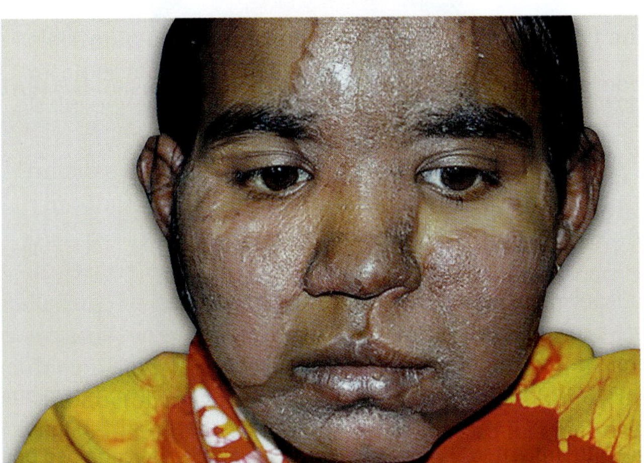

Fig. 2: Leprosy BT.
Courtesy: Dr Koushik Lahiri.

- *Course*: Prone to develop type 1 lepra reaction; deformities are common.

MID-BORDERLINE LEPROSY

- Unstable form, very rarely seen clinically
- Multiple lesions
- Symmetric lesions
- Lesions range from papules, macules and plaques. Plaques show well-demarcated edges with characteristic punched out center. Face may show infiltration with nodules on ears

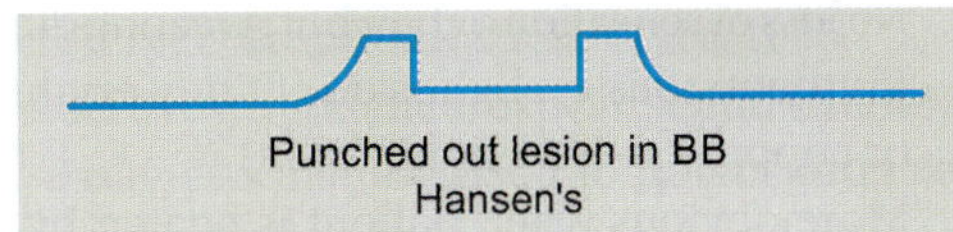

- *Anesthesia*: Moderate
- *Surface*: Normal to shiny
- *Nerve involvement*: Variable and depends on reversal/ downgrading and whether any reaction occurs
- No systemic involvement
- *Skin smears*: Positive
- *Lepromin test*: Negative
- *HPE*: There is a diffuse epithelioid cell granuloma
- *Course*: Upgrades or downgrades; prone to type 1 lepra reaction

BORDERLINE LEPROMATOUS LEPROSY

- Multiple lesions
- Symmetric (less symmetric than LL)
- This type classically starts as macule, widespread and symmetrical, later become infiltrated centrally → Papules, nodules and plaques with sloping edges

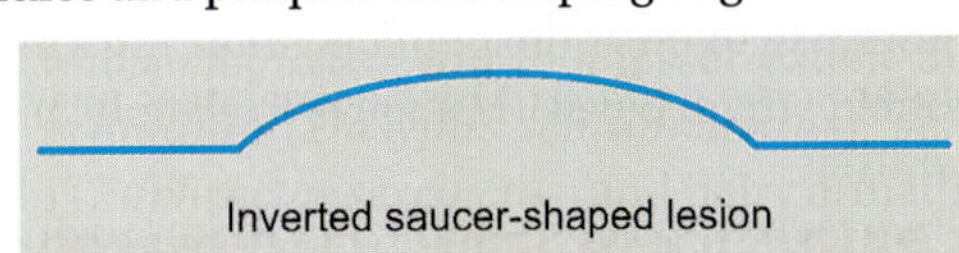

If the patient is downgrading from BT → BL many features of BT may be present.

- *Anesthesia*: Variable; glove and stocking hypoesthesia occurs late
- *Surface*: Shiny and infiltrated
- *Nerve involvement*: Widespread and asymmetrical; eyebrows not involved (or lost partially)
- Eyebrows not involved (or lost partially); systemic involvement associated with type-2 lepra reaction
- *Skin smear*: Positive
- *Lepromin test*: Negative
- *HPE*: There is a granuloma composed of macrophages with lymphocytes in dense clumps or sheets.
- *Course:*
  - Patients prone to develop type 2 lepra reaction
  - Type 1 reaction may occur.

LEPROMATOUS LEPROSY (FIGS. 3A TO C)

- *Two early symptoms:*
  - *Nasal symptoms*: Stuffiness, crusting, blood-stained discharge
  - *Edema of legs*: Bilateral edema of feet, toward end of the day. Disappear after night rest.
- Numerous lesions
- *Lesions:*
  - *Macules*: The early lesions—Small, numerous, shiny surface vague edge, symmetrical
    - No loss of sensation or hair but sweating diminished
    - Erythematous on light skin (faintly erythematous or coppery sheen on dark skin)
    - More obvious when patient is heated by exercise or hot bath
  - *Papules or nodules*:
    - May be of normal skin color or pigmented
    - Usually erythematous, coppery
    - In skin not in subcutis, therefore skin cannot be moved over them
    - Firm on palpation
    - When all the three lesions are present → nodules are present on face and limbs, macular lesions on trunk
- *Anesthesia*: Glove and stocking
- Dry skin, ichthyosis present
- Nerve involvement → Evidence of nerve damage is late in LL. Therefore, skin manifestation always present along nerve thickening
  - Thickened nerves are → firm, smooth
  - Thickening being localized to superficial part of nerve
  - Nerve damage is bilaterally symmetrical thus leading to bilateral glove and stocking anesthesia.
  - Fibrosis of nerve is due to reaction to dead bacilli
  - *Motor nerve damage*: Muscle weakness or wasting or paralysis
  - *Ulnar nerve*: Earliest—difficulty in approximation of ring with little finger when outstretched
  - *Facial nerve*: 1st involvement in lower eyelid (due to selective involvement of zygomatic branch) (this differentiates it from Bell's palsy) **(Fig. 4)**
- *Mucosal and systemic involvement:*
  - Leonine facies
  - Madarosis and milphosis
  - Xanthelasma palpebrarum (yellow tinge due to fat liberated by destroyed lepra cells)
  - *Nails finger toes*: Lusterless, shrunken, narrowed, longitudinally ridged
  - Digits become narrowed distally due to bone deformity
  - *Advanced*: Shortened digits retain the nail in much shrunken form.
  - *Ears*: Thickening and nodulation of ears (*Buddha ears*)
  - *Nose*: Anosmia, nasal stuffiness, discharge, epistaxis, perforation of nasal septum (destruction of nasal cartilage)

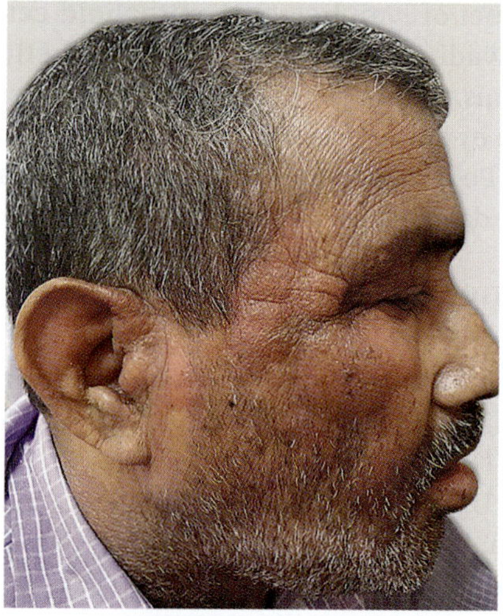

Fig. 3A: Lepromatous Leprosy.
Courtesy: Dr Aarti Sarda.

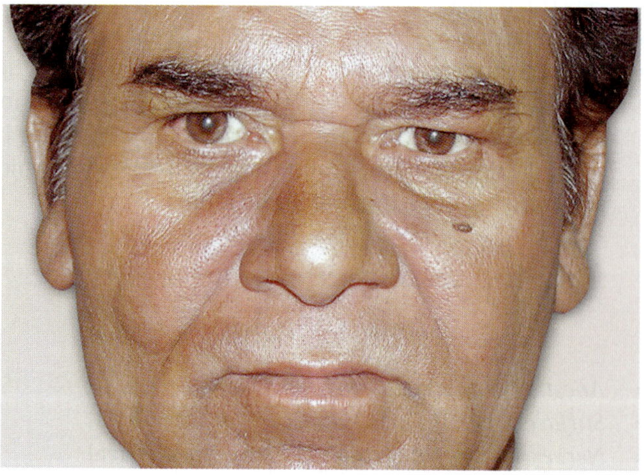

Fig. 3B: Lepromatous Leprosy.
Courtesy: Dr Koushik Lahiri.

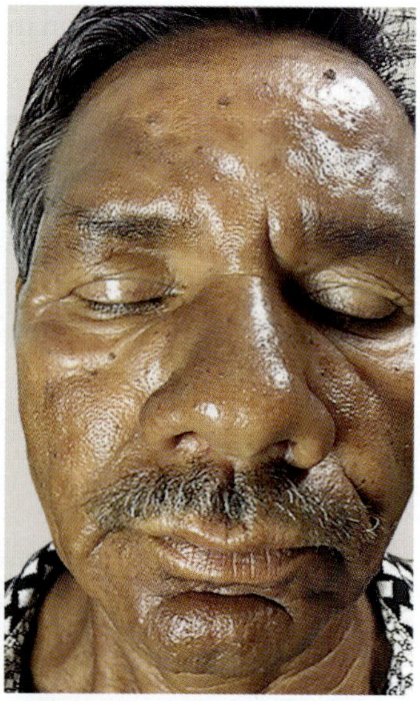

Fig. 3C: Lepromatous Leprosy.
Courtesy: Dr Koushik Lahiri.

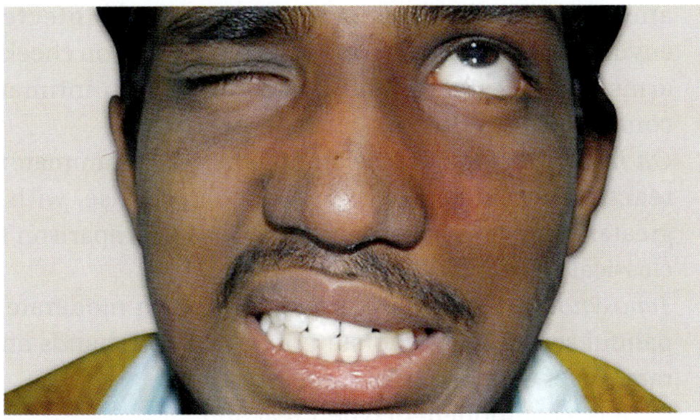

Fig. 4: Bell's palsy.
Courtesy: Dr Koushik Lahiri.

- *Face*: Skin becomes thickened, deepening of natural lines
- *Mouth, pharynx, larynx*: Papules on mucosal surface of lips: Nodules-tongue, palate, uvula ulcerate
- Hard palate may perforate
- Larynx → fibrosis of vocal cord → immobile → hoarseness of voice
  - Later-stridor-glottis becomes narrowed, coarse cough may be present
- *Bones and fingers*: Periostitis of bones (of forearm and lower legs)
  - Bone damage
  - *Metacarpals and carpals not involved*
  - Atrophic changes in tarsal, metatarsal and phalanges
  - *Distal phalanx*: Slow atrophy and absorption via concentric bone atrophy finally only needle of bone left
  - Shortening of fingers
  - *Penciling/sucked candy store*: Thinned and pointed metatarsals beginning in 5th ones
- *Skull:*
  - Atrophy of anterior nasal spine → Nasal collapse
  - Maxillary alveolar process → Loosening of upper central incisors
  - Leads to *facies leprosa*
- *Eye involvement:*
  - *Anterior eye most commonly involved (cooler)*: Superficial punctate keratitis
  - Milky haze over the upper part of each cornea
  - *Punctated by tiny lepras, cake grains of chalk*: Aggregation of leprosy bacilli (miliary lepromata)
  - Accompanied by pannus formation. Leads to sclerosing keratitis
  - Pannus in Hansen's commences on superior limbus → spreads all round cornea (*in trachoma: pannus is confined to upper region)*
  - Yellowish gelatinous nodules at 3 and 9 o'clock position at sclerocorneal junction
  - *Insidious iritis*: No ocular discomfort/redness (if undiagnosed → can cause iris atrophy and blindness)
  - Earliest manifestation → Miliary lepromata/iris pearls
  - *Iris pearls*: Deposits of tightly packed bacilli within macrophages and present in autonomic nerve plexus of iris
  - Gradually miosis and unresponsive to atropine
  - *Other eye complication(s):*
    - Cataract
    - Glaucoma
    - Herniation of ciliary body
  - *Posterior segment*: Rare, yellowish retinal bodies
  - *Involvement outside skull*:
    - 5th-corneal anesthesia
    - 7th nerve-facial palsy, lagophthalmos
    - Exposure keratitis can occur
- *Muscle*: Extensive interstitial myositis with granular bacilli between muscle bundle.
- *Kidney*: Renal amyloidosis, glomerulonephritis, nonspecific self-limiting and interstitial nephritis resolve with correct treatment. Pyelonephritis may occur
- *Testes:* Testicular atrophy
  - Neglected cases repeated epididymo-orchitis during lepra reaction
  - Early stages-potent but semen devoid of spermatozoa
  - Impotence and gynecomastia → develop late
- Female reproductive organs → not affected

- *Skin smears*: Positive always
- *Lepromin test*: Negative
- *HPE*: Thinned epidermis and flattened rete ridge. Diffuse leproma of foamy macrophages with few lymphocytes and plasma cells. Comparing LLs (sub-polar) with LLp (polar), foamy change is decreased or absent, lymphocytes are increased, and cutaneous nerves may show slight cellular infiltrate.

Differences between BL and LL Nodules

The lesions in BL lesions are:

- More distinct
- More variable in shape
- Asymmetrical
- Scantier

As compared to LL:

LLp and LLs[7]	*BBp and BBs*[8]
• LLp → *(LL polar):* Patient having features of LL leprosy from beginning throughout the course of disease • LLs → *(LL subpolar):* Patient who degraded to LL	• BBp → *(BB primary):* Display only the lymphocytic immune process lymphocytes ++ on HPE) These patients have never passed through a borderline phase • BBs → *(BB secondary):* (Langerhans cells ++ on HPE) less-well-developed mixed type of response. It has evolved as a result of reactional processes

INDETERMINATE LEPROSY[5,9]

No cardinal signs of leprosy.
First sign of disease 20–80% → of patients.

- Usually solitary lesion
- Asymmetrical
- Hypopigmented or slightly erythematosus poorly-defined macule usually on face (1–5 cm)
- Anesthesia is absent over lesion
- *Surface*: Hair growth is normal and the lesions are slightly dry
- No nerve involvement
- *Skin smear*: Negative
- Lepromin test → Variable weakly positive/negative or negative to positive transformation
- *HPE*: Nonspecific cellular reaction with tendency to surround skin appendages. Occasionally bacilli within cutaneous nerve in biopsy can be seen
- *Course:*
  - Heal spontaneously [30% → progress to determinate type (Lepromatous pole)]
  - *Signs of movement toward tuberculoid pore:*
    - Increasing definition of margins
    - Increasing hypopigmentation or erythema and anesthesia

CLINICAL FEATURES OF ATYPICAL FORMS OF LEPROSY

Atypical Types of Tuberculoid Leprosy

- Inoculation leprosy
- Childhood nodular leprosy
- Tenosynovitis with type 1 lepra reaction
- Lazarine leprosy
- Spontaneous skin ulceration
- Pure neural leprosy

Atypical Types of Lepromatous Leprosy

- Localized lepromatous leprosy
- Histoid leprosy
- Lucio leprosy
- Autoaggressive hanseniasis
- Silent/invisible lepromatous
- Spontaneous skin ulceration
- Pure neural

Atypical type of tuberculoid leprosy:

- *Inoculation leprosy*: The development of leprosy lesions at sites of tattooing, wounds or minor abrasions (over trauma prone areas) is usually a single lesion. The lesion(s) of inoculation leprosy manifests itself either in the form of tuberculoid (TT), BT, or maculoanesthetic (MA).[10]
- *Childhood nodular leprosy*: Benign clinical variant of tuberculoid leprosy affects breastfeeding infants and younger children inhabiting a highly infected environment. The lesions are usually localized on cheeks, arms, buttocks, and limbs. May result from intimate contact with lepromatous patients or relatives.
- *On histopathology*: Dense granulomatous inflammatory reaction associated with neural compromise, with a greater number of confluent tubercles in comparison to classical tuberculoid lesion.[11]
- *Tenosynovitis*: Synovial inflammation with moderately painful swelling over dorsum of one or both hands and rarely over the dorsum of the feet.[3]
  - It is a component of type 1 reaction.
  - Associated with other evidence of BT.
  - Occurs rarely in BL
  - *Treatment:* Controlling type 1 reaction, treatment of leprosy.
- *Lazarine leprosy*: Lazarine leprosy is the term used for severe ulceration, seen usually in patients at the tuberculoid end with underlying malnutrition or other debilitating illness.

  Clinically, it presents as slow healing ulcers that are preceded by edema and subsequent blister formation and later ulceration. These ulcers may go deep up to the tendons and bones. The blisters and ulcers show large number of lepra bacilli. The exact pathogenic mechanism underlying this rare phenomenon are not known, but factors such as breakdown of local cellular immunity, increased proliferation of the pathogen and tissue edema have been implicated. Protein malnutrition has been suggested to be the main event in the pathogenesis of ulceration. However. It has also been seen in BT leprosy without any underlying malnutrition or immunosuppression. It differs from Lucio phenomenon, which occurs in lepromatous patients and is due to thrombosis of vessels leading to ischemic necrosis.[12,13]

	Lazarine leprosy	*Lucio leprosy*
Onset	First few months	After 3–4 years
Patient's general condition	Usually healthy	Immunodepressed
BL at four sites	Negative or weakly positive	Highly positive
BL in the bullae	Positive	Positive
Sign and symptoms of a lepra reaction	Absent	Present
Spectrum of disease	TT/BT	LL
Lepromin reaction	Positive	Negative

Atypical Types of Lepromatous Leprosy

- *Localized lepromatous:*
  - There is a single nodule/localized area of nodules or papules, while most of the body surface area is normal.
  - The nodule/papules have a high bacterial index while the rest of the skin is negative (or nearly so, to standard methods of examination of *M. leprae*).

- *Treatment*: Treatment of multibacillary leprosy.[3]
- *Spontaneous skin ulceration*: In patients with severe, long standing, untreated LL.
- These lesions appear in an area of chronic panniculitis.
- The skin is fixed to underlying muscle or bone by dense bracony inflammatory tissue.
- Most commonly seen over anterior thigh, the calf, the triceps area or dorsum of forearm.
- The ulcers are not due to trauma rather skin dies and sloughs away leaving irregular, often triangular defects that look like third degree burns.[3]

- *Autoaggressive hanseniasis:*
  - This is a distinct clinical and immunological syndrome occurring in the lepromatous leprosy or infrequently in the borderline leprosy that has features resembling autoaggressive connective tissue diseases such as systemic lupus erythematosus.
  - The patients present with fever that is variable in intensity and chronology, anorexia, weight loss, asthenia, arthralgia, neuralgia, photosensitivity, malar rash, erythema nodosum, and erythema multiforme-like and necrotizing vasculitis-like skin lesion.
  - Generalized lymphadenopathy, arthritis, nephritis, orchitis, epididymitis, iritis, uveitis, and hepatitis may also be seen.
  - In addition, patients have hypergammaglobulinemia and one or more autoantibodies, such as antinuclear antibodies, present in their serum.
  - It has rarely been described in patients from India.
  - The exact etiology of this distinct presentation is not known, but it is speculated that antigen complexes of *M. leprae* and autologous tissue stimulate B-cells and also cause dysfunction of T-suppressor lymphocytes.
  - It is difficult to distinguish this entity from a type 2 lepra reaction due to overlapping features. Autoimmune connective tissue diseases like systemic lupus erythematosus, rheumatoid arthritis, necrotizing vasculitis, and dermatomyositis should also be considered in the different diagnosis.
  - It usually responds to thalidomide 100–300 mg/day in combination with antileprosy drugs.
  - Clofazimine is preferred in female patients of childbearing age.
  - The response to corticosteroids alone is usually poor.[13]
- *Silent/invisible lepromatous*: Rarely patients have imperceptible or apparently no skin infiltration and are detected incidentally when they develop peripheral anesthesia or nasal symptoms, or a type 2 reaction. A slit skin smear is positive from all sites, but the patient may virtually refuse to believe the diagnosis as the disease is almost asymptomatic.[13]
- *Spontaneous skin ulceration*: Presumably result of exaggerated hypersensitivity in type 1 reaction.
  - Rarely this occurs without any history or evidence of pre-existing lesions or nerve pathology.
  - *HPE*: Necrosis due to extreme cellular hypersensitivity in BT leprosy.
  - *Treatment*: Corticosteroids and treatment of Hansen's.[3]

PURE NEURAL LEPROSY

- The majority of patients present with sensory impairment, 5–10% present with nerve pain or deformity, and rarely as a nerve abscess. The deformity rate is up to 25–30%.
- The majority of cases are mononeuritic. The ulnar, median, and lateral popliteal nerves are commonly involved. Cutaneous nerves like sural, mucocutaneous, superficial radial, and greater auricular nerves can be involved.
- Pure neuritic leprosy can be diagnosed on the finding of thickened nerve and sensory impairment, negative slit skin smears, and absence of skin lesions.
- A nerve biopsy is diagnostic and on histology the entire spectrum from TT to BL leprosy may be seen.
- A singly thickened nerve that is firm in consistency with a strongly positive lepromin response indicates TT-BT leprosy. Abscess formation may be presenting feature and suggest tuberculoid leprosy.
- If two or more nerves are thickened and the lepromin and the lepromin test is negative or doubtful, BL leprosy may be suspected and confirmed by a nerve biopsy.
- Pure neuritic leprosy (or polyneuritic as it was referred to) was conventionally included under nonlepromatous leprosy. However, the finding BL-like histology and large number of AFB in a single nerve biopsy has thrown doubt on its being classified as nonlepromatous leprosy and being treated as paucibacillary leprosy.
- Recent recommendations suggest that if two or more nerves are thickened, MDT for multibacillary leprosy may be given.
- Follow-up of patients with pure neuritic leprosy shows the development of skin lesions in 35% of cases over 3–5 years or without treatment.[13,14]
- *Histoid leprosy*: It is an expression of multibacillary leprosy. Characterized by occurrence of nodules and/or plaques on skin and/or subcutaneous tissue. Well-demarcated cutaneous nodule is its cardinal feature. The lesions are present over normal looking skin. Reactional episodes are seldom encountered. The lesions are small soft and on scraping the cut surface they look pulpy. Most striking feature on histopathology is presence of numerous thin spindle-shaped histiocytes. Histoid habitus refers to the arrangement of lepra bacilli in groups or parallel bundles along the long axis of histiocytes.[3,15,16]
- *Lucio leprosy*: Also known as pretty leprosy or leprosy bonita. First described by Lucio and Alvarado and later redefined by Latapi. Commonly seen in Mexico and Costa Rica. It is a non-nodular and diffuse form of leprosy.

Clinically Lucio leprosy presents as slowly progressive diffuse infiltration of the skin without any evidence of discrete lesions. As a result the skin looks waxy and has shiny appearance. The wrinkles are obliterated. Due to these clinical findings Lucio leprosy is also called as pretty leprosy or leprosy bonita. There is loss of body hair except the scalp hair. Widespread sensory loss is present. Thickening of upper eyelids gives a sleepy look.[3,17,18]

KEY POINTS

- Clinical features of leprosy vary with basic interplay between CMI and bacterial load.
- When CMI is high lesions of leprosy are less in number, well-defined and bacterial load is nominal.
- With low CMI leprosy, lesions are widespread, more in number and with very high bacterial load.
- That's how they are divided into tuberculoid or lepromatous.
- Few rare varieties of leprosy such as indeterminate, lucio, and pure neuritic are also to keep in mind while dealing with leprosy patient.

REFERENCES

1. Pardillo FEF, Fajardo TT, Abalos RM, Scollard D, Gelber RH. Methods for the classification of leprosy for treatment purposes. Clin Infect Dis. 2007;44(8):1096-9.
2. Ridley DS, Jopling WH. Classification of leprosy according to immunity a five-group system. Int J Lepr. 1966;34(3):255-73.
3. Pfaltzgraff RE, Bryceson A. Clinical leprosy. In: Leprosy. London, United Kingdom: Churchill Livingstone; 1985. pp. 134–76.
4. Bhushan P, Thatte SS. Saucer lesions in leprosy: anatomy of the controversy. Indian J Dermatol. 2016;61(1):100.
5. Jopling WH, McDougall AC. The Disease. In: Handbook of Leprosy, 5th edition. New Delhi: CBS Publishers & Distributors; 1996. pp. 10-53.
6. Kumarasinghe SPW, Kumarasinghe MP, Amarasinghe UTP. "Tap sign" in tuberculoid and borderline tuberculoid leprosy. Int J Lepr Mycobact Dis Off Organ Int Lepr Assoc. 2004; 72(3):291-5.
7. Ridley DS, Waters MF. Significance of variations within the lepromatous group. Lepr Rev. 1969;40(3):143-52.
8. Ridley DS. The pathogenesis and classification of polar tuberculoid leprosy. Lepr Rev. 1982;53(1):19-26.
9. Findlay GH. Indeterminate leprosy. Br J Dermatol. 1951;63(3): 100-4.
10. Sehgal V. Inoculation leprosy. Int J Dermatol. 1988;27(1):6-9.
11. Singal A, Chhabra N. Childhood leprosy. In: IAL Textbook of Leprosy, 2nd edition. New Delhi, India: Jaypee Brothers Medical Publishers; 2015. pp. 364-5.
12. Pardo-Castello V, Caballero GM. Lazarine leprosy: a peculiar monosymptomatic form of leprosy. Arch Dermatol Syphilol. 1931;23(1):1-11.
13. Sharma VK, Malhotra AK. Leprosy: classification and clinical aspects. In: IADVL Textbook of Dermatology, 3rd edition. Mumbai: Bhalani Publishing House; 2008. pp. 2032-88.
14. Rao PN, Suneetha S. Pure neuritic leprosy: current status and relevance. Indian J Dermatol Venereol Leprol. 2016;82(3):252-61.
15. Sehgal VN. Histoid leprosy. In: IAL Textbook of Leprosy, 2nd edition. New Delhi: Jaypee Brothers Medical Publishers; 2017. pp. 268-77.
16. Karthikeyan K. Histoid leprosy. Am J Trop Med Hyg. 2015;92(6): 1085-6.
17. Saoji V, Salodkar A. Lucio leprosy with lucio phenomenon. Indian J Lepr. 2001;73(3):267-72.
18. Kaur C, Thami GP, Mohan H. Lucio phenomenon and Lucio leprosy. Clin Exp Dermatol. 2005;30(5):525-7.

EXAMINATION QUESTIONS

1. What are the atypical types of leprosy?
2. Describe the indeterminate leprosy.
3. What are the effects of pregnancy on leprosy?

Write short notes on the following:

4. Neuritic leprosy.
5. Histoid leprosy.
6. Ocular leprosy.
7. Various bone changes in leprosy.
8. Lucio leprosy.
9. TT Hansen's disease.
10. Lazarine leprosy.
11. Childhood leprosy.

115 CHAPTER Systemic Involvement in Leprosy

Suresh Joshipura, Deep Joshipura, Vivek V Pai

INTRODUCTION

Leprosy is a chronic multisystem disease caused by *Mycobacterium leprae*. Although it has a predilection for skin and peripheral nerves, it is known to cause systemic involvement. Based on the hosts' immunity, leprosy can be broadly divided into lepromatous, borderline, and tuberculoid leprosy. Systemic involvement usually occurs in lepromatous leprosy (LL) with some involvement in tuberculoid. Hematogenous spread of bacilli, secondary amyloidosis, direct invasion of the bacilli or lepra reaction can result in major involvement and dysfunction of peripheral nerves, eyes, nasopharynx, bones, kidney, liver, and testes.[1]

HISTORY

Leprosy has been a historic disease studied for centuries. Its initial descriptions were found in India (600 BC), China and Japan (200 BC).[2] In 1873, Norwegian Physician GA Hansen introduced the microbiology of *M. leprae* leading to advances in understanding pathogenesis of leprosy. In 1966, Ridley and Jopling introduced a classification of leprosy which is widely used to date. In 1953, Møller-Christensen, a Danish medical historian, and a paleopathologist pioneered study of bone involvement in leprosy.

ORGAN INVOLVEMENT

Ocular Leprosy

- An estimated 70–75% worldwide occurrence, with 10–50% patients with severe dysfunctional ocular lesions, with 5% estimated rate of blindness **(Table 1)**.[3]
- Ocular manifestations are secondary to either infiltration of colder anterior part of the eyeball by *M. leprae* or due to nerve damage.
- Leprosy affects extraocular structures as well as ocular structures, mostly anterior half of the ocular structures.
- Extraocular lesions include madarosis, lagophthalmos, ectropion, entropion, trichiasis, chronic dacryoadenitis, and nasolacrimal duct block.
- Ocular lesions consist of conjunctivitis, corneal anesthesia, and ulcers, superficial punctate keratitis, corneal nerve beading, scleritis, episcleritis, and uveitis—acute and chronic.

Extraocular Lesions

Madarosis **(*Fig. 1*)**

- Madarosis is loss of eyebrows. It is pathognomonic of LL, and can be unilateral in tuberculoid leprosy in presence of overlying patch or bilateral in temporal two-thirds in LL.
- *Etiology*: Direct invasion of hair bulbs by *M. leprae*, causing loss of hair bulbs and subsequent atrophy.[3]
- *Clinical features (C/F)*: Loss of eyebrows in outer two-thirds of eyelashes later progresses nasally with total loss of eyelashes and eyebrows in advanced disease.
- *Treatment*: Cosmetic surgery such as skin grafting.

Lagophthalmos **(*Figs. 2 and 3*)**

- *Definition*: Lagophthalmos is the inability to close eyes properly.
- *Etiology*: Paralysis of seventh cranial nerve, occurs in PB and MB leprosy.
- *C/F*: Inability to close eyelids, along with corneal anesthesia secondary to trigeminal nerve involvement predisposes to exposure keratitis, corneal ulcers, corneal

TABLE 1: Ocular lesions potentially causing blindness.

Ocular lesion	*Mechanism*	*Cause of blindness*
Corneal anesthesia	Loss of corneal reflex and anesthesia due to involvement of ophthalmic division of trigeminal nerve	When associated with lagophthalmos, entropion, and trichiasis, it causes corneal ulcers and perforation leading to blindness
Lagophthalmos	Involvement of fibers of facial nerve	Excessive exposure, dryness of cornea leading to keratitis, ulcers, perforation, and blindness
Uveitis	Direct invasion from *Mycobacterium leprae* or part of lepra reactions	Chronic iridocyclitis may be insidious and could be a cause of blindness
Cataract	Age-related, secondary to chronic uveitis, chronic steroid therapy	Decreased vision secondary to opacity of lenses

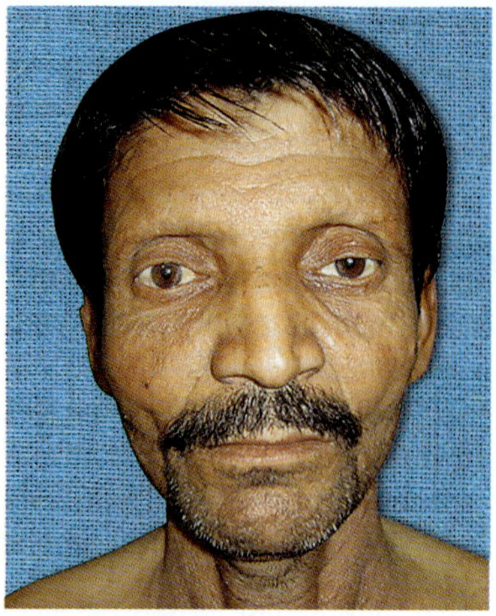

Fig. 1: Madarosis.
Courtesy: Dr Bela Shah, Department of Dermatology, BJ Medical College and Civil Hospital, Ahmedabad.

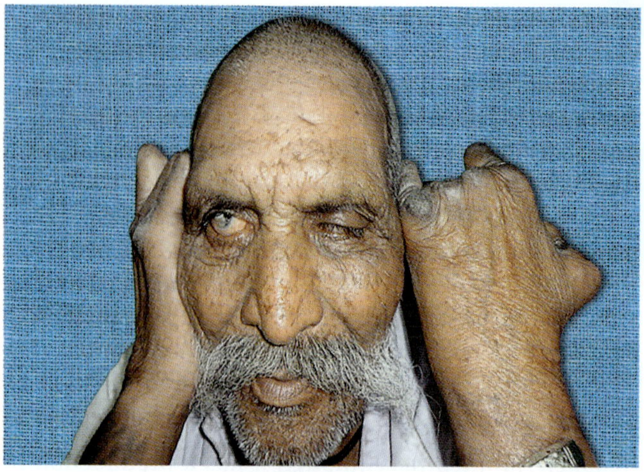

Fig. 2: Ophthalmic manifestations: lagophthalmos with corneal opacity over right eye.
Courtesy: Department of DVL, PDU Government Medical College and Hospital, Rajkot, Gujarat.

perforation, and blindness, if not medically or surgically intervened.

- *Treatment*: Lagophthalmos with lid-gap of 5 mm or less and <6 months early onset can be managed conservatively with sunglasses, physiotherapy measures such as blinking exercises and muscle stimulation, systemic steroids, and artificial tears. More than 6 months duration with large lid-gap (5–6 mm) needs surgical correction.[3]

Ectropion and entropion

- Ectropion or outward turning of the eyelid, commonly of the lower eyelid, is seen in chronic patients, and is caused due to damaged tarsal plate and orbicularis oculi muscle secondary to facial nerve palsy.
- Entropion is a term used for inversion or in rolling of the eyelids, particularly lower eyelids.
- *Treatment*: Treatment of ectropion and entropion is mostly surgical.

Trichiasis

- Trichiasis is inward misdirection of the eyelashes.
- *Etiology*: *Mycobacterium leprae* infiltration in the follicles causes loss of support.
- It can cause corneal irritation from constant striking of eyelashes against likely anesthetized cornea causing punctate epithelial erosions and pannus formation in chronic cases.[3]
- *Treatment*: Epilation in early cases.

Ocular Lesions

Conjunctivitis

- Conjunctivitis is caused by primary infection from *M. leprae* along with inflammation and edema.
- It can be complicated by pterygium, which can cause astigmatic refractive errors and conjunctival scarring.[3]

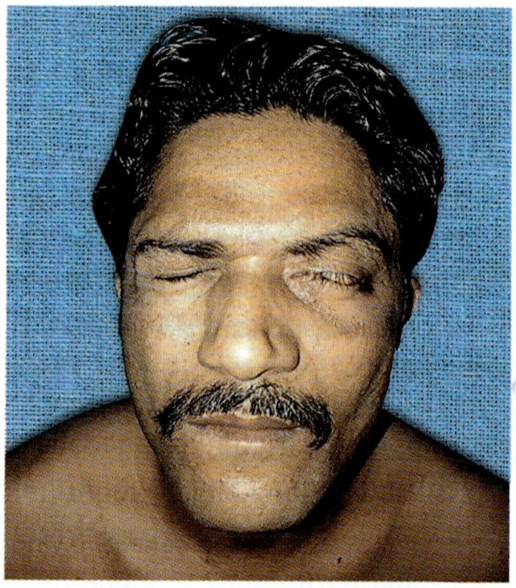

Fig. 3: Facial nerve palsy manifesting as lagophthalmos of left eye in a patient of lepromatous leprosy.
Courtesy: Department of DVL, PDU Government Medical College and Hospital, Rajkot, Gujarat.

- Conjunctival crystalline deposits from clofazimine can cause ocular toxicity in patients on chronic multidrug therapy.[3]

Cornea

- Involvement of cornea is one of the prime manifestations of ocular leprosy. Cornea being anesthetized in severe disease due to fifth nerve palsy is affected indirectly due to increased rubbing, friction, and exposure keratitis or can be directly infiltrated by *M. Leprae* resulting in punctate avascular keratitis and corneal nerve beading.
- Corneal nerve beading or swellings are seen in LL with high bacterial loads. It is caused by calcified collections of *M. leprae* on unmyelinated corneal stroma of the corneal nerve leading to appearance of "beads on a string."[3,4]

- Corneal anesthesia can occur in patients with long-standing and poorly treated leprosy. It is caused by direct invasion of *M. leprae* into corneal nerves. When associated with lagophthalmos and other lid abnormalities, it can predispose to corneal irritation leading to keratitis, ulcers, and scarring. Additionally, corneal anesthesia is often associated with a decrease in tear secretion and dry eyes.
- Punctate avascular keratitis caused by direct infiltration of *M. leprae* presents clinically as chalky white, punctate subepithelial opacities occurring mostly in an upper temporal quadrant of the cornea. These opacities can complicate to interstitial keratitis and pannus formation.
- A number of bacteria such as *Pseudomonas aeruginosa, Staphylococcus epidermidis, Streptococcus pneumoniae, Enterococci,* and *Nocardia* asteroids can cause infectious keratitis in patients with leprosy.[3]
- Examination of corneal reflex should be included as part of routine eye examination in patients with leprosy.
- *Treatment*: Corneal ulcer is treated with antibiotic eye ointment along with atropine and systemic steroids if necessary. Concomitant treatment of lagophthalmos is often required along with generous use of artificial tears. Keratoplasty may be required in healed corneal ulcers.

Episcleritis and scleritis

Episcleritis and scleritis could be caused either by direct invasion of *M. leprae* or part of type II lepra reactions.

Iridocyclitis and uveitis

- Iridocyclitis, either acute or chronic is seen in about 2.3–4% leprosy patients, caused by infiltration of *M. leprae* into cooler anterior areas of eyeball and during lepra reaction.[3]
- The onset of iritis may be insidious and asymptomatic in the beginning which can be diagnosed by slit-lamp examination.
- *Etiology*: Invasion of *M. leprae*, neuroparalytic or autoimmune,[5] causing acute or chronic iridocyclitis, or iris pearls
- Iris pearls, which are pathognomonic for chronic ocular leprosy, are a collection of bacilli and stromal mononuclear cells.
- Chronic iridocyclitis is caused by cell-mediated immune reaction forming iris granuloma comprising macrophages, epithelioid cells along with T-lymphocytes.[3]
- *C/F*: Red watery eye, photophobia, myosis along with eye pain, and difficulty in vision. Acute iridocyclitis often occurs as part of lepra reaction.
- *Complications*: Anterior chamber flare and cells, keratic precipitates, synechiae formation causing occlusion of papillae and secondary glaucoma, iris atrophy, and pupillary defects. Uveitis can also cause secondary complicated cataract of central posterior subcapsular region.
- *Treatment*: Local steroid and atropine drops and oral steroids as indicated along with clofazimine and thalidomide if associated erythema nodosum leprosum (ENL).

Cataract

- Cataract, which is opacification of lens, is a commonly seen ocular lesion in leprosy, with thrice the risk of development of cataract in leprosy.
- *Etiology*: Age-related, related to chronic uveitis, and long-term steroid therapy for lepra reactions. Leprosy may predispose to early onset cataract due to changes in aqueous humor physiology due to ciliary body involvement.
- *Treatment*: Surgical intervention such as phacoemulsification, simple extracapsular cataract extraction (ECCE) with sclerocorneal stitches and manual small-incision cataract surgery (SICS).[6] In patients with severe chronic eye involvement, cataract surgery may be difficult due to lesions in anterior chamber.

Prevention of blindness

- Regular ophthalmic examinations of all leprosy patients even after completion of therapy.
- Eye examinations should include at the least corneal reflex, checking for lagophthalmos, tenderness, and visual acuity.

Nasopharynx (Figs. 4 and 5)

- Involvement of nose and upper pharynx are common since *M. leprae* tend to gain access via respiratory droplets. Trachea, bronchi, and lung parenchyma seems to be spared.
- *Nasal involvement*: Anterior aspect of inferior turbinate and nasal septum are involved with edema and mucosal thickening along with nasal septum perforation, collapse of septal cartilage (saddle nose) and paranasal sinus involvement in severe multibacillary (MB) leprosy.
- *Oropharynx*: Ulceration of tongue, tonsillar pillars, and palatal perforation. Involvement of Eustachian tube and cochlea may cause difficulty in hearing.
- *Larynx*: Ulceration, nodules, and fibrosis in severe disease resulting in tracheostomy in severe cases. Impaired mobility of vocal cords can lead to difficulty in speech or respiration. Aspiration of food and secretion can cause aspiration pneumonia.
- There have been some reports of development of pulmonary tuberculosis in patients with leprosy. Since most patients are treated with multidrug therapy, a risk of rifampin-resistant pulmonary tuberculosis may develop.[1]
- *C/F*: Earliest sign or vital clue for nasal involvement is history of epistaxis in a patient with LL with or without additional brownish nasal crusting. Epiglottis may be involved and can become nodular or edematous.[1] Laryngeal involvement can cause hoarseness, cough, pain, and even acute respiratory distress.

Musculoskeletal and Bones (Figs. 6 to 8)

- Musculoskeletal involvement generally occurs following involvement of peripheral nerves in leprosy.

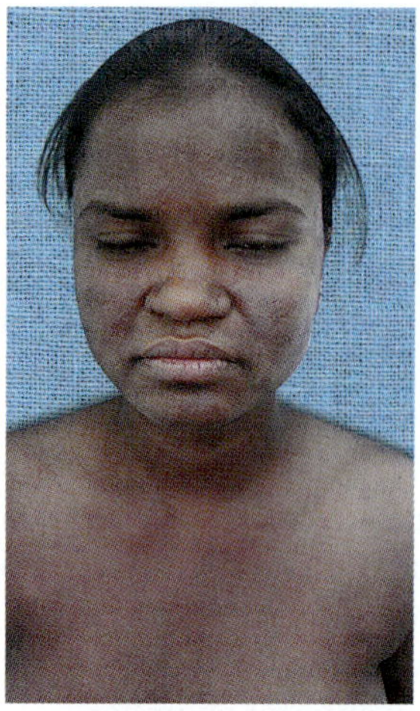

Fig. 4: Depressed nasal bridge.
Courtesy: Dr Bela Shah, Department of Dermatology, BJ Medical College and Civil Hospital, Ahmedabad.

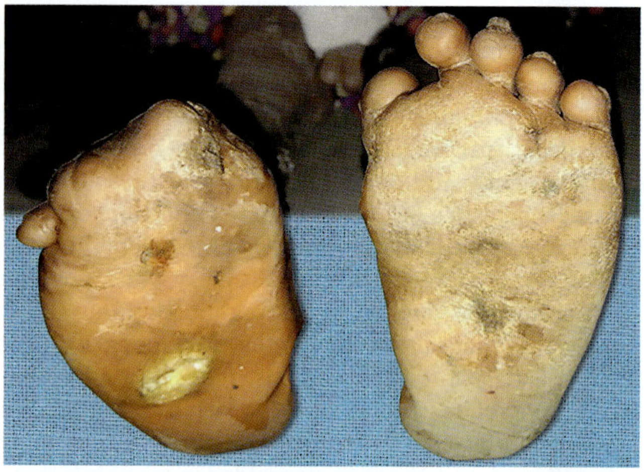

Fig. 6: Resorption of toes along with trophic ulcer and callosities over sole.
Courtesy: Department of DVL, PDU Government Medical College and Hospital, Rajkot, Gujarat.

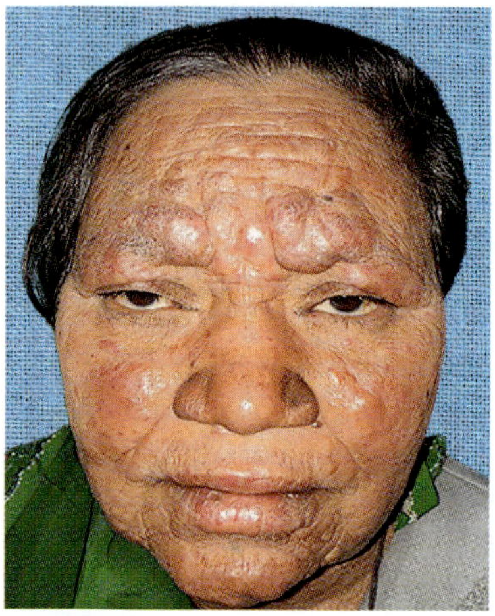

Fig. 5: Leonine face of lepromatous leprosy with papulonodular lesions, madarosis, and depressed nasal bridge.
Courtesy: Department of DVL, PDU Government Medical College and Hospital, Rajkot, Gujarat.

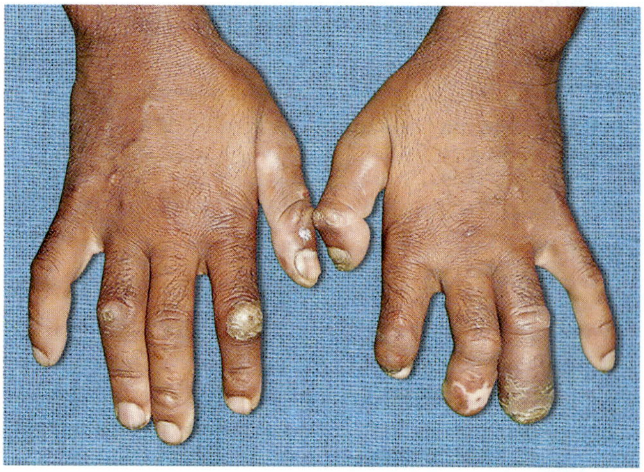

Fig. 7: Complete claw hand deformity with resorption of terminal phalanges.
Courtesy: Department of DVL, PDU Government Medical College and Hospital, Rajkot, Gujarat.

- Loss of sensations secondary to nerve palsies predisposes to repeated trauma leading to osteomyelitis. Other bone changes occur due to disuse atrophy of muscles.
- Bone changes in leprosy are of two types: (1) nonspecific and (2) specific.
- Nonspecific changes include atrophy and absorption of bones, osteoporosis and osteomyelitis.[7] These changes are secondary to nerve palsies and deranged blood supply.
- *Absorption of bones*: Necrosis and bone resorption are especially seen in fingers, toes, and proximal bones, mainly in LL. Atrophy and resorption begin distally and extend proximally. Metatarsals assume a shape of a "pencil" or "sucked candy stick" due to thinning of the bone distally.[7]
- *Osteoporosis*: It is common in females and males with testicular involvement leading to hypogonadism. It is particularly crucial in elderly patients who are at a risk of

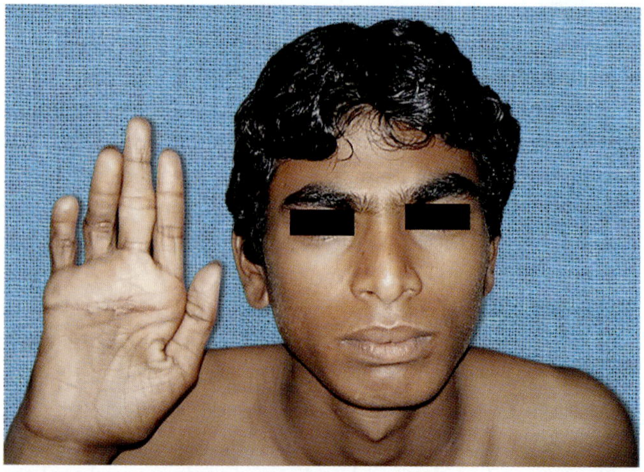

Fig. 8: Partial (ulnar) claw hand with flattening of hypothenar eminence.
Courtesy: Department of DVL, PDU Government Medical College and Hospital, Rajkot, Gujarat.

pathological fractures of the spine if they have a fall. These chronic leprosy patients may have ocular involvement such as cataract which may predispose them to increased risk of falls.

- *Osteomyelitis*: Osteomyelitis occurs following a long-term trophic ulcer due to neuropathy.
- Specific changes are due to direct invasion and deposits of *M. leprae* into bones or their blood vessels and include osteitis, periostitis, lytic lesions, erosions, and bone cysts.[7]
- Facial bones are involved in leprosy and give rise to characteristic, "facies leprosa" consists of atrophy of the anterior nasal spine, atrophy and recession of the maxillary alveolar processes, and endonasal inflammatory change.[8]
- Inflammatory arthritis of small hands and feet is not uncommon. Skeletal muscle involvement is rare and does not affect function.

Cardiovascular System

- Cardiovascular involvement is commonly seen in MB patients than paucibacillary (PB)
- Multiple signs and symptoms such as tachycardia, arrhythmias, and palpitations are reported which can be attributed to autonomic nervous dysfunction.[1]
- Autonomic dysfunction, including both sympathetic and parasympathetic chain is likely secondary to acid-fast bacilli (AFB) infiltration or involvement of baroreceptors.[1]
- Acid-fast bacilli have been demonstrated by various stains in vessel walls indicating involvement of arteries and veins along with arteriographic evidence of abnormalities in patients with leprosy.
- Vascular derangements along with neuropathy may play a role in pathogenesis of bony deformities.[1,7]

Gastrointestinal Tract

- Oropharyngeal structures, liver and spleen are mainly involved.
- Esophagus, stomach, pancreas, gallbladder, and intestines do not seem to be involved.
- Spleen involvement includes infiltration by lepra bacilli along with foam cells and granuloma formation, especially in MB patients.[1]
- Hepatic involvement is extensive via hematogenous spread and can lead to functional impairment including hepatitis.
- Hepatic parenchymal infiltration with leprous granulomata along with steatosis and Kupffer cell hyperplasia have been noted.[9]
- "Lepromatous hepatitis" is a term used for well-defined granuloma consisting of Virchow cells with or without lymphocytes, with multiple AFBs and minimal fibrosis, more commonly seen in LL.[1]
- The drug-induced hepatic injury is also not uncommon, given long-term treatment with medications such as rifampicin.
- Hepatitis B and hepatitis C coinfection (to a lesser extent) is frequently observed in LL. Secondary amyloidosis in liver is also seen in patients with leprosy.

Nervous System[1]

- Brain, meninges, cerebellum, and spinal cord are not affected by leprosy with no direct infiltration.
- However, a study has shown autopsies showing vacuolar changes in motor neurons of medulla oblongata and spinal cords in selected patients of LL.
- Conduction abnormalities in brain stem, depression and dementia have been observed in selected studies.
- Peripheral nerves are usually affected by infiltration of *M. leprae*. It is the sensory compartment of the nerve that is largely affected in leprosy. Motor fiber involvement occurs as a result of the damage to the mixed nerve.
- The three main factors that contribute to nerve damage in leprosy are: (1) infection, (2) immune response of the host, and (3) special anatomical and physiological dispositions of the nervous system.[10]
- Pathological changes in the nerves include demyelination, fiber loss, infarcts, necrosis, and edema, which lead to both sensory and motor nerve palsies resulting in disabilities.

Renal[7]

- Renal involvement is frequent with possible functional abnormalities seen in patients with leprosy.
- Glomerulonephritis resulting in proteinuria, microscopic hematuria, granular, hyaline, and red blood cell (RBC) casts are seen.
- Functional impairment with regards to reduced glomerular filtration rate (GFR) and increased blood urea nitrogen (BUN) and creatinine has been seen.
- Reactional states can predispose to acute renal failure. Chronic involvement with glomerulonephritis or secondary to renal amyloidosis can cause chronic renal failure often requiring hemodialysis.

Endocrine System

Male Reproductive

- Lepromatous leprosy is commonly associated with testicular involvement due to infiltration of *M. leprae* as well as orchitis due to recurrent type 2 immune reactions.
- Testicular involvement consists of involvement of both seminiferous tubules and interstitial cells.[7]
- *C/F*: Testicular pain and swelling is the initial presentation followed by change in texture of the testes.
- *Complications*: Infertility, reduced testicular size likely secondary to atrophy, increased follicle-stimulating hormone/luteinizing hormone (FSH/LH), and reduced testosterone leading to gynecomastia, impotence, and hypogonadism leading to osteoporosis in men

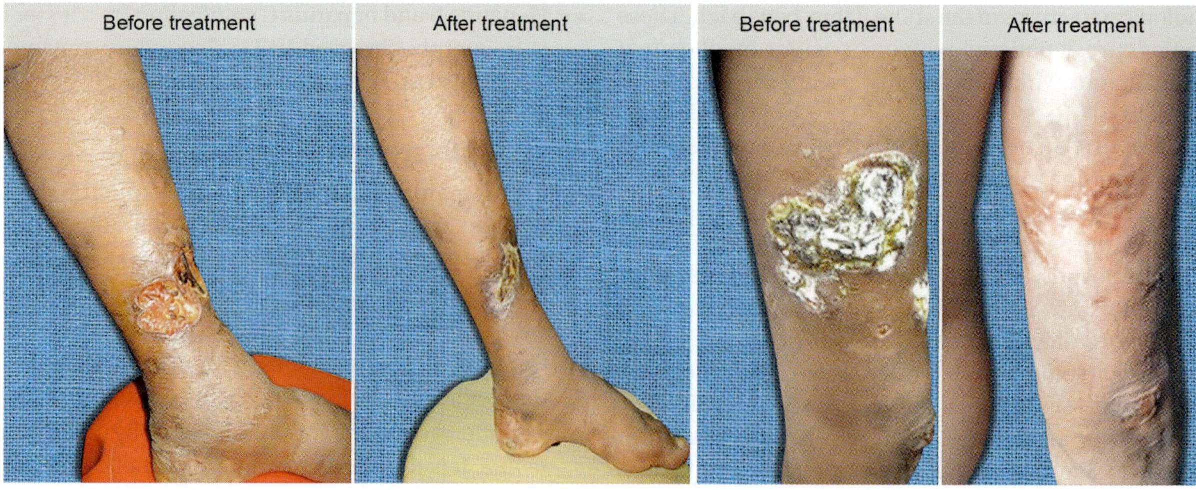

Fig. 9: Ulcerative erythema nodosum leprosum (ENL) reactions in lepromatous leprosy.
Courtesy: Dr VV Pai, Director, Bombay Leprosy Project, Mumbai.

- *Treatment*: Testosterone replacement therapy has been satisfactorily been utilized.[1]

Female Reproductive[1,7]

- Little or no involvement of female reproductive system with no effect on menarche, menstruation, or fertility or menopause
- Transplacental transmission is rare, low birth weight and prematurity has been seen in mothers with LL.

Hematopoietic System

- Anemia is seen in patients with leprosy, which may be a combination of hemolytic and megaloblastic anemia.
- There is reduction in RBC and hemoglobin probably due to increased activation of reticuloendothelial system (RES) secondary to increased RBC destruction.
- Megaloblastic anemia is attributed to nutritional deficiencies as well as bacillary infiltration of bone marrow and formation of leprous granulomata in bones.

Lepra Reactions[11]

- Lepra reactions, such as ENL, are a severe, inflammatory, painful, and multisystem complication of LL, causing multiple comorbidities and affecting quality of life.
- Besides cutaneous lesions, it is associated with fever, pain, presence of edema of hands or/and feet, dactylitis, arthritis, orchitis, lymphadenitis, neuritis, and periostitis.
- *Treatment*: Systemic corticosteroids, clofazimine, and thalidomide
- As ENL is a multisystem disorder characterized by crops of painful skin lesions, fever, and systemic manifestations, a 10-item clinical severity score for ENL, the ENLIST ENL Severity Score (EESS), has been developed and recently validated by the ENLIST Group. The range of scores possible is 0–30. The higher the score the more severe the ENL. A score of 9 or more has been shown to be associated with more severe ENL **(Fig. 9)**.

Psychiatry

- Psychiatric involvement is almost always present is a patient with leprosy, especially LL.
- *Causes*: Psychological trauma from disease, fear of social stigma, and anticipation of a long chronic course of treatment
- Psychiatric involvement increases with poor knowledge about the course of the disease and available treatments.
- Psychiatric counseling is an integral part of the treatment and should include counseling about the disease and modes of transmission. Emphasis should be made on preventative aspects such as regular eye examinations, examinations of hands and toes, and importance of medication compliance.

Nail Involvement[7]

Changes in nails in leprosy are often nonspecific and nails may appear dystrophic which are observed more frequently in MB leprosy.

Affection of nails could be due to multifactorial that include neuropathy, trauma, vascular changes, chronicity of the disease, and infections.

KEY POINTS

- Madarosis is diagnostic of LL, caused by destruction of hair bulbs from *M. leprae* infiltration.
- Lagophthalmos is due to seventh nerve palsy and along with ectropion and corneal anesthesia, could predispose to exposure keratitis, dry eye, and blindness.

- Cornea is commonly affected as ocular manifestation of leprosy and it could lead to serious ocular dysfunction including corneal ulcers and keratitis, which, if not intervened medically or surgically, could be a cause of blindness.
- Iridocyclitis, both acute and chronic are common in leprosy, needs to be treated or else could lead to serious complications such as blindness.
- "Facies leprosa", a peculiar appearance of face as seen in patients with untreated LL, is due to involvement of nasal bones.
- Bone changes are specific and nonspecific, later being more common. Absorption of bones likely due to neuropathic and vascular involvement and affects distal phalanges of hands along with toes.
- Testes often always get involved in lepra reactions leading to orchitis along with direct infiltration of *M. leprae*. This leads to subsequent testicular atrophy leading to low levels of testosterone causing osteoporosis, impotence, and gynecomastia.
- Hepatic involvement is common and could lead to functional hepatitis. Hepatitis B and C are found to be associated with leprosy.
- Renal involvement can lead to functional impairment in GFR, BUN, or creatinine.

REFERENCES

1. Klioze AM, Ramos-Caro FA. Visceral leprosy. Int J Dermatol. 2000;39(9):641-58.
2. Ramos-e-silva M, Ribeiro de Castro MC. Mycobacterial infections. In: Bolognia J, Schaffer J, Cerroni L (Eds). Dermatology, 4th edition. China: Elsevier; 2018. pp. 1296-316.
3. Grzybowski A, Nita M, Virmond M. Ocular leprosy. Clin Dermatol. 2015;33(1):79-89.
4. Khandpur S, Ashwin R. Systemic Involvement. In: Sacchidanand S, Oberai C, Inamadar A (Eds). IADVL Textbook of Dermatology, 4th edition. Mumbai: Bhalani Publishing House; 2015. pp. 3120-32.
5. Ffytche TJ. Role of iris changes as a cause of blindness in lepromatous leprosy. Br J Ophthalmol. 1981;65(4):231-9.
6. Samanta SK, Singh MD. Ocular leprosy. In: Kumar B, Kar HK (Eds). IAL Textbook of Leprosy, 1st edition. New Delhi: Jaypee Brothers Medical Publishers (P) Ltd; 2010. pp. 503-19.
7. Ramesh V, Kumar J. Systemic manifestation. In: Kumar B, Kar HK (Eds). IAL Textbook of Leprosy, 1st edition. New Delhi: Jaypee Brothers Medical Publishers (P) Ltd; 2010. pp. 293-301.
8. Möller-Christensen V. Changes in the anterior nasal spine and the alveolar process of the macillae in leprosy a clinical examination. Int J Lepr Other Mycobact Dis. 1974;42(4):431-5.
9. Singh N, Bhatia A, Lakra A, Arora VK, Bhattacharya SN. Comparative cytomorphology of skin, lymph node, liver and bone marrow in patients with lepromatous leprosy. Cytopathology. 2006;17(5):257-61.
10. P Shetty VP. Systemic Manifestation. In: Kumar B, Kar HK (Eds). IAL Textbook of Leprosy, 2nd edition. New Delhi: Jaypee Brothers Medical Publishers; 2016.
11. Walker SL, Sales AM, Butlin CR, Shah M, Maghanoy A, Lambert SM, et al. A leprosy clinical severity scale for erythema nodosum leprosum: an international, multicentre validation study of the ENLIST ENL Severity Scale. PLoS Negl Trop Dis. 2017;11(7):e0005716.

EXAMINATION QUESTION

1. What are the systemic features of LL Hansen's disease?

116 CHAPTER

Nerve Involvement in Leprosy and Pure Neuritic Leprosy

Abhishek De, Aarti Sarda

INTRODUCTION

- The most important consequences of leprosy are the direct result of the involvement of peripheral nerves.
- Leprosy is one of the most common treatable peripheral neuropathies in the world.
- Neuritis in leprosy is usually a subacute, demyelinating, and nonremitting event involving cutaneous nerves and larger peripheral nerve trunks.
- The pathogenic bacterium, *Mycobacterium leprae* has the unique ability to infect Schwann cells and axons.
- The antigenic products of *M. leprae* initiate an immunological recognition and response.[1]

HISTORY OF NEURAL LEPROSY

- Albert Neisser, in 1903 for the first time mentioned a "neural type of leprosy."
- Wade in 1952 first proposed the term "neural leprosy" with only nerve involvement without skin lesions as a separate type of leprosy.
- The Indian Association of Leprologists (IAL) included "neural leprosy" in their six group classification in 1955 and named it "polyneuritic leprosy."
- In 1982, IAL updated its classification of leprosy by naming it "pure neuritic type of leprosy", avoiding the term "poly."[2]

PATHOMECHANISM OF NERVE DAMAGE IN LEPROSY

- Schwann cells are the main target cells of *M. leprae*.
- In leprosy sensory nerves followed by nerves for autonomic and motor functions.
- There are two hypotheses how leprosy bacilli reach nerves. Most likely it reaches via lymphatics and blood stream to perineural and endoneural blood vessels, endothelial cells and then to Schwann cells. It was also postulated to reach nerves via dermal nerves as an ascending infection through "schwannian relay."
- Mycobacterial antigens such as phenolic glycolipid 1 (PGL-1) and laminin-2-binding protein (LBP21) specifically bind to the G domain of the laminin 2-chain on the Schwann cell surface. This complex subsequently binds to the dystroglycan (DG) in the basal lamina of the Schwann cell leading to endocytosis of the bacilli into the Schwann cells.
- The infection can cause nerve damage by the following mechanisms:
  - Obstruction of vasa nervorum by endothelial proliferation (leprous vasculitis).
  - Interference with Schwann cell metabolism leading to demyelination while *M. leprae* cell.
  - Biochemical reactions such as hypophosphorylation of axonal neurofilaments.
  - Immunological reactions such as cell-mediated type 1 reaction, immune complex mediated type 2 reaction or by cytokine released from leprosy granuloma.
  - Pressure effect by leprosy granuloma
  - Fibrosis[3,4]

CLINICAL PRESENTATIONS OF LEPROSY NEUROPATHY

- *Classical leprosy neuropathy:*
  - Cutaneous lesions mostly in low-temperature body regions
  - *Types*: Mononeuritis, mononeuritis multiplex and polyneuropathy with "glove and stocking" type
  - It may also have cranial neuropathies.
  - Thickening of nerve trunks is present.
  - Features of peripheral autonomic dysfunctions (ulcers, anhidrotic dry skin, compromised sudomotor and vasomotor responses) are also associated.
  - Skin biopsy
  - *Treatment*: MDT ± immunosuppression
- *Pure neuritic leprosy:*
  - No detectable cutaneous lesions
  - *Types*: Mononeuritis; mononeuritis multiplex; overlapping neuritis (polyneuropathy) with a "glove and stocking" type.
  - Nerve thickening is present and demonstrable.
  - Peripheral autonomic dysfunctions (sudomotor and vasomotor responses compromised distally)
  - It can be painful.
  - Nerve biopsy is "gold standard" for diagnosis.

- *Reactional leprosy neuritis:*
    - *Type 1 reaction*: Seen usually in the first month of treatment, painful, skin lesions worsening ulcers; fever, malaise; facial and limbs swelling, nerve trunks thickening
    - *Type 2 (erythema nodosum)*: Common in high bacterial index cases; nodules and painful red papules; uveitis, arthritis; fever, etc.
    - *Treatment*: Corticosteroid
- *Leprosy painful small-fiber neuropathy:*
    - Severe neuropathic pain
    - Small-fiber neuropathy, including overlapping neuritis (polyneuropathy) with a "glove and stocking" type
    - Rarely presents as complex regional pain syndrome
    - *Management*: Pain therapy; immunosuppression or immunomodulation
- *Leprosy late-onset neuropathy:*
    - Presents late, usually many years after a previous leprosy treatment
    - Presents as mononeuritis or mononeuritis multiplex
    - May present as ataxic, overlapping neuritis (polyneuropathy) with a "glove and stocking" type
    - Usually painful
    - Nerve biopsy is the "gold standard" for diagnosis.
    - *Management*: Responsive to immunosuppression or immunomodulation
- *Arthritic leprosy:*
    - Simulates rheumatoid arthritis
    - Painful
    - Nerve thickening is present.
    - Antinuclear antibody and Rheumatoid factor may be false positive.
    - *Management*: MDT, immunosuppression or immunomodulation
- *Autonomic neuropathy:*
    - Commonly involves regional skin
    - Sweating and vasomotor reflexes are compromised.[5]

PURE NEURITIC LEPROSY

Pure Neuritic Leprosy as an Entity

- Indian association of leprosy in their original definition of pure neuritic leprosy in the five-type classification of leprosy of 1982 stated: "In this type of leprosy, there are no skin lesions. Larger nerve trunks or their branches are enlarged. There is a sensory loss in the areas of distribution of the nerves."
- Synonyms for pure neuritic leprosy used in the literature include neural, neuritic, pure neural, primary neural, primary neuritic, purely neural, or polyneuritic leprosy.
- Though there is a worldwide acceptance of pure neuritic leprosy as a distinct type of leprosy, this subtype of leprosy remains an enigma.[6]

Prevalence

- Pure neuritic leprosy constitutes about 4–18% of leprosy patients.
- It is more common in men and it is most common in the 15–30 age group.
- It is less commonly reported in some parts of the world such as Africa.[7]

Clinical Features

- There are no skin lesions as a rule in pure neuritic leprosy, most patients present either with sudden appearance of numbness with or without ulcers, or with deformity or muscle weakness in a limb.
- *Pattern of nerve involvement:*
    - Upper limb nerves are more commonly involved, of which ulnar nerve is the most common, followed by the posterior tibial and sural nerves.
    - Selective involvement of the facial nerve branches was also reported.
    - Mononeuritis is the most common presentation of pure neuritic leprosy.
    - Mononeuritis multiplex where there is involvement of multiple unrelated and distant nerve trunks is also seen.
    - Symmetrical polyneuritis is rarely reported.
- *Skin changes in pure neuritic leprosy:*
    - Classical leprosy skin lesions/patches should be essentially absent for the diagnosis of pure neuritic leprosy.
    - Skin along the distribution of the affected nerve is usually hypoanesthetic or anesthetic.
    - There can also be a hypo or anhidrosis, xerosis, fissuring and ulcers along the distribution of the affected nerve.
- *Nerve changes in pure neuritic leprosy:*
    - Affected nerve in pure neuritic leprosy is significantly thickened.
    - It can be nodular or beaded and occasionally, there can be abscess formation.
    - Nerve pain usually precedes clinical diagnosis of pure neuritic leprosy.
    - Most experts believe pure neuritic leprosy shows a narrow histological spectrum, ranging from tuberculoid to mid-borderline leprosy only. However, many others demonstrated presence of lepromatous spectrum in nerve biopsy of pure neuritic leprosy.
- *Reaction in cases of pure neuritic leprosy:*
    - A study from India reported reactions in the form of neuritis in 30.8% at the time of initial presentation, and 21.5% developed it later during treatment.
    - The true incidence of type 1 reactions in pure neuritic leprosy is not known.

- There can be "silent neuritis" or "quiet nerve paralysis" with low-grade inflammation in the nerve leading to incessant nerve damage and deficits.
- *Subsequent development of skin lesions in pure neuritic leprosy:*
  - There are many reports of patients with pure neuritic leprosy developing classical leprosy skin lesions later.
  - In a study of 182 pure neuritic leprosy patients, 29 patients developed visible skin lesions during follow-up of 2 years.
  - It is believed that leprosy is primarily neural in origin and that a neuritic phase precedes the development of cutaneous lesions.[6]

Complications

- *Nerve abscess*: Nerve abscesses could be single or multiple, noted in 12.5% of cases. Nerve abscesses in leprosy are usually "cold abscesses", and are relatively painless.
- *Segmental necrotizing granulomatous neuritis (SNGN)*: Single or multiple nodules along the course of a thickened peripheral nerve. Nerve biopsy shows multiple foci of caseous necrosis bordered by epithelioid cells and lymphocytes.
- Sensory impairment commonly along ulnar, lateral popliteal and posterior tibial nerves distribution
- *Disabilities and deformities*: Claw hand, foot drop
- Trophic changes

Investigations

- *When to suspect*: In endemic countries such as India, the presence of "mononeuritis" or "mononeuritis multiplex", along with tender enlarged nerves should always raise a suspicion of the diagnosis.
- *Clinical diagnosis*: Thickened peripheral nerve trunk, tenderness and sensory impairment associated with absence of skin lesions and negative skin smears for acid fast bacilli.
- *Nerve biopsy*:
  - Nerve biopsy when possible, is the gold standard for confirmation of pure neuritic leprosy.
  - It is prudent to biopsy a branch of a sensory nerve.
  - The common nerves where nerve biopsy is performed are:
    - Superficial sensory radial nerve branch at the wrist
    - Ulnar cutaneous nerve near the ulnar border of base of the hand
    - Sural nerve near the ankle.
- *Fine-needle aspiration cytology (FNAC):*
  - FNAC is a safe, less invasive, and briefer procedure as compared to nerve biopsy for the diagnosis of pure neuritic leprosy.
  - FNAC can be done both from pure sensory as well as in mixed nerves.
  - Aspirates are examined for cellularity, their arrangement, and presence of acid-fast bacilli.
  - Limitation of this technique is that a negative aspirate does not rule out leprosy.[8,9,10]
- *Polymerase chain reaction (PCR)*: The authors have performed both cytological examination as well as PCR on the nerve aspirates and proved its value as a diagnostic tool of pure neuritic leprosy in a series of publications.
- *Nerve conduction studies*:
  - Marked slowing of conduction can occur in leprosy-affected nerves.
  - Pattern of neuropathy described is the impairment of conduction of nerve impulse and decreased amplitude of sensory-motor potentials.
  - Results can be nonspecific.
- *Imaging of nerves in pure neuritic leprosy*:
  - High-resolution ultrasonography can visualize structural changes of nerves in leprosy.
  - It objectively confirms nerve thickening in cases of pure neuritic leprosy.

Management

- National Leprosy Eradication Programme (NLEP) guidelines suggest when one nerve trunk is involved in leprosy, it can be considered as paucibacillary, and when more than one nerve trunk is involved, it is considered as multibacillary for therapeutic purposes and treated accordingly along standard WHO regimen.
- In case of ambiguity regarding the number of nerves involved, it is advisable to treat it as multibacillary leprosy.
- In pure neuritic leprosy, there can be some neuritis associated with the disease.
- Evident or silent neuropathy associated with pure neuritic leprosy is managed with tapering doses of systemic corticosteroids.

CRANIAL NERVE INVOLVEMENT IN LEPROSY

- Though the peripheral nerves are most commonly affected in leprosy, cranial nerves, especially, facial and trigeminal nerves, are also commonly involved in leprosy.
- There are other reports highlighting involvement of multiple cranial nerves (polyneuritis cranialis).
- Cranial nerve involvement may vary from 17 to 22%.
- The involvement tends to be more common in patients with lepromatous type of leprosy of longer duration. But it can occur in other forms of leprosy and in short-duration disease also.
- Facial or trigeminal nerve involvement were most common amongst cranial nerves.
- Other cranial nerve reported to be involved with leprosy are olfactory, oculomotor, auditory, vagus, spinal accessory, glossopharyngeal, and hypoglossal nerves.
- Facial nerve involvement in leprosy is reported to occur in about 10% of the patients and is the most common nerve affected. Leprosy affects facial nerves in a scattered

distribution from the main trunk to all peripheral branches.

- Trigeminal nerve is the second most common cranial nerve to get affected in leprosy, and anesthesia in the maxillary divisions of the trigeminal nerve is a finding on those.
- Other symptoms are cochlear type of hearing impairment, loss of taste, etc.
- Associated features of leprosy such as madarosis, resorption of digits and toes and trophic ulcers are seen in the majority of cases with leprous cranial neuropathy.[11,12]

KEY POINTS

- Classical leprosy neuropathy is usually either mononeuritis or mononeuritis multiple.
- Pure neuritic leprosy constitutes about 4–18% of leprosy patients and there is no skin lesion as a rule in this type of leprosy.
- Upper limb nerves are more commonly involved, of which ulnar nerve is the most common, followed by the posterior tibial and sural nerves in PNL.
- Facial or trigeminal nerve involvements are the most common amongst cranial nerves involved in leprosy.

REFERENCES

1. Agrawal A, Pandit L, Dalal M, Shetty JP. Neurological manifestations of Hansen's disease and their management. Clin Neurol Neurosurg. 2005;107(6):445-54.
2. Couto Dal Secco RG, França K, Castillo D, alHarbi M, Lotti T, Fioranelli M, et al. A synopsis of the history of Hansen's disease. Wien Med Wochenschr. 2017;167(Suppl 1):27-30.
3. Wilder-Smith EP, Van Brakel WH. Nerve damage in leprosy and its management. Nat Clin Pract Neurol. 2008;4(12):656-63.
4. Aarão TLS, de Sousa JR, Falcão ASC, Falcão LFM, Quaresma JAS. Nerve growth factor and pathogenesis of leprosy: review and update. Front Immunol. 2018;9:939.
5. Nascimento OJ. Leprosy neuropathy: clinical presentations. Arq Neuropsiquiatr. 2013;71(9B):661-6.
6. Rao PN, Suneetha S. Pure neuritic leprosy: current status and relevance. Indian J Dermatol Venereol Leprol. 2016;82(3): 252-61.
7. Forgione P, Barabino G, Cavalchini A, Clapasson A, Reni L, Parodi A. Pure neuritic leprosy. G Ital Dermatol Venereol. 2018;153(1):124-6.
8. Bezerra Da Cunha FM, Werneck MC, Scola RH, Werneck LC. Pure neural leprosy: diagnostic value of the polymerase chain reaction. Muscle Nerve. 2006;33(3):409-14.
9. De A, Hasanoor Reja AH, Aggarwal I, Sen S, Sil A, Bhattacharya B, et al. Use of fine needle aspirate from peripheral nerves of pure-neural leprosy for cytology and polymerase chain reaction to confirm the diagnosis: a follow-up study of 4 years. Indian J Dermatol. 2017;62(6):635-43.
10. Reja AH, De A, Biswas S, Chattopadhyay A, Chatterjee G, Bhattacharya B, et al. Use of fine needle aspirate from peripheral nerves of pure-neural leprosy for cytology and PCR to confirm the diagnosis: a pilot study. Indian J Dermatol Venereol Leprol. 2013;79(6):789-94.
11. Kumar S. Cranial nerve involvement in leprosy. Indian J Lepr. 2005;77(2):177-8.
12. Gopinath DV, Thappa DM, Jaishankar TJ. A clinical study of the involvement of cranial nerves in leprosy. Indian J Lepr. 2004;76(1):1-9.

EXAMINATION QUESTIONS

1. Write a note on pure neural Hansen's disease.
2. Write a note on cranial nerve involvement in leprosy.
3. Write a note on trophic ulcer in leprosy and discuss its management.
4. Discuss the management of claw hand in leprosy.

Lepra Reactions

Balachandra S Ankad, Mahajabeen S Madarkar

INTRODUCTION

Lepra reactions occur due to possible alterations in the immunological status of leprosy patients. These are hypersensitivity expressions involving components of leprosy bacilli and host immunity. Why should we know reactions in leprosy? Considering all aspects of leprosy, lepra reactions epitomize effects of leprosy with inflammation and disturbed immunity and also mechanisms of hypersensitivity are central to the problems of leprosy.[1]

From an immunological point of view, lepra reactions are unpredictable and progressive. Clinicians should be aware to predict, treat, and to prevent these lepra reactions. Lepra reactions constitute an important problem both for the patient and the treating physician. Lepra reactions can develop at anytime; at first presentation, before starting the treatment, during the treatment, and after completion of treatment. Patients developing reactions are at higher risk of developing disabilities and deformities, compared to people who do not develop reactions.[2]

HISTORY

Ridley was the first to differentiate reversal reaction from erythema nodosum leprosum (ENL) and downgrading reactions.[2,3] Jopling also had clarified it. Hence, the confusion was cleared in the terminology of reactional states in leprosy. Earlier they were called as "acute infiltration reactions" or "reactional tuberculoid."[3] Some authors still use the term ENL as synonym for type 2 lepra reaction.

CLASSIFICATION

Three types of lepra reactions **(Box 1)** are:[4]

1. Type 1 lepra reaction (T1R)
2. Type 2 lepra reaction (T2R)
3. Lucio phenomenon

BOX 1: The signs of reaction in a patient of leprosy.

- Sudden appearance of symptoms
- Inflammation of existing skin lesions (T1R)
- Appearance of painful tender nodules (T2R)
- Inflammation of nerves
- Involvement of ocular tissue
- Swelling of hands, feet, and pain in small joints

These types should not be confused with I-IV types of hypersensitivity reactions described by Coombs and Gel.

TYPE 1 LEPRA REACTION

A type 1 lepra reaction (T1R) is characterized by the development of acute inflammation in skin lesions or nerves or both. Borderline leprosy is a strong risk factor for the occurrence of T1Rs but individuals with polar forms of leprosy may also experience T1Rs. The onset of a T1R may be very rapid. T1Rs are frequently recurrent and this can lead to further nerve damage.[5]

Upgrading or Reversible Reaction

If there is increase in immunity, shift is from borderline spectrum toward tuberculoid pole, this is called as upgrading or reversal reaction. The term reversal reaction is because of natural tendency for subpolar tuberculoid and borderline leprosy to downgrade slowly toward lepromatous pole, without treatment, which is reversed with treatment.

Downgrading Reaction

Sudden shift toward the lepromatous pole with reduction of immunity, it is called as downgrading reaction. This is due to immunity against antigenic determinants of secreted antigens, remnants of dead and dying bacteria or against antigenic determinants of host that has in common with *Mycobacterium leprae*.[6] However, distinction between two is difficult and for management purpose all T1Rs reactions are regarded as reversal reactions.

Epidemiology

The measured prevalence rates of T1R vary depending on whether the studies are conducted in hospital or field settings. Prevalence ranges from 19.8 to 30% in various studies.[4]

Pathogenesis

T1Rs are caused by upregulation of cell-mediated immunity (CMI) to *M. leprae* antigen in skin and nerves, which is delayed type of hypersensitivity (DTH). *M. leprae* antigens have been demonstrated in the skin and nerves of patients with T1R. *M. leprae* infection may lead to the expression of major histocompatibility complex-II on the surface of the cells and this may give rise to antigen presentation, which triggers CD4+ T-cells killing the cell mediated by cytokines such as tumor necrosis factor.[4]

Risk Factors for T1R[4,7]

- Borderline group of patients [borderline tuberculoid (BT), borderline-borderline (BB), and borderline lepromatous (BL)] are the most vulnerable to develop T1R.
- Patients with one episode of reaction are more likely to develop second episode.
- Females carry higher risk than men.
- Older age group is at higher risk than younger age group.
- Multiple disseminated patches, large facial patches, and multiple nerve involvement.
- Neuritis or previous history of nerve pain.

Clinical Features[4]

Clinical features are result of increased immune response, particularly cell-mediated immunity against lepra bacilli or its remnants. Systemic symptoms such as fever, weakness, or myalgia are absent.

- Some or all pre-existing lesions become redder, shiny, prominent, swollen, warm, and resemble erysipelas **(Fig. 1)**. Lesions are usually not painful but tender. Lesions subside with desquamation.
- Some previously unnoticed lesions may become visible **(Figs. 2 and 3)**. Fresh lesion can be seen.
- Edema of extremities or face, frequently accompanied by nerve involvement **(Fig. 4)**.
- Peripheral nerves manifest with sudden swelling and severe pain/tenderness of one or more nerves. The nerves affected are in the vicinity of inflamed lesions. Nerve abscess are observed in severe form of T1R.

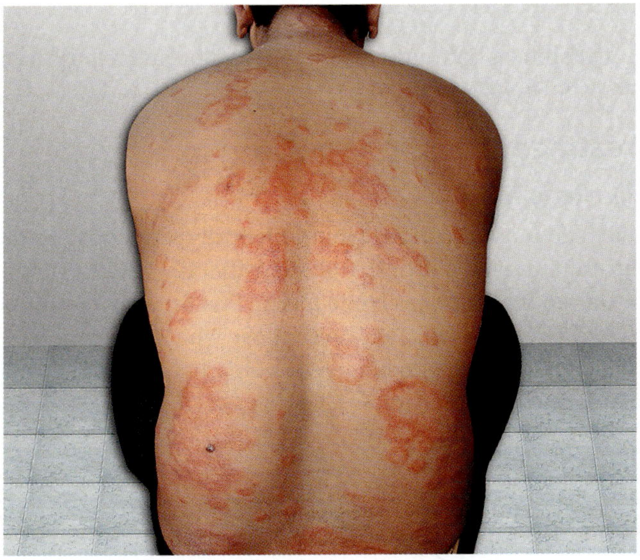

Fig. 1: Clinical image of borderline tuberculoid leprosy with type 1 reaction showing erythematous and indurated plaques on the back. Note that lesions are looking similar to erysipelas.

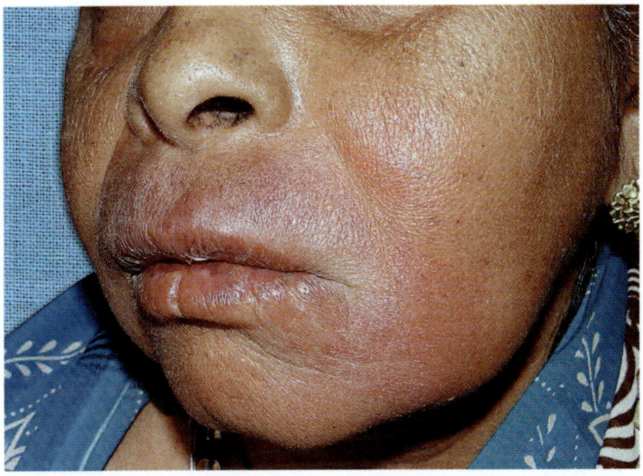

Fig. 2: Clinical image of borderline tuberculoid leprosy with type 1 reaction showing erythematous and indurated plaque on the face.

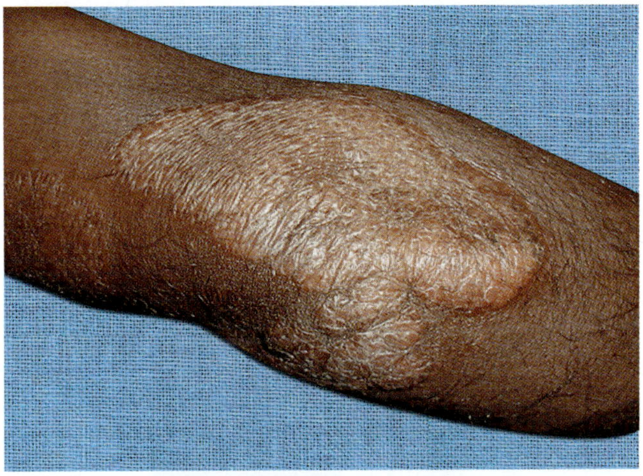

Fig. 3: Clinical image of type 1 reaction occurring in borderline tuberculoid leprosy plaque on the elbow. Note the characteristic induration of patch.
Courtesy: Dr Aparna Palit, AIIMS, Kalyani, West Bengal, India.

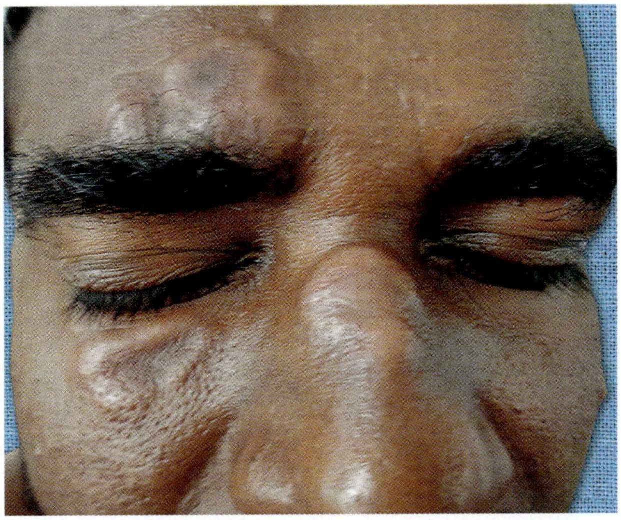

Fig. 4: Clinical image of borderline lepromatous leprosy presenting with indurated plaques on the face in type 1 reaction.
Courtesy: Dr Aparna Palit, AIIMS, Kalyani, West Bengal, India.

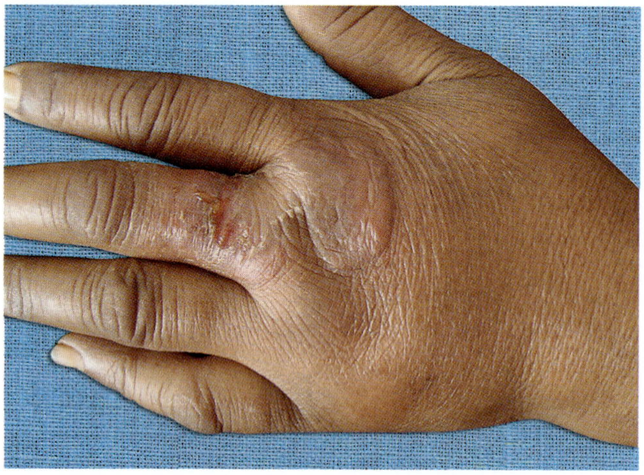

Fig. 5: Clinical image of type 1 reaction presenting with vesiculation and ulcer on the indurated patch on the dorsum of hand.

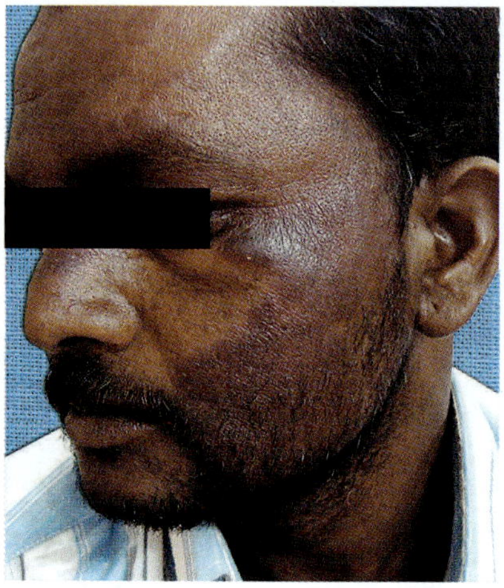

Fig. 6: Clinical image of type 1 reaction shows flattened and bluish-colored patch after treatment.

BOX 2: Naaf's criteria for type 1 reaction.[4]

Major: Pre-existing and/or new skin lesions become inflamed, red, and swollen.

Minor:
- Tender and thickened peripheral nerves
- Crops of new (painless) lesions
- Sudden edema of face and extremities
- Recent loss of sensation in hands and feet or signs of recent nerve damage (loss of sweating, sensation, muscle strength) in an area supplied by particular nerve

TABLE 1: Differences between type 1 lepra reaction and relapse.[4]

Criteria	*Type 1 reaction*	*Relapse*
Type of leprosy	Observed in BT, BB, BL and subpolar leprosy	Can occur in all types of leprosy after it becomes inactive with treatment
Onset	Sudden	Insidious
Time	Any time during treatment and within 3 years after release from treatment	>3 years after released from treatment (RFT)
Progression of signs and symptoms	Fast	Slow
Sites of skin lesions	Over old patches	In new places
Pain, tenderness or swelling	Present over skin lesions and nerves	Not usually present, however, rarely relapse may present with clinical manifestation of reversal reaction (RR)
Nerve damage	Sudden onset	Occurs slowly
General conditions	May be there	Not affected
Response to steroid	Good	Not effective

(BB: borderline-borderline; BL: borderline lepromatous; BT: borderline tuberculoid)

- *Silent neuritis*: Loss of nerve function in the absence of signs of inflammation is called as "quiet" or "silent" nerve paralysis. Foot or wrist drop and facial palsy are noted in this form of neuritis.
- *Tinel's sign*: Tingling sensation at distal part of limb on applying pressure on nerves.
- Rarely, tenosynovitis can present with painful swelling on the dorsa of hands.
- Severe reaction can produce deep ulceration and necrosis **(Fig. 5)**.
- In subsiding lesions, patches desquamate and turn into bluish in color **(Fig. 6)**.

Diagnosis

Clinical features with tender erythematous patches and nerve involvement are characteristic of T1R. Naaf et al. proposed criteria which are aimed for research and operation at field level **(Box 2)**. It includes one major criterion or, at least two minor criteria (without signs of ENL).

Differences between type 1 lepra reaction and relapse have been shown in **Table 1**.

Treatment

Mild Reaction

Mild reactions are treated symptomatically with nonsteroidal anti-inflammatory drugs. Multidrug therapy (MDT) should be started if person has come for the first time and continue MDT if already taking. However, those who have completed their course of MDT do not need antileprosy treatment while on treatment for reaction.

Severe Reaction

Prednisolone

- It is the drug of choice treatment of severe reactions.
- It relieves pain and inflammation in the nerve and the skin. Reduction in pain, tenderness and edema helps in gradual restoration to normalcy. It is a very effective

drug and its affect starts in a few days. It should never be stopped abruptly.

- Start with 1–2 mg/kg and duration of treatment is 12–24 weeks depending on the severity of reaction and response to the therapy.
- If inflammation of skin and nerve subsides and there is no new nerve involvement, the dose of prednisolone is gradually reduced by 5 mg at every fortnightly interval.
- Duration of treatment should be long to prevent nerve function impairment. It is 4–9, 6–12, and 6–24 months in BT, BB, and BL, respectively.

Other immunosuppressive drugs: When systemic steroids intolerance or side effects are present, immunosuppressive drugs can be given.

Methotrexate: As it reduces the Th1 cytokine, it may be useful in T1R when given in a dose of 5–7.5 mg/week.

Cyclosporine: By inhibiting transcription of IL-2 mRNA, it blocks the proliferation of T-cell which in turn antinerve growth factor antibodies. It is proven to be efficacious in chronic neuritis. Dose ranges from 3 to 5 mg/kg for up to 1 year with tapering.

Azathioprine and *Mycophenolate mofetil* are also useful in T1R.

Rest to the affected nerve using splint: Rest to the affected nerves is provided by use of static splint. Splint is applied for 24 hours and removed only for exercise. Initially, gentle passive exercises are allowed till inflammation subsides. Active exercises can be advised in the later stages to restore the strength of affected muscle.

TYPE 2 LEPRA REACTIONS

Type 2 lepra reaction (T2R) is humoral immunity-mediated reactional stage of leprosy exclusively seen in lepromatous leprosy (LL), sometimes in borderline lepromatous leprosy (LLp and LLs). It differs from T1R in several ways.[8]

Epidemiology

Incidence of T2R ranges from 2.1 to 10.5% in BL and 2.1 to 47.5% in LL. These figures are after introduction of MDT which played a significant role in the reduction of T2R.[4]

Pathogenesis

Mycobacterium leprae antigens, IgM, IgG, complement (C3d) and IL-4 mRNA are all identified as responsible factors in ENL lesions. Initially, lymphocytes increase in number around the blood vessels. Majority of them are CD4+Th2 cells. Antibodies are formed against *Mycobacterium* antigens which produce immune complexes. These attach endothelium of vessels and activate cascade of immune reactions. Hence, in T2R both cell mediated and humoral immune systems play a role.[9]

Salient Features of T2R[10]

- Systemic disturbances are pronounced as compared to T1R.
- No change in the pre-existing lesions.
- Painful and evanescent erythematous nodules appear which are called as ENL.
- Commonly occurs after 6 months of MDT.
- It should be remembered that patients can present with ENL for the first time.
- ENL was first described by Japanese leprologist Murata in 1912, who was not referring ENL to whole symptom complex of T2R. Hence, the term ENL is not synonym of T2R; rather ENL is a part of T2R.

Risk factors for T2R have been shown in **Box 3**.

Clinical Features

Type 2 lepra reaction is characterized by clinical features which are analogous to serum sickness. ENL are considered as most specific lesions of T2R **(Fig. 7)**. T2R presents with crops of red painful cutaneous lesions (cutaneous onset) or only with swollen and tender joints with fever (rheumatic onset) or with fever, joint pain, skin lesions (mixed onset).

BOX 3: Risk factors for type 2 reaction.[11]

- Antileprosy drugs except clofazimine
- Lepromatous leprosy
- Bacterial index more than 4+
- Intercurrent infections
- Trauma
- Immunization
- Pregnancy and lactation
- Physical and mental stress

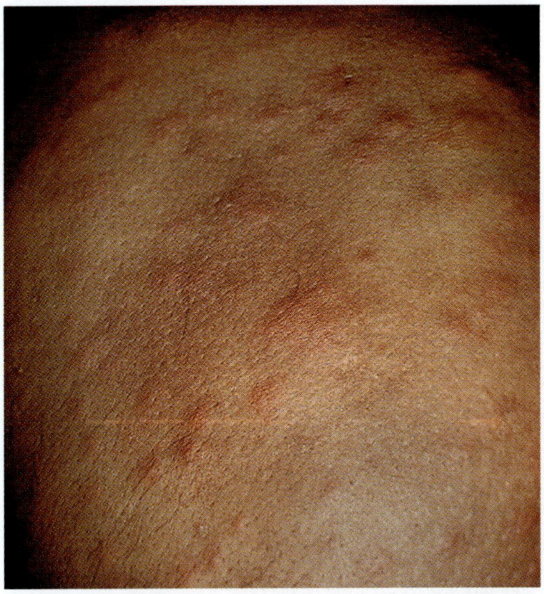

Fig. 7: Clinical image of crops of erythema nodosum leprosum on the back in type 2 reaction.
Courtesy: Dr Aparna Palit, AIIMS, Kalyani, West Bengal, India.

Erythema nodosum leprosum appears suddenly as pink-red nodules with tenderness. They are present in the deep dermis and subcutaneous tissue; sometimes, may not be evident on skin surface. Extensor aspects of arms, thighs, legs, and face are predilected sites. They can be seen anywhere on the body except hairy scalp, axillae, groin and perineum. Individual ENL persist for 24–48 hours after which they subside with bluish hue in 10 days **(Figs. 8 and 9)**. Rarely ENL may become pustular and break down to producing ulceration. This entity is called as erythema nodosum necroticans **(Fig. 10)**. T2R manifests with inflammatory edema of dorsum of hands with subcutaneous nodules and arthritis of interphalangeal joints. This is called as "reaction hand" **(Fig. 11)**. Due to repeated reactional episodes, subcutaneous tissue becomes fixed to underlying muscles and bones.

Systemic Manifestations

Fever, weakness, joint pain, myalgia are common in T2R and may precede appearance of ENL. Acute myositis, arthritis, nose involvement, bone changes, epididymo-orchitis are other features seen in T2R **(Box 4)**.

Clinical Tests

Ryrie test: Stroking of skin on the sole produces burning pain.
Ellis test: During ENL, squeezing the wrist causes pain.

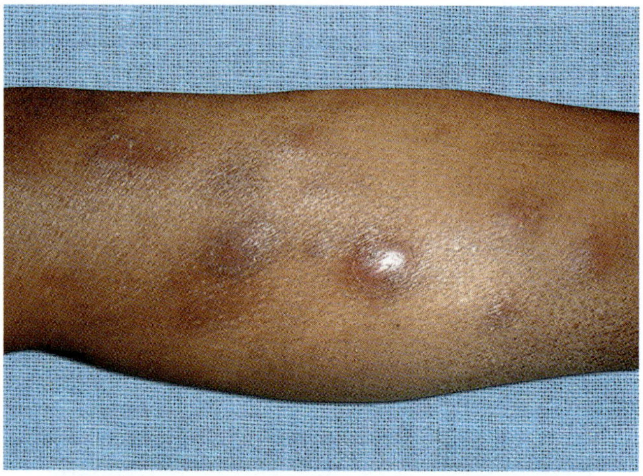

Fig. 8: Clinical image of erythema nodosum leprosum subsiding with hyperpigmentation.
Courtesy: Dr Aparna Palit, AIIMS, Kalyani, West Bengal, India.

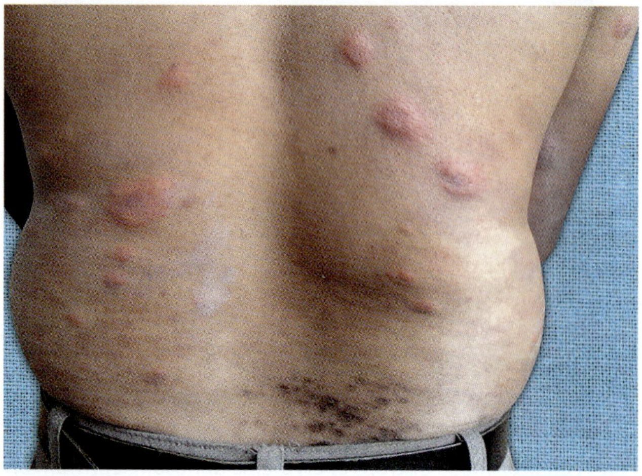

Fig. 9: Clinical image of erythema nodosum leprosum on the back showing erythematous plagues.

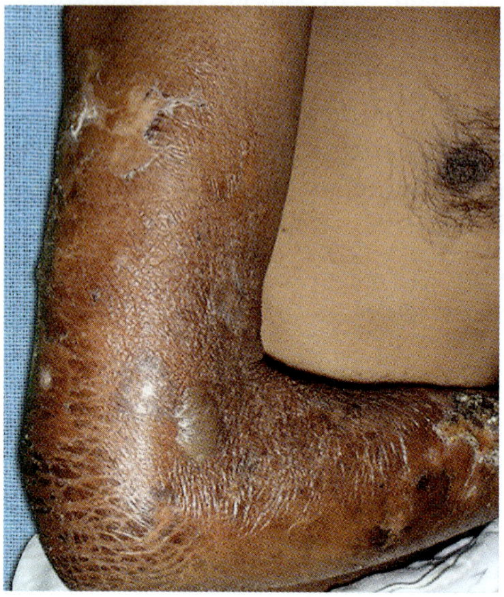

Fig. 10: Clinical image of vesicular and necrotic erythema nodosum leprosum.
Courtesy: Dr Aparna Palit, AIIMS, Kalyani, West Bengal, India.

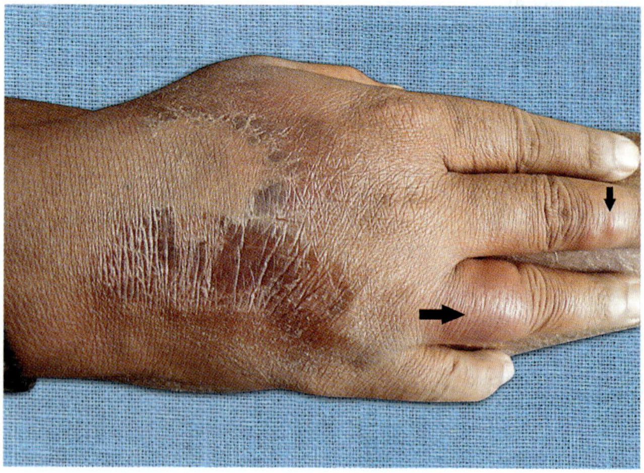

Fig. 11: Clinical image of "reaction hand" in type 2 reaction with edema of hand and subcutaneous nodules (black arrows).

BOX 4: Naaf's criteria for type 2 reaction.[12]

Major: Sudden appearance of tender, red papules, nodules which may ulcerate
Minor:
- Mild fever, the patient is unwell
- Tender enlarged nerves
- Arthritis, lymphadenitis, epididymo-orchitis, irido-cyclitis, episcleritis, edema of hands or face, positive Ryrie and Ellis test

Laboratory tests: Leukocytosis, elevation of ESR and C-reactive proteins, deranged liver function tests.

Treatment

Multidrug therapy should be continued if already taking or should be started along with antireaction treatment.

Aspirin is given for milder cases.

In moderate T2R, colchicine is given in a dose of 0.5 mg three times a day. It reduces nerve and joint pain well controlled by colchicine as compared to aspirin.

Corticosteroids: These are the mainstay of treatment for severe T2R. One (1) mg/kg should be started. Maintenance of 20–30 mg per day is a must for several weeks to prevent recurrences of ENL. Then it is tapered over 6–9 months duration.

Clofazimine: It is given in the dose of 300 mg daily for 1–3 months, then 200 mg daily for 3 months and 100 mg daily for a period until symptoms subside. It is slower in action; however, it can prevent recurrences of T2R and also acts as steroid sparing drug.

Thalidomide: Dose is 400 mg at night or 100 mg four times a day. Dose is reduced slowly, 100 mg every month and lowest dose that controls symptoms must be continued for at least 2–3 months. Its derivative, lenalidomide which is more potent and specific in nature is expected to be good.

Azathioprine: It is given in a dose of 2–3 mg/kg/day for 3 months. Later it should be tapered to a dose of 50 mg per day for another 6 months or until symptoms subside.

For chronic and recurring ENL, combinations of prednisolone and clofazimine or prednisolone and thalidomide are better choices.

Recently, anti-TNF-α agents such as etanercept, infliximab, and adalimumab have promised to give better results.

Differences between T1R and T2R have been shown in **Table 2**.

TABLE 2: Summary of differences between type 1 and type 2 lepra reactions.[4]

Type 1	*Type 2*
Delayed type of Coombs and Gel reaction: Type I	Immunocomplex-mediated reaction: Type III
Usually starts within first 6 months of antileprosy treatment	Usually starts in the late phase of antileprosy treatment
Seen in borderline types BT, BB, BL	Seen exclusively in LL, rarely in BL
Pre-existing lesions become indurated, erythematous and tender, but few fresh lesions may be seen	No change in the pre-existing lesions. New lesions in the form of ENL are characteristic
Severe nerve involvement is the hallmark	Nerves are affected with lesser severity
Systemic disturbances are the hallmark	Very minimal systemic disturbances
Lagophthalmos and corneal anesthesia are seen due to 7th and 5th cranial nerves affection	Internal eye involvement such as iritis, iridocyclitis, episcleritis, glaucoma and cataract are common

(BB: borderline-borderline; BL: borderline lepromatous; BT: borderline tuberculoid; ENL: erythema nodosum leprosum; LL: lepromatous leprosy)

LUCIO PHENOMENON

This is special type of reaction seen in Lucio leprosy which is mainly observed in Mexicans. Lucio phenomenon occurs due to the vascular compromisation to the deposition of unusually large lepra bacilli in vessel walls.

It begins as indurated reddish plaque on the skin of limbs. Later, center of the lesion develops hemorrhagic infarct or blister. This results in necrotic eschar which leaves behind irregular shaped ulcer. It takes 3 weeks to for a lesion to develop an ulcer from the initial lesion **(Box 5)**.

BOX 5: Salient features of Lucio phenomenon.[13,14]

- It occurs in Lucio leprosy
- It is seen in untreated leprosy patients
- Presents with 1 cm lesions
- Starts with irregular purpuric maculae and patches which form ulcers
- It does not affect nerves
- Patients are usually afebrile (if severe necrosis present, patients are acutely ill)
- No systemic involvement
- Histopathology is characterized by ischemic epidermal necrosis and necrotizing vasculitis of small blood vessels
- It does not respond to thalidomide

Diagnosis

Classical clinical features are usually sufficient to make diagnosis. Histopathology shows changes that are unique to Lucio phenomenon. Medina test is positive which is similar to Lepromin test but for the antigens taken from lesions of Lucio leprosy.

Treatment

Patients respond very well to MDT. Systemic corticosteroids are also helpful.

KEY POINTS

- Once the patients acquires leprosy bacillus in the body, he or she is bound to be affected by lepra reactions, although it depends on in which spectrum, the patient falls.
- Type 1 reaction mainly occurs in the borderline spectrum of the disease, i.e., BT, BB, and BL types.

- Type 1 reaction is due to delayed hypersensitivity immunity mounted upon the antigens of *M. leprae.*
- In T1R, nerve involvement is significant while systemic disturbance in almost absent. Classically, pre-existing lesions become indurated and tender.
- T2R is like serum sickness seen in LL and BL with florid systemic affection manifesting with fever, weakness, myalgia, joint pain, eye and testicles involvement and lymphadenopathy.
- ENL are specific to T2R; however, T2R can present without ENL.
- Lucio phenomenon is exclusively seen in Lucio leprosy which can be diagnosed with high index of suspicion.
- T1R and T2R respond very well to systemic corticosteroids whereas Lucio phenomenon is managed with MDT.

REFERENCES

1. Pfaltzgraff RE, Ramu G. Clinical leprosy. In: Hastings RC (Ed). Leprosy, 2nd edition. Edinburgh: Churchill Livingstone; 1994. pp. 237-90.
2. Klenerman P. Aetiological factors in delayed-type hypersensitivity reactions in leprosy. In: Ryan TJ, McDougall AC (Eds). Essays on Leprosy-by Oxford Medical Students. Oxford: Alden Press; 1988. pp. 52-63.
3. Ridley DS. Reactions in leprosy. Lep Rev. 1969;40:77-81.
4. Kar HK, Chauhan A. Leprosy reactions: Pathogenesis and clinical features. In: Kumar B, Kar HK (Eds). IAL Textbook of Leprosy, 2nd edition. New Delhi: Jaypee Brothers Medical Publishers; 2016. pp. 416-37.
5. Kumar B, Dogra S, Kaur I. Epidemiological characteristics of leprosy reactions: 15 years experience from North India. Int J Lepr Other Mycobact Dis. 2004;72:125-33.
6. Nery JA, Vieira LM, de Matos HJ, Gallo ME, Sarno EN. Reactional states in multibacillary Hansen's disease patients during multidrug therapy. Rev Inst Med Trop Sao Paulo. 1998;40:363-70.
7. Anderson AK, Chaduvula M, Atkinson SE. Effects of prednisolone treatment on cytokine expression in patients with leprosy type 1 reactions. Infect Immun. 2005;73(6): 3725-33.
8. Jopling WH, McDougall AC. Leprosy reactions (Reactional states). In: Jopling WH, McDougall AC (Eds). Handbook of Leprosy, 5th edition. New Delhi: CBS Publishers and Distributors; 1996. pp. 2-91.
9. Modlin RL, Mehra R, Bloom BR. In situ and in vitro characterization of cellular immune-response in erythema nodosum leprosum. J Immunol. 1986;123:1813-7.
10. Saunderson P, Gebre S, Byass P. ENL reactions in the multibacillary cases of AMFES cohorts in central Ethiopia: Incidence and risk factors. Lepr Rev. 2000;71:318-24.
11. Manandhar R, LeMaster JW, Roche PW. Risk factors for erythema nodosum leprosum. Int J Lepr. 1999;67:270-8.
12. Naafs B. Symposium paper "Current views on reaction in leprosy". Ind J Lepr. 2000;72:97-122.
13. Leticia F, Elemir MS, Maria LC, Paulo ENFV. Vasculonecrotic reactions in leprosy. Brazilian J Infect Dis. 2007;11:378-82.
14. Saoji V, Salodkar A. Lucio leprosy and Lucio phenomenon. Indian J Lepr. 2001;73:267-72.

EXAMINATION QUESTIONS

Write a short note on following:
1. Type 1 lepra reaction.
2. Type 2 lepra reaction.
3. Lucio phenomenon.
4. Immunopathogenesis of lepra reactions.

118 CHAPTER

Laboratory Tests in Leprosy

Subhra Sankar Sahoo, Abhishek De, Aarti Sarda

INTRODUCTION

Diagnosis of leprosy is most often clinical and a thorough history and physical examination is often all that one needs. However, with a decreasing number of cases, the expertise to diagnose leprosy clinically is gradually getting diminished. Moreover, laboratory tests have an important role in early diagnosis as well as in monitoring the response to treatment. Contacts of multibacillary (MB) leprosy patients also require screening for early and subclinical infections. Laboratory tests are also important for research purposes **(Box 1)**.[1-4]

SLIT-SKIN SMEAR (SSS) EXAMINATION[5,6]

History

- First described by Wade in 1935
- It was standardized by Cochrane in 1947.

Role of SSS Examination

- Confirmation of the diagnosis of leprosy
- Classification of disease
- Determine the disease activity
- Prognostication
- Early identification of reaction
- Follow-up and treatment response
- Diagnosis of relapse

BOX 1: Laboratory tests that can be helpful in leprosy.

- Slit-skin smear examination
- Nasal mucosal smears
- Skin biopsy for histopathology and special stain (will be dealt with elsewhere in the book)
- Fluorescent microscopy to detect *Mycobacterium leprae*
- Immunochemical staining to demonstrate mycobacterial antigens
- S-100 stain for Schwann cells
- Nerve biopsy
- Lepromin test
- Histamine test
- The Sweat test
- Fine-needle aspiration cytology (FNAC) for cutaneous lesions of leprosy
- FNAC for nerve lesions of leprosy
- Humoral immune response evaluation
- Molecular diagnosis of leprosy
- Tests for viability of *M. leprae*

Indications for SSS Examination

- In cases of diagnostic dilemma especially in atypical presentations like:
  - Diffuse skin infiltration with minimal sensory impairment; indeterminate leprosy; numerous, bilaterally symmetrical
  - Ill-defined macular lesions with minimal sensory impairment
  - Ill-defined papules, plaques, and nodules on the earlobes, face, trunk back, and extensor aspects of limbs, with minimal sensory impairment
- In cases of uncertain diagnosis of paucibacillary (PB) or MB leprosy before starting treatment
- Patient presenting with fresh lesions after release from treatment
- To rule other differentials including other causes of chronic granulomatous diseases
- For research purposes

At present suggested routine sites are:

- Right earlobe
- Forehead
- Chin
- Left buttock in men and left upper thigh in women
- Active or suspicious lesions

Sites for SSS

- Earlier, smears were obtained from multiple sites including both ear lobes, both cheeks, forehead, chin, buttocks, and an additional six active/suspicious sites.
- Presently, the suggested four sites for routine SSS are:
  1. Right earlobe
  2. Forehead
  3. Chin
  4. Left buttock in men and left upper thigh in women

  (However, other active or suspicious lesions are included when the disease is PB.)
- In borderline leprosy, smears should be obtained from eight sites to include four active lesions in addition to the four routine sites, as the bacterial load is variable.

General Principles of SSS

- Initial SSS should be done from the recommended sites as mentioned above.
- Repeat smears may be done annually once from 3 to 4 of the most active sites to evaluate progress and rule out chances of any evidence of relapse.
- All microscopic slides on which skin smears are made should be precleaned in 70% alcohol, acetone, or alcohol-acetone to remove amorphous debris. The slides are wiped dry with a clean hand towel. Blades that are used in smear taking are likewise cleaned.

Equipment Used for SSS

- Glass slides for microscopy
- Sterile surgical gloves
- Surgical scalpel with detachable sterile blades (15 Bard-Parker blade)
- Cotton swabs soaked in methyl alcohol
- Tincture benzoin
- Methyl alcohol
- Spirit lamp

Technique of SSS

- Universal precautions should be observed in obtaining skin smears.
- The skin is cleansed with 70% alcohol and air-dried or wiped dry with cotton.
- A portion of the skin of the site is gripped between the thumb and forefinger of the left hand to drive out the blood.
- Local anesthesia is generally unnecessary
- An incision is made between the fingers of the left hand about 5 mm long and 3 mm deep with a small-bladed scalpel (usually the number 15 Bard-Parker blade) while maintaining the pressure of the fingers.
- The blade is then turned at right angles to the cut, and the wound is scraped several times in the same direction, so that tissue fluid and pulp (not blood) collects on one side of the blade
- The material is then transferred to the cleaned microscope slide and smears are prepared. Two or more smears can be made on one slide, each being numbered with a marking pencil.
- A moderately thick smear, with a visible uniform opacity, is made. The smear is made circularly on the slide, no larger than a pencil eraser (5–7 mm), beginning peripherally and ending in the center, leaving a central "button" (2–4 mm) which can be easily focused upon with the microscope.
- The smear is fixed over a flame before being sent for staining. The heating of slides should be gentle as excess heat will likely destroy the smear tissue.
- Slides used once should never be used again.
- A Band-Aid is generally sufficient to protect the smear site.

WHO Recommendations on the Use of SSS in Leprosy Programs

- *1982*: MB leprosy was defined by a BI of 2+ or more at any site in the initial skin smears. PB leprosy was defined with a bacteriological index of <2 at all sites in initial slit smears.
- *1988*: All smear-positive cases were classified as MB leprosy for MDT programs.
- *1994*: WHO concluded that where skin smears are not available, cases can be classified based on clinical examination alone as either PB leprosy (one to five skin lesions) or MB leprosy (six or more skin lesions).

Staining Procedure: Modified Ziehl–Neelsen Method[5]

- Chemicals required for Ziehl–Neelsen method are:
  - Basic fuchsin
  - Decolorizing agent
  - Methylene blue (counterstain)
- Not more than six slides with fixed smears are placed on rods over a sink.
- The slide with the smear is flooded with freshly prepared or filtered carbol fuchsin.
- Heat is applied gently beneath it, usually with a spirit lamp till a point to cause steam to rise from all parts of the slide, but boiling is avoided. More stain is added when needed. The stain is not allowed to evaporate to dryness.
- The slide is left for 15 minutes without any further heating.
- The stain is tipped away and the slide is washed under a gentle stream of tap water.
- An acid-alcohol mixture consisting of 1% hydrochloric acid in 70% alcohol is poured onto the slide and left for 3 seconds if the smear is thin or for 5 seconds if the smear is thick.
- It is then washed in running tap water.
- The slide is then inspected to see the degree of pinkness; if faintly pink, proceed to the next stage, but if deeply pink, treat again with acid-alcohol for 2 seconds and wash with running water.
- The slide is then flooded with the counterstain (1% methylene blue) for about 1 minute.
- It is then washed in tap water. A blotting paper is used at last to allow the water to drain off and to make the smears to dry.

Microscopic Examination of Skin Smears

- The stained smears are examined with a quality microscope using the oil immersion objective (×100) to determine the total number of bacilli.
- The same individual should read all smears for consistency.
- The smear will have similar numbers of bacilli throughout. However, four separate quadrants of the smear are

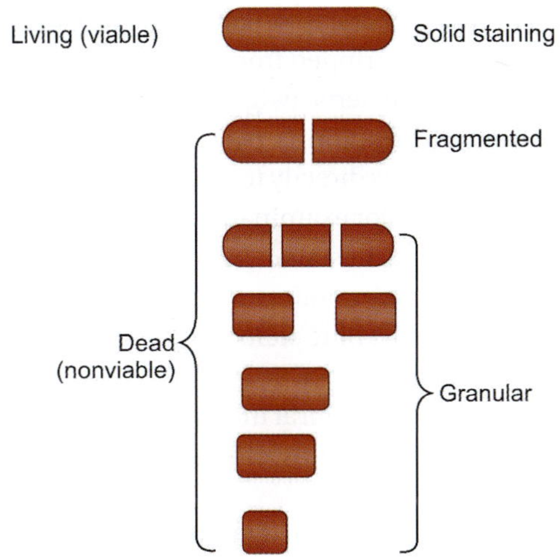

Fig. 1: Diagrammatic representation of variable staining patterns of *Mycobacterium leprae* stained by the modified Ziehl–Neelsen method.

examined and averaged to establish the bacterial (bacteriological) index (BI).

- First, we have to differentiate live bacilli from dead bacilli. Living bacilli appear as uniformly stained rods (solid-staining) and dead bacilli appear irregularly stained (fragmented bacilli) or as granules (granular bacilli) **(Fig. 1)**.[7]

Interpretation of Smears

Bacterial (Bacteriological) Index

- The density of bacilli in smears is known as the BI and includes both living and dead bacilli.
- Ridley's logarithmic scale is used to express BI. This is based on the number of bacilli seen in an average microscopic field using an oil-immersion objective.
- The mean index is calculated where multiple smears are taken.

Bacteriological index (BI)	*No. of bacilli seen*
0	0 bacilli in 100 fields
1+	1–10 bacilli in 100 fields
2+	1–10 bacilli in 10 fields
3+	1–10 bacilli, on average, in each field
4+	10–100 bacilli, on average, in each field
5+	100–1,000 bacilli, on average, in each field
6+	Many clumps of bacilli in an average field (over 1,000)

The Morphological Index[8-10]

- Morphological index (MI) is a tedious but useful measure of the viability of bacilli based on the concept that solid staining bacilli are viable organisms.
- This has been shown to correlate with infectivity in mice and with bacillary ATP content.
- MI is measured by calculating the proportion or percentage of solid stained (uniformly and brightly stained down their length) bacilli, after examining preferably 200 red staining elements, lying singly.
- Bacilli are considered solid staining if they satisfy the following criteria:
  - The entire organism must be uniformly stained
  - The longitudinal sides are parallel
  - Both ends are rounded
  - The length is five times its width.
- *Utility of MI:*
  - Suggests if the disease is active or not
  - Gives important information as to treatment response
  - Suggests defaulter to treatment
- *Limitations:*
  - Zero MI values have been recorded from untreated cases with positive mouse uptake
  - Significantly dependent on the staining methods
  - There is subjective variation in determining nonsolid staining bacilli
  - There is little correlation between the initial value of MI with initial BI in general
  - Besides the skin, bacilli are also lodged in other tissues like nerves, skeletal and smooth muscles, internal organs, etc., that cannot be bacteriologically examined routinely.

The SFG Index

- SFG index divides bacilli further into three classes:
  1. "Solid" (S) is used to describe solid-staining unbroken rods
  2. "Fragmented" (F) is used to describe bacilli in which the acid-fast substance is interrupted at one or more points, but at least one fragment displays an elongated form; also single very short rods;
  3. "Granular" (G) is used to describe bacilli in which the acid-fast substance is round granules either linear or in clumps.

NASAL MUCOSAL SMEARS[11]

- The nasal mucosal is the most common site from where *M. leprae* are disseminated into the environment.
- About 10 million bacilli per day are discharged from the nasal secretion of a lepromatous leprosy patient.
- The nasal smear helps assess the response of a patient to treatment and his infectivity.
- The nasal smear is collected using a nasal scraper gently and aseptically, under direct vision of the nasal cavity, avoiding bleeding as much as possible.
- The material thus obtained is smeared onto a glass slide and processed similarly as SSS.
- Alternatively, an early morning nasal blow can be collected before the patient has cleared his nose.
- Staining of nasal smear/blow should be done carefully using acid-alcohol decolorizing solution to avoid false-positive staining "artifact" of acid-fast saprophytes present in the nose.
- Use is limited, presently mostly used for research purposes.

FLUORESCENT MICROSCOPY TO DETECT *M. LEPRAE*

- Though Fite-Faraco staining is very sensitive to diagnosing *M. leprae* in tissue sections, it is not free from flaws. The density of the bacilli should be about 1,000 per cubic millimeter of the tissue to pick single bacilli in the section.
- Fluorescent method using Auramine-Rhodamine is more sensitive than the modified Fite-Faraco method in detecting lepra bacilli in tissue sections especially in cases with bacillary index less than three.

IMMUNOCHEMICAL STAINING TO DEMONSTRATE MYCOBACTERIAL ANTIGENS

Some studies suggest that finding mycobacterial antigens by immunostaining using polyclonal Bacillus Calmette-Guerin (BCG) antibodies can have an advantage over Fite-Faraco staining especially in early leprosy cases.

S-100 STAIN FOR SCHWANN CELLS

- S-100 stain which selectively stains Schwann cells.
- This is sometimes used to demonstrate the remnants of the destroyed nerves inside tuberculoid granulomas.
- This can be especially helpful in PB leprosy where demonstration of acid-fast bacilli (AFB) is not always possible.

NERVE BIOPSY[12]

- Nerve biopsy is essential in the diagnosis of pure neural leprosy.
- Nerves suitable for skin biopsy are thickened sensory nerves that do not contain motor fibers and therefore there is no risk of motor damage. Examples of such nerves include:
  - Supraorbital branch of the 5th cranial nerve
  - Supraclavicular nerve
  - Great auricular nerve
  - Branch of radial cutaneous nerve at the wrist region
  - Branch of sural nerve at the level just above the ankle
  - Superficial peroneal nerve on the dorsum of the foot
  - A cutaneous nerves adjacent to a skin lesion
  - The cutaneous nerve of the forearm or thigh
- The nerve deficit resulting from nerve biopsy is rare and minimal.
- Method of nerve biopsy:
  - Choose a thickened sensory nerve
  - Standard sterilization of the area
  - 2% lignocaine is injected around the nerve for anesthesia.
  - A transverse skin incision over the nerve is made.
  - The nerve is identified and then separated from the surrounding by blunt dissection.
  - A small nick is made to separate one or two fasciculi, which are then stripped from the nerve bundle.
  - About 2 cm long nerve twig is then dissected out.
  - 10% neutral formalin is used as a fixative and the dissected nerve is directly transferred into the fixative.
- Stains that are used for examination of a nerve biopsy are:
  - Hematoxylin-eosin stain
  - *AFB*: Job-Chacko modification of Fite-Faraco stain
  - *Myelin*: Luxol fast blue stain
  - *Axons*: Bodian stain
- Suggestive features of neural involvement in leprosy are:
  - Job-Chacko modification of Fite-Faraco stain showing AFB inside nerves
  - Hematoxylin-eosin stain demonstrating granuloma in nerve parenchyma
  - Luxol fast blue stain showing patchy demyelination
  - Bodian stain showing fragmentation of axons.

THE LEPROMIN TEST[13]

Introduction:

- The lepromin skin test was used to determine what type of leprosy a person has. It involves intradermal injection of a standardized extract of the inactivated "leprosy bacillus."
- It is a nonspecific test and not recommended as a primary mode of diagnosis.
- It is a delayed-type hypersensitivity reaction to *M. leprae* or its antigens.
- *History:* Kensuke Mitsuda first described the lepromin reaction.
- *Types of lepromin antigen:*
  - *Dharmendra antigen*: Evokes a stronger early positive reaction
  - *Mitsuda antigen*: Provokes a stronger late reaction
- *Methods:*
  - Inactivated *M. leprae* antigen is extracted from lepromas.
  - Intradermal injection of 0.1 mL of the lepromin antigen is given in the flexor surface of the forearm.
  - The reaction is interpreted at 2 moments. One inspection looks for an early (Fernandez) reaction at 48 hours. The other is for a late (Mitsuda) reaction at 21 days.
  - Positive reaction means: (A) 10 mm or more induration after 48 hours; (B) 5 mm or above nodule after 21 days.
- *Types of reaction:*
  - *The early (Fernandez) reaction*: Read at 48 hours. It appears within 2 days and is roughly equivalent to the tuberculin test. Induration of 5 mm or more with erythema (redness), or 10 mm without, 48 hours postinjection are positive Fernandez reactions. This reaction is demonstrated best with Dharmendra antigen.

- *The late (Mitsuda) reaction*: The Mitsuda reaction is read at 21 days and indicates resistance to the bacillus. A nodule measuring more than 5 mm indicates positivity.
- It is important to note that neither of these tests are diagnostic; rather, they are used for classification and prognostic purposes.

- *Risk*: There is an extremely small risk of an allergic reaction which may include itching and rarely hives.

THE SWEAT TEST[14]

- *The principle:*
  - This evaluates the function of autonomic nerves in the skin which is impaired early in leprosy.
  - The parasympathetic nerves supply the sweat glands, and anhidrosis is characteristic of skin lesions in tuberculoid leprosy.
  - In leprosy, because of loss of function of the autonomic nerves, sweating response chemical (injection of pilocarpine nitrate) or physical challenges (exposure to sun in tropical summer) is lost in the leprosy patches in tuberculoid leprosy.
- *Method of performing the test:*
  - 0.2 mL of a 1 in 1,000 solution of pilocarpine nitrate is injected intradermally into the lesion to be tested.
  - The area is painted with a tincture of iodine and then to dusted with starch powder (alternatively, Quinizarin powder can be used obviating the need of iodine).
  - The blue color created by sweating is absent due to damage to autonomic cutaneous nerves in leprosy.
- Nonspecific test. Not regularly done nowadays.

THE HISTAMINE TEST[15]

- *The principle:*
  - Histamine elicits weal and flare reactions in normal skin when the cutaneous nervous system is intact.
  - In the skin affected by leprosy, flare may be impaired or absent, due to malfunctioning of the nervous system and only a weal is seen.
  - This helps decide if a hypopigmented patch is due to leprosy.
- *Method of performing the test:*
  - One drop of histamine acid phosphate (diphosphate) 1 in 1,000 (1 mg in 1 mL) is placed on the area of skin to be tested and another on a control site.
  - A superficial prick is made through each drop.
  - In the control area where the dermal nerves are intact, a bright flare will appear.
  - In a leprosy macule, the flare is delayed, feeble (indeterminate and borderline leprosy), or absent (tuberculoid leprosy).
- Nonspecific test. Depression of histamine flare can occur in all types of peripheral neuropathy. Not regularly done nowadays.

CYTOLOGICAL DIAGNOSIS OF LEPROSY

- FNAC is a simple and effective tool for diagnosing Hansen's disease from both skin and nerve lesions.
- It requires less infrastructure and can be used in field conditions.
- It is an especially important tool for the diagnosis of pure neural leprosy (PNL) where nerve biopsy needs specialized infrastructure and expertise.

FINE-NEEDLE ASPIRATION CYTOLOGY FOR CUTANEOUS LESIONS OF LEPROSY

Singh et al. suggested cytology criteria for subclassification of leprosy **(Table 1)**.[16]

FINE-NEEDLE ASPIRATION CYTOLOGY FOR NEURAL LESIONS OF LEPROSY

- FNAC of affected nerves can be a valuable and less invasive procedure for the diagnosis of PNL.
- Vijaikumar et al. have proposed a set of criteria for interpreting the cytology of nerve aspirates **(Table 2)**.[17]
- Some of the authors of this chapter have done a series of work to demonstrate improved sensitivity, specificity, and objectivity of diagnosis of pure neural leprosy

TABLE 1: Cytology criteria for subclassification of leprosy from skin lesion.

Type of leprosy	*Cytology criteria*
Tuberculoid leprosy (including TT and BT)	• Cellular smears • Cohesive epithelioid cell granulomas • Numerous lymphocytes not infiltrating the granuloma • No stainable AFB (BI = 0)
Mid-borderline (BB)	• Fair cellular yield • Poorly cohesive granulomas composed of an admixture of epithelioid cells and macrophages • Few lymphocytes infiltrating the granulomas • BI = 1+ to 2+
Borderline lepromatous (BL)	• Moderate cellularity • Singly dispersed macrophages with "negative images"; no epithelioid cells • Numerous lymphocytes (predominant cell type) diffusely admixed with macrophages • BI = 3+ to 4+
Lepromatous leprosy (LL)	• Heavy cellularity • Numerous foamy macrophages (predominant cell type) in a fatty background with intracellular and extracellular negative image • Few lymphocytes • BI = 5+ to 6+ (globi)

TABLE 2: Cytology criteria for subclassification of leprosy from nerve lesion.

Type of leprosy	*Cytology criteria of nerve lesion*
Paucibacillary (indeterminate, TT and BT)	• Good number of inflammatory cells in the aspirate • Predominantly epithelioid cell granulomas and moderate numbers of lymphocytes • Occasional giant cells and neutrophils • BI 0 to 1+
Mid borderline (BB)	• Fair number of inflammatory cells in the aspirate • Predominantly non-foamy macrophages, a moderate number of epithelioid cells, and lymphocytes. • BI 2+ to 3+
Borderline lepromatous (BL)	• Fair number of inflammatory cells in the aspirate • Predominantly lymphocytes and moderate numbers of foamy macrophages • BI 4+ to 5+
Lepromatous leprosy (LL)	• Fair to poor cellularity • Predominantly foamy macrophages and a few lymphocytes • BI 6+

by combining fine needle aspiration with multiplex polymerase chain reaction (PCR).[18,19]

HUMORAL IMMUNE RESPONSE EVALUATION

- ELISA is the most commonly studied serological tests used in leprosy.
- ELISA is 64% sensitive and 91% specific.
- *Other serological tests studied are*: (1) Lateral flow test (sensitivity 68% and specificity 87%) and (2) agglutination test (sensitivity of 73% and specificity of 90%).
- Phenolic glycolipid 1 (PGL-1) was the most frequently studied antigen, and the most detected are IgM antibodies.
- ELISAs targeting PGL-1 antigen have in general lower sensitivity than the other antigens (e.g., LID-1, ND-O-HSA, GPF-C), but it did not affect the specificity.
- A combined detection of antibodies and cytokine biomarkers significantly improves the diagnostic potential.[20]

MOLECULAR DIAGNOSIS OF *M. LEPRAE*

- Molecular diagnosis of *M. leprae* is required in the following situations:
  - Early leprosy
  - Indeterminate
  - Paucibacillary leprosy with diagnostic dilemma
  - Pure neural leprosy
  - Detection of drug resistance
  - Relapse
  - Research purposes
- Two major methods of molecular diagnosis of *M. leprae* include: (1) PCR methods to detect *M. leprae* in biopsies or skin smears or nerve aspirates; (2) *M. leprae* genotyping.
- PCR improves identification of PB leprosy or neural leprosy as complementary to histological analysis.
- PCR also has found an important role in identifying drug resistance.
- The sensitivity of conventional PCR varied from 50 to 93% and its specificity from 90 to 100%.
- Quantitative PCR (qPCR) showed a higher sensitivity than conventional PCR (79%), with a lower specificity (89%).
- Conventional PCR studies usually target the *M. leprae*-specific repetitive element (RLEP).
- qPCR improved the sensitivity of the molecular diagnosis of PB patients.
- The use of molecular-based techniques in finding mutations in drug-resistant determining regions (DRDR) of *M. leprae* is opening up a new dimension in leprosy therapeutics.[20]

KEY POINTS

- Sites for routine SSS are right earlobe, forehead, chin, and left buttock in men and left upper thigh in women.
- Staining procedure used for SSS is modified Ziehl–Neelsen method.
- The density of bacilli in smears is known as the bacterial BI and includes both living and dead bacilli.
- The MI is measured by calculating the proportion or percentage of solid stained (uniformly and brightly stained down their length) bacilli, after examining preferably 200 red staining elements, lying singly.
- Staining of nasal smear/blow should be done carefully using acid-alcohol decolorizing solution to avoid false-positive staining "artifact" of acid-fast saprophytes present in the nose.
- The lepromin test, is a nonspecific delayed-type hypersensitivity reaction to *M. leprae* or its antigens and not recommended as a primary mode of diagnosis.
- In lepromin test, the Dharmendra antigen evokes a stronger early positive reaction and the Mitsuda antigen provokes a stronger late reaction
- FNAC is a simple and effective tool for diagnosing Hansen's disease from both skin and nerve lesions.
- Two major methods of molecular diagnosis of *M. leprae* include: (1) PCR methods to detect *M. leprae* in biopsies or skin smears or nerve aspirates; (2) *M. leprae* genotyping.

REFERENCES

1. De A, Surana TV, Biswas S, Reja AH, Chatterjee G. Isolated tenosynovitis as a sole manifestation: the great mimicker still continues to surprise us. Indian J Dermatol. 2015; 60(2):213.

2. Das NK, De A, Naskar B, Sil A, Das S, Sarda A, et al. A quality of life study of patients with leprosy attending the dermatology OPD of a tertiary care center of eastern India. Indian J Dermatol. 2020;65(1):42-6.
3. Reja AHH, De A, Patra PK, Biswas S, Duttagupta U, Sil A, et al. Genomic reduction at TTC repeats in the bacterial genome of treated cases of Hansen's disease: a possible survival mechanism of *Mycobacterium leprae*. Indian J Dermatol. 2018;63(6):449-54.
4. De A, Reja AH, Biswas S, Bhattacharya B, Chatterjee G, Basu K, et al. Unique TTC repeat base pair loss mutation in cases of pure neural leprosy: a survival strategy of *Mycobacterium leprae*? Indian J Dermatol. 2015;60(4):351-5.
5. Sehgal VN, Joginder. Slit-skin smear in leprosy. Int J Dermatol. 1990;29(1):9-16.
6. Mahajan VK. Slit-skin smear in leprosy: lest we forget it! Indian J Lepr. 2013;85(4):177-83.
7. Ridley DS. The SFG (solid, fragmented, granular) index for bacterial morphology. Lepr Rev. 1971;42:96-7.
8. Ridley DS. The morphological index. Lepr Rev. 1971;42:75-7.
9. Browne SG. Some observations on the morphological index in lepromatous leprosy. Lepr Rev. 1966;37:23-5.
10. Desikan KV. Correlation of morphology with viability of *Mycobacterium leprae*. Lepr India. 1976;48:391-7.
11. Jaffé L. Value and worthlessness of the nasal smear in the diagnosis of leprosy. Dtsch Med Wochenschr. 1968;93(7):308-9.
12. Kulshreshtha D, Malhotra KP, Malhotra HS, Thacker AK, Garg RK, Singh AK, et al. Mandating nerve biopsy: a step towards personalizing therapy in pure neuritic leprosy. J Peripher Nerv Syst. 2018;23(3):190-6.
13. Chatterjee BR. The lepromin test. Lepr India. 1976;48(2):114-8.
14. Dogra S, Saraswat A, Kaur I, Kumar B. "A natural sweat test" in leprosy. Int J Lepr Other Mycobact Dis. 2002;70(1):36-7.
15. Orsini O. Histamine test in the diagnosis of leprosy. Arq Min Leprol. 1952;12(2):124-6.
16. Singh N, Bhatia A, Gupta K, Ramam M. Cytomorphology of leprosy across the Ridley-Jopling spectrum. Acta Cytol. 1996;40:719-23.
17. Vijaikumar M, D'Souza M, Kumar S, Badhe B. Fine needle aspiration cytology (FNAC) of nerves in leprosy. Lepr Rev. 2001;72(2):171-8.
18. De A, Hasanoor Reja AH, Aggarwal I, Sen S, Sil A, Bhattacharya B, et al. Use of fine needle aspirate from peripheral nerves of pure-neural leprosy for cytology and polymerase chain reaction to confirm the diagnosis: a follow-up study of 4 years. Indian J Dermatol. 2017;62(6):635-43.
19. Reja AH, De A, Biswas S, Chattopadhyay A, Chatterjee G, Bhattacharya B, et al. Use of fine needle aspirate from peripheral nerves of pure-neural leprosy for cytology and PCR to confirm the diagnosis: a pilot study. Indian J Dermatol Venereol Leprol. 2013;79(6):789-94.
20. de Oliveira ALG, Fraga VG, Sernizon-Guimarães N, Cardoso MS, Viana AG, Bueno LL, et al. Diagnostic accuracy of tests using recombinant protein antigens of *Mycobacterium leprae* for leprosy: a systematic review. J Infect Public Health. 2020;13(8):1078-88.

EXAMINATION QUESTIONS

Write short notes on the following:

1. Laboratory diagnosis of Hansen's disease.
2. Slit skin smear.
3. Bacteriological and morphological index.
4. Newer advances in the laboratory diagnosis of leprosy.

119 CHAPTER Management of Leprosy

Swetalina Pradhan, Sabha Mushtaq, Kananbala Sahu

INTRODUCTION

Leprosy is a chronic infectious disease caused by mycobacterium *Mycobacterium leprae.* Despite the social stigma surrounding it, leprosy is curable if adequate World Health Organization multidrug therapy (WHO-MDT) is taken. The management of leprosy involves not only the treatment of the infection but also the complications arising thereof and the special scenarios such as resistance, relapse, etc. Identifying the early signs and symptoms of the disease, making a timely diagnosis, and adherence to the treatment are decisive for the success of leprosy control program.

NEW CASE

According to WHO, a case of leprosy is defined as a person who has not completed the prescribed course of MDT and is having at least one of the three "cardinal signs" of the disease:[1]

1. Hypopigmented or reddish skin lesion(s) with definite sensory loss/impairment.
2. Thickened peripheral nerve(s) with impairment of sensation in the distribution of nerve and/or weakness of muscles supplied by that nerve.
3. Acid fast bacilli in the slit skin smear.

Treatment Regime for a New Leprosy Case

The treatment of leprosy has slowly evolved over time from the era of chaulmoogra oil and dapsone monotherapy to the present day MDT recommended by the WHO **(Table 1)**.[2] For treatment purposes, WHO classifies leprosy patients into: paucibacillary (PB) and multibacillary (MB) cases to administer MDT. The latest WHO guidelines recommend the same three drug regimen for all leprosy patients with the total duration of 6 months for PB and 12 months for MB **(Tables 2 and 3)**.[3]

Clinical Response with MDT

Clinical response is rapid with rifampicin. In lepromatous leprosy, nasal symptoms regress within 2–3 weeks, and skin lesions in 2–3 months. Infiltration also begins to clear in 2–3 months but complete regression of infiltration takes a long time. With dapsone, mucosal and skin ulcers are first to heal like rifampicin. Regression of skin nodules and skin thickening starts later which may take around 2–3 years to regress completely. Nerve thickening shows slow and incomplete regression. The nerve deficit mostly remains unaffected with MDT. Paucibacillary patients (TT and BT) show complete recovery within 6 months in two-thirds of cases while the other types may take more than a year to regress completely.[2]

Treatment of Leprosy in Special Clinical Scenarios

In certain situations, a modification of the standard WHO-MDT[2,7] is required as discussed in **Table 4**.

Alternative and Newer Treatment Regimens

With the introduction of newer antileprosy drugs and to increase the compliance with the treatment, many treatment regimens have been tried and tested over the years with variable results **(Table 5)**.[2,4,8-10]

Characteristics of Antileprosy Drugs

Over the years; many drugs have made way into the therapeutic arsenal of leprosy. The role, mechanism of action, pharmacokinetics and side-effects of these drugs[2,4,7,11] are given in **Tables 6 and 7**.

DRUG-RESISTANT LEPROSY

The problem of drug resistance is almost as old as leprosy treatment itself with dapsone resistance reported as early as 1964. Since then reports of resistance to several other drugs have emerged. The features of drug resistance to various antileprosy drugs are given in **Table 8**. Patients on MDT who are found to have resistance to rifampicin alone with or without resistance to dapsone, should be restarted on a full course of second-line treatment **(Table 9)**.[3]

RELAPSE

Diagnostic criteria and treatment of relapse have been shown in **Tables 10 and 11**, respectively.

DEFAULTER

Defaulter refers to a patient who fails to complete the treatment, either by failing to take the drugs regularly or by not attending

TABLE 1: History of antileprosy drugs and evolution of MDT.[2]

Year	*Drug/treatment regime/MDT*	*Components*	*Duration*
1946	Dapsone monotherapy	–	*MB*: Lifelong *PB*: 10 years
1971	Rifampicin	–	–
1962	Clofazimine	–	–
1972	MDT-Malta project	*Isoprodian:* Isoniazid, prothionamide, dapsone *Isoprodian-R:* Isoprodian + rifampicin	5–89 months
1982	WHO MDT-FDT	*MB*: • Rifampicin 600 mg MS* • Clofazimine 300 mg MS and 50 mg daily • Dapsone 100 mg daily *PB*: • Rifampicin 600 mg MS • Dapsone 100 mg daily **NLEP modification:* Rifampicin was initially given as 21 days intensive therapy; later modified to 14 days therapy and finally to monthly supervised dose	*MB:* 24 months or till smear negative *PB*: 6 months
1994	WHO MDT-FDT	*MB*: • Rifampicin 600 mg MS • Clofazimine 300 mg MS and 50 mg daily • Dapsone 100 mg daily *PB*: • Rifampicin 600 mg MS • Dapsone 100 mg daily	*MB*: 24 months *PB*: 6 months
1997	WHO MDT-FDT	*MB*: • Rifampicin 600 mg MS • Clofazimine 300 mg MS and 50 mg daily • Dapsone 100 mg daily *PB*: • Rifampicin 600 mg MS • Dapsone 100 mg daily	*MB*: 12 months *PB*: 6 months
2018	WHO MDT-FDT	*MB/PB:* • Rifampicin 600 mg MS • Clofazimine 300 mg MS and 50 mg daily • Dapsone 100 mg daily	*MB*: 12 months *PB*: 6 months

(WHO MDT-FDT: World Health Organization multidrug therapy fixed duration therapy; MS: monthly supervised; MB: multibacillary; PB: paucibacillary)

TABLE 2: WHO classification and treatment regimen for PB and MB cases.[3]

Feature	*MB**	*PB*
Skin lesions	>5	1–5
Smear for AFB	Positive	Negative
MDT (adults)	• *Rifampicin:* 600 mg MS • *Clofazimine:* 300 mg MS; 50 mg daily • *Dapsone:* 100 mg daily	Same as MB
MDT (children)	*10–14 years:* • Rifampicin 450 mg MS • Clofazimine 150 mg MS, 50 mg daily • Dapsone 50 mg daily *<10 years or <40 kg:* • Rifampicin 10 mg/kg MS • Clofazimine 6 mg/kg MS and 1 mg/kg daily • Dapsone 2 mg/kg daily	Same as MB
Duration	12 months course completed in 18-month period	6 months course completed in 9-month period

**As per NLEP 2009:* Patient with more than one thickened nerve is also classified as MB.
(MB: multibacillary; PB: paucibacillary; MDT: multidrug therapy; MS: monthly supervised; AFB: acid-fast bacilli)

TABLE 3: Drug interactions, contraindications, and monitoring of patients on MDT.[2,4-6]

MDT drug	*Drug interactions*	*Contraindications*	*Lab monitoring*	*Pregnancy category*
Rifampicin	Rifampicin is a potent inducer of multiple CYP isoforms resulting in reduced level and therapeutic efficacy of various drugs: • OCPs, CSs, OHDs • Warfarin • Azole antifungals • CCBs, BZDs • Statins • Cyclosporine • Theophylline • Anticonvulsants phenytoin, lamotrigine	*Absolute:* Hypersensitivity to rifampicin *Relative:* • Pregnancy • Severely impaired liver function	*Baseline:* CBC, LFT, RFT, Urinalysis, G6PD level *Follow-up:* • CBC weekly for 4 weeks then every 2 weeks for 3 months, thereafter every 3–4 months • LFT, RFT and urinalysis every 3–4 months	C
Dapsone	• ↓ *dapsone serum levels:* Antacids, rifampicin, anticonvulsants, griseofulvin, nevirapine • ↑ *dapsone serum levels:* Probenicid • ↑ *hematologic risk:* Sulfonamide antibiotics, methotrexate, pyrimethamine, trimethoprim	*Absolute*: Hypersensitivity to dapsone *Relative:* • G6PD deficiency • Allergy to sulfonamide antibiotics • Significant hepatic or renal impairment • Significant cardiopulmonary disease • Pre-existing peripheral neuropathy	*Baseline*: CBC, LFT, RFT, urinalysis, G6PD level *Follow-up:* • CBC weekly for 4 weeks then every 2 weeks for 3 months, thereafter every 3–4 months • LFT, RFT and urinalysis every 3–4 months *(Methemoglobin levels and reticulocyte count wherever indicated)*	C
Clofazimine	Minimal	*Absolute*: Hypersensitivity to clofazimine *Relative*: • Pregnancy and lactation • Pre-existing GI disease • Patients prone to electrolyte disturbance	Periodic LFT evaluation if dose exceeds 100 mg	C

(CBC: complete blood count; LFT: liver function test; RFT: renal function test; CYP: cytochrome P; OCPs: oral contraceptives; CCBs: calcium channel blockers; OHD: oral hypoglycemic drugs; BZD: benzodiazapine drugs; CS: corticosteroids)

TABLE 4: Management of leprosy in different clinical scenarios.[2,7]

Clinical scenarios	*Treatment modification/adjustment*
Coexistent tuberculosis and leprosy	• Start treatment of tuberculosis first • Make the necessary additions or adjustments in the antileprosy treatment such that during the treatment course, patient is on at least three antileprosy drugs in case of MB leprosy and at least two antileprosy drugs in case of PB leprosy
Nonacceptance of clofazimine	Ofloxacin 400 mg daily, or minocycline 100 mg daily as substitutes for clofazimine or Monthly ROM (Rifampicin, ofloxacin, minocycline) for 24 months
Pregnancy	• *First time diagnosed:* Start MDT irrespective of the trimester • *Already on MDT:* Continue MDT
Severe dapsone toxicity	• Stop dapsone immediately • For MB leprosy, no further modification is required • For PB leprosy, clofazimine may be substituted for dapsone for a period of 6 months

(MB: multibacillary; PB: paucibacillary; MDT: multidrug therapy)

treatment centers.[14] As per the WHO, a multibacillary (MB) case should take the 12 pulses within 18 months and a PB case should take 6 pulses in 9 months period. At any point of time during treatment, the patient should have ingested two-thirds of the pulses till that time. If the patient fails to do so, the treatment course is restarted.[13,14]

TABLE 5: Newer/alternative drug regimens in leprosy.[2,4,8-10]

Regime	*Year*	*Component*	*Duration*	*Drawbacks/Remarks*
Treatment regimens not in frequent use				
RO trial	1992	**R**ifampicin 600 mg daily **O**floxacin 400 mg daily	*PB/MB:* 28 days	High relapse rate
ROM trial: Single dose	1997	**R**ifampicin 600 mg **O**floxacin 400 mg **M**inocycline 100 mg	*SSL-PB*: Single dose	Initial observation showed equal efficacy to WHO PB MDT for SSL-PB *(Later withdrawn due to operational reasons)*
ROM trial: Intermittent	1995	**R**ifampicin 600 mg **O**floxacin 400 mg **M**inocycline 100 mg *(All drugs given once a month)*	*PB*: 6 months *MB*: 12 months	An RCT assessed the addition of clarithromycin to ROM but found no significant difference[8]
Newer treatment regimens				
PMM	2000	Rifa**P**entine 900 mg **M**oxifloxacin 400 mg **M**inocycline 100 mg *(All drugs given once a month)*	*MB:* 12 months	Moxifloxacin is the most powerful bactericidal drug
Six-week quadruple regimen	2000	Daily supervised rifampicin 600 mg, ofloxacin 400 mg and clofazimine 100 mg for 6 days a week Minocycline 100 mg weekly	*MB*: 6 weeks	In a 10 years follow-up study, late relapses after more than 5 years were observed[9]
Accompanied MDT (A-MDT)	2000	WHO-MDT MB/PB	*MB*: 1 year *PB*: 6 months	Full course of WHO-MDT is provided at first visit to leprosy patients living in remote areas, mobile populations and areas affected by civil strife
Uniform MDT (U-MDT)	2002	*MB*: • Rifampicin 600 mg MS • Clofazimine 300 mg MS and 50 mg daily • Dapsone 100 mg daily *PB*: • Rifampicin 600 mg MS • Dapsone 100 mg daily	*PB/MB*: 6 months	Effective and well tolerated in patients with PB leprosy but it was found to be too short to adequately treat MB patients[10]

(MB: multibacillary; PB: paucibacillary; MDT: multidrug therapy; SSL: single skin lesion; RCT: randomized controlled trial)

TABLE 6: Profile of drugs used in leprosy.

Drug	*Source/class*	*Mechanism of action*	*Activity against M. leprae*	*Side effects*
Rifampicin (Rifampin)	Ansamycin derived from *Streptomyces mediterranei*	• Inhibits deoxyribonucleic acid dependent • (DNA-dependent) ribonucleic acid (RNA) polymerase by binding to its β-subunit thereby inhibiting RNA synthesis and subsequent translation to proteins	• Bactericidal • A single dose of 1,500 mg or 3 doses of 600 mg kill 99.99% of viable *M. leprae* • MI becomes negative in 4–6 weeks	• Orange discoloration of urine and other body fluids • Nausea, vomiting, diarrhea • Hepatitis *Common with once/twice weekly administration*: • Flu-like syndrome (fever, headache, bone and joint pains) • Thrombocytopenia • Acute renal failure due to interstitial nephritis
Dapsone (Diaminodiphenyl sulfone; DDS)	Sulfonamide	Blocks the enzyme dihydropteroate synthetase thereby inhibiting the synthesis of dihydrofolic acid	• Weakly bactericidal • Reduces MI to <1% of the baseline value over a period of 3 months	• Hemolytic anemia • Methemoglobinemia • Hepatitis • Dapsone syndrome • Leukopenia, agranulocytosis • Morbilliform eruption • Peripheral neuropathy • Psychosis

Contd...

Contd...

Drug	*Source/class*	*Mechanism of action*	*Activity against M. leprae*	*Side effects*
Clofazimine (Lamprene; B663)	Iminophen-azine dye	Not clearly known *Possible modes of action:* • Iron chelation with production of nascent oxygen radicals intracellularly • Interference with guanine bases during mycobacterial DNA replication	Weakly bactericidal	• Orange-brown skin and conjunctival discoloration • Red discoloration of body secretions • Xerosis, ichthyosis • Abdominal pain, nausea and diarrhea • Splenic infarction • Eosinophilic enteritis
Ofloxacin	Fluoroquino-lone	Inhibition of enzyme DNA gyrase	• Bactericidal • Single dose kills 60.2% of *M. leprae*. Over 99% to 99.99% are killed with only 22 doses given over 28 days	• Nausea, diarrhea • Pruritus • Photosensitivity • Headache, insomnia, dizziness • Tendinitis and tendon rupture
Moxifloxacin	Fluoroquino-lone	Inhibition of enzyme DNA gyrase	• Bactericidal • Single dose kills 92.1% of *M. leprae*	• Nausea, diarrhea • Dizziness • Electrolyte disturbances • Hepatitis • Bradycardia • Peripheral neuropathy • Tendinitis and tendon rupture • Mucocutaneous pigmentation
Minocycline	Tetracycline	Binds to 30S ribosomal subunit blocking the binding of aminoacyl transfer RNA to the messenger RNA ribosomal complex thereby inhibiting protein synthesis	Bactericidal	• Nausea, diarrhea, abdominal pain • Headache, dizziness • Photosensitivity • Discolored teeth in children
Clarithromycin	Macrolide	Inhibits protein synthesis by binding to 50S	• Bactericidal • Single dose kills 74.9% of *M. leprae.* 28 and 56 days of treatment kill 99% and 99.9% of viable bacilli respectively	• Nausea, abdominal pain, diarrhea • Altered taste • Headache, psychosis • Hepatitis • QT prolongation
Rifabutine/ Rifapentine	Ansamycin	Inhibit DNA dependent RNA synthesis	• Bactericidal • Single dose of rifapentine kills 99.6% of *M. leprae* • Effective against rifampi-cin resistant strains • It has longer half-life and lesser MIC than rifampicin	Uveitis
Linezolid	Oxazolidinone	Inhibits protein synthesis	Bacteriostatic at lower doses and bactericidal at high doses (≥50 mg/kg)	–
Fusidic acid	Fusidanes	Inhibits protein synthesis by binding to elongation factor G	Bacteriostatic	–
Cephaloridine, cefuroxime and amoxicillin plus clavulanic acid	Beta-lactam antibiotics	Inhibits the synthesis of the peptidoglycan layer of bacterial cell wall	Bactericidal	–
Bedaquiline	Diarylquinoline	Targets the subunit C of mycobacterial ATP synthase	Bactericidal	–
Deoxyfructo-serotonin (DFS)	–	Not known	–	–

(ATP: adenosine tri phosphate; MI: morphological index; MIC: minimum inhibitory concentration)

TABLE 7: Pharmacokinetics of antileprosy drugs.

Antileprosy drug	*Oral bioavailability*	*Time to peak serum level*	*Elimination half-life*	*Metabolism*	*Excretion*	*Standard daily dose (mg)*
Rifampicin	90% Food reduces absorption by one-third	2–3 h (45–70 times the MIC)	12 h	De-acetylation and oxidation in liver	Urine, feces	600
Dapsone	70–80%	4–6 h (500–600 times the MIC)	10–50 h (mean: 28)	N-acetylation and N-hydroxylation in liver	Feces	100
Clofazimine	20–70%	1–6 h	*Short course:* 7 days *Long course:* 70 days	Hepatic	Urine, sebum, tears, sweat	300 mg MS 50 mg daily
Ofloxacin	98%	1–3 h	8–9 h	Hepatic	Urine	400
Moxifloxacin	86%	1–2.5 h	12 h	Hepatic	Urine, feces	400
Clarithromycin	50%	1–4 h	3–4 h	Hepatic	Urine, feces	500
Minocycline	95–100%	1–4 h (10–20 times the MIC)	11–22 h	Hepatic	Urine, feces	100

(MIC: minimum inhibitory concentration; MS: monthly supervised)

TABLE 8: Drug resistance to various antileprosy drugs.[4,12]

Drugs	*Year first reported*	*Mechanism*	*Frequency of drug-resistant mutants*	*Criteria for diagnosis in mouse foot pad studies [concentration in the diet (%)]*
Dapsone	1964	Missense mutations at codon 53 or 55 in *folP1* gene coding for enzyme dihydropteroate synthetase	1 in 10^6	• 0.0001 (low) • 0.001 (intermediate) • 0.01 (high)
Rifampicin	1976	Missense mutations within highly conserved regions in the *rpoB* gene which hinder rifampicin binding to the beta subunit of DNA dependent RNA polymerase	1 in 10^7	0.003–0.01
Clofazimine	1982	–	Extremely low	0.0001–0.001
Ofloxacin	1994	Mutations in *gyr A* gene which codes for enzyme gyrase	1 in 10^8	0.15

TABLE 9: Treatment regimens for drug-resistant leprosy.

	Treatment	
Resistance type	*First 6 months*	*Next 18 months*
Rifampicin	Ofloxacin 400 mg + Clarithromycin 500 mg or Minocycline 100 mg + Clofazimine 50 mg	Ofloxacin 400 mg or Minocycline 100 mg + Clofazimine 50 mg
Rifampicin and ofloxacin	Clarithromycin 500 mg + Minocycline 100 mg + Clofazimine 50 mg	Clarithromycin 500 mg or Minocycline 100 mg + Clofazimine 50 mg

Source: Adapted from WHO guidelines for the diagnosis, treatment and prevention of leprosy; 2018.[3]

MANAGEMENT OF LEPRA REACTION

Leprosy reactions are immune-mediated complications, seen in up to 50% of leprosy patients.[15] There are two types of reactions: type 1 (T1R, reversal or downgrading) and type 2 reactions [erythema nodosum leprosum (ENL)]. Reactions can cause rapid nerve damage resulting in anesthesia and weakness, which in turn increases risk of injury and deformity.[16]

Reactions can occur at presentation of disease, during treatment with MDT and sometimes following completion of MDT.[17]

TABLE 10: Diagnostic criteria for relapse.[13]

*Criteria**	*Definition*
Clinical	• Increase in size and extent of existing lesion(s) • Appearance of new lesion(s) • Erythema and infiltration in lesions that had completely subsided • Nerve involvement (thickening or tenderness)
Bacteriological	• *Baseline smear positive*: Increase in BI by 2+ over previous smears at any two sites at two examinations • *Baseline smear negative*: Positivity at any site at two examinations
Therapeutic	• If reversal reaction is suspected, administration of prednisolone at dose of 1 mg/kg/day results in subsidence of reaction in 2 months • But if symptoms do not subside or only partially subside or lesions persist or increase under the cover of steroids, then relapse should be suspected
Histopathological	• *PB cases*: Reappearance of already regressed/regressing granuloma • *MB cases*: Increased macrophage infiltration with solid staining bacilli and increasing BI
Serological	In LL cases, the measurement of PGL-1 IgM antibodies is a good indicator of relapse

*The first three criteria are sufficient to make a diagnosis of relapse; criteria 4 and 5 are additional, and may be used wherever facilities are available.
(MB: multibacillary; PB: paucibacillary; LL: lepromatous leprosy PGL: phenolic glycolipid 1; IgM: immunoglobulin M)

TABLE 11: Treatment of relapse.[13]

Previous treatment	*Scenario*	*Treatment plan*
Relapse after previous cure with dapsone monotherapy	Relapse with dapsone-resistant *M. leprae*	Standard WHO-MDT
Relapse after previous treatment with clofazimine monotherapy	Relapse with *M. leprae* sensitive to all standard drugs	Standard WHO-MDT
Relapse after a course of MB-MDT	Relapse with *M. leprae* sensitive to all standard drugs	Retreatment with WHO-MDT depending on the type of disease (PB or MB-MDT)
Primary or secondary dapsone-resistant MB cases who received standard WHO-MB-MDT but did not take clofazimine (equivalent to rifampicin monotherapy)	Relapse with rifampicin-resistant or rifampicin- and dapsone-resistant *M. leprae*	*First 6 months*: Ofloxacin 400 mg + Clarithromycin 500 mg or Minocycline 100 mg + Clofazimine 50 mg *For next 18 months:* Ofloxacin 400 mg or Minocycline 100 mg + Clofazimine 50 mg

BOX 1: Assessment of severity of type 1 reaction.

Mild reaction: No evidence of neuritis (pain, loss of sensation or function)

Severe reaction:
- Involvement of more number of existing skin, lesions
- Nerve pain, tenderness or paresthesia or nerve impairment
- Red skin plaques on the face, or overlying major trunk
- Fever, discomfort or arthralgia
- Edema of hands and/or feet
- Ulcerative skin lesion
- Reaction persisting for more than 6 weeks with usual dose of analgesics

TABLE 12: Dose of steroid recommended as per WHO in field purpose.

Dose of prednisolone	*Weeks of treatment*
40 mg daily	1st and 2nd week
30 mg daily	3rd and 4th week
20 mg daily	5th and 6th week
15 mg daily	7th and 8th week
10 mg daily	9th and 10th week
5 mg daily	11th and 12th week

Assessment of severity of type-1 reaction has been shown in **Box 1**.

Management of Type 1 Reaction

Mild reaction should be treated with analgesics, such as acetylsalicylic acid or paracetamol.

If there is nerve involvement, type 1 reactions should be treated with analgesics and corticosteroids, such as oral prednisolone.

Treatment of Type 1 Reaction

Treatment of type 1 reaction has been shown in **Table 12**.

- *Steroid dose in referral centers*:
  Start dose—40–60 mg daily (up to a maximum of 1 mg/kg).
  Tapering—reduced by 5 mg weekly or fortnightly after improvement of skin lesions and nerve tenderness subsides.
  Maintenance dose—15–20 mg for several months, then reduced by 5 mg for every 2–4 months.

Duration: BT—4-9-month, BB—6-12 month, BL—6-24 month

Adverse events:

- Skin changes—striae, steroid acne, purpura, ecchymosis, xerosis cushingoid features, hair loss
- GIT side effect such as hematemesis, peptic ulcer
- Metabolic complication—hypertension, hypokalemia, hyperlipidemia, secondary amenorrhea
- Ocular side effect—cataract, glaucoma
- Bone changes—osteoporosis, pathological fracture, and aseptic necrosis of bone
- CNS complication—psychosis and *Pseudotumor cerebri*
- Opportunistic infection—TB, chromoblastomycosis

Neuritis:

- Rest
- Splinting and padding
- Oil massage
- Short wave diathermy (SWD) or ultrasonic therapy (UST)
- Surgical decompression

Treatment of late reversal reaction: Prednisolone 1 mg/kg body weight per day for 4–6 weeks and steroid should be continued till complete subsidence of lesion

Type 2 lepra reactions (erythema nodosum leprosum), are associated with circulation and tissue deposition of immune complexes. They are an antibody response or immune complex response to *M. leprae* antigenic determinants which occur only in multibacillary leprosy.

Assessment of type 2 lepra reaction has been given in **Boxes 2 and 3** and treatment has been shown in **Tables 13 to 15**.

Neuritis: Neuritis is an acute inflammation of the nerves with nerve pain, local edema and rapid loss of function. Neuritis may occur before leprosy is diagnosed, during leprosy treatment, or up to several years after leprosy treatment has been completed.

Types and diagnosis of lepra neuritis have been shown in **Boxes 4 and 5**.

MANAGEMENT

Early detection and appropriate treatment of neuritis and lepra reactions is the key issue in leprosy management.

The principles of management of neuritis are:

- Continuing the treatment of leprosy (MDT)
- Treating complicating reactional states, i.e., type 1 and type 2 reactions
- Effective and prolonged anti-inflammatory therapy **(Table 16)**

BOX 2: Management of type 2 lepra reaction.

- *A:* Severity grading
- *B:* Treat precipitating factor such as intercurrent infection such as sore throat (streptococcal), viral, malaria, filaria or stress or medication
- *C:* Continue multidrug therapy (MDT)
- *D:* Specific treatment of type 2 reaction

BOX 3: Assessment of severity of type 2 lepra reaction.

Mild reaction: Only few erythema nodosum leprosum (ENL) lesions with no other organ involvement

Severe reaction:

- High fever, body pain, myalgia
- Extensive ENL with or without pustular/necrotic lesion
- Pain/tenderness of one or more nerve or loss of function
- Recent nerve function impairment
- Painful swelling of testes (Orchitis)
- Marked arthritis or lymphadenitis

TABLE 13: Treatment options for type 2 lepra reaction.

	Treatment	
Type 2 reaction	*Mild reaction*	*Severe reaction*
First episode For recurrent or chronic ENL	• Aspirin • Colchicine • Paracetamol	*Option-1: Prednisolone* (1 mg/kg body-weight till clinical improvement, then taper by 5–10 mg over 6–8 weeks) Maintenance dose of 20–40 mg needed for several weeks to prevent recurrence. OR *Prednisolone with clofazimine:* Not responding corticosteroid or whom corticosteroids are contraindicated *Option-2: Thalidomide* 200 mg BD for 3–7 days or till reaction is under control, followed by tapering within 3–4 weeks or slow tapering *Combination treatment is preferred:* • *Option-1:* Clofazimine + prednisolone • *Option-2:* Thalidomide + prednisolone

TABLE 14: Drugs used for type 2 lepra reaction.

Immunosuppressants	*Mechanism of action*	*Dose*	*Adverse effects*
Prednisolone	• Genomic—by modulating gene and protein synthesis • Non-genomic—by interacting cell surface receptors (responsible for early and anti-inflammatory effect)	• *Start dose:* 1 mg/kg bodyweight till clinical improvement, then taper by 5–10 mg over 6–8 weeks • *Maintenance dose:* 20–40 mg needed for several weeks to prevent recurrence	Striae, steroid acne, purpura, peptic ulcer, hematemesis cushingoid features glaucoma osteoporosis
Clofazimine	• Blocking DNA template function, by increasing lysosomal enzyme synthesis, and by increasing phagocytosis by macrophage • Stimulation of PGE2 synthesis, inhibition of neutrophilic motility and also inhibiting NFAT pathway	• *Start dose:* 300 mg daily (3 doses of 100 mg each) • Duration should not more than 12 months	Gastritis, skin hyperpigmentation, ichthyosis
Thalidomide	• Reduction of transcription of TNF-α, chemotactic factors and IgM synthesis • Reduction in CD4 lymphocytes and normalizes CD4/CD8 ratio • Inhibits inflammatory cytokines like IFN-, VEGF and FGF, IL-2 receptors, ICAM-1 expression on keratinocytes, inhibit NF-κβ activation	• *Start dose*: 200 mg BD for 3–7 days or till reaction is under control • *Maintenance dose*: Tapering within 3–4 weeks 100 mg morning + 200 mg evening for 4 weeks; 200 mg evening for 4 weeks f/b; 100 mg evening for 4 weeks; 50 mg daily evening or 100 mg alternate day for 8–12 weeks	Teratogenicity, neuropathy, thromboembolism, somnolence and rare cutaneous adverse reactions like erythema multiforme, erythroderma and toxic epidermal necrolysis

(NFAT: nuclear factor for activated T-cells; FGF: fibroblast growth factor; ICAM: intercellular adhesion molecule)

TABLE 15: Immunosuppressants used in treatment of lepra reaction.

Immunosuppressants	*Mechanism of action*	*Dose*
Methotrexate	Reduce production of Th1 cytokines and increase expression of anti- inflammatory Th2 cytokines	5–7.5 mg/week
Cyclosporine A	Inhibits transcription of interleukin 2 mRNA, there by blocking proliferation of T-cells Decrease anti-nerve factor antibody	5 mg/kg/day
Azathioprine	Inhibits T- and B-cell proliferation, antibody synthesis and TNF-α	0.5–1 mg/kg daily then increased to 2–2.5 mg/kg daily over 3–4 weeks
Mycophenolate mofetil	Reversible inosine monophosphate dehydrogenase responsible for T- and B-cell proliferation	1 g/day, may be increased to 2 g/day

BOX 4: Types of lepra neuritis.

- *Acute neuritis*: Neuritic pain or tenderness and/or swelling due to nerve access and/or recent onset neurological deficit of usually less than 6 months duration.
- *Chronic neuritis*: Neuritis presenting more than 6 months duration and presents with progressive neurological deficit with nerve tenderness or pain.
- *Recurrent neuritis*: An episode of neuritis recurring after a symptom-free interval of at least 3 months. It indicates poor prognosis.
- *Silent neuropathy*: Only neurological deficit, which is mostly progressive in the absence of nerve pain and tenderness with no evidence of reaction.
- *Subclinical neuropathy*: Patients have normal values for voluntary muscle testing and monofilament testing, but have impaired nerve conduction studies and/or warm detection threshold.[18] In a study, 16% of such patients subsequently developed clinical nerve function impairment.[19]
- *Catastrophic paralysis*: It is an emergency where development of sudden paralysis occurs.

BOX 5: Diagnosis of neuritis.

Clinical examination: Nerve examination—
- Nerve palpation is done to look for tenderness, thickening, consistency, and abscess formation.
- Nerve function assessment (NFA): Sensory function evaluation in the distribution of nerves for touch, pain and temperature. John et al. demonstrated that using 0.2 g and 4 g Semmes Weinstein filaments for sensory testing in the field would be a cost-effective method to enhance the prevention of disability by detecting nerve function impairment at an earlier stage.[20]

Investigations:
- *Fine needle aspiration (FNA):* A simple, quick, less invasive procedure which does not affect the nerve adversely and, therefore, can be done from any accessible nerve. It provided diagnostic aspirate in 67–92% patients in different studies.[21,22]
- Nerve biopsy.
- Electrophysiological studies.
- Laser Doppler flowmetry.
- *Nerve imaging:* High resolution sonography ultrasonography and color Doppler imaging provide objective measure of nerve dimensions and structural changes resulting from nerve damage and inflammation in leprosy.

TABLE 16: Anti-inflammatory therapy for neuritis.

Drugs	*Mechanism of action*	*Dose*
Corticosteroid	All neuritis <6 weeks should be treated	40–60 mg/day up to maximum 1 mg/kg body- weight
Clofazimine[23-25]	Reduces granulocyte chemotaxis and stabilizing lysosome membranes	300 mg in three divided doses for a maximum period of 12 weeks followed by gradual tapering
Thalidomide	Antitumor necrosis factor alpha (TNF-alpha) with immunomodulatory, anti-inflammatory effect	200 mg BD for 3–7 days followed by gradual tapering
Azathioprine	Inhibits T- and B-cell proliferation, antibody synthesis and TNF-α	3 mg/kg/day for 3 weeks

BOX 6: Chronic neuropathic pain management.

Tricyclic antidepressants (TCAs):
- Amitriptyline and nortriptyline
- Started at doses of 10–25 mg
- Escalation is done every 3–7 days till adequate pain relief

Anticonvulsants:
- *Carbamazepine:* Started at dose of 100 mg daily and escalation of drug dose is by 100 mg after every 3–5 days.
- Adequate pain relief is usually attained at doses of 400–600 mg daily
- *Gabapentin:* Started at dosage of 300 mg daily at bed time. The dose is escalated by 300 mg every 1–3 days till a maximum dose of 3,600 mg. The most common adverse effects are vertigo, tiredness and edema.
- *Pregabalin*: Started at dose of 150 mg daily at bed time and the dose can be up to 450 mg/day. Dizziness, drowsiness, ataxia and peripheral edema are uncommon side effects. Rarely neutropenia has been reported.
- *Opioids:* Tramadol is a weak opioid with proven efficacy in neuropathic pain. It produces little dependence and tolerance.

- Physical therapy and rest during the phase of active neuritis
- Surgery when indicated
- Physiotherapy during recovery phase **(Box 6)**.

SURGERY

The important indications are:[26]
- No improvement or deterioration while on steroids for several weeks, particularly in cases presenting with symptoms of more than 3 months duration.
- Nerve abscess.
- Intractable pain despite adequate dose of anti-inflammatory drugs and vigorous immunosuppressive therapy.
- Increasing pain while receiving MDT and corticosteroid treatment for NFI.

Mechanism: Axonal damage is due to the inflammatory response of the body against *M. leprae* and ischemia. Ischemia is the result of increased intraneural pressure compromising the blood flow in vasa nervorum. The affected nerve is swollen and is unable to accommodate edema in the rigid fibro-osseous channels with limited space, resulting in increased external pressure and obstructing the axoplasmic flow. Surgeries relieve the mechanical compression, restoring the blood flow and functioning of nerve axonal cylinders. Intervention with surgery and early steroid use results in complete recovery or arrest of progression of damage **(Box 7)**.[28]

NEWER APPROACHES OF TREATMENT

- Drugs and vaccines blocking the attachment of mycobacteria to the Schwann cell-axon unit: With the identification of neural targets on Schwann cells and the specific bacterial component responsible for neural tropism, agents blocking the attachment of the two can be designed.[27] These agents would prevent the entry of bacilli into the nerve.

BOX 7: Types of surgeries.[29,30]

- *Extra-neural neurolysis*: It is a decompression surgery in which constricting fibrous bands and ligaments are excised and rigid fibro-osseous channels opened.
  It relieves the external pressure only.
  All the vessels supplying nerve should be carefully saved and the nerve should not be subjected to undue trauma or tension or traction or displacement from its bed.
- *Intraneural neurolysis or longitudinal epineurotomy:* Longitudinal incisions are given in the sheath of the nerve trunk, i.e., epineurium taking care not to injure the vasa nervorum. It has to be preceded by extra-neural neurolysis.
- *Interfascicular neurolysis*: Individual nerve bundles are dissected and separated. It is now almost abandoned as it damages the nerve tissue and its vascularity producing fibrosis.[26,27]
- *Nerve abscess drainage*: Nerve abscess should always be drained. Longitudinal incision is given over abscess and then all the caseous liquid material is drained.
- *Nerve transposition by means of medial epicondylectomy*: It is done for the ulnar nerve at elbow. The objective is to avoid stretching of the nerve with movement of the elbow joint to increase the blood supply and protecting it from injury by burying it into the muscles.

- *Neurotropic factors (NTFs):* Schwann cells play significant role in the maintenance and regeneration of axons of the neurons in the peripheral nervous system. These cells are regulated by NTFs.

KEY POINTS

- Management of leprosy involves treatment of the infection, complications, and the special situations such as resistance, relapse, etc.
- History of antileprosy drugs includes from dapsone monotherapy to fully evolved MDT.
- WHO classifies leprosy patients into: Paucibacillary (PB) and multibacillary (MB) cases. The latest WHO guidelines recommend MDT for all leprosy patients with the total duration of 6 months for PB and 12 months for MB cases.
- Rifampicin, dapsone, and clofazimine are first line drugs used as multidrug therapy (MDT).
- Newer antileprosy drugs increase the compliance with the treatment, e.g., ROM trial (**R**ifampicin 600 mg, **O**floxacin 400 mg, **M**inocycline 100 mg), and PMM trial (Rifa**P**entine 900 mg **M**oxifloxacin 400 mg **M**inocycline 100 mg).
- Recently uniform MDT (U-MDT) has been proposed by WHO. for 6 months in both PB and MB cases.
- Leprosy reactions are immune-mediated complications that may develop before, during or after MDT. They are type 1 and type 2 reactions and can present as mild or severe reaction.
- Treatment of reactions includes MDT along with control of reaction by immunosuppressants such as corticosteroid, thalidomide and rarely methotrexate, clofazimine, and azathioprine.
- Treatment of neuritis includes physical therapy and rest during the phase of active neuritis, effective and prolonged anti-inflammatory therapy (corticosteroid), chronic pain management by tricyclic anti-depressants (nortriptyline), surgery when indicated and physiotherapy during recovery phase.

REFERENCES

1. World Health Organization (WHO). WHO expert committee on leprosy: Eighth report. World Health Organ Tech Rep Ser. 2012;968:1-61.
2. Pai VV, Rao RR, Halwai V. Chemotherapy: development and evolution of WHO-MDT and newer treatment regimens. In: Kumar B, Kar KH (Eds). IAL Textbook of Leprosy, 2nd edition. New Delhi: Jaypee Brothers Medical Publishers; 2016. pp. 448-62.
3. World Health Organization (WHO). Guidelines for the diagnosis, treatment and prevention of leprosy; 2018.
4. Kar HK, Gupta R. Treatment of leprosy. Clin Dermatol. 2015;33:55-65.
5. Edhegard K, Hall PR. Dapsone. In: Wolverton SE (Ed). Comprehensive Dermatology Drug Therapy, 3rd edition. Philadelphia: WB Saunders; 2007. pp. 228-40.
6. Kim S, Michel DB, Kim KG, Rosso DQJ. Systemic antibacterial agents. In: Wolverton SE (Ed). Comprehensive Dermatology Drug Therapy, 3rd edition. Philadelphia: WB Saunders; 2007. pp. 67-97.
7. Jopling WH, McDougall AC. Chemotherapy. In: Jopling WH, McDougall AC (Eds). Handbook of Leprosy, 5th edition. New Delhi: CBS Publishers and Distributors; 2008. pp. 101-14.
8. Girdhar A, Kumar A, Girdhar BK. A randomised controlled trial assessing the effect of adding clarithromycin to rifampicin, ofloxacin and minocycline in the treatment of single lesion paucibacillary leprosy in Agra District, India. Lepr Rev. 2011;82(1):46.
9. Pattyn S, Grillone S. Relapse rates and a 10-year follow-up of a 6-week quadruple drug regimen for multibacillary leprosy. Lepr Rev. 2002;73:245-7.
10. Pratap D. Comparative study of uniform-MDT and WHO-MDT in pauci- and multibacillary leprosy patients over 24 months of observation. Lepr Rev. 2009;80:143-55.
11. Saunderson RP. Chemotherapy of leprosy. In: Kumar B, Kar KH (Eds). IAL Textbook of Leprosy, 2nd edition. New Delhi: Jaypee Brothers Medical Publishers; 2016. pp. 441-7.
12. Matsuoka M. Drug resistance in leprosy. In: Kumar B, Kar KH (Eds). IAL Textbook of Leprosy, 2nd edition. New Delhi: Jaypee Brothers Medical Publishers; 2016. pp. 573-9.
13. Thappa DM, Kaimal S, Gupta D. Relapse in leprosy. In: Kumar B, Kar KH (Eds). IAL Textbook of Leprosy, 2nd edition. New Delhi: Jaypee Brothers Medical Publishers; 2016. pp. 562-71.
14. Rao PSS. A study on non-adherence to MDT among leprosy patients. Indian J Lepr. 2008;80:149-54.

15. Scollard DM, Adams LB, Gillis TP, Krahenbuhl JL, Truman RW, Williams DL. The continuing challenges of leprosy. Clin Microbiol Rev. 2006;19:338-81.
16. Saunderson P. How to Recognise and Manage Leprosy Reactions. International Federation of Anti-Leprosy Associations; 2002. p. 52.
17. Britton WJ, Lockwood DNJ. Leprosy. Lancet. 2004;363:1209-19.
18. Wagenaar I, Brandsma W, Post E, Brakel WV, Lockwood D, Nicholls P, et al. Two randomized controlled clinical trials to study the effectiveness of prednisolone treatment in preventing and restoring clinical nerve function loss in leprosy: the TENLEP study protocols. BMC Neurol. 2012;12:159.
19. Van Brakel WH, Nicholls PG, Wilder-Smith EP, Das L, Barkataki P, Lockwood DNJ, et al. Early diagnosis of neuropathy in leprosy—comparing diagnostic tests in a large prospective study (the INFIR cohort study). PLoS Negl Trop Dis. 2008;2:e212.
20. John AS, Rao PS, Pitchaimani G. Early detection of sensory nerve function impairments in the field. International Leprosy Congress: Hidden challenges; 2013 September 16 - September 19; Brussels, Belgium.
21. Vijaikumar M, D'Souza M, Kumar S, Badhe B. Fine needle aspiration cytology (FNAC) of nerves in leprosy. Lepr Rev. 2001; 72:171-8.
22. Jayaseelan E, Shariff S, Rout P. Cytodiagnosis of primary neuritic leprosy. Int J Lepr Other Mycobact Dis. 1999;67:429-34.
23. Ross WF. Does clofazimine have any value in the management of reversal reaction? Lepr Rev. 1980;51:92-3.
24. Imkamp FM. Clofazimine (lamprene or B663) in lepra reactions. Lepr Rev. 1981;52:135-40.
25. Pfaltzgraff RE. The control of neuritis in leprosy with clofazimine. Int J Lepr Other Mycobact Dis. 1972;40:392-8.
26. Nickerson DS, Nickerson DE. A review of therapeutic nerve decompression for neuropathy in Hansen's disease with research suggestions. J Reconstr Microsurg. 2010;26:277-84.
27. Husain S, Mishra B, Prakash V, Malaviya GN. Results of surgical decompression of ulnar nerve in leprosy. Acta Leprol. 1998;11:17-20.
28. Rambukkana A. Molecular basis of the interaction of *Mycobacterium leprae* with peripheral nerve: implications for therapeutic strategies. Lepr Rev. 2000;71(Suppl):S168-9.
29. Malaviya GN. Shall we continue with nerve trunk decompression in leprosy? Indian J Lepr. 2004;76:331-42.
30. Virmond M, Garbino JA, Cury Filho M. Proposal for a prospective, randomized trial to determine the role of nerve decompression in leprosy neuropathy. Manila: International Leprosy Congress; 2013. p. 304.

EXAMINATION QUESTIONS

Describe the following (Long answers):

1. Describe the treatment guideline for management of leprosy cases. Describe mechanisms and side effects of antileprosy drugs.
2. What is definition of relapse? Describe treatment of a relapse case of leprosy.
3. What is U-MDT? Describe newer drugs in leprosy.
4. What is type 1 reaction? Discuss the management of type 1 reaction.
5. What is erythema nodosum leprosum? Describe the management of type 2 reaction.
6. Discuss types and management of leprosy neuritis.

Write short notes on the following:

7. ROM regimen.
8. Uniform MDT (U-MDT).
9. Erythema nodosum leprosum.
10. Newer antileprosy drugs.
11. Thalidomide.
12. Clofazimine.
13. Drug-resistant leprosy.
14. Dapsone.
15. Lepra reaction.

120 CHAPTER

Newer Drugs and Regimens in Leprosy

Dipayan Sengupta

INTRODUCTION

After the introduction of multidrug therapy (MDT) by World Health Organization (WHO) in 1982, it has become the default treatment in India and many other countries for the management of leprosy. MDT achieved its most significant milestone in 2005 when leprosy elimination target was met in India. However, research on newer treatment regimen did continue because certain limitations on MDT such as long treatment duration and compliance-related issues were widely understood. Also like any infectious disease, the possibility of a vaccine has received significant attention in the recent past.

Apart from the drugs used in standard WHO MDT regimens, few other drugs have been proved to be efficacious in various trials. Few of them are:

- *Bacteriostatic:* Brodimoprim, K 130, fusidic acid, etc.
- *Bactericidal:* Fluoroquinolones such as moxifloxacin or ofloxacin, minocycline, clarithromycin, rifapentine, amoxicillin, and clavulanic acid.

However, as because MDT has been so widely adopted and successful, any new drug or regimen must go through proper evaluation in order to be adopted mainstream. In this chapter, we will briefly discuss some of the successful regimens that have been compared with standard MDT either as alternative or as an adjuvant and the relative merits of each of the regimens. We have excluded regimens from the pre-MDT era from our discussion because they no longer have any practical importance.

PAUCIBACILLARY LEPROSY

Among the various new regimens tried for paucibacillary (PB) leprosy, rifampicin, ofloxacin, and minocycline (ROM) therapy has been most widely studied. Some other notable regimens are also discussed.

Rifampicin, Ofloxacin, and Minocycline Therapy

A well-tested alternative to WHO MDT for PB leprosy is ROM therapy which consists of only one single dose of rifampicin (600 mg), ofloxacin (400 mg), and minocycline (100 mg). It is an attractive option, especially in rural settings where disease-related stigma is high. Multiple studies have shown comparable clinical cure with WHO regimen at least for single lesion PB leprosy,[1] one to three lesions,[2] and two to three lesions.[3] Though one study found more relapse rate in ROM regimen.[4] However, no such difference was observed in subsequent studies with much longer follow-up period.[5] It is worth noting that one Indian study found that ROM is somehow less effective if the number of lesions is three or more.[1]

In conclusion, ROM therapy seems to have similar efficacy compared to WHO MDT and can be considered as an operationally much simpler option at least when the number of lesions is less than three.

Other Notable Regimens

Some other regimens that have been tried in various trials to compare them with standard WHO MDT are discussed here.[6]

- Universal MDT (U-MDT) is a regimen that takes the WHO multibacillary (MB) leprosy regimen, but continues it only for 6 months. It is supposed to cover both PB and MB cases. For PB cases, U-MDT has shown better results compared to WHO MDT but it was not statistically significant.
- A regimen was tried consisting of rifampicin 1,500 mg at the onset supervised, and repeated after 3 months and dapsone 100 mg daily for 6 months. It has shown slightly faster clinical resolution compared to standard regimen though it was not statistically significant.
- A daily rifampicin (600 mg) plus ofloxacin (400 mg) for 28 days regimen was shown to have similar efficacy compared to WHO regimen for PB leprosy.
- Addition of daily clofazimine 50 mg to existing MDT PB regimen did not improve the outcome significantly.

MULTIBACILLARY LEPROSY

Because of so many regimens have been compared with WHO MDT, we have classified them according to their results (in terms of whether they have shown better, similar, or inferior clinical outcomes that was measured).[6]

No Significant Difference

- Additional clofazimine 100 mg/day for 12 months did not decrease the chances of erythema nodosum leprosum (ENL). However, steroid-related deaths decreased though it was not statistically significant.

- 600 mg rifampicin and 300 mg of clofazimine given under supervision on two consecutive days monthly, 225 mg injection of acedapsone bimonthly, and dapsone 100 mg daily.
- Additional 1 month of daily ofloxacin therapy.
- 24 months of MDT. However, it has shown less severe reactions notably ENL.
- Clarithromycin 2,000 mg can be used instead of rifampicin 600 mg. One study showed more reduction of bacteriological index at the initial 3 months.
- Ofloxacin can also be used in places of rifampicin.
- Daily rifampicin therapy can result in greater reduction of bacillary indices (BI), but it is difficult to put into practice because of its higher cost.
- Addition of levamisole does not have any additional positive effect over standard MDT regimen.

Inferior Result

Once daily rifampicin and ofloxacin for only 1 month. It resulted in higher chances of relapse even after 5 years after therapy.

Similar Efficacy to WHO MDT but Operationally Simpler

- Daily rifampicin 600 mg, sparfloxacin 200 mg, clarithromycin 500 mg, and minocycline 100 mg for 12 weeks.
- Monthly ROM therapy for 24 months (compared with 24 months of WHO MDT). It has shown similar result to that of WHO MDT.

Results were Controversial in Different Studies

A U-MDT regimen similar to WHO MDT (MB) regimen, but only for 6 months duration has been tried also for MB leprosy. Though the relapse was more, it was not statistically significant. The chances of reaction were also comparable. However, an Indian study shown that the result was significantly poor compared to WHO MDT.

CHEMOPROPHYLAXIS

In the post-MDT era, the most studied chemoprophylaxis is single-dose rifampicin (SDR). It has been started as a leprosy post-exposure prophylaxis (LPEP) program in multiple countries including India. As per interim report, it seems to be safe and effective.[7] Also a recent randomized controlled trial (RCT) (MALTALEP trial) has shown reduced incidence of leprosy (by 42%) when SDR was given after Bacillus Calmette-Guérin (BCG) vaccination.[8] Other possible candidates for chemoprophylaxis trial are rifapentine, moxifloxacin, and clindamycin though each of them has their own set of drawbacks.

IMMUNOPROPHYLAXIS AND FUTURE PROSPECTS

Several vaccines have been proposed and tried in the past and some interesting ones are in the pipeline. Some notable candidates worth mentioning are discussed here in brief.

- *International Committee of the Red Cross (ICRC) vaccine*: The oldest "leprosy vaccine" was derived from ICRC bacillus that showed cross reactivity with *Mycobacterium leprae*. When given at the initiation of MDT therapy, it resulted in more reduction of bacteriological index in a small trial.[9]
- *Mycobacterium indicus pranii (MIP) vaccine*: It was based on the antigens from MIP (previously known as *Mycobacterium w*) and has been successfully used as an adjuvant therapy along with MDT MB.[10] It is now commercially available as Immuvac. Apart from its effect on leprosy, it has shown to have a positive effect on some other diseases such as verruca. It has also been used for immunoprophylaxis. The protection seems to sustain around 7–8 years.[11]
- *BCG and similar*: Because *Mycobacterium tuberculosis* and *M. leprae* contain similar genetic regions. A single vaccine could theoretically protect against both diseases. In the past, BCG vaccine was thought to be such a candidate but the result was insufficient. A meta-analysis of various studies involving BCG as a protective agent showed 20–90% results and the effect seems to be diminishing with age.[12] However, a number of possible tuberculosis (TB) vaccine candidates are in the pipeline (most notably Ag85A and Ag85B) and most of them shares orthologous genetic region with *M. leprae*. A detailed discussion about them can be found here.[13]
- *LepVax*: It is a recombinant protein composed of four *M. laprae* antigens[13] and another strong candidate for leprosy vaccine. It has recently completed phase 1 safety trial and now considered to be both safe and adequately immunogenic for healthy individuals.[14]

CONCLUSION

In this chapter, we have briefly discussed some interesting new regimen that can be tried instead of or as an adjuvant with standard WHO MDT. Some of them seem to be quite effective and operationally simpler, though more studies are required to confirm their effectiveness and long-term results. Of course, ROM therapy needs special mention as it is probably the most studied regimen and is proved to be quite useful in PB leprosy with small number of lesions. However, most regimens could not offer any significant benefit over standard MDT regimen. Several vaccines also have been tried and some exciting ones like LepVax is currently under trial.

KEY POINTS

- Though MDT is mostly successful, it is operationally complex. To overcome this, newer regimens have been tried for both PB and MB leprosy.
- Among the paucibacillary regimens, ROM therapy is most well studied and simple to administer. Efficacy is comparable to WHO MDT regimen.
- Among multibacillary regimens, some are at least of equal efficacy but operationally simpler. However, more studies are required to confirm long-term result.
- In the post-MDT era, the most promising chemoprophylaxis is single dose rifampicin.
- Several vaccines including BCG have been tried for immunoprophylaxis. Newer vaccine candidates like LepVax is under trial.

REFERENCES

1. Efficacy of single dose multidrug therapy for the treatment of single-lesion paucibacillary leprosy. Single-lesion Multicentre Trial Group. Indian J Lepr. 1997;69(2):121-9.
2. Deshmukh AR, Dhurat RS, Jerajani HR. A comparative clinico-pathological study of single dose ROM in paucibacillary leprosy patients with 1–3 skin lesions. Indian J Lepr. 2003;75(3):209-17.
3. Emmanuel M, Gupte MD. Lesional characteristics and histopathology in paucibacillary leprosy patients with 2 or 3 skin lesions: comparison between ROM and PB-MDT regimens. Indian J Lepr. 2005;77(1):19-25.
4. Manickam P, Nagaraju B, Selvaraj V, Balasubramanyam S, Mahalingam VN, Mehendale SM, et al. Efficacy of single-dose chemotherapy (rifampicin, ofloxacin and minocycline-ROM) in PB leprosy patients with 2 to 5 skin lesions, India: randomised double-blind trial. Indian J Lepr. 2012;84(3): 195-207.
5. Kumar A, Girdhar A, Girdhar BK. A randomized controlled trial to compare cure and relapse rate of paucibacillary multidrug therapy with monthly rifampicin, ofloxacin, and minocycline among paucibacillary leprosy patients in Agra District, India. Indian J Dermatol Venereol Leprol. 2015;81:356-62.
6. Lazo-Porras M, Prutsky GJ, Barrionuevo P, Tapia JC, Ugarte-Gil C, Ponce OJ, et al. World Health Organization (WHO) antibiotic regimen against other regimens for the treatment of leprosy: a systematic review and meta-analysis. BMC Infect Dis. 2020;20(1):62.
7. Steinmann P, Cavaliero A, Aerts A, Anand S, Arif M, Ay SS, et al. The Leprosy Post-Exposure Prophylaxis (LPEP) programme: update and interim analysis. Lepr Rev. 2018; 89:102-16.
8. Richardus R, Alam K, Kundu K, Roy JC, Zafar T, Chowdhury AS, et al. Effectiveness of single-dose rifampicin after BCG vaccination to prevent leprosy in close contacts of patients with newly diagnosed leprosy: a cluster randomized controlled trial. Int J Infect Dis. 2019;88:65-72.
9. Bhatki WS, Chulawala RG. Immunotherapeutic potential of ICRC vaccine: a case control study. Lepr Rev. 1992;63(4): 358-64.
10. Talwar GP, Gupta JC. Launching of immunization with the vaccine *Mycobacterium indicus pranii* for eradication of leprosy in India. Int J Vaccine Res. 2017;2(3):1-5.
11. Talwar G, Sarathchandra K, Walia R, Parida S, Pandey R, Rani R, et al. Immunoprophylactic effects of the anti-leprosy Mw vaccine in household contacts of leprosy patients: clinical field trials with a follow up of 8–10 years. Lepr Rev. 2005;76:127-43.
12. Merle CS, Cunha SS, Rodrigues LC. BCG vaccination and leprosy protection: review of current evidence and status of BCG in leprosy control. Expert Rev Vaccines. 2010;9(2): 209-22.
13. Coppola M, van den Eeden SJ, Robbins N, Wilson L, Franken KL, Adams LB, et al. Vaccines for leprosy and tuberculosis: opportunities for shared research, development, and application. Front immunol. 2018;9:308.
14. Duthie MS, Frevol A, Day T, Coler RN, Vergara J, Rolf T, et al. A phase 1 antigen dose escalation trial to evaluate safety, tolerability and immunogenicity of the leprosy vaccine candidate LepVax (LEP-F1 + GLA-SE) in healthy adults. Vaccine. 2020;38(7):1700-7.

EXAMINATION QUESTIONS

1. Describe the newer regimens in leprosy.

Write short notes on the following:

2. Chemoprophylaxis in leprosy.
3. ROM therapy.
4. Leprosy vaccines.

121 CHAPTER

National Leprosy Eradication Programme

Arnab Dutta, Abhishek De, Aarti Sarda

INTRODUCTION

In India, the National Leprosy Eradication Programme (NLEP) is the centrally sponsored health scheme of the Ministry of Health and Family Welfare, Government of India. While the NLEP strategies and plans are formulated centrally, the program is implemented by states and union territories (UTs). The program is also supported by World Health Organization (WHO), International Federation of Anti-Leprosy Associations (ILEP), and few other nongovernmental organizations (NGOs).

HISTORY

The National Leprosy Control Programme (NLCP) has been in operation since 1955, as a centrally aided program to achieve control of leprosy. In 1980, the Government of India declared its resolve to "eradicate" leprosy by the year 2000 and constituted a Working Group to advise accordingly. Multidrug therapy (MDT) was introduced in 1982. In 1983, the strategies for leprosy control were changed and NLEP was launched. A revised strategy has been recommended based on multidrug chemotherapy aimed at leprosy "eradication" through reduction in the quantum of infection in the population.[1]

In 1991, the World Health Assembly resolved to eliminate leprosy at a global level by the year 2000. In order to strengthen the process of elimination in the country, the first World Bank-supported project was introduced in India in 1993 and completed in 2000. The second World Bank-supported project happened between 2001 and 2002. In 2005, due to the declining number of leprosy cases, the goal of NLEP was declared as elimination of leprosy at the national level. In 2009, a special action plan for 209 high endemic districts in 16 states/UTs was made. Timeline for NLEP is given in **Box 1**.

GLOBAL LEPROSY SITUATION

The WHO launched a 5-year "Global Leprosy Strategy 2016–2020" in April 2016 titled "accelerating towards a leprosy-free world".[2] Challenges that remains in global leprosy elimination are focus of high leprosy prevalence in subnational level, continued delay in detecting new patients, persisting discrimination against people affected by leprosy, and limited impact on transmission of leprosy.

The strategy is built around three pillars: (1) to strengthen government ownership, coordination, and partnership; (2) to stop leprosy and its complications; and (3) to stop discrimination and promote inclusion.

The global prevalence at the end of 2016 was 171,948 with a registered prevalence rate (PR) of 0.23 per 10,000 population, a decrease from that in 2015. The new case detection in the year, however, was 214,783, a marginal increase compared to 2015.[3]

BOX 1: Timeline for NLEP.

- 1955—National Leprosy Control Programme (NLCP)
- 1982—Launch of multidrug therapy (MDT)
- 1983—Launch of National Leprosy Eradication Programme (NLEP)
- 2005—The goal of NLEP was declared as elimination of leprosy
- 2009—Special action plan for 209 high endemic districts

CURRENT ELIMINATION STATUS IN INDIA

The program in India saw a reduction from a PR of 57.8/10,000 in 1983 to less than 1/10,000 by the end of 2005 when India declared to have reached the WHO target of elimination as a public health problem.

A total of 34 states/UTs achieved the status of leprosy elimination. Only two states/UTs viz. Chhattisgarh and Dadra and Nagar Haveli are yet to achieve elimination. Bihar, Goa, Chandigarh, and Odisha, who have achieved elimination status earlier, show PR > 1 per 1,000 population.[3]

COMPONENTS OF NATIONAL LEPROSY ERADICATION PROGRAMME[1]

- Decentralized integrated leprosy services through general healthcare system.
- Capacity building of all general health services functionaries.
- Intensified information, education, and communication.
- Prevention of disability and medical rehabilitation.
- Intensified monitoring and supervision.

MAJOR INITIATIVES IN NATIONAL LEPROSY ERADICATION PROGRAMME

- More focus has now been given to new case detection.
- Treatment completion rate has been taken as an important indicator.

- Dressing materials, supportive medicines, and ulcer kits are provided to leprosy affected persons with ulcers and wounds.
- Microcellular rubber footwear is provided for protection of insensitive feet.
- An amount of ₹ 5,000/- is provided as incentive to each leprosy affected person from Below Poverty Line (BPL) family undergoing reconstructive surgery.
- Support is also provided to government institutions/Physical Medicine and Rehabilitation (PMR) centers in the form of ₹ 5,000/- per reconstructive surgery conducted.
- To facilitate the involvement of Accredited Social Health Activist (ASHA)[1] in the program, they are being paid incentive money as below: (1) On confirmed diagnosis of case brought by them—₹ 250/-; (2) On completion of full course of treatment of the case within specified time—paucibacillary (PB) leprosy case—₹ 400/-; and multibacillary (MB) leprosy case—₹ 600/-, (3) An early case before onset of any visible deformity—₹ 250/-; (4) A new case with visible deformity in hands, feet or eye—₹ 200/-.

REFERRAL SYSTEM IN NATIONAL LEPROSY ERADICATION PROGRAMME

The primary level care institutions are all Primary Health Centers (PHCs), Community Health Centers (CHCs), subdivisional hospitals, and urban leprosy centers/dispensaries.

The secondary level care institutions are all District Headquarter Hospitals and District Nucleus Units.

The tertiary level care institutions are:

- Central Government Institutes [Central Leprosy Teaching and Research Institute (CLTRI) Chengalpattu and Regional Leprosy Training and Research Institute (RLTRI) at Aska/Gauripur/Raipur).
- Indian Council of Medical Research (ICMR) institute JALMA, Agra.
- ILEP supported leprosy hospitals.
- All PMR institutes and departments of medical colleges.

PROGRAM IMPLEMENTATION PLAN FOR 12TH PLAN PERIOD (2012–2013 TO 2016–2017) (TABLE 1)[2]

As the disease is still prevalent with moderate endemicity in about 15% of the country, the plan objectives are set as follows:

- Elimination of leprosy, i.e., prevalence of less than 1 case per 10,000 population in all districts of the country.
- Strengthen disability prevention and medical rehabilitation of persons affected by leprosy.
- Reduction in the level of stigma associated with leprosy.[4,5]

NIKUSTH

National Leprosy Eradication Programme has launched "Nikusth," a web-based reporting system for the ease of reporting and data management of registered leprosy cases.[3] In addition, "Nikusth" will be helpful in keeping track of all the activities being implemented under the NLEP.[6]

CHEMOPROPHYLAXIS OF CONTACTS

Studies have shown that the chance of finding an undetected leprosy patient is 10 times higher in household contacts of leprosy patients than in the general population. Leprosy post-exposure prophylaxis (LPEP) was launched globally in the year 2014. The program has three prime components—contact tracing, screening, and single-dose rifampicin (SDR) administration.[7]

Chemoprophylaxis with SDR has a 57% overall risk reduction in preventing the development of leprosy for household contacts at least for the first 2 years.

MYCOBACTERIUM INDICUS PRANII IMMUNOPROPHYLACTIC VACCINE

Mycobacterium indicus pranii (MIP) vaccine has both immunotherapeutic and immunoprophylactic effects in MB leprosy patients.

TABLE 1: Targets for the plan period 2012–2013 to 2016–2017.

Indicators	*Baseline (2011–2012)*	*Targets (by March 2017)*
Prevalence rate (PR) < 1/10,000	543 districts (84.6%)	642 districts (100%)
Annual new case detection rate (ANCDR) < 10/100,000 population	445 districts (69.3%)	642 districts (100%)
Cure rate multibacillary (MB) leprosy cases	90.56%	>95%
Cure rate paucibacillary (PB) leprosy cases	95.28%	>97%
Grade II disability rate in percentage of new cases	3.04%*	2% (35% reduction)
Stigma reduction	Percentage reported (NSS 2010–2011)**	50% reduction over the percentage reported by NSS

*Grade II disability rate among new cases per million population to be reduced by 35%, i.e., from 3 (2011–2012) to 2 per million population by end of the 12th plan.
**Based on the National Sample Survey (NSS) report, 2010–2011.

The ICMR and NLEP has started a new project where an index leprosy patient will receive the MIP vaccine over and above the MDT and also his family members and contacts would be immunized with MIP twice at an interval of 6 months.

AREAS OF CONCERN

- The use of term "elimination" is somewhat confusing among common public and even among medical professional.
- There is no decline in occurrence of new leprosy cases in India over last decade.
- Over the last two decades, there was reallocation of resources and a gradual decline in funding for leprosy related programs.
- Leprosy health workers were made multipurpose workers with additional responsibilities of human immunodeficiency virus (HIV) and tuberculosis control.
- Inadequate monitoring could lead to a reduction in early diagnosis, a delay in initiation of MDT, and an increase in disability rates.
- Doing away with skin smear services, efforts towards further reducing the duration of therapy and reduced attention to research can reverse some of the program's achievements.

CONCLUSION

National Leprosy Eradication Programme is aimed at increase in coverage for leprosy services to one of sustaining quality services, and from centralization to decentralization.[5]

KEY POINTS

- Main component of NLEP is decentralized integrated leprosy services through general healthcare system.
- Treatment completion rate has been taken as an important indicator.
- Objective of NLEP is elimination of leprosy, i.e., prevalence of less than 1 case per 10,000 population in all districts of the country.
- Dressing materials, supportive medicines, and ulcer kits are provided to leprosy affected persons with ulcers and wounds under NLEP scheme.

REFERENCES

1. Park K. Health programmes in India. In: Park K (Ed). Park's Textbook of Preventive and Social Medicine, 25th edition. Jabalpur: M/s Banarsidas Bhanot Publishers; 2019. pp. 454-7.
2. World Health Organization. Global Leprosy Strategy 2016–2020: Accelerating towards a leprosy-free world. New Delhi: World Health Organization, Regional Office for South-East Asia; 2016.
3. Rao PN, Suneetha S. Current situation of leprosy in India and its future implications. Indian Dermatol Online J. 2018;9: 83-9.
4. Ministry of Health and Family Welfare. NLEP Annual Report 2015–2016. New Delhi: Central Leprosy Division, Directorate General of Health Services, Ministry of Health and Family Welfare, Government of India; 2017.
5. NLEP DDG Leprosy: Office Memorandum on 3 pronged strategies for Early Case Detection; 2016.
6. Sasakawa Health Foundation (2016). WHO Goodwill Ambassador's Newsletter No 80. [online] Available from https://www.shf.or.jp/wsmhfp/wp-content/uploads/2019/03/nl080.pdf?lang=en [Last accessed January, 2021].
7. Novartis foundation. Leprosy Post-Exposure Prophylaxis (LPEP) Program. [online] Available from https://www.novartisfoundation.org/sites/arctic_novartisfoundation/files/2020-11/novartis-foundation-factsheet-september.pdf [Last accessed January, 2021].

EXAMINATION QUESTIONS

1. Write a short note on NLEP.
2. Discuss newer treatment advances of NLEP.

122 CHAPTER

Deformity, Disability, and Rehabilitation in Leprosy

Deepika Halder, Abhishek De, Aarti Sarda

INTRODUCTION

Leprosy causes deformity and disabilities but seldom kills. These deformities cause an impact on personal, family, and social life as a whole like aversion, hatred, fear, stigma, and discrimination, and ultimately socioeconomic dehabilitation. Newer drugs and new treatment regimens can completely cure leprosy patients in 6–12 months without any disabilities. The most serious consequences of cured leprosy patients are caused by permanent peripheral nerve function impairments. Deformity is defined as visible impairment or visible consequence of impairment inside the body. Primary impairments are specific and paralytic deformities whereas "anesthetic deformities" are secondary impairments. Disability is the functional consequence of deformity. Limitation and prevention from fulfilling the normal daily activities is known as handicaps. Rehabilitation is the process intended to enable people to maintain optimal physical, psychological, and social functions with disabilities.

DEFORMITIES

Introduction

- *Definition of deformity*: A deformity is a structural, usually visible impairment **(Box 1)**.
- Deformities are found in approximately 20–25% of leprosy patients.
- The factors implicated in the development of deformities include:
  - The type of leprosy—incidence is higher in multibacillary (MB) leprosy
  - The duration of active disease—more the duration chances or nerve damage is more so the chance of deformities
  - The number of nerve trunks—it can be involved by the disease itself or during reaction. More the number of involvement of the nerve trunk increases the chance of deformities
- *Types of deformities in leprosy*:
  - *Primary*: It can be specific (due to local leprosy-related pathology) and paralytic (due to motor nerve palsy).
  - Secondary is anesthetic (due to damage of sensory nerves).

BOX 1: WHO definitions.

- *Impairment*: Problems in body structure or functions, such as significant deviation or loss. Impairment may be either structural or functional.
- *Deformity*: A deformity is a structural, usually visible impairment.
- *Activity limitation*: Difficulties one individual may have in executing a task or action.
- *Participation restrictions*: Problems an individual may experience in involvement in a life situation.
- *Disability*: Disability is the umbrella term for impairments, activity limitations, and participation restrictions, referring to the negative aspects of the interaction between an individual (with a health condition) and that individual's contextual factors (environmental and personal factors).

Specific Changes

Face

- *Madarosis*: Loss of eyebrows (superciliary madarosis) and eyelashes (ciliary madarosis) occur due to heavy infiltration of skin with lepromatous granuloma which results in atrophy of hair follicles.
- *Premature senile appearance*: Elastic fibers are destroyed by leprous granulomatous infiltration so skin hangs in redundant folds and results in a deeply wrinkled appearance also known as "sagging face."
- *Buddha ears*: Loose skin in the external ear gives rise to this mega lobule deformity resembling Buddha ear.
- *"Rat-bitten" ears*: Type II lepra reaction can form irregularly scalloped rim of pinna due to ulceration and chondritis.
- *Collapsed pinna*: The cartilaginous skeleton of the pinna can be extensively destroyed rarely.
- *"Sunken nose" deformity*: This deformity is typical of leprosy. Nasal septal perforation along with atrophy of anterior nasal spines gives rise to "Sunken nose" deformity. The most common facial deformity was nasal septal involvement was in a Korean study.[1]
- *Facies leprosa*: Resorption of maxillary anterior alveolar bone and the anterior nasal spine in patients with lepromatous leprosy.

Hands

- *Banana fingers*: This is due to heavy infiltration by the bacteria of the skin and subcutaneous tissue of fingers followed by atrophy and deposition of fat under the skin.

- Nonparalytic clawing and "straight stiff finger"
- *"Reaction hand" or frozen hand*: It is the most disabling deformity that occurs after an episode of ENL. "Reaction hand" refers to severe edematous dorsum of hands, interphalangeal joint arthritis, and functional inabilities due to type II lepra reactions.[2] "Frozen hand" occurs due to repeated lepra reactions which lead to fibrosis of the skin and subcutaneous tissue which shows a hyperpigmented and leathery look. The hand is universally flexed with nails digging into the palm due to the formation of scar-like tissue and forms bizarre deformity. Ring and little fingers sometimes show severe clawing without any paralysis of intrinsic muscles. There is marked hyperextension at metacarpophalangeal (MCP) joints which may get dislocated; this deformity is usually impossible to correct.
- *Swan neck deformity*: Fibrosis and contracture of intrinsic muscles due to repeated lepra reactions leads to flexion at basal joint and hyperextension at proximal interphalangeal (PIP) joint, which is opposite of frozen hand. "Swan-neck" deformity is also found in rheumatoid arthritis.[3] It may also occur in isolation or along with a reaction hand.
- *Twisted fingers*: Decalcification of pathological fractured juxta-articular zones in small bones of hands during lepra reaction leads to malunion during healing giving rise to bizarre deformities. So the finger is twisted in an odd direction.

Feet

Reaction foot and "intrinsic plus toes" are specific changes of the foot that are not very common.

Paralytic Changes

Face

- The paralytic deformity is caused by the involvement of the facial nerve.
- Partial paralysis, especially of the upper (zygomatic) branches of the facial nerve is more common than lower branch paralysis.
- Bell's palsy as damage to the facial nerve trunk is quite rare.
- Zygomatic branches are more commonly affected as it is in a more superficial and cooler location and constricted within the osteofascial tunnels.
- Upper facial paralysis produces paralysis of the eyelids (lagophthalmos) or even the upper part of the face.
- Most of the cases occur in borderline leprosy with reactions and with prompt and adequate treatment with steroids, so facial nerve paralysis may be reversed and permanent deformities can be avoided.

Hands (Figs. 1A to C)

- *Ulnar nerve palsy*:
  - The most common paralytic changes associated with leprosy is an isolated low ulnar nerve palsy which usually presents as an ulnar claw hand involving mainly the little and ring fingers.
  - The ulnar nerve is usually the first and most severely involved followed by median and less frequently by radial nerve.
  - The earliest feature of ulnar palsy is persistent abduction of the little finger due to paralysis of the third palmar interossei.
  - Flattening of the hypothenar eminence
  - When the ring and little fingers are completely deprived of functioning intrinsic muscles in ulnar nerve palsy it is referred to as "intrinsic zero" finger.
  - Wasting of bulky first dorsal interossei muscles forms characteristic depression over the dorsum of the hand, known as "Guttering sign."
  - Thenar eminence may sometimes flatten due to paralysis of the distal part of flexor pollicis brevis as supplied by the deep branch of the ulnar nerve.
  - Straightening of thumb at MCP joint occurs if flexor pollicis brevis is paralyzed.
  - High ulnar paralysis causing wasting of flexor carpi ulnaris manifests as flattening of the normally slightly bulging medial border of the forearm.

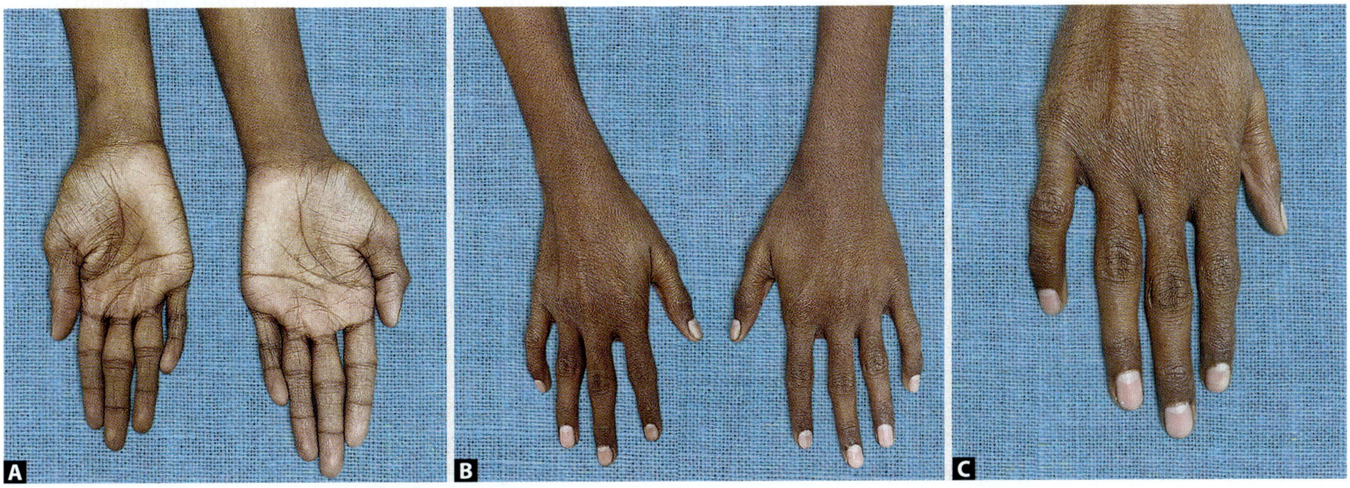

Figs. 1A to C: Ulnar nerve palsy in a patient of pure neural Hansen's disease.

- *Median nerve palsy*:
  - It can be of two types either low or high, the former being commoner.
  - *Low median paralysis*: Only intrinsic muscles of the hand are paralyzed and sometimes associated with anesthetic sequelae.
  - *High median paralysis (injury above the level of the elbow)*: The intrinsic muscles of the hand plus muscles of the front of the forearm are paralyzed. The fingers lose all power of flexion and any movement becomes impossible after this.
- *Combined ulnar and median nerve palsy*: A combined ulnar and median palsy causes clawing of all five fingers. The thumb comes to lie in the same plane with the other fingers and is also clawed which means it is adducted, hyperextended, and externally rotated at the carpometacarpal joint, and flexed at the MCP and IP joints. There is flattening of the thenar eminence and the deformity is known as "Ape thumb" deformity.
- *Radial nerve paralysis*: It is a rare occurrence and when it occurs, it is always with or after ulnar and median nerve palsy and known as triple nerve palsy. Clawing due to intrinsic paralysis is not manifested because of the paralysis of digital extensors which normally cause hyperextension of MCP joints. The radial nerve often recovers with treatment and so the patient suffers temporary disability only.

Feet

- Anesthetic and paralytic deformities are of main concern of the foot. Though specific deformities are uncommon sometimes lepromatous nodules may breakdown or during intense inflammatory reactions, ulceration can occur.
- *Clawfoot*: Clawing of toes is paralysis of intrinsic muscles of the toes resulting in an imbalance of forces around the metatarsophalangeal and interphalangeal joints. These intrinsic muscles are supplied by the terminal medial and lateral plantar branches of the posterior tibial nerve. Clawing of toes is not as common as claw hands.
- Claw toe has been defined into the following third degree of severity:
  1. *Mild (first degree)*: Toe can be actively straightened when proximal phalanx is pressed down as the metatarsophalangeal joints and IP joints are mobile.
  2. *Moderate (second degree)*: There is flexion contracture at the PIP joint and toe cannot be actively or passively straightened.
  3. *Severe (third degree)*: Toes cannot even be straightened at the metatarsophalangeal.
- Joints because of the stiffness of this joint too. Eventually, there is dislocation of the proximal phalanx and the severely clawed toe gets high up on the dorsum of the foot and the toe-tip no longer touches the ground.
- Claw toes in severe cases may cause toe-tip ulceration though mild cases usually do not produce any disabilities.
- *Foot drop*: The lateral popliteal nerve (common peroneal) is also commonly
- *Involved like the ulnar nerve:* The lateral popliteal nerve supplies the anterior group of muscles (dorsiflexion) through its deep branch and the lateral group of muscles of the leg (evertors) by the superficial branch. Thus damage to this nerve, makes the patient unable to lift up the foot which drops down with its own weight.

Anesthetic Deformities

- They are largely characterized by neuropathic plantar ulcers. The ulcer has its own natural history.
- *Sites of ulceration*:
  - The sole of the foot remains the most common site.
  - *Forepart of foot (ball of foot)*: 70–90% of ulcers involve the forefoot, of which most occur in relation to the metatarsal of the big toe.
  - *Heel and mid-lateral border (in relation to fifth metatarsal) of sole*: 5–10% cases each.
  - *Toe-tips*: 1–5% cases, especially with claw toes.
- *Pathogenesis of plantar ulcer*:
  - External injury with subsequent infection.
  - Infection through cracks and fissures.
  - Internal injury caused by walking and other activities of the anesthetic foot (most common).
- *Stages of plantar ulcers*:
  - *Stage of threatened ulcer*: Tenderness on deep pressure over the metatarsal head, slight puffiness, and warmth, splaying of digits.
  - *Stage of concealed ulcer*: Necrosis occurs and blister forms.
  - *Stage of overt, manifest, or visible ulcer*: Underlying bone and open ulceration muscles may be affected.
- *Types of plantar ulcers*:
  - *Acute*: Acute infection and acute inflammation
  - *Chronic*: Less or scanty discharge, with heaped-up hyperkeratotic edges and a hard fibrosed base
  - *Complicated*: Involves the bones, joints, and tendon sheaths
  - *Recurrent*: Due to lack of care on the patient's part or other factors
- *Management of plantar ulcers*:
  - *Acute ulcer*:
    - Absolute rest (in bed)
    - Elevate foot, Eusol bath, irrigation, dressing
    - Limit surgery to drainage procedures
    - Antibiotics if needed and treat as chronic ulcer after acute phase subsides
  - *Chronic ulcer*:
    - Simple scraping floor of ulcer
    - Sticking plaster or Vaseline gauze dressing

- Below knee POP cast or bulky dressing
- Protective footwear + foot-care training
- *Complicated ulcer:*
  - Debridement
  - Physiological rest by below-knee POP cast
  - Protective footwear on POP removal
  - Correct deformity, if necessary
  - Identify other complications and treat them accordingly
  - Skin graft large ulcers
- *Recurrent ulcer:*
  - Improve quality of scar (scar revision using excision and suture, local flaps, distant flaps, free flaps, etc.)
  - Reduce load on scar by footwear modification or corrective surgery
  - Eradicate infection

DISABILITY

Introduction

- Disability is the umbrella term for impairments, activity limitations, and participation restrictions, referring to the negative aspects of the interaction between an individual (with a health condition) and that individual's contextual factors (environmental and personal factors).
- United Nations Convention on the Rights of Persons with Disabilities (CRPD) acknowledges that disability is "an evolving concept," but also stresses that "disability results from the interaction between persons with impairments and attitudinal and environmental barriers that hinder their full and effective participation in society on an equal basis with others." Defining disability as an interaction means that "disability" is not an attribute of the person.
- Prevention of impairments and disability (POID) is integral to the success of management of Leprosy-affected persons. The objectives of managing disabilities in leprosy, therefore, are to prevent:
  - Onset of new disabilities
  - Worsening of existing disabilities

Evaluation of a Patient and Assessment of Disability

The patient is evaluated for his disabilities and deformities and the assessment is recorded before starting the treatment. This baseline information is helpful to assess the response to therapy and nerve functions.[4,5]

Methods to Assess Sensory Functions

Testing for Touch Sensation

- Semmes-Weinstein monofilaments have been found to be fairly reliable for screening and monitoring peripheral sensory function.
- The staircase method is followed.[6] In this technique, a series of stimuli are presented. If a stimulus is detected, subsequent stimuli are continuously reduced in magnitude until these can no longer be detected. When the subject fails to detect a stimulus, subsequent stimuli are gradually increased until the subject once again detects the stimulus. The mean of the two is taken for further averaging the perception. Two positive responses out of three are taken as a confirmed sensibility to the nylon number.
- One of the problems with monofilament nylons is the difference in fiber diameter, however, it is reproducible and convenient. Normal perception thresholds for nylons at the finger pulps are 0.217 g/mm^2; levels of protective sensations are double the normal thresholds, i.e., 0.434 g/mm^2. For the sole, these values are 2.35 g/mm^2 and 5 g/mm^2, respectively.[7,8]
- The perception of touch sensation decreases with age, however, the perception of pain remains the same **(Table 1)**.[9]

Testing for Pinprick Pain

- In its basic form, it is a nongraded test ("yes" or "no" replies).
- The ballpoint pen test is the most widely used sensory test in the field. It is universally available and simple to use.
- Static two-point discrimination, a test for innervations density, is reliable but slow to respond to changes as compared to monofilament nylons.

TABLE 1: Tests for evaluation of motor functions of nerve trunks affected in leprosy.

Nerve trunk	*Site of damage*	*Test procedure*
Ulnar	Forearm	Flexion of the DIP joint of the little finger
	Wrist	• Abduction and adduction of the little finger • Flexion of the MCP joint of the little finger keeping the IP joint neutral • Adduction of the thumb
Median	Forearm	• Weakness of all extrinsic flexors of the fingers • Wrist loss of abduction opposition of the thumb
Radial	Upper arm	Wrist dorsiflexion
	Forearm	Independent extension of the index finger
Common peroneal	Just below knee	Dorsiflexion of the ankle Dorsiflexion of the great toe
Posterior tibial	At ankle	Spreading of the toes Tests for abductor/flexor hallucis
Facial	At the stylomastoid foramen	Total facial paralysis
	Over the zygomatic bone	Eye closure test

(DIP: distal interphalangeal joints)

BOX 2: Grades of muscle power.

- *Grade 0:* No contraction of muscle
- *Grade 1:* Flickering contraction of muscle but no actual movement of the part
- *Grade 2:* Active movement of the part occurs but full range not possible against gravity
- *Grade 3:* Full range of movement against gravity but not against any external resistance
- *Grade 4:* Full range of movement against mild external resistance
- *Grade 5:* Full range of movement against full external resistance (normal power)

Testing for Temperature Sensation

It is important to detect early cases.

Assessment of Motor Functions

- The muscle power is graded according to Medical Research Council (MRC) grades **(Box 2)**.[10]
- For muscles of the face and intrinsic muscles of the foot where it not possible to assess muscle grades as above, the muscle strength is recorded as normal, weak, or paralyzed.
- A simplified version of voluntary muscle testing (VMT) can be used in a busy practice to quickly assess the muscle strength.

Rapid Neurological Evaluation

A rapid neurological evaluation must test sensibility, mobility, and trophicity. Only six main nerve trunks are affected (on each side) in leprosy. The tests should be performed on each side, but in a sequence to save time.[11]

Examination of Joints

- The joints of the hand and foot must be examined individually for appearance, movement (both active and passive), stability, and any other abnormality.
- The patient is asked to hold his fingers in the lumbrical position, i.e., metacarpophalangeal joint (MCPJ) flexed at 90° and proximal interphalangeal joint (PIPJ) fully extended. Such a posture is not possible if the intrinsic muscles of the hand are paralyzed.

Grading of Deformities and Disabilities

Disability grading for every very new case of leprosy must be assigned a "Disability grade", which must be recorded at the time of diagnosis. The grade is on a scale of 0, 1 or 2. Each eye, each hand and each foot is given its own grade, the highest grade given is used as the disability grade for that patient **(Box 3)**.

EHF Score (Eyes, Hands, Feet) Sum-score or the Impairment Summary Form (ISF)

- The EHF score is calculated from data already being recorded routinely. It is the sum of all the individual disability grades for the two eyes, two hands, and two feet. EHF score ranges from 0 to 12.

BOX 3: Disability grading for a case of leprosy.

Hands and feet:
- *Grade 0:* No anesthesia, no visible deformity or damage
- *Grade 1:* Anesthesia present, but no visible deformity or damage
- *Grade 2:* Visible deformity or damage present

Eyes:
- *Grade 0:* No eye problem due to leprosy; no evidence of visual loss
- *Grade 1:* Eye problems due to leprosy present, but vision not severely affected as a result of these (vision: 6/6 or better; can count fingers at 6 m)
- *Grade 2:* Severe visual impairment (vision: worse than 6/60; inability to count fingers at 6 m) also includes (corneal anesthesia, lagophthalmos, and iridocyclitis)

- The EHF score has been shown to be more sensitive to change over time than the disability grade itself. The simplest way to use the EHF score to measure the development of new or additional disability during MDT is to calculate the score at diagnosis (this examination is already done in the initial assessment of the disability grade) and then repeat the examination at the time treatment is completed. The two scores can then be compared.

Stages of Disability

Three major stages are recognized in the process of disablement in a patient of leprosy:

1. *Impairment*: This refers to changes or abnormalities (including losses) in body parts and functions (including the mind) as a consequence of a disease or disorder.
    - Primary impairments in leprosy include thickening and nodulation of the skin and subcutaneous tissue due to granulomatous infiltration and damage to peripheral nerves, giving rise to loss of sensation and motor paralysis in the hands, feet, and eyes.
    - Secondary impairments in leprosy include ulceration, contractures of extremities corneal ulceration and vision loss due unprotected use of insensitive structures.
2. *Activity limitation*: The affected person finds it difficult or impossible to do activities of daily living because of some impairment. Examples are difficulty in the skillful use of the hand, walking and running difficulty, and poor vision, restricting mobility and communication.
3. *Participation restriction*: Persons with leprosy-related disabilities experience disadvantages, social stigma, social rejection, isolation.

Nerve Involvement and Damage

- Nerve involvement in leprosy can be said to occur in five stages:
    1. *Parasitization*: A few *M. leprae* found in the nerve, but no other change.
    2. *Tissue response*: This stage is characterized by host tissue response.

TABLE 2: Nerve tenderness scale.

Grade	*Clinical features*
0: No tenderness	Palpation of the nerve is not painful even when asked about it
1: Mild tenderness	Palpation of the nerve hurts only when asked about it
2: Moderate tenderness	Indicates nerve palpation is painful even without being asked about it, but says it is not very painful when asked about it
3: Severe tenderness	Indicates or says palpation is very painful even without being asked about it
4: Very severe tenderness	Is apprehensive of palpation; or, does not allow palpation of the nerve trunk

TABLE 3: Nerve pain scale.

Grade	*Clinical feature*
0: No nerve pain	Says no nerve pain even when asked about it
1: Mild nerve pain	Says has nerve pain only when asked about it
2: Moderate nerve pain	Complaints of nerve pain even without asking about it; but sleep/joint movement not affected
3: Severe nerve pain	Complaints of severe nerve pain; sleep affected; and/or, joint movement restricted by pain

3. *Clinical involvement*: Nerve clinically thickened with or without associated pain or tenderness **(Tables 2 and 3)**.
4. *Nerve damage*: This stage is characterized by clinically detectable nerve function deficit.
5. *Nerve destruction*: This stage is indicated by irreversible nerve function deficit, muscle paralysis with muscle wasting.

- In leprosy, the damaged nerves can recover with treatment but the potential for recovery varies with the involved nerve.
- Nerve care involves:
    - Recognizing and treating acute or subacute "clinical neuritis" early
    - Recognizing and treating nerve function deficit early which may involve surgical decompression of the concerned nerve trunk when necessary.
- Categorization of leprosy patients according to presence of "clinical neuritis" and nerve function deficit (NFD):
    - *Category A patients*: No neuritis, no NFD
    - *Category B patients*: Neuritis present; no NFD
    - *Category C patients*: No neuritis, NFD present
    - *Category D patients*: NFD present, neuritis present

REHABILITATION

Purview of Rehabilitation

- It is estimated that over three million people live with disability due to leprosy, and every year, there is an addition of 30–40% of newly diagnosed patients with leprosy presenting with disabilities[12]

BOX 4: Simple self-care steps to preventing corneal damage in long-standing lagophthalmos.

- Wear protective glass (sunglasses) or cover eye with the help of cloth to prevent dust and insects from damaging the eye and prevent dryness on the surface of the eye during the day
- While sleeping, cover your eyes with the help of a towel or bedsheet to prevent damage to the cornea
- Wash the eye with clean lukewarm water to flush out dirt (avoid splashing). After face washing, inspect the eye in the mirror to see early signs of damage such as red eyes
- Avoid rubbing the eyes and use soft cloth to wipe the watering

- Rehabilitation usually includes the following types of services:
    - Early detection, diagnosis and intervention
    - Medical care and treatment
    - Social, psychological and other types of counseling and assistance
    - Training in self-care activities, including mobility, communication and daily living skills, with special provisions as needed, e.g., for the hearing impaired, the visually impaired and the mentally retarded
    - Provision of technical and mobility aids, and other devices
    - Specialized education services
    - Vocational rehabilitation services (including vocational guidance), vocational training, placement in open or sheltered employment
    - Follow-up

Principles of Self-Care

All patients with the impairments in eyes, hands and feet need to be educated about self-care to prevent secondary impairments.

Care of Eyes

- The loss of sensation in the cornea, absence of blink reflex and lagophthalmos are serious eye-related impairments which if not taken care of may lead to damage to cornea and decreased vision **(Box 4)**
- *Management of lagophthalmos*:
    - In long-standing lagophthalmos (>6 months duration and eyelid gap <6 mm), the following must be taught and practiced:
        - "Blinking exercises" (blinking three times daily, with 20 blinks each time) to reinforce the orbicularis function.
        - *"Think blink"*: By making use of the Bell's phenomenon, this exercise leads to moistening of cornea behind the upper eyelids in a kind of "reverse blinking."
        - Preventing corneal damage by passive exercises if the patient is unable to close the eye actively

- Surgery is indicated when duration of lagophthalmos >6 months, eyelid gap more than 6 mm and any of the following is present:
  - Exposure keratitis is present
  - Exposed cornea in sleeping position
  - Corneal anesthesia
  - Bilateral involvement
  - Continuous epiphora or intermittent redness
- *Vision testing*: Regularly check vision by looking at the fixed objects as available in the field setting.
- *Management of redness of eyes:*
  - High doses of clofazimine (for type 2 reaction) cause gradual redness of the eyes, which will gradually disappear after clofazimine treatment is stopped.
  - In case of sudden redness or pain of eye, an immediate referral to ophthalmic consultant is mandated.

Care of Hands and Feet

- The anesthetic hands or feet may get repeatedly injured; so regular care of anesthetic hand or feet is of utmost importance to prevent deformity and limiting disability **(Box 5)**.
- *Appropriate footwear*:
  - An appropriate footwear should be worn throughout the day. If shoes are worn, they should be strong, comfortable, free from nails, broad at the toes and without toecap. Laces should be avoided if the patient has deformed fingers. Velcro is the ideal alternative. The patient must be advised about "wearing" new shoes before they can be worn all day.
  - A sandal with a strong stiff outer-sole, lined by a Plastazote insole which is glued in position to prevent shifting, is ideal. Alternatively, insoles can be made of microcellular rubber (MCR).
  - Plastazote insoles can play an important part in the prevention of plantar ulceration as they are molded to the shape of each sole and it is even possible to have shoes made entirely of this material.
  - Where expertise is available, the podiatry assessment should be done to assess the foot alignment and provide appropriate orthoses along with the footwear.[13-15]
- *Common indications of splinting on leprosy:*
  - Proximal interphalangeal flexion contractures and claw hand
  - Interphalangeal flexion contracture of the thumb
  - Thumb-web contracture
  - Paralysis of short muscles of the thumb
  - The reaction hand
  - Open wounds at the finger flexion creases
  - Foot ulcers, foot drop
  - Wrist drop
- Common orthoses for deformities in leprosy **(Table 4)**

BOX 5: Instructions to minimize damage to anesthetic hands/feet.

- The anesthetic hands/feet should be soaked in cool water and scraped thoroughly with stone or commercially available skin scrapers to remove any thickened skin or callosities. The foot is then wiped dry particularly in between toes to prevent fungal infection
- The moisture should then be retained by applying a thin coat of oil or moisturizer
- Hands/feet should be daily inspected for hot spots, blisters, wounds or swelling
- Utmost caution should be practiced in handling hot or sharp objects.
- Wounds should be properly cared and rested to prevent further progression. This is especially important for plantar blisters/ulcers. This can be achieved by walking with the help of crutch or canes
- Ulcers should be appropriately dressed
- Regular exercises needed to be performed to prevent damage to the joints (contractures)
- Use of footwear with soft insoles such as microcellular rubber (MCR) and rigid outer soles should be encouraged
- The footwear needs to be inspected regularly for excessive wear and tear or for the presence of any embedded sharp objects
- To avoid plantar ulceration, the patient must learn to take short steps while walking
- Callosities should be pared down regularly
- In the presence of a crack, it is advisable to thin the edges of the crack by rubbing along the line of the edge and not across the edge

Common Assistive Devices Used in Leprosy

- When patients with impairment have difficulty in performing activities of daily living (ADL) as well as work and leisure-related activities, provision of adaptive devices improves their ability to perform the daily activities, such as those related to personal hygiene, brushing, bathing, feeding and dressing **(Box 6)**.[16]
- *Assistive devices for protection of eyes*: Eye-glasses, head clothes, hats and caps, pads, cloths, mosquito nets and bedsheets to cover eyes while sleeping
- *Assistive devices protection of hands*: Adapting tools, splints, gloves, pot holders and cooking gloves, padding around handles, long handles, sticks and prongs

TABLE 4: Common orthoses for deformities in leprosy.

Deformity	*Dynamic splint*	*Static splint*
Claw hand	• Dynamic ulnar nerve palsy splint • Knuckle bender splint • Wrist driven wrist hand orthoses splint • Hand orthoses with MCP extension stop • Lumbrical bar	• Static ulnar nerve palsy splint • Static WHO (wrist–hand orthoses)
Wrist drop	• Dorsal wrist cock-up splint with dynamic finger extension • Wrist action wrist hand orthoses • Tenodesis splint	• Static volar wrist cock up splint • Static WHO splint

BOX 6: Common adaptive/assistive devices used in leprosy.

- *Adapted spoon*: For patient who has no grasp
- *Built-up spoon*: For patient who has some grasp but are unable to hold thin items
- Nail-cutting device
- Button hook
- *Writing aid*: For patient with poor prehension function with some pinch power
- *Grip-aids*: For patient with absorbed digits with some grasp/prehension function
- *Universal cuff*: For patients with poor or no grasp

- *Assistive devices protection of feet*: Footwear, orthoses, splints, foot-drop splints, drop-foot supports, crutches, walking sticks

Rehabilitation Schemes

- These include surgical rehabilitation and vocational training.
- Under the NLEP, 75 reconstructive surgery units and 13 leprosy rehabilitation approaches for leprosy rehabilitation promotion units (LPRU) have been functioning.
- It has been realized that rehabilitation approaches for leprosy done exclusively or in isolation can be distressful and may cause dissatisfaction among the leprosy disabled. This has prompted an integrated rehabilitation service and community-based rehabilitation (CBR) program for the general handicapped persons along with the leprosy disabled.[17]

Social Dimensions of Leprosy

- The community needs to change its attitude by accepting leprosy-affected persons and giving those equal rights and the dignity that they deserve.
- Community participation, either active or passive, in the leprosy control program is a central theme. Active participation is most desired for welfare programs. On the other hand, passive participation helps in strengthening services-related programs.
- WHO propagates the concept of CBR which encourages active participation of the community in the rehabilitation process of leprosy patients. Community health volunteers have an important role to play in disease prevention, health promotion, and rehabilitation activities.

KEY POINTS

- A deformity is a structural, usually visible impairment.
- Disability is the umbrella term for impairments, activity limitations, and participation restrictions, referring to the negative aspects of the interaction between an individual (with a health condition) and that individual's contextual factors (environmental and personal factors).
- Deformities can be primary or secondary/anesthetic.
- Primary deformities can be specific and paralytic.
- Facies leprosa is seen in patients with lepromatous leprosy characterized by resorption of maxillary anterior alveolar bone and the anterior nasal spine.

REFERENCES

1. Kim JH, Lee OJ, Lee JJ, Park CH. Analysis of facial deformities in Korean leprosy. Clin Exp Otorhinolaryngol. 2013;6:78-81.
2. Ramu G, Dharmendra. Acute exacerbations (reactions) in leprosy. In: Dharmendra (Ed). Leprosy, Vol. I. Bombay: Kothari Medical Publishing House; 1978. pp. 108-39.
3. Srinivasan H, Dharmendra. Deformities of hands. In: Dharmendra (Ed). Leprosy. Mumbai: Kothari Medical Publishing House; 1978. pp. 205-17.
4. Srinivasan H, Dharmendra. Deformities of feet. In: Dharmendra (Ed). Leprosy. Mumbai: Kothari Medical Publishing House; 1978. pp. 218-23.
5. Pearson JM. The evaluation of nerve damage in leprosy. Lepr Rev. 1982;53:119-30.
6. Conomy JP, Barnes KL. Quantitative assessment of cutaneous sensory function in subjects with neurologic diseases. J Neuro Sci. 1976;30:221-35.
7. Malaviya GN, Husain S, Girdhar A, Girdhar BK. Sensory functions in limbs of normal persons and leprosy patients with peripheral trunk damage. Ind J Lepr. 1994;66:157-64.
8. Saltzman CL, Rashid R, Hayes A, Fellner C, Fitzpatrick D, Klapach A, et al. 4.5-gram monofilament sensation beneath both first metatarsal heads indicates protective foot sensation in diabetic patients. J Bone Joint Surg. 2004;86:717-23.
9. Horch KH, Hardy M, Jiminez S, Jabaley M. An automated tactile tester for evaluation of cutaneous sensibility. J Hand Surg. 1992;17:829-37.
10. Medical Research Council War Memorandum. Aids to the Investigation of Peripheral Nerve Injuries, [Memo no. 7], 2nd edition. London: HMSO; 1962.
11. Palande DD, Bowden REM. Early detection of damage to nerves in leprosy. Lepr Rev. 1992;63:60-72.
12. Lockwood DN. Chronic aspects of leprosy—neglected but important. Trans R Soc Trop Med Hyg. 2019;113:813-7.
13. Lal V, Sarkar D, Das S, Mahato M, Srinivas G. A study to assess the usage of MCR footwear in West Bengal, India. Lepr Rev. 2015;86:273-7.
14. Gupta P, Karthikeyan, Nathan RJ. Footwear for the person with an anesthetic foot: what options are available? Lepr Rev. 2017; 88(2):265-9.
15. Govindharaj P, Mani S, Darlong J, John AS. Acceptance and satisfaction of microcellular rubber ready-made footwear among patients with insensitive feet due to leprosy. Lepr Rev. 2017;88:381-90.
16. Borg J, Larsson S. Assistive devices for people affected by leprosy: underutilised facilitators of functioning? Lepr Rev. 2009;80:13-21.
17. Ganapati R, Pai VV, Kingsley S, Dhamale CB. Prevalence of disability in an urban slum: an assessment with reference to rehabilitation (Absract: Sept. 7-12). Beijing, China: 15th International Leprosy Congress; 1998.

EXAMINATION QUESTIONS

1. What is a deformity ? Classify and describe the types of deformities in leprosy.
2. Describe rehabilitation in leprosy.

13 SECTION | Sexually Transmitted Disease

123 CHAPTER Introduction and Overview of STD

Yogesh S Marfatia, Ruchi Shah

INTRODUCTION

The origin of the term "Venereal" is from "Venus", the Roman goddess of love, beauty, and creativity.

Venereal diseases include first generation bacterial infections while "sexually transmitted diseases" (STD) includes many more conditions but does not include asymptomatic infections which are transmissible through sexual contact. Thus currently, the term "sexually transmissible infections (STIs)" is preferred. More than 30 different pathogens are known to be transmitted through sexual contact. Eight out of these pathogens are linked to the greatest incidence of STDs which includes 4 curable infections-syphilis, gonorrhea, chlamydia, and trichomoniasis and 4 incurable viral infections—Herpes simplex virus (HSV), human papilloma virus (HPV), HIV, hepatitis B virus (HBV).

REPRODUCTIVE TRACT INFECTIONS

They may start as lower reproductive tract infection (RTI) which can disseminate to upper reproductive tract if appropriate treatment is not given.

It is responsible for a large amount of mortality and morbidity mainly in females, but also in males as well as infants.

Causes of RTIs have been shown in **Table 1**.

Changing Profile of Sexually Transmissible Infections (Table 2)

Over decades, the etiologic profile of STIs have drastically changed in favor of persistent, recurrent and incurable viral infections associated with morbidity, malignancy, and mortality.

Sexually Transmissible Infections: Global Estimates[1]

More than 1 million STIs are acquired daily.

Annual incidence of 4 curable STIs	*357 million*
Trichomoniasis	143 million
Chancroid	131 million
Gonorrhea	78 million
Syphilis	5.6 million

Sequelae of Sexually Transmitted Diseases

Sexually transmitted diseases take their toll through complications and sequelae.

Untreated STDs disseminate locally in genitourinary tract and causes complications.

The impact of STD on pregnancy ***(Table 3)****:* Many STIs can be transmitted vertically and have impact on outcome of pregnancy.

Sequelae of STDs:

- Pelvic inflammatory disease
- Ectopic pregnancy and infertility

TABLE 1: Causes of reproductive tract infections (RTIs).

RTIs	*Cause*	*Female*	*Male*
Endogenous: Occur irrespective of sexual contact, but can be transmitted sexually	Candidiasis (due to diabetes, pregnancy, etc.), bacterial vaginosis (linked with inadequate hygienic practices)	+	–
Exogenous: Mainly sexually transmitted pathogens	STD Tampon	+ ++	+ –
Iatrogenic	Unsafe delivery/ abortion/IUD insertion	+	–

TABLE 2: Changing profile of sexually transmissible infections (STIs).

	Sexually transmitted disease (STD)	*Characteristics*
First generation STDs (Bacterial infections)	• Syphilis • Chancroid • Gonorrhea • LGV • Donovanosis	• Clinically apparent • Easy to diagnose • Contagiousness is limited • Curable • Antibiotic resistance is an important issue
Second generation STDs (Viral infections)	• Anogenital warts • Genital herpes • *Chlamydia*	• Usually asymptomatic • Latent • Persistent and recurrent • Associated with risk of malignancy (HPV) • Capable of transmission from asymptomatic carriers
Third generation STDs	• HIV/AIDS • Hepatitis B	• Lifelong infection • Highly virulent and mutations are common • Potential causes of high morbidity and mortality

TABLE 3: The impact of STD on pregnancy.

Agent	Transmission	Sequelae
Treponema pallidum	• Antepartum • Perinatal	• Spontaneous abortion • Prematurity/PROM • Neurological involvement • Congenital syphilis
HIV	Highest chances during intrapartum period, can occur in antepartum and through breast milk in postpartum period	Parent to child transmission of HIV infection
Neisseria gonorrhoeae	Intrapartum	• Conjunctivitis (ophthalmia neonatorum) • Chorioamnionitis • Spontaneous abortion • Postpartum endocarditis
Chlamydia trachomatis	Intrapartum	• Conjunctivitis • Sepsis/death
HSV-2	Intrapartum	• Spontaneous abortion/ miscarriage • TORCH syndrome • Neonatal herpes with neurological involvement

(HSV: herpes simplex virus; PROM: premature rupture of membranes)

- Anogenital carcinoma due to oncogenic strains of HPV

Sequelae are more frequent in females. Moreover, the presence of STDs facilitates HIV transmission.

STDs and Females

Factors responsible for vulnerability of females to contract STDs:

Biologic Vulnerability

Anatomy:
- Large vaginal mucosa to interact with infected material
- Cervical ectopy—immature cervix with low vaginal mucous production in younger females facilitates STD/HIV transmission

Physiology:
- Menarche to menopause (pregnancy/delivery/abortion) provides ample chances for iatrogenic infections
- Menstrual cycle—inadequate hygiene and tampon use increases chances of RTIs

Other factors:
- Lack of power to negotiate about the type of sexual activity, conception, contraception, and prevention of RTI/STD/HIV infection
- Socioeconomic inequities responsible for engaging them in commercial sexual activity

STDs and Children[2]

Modes of transmission:
- Transplacental (syphilis)
- Intrapartum during delivery (gonorrhea/HIV/HSV/HPV)
- Postnatal transmission (during breast feeding)(HIV)
- Sexual abuse during prepubertal age

The Protection of Children from Sexual Offences (POCSO) Act, 2012 defines a child as any person below 18 years of age and provides protection to all children under the age of 18 years from sexual abuse.

STDs and MSM (Men Who have Sex with Men)

Prevalence of MSM activity is 2–12%.

Factors responsible for STDs in MSM are:
- Risky sexual practices with more sexual partners
- Infrequent use of condoms
- Improper treatment seeking behavior
- Anal mucosa is more fragile as compared to vaginal mucosa
- Anogenital sex is the riskiest activity as far as HIV transmission is concerned.

STDs in MSM predominantly have anorectal presentations, e.g., proctitis, ulcerative lesions, tumor, and Kaposi's sarcoma (rare in India) and are not easily picked up on clinical grounds.

HIV and STDs

HIV and STDs are perfect examples of epidemiologic synergy and they are core transmitters of each other:
- STD increases the risk of sexual transmission of HIV by 2–10 folds.
- HIV seroconcordance rate is found to be higher if one of the partners had STD.
- Many of the STDs can accelerate HIV disease progression, e.g., HSV and HPV infections.
- Coexistent HIV infection alters the natural history, diagnostic accuracy, and response to therapy of classic major and minor STDs. AIDS leads to poor prognosis of STDs, thus increasing the chances of recurrence. Potential of neurosyphilis is increased in HIV-infected cases. HIV-infected cases are at increased risk for anogenital and oral carcinoma due to HPV.
- Early detection and treatment of STDs must be undertaken in HIV patients to reduce their infectiousness and prevent their sequelae.

Healthcare Seeking Behavior[3]

- Only 5% of STI cases visit STD clinics and up to 15% uses public health facilities, the rest take treatment from non-STD clinic or traditional healers or even indulge in self-medication. Most of the STD cases receive delayed or inadequate treatment, thus increasing the potential for dissemination of STDs/HIV and their complications.

Improper healthcare seeking behavior is probably due to lack of awareness and stigma attached to STDs. STD is still not perceived as a public health problem by patients and practitioners.

- Other crucial components of STD management like education and counseling are not duly taken care of in majority of cases treated beyond public healthcare facilities.

APPROACH TO STD MANAGEMENT[4]

Sexually transmitted disease is a public health problem. Early diagnosis and prompt treatment is crucial in preventing local dissemination of infection, complications and sequelae as well as to interrupt the chain of transmission including potential vertical transmission. This can be achieved only if primary care physician is trained and equipped with STD management.

The ideal approach to STD case management is etiology-based treatment.

Etiological approach: Based on identification of the causative organism and its treatment.

There are more than 30 different sexually transmitted pathogens causing overlapping clinical features. The chances of mixed infection are higher. Laboratory facilities for diagnosis are not easily available. Patient cannot be treated in first visit and continues to disseminate the infection. This approach places constraints on time, resources, cost, and access to treatment as well as decrease compliance.

Syndromic approach means treatment based on easily identifiable symptoms and signs (syndrome). The basis of this approach is the fact that many STD pathogens are known to produce similar clinical features. Any primary care physician with proper training and provision of flowcharts as well as medicines can treat cases of STD at first contact.

Its *essential components* include the following:

- Diagnosis and treatment based on syndromes
- Education and counseling on treatment compliance, risk reduction, and condom use
- Promotion and provision of condoms
- Partner notification, treatment, and follow-up.

The syndromes included under this approach are:

- Urethral discharge
- Genital ulcer disease (herpetic and nonherpetic)
- Scrotal swelling
- Vaginal discharge
- Inguinal bubo
- Lower abdominal pain
- Neonatal conjunctivitis.

Advantage: Any doctor trained in the syndromic approach can treat a patient with the help of a flowchart, and an STD case is offered comprehensive care package on first contact with the trained physician.

Disadvantage: Exposure to multiple antimicrobial agents and thereby their adverse drug reactions and potential for increased antimicrobial resistance.

STD Prevention

Existing prevention options for STD:

- Sexual abstinence
- Behavioral changes (monogamy)
- Male condoms
- Screening for STDs in high-risk groups and during pregnancy
- Early diagnosis and prompt treatment along with the treatment of partner
- Promotion of syndromic approach
- Promotion of circumcision

Male condom: Correct and consistent use of good quality lubricated latex condom at every coital act offers high degree of protection. Protective efficacy of male condom varies against different sexually transmitted pathogens **(Table 4)**.

Pitfalls in STD prevention: The acceptance of male condom-based preventive measure is not very high and hence, it is crucial to promote female-driven protective measures.

Female-driven protective devices:

- Female condoms which are prelubricated polyurethane sheath and cover introitus in toto. However, they are less acceptable and there is a potential for reuse.
- Vaginal microbicides (Tenofovir 0.1% gel) has mixed results in terms of the ability to prevent HIV acquisition, but has shown some effectiveness against HSV-2.
- Pre- and postsexual exposure prophylaxis with antiretroviral drugs for prevention of HIV transmission.

TABLE 4: Protective efficacy of male condoms against sexually transmitted pathogens.

Pathogen	*Estimated efficacy*
Human immunodeficiency virus	>90% protection
Hepatitis B virus	>90% protection
*Human papilloma virus**	Not significant
Herpes simplex virus type 2	10–50% protection
Cytomegalovirus	50–90% protection
Chlamydia trachomatis	50–90% protection
Neisseria gonorrhoeae	>90% protection
*Trichomonas vaginalis**	>90% protection
Treponema pallidum	50–90% protection
Haemophilus ducreyi	10–50% protection
Pthirus pubis	Not significant

*Latest data—condoms provide no reduction in the transmission of the human papilloma virus (HPV) or Trichomonas vaginalis.

STD Vaccines

Genital tract mucosa *lacks organized lymphoid structures* leading to poor ability to counter sexually transmitted pathogens and some pathogens have the ability to evade the immune system. The goal of STD vaccine is to *enhance mucosal immune response.* Systemic immunization may induce weak mucosal immune response.

Vaccines are available against:

- Hepatitis B.
- HPV (bivalent, quadrivalent and nonavalent) for prevention of anogenital warts and carcinoma.
- HIV vaccine (under trial) is a difficult task due to following factors:
  - No natural immunity
  - Mutation
  - Genetic variability of the virus as well as human population
  - Viral latency
  - Antibodies elicited by immune system during natural infection with HIV do not prevent the progression in the long-term
  - Superinfection with different strain
  - Social challenges.

STD Vaccines—Issues and Challenges

- The ideal target for STI immunization is adolescent group before their coital debut, hence it is difficult to implement and promote due to social and parental resistance.
- Acceptance:
  - Vaccine availability may not ensure vaccine acceptance
  - Acceptance is an explicit acknowledgement of STI risk.
- Postimmunization behavioral change.

Male Circumcision[5]

It provides protection against subsequent development of malignancy as well as STDs.

Lack of circumcision causes increased chances of STDs due to following factors:

- Large surface area of prepuce as well as secretions provide optimal infective inoculums for establishing infection.
- Poor hygiene.
- Increased chances of trauma.
- Inner mucosal surface contains less protective keratin and is also rich source of Langerhans cells with HIV receptors.

Uncircumcised males are at 8 times higher risk of HIV infection and 3 times higher risk of developing STIs like chancroid and herpes genitalis.

STDs and Alternate (Anogenital and Orogenital) Sexual Practices

STDs in cases practicing alternate sexual practices are often underdiagnosed due to subtle, atypical manifestations, and lack of guidelines for clinical diagnosis and management.

Also, condom usage is inconsistent in such practices. The prevalence of consistent condom use for oral sex was 70.4% compared to 96.8% for vaginal sex. HPV infection of the oral mucosa is believed to affect 1–50% of the general population, with HPV-induced oral carcinogenesis being the second most common cause of oral carcinoma following tobacco usage-induced carcinoma.

APPROACH TO STD PATIENT[6-9]

- Ensure privacy and reinforce confidentiality.
- Avoid judgmental and moralistic attitude toward the patient.
- STD preventive counseling should be an integral part and must include promotion of safe sex, condoms, and partner management.
- *History taking*: Demographic details along with marital status.
- *Present illness*:
  - *Discharge:*
    - *In males:*

Urethral discharge Pus or matter coming out of penis
↓
• Whether from urethral opening or foreskin? • Duration? • Foul smelling? Color?

    - *In females:*

c/o excessive vaginal discharge?
↓
• Causes irritation/itching? • Duration? • Color? • Foul smelling/offensive odor? • Blood stained? • Related to menstrual cycles? • Associated c/o lower abdominal pain? Dyspareunia?

  - *Urinary symptoms:* c/o difficulty passing urine?

↓
• Burning sensation? While passing urine or while urine comes in contact with surrounding inflamed area in females? • Blood stained? • Frequency? • h/o urgency/strangury /loin pains/ fever and rigors (s/o pyelonephritis)?

  - *Genital lesions:*

Any sores/eruptions/erosions over external genitalia?
↓
• Painful? • Onset and duration? Recurrent? • Location?

- *Inguinal bubo:*

  Any swelling over groin?
  ↓
  - Duration?
  - Painful?
  - Associated with Genital ulcer?

- *Other symptoms:* Details should be obtained of any associated fever, itch, pain, skin rash, aching or swelling in joints, pain or redness in eyes, and oral lesions.
- *Treatment taken:*
  - History of topical or systemic treatment?
  - History of drug allergy?

- *Past medical history of:* Any illness or operation requiring hospitalization/venereal disease/jaundice/blood transfusion?
- *Sexual history:* A detailed sexual history:
  - Number and types of sexual contacts (viz. genito-genital, oro-genital, ano-genital, oro = anal) with dates
  - Partners (whether regular or casual)
  - Use of condoms or other forms of contraception.
- *Other history:* Enquire about:
  - Venereal diseases research laboratory (VDRL) and HIV testing results
  - Hepatitis B vaccination status.
- *In females:*
  - *Menstrual history:*
    - Last menstrual period?
    - Regular? Painful?
    - Intermenstrual/intercoital bleeding?
  - *Gynecological and obstetric history:*
    - Methods of contraception used
    - Details of previous conceptions
    - History of dyspareunia?
    - History of gynecological problems?
    - Last Pap smear?

Examination: Prerequisites are privacy and a good source of light. Expose the patient adequately form chest down to knees **(Table 5)**.

- *Genital examination:*

  Males:
  - Palpate the *scrotum* and feel for *testis, epididymis, and spermatic cord.* Note any asymmetry, erythema, and superficial lesions (e.g., scrotal cysts and varicocele).
  - *Penis, coronal sulcus, and frenulum* should be inspected for any rashes or sores. Retract the *foreskin* and inspect *the subpreputial area* for evidence of balanitis, posthitis or other abnormality.
  - Inspect the *external urinary meatus* for meatitis, urethral lesions or discharge, and congenital abnormalities like hypospadias. Examination of the inner surface of the underpants or milking of urethra may also provide evidence of urethral discharge.

  Females:
  - In lithotomy position, examine the vulva, anus, and perineum.
  - Palpate the abdomen for pelvic masses and tenderness.
  - Record the presence or absence of rashes, nits, lice, lymphadenopathy, buboes, ulcers, and vaginal discharge (noting the type, color, odor, and amount).
  - Bartholin's glands must be identified and examined.
  - Cervix should be inspected for ulceration, discharge, bleeding and ectopy and the walls of the vagina for condylomata.
  - Bimanual pelvic examination is performed to elicit adnexal tenderness or masses, cervical tenderness and to assess the position, size, and mobility of the uterus.

TABLE 5: Investigations for sexually transmitted infections.

Presenting complaints	*Organisms*	*Investigations*
Genital ulcer—herpetic	Herpes simplex virus	• Tzanck smear • Multinucleated epithelial giant cells on Wright's stain • Antibodies against HSV-1 and 2 (IgG and IgM) • Polymerase chain reaction • Western Blot
Genital ulcer—nonherpetic	*Haemophilus ducreyi* *T. pallidum* *Calymmatobacterium granulomatis*	• Gram stain for Gram negative bacilli in parallel chains (School of fish/Railroad track appearance) • Dark ground illumination • VDRL/RPR and TPHA* • Wright's stain-coccobacilli within macrophage
Urethral discharge	*Neisseria gonorrhoeae* *Chlamydia trachomatis*	• Smear examination (Gram's stain) and culture-sensitivity • Urethral swab for culture
Vaginal discharge	*Gardnerella vaginalis* *Candida albicans* *Neisseria gonorrhoeae* *Trichomonas vaginalis*	• Whiff test (KOH amine test), saline preparation for clue cells and pH • KOH examination for fungal elements • Gram stain and culture • Wet mount
Additional serological testing	HIV Hepatitis B Hepatitis C	

*(RPR: rapid plasma regain; TPHA: *T. pallidum* hemagglutination assay; VRDL: venereal disease research laboratory).

- *Lymph nodes*: Palpate anterior and posterior triangles of neck, submental and suboccipital areas, axillae, and epitrochlear area. Note their size, consistency, number and whether they are painful.
- Look for *rashes* by inspecting the face, trunk, abdomen, palms, soles, and thighs.
- Examine the *oral cavity* for any ulceration.
- Examine the *pubic hair* for nits, lice, folliculitis, and other skin lesions.
- Inspect the *inguinal region and then palpate it for lymphadenopathy*; note its distribution, consistency, and tenderness.
- Inspect the anus (rectal examination/proctoscopy) and the perineum.

INVESTIGATIONS FOR STIs (TABLE 5)

Bedside tests like smear examination and serologic tests as well as culture can be used to confirm clinical diagnosis.

KEY POINTS

- The term STIs is preferred as it covers both symptomatic as well as asymptomatic infections.
- Over decades, etiologic profile of STIs have drastically changed in favor of persistent, recurrent and incurable viral infections like HIV, HPV, HSV, and HBV.
- Commonly prevalent bacterial STDs include syphilis, gonorrhea, chlamydia, and trichomoniasis.
- STDs take their toll through complications and sequelae. Important sequelae include pelvic inflammatory disease, ectopic pregnancy, infertility, and anogenital carcinoma.
- *T. pallidum*, HIV, HSV, *N. gonorrhoeae* and *Chlamydia* have an impact on pregnancy as well as fetus in utero.
- Females are biologically and socioeconomically more susceptible to STIs and their sequelae.
- STDs in MSM predominantly have anorectal presentations and are likely to be underdiagnosed.
- HIV infection alters the natural history, diagnostic accuracy, and response to therapy of STD, and STD increases the chances of HIV transmission and disease progression.
- Health care seeking behavior of STD patients is far from satisfactory. Around 80% cases are treated at non-STD clinics or by traditional healers and thereby, are likely to be improperly treated.
- Approach to STD management can be etiology based or syndromic. Etiological approach places constraints on the time, resources, cost, and access to treatment as well as decrease compliance.
- Syndromic approach means treatment based on easily identifiable symptoms and signs and the patient is treated at the first contact. It also includes education and counseling on treatment compliance, risk reduction, and condom use; promotion and provision of condoms; partner notification, treatment, and follow-up.
- Male condom is highly protective against HIV, HBV and gonorrhea but not against HPV, HSV, and syphilis.
- As acceptance of male condoms is not very high, it is essential to promote female-driven preventive devices such as female condoms and vaginal microbicides.
- The goal of STD vaccine is to *enhance mucosal immune response but* systemic immunization may induce weak mucosal immune response.
- Currently, vaccines against HPV and HBV are available.
- Male circumcision provides protection against HIV and STD and it must be promoted.

REFERENCES

1. Marfatia YS, Sharma A, Joshipura S. Overview of sexually transmitted diseases. In: Valia RG. IADVL Textbook of Dermatology, 3rd edition. Vol 3 . Mumbai: Bhalani; 2010. pp. 1766-78.
2. Murugan S. Sexually transmitted diseases in children. In: Sharma VK (Ed). Textbook of STDs and AIDS, 1st edition. New Delhi: Viva Books; 2003. pp. 353-4.
3. Marfatia YS, Sharma A, Singla M. Health care seeking behavior of STD patients. Indian J Sex Transm Dis. 2005;26:23-5.
4. Using flowcharts for syndromic management. Management of STD patients, Training Module 1-6; National AIDS Control Organization, Ministry of Health and Family Welfare, Government of India, New Delhi.
5. Szabo R, Short RV. How does male circumcision protect against HIV infection? BMJ. 2000;320:1592-4.
6. Schmid GP. Approach to the patient with genital ulcer disease. Med Clin North Am. 1990;74:1559-72.
7. Wilcox Rr, Wilcox JB. Venereological medicine. London: Grant McIntyre; 1992. p. 22-32.
8. Farthing MJG, Jeffrie DJ. Sexually transmitted diseases. In: Kumar P, Clark M (Eds). Clinical Medicine, 4th edition. London: WB Saunders; 1998. p. 97-9.
9. Ministry of Health and Family Welfare. History taking and examination. Management of STD patients. New Delhi: NACO; 1994. pp. 1-19.

EXAMINATION QUESTIONS

1. Classify the reproductive tract infections.
2. Describe STD in female.
3. What is the impact of STD on pregnancy?
4. Explain the STD prevention.
5. Write briefly on STD vaccine.

Write short notes on the following:

6. Circumcision.
7. Condom.
8. Laboratory diagnosis of genital ulcer in young sexually active cases.
9. Laboratory diagnosis of vaginal discharge.
10. HIV and STD.

124 CHAPTER

Anatomy of Male and Female Genitalia

Nishant Choudhary

MALE REPRODUCTIVE SYSTEM

- Testes
- Epididymis
- Spermatic cord
- Scrotum
- Vas deferens
- Prostate
- Seminal vesicle
- Male urethra
- Penis.

Male Urethra

Membranous channel for discharge of seminal fluids and urine.

Length: 18–20 cm (extends from neck of the bladder to external meatus).

Parts:
- Posterior →
  - *Prostatic*: ~3 cm
    Lining: Transitional epithelium
    Receives secretion of ejaculatory duct and prostate
  - *Membranous*:~ 2 cm (shortest part)
    Lining: Transitional epithelium
- Anterior → *Penile*: ~15 cm
  Lining: Pseudostratified columnar epithelium except distal 1–1.2 cm, therefore sample for gonorrhea to be collected 1–2 cm proximal to meatus

Sphincter:
- → *Internal*: Involuntary, at neck of bladder above opening of ejaculatory duct
- → *External*: Voluntary, supplied by perineal branch of pudendal nerve

Penis: *Parts*: roots + body
Shaft/body: 1 corpora spongiosa + 2 corpora cavernosa
Erectile tissue
Glans: Bulb like distal end
Coronal sulcus: Circular groove separating from shaft of penis
Prepuce: Fold of skin covering glans
Preputial sac: Space between glans and prepuce
Frenulum: Fold of skin which serves as attachment to glans on its ventral surface

Scrotum: Loose, thin, rugose sac of skin containing testes, epididymis, vas deferens and loose areolar tissue. No subcutaneous adipose tissue present.

Testes: Primary reproductive organs in male, responsible for sperm production.

- Contain seminiferous tubules which have spermatogenic cells and Sertoli cells.

Seminiferous tubules → rete testes → efferent ducts → epididymis → vas deferens → Ejaculatory ducts → urethra.

Vas deferens: ~45 cm (2 in number).

Ejaculatory duct: Formed by union of duct of seminal vesicle and vas deferens. Opens in prostatic urethra.

Seminal vesicle: Secrete alkaline fluid. Constitute about 60–70% of ejaculatory volume.

Prostate: Compound tubuloalveolar exocrine gland 30–35% of the semen ejaculate-alkalinity helps the sperm survive in the acidic vaginal environment.

Contains 5-alpha-reductase which converts testosterone to DHT (responsible for BPH, prostate ca—PSA).

Prostate consists of:

Peripheral zone	The subcapsular portion. About 70–80% of prostatic cancer originate from this region
Central zone	Surrounds ejaculatory ducts
Transitional zone	Grows throughout life and causes benign prostatic enlargement. About 10–20% of prostatic cancer originate from this region
Stroma	Fibromuscular zone, usually devoid of glandular elements

Cowper's gland: 2 in number. Located on sides of membranous urethra.

Littre's glands: Mucus glands. Located on sides of penile urethra.

Tysons gland: Sebaceous glands. Located on sides of frenulum.

Lymphatic drainage:
Skin of penis → Superficial inguinal lymph nodes
Anterior urethra → Deep inguinal lymph nodes
Posterior urethra → Iliac lymph nodes
Glans → Deep inguinal lymph nodes

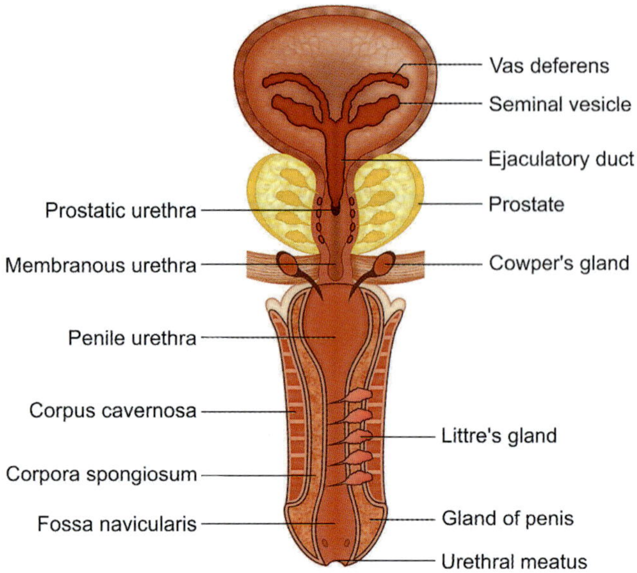

Fig. 1: Male urethra (coronal section).

Skin of scrotum → Superficial inguinal lymph nodes
Testes and epididymis → pre- and para-aortic group of lymph nodes

Prostate: Internal iliac and sacral lymph nodes.

Applied:

- Due to long course of male urethra it is more subjected to trauma than female urethra.
- Columnar epithelium lining makes male urethra more vulnerable for gonococci infection than female urethra.
- Prostate, Cowper's, and Littre's gland have columnar epithelium lining thus making them vulnerable for gonococci infection.
- Some diseases over glans are rare in circumcised individual like Zoons balanitis, lichen sclerosus et atrophicus, psoriasis, and lichen planus.[1]
- Circumcised individual have less chance of acquiring HIV following sexual exposure **(Fig. 1)**.

ANATOMY OF FEMALE GENITAL TRACT

Female genital tract

External
- Vulva
- Mons pubis
- Labia majora
- Labia minora
- Clitoris
- Hymen
- Vestibule
- Urethral opening
- Bartholin's gland
- Paraurethral glands of skene

Internal
- Vagina
- Uterus
- Fallopian tube
- Ovaries

Mons pubis: Triangular mound of subcutaneous adipose connective tissue over:

- Pubic symphysis
- Hair bearing skin

Labia majora: Female counterpart of scrotum.

- It is 2 longitudinal folds of skin with subcutaneous tissue covering vaginal opening.
- Outer surface has hair, inner surface do not.
- Folds join anteriorly to form anterior commissure and posteriorly to form posterior commissure.

Labia minora: Thin cutaneous folds lying medial to labia majora

- Fuse superiorly to form prepuce of clitoris
- Fuse inferiorly to form fourchette

Clitoris: Erectile tissue located beneath prepuce and above urethra

- Principal female erogenous organ
- Consists of glans, body, and 2 crura

Vestibule: It is space between two minora **(Fig. 2)**.

- Has openings of:
  - Vagina
  - Urethral meatus
  - Paraurethral glands of skene
  - Bartholin's glands duct

Urethral opening: Located below clitoris and above vaginal opening

- Ducts of paraurethral glands usually open on each side of urethral opening

Female urethra: ~4 cm in length

- Lined by transitional epithelium proximally and stratified squamous distally.

Applied: Lack of columnar epithelium provides resistance from gonococci infection.

Bartholin's gland: Also known as greater vestibular glands.

- Ducts of the glands open between hymen and labia minora.
- Homologous to Cowper's gland.

Applied: Ducts of glands have columnar epithelium thus prone for gonococci infection.

Paraurethral glands of skene: Homologous to prostate. Involved less in sexually transmitted diseases (STDs)

Vagina: A fibromuscular tube from vulva to uterus

Length: Anterior wall—8–9 cm
Posterior wall—10–11 cm

Lined by stratified squamous epithelium.

Arterial supply: Mostly from vaginal artery (a branch of Internal Iliac Artery).

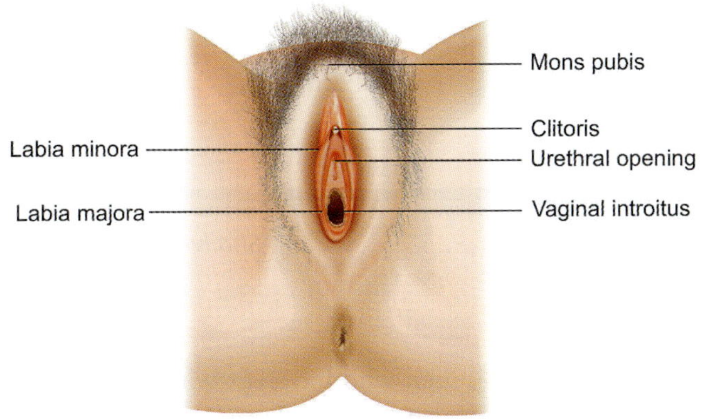

Fig. 2: External genitalia (female).

Applied: Epithelial cells rich in glycogen which helps in maintaining acidic environment and thus offers some protection from STDs.

Uterus: Hollow muscular organ.
Consists of—Body (lies above internal os).

- Cornu (near insertion fallopian tubes)
- Fundus (above insertion of fallopian tubes).

Lymphatic Drainage of Female Genitalia

Vulva: Superficial group of inguinal lymph nodes and femoral lymph nodes.

Vestibule: Common iliac and sacral lymph nodes.

Vagina: Upper one-third—external iliac lymph nodes.
Middle one-third—internal iliac lymph nodes.
Lower one-third—superficial inguinal lymph nodes.

Cervix: External iliac, internal iliac, and sacral lymph nodes. To some extent also in common iliac and para-aortic lymph nodes.

Uterus: *Upper part*—para-aortic lymph nodes

Middle part—External iliac lymph nodes

Lower part—Superficial inguinal lymph nodes

Fallopian tubes: Para-aortic lymph nodes
Isthmus drains in superficial inguinal lymph nodes

Ovaries: Para-aortic and pre-aortic lymph nodes

Some useful points in lymphatics: Enlargement of lymph nodes is seen in various STDs and is useful in diagnosing genital ulcer diseases.

Various morphology is observed in various diseases.

Example:

Syphilis: Discrete, shotty, nontender, bilateral

Herpes: Firm, tender, often bilateral

Chancroid: Tender, may suppurate, usually unilateral.

Lymphogranuloma venereum: Tender, may suppurate, usually unilateral.

Donovanosis: No lymphadenopathy, pseudobuboes may be present.

Destruction of lymph nodes can lead to lymphedema and elephantiasis (LGV, filariasis, and donovanosis).

Lymphatics from perianal skin and anal canal below the pectinate line drains into superficial inguinal group of lymph nodes.

Lymphatics from rectal mucosa drains into internal iliac group of lymph nodes.

What to examine in a case for genital lesion:

- Site, size, number and discharge from lesion
- Erythema, swelling, erosion, ulcer or pigmentary changes
- Inspect the scrotum and shaft of penis
- Inspect labia and folds between them
- Look for any deviation from normal anatomy and scarring
- Inspect the perianal skin
- Look for any discharge from urethra or vagina
- Palpate to assess induration and tenderness
- Palpate for any lymphadenopathy
- Also examine oral mucosa and eyes
- Look for lesion anywhere else in the body
- Ask for history of sexual exposure and past medical history
- Elicit history of similar lesions in the partner also

KEY POINTS

- Due to long course of male urethra, it is more subjected to trauma than female urethra.
- Columnar epithelium lining makes male urethra more vulnerable for gonococci infection than female urethra.
- Enlargement of lymph nodes is seen in various STDs and is useful in diagnosing genital ulcer diseases.

REFERENCE

1. Read SI, Abell E. Pseudoepitheliomatous, keratotic balanitis. Arch Dermatol. 1981;117:435-7.

EXAMINATION QUESTIONS

1. Discuss the anatomy of male urethra. Explain with diagram.
2. Write the anatomy of external female genitalia. Explain with diagram.
3. Describe the lymphatic drainage of male genital tract.
4. Discuss the lymphatic drainage of female genital tract.

125 CHAPTER Syphilis

Shailvi Banka Biyani

INTRODUCTION

Syphilis (synonyms: lues) is a chronic multistage infection caused by a microaerophilic spirochete called *Treponema pallidum* (ssp. pallidum). It is predominantly transmitted sexually although it can also pass through the placenta and by blood transfusion. Sir William Osler called it "a great imitator" because of its vivid clinical manifestations.

HISTORY

The disease was named after an afflicted shepherd named Syphilus, from a poem "Syphilis sive morbus gallicus," in 1530.[1,2] The "pre-Columbian hypothesis" and its variant the "unitarian hypothesis" states that all treponemal diseases had a global distribution.[2,3] The "Columbian hypothesis" proposes that Columbus brought syphilis with him.[3,4] Thus, the origins of syphilis have been the subject of several debates.

In 1928, Alexander Fleming (1881–1955) **(Fig. 1)** discovered penicillin and from 1943, it became the main treatment of syphilis.[5,6]

EPIDEMIOLOGY

The distribution of syphilis is worldwide, predominately in areas of high sexual promiscuity. Low- and middle-income countries (LMICs), men who have sex with men (MSM), transgender women, and sex workers are the vulnerable sector.[7-11] The advent of serologic testing, contact tracing, penicillin treatment, and stringent public measures has reduced the incidence dramatically.[12]

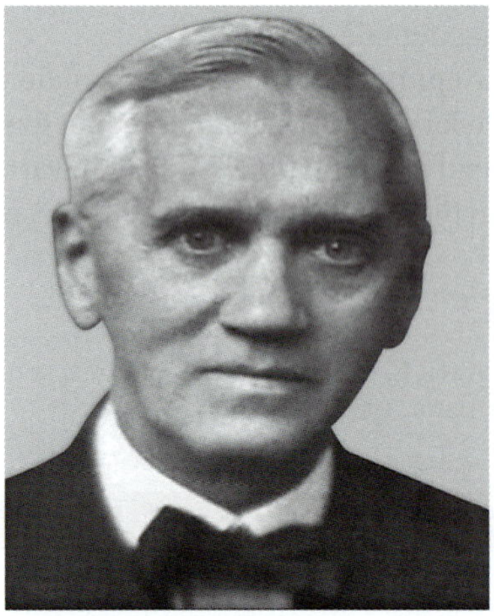

Fig. 1: Alexander Fleming.
Source: https://www.nobelprize.org/prizes/medicine/1945/fleming/biographical/.

ETIOLOGY

Treponema pallidum is a member of the genus *Treponema* of the order Spirochaetales. It was identified by Schaudinn and Hoffmann.[13] The characteristics of this microorganism are outlined in **Box 1**.

NATURAL COURSE OF DISEASE

The organism enters the body via mucosal surfaces and abraded skin, followed by attachment to host cells and multiplication. Within a few hours, treponemes disseminate to the regional lymph nodes and internal organs.

CLINICAL FEATURES

Syphilis is a multistage disease with primary, secondary, tertiary, and latent stage. Early syphilis includes primary, secondary, and early latent phase (<2 years). Late syphilis includes late latent (>2 years) and tertiary stage **(Flowchart 1)**. The clinical features are given in **Table 1**.

Latent Syphilis

There are no clinical signs of syphilis, but the serologic tests for syphilis are reactive.

BOX 1: Characteristics of *Treponema pallidum*.

- 6–20 μm in length, 0.1–0.18 μm in diameter
- Actively motile due to tight spirals
- Inability to survive outside of an animal host
- Cannot be cultured in vitro for extended time period
- Demonstrated by dark-field microscopy or by fluorescent antibody techniques:
  - *Outer membrane:* Lipid-rich—contains uniform-sized trans-membrane rare outer membrane proteins (TROMPs)—lacks lipopolysaccharide
- Periplasmic flagella—movements are pathognomonic

Source: Bolognia J, Schaffer J, Cerroni L. Dermatology: 2-Volume Set, 4th Edition. Gurugram: Elsevier India; 2017.

Flowchart 1: Natural history of untreated syphilis.

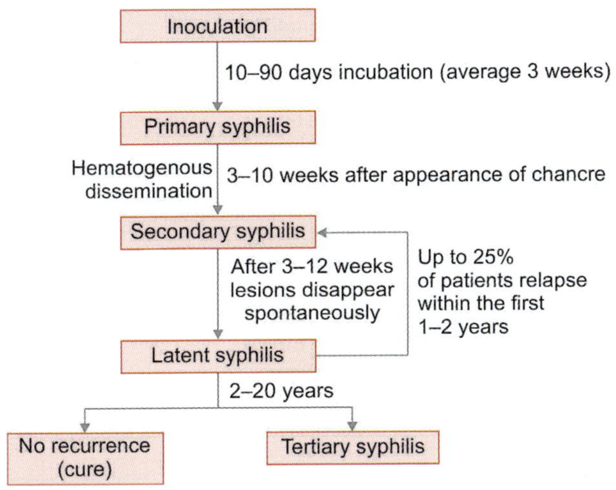

Source: Bolognia J, Schaffer J, Cerroni L. Dermatology: 2-Volume Set, 4th Edition. Gurugram: Elsevier India; 2017.

HISTOPATHOLOGY[5]

- Perivascular infiltration of lymphocytes and plasma cells
- Endarteritis obliterans
- Organisms in the walls of capillaries and lymphatic vessels, demonstrated by Levaditi's silver stain or by the fluorescent antibody technique
- Heubner's arteritis occurs in cardiovascular and meningovascular syphilis.

DIAGNOSIS

Investigation

Different investigations are shown in **Figure 6**.

TREATMENT (BOXES 2 AND 3)

Penicillin G is the treatment of choice all stages of syphilis.

TABLE 1: Clinical features of different stages of syphilis.

Stage of syphilis	*Incubation period*	*Prodromal symptom*	*Cutaneous lesion*	*Extracutaneous manifestation*	*Differential diagnosis*	*Signs in syphilis*
Primary syphilis	9–90 days	Absent	*Morphology:* "Hunterian chancre" **(Figs. 2A and B)**—round or oval ulcer, nontender, raised, indurated, firm and rubbery border, hemorrhagic necrotic base with yellowish slough, approximately 1 cm in diameter *Fate:* Persists for 1–6 weeks; heals without scarring *Site:* Glans, coronal sulcus and the foreskin in males labia, fourchette, urethra, perineum in females Extragenital—lips, oral cavity, fingers, breasts, trunk, abdomen, and extremities	Enlarged, rubbery, movable, nontender, nonsuppurative, discrete lymph nodes	• Chancroid • Herpes simplex • Granuloma inguinale • Traumatic erosion ulcer • Aphthous ulcer • Squamous cell carcinoma • Basal cell carcinoma • Fixed-drug eruption	Retraction of the foreskin with a chancre in its mucosal surface causes the foreskin to flip briskly, a sign known as the *dory flop*
Secondary syphilis	3–12 weeks	Malaise, appetite loss, fever, headache, stiff neck, lacrimation myalgias, arthralgias, nasal discharge, depression Hepato-splenomegaly	Lesions are called "syphilids". *Early (10%):* Nonpruritic, roseola-like, discrete, generalized macules, on the flanks and shoulders *Late (70%):* Generalized maculopapular, papulosquamous infiltrated, copper-colored lesions **(Figs. 5A and B)** Annular plaques on face; corymbose, polymorphic palms and soles: symmetric papules and plaques with a collarette of scale *(collarette of Biett)*	• Generalized lymphadenopathy • Syphilitic perlèche • Split papules • Mucous patches: "plaques muqueuses" **(Figs. 4A and B)** in the oropharynx • Syphilitic sore throat • Hair: "moth-eaten"—alopecia • Toxic telogen effluvium • Nail-fissuring, onycholysis, Beau's lines, and onychomadesis	• Pityriasis rosea • Condyloma lata • Drug eruption • Viral eruption • Psoriasis • Lichen planus • Eczema • Sarcoid • Cutaneous T-cell lymphoma • Erythema multiforme	• *Crown of Venus (corona veneris):* Lesion in a crown-like pattern • *Necklace of Venus:* Hypopigmented macule on neck • *Condyloma lata* ***(Figs. 3A and B):*** Anogenital area • *Nickels and dimes:* Annular papules and plaques around mouth and nose

Contd...

Contd...

Stage of syphilis	*Incubation period*	*Prodromal symptom*	*Cutaneous lesion*	*Extracutaneous manifestation*	*Differential diagnosis*	*Signs in syphilis*
Tertiary syphilis	2–20 years		*Morphology:* Gummas **(Figs. 5A and B)**—nodular or noduloulcerative, superficial, firm, painless, dull-red, shiny, flat cutaneous nodules that measure several millimeters and coalesce to plaque, locally destructive often with an arciform pattern, heals with scarring *Site:* Arms, back, forehead, buttocks, prestemal, supraclavicular, or pretibial area	Gumma in bone, liver, oral cavity, respiratory tract, myocardium, digestive, and nervous system *Nervous system:* • *Asymptomatic:* Early *Late:* • *Meningeal:* Acute syphilitic meningitis Meningovascular Cerebrovascular Spinal form • *Parenchymatous:* General paresis Tabes dorsalis Taboparesis Optic atrophy • *Gummatous:* Cerebral form Spinal form Both *CVS:* Transmural inflammatory lesions, which lead to endarteritis of the vessels	• Sarcoid • Metastatic carcinoma • Sarcomas • Lymphoma • Wegener's granulomatosis • Leishmaniasis • Vasculitis • Deep fungal infections • Lupus vulgaris • Psoriasis	• Saddle nose • Chronic interstitial glossitis • Osteitis • Periostitis • Sclerosing osteitis
Congenital syphilis	*Early:* <2 years of age *Late:* >2 years of age	*Early:* Marasmic, fretful, dehydrated *Late:* Stigmata	*Early:* Similar to secondary syphilis, syphilitic pemphigus—bulla rupturing to form erosion in ankle, wrist, etc., fissured lesions in intertriginous sites resulting in radial scarring called rhagades	*Early:* • "Snuffles" (bloody or purulent mucinous nasal discharge) • Perioral and perianal fissures • Lymphadenopathy • Hepatosplenomegaly • Osteochondritis • Anemia, thrombocytopenia, pneumonitis (pneumonia alba), hepatitis, nephropathy, and neurosyphilis *Late:* Interstitial keratitis, perisynovitis *(Clutton's joint)*, gumma in bones, tabes dorsalis, and general paralysis of insane		*Early:* • *Parrot pseudoparalysis*—epiphysitis of long bones *Late:* • *Hutchinson's teeth* (peg-shaped, notched permanent incisors) • *Mulberry molars* (rudimentary cusps on the permanent first molars) • *Higouménakis' sign* (thickening of the medial clavicle) • *Scaphoid scapulae* • *Saber shins* (anterior tibial bowing) • *Saddle nose* (depression of nasal root) • *Olympian brow* (frontal bossing of Parrot) • *Hypoplastic maxilla* • *High palatal arch* ± perforation

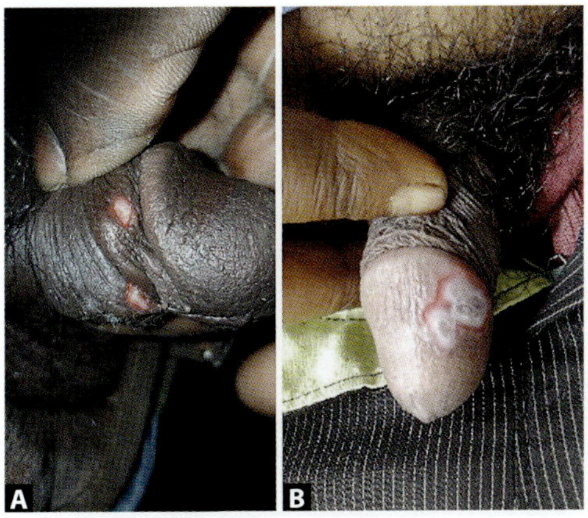

Figs. 2A and B: Chancres of primary syphilis in penis.
Courtesy: Dr Jayanti Dutta, PGT, Bankura Sammilani Medical College and Hospital (BSMCH), Bankura, West Bengal, India.

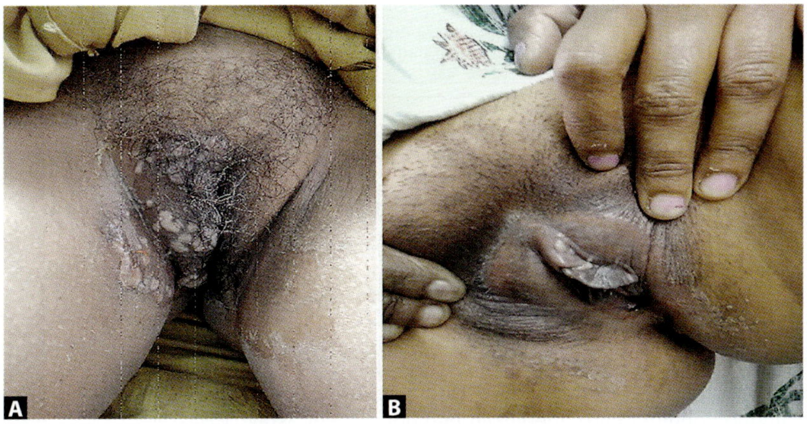

Figs. 3A and B: Condyloma lata.
Courtesy: Dr Jayanti Dutta, PGT, Bankura Sammilani Medical College and Hospital (BSMCH), Bankura, West Bengal, India.

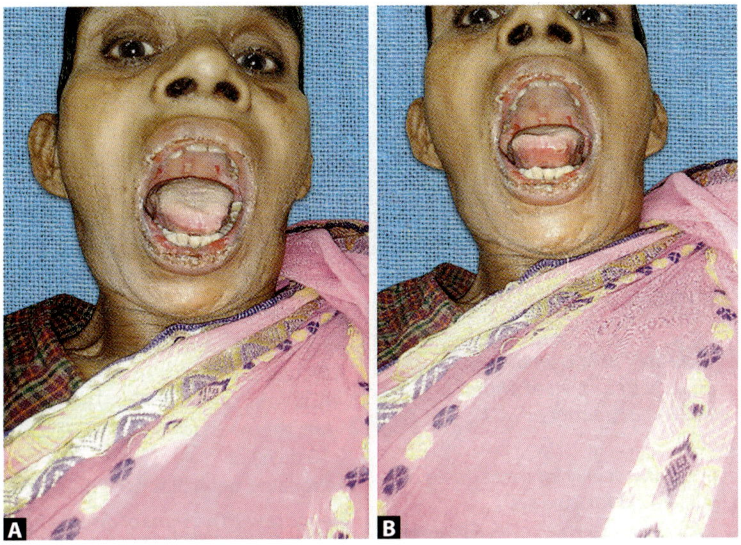

Figs. 4A and B: *Mucous patches:* Plaques muqueuses.
Courtesy: Dr Jayanti Dutta, PGT, Bankura Sammilani Medical College and Hospital (BSMCH), Bankura, West Bengal, India.

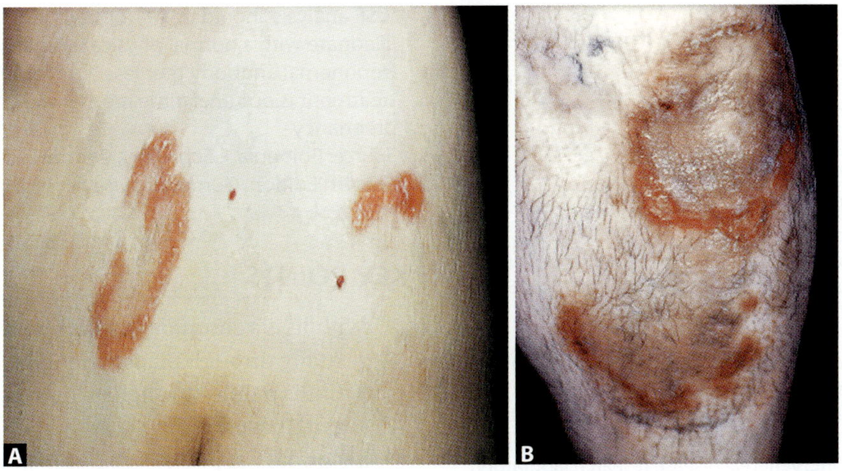

Figs. 5A and B: Cutaneous gumma of tertiary syphilis.
Source: Bolognia J, Schaffer J, Cerroni L. Dermatology: 2-Volume Set, 4th Edition. Gurugram: Elsevier India; 2017.

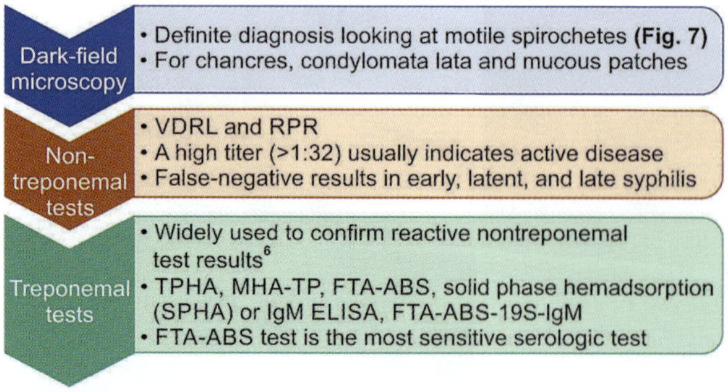

Fig. 6: Investigations of syphilis.
(FTA-ABS: fluorescent treponemal antibody absorption; IgM ELISA: immunoglobulin M enzyme-linked immunosorbent assay; MHA-TP: microhemagglutination assay-*Treponema pallidum*; RPR: rapid plasma regain; TPHA: *Treponema pallidum* hemagglutination; VDRL: venereal disease research laboratory)

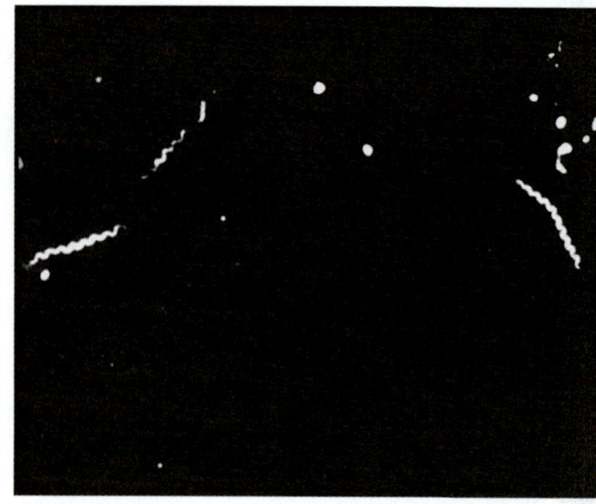

Fig. 7: Dark-field microscopy showing spiral treponemes 98.
Source: Centers for Disease Control and Prevention Public Health Image Library (CDC/Renelle Woodall, 1969).

BOX 2: Treatment recommendations for syphilis.

Early syphilis [primary, secondary, and early latent (acquired <1 year previously)]

Recommended:
- Benzathine penicillin, 2.4 million units* IM as a single dose or
- Procaine penicillin, 1.2 million units IM qd for 10 days†

Alternative regimens for penicillin-allergic patients.‡
- Doxycycline, 200 mg qd (100 mg po bid preferred over a single 200 mg dose) for 14 days or
- Tetracycline, 500 mg po qid for 14 days or
- Ceftriaxone, 1 g IM or IV qd for 8–10 days or
- Azithromycin, 2 g po as a single dose$

Late latent (acquired >1 year previously or of unknown duration), cardiovascular and gummatous syphilis; retreatment of primary, secondary or latent syphilis after failed initial treatment¶

Recommended:
- Benzathine penicillin, 2.4 million units* IM weekly for three doses or
- Procaine penicillin, 1.2 million units IM qd for 20 days†

Alternative regimens for penicillin-allergic patients:‡
- Doxycycline, 200 mg qd (100 mg po bid preferred over a single 200 mg dose) for 28 days or
- Tetracycline, 500 mg po qid for 28 days

Neurosyphilis and ocular syphilis

Recommended:
- Aqueous penicillin G, 3–4 million units IV q4h (18–24 million units daily) for 10–14 days or
- Procaine penicillin, 2.4 million units IM qd plus probenecid, 500 mg po qid, both for 10–14 days

Alternative regimens for penicillin-allergic patients:
- Ceftriaxone, 2 g IM or IV qd for 10–14 days or
- Consider desensitization

*In children, 50,000 U/kg up to the adult dose.
†Alternative treatment regimen in the World Health Organization (WHO) guidelines (http://whqlibdoc.who.int/publications/2003/9241546263.pdf).
‡Limited data.
$Resistance reported.
¶E.g. if RPR/VDRL titers fail to decrease four-fold or symptoms persist/progress; must first examine the CSF to exclude neurosyphilis.
(bid: twice daily; H: hours; CSF: cerebrospinal fluid; IM: intramuscularly; IV: intravenously; po: orally; q: every; qd: daily; qid: four times daily; RPR: rapid plasma regain; VDRL: venereal disease research laboratory)
Source: Bolognia J, Schaffer J, Cerroni L. Dermatology: 2-Volume Set, 4th Edition. Gurugram: Elsevier India; 2017.

BOX 3: Treatment recommendations for syphilis in special situations.

Recommended:
- Benzathine penicillin, 2.4 million units IM weekly for two (early syphilis) or three (late syphilis) doses or
- Procaine penicillin, regimen appropriate for the stage of syphilis

In the case of penicillin allergy:
- Desensitization to penicillin or
- Alternative regimens:*
  - Azithromycin, 500 mg qd for 10 days or
  - Ceftriaxone, 1 g IM or IV qd for 10–14 days

Congenital

Neonate with proven or highly probable disease or born to mother with untreated early syphilis:†
- Aqueous penicillin G, 50,000 U/kg IV q12h for the first 7 days of life, then q8h for 3 days (100,000–150,000 U/kg/day for a total of 10 days) or
- Procaine penicillin, 50,000 U/kg IM qd for 10–14 days

Neonate with no signs of disease born to mother with treated syphilis:‡
Benzathine penicillin, 50,000 U/kg IM in a single dose

*Limited data; not recommended by the centers for disease control (CDC) but included in the World Health Organization (WHO) and European Branch of the International Union against Sexually Transmitted Infections (IUSTI) guidelines.
†CSF analysis should be performed prior to therapy.
‡Neonate with a normal physical examination and serum non-treponemal antibody titer less than four-fold the maternal titer; treatment is optional if the mother was fully treated before pregnancy.
Source: Bolognia J, Schaffer J, Cerroni L. Dermatology: 2-Volume Set, 4th Edition. Gurugram: Elsevier India; 2017.

KEY POINTS

- Syphilis is a chronic systemic infection which is transmitted sexually through placenta and by blood transfusion.
- Syphilis passes through primary, secondary, tertiary, and latent phases.
- Secondary syphilis is called "a great imitator" because of its various clinical presentation.
- Syphilis increases the chance of transmission of HIV.

- The cure rate of syphilis is >95% and is favored by a long period of incubation.
- Nontreponemal tests have a low sensitivity and specificity.
- Treponemal tests have high sensitivity and specificity and are confirmatory.
- Biologic false positive (BFP) is when nontreponemal test is positive and treponemal test negative.
- Stigmata of syphilis persist throughout life and enable a diagnosis of congenital syphilis.

REFERENCES

1. Franzen C. Syphilis in composers and musicians—Mozart, Beethoven, Paganini, Schubert, Schumann, Smetana. Eur J Clin Microbiol Infect Dis. 2008;27(12):1151-7.
2. Rothschild BM. History of syphilis. Clin Infect Dis. 2005;40(10):1454-63.
3. Forsea D, Popescu R, Popescu CM. Compendiu de dermatologie si venerologie/Dermatology and Venerology Compendium. Iasi: Ed Tehnica; 1996.
4. Baker BJ, Armelagos GJ. The origin and antiquity of syphilis: paleopathological diagnosis and interpretation. Curr Anthropol. 1988;29(5):703-38.
5. Forrai J. History of Different Therapeutics of Venereal Disease before the Discovery of Penicillin, Syphilis—Recognition, Description and Diagnosis (Dr Neuza Satomi Sato). Bengaluru: Intech Solutions; 2011.
6. Sefton AM. The great pox that was...syphilis. J Appl Microbiol. 2001;91(4):592-6.
7. Lurie P, Fernandes ME, Hughes V, Arevalo EI, Hudes ES, Reingold A, et al. Socioeconomic status and risk of HIV-1, syphilis and hepatitis B infection among sex workers in São Paulo State, Brazil. Instituto Adolfo Lutz Study Group. AIDS. 1995;9(Suppl 1):S31-7.
8. Uribe-Salas F, Del Río-Chiriboga C, Conde-Glez CJ, Juárez-Figueroa L, Uribe-Zúñaga P, Calderón-Jaimes E, et al. Prevalence, incidence, and determinants of syphilis in female commercial sex workers in Mexico City. Sex Transm Dis. 1996;23(2):120-6.
9. Ahmed HJ, Omar K, Adan SY, Guled AM, Grillner L, Bygdeman S. Syphilis and human immunodeficiency virus seroconversion during a 6-month follow-up of female prostitutes in Mogadishu, Somalia. Int J STD AIDS. 1991;2(2):119-23.
10. Killewo JZ, Sandstrom A, Bredberg Raden U, Mhalu FS, Biberfeld G, Wall S. Prevalence and incidence of syphilis and its association with HIV-1 infection in a population-based study in the Kagera region of Tanzania. Int J STD AIDS. 1994;5(6): 424-31.
11. Kunawararak P, Beyrer C, Natpratan C, Feng W, Celentano DD, de Boer M, et al. The epidemiology of HIV and syphilis among male commercial sex workers in northern Thailand. AIDS. 1995;9(5):517-21.
12. Clement ME, Hicks CB. Syphilis on the rise: what went wrong? JAMA. 2016;315(21):2281-3.
13. Smibert RM. Genus III: Treponema Schaudinn 1905,1728. In: Krieg NR, Holt JG (Eds). Bergey's Manual of Systematic Bacteriology. Baltimore: Williams and Wilkins; 1984. pp. 49-57.

EXAMINATION QUESTIONS

1. Discuss different types of cutaneous manifestation of secondary syphilis.
2. Write a short note on congenital syphilis.
3. What are the treponemal and the nontreponemal tests for syphilis? Discuss the nontreponemal tests of syphilis.
4. Describe the treatment of primary and secondary syphilis.
5. Write the differential diagnosis of primary and secondary syphilis.
6. Explain briefly "gumma of syphilis."
7. Describe "stigmata of congenital syphilis".
8. Write a short note on VDRL.
9. Describe approach to a case of genital ulcer.
10. How will you approach a case of inguinal bubo?
11. What is the management of congenital syphilis?
12. Discuss syphilis and pregnancy.
13. What is Jarisch-Herxheimer reaction?
14. Describe point of care test for STIs and diagnosis of congenital syphilis.

126 CHAPTER Nonvenereal Treponematosis

Somodyuti Chandra

INTRODUCTION

The human treponematoses comprise the venereal syphilis and the nonvenereal endemic treponematoses: Yaws, bejel and pinta. The etiological agents include four closely-related gram-negative spirochetal bacteria belonging to the order *Spirochaetales*, family *Spirochaetaceae*, genus *Treponema*, and species *pallidum*. *Treponema pallidum* subspecies pallidum is responsible for venereal syphilis, whereas *T. pallidum* subspecies pertenue causes yaws, *T. pallidum* subspecies endemecium causes bejel (endemic syphilis), and *T. pallidum* subspecies carateum is responsible for pinta.

Between 1952 and 1964, the number of endemic treponematoses cases was reduced from an estimated 50 million to 2.5 million as a result of mass treatment campaigns led by the World Health Organization (WHO) and the United Nations Children's Emergency Fund (UNICEF) in 46 countries. In some regions, disease was eliminated, as bejel was eliminated in Bosnia, and yaws in Malaysia and Brazil. Yaws was declared eliminated from India on 19 September 2006.[1-3] Nevertheless, some endemic foci still persist in the Globe.

In 2012, the WHO officially set a goal for yaws eradication by 2020. This challenging but potentially feasible endeavor is favored by the adoption of oral azithromycin for mass treatment and the currently focused distribution of yaws and endemic treponematoses.

YAWS

- *AKA:* Framboesia tropica, thymosis, polypapilloma tropicum, parangi and paru (Malay), bouba (Spanish), pian (French), madia roga, or gondi roga (India)
- *Etiological agent: Treponema pallidum* subspecies pertenue
- *Epidemiology:*
  - *Geographical distribution:* Hot humid tropical regions, particularly parts of Africa, Asia, South America, Pacific Islands
  - *Age group:* Children younger than 15 years age; peak age group 6–10 years
  - Both genders are affected
  - Overcrowding, poor sanitation, poor hygiene, lack of water supply, lack of protective clothing facilitates spreading.[4]
- *Transmission:* Mainly through direct skin-to-skin contact with infectious lesion, wherein treponemes enter through a breech in skin continuity. Transmission through vectors (flies) has been reported.
- *Incubation period:* 9–90 days (mean 21 days)
- *Clinical features:*
  - *Primary stage:* Also called the primary yaw or mother yaw.
    - *Common sites:* Buttocks and lower extremities
    - Begins at the site of inoculation as a painless but pruritic papule → Spreads by peripheral extension or by coalescence of adjacent satellite papules to form a papilloma, 2–5 cm in diameter → Breaks down into a nontender ulcer covered by honey-brown crust → On removal of the crust, a round-oval, soft, red, moist ulcer (resembling a raspberry) is revealed with the highly infectious exudate teeming with treponemes.
    - Left untreated, the lesion resolves spontaneously in 3–6 months leaving a depigmented atrophic scar with hyperpigmented margin.
    - May be associated with fever, arthralgia, and lymphadenopathy.[5]
  - *Secondary stage:* Occurs within months to years, due to widespread dissemination via blood and lymphatics producing multiple smaller lesions resembling the mother yaw, called the daughter yaws. These lesions heal without scarring but tends to frequently relapse.
    - *Cutaneous lesions:* Commonly occurs in the periorificial sites (mouth and nose), axillae and groins → Multiple daughter yaws or "pianomas" spread diffusely and ulcerate, with the exudate containing numerous treponemes → Annular lesions can occur due to central healing of the papilloma or coalescence of multiple lesions, known as "tinea yaws" → Condyloma lata on moist surfaces such as axillae and groins and measles-like morbilliform eruption can also occur.[6]
    - *Palmoplantar lesions:* Characterized by thick hyperkeratotic plaques with ulceration and secondary infection, producing a painful crab-like gait. Hence, called "wet crab yaws." Macules and hyperkeratotic papules can also occur.[7]

- *Nail lesions:* Hyperkeratotic macules and papules affecting nail-fold results in paronychia, called "pianic onychia."
- *Bone and cartilage lesions:* Painful periostitis and osteitis affect the fingers resulting in dactylitis, and the long bones of forearm and leg, resulting in pain and swelling. Multiple bones are usually affected.
- Constitutional symptoms including headache, malaise, lymphadenopathy, arthralgia are commonly present.[8]

- *Latent stage:* It is an asymptomatic noninfectious stage where only the positive serology is the evidence of infection.
- *Tertiary stage:* Rarely seen now, around 10% of the untreated patients can progress to this stage, several years after the primary infection.
    - *Cutaneous lesions:* Characterized by diffuse subcutaneous gummatous nodules that suppurate in the center and break into large, serpiginous ulcers with massive tissue necrosis → Heals with scarring, contracture, and sometimes keloid.
    - Palmoplantar keratoderma with fissuring (called "dry crab yaws") is common.
    - *Bone and joint lesions:* Characterized by hypertrophic periostitis, gummatous periostitis, osteitis, and osteomyelitis. Hydrarthrosis, synovitis, and bursitis can result in joint contractures. Rare manifestations include destructive osteitis of long bones causing bowing of the shin (saber tibia), destruction of the bones of the central face, i.e., maxilla, ethmoid, nasal, and palate (gangosa), and hypertrophic periostitis causing exostosis of the paranasal maxilla (gondou).[4]
    - *Neurologic/ophthalmologic lesions:* Rarely damage to pyramidal tract and posterior columns of spinal cord, retrobulbar neuropathy, and nerve deafness can occur.[9,10]

- *Differential diagnosis:*
    - Venereal syphilis
    - *Skin lesions:* Ecthyma, Hansen, leishmaniasis, tropical ulcer, eczema, psoriasis, sarcoidosis
    - *Palmoplantar lesions:* Idiopathic keratoderma, calluses, Norwegian scabies
    - *Late yaws:* Tuberculosis verrucosa cutis (TBVC), deep mycoses, blastomycosis-like pyoderma, Hansen, osteomyelitis, rhinoscleroma, rhinosporidiosis, African histoplasmosis
- *Attenuated yaws:* Vorst described a "clinically attenuated variant." In areas of lesser prevalence of yaws, patients often present with milder disease characterized by transient, single or few, dry, flat, gray lesions limited to the intertriginous area.[11]

ENDEMIC SYPHILIS

- *AKA:* Bejel, belesh, firjal, loath (Middle East), njovera (Zimbabwe), dichuchwa (Botswana).
- *Etiological agent: T. pallidum* subspecies endemicum
- *Epidemiology:*
    - *Geographical distribution:* Hot dry climate. Although once prevalent in northern Europe, northern Asia, eastern Mediterranean, and southern Africa, it is now found predominantly in the Arabian-peninsula and the Sahel (southern border of the Sahara desert).
    - *Age group:* Children 2–15 years age
    - Both genders are affected
    - Infection tends to run in families
    - Overcrowding, poor sanitation, poor hygiene, lack of water supply, lack of protective clothing facilitates spreading.
- *Transmission:* Mainly through skin-to-skin contact, kissing and fomites, as in contaminated drinking vessels and pipes.
- *Incubation period:* 9–90 days
- *Clinical features:*
    - *Primary stage:* Characterized by inconspicuous tiny, painless papule or ulcer in the mouth or nasopharynx, that is often missed. Rarely lesion on nipple of nursing women and genitalia of adults have been reported.[12]
    - *Secondary lesions:* Develops 3–6 months after infection.
        - *Mucosal lesions:* Mucosal patches are the earliest lesions characterized by shallow, painless ulcers on the tongue, lips, fauces, tonsils, and buccal mucosa. Split papules at the oral commissures (angular stomatitis), and laryngitis causing hoarseness can also occur.
        - *Skin lesions:* A variety of secondary skin lesions have been reported to occur—maculopapular, papulosquamous, macular erythema, annular and pigmented lesions, ecthyma, psoriasiform lesions, and condyloma lata on intertriginous areas. There may be associated generalized lymphadenopathy with characteristically firm, discrete, mobile, nontender nodes.
        - *Bone/cartilage lesions:* Osteitis and periostitis of long bones are common causing arthritis and nocturnal bone pain.[13]
    - *Latent stage:* Occurs within 4 years of onset. Approximately 1/3rd of the patients in secondary stage spontaneously recover, 1/3rd go into latency and the rest 1/3rd progresses to tertiary stage.
    - *Tertiary stage:* Gummatous lesions resembling gangosa and gondaou occur on the skin, mucosa and bones that often progresses to form destructive ulcers. These skin lesions often spontaneously resolve with atrophic depigmented scars surrounded by hyperpigmentation. Destruction of the palate and nasal septum can

cause difficulty in speech and swallowing. Ocular involvement in the form of uveitis, chorioretinitis, and optic atrophy have been reported.[5]

- *Differential diagnosis:*
  - Syphilis
  - *For early skin lesions:* Psoriasis, pityriasis rosea, eczema, lichen planus
  - *For oral lesions:* Aphthous stomatitis, perleche, vitamin deficiency, herpetic stomatitis
  - *For rhinopharyngeal lesions:* TB, leprosy, rhinosporidiosis, rhinoscleroma, mucocutaneous leishmaniasis (such as espundia), histoplasmosis.
  - *For late-stage lesions:* Malignancies (such as squamous cell carcinoma), lupus vulgaris, bromoderma tuberosum, iododerma, facial granuloma.[14,15]

PINTA

- *AKA:* Enfermedad Azul (Chile, Peru), Carate (Colombia, Venuzuela), Mal del Pinto (Mexico, Cuba), Empeines (Spain), Lota (South and Central America)
- *Etiological agent: T. pallidum* subspecies carateum
- *Epidemiology:*
  - *Geographical distribution:* Hot dry climate. Although once prevalent in northern Europe, northern Asia, Colombia, eastern Mediterranean, and southern Africa, it is now found predominantly in the Arabian-peninsula and the Sahel (southern border of the Sahara Desert)[6]
  - *Age group:* Peak age group affected 15–30 years
  - Both genders are affected.
  - Overcrowding, poor sanitation, poor hygiene, lack of water supply, lack of protective clothing facilitates spreading.
- It is the mildest form of treponematoses as the lesions are limited to the skin, and there is no evidence of systemic involvement or vertical transmission.
- *Transmission:* Mainly through skin-to-skin contact
- *Incubation period:* 1 week–2 months
- *Clinical features:*
  - *Primary stage:* Characterized by small erythematous macule or papule that progresses into patches or plaque with a pale center. Exposed areas such as face and extremities are the most common sites; rarely neck, chest and abdomen may be involved. Rarely, there may be pruritus and regional lymphadenopathy; however, constitutional symptoms are absent. Lesions resolve with hyperpigmentation or depigmentation or persist into the secondary stage.[16]
  - *Secondary stage:* Occurs 3–5 years postinoculation. Characterized by generalized eruption of small, red, scaling papules called "pintids" → These expand and coalesce together to form psoriasiform plaques → Pintids change their color from red to shades of brown, slate-blue, gray, or black. The lesions tend to have a waxing and waning course over several years, resulting in oval, circinate or polycyclic lesions within larger lesion which later heal with depigmentation or hyperpigmentation.
  - *Tertiary stage:* Characterized by depigmented lesions over body prominences, wrists, elbows, and ankles. Periarticular cutaneous atrophy and hyperkeratotic plaques on extensor surface are characteristic. Unlike the other treponematoses, in pinta, neither destructive skin and bone lesions nor cardiovascular and neurological manifestations occur.[5]
- *Differential diagnoses:*
  - Yaws, bejel, syphilis
  - *Early skin lesions:* Eczema, psoriasis, pityriasis alba, EDP, atrophic LP, lupus erythematosus, vitamin deficiency, pellagra, tinea corporis, pityriasis versicolor, leprosy.
  - *Pigmentary change:* Vitiligo, chemical leukoderma, leprosy, hypopigmented mycosis fungoides.

DIAGNOSIS

- Clinical features
- *Direct microscopy:* Direct microscopic identification of treponemes from lesion fluids by either dark-field microscopy or direct fluorescent antibody is the initial step in diagnosing a treponemal infection. This is most helpful during the primary stage of infection because treponemal antibodies do not usually appear until 1–4 weeks after the lesion has formed.
- *Nontreponemal tests:* These include VDRL and RPR tests. These tests usually become positive within 2–4 weeks of the appearance of the primary lesion and can be used as "tests of cure" because they usually become negative after treatment.
- *Treponemal tests:* Tests such as fluorescent treponemal antibody absorption (FTA-ABS) test, *T. pallidum* hemagglutination assay (TPHA), and *T. pallidum* particle agglutination assay (TPPA) are used to confirm the diagnosis. Once positive, these tests usually remain positive for life.
- *Radiological studies:* To note bone, cartilage, and periosteal changes.

TREATMENT

- Single dose intramuscular benzathine penicillin or single oral dose of azithromycin (30 mg/kg) is the drug of choice for all nonvenereal treponematosis.[17]

Age	*Dosage of penicillin*
Less than 6 years	600,000 units
6–14 years	1.2 million units
Above 14 years	2.4 million units

- Penicillin kills treponemes within minutes and the lesions become non-infectious within 18–24 hours.
- In penicillin allergic patients, tetracycline (25 mg/kg/day), chloramphenicol (25 mg/kg/day), erythromycin (8 mg/kg/day) or doxycycline (2.5 mg/kg/day) can be given for 10–15 days.
- Other important measures include avoiding contact with others with cutaneous lesions and careful follow-up care to identify and to retreat initial treatment failures.

CONCLUSION

Nonvenereal treponematoses remain a considerable burden on local healthcare systems. Though they share considerable similarity with venereal syphilis in being chronic multistage disease, overlapping serological findings and similar therapeutic responsiveness, the former has much less prevalence, and less severe late manifestations. As with syphilis, penicillin has been the mainstay of treatment, but azithromycin has recently been shown to be effective in the treatment of yaws, prompting renewed efforts to eradicate it.

KEY POINTS

- Largely forgotten in industrialized countries, but not lost elsewhere, endemic nonvenereal treponematoses cause dramatic morbidity in many regions of the third world.
- Although antigenically and morphologically identical, the causative organisms of treponematosis behave so distinctly as to warrant subspecies designations.
- All of them share impressive similarities in pathogenesis and natural history.
- All are transmitted by direct contact with infectious lesions.
- All are chronic infections that manifest in multiple stages involving the skin.
- Like venereal syphilis, these infections are clinically characterized by three successive stages separated by periods of latency.
- All except pinta can progress to cause serious and destructive lesions of skin, bone, and cartilage.
- Congenital infection has not been reported.
- The means of investigation and diagnosis is same as venereal syphilis.
- Penicillin is highly effective for both cutaneous and systemic lesions.

REFERENCES

1. Arslanagić N, Bokonjić M, Macanović K. Eradication of endemic syphilis in Bosnia. Genitourin Med. 1989;65:4.
2. Lo EK. Yaws in Malaysia. Rev Infect Dis. 1985;7(Suppl 2):S251.
3. Muniz ES. "Is a shot alone enough?": concepts of health, hygiene, and nutrition and the Program to Eradicate Yaws in Brazil, 1956-1961. Hist Cienc Saude Manguinhos. 2012;19:197.
4. Perine PL, Hopkins DR, Niemel PLA, St. John RK, Causse G, Antal GM. Handbook of endemic treponematoses: yaws, endemic syphilis and pinta. Geneva: World Health Organization; 1984.
5. Giacani L, Lukehart SA. The endemic treponematoses. Clin Microbiol Rev. 2014;27(1):89-115.
6. Koff AB, Rosen T. Nonvenereal treponematoses: yaws, endemic syphilis, and pinta. J Am Acad Dermatol. 1993;29:519-35.
7. Walker SL, Hay RJ. Yaws: a review of the last 50 years. Int J Dermatol. 2000;39:258-60.
8. Farnsworth N, Rosen T. Endemic treponematosis: review and update. Clin Dermatol. 2006;24(3):181-90.
9. Roman GC, Roman LN. Occurrences of congenital, cardiovascular, visceral, neurologic, and neuro-ophthalmologic complications of late yaws: a theme for future research. Rev Infect Dis. 1986;8:760-70.
10. Mohammed KN. Late yaws and optic atrophy. Ann Trop Med Parasitol. 1990;84:637-9.
11. Verst FA. Clinical diagnosis and changing manifestations of treponemal infection. Rev Infect Dis. 1985;7:S327-31.
12. Grin EI. Endemic syphilis in Bosnia; clinical and epidemiological observations on a successful mass-treatment campaign. Bull World Health Organ. 1952;7:1-74.
13. Seghal VN. Leg ulcers caused by yaws and endemic syphilis. Clin Dermatol. 1990;8:166-74.
14. Kanan MW, Abbas M, Girgis HY. Late mutilating bejel in the nomadic Bedouins of Kuwait. Dermatologica. 1971;143:277-86.
15. Engelkens HJ, Vuzevski VD, Stolz E. Nonvenereal treponematoses in tropical countries. Clin Dermatol. 1999;17:143-52.
16. Marquez F, Rein CR, Arias O. Mal de pinto in Mexico. Bull Org Mond Sante; Bull Wld Hlth Org. 1955;13:299-322.
17. Mitja O, Hays R, Ipai A, Penias M, Paru R, Fagaho D, et al. Single-dose azithromycin versus benzathine benzylpenicillin for treatment of yaws in children in Papua New Guinea: an open-label, non-inferiority, randomised trial. Lancet. 2012;379:342-7.

EXAMINATION QUESTION

1. Write a short note on nonvenereal trepanomatoses.

127 CHAPTER

Chancroid

Akhilesh Shukla, Sanjay K Rathi

INTRODUCTION

Chancroid is a bacterial sexually transmitted disease (STD) characterized by painful genital ulcer and inguinal lymphadenopathy. It is caused by *Haemophilus ducreyi*. Its prevalence has gradually declined over the years in the western world, but it remains prevalent in some underdeveloped regions of Asia and Africa. The disruption of mucosal barrier due to ulcer increases the risk of human immunodeficiency virus (HIV) transmission among patients of chancroid.

HISTORY

Synonym: *Ulcus molle*, soft chancre, Ducrey's chancre, soft sore, chancre mou.

The first person to describe the soft ulcer of chancroid as a separate clinical entity from the hard indurated chancre of syphilis was Leon Bassereau in 1852.[1] It was Augusto Ducrey who in 1889 reported finding short streptobacillary rods with rounded ends in genital ulcers, and proposed this organism to be causing chancroid.[2]

EPIDEMIOLOGY

World Health Organization (WHO) estimates that nearly 7 million cases of chancroid occur annually. Though true global estimates are difficult because of lack of readily available diagnostic tests for chancroid in resource-poor settings and clinical difficulties differentiating from other genital ulcerative diseases (GUDs). Chancroid is prevalent in Asia, Africa, and the Caribbean, because of weak public health infrastructure. It is prevalent in areas with high HIV transmission (>8%)[3] and among drug addicts, particularly crack cocaine.

Chancroid is endemic in some parts of India, and its prevalence has varied from 1.6 to 51.9% based on reports from various sexually transmitted infection (STI) clinics.[4-6]

Recent studies have showed changing patterns in GUDs with increasing viral infections and decreasing bacterial STDs, attributable to wide application of syndromic management, use of broad-spectrum antibiotics, and safer sexual practices.

Chancroid is primarily a disease of sexually active and promiscuous individual, with males being affected more commonly because foreskin environment makes males more susceptible to *H. ducreyi* and moreover ulcers are usually asymptomatic in females (females act as carrier). Commercial sex workers are the major reservoir, and disease spreads from person-to-person mainly by sexual contact, fomites do not play any role in transmission. There is no nonhuman reservoir for *H. ducreyi*. Autoinoculation is reported to occur in chancroid.

ETIOLOGY

Chancroid is caused by *H. ducreyi*, a small (1.2 μm × 5 μm) gram-negative nonmotile, nonspore forming facultative anaerobic streptobacillus. It is pathogenic to only humans with no intermediate environment or animal host. They are often found in chains giving "*school of fish*" appearance or in whorls like "*fingerprints*" on solid agar medium whereas in liquid culture or tissue they form parallel chains giving "*railroad track appearance.*"[7] It is a fastidious organism with unique nutritional requirements, e.g., it requires hemin "X factor" for growth. They are oxidase and alkaline phosphatase positive, reduces nitrate to nitrite and catalase negative.

PATHOGENESIS

The exact pathogenesis of genital ulcer in chancroid is unknown. Organisms enter the sites of abrasion or trauma. The size of the inoculum has to be $>10^4$ to produce an infection.[8] Once bacteria adhere to epithelial cells via pili and hemagglutinins, there is release of hemolysins and cytotoxins leading to tissue damage and ulcer formation **(Flowchart 1)**.

Other virulence factors produced by *H. ducreyi* is lipo-oligosaccharide (LOS) (may play a role in pathogenesis of bubo), soluble cytolethal distending toxin (Hd-CDT) (causes host cell cycle arrest at G2), delaying specific host response

Flowchart 1: Pathogenesis of ulcer formation in chancroid by hemolysin and cytotoxin.

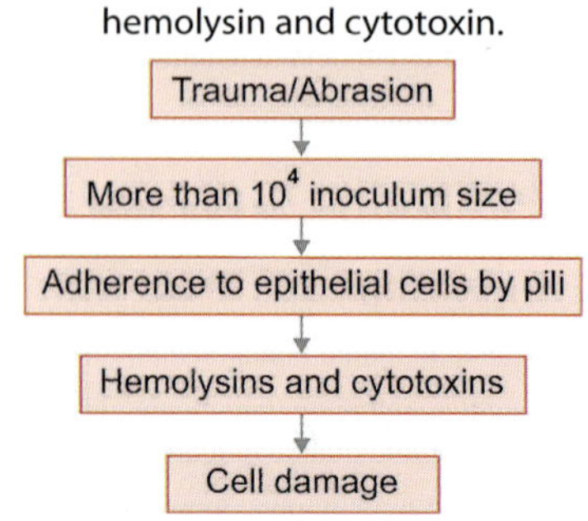

and persistence of chancroid ulcer, Cu-Zn superoxide dismutase (causes host immune system avoidance by *H. ducreyi)*; Hemolysins (contributes to ulcer formation and epithelial cell damage); Hb-binding outer membrane protein (OMP) (responsible for pustular stage of ulcer).

Lymphadenitis secondary to chancroid ulcer is a pyogenic inflammatory response with predominant neutrophils and paucity of organism in the bubo, though exact pathogenesis of lymphadenitis is unknown.

Chancroid elicits both cell-mediated and humoral responses. Delayed hypersensitivity reaction with recruitment of peripheral blood mononuclear cells occurs to antigens of *H. ducreyi*. Cell-mediated response is predominantly Th-1, mononuclear infiltrate consists mainly of CD4+ and CD8+ T-lymphocytes, and monocytes with paucity of B-lymphocytes. A humoral response with production of immunoglobulin G (IgG), IgM, and IgA occur but do not confer lifelong immunity.

CLINICAL FEATURES

The incubation period of chancroid ranges between 3 and 7 days, except in patient of HIV, where it may be longer. There is no prodromal stage. A papule with erythematous halo appears at the site of entry of organism, which is followed 24–48 hours later by a pustular stage, which undergoes central necrosis to form the characteristic, small, necrotic, tender, bleeding, nonindurated base (soft sore) with ragged or undermined edges **(Fig. 1)**. Autoinoculation may lead to formation of kissing ulcer or multiple ulcers **(Figs. 2 and 3)**.

Males usually present with painful genital ulcer with **(Fig. 4)** or without inguinal bubo. Edema of the preputial skin is common and phimosis as well as paraphimosis can sometime be the initial presentation. Females often present with less symptoms such as dyspareunia, pain in voiding or defecation, vaginal discharge, or rectal bleeding depending on site of lesion.

Sites of ulcers in decreasing order of frequency in males are prepuce (**Fig. 5**), frenulum (**Fig. 6**), coronal sulcus, glans,

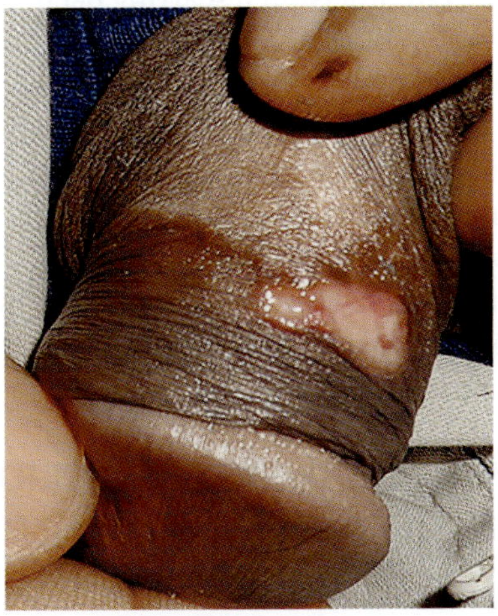

Fig. 1: Irregular necrotic ulcer with undermined margins surrounded by an inflammatory margin over preputial skin.

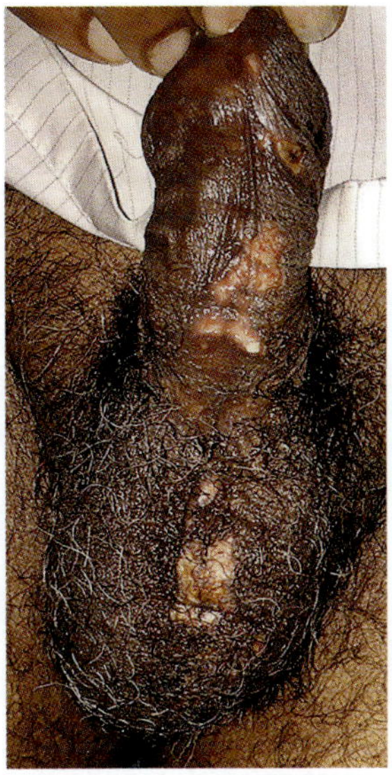

Fig. 2: Multiple necrotic ulcers with ragged borders over the penile shaft with kissing chancroidal ulcer over scrotal skin in a human immunodeficiency virus (HIV) positive male.

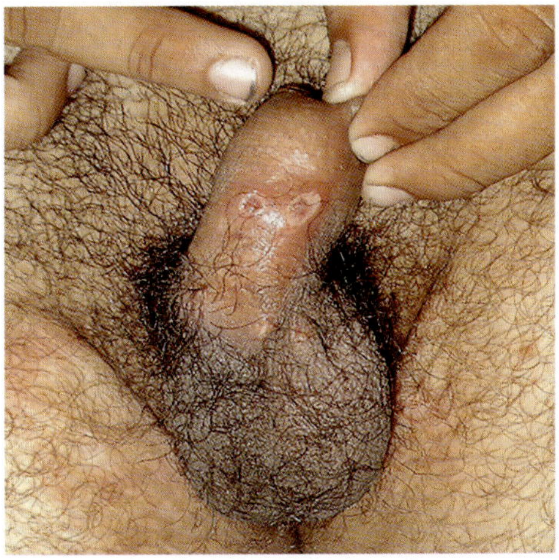

Fig. 3: Kissing chancroid ulcer over penis shaft and scrotum.

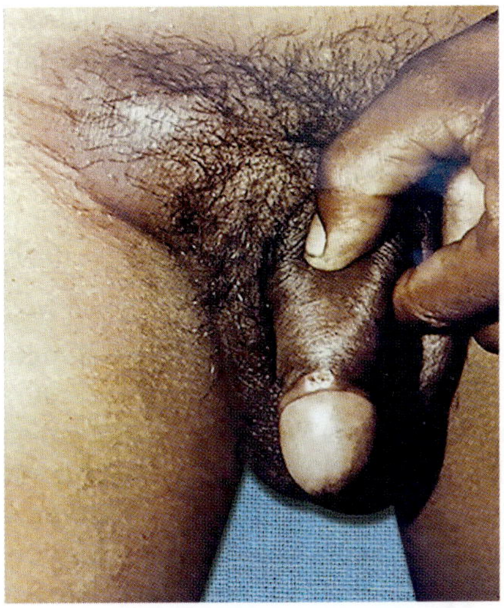

Fig. 4: Chancroid ulcer with inflamed inguinal bubo.

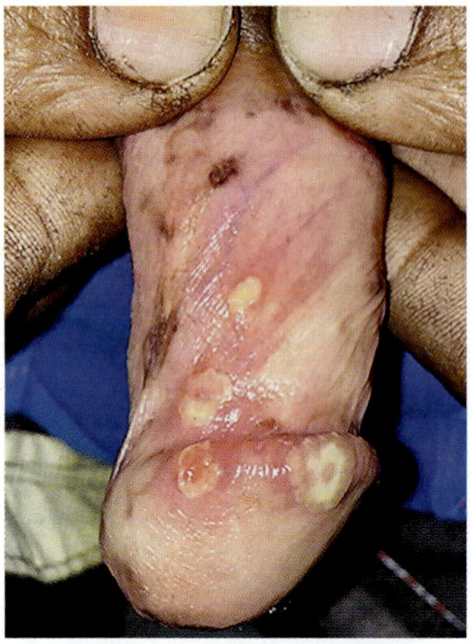

Fig. 5: Multiple necrotic chancroid ulcers with surrounding inflammation on glans and prepuce.

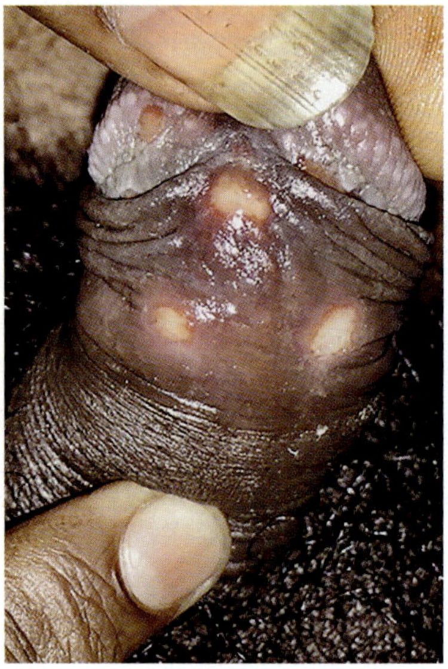

Fig. 6: Multiple chancroid ulcers over glans, frenulum, and prepuce.

meatus, shaft of penis while in female's vulva, fourchette, labia minora, vestibule, and clitoris are commonly involved. Rarely, the ulcer may be localized in urethra causing purulent urethritis. Vaginal, cervical, and perianal ulcers have also been described in chancroid.

Extragenital lesions have been reported from tongue, fingers, breasts, lips, oral mucosa, and thighs; they are thought to occur secondary to autoinoculation.

Bubo: Subsequent to genital ulcer regional inguinal lymph nodes become tender and enlarged. Unilateral inguinal lymphadenopathy occurs in around 30–60% patients after 1–2 weeks of ulcer. A classical bubo consists of matted inguinal lymph nodes secondary to periadenitis forming a unilocular swelling with erythematous overlying skin. The bubo softens and undergoes suppuration to form unilocular fluctuant swelling which may rupture to form ulcer. The margins of the ulcer are inflammatory and necrotic. In almost half of the patients the inguinal lymphadenitis subsides without suppuration.

TABLE 1: Differentiating features of lymphadenopathy in chancroid and lymphogranuloma venereum (LGV).[3]

Characteristics	*Chancroid*	*LGV*
Frequency of bubo	30–60%	Almost all cases (~100%)
Unilateral	75%	66.7%
Incubation period	7–14 days	10–30 days
Presence of primary genital ulcer when patient present with bubo	Present	Absent
Sinus formation after rupture of bubo	Single	Multiple
Constitutional symptoms	Absent	Present
Systemic spread	Absent	Present
Groove sign	Absent	Present (20% cases)
Loculation	Unilocular	Multilocular

Mild constitutional symptoms such as low-grade fever and malaise may accompany ulcer. Systemic spread and adverse effects on pregnancy or fetus has not been described with chancroid.

Features differentiating the bubo of chancroid from that of lymphogranuloma venereum (LGV) are summarized in **Table 1**.

Chancroid has several clinical variants described in **Table 2**.

CLINICAL COURSE AND COMPLICATION

Chancroid is a self-limiting disease and most patients' only complaint is pain. Primarily, lesion heals without scar formation in most cases and inguinal lymphadenitis resolves. Complications are more common in men. Following complications are described in chancroid:

- *Rupture of inguinal bubo*: Most common complication, leading to sinus or ulcer formation
- *Phimosis or paraphimosis*: Due to preputial ulceration, may require circumcision if scarring occurs
- *Balanitis and balanoposthitis*: Especially seen in uncircumcised men
- *Secondary infection*: Due to anaerobes such as *Fusobacterium* or *Bacteroides* lead to phagedenic ulceration
- Formation of urethral or rectovaginal fistula secondary to destructive ulceration
- Hemorrhage due to rupture of underlying blood vessels
- Esophageal lesions in HIV patients
- Acute conjunctivitis (rare)

HUMAN IMMUNODEFICIENCY VIRUS AND CHANCROID

Chancroid facilitates the transmission of HIV by increasing both the infectiousness of HIV and the susceptibility to

TABLE 2: Clinical types or variants of chancroid.

Dwarf chancroid	Single or multiple small superficial herpes genitalis such as ulcers, relatively painless and with or without inguinal lymphadenopathy
Giant chancroid	Starts as small ulcer with rapid peripheral extension associated with inguinal lymphadenopathy
Transient chancroid (*chancre mouvolant*)	Initial chancre resolves within 4–6 days followed by acute inguinal lymphadenopathy with suppuration
Papular chancroid (*ulcus molle elevatum*)	Starts as an ulcer but later becomes raised especially at edges (resembles donovanosis or condyloma lata)
Follicular chancroid	Arise in the hair follicle over the hairy surface around genitalia
Serpiginous chancroid (*ulcus molle serpiginosum*)	Multiple small ulcers coalesce to form large ulcers in serpiginous pattern through autoinoculation
Phagedenic chancroid (*ulcus molle gangrenosum*)	Extensive necrosis with deep and widespread destruction of genitalia, caused by superinfection with fusospirochetes
Intraurethral chancroid	Presents as nongonococcal urethritis
Mixed chancroid	Tender nonindurated chancre together with nontender indurated ulcer of syphilis

infection by the virus.[3] Following factors are responsible for increased infectiousness:

- Increased HIV shedding into the genital tract from ulcer exudates.
- Genital ulcers bleed during intercourse leading to increase in viral shedding and HIV infectiousness.
- In men with genital ulcer, there is increased concentration of virus in seminal fluid.

Concomitant HIV infection with chancroid modifies the clinical presentation. The ulcers may present with large size, multiple lesions **(Fig. 2)**, and extragenital lesions. The ulcers may take long time to resolve. The response to single-dose treatment is inadequate in patients of HIV, requiring treatment for longer duration and/or increase dosage.

LABORATORY DIAGNOSES

The laboratory confirmation of chancroid is essential for accurate diagnoses, epidemiological data, and appropriate management. Diagnoses of chancroid solely on clinical appearance of ulcer are accurate only in 30–50% cases. It is interesting to note that the accurate diagnoses of chancroid on clinical grounds are directly related to prevalence of disease.

Examination of the Smears

After cleaning the ulcer base with saline, a direct swab is taken from the undermined edge with cotton or calcium alginate swab and stained with Gram or Giemsa stain. Swab can also be taken from pus aspirate of bubo. Typically, streptobacilli are seen lying in clusters, either inside the leukocytes or outside in chains paralleling the shreds of mucus with appearance of "school of fish" (**Fig. 7**), "railroad tracks", and "fingerprints." Organism is rarely seen in aspirate from bubo. Other useful stains are Unna–Pappenheim, Wright's, and pyronin methyl green stains. Because of presence of polymicrobial flora in genital area, direct smear examination lacks sensitivity and specificity.

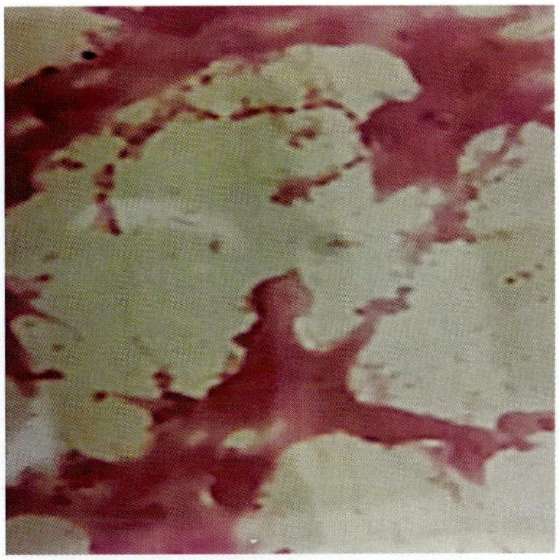

Fig. 7: Smear from chancroid ulcer showing typical "school of fish appearance."
Courtesy: Professor Paschal D'Souza (New Delhi).

Culture

This remains the "gold standard" for diagnoses of chancroid, though the organism is fastidious in nature. Because of fastidious nature of *H. ducreyi* it is essential to directly plate the swab from ulcer or bubo aspirate on to the culture medium. *H. ducreyi* survives for 2–4 hours on a swab unless refrigerated. Most widely used culture media is gonococcal agar base enriched with 1% hemoglobin, 1% IsovitaleX, and 5% fetal calf serum; Mueller–Hinton agar enriched with 5% horse blood and IsovitaleX; Columbia agar enriched with 5% lyzed horse blood. *H. ducreyi* grows best at 33°C in a microaerophilic, water saturated atmosphere containing 5% carbon dioxide. Characteristic colonies are small, nonmucoid, yellow-gray, semiopaque, or translucent colonies appear 2–4 days after inoculation **(Fig. 8)**. Sensitivity at best is ~75%. Testing for antibiotic susceptibility is recommended for chancroid, as clinically significant antibiotic resistance has been reported with chancroid.

Recent Diagnostics

Diagnoses of chancroid is mainly clinical, however recent diagnostic development has led to following new techniques:

- *DNA amplification techniques*: Polymerase chain reaction (PCR) has been developed to increase the sensitivity of diagnoses with following primers: *H. ducreyi* 16S ribosomal *RNA* gene, the rrs (16S)-rrl (23S) ribosomal intergenic spacer region, and *groEL* gene.

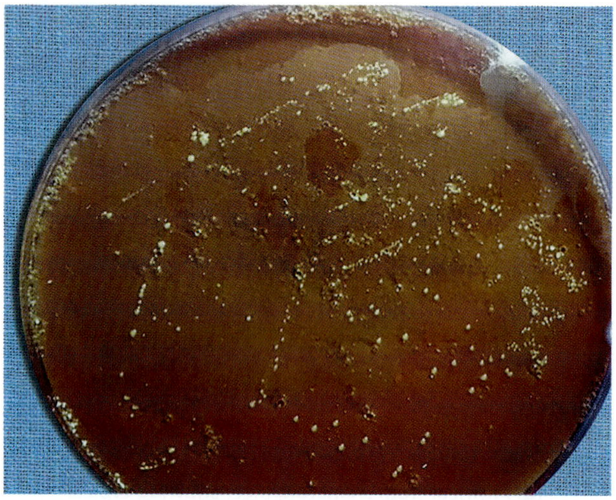

Fig. 8: Characteristic yellow-gray nonmucoid semiopaque colonies of *H. ducreyi* on gonococcal agar base. *Courtesy*: Professor Paschal D'Souza (New Delhi).

- *Antigen detection*: Monoclonal antibodies (Mabs) against 29 kDa OMP or against LOS of *H. ducreyi* have been used for antigen detection using immunofluorescence.
- *Nucleic acid probe technology*: DNA-DNA hybridization using *H. ducreyi* probes have been used to detect the DNA of *H. ducreyi.*
- *Serological tests*: Enzyme immunoassays (EIAs), dot immunobinding, agglutination, compliment fixation, and precipitation techniques can be used to detect the serological responses to *H. ducreyi.*
- *Mass spectrometric methods*: Matrix-assisted laser desorption/ionization time of flight mass spectrometry (MALDI/TOF-MS) can rapidly identify *Haemophilus* bacteria and determine strain differences.

Histopathology

Chancroid lesions have three vertical zones with characteristic vascular changes:

1. *Surface zone at floor*: Narrow, consists of neutrophils, fibrin, erythrocytes, and necrotic tissues
2. *Middle zone*: Wide, newly formed blood vessels with marked proliferation of endothelial cells, and thrombosis and degenerative changes in the vessel wall
3. *Deep zone*: Dense infiltrate of plasma and lymphoid cells

DIAGNOSES

A *definitive diagnosis* of chancroid requires the identification of *H. ducreyi* on special culture media.

The combination of a painful genital ulcer and tender suppurative inguinal adenopathy *suggests* the diagnosis of chancroid.

For both clinical and surveillance purposes, a *probable diagnosis* of chancroid can be made if all of the following criteria are met:

- The patient has one or more painful genital ulcers.
- The clinical presentation, appearance of genital ulcers and, if present, regional lymphadenopathy are typical for chancroid.
- The patient has no evidence of *Treponema pallidum* infection by dark-field examination of ulcer exudate or by a serologic test for syphilis performed at least 7 days after onset of ulcers.
- A herpes simplex virus polymerase chain reaction (HSV PCR) test or HSV culture performed on the ulcer exudate is negative.

CHANCROIDAL ULCER

Chancroid means "like a chancre" similarly chancroidal means "like chancroid." Few authors use these terms synonymously, but current understanding labels those chancroid-like ulcers in which *H. ducreyi* cannot be demonstrated. These ulcers (especially genital herpes) are those ulcers in which there is secondary invasion by pyogenic bacteria. The accurate diagnoses of chancroid now require the isolation and identification of *H. ducreyi.*

DIFFERENTIAL DIAGNOSES

Chancroid should be differentiated from other sexually transmitted genital ulcerative diseases such as genital herpes, primary syphilis, granuloma inguinale, LGV, candidial balanitis, and other non-STDs such as fixed drug eruptions, Behçet's disease, secondarily infected traumatic ulcer, extracutaneous Crohn's disease, and carcinoma.

TREATMENT

General measures: Bed rest is recommended early in course to avoid pain in ulcer and rest helps in decreasing the chances of development of inguinal lymphadenopathy. Patient should be advised to avoid unprotected sexual intercourse until they and their sexual partner(s) have completed treatment and follow-up.

Local Treatment

Local and subpreputial cleansing with normal saline is recommended. Local antiseptics are contraindicated, because that interferes with diagnoses of syphilis with disseminated gonococcal infection (DGI). The conventional treatment of bubo is by aspiration with a wide-bore needle from a nondependent position so as to not form sinus. However, as per the latest WHO guidelines, incision and drainage or excision of bubo delays healing and is contraindicated.

Systemic Treatment

The Centers for Disease Control and Prevention (CDC) 2015 Sexually Transmitted Diseases Treatment Guidelines for the management of chancroid recommend the following antibiotic options:[9]

- *Azithromycin*: 1 g orally (PO) as a single dose

- *Ceftriaxone*: 250 mg intramuscularly as a single dose
- *Erythromycin base*: 500 mg PO 3 times daily for 7 days
- *Ciprofloxacin*: 500 mg PO twice daily for 3 days

Azithromycin and ceftriaxone as single-dose treatments have the advantage of observed compliance.

Re-examination of the patient should be carried out 7th day after initiation of therapy.

With administration of proper treatment, the ulcers should show improvement symptomatically 3 days followed by substantial re-epithelialization after 7 days.

Ceftriaxone is the treatment of choice in pregnant women, although data have suggested that ciprofloxacin presents a low risk to the fetus during pregnancy with potential toxic effects during breastfeeding.[10]

In patients with concomitant HIV infection, these regimens are often found to be inadequate. Increased dose and a more prolonged duration of therapy might be necessary. Patients should be followed up weekly till there is complete clearance of chancroid lesions. CDC recommends to treat HIV patients with single-dose regimens only if follow-up can be assured.

In phagedenic chancroid, benzylpenicillin 1 million units 8 hourly along with oral metronidazole 200 mg TID for 7–10 days should be given in addition to the standard treatment of chancroid.

Sexual partners of patients with chancroid should be examined and treated regardless of the presence of symptoms if they had sexual contact within 10 days preceding the onset of symptoms. Serological tests for syphilis and HIV should be offered to all patients and their contacts.

KEY POINTS

- Primarily, an STD is caused by the fastidious and gram-negative coccobacillus *H. ducreyi*.
- Common in Africa, Asia, and Latin America, but rare in developed countries.
- Classically presents with the acute onset of a painful genital ulcer with fluctuant lymphadenitis (bubo formation).
- An important cofactor in HIV transmission and HIV status must be assessed.
- Most cases resolve with antibiotic therapy (single-dose regimen of azithromycin or ceftriaxone); recurrence is rare.
- Sexual partners within 10 days prior to onset of symptoms must be traced and treated, even if asymptomatic.

REFERENCES

1. Bassereau PI. Symptomatic Treatment of Syphilis. Paris: JB Bailliere; 1852.
2. Ducrey A. Experimental studies of the infectious agent of soft chancre and about the bubos. Monatsh Prakt Dermatol. 1889;9:387-405.
3. Nanda S, Reddy BV, Reddy BSN. Chancroid. In: Gupta S, Kumar B (Eds). Sexually Transmitted Infections, 2nd edition. Gurugram, India: Elsevier; 2011. pp. 522-32.
4. Hira SK. Sexually transmitted diseases in era of AIDS. AIDS Watch—WHO South-East Asia Region Newsletter. 1997;2:1-2.
5. Reddy BSN, Garg BR, Rao MV. An appraisal of trends in sexually transmitted disease. Indian J Sex Transm Dis. 1993;14:1-4.
6. Kura MM, Hira S, Kohli M, Dalal PJ, Ramnani VK, Jagtap MR. High occurrence of HBV among STD clinic attenders in Bombay, India. Int J STD AIDS. 1998;9:231-3.
7. Albritton WL. Biology of *Haemophilus ducreyi*. Microbiol Rev. 1989;53:377-89.
8. Ronald AR, Albritton WL. Chancroid and *Haemophilus ducreyi*. In: Holmes KK, Sparling PF, Mardh PA (Eds). Sexually transmitted diseases. New York: McGraw Hill; 1999. pp. 515-23.
9. O'Farrell N, Lazaro N. UK National Guideline for the Management of Chancroid 2014. Int J STD AIDS. 2014; 25(14): 975-83.
10. Breau C, Cameron DW, Desjardins M, Lee BC. Oral immunization using HgbA in a recombinant chancroid vaccine delivered by attenuated *Salmonella typhimurium* SL3261 in the temperature-dependent rabbit model. J Immunol Methods. 2012;375(1-2):232-42.

EXAMINATION QUESTIONS

1. Describe etiopathogenesis and clinical features of chancroid.
2. Outline the CDC recommendations for treatment of patient with chancroid and his/her partner.
3. Tabulate the differences between bubo of chancroid and lymphogranuloma venereum.

128 CHAPTER

Lymphogranuloma Venereum

Jayadev Betkarur, Chethana S Gurumurthy

INTRODUCTION

Lymphogranuloma venereum (LGV) is a sexually transmitted disease caused by *Chlamydia trachomatis* infecting the lymphatic channels. (Synonyms—climatic bubo, tropical bubo, lymphopathia venereum, Durand–Nicolas–Favre disease, strumous bubo, poradenitis inguinalis, lymphogranuloma inguinale, and the fourth, fifth, or sixth venereal disease).

HISTORY

Rudolph Kampmeir's review[1] (1939) on human chlamydial infection and Rajam and Rangiahs[2] (1955) monograph details the history of LGV. Nelaton (1890) and L Hardy (1894) documented the genital portal of entry and transmission by sexual contact. Caddy (1902) called it climatic bubo while recording the first case in India. Durand, Nicholas, and Favre named it lymphogranuloma inguinale and detailed the clinical and histopathological features and distinguished it from syphilis and tuberculosis. Frei (1925) described an intracutaneous test from bubo material and described that climatic bubo and LGV have the same etiology. Miyagawa (1935) first grew the organism in embryonated eggs.[3]

EPIDEMIOLOGY

Lymphogranuloma venereum has a global distribution and affects all races. It is commonly found in tropical and semi-tropical environment and is endemic in India, East and West Africa, parts of South East Asia, South America, and Caribbean.[4] In India, the incidence varies from 0.2 to 11.5%.[5] It is commonly seen in adult men and women (20–40 years) with male to female ratio of 5:1, however late complications are more in women.[6]

ETIOLOGY

Chlamydia are obligate intracellular anaerobic, gram-negative organisms with no cytochrome system, no adenosine triphosphate (ATP) production and do not utilize glutamate. They multiply by binary fission and produce intracytoplasmic inclusion bodies. It has features of both bacteria and virus. There are different serotypes (A–L3) causing various diseases in human beings **(Table 1)**.

STAINS AND CULTURE

They can be stained using Giemsa stain, Brown Hopps tissue Gram stain, hematoxylin, and eosin-appearing faintly blue with Warthin–Starry silver impregnation stain they appear black.[7] Chlamydia organisms do not grow on artificial media. They grow on yolk sac of chick embryos, HeLa cells, and live cell cultures and can be preserved indefinitely at –20 to –70°C.[2] A trilaminar outer membrane contains at 36–43 kDa, cysteine-rich major outer membrane protein (MOMP) which plays an important role in attachment of elementary body to host cells. Nine polymorphic MOMP genes are identified in genome of serovar L2.

PATHOGENESIS

Humans are the sole natural host for *C. trachomatis*, but can be experimentally transmitted to monkeys, mice, and guinea pig. Chlamydia does not penetrate intact skin or mucous membrane; it requires minute disruption. The organism predominantly infects the lymphatic tissue leading to thrombolymphangitis and perilymphangitis.[4] It spreads to adjacent lymph nodes by contiguous spread, later causing necrosis, and forming triangular or quadrangular stellate loculated abscess.

Rupture of these abscesses produces fistulae and sinus tracts. Healing occurs by fibrosis causing destruction of the normal structures of lymph nodes and blocks the subcutaneous and submucosa lymph vessels. This results in chronic edema and sclerosing fibrosis leading to induration, enlargement, and ulceration of affected part. Dissemination and local extension is limited by host immunity, which may not eliminate the organism permanently, hence leads to persistent and latent infection and development into systematic disease.

TABLE 1: Strains of chlamydia and diseases.

Serotypes	*Diseases*
A, B, Ba, and C	Trachoma
D–K	Urethritis, cervicitis, and salpingitis
L1, L2, and L3	Lymphogranuloma venereum

CLINICAL MANIFESTATION

The clinical manifestations depend on the sex of the patient, mode of sexual contact, and the stage of the disease.

Course

- Primary stage
- Secondary stage (inguinal syndrome)
- Tertiary stage (anogenitorectal syndrome)

Primary Stage

Incubation period varies from 7 to 12 days. In majority, (68.7% males and 50% females) no primary lesion is observed. This stage varies according to sex, mode of sexual contact, and stage of disease **(Table 2)**.

Inguinal Syndrome (Bubo)

Time of exposure to the secondary stage varies from 30 days to 6 months. Inguinal syndrome is characterized by an inflammatory swelling of the inguinal lymph nodes and their corresponding tributaries and branches **(Table 3)**. LGV is predominantly seen in males and is unilateral in two-thirds of cases.[2]

Constitutional symptoms such as fever, chills, sweating, lassitude, anorexia, arthralgia, myalgia, and malaise often precede or are associated with the onset of bubo. The fever is usually of a hectic type and subsides with the formation of periadenitis and adhesion of the glands to the skin.[2,4] Adenitis may terminate by suppuration (60–70%) (inguinal lymph nodes), spontaneous resolution (25–30%) or may persist as stationary mass (5%).[2]

Suppuration occurs in multiple foci, giving rise to multiple sinuses discharging grayish-white, thick, and gluey pus. The sinuses may persist for a few weeks to many months. Secondary pyogenic infection, a rapidly spreading phagedenic inflammation caused by fusospirillary organisms, or infestation by maggots may complicate unsealed sinuses in tropical countries.[2] Healing is very slow and leaves behind contracted scars in the inguinal region. When there is bilateral inguinal lymphadenitis of this type, elephantiasis of the genitalia gradually sets in.[2]

TABLE 2: Types and signs and symptoms of lymphogranuloma venereum (primary stage).

Type	*Signs and symptoms*
Genital	Herpetiform, superficial, painless, ulcer, papule, nodule, and evanescent lesion that heals with no scar Rarely in men; phimosis, balanitis or balanoposthitis, bubonulus, and nongonococcal urethritis and in females; genital swelling,[7] cervicitis, endometritis, parametritis or salpingitis is seen
Anorectal	Proctitis (*symptoms:* rectal pain, anorectal bleeding, mucoid and/or hemopurulent rectal discharge, tenesmus, and constipation)
Extragenital	Lesions are seen on the lip, mouth, pharynx, or tonsils due to oral sexual exposure

Dissemination may cause systemic disease such as hepatitis, pneumonitis, arthritis, endocarditis, spondylitis, Reiter's syndrome, erythema nodosum, erythema multiforme, and ocular affections.[1,4]

The localization of disease differs in men and women due to the different lymphatic drainage of genitalia.[2] Lymphatic involvement depends on the site of primary infection **(Table 4)**.

Anogenitorectal Syndrome

The genitals in both the sexes, but more frequently in women, may be the seat of hyperplastic ulcerative changes **(Table 5)**. These lesions occur alone or more often in association with anorectal changes, and together are known as the genito-ano-rectal syndrome of LGV.[2] Elephantiasis of the genitalia may occur due to lymphatic obstruction.

Genital Manifestations

Anorectal Syndrome

The majority of patients with the anorectal syndrome are women or homosexual men.[5] Inoculation of the rectal mucosa

TABLE 3: Lymph node involvement and signs and symptoms of inguinal syndrome.

Lymph node involvement	*Signs and symptoms*
Inguinal	In majority, the superomedial group is involved first. Patient will have severe pain in the groin and as the bubo enlarges walks with a limp bent at the waist in an attempt to limit pain In 1–2 weeks, bubo gets fluctuant leading to periadenitis and matting of glands to overlying skin and fixing to the adjacent tissue The overlying skin gets thickened and in fair skin violaceous hue may appear that predicts an impending rupture
Femoral	In 20% of cases, there is enlargement of femoral lymph nodes. When these and inguinal lymph nodes are enlarged they are separated by Poupart's or Inguinal ligament producing a pathognomonic sign *(Groove sign of Greenblatt)*
Iliac	Sometimes the iliac lymph nodes take the main brunt of infection leading to a tender, firm swelling, size of a closed fist, occupying greater part of iliac fossa[1]
Pelvic lymph nodes	Cystitis and urinary retention
Submandibular, cervical, and axillary	When primary lesion is in the mouth, tonsil, or pharynx

TABLE 4: Lymphatic involvement and site of primary infection.

Lymphatic nodes involved	*Site of primary infection*
Inguinal	Penis, anterior urethra, vulva, and anus
Deep iliac and perirectal	Posterior urethra and rectum
Deep iliac, perirectal, retrocrural, and lumbosacral	Vagina and cervix

TABLE 5: Anogenitorectal syndrome.

Males	Bubonuli, urethral stricture, prostatitis, seminal vesiculitis, and epididymo-orchitis penile and scrotal elephantiasis lead saxophone or ramrod penis
Females	Esthiomene is seen mainly in women. It is characterized by elephantiasis of vulva, clitoris, and perianal area with chronic, indolent, superficial, and spreading ulcers. They are commonly seen on the inner surface of the labia minora, fourchette, around the urethral orifice, and the root of the clitoris[2] Vaginal stenosis and urethral strictures. Rectovaginal, urethrovaginal, cervicovaginal, or vulval fistulae may be produced by localized perforating ulcers Triple syndrome is esthiomene associated with similar pathology in the anus and rectum

may occur directly during receptive anal intercourse or by lymphatic spread in men whereas in women, it could also be by spread of infectious vaginal secretions.

Anorectal syndrome is the consequences of a chronic inflammatory infection of the pelvic, perirectal, and anorectal tissues. The infection is usually confined to the lower 3–4 inches of the bowel, occasionally spreads to the transverse colon and rarely to the parametrial tissues in females. The duration of the disease may vary from a few months to many years.[2]

The earliest change is perianal edema followed by diffuse edema of the anorectal mucosa. Multiple fissures radiating from the anal margin and involving the edematous skin appear as the disease progresses. At chronic proctocolitis stage, the patient complains of tenesmus, fever, and a mucoid bloodstained discharge that may become mucopurulent due to secondary infection by endogenous bowel flora.[2]

After a variable period of 3–6 months, the anorectal mucosa acquires rigidity with an annular or tubular stricture due to replacement by fibrous tissue.[2] The patient experiences increasing difficulty in defecation, with tenesmus, bloodstained rectal leukorrhea. In women, the destructive ulcerative process may result in a rectovaginal fistula.[2]

Rectal strictures can be annular in 64% (most common), tubular in 24%, or funnel shaped in 12%.[2] Rectal cancer is reported in 2.5% of rectal stricture patients due to LGV. Death may occur due to pyemia, peritonitis (rupture of intestine), intercurrent tuberculosis of lungs, or terminal intestinal obstruction.[2]

OTHER MANIFESTATIONS

Table 6 depicts other manifestations of lymphogranuloma venereum.

INVESTIGATIONS

Laboratory diagnosis is based on positive chlamydial serology, isolation of *C. trachomatis* from infected site, and histological identification in infected tissue (**Table 7**).

TABLE 6: Other manifestations of lymphogranuloma venereum.

Cutaneous manifestations	• Transient generalized exanthemata, papular, papulopustular, nodular, erythema nodosum, and erythema multiforme • Itchy papular and papulovesicular eruptions due to photosensitivity[1]
Ocular manifestations	Follicular conjunctivitis, Parinaud's oculoglandular syndrome, bilateral conjunctivitis, episcleritis, keratitis, iritis, and blindness[2]
Systemic manifestations	Chronic cholecystitis, fibrous adhesion of liver capsule (Fitz–Hugh–Curtis syndrome),[7] abdominal and pelvic wall adhesions, psoas abscess, and urinary bladder involvement

TABLE 7: Laboratory diagnosis of lymphogranuloma venereum.

Hematology	Mild leukocytosis with increase in monocytes and eosinophils
Serology	Various tests such as complement fixation test, Single L-type immunofluorescence, microimmunofluorescence, ELISA, immune dot blot, radioisotope precipitation test, neutralizing antibody test, immunoperoxidase test, single plasmid PCR, nested MOMP PCR, restriction fragment length polymorphism, nucleic acid amplification tests (NAATs),[8] and counter immunoelectrophoresis have been used
Histology	• Demonstration of elementary and reticulate bodies in secretions, infected tissue, and bubo pus • Stains—Giemsa–Romanowsky, iodine, or Macchiavello stains • Electron microscopic demonstration of organism • Lymph node biopsy—stellate abscess and chronic granuloma
Isolation of chlamydia	They can be cultivated by inoculation into mouse brain, yolk sac, or tissue culture Cell culture such as McCoy cells, irradiated McCoy cells, and DEAE-treated HeLa 229 cells can be used for chlamydial growth
Intradermal test	Frei test (commercial lygranum antigen) and inverse Frei test (patient's own bubo pus)(now obsolete)
Biochemical tests	Hypergammaglobulinemia, reversal of A/G ratio, increase in IgA, IgM, and IgG
Radiological investigations	Lymphography and barium enema (rectal strictures)[3]

(A/G: albumin/globulin; ELISA: enzyme-linked immunosorbent assay; DEAE: diethylaminoethyl; Ig: immunoglobulin; MOMP: major outer membrane protein; PCR: polymerase chain reaction)

DIFFERENTIAL DIAGNOSIS

While examining and investigating patients with a sexually transmitted disease (STD), it should be kept in mind that more than one STD may coexist in the same patient.[3] Differential diagnosis of lymphogranuloma venereum has been presented in **Table 8**.

TREATMENT

Medical Management

Many drugs are used for treating LGV, but there is no single universally effective drug that produces bacteriologic cure. Prolonged treatment for up to 3 weeks and more than one course, alternating with some known effective antibiotics is advised in chronic cases **(Table 9)**.[9]

Tetracycline group is the drug of choice. Penicillin and streptomycin are ineffective. Azithromycin 1 g orally as a single dose along with doxycycline 100 mg bid orally for 7 days can be used as an alternative regimen.

Surgical Management

Bubo-hot fomentation and aseptic aspiration from nondependent area.[1]

TABLE 8: Differential diagnosis of lymphogranuloma venereum.

Primary lesion (transient ulcer)	Herpes genitals, traumatic ulceration, chancroid, and syphilis
Intraurethral primary lesion	Gonorrhea and other causes for urethritis
Inguinal adenitis	Chancroidal inflammatory bubo, syphilitic indolent bubo, filarial lymphadenitis, pseudo bubo of donovanosis, tuberculous lymphadenitis, cat-scratch disease, septic lymphadenitis, and incarcerated inguinal hernia
Vulval or genital elephantiasis	Filariasis, tuberculosis, and surgical excision of lymph nodes
Anorectal syndrome	Condyloma lata, condyloma acuminatum, amoebic ulcer of the rectum and anus with or without stricture, fistula-in-ano, and tuberculosis of rectum and anus
Rectal strictures	Inflammatory or malignant

TABLE 9: Medical management of lymphogranuloma venereum.

Drug	*Dose*	*Duration*
Sulfadiazine	500 mg qid	2–3 weeks
Cotrimoxazole	2 tablets bd	2 weeks
Tetracycline hydrochloride	500 mg qid	2–3 weeks
Doxycycline	100 mg bid	3 weeks
Minocycline	300 mg initially followed by 200 mg	10 days
Erythromycin stearate (in pregnant and children below 8 years)	As per body weight or 500 mg qid	3 weeks
Azithromycin	1 g	Single dose
Rifampicin	450 mg OD	10 days
Moxifloxacin	400 mg OD	3 weeks

Strictures

Hegar dilators, internal proctotomy, or resection of rectum after preparatory ileocolostomy for rectal stricture. Urethral strictures are dilated with Lister's or Glutton's bougies.[1]

Other indications for surgery are bowel obstruction, persistent rectovaginal and other fistulae, gross destruction of anal canal, anal sphincter, and perineum. Plastic surgery may be required for esthiomene and genital elephantiasis.

Partner Management

The patient who has sexual contact with LGV within 30 days of onset of symptoms should be examined and investigated for cervical and urethral infections and treated for 3–6 weeks with follow-up till clearance of signs and symptoms.

LYMPHOGRANULOMA VENEREUM AND HUMAN IMMUNODEFICIENCY VIRUS

Lymphogranuloma venereum is more common in patients with human immunodeficiency virus (HIV). In most cases, the presentation and course are same as in non-HIV patients except that the treatment may be prolonged. There are some reports of atypical presentations like Parinaud's oculoglandular syndrome with associated inguinal lymphadenopathy. Latent LGV may be reactivated in HIV patients and present with multiple abscesses. They may acquire multiple STDs including LGV and hepatitis C.[10]

CONCLUSION

Lymphogranuloma venereum is an uncommon STD that has both local and systemic manifestations. It runs a chronic course, leading to local and systemic complications that may be debilitating and disfiguring. Early recognition and prompt treatment will prevent these complications.

KEY POINTS

- LGV is caused by a sexually transmitted *C. trachomatis* L1, L2, and L3.
- LGV course is characterized by three stages, i.e., primary stage, secondary stage (inguinal syndrome), and tertiary stage (anogenitorectal syndrome).
- LGV is associated with various complications such as strictures, fistulae, perforation, esthiomene, and carcinoma.
- Investigations are based on chlamydial serology, isolation of *Chlamydia trachomatis*, and demonstration of chlamydia in infected tissue.
- Tetracycline group for 3 weeks is the drug of choice through a single dose of azithromycin is also effective.
- Surgical management may be considered in case of complications.

REFERENCES

1. Kampmeir RH, Smith DW, Larsen RM. Human chlamydial infection. Am J Med Sci. 1939;198:516.
2. Rajam RV, Rangiah PN. Lymphogranuloma venereum. Indian J Dermatol. 1955;21(4, Suppl 1):1-65.
3. Ravindra K, Siddappa K. Lymphogranuloma venereum. In: Sacchidanand S, Oberai C, Inamadar AC (Eds). IADVL Textbook of Dermatology, 4th edition. Mumbai: Bhalani Publishing House; 2015. pp. 2894-907.
4. Perine PL, Osoba AO. Lymphogranuloma venereum. In: Holmes KK, Mardh PA, Sparling PF, Weisner PJ (Eds). Sexually Transmitted Diseases, 2nd edition. New York: McGraw Hill; 1990. pp. 195-204.
5. Chopra A, Mittal RR, Singh P, Sharma P. Pattern of sexually transmitted diseases at Patiala. Indian J Sex Transm Dis. 1990;11:43-5.
6. Annamuthodo H. Rectal lymphogranuloma venereum in Jamaica. Ann R Coll Surg Engl. 1961;29:141-59.
7. Hadfield TL, Lamy Y, Wear DJ. Demonstration of *Chlamydia trachomatis* in inguinal lymphadenitis of lymphogranuloma venereum: a light microscopy, electron microscopy and polymerase chain reaction study. Modern Pathol. 1995;8: 924-9.
8. White J, O'Farrell N, Daniels D. 2013 UK national guideline for the management of lymphogranuloma venereum. Int J STD AIDS. 2013;24(8):593-601.
9. Bajaj AK, Rajeev S. Lymphogranuloma venereum. In: Sharma VK (Ed). Sexually Transmitted Diseases and HIV/AIDS, 2nd edition. New Delhi: Viva Books; 2009. pp. 388-94.
10. Vries HJC, Reddy BSN, Khandpur S. Lymphogranuloma venereum. In: Gupta S, Kumar B (Eds). Sexually Transmitted Infections. 2nd edition. New York: Elsevier; 2012. pp. 506-16.

EXAMINATION QUESTIONS

1. What are the etiopathogenesis and cutaneous manifestations of LGV?
2. Discuss extragenital manifestations of LGV.

129 CHAPTER Donovanosis

Savitha AS, Shashi Kumar BM

INTRODUCTION

Donovanosis is a chronic and progressive bacterial infection involving the genitalia caused by *Calymmatobacterium granulomatis*, now reclassified as *Klebsiella granulomatis.*[1] McLeod, Professor of Surgery at the Medical College of Calcutta, India, in 1882 was the first to describe donovanosis. The causative organism was first described in 1905 by Donovan in Madras.[2]

SYNONYMS[3]

- Serpiginous ulceration of the groin
- Lupoid form of groin ulceration
- Ulcerating granuloma of the pudenda
- Granuloma genitoinguinale
- Granuloma inguinale tropicum
- Chronic venereal sores
- Ulcerating sclerosing granuloma
- Granuloma inguinale
- Granuloma venereum

ETIOLOGY

Klebsiella granulomatis is a gram negative, encapsulated, nonmotile, and facultative anaerobic intracellular bacteria, identified as Donovan bodies within macrophages. It is pleomorphic when observed in a single plane, i.e., curved or straight rods, coccoid, diplococcoid, ovoid, or elliptical in shape. Immature and noncapsulated forms may appear like closed safety pins with certain stains due to bipolar chromatin densities. *K. granulomatis* cannot be routinely cultured on conventional media. It has been cultured in human epithelial type 2 (HEp-2) cells and monocyte coculture from the biopsy specimens.[4]

EPIDEMIOLOGY

The incidence of donovanosis has drastically reduced in the postantibiotic era. It has a predominantly tropical distribution. It is most well-known in Southeast India, where it was first described, in New Guinea, the Caribbean and neighboring parts of South America, particularly the Guiana and Brazil. Moderate relative humidity and consistently high temperature are influencing factors in the prevalence. Most of the established infections are associated with poor personal genital hygiene. The majority of cases are in the 20- to 40-year age group, i.e., the most sexually active. Higher male-to-female ratios of more than 6:1 have been reported.[5] The incubation period is uncertain ranging from 1 to 360 days. Infection rates among conjugal partners have varied from 0.4 to 52%. This wide range can be explained by the long incubation period and relatively low infectivity of *K. granulomatis.*[6]

Due to the following points, questions have been raised regarding the sexual transmission of the disease:

- Uncertainty of incubation period
- Low incidence of the disease
- Differences in racial and sex distribution
- Infrequency of cases of conjugal infection
- Occurrence of primary extragenital lesions

Other suggested modes of transmission are:

- Fecal contamination of abraded skin
- Infection in children due to sitting on the laps of infected adults
- During birth, neonates acquiring infection from the mother

CLINICAL FEATURES

About 90% of the infections occur over the genitalia. In men, the common sites are the prepuce, coronal sulcus, frenum, and glans penis. In women, the lesions are seen over the labia minora and fourchette. The lesion begins as a firm papule or nodule, which eventually ulcerates. The primary lesions expand slowly by direct extension, however, autoinoculation, which produces new lesions from contact with adjacent skin ("kissing" lesions), is a common feature.

Four types of donovanosis are described classically:[1]

1. Ulcerogranulomatous—the most common variant. It is characterized by nontender, fleshy, exuberant, single or multiple, and beefy-red ulcers that bleed readily when touched.

2. Hypertrophic or verrucous type—an ulcer or growth with a raised, irregular edge, sometimes completely dry with a walnut-like appearance.
3. Necrotic, usually a deep, foul-smelling ulcer causing tissue destruction.
4. Sclerotic or cicatricial, characterized by extensive formation of fibrous and scar tissue.

Extragenital sites of infection include the lip, gums, cheek, palate, pharynx, neck, nose, larynx, and chest. There are numerous reports of oral donovanosis, which is probably the most common manifestation of extragenital involvement.

Lymphadenopathy is not a common association in donovanosis. The prominent inguinal swellings seen in patients with donovanosis have been called pseudobuboes, because they are subcutaneous granulomata that occur superficially in the area of inguinal lymph nodes.

Concomitant infection with other sexually transmitted infection is frequently seen. Primary syphilis, lymphogranuloma venereum (LGV), and gonorrhea are the frequent associations.

COMPLICATIONS

The following are the complications:

- Phimosis and paraphimosis
- Pseudoelephantiasis is more common in women due to the mechanical pressure of scar tissue over the local lymphatics.[7]
- Polyarthritis and osteomyelitis
- Dissemination to liver and bone can occur rarely. The cervix is the most common primary site in cases of disseminated bone disease.
- Carcinoma in long-standing lesions
- Stenosis of the urethra, vagina, or anus may occur in the sclerotic variant.

DIAGNOSIS

Most of the cases of donovanosis are clinically obvious; however, demonstration of Donovan bodies in smear or tissue sections is diagnostic.

Preparation of Tissue Smear

Tissue smears remain the gold standard method of diagnosis. An active area of ulceration should be selected and cleansed with saline. A specimen from the edge of the lesion can be obtained using a curette, forceps or scissors, and crushed between two glass slides. The slide is then stained with Leishman and Giemsa stain or Wright's stain to look for Donovan bodies. When dry, flat, or necrotic lesions are present, a punch biopsy specimen is to be taken. Donovan bodies may be difficult to demonstrate in early lesion, necrotic, and sclerotic type of donovanosis, if inadequate smear is taken or patient has taken antibiotics.

BOX 1: Pathognomonic histopathological features of Donovanosis.

- Massive cellular infiltrate formed predominantly by plasma cells
- Paucity of lymphocytes
- Diffuse sprinkling of polymorphonuclear leukocytes with focal collections
- Pronounced epithelial proliferation at the margins
- Large and mononuclear cells in the infiltrate

The large mononuclear cells containing typical intracellular Donovan bodies, 25–90 mm in diameter, with a vesicular or pyknotic nucleus are the Greenblatt and Pund cells.

Biopsy

Biopsy is performed if the tissue smear is negative and to rule out other differentials. The histopathological features include:[8]

- Ulceration and acanthosis with focal collections of polymorphonuclear leukocytes in the epidermis.
- Elongation of rete ridges occurs in association with the hypertrophic variant.
- Infiltration of plasma cells and polymorphonuclear leukocytes in the dermis.
- A few large cells containing cystic spaces, often with nuclei pushed to one side, and darkly staining inclusions (cells of Greenblatt) are characteristic.
- Donovan bodies may be easily identified in Giemsa-stained tissue sections, but difficult to identify in hematoxylin and eosin-stained sections.

Pathognomonic histopathological features of Donovanosis are listed in **Box 1**.

Serological Tests

Complement-fixation tests are found to be quite sensitive. An indirect immunofluorescent technique had a high sensitivity for established lesions but was not deemed suitable for early donovanosis ulcers. However, this test could be of use as an epidemiologic tool in population studies.[9]

Culture

Klebsiella granulomatis cannot be cultured on conventional cell-free media, although occasionally successful growth in embryonated eggs, and more recently in a monocyte coculture system, has been achieved.[4]

Other Tests

Carter J et al. developed the first polymerase chain reaction (PCR) for the detection of *K. granulomatis*, which could be performed on surface swabs of lesions.[10] It was successfully incorporated into a colorimetric detection system for use in routine diagnostic laboratories. No serological tests are currently in use.

BOX 2: Control and prevention recommendation for treatment of donovanosis.

Recommended regimen: Azithromycin 1 g orally once per week or 500 mg daily for at least 3 weeks and until all lesions have completely healed

Alternative regimens:
- Doxycycline 100 mg orally twice a day for at least 3 weeks and until all lesions have completely healed, OR
- Ciprofloxacin 750 mg orally twice a day for at least 3 weeks and until all lesions have completely healed, OR
- Erythromycin base 500 mg orally four times a day for at least 3 weeks and until all lesions have completely healed, OR
- Trimethoprim-sulfamethoxazole one double-strength (160 mg/800 mg) tablet orally twice a day for at least 3 weeks and until all lesions have completely healed

TABLE 1: Differential diagnosis of donovanosis.

Genital ulcer/bubo	Primary and secondary syphilis, ulcerated genital warts, and chancroid
Lymphatic obstruction (pseudoelephantiasis)	Elephantiasis due to LGV
Necrotic form of donovanosis	Squamous carcinoma, tuberculosis, or amebiasis
Disseminated donovanosis (of bones)	Tuberculosis
Histopathological differential diagnosis	Rhinoscleroma, leishmaniasis, and histoplasmosis

(LGV: lymphogranuloma venereum)

TREATMENT

Antimony compounds were used successfully in preantibiotic era. The Centers for Disease Control and Prevention (CDC) recommendation is given in **Box 2**.[11]

Children with donovanosis should receive a short course of azithromycin 20 mg/kg. Children born to mothers with untreated donovanosis should receive prophylaxis with a 3-day course of azithromycin 20 mg/kg once daily.[12]

Management of Sex Partners

Persons who have had sexual contact with a patient who has granuloma inguinale within the 60 days before onset of the patient's symptoms should be examined and offered therapy.

DIFFERENTIAL DIAGNOSIS (TABLE 1)

The lesions which are most likely to cause confusion are primary and secondary syphilis, ulcerated genital warts, and chancroid. The condylomata lata of secondary syphilis usually appear as white or pale moist plaques in the anogenital area and are readily distinguished from the bright-red lesions of donovanosis. If the patient cannot be investigated, a single dose of benzathine penicillin may be given which will resolve condyloma lata in a week. A variant of chancroid with a strong resemblance to donovanosis is called "pseudogranuloma inguinale".

The late manifestation of LGV due to lymphatic obstruction closely mimics pseudoelephantiasis of donovanosis.

The necrotic form of donovanosis may resemble squamous carcinoma, tuberculosis, or amebiasis. Disseminated donovanosis lesions of bones, particular the bones in the lower spine, can mimic tuberculosis.

DONOVANOSIS AND HUMAN IMMUNODEFICIENCY VIRUS

Donovanosis is a risk factor for the acquisition of human immunodeficiency virus (HIV) like any other genital ulcer. HIV-positive patients with donovanosis had high failure rate to first-line antibiotic therapy such as cotrimoxazole and tetracycline.[13] The treatment has to be modified according to the degree of immunosuppression.

CONCLUSION

In endemic areas, donovanosis is clinically recognizable easily and effectively treated with antibiotics. It is associated with significant morbidity if patients delay in seeking treatment due to significant tissue destruction. Source of contact of index cases have to be recognized and treated. Patients with donovanosis may need prolonged courses of antibiotics and require careful explanation and reassurance about a condition that they may have had for a long time.

KEY POINTS

- Donovanosis is a chronic and progressive bacterial infection involving the genitalia caused by *Klebsiella granulomatis*.
- Diagnosis is by clinical features and observation of Donovan bodies on histopathology.
- Treatment is Azithromycin 1 g orally once per week or 500 mg daily for at least 3 weeks and until all lesions have completely healed.

REFERENCES

1. O'Farrel N. Donovanosis. In: Holmes K, Sparling P, Stamm E, Piot P, Wasserheit N, Corey L, (Eds). Sexually Transmitted Diseases, 4th edition. Washington: McGraw Hill; 2008. pp. 701-9.
2. Donovan C. Medical cases from Madras General Hospital. Ind Med Gaz. 1905;40:411-4.
3. Rajam RV, Rangiah PN. Donovanosis (Granuloma Inguinale, Granuloma Venereum). Geneva: World Health Organization, WHO Monograph Series No 24; 1954. pp. 1-72.
4. Veeranna S. Donovanosis. In: Sacchidanand S (Ed). IADVL Textbook of Dermatology, 4th edition. Mumbai: Bhalani Publishing House; 2014. pp. 1884-92.
5. Sehgal VN, Jain MK. Pattern of epidemics of donovanosis in the "nonendemic" region. Int J Dermatol. 1988;27:396-9.
6. Lal S, Nicholas C. Epidemiological and clinical features in 165 cases of granuloma inguinale. Br J Vener Dis. 1970;46:461-3.

7. Lal S. Continued efficacy of streptomycin in the treatment of granuloma inguinale. Br J Vener Dis. 1971;47:454-5.
8. Goldzieher M, Peck SM. Das venerische granulom. Virchows Arch. 1926;259:795-814.
9. Freinkel AL, Dangor Y, Koornhof HJ, Ballard RC. A serological test for granuloma inguinale. Genitourin Med. 1992;68: 269-72.
10. Carter J, Bowden FJ, Sriprakash KS, Bastian I, Kemp DJ. Diagnostic Polymerase Chain Reaction for Donovanosis. Clin Infect Dis. 1999;28:1168-9.
11. Centers for Disease Control and Prevention (2015). Granuloma Inguinale (Donovanosis). [online]Available from http://www.cdc.gov/std/tg2015/donovanosis.htm. [Last accessed January, 2021].
12. Bowden FJ, Bright A, Rode JW, Brewster D. Donovanosis causing cervical lymphadenopathy in a five month-old boy. Pediatr Infect Dis J. 2000;19:167-9.
13. Veeranna S, Raghu TY. A clinical and investigational study of donovanosis. Indian J Dermatol Venereol Leprol. 2003;69:159-62.

EXAMINATION QUESTION

1. Write a short note on donovanosis.

130 CHAPTER Gonorrhea

Nina Madnani, Kaleem Khan, Nisha Chaturvedi

INTRODUCTION

Gonorrhea, a disease known since ancient times, still remains one of the most common sexually transmitted diseases after chlamydia.[1] Today, the rates of gonorrhea in MSM (men who have sex with men) parallel those of syphilis.

NOMENCLATURE

Gonorrhea (Greek *gonos*: seed, *rhoia*: flow) was previously termed as "clap" following various hypothesis. It was believed that the patient suffering with the disease would experience a clapping sensation during urination. Others believed the term was coined by the process of milking the urethra by clapping the shaft between the two hands. Yet another explanation is that the name refers to the Parisian red-light district "Les Clapiers" of ancient times where the disease was highly prevalent.[2]

HISTORY

The exact period when gonorrhea was first detected is not known. It has been described by Galen in the second century. England and France laid down laws in 1161 and 1256 respectively to control the spread of the disease. In 1879, Albert Neisser described the causative organism, which was grown in pure culture by 1885. Initially, heavy metals (arsenic, antimony, bismuth, gold, and mercury) were tried in its treatment but were replaced by sulfur compounds in the 1930s. Penicillin was introduced in 1940s, but rapid development of resistant strains by 1980 stopped its use as an effective treatment drug.

CAUSATIVE ORGANISM

Neisseria gonorrhoeae is a gram-negative paired Diplococcus found intracellularly in neutrophils. It has a preference of attaching to columnar epithelium.

METHOD OF TRANSMISSION

Sexual: Vaginal, anal, or oral sex with an infected partner.

Perinatal: From mother to child during childbirth.

Anal sex is the most efficient means of transmission whereas the stratified squamous epithelium of the vaginal wall is not susceptible to this infection.

INCUBATION PERIOD

1–14 days; average of 2–7 days

CLINICAL SYMPTOMATOLOGY

About 55% of episodes of gonorrhea in men and 86% of episodes in women remain asymptomatic.[3] An overview of symptoms and associated complications are mentioned in **Table 1**. Most complications arise from delay in seeking treatment and the resulting spread of infection as its ascends the anatomical tract. Associated coinfections must be suspected in evaluating patients with urethral discharge. The presence of gonococcal urethritis can increase seminal human immunodeficiency virus (HIV) shedding eight-fold in coinfected men.

Systemic involvement is due to hematogenous spread and is described as dermatitis-arthritis syndrome. Patients present with mild fever, transient petechial or pustular eruptions distributed acrally. Joint pains present as septic oligoarthritis or migratory polyarthralgia involving the knees, elbows, and small joints of the hands and feet.[4] Blood cultures are highly sensitive for detecting the infection. Joint aspirate may show the organism on Gram stain. Rarely, cases of endocarditis and meningitis have been reported.

Pregnancy and neonate: Pregnant women may have symptoms of acute infection but they are at a higher risk of hematogenous spread and developing systemic symptoms. They have a risk of preterm labor. Neonates can get the infection during the birth passage and present with ophthalmia neonatorum. Purulent discharge from the eyes on day 2–5 postpartum should prompt the diagnosis and immediate treatment must be instituted to prevent possible blindness.[5]

INVESTIGATIONS

Direct microscopy of smears with Gram stain is an inexpensive and rapid test with a high positive predictive value. Samples can be collected from urethra, endocervix, pharynx,

TABLE 1: Clinical presentations and complications associated with ascending infection.

	Men	*Women*	*Neonates*
Sites of infection	Anterior urethra, Tyson's glands, paraurethral glands, epididymis, rectum, throat, eyes	Endocervix, urethra, paraurethral gland, Bartholin's glands, rectum, throat, eyes	Eyes (gonococcal ophthalmia neonatorum)
Clinical presentation	• Usually symptomatic • Urethral discharge—thick, yellow **(Fig. 1)** • Dysuria, meatitis **(Fig. 2)**, and burning	• Usually asymptomatic • Vaginal discharge—odorless, thin, greenish or yellow • Postcoital vaginal bleeding • Dyspareunia • Increased urinary frequency	• Conjunctivitis—bilateral, purulent discharge with redness • Keratitis • Conjunctival scarring
Complications due to ascending infection	• Periurethral abscess • Acute epididymo-orchitis—unilateral pain or tenderness in the scrotum • Prostatitis • Seminal vesiculitis	• Bartholinitis • Bartholin's abscess • Cervicitis • Salpingitis • Acute PID	
Chronic and repeated infection complications	• Urethral strictures • Saxophone penis	• Chronic PID • Tubo-ovarian mass • Infertility	
Complications due to hematogenous spread	• Dermatitis-arthritis syndrome • Fitz-Hugh–Curtis syndrome (perihepatitis) • Endocarditis • Meningitis		
Complications during pregnancy		• First trimester abortions • Premature delivery	

(PID: pelvic inflammatory disease)

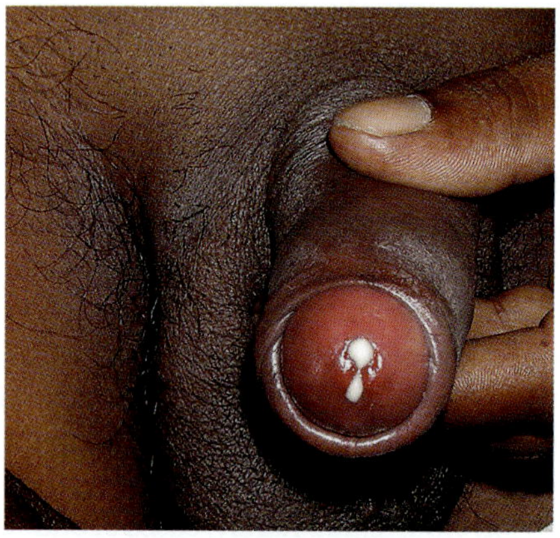

Fig. 1: Yellowish discharge described as a "bead of pus" seen at the meatal opening.

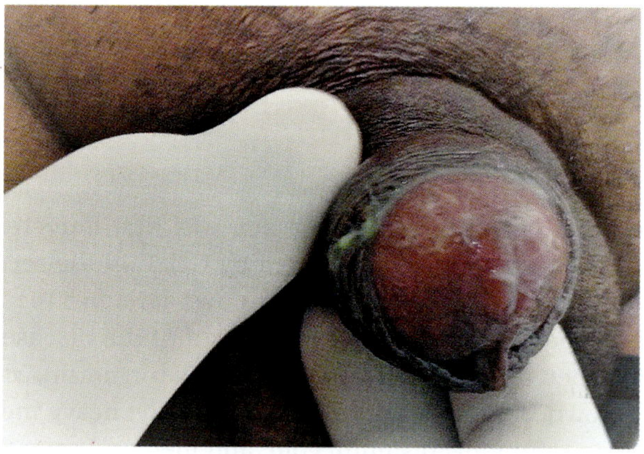

Fig. 2: Meatal edema with yellowish discharge.

rectum, conjunctiva, or urine for Gram stain. Specificity and sensitivity from rectal smears are low, hence not routinely done. Pharyngeal smear can show false positive results as oropharynx can be colonized by other *Neisseria* species. The presence of typical gram-negative intracellular diplococci and polymorphonuclear neutrophils on Gram stain establishes the diagnosis of gonorrhea **(Fig. 3)**. The sensitivity in men is up to 95% while specificity ranges from 95 to 99% for urethral smears, and in females the sensitivity vary from 40 to 60% and specificity from 90 to 100% for endocervical smears.[6]

Culture of the discharge is the gold standard in the diagnosis of infection at all potential sites. Culture swabs should be inserted 2–3 cm into the male urethra or 1–2 cm into the female endocervical canal with 2–3 rotations of the swab.

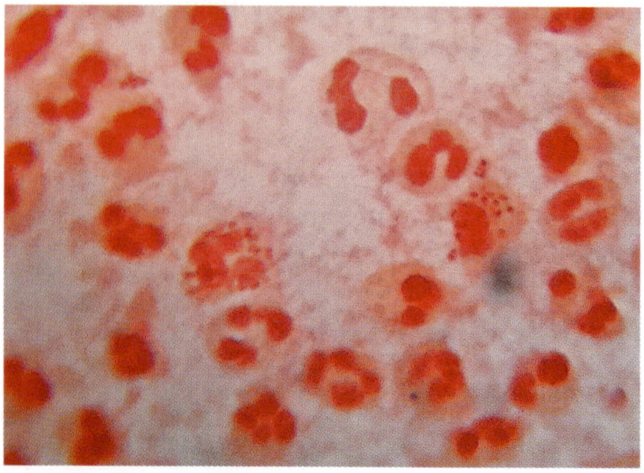

Fig. 3: Gram-negative diplococci seen intracellularly within neutrophils.

TABLE 2: Treatment recommendations as per the Centers for Disease Control and Prevention (CDC).

	Recommended treatment	*Resistant infection*
Uncomplicated Infection		
• Urogenital • Rectal • Pharyngeal	Ceftriaxone 250 mg IM + azithromycin 1 g PO single dose	Ceftriaxone 500 mg IM + azithromycin 2 g PO single dose OR Gentamicin 240 mg IM + azithromycin 2 g PO single dose
Ophthalmia neonatorum	Ceftriaxone 25–50 mg/kg IM single dose (maximum 125 mg)	
Disseminated infections		*Alternate regimes*
Dermatitis-arthritis syndrome	Ceftriaxone 1 g IV OD + azithromycin 1 g PO single dose	Cefotaxime 1 g IV every 8 hourly + azithromycin 1 g PO single dose
Gonococcal meningitis/ endocarditis	Ceftriaxone 1–2 g IV every 12–24 hourly + azithromycin 2 g PO single dose	
Pelvic inflammatory disease (PID)	Cefotetan 2 g IV every 12 hourly OR Cefoxitin 2 g IV every 6 hourly + doxycycline 100 mg PO 12 hourly	Ceftriaxone 250 mg IM single dose + doxycycline 100 mg PO BD × 2 weeks + metronidazole 500 mg PO BD × 2 weeks

In case of urethral discharge, exhumation collection is adequate. Enriched media such as modified Thayer–Martin or Martin–Lewis medium is required for growth of fastidious organism such as *N. gonorrhoeae*. It must be incubated at 35–36.5°C with 5% CO_2. Gonococci form small, round, soft, translucent, and convex colonies with granular surface. The sensitivity of culture is 80–95% and is affected by poor technique, slow transport and failure to store the collected specimen.

Nucleic acid amplification test (NAAT) is very sensitive, more rapid than culture, and does not require viable organism.[7] NAAT amplify genetic sequences from a few copies to millions in short time span. This test can be performed on swabs from endocervix, vagina, urethra, and urine. The disadvantage of these tests are that they are expensive, needed to be interpreted carefully, and inability to provide knowledge on antibiotic sensitivity.

TREATMENT

The Center for Disease Control and Prevention (CDC) has updated its treatment recommendations repeatedly over the last two decades in view of development of antibiotic resistance.[8] It now recommends dual therapy in an attempt to improve treatment outcomes and potentially slow down the emergence of resistance. The latest recommendations are mentioned in **Table 2**.

Most relapses are due to reinfection and must be treated as such. Resistance must be documented by culture and antibiotic testing and then treated accordingly. Sex partners should also be treated simultaneously and instructed to abstain from unprotected sexual intercourse for 7 days after completing therapy.

The CDC recommended treatment can be given in HIV-positive individuals without any dose modifications. It is also safe in pregnancy and can be administered to expecting mothers. To prevent (gonococcal) ophthalmia neonatorum, erythromycin ointment (0.5%) must be instilled in both eyes of the newborn immediately after delivery.

KEY POINTS

- Gonorrhea is the most prevalent STI after chlamydia.
- Gonococci have a preference for columnar epithelium.
- Transmission may be sexual, hematogenous, or perinatal during vaginal delivery.
- Infected women may be asymptomatic.
- Swab culture is the gold standard for diagnosis.
- Nucleic acid amplification test is very sensitive; more rapid than culture and do not require viable organism.
- All people tested positive for gonorrhea should also be tested for other sexually transmitted disease such as chlamydia, syphilis, and HIV.

REFERENCES

1. Unemo M, Shafer WM. Antibiotic resistance in *Neisseria gonorrhoeae*: origin, evolution, and lessons learned for the future. Ann NY Acad Sci. 2011;1230:E19-28.
2. Unemo M, Shafer WM. Antimicrobial resistance in *Neisseria gonorrhoeae* in the 21st century: past, evolution, and future. Clin Microbiol Rev. 2014;27(3):587-613.
3. Hook EW III, Handsfield HH. Gonococcal infections in the adult. In: Holmes KK, Sparling PF, Stamm WE, Piot P, Wasserheit JN, Corey L (Eds). Sexually Transmitted Diseases, 4th edition. New York, NY: McGraw-Hill; 2008.
4. Beatrous SV, Grisoli SB, Riahi RR, Matherne RJ, Matherne RJ. Cutaneous manifestations of disseminated gonococcemia. Dermatol Online J. 2017;23(1):13030/qt33b24006.
5. Comunián-Carrasco G, Peña-Martí GE, Martí-Carvajal AJ. Antibiotics for treating gonorrhoea in pregnancy. Cochrane Database Syst Rev. 2018;2(2):CD011167.
6. Thorley N, Radcliffe K. The performance and clinical utility of cervical microscopy for the diagnosis of gonorrhoea in women in the era of the NAAT. Int J STD AIDS. 2015;26: 656-60.
7. Meyer T, Buder S. The laboratory diagnosis of *Neisseria gonorrhoeae*: current testing and future demands. Pathogens. 2020;9(2):91
8. Centers for Disease Control and Prevention (2020). Gonorrhea. [online] Available from: https://www.cdc.gov/std/gonorrhea/arg/basic.htm [Last accessed January, 2021].

EXAMINATION QUESTIONS

1. Describe the investigations and management of gonococcal urethritis.
2. What are the long-term complications of untreated gonococcal urethritis in men and women?
3. Draw structure of:
   (a) *Neisseria gonorrhoeae*
   (b) Management of PPNG
   (c) Complications of gonorrhoea in females.
4. Write the microbiological characteristics of *Gonococcus.*
5. Discuss the treatment of uncomplicated gonococcal urethritis.
6. What is dermatitis-arthritis syndrome?
7. Explain the treatment of systemic complications of gonococcal urethritis.
8. Discuss the management of gonococcal urethritis in pregnancy.
9. What are the clinical characteristics of gonococcal urethritis?
10. Explain bedside investigation of urethral discharge in a suspected case of gonococcal urethritis.
11. Write a short note on ophthalmia neonatorum.
12. What is disseminated gonococcal infection?

131 CHAPTER Nongonococcal Urethritis

Sudip Das, Sudip Sarkar

INTRODUCTION[1]

Urethritis, or urethral inflammation, is in the majority of cases caused by sexually transmitted agents. Typical symptoms are discharge, dysuria, urethral stinging/itching, but urethritis is often asymptomatic.

Urethritis may be gonococcal, when *Neisseria gonorrhoeae* is detected or nongonococcal when examination findings or microscopy indicate inflammation without gram negative intercellular diplococci.

Mucopurulent nongonococcal cervicitis and urethritis is the female equivalent of urethral discharge. However, the definition of cervicitis and female urethritis is controversial.

ETIOLOGY[2-4]

Etiological agent	*Isolate in percentage of cases*
Chlamydia trachomatis (serovars D to K)	20–50%
Mycoplasma genitalium	10–30%
Trichomonas vaginalis	2.5–17%
Herpes simplex, adenovirus, candida	-
Noninfective causes such as trauma, chemical, neoplasm, foreign body	-

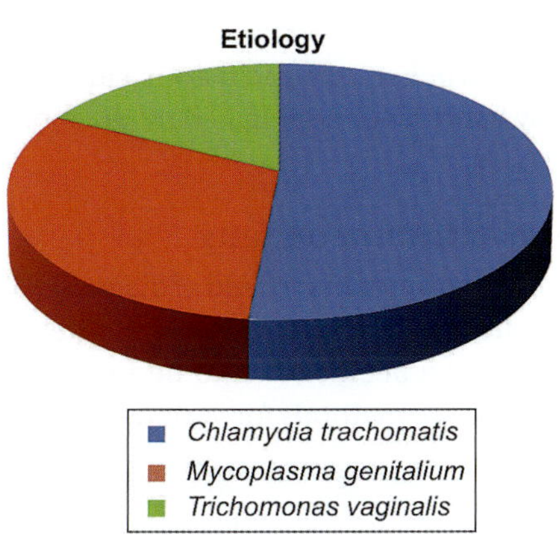

CHLAMYDIA TRACHOMATIS[5,6]

- *Chlamydia trachomatis* is an obligate intracellular parasite and cannot be cultured on artificial media.
- Chlamydia lack the ability to synthesize high energy compounds, amino acids, vitamins, and cofactors. Thus, they depend on the host cell to supply them with ATP.

Pathogenesis

Figure 1 shows pathogenesis of *Chlamydia trachomatis*.

Clinical Features[5,6]

- *Incubation period*: Varies from 1 to 3 weeks.
- Men: There is usually scanty mucoid or mucopurulent discharge, less purulent than the typical discharge in gonorrhea.
- Women: Chlamydial infection of the lower genital tract occurs in the endocervix. It can cause an odorless, mucoid vaginal discharge, generally not associated with pruritus, although some women may have symptoms.
- Postgonococcal urethritis usually develops 2 weeks after in men who have received adequate treatment for gonorrhea, but not for *Chlamydia* or other causes of urethritis.

Diagnosis[8,9]

The diagnosis of urethritis must be confirmed by demonstrating polymorphonuclear leukocytes (PMNLs) in the anterior urethra.

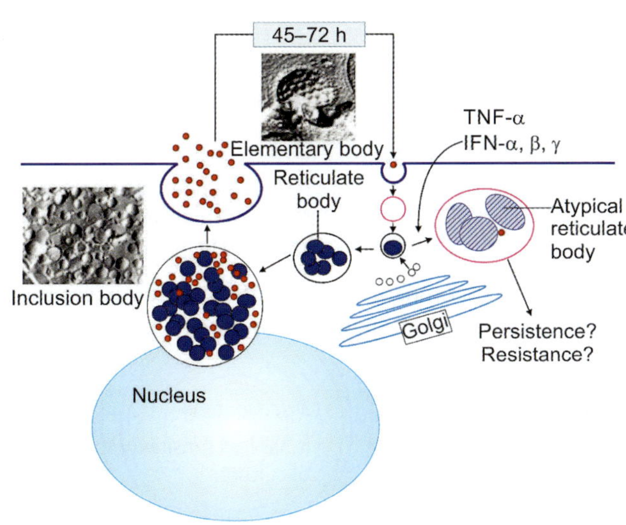

Fig. 1: Pathogenesis of *Chlamydia trachomatis*.[7]
Source: Adapted from Gross G, Tyring SK. Sexually transmitted infections and sexually transmitted diseases. New Delhi: Elsevier; 2011. pp. 93-4.

Methods of Collection of the Specimen

- *Urethral swab*:

Collect specimen at least 2 hours after urination as voiding decreases the amount of exudate

↓

If no urethral discharge is seen
Milk/strip the urethra from the root

↓

If no discharge is obtained, insert a sterile cotton tipped/thin calcium alginate swab with a flexible wire shaft 2–3 cm into the urethra and rotate for 5–10 seconds

- *Urine sample* : The first 10–15 mL of the early morning first void urine is collected in a sterile plastic container with a wide mouth and processed immediately.

Direct Microscopy

- *Gram stain*: A Gram-stained urethral smear containing 5 PMNL per high-power (×1000) microscopic field (averaged over five fields with the greatest concentration of PMNLs), and/or
  A Gram-stained preparation from a first-void urine specimen, containing 10 PMNL per high-power (×1000) microscopic field (averaged over five fields with the greatest concentration of PMNLs).
- *Giemsa stain*: Not sensitive. Shows intracytoplasmic (of epithelial cells) basophilic bodies in epithelial cells.
- *Iodine stain*: Shows brown intracytoplasmic bodies.
- *Fluorescent antibody technique*: Fluorescent-labelled polyclonal or monoclonal antibodies are used to detect infected cells in smears (75–85% sensitivity, 98–99% specificity) **(Figs. 2 and 3)**.

Advantages	*Disadvantage*
Much cheaper, less time	Less sensitive than nucleic acid amplification tests (NAATs)

Serology

- *Complement fixation titers*: 1:64 can support the diagnosis of chlamydia in appropriate clinical context.

Advantages	*Disadvantages*
Much cheaper, less time	It is not standardized, and requires a high level of expertise to interpret

- *Enzyme immunoassay*: In this, the antigen is captured with antibodies, but signal generation is amplified by two mechanisms.

Advantage	*Disadvantage*
More specificity (97%)	It has less sensitivity than that of culture.

Cell Culture

- *Cycloheximide*: Treated McCoy/BHK2/HeLa cell. Lines are used for *C. trachomatis* culture.

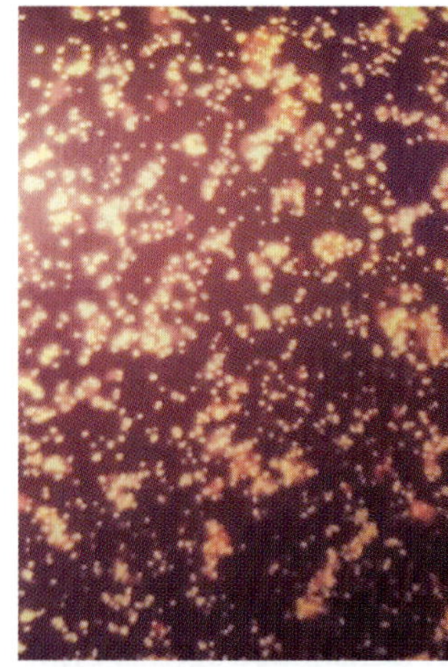

Fig. 2: Microphotograph by fluorescent microscopy showing Chlamydial antibody as greenish refractile particles (Magnification 100×).

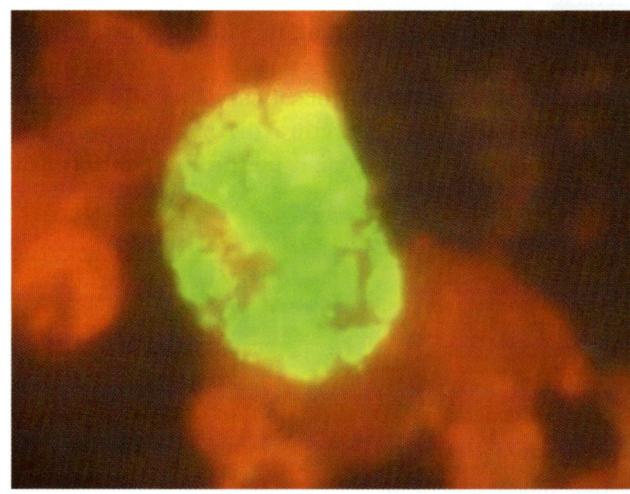

Fig. 3: Immunofluorescent staining of an inclusion body of McCoy cells infected with *Chlamydia trachomatis*.[7]
Source: Adapted from Gross G, Tyring SK. Sexually Transmitted Infections and Sexually Transmitted Diseases. New Delhi: Elsevier; 2011. pp. 93-4.

- *Chlamydia trachomatis* inclusions can be detected in culture by fluorescein-conjugated monoclonal antibodies **(Fig. 4)**.

Nucleic Acid Amplification Tests

The most recent advance in the field of diagnosis of chlamydia infections during the last 20 years is the development of NAATs, which have been shown to be more accurate than any other diagnostic methods for various genital pathogens.

Advantages	*Disadvantages*
• NAATs is their high sensitivity (80–95%) • It can detect organism with a low target concentration • Helpful for asymptomatic individuals or contact persons	The major limitation is cost; these tests are more expensive than other nonculture laboratory tests

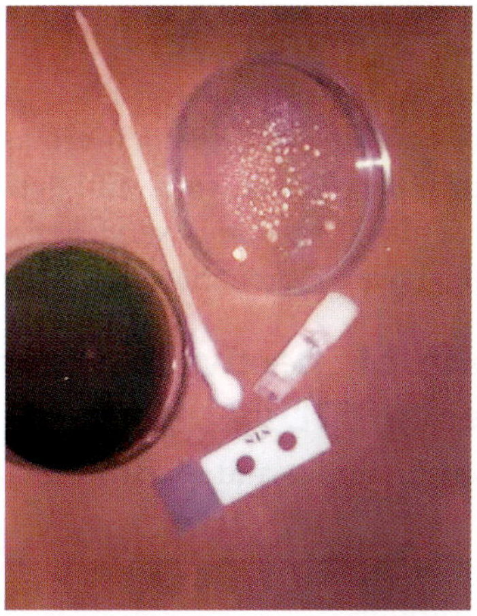

Fig. 4: Essential kits for investigation of urethral discharge in an OPD setup. [Shows chocolate agar (for gonococcal culture), 2 SP tubes (Chlamydial culture), Teflon-coated slide (for chlamydial antigen), and chlamydial swab].

Treatment[10]

Regimens

- Centers for Disease Control and Prevention (CDC), 2010 recommended regimen:
  Azithromycin 1g orally in a single dose,
  OR
  Doxycycline 100 mg twice a day for 7 days
- Alternative regimens:
  Erythromycin base 500 mg four times daily for 7 days
  OR
  Erythromycin ethyl succinate 800 mg four times a day for 7 days
  OR
  Levofloxacin 500 mg orally once a day for 7 days
  OR
  Ofloxacin 300 mg twice a day.

Prevent Transmission

- Men treated for nongonococcal urethritis (NGU) should be instructed to abstain from sexual intercourse for 7 days after single-dose therapy or until completion of a 7-day regimen, provided their symptoms have resolved.
- Persons who have been diagnosed with a new STD should receive testing for other infections, including syphilis and HIV.

Management of Partner

All sex partners within the preceding 60 days should be referred for evaluation, testing, and empiric treatment against chlamydia.

Follow-up

- Unless a patient's symptoms persist or therapeutic noncompliance or reinfection is suspected by the provider, a test-of-cure (Repeat testing 3–4 weeks after completing therapy) is not recommended for persons with documented chlamydia or gonococcal infections who have received with recommended or alternative treatment regimens.
- However, because men with documented chlamydial or gonococcal infections have a high rate of reinfection within 6 months after treatment, repeat testing of all men diagnosed with chlamydia or gonorrhea is recommended 3–6 months after treatment, regardless of whether sex partners were treated.

NONCHLAMYDIAL NONGONOCOCCAL URETHRITIS[11]

A significant fraction of urethritis patients (up to 50%), however, are not infected by *Neisseria gonorrhoeae* or *C. trachomatis*. In these cases the clinical syndrome is referred to as nonchlamydial nongonococcal urethritis (NCNGU) or nonspecific urethritis.

Mycoplasma Genitalium[12-14]

- *Mycoplasmas* commonly colonize the genital tracts of men and women. At least 13 species of *Mycoplasma* and two species of *Ureaplasma* are common commensals of the human urogenital tract.
- *Clinical features*: These diminutive microbes are transmitted efficiently by sexual contact. Most colonized individuals remain asymptomatic, but there are evidence of symptomatic urethritis due to *M. genitalium*, *M. hominis*, and the *Ureaplasmas.*

Culture

- *Mycoplasma*: It can be cultured on pleuropneumonia-like organisms (PPLO) broth containing arginine. The colonies show a "fried egg appearance."
- *Ureaplasma*: A sample should be taken in PPLO broth containing urea, which will identify *Ureaplasma urealyticum*, another cause of NCNGU. Serological tests for *Mycoplasmas* are not standardized.
- *Treatment:* Tetracycline resistance is reported in *Mycoplasma*. Azithromycin 1 g in a single dose appears to be the drug of choice for this infection.

Trichomonas Vaginalis[10,15]

Trichomonas vaginalis is a flagellated parasitic protozoan of the human urogenital tract, and remains the leading causative agent of nonviral, sexually transmitted infections (STIs) worldwide.

A recent study has shown that nearly 20% of men with NGU were infected with *T. vaginalis* and coinfection of gonorrhea in western Europe, *T. vaginalis* as a cause of male urethritis is uncommon. In the United States, *T. vaginalis* is associated with Afro-American race.

- *T. vaginalis* is an important cause of persistent or recurrent urethritis.

- Therefore, a patient whose symptoms persist after adequately treating for gonorrhea and chlamydia, should be investigated for *T. vaginalis* infection or treated syndromically with metronidazole, assuming TV as the cause **(Fig. 5)**.

Diagnosis

Wet mount: A wet mount under 40× shows pear-shaped flagellate motile (jerky movements) organisms **(Fig. 6)**.

Serology

A PCR-based assay is more sensitive than culture for diagnosis of *Trichomonas* urethritis.

Treatment

Two regimens are used for the treatment of urethritis due to *T. vaginalis*. Secnidazole or Tinidazole may be given in a single dose of 2 g orally.

SYNDROMIC MANAGEMENT

Early diagnosis and treatment of STIs is very important to prevent late complications, which are associated with significant morbidity, loss of work, and even mortality. In resource-poor settings, laboratory services are not equipped with tools to diagnose STIs reliably **(Table 1)**.

Requirements of Effective Syndromic Management of STDs

- Recognition of common and effective signs and symptoms of STIs
- Knowledge of most common causative organisms for various syndromes
- Knowledge of social behavior and health seeking behavior of STI patients
- Local antibiotic susceptibility patterns

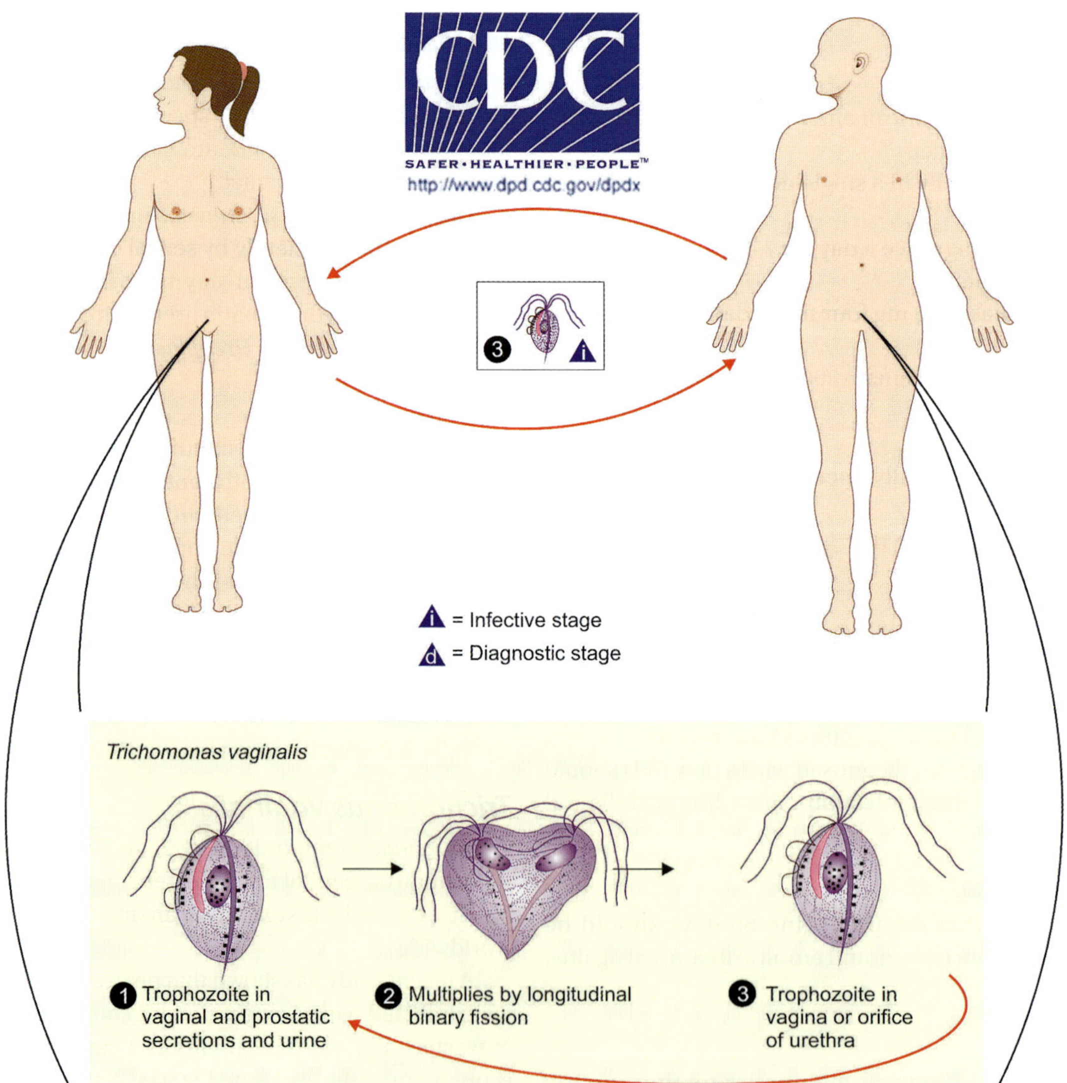

Fig. 5: Life cycle of *Trichomonas vaginalis*.
Source: Adapted from Centers for Disease Control and Prevention. Trichomoniasis. [online] Available from: https://www.cdc.gov/std/trichomonas/stdfact-trichomoniasis.htm [Last accessed March, 2021].

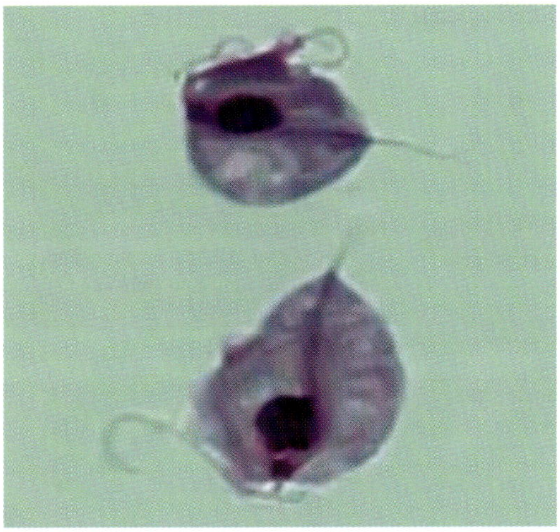

Fig. 6: Two trophozoites of *Trichomonas vaginalis* obtained from in vitro culture. Smear was stained with Giemsa.[7]
Source: Adapted from Gross G, Tyring SK. Sexually transmitted infections and sexually transmitted diseases. New Delhi: Elsevier; 2011. p. 603.

- Cooperation of partners of people with STIs
- Data on drug availability, cost and drug distribution patterns
- Choice of algorithm appropriate for residents and level of clinical staff
- Regular monitoring and evaluation of management protocols

Therefore, the World Health Organization (WHO) has introduced treatment algorithms for syndromic management of STI syndromes **(Flowcharts 1 and 2)**.

Persistent and Recurrent Urethritis[3,14]

- The etiology of persistent NGU is probably multifactorial with an infectious agent being identified in <50% of cases.
- *M. genitalium* has been identified in 20–40% and *C. trachomatis* in 10–20% in men treated with azithromycin 1 g.
- *U. urealyticum* may also play a role in some men.

TABLE 1: Advantages and disadvantages of syndromic case management.[7]

Criteria	*Advantages*	*Disadvantages*
Algorithm	• Simple • Problem-oriented, based on presenting symptoms	Low sensitivity and specificity for cervical gonococcal and chlamydial infections in women
Initiation of therapy	Rapid. Patients are treated at first visit without need for laboratory confirmation	• Risk scores are not highly sensitive or specific • Not easily a accepted by doctors
Treatment outcome	High rates of cure	• Requires surveillance of antibiotic susceptibility profiles • Some algorithms do not provide for second or third line treatment
Cost	• Saves money on laboratory tests • Cost-effective	Leads to over treatment, which may be costly
Coverage	Can achieve high population coverage	Does not detect asymptomatic cases
Implementation of approach	• Can be easily integrated into the PHC system • Can rely on nonmedical staff to manage cases	Needs to be adapted to specific settings
Management support system	• Simplifies reporting, supervision and ordering of drugs • Facilitates data collection for surveillance and planning	May have to setup a modified information system in order to monitor trends in etiology of conventional STDs

Flowchart 1: Syndromic management of sexually transmitted infection (STI) syndromes.[16]

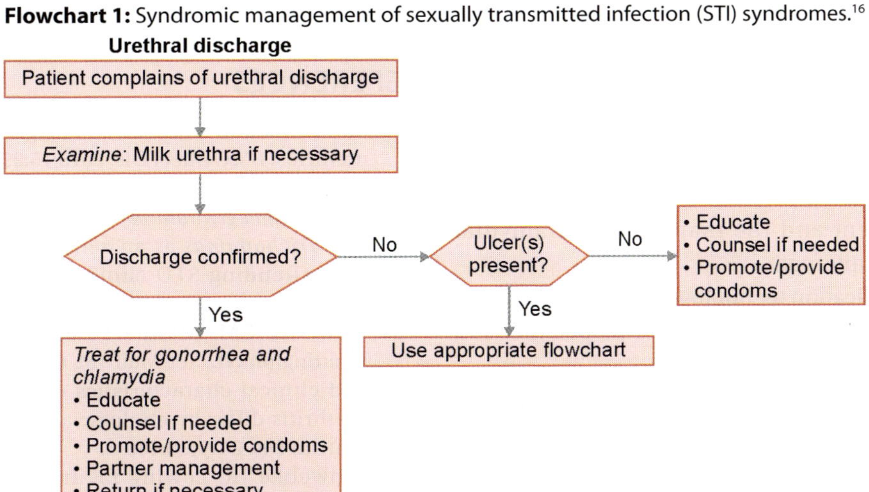

Source: Adapted from World Health Organization. Guidelines for the Management of Sexually Transmitted Infections. Geneva: WHO; 2001. pp. 18-20.

Flowchart 2: Treatment of *Trichomonas vaginalis*.[16]

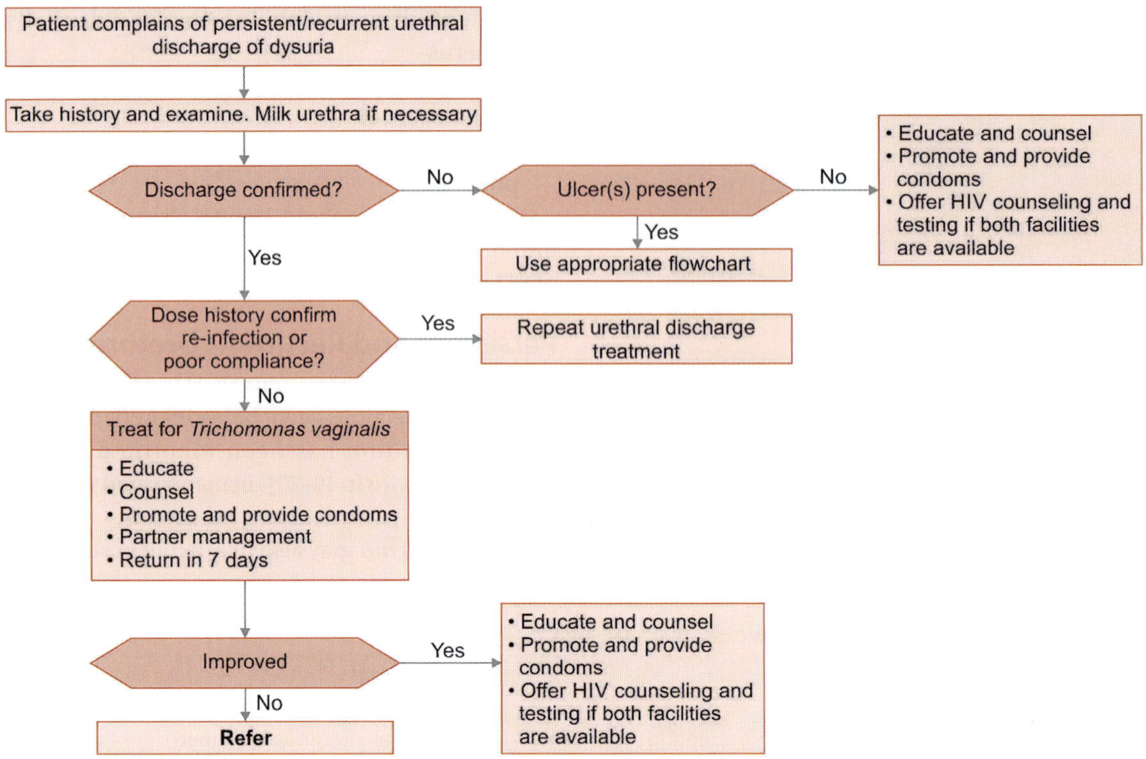

Source: Adapted from World Health Organization. Guidelines for the Management of Sexually Transmitted Infections. Geneva: WHO; 2001. pp. 18-20.

- *Trichomonas vaginalis* can be identified in up to 10% in populations where it is endemic, but is rare in Western Europe.
- Recurrent herpes simplex virus infection should be considered, as this can cause dysuria without signs outside the urethra.
- Any treatment of persistent NGU should cover *M. genitalium*, *T. vaginalis* and anaerobes, if not tested and treated for an initial presentation.

KEY POINTS

- *Chlamydiae* are bacteria that are highly adapted to an intracellular life cycle in eukaryotic host cells.
- *Chlamydia trachomatis* is an important genital pathogen and the most common bacterial cause of STIs.
- Most clinical manifestations of *C. trachomatis* genital infections are silent and the majority of chlamydial infections are asymptomatic.
- Nucleic acid amplification technologies enable chlamydia diagnosis from invasive and noninvasive specimens in both men and women.
- Azithromycin is the best single-dose agent for treatment of chlamydial infections.
- Screening programs remain important in limiting the upper genital tract complications of chlamydial infection.
- *M. hominis* and *Ureaplasma urealyticum* (*Ureaplasmas*) are two of the most frequent microorganisms isolated from the genitourinary tract.
- *Mycoplasma genitalium* has recently been detected and associated with pelvic inflammatory disease (PID) in women.
- *Trichomonas vaginalis* is the leading causative agent of nonviral, STIs worldwide.
- Infection with *T. vaginalis* is a marker of high-risk sexual behavior as it is frequently seen concomitantly with other STIs.

REFERENCES

1. Moi H, Blee K, Horner PJ. Management of non-gonococcal urethritis. BMC Infect Dis. 2015;15:294.
2. Gaydos C, Maldeis NE, Hardick A, Hardick J, Quinn TC. *Mycoplasma genitalium* compared to chlamydia, gonorrhoea and *Trichomonas* as an aetiological agent of urethritis in men attending STD clinics. Sex Transm Infect. 2009;85:438-40.
3. Wetmore CM, Manhart LE, Lowens MS, Golden MR, Whittington WL, Xet-Mull AM, et al. Demographic, behavioral, and clinical characteristics of men with nongonococcal urethritis differ by etiology: a case-comparison study. Sex Transm Dis. 2011;38:180-6.
4. Schwebke JR, Lawing LF. Improved detection by DNA amplification of *Trichomonas vaginalis* in males. J Clin Microbiol. 2002;40:3681-3.

5. Ndowa F, Dludlu S. Urethral discharge. In: Kumar B, Gupta S (Eds.) Sexually Transmitted Infections. New Delhi: Elsevier; 2005. pp. 502-8.
6. Miller KE. Diagnosis and treatment of *Neisseria gonorrhoeae* infections. Am Fam Phys. 2006;73:1411-6.
7. Gross G, Tyring SK. Sexually transmitted infections and sexually transmitted diseases. New Delhi: Elsevier; 2011. pp. 93-94, 112, 604.
8. Swartz SL, Kraus SJ, Herrmann KL, Stargel MD, Brown WJ, Allen SD. Diagnosis and etiology of nongonococcal urethritis. J Infect Dis. 1978;138:445-54.
9. Cheng H, Macaluso M, Vermund SH, Hook EW. Relative accuracy of nucleic acid amplification tests and culture in detecting *Chlamydia* in asymptomatic men. J Clin Microbiol. 2001;39:3927-37.
10. Centers for Disease Control and Prevention. Sexually Transmitted Diseases Treatment Guidelines, 2010. MMWR. 2010;59(RR-12):40-55.
11. Riemersma WA, van der Schee CJC, van der Meijden WI, Verbrugh HA, van Belkum A. Microbial population diversity in the urethras of healthy males and males suffering from nonchlamydial, nongonococcal urethritis. J Clin Microbiol. 2003;41:1977-86.
12. Yoshida T, Maeda SI, Deguchi T, Ishiko H. Phylogeny based rapid identification of *Mycoplasmas* and *Ureaplasmas* from urethritis patients. J Clin Microbiol. 2002;40:105-10.
13. Robertson JA, Stemke JW, Davis JW Jr, Harasawa R, Thirkell D, Kong F, et al. Proposal of *Ureaplasma parvum* spp. nov. and amended description of *Ureaplasma urealyticum*. Int J Syst Evol Microbiol. 2002;52:587-97.
14. Povlsen K, Bjornelius E, Lidbrink P, Lind I. Relationship of *Ureaplasma urealyticum* biovar 2 to nongonococcal urethritis. Eur J Clin Microbiol. 2002;21:97-101.
15. David MH. Urethritis in males. In: King HK (Ed). Sexually Transmitted Diseases, 4th edition. New York: McGraw Hill; 2008. pp. 1107-26.
16. World Health Organization. Guidelines for the Management of Sexually Transmitted Infections. Geneva: WHO; 2001. pp. 18-20.

EXAMINATION QUESTIONS

1. How will you approach to a female patient with urethritis?
2. What is nongonococcal urethritis?
3. Describe the evaluation of urethral discharge.
4. What is the diagnosis of nongonococcal urethritis?

132 CHAPTER Viral Sexually Transmitted Diseases

Sudip Das, Yashpal Manchanda

INTRODUCTION

The landscape of sexually transmitted diseases has been changing constantly. In the early part of 20th century, it was the bacterial venereal diseases which caused havoc all over the world, and even lead to countries losing battles in the World War II. However, toward the later part of the century with the discovery of penicillin and other effective antimicrobial agents classical venereal diseases such as syphilis and gonorrhea were brought under control to some extent. But, it was during same period that viral sexually transmitted infections had started creeping up, to the extent that they soon became enormous public health issue. The most significant of all, was the emergence of human immunodeficiency virus infection. It was not only a newer infection with no known treatment. But, it also altered the course of other classical venereal diseases, making both their diagnosis as well as treatment very difficult. The surge in cases of viral venereal diseases could possibly have been caused by the false sense of security in the minds of general population, with the reducing number of conventional sexually transmitted infections due to effective treatment. Coupled with the more liberal societal attitude toward sexual freedom and easy availability of birth control pills, the greatest fears of sexual intimacy, pregnancy and venereal disease, were no more a major concern. Thus, the world experienced resurgence of sexually transmitted diseases. Albeit, this time it was because of viruses including herpes simplex viruses (HSV), human papillomaviruses (HPV), human immunodeficiency virus (HIV), hepatitis B virus, and cytomegalovirus. With infections with HSV, HPV, and HIV having reached epidemic proportions and posed a significant global health challenge. The situation got further complicated by the emergence of resistance strains of bacterial STDs, and the experts worldwide are struggling to control this menace. The two most common of the viral venereal diseases (HSV and HPV) are notorious to recur in large number of patients, in spite of all treatments. With no effective permanent cure in sight, the only hope lies in vaccine. Some definite progress has been made in developing vaccine against both these viruses, and once again there is a hope amongst the scientific community of getting good control over them in near future.[1-3]

HERPES GENITALIS

Epidemiology: According to one report, it is estimated to have infected 417 million people worldwide till 2012, between the ages of 15 and 49 years. And with just over 19 million new infections being reported every year, the prevalence would be around 600 plus million by now.[4,5]

Organism: Herpes simplex virus 2 (HSV2; also called HHV 2) and to some extent, also herpes simplex virus 1 (HSV 1; or HHV 1) are responsible for causing herpes genitalis, a leading cause of genital ulcer disease worldwide **(Fig. 1)**. They are both relatively large, enveloped DNA viruses belonging to the subfamily of alpha-herpesvirinae. They have a peculiar tendency to remain dormant in the sacral ganglion after primary infection, and can reactivate anytime, leading to multiple relapses.[6] Due to its tendency to replicate inside the nucleus. The virus typically leads to formation of large intranuclear inclusion bodies, which are visible under microscope in the stained preparations of the smears taken from the lesions.

Mode of transmission: Through intimate genital tract contact during unprotected sexual exposure

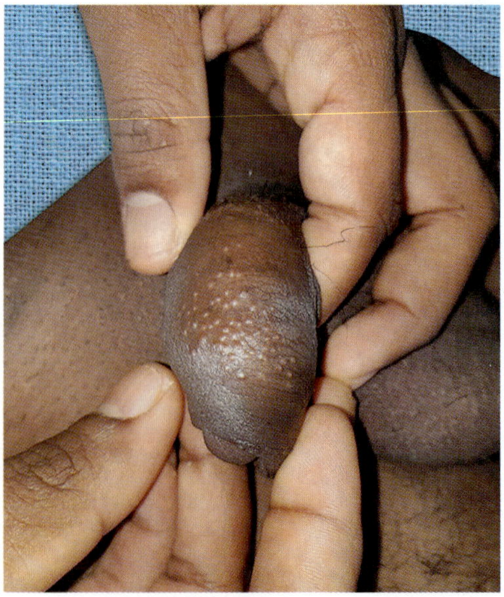

Fig. 1: Characteristic grouped multiple vesicular lesions of herpes genitalis.

Type of infection[7]:
- Primary infection: In most cases caused by HSV2 are symptomatic
- Recurrent infection
- Asymptomatic viral shedding

Clinical features: It is characterized by multiple, grouped, small, superficial painful ulcers. There may be a preceding prodrome of general malaise and fever in some cases. In few cases, it may also lead to dysuria. The lesions if left untreated can last for 2–3 weeks in cases with primary infection. The lesions are commonly located on glans, prepuce and shaft of penis in males. Anal mucosal involvement can be seen in homosexual males.[8] Whereas in females, the lesions are located on external genitalia and vulvovaginal mucosa. In cases with associated HIV disease, the lesion may appear chronic and verrucous.

Investigations: Tzanck smear from ulcer floor scraping is a simple bedside procedure helpful in making rapid diagnosis. It shows multinucleate giant cells in classical cases, and cannot differentiate between HSV 1 and HSV 2.[9] However, confirmation of the diagnosis can be done by viral culture from the vesicular fluid or scraping from the base of the ulcers. But, the culture results may take up to 5 days. For rapid diagnosis, detection of viral antigen from the scraping of ulcer floor or in vesicular fluid under electron microscope can be done, immunofluorescence test and/or PCR from the scraping can also give faster results.[10] Serology for type specific HSV antibodies can also be done.[11]

Management: Prevention of infection in seronegative cases is possible by vaccination at early age or by using barrier contraceptive methods.[12] Acute infection in immunocompetent cases can be managed by conventional antiviral drugs such as acyclovir, famciclovir or valacyclovir given in standard dosing schedule **(Table 1)**. However, in case of immunosuppression due to HIV or other reasons, the drugs have to be given in higher doses and for longer duration. Subset of immunocompromised patient may not respond to conventional agents, and may require to be given combination of imiquimod and cidofovir, or parental foscarnet. In cases of too frequent recurrences, the conventional antiviral drugs can also be given in suppressive doses to improve the quality of life, reduce viral shedding as well as to minimize the chance of its transmission to sexual partner.[13]

HUMAN PAPILLOMAVIRUS INFECTIONS

Human papillomaviruses (HPVs) are another common sexually transmitted viral infections in the world. Although, genital warts have been recognized as venereal disease since Greek and Roman times. However, it was not until 1949, when the virus was first identified under electron microscope and true etiology of genital warts was ascertained.[14] Because the virus could not be cultured. Even two decades after its identification, it was not known that the HPV responsible for causing cutaneous warts was different from the one causing genital warts.[15] Major advancement in our understanding of HPV was made possible only after the advent of DNA sequencing technology. At least 150 different types of HPV have been identified now, of which at least 7 different types are known to affect the genital tract.[16] They are known to be responsible for causing wide spectrum of genital diseases, including condylomas, intraepithelial neoplasia, and squamous cell carcinomas of genital tract.

ANOGENITAL WARTS (CONDYLOMA ACUMINATA)

Epidemiology: Worldwide, the overall incidence of genital warts is around 200 of 100,000, and is highest amongst young adults of ages between 16 and 24 years, which is about 700 of 100,1000.[17]

Transmission: HPV transmission in genital warts occurs mostly through sexual contact. However, there is consensus that not all the cases of genital warts are transmitted sexually. The latent period between the contact and diagnosis of genital warts can vary from 3 weeks to up to 24 months.[18]

Organism: HPV are small non-enveloped double-stranded DNA viruses capable of infecting and causing disease at any site with stratified squamous epithelial lining. Genital warts are most commonly caused by HPV 6 (up to 90%) or HPV 11, and very rarely other types of HPV may be indicated.[19]

TABLE 1: Antiviral drug dosages in various genital herpes virus infections.

Indications	*Acyclovir*	*Valacyclovir*	*Famciclovir*
• Immunocompetent • Primary genital herpes • Immunocompromised	200 mg 5 times a day for 10 days or 400 mg 3 times a day for 7–10 days	1 g BD for 10 days	250 mg 3 times daily for 7–10 days
• Immunocompetent • Recurrent genital herpes • Immunocompromised	200 mg 5 times a day or 400 mg three times a day for 5 days	1 g BD for 3 days	1000 mg BD for 1 day started within 6 hours of first symptom 500 mg BD for 5–10 days
• Immunocompetent • Suppressive dose in genital herpes • Immunocompromised	400 mg 2 times a day for 1 year	1 g OD for 1 year 500 mg BD for 1 year	250 mg 2 times a day for 1 year 500 mg BD for 1 year

Clinical features: The lesions are usually asymptomatic soft pinkish papules. They classically appear as discreet flat, papular, or pedunculated lesions on the genital mucosa. However, sometimes multiple close lesions merge to appear as a single large plaque. Occasionally, they can be painful or itchy depending upon their size and location, and in case of secondary infection they can have foul discharge and at times bleed.[20] The immune status of the patient plays a significant role in the progression of HPV infection as well as the response to treatment. The prevalence of HPV infection is noted in more than half of HIV positive cases. It could be because of their reduced ability to clear HPV infection due to impaired cytotoxic T-cell response to the oncoprotein E6 and E7.

- Bowenoid papulosis presents as multiple reddish brown discreet papules or confluent plaques, clinically resembling condyloma acuminata **(Fig. 2)**, but it is usually caused by high-risk HPV types such as HPV 16 and appears as squamous cell carcinoma (SCC) in situ on histopathology.
- *Erythroplasia of Queyrat*: Another distinct clinical entity caused by high-risk HPV 16, usually presents as well-defined erythematous, velvety flat plaque on the glabrous skin. Histologically, again it is SCC in situ.
- *Buschke–Lowenstein tumor (Giant condyloma acuminata)*: It is a rare tumor caused by low-risk HPV types 6 and 11, but considered as premalignant lesion unlike condyloma acuminata. The histopathological features are similar to condyloma acuminata, but may have focal frank areas of malignant transformation **(Fig. 3)**.

Diagnosis: The diagnosis of anogenital warts is mostly made clinically. However, in certain situations such as pigmented, indurated, ulcerated, bleeding, large sized lesions, biopsy can be done to confirm the diagnosis. Skin biopsy is also indicated if the patient does not improve or worsens with treatment, or has an associated underlying condition like HIV infection, leading to immunocompromised state. Carcinoma is associated with high-risk type 16 and 18. The most characteristic histological finding seen in all types of HPV-induced lesions is the presence of numerous koilocytes (epithelial cells with vacuolated cytoplasm) **(Fig. 4)**.[21]

Prevention: Although, use of barrier methods (like condoms) during sexual contact, does give some protection against HPV infection. But, prophylactic vaccination against HPV types 6, 11, 16 and 18 has shown clear evidence. Prophylactic use of tetravalent vaccine by many countries has led to reduced incidence of anogenital warts **(Fig. 5)**.[22-24] Vaccines covering other uncommon HPV types are also being developed.

Treatment: Around one-third of the cases are known to resolve on their own even without any treatment within 2 years.[25] As of now, there is not even a single antiviral drug available that can cure HPV infection. All existing therapies primarily result in physical destruction of the visible lesion or at the most cause cell death of the infected epithelial cells. The treatment can be done using various drugs such as podophyllin/podophyllotoxin, trichloroacetic acid, and imiquimod. Topical podophyllotoxin is the most commonly used agent, it is applied as 0.15% cream or 0.5% solution twice daily for 3 consecutive days every week for at least 4 weeks. However, it should be avoided in pregnant females. Imiquimod is used as 5% cream, to be applied twice daily on alternate days for up to 16 weeks. It is a Toll-like receptor 7 agonist, which activates nuclear factor kappa-beta (NF-Kb) and induces proinflammatory cytokines such as IFN-gamma, TNf-alfa.Il6, and Il 8.

Other modalities used are electrocautery, cryotherapy, photodynamic therapy, ablative lasers, and surgical excision. Interferons have also been used either intralesionally or systemically in cases with extensive or very large lesions, especially in immunocompromised patients.

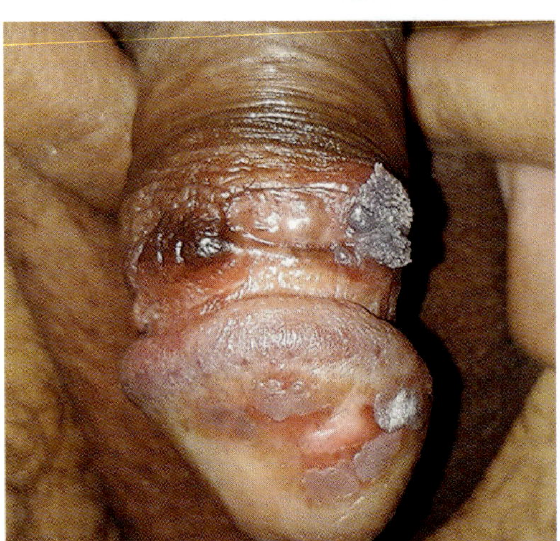

Fig. 2: Multiple condyloma acuminata.

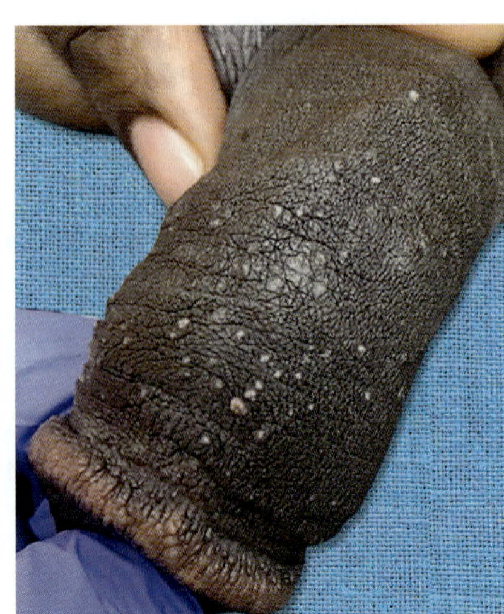

Fig. 3: Pearly white papules of molluscum contagiosum on penile shaft.

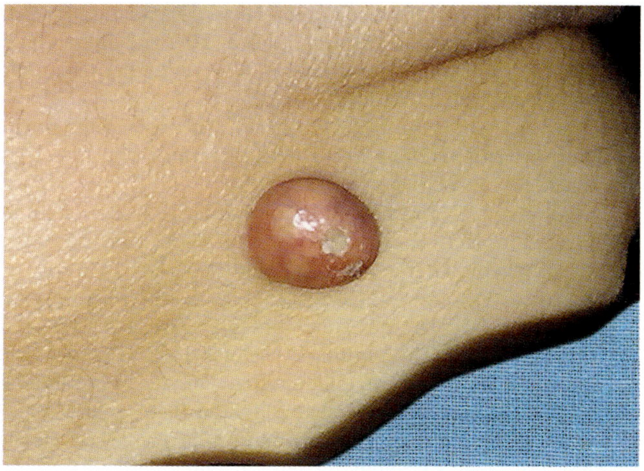

Fig. 4: A giant molluscum contagiosum.

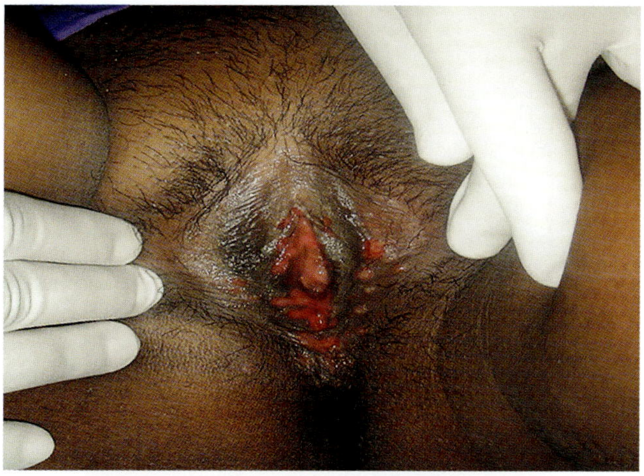

Fig. 5: Herpes genitalis in a young lady.

GENITAL MOLLUSCUM CONTAGIOSUM

Epidemiology: Molluscum contagiosum is a relatively common skin infection, usually seen in school going children and occasionally in adults and immunocompromised individuals. It is associated with high risk of transmission and with an increasing frequency in worldwide populations **(Fig. 6)**.[26]

Transmission: In adults, the transmission generally occurs through sexual contact. However, in cases of children, child abuse should be considered. Although, autoinoculation is also a potentially possible mode of transmission in children with genital molluscum contagiosum.[27]

Organism: It is caused by another double-stranded DNA virus belonging to Pox viruses, "Molluscum Contagiosum Virus." The typical incubation period varies from 2 to 7 weeks, but can be as long as 6 months in some cases.[28]

Clinical features: The lesions are usually asymptomatic pearly white to skin colored, discreet, firm, smooth, shiny, dome-shaped 2–5 mm papules with central umbilication. The lesions are usually located on and around the anogenital area including the external genital organs, groins, inner thighs and the suprapubic area.[29] On puncturing the lesion, a cheesy material comes out. It usually follows a benign and self-limiting course, except in immunocompromised patients which can have persistent lesions.

Diagnosis: The diagnosis is essentially clinical, except in rare cases of atypical lesions. In which case, dermoscopy and skin biopsy can be helpful in making the diagnosis. Dermoscopic features of typical molluscum papule include polylobular, pinkish-white, amorphous structure in the center with a surrounding crown of vessels.[30] Classical histopathological picture reveals keratinocytes containing large intracytoplasmic, faintly granular eosinophilic inclusions (Henderson–Patterson bodies) with a peripherally-pushed nuclei, giving it a signet ring appearance **(Fig. 7)**.[31]

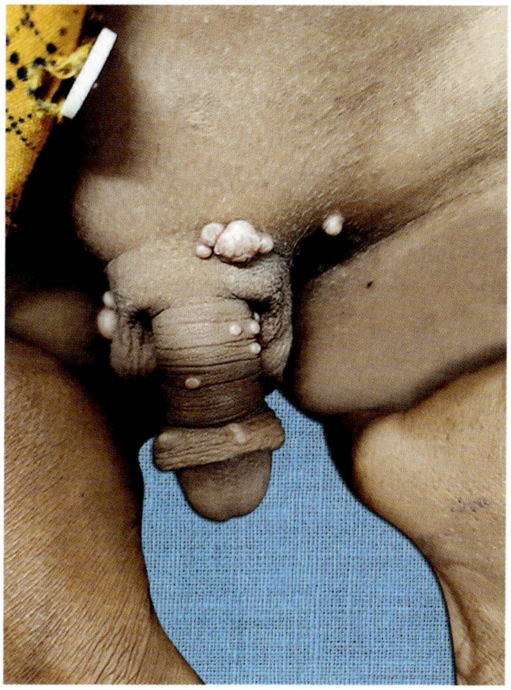

Fig. 6: Genital warts.

Treatment: Although, it is a self-limiting condition and can as well be left to heal spontaneously by itself, at least in immunocompetent cases.[32] The indications for active intervention include high risk of transmission, patients request, persistent lesions, and extensive involvement, to name a few. Various forms of medical and surgical therapies have been used with variable success. They all act by one of the following modes that includes destruction of infected cells, stimulation of an immune response, and direct action against the virus. Physical treatment modalities include curettage, cryotherapy, electrocautery, ablative lasers. Podophyllotoxin, cantharidin, silver nitrate, potassium hydroxide, and alpha-hydroxy acids such as salicylic acid, lactic acid, glycolic acid, and trichloroacetic acid are some of the chemical agents used.

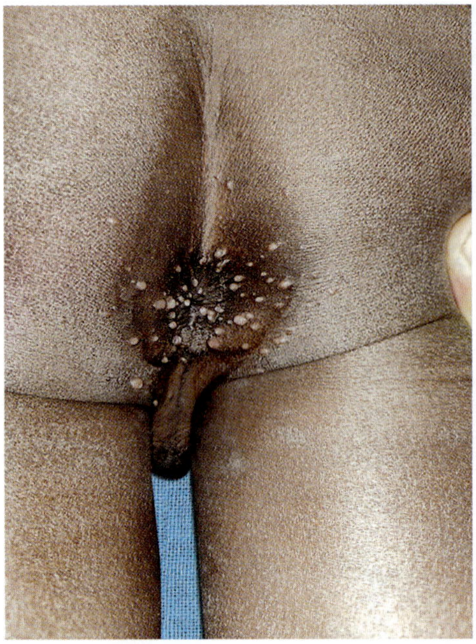

Fig. 7: Perianal molluscum in a men who have sex with men (MSM).

These are applied twice daily for three consecutive days every week. Others, which act by enhancing the immune response include imiquimod, intralesional or systemic interferons, cimetidine, intralesional *Candida* antigen.

REFERENCES

1. Dhawan J, Khandpur S. Emerging trends in viral sexually transmitted infections in India. Indian J Dermatol Venereol Leprol. 2009;75:561-5.
2. Ray K, Bala M, Gupta SM, Khunger N, Puri P, Muralidhar S, et al. Changing trends in sexually transmitted infections at a regional STD centre in North India. Indian J Med Res. 2006;124:559-68.
3. Paz-Bailey G, Rahman M, Chen C, Ballard R, Moffat HJ, Kenyon T, et al. Changes in the etiology of sexually transmitted diseases in Botswana between 1993 and 2002: implications for the clinical management of genital ulcer disease. Clin Infect Dis. 2005;41:1304-12.
4. Johnston C, Corey L. Current concepts for genital herpes simplex virus infection: diagnostics and pathogenesis of genital tract shedding. Clin Microbiol Rev. 2016;29(1):149-61.
5. Looker KJ, Magaret AS, Turner KME, Vickerman P, Gottlieb SL, Newman LM. Global estimates of prevalent and incident herpes simplex virus type 2 infections in 2012. PLoS One. 2015;10:e114989.
6. Mark KE, Wald A, Magaret AS, Selke S, Olin L, Huang ML, et al. Rapidly cleared episodes of herpes simplex virus reactivation in immunocompetent adults. J Infect Dis. 2008;198:1141-9.
7. Hofstetter AM, Rosenthal SL, Stanberry LR. Current thinking on genital herpes. Curr Opin Infect Dis. 2014;27(1):75-83.
8. Bissessor M, Fairley CK, Read T, Denham I, Bradshaw C, Chen M. The etiology of infectious proctitis in men who have sex with men differs according to HIV status. Sex Transm Dis. 2013; 40:768-70.
9. Folkers E, Oranje AP, Duivenvoorden JN, van der Veen JP, Rijlaarsdam JU, Emsbroek JA. Tzanck smear in diagnosing genital herpes. Genitourin Med. 1988;64(4):249-54.
10. Kuypers J, Boughton G, Chung J, Hussey L, Huang ML, Cook L, et al. Comparison of the simplex a HSV1 & 2 direct kit and laboratory-developed real-time PCR assays for herpes simplex virus detection. J Clin Virol. 2015; 62:103-5.
11. Wald A, Ashley-Morrow R. Serological testing for herpes simplexvirus (HSV)-1 and HSV-2 infection. Clin Infect Dis. 2002;35:S173-82.
12. Stanberry LR, Spruance SL, Cunningham AL, Bernstein DI, Mindel A, Sacks S, et al. Glycoprotein-D-adjuvant vaccine to prevent genital herpes. N Engl J Med. 2002; 347:1652-61.
13. Martinez V, Caumes E, Chosidow O. Treatment to prevent recurrent genital herpes. Curr Opin Infect Dis. 2008;21(1):42-8.
14. Strauss MJ, Shaw EW, Bunting H, Melnick JL. "Crystalline" virus-like particles from skin papilloma characterized by intranuclear inclusion bodies. Proc Soc Exp Biol Med.1949;72:46-50.
15. Howley PM, Lowy DR. Papillomaviruses. In: Knipe DM, Howley PM (Eds). Fields Virology, 5th edition. Philadelphia: Lippincott Williams & Wilkins; 2001. pp. 2299-354.
16. Bernard HU, Burk RD, Chen Z, Doorslaer KV, Hausen HZ, de Villiers EM. Classification of papillomaviruses (PVs) based on 189 PV types and proposal of taxonomic amendments. Virology. 2010;401:70-9.
17. Patel H, Wagner M, Singhal P, Kothari S. Systematic review of the incidence and prevalence of genital warts. BMC Infect Dis. 2013;13:39.
18. Winer RL, Kiviat NB, Hughes JP, Adam DE, Lee SK, Kuypers JM, et al. Development and duration of human papillomavirus lesions, after initial infection. J Infect Dis. 2005;191:731-8.
19. Ball SL, Winder DM, Vaughan K, Hanna N, Levy J, Sterling JC, et al. Analyses of human papillomavirus genotypes and viral loads in anogenital warts. J Med Virol. 2011;83:1345-50.
20. Bolognia J, Schaffer J, Cerron L. Bolognia Textbook of Dermatology, 4th edition. New York: Elsevier; 2017.
21. Gilson R, Nugent D, Werner RN, Ballesteros J, Ross J. 2019 IUSTI-Europe Guideline for the Management of Anogenital Warts. J Eur Acad Dermatol Venereol. 2020;34:1644-53.
22. Dillner J, Kjaer SK, Wheeler CM, Sigurdsson K, Iversen OE, Hernandez-Avila M, et al. Four years efficacy of prophylactic human papillomavirus quadrivalent vaccine against low grade cervical, vulvar, and vaginal intraepithelial neoplasia and anogenital warts: randomized controlled trial. BMJ. 2010;341:c3493.
23. Garland SM, Hernandez-Avila M, Wheeler CM, Perez G, Harper DM, Leodolter S, et al. Quadrivalent vaccine against human papillomavirus to prevent anogenital diseases. N Engl J Med. 2007;356:1928-43.
24. Donovan B, Franklin N, Guy R, Grulich AE, Regan DG, Ali H, et al. Quadrivalent human papillomavirus vaccination and trends in genital warts in Australia: analysis of national sentinel surveillance data. Lancet Infect Dis. 2011;11:39-44.
25. Juckett G, Hartman-Adams H. Human papillomavirus: clinical manifestations and prevention. Am Fam Phys. 2010; 82(10):1209-13.
26. Villa L, Varela JA, Otero L, Sánchez C, Junquera ML, Sánchez-del Río J, et al. Molluscum contagiosum: a 20-year study in a sexually transmitted infections unit. Sex Transm Dis. 2010;37:423-4.
27. Brown J, Janniger CK, Schwartz RA, Silverberg NB. Childhood molluscum contagiosum. Int J Dermatol. 2006;45:93-9.
28. Chen X, Anstey AV and Bugert JJ. Molluscum contagiosum virus infection. Lancet Infect Dis. 2013;13:877-88.
29. Hanson D, Diven DG. Molluscum contagiosum. Dermatol Online J. 2003;9.

30. Ianhez M, Cestari Sda C, Enokihara MY, de Paiva Melo Seize MB. Dermoscopic patterns of molluscum contagiosum: a study of 211 lesions confirmed by histopathology. An Bras Dermatol. 2011;86:74-9.
31. Ishikawa MK, Arps DP, Chow C, Hocker TL, Fullen DR. Histopathological features of molluscum contagiosum other than molluscum bodies. Histopathology. 2015;67:836-42.
32. Edwards S, Boffa MJ, Janier M, Calzavara-Pinton P, Rovati C, Salavastru CM, et al. 2020 European Guideline on the Management of Genital molluscum Contagiosum. J Eur Acad Dermatol Venereol. 2021;35(1):17-26.

EXAMINATION QUESTIONS

1. Write a short note on imiquimod.
2. Write a short note on molluscum contagiosum.
3. Draw a labelled structure of HPV virus.
4. Write a short note on HPV vaccine.

133 CHAPTER

Reactive Arthritis

Anil Ganjoo, Astha Sharma

INTRODUCTION

Reiter's syndrome (RS), now known as "reactive arthritis," is a classical triad of arthritis, urethritis and/or cervicitis, and conjunctivitis. However, a majority of patients do not present with the classic triad. It is a disease of the young and happens in those with a genetic predisposition. This inflammatory arthritis usually follows a gastrointestinal or urogenital infection.

The name, Reiter's syndrome is now an obsolete term because it is believed that Hans Reiter, after whom it has been named, was a member of The National Socialist German Workers' Party or the "Nazis."[1]

EPIDEMIOLOGY

Reiter's syndrome is more common in adults than in children. Mean age of onset is between 20 and 30 years and it is more common in sexually active males.[2] Incidence of reactive arthritis is more in patients with HIV infection.[3] Epidemiological data from India is lacking.

ETIOPATHOGENESIS

Pathogenesis of RS is associated with two factors:

1. Genetic, i.e., presence of HLA-B27[4]
2. *Infection*:
   i. *Enteric*: *Salmonella*, *Shigella*, *Yersinia* or *Campylobacter*
   ii. *Genitourinary/sexually-acquired reactive arthritis (SARA)*: *Chlamydia* or *Ureaplasma*

The prevalence of HLA-B27 in reactive arthritis is estimated at 30–50% in patients with reactive arthritis. It is believed that HLA-B27 potentiates reactive arthritis by presenting bacterial antigens to T-cells, altering self-tolerance of the host immune system, increased tumor necrosis factor-α (TNF-α) production, and delayed clearance of causative organisms.

CLINICAL FEATURES

The clinical picture consists of involvement of skin, nails, mucous membranes, and joints. Typical triad of urethritis, conjunctivitis, and arthritis is rarely seen. Symptoms generally appear after about 2–4 weeks of genitourinary or gastrointestinal infection. This may, however, vary extensively. A woman exhibited mucocutaneous symptoms 4 years before arthritic symptoms.[5] In some patients, certain symptoms may not manifest until years later. In one patient, onset of disease exhibited skin manifestations 12 years after the initial onset of disease.[6]

Skin lesions resemble those seen in psoriasis and involve the palms, soles, and the glans penis. *Keratoderma blennorrhagicum* is the name given to the palmoplantar lesions and they consist of brownish-red maculopapular lesions topped by pustules. These enlarge and become hyperkeratotic and crusted.[7] Pustular lesions resembling those seen in psoriasis can appear on the penile shaft and also the shaft of the penis. Balanitis is seen in the form of shallow ulcers with serpiginous pustular borders—*circinate balanitis.* It is the most common skin manifestation of RS, occurring in up to 50% patients **(Figs. 1A to C)**.[8]

Nails show subungual pustulosis, hyperkeratosis, and finally onycholysis.

Genitourinary involvement occurs in the form of urethritis/cervicitis, which occurs in about 90% of patients as a result of either direct infection to the genitourinary system or as a postdysenteric phenomenon that causes urethral inflammation by other mechanisms.[8,9] The latter is associated with sterile discharge. Prostatitis may also occur in men. The duration and severity of urethritis is variable, ranging from asymptomatic to mild painless urethral discharge to dysuria with mucopurulent discharge. Meatal inflammation may be the only sign of urethritis.[8,10]

The *mucosae* of mouth and eyes can also be involved with erosive lesions in the mouth, resembling migratory glossitis or in the form of conjunctivitis or anterior uveitis. Conjunctivitis is the most common eye symptom, observed in 30–60% of patients. Uveitis and keratitis also occur, but with lower frequencies at 12–37% and 4%, respectively.[11]

Arthritis is usually polyarticular and asymmetric, and most commonly involves the knees, ankles, and small joints of the hands and feet. Diffuse swelling of the fingers and toes is seen. In the 1981 study of patients with typical Reiter's syndrome by Willkens et al.,[12] almost all 249 patients had peripheral or spinal arthritis as part of the initial episode. *Enthesitis* is a characteristic feature and presents as heel pain due to Achilles tendonitis.

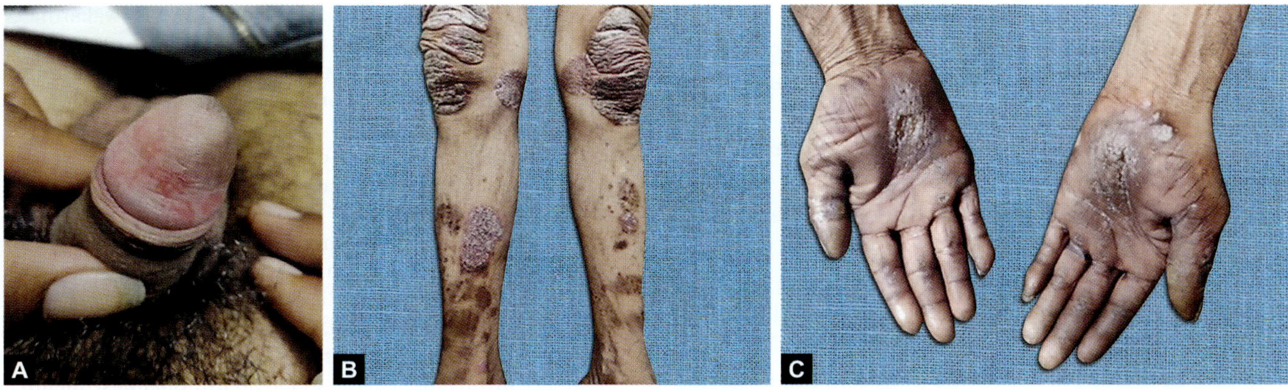

Figs. 1A to C: Cutaneous lesions of RA: (A) Circinate balanitis; (B) Psoriasiform plaques; and (C) Keratoderma blennorrhagicum.
Courtesy: Dr Utkrist Lahoria.

DIAGNOSIS

American College of Rheumatology came up with diagnostic guidelines for reactive arthritis in 1999.[13] The criteria were divided into two major and two minor criteria:

Major Criteria

- *Arthritis:* Asymmetric, mono- or oligoarthritis with lower limb involvement.
- Symptomatic infection, either enteritis or urethritis, preceding the onset of arthritis by a time interval of 3 days to 6 weeks.

Minor Criteria

- *Evidence of triggering infection*:
  - Positive urine ligase reaction or urethral/cervical swab for *Chlamydia trachomatis*
  - Positive stool culture for enteric pathogens associated with reactive arthritis.
- Evidence of persistent synovial infection [positive immunohistology or polymerase chain reaction (PCR) for *Chlamydia*].

A "definite" diagnosis of reactive arthritis is based on the fulfilment of both major criteria and a relevant minor criterion, while a "probable" diagnosis is characterized by both major criteria but no relevant minor criterion or one major criterion and one or more of the minor criteria.

The positivity of HLA-B27 in reactive arthritis is not considered useful for the diagnosis of the chronic forms of reactive arthritis. Other elements that can help in the diagnosis are the elevation of inflammatory parameters [erythrocyte sedimentation rate (ESR), C-reactive protein CRP] and an elevated number of leukocytes in the synovial fluid. It has been estimated that the combination of elevated CRP, genitourinary symptoms, metatarsophalangeal joint involvement, and HLA-B27 positivity can predict the diagnosis of reactive arthritis with a 69% sensitivity and a 93.5% specificity.[14]

TREATMENT

If an infectious agent has been identified as a trigger for reactive arthritis, antimicrobial therapy is strongly recommended. For SARA, azithromycin, tetracyclines, and rifampicin or a combination of these is usually given for long periods. Psoriatic skin lesions and balanitis are treated with coal tar or topical steroid and salicylic acid preparations. Methotrexate, acitretin, and cyclosporine may be beneficial in treating resistant cutaneous manifestations that do not respond to conservative therapy.[15,16]

The goal of therapy in reactive arthritis is to provide symptomatic relief and prevent chronic complications. For arthritis and spondyloarthritis manifestations, the use of nonsteroidal anti-inflammatory drugs (NSAIDs) and glucocorticoid injections is the most effective treatment in patients with mono- or oligoarticular disease. Disease-modifying antirheumatic drugs (DMARDs), such as sulfasalazine and methotrexate, have been shown to be effective in chronic reactive arthritis patients who have failed NSAID therapy. Biologicals such as TNF blocking agents (e.g., adalimumab, infliximab, and etanercept) have been suggested in the treatment of reactive arthritis.[17] However, further studies are needed to determine their efficacy.

PROGNOSIS

Rheumatoid arthritis usually has a self-limited course and the symptoms resolve within 3–6 months. Symptoms lasting beyond 6 months indicate a chronic element of the disease. Sacroiliitis is the most common chronic joint involvement. Patients who are HLA-B27 positive have a higher risk of recurrence of reactive arthritis. About 15–30% of patients with reactive arthritis can develop long-term arthritis or other joint abnormalities.

KEY POINTS

- RA is a classical triad of arthritis, urethritis and/or cervicitis, and conjunctivitis.

- Common in young men, 20–30 years of age.
- Happens in those with a genetic predisposition, particularly HLA-B27 positive, coupled with enteric or genital infections.
- Skin lesions resemble that of psoriasis and involve the palms, soles, and glans.
- Genitourinary involvement happens in the form of urethritis or cervicitis.
- Arthritis is usually polyarticular and asymmetric, and most commonly involves the knees, ankles, and small joints of the hands and feet.
- The goal of therapy is to provide symptomatic relief and prevent chronic complications and to treat the underlying infection if present.

REFERENCES

1. Panush RS, Paraschiv D, Dorff RE. The tainted legacy of Hans Reiter. Semin Arthritis Rheum. 2003;32(4):231-6.
2. Butler MJ, Russell AS, Percy JS, Lentle BC. A follow-up study of 48 patients with Reiter's syndrome. Am J Med. 1979;67: 808-10.
3. Winchester R, Bernstein DH, Fischer HD, Enlow R, Solomon G. The co-occurrence of Reiter's syndrome and acquired immunodeficiency. Ann Intern Med. 1987;106:19-26.
4. McClusky OE, Lordon RE, Arnett FC Jr. HL-A 27 in Reiter's syndrome and psoriatic arthritis: a genetic factor in disease susceptibility and expression. J Rheumatol. 1984;11:571.
5. Lotery HE, Galask RP, Stone MS, Sontheimer RD. Ulcerative vulvitis in atypical Reiter's syndrome. J Am Acad Dermatol. 2003;48:613-6.
6. Sehgal VN, Koranne RV, Basumatary RK, Vishwakarma GK, Singh AK, Raj GA. Reiter's disease. J Dermatol. 1982;9:145-8.
7. Chogle AR, Verma SC, Sthalekar BS, Sahu D. Reiter's syndrome with keratoderma blennorrhagica. J Assoc Physicians India. 1999;47:416.
8. Callen JP, Mahl CF. Oculocutaneous manifestations observed in multisystem disorders. Dermatol Clin. 1992;10: 709-16.
9. Amor B. Reiter's syndrome: diagnosis and clinical features. Rheum Dis Clin North Am. 1998;24:677-95.
10. Arora S, Arora G. Reiter's disease in a six-year-old girl. Indian J Dermatol Venereol Leprol. 2005;71:285-6.
11. Banares A, Hernandez-Garcia C, Fernandez-Gutierrez B, Jover JA. Eye involvement in the spondyloarthropathies. Rheum Dis Clin North Am. 1998;24:771-84.
12. Willkens RF, Arnett FC, Bitter T, Calin A, Fisher L, Ford DK, et al. Reiter's syndrome: evaluation of preliminary criteria for definite disease. Arthritis Rheum. 1981;24:844-9.
13. Inman RD. Classification criteria for reactive arthritis. J Rheumatol. 1999;26:1219-21.
14. Selmi C, Gershwin ME. Diagnosis and classification of reactive arthritis. Autoimmun Rev. 2014;13(4-5):546-9.
15. Owen ET, Cohen ML. Methotrexate in Reiter's disease. Ann Rheum Dis. 1979;38:48-50.
16. Kiyohara A, Takamori K, Niizuma N, Ogawa H. Successful treatment of severe recurrent Reiter's syndrome with cyclosporine. J Am Acad Dermatol. 1997;36:482-3.
17. Meyer A, Chatelus E, Wendling D, Berthelot JM, Dernis E, Houvenagel E, et al. Safety and efficacy of anti-tumor necrosis factor α therapy in ten patients with recent-onset refractory reactive arthritis. Arthritis Rheum. 2011;63(5): 1274-80.

EXAMINATION QUESTION

1. Write a short note on reactive arthritis.

134 CHAPTER Cervicitis and Vulvovaginitis

Sujata Sengupta

CERVICITIS

Cervicitis is the inflammation of the uterine cervix. It may affect the endocervix as well as the ectocervix. The involvement of the columnar epithelial cells of the endocervical glands is more common, but the squamous epithelial cells of the ectocervix can also be involved. Cervicitis may be acute or chronic. Acute cervicitis is usually of an infectious origin while chronic cervicitis has a noninfectious origin. The female genital tract extends from the vulva to the fallopian tubes. So, there is some overlap between vulvovaginitis and cervicitis. Both conditions are commonly categorized as lower genital tract infections.

Etiology

The infectious etiologies of cervicitis are significantly more common than the noninfectious ones.[1] All of these are sexually transmitted infections (STIs). *Chlamydia trachomatis* (commonly serovars D-K) and *Neisseria gonorrhoeae* are the most common organisms identified **(Table 1)**. Chlamydial cervicitis occurs more often than gonococcal, and both primarily affect the columnar epithelium of the endocervix. Other organisms include *Trichomonas vaginalis (TV)* and herpes simplex virus (HSV), especially primary type 2 HSV. *Mycoplasma* and group A *Streptococcus* are rarely reported. Tuberculosis involves the cervix in a small proportion of women with tuberculous endometritis.[2]

The risk factors for cervicitis include young age, multiple sexual partners, single marital status, low socioeconomic status, and drug and alcohol abuse. In addition, genetic predispositions leading to variable immune responses are additional risk factors.[3]

TABLE 1: Causes of acute cervicitis.

Infectious causes	*Noninfectious causes*
• *Chlamydia trachomatis* • *Neisseria gonorrhoeae* • *Trichomonas vaginalis* • *Herpes simplex virus* • *Mycoplasma genitalium* • Group A *Streptococcus* • Tuberculosis	• *Mechanical irritation:* Surgical instruments, foreign bodies, e.g, pessary, diaphragm, tampon, and cervical cap • *Chemical irritation:* Vaginal douches, contraceptive creams, and latex • Radiation therapy • Systemic diseases, e.g., Behçet's disease • Malignancy

Clinical Features

All sexually active women should be asked for complete gynecological and sexual history at the initial evaluation and on subsequent visits. Females with cervicitis are most often asymptomatic and do not seek evaluation or treatment. Cervicitis in these women may be detected incidentally during physical examination. Nonspecific symptoms such as a mucopurulent vaginal discharge and a postcoital or intermenstrual bleeding are the most common symptoms. A concomitant urinary tract infection may cause dysuria, increased frequency of micturition, and dyspareunia. Fever and pain may be present in primary attacks of herpes simplex.

Cardinal Signs

- Mucopurulent or purulent discharge on the ectocervix or coming out of the endocervical canal
- Bleeding on minor contact like that of a cotton swab.

Erythema, edema, and tenderness to motion may be the other signs. The clinical features may vary according to the infecting organism **(Table 2)**.[4] A high organism load leads to more severe signs of inflammation. Noninfectious causes of cervicitis do not show any specific manifestations to distinguish them from the infectious causes.

Diagnosis

Once a clinical diagnosis of cervicitis is made, there should be further evaluation to detect the cause and rule out pelvic inflammatory disease. In a study from India, it was found that histology of 613 cases of cervicitis showed nonspecific changes in 547 (89.23%) cases.[5] The Centers for Disease Control and Prevention (CDC) recommends that endocervical

TABLE 2: Signs of acute infectious cervicitis.

Organism	*Signs*
Gonococcus	Mucopurulent cervical discharge, friable cervix, and edema
Chlamydia	Mucopurulent cervical discharge, friable cervix, and edema
Herpes simplex virus (HSV)	Diffuse vesicular lesions, ulcerations, erosive inflammation, and hemorrhagic lesions
Trichomonas	Punctate hemorrhages (strawberry cervix), erosive inflammation, and hemorrhagic lesions
Mycoplasma	Ill-defined lesions

and vaginal swabs as well as urine samples are tested. In a Gram's stain, the presence of >10 polymorphonuclear cells per oil immersion field (i.e., high-power field) is indicative of mucopurulent cervicitis and suggests chlamydia or gonorrhea infection. But it has a low sensitivity and does not confirm a specific organism. Nucleic acid amplification test (NAAT) is the most sensitive and specific test for gonorrheal and chlamydial infections. It has replaced culture as the "gold standard" test, but is expensive and takes time to yield results. When *Trichomonas* is suspected, the presence of the motile organisms on wet mount is diagnostic of infection but found in only 60–70% of culture-confirmed cases.[6] So further testing by culture, antigen-based methods, or ideally NAAT should be done. Viral culture, polymerase chain reaction (PCR), direct fluorescence antibody, and type-specific serologic tests are used to confirm herpes genitalis infections.[7]

Treatment

The aims of therapy are relief of symptoms, stopping the transmission to sexual contacts, and prevention of upper genital tract involvement. Medical therapy is the treatment of choice in all types of cervicitis and can be done presumptively or with specific antibiotic treatment if the etiology is known. Treatment must be extended to the sexual partners and abstinence is advised till a week after both patient and partner are treated. The CDC's Sexually Transmitted Diseases Treatment Guidelines recommend empirical therapy for *Chlamydia* as well as *Gonococcus*. The CDC guidelines for individual diseases are summarized in **Table 3**. For pregnant women, tetracyclines and quinolone groups are not prescribed. Macrolides and amoxicillin are safer alternatives. Metronidazole may also be used. For women with human immunodeficiency virus (HIV) and cervicitis, the therapy is similar to non-HIV women. Treatment of cervicitis in this group significantly decreases HIV shedding and transmission to partner.[1] Persistent infections should prompt a gynecological referral and evaluation. Chronic cervicitis usually has a noninfectious source and should be treated according to its cause.

TABLE 3: Treatment recommendations for acute cervicitis [Centers for Disease Control and Prevention (CDC) guidelines].

Disease	*Treatment recommendations*
Gonococcus	• Ceftriaxone 250 mg intramuscularly (IM) in a single dose Plus • Azithromycin 1 g orally in a single dose or doxycycline 100 mg orally twice daily for 7 days
Chlamydia	• Azithromycin 1 g orally once Or • Doxycycline 100 mg orally twice daily for 7 days
Trichomonas	• Metronidazole 2 g orally in a single dose Or • Tinidazole 2 g orally in a single dose Or • Metronidazole 500 mg PO bid for 7 days
Mycoplasma	Azithromycin 1 g single dose
Herpes simplex virus	• *Acyclovir*: 400 mg orally three times per day or 200 mg orally five times a day for 7–10 days Or • *Famciclovir*: 250 mg orally three times a day for 7–10 days Or • *Valacyclovir*: 1,000 mg orally twice daily for 7–10 days

VULVOVAGINITIS

Vulvar and vaginal inflammation is a very common problem encountered by the gynecologist as well as the dermatologist. Like cervicitis, vulvovaginitis may be of infectious and noninfectious origin and differentiating the two can often be very difficult **(Table 4)**. The symptoms of vulvovaginitis are mostly nonspecific **(Box 1)**.

Clinical examination may show atrophy, excoriations, and fissures in the vulvovaginal areas. Distinguishing the infectious from noninfectious causes is of utmost importance to prevent the unnecessary use of antimicrobials. Often, successful treatment is possible only if a correct diagnosis is made.

Since vaginal discharge is present in most cases of vulvovaginitis, examination of the discharge is one of the earliest investigations done. **Table 5** lists a summary of the results for normal vagina and in some common causes

TABLE 4: Causes of vulvovaginitis.[8]

Infectious causes	*Noninfectious causes*
• Bacterial vaginosis • Vulvovaginal candidiasis • Trichomoniasis • Herpes simplex virus infection • Cervicitis	• Desquamative inflammatory vaginitis • Atrophic vaginitis • Aphthous ulcers • Behçet's disease • Lichen planus • Lichen sclerosus • Contact, chemical, and radiation dermatitis • Vulvovaginal malignancies • Vulvar intraepithelial neoplasia • Parasitic infestations • Vulvodynia • Foreign body (e.g., tampon) • Sexual abuse • Eczema • Psoriasis • Plasma cell vulvitis

BOX 1: Symptoms of vulvovaginitis.

- Pruritus
- *Vaginal discharge*: Change in volume, color, and odor
- Burning
- Irritation
- Erythema
- Dyspareunia
- Spotting
- Dysuria

TABLE 5: Vaginal secretion test results for common causes of vulvovaginitis.[8]

Condition	*pH*	*Saline microscopy*	*10% KOH*	*Others*	*Gold standard*
Normal	<4.5	Normal flora, lactobacillus +, WBC +/–	Not applicable	Clinical diagnosis	None
Candidiasis	<4.5	Hyphae, blastospores ±, and WBCs abundant	Fungal elements +	Vaginal DNA probe	Fungal culture
Bacterial vaginosis	>4.5	Clue cells, lactobacillus –/↓ coccobacillary flora	Whiff test +	Vaginal DNA probe	Gram stain
Trichomoniasis	Normal or >4.5	Trichomonads may be seen, and WBCs abundant	Variable	Vaginal DNA probe Trichomonas culture	PCR for *Trichomonas vaginalis*
Atrophic vaginitis	>4.5	Parabasal cells and decreased flora	Not applicable	Vaginal maturation index	Vaginal maturation index
Desquamative inflammatory vaginitis	>4.5	Parabasal cells, sheets of WBCs and mixed flora	Not applicable	Clinical diagnosis	Clinical diagnosis

(DNA: deoxyribonucleic acid; KOH: potassium hydroxide; PCR: polymerase chain reaction; WBC: white blood cell)

of vulvovaginitis.[8] A literature review concluded that this initial office evaluation correctly diagnosed 60% of candidal vulvovaginitis, 70% of trichomoniasis, and 90% of bacterial vaginosis (BV).[9]

Bacterial Vaginosis

Bacterial vaginosis is one of the most common causes of abnormal vaginal discharge worldwide. It is characterized by:

- A shift in vaginal microbe environment from *Lactobacillus* species to multiple bacterial colonization, including facultative anaerobes
- Production of volatile amines by the new bacterial colony
- Rise in vaginal pH to >4.5

The major bacteria found in women with BV are *Gardnerella vaginalis*, *Prevotella* species, *Porphyromonas* species, *Bacteroides* species, *Peptostreptococcus* species, *Mycoplasma hominis*, and *Ureaplasma urealyticum*, as well as *Mobiluncus*, *Megasphaera*, *Sneathia*, and *Clostridia* species.[10] *Fusobacterium* and *Atopobium vaginae* are also common. *G. vaginalis* is the key player in the pathogenesis of BV and acts via the development of a biofilm.

Diagnosis

- *Amsel's criteria*: Its a cheap and quick test to diagnose BV. Four of the following criteria have been laid down of which three need to be present to diagnose BV:
  1. Homogeneous discharge
  2. pH > 4.5%
  3. Positive whiff test
  4. Clue cells
- Nugent score or Hay/Ison criteria that is used to asses a Gram-stained smear, is the standard test adopted by many laboratories.
- Food and Drug Administration (FDA)-approved tests with acceptable performance include a deoxyribonucleic acid (DNA) probe-based test (BD Affirm VPIII), vaginal fluid sialidase activity test (OSOM BVBlue test), and two PCR-based assays (BD MAX, Aptima BV).[11]

Treatment Recommendations

The European guideline [International Union against Sexually Transmitted Infections/World Health Organization (IUSTI/WHO)] for the management of BV, 2018, is as follows:

- Topical or oral metronidazole 500 mg for 5–7 days or intravaginal clindamycin for 7 days as first-line of therapy (strength of recommendation: Grade A; quality of evidence: Grade 1)
- *Therapy for recurrence*: Intravaginal metronidazole (strength of recommendation: Grade B; quality of evidence: Grade 2)
- *Partner treatment*: Only for female sexual partners if they have BV (strength of recommendation: Grade B; quality of evidence: Grade 2)
- *Pregnant women*: Clindamycin (strength of recommendation: Grade B; quality of evidence: Grade 2)

Vulvovaginal Candidiasis

Candidiasis is one of the most common causes of vaginal itching and discharge. Besides these, a cottage cheese-like white curdy discharge, pain, swelling and redness, excoriations and fissures on examination, may also be encountered. The mere presence of the yeast does not confirm disease because the vagina may be its normal habitat in 25% women.[8] A spontaneous phenotypical switch is postulated to cause symptomatic vaginitis. The *Candida* species does not require any receptors to attach itself to the vaginal epithelium. Although *Candida albicans* is known to cause about 90% cases of vulvovaginitis, some investigators have reported a rise in *Candida glabrata* infection.[12] The yeast probably gains access to the vagina by migration from the rectum via anal opening. Recurrent vulvovaginal candidiasis is due to persistent gastrointestinal (GI) carriage and a locally acquired defect in cell-mediated immunity of the vagina. Vulvovaginal candidiasis is traditionally not considered as an STI.

Diagnosis

- *Saline microscopy*: 10% potassium hydroxide is added to a vaginal sample and microscopy reveals fungal hyphae and pseudohyphae. The sensitivity is around 50%. It can also identify clue cells and motile *Trichomonas* and thereby helps in ruling out a coinfection.
- Fungal culture is considered the gold standard. It aids in the decision of antifungal use also.
- Other tests include a DNA probe test and PCR (high sensitivity and specificity). In a study by Cartwright, real-time PCR was found to be more sensitive but less specific than DNA probe test.[13]

Treatment Recommendations

The European guideline (IUSTI/WHO) for the management of vulvovaginal candidiasis, 2018 is as follows:

- Single dose (oral/vaginal) of azole for uncomplicated *Candida* (strength of recommendation: Grade A; quality of evidence: Grade 1)
- *Recurrent candidiasis*: Fluconazole 150–200 mg for 3 days, followed by once a week for 6 months (strength of recommendation: Grade B; quality of evidence: Grade 2)
- *Partner treatment*: Not required (strength of recommendation: Grade A; quality of evidence: Grade 2)
- *Pregnancy*: Topical azole (strength of recommendation: Grade A; quality of evidence: Grade 2).

Trichomoniasis

Trichomoniasis, caused by the protozoan *TV*, is the most common nonviral sexually transmitted disease. In women, it affects the vagina, urethra, and paraurethral glands but may also affect the cervix and bladder.

Common symptoms of acute infection include a purulent, greenish-yellow malodorous, thin discharge associated with burning, pruritus, dysuria, frequency, lower abdominal pain, or dyspareunia. Some patients may be in an asymptomatic carrier state. Examination reveals an erythematous vulvovaginal area. Punctate hemorrhagic spots may be visible on the vagina and cervix, a condition described as "strawberry cervix".

Diagnosis

- Vaginal pH may be normal or >4.5.
- *Direct microscopy*: Saline suspension shows motile *Trichomonas* with their characteristic jerky movements. Though the test's sensitivity is about 50%, the specificity is 100%. Delay in smear examination reduces the sensitivity further.
- *Culture*: Before the advent of molecular diagnostic tests, culture had been the gold standard with both sensitivity and specificity above 90%. But the reports may take about a week to be available and this test lost popularity.
- *Nucleic acid amplification test*: NAATs detect ribonucleic acid (RNA) by transcription-mediated amplification (PCR or reverse transcriptase). These tests are highly sensitive and specific and are now the accepted gold standard for the diagnosis of trichomonads.
- The FDA-approved BD MAX vaginal panel tests for *Trichomonas*, BV, and *Candida* species.[14]

Treatment Recommendations

The European guideline (IUSTI/WHO) for the management of trichomoniasis, 2018 is as follows:

- Metronidazole or tinidazole, 500 mg BD (strength of recommendation: Grade A; quality of evidence: Grade 1)
- *Recurrent TV*: Nitroimidazole in higher doses (strength of recommendation: Grade B; quality of evidence: Grade 2)
- *Partner treatment*: Treatment for TV (strength of recommendation: Grade A; quality of evidence: Grade 2)
- *Pregnancy*: Metronidazole (strength of recommendation: Grade A; quality of evidence: Grade 1).

Herpes Simplex Virus-associated Vulvovaginitis

Herpes simplex virus is a common sexually transmitted disease worldwide. With the change in sexual practices, HSV-1 is increasingly being associated with genital herpes. Three types of infection may occur namely; primary, nonprimary first episode, and recurrent. Primary infection occurs in a patient who has no preexisting antibodies to either strain of HSV. In nonprimary infection, the patient during the first episode already has antibodies to the strain he or she is infected with. Recurrent herpes simplex refers to the reactivation of genital HSV where the type remains the same as before. Primary infection presents as painful multiple genitals ulcers along with fever, malaise, dysuria, and tender local lymphadenopathy. There are fewer lesions and less systemic symptoms. Clinical course and infectivity periods are shorter during recurrent episodes than the other two types. Vulvovaginal hidradenitis suppurativa (HS) infection can be transmitted to the baby during delivery.

Diagnosis

- *Tzanck smear, direct immunofluorescence*: Nonspecific tests with poor sensitivity and specificity
- *Culture*: Newer lesions increase the sensitivity
- *PCR*: Real-time HSV PCR tests are more sensitive and the best tests for asymptomatic HSV shedding
- Immunoglobulin M (IgM) testing for HSV-1 or -2 is not diagnostic or type-specific and can show positive results during recurrent episodes also.

Treatment Recommendations

- In general, there is no role of topical therapy.
- Oral therapy is best started within 72 hours of skin lesions. The 2015 United States CDC guidelines for primary and

nonprimary first episodes are as follows (with normal renal function):
- Acyclovir 400 mg three times a day or 200 mg five times a day for 7–10 days or
- Famciclovir 250 mg three times a day for 7–10 days or
- Valacyclovir 1,000 mg twice a day for 7–10 days

- Intravenous (IV) therapy is given when other complications such as urinary retention due to sacral nerve involvement, central nervous system (CNS), chest, or liver involvement and disseminated HSV infections. Acyclovir can be given in the dose of 5–10 mg per kg body weight three times a day for as long as clinical improvement is desired.
- *Recurrent infections*: The median recurrence rate after the first episode of HSV-2 infection is about 4 recurrences per year, with about 40% of patients having at least 6 recurrences and 20% having more than 10 recurrences in the first year.[15] Suppressive therapy is prescribed to these patients. Chronic suppressive therapy reduces the risk of HSV reactivation and decreases the shedding of virus. Acyclovir 400 mg twice a day or valacyclovir 500 mg once a day are more commonly used than famciclovir. There are safety studies for up to 8 years for acyclovir and 1 year for the other two.

Of the noninfectious causes of vulvovaginitis, the ones which deserve special mention are atrophic vaginitis (AV), desquamative inflammatory vaginitis (DIV), lichen planus, contact dermatitis (CD), and lichen sclerosus (LS).[8]

Atrophic Vaginitis

Atrophic vaginitis is seen in postmenopausal and hypo-estrogenic women. In the former, the prevalence of AV is approximately 50%.[16] The common symptoms are dryness, dyspareunia, and introital burning. Clinical examination can show a near normal to an atrophic vagina with pallor, dryness, loss of elasticity, and narrowing of the introitus with loss of vaginal rugosity. The vaginal pH is elevated. Saline microscopy shows parabasal cells which are immature round squamous epithelial cells which have replaced the mature fat cuboidal epithelial cells. Lactobacillus is absent which makes *Candida* infection rare in AV. Hormone replacement or topical estrogen can produce dramatic results. The risk of systemic absorption following topical estrogen therapy is low. But the patients should be counseled that recurrences after treatment withdrawal are common.

Desquamative Inflammatory Vaginitis

Desquamative inflammatory vaginitis is a chronic vaginal disorder, which may be seen in pre- or postmenopausal women and is a disease of exclusion. The patient presents with copious greenish-yellow mucoid discharge, an erythematous vulva and complains of vaginal pain and dyspareunia. The vaginal pH is elevated. The diagnosis is based on the presence of all of the following criteria:[17]

- At least one symptom (i.e., vaginal discharge, dyspareunia, pruritus, pain, irritation, or burning)
- Vaginal inflammation on examination
- pH more than 4.5
- Presence of parabasal cells and leukorrhea on microscopy (a ratio of leukocytes to vaginal epithelial cells > 1:1)

Treatment

The treatment of DIV consists of either clindamycin 2% cream or topical corticosteroids like hydrocortisone 10% cream for vaginal use. The duration of therapy is usually 2–4 weeks and sometimes both medications are used at a time. Patients who do not respond should be evaluated for estrogen deficiency and other causes of vulvovaginitis that may be coexistent.

Vulvovaginal Lichen Planus

Vulvovaginal lichen planus is a chronic condition that may be asymptomatic or may present with severe pruritus or pain. Erosive vulvovaginal lichen planus may be commonly seen affecting the oral mucosa, vulva, and vagina. Perianal or esophageal involvement may also occur. The findings may range from erythema, erosions, and white striae to severe scarring. Severe disease may result in narrowing of vaginal introitus and synechia of its walls making sexual intercourse impossible. The women are mostly postmenopausal and a wet mount of vaginal secretions show nonspecific inflammatory changes with leukocytes, parabasal cells, and absent lactobacilli. Biopsy from the whitish epithelium or the edge of an erosion shows lichenoid dermatitis. The treatment consists of high potency topical corticosteroids like clobetasol propionate 0.5% as the first line of therapy. They are initially used twice a day and then tapered off gradually. Hydrocortisone rectal suppositories (25 mg) are used and some preparations are available for vaginal insertion as well. In severe cases intralesional triamcinolone acetonide injections or systemic corticosteroids are prescribed. Topical calcineurin inhibitors such as tacrolimus and pimecrolimus are also used. Systemic medications such as dapsone, hydroxychloroquine, retinoids, cyclosporine, azathioprine, mycophenolate mofetil, etanercept, adalimumab, and thalidomide have produced variable results.[18]

Lichen Sclerosus

Lichen sclerosus (LS) is a complex chronic inflammatory autoimmune skin disease with a predilection for the genital skin. Though vulvar LS commonly affects women in their fifth or sixth decade, it may affect children as well. Young girls present with irritation and soreness and may complain of constipation and urinary symptoms. Older women complain of vulvar irritation, pain, erosions, and fissures. Clinically, ivory-white plaques with atrophic or thickened skin are seen and are often enough for diagnosis. Biopsy shows inflammation, thinned epidermis, and distinctive dermal changes of a wide band of homogenized collagen below the dermoepidermal junction. Topical therapy consists of clobetasol propionate 0.5% creams in tapering doses.[19] Topical calcineurin inhibitors such as tacrolimus and pimecrolimus are safe and effective too. LS is generally a steroid responsive disease and absence of improvement after compliant therapy is an indication for a biopsy to rule out squamous cell carcinoma.

Vulvovaginal Contact Dermatitis

Contact dermatitis (CD) of the vulva is a common entity with irritant CD being more common than allergic CD. Common vulvar irritants include body fluids (abnormal vaginal discharge, semen, urine, and feces), feminine hygiene products (washes, soaps, wipes, lubricants, sanitary napkins, and depilators), and commonly used medications such as alcohol-based creams and gels, imiquimod, fluorouracil, trichloroacetic acid, podophyllin, and spermicides.[20] Allergic CD results from exposure to an allergen to which the patient has been sensitized previously and medications, preservatives, and fragrances are the most common culprits here. Patch tests are done to identify the relevant contact allergens. Other than symptomatic treatment with antihistamine medications, topical steroids need to be chosen and used judiciously. Systemic corticosteroids may be necessary in some cases. In addition, comprehensive patient education is essential for favorable results.

KEY POINTS

- Cervicitis, the inflammation of the cervix, may involve both the ectocervix and endocervix.
- Acute cervicitis is mostly of infectious origin and chronic cervicitis is of noninfectious origin.
- Vulvovaginitis may be of infectious and noninfectious origin which can be difficult to distinguish.

REFERENCES

1. Centers for Disease Control and Prevention. Sexually Transmitted Diseases Treatment Guidelines, 2015: Diseases Characterized by Urethritis and Cervicitis. MMWR Recomm Rep. 2015;64(3):51-3.
2. Samantaray S, Parida G, Rout N, Giri SK, Kar R. Cytologic detection of tuberculous cervicitis: a report of 7 cases. Acta Cytol. 2009;53:594-6.
3. Taylor BD, Darville T, Ferrell RE, Kammerer CM, Ness RB, Haggerty CL. Variants in toll-like receptor 1 and 4 genes are associated with *Chlamydia trachomatis* among women with pelvic inflammatory disease. J Infect Dis. 2012;205(4):603-9.
4. Marrazzo JM, Handsfield HH, Whittington WL. Predicting chlamydial and gonococcal cervical infection: implications for management of cervicitis. Obstet Gynecol. 2002;100(3):579.
5. Jayakumar NKB. Cervicitis: how often is it non-specific? J Clin Diagn Res. 2015;9:EC11-2.
6. Krieger JN, Tam MR, Stevens CE, Nielsen IO, Hale J, Kiviat NB, et al. Diagnosis of trichomoniasis. Comparison of conventional wet-mount examination with cytologic studies, cultures, and monoclonal antibody staining of direct specimens. JAMA. 1988;259:1223-7.
7. Gupta R, Warren T, Wald A. Genital herpes. Lancet. 2007;22: 2127-37.
8. Goje O, Munoz LJ. Vulvovaginitis: find the cause to treat it. Cleve Clin J Med. 2017;84:215-24.
9. Carr PL, Rothberg MB, Friedman RH, Felsenstein D, Pliskin JS. "Shotgun" versus sequential testing. Cost-effectiveness of diagnostic strategies for vaginitis. J Gen Intern Med. 2005;20:793-9.
10. Hill GB. The microbiology of bacterial vaginosis. Am J Obstet Gynecol. 1993;169:450-4.
11. Briselden AM, Hillier SL. Evaluation of affirm VP microbial identification test for *Gardnerella vaginalis* and *Trichomonas vaginalis*. J Clin Microbiol. 1994;32:148-52.
12. Vermitsky JP, Self MJ, Chadwick SG, Trama JP, Adelson ME, Mordechai E, et al. Survey of vaginal-flora *Candida* species isolates from women of different age groups by use of species-specific PCR detection. Clin Microbiol. 2008;46: 1501-3.
13. Cartwright CP, Lembke BD, Ramachandran K, Body BA, Nye MB, Rivers CA, et al. Comparison of nucleic acid amplification assays with BD Affirm VPIII for diagnosis of vaginitis in symptomatic women. J Clin Microbiol. 2013;51:3694-9.
14. Schwebke JR, Gaydos CA, Nyirjesy P, Paradis S, Kodsi S, Cooper CK. Diagnostic performance of a molecular test versus clinician assessment of vaginitis. J Clin Microbiol. 2018;56: e00252-18.
15. Corey L, Adams HG, Brown ZA, Holmes KK. Genital herpes simplex virus infections: clinical manifestations, course, and complications. Ann Intern Med. 1983;98:958-72.
16. MacBride MB, Rhodes DJ, Shuster LT. Vulvovaginal atrophy. Mayo Clin Proc. 2010;85:87-94.
17. Bradford J, Fischer G. Desquamative inflammatory vaginitis: differential diagnosis and alternate diagnostic criteria. J Low Genit Tract Dis. 2010;14:306-10.
18. Neil SM, Lewis FM. A disease in need of a unified approach. Arch Dermatol. 2008;144:1502-3.
19. Lewis FM, Tatnall FM, Velangi SS, Bunker CB, Kumar A, Brackenbury F, et al. British Association of Dermatologists guidelines for the management of lichen sclerosus, 2018. Br J Dermatol. 2018;178:839-53.
20. Nardelli A, Degreef H, Goossens A. Contact allergic reactions of the vulva: a 14-year review. Dermatitis. 2014;15:131-6.

EXAMINATION QUESTIONS

1. What are the cardinal signs of cervicitis? How to approach a case of acute cervicitis?
2. Discuss the noninfectious causes and management of vulvovaginitis.

135 CHAPTER Pelvic Inflammatory Disease

Aditi Chakrabarti

INTRODUCTION

Pelvic inflammatory disease (PID) is a clinical syndrome resulting from infection and inflammation of the upper reproductive tract occurring most commonly in single and sexually active young women. This can lead to endometritis, salpingitis, tubo-ovarian abscess, and pelvic peritonitis either alone or in any combination.[1] The long-term sequelae result from tubal scarring which may cause infertility, ectopic pregnancy, or chronic pelvic pain.

Pelvic inflammatory disease is the most common gynecological reason for admission to hospital in the USA. In resource-poor countries, it accounts for 17–40% of gynecological admissions in sub-Saharan Africa, 15–37% in Southeast Asia, and 3–10% in India.[2]

RISK FACTORS

- *Age and age of sexual debut*: Age less than 20 years is a major risk factor as it is a younger sexual debut, which correlates with a higher incidence of chlamydia and gonorrhea infections in adolescents and young adults. Cervical ectopy often present in adolescents enables pathogens to efficiently infect the upper reproductive tract.[3]
- *Number of sexual partners*: The greater the number of sexual partners greater is the risk of PID.
- *History of PID*: The tubal damage caused by an episode of PID makes a woman more susceptible to recurrent infections as does the presence of chlamydia or gonorrhea infection in the male partner.[4]
- *Vaginal douching*: Increases the risk by changing the vaginal flora, damaging the cervical epithelium, and altering the composition of cervical mucosal plug.
- *Intrauterine device*: The risk increases by nearly six-fold within the first 21 days of placement but thereafter declines to baseline.[5]
- *Oral contractive use*: May increase the risk for chlamydia infection by inducing cervical ectopy whilst it can also afford some protection against ascending infection by thickening the cervical mucosal plug.[5]

MICROBIOLOGY AND PATHOGENESIS

- Etiology of PID is polymicrobial **(Table 1)**.[6]
- There is ascending spread of organisms from vagina/cervix to the upper reproductive tract.
- The most common pathogens are *Neisseria gonorrhoeae* and *Chlamydia trachomatis*. Studies suggest that 15% of untreated *C. trachomatis* infection can progress to PID and it is possibly higher with *Gonococcus*.[7]
- Sexual intercourse and retrograde menstruation may play a role in the ascending infection.[6]
- The presence of concomitant bacterial vaginoses may help in the ascent of organisms by producing enzymes that degrade the cervical mucus plug.[8]
- Clinically, PID may be acute, subacute, or chronic depending on the duration of the signs and symptoms.
- The pathogens are also different in acute and chronic PID. Acute and subacute PID will be discussed in this chapter.

CLINICAL MANIFESTATIONS

- PID may be asymptomatic or symptoms may vary from mild to severe.
- Symptoms may be nonspecific and an evaluation of the urinary tract and gastrointestinal system should be carried out during gynecological examination.

TABLE 1: Pelvic inflammatory disease (PID)—clinical classification and possible pathogens.

Clinical presentation	*Causes*
Acute PID—less than 30 days duration	• *Cervical microbes: Neisseria gonorrhoae, Chlamydia trachomatis, Mycoplasma genitalium* • *Bacterial vaginosis microbes: Bacteroides* species, *Peptostreptococcus* species, *M. hominis, Ureaplasma urealyticum, Clostridia* species, *Leptotrichia* species, *Atopobium* species • *Respiratory microbes: Streptococcus pneumonia, Haemophilus influenzae, Staphylococcus aureus,* group A streptococci • *Enteric microbes: E. coli, Bacteroides fragilis, Campylobacter* species, group B streptococci
Subclinical PID	*Chlamydia trachomatis, Neisseria gonorrhoae*
Chronic PID—more than 30 days	*Mycobacterium tuberculosis* and *Actinomycetes* species

Source: Brunham RC, Gottlieb SL, Paavonen J. Pelvic inflammatory disease. N Engl J Med. 2015;372:2039-48.

- The common symptoms of PID are:
  - Lower abdominal or pelvic pain
  - Abnormal vaginal discharge
  - Dysuria and cramping
  - Irregular menstrual bleeding and postcoital vaginal bleeding
  - Dyspareunia
  - Fever > 38°C
  - In severe PID, there is high fever, chills, purulent vaginal discharge, nausea, and vomiting.
- Clinical examination may detect uterine tenderness, cervical motion pain, or adnexal tenderness.
- Silent PID is the development of asymptomatic upper genital tract infection, which can lead to long-term complications and remain a diagnostic and therapeutic challenge.[1]

Acute Complications

- The inflammation resulting from the infection causes local tissue damage leading to tubal swelling, occlusion, and adhesion formation.
- Adhesions involving the liver capsule cause perihepatitis. It is an uncommon occurrence termed Fitz-Hugh–Curtis syndrome.
- Tubo-ovarian abscess can develop as a subacute complication.

Chronic Complications

- Ectopic pregnancy, infertility, and chronic pelvic pain can occur even after a single episode of symptomatic PID.[9]
- The risk increases manifold with recurrent or severe episodes.
- Institution of appropriate treatment decreases the chances of long-term sequelae.

DIAGNOSIS

- There is no single clinical finding, laboratory test, or imaging study which can make a definitive diagnosis of PID.
- A low threshold is necessary for the diagnosis of PID in young sexually active women.

CRITERIA FOR INITIATING PRESUMPTIVE TREATMENT

Presumptive treatment for PID is started in sexually active young women and other women at risk for sexually transmitted diseases (STDs) if they are experiencing pelvic or lower abdominal pain, if no other cause for the illness can be identified, and if one or more of the following minimum clinical criteria are present on pelvic examination:

- Cervical motion tenderness,
- Uterine tenderness, or
- Adnexal tenderness

Additional Criteria

One or more of the following additional criteria can be used to increase the specificity of the minimum clinical criteria and support a diagnosis of PID:

- Oral temperature > 101°F (>38.3°C)
- Abnormal cervical mucopurulent discharge or cervical friability
- Presence of abundant numbers of white blood cell (WBC) on saline microscopy of vaginal fluid*
- Elevated erythrocyte sedimentation rate
- Elevated C-reactive protein
- Laboratory documentation of cervical infection with *N. gonorrhoeae* or *C. trachomatis*.

Most Specific Criteria for the Diagnosis of PID[1]

One or more of the following more extensive procedures might be required in some cases:

- Endometrial biopsy with histopathologic evidence of endometritis;** or
- Transvaginal sonography or magnetic resonance imaging techniques showing thickened, fluid-filled tubes with or without free pelvic fluid or tubo-ovarian complex, or Doppler studies suggesting pelvic infection (e.g., tubal hyperemia); or
- Laparoscopic findings consistent with PID.[1]

TREATMENT

- Treatment regimens should provide empiric, broad-spectrum coverage of possible pathogens such as *N. gonorrhoeae*, *C. trachomatis*, anaerobes, gram-negative facultative bacteria, and streptococci.
- Prompt administration of antibiotics has been shown to improve outcomes, prevent progression of disease, and decrease long-term sequelae.[10]
- Women with mild-to-moderately severe acute PID can be treated with intramuscular/oral therapy as outpatients (**Box 1**, CDC recommendations and **Box 2**, Indian National Guidelines on Prevention, Management, and Control of Reproductive Tract Infections including Sexually Transmitted Infections recommendations).
- Oral antibiotic regimens are for a period of 14 days. The patients should show significant improvement at 72 hours follow-up.
- If there is no improvement, the patient should be reevaluated to confirm the diagnosis and switched to

* Most women with PID have either mucopurulent cervical discharge or evidence of WBCs on a saline wet preparation of vaginal secretions. If no WBCs are found on the wet preparation, the diagnosis of PID is unlikely.

** Endometrial biopsy is warranted in women undergoing laparoscopy who do not have visual evidence of salpingitis, because endometritis is the only sign of PID for some women.

BOX 1: Treatment guidelines recommended by the CDC.

Outpatient regimen for mild-to-moderate PID†:
- Doxycycline (100 mg orally twice a day for 2 weeks) *with or without metronidazole* (500 mg orally twice daily for 2 weeks)

Plus one of the following:
- Ceftriaxone (250 mg intramuscularly in a single dose)
  or
- Cefoxitin (2 g intramuscularly) *with* probenecid (1 g orally) concurrently in a single dose
  or
- Other parenteral third-generation cephalosporin (cefotaxime or ceftizoxime)

Alternative intramuscular/oral regimen:
Azithromycin 500 mg IV daily for one to two doses followed by 250 mg orally once a day for 12–14 days alone or with metronidazole

†Transition to oral therapy can usually be initiated within 24–48 hours after clinical improvement, and oral therapy should be continued to complete 2 weeks of therapy.

(CDC: Centers for Disease Control and Prevention; PID: pelvic inflammatory disease)

Source: Workowski KA, Bolan GA. Sexually transmitted diseases treatment guidelines, 2015. MMWR Recomm Rep. 2015;64(3):1-137.

BOX 2: Outclient treatment of mild or moderate PID recommended by Indian National Guidelines on Prevention, Management, and Control of Reproductive Tract Infections including Sexually Transmitted Infections.

Therapy should cover *Neisseria gonorrhoeae, Chlamydia trachomatis,* and anaerobes.
- Tablet cefixime 400 mg orally BD for 7 days + tablet metronidazole 400 mg orally BD for 14 days
- Doxycycline 100 mg orally BD for 14 days
- Tablet ibuprofen 400 mg orally TDS for 3–5 days
- Tablet ranitidine 150 mg orally BD to prevent gastritis
- Remove IUD, if present, under antibiotic cover of 24–48 hours
- Advise abstinence during course of treatment and educate on correct and consistent use of condoms
- Observe for 3 days and if no improvement (i.e., absence of fever, reduction in abdominal tenderness, reduction in cervical motion, and adnexal and uterine tenderness) or if symptoms worsen, refer for inclient treatment

(IUD: intrauterine device; PID: pelvic inflammatory disease)

parenteral therapy.[1] CDC recommends three regimens for initial parenteral therapy **(Box 3)**.
- If there is satisfactory clinical improvement after 24–48 hours of parenteral therapy, patients may be given oral therapy.[1]
- Metronidazole can be added, as anaerobic organisms are suspected in many cases and will also treat bacterial vaginosis, which is a frequent association.

HOSPITAL ADMISSION CRITERIA WITH ACUTE PID

The following criteria suggested by the STD guidelines are useful to decide which patients need hospitalization:
- Inability to exclude surgical emergencies such as appendicitis and ectopic pregnancy

BOX 3: Treatment guidelines recommended by CDC—parenteral regimens for moderate-to-severe PID with or without tubo-ovarian abscess.

- Cefotetan (2 g IV every 12 hours) + doxycycline (100 mg orally/IV every 2 hours)
- Cefoxitin (2 g IV every 6 hours) + doxycycline (100 mg orally/IV every 12 hours)

Because of the pain associated with intravenous infusion, doxycycline should be administered orally when possible. Oral and IV administration of doxycycline provide similar bioavailability.

Note: Oral therapy with doxycycline 100 mg twice daily can be used 24–48 hours after clinical improvement to complete the 14 days of therapy.
- Clindamycin (900 mg IV every 8 hours) + gentamicin (loading dose of 2 mg/kg, IV or IM followed by a maintenance dose of 1.5 mg/kg every 8 hours). Single daily dosing (3–5 mg/kg) can be substituted.

Note: Oral therapy with clindamycin (450 mg orally four times daily) or doxycycline (100 mg twice daily) can be used to complete the 14 days of therapy.

When tubo-ovarian abscess is present, clindamycin (450 mg orally four times daily) or metronidazole (500 mg twice daily) should be used to complete at least 14 days of therapy with doxycycline to provide more effective anaerobic coverage than doxycycline alone.

Alternative parenteral regimen:
Ampicillin-sulbactam (3 g IV every 6 hours) + doxycycline (100 mg oral/IV every 12 hours)

(CDC: Centers for Disease Control and Prevention; IM: intramuscular; IV: intravenous; PID: pelvic inflammatory disease)

Source: Workowski KA, Bolan GA. Sexually transmitted diseases treatment guidelines, 2015. MMWR Recomm Rep. 2015;64(3):1-137.

- Tubo-ovarian abscess
- Pregnancy
- Severe illness, nausea and vomiting, or high fever
- Nonresponse to oral therapy or the inability to tolerate an outpatient oral regimen
- Current immunodeficiency [human immunodeficiency virus (HIV) infection with low CD4 cell count and immunosuppressive therapy]

MANAGEMENT OF PID IN WOMEN WITH HIV INFECTION

- The antimicrobial management in women with HIV remains the same.
- They may show a reduced response to antibiotics, require a longer hospital stay, and increased surgical interventions.

Partner Management

- Treat all male sex partners who had come in contact with a patient during 60 days prior to the diagnosis. The patient's most recent sex partner should be treated in case the last sexual intercourse was more than 60 days before onset of symptoms or diagnosis.
- Treat male partners for urethral discharge (gonorrhea and chlamydia).

- Advise sexual abstinence during course of the treatment.
- Provide condoms and educate on correct and consistent use.
- Refer for voluntary counseling and testing for HIV, syphilis, and hepatitis B.
- Inform about complications if left untreated and sequelae.
- Schedule return visit in 3, 7, and 14 days to ensure compliance.

Management of Pregnant Women

Pregnancy is rare in PID:

- Any pregnant woman suspected to have PID should be referred to district hospital for hospitalization and treated with a parenteral regimen which would be safe in pregnancy.
- Doxycycline is contraindicated in pregnancy.
- Metronidazole is generally not recommended during the first 3 months of pregnancy. However, it should be not withheld for a severely acute PID which is an emergency.

PATIENT COUNSELING AND EDUCATION

- Patient should be counseled and educated about the nature of the disease, transmission issues, and risk reduction.
- Sexual abstinence should be practiced for at least 7 days after completing therapy and until both partners are asymptomatic.

KEY POINTS

- PID is a clinical syndrome characterized by ascending spread of organisms from the vagina or cervix to the structures of the upper genital tract most commonly in single, sexually active, and young women.
- Most cases are polymicrobial, the most common pathogens being *N. gonorrhoeae* or *C. trachomatis* or both. Other pathogens may be associated.
- Ectopic pregnancy, infertility, or chronic pelvic pain is the long-term sequelae.
- CDC diagnostic criteria should be used for decisions to initiate presumptive treatment as no single physical examination finding, image, or laboratory test can reliably make a definitive diagnosis.
- Treatment regimens (oral or parenteral) must ensure empiric, broad-spectrum coverage of likely pathogens (*N. gonorrhoeae*, *C. trachomatis*, anaerobes, gram-negative facultative bacteria, and streptococci).

REFERENCES

1. Workowski KA, Bolan GA. Sexually transmitted diseases treatment guidelines, 2015. MMWR Recomm Rep. 2015;64(3): 1-137.
2. Ross JDC. Pelvic inflammatory disease. BMJ Clin Evid. 2008; 2008:1606.
3. Hay PE, Kerry SR, Normansell R, Horner PJ, Reid F, Kerry SM, et al. Which sexually active young female students are most at risk of pelvic inflammatory disease? A prospective study. Sex Transm Infect. 2016;92:63-6.
4. Washington AE, Aral SO, Wølner-Hanssen P, Grimes DA, Holmes KK. Assessing risk for pelvic inflammatory disease and its sequelae. JAMA. 1991;266:2581-6.
5. Carr S, Espey E. Intrauterine devices and pelvic inflammatory disease among adolescents. J Adolesc Health. 2013;52:S22-8.
6. Brunham RC, Gottlieb SL, Paavonen J. Pelvic inflammatory disease. N Engl J Med. 2015;372:2039-48.
7. Price MJ, Ades AE, De Angelis D, Welton NJ, Macleod J, Soldan K, et al. Risk of pelvic inflammatory disease following *Chlamydia trachomatis* infection: analysis of prospective studies with a multistate model. Am J Epidemiol. 2013;178:484-92.
8. McGregor JA, French JI, Jones W, Milligan K, McKinney PJ, Patterson E, et al. Bacterial vaginosis is associated with prematurity and vaginal fluid mucinase and sialidase: results of a controlled trial of topical clindamycin cream. Am J Obstet Gynecol. 1994;170:1048-59.
9. Chayachinda C, Rekhawasin T. Reproductive outcomes of patients being hospitalised with pelvic inflammatory disease. J Obstet Gynaecol. 2017;37(2):228-32.
10. Hillis SD, Joesoef R, Marchbanks PA, Wasserheit JN, Cates W Jr, Westrom L. Delayed care of pelvic inflammatory disease as a risk factor for impaired fertility. Am J Obstet Gynecol. 1993; 168:1503-9.

EXAMINATION QUESTIONS

1. What is the etiology and pathogenesis of PID? What are the symptoms and clinical manifestations of PID?
2. Describe the complications of PID. Outline the principles of management for PID.

136 CHAPTER Balanoposthitis

Mamatha George, Fibin Thanveer

INTRODUCTION

Balanitis refers to inflammation of the glans penis, while posthitis refers to inflammation of the prepuce. In practice, as both are often affected together, the term balanoposthitis is used. This is a collection of diverse conditions, with similar clinical presentation and varying etiologies, affecting the same anatomical site.[1]

Balanoposthitis is reported to account for 11% of males attending genitourinary clinics.[2] It can be recurrent or persistent.

ETIOLOGY

Various infectious and noninfectious conditions can cause balanoposthitis **(Table 1)**. Of the identifiable causes, candidiasis is the most common.[3] Most cases are related to inadequate hygiene in uncircumcised men leading to accumulation of smegma, debris, and bacteria or fungi, resulting in inflammation.

CLINICAL MANIFESTATIONS

Symptoms: Often present as pruritus, pain, or tenderness of the glans and/or foreskin.

Signs: Vary according to etiology.

Complications:

- Localized edema may develop if balanitis progresses without treatment. The combination of inflammation and edema can result in adherence of the foreskin to the glans. Persistent inflammation may result in scarring. Ultimately, this process can evolve to phimosis.
- Balanitis may be severe in patients with diabetes mellitus, where candidiasis is especially common. It has been reported as a source of fever and bacteremia in neutropenic men.[4]
- Manifestation of balanoposthitis irrespective of etiology is much more severe when associated with human immunodeficiency virus (HIV) infection, particularly in advanced stage.

TABLE 1: Causes of balanoposthitis.[1,2]

Infectious	*Inflammatory*	*Premalignant*
• *Fungal: Candida albicans* (most common) • *Anaerobic bacterial:* Bacteroides • *Aerobic bacterial:* – *Gardnerella vaginalis* – *Mycoplasma genitalium* – *Neisseria gonorrhoeae* – *Staphylococcus aureus* – *Streptococci* – *Haemophilus ducreyi* – *Chlamydia* – *Calymmatobacterium granulomatis* • *Parasitic*: – Scabies – Creeping eruption • *Mycobacterial* • *Protozoal:* – *Trichomonas vaginalis* – *Entamoeba histolytica* • *Spirochaetal:* – Syphilitic balanitis – Nonsyphilitic spirochaetes • *Viral:* – Herpes simplex virus – Human papillomavirus	• Lichen sclerosus et atrophicus/balanitis xerotica obliterans • Zoon's balanitis • Circinate balanitis • Fixed drug eruption • Irritant and allergic balanitides • Pemphigus and cicatricial pemphigoid • Psoriasis • Lichen planus • Erythema multiforme • Stevens–Johnson syndrome • Behçet's disease • *Inflammatory bowel disease:* Ulcerative colitis and Crohn's disease • Dermatitis artefacta • Trauma	• Erythroplasia of Queyrat • Bowen's disease • Bowenoid papulosis • Pseudoepitheliomatous micaceous and keratotic balanitis (PMKB)

DIAGNOSIS

The history, clinical examination findings, and tailored investigations will help to guide the clinical diagnosis and are mentioned under the individual conditions below. It is worth noting that the etiology of many balanitides proves difficult to diagnose and any condition which persists despite treatment warrants further investigations and may require biopsy from the lesion.

SPECIFIC CAUSES OF BALANITIS

Infectious Causes

Description of clinical features of infectious causes are discussed in **Table 2.**[4]

Noninfectious Inflammatory Causes

Balanitis Xerotica Obliterans

Balanitis xerotica obliterans (BXO) refers to a chronic scarring balanitis first described by Stuhmer, which is most commonly caused by lichen sclerosus et atrophicus (LSA). Other rare causes include pemphigus vulgaris, lichen planus, cicatricial pemphigoid, and chronic nonspecific bacterial balanitis.[2]

Lichen sclerosus et atrophicus is a chronic inflammatory scarring skin disease with a predilection for anogenital skin. Association between BXO and LSA was made by Laymon and Freeman.[2]

Clinical features:

- Pain, irritation, disturbance of sexual function, or urinary symptoms including obstruction.
- Examination shows porcelain white plaques on the glans, often with involvement of the prepuce which becomes thickened and nonretractile. Hemorrhagic vesicles can occur in active disease.
- Rarely this can present as a recurrent bullous balanitis, leading to ulceration which may be precipitated by local trauma.
- Urethral stenosis and phimosis can occur due to atrophy and scarring of glans.

Histopathological examination (HPE):

- Hyperkeratosis, follicular plugging, thinning of the epidermis, and vacuolar degeneration of the basal layer.

TABLE 2: Clinical features of infectious causes of balanitis.

Organism	*Clinical features*	*Diagnosis*	*Management*
Candidal balanitis	Eroded papules with collarette of whitish scales or dull red areas with glazed appearance **(Fig. 1)**. Maceration and fissuring may occur in chronic cases **(Fig. 2)**	Subpreputial swab for potassium hydroxide (KOH) mount shows pseudohyphae, fungal culture urinalysis for glucose, and blood sugar	Clotrimazole cream 1% or miconazole cream 2% *Alternative regimens:* • Fluconazole 150 mg orally as a single dose • Nystatin cream—if resistance suspected *Notes:* • Topical 1% hydrocortisone may be combined only if marked inflammation is present • Treat sexual partners
Anaerobic infection—Bacteroides	• Foul smelling subpreputial discharge • Preputial edema, superficial erosions; with associated inguinal adenitis in severe cases. A severe erosive and gangrenous form (fourth venereal disease of Corbus) has been described with coinfection of anaerobes and *Fusobacterium* species[2]	• Gram stain may show gram-negative bacilli or a mixed pattern • Subpreputial culture	Metronidazole 400 mg twice daily for 1 week *Alternative regimen:* Clindamycin cream applied twice daily until resolved
Gonococcal infection	Presents as erosions on glans with thick purulent discharge per urethra **(Fig. 3)**	• *Gram stain:* Intracellular gram-negative diplococci • Subpreputial culture	• Cefixime 400 mg orally as single dose • Ceftriaxone 125 mg intramuscular (IM) as a single dose • Ciprofloxacin 500 mg orally as a single dose
Gardnerella vaginalis	Macular erythema and subpreputial discharge with fishy odor	*Gram stain:* Variable	• Metronidazole 400 mg twice daily for 7 days • Clindamycin 300 mg twice day for 7 days • Clindamycin 2% vaginal cream
Trichomonas vaginalis	Superficial erosive balanitis which may lead to phimosis	• Wet mount demonstrates the organism • Polymerase chain reaction (PCR)	• Metronidazole 2 g orally as a single dose • Tinidazole 2 g orally as a single dose *Alternative regimen:* Metronidazole 400 mg orally twice daily for 7 days

Contd...

Contd...

Organism	*Clinical features*	*Diagnosis*	*Management*
Syphilitic balanitis of Follmann (SBF)	Erosive balanitis, may be associated with chancre	Dark field microscopy Serological tests for syphilis	• Single IM administration of 2.4 MU of benzathine penicillin, or • Doxycycline 100 mg orally BID for 2 weeks, or • Tetracycline 500 mg orally QID for 2 weeks
Viral—Herpes simplex	Grouped vesicles on erythematous base over glans, prepuce and shaft which rupture to form shallow erosions. Rarely primary herpes can cause a necrotizing balanitis **(Fig. 4)**	• Tzanck smear • Immunoglobulin G (IgG) and IgM for herpes simplex virus (HSV) • Cell culture PCR	• Acyclovir 400 mg orally three times a day for 7–10 days, or • Famciclovir 250 mg orally three times a day for 7–10 days • Valacyclovir 1 g orally twice a day for 7–10 days
Viral—Human papillomavirus	Chronic balanitis	Aceto-whitening after the application of 5% acetic acid	*Patient applied:* • Podophyllotoxin (podofilox) 0.5% solution or gel twice daily for three consecutive days, but no more than 4 weeks, or • Imiquimod 5% cream—applied at bedtime three times/week for a maximum of 16 weeks, and must be left in place for 6–10 hours following application, or *Provider administered:* • Podophyllin resin 10%–25% in a compound tincture of benzoin—once a week for 6–8 weeks, or • Cryotherapy, chemical cautery using trichloroacetic acid—80–90%

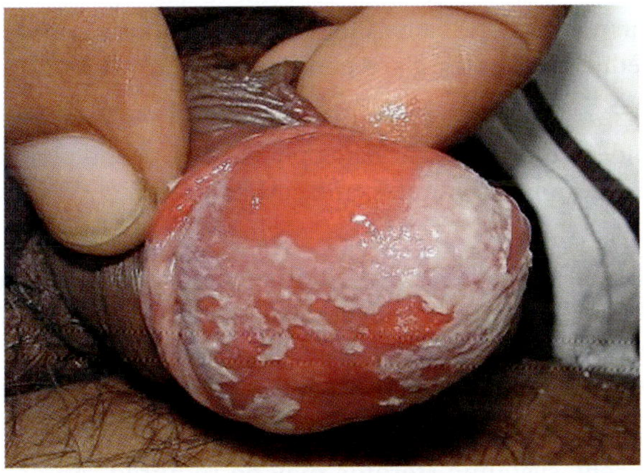

Fig. 1: Candidal balanoposthitis.
Courtesy: Dr Rakesh SV, Kozhikode, Kerala.

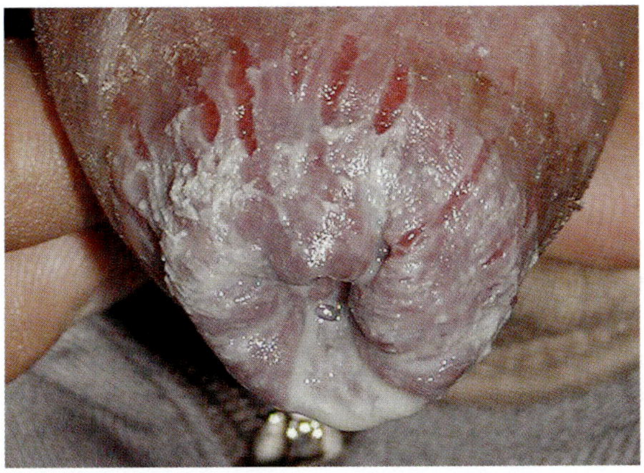

Fig. 2: Chronic candidal balanoposthitis with fissuring.
Courtesy: Dr Sugathan P, Kozhikode, Kerala.

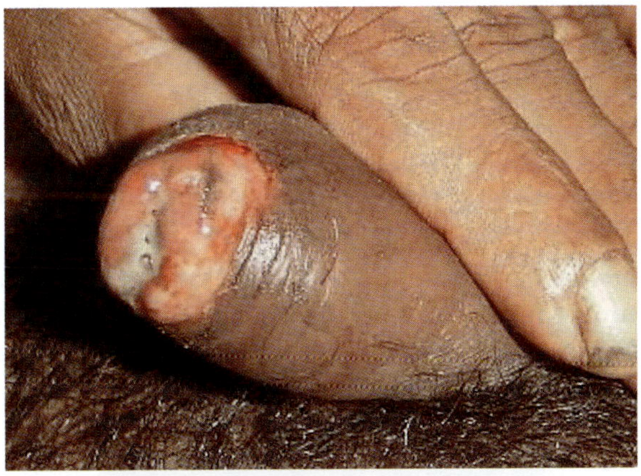

Fig. 3: Gonococcal balanoposthitis.
Courtesy: Dr Sugathan P, Kozhikode, Kerala.

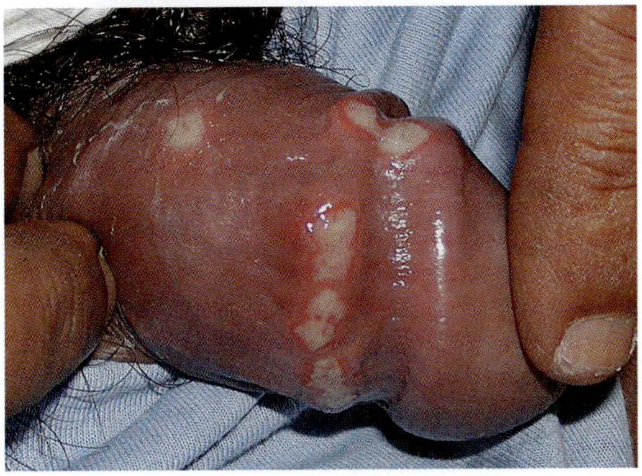

Fig. 4: Herpes genitalis.
Courtesy: Dr Sugathan P, Kozhikode, Kerala.

- A zone of subepidermal edema with homogeneous collagen which becomes eosinophilic and more sclerotic in older lesions.
- A band of mononuclear cells just beneath the homogeneous zone and is most evident in the mid-dermis, although sparse in established lesions.[5]

Course: Chronic and relapsing. Development of squamous cell carcinoma (SCC) has been reported in BXO.

Treatment:

- Potent topical steroids are the most accepted and recommended treatment.[5]
- Testosterone 2%, topical tacrolimus and intralesional steroids are other options.
- If phimosis is present, circumcision may be required, or meatotomy for meatal stenosis.

Plasma Cell Balanitis of Zoon (PCB)

Synonym: Balanitis circumscripta plasmacellularis.

Benign idiopathic condition of uncircumcised male first described by Zoon in 1952.

Etiology: Unclear, though chronic infection with *Mycobacterium smegmatis* has been proposed.[2]

Clinical features:

- Usually asymptomatic, may be associated with mild pruritus, irritation, and discharge.
- Well-circumscribed bright red areas with characteristic glazed appearance and multiple pinpoint red spots—"cayenne pepper spots" on the glans and/or the prepuce **(Fig. 5)**.[1]

Histopathological examination: Epidermal atrophy, loss of rete ridges, diamond-shaped "lozenge keratinocytes", and spongiosis. Subepidermal infiltrate with predominantly plasma cells is characteristic.

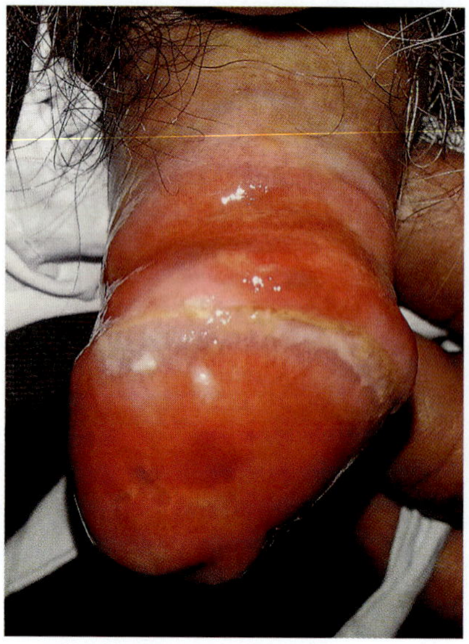

Fig. 5: Zoon's balanitis.
Courtesy: Dr Muhammed Razmi, Kozhikode, Kerala.

Treatment: Circumcision is curative. Topical corticosteroids, tacrolimus, and CO_2 laser have also been tried with variable results.

Circinate Balanitis

Circinate balanitis occurs in 20–40% of patients with sexually acquired reactive arthiritis,[2] being the most common mucocutaneous manifestation. Incidence in enteric reactive arthiritis is rare.

Circinate balanitis may occur with or without other features of reactive arthiritis.

Clinical feature: Grayish white areas on the glans, which coalesce to form larger "geographic" areas with a white margin.

Histopathological examination: Spongiform pustules in upper epidermis with parakeratosis, acanthosis, and elongation of rete ridges, increased and enlarged dermal capillaries with a mononuclear cell infiltrate. The HPE appearance is similar to pustular psoriasis.

Treatment: It is primarily directed at the underlying infection.

Fixed Drug Eruptions

Fixed drug eruption (FDE) is a specific reaction pattern where lesion recurs at the same sites with each exposure, and have a predilection for the glans penis.

Drugs associated: Antibiotics—tetracyclines and sulphonamides (common), salicylates, phenacetin, phenolphthalein, paracetamol, barbiturates, and carbamazepine.

Clinical features:

- Usually well-demarcated erythematous areas which may be bullous and subsequently ulcerated **(Figs. 6 and 7)**.[1]
- Can occur on the first exposure to a drug and repeated exposure will precipitate new lesions at the initial site.

Treatment: The offending drug should be withdrawn. Topical, or rarely, systemic steroids may be required. An area of residual hyperpigmentation may remain.

Irritant and Allergic Balanitides[2]

This is a common nonspecific entity. A precipitant may be evident only in some of the cases.[1]

Etiology:

- Common agents include perfumed soap, condoms, vaginal spermicides, lubricants, and irritants from vaginal secretion.
- May be associated with a history of atopy and more frequent washing of genitalia with soap.
- Topical agents used for treatment can also result in allergic reactions. Severe irritant reaction may follow use of podophyllin for genital warts.

Clinical feature: Wide spectrum of clinical manifestations varying from balanitis to edema of the whole penis extending to the groins (**Fig. 8**).

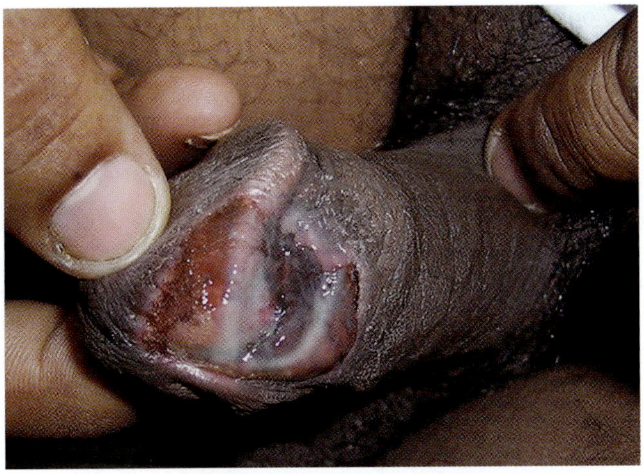

Fig. 6: Fixed drug eruption.
Courtesy: Dr Abhay Mani Martin, Kozhikode, Kerala.

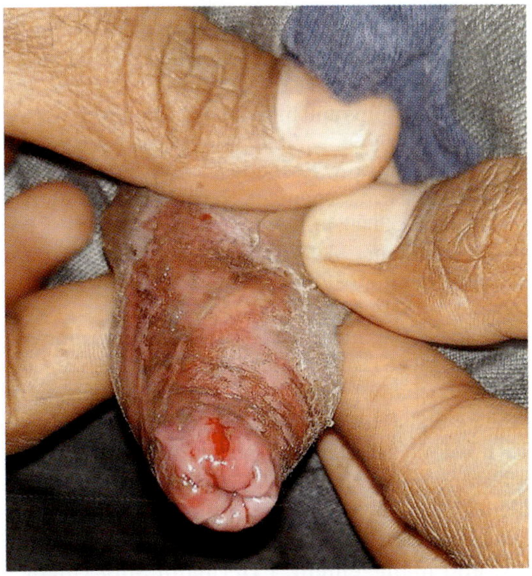

Fig. 7: Candidiasis with fixed drug eruption (FDE).
Courtesy: Dr Bishurul Hafi NA, Kozhikode, Kerala.

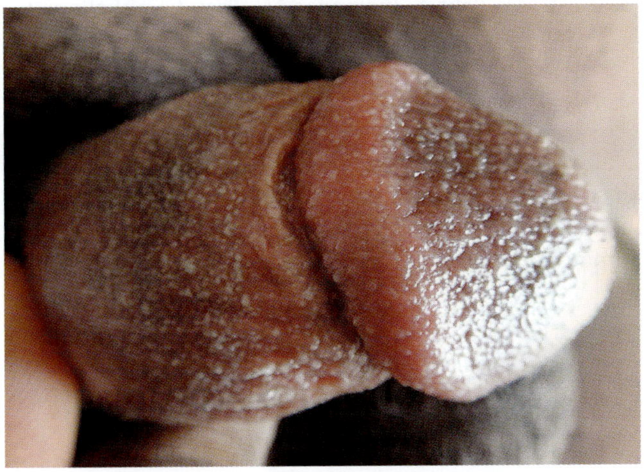

Fig. 8: Allergic balanoposthitis to condom.
Courtesy: Dr Sugathan P, Kozhikode, Kerala.

Treatment: Depending on the severity of the reaction, topical, or systemic steroids may be used. Patch testing may help to identify the agent and avoidance of the precipitant is required.

Miscellaneous Causes

Dermatological diseases such as lichen planus, psoriasis, pemphigus, and erythema multiforme can present with lesion on the glans penis. Crohn's disease, ulcerative colitis, chronic lymphocytic as well as acute promyelocytic leukemia have been reported as rare causes of balanoposthitis.[6]

Premalignant Conditions

There are three clinical presentations of penile carcinoma in situ (PCIS): (1) Erythroplasia of Queyrat, (2) Bowen's disease, and (3) bowenoid papulosis.

Erythroplasia of Queyrat and Bowen's disease are considered together as they are similar but affect the nonkeratinized and keratinized skin, respectively. Erythroplasia of Queyrat represents Bowen's disease on genital mucosa. All three may progress to SCC, but the risk is much less in bowenoid papulosis.

Erythroplasia of Queyrat (Penile Carcinoma in situ of the Glans)[7]

- Described by Queyrat in 1911.
- Usually occurring in the uncircumcised male over 40 years of age.

Clinical features:

- Well-defined erythematous velvety plaque. May be single or multiple. Induration on the plaque suggests the development of SCC.
- Diagnosis should be confirmed by biopsy.

Treatment:

- 5-fluorouracil, topical imiquimod 5% cream, Mohs microsurgery, cryotherapy, laser treatment, photodynamic therapy (PDT), or surgical excision.
- Circumcision is recommended and close follow-up is advised.

Bowenoid Papulosis[1]

Clinical features:

- Multiple discrete warty lesions often pigmented on keratinized skin, more inflammatory at the mucosal sites. Clinically very similar to genital warts.
- Diagnosis should be confirmed by biopsy.

Treatment:

- Imiquimod 5% cream and laser resection
- Alternative treatment options are PDT, fluorouracil cream, cryotherapy, curettage and cautery, and surgical excision.

Pseudoepitheliomatous, Keratotic and Micaceous Balanitis[8,9]

This is a rare entity, described by Lortat-Jacob and Civatte in 1961.

Clinical feature: Well-demarcated hyperkeratotic plaque on the glans penis with micaceous scaling. Pseudoepitheliomatous keratotic and micaceous balanitis (PKMB) is generally asymptomatic, may be associated with irritation, burning sensation, fissuring, or maceration.

Histopathological examination: Hyperplastic epidermis with massive hyperkeratosis and elongation of rete ridges with a polymorphonuclear infiltrate.

Course: Originally considered to be benign but reports suggest that the lesion may be locally invasive or synonymous with verrucous carcinoma.

Treatment: Topical 5-fluorouracil, cryotherapy, and Mohs microsurgery.

KEY POINTS

- Balanitis refers to inflammation of the glans penis, while posthitis refers to inflammation of the prepuce. In practice, as both are often affected together, the term balanoposthitis is used.
- Most cases are related to inadequate hygiene in uncircumcised men.
- Various infectious and noninfectious conditions can cause balanoposthitis. Of the identifiable causes, candidiasis is the most common.
- The etiology of many balanitides proves difficult to diagnose and any condition which persists despite simple treatment warrants further investigation.
- Ulcerative venereal diseases such as syphilis, chancroid, donovanosis, lymphogranuloma venereum, and herpes genitalis can cause erosions and ulcers on genital mucosa with inflammation.
- Balanitis xerotica obliterans is most commonly caused by LSA. Potent topical steroids (clobetasol propionate) remain the accepted and recommended treatment.
- Zoon's plasma cell balanitis is a benign idiopathic condition of uncircumcised male with a well-circumscribed smooth plaque with a characteristic glazed appearance with multiple pinpoint red spots—"cayenne pepper spots" on the glans and/or the prepuce. Treatment of choice is circumcision.
- Circinate balanitis is a common mucocutaneous manifestation of Reiter's syndrome.
- There are three clinical presentations of PCIS: (1) Erythroplasia of Queyrat, (2) Bowen's disease, and (3) bowenoid papulosis.
- PMKB presents as demarcated hyperkeratotic plaque on the glans penis with micaceous scaling. Though considered to be benign, the lesion may be locally invasive, or synonymous with verrucous carcinoma.

REFERENCES

1. Edwards SK, Bunker CB, Ziller F, van der Meijden WI. 2013 European guideline for the management of balanoposthitis. Int J STD AIDS. 2014;25:615-26.
2. Edwards S. Balanitis and balanoposthitis: a review. Genitourin Med. 1996;72:155-9.
3. Lisboa C, Ferreira A, Resende C, Rodrigues AG. Infectious balanoposthitis: management, clinical and laboratory features. Int J Dermatol. 2009;48:121-4.
4. Pandya I, Shinojia M, Vadukul D, Marfatia YS. Approach to balanitis/balanoposthitis: current guidelines. Indian J Sex Transm Dis. 2014;35:155-7.
5. Yesudian PD, Sugunendran H, Bates CM, O'Mahony C. Lichen sclerosus. Int J STD AIDS. 2005;16(7):465-73.
6. Grewal RS, Chatterjee M, Das AL. NonVenereological disorders of the genitalia. In: Sacchidanand S, Oberai C, Inamadar AC (Eds). IADVL Textbook of Dermatology. Mumbai: Bhalani Publishing House; 2015. pp. 1779-802.
7. Mikhail GR. Cancers, precancers and pseudocancers on the male genitalia: a review of clinical appearances, histopathology, and management. J Dermatol Surg Oncol. 1980;6:1027.
8. Read SI, Abell E. Pseudoepitheliomatous, keratotic and micaceous balanitis. Arch Dermatol. 1981;117:435-7.
9. Adya KA, Palit A, Inamadar AC. Pseudoepitheliomatous keratotic and micaceous balanitis. Indian J Sex Transm Dis AIDS. 2013;34:123-5.

EXAMINATION QUESTIONS

1. Enumerate the noninfectious causes of balanoposthitis and describe the clinical features, diagnosis, and management of Zoon's balanitis.
2. Write a note on Follmann balanitis. Describe pseudoepitheliomatous, keratotic, and micaceous balanitis (PKMB).

137 CHAPTER

Nonvenereal Diseases of Genitalia

SK Shahriar Ahmed

INTRODUCTION

Dermatoses involving genitalia are not exclusively sexually transmitted. They can be venereal as well as nonvenereal. Nonvenereal genital dermatoses, are not sexually transmitted, and are referred to a wide array of diseases with varied etiology. They can either affect solely genitalia or may be a part of other dermatological condition occurring elsewhere over the skin.[1] A comprehensive understanding of various nonvenereal genital dermatoses, their cause and appropriate management options is indispensable.

CLASSIFICATION

There is no distinct classification of such diseases. However, we can classify it into three major groups:

1. *Physiological abnormalities:* Fordyce spots, pearly penile papule
2. *Genital lesion exclusively or as a part of other dermatological condition:*

Papulosquamous diseases	Psoriasis, lichen planus, seborrheic dermatitis
Disorder of keratinization	Porokeratosis
Congenital	Median raphe cyst, epidermal nevi
Disorder of pigmentation	Vitiligo, lentigines
Bullous disorders	Pemphigus or pemphigoid group of disease
Drug reaction	Fixed drug eruption (FDE), Stevens-Johnson syndrome-toxic epidermal necrolysis (SJS-TEN)
Infective	Scabies, impetigo, tubercular chancre, dermatophytosis, phthiriasis
Malignancy	Erythroplasia of Queyrat, squamous cell carcinoma (SCC), basal cell carcinoma (BCC), melanoma, sarcoma
Premalignant conditions	Bowen's disease, Bowenoid papulosis, extramammary Paget's disease, lichen sclerosus et atrophicus (LSA), pseudoepitheliomatous keratotic micaceous balanitis (PKMB)

3. *Disease peculiar to genitalia:* Circinate balanitis, Peyronie's disease, Zoon's plasma cell balanitis, Fournier's gangrene, phimosis and paraphimosis, angiokeratoma of Fordyce, nonvenereal sclerosing lymphangitis.

PHYSIOLOGICAL ABNORMALITIES

Fordyce Spots[2]

- *Introduction:* Ectopic sebaceous glands
- *Synonym:* Fordyce granules
- *History:* Named after John Addison Fordyce, an American dermatologist
- *Epidemiology:* Male > Female, prominent at puberty
- *Clinical features:* Multiple, asymptomatic, discrete, tiny whitish-yellow papules
- *Site:* Subpreputial area of penis, scrotum or over vulva
- *Other sites:* Vermilion border of lips (MC), oral mucosa
- *Differential diagnosis:* Sebaceous hyperplasia, epidermoid cyst
- *Treatment:* Counseling about benign nature of the disease.

Pearly Penile Papule[3]

- *Introduction:* A form of acral angiofibroma.
- *Synonym:* Hirsute coronae glandis, hirsutoid papillomas
- *Epidemiology:* Incidence around 8–48% of all men, uncircumscribed>circumscribed male
- *Clinical features:* One or several rows of small (1–2 mm), pearly-white or flesh-colored, spiny papules
- *Site:* Corona or sulcus of the glans penis
- *Differential diagnosis:* Condyloma acuminata
- *Histopathological Differential diagnosis:* Adenoma sebaceum, sub- or periungual fibroma, fibrous papule of nose, acquired acral angiofibroma
- *Treatment:* Reassurance about physiological nature of the disease
- Electrosurgery, CO_2 laser **(Fig. 1)**.

GENITAL LESION EXCLUSIVELY OR AS A PART OF OTHER DERMATOLOGICAL CONDITION

Psoriasis

- *Introduction:* Mostly occurs along with typical lesions elsewhere on the body

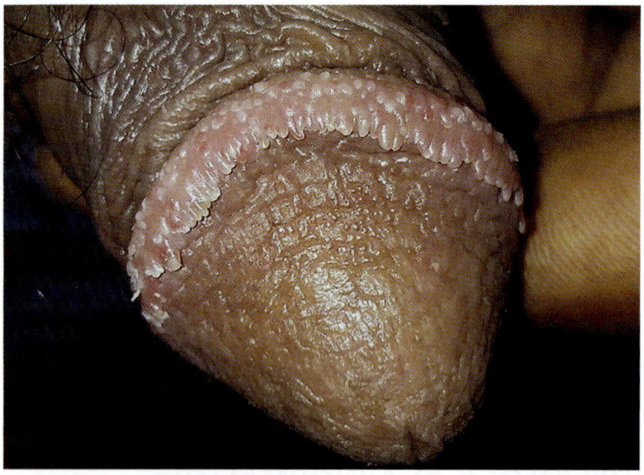

Fig. 1: Pearly penile papule.

- *Epidemiology:* Not as common as over trunk
- *Clinical features:* Erythematous, smooth, clearly demarcated plaques
- The silvery scales are lost as over flexural sites.
- *Site:* Glans penis and shaft of the penis of male; labia majora and the mons pubis of female
- *Complication:* Fissuring and bleeding can occur.
- *Differential diagnosis:* Seborrheic dermatitis, tinea, erythrasma, circinate balanitis
- *Treatment:* Poor response to treatment
    - Moderately potent topical corticosteroid, vitamin D derivatives, topical calcineurin inhibitors. Systemic therapy (e.g., methotrexate, cyclosporine, TNF inhibitors), usually for widespread disease

Lichen Planus

- *Introduction:* Can occur exclusively over genitalia or as a part of cutaneous involvement.
- *Epidemiology:* 15% cases lichen planus (LP) occurs exclusively over mucosa either oral or genital.
- *Clinical features:*
    - Annular lesion occurs most commonly over glans.
    - Classical violaceous, flat-topped papules seen over shaft of the penis
    - Erosion or ulceration of male genital LP is uncommon.
    - Erosive vaginal LP is common causes severe itching and pain.
- *Site:* Glans and shaft of the penis, scrotum for male and vulval skin, both labia majora and minora for female
- *HPE:* Same as histopathology of classical LP except epidermis is less or nonkeratinized with parakeratosis, dermis rich in plasma cells, and less of cytoid bodies.
- *Complication:* Erosive vaginal LP may lead to dyspareunia and adhesion.
- *Differential diagnosis:*
    - Annular LP can be confused with porokeratosis.
    - Erosive LP can be confused with genital herpes or fixed drug eruption.
- *Treatment:*
    - Poor response to treatment and chronic and recurrent than classical LP
    - Topically moderately potent topical corticosteroid, vitamin D derivatives, topical calcineurin inhibitors can be used. Immunosuppressive can be used in severe cases.

Fixed Drug Eruption

- *Introduction:* A specific manifestation of drug reaction where lesion appears over the exact same site on exposure of a particular drug.
- *Pathogenesis:* Intraepidermal CD8+ T-cell releases IFN-γ
- *Clinical features:* Over genitalia, it occurs mostly over glans as erosion. The classical well-circumscribed erythematous plaques or sometimes bulla can be present elsewhere in the body. It heals with dark brown pigmentation
- *Drug responsible:* Common culprits are acetaminophen (paracetamol), tetracyclines, trimethoprim–sulfamethoxazole, and nonsteroidal anti-inflammatory drugs
- *Complication:* Ulceration
- *Differential diagnosis:* Ulcerative STDs
- *Treatment:* Systemic/topical corticosteroid can be used **(Fig. 2)**.

Erythroplasia of Queyrat[4]

- *Introduction:* It is a squamous cell carcinoma in situ of genitalia.
- *History:* Vincent Jules Louis Queyrat, a French dermatologist
- *Epidemiology:* Most common among uncircumscribed male
- *Clinical features:* Red shiny patches or plaques over the glans and prepuce of the penis usually without scaling.
- *HPE:* Nuclear hyperchromasia, disordered maturation of keratinocytes, coarse nuclear chromatin. Multiple mitotic figures usually do not cross beyond the basal layer.

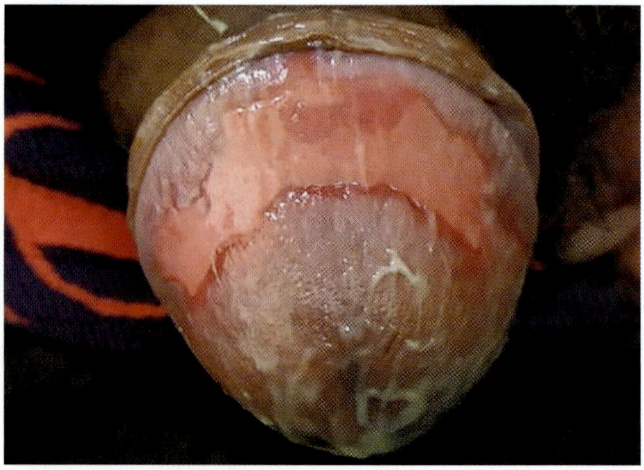

Fig. 2: Fixed drug eruption (FDE) over glans.

- *Complication:* Turns into invasive SCC
- *Differential diagnosis:* Bowen's disease, LSA, PKMB, Zoon balanitis
- *Treatment:* Topical 5% 5-fluorouracil cream, cryosurgery, curettage and electrocautery, excisional surgery, glans resurfacing, Mohs micrographic surgery, laser, etc.

PREMALIGNANT CONDITIONS OF GENITALIA

Bowen's Disease[5]

- *Introduction:* Precancerous form of SCC
- *History:* First described by JT Bowen in 1912
- *Pathogenesis:* Immunosuppression (HIV, organ transplantation etc.), HPV infection, radiotherapy
- *Clinical features:* Slowly enlarging well-defined erythematous scaly or crusted plaque
- *Site:* Glans most commonly, can spread to prepuce, perianal region; vulva in case of female
- *HPE:* Haphazardly arranged keratinocytes with loss of polarity (Windblown appearance), keratinocyte atypia, hyperchromatic nucleus, dyskeratotic and apoptotic cells; sparing the basal layer (eyeliner sign-line of normal basal layer under layers of atypical keratinocytes)
- *Complication:* Malignant transformation mostly in SCC (10% cases in genital Bowen's)
- *Differential diagnosis:* Erythroplasia of Queyrat, PKMB, genital psoriasis
- *Treatment:* Topical 5% 5-fluorouracil cream, imiquimod, cryosurgery, photodynamic therapy. Excision is the definitive treatment **(Fig. 3)**.

Bowenoid Papulosis[6]

- *Introduction:* Rare condition of genitalia which clinically resembles wart and histopathologically Bowen's disease
- *History:* First described by Kopf and Bart
- *Epidemiology:* Mostly affects younger age groups
- *Pathogenesis:* HPV infection, immunosuppression
- *Clinical features:* Multiple, small, skin colored or reddish-brown asymptomatic papules. Surface may be verrucous or smooth. Sometimes they coalesce to form plaque. Spontaneous regression can occur.
- *Site:* Penile shaft or glans for male, vulva or perianal area for female
- *HPE:* Hyperkeratosis with focal parakeratosis, dyskeratosis, hyperchromatic and pleomorphic nuclei of keratinocytes.
- *Complication:* Invasive SCC, though rare, can occur
- *Differential diagnosis:* Condyloma acuminata
- *Treatment:* Electrocautery, cryosurgery, chemical cautery (podophyllin, trichloroacetic acid), laser. Topical cidofovir, imiquimod **(Fig. 4)**

Extramammary Paget's Disease[7]

- *Introduction:* Extremely are condition represents as intraepidermal adenocarcinoma.
- *History:* First described Sir James Paget in 1874
- *Epidemiology:* Mostly affects elderly population; F>M
- *Pathogenesis:* Primary EMPD arises from intraepithelial adenocarcinoma. Secondary EMPD occurs due to extension of underlying adnexal or visceral adenocarcinoma (12% cases).
- *Clinical features:* Sharply demarcated itchy erythematous scaly plaque. Scattered areas of white scale and erosion can give rise to a "strawberries and cream" appearance.
- *Site:* The vulva in women and the perianal region in men.
- *HPE:* Vacuolated pagetoid cells with ample mucin in the epidermis are classical. Primary Paget's disease is GCDFP-15 positive, CK7 positive, CK20 negative.
- *Complication:* Adenocarcinoma
- *Differential diagnosis:* Bowen's disease, LSA, PKMB, Zoon balanitis, psoriasis
- *Treatment:* Topical imiquimod, 5-fluorouracil, radiotherapy, photodynamic therapy, CO_2 laser ablation. Wide local excision or Mohs micrographic surgery is

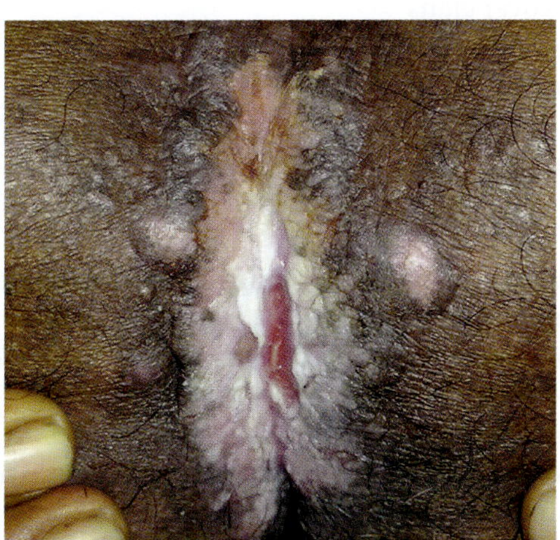

Fig. 3: Perianal Bowen's disease.

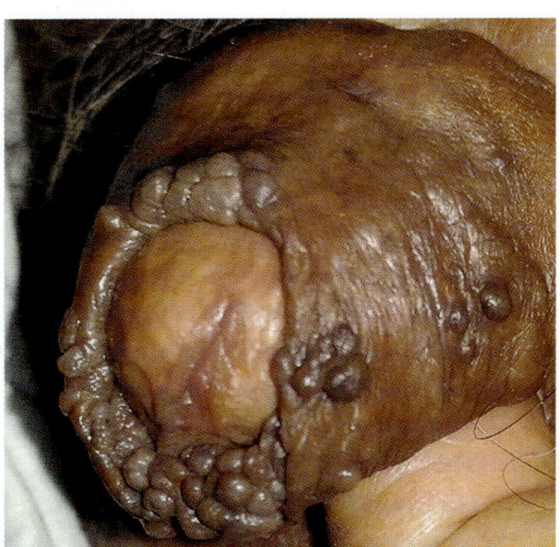

Fig. 4: Bowenoid papulosis.

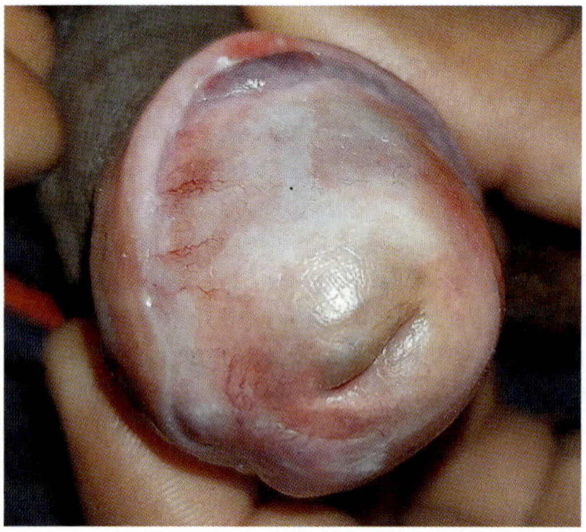

Fig. 5: Lichen sclerosus et atrophicus.

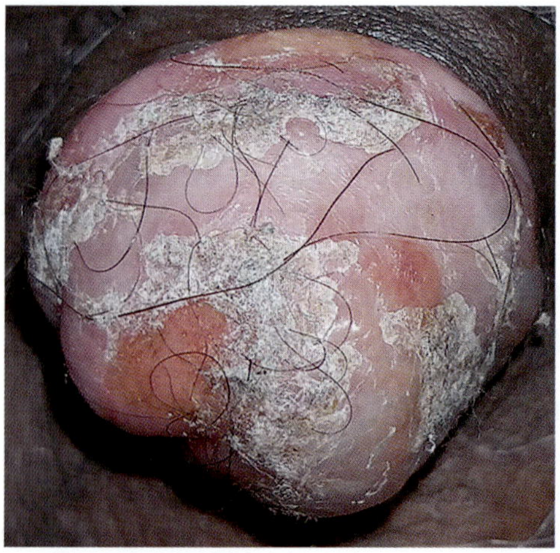

Fig. 6: Pseudoepitheliomatous keratotic micaceous balanitis.

recommended. Search for internal malignancy and long-term follow-up is necessary.

Lichen Sclerosus et Atrophicus

- *Introduction:* A chronic inflammatory disease that preferentially affects the anogenital region.
- *History:* Clinical description by Hallopeau in 1889 and histologic features described by Darier in 1892
- *Epidemiology:* Two peaks of onset—at childhood and after menopause. F>M. Asians and Africans commonly affected
- *Pathogenesis:* Familial (HLA-DRB1*12), autoimmune, infection (Borrelia or other spirochetal infection, HPV), friction, microurinary incontinences
- *Clinical features:* Vulvar hypopigmentation and atrophic skin in a figure-of-eight distribution encircling the vulvar and perianal region. Focal areas of erosion, fissure, purpura, telangiectasias, hemorrhagic bulla. Pruritus and pain is common
- *HPE:* Compact orthokeratosis, follicular plugging (in non-mucosal sites), epidermal thinning, vacuolization of the basal layer, and band-like lymphocytic infiltrate with hyalinization of the papillary dermis
- *Complication:* Fusion of the labia minora to the labia majora may occur leading to narrowing of the introitus. Dyspareunia, constipation, difficulty in micturition, malignant changes
- *Differential diagnosis:* Erosive lichen planus, vulvar eczema, lichen simplex chronicus, and vitiligo
- *Treatment:* Potent topical corticosteroid (for 3 months), topical calcineurin inhibitor, circumcision, and corrective surgery **(Fig. 5)**.

Pseudoepitheliomatous Keratotic Micaceous Balanitis[8]

- *Introduction:* An extremely rare premalignant condition
- *History:* Described by Lortat-Jacob and Civatte in 1961
- *Epidemiology:* Mostly occurs among elderly circumcised men.
- *Pathogenesis:* unknown; maybe infection (pyodermatitis, HPV), autoimmune (Reiter's)
- *Clinical features:* Well defined, dry, mica-like scaly, rough verrucous plaque mostly over the glans
- *HPE:* Massive hyperkeratosis, parakeratosis, epithelial hyperplasia without atypia and mild dermal lymphocytic infiltrate
- *Complication:* SCC.
- *Differential diagnosis:* Giant condyloma, psoriasis, SCC, erythroplasia of Queyrat
- *Treatment:* Topical 5FU, Imiquimod, cryotherapy. Surgical excision, if malignant transformation **(Fig. 6)**.

DISEASE PECULIAR TO GENITALIA

Circinate Balanitis

- *Introduction:* One of the most common mucocutaneous manifestations of reactive arthritis.
- *Pathogenesis:* Associated with reactive arthritis.
- *Clinical features:* Serpiginous ring-shaped erythematous lesion over glans
- *Complication:* Nothing such
- *Differential diagnosis:* Candidiasis
- *Treatment:* Topical corticosteroids and calcineurin inhibitors

Peyronie's Disease[9]

- *Introduction:* Acquired benign condition causes penile fibromatosis.
- *History:* First described by Francois Gigot de la Peyronie in 1743
- *Epidemiology:* Mostly among middle-aged men
- *Pathogenesis:* Unknown. May be associated with other fibromatous disease, genetic, atherosclerosis, veno-occlusive disease, sexual trauma, after reconstructive surgery. Fibrosis, calcification of the shaft occurs

- *Clinical features:* Cord-like subcutaneous plaques or palpable induration in the penile shaft. May present as curvature or indentation of erect penis, bending, penile pain, and erectile dysfunction
- *Complication:* Calcification and rarely ossification
- *Treatment:* Conservative therapy, spontaneous recovery in 20–30% cases. Intralesional corticosteroid, verapamil, interferon, clostridial collagenase injection; systemic vitamin E, colchicines, tamoxifen, acetyl-L-carnitine; surgical correction (Nesbit's operation), penile prosthesis.

Zoon's Plasma Cell Balanitis[10]

- *Introduction:* A benign nonvenereal dermatosis
- *Synonym:* Balanitis circumscripta plasmacellularis.
- *History:* Described by Zoon's in 1952
- *Epidemiology:* Mostly among uncircumscribed middle or old-aged men
- *Pathogenesis:* Trauma, friction, heat, infection (*Mycobacterium smegmatis*, HPV)
- *Clinical features:* Solitary, shiny, well-defined persistent erythematous plaque over glans. Pinpoint-speckled red spots over it—"cayenne pepper spot"
- *HPE:* Absence of horny and granular layer, spongiosis, necrotic keratinocytes, band-like infiltrate predominantly plasma cells, extravasated RBC.
- *Complication:* Superadded candidiasis
- *Differential diagnosis:* Lichen planus, erythroplasia of Queyrat, FDE, herpes.
- *Treatment:* Topical corticosteroid and calcineurin inhibitors. Relapse is common, circumcision is curative **(Fig. 7)**.

Fournier's Gangrene

- *Introduction:* A rare but life-threatening condition of genitalia
- *Synonym:* Idiopathic scrotal edema, synergistic gangrene, necrotizing fasciitis of perineum

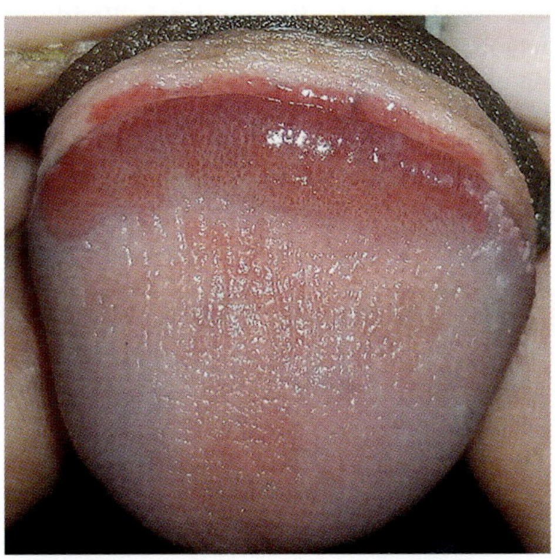

Fig. 7: Zoon's plasma cell balanitis.

- *History:* Named after French venereologist Jean Alfred Fournier
- *Pathogenesis:* Vascular compromise occurs following minor trauma due to any intervention topped with bacterial infection (*Streptococcus*, *Staphylococcus*, *E. coli*, *Clostridium*, Bacteriods). Diabetes, alcoholism, malnutrition old age, and HIV are the risk factors
- *HPE:* Huge inflammation, neutrophilic infiltration, necrosis, endarteritis obliterans
- *Clinical features:* Sudden onset pain and swelling of scrotum and prostration, pallor, and fever. Rapidly progresses to extensive necrosis
- *HPE:* Huge inflammation, neutrophilic infiltration, necrosis, endarteritis obliterans
- *Complication:* Rapidly worsens, sloughing off of the scrotal coverings, infection spreads in fascial planes, sepsis, multiorgan failure. Mortality is high (20–40%).
- *Differential diagnosis:* Cellulitis, vascular occlusive syndromes, PAN, and ecthyma gangrenosum
- *Treatment:* Broad-spectrum antibiotics initially then according to culture-sensitivity. Debridement of necrotic tissue, transplantation of testis, and skin grafts are absolutely necessary.

Angiokeratoma of Fordyce

- *Introduction:* It is a rare benign vascular lesion over scrotum.
- *History:* Described by Fordyce in 1896
- *Pathogenesis:* Degeneration of vascular elastic tissue, venous hypertension
- *Clinical features:* Multiple, tiny, discrete, reddish purple-colored soft compressible papules
- *Sites:* Scrotum (MC), penis, thigh, groin, abdomen, vulva.
- *HPE:* Epidermal hyperkeratosis, acanthosis. Numerous dilated and congested thin-walled blood vessels at papillary dermis
- *Complication:* Bleeding can occur due to trauma
- *Differential diagnosis:* Genital wart, melanoma
- *Treatment:* Electrocautery, cryosurgery, CO_2, laser ablation **(Fig. 8)**.

Balanitis Xerotica Obliterans (Fig. 9)

Introduction: Common penile disease mostly associated with lichen sclerosus.

History: First described in 1928 by Stuhmer.

Epidemiology: Mostly among child and middle-aged men.

Pathogenesis: Not clear but commonly associated with lichen sclerosus. It can be a consequence of other scarring dermatoses as lichen planus and cicatricial pemphigoid, causing chronic damage to glans and prepuce (Posthitis xerotica obliterans).

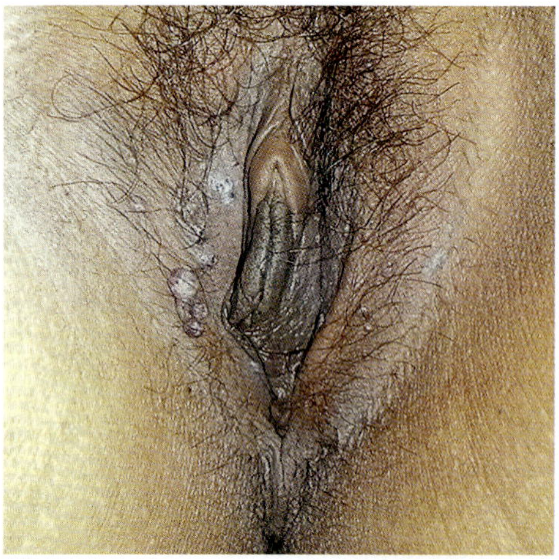

Fig. 8: Angiokeratoma of Fordyce over vulva.

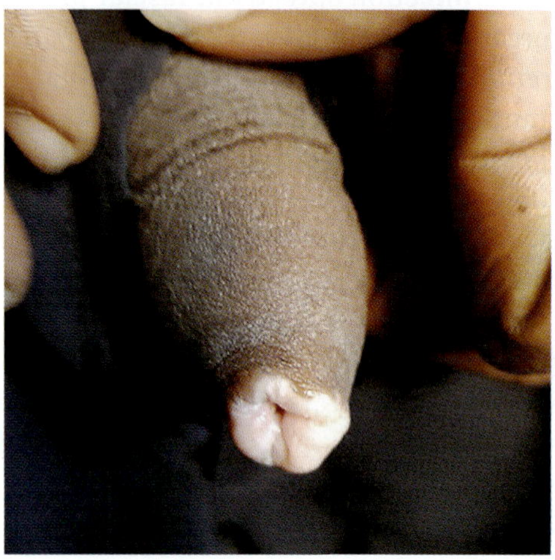

Fig. 9: Balanitis xerotica obliterans.
Courtesy: Dr Abhijit Saha.

Clinical features: Initially presents with grey-white skin discolouration, blistering and fissuring. In late stage, it causes phimosis, paraphimosis meatal stenosis, urethral strictures.

Complication: Secondary infection, urinary retention, chronic penile edema, chronic renal failure.

Differential diagnosis: Vitiligo and other causes of phimosis like non-specific balanoposthitis (e.g. in diabetes), lichen sclerosus, chronic penile lyphoedema, candidiasis.

Treatment: Potent topical steroid can be used initially. Circumcision can be a curative procedure. Meatoplasty, urethrotomy, urethral dilatation or urethroplasty maybe required, if complicated.

KEY POINTS

- Though dermatosis involving genitalia is mostly sexually transmitted, nonveneral genital dermatosis is not uncommon.
- They can either effect only genitalia or may be as a part of other dermatological condition occurring elsewhere, can be congenital also.
- They can affect any age group or sex.
- Diagnosis is sometimes difficult due to overlapping clinical features.
- Histopathological examination should be performed, whenever appropriate to diagnose the condition and to exclude malignancy.
- Early diagnosis and treatment are utmost necessary.
- Some are benign condition, reassurance is necessary.
- Treatment is mostly topical, but surgical interventions are required in some cases.

REFERENCES

1. Khaitan BK. Non-venereal diseases of genitalia. In: Sharma VK, (Ed). Sexually Transmitted Diseases and AIDS, 1st edition. New Delhi: Viva Books Pvt Ltd; 2003. pp. 413-21.
2. Lee JH, Lee JH, Kwon NH, Yu DS, Kim GM, Park CJ, et al. Clinicopathologic manifestations of patients with Fordyce's spots. Ann Dermatol. 2012; 24(1):103-6.
3. Agrawal SK, Bhattacharya SN, Singh N. Pearly penile papules: a review. Int J Dermatol. 2004;43:199-201.
4. Fanning DM, Flood H. Erythroplasia of Queyrat. Clin Pract. 2012;2(3):e63.
5. Dandale A, Mantri MD, Thakkar V, Dhurat RS, Ghate S. Bowen's disease: an unusual clinical presentation. Indian Dermatol Online J. 2014;5(4):526-8.
6. Shastry V, Betkerur J, Kushalappa. Indian J Dermatol. 2009; 54(3):283-6.
7. Ekwueme KC, Zakhour HD, Parr NJ. Extramammary Paget's disease of the penis: a case report and review of the literature. J Med Case Rep. 2009:3:4.
8. Murthy PS, Kanak K, Raveendra L, Reddy P. Pseudo-epitheliomatous, keratotic, and micaceous balanitis. Indian J Dermatol. 2010;55:190-1.
9. Jalkut M, Cadavid NZ , Rajfer J. Peyronie's disease: a review. Rev Urol. 2003; 5(3):142-8.
10. Dayal S, Sahu P. Zoon balanitis: a comprehensive review. Indian J Sex Transm Dis AIDS. 2016; 37(2):129-38.

EXAMINATION QUESTIONS

Write short notes on the following:
1. Non-veneral diseases of genitalia.
2. Premalignant condition of genitalia.
3. Balanitis xerotica obliterans.
4. Lichen sclerosus et atrophicus.
5. Zoon's plasma cell balanitis.

138 CHAPTER

Syndromic Management in Sexually Transmitted Infection

Devinder Mohan Thappa, Mary Zothanpuii Chhangte

INTRODUCTION

A syndrome is defined as a group of common symptoms and signs caused by more than one organism. A sexually transmitted infection/reproductive tract infection (STI/RTI) syndrome is a combination of symptoms and signs typically associated with sexually transmitted micro-organisms.[1]

In 1991, syndromic management approach was developed by World Health Organization (WHO) to address the limitation of etiological and presumptive diagnosis. Syndromic approach uses clinical algorithms based on a sexually transmitted disease (STD), constellation of symptoms and clinical signs, to determine therapy.[2]

The aim of STI/RTI syndromic case management is to identify the syndrome correctly and manage them accordingly. While clinical diagnosis is based on identifying the specific causative agent, syndromic diagnosis leads to immediate treatment for all of the most important possible causative agents. This is important because mixed infections occur frequently in STI/RTI. Besides, syndromic management of STI/RTI can effectively treat cases in settings with limited or no laboratory facilities. This means syndromic treatment can quickly render the patient noninfectious.[1]

It is important to understand that in our country, where diagnostic services are limited, the only reliable way to manage STIs is through syndromic management approach.[3]

Syndromic approach overcomes the problems associated with etiological diagnosis as:

- Many of the tests for STIs are expensive and time consuming
- Frequent visits of patients are required
- Patients have to travel long distances, which may lead to them not reporting for subsequent follow-ups.
- Delay in starting treatment leads to prolonged period of infectivity.

Advantages of syndromic management are given in **Box 1**.

BOX 1: Advantages of syndromic management.

- Current requirement at present
- Less dependent on laboratory tests
- Readymade tool in the hands of healthcare provider
- Helps to provide wide scale sexually transmitted infection (STI) clinic services reducing STI burden
- Treatment at first contact reduces the period of infection and reduces chances of losing the patient for treatment
- Waiting time in STI clinic is reduced
- More successful cure rates
- General practitioners can also treat STIs using syndromic approach
- Provides opportunities for promoting preventive measures such as condom use
- Quickly render patients noninfectious and takes care of mixed infections that are common in STIs[4]

OBJECTIVES OF STI/RTI SYNDROMIC MANAGEMENT[5]

- Enhance access to STI/RTI control and prevention services to all, especially for pregnant and nonpregnant women, adolescents, and high-risk group population who are constrained to seek services and face several access-related barriers.
- Focus on prevention, with special reference to counseling, partner management, condom demonstration, and provision; follow-up and management of side effects.
- Emphasis mostly on single-dose regimens and directly observed therapy (DOT) for better treatment adherence and outcomes.
- Reinforce behavior change communication—interpersonal communication leading to improved knowledge on causation, transmission, and prevention of STI/RTI.
- Ensure good linkages with obstetrics and gynecology, antenatal clinic (ANC), and cross-referral linkages with integrated counseling and testing centers (ICTC), prevention of parent to child transmission centers, antiretroviral therapy (ART) centers, blood banks, adolescent reproductive sexual health (ARSH) clinic, designated microscopy centers [Revised National Tuberculosis Control Program (RNTCP)], and community support centers including people living with HIV (PLHIV) networks and targeted intervention projects. Ensure linkages also with regional and state STI training and reference laboratories, especially for managing suspected treatment failure and persistent cases.
- Screen all attendees of designated STI/RTI clinic and ANC clinic for syphilis and HIV preferably through single window and single-prick testing.
- Ensure nonjudgmental STI/RTI control and prevention service provision for high-risk groups such as male and

female sex workers, men who have sex with men, transsexuals/transgenders, and people who inject drugs (PWID).

- Offer interactive counseling to clients by all healthcare providers, counselors, and other clinical staffs. Client-centered STI/RTI/HIV counseling can increase the likelihood that the patient undertakes or enhances risk-reduction practices.

ESSENTIAL STEPS OF STI/RTI SYNDROMIC CASE MANAGEMENT

The essential steps of STI/RTI syndromic case management are given in **Box 2**.

BEHAVIORAL RISK ASSESSMENT

If the patient is to receive proper education and counseling, these must be preceded by behavior risk assessment. Make sure that the patient is aware that the history will be kept strictly confidential. Inquire about the following risk factors:

- *Marital status*: Married, living together, single, separated, and widowed
- *Occupation*: Sex workers (male and female), seamen, workers in the hospitality industry, transport workers, migrant workers, etc.
- *Travel*: Frequent traveler (holidays, business, or employment)
- Unprotected casual sexual encounters (other than with regular partner)
- Previous history of STI
- History of injections or blood transfusions
- *Substance use*: Alcohol and drugs (e.g., heroin)
- Tattooing
- Partner with symptoms suggestive of STI
- Multiple sexual partners

BOX 2: Essential steps of STI/RTI syndromic case management.

- History taking
- *Clinical examination*: Genital/oral and anorectal apart from general examination
- Appropriate syndromic diagnosis as per syndromic flowcharts
- Minimal laboratory tests (VDRL and HIV testing), wherever available
- Early and effective treatment, preferably single dose and directly observed
- Promotion and provision of condoms
- Counseling for behavior change and risk reduction
- Referral for syphilis screening and HIV counseling and testing
- Partner(s) notification and management
- Follow-up as per schedule
- Documentation of case details and laboratory results

(HIV: human immunodeficiency virus; STI/RTI: sexually transmitted infection/reproductive tract infection; VDRL: venereal disease research laboratory)

SEXUAL HISTORY

A sexual history must be taken from all patients before examining them and managing their sexual health problems. All individuals should be asked about the following:

- Sex of the partner
- Type of exposure (oral, vaginal, and anal)
- Use of condoms with any type of partner
- Relationship to partner/s (spouse, regular nonspouse, and casual)
- Problems or symptoms in the partner/s
- Date of last sexual intercourse
- Number of partners in the past 3 months

CLINICAL EXAMINATION

This is an important step to arrive at a probable syndromic diagnosis and avoids making an incorrect diagnosis based on the patient's history alone. Inform the patient that you will do a genital examination and obtain the patient's permission to do so. Ensure privacy during the examination. Always have a female attendant when examining a female patient (particularly if the healthcare provider is a male).

Genital examination includes a bimanual and speculum examination of the genital tract for all female patients, and rectal examination (including proctoscopy, if indicated and available) for patients (male and female) practicing receptive anal sex.[1]

The commonly encountered STI syndromes are given in **Box 3**.[3]

Table 1 will guide on how to approach any of the below-mentioned syndromes.[1] It is based on history, causative organisms and examination findings Treatment is based on STI syndrome.

MANAGEMENT

Management is based on the STI syndrome and accordingly supported by relevant flowcharts.

Urethral Discharge

Approach to the management of urethral discharge is shown in **Flowchart 1**.

Genital Ulcer

Approach to the management of genital ulcer is shown in **Flowchart 2**.

BOX 3: The commonly encountered STI syndromes.

- Urethral discharge in men
- Genital ulcer—herpetic and nonherpetic
- Vaginal discharge
- Cervical discharge
- Lower abdominal pain in women
- Inguinal bubo
- Scrotal swelling
- Neonatal conjunctivitis

TABLE 1: Approach of sexually transmitted infection (STI) syndromes.

Syndrome	*History*	*Causative organisms*	*Examination findings*	*Treatment*
Vaginal discharge syndrome (vaginitis/ vaginosis)	• Nature and type of discharge (quantity, smell, color, and consistency) • Genital itching • Burning while passing urine, increased frequency • Any ulcer, swelling on the vulval or inguinal region • Genital complaints in sexual partners • Low backache • Menstrual history to rule out pregnancy	*Trichomonas vaginalis* (TV), *Candida albicans*, *Gardnerella vaginalis*, *Mycoplasma*, *Urea-plasma*, and other fastidious and unculti-vated anaerobes	• Differentiate between vaginitis and cervicitis • Trichomoniasis—greenish frothy discharge • Candidiasis—curdy white discharge • Bacterial vaginosis—adherent discharge • Mixed infections may present with atypical discharge	Tablet secnidazole 2 g orally, single dose *OR* Tablet tinidazole 500 mg orally, twice daily for 5 days *OR* Tablet metronidazole 400 mg, twice daily for 7 days plus tablet fluconazole 150 mg orally single dose
Cervical discharge syndrome (cervicitis)	• Nature and type of discharge (quantity, smell, color, and consistency) • Genital itching • Burning while passing urine, increased frequency • Any ulcer and/or swelling on the vulval or inguinal region • Low backache • Menstrual history to rule out pregnancy • Problems or symptoms in the sexual partners	• *Neisseria gonorrhoeae* • *Chlamydia trachomatis* • Others: – *Trichomonas vaginalis* – Herpes simplex virus – Human papillomavirus	Two major diagnostic signs characterize cervicitis: 1. A purulent or mucopurulent endocervical exudate visible in the endocervical canal or on an endocervical swab specimen 2. Sustained endocervical bleeding easily induced by gentle passage of a cotton swab through the cervical os Following are features suggestive of cervicitis: – Erythematous cervix – Mucopurulent cervical discharge Bimanual pelvic examination to rule out pelvic inflammatory disease (PID)	Tablet cefixime 400 mg orally, single dose *PLUS* Tablet azithromycin 1 g, 1 hour before food
Urethral discharge/ burning micturition	• Sexual exposure including high-risk practices like orogenital sex in the previous two months/urethral discharge • Pain or burning while passing urine • Increased frequency of urination	• *Neisseria gonorrhoeae* • *Chlamydia trachomatis* • *Trichomonas vaginalis* • Other organisms such as *Mycoplasma genitalium*, herpes simplex virus, enteric bacteria, and adeno-virus	• Redness and swelling of the urethral meatus • Presence of urethral discharge • If urethral discharge is not seen, then gently massage the urethra from the ventral part of the penis toward the meatus and look for thick, creamy greenish-yellow or mucoid discharge	Tablet cefixime 400 mg orally, single dose *PLUS* Tablet azithromycin 1 g orally single dose under supervision *OR* Capsule doxycycline 100 mg twice a day for 7 days • When symptoms persist (discharge or only dysuria persists after 7 days) after adequate treatment in the index client and partner(s), they should be treated for *T. vaginalis* with tablet secnidazole 2 g orally, single dose (to treat for *T. vaginalis*) • Even after the above treatment, if symptoms persist, refer the patient to higher center

Contd...

Contd...

Syndrome	*History*	*Causative organisms*	*Examination findings*	*Treatment*
Genital ulcer disease (nonherpetic)	• Genital ulcer • Burning sensation in the genital region • Sexual exposure of either partner including high-risk practices like orogenital sex	• *Treponema pallidum* (syphilis) • *Haemophilus ducreyi* (chancroid) • *Klebsiella granulomatis* (granuloma inguinale) • *Chlamydia trachomatis* (lymphogranuloma venereum)	• Presence of genital ulcer—single or multiple • *Ulcer characteristics:* – Painless ulcer with firm lymph nodes—syphilis – Painless ulcer without inguinal lymph nodes—granuloma inguinale – Transient painless penile ulcer with painful, enlarged inguinal lymph nodes—lymphogranuloma venereum (LGV) – Painful ulcers usually multiple and associated with painful bubo—chancroid	Injection benzathine penicillin 2.4 million IU IM single dose after test dose in two divided doses (with emergency tray ready) (for syphilis) *PLUS* • Tablet azithromycin 1 g orally single dose/ erythromycin 500 mg four times a day for 7 days *OR* • Tablet ciprofloxacin 500 mg orally, twice a day for 3 days (for chancroid) In individuals allergic or intolerant to penicillin • Capsule doxycycline 100 mg orally, twice daily for 15 days *OR* • Tablet azithromycin 2 g as a single dose to treat early syphilis
Genital ulcer disease (herpetic)	• Genital ulcer/vesicles • Burning sensation in the genital region • Sexual exposure of either partner including practices like orogenital sex • Recurrent lesions or history of similar lesions in the past	Herpes simplex virus (genital herpes)	• Presence of vesicles • Presence of multiple genital erosions/ulcer	• *In primary episodes (first episodes):* Tablet acyclovir 400 mg three times a day for 7 days • *For recurrences:* Tablet acyclovir 400 mg orally, three times a day for 7 days. • *For further investigations* refer to higher center, if not responding to treatment
Painful scrotal swelling	• Swelling and pain in scrotum • Pain or burning while passing urine • Urethral discharge • Systemic symptoms such as malaise and fever	• *Neisseria gonorrhoeae* • *Chlamydia trachomatis* • Also caused infrequently by: – Non-STI such as tuberculosis, filariasis, coliforms, pseudomonas, mumps virus infection – Noninfectious such as trauma with or without hematoma and torsion	• Redness and edema of the overlying skin and raised local temperature • Tenderness of the epididymis and vas deferens • Associated urethral discharge/ genital ulcer/inguinal lymph nodes—if present, refer to the respective flowchart • A transillumination test to rule out hydrocele	Tablet cefixime 400 mg orally, single dose *PLUS* • Tablet azithromycin 1 g orally single dose under supervision • Advise the client to return after 7 days of start of therapy • Supportive therapy to reduce pain (bed rest, scrotal elevation with T-bandage and analgesics)

Contd...

Contd...

Syndrome	*History*	*Causative organisms*	*Examination findings*	*Treatment*
Lower abdominal pain	• Fever • Vaginal discharge • Menstrual irregularities such as heavy and irregular vaginal bleeding • Dysmenorrhea • Dyspareunia • Dysuria, tenesmus • Low backache • Contraceptive use like intrauterine device (IUD)	• *Neisseria gonorrhoeae* • *Chlamydia trachomatis* • *Mycoplasma, Gardnerella,* anaerobic bacteria (*Bacteroides* spp., gram-positive cocci)	• *General examination:* Temperature, pulse, and blood pressure • *Per speculum examination:* Vaginal/cervical discharge, congestion or ulcers • *Per abdominal examination:* Lower abdominal tenderness or guarding • *Pelvic examination:* – Uterine/adnexal tenderness – Cervical movement tenderness	In mild or moderate PID (absence of tubo-ovarian abscess), outpatient treatment can be given • Tablet cefixime 400 mg orally STAT *PLUS* • Tablet metronidazole 400 mg orally, twice daily for 14 days (to treat anaerobic infection) *PLUS* • Capsule doxycycline 100 mg orally, twice a day for 14 days (to treat chlamydial infection) • Tablet ibuprofen 400 mg orally, three times a day for 3–5 days • Tablet ranitidine 150 mg orally, twice daily to prevent gastritis • Remove intrauterine device, if present, under antibiotic cover of 24–48 hours • Observe for 3 days. If no improvement (i.e., absence of fever, reduction in abdominal tenderness, reduction in cervical movement, adnexal, and uterine tenderness) or if symptoms worsen, refer for inpatient treatment
Inguinal bubo	• Swelling in inguinal region which may be painful • Preceding history of genital ulcer • Sexual exposure of either partner including practices such as orogenital sex • Systemic symptoms such as malaise and fever	• *Chlamydia trachomatis* (L1, L2, and L3) • *Klebsiella granulomatis* (donovanosis) • *Treponema pallidum* • *Haemophilus ducreyi*	• Localized enlargement of lymph nodes in the groin which may be tender and fluctuant • Inflammation of skin over the swelling • Presence of multiple sinuses • Edema of genitals and lower limbs • Presence of genital ulcer or urethral discharge	Capsule doxycycline 100 mg orally twice daily for 21 days *PLUS* • Tablet azithromycin 1 g orally *OR* • Tablet ciprofloxacin 500 mg orally, twice a day for 3 days to cover chancroid A bubo should never be incised and drained at the primary health center, even if it is fluctuant, as there is a high risk of a fistula formation and chronicity. If a bubo becomes fluctuant always aspirate
Neonatal conjunctivitis	• Maternal infection with STI • Exposure of the infant to infectious organisms • Inadequacy of ocular prophylaxis immediately after birth • Premature rupture of membrane • Ocular trauma during delivery • Mechanical ventilation • Prematurity	• *Neisseria gonorrhoeae* • *Chlamydia trachomatis* • *Streptococcus pneumoniae* • *Haemophilus influenzae* • *Staphylococcus aureus*	• Red and edematous conjunctiva • Edematous eye lid • Discharge which may be purulent • Orbital cellulitis in more serious cases	• Ceftriaxone 50 mg/kg IM stat maximum dose 125 mg/kg body weight • Spectinomycin 25 mg/kg IM stat maximum dose 75 mg plus erythromycin 50 mg/kg orally in four divided doses for 14 days

Flowchart 1: Urethral discharge.

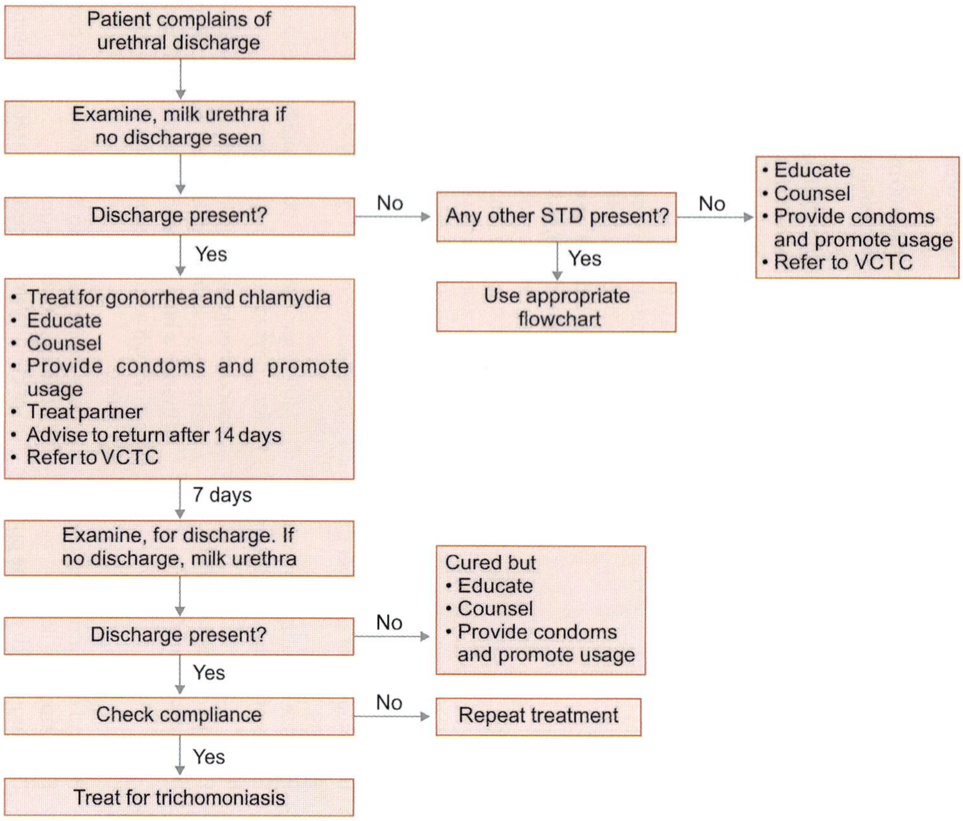

(STD: sexually transmitted disease; VCTC: voluntary counseling and testing centers)

Flowchart 2: Genital ulcer.

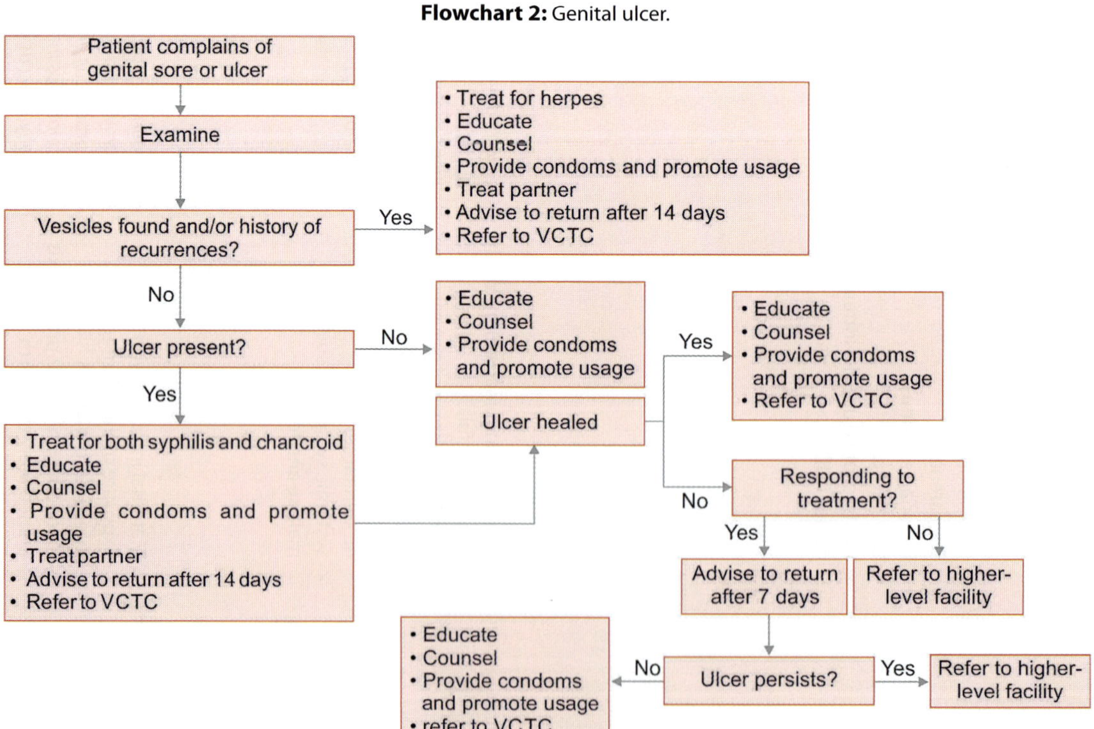

(VCTC: voluntary counseling and testing centers)

Flowchart 3: Vaginal discharge syndrome (without speculum examination).

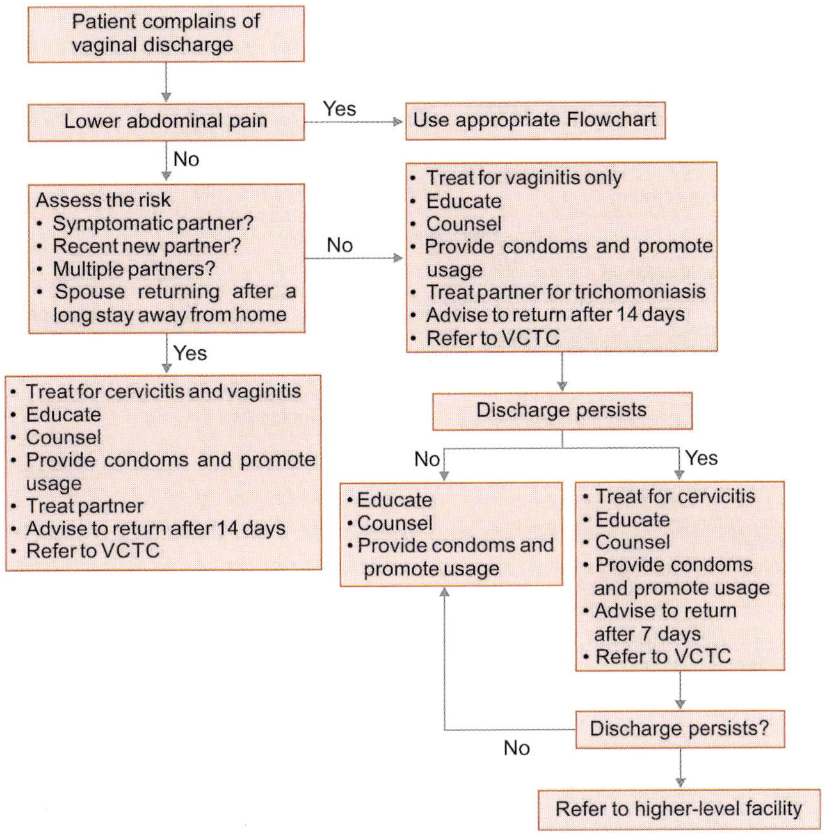

Flowchart 4: Vaginal discharge syndrome (with speculum examination).

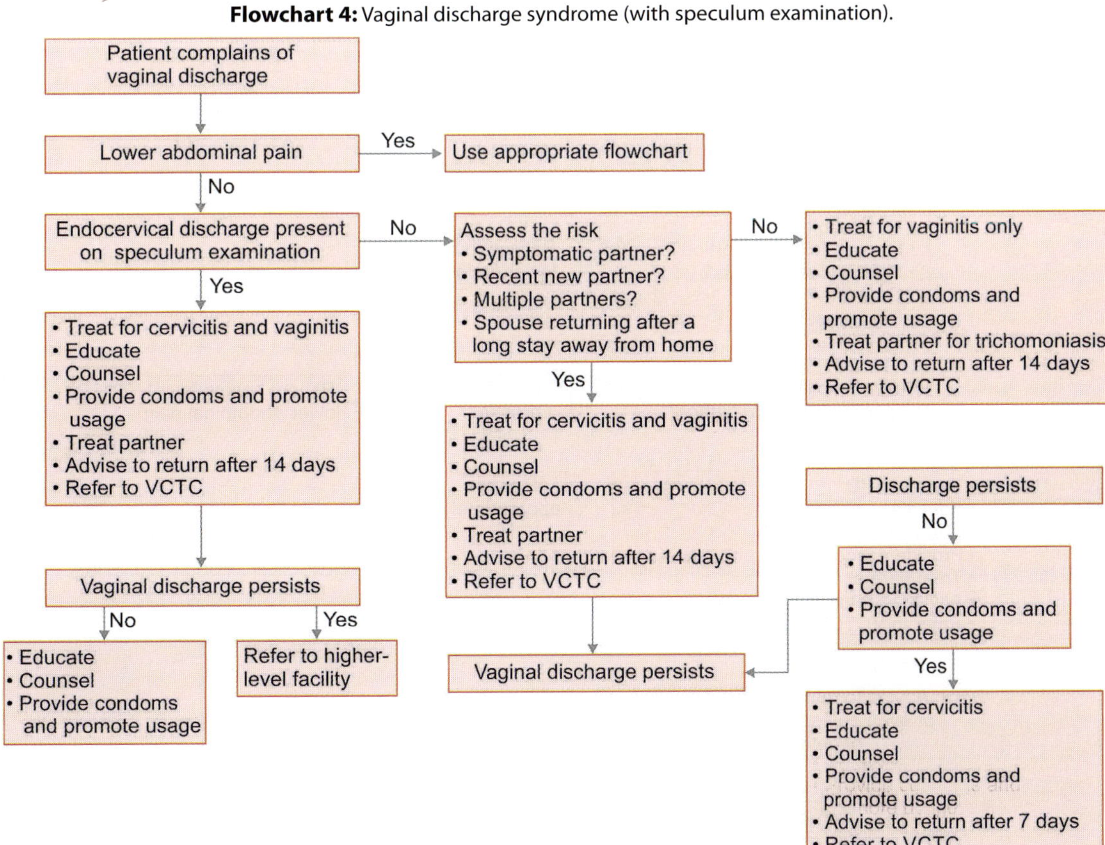

Flowchart 5: Scrotal swelling.

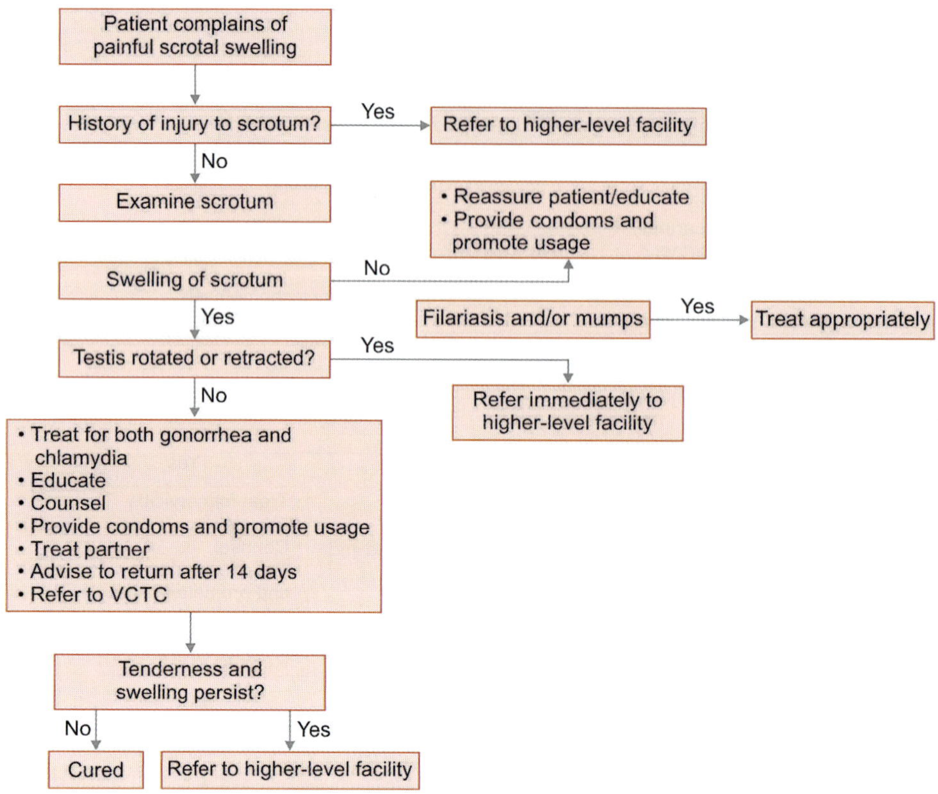

Flowchart 6: Lower abdominal pain in the female.

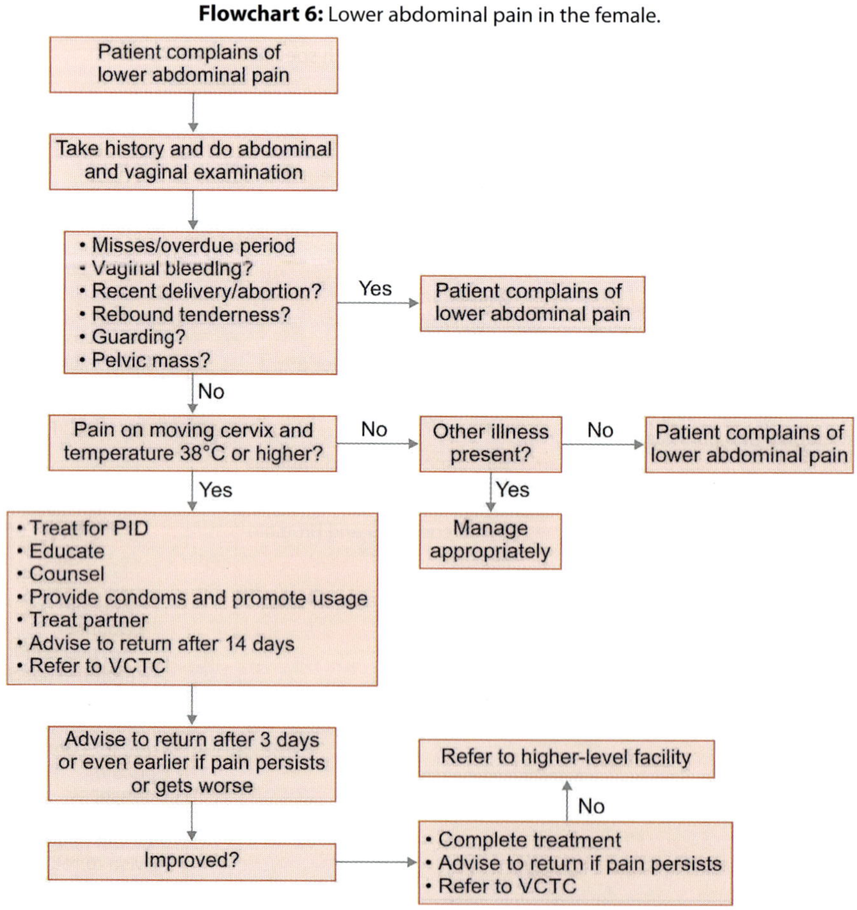

Flowchart 7: Inguinal bubo.

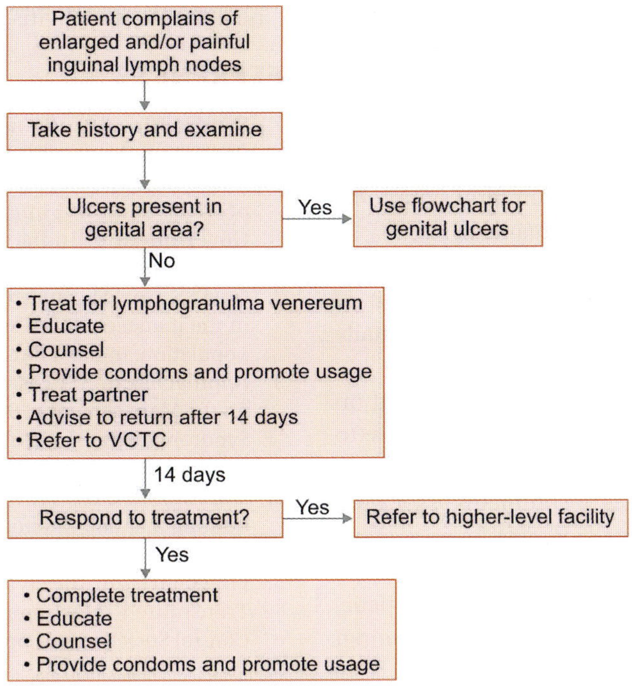

Flowchart 8: Ophthalmia neonatorum (neonatal conjunctivitis).

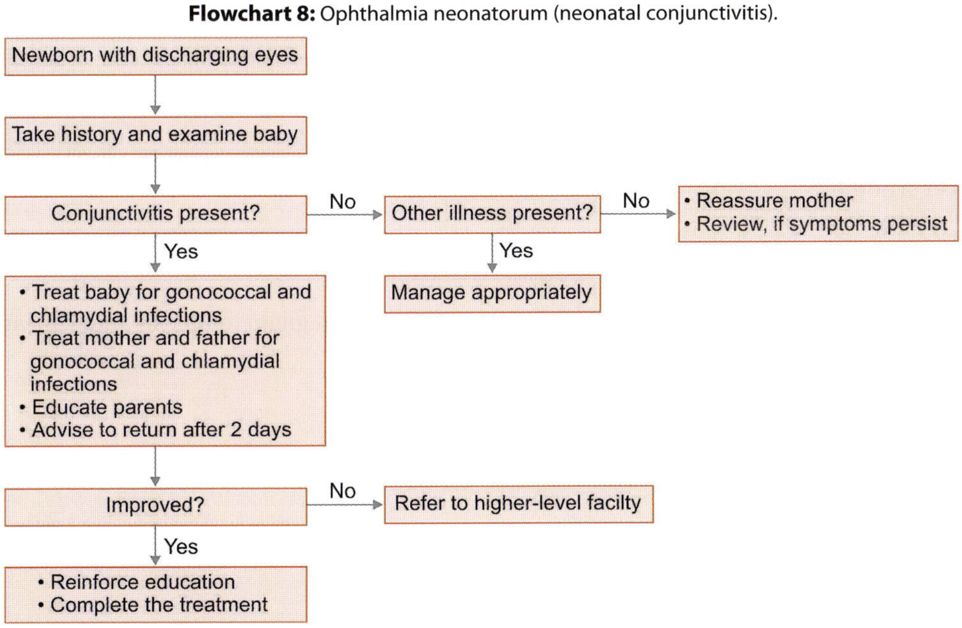

Vaginal Discharge Syndrome

Approaches to the management of vaginal discharge syndrome (without speculum examination and with speculum examination) are shown in **Flowcharts 3 and 4,** respectively.

Vaginal Discharge Syndrome (With Speculum Examination)

Approach to the management of vaginal discharge syndrome (with speculum examination) is shown in **Flowchart 4**.

Scrotal Swelling

Approach to the management of scrotal swelling is shown in **Flowchart 5**.

Lower Abdominal Pain in the Female

Approach to the management of lower abdominal pain in the female is shown in **Flowchart 6**.

Inguinal Bubo

Approach to the management of inguinal bubo is shown in **Flowchart 7**.

Ophthalmia Neonatorum

Approach to the management of ophthalmia neonatorum is shown in **Flowchart 8**.

KEY POINTS

- A syndrome is defined as a group of common symptoms and signs caused by more than one organism.
- A sexually transmitted infection/reproductive tract infection (STI/RTI) syndrome is a combination of symptoms and signs typically associated with sexually transmitted microorganisms.
- Syndromic approach uses clinical algorithms based on a STD, constellation of symptoms and clinical signs, to determine therapy.
- Syndromic approach overcomes the problems associated with etiological diagnosis.
- The commonly encountered STI syndromes are urethral discharge in men, genital ulcer—herpetic and nonherpetic, vaginal discharge, cervical discharge, lower abdominal pain in women, inguinal bubo, scrotal swelling, and neonatal conjunctivitis.

REFERENCES

1. Syndromic case management. National Guidelines on Prevention, Management and Control of Reproductive Tract Infections and Sexually Transmitted Infections. Department of AIDS Control, Ministry of Health and Family Welfare, Government of India, July 2014. National AIDS Control Organization; 2014. pp. 6-36.
2. Goel SS, Goel SS. Study of syndromic management approach in the management of sexually transmitted diseases in rural population. Indian J Sex Transm Dis AIDS. 2012;33(2):146-7.
3. Approaches to STI case management. National Guidelines for the Management of Sexually Transmitted Infections Using Syndromic Approach, July 2015. Federal Democratic Republic of Ethiopia Ministry of Health; 2015. pp. 6-7.
4. CAPACS. STI/HIV/AIDS Prevention Education—Doctors training manual. Chennai: Corporation AIDS Prevention and Control Society; 2006. pp. 48-61.
5. Flowcharts on the Syndromic Management of Sexually Transmitted Infections. Chennai: Tamil Nadu State AIDS Control Society; 2007. pp. 1-11.

EXAMINATION QUESTIONS

1. Name the commonly encountered STI syndromes. Write the steps involved in STI syndromic management.
2. With a flowchart, show the syndromic management of vaginal discharge.
3. What are the advantages and disadvantages of syndromic management?
4. Write short notes on the following:
   a. Genital ulcer syndrome
   b. Urethral discharge syndrome
   c. Inguinal bubo
   d. Scrotal swelling—syndromic management
5. How will you approach a case of genital ulcer disease in a 25-year-old pregnant female in 2nd trimester?

139 CHAPTER HIV: Introduction and Virology

Jayadev Betkerur, Vinutha Rangappa

INTRODUCTION

The natural course of human immunodeficiency virus (HIV) infection varies widely ultimately leading to death, if left untreated. Hence, a brief knowledge about HIV structure and its replication is necessary for better understanding and control of the disease.

This chapter focuses on the structure and replication of the virus.

HISTORY[1]

In 1983, Barré-Sinoussi et al. detected retroviral particles in a patient with lymphadenopathy. During the next year, Luc Montagnier of France and Robert Gallo of USA independently isolated and cultured the virus from affected patients and was named as Human T-cell lymphotropic virus III (HTLV-III) by Gallo. In the same year, Levy et al. isolated the virus from acquired immunodeficiency syndrome (AIDS) patient and called it AIDS-related virus (ARV). An international committee in 1986 finally named the causative agent as HIV-1. A new lentivirus, sub-related but distinct from HIV-1, was isolated from western Africa and was named as HIV-2.

TRANSMISSION[1]

There are three routes through which HIV can be transmitted. This includes:

1. *Sexual*: This is the most common route. The sexual contact may be heterosexual, homosexuals, bisexuals, and also through artificial insemination. The chances seem to be high among men who have sex with men (MSM). Presence of genital ulcers increases the risk of transmission.
2. *Perinatal*: From infected mother to the newborn either transplacentally, at time of birth and/or through breast milk
3. *Parenterally*: Through infected needles among intravenous drug users (IDUs), blood transfusion or other contaminated body fluids

VIRUS

Human immunodeficiency virus is a single-stranded RNA virus belonging to family Retroviridae. Retroviruses possess a specific enzyme called RNA-dependent DNA polymerase or reverse transcriptase (RT), which has the ability to reverse the ordinary flow of genetic information. HIV is grouped as HIV-1 and 2.

Characteristics of Classification HIV-1 and HIV-2[2,3]

Group M is the predominant circulating HIV-1 group. It has been divided into subtypes, denoted with letters, and sub-subtypes, denoted with numerals. This includes A1, A2, A3, A4, B, C, D, F1, F2, G, H, J, and K. HIV-1 subtypes, also called clades, are phylogenetically linked strains of HIV-1 and are also linked geographically or epidemiologically **(Table 1)**.

Structure

The structure of human immunodeficiency virus is shown in **Figure 1**.

The mature HIV particle under electron microscope is round with central electron dense core region surrounded by lipid envelope.

HIV-1 Genome[4,5]

The structure of HIV-1 genome is shown in **Figure 2**.

It consists of 8.5–9 kb of protein coding information. It encodes for at least nine genes.

Structural genes:

- *Gag*: It encodes for proteins:
  - p17 forming the symmetrical outer capsid membrane
  - p24 forming the inner icosahedral capsid
  - Nucleocapsid (p9) is a small protein found in association with viral genome.
- *Pol*: This gene encodes for viral enzymes RT, integrase (IN), and protease (PR) (discussed later).
- *Env*: This gene encodes for surface gp120 and transmembrane gp41 protein.

TABLE 1: Characteristics of *HIV-1* and *HIV-2*.

	HIV-1	*HIV-2*
Types and subtypes	M, N, O M—A, B, C, D, F, G, H, K	
Transmission	Chimpanzee	Sooty mangabey monkeys
Distribution	Worldwide	Central and western Africa
Virulence	High	Low

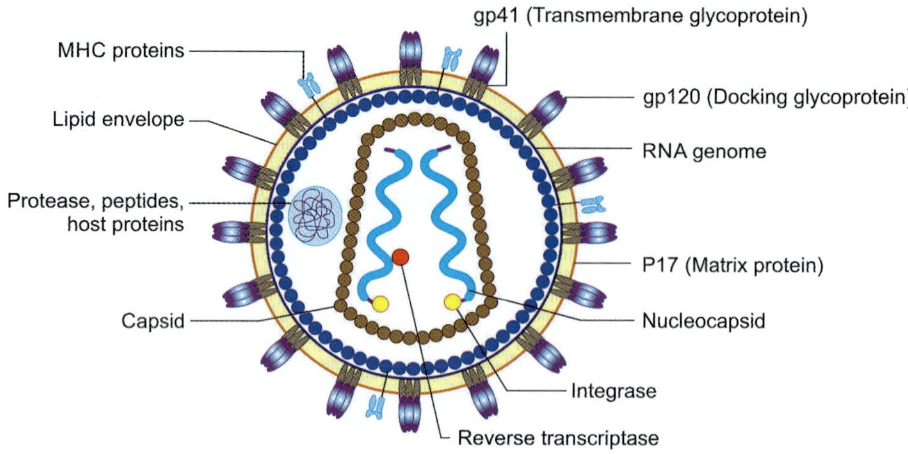

Fig. 1: Structure of human immunodeficiency virus.
Source: https://mappingignorance.org/10.01.2013/towards-a-vaccine-against-hiv.

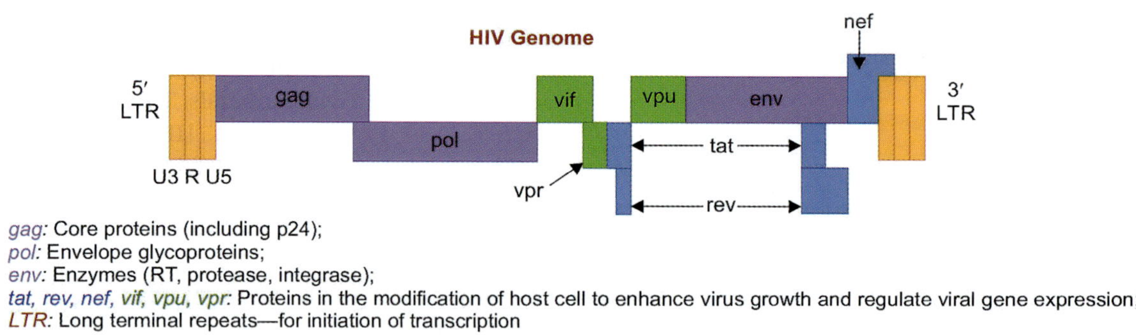

Fig. 2: Genomic representation of HIV-1.
Source: https://www.slideshare.net/129109141918/lecture-on-aids-for-mbbs.

Regulatory genes:

- *Tat*: Transactivator of transcription, accelerates the availability of viral RNA, and transactivates additional HIV genomes.
- *Nef*: Negative regulation factor, reduces rate of RNA initiation.
- *Rev*: Regulation of expression, helps to maintain the full length unspliced RNA in the nucleus.

Accessory genes: They are *vpu, vpr,* and *vif* genes. They regulate the rate of viral replication.

Viral enzymes[6]*:* The RNA genome encodes for three different enzymes necessary for viral replication.

1. *Reverse transcriptase*: It is responsible for conversion of single-stranded genomic RNA to double-stranded proviral DNA. It is a heterodimer composed of two subunits—66 kDa and 51 kDa. They are devoid of 3′-5′ exonucleolytic proofreading activity. Thus an error-prone enzyme resulting in error frequency. This corresponds to one new nucleotide substitution per genome per replication cycle. RTs have two distinct activities, DNA polymerase which uses viral RNA as a template to produce double-stranded DNA, an essential step in viral replication and RNase H activity which degrades the synthesized genomic hybrids to form single-stranded DNA. Most of the antiretroviral therapy (ART) drugs act by inhibiting this enzyme.
2. *Integrase (IN)*: After formation of viral DNA by RT, IN recognizes the two viral DNA ends and through 3′ processing transports to host cell chromosomal DNA to form provirus. The site of integration is usually random. Drugs such as raltegravir, dolutegravir act by inhibiting this enzyme.
3. *Viral protease (PR)*: PR plays a critical role at the last stage of viral replication. In the absence of effective viral PR, the virus remains noninfectious. It cleaves newly synthesized polyprotein at the appropriate sites to create mature protein components. There exist two different types of cleavage sites. Knowing this helps in developing broad-spectrum inhibitors for HIV. The ART drugs belonging to protease inhibitors, which form the second line of highly active antiretroviral therapy (HAART), act at this level.

HIV Co-receptors[7]

The primary receptors for HIV are identified as CD4+ T-cells. HIV-1 virion has affinity toward CXCR4 and CCR5 co-receptors expressed on the CD4 cells. These co-receptors have a key role in immune signaling and T-cell function. CCR5 antagonists such as maraviroc are effective at this level. Many CXCR4 antagonists are under investigation.

Complex expression pattern for HIV receptor, co-receptors, surface adhesion molecules, and alternate receptors that individually or collectively could support extension and stable virion binding.

HIV Replication Cycle (Fig. 3)[8,9]

The life cycle of retrovirus is divided into two distinct phases:

1. *Early phase*: It starts from binding of virus to the host cell surface till integration of the viral genome to host cell DNA.
2. *Late phase*: It begins with the expression of viral genes till the release and maturation of viral progeny.

Retroviruses face multiple obstacles during their entire journey from cell surface binding to the release of provirus. They will have to cross two main barriers—the plasma and nuclear membrane. The surge of HIV research in order to identify new therapeutic targets has led to better understanding of each step of the viral life cycle. However, few steps are still poorly understood.

Binding

The virus binds to the CD4 receptors and co-receptors (CXCR 4 and CCR 5) by way of gp120 protein. The virus can also infect several cell types of glial and neuroblastoma cell lines. Other modes of binding to cells include binding of antibody coated to Fc receptors of macrophages.

Entry

The initial step of binding of gp120 to CD4 receptors and co-receptors triggers conformational shifts in the env proteins leading to insertion of gp41 fusion peptide into target membrane. This fusion of viral to cellular membrane results in release of the viral core into the cytoplasm.

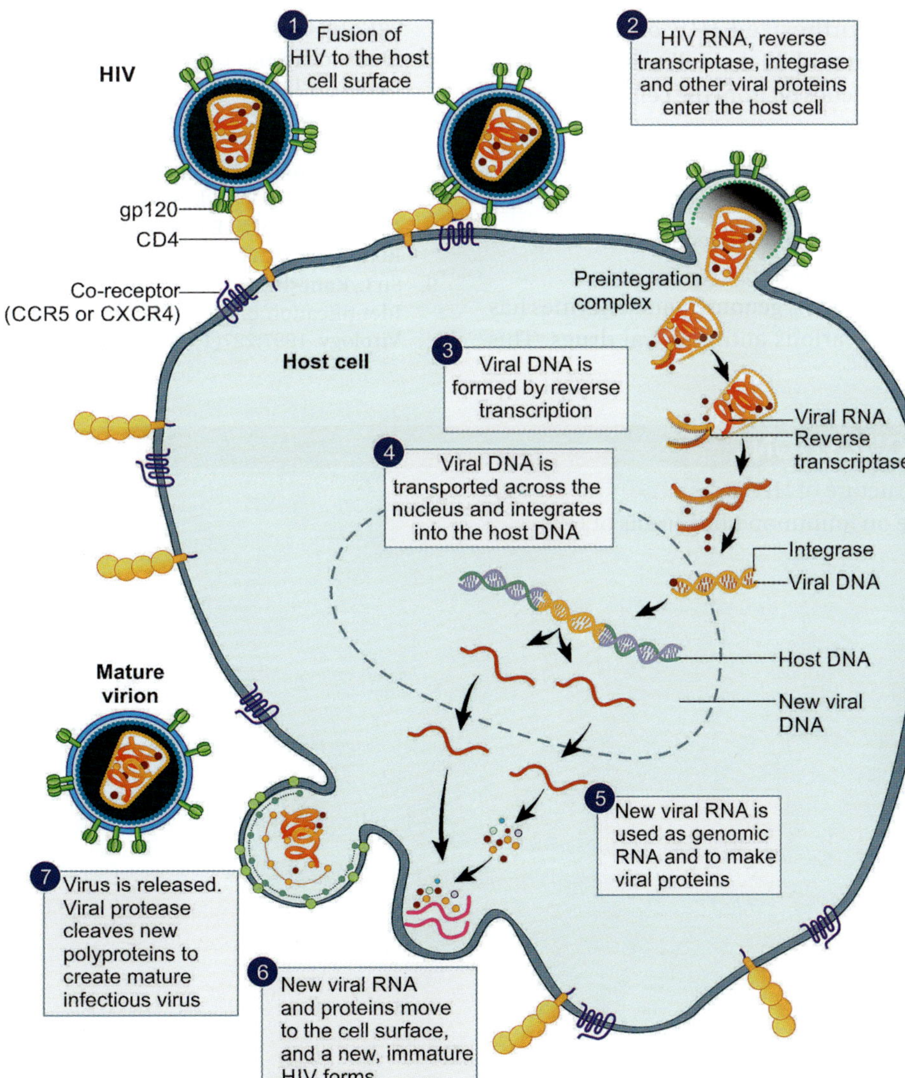

Fig. 3: Human immunodeficiency virus (HIV) replication cycle.
Source: https://niaid.nih.gov/10.06.2010/diseases-conditions/hiv-replication-cycle.

Uncoating and Reverse Transcription

The viral RNA is reverse transcribed into linear double-stranded DNA molecule. This step requires coordinated activities of enzyme RT, an RNA- and DNA-dependent polymerase. Immediately after the release of viral core into the cytoplasm, it undergoes a partial and progressive disassembly known as uncoating. The process of reverse transcription is coupled with uncoating.

Nuclear Entry and Integration

The reverse transcribed DNA along with viral proteins are able to pierce intact cellular nuclear membrane, mediated by various viral proteins. This is followed by integration of viral DNA into host cell chromosomal DNA to form a provirus. This occurs in a nonsequence specific pattern.

Viral Protein Expression and Assembly

The host cell transcription machinery and viral regulatory proteins together lead to expression of viral genes and core proteins. Newly synthesized HIV core proteins, enzymes and RNA gather within the cell membrane. An immature viral particle pinches off from the cell and acquires an envelope.

KEY POINTS

- HIV-1 is the common cause of AIDS epidemic.
- Complex structure and replication.
- Understanding the receptors, genomes, and enzymes has helped in developing various antiretroviral drugs. This has helped in providing quality care to the patients and controlling the disease epidemic.
- Further understanding of all these is necessary to develop an effective vaccine for complete control of AIDS.

REFERENCES

1. Singh R, Singh S, Kaur V. Human immunodeficiency virus. Indian J Dermatol Venereol Leprol. 1992;58:233-42.
2. Fanales-Belasio E, Raimondo M, Suligoi B, Buttò S. HIV virology and pathogenetic mechanisms of infection: a brief overview. Ann Ist Super Sanita. 2010;46(1):5-14.
3. Taylor BS, Sobieszczyk ME, McCutchan FE, Hammer SM. The challenge of HIV-1 subtype diversity. N Engl J Med. 2008; 358(15):1590-602.
4. German Advisory Committee Blood (Arbeitskreis Blut), Subgroup 'Assessment of Pathogens Transmissible by Blood.' Human Immunodeficiency Virus (HIV). Transfus Med Hemother. 2016;43(3):203-22.
5. Engelman A, Cherepanov P. The structural biology of HIV-1: mechanistic and therapeutic insights. Nat Rev Microbiol. 2012;10(4):279-90.
6. Menéndez-Arias L. Special issue: retroviral enzymes. Viruses. 2010;2(5):1181-4.
7. Kumar RB, Maher DM, Herzberg MC, Southern PJ. Expression of HIV receptors, alternate receptors and co-receptors on tonsillar epithelium: implications for HIV binding and primary oral infection. Virol J. 2006;3:25.
8. Nisole S, Saïb A. Early steps of retrovirus replicative cycle. Retrovirology. 2004;1:9.
9. Su L, Kaneshima H, Bonyhadi ML, Lee R, Auten J, Wolf A, et al. Identification of HIV-1 determinants for replication in vivo. Virology. 1997;227(1):45-52.

EXAMINATION QUESTIONS

1. Draw a labeled structure of HIV virus.
2. Write a short note on immunopathogenesis of HIV.

140 CHAPTER

Cutaneous Manifestations of HIV-AIDS

Sumit Sen

INTRODUCTION

Mucocutaneous presentations of human immunodeficiency virus (HIV) have profound importance in the diagnosis of this morbid disease.

Understanding the various cutaneous disorders can help a physician to assess the severity of the patient's condition. Many of these cutaneous features correlate with CD4 counts **(Table 1)**. Some of the cutaneous manifestations may also result from the drugs used to treat the disease. Many cutaneous features show atypicality while manifesting in AIDS patient.[1]

Other skin manifestations may resemble those found in immunocompetent patients. Some dermatological conditions are more common among patients suffering from this disease. Importance of such skin manifestations are:

- The dermatological disorders themselves may cause significant morbidity as HIV progresses. Number of mucocutaneous disorders may coexist and is directly related to overall survival in AIDS.[1]
- Many mucocutaneous disorders are very disturbing to the patient.
- Earliest diagnosis of HIV-AIDS is possible if a thorough knowledge is present about the dermatological manifestations.
- Cutaneous dendritic cells and Langerhans cells may be the principal target in acute HIV infection and contribute to the pathogenesis of the disease.[2]
- Sexually transmitted ulcerative genital diseases like syphilis facilitate the spread of HIV and need to be diagnosed early for control of HIV.[3]

STAGES OF HIV

- Acute primary HIV infection
- Symptomatic infection
- Early symptomatic state
- Late symptomatic state and advanced disease

It is important to diagnose HIV infection in the acute primary stage with the help of the dermatological manifestations as early detection of HIV can prevent complications. This early stage starts 1–6 weeks after exposure and lasts from a fortnight to several months.

The cutaneous manifestations may resemble many diseases at this initial stage. They are:

- Erythematous symmetrical maculopapular rash on the face palms and soles.
- Urticarial and vesicular rash.

TABLE 1: Mucocutaneous manifestations of HIV patients with their corresponding CD4 counts.

<50 CD4 cells/mm³	*>50–250 CD4 cells/mm³*	*>250–500 CD4 cells/mm³*	*>500 CD4 cells/mm³*
Herpes simplex infection	Eosinophilic folliculitis	Oral thrush	Acute retroviral syndrome
Papular pruritic eruption	Recalcitrant seborrheic dermatitis	Herpes zoster	Oral hairy leukoplakia (but patient develops AIDS within 2–3 years)
Giant molluscum contagiosum	Extensive molluscum contagiosum	Psoriasis, severe or refractory	Vaginal candidiasis
Cytomegalovirus perianal ulcers	Bacillary angiomatosis	Severe form of psoriasis	Seborrheic dermatitis
Ichthyosis	Disseminated herpes simplex virus	Melanoma	Bullous impetigo
Aspergillosis	Disseminated cryptococcosis and disseminated histoplasmosis	Kaposi sarcoma	
Major aphthae	Botryomycosis		
Necrotizing gingivitis	Non-Hodgkin lymphoma		
Mycobacterium avium intracellulare infection	Oral hyperpigmentation		
	Proximal subungual onychomycosis		

- Steven Johnson syndrome and acute erosive genitocrural intertrigo has also been described. Lymphopenia, thrombocytopenia, and features of hepatitis and cholestasis may also occur. Nonspecific symptoms like fever, arthralgia, myalgia, diarrhea, and lymphadenopathy usually accompanies the skin rash.

The dermatological disorders in HIV patients are outlined in the following sections.

INFECTIONS AND INFESTATIONS

Superficial Fungal Infections

Disease	Important characteristics of dermatological features
1. Oropharyngeal candidiasis (CM) *[cutaneous marker of HIV (CM)]*	This condition is a sign of transmission to AIDS. Pseudomembranous **(Fig. 1)** atrophic, hyperplastic and angular cheilitis types. It is more common among men who have sex with men.[4] Single dose oral fluconazole is effective but some may not respond to this dose. Disseminated candidiasis is uncommon.
2. Dermatophytosis	Present in one-third of HIV patients. Tinea incognito is a cutaneous marker (*CM*) of HIV. Typical as well as atypical lesions of Tinea may be present. Widespread Tinea infection is uncommon in HIV affected persons. Atypical lesions without border or central clearing may create confusion **(Fig. 2)**. Deep lesions and Majocci's granuloma occur.[5,6] Itraconazole or oral terbinafine are necessary to control the infection.
3. Pityriasiform infections	Seborrheic dermatitis is seen in 80% of HIV infected individuals. It is caused by *P. ovale*. Ketoconazole 200 mg/day is effective in severe seborrheic dermatitis. Itraconazole 100 mg/day is an alternative. Tinea versicolor can be extensive in HIV infections. *P. folliculorum* infection affects the upper trunk and proximal parts of the arms.
4. *Pneumocystis jiroveci* infection	It has been currently included in the fungi family. Though *Pneumocystis pneumonia* is common in AIDS, skin manifestations are rare and include necrotic plaques, molluscum-like lesions and erythematous nodular eruptions of external ear.[7] Treatment is with intravenous cotrimoxazole or pentamidine.

Deep Fungal Infections

Disease	Dermatological features
1. Cryptococcosis [CM]	Presents as pink papules, ulcerated nodules or pustules. Centers have hemorrhagic or necrotic crusts. Occurs in 10% of AIDS patients. Mucicarmine stain outlines the capsule of the organism. Meningitis is its most frequent complication and carries a poor prognosis. Cryptococcosis responds to IV Amphotericin B and oral Fluconazole (400–800 mg/day).

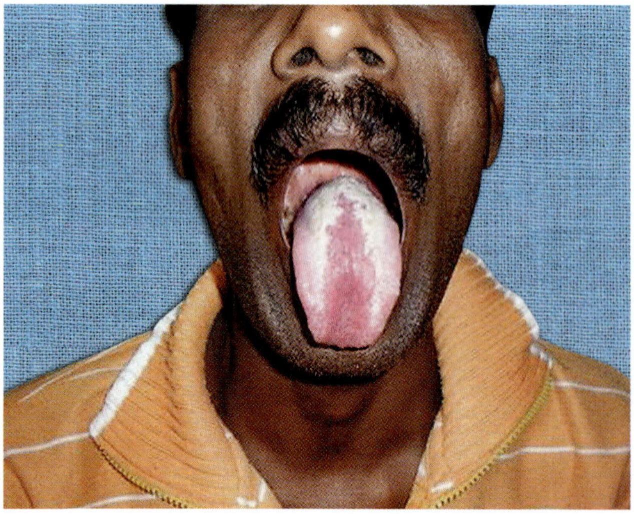

Fig. 1: Oral thrush.

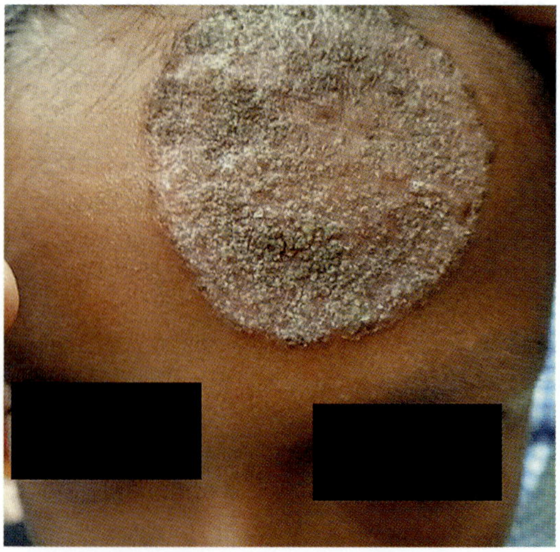

Fig. 2: Atypical tinea in child.

2. Penicilliosis	AIDS defining opportunistic infection. The various morphological conditions of this disease are umbilicated papules, nodules, folliculitis-like lesions, oral, and genital ulcers.[8] Amphotericin B followed by Itraconazole is effective in treating this condition.
3. Histoplasmosis [CM]	Appears as molluscum contagiosum-like papules **(Figs. 3A and B)** and plaques. Warty lesions, ulcers, or erythema nodosum-like lesions can be other manifestations of this disorder in AIDS patients. Oral mucosa may show varied manifestations like nodules, vegetations or ulcerations.[9] Polymorphic morphology on presentation indicates a higher CD4 count in this condition where extrapulmonary manifestation is an AIDS defining condition. Itraconazole is effective in treating this condition.

Viral Infections

1. Herpes simplex [CM]	It can be self-limited in early stages of HIV. Anogenital involvement is frequent. Mucocutaneous HSV infection present for more than 1 month is seen in advanced HIV. Tender painful ulcerative lesions of penis, perianal area, and lips occur. Odynophagia, progressive herpetic whitlow, persistent necrotic digits[10] and folliculitis occur. Lesions of herpes genitalis become more painful and increase in number. These can present with atypical morphology and in atypical sites such as buttocks and lower back. Severity of lesions are often increased and they are usually slow to heal. Acyclovir 800 mg five times daily is effective but in resistant cases foscarnet, cidofovir and imiquimod may be tried.
2. Varicella zoster infection	It can recur, disseminate, can be prolonged and can cause death by bacterial superinfection.
3. Herpes zoster infection [CM]	It is usually unidermatomal but may be multidermatomal **(Fig. 4)**. It may be bullous, hemorrhagic, necrotic with severe persistent pain. Increased chance of neurologic and ophthalmic complications. Acyclovir 10 mg/kg 8 hourly is to be administered in complicated cases. Pain can be managed by additional use of carbamazepine and dosulepin. Complicated zoster with involvement of eyes, sphincters of the urogenital system, pulmonary. and neurological system need parenteral acyclovir. Acyclovir resistant cases are to be treated with vidarabine or recombinant interferon-α.[11]
4. Cytomegalovirus infection	Skin is rarely affected. When involved the CD4 count is usually below 50/mm^3 and there is a 85% chance of mortality within 6 months.[12] The various presentations are perianal ulcer, hyperkeratotic lesions indurated pigmented nodules and plaques, lesions of vasculitis and mucosal ulcers. Effective drugs are IV foscarnet, ganciclovir, and cidofovir.

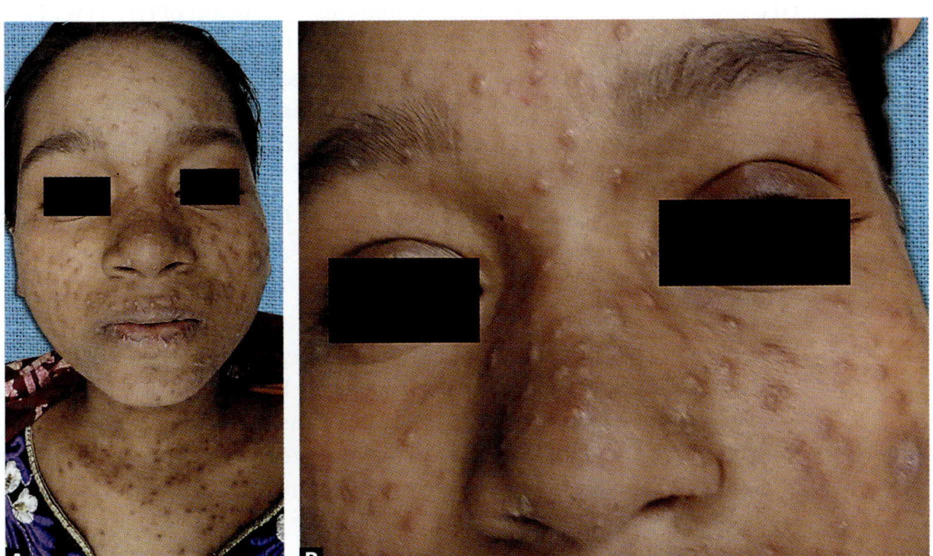

Figs. 3A and B: Histoplasmosis.

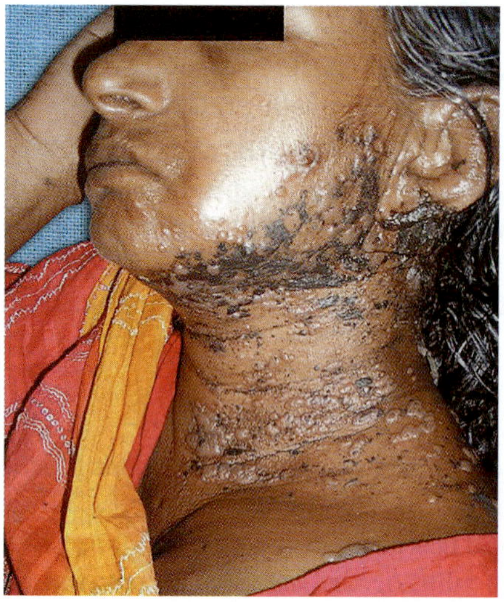

Fig. 4: Multidermatomal herpes zoster.

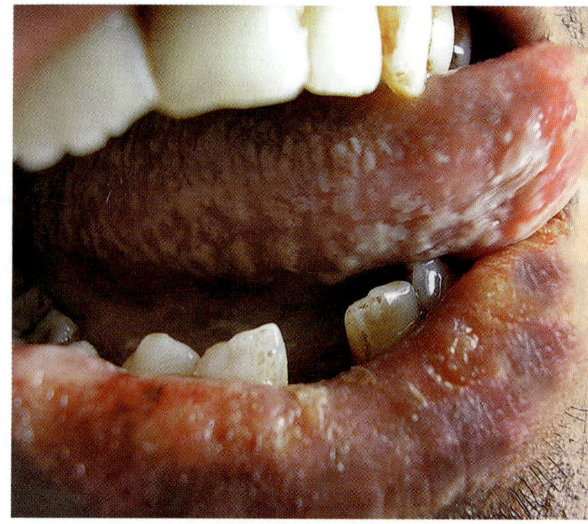

Fig. 5: OHL.

5. Epstein–Barr virus (EBV) infection
   Oral hairy leukoplakia (OHL) associated with EBV is an early sign of HIV though it can present in any stage of HIV and can forecast rapid progression of the disease.[13] OHL changes daily. It presents as corrugated white plaque on lateral side of tongue **(Fig. 5)**. Its reappearance after resolution while on antiretroviral regime indicates ineffectiveness of antiretrovirals in the patient and needs change of regime.

6. Molluscum contagiosum [CM]
   HIV patient usually has very low CD4 count when seen with MC lesions. The causative organisms are MCV 1–4 molluscipox viruses. The lesions can be numerous, conglomerated (agminate) **(Fig. 6)**, giant and can be clustered around the genitalia. The lesions may not show central umbilication. Resolution of giant molluscum after antiretroviral therapy has been reported.[14] Topical imiquimod, cidofovir (both topical and systemic), diphencyprone and electron beam therapy have been found to be effective.[15]

7. Human papillomavirus infection
   It may be numerous and may coexist with other conditions such as molluscum contagiosum (MC). HPV 6 and HPV 11 are the most frequent types isolated among seropositive.[16] Seen more on the genital area. Intravenous drug abusers who are seropositive are found to be frequently affected with genital warts. In general warts may suffer recalcitrant and protracted course in HIV patients. Huge perianal wart should raise suspicion of HIV **(Fig. 7)**. Oral warts are seen among seropositives who indulge in oral sex **(Fig. 8)**. Higher rates of cervical, anal, genital carcinomas have been recorded. Epidermodysplasia verruciformis occurs more frequently among the seropositives especially in children.[17] Development of useful vaccines against the HPV virus is increasingly improving the outlook of treatment of warts and malignancies associated with the HPV virus.[18]

8. Hepatitis B and C infection
   The two usually coexist among seropositives. Chance of sexual transmission is more with hepatitis B virus than hepatitis C virus.

Bacterial Infections

1. Staphylococcal infection
   Most common bacterial infection. It can present as impetigo, bullous ecthyma, folliculitis, furunculosis, carbuncles, or pyomyositis. Pyoderma is a *CM*. Methicillin-resistant *Staphylococcus aureus* (MRSA) skin infections are cause of concern in HIV patients but their incidence is on the decline. Cotrimoxazole, doxycycline, minocycline, levofloxacin, and linezolid are all effective. Ecthyma gangrenosum due to pseudomonas also is cause for concern in the seropositives.

2. Bacillary angiomatosis
   Widespread cherry angioma like lesions or pyogenic granuloma like lesions are the usual presentations. May represent first clinical sign of AIDS. The causative organism *B. bacilliformis* may be identified by Warthin-Starry silver staining. Erythromycin and doxycycline are effective.

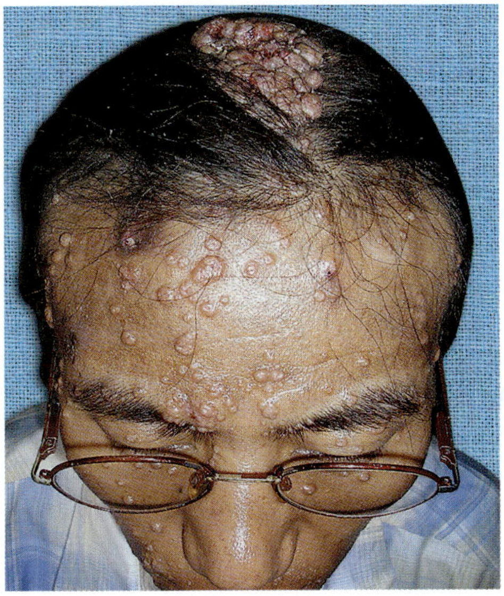

Fig. 6: Agminate molluscum contagiosum.

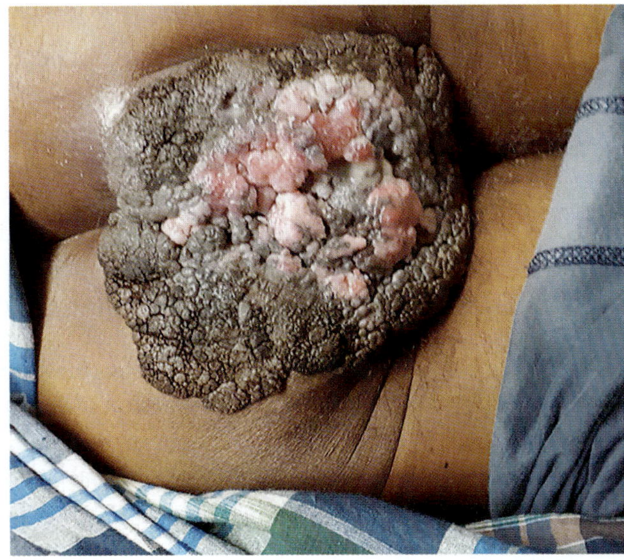

Fig. 7: Huge wart on perianal area of seropositive person.

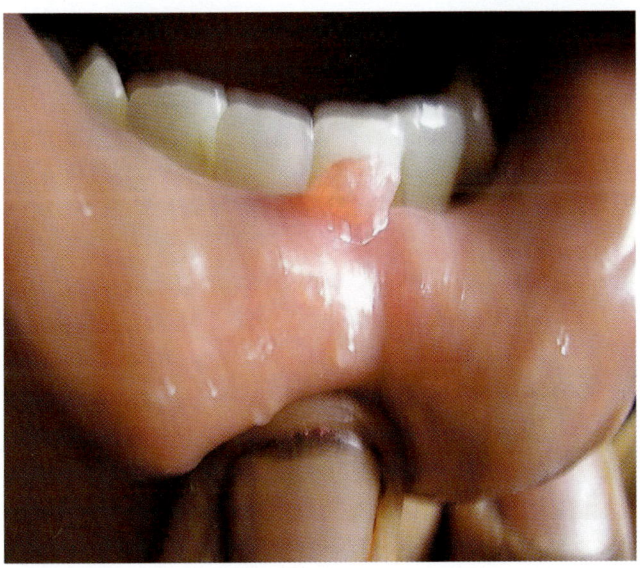

Fig. 8: Oral wart.

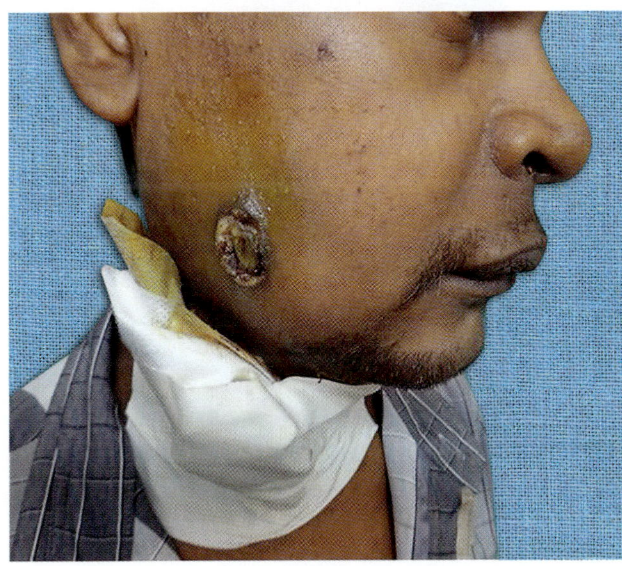

Fig. 9: Scrofuloderma in HIV patient.

3. *Mycobacterium* infection [CM] — The most common opportunistic infection among seropositives in India. Presents as scrofuloderma **(Fig. 9)** which may have multiple lesions **(Fig. 10)**, scattered violaceous papules, keratotic papules and nodules, tuberculids, or tubercular lymphadenitis. There is higher prevalence of extrapulmonary and disseminated disease. The usual regimes for pulmonary tuberculosis are effective. Biopsy and histopathology of skin tissue often reveals a noncaseating granuloma due to diminished cell mediated immunity.[19] Atypical mycobacterium infection among those positive for HIV is usually caused by *M. avium-intracellulare*. This infection is treated with combination of macrolide and ethambutol.
4. Leprosy — HIV does not lead to serious forms of leprosy. Less number of sites are chosen now for slit skin smear to prevent chance of transmission of HIV.
5. Anaerobic bacterial infection — Cancrum oris or Noma can occur in HIV AIDS patients. It is a type of orofacial gangrene occurring in the debilitated patient **(Fig. 11)**.

Sexually Transmitted Infections

1. Syphilis	Atypical morphological forms may occur **(Fig. 12)**. Multiple or giant painful chancres with slow resolution are seen. Secondary syphilis can present as lues maligna which is a virulent form. There may be rapid progression from the secondary to the tertiary phase. There may be high RPR titer or absent antibody response, increased chance of Jarisch-Herxheimer reaction and of relapse. There is also increased chance of treatment failure and more chance of syphilitic aortitis. Long acting Benzathine penicillin is given in the dose of 2.4 million units deep IM weekly for 3 weeks.
2. Chancroid	Manifests after an increased incubation period. Ulcers persist for long duration and are more in number than in immunocompetent individuals. Necrotizing forms and those with multilocular buboes may occur. Treatment has to be given for a longer period than is usually given for resolution of lesions.
3. Donovanosis	Destructive beefy red granulomatous ulcer is the usual manifestation over genital area, buttocks, and perianal area **(Fig. 13)**. Responds to parenteral gentamycin.
4. Lymphogranuloma venereum	Coinfection with HIV may not have any effect on the cutaneous presentation of this disease.

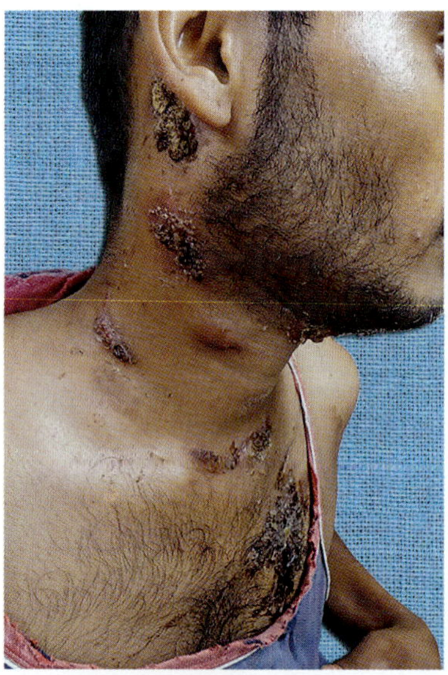

Fig. 10: Scrofuloderma in HIV patient with multiple lesions.

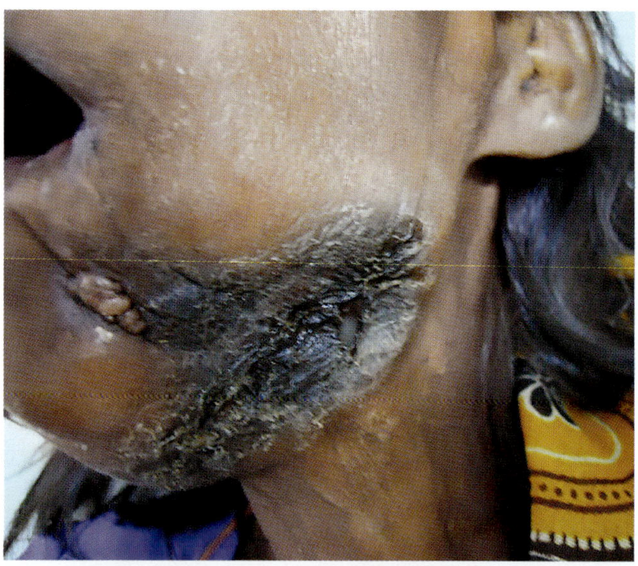

Fig. 11: Cancrum oris.

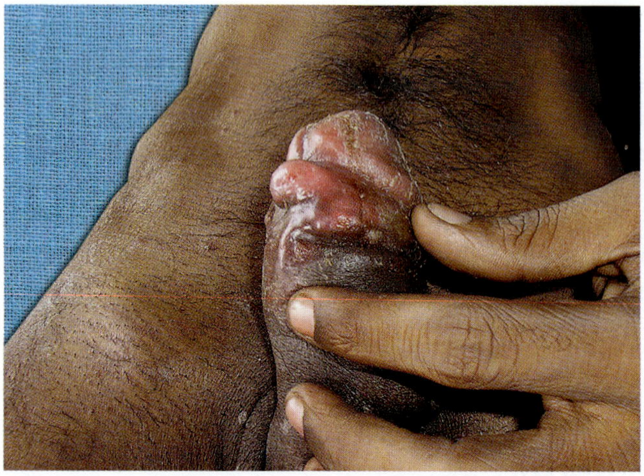

Fig. 12: Atypical form of syphilis.

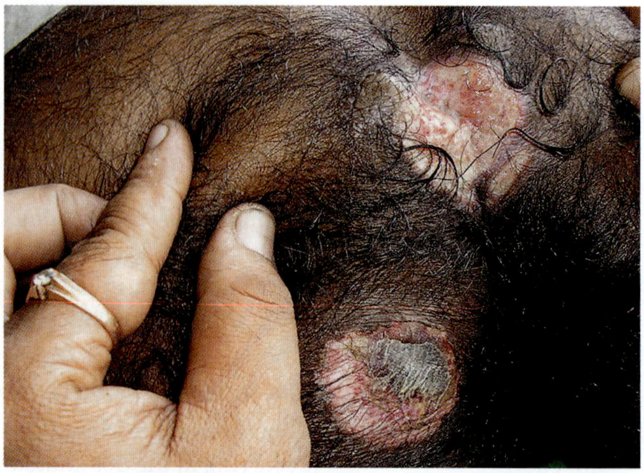

Fig. 13: Donovanosis in seropositive male.

Parasitic Infections

1. Scabies [*CM*]	In severe immunodeficiency state involvement of the head and neck can occur. Crusted form of scabies also occurs. Papular extremely itchy variety is seen as are bullous forms. Treatment is with a combination of topical 5% permethrin, salicylic acid (to remove crusts when they occur) sulfur ointment and oral ivermectin.
2. Demodicidosis [*CM*]	Presents as pruritic papulonodular eruption of face, neck and upper trunk. 5% benzoyl peroxide topical application is effective.
3. Leishmaniasis	This can present as a submerged nodule resembling a dermatofibroma or even may appear like lesion of Kaposi sarcoma. Atypical disseminated forms may also occur.
4. Extraintestinal strongyloidiasis	Reticulated petechial and purpuric lesions are seen in a centripetal distribution and is included as a marker in the case definition of AIDS.

INFLAMMATORY DISEASES

1. Seborrheic dermatitis [*CM*]	It is seen in all stages of HIV infection.[20] Presentation is more severe. It is one of the commonest dermatological manifestations seen in the HIV patient. A histopathology usually shows keratinocyte necrosis and dermoepidermal junction inflammation. This condition is often resistant to treatment.
2. Psoriasis [*CM*]	Benign guttate and plaque forms are seen as is the diffuse form. It may appear for the first time in a severe form.[21] The disease may present with generalized palmoplantar keratoderma. Psoriatic arthritis is more common among seropositives than their immunocompetent counterparts. Langerhans cells known to play a key role in pathogenesis of Psoriasis are found to be infected with HIV virus.[22] Moderate-to-severe psoriasis in HIV affected person is an indication to start antiretroviral drugs. Drugs effective in controlling psoriasis in HIV are acitretin, PUVA (superior to UVB) and etanercept. Cyclosporin and methotrexate are contraindicated for fear of precipitation of severe leucopenia.
3. Reiter's syndrome [*CM*]	Presents with facial seborrheic dermatitis like features. Another presentation is flexural psoriasis type. Acral involvement with severe pustules of palms and soles may also be seen. Acitretin or PUVA is useful in treating this condition which is often resistant to treatment.
4. Ichthyosis	Seen in 23–30% of seropositives.

PRURITIC CONDITIONS IN HIV

1. Papular pruritic eruption [CM]	Occurs over the head, neck and upper trunk as excoriated reddish urticarial rash. It may also occur over the extremities **(Fig. 14)**. It is associated with peripheral eosinophilia and a raised serum IgE level. The lesions heal with scarring which may be unsightly and depressing to the patient. Hypothesized to be result of exaggerated response to insect bite.[23] Histopathology

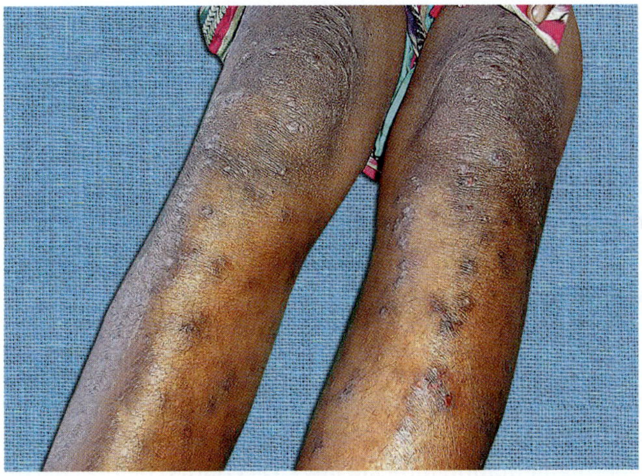

Fig. 14: Papular pruritic eruption.

reveals perivascular infiltrate of lymphocytes and eosinophils. Immunohistochemistry is diagnostic of the condition. It is a sign of advanced HIV. Treatment is phototherapy. The condition is an indication to start antiretroviral drugs.

2. Eosinophilic folliculitis — A rare condition. This entity is specific for the HIV disease,[24] seen as pruritic perifollicular papules and pustules present over face, trunk and on the back extending down to the lumbar spine. The pustules are sterile. It is uncommon in women. The condition often proclaims onset of opportunistic infection as it is seen in those with low CD4 counts. Morphologically it resembles immune reconstitution inflammatory syndrome (IRIS) papular pruritic eruption of HIV though the two are different entities as has been proven immunohistochemically. Perifollicular degranulating eosinophils and mast cells are found histopathologically. It can be a part of IRIS. Phototherapy is effective.

Neoplasms

1. Kaposi sarcoma [CM] — Associated with Herpes virus 8. It is derived from the endothelium and is the most common tumor in HIV. It is more common among men who practice sex with men. The trunk, lower limbs, arms, face, and hard palate are commonly affected. Genitalia too may be involved. Neoplasm usually presents as a purple colored plaque or nodule which ulcerates. Lesions may be present along the skin creases, may coalesce or be present in linear fashion. It may spread to involve the gastrointestinal tract and the lungs. The outcome of this condition is related to HIV activity in the patient. Histopathology showing irregularly shaped vessels followed by immunohistochemistry is to be performed for a definitive diagnosis. Treatment is offered for troublesome lesions. Radiotherapy, chemotherapy and cryotherapy are effective in managing the disorder. Liposomal anthracycline is recommended for rapidly disfiguring disease.[25] Combination of antiretroviral therapy and paclitaxel is used for cases resistant to anthracycline. Thrombocytopenic purpura of HIV may be mistaken for Kaposi sarcoma.
2. Lymphoma — Non-Hodgkin lymphoma can occur. A polymorphic morphology is usually seen in those lymphoma patients who have undergone kidney transplantation.[26] Cutaneous T-cell lymphoma and Sezary syndrome too can occur albeit rarely. Plasmablastic lymphoma which is associated with Epstein-Barr virus and which affects the skin and oral cavity have been reported in HIV-AIDS. It is self-healing. Multiple myeloma too has been reported.
3. Melanoma and nonmelanoma skin cancers — The incidence of AIDS defining cancers is decreasing but those malignancies such as melanoma, squamous cell and basal cell cancers are being increasingly identified in HIV-AIDS patients. These are known as NADCs or non-AIDS defining cancers. Melanoma may present with atypical manifestations such as a benign looking naevi or pigmented macule. Treatment for all these malignancies remain the same as in non-HIV patients but greater care must be exercised after excision with adequate follow-up.
4. Adverse cutaneous drug reactions [CM] — HIV patients are more susceptible to drug reactions. Some antiretroviral drugs such as Abacavir cause a discrete rash without eosinophilia and this can be life-threatening. The adverse drug reactions are seen mostly with sulfonamides, amoxicillin, antitubercular drugs. Any sort of drug rash can occur such as morbilliform, fixed drug rash, SJS, TEN, and DRESS. The most common type of drug reaction is a morbilliform erythematous rash associated with fever, arthralgia abnormal liver function tests, and eosinophilia. Adverse reaction to Lamivudine is rare. Zidovudine can cause hyperpigmentation of the nails. Most adverse reactions to antiretroviral drugs are noted to resolve and hence the antiretroviral may not be stopped.

MISCELLANEOUS CUTANEOUS DISORDERS

1. Hyperpigmentation — Reasons for hyperpigmentation may be drugs such as zidovudine and indinavir and opportunistic infections such as toxoplasmosis. Hypoadrenalism may also lead to hyperpigmentation. Late HIV infection may produce hyperpigmentation.[27] Oral and anal hyperpigmentation indicate low CD4 counts (below 200/mm^3).

2. Hidradenitis suppurativa	Seen in the apocrine gland bearing areas such as the axillae, inguinal region and anogenital regions.
3. Hair alterations	Hypertrichosis of eyelashes and long eyelashes are seen. Alopecia areata and premature graying of hair are seen.
4. Nail changes [CM]	Proximal subungual onychomycosis is a cutaneous marker of AIDS. Nail dyschromia due to antiretroviral drugs **(Fig. 15)** also occur and the nails may also be affected by such diseases such as psoriasis and severe herpes infection occurring in the course of HIV-AIDS infection.
5. Aphthae	Recurrent aphthae (*CM*) are common. Larger ulcers are seen in those with advancing HIV. Ulcers are painful.
6. Erythroderma [CM]	This can occur due to several conditions prevalent in a HIV patient such as seborrheic dermatitis, Norwegian scabies, dermatophytosis, ichthyosis, etc. It is to be considered a cutaneous marker among the dark skinned.[28] Besides the above mentioned disorders porphyria cutanea tarda, granuloma annulare, atopic dermatitis, rosacea, cutaneous vasculitis, pityriasis rosea, acanthamebiasis, photosensitivity reactions, venous and arterial thrombosis leading to leg ulcers, xerosis, ichthyosis, HIV-associated lipodystrophy and skin infarcts have been noted with increased frequency among HIV infected persons. HIV may be a cause of severe pruritus but the antiretroviral drugs may also cause pruritus. Prurigo nodularis occurs among such diseased persons but it often responds to Thalidomide. Raltegravir is also found to be effective.[29]
7. IRIS	It is a unique condition seen in persons affected with HIV. Cutaneous manifestations and signs and symptoms of coexisting disease in the seropositive individual are seen to exacerbate though the immunological status is seen to improve as shown by rising CD4 counts usually after treatment. The diseases associated with IRIS are viral infections caused by Herpes, Varicella-zoster, Epstein-Barr (hairy leukoplakia), Cytomegalo and HHV8 (Kaposi sarcoma), HPV viruses and molluscum contagiosum causing virus; tuberculosis, atypical mycobacteria and leprosy, candidiasis, tinea versicolor, tinea corporis, opportunistic deep fungal infections, leishmaniasis, crusted scabies; demodicidosis, eosinophilic folliculitis, papular pruritic eruption, photosensitivity, lupus erythematosus, granulomatous diseases like sarcoidosis; Common conditions such as vitiligo, acne vulgaris and rosacea; Tumors such as non-Hodgkin lymphoma, squamous cell carcinoma and eruptive dermatofibroma.

HIV infections in children usually occur from mothers. Oral candidiasis is seen in one-third of children affected with HIV. Signs of sexual abuse with perianal and perigenital ulcerations should prompt testing the child for HIV infection **(Fig. 16)**. Pruritic papular eruptions, eczematous lesions, and drug eruptions are seen with increased frequency in this group. Extensive tinea infections, disseminated forms of herpes zoster, atypical measles rash may pose problems in children with HIV-AIDS. Molluscum contagiosum lesions are seen mostly on the face and extensive viral warts may occur. Fifty

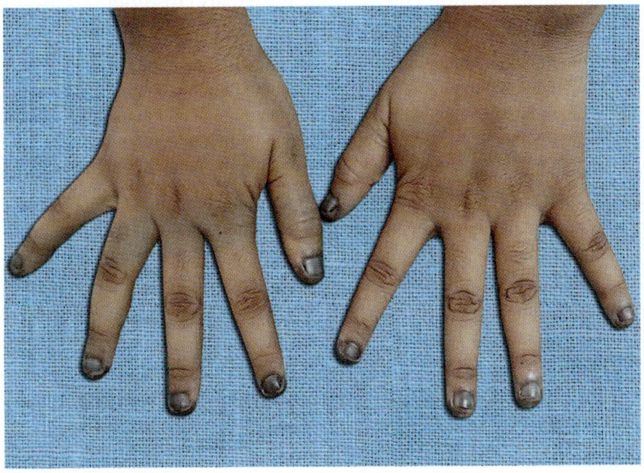

Fig. 15: Dyschromia of nails due to zidovudine.

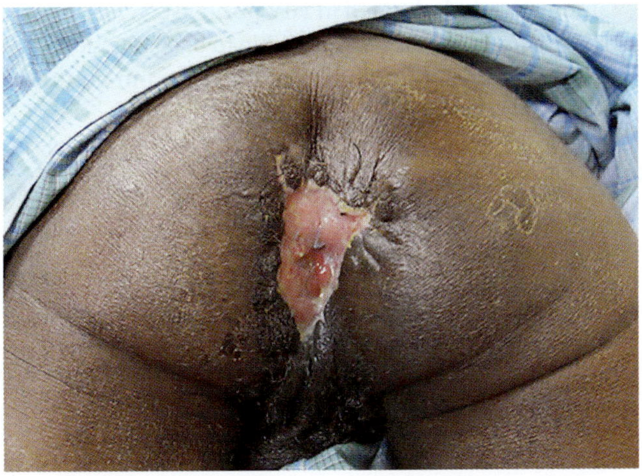

Fig. 16: Perianal ulceration in teenage child due to sexual abuse.

percent of HIV-positive children with varicella develop herpes zoster or a disseminated varicella like eruption within 2 years of the initial varicella eruption.[30] Skin tumors are uncommon. The skin lesions respond well to antiretroviral drugs.

Recent reports suggest the finding of linear streaks of telangiectasias on the chest of HIV persons among males who have sex with males.[31]

Regional and global variations in the mucocutaneous manifestations have been recorded.[32]

CONCLUSION

Significant number of HIV-AIDS cases can be diagnosed early with knowledge about the specific dermatological manifestations of the disease and most of these mucocutaneous features can help the physician place a specific case of HIV-AIDS in a particular CD4 spectrum. This can allow initiation of antiretroviral therapy at the appropriate time.

KEY POINTS

- Mucocutaneous presentations of HIV can help in diagnosis of this disease.
- Most of the mucocutaneous manifestations correlate with the CD4 count of the patient.
- Oropharyngeal candidiasis is an important common cutaneous marker of HIV-AIDS.
- Dermatophytes may manifest with typical and atypical cutaneous lesions in HIV.
- Cryptococcosis in HIV affected persons respond to IV amphotericin B and oral fluconazole.
- Lesions of herpes genitalis become more painful and increase in number and can present with atypical morphology in seropositives.
- OHL can present in any stage of HIV.
- There may be rapid progression from the secondary to the tertiary phase in syphilis in HIV positive patients.
- Erythroderma is to be considered a cutaneous marker among the dark skinned in HIV positives.
- HIV patients are more susceptible to drug reactions.
- HIV infections in children usually occur from mothers.
- Kaposi sarcoma is associated with IRIS in HIV.

REFERENCES

1. Kahn JO, Walker BD. Acute human immunodeficiency virus type 1 infection (review). N Engl J Med. 1998;339:33-9.
2. Ho DD, Neumann AU, Perelson AS, Chen W, Leonard JM, Markowitz M. Rapid turnover of plasma virions and CD4 lymphocytes in HIV-1 infection. Nature. 1995;373:123-6.
3. Calza AM, Kinloch S, Mainetti C. Primary human immunodeficiency virus infection mimicking syphilis. J Infect Di. 1991;164:615-6.
4. Reynaud-Mendel B, Janier M, Gerbaka J, Hakim C, Rabian C, Chastang C. Dermatologic findings in HIV-1 infected patients: a prospective study with emphasis on CD4 cell count. Dermatology. 1996;192:325-8.
5. Johnson RA. HIV disease: mucocutaneous fungal infections in HIV disease. Clin Dermatol. 2000;18:411-22.
6. Munoz-Perez MA, Rodriguez-Pichardo A, Camacho F, Rios JJ. Extensive and deep dermatophytosis caused by Trichophyton var. interdigitalis in an HIV-1 positive patient. J Eur Acad Dermatol Venereol. 2000;14:61-3.
7. Hennessey NP, Parro EL, Cockerell CJ. Cutaneous *Pneumocystis carinii* infections in patients with acquired immunodeficiency syndrome. Arch Dermatol. 1991;127:1699-1701.
8. Kullavanijaya P. Penicillosis in AIDS. J Dermatol. 2001;28: 667-70.
9. Mehta V, De A, Balachandran C, Monga P. Mucocutaneous histoplasmosis in HIV with an atypical ecthyma like presentation. Dermatol Online J. 2009;15:10.
10. Baden LA, Bigby M, Kwan T. Persistent necrotic digits in a patient with the acquired immunodeficiency syndrome. Herpes simplex virus infection. Arch Dermatol. 1991;127:113-6.
11. Vafai A, Berger M. Zoster in patients treated with HIV: a review. Am J Med Sci. 2001;321:372-80.
12. Lee JY. Cytomegalovirus infection involving the skin in immunocompromised hosts. A clinicopathologic study. Am J Clin Pathol. 1989;92:96-100.
13. Rigopoulos D, Paparizos V, Katsambas A. Cutaneous markers of HIV infection. Clin Dermatol. 2004;22:487-98.
14. Sen S, Bhaumik P. Resolution of giant molluscum contagiosum with antiretroviral therapy. Indian J Dermatol Venereol Leprol. 2008;74:267-8.
15. Scolaro MJ, Gordon P. Electron beam therapy for AIDS-related molluscum contagiosum lesions: preliminary experience. Radiology. 1999;210:479-82.
16. Silverberg MJ, Ahdieh L, Monoz A. The impact of HIV infection and immunodeficiency on human papilloma virus type 6 or 11 infection and on genital warts. Sex Transm Dis. 2002;29:427-35.
17. Lowe SM, Katsidzira L, Meys R. Acquired epidermodysplasia verruciformis due to multiple and unusual HPV infection among vertically-infected, HIV positive adolescents in Zimbabwe. Clin Infect Dis. 2012;54:e119-23.
18. Deny LA, Franceschi S, deSanjose S, HeardI, Moscicki AB, Palefsky J. Human papilloma virus, human immunodeficiency virus and immunosuppression. Vaccine. 2012;30(Suppl 5):F168-74.
19. Smith KJ, Skelton HG III, Angritt P. Histopathologic features of HIV-associated skin disease. Dermatol Clin. 1991;9:551-8.
20. Mathes BM, Douglass MC. Seborrheic dermatitis in patients with acquired immunodeficiency syndrome. Am Acad Dermatol. 1985;13:947-51.
21. Mallon E, Bunker CB. HIV-associated psoriasis. AIDS patient Care STDS. 2000;14:239-46.
22. Kalter DC, Gendelman HE, Meltzer MS. Monocytes, dendritic cells, and Langerhans cells in immunodeficiency virus infection. Dermatol Clin. 1991;9:415-28.
23. Resnek JS Jr, Van Beek M, Furmanski L. Etiology of pruritic popular eruption with HIV infection in Uganda. JAMA. 2004;292:2614-21.
24. Fernandez C, Ribera M, Barranco JC. Eosinophilic pustular folliculitis in patients with acquired immunodeficiency syndrome. Int J Dermatol. 1992;31:193-5.

25. Bunker CB, Staughton RCD. HIV-associated disease: dermatology. In: Gazzard BG (Ed). AIDS Care Handbook. London: Mediscript; 2002. pp. 115-39.
26. Nador RG, Chadburn A, Gundappa G. Human immunodeficiency virus (HIV)-associated polymorphic lymphoproliferative disorders. Am J Surg Pathol. 2003;27:293-302.
27. Grover C, Kubba S, Bansal S. Pigmentation: a potential cutaneous marker for AIDS? J Dermatol. 2004;31:756-60.
28. Morar N, Dlova N, Gupta AK. Erythroderma: a comparison between HIV positive and negative patients. Int J Dermatol. 1999;38:895-900.
29. Unemori P, Leslie KS, Maurer T. Persistent prurigo nodularis responsive to initiation of combination therapy with raltegravir. Arch Dermatol. 2010;146:682-3.
30. Gnann JW. Varicella-zoster virus: atypical presentations and unusual complications. J infect Dis. 2002;186(Suppl 1):S91-8.
31. Fallon T, Abell E, Kingsley L. Telangiectases of the anterior chest in homosexual men. Ann Inten Med. 1986;105:679-82.
32. Sen S, Halder S, Mandal S, Pal PP, Halder A, Bhaumik P. Clinico-epidemiological profile of cutaneous manifestations among human immunodeficiency virus positive patients in the sub Himalayan region. Indian J Dermatol Venereol Leprol. 2009;75:403-5.

EXAMINATION QUESTIONS

1. Describe the mucocutaneous manifestations of HIV-AIDS patients.
2. Write briefly about the "fungal infections in AIDS."
3. Briefly describe the "pruritic conditions in HIV-AIDS."
4. Write short note on Kaposi sarcoma in AIDS.
5. Write short note on IRIS.
6. Describe viral infections associated with HIV.

141 CHAPTER

Laboratory Diagnosis of HIV

Neha Bhardwaj, Ashish Amrani

INTRODUCTION

Human immunodeficiency virus (HIV) is a *Lentivirus* (slow virus) which is grouped under retroviruses.[1] It infects human helper T-cells, thus destroying the immune system.[2]

About 35 million people have been infected with HIV worldwide by 2013.[1] In India, it is estimated that there are about 1.16 lakh new cases of HIV annually in adults, and around 14,500 new infections among children in 2011.[1] HIV and acquired immunodeficiency syndrome (AIDS) pose a public health risk, and prompt and accurate diagnosis is critical for starting the treatment, decreasing the transmission as well as improving the prognosis of the disease in an individual.

There are two types of HIV: HIV-1 and HIV-2. HIV-1 is the most common type worldwide whereas HIV-2 is limited to certain geographic areas. HIV-2 is endemic in West Africa, but new cases have also been found in India and Europe over the last decade.[1]

Laboratory diagnosis is the only modality to find out the HIV status of a person.[1] There are various tests, aimed at identifying the viral antibodies, antigen, or the viral nucleic acid. This chapter discusses these tests, the principle behind them, and the algorithm to be followed to get the most accurate results.

OBJECTIVES OF TESTING[1]

- To ensure blood transfusion and organ transplantation safety
- To screen sperm and tissue donors
- To diagnose HIV infection in symptomatic individuals
- To determine the HIV status of voluntary clients
- To prevent parent to child transmission
- To differentiate between HIV-1 and HIV-2 infection
- For postexposure prophylaxis
- For epidemiological surveillance
- Research purposes

CONSIDERATIONS BEFORE TESTING OF HIV

To test for the HIV status of a person it is important to counsel them before the test and take an informed consent. The pre- and post-test counseling prepares the individual mentally for what is to come. Maintaining confidentiality to protect the individuals from any stigmatization is also very critical. Ensure that the test results are handed directly to the individual or to the authorized person.[1]

LABORATORY MARKERS OF HIV INFECTION

It is important to have a basic knowledge about the sequence of emergence of various laboratory markers in order to have a better understanding of the diagnostic tests **(Fig. 1)**.[3]

- *HIV-1 ribonucleic acid (RNA)*: This is the first laboratory marker that can be detected in the serum or plasma, approximately 10 days after the infection. The test that can be used is nucleic acid test (NAT).[4]
- *HIV-1 p24 antigen (Ag)*: This marker is detectable by fourth-generation immunoassay within 4–10 days after the initial detection of HIV-1 RNA. Its detection window in the blood is transient because as antibodies begin to develop, they bind to this antigen and interfere with its detection.[5,6]
- *Immunoglobulin M (IgM) antibodies*: These become detectable 3–5 days after p24 Ag first becomes detectable. The tests that can be used are third- or fourth-generation immunoassays.[5]
- *IgG antibodies*: Finally IgG antibodies emerge and persist throughout the course of HIV infection.

This pattern of emergence of HIV markers is quite consistent and allows classification of HIV into the following laboratory stages:[3]

- *Eclipse period*: This period begins right after acquiring the HIV infection till the HIV-1 RNA can be first detected.
- *Seroconversion window period*: This is the period between acquiring the HIV infection and first detection of antibodies.
- *Acute HIV infection*: The period between the first emergence of detectable levels of HIV-1 RNA and the first detection of antibodies.
- *Established HIV infection*: This is the stage of fully developed IgG antibody response sufficient to be interpreted by Western blot (WB) or immunofluorescent assay (IFA).

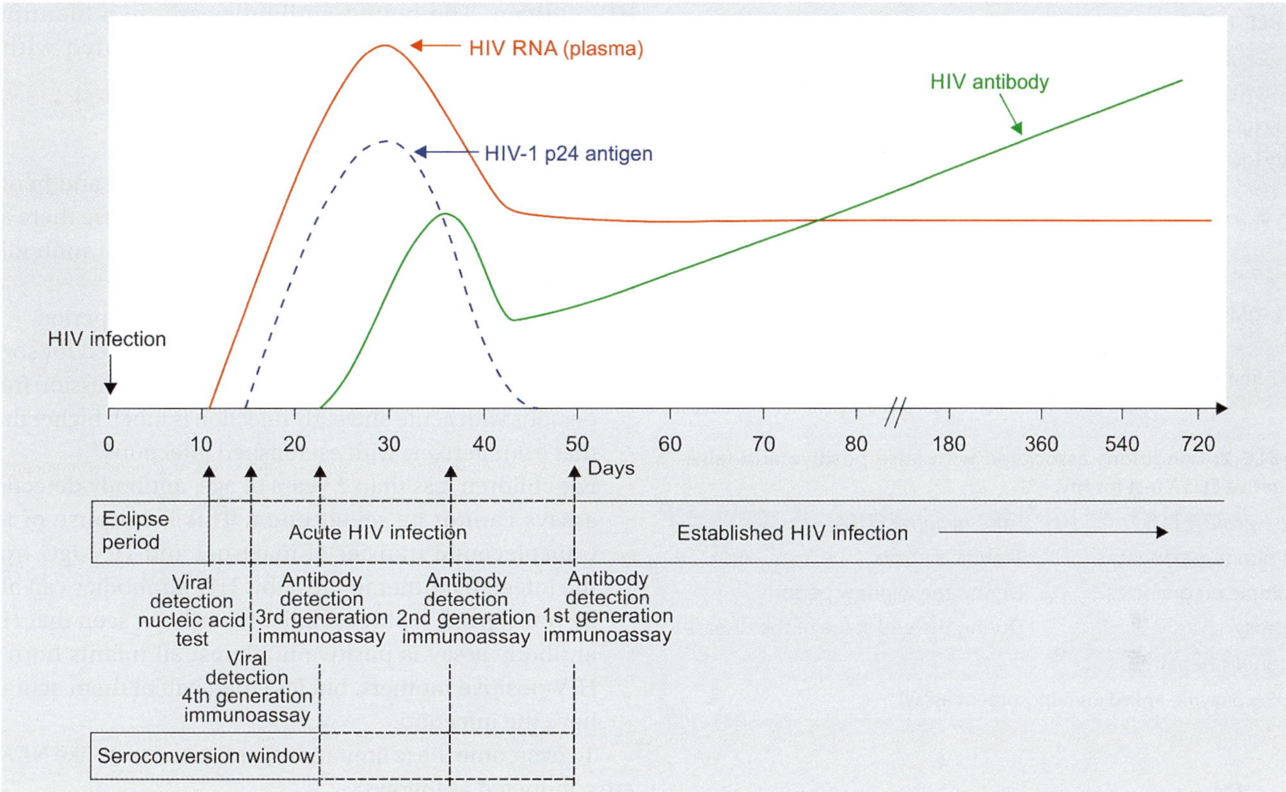

Fig. 1: Appearance of laboratory markers with respect to duration of HIV infection.

Source: Centers for Disease Control and Prevention (2014). Laboratory Testing for the Diagnosis of HIV Infection: Updated Recommendations. [online] Available from: https://stacks.cdc.gov/view/cdc/23447 [Last accessed February, 2021].

LABORATORY TESTS

- Screening tests should be the test with highest sensitivity:[7]
  - Enzyme-linked immunosorbent assay (ELISA)
  - *Rapid tests*:
    - Immunoconcentration assay (vertical flow)
    - Agglutination assay
    - Immunochromatographic assay (lateral flow)
    - Dipstick and comb assay based on enzyme immunoassay (EIA)
- Confirmatory tests:
  - Western blot
  - IFA
  - Molecular tests to detect HIV RNA or deoxyribonucleic acid (DNA) like nucleic acid amplification tests (NAATs)
  - Viral isolation
  - HIV p24 Ag detection
- Tests for monitoring progression of HIV infection and response to therapy:
  - Immunologic tests—CD4 T-cell count
  - Virological assays—HIV RNA viral load assays and reverse transcriptase (RT) activity assay

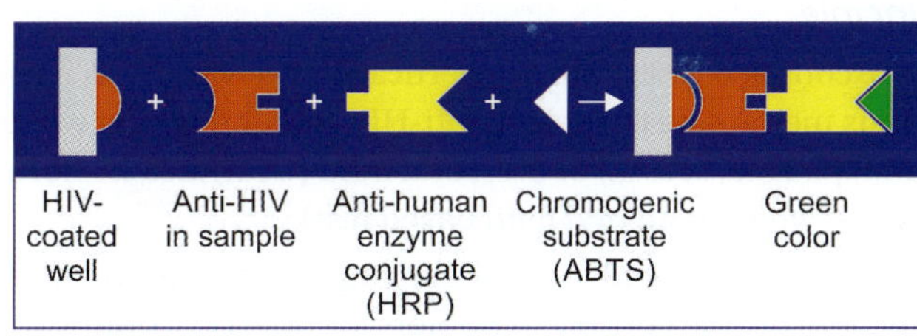

Fig. 2: Diagrammatic illustration of ELISA test in HIV.
(ABTS: 2,2′-azino-bis(3-ethylbenzthiazoline-6-sulfonic acid; ELISA: enzyme-linked immunosorbent assay; HIV: human immunodeficiency virus; HRP: horseradish peroxidase)

Enzyme-linked Immunosorbent Assay

Principle

Enzyme-linked immunosorbent assay consists of HIV antigen or antibody, attached to a solid phase and incorporated with a conjugate and substrate detection system **(Fig. 2)**. If the specimen contains HIV antibody, a color reaction (if the conjugate is an enzyme) or fluorescence takes place (if the conjugate is a fluorochrome).[1]

Over the period of time, various modifications and improvements have been made resulting in dividing the EIA into generations. Fourth-generation EIA is preferred because it can detect both IgM and IgG as well as p24 Ag **(Table 1)**.

Various conditions associated with false positive and false negative ELISA test for HIV has been depicted in **Table 2**.

TABLE 1: Different generations of antibody tests for HIV.

Nature of antibodies and antigens identified	*Generation*	*Description of antigens/ antibodies*
Only IgG	First	Antigens from HIV lysates
Only IgG	Second	Recombinant or synthetic peptides
IgG and IgM	Third	Recombinant or synthetic peptides in sandwich configuration
IgG, IgM and p24	Fourth	Detects p24 antigen and IgG and IgM simultaneously

(IgG: immunoglobulin G; IgM: immunoglobulin M)

TABLE 2: Conditions associated with false-positive and false-negative ELISA test for HIV.

False-positive ELISA	*False-negative ELISA*
Autoimmune diseases	Technical errors
Multiple pregnancies	During the window period
Leprosy	During the end stage of the disease
Alcoholic hepatitis	

(ELISA: enzyme-linked immunosorbent assay)

Rapid Tests

Rapid HIV tests are easy to do, give quick results and do not require any special equipment or expertise.

Principle

These consist of lateral flow or vertical flow devices which use porous membranes to detect anti-HIV IgG and IgM in whole blood, plasma, serum, or even oral fluid (OraQuick In-home HIV test which is an oral fluid based test).[7,8]

Even though rapid tests are no longer the recommended screening tests according to Centers for Disease Control and Prevention (CDC) 2014 guidelines,[3] these are particularly useful in resource limited setting or when immediate results are needed like women presenting in labor and patients with poor follow-up.[7]

Western Blot

Principle

Western blot detects HIV antibodies which bind to HIV proteins adsorbed onto a nitrocellulose paper, which then create a specific pattern when exposed to a substrate.[1,7]

Western blot is a highly specific test used for confirmation of HIV infection.[1]

Immunofluorescent Assay

Principle

Human immunodeficiency virus antibodies are detected by mixing serum or plasma sample with T-cells expressing HIV antigen. The bound antibodies are then identified using antihuman immunoglobulin conjugated with a fluorochrome.[7]

Molecular Tests

Molecular tests are used to detect viral genome and hence, are highly specific tests. These are needed because there are certain limitations of the tests which detect HIV antibodies (ELISA, rapid tests, WB, and IFA):

- Cannot diagnose the patients in the window period
- Acute HIV infections may remain undiagnosed for some time. It has been proven that the risk of transmission from persons with acute and early infection is much higher than that from persons with established infections.[9]
- For children less than 2 years of age, antibody detection assays cannot be relied upon. This is because of the transplacental transfer of maternal anti-HIV IgG from the infected mother to the baby. HIV antibodies can also be transferred via breast milk. It has been seen that HIV antibody assay is positive in almost all infants born to HIV-positive mothers, but less than half of them actually have the infection.

To overcome these limitations, molecular tests like NAATs are conducted as follows:

Qualitative Polymerase Chain Reaction of HIV DNA

Principle: HIV uses RT enzyme to produce DNA from the RNA genome of the virus. Then the viral DNA polymerase produces a complementary strand of DNA to make double-stranded viral DNA. This viral double-stranded DNA (dsDNA) can either integrate into the host's genome or lie freely in the cytoplasm. Polymerase chain reaction (PCR) is used to amplify and detect this HIV DNA.

The National AIDS Control Organization (NACO) first choice in detecting HIV infection in infants and children < 18 months is the HIV-1 DNA PCR test.[1] There are NAATs to detect HIV-2 nucleic acid, but they lack United States Food and Drug Administration (USFDA) approval.[3]

Quantitative HIV-1 RNA Assay

Principle: This test detects plasma viral RNA using various techniques like PCR. This is mainly used to identify the viral load, which is largely significant in monitoring the progression of the disease.

Viral Isolation

Isolating HIV requires peripheral blood mononuclear cells (PBMCs) cultivation from an infected individual with the mitogen stimulated PBMCs of an HIV-uninfected person. These are cultured together for about 6 weeks in a medium containing interleukin-2 (IL-2), at 37°C in 5% CO_2 for up to 28 days. The replication of HIV can be measured by p24 Ag detection by fourth-generation ELISA or by RT activity.[1]

This has significance only as a research tool since it is labor intensive, time consuming, expensive, and requires expertise.

Antigen Detection

Detection of p24 Ag in the specimen confirms the diagnosis of HIV-1 infection. But its absence does not rule out HIV, as mentioned earlier in the chapter that the presence of detectable levels of p24 Ag is only transient till the HIV antibodies production takes place.[1] HIV p24 Ag can now be detected by ELISA using the fourth-generation EIA.[3]

LABORATORY TESTING ALGORITHMS (FLOWCHART 1)

Human immunodeficiency virus testing algorithms involve a logical sequence of the above mentioned tests in order to arrive at an accurate HIV status of the individual in short time using minimum resources.

The latest CDC recommendations on laboratory testing for HIV will be discussed in a precise yet informative manner here. These guidelines are for adults and children of 2 years of age and more, and the specimen to be used is freshly collected serum or plasma. These recommendations do not address the tests for screening blood or organ donors. Special emphasis has been made on using USFDA approved tests as much as possible.[3]

- The testing begins with an FDA-approved fourth-generation immunoassay, which can detect both HIV-1 and HIV-2 antibodies as well as HIV-1 p24 Ag. No further testing is required if the specimen comes out to be nonreactive on this assay.
- Specimens coming out as reactive for the initial EIA should undergo testing with an FDA-approved antibody immunoassay that differentiates HIV-1 antibodies from HIV-2 antibodies. Accurate diagnosis of HIV-2 is clinically significant as some antiretroviral agents which are effective against HIV-1 [nucleoside reverse transcriptase inhibitor (NRTIs) and some protease inhibitors (PIs)] are not effective against HIV-2.[10]
- Specimens, which are reactive for the initial immunoassay but nonreactive or indeterminate for the HIV-1/HIV-2 antibody differentiation immunoassay, should be tested with the FDA-approved HIV-1 NAT.
    - HIV-1 NAT reactive but HIV-1/HIV-2 antibody differentiation assay nonreactive—acute HIV infection.
    - HIV-1 NAT reactive but HIV-1/HIV-2 antibody differentiation assay indeterminate—HIV infection positive.
    - HIV-1 NAT nonreactive and indeterminate/nonreactive HIV-1/HIV-2 antibody differentiation assay—negative for HIV infection.
- Positive results from the recommended algorithm require the need for additional tests such as HIV viral load, CD4 T-cell count, antiretroviral resistance assay to stage the disease, and choose the antiretroviral therapy (ART) regimen.[11]

HIV TESTING IN SPECIAL SITUATIONS

- *HIV diagnosis in pediatric population*: As mentioned earlier, detection of HIV antibodies in children less than 2 years of age is not a ground for diagnosis of HIV as IgG antibodies can be transmitted transplacentally from mother to the fetus.[12] In such cases, HIV-1 NAT becomes the test of choice.[1]
- *For blood transfusion and transplant safety:* As advised in NACO guidelines,[1] only one test with high sensitivity is required (third- or fourth-generation ELISA or rapid tests). If nonreactive, the specimen is considered HIV negative, and if it comes out to be reactive, the specimen is labeled as HIV positive and the blood unit is discarded. No further testing is necessary.

Flowchart 1: Algorithm for HIV testing of serum or plasma specimens.

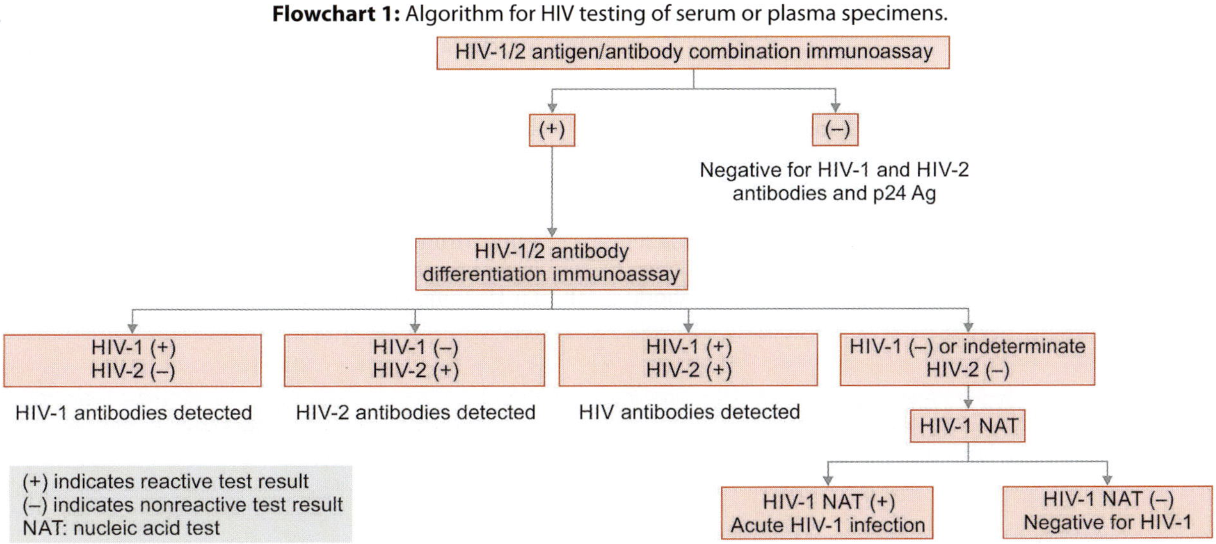

Source: Centers for Disease Control and Prevention (2014). Laboratory Testing for the Diagnosis of HIV Infection: Updated Recommendations. [online] Available from: https://stacks.cdc.gov/view/cdc/23447 [Last accessed February, 2021].

- *HIV vaccine recipients testing*: HIV vaccine recipients who test positive with the initial EIA should contact the vaccine trial site for specialized testing.[13]

FUTURE OF HIV DIAGNOSTICS

- Simultaneous detection of HIV-1 viral load and RNA based on a novel pH-mediated complementary metal-oxide semiconductor (CMOS) chip.[14]
- Biosensor is an upcoming technology which can be used for molecular diagnosis of HIV. The principle is molecular interaction between the surface-linked oligonucleotides and hybridization with complementary target nucleotides present in the specimen.[15]
- Better diagnostics for HIV-2 infection determination. Need for a USFDA approved HIV-2 NAT and tests for HIV-2 Ag p26/27 (the core protein counterpart of p24 Ag in HIV-1).[16]

KEY POINTS

- Fourth-generation EIA that detects HIV-1 and HIV-2 antibodies as well as HIV-1 p24 Ag is the first test to be done in most situations.[17]
- HIV-1 NAT can diagnose an acute HIV-1 infection and distinguish it from a false-positive initial immunoassay.
- HIV-1 NAT does not detect HIV-2.
- *Myth buster*: HIV-1 NAT is not the test of choice when it comes to detecting HIV status of the general population. It is, however, the test of choice in certain situations like in children less than 2 years of age and transplant recipients.[18]
- *Myth buster*: The rapid tests for HIV do not have anything to do with the early diagnosis of HIV infection. The "rapid" refers to the fact that the test procedure and results take a short time.[18]
- The tests suggested in the chapter are for plasma/serum and not recommended for oral fluids or dried blood spots.

REFERENCES

1. National AIDS Control Organization. Serological diagnosis of HIV infection. In: National Guidelines for HIV Testing. New Delhi: National AIDS Control Organization; 2015.
2. James WD, Berger TG, Elston DM. Viral diseases. In: James WD, Berger TG, Elston DM (Eds). Andrews' Diseases of the Skin, 12th edition. Philadelphia: Elsevier; 2016. pp. 359-417.
3. Centers for Disease Control and Prevention (2014). Laboratory Testing for the Diagnosis of HIV Infection: Updated Recommendations. [online] Available from: https://stacks.cdc.gov/view/cdc/23447 [Last accessed February, 2021].
4. Keele BF, Giorgi EE, Salazar-Gonzalez JF, Decker JM, Pham KT, Salazar MG, et al. Identification and characterization of transmitted and early founder virus envelopes in primary HIV-1 infection. Proc Natl Acad Sci USA. 2008;105(21):7552-7.
5. Masciotra S, McDougal JS, Feldman J, Sprinkle P, Wesolowski L, Michele Owen S. Evaluation of an alternative HIV diagnostic algorithm using specimens from seroconversion panels and persons with established HIV infections. J Clin Virol. 2011;52(Suppl 1):S17-22.
6. Goudsmit J, de Wolf F, Paul DA, Epstein LG, Lange JM, Krone WJ, et al. Expression of human immunodeficiency virus antigen (HIV-Ag) in serum and cerebrospinal fluid during acute and chronic infection. Lancet. 1986;2(8500):177-80.
7. Cornett JK, Kirn TJ. Laboratory diagnosis of HIV in adults: a review of current methods. Clin Infect Dis. 2013;57(5):712-8.
8. Food and Drug Administration (2012). OraQuick In-Home HIV Test. [online] Available from: http://www.fda.gov/downloads/AdvisoryCommittees/CommitteesMeetingMaterials/Blood VaccinesandOtherBiologics/BloodProductsAdvisoryCommittee/UCM303652.pdf [Last accessed February, 2021].
9. Hollingsworth TD, Anderson RM, Fraser C. HIV-1 transmission, by stage of infection. J Infect Dis. 2008;198(5):687-93.
10. Ntemgwa ML, d'Aquin TT, Brenner BG, Camacho RJ, Wainberg MA. Antiretroviral drug resistance in human immunodeficiency virus type 2. Antimicrob Agents Chemother. 2009;53(9):3611-9.
11. Panel on Antiretroviral Guidelines for Adults and Adolescents. Guidelines for the use of antiretroviral agents in HIV-1-infected adults and adolescents. Washington, DC: Department of Health and Human Services; 2013.
12. Jendis JB, Tomasik Z, Hunziker U, Nadal D, Seger R, Wetzel JC, et al. Evaluation of diagnostic tests for HIV infection in infants born to HIV-infected mothers in Switzerland. AIDS. 1988;2(4): 273-9.
13. HIV Vaccine Trials Network. HIV vaccine study participants need to get the right test for HIV. [online] Available from: http://www.hvtn.org/en/participants/visp-hiv-testing.html [Last accessed February, 2021].
14. Gurrala R, Lang Z, Shepherd L, Davidson D. Novel pH sensing semiconductor for point-of-care detection of HIV-1 viremia. Sci Rep. 2016;6:36000.
15. Arya S, Lal P, Singh P, Kumar A. Recent advances in diagnosis of HIV and future prospects. Indian J Biotechnol. 2015;14:9-18.
16. Masciotra S, Luo W, Youngpairoj AS, Kennedy MS, Wells S, Ambrose K, et al. Performance of the Alere Determine HIV-1/2 Ag/Ab Combo Rapid Test with specimens from HIV-1 seroconverters from the US and HIV-2 infected individuals from Ivory Coast. J Clin Virol. 2013;58(Suppl 1):e54-8.
17. Suligoi B, Rodella A, Raimondo M, Regine V, Terlenghi L, Manca N, et al. Avidity Index for anti-HIV antibodies: comparison between third and fourth-generation automated immunoassays. J Clin Microbiol. 2011;49(7):2610-3.
18. Lu H, Tang YW. Myths in the laboratory diagnosis of HIV infection. Emerg Microbes Infect. 2019;8(1):1240-2.

EXAMINATION QUESTION

1. Write a short note on laboratory diagnosis of HIV.

142 CHAPTER

Antiretroviral Therapy

Arnab Dutta, Abhishek De, Aarti Sarda

INTRODUCTION

- Antiretroviral therapy (ART) denotes the use of pharmacological agents effective against the HIV virus.
- Highly active antiretroviral therapy (HAART) is a treatment regimen typically comprised of a combination of three or more antiretroviral drugs. HAART may be called interchangeably ART or combination antiretroviral therapy (cART).
- The dramatic decline in annual AIDS-related mortality has largely been attributed to the use of HAART. Several effective antiretroviral (ARV) agents are available and many more are in the pipeline.[1]
- ART suppresses replication of the HIV virus and with the virological suppression that ensues, CD4 lymphocyte depletion is halted and patients develop slow but definite immune restoration.
- Advances in modern ART have dramatically reduced morbidity and mortality for persons living with HIV (PLWH).
- Studies have found that 3-drug therapy has led to a 60% to 80% decline in rates of AIDS, hospitalization, and death. By 2030 the CDC plans to implement a 90-90-90 plan (90% HIV diagnosed, 90% on therapy, and 90% suppressed).[2]

HISTORY OF ART[3]

- The first therapy to work against HIV was the nucleoside reverse transcriptase inhibitor zidovudine (1987).
- In short succession, three other nucleoside reverse transcriptase inhibitors (NRTIs) were approved for use in HIV-1 infection: zalcitabine (ddC), didanosine (ddI), and stavudine (d4T).
- The first protease inhibitor to be approved was saquinavir in 1995.
- Indinavir is a protease inhibitor, approved in 1996, which substantially changed the treatment landscape, ushering in the HAART era.
- During the Vancouver AIDS Conference in 1996, the successful impact of triple combination therapy was reported.
- Over the past years, progress in ART has been characterized by the availability of new potent, and relatively safer ARV drugs belonging to old classes (NRTI, NNRTI, and protease inhibitor) and to new classes (entry/attachment inhibitors and integrase inhibitors).

INITIATING ART

- This decision of starting ART should be based on CD4 cell count, presence of symptoms, and viral load.
- The CD4 count is the most important indicator and there is a general consensus treatment is indicated for all patients with a CD4 count <200 cells/mm^3.
- Symptomatic HIV infection is an indication for ART, irrespective of the CD4 counts.
- Whether to initiate therapy in the CD4 stratum between 200 and 350 cells/mm^3 in an asymptomatic patient is a controversial issue. ART should probably be started within this range depending on the symptoms, viral load, CD4 slope, patient preference, and associated comorbidities.[2]
- According to recent guidelines, ART is recommended for all individuals with HIV to reduce the morbidity and mortality associated with HIV infection and to prevent HIV transmission to sexual partners and infants. ART should be initiated as soon as possible after HIV diagnosis. When initiating ART, it is important to educate patients about the goals and benefits of ART and to identify and address barriers to care engagement and treatment adherence.[4]
- The TEMPRANO study showed that starting ART at CD4 >500 in the absence of any of the existing clinical criteria for starting therapy reduced severe HIV morbidity.[5]
- Another advantage of early initiation of ART in countries like India is the reduction in chance of tuberculosis.
- Early initiation of ART was also found to be more cost effective as there is future reduced costs of future hospitalizations and improved quality of life, as well as costs saved due to reduction in number of new infections.[3]

GOALS OF THERAPY

- Durable suppression of HIV viral load to less than 50 copies/mL
- Reduce morbidity and mortality (AIDS and non-AIDS associated causes)
- Restoration of immune function as evidenced by CD4 cell count increase

- Prevention of HIV transmission
- Prevention of drug resistance
- Improvement in quality of life.

PRETREATMENT EVALUATION[6]

- A complete history and physical examination
- *Eye:* Fundus examination
- Complete blood count with differential
- Biochemistry profile
- Fasting glucose and hemoglobin A1C
- Urinalysis
- Pregnancy test
- CD4/CD8 T-cell count/ratio
- Plasma HIV-1 RNA measurement (viral load)
- Supplementary tests including the venereal disease research laboratory (VDRL), Mantoux test, chest X-ray, and serology for hepatitis C and B
- HLA-B*5701 testing

MONITORING

Every 3–6 months:

- CD4 count for the first 2 years of ART or if viremia develops
- HIV viral load
- Basic chemistry
- Alanine transaminase (ALT)/aspartate transaminase (AST)/bilirubin
- Complete blood count (CBC) with differential
- Fasting glucose and hemoglobin A1C if abnormal before
- Urinalysis

Every 12 months:

- After 2 years, if the CD4 count is 300–500, then every 12 months; if CD4 is greater than 500, monitoring is optional
- Hepatitis B serology may get repeated unless immunized
- Hepatitis C screen if the patient is at risk
- Fasting lipid profile
- Fasting glucose and hemoglobin A1C
- Urinalysis
- QuantiFERON TB test

For treatment failure/modification:

- CD4 count
- HIV viral load
- Resistance testing
- Tropism testing
- Hepatitis B serology
- Hepatitis C screening
- Basic chemistry
- ALT/AST/bilirubin
- CBC with differential
- Fasting lipid profile
- Fasting glucose and hemoglobin A1C
- Urinalysis
- Pregnancy test

ANTIRETROVIRAL MEDICATIONS

The goal of HIV medicines is to prevent HIV from multiplying. These drugs generally fall into classes according to the phase of the HIV life cycle inhibited by them **(Box 1)**.

More common combinations include two nucleoside reverse transcriptase inhibitors (NRTIs) and one non-nucleoside reverse transcriptase inhibitor (NNRTI), a protease inhibitor (PI), or an integrase inhibitor (II) **(Box 2)**.

MECHANISM OF ACTION OF ANTIRETROVIRAL MEDICATIONS

Antiretroviral drugs target different stages in the viral life cycle **(Fig. 1)**.[7-9]

NRTIs:

- NRTIs are administered as prodrugs, which require host cell entry and phosphorylation by cellular kinases before enacting an antiviral effect.

BOX 1: List of FDA-approved antiretroviral (ARV) medications.

- *NRTIs:* Abacavir, emtricitabine, lamivudine; tenofovir disoproxil fumarate, zidovudine
- *NNRTIs:* Efavirenz, etravirine, nevirapine, rilpivirine
- *Fusion inhibitors (FIs):* Enfuvirtide
- *Protease inhibitors (PIs):* Atazanavir, darunavir, fosamprenavir, ritonavir, saquinavir, tipranavir
- *CCR5 antagonist:* Maraviroc
- *IIs:* Dolutegravir, raltegravir, elvitegravir, bictegravir
- *Postattachment inhibitors:* Ibalizumab
- *Pharmacokinetic enhancers:* Cobicistat

(CCR5: C-C motif chemokine receptor; NRTIs: nucleoside reverse transcriptase inhibitors; NNRTIs: non-nucleoside reverse transcriptase inhibitors; PIs: protease inhibitors)

BOX 2: FDA-approved HIV combination medicines.

- Abacavir and lamivudine
- Abacavir, dolutegravir, and lamivudine
- Abacavir, lamivudine, and zidovudine
- Atazanavir and cobicistat
- Bictegravir, emtricitabine, and tenofovir alafenamide
- Darunavir and cobicistat
- Dolutegravir and rilpivirine
- Efavirenz, emtricitabine, and tenofovir disoproxil fumarate
- Efavirenz, lamivudine, and tenofovir disoproxil fumarate
- Elvitegravir, cobicistat, emtricitabine, and tenofovir alafenamide fumarate
- Elvitegravir, cobicistat, emtricitabine, and tenofovir disoproxil fumarate
- Emtricitabine, rilpivirine, and tenofovir alafenamide
- Emtricitabine, rilpivirine, and tenofovir disoproxil fumarate
- Emtricitabine and tenofovir alafenamide
- Emtricitabine and tenofovir disoproxil fumarate
- Lamivudine and tenofovir disoproxil fumarate
- Lamivudine and zidovudine
- Lopinavir and ritonavir

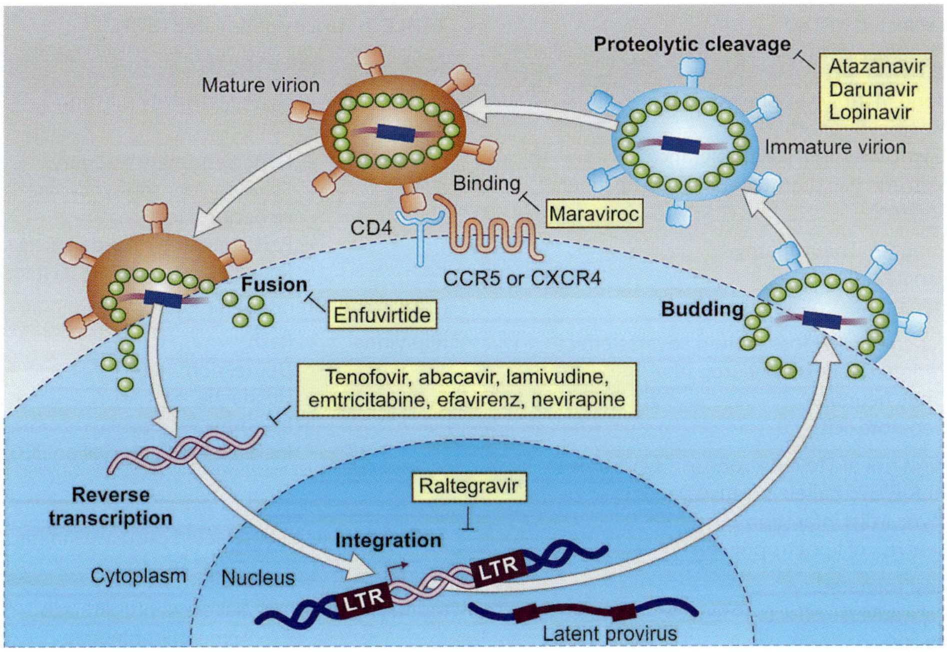

Fig. 1: Mechanism of action of antiretroviral drugs and their targets of action.

- NRTIs compete with natural deoxy-nucleotides to get incorporated into a growing viral DNA strand.
- However, NRTIs lack a 3'-hydroxyl group on the deoxy-ribose moiety.
- This difference results in the incorporation of an NRTI, and the next incoming deoxynucleotide cannot form the following 3'-5' phosphodiester bond needed to extend the DNA chain.
- This results in chain termination.
- All NRTIs are excreted by the kidney except abacavir and zidovudine.
- HIV resistance occurs through nucleotide associated mutations that remove NRTIs from the 3' end.

NNRTIs:

- Block reverse transcriptase (RT) by directly binding to the enzyme.
- Though NNRTIs do not get incorporated into the viral DNA, they inhibit the movement of protein domains of RT that are essential to carry out the DNA synthesis.
- They inhibit reverse transcriptase enzyme by non-competitive inhibition and are active only against HIV-1 and not against HIV-2.

Protease inhibitors:

- Bind HIV-1 protease and block proteolytic cleavage of protein precursors that are necessary for the production of viral particles.
- PI inhibits post-transcriptional cleavage of gag polyprotein, preventing processing of viral proteins into functional conformations.
- This results in the production of immature non-infectious viral particles.
- Protease inhibitors are metabolized by CYP3A4 except nelfinavir metabolized by CYP2C19. Ritonavir is the most potent CYP3A4 inhibitor. Most PIs are substrate for P-glycoprotein efflux pumps.

Integrase inhibitors:

- Block the action of integrase, preventing the viral genome from inserting itself into the DNA of a host cell.
- Raltegravir is active against both HIV-1 and 2.

Fusion inhibitors:

- Disrupt binding, fusion, and entry of HIV virions into a human cell.
- Enfuvirtide binds to gp41 and disrupts membrane attachment.

CCR5 antagonist: Maraviroc blocks the CCCR receptor on the T-cell to prevent viral attachment.

Postattachment inhibitors: This is a monoclonal antibody that binds CD4 inhibiting viral entry into the cell.

Pharmacokinetic enhancers: Inhibition of human CYP3A protein, increasing plasma concentration of other anti-HIV drugs.

ADVERSE EFFECTS

NRTIs:

- Adverse effects of NRTIs are due to inhibition of mito-chondrial DNA polymerase gamma.
- NRTIs are known to cause mitochondrial toxicity that may present as peripheral neuropathy and lactic acidosis that can be fatal.
- Some NRTIs may also cause bone marrow suppression, anemia, and lipodystrophy **(Table 1)**.

TABLE 1: Toxicity of selected NRTIs.[4]

Drug	*Adverse effect*
Zidovudine (AZT)	• Bone marrow suppression • Macrocytic anemia • Gastrointestinal (GI) intolerance • Skin and nail pigmentation—azure lunula • Steatosis
Stavudine	• Peripheral neuropathy • Pancreatitis • Hepatic steatosis
Didanosine	• Pancreatitis—dose limited adverse effect • Peripheral sensory neuropathy • Optic neuritis • Hepatotoxicity
Abacavir	• High risk of Stevens–Johnson syndrome in HLA-B*5701 allele positive patients • Myocardial infarction • Less risk of lipoatrophy
Lamivudine	• Best tolerated • Rare adverse effects—neutropenia, headache, nausea • Safe in pregnancy
Emtricitabine	• GI toxicity • Hyperpigmentation of palms
Tenofovir	• Renal insufficiency • Fanconi syndrome • Asthenia headache • Diarrhea, nausea, vomiting • Flatulence

- Abacavir is associated with a CD8 mediated hypersensitivity reaction in patients with the HLA-B*5701 mutation.
- Tenofovir may cause renal toxicity or decreased bone mineral density.
- Didanosine is seldom used these days due to the high risk of pancreatitis and hepatomegaly.[10-12]

NNRTIs:

- NNRTIs may cause skin rashes from transient hypersensitivity to Stevens–Johnson syndrome.
- Hepatitis can occur as early as 6 weeks into starting therapy.
- There is some evidence of teratogenicity in some of the NNRTIs including a risk of neural tube defects.
- QT prolongation may occur with the use of NNRTIs, especially rilpivirine.
- NNRTIs also cause a range of interactions with hepatic cytochrome P450 enzymes, so concurrent medications must be checked closely for dosage adjustments or interaction concerns.[10-12]
- Efavirenz is known to cause a range of neuro-psychiatric effects including vivid dreams, delusions, sleep disturbances, dizziness, headaches, increased suicidal tendency, psychosis, and mania **(Table 2)**.[10-12]

TABLE 2: Toxicity of selected NRTIs.[5]

Drug	*Adverse effect*
Nevirapine (NVP)	• Hypersensitivity reaction • Rash
Efavirenz (EFV)	• Hypersensitivity reaction • Stevens–Johnson syndrome • Hepatic toxicity • Persistent and severe CNS toxicity • Potential teratogenicity (first trimester of pregnancy)
Delavirdine	Teratogenic
Rilpivirine	• Rash • Depression • Headache • Insomnia • Increase in QT interval on ECG

TABLE 3: Toxicity of selected protease inhibitors.

Drug	*Adverse effect*
Indinavir	• Severe nephrolithiasis • Hyperbilirubinemia • Insulin resistance • Increased incidence of myocardial infarction • Elevated liver enzymes • Insomnia • Sicca syndrome • Increased risk of pyogenic granuloma
Ritonavir	• GI upset • Circumoral paresthesia • Asthenia • Hepatitis • Dysgeusia
Amprenavir	Contraindicated in – young children, pregnancy, renal and hepatic failure
Fosamprenavir	• GI upset • Hyperglycemia • Deranged lipid profile
Saquinavir	• GI upset • Increase in QT interval on ECG • Lipodystrophy
Atazanavir	• Hyperbilirubinemia • GI toxicity • Peripheral neuropathy • No insulin resistance, lipodystrophy
Nelfinavir	• Diarrhea and flatulence • Glucose intolerance
Lopinavir	• Hepatotoxic • Increase in QT interval on ECG
Tipranavir	• Hepatotoxicity • Increased risk of intracranial hemorrhage

Protease inhibitors:

- PI can cause hepatotoxicity, insulin resistance, hyperglycemia, hyperlipidemia, lipodystrophy, and PR interval prolongation **(Table 3)**.
- Indinavir is no longer used regularly due to inefficiency, increased resistance, and an increased risk of nephrolithiasis.[10-12]

Integrase inhibitors:

- IIs are generally well-tolerated, and overall they have neutral effects on lipid profile.
- Some patients may experience dizziness, sleep disturbances, or depression.
- Rhabdomyolysis and myopathy are rarely reported in patients taking raltegravir and dolutegravir. Raltegravir is also reported to cause DRESS syndrome.
- Dolutegravir can occasionally cause a decrease in the glomerular filtration rate (GFR). It can also have interactions with several medications, including those that inhibit/induce CYP3A4 enzymes, metformin, rifampin, and antiepileptics.
- Elvitegravir has substantial pharmacokinetic benefit with cobicistat which is a ritonavir analogue that lacks ARV action.[10-12]

Fusion inhibitors: Enfuvirtide is generally well tolerated though some patients may experience injection site reactions.[10-12]

Chemokine receptor antagonists (CCR5 antagonists):

- Maraviroc is generally well tolerated though some patients may experience dizziness or skin rashes.
- There is a risk of hepatotoxicity with allergic features, so patients should be monitored closely for symptoms of allergic reactions or hepatic dysfunction.
- Drug-drug interactions should be a consideration if patients are taking concurrent CYP3A4 inhibitors or inducers.[10-12]

CONTRAINDICATIONS

- There are no outright contraindications to HAART therapy; all patients clinicians find to be HIV positive should start a treatment regimen immediately, regardless of their CD4 count.
- There are, however contraindications to specific ARV medications, but healthcare providers should find a different HAART combination for patients with these specific comorbidities **(Box 3)**.[10-12]

BOX 3: Contradiction of various antiretroviral (ARV) drugs in comorbidities.

- *Hepatic dysfunction:* Avoid efavirenz, tenofovir-disoproxil fumarate (TDF), and maraviroc.
- *Renal dysfunction:* Avoid or adjust dosages of tenofovir, maraviroc, and atazanavir.
- *Psychiatric illnesses:* Avoid efavirenz and dolutegravir.
- *Pregnancy, or Lactation:* Should avoid NNRTIs, dolutegravir, bictegravir, stavudine, didanosine, and ritonavir. Preferred regimen in pregnancy is usually a combination of NRTIs plus a protease or integrase inhibitor.
- *Torsades de pointes or cardiovascular disease:* Avoid efavirenz and abacavir
- *Concurrent tuberculosis:* Rifampin should be replaced with rifabutin
- *HLA-B*5701 positive patient:* Should avoid abacavir

ANTIRETROVIRAL THERAPY GUIDELINES (NACO 2018)[13]

1. *First-line regime:* Tenofovir + Lamivudine + Efavirenz
2. In patients with: (a) Known renal disease; (b) HIV-2 or HIV-1 and 2 infection; (c) Women with single dose Nevirapine exposure in past pregnancy; (d) Renal disease: Abacavir + Lamivudine + Efavirenz
3. *HIV-1 and HIV-2 coinfection:* Tenofovir + Lamivudine + Lopinavir/ritonavir
4. ART regimen for pregnant women having prior exposure to NNRTI for PPTCT - TDF + 3TC and LPV/r
5. Postexposure prophylaxis – (to be continued for 4 weeks): (a) Tenofovir (300) + Lamivudine (300)—One tablet once daily (OR); (b) Lopinavir (200) + Ritonavir (50)—Two FDC tablets twice daily
6. Cotrimoxazole preventive therapy: (a) One double strength tablet – 800 sulfamethoxazole + 160 mg trimethoprim (b) START – CD4 < 350/mm^3; (c) STOP - CD4 > 350 on two occasions 6 months apart + ascending trend of CD4 + no WHO stage 3, 4.

ADHERENCE TO ART

- Before starting ART, it is imperative that the patient has a fair idea that therapy is long-term, i.e., life-long; and that compliance with the drug regimen is most important for good virologic response.
- At least 95% adherence is required for durable and optimal viral suppression.
- There should be an adequate discussion regarding childbearing, treating other affected family members like a spouse or a child.[14]

TREATMENT FAILURE

- Treatment failure is defined using the same variables that define the goals of ART.
- Virologic failure is viral load (VL) >200 c/mL or a sustained VL > 50 c/mL, after 24 weeks of therapy. Immunologic failure is arbitrarily defined as failure of the CD4 count to rise by 25–50 cells/mm^3 in the first year after HAART.
- Clinical failure is defined as the occurrence of an AIDS-defining opportunistic complication after three months of HAART, when immune reconstitution inflammatory syndrome (IRIS) has been excluded.[14]

NATIONAL STRATEGIC PLAN FOR HIV/AIDS (2017–2024)

- *Objective 1:* Reduce 80% new infections by 2024 (Baseline 2010).
- *Objective 2:* Ensure 95% of estimated PLHIV know their status by 2024.

- *Objective 3:* Ensure 95% PLHIV have ART initiation and retention by 2024 for sustained viral suppression.
- *Objective 4:* Eliminate mother-to-child transmission of HIV and syphilis by 2020.
- *Objective 5:* Eliminate HIV/AIDS-related stigma and discrimination by 2020.
- *Objective 6:* Facilitate sustainable NACP service delivery by 2024.

PREDICTORS OF INADEQUATE RESPONSE TO ART

There are some factors that predict poor adherence:[15]

- Poor interpersonal relation between the patient and the treating physician
- Active psychiatric illness (e.g., depression)
- Inability of illiterate patients to identify medications
- Restricted access to primary medical care or medications

STRATEGIES TO IMPROVE ADHERENCE TO THERAPY

- Education of the patient about the disease and its course.
- Assessment and establishment of the patient's readiness to take medication.
- Discussion of the goals of therapy, need for adherence, and the outcome with the patient.
- Making him understand that the initial regimen has the best chance for long-term success.
- Implementation of a treatment plan that the patient understands and to which he/she commits.

NEED FOR A LONG-TERM VIEW

- ART provides a lifeline to those infected by the virus. Judicious use of these drugs is essential to ensure delayed development of resistance, and durable viral suppression.
- In resource-poor settings, ART drug regimens have often not been chosen with long-term treatment as the first priority.
- An initial choice of the cheapest combination will come at a high cost later on.
- Although price considerations remain important, regimen choices should be driven mainly by data demonstrating durability of therapy, which is determined by antiviral potency, a high barrier against the development of viral resistance, and good short- and long-term tolerability.
- In combination with adherence support, this will lead to near universal treatment success, allowing for a reversal of the downward spiral of socioeconomic development that HIV/AIDS has caused in resource-poor settings.[15]

KEY POINTS

- ART denotes the use of pharmacological agents effective against the HIV virus.
- ARV drugs delay progression of HIV disease and improve the quality of life in the HIV infected.
- The pretreatment evaluation should include a complete history and physical examination, fundus examination, complete blood count, biochemistry profile, lipid profile, CD4/CD8 T-cell count/ratio, plasma HIV-1 RNA measurement (viral load) and supplementary tests including VDRL, Mantoux test, chest X-ray, and serology for hepatitis C and B.
- ART drugs are distributed into six distinct classes based on their molecular mechanism and resistance profiles: (1) nucleoside-analog reverse transcriptase inhibitors (NNRTIs), (2) non-nucleoside reverse transcriptase inhibitors (NNRTIs), (3) integrase inhibitors, (4) protease inhibitors (PIs), (5) fusion inhibitors, and (6) coreceptor antagonist.
- Regimen choices should be driven mainly by data demonstrating durability of therapy, which is determined by antiviral potency, a high barrier against the development of viral resistance, and good short- and long-term tolerability.

REFERENCES

1. Nischal KC, Khopkar U, Saple DG. Improving adherence to antiretroviral therapy. Indian J Dermatol Venereol Leprol. 2005;71:316-20.
2. Grobler A, Cawood C, Khanyile D, Puren A, Kharsany ABM. Progress of UNAIDS 90-90-90 targets in a district in KwaZulu-Natal, South Africa, with high HIV burden, in the HIPSS study: a household-based complex multilevel community survey. Lancet HIV. 2017;4(11):e505-13.
3. Pau AK, George JM. Antiretroviral therapy: current drugs. Infect Dis Clin North Am. 2014;28(3):371-402.
4. García-Deltoro M. Rapid initiation of antiretroviral therapy after HIV diagnosis. AIDS Rev. 2019;21(2):55-64.
5. Lundgren JD, Borges AH, Neaton JD. Serious non-AIDS conditions in HIV: benefit of early ART. Curr HIV/AIDS Rep. 2018;15(2):162-71.
6. Boffito M, Acosta E, Burger D, Fletcher CV, Flexner C, Garaffo R, et al. Therapeutic drug monitoring and drug-drug interactions involving antiretroviral drugs. Antivir Ther. 2005; 10:469-77.
7. Taylor BS, Tieu HV, Jones J, Wilkin TJ. CROI 2019: advances in antiretroviral therapy. Top Antivir Med. 2019;27(1):50-68.
8. Pau AK, George JM. Antiretroviral therapy: current drugs. Infect Dis Clin North Am. 2014;28(3):371-402.
9. Lu DY, Wu HY, Yarla NS, Xu B, Ding J, Lu TR. HAART in HIV/AIDS treatments: future trends. Infect Disord Drug Targets. 2018;18(1):15-22.
10. Sharma A, Vora R, Modi M, Sharma A, Marfatia Y. Adverse effects of antiretroviral treatment. Indian J Dermatol Venereol Leprol. 2008;74:234-7.
11. Lucas GM, Chaisson RE, Moore RD. Highly active antiretroviral therapy in a large urban clinic: risk factors for

virologic failure and adverse drug reactions. Ann Intern Med. 1999;131:81-7.
12. Fellay J, Bousaker K, Ledergerber B, Bernasconi E, Furrer H, Battegay M, et al. Prevalence of adverse drug events associated with potent antiretroviral treatment: Swiss HIV cohort study. Lancet. 2001;358:1322-7.
13. Mitruka K, Bamrotiya M, Agarwal R, Parvez A, Allam RR, Sivalenka S, et al. Implementation of the treat all policy among persons with HIV infection enrolled in care but not on antiretroviral therapy - India, May 2017-June 2018. Morb Mortal Wkly Rep. 2018;67(47):1305-9.
14. O'Brien ME, Clark RA, Besch CL, Myers L, Kissinger P. Patterns and correlates of discontinuation of the initial HAART regimen in urban outpatient cohort. J Acquir Immune Defic Syndr. 2003;34:407-14.
15. Maniar J, Desai S. Antiretroviral therapy: Real challenges for developing World. Int Cong Drug Ther HIV. 2000; 5:249.

EXAMINATION QUESTIONS

Write a short note on the following:

1. ART.
2. HAART.
3. Adverse effects of ART drugs.
4. ART recent guidelines.
5. Pre-exposure prophylaxis in HIV.
6. Post-exposure prophylaxis in HIV.
7. HIV and pregnancy.
8. HIV and leprosy.

14 SECTION | Therapeutics in Dermatology

143 CHAPTER Principles and Advances in Topical Therapy

Sujata Sengupta, Arijit Coondoo

INTRODUCTION

Skin being the largest organ of the body is exposed to the perils of different harmful external agents. This easy accessibility of skin also makes topical therapy one of the two biggest pillars of treatment of dermatological diseases. A large number of dermatologic disorders can be well managed with topical therapy alone thus bypassing the side-effects of systemic use. Sometimes, a combination of both topical and systemic therapy gives faster and sustained results. Along with several advantages, topical therapy has certain drawbacks also **(Table 1)**.

TABLE 1: Advantages and disadvantages of topical therapy.

Advantages	*Disadvantages*
Lesser doses needed than systemic routes, so economical	Time-consuming
Bypass of hepatic first pass metabolism	Can be messy
Elimination of GI adverse effects	Multiple medications can make application complicated and impractical
High concentrations of drugs may be used locally without internal organs getting exposed	Cutaneous side effects can be troublesome, e.g., topical steroids
Newer formulations make slow and sustained release possible	
Improved patient compliance	

PERCUTANEOUS ABSORPTION OF DRUGS

The percutaneous absorption of drugs follows three steps:[1]

1. *Penetration*: Drug entry through a skin layer
2. *Permeation*: Passage of drug from one layer to another
3. *Resorption*: Drug uptake by vascular system.

So, a drug has to go through these steps before exerting its final effect. The active ingredient is usually incorporated in a vehicle. A vehicle facilitates the drug delivery and in certain cases the vehicle itself is applied onto the skin. Usually, the first step is the dissociation of the drug from the vehicle. Then the ingredient passes through the stratum corneum (penetration) and is either bound superficially to the skin (adsorption), or is taken up by different layers of the skin (absorption). The drug may permeate through the different layers of the skin or the follicular and eccrine pathways before entering blood vessels and lymphatics.[2] The pharmacokinetic factors affecting the action of a drug depend on both the drug factors and the host factors **(Table 2)**.[3]

TABLE 2: Drug and host factors determining action of a drug.

Drug factors	*Host factors*
Percutaneous penetration	Patient's age
Percutaneous absorption	Site of application
Vehicle	Water content of skin
Type of topical agent	Temperature of skin
Amount of drug	pH of skin
Frequency of application	Integrity of stratum corneum
Drug reactions	Circulation

Percutaneous drug delivery is governed by the Fick's law which states that the rate of absorption or flux (J) of any substance across a barrier is proportional to its concentration difference across that barrier. The formula that follows is $J = K_pC_v$ where K_p stands for permeability coefficient and Cv is the concentration of the drug in the vehicle.[1] The skin barrier which is altered by trauma, diseases or by the drug formulation, allows easier penetration of the drug. The penetration of drugs is inversely proportional to the thickness of the stratum corneum. So it is maximum on the mucous membranes and minimum on the soles. Certain formulations such as alcohol, surfactants and solvents may cause increased absorption of the drug by denaturation of the stratum corneum. Application under occlusion facilitates increase in temperature and hydration while preventing removal of the drug. While this leads to increased efficacy, it can cause more local side-effects too. Skin atrophy or HPA axis suppression may be caused by topical corticosteroid application under occlusion. Other penetration enhancers include propylene glycol, urea, azones, dimethylsulphoxide (DMSO), and salicylic acid. The barrier may also be physically altered by ionto-or-photopheresis.[4]

Vehicles

A vehicle is a substance which is incorporated into a topical preparation in order to facilitate drug delivery to the skin.

TABLE 3: Types of vehicles.

Vehicle	
Lipids	Petrolatum, glycerine, cetyl alcohol, stearyl alcohol, isopropyl myristate, squalene, stearic acid, lanolin, shea butter
Emulsifying agents	Cholesterol, polysorbates, lanolin, sodium lauryl sulphate, sodium laureth sulphate, polyethylene glycol
Humectants	Propylene glycol, glycerine, sorbitol
Solvents	Alcohol, acetone, ether, glycerine, water
Stabilizers and preservatives	Benzyl alcohol, chlorocresol, parabens, potassium sorbate, glycerine
Thickening agent	Beeswax, carbomer, polyethylene

An ideal vehicle should be physically and chemically stable, nonirritating, nonallergenic, cosmetically elegant, easy to use, and should not interfere with the potency of the drug. According to functions, vehicles may be of different categories **(Table 3)**.[5]

Types of Topical Formulations and Instructions for Topical Therapy

Topical formulations may be solids, semisolids, or liquids **(Table 4)**.

The aim of topical therapy is to achieve the maximum efficacy with minimum side effects. To ensure this, proper instruction for application is of utmost importance. One gram of cream usually covers a surface area of roughly 100 cm^2 as a 100 μm thick layer, while an ointment covers 5–10% more. One standard of measurement widely used is the Fingertip Unit (FTU). The amount of cream that is squeezed out of a tube with a nozzle of 5 mm, over the distal part of the index finger from the distal skin crease to the tip, is roughly 0.5 g and is designated as 1 FTU. FTU is useful in assessing the amount of topical agent required for a single application according to the body parts involved **(Table 5)**. The frequency of application ensures the adequate pharmacological response to the drug and the physicians' advice in this regard has to be adhered to strictly. Increased frequency usually does not increase effectiveness but on the other hand may cause systemic toxicity. For example, emollients can be applied many times a day to but corticosteroids are to be applied only once or twice a day.[6-8]

Advances in Topical Therapy

There have been many advances in topical therapy due to modern techniques of improved drug delivery. While some of them are already in use, others are still at investigational level **(Box 1)**. Modern drug delivery aims at a targeted response of the drug and a sustained release that improves the efficacy as well as tolerability and causes fewer side effects. Transdermal drug delivery systems are methods of controlled delivery of the drugs directly into the circulation via topical route, e.g., permeation enhancers, transdermal patches, occlusion, iontophoresis, and needleless jet injectors.[1]

TABLE 4: Classification of topical formulations.[2]

Liquids	**Solutions** • *Aqueous solutions*: Wet dressings—soaks and baths • *Alcoholic solutions*: Tinctures, paints, varnishes, sprays
	Lotions: Solid in liquid (Shake lotions); liquid in liquid
Semisolids	**Liniments:** *Creams*: Lipophilic creams, hydrophilic creams, ambiphilic creams, barrier creams
	Ointments: Hydrophobic water-absorbing, hydrophilic
	Gels: Lipophilic gels, hydrophilic gels
	Pastes: Hard pastes, soft pastes, drying pastes
Solids	Powders Poultice Tapes and plasters

TABLE 5: Fingertip units (FTUs).[6]

Body part	*Number of FTUs required*
Face and neck	2.5
One arm	4
One hand	1
One leg	8
One foot	2
Front and back of trunk	14

BOX 1: Newer drug delivery techniques.[7,8]

- Microemulsions
- Microsponges
- Liposomes
- Transferosomes
- Aerosols
- Niosomes
- Ethosomes
- Solid–lipid nanoparticles
- Nanostructured lipid carriers
- Cyclodextrin
- Sol–gel microcapsules peptides and growth factors

Microemulsions: A microemulsion is a combination of water, oil, and amphiphilic compounds that is thermodynamically stable. The size of particles dispersed in an microemulsion is 1–20 nm in contrast to an emulsion where it is 1–20 μ. Microemulsions are more stable than emulsions. As compared to other topical formulations, microemulsions cause increased absorption of both hydrophilic and lipophilic drugs.[9]

Microsponge: Microsponge is a technique that allows controlled drug delivery to the skin which increases efficacy while minimizing side effects. Microsponges are macroporous beads containing the active drug which is released at a particular time span. An ideal microsponge is nonirritating, nonmutagenic, nonallergenic, and nontoxic. This technique is used to reduce the irritant potential of drugs such as topical retinoids.[10]

Liposome: A liposome is a vesicle consisting of a lipid bilayer surrounding an aqueous base. This lipid bilayer attaches itself to the cell membrane and the drug is delivered by diffusion or endocytosis. Retinoids, benzoyl peroxide, and dithranol delivered in this way cause reduced irritation. Liposomal drug delivery is very useful in delivering drugs into sebaceous glands and hair follicles. Many cosmetics have liposomes as vehicles.[11]

Transferosome: Transferosomes are vesicle-like drug carrier systems that consist of phospholipid, surfactant, and water to facilitate transdermal delivery. They can pass in intact form to deeper skin layers.[12]

Aerosol: In the aerosol system, the drug is in the form of a solution with a pure propellant which is usually a mixture of nonpolar hydrocarbons. Topical steroids are often used as aerosol foams to increase their potency.[13]

Ethosomes: They are modified forms of liposomes that have a high ethanol content. They contain phospholipids, alcohol, and water. Compared to lipososmes they have an increased penetration rate in the skin and are used for delivery of antifungal drugs, HIV drugs, and NSAIDs.[14]

Novasome: Novasomes are a recent modification of the liposomal technology. They are nonphospholipid vesicles which show sustained release of active ingredients.[15]

Topical Therapy in Pregnancy and Lactation

While women during pregnancy commonly develop dermatological issues, women with pre-existing skin problems may become pregnant and seek assistance of the dermatologist.

Any medication given to a pregnant mother can affect the unborn baby and all dermatologists need to be cautious while prescribing topical drugs for a woman of child-bearing age. The risk benefit ratio has to be carefully weighed and topical therapy remains the first line of treatment. US FDA has specified guidelines to monitor drug use in pregnancy.[16] There is very little data assessing the safety of dermatological medications during lactation.[17]

Topical Therapy in Neonates

The essence of skin care in newborn babies, infants, and children is to preserve skin integrity, prevent toxicity, and to avoid exposure to harmful chemical agents.[18] Topical medications applied on neonatal skin can lead to systemic toxicity due to increased surface area, decreased hepatic metabolism and renal excretion, widespread distribution of the drug, and decreased plasma protein binding. Clinicians should be aware of the adverse effects of different topical agents on neonatal skin.

KEY POINTS

- A large number of dermatologic disorders can be well managed with topical therapy alone thus bypassing the side-effects of systemic use.
- A thorough knowledge of the principles of topical therapy is required to make it maximally effective yet safe.
- Both the active ingredient and the vehicle are important to optimize therapy.
- Novel drug delivery techniques help in targeted therapy to achieve maximum results and minimum side-effects.
- Special populations such as pregnant and lactating mothers and neonates need individualized therapeutic approach to avoid adverse reactions.

REFERENCES

1. Viswanath V, Pund P. Principles of topical therapy. In: Sarma N (Ed). Skin Clinical Dermatology, 1st edition. New Delhi: Jaypee Brothers Medical Publishers; 2019. pp. 610-9.
2. Berth-Jones J. Principles of topical therapy. In: Griffith C, Barker J, Bleiker T, Chalmers R, Creamers D (Eds). Rook's Textbook of Dermatology, 9th edition. Oxford: Wiley Blackwell; 2016. pp. 18.1-18.4.
3. Coondoo A, Sengupta S. Topical therapy in dermatology. In: Sacchidanand S, Oberoi C, Inamdar AC (Eds). IADVL Textbook of Dermatology, 4th edition. Mumbai: Bhalani Publishing House; 2016. pp. 2243-313.
4. Thong HY, Zhai H, Maibach HI. Percutaneous penetration enhancers: an overview. Skin Pharmacol and Physiol. 2007;20:272-82.
5. Surber C, Smith EW. The mystical effects of dermatological vehicles. Dermatology. 2005;210:157-68.
6. Long CC, Finlay AY. The finger-tip unit: a new practical measure. Clinical Exp Dermatol. 1991;16;444-7.
7. Fireman S, Toledano O, Neimann K, Loboda, Dayan N. A look at emerging delivery systems for topical drug products. Dermatol Ther. 2011;24:477-88.
8. Katare OP, Raza K, Singh B, Dogra S. Novel drug delivery systems in topical treatment of psoriasis: rigors and vigors. Indian J Dermatol Venereol Leprol. 2010;76:612-2.
9. Bagwe RP, Kanicky JR, Palla BJ, Patanjali PK, Shah DO. Improved drug delivery using microemulsions: rationale, recent progress and new horizons. Crit Rev Therap Drug Carrier Syst. 2001;18:77-140.
10. Kaity S, Maiti S, Ghosh AK, Pal DK, Ghosh A, Banerjee S. Microsponges: a novel strategy for drug delivery system. J Adv Pharm Technol Res. 2010;1:283-90.
11. Pierre MB, Dos Santos Miranda Costa I. Liposomal systems as drug delivery vehicles for dermal and transdermal applications. Arch Dermatol Res. 2011;303:607-21.
12. Cevc G. Transfersomes, liposomes and other lipid suspensions on the skin: permeation enhancement, vesicle penetration, and transdermal drug delivery. Crit Rev Ther Drug Carrier Syst. 1996;13:257-388.

13. Popli H, Collett JH. Aerosol drug delivery systems for topical medication. Proc Int Symp Control Release. 1997;24:31-2.
14. Touitou E, Dayan N, Bergelson L, Godin B, Eliaz M. Ethosomes - novel vesicular carriers for enhanced delivery: characterization and skin penetration properties. J Control Release. 2000;65: 403-18.
15. Singh A, Malviya R, Sharma PK. Novasome—a breakthrough in pharmaceutical technology: a review article. Advan Biol Res. 2011;5:184-9.
16. Hale EK, Pomeranz MK. Dermatologic agents during pregnancy and lactation and clinical review. Int J Dermatol. 2002; 14:197-203.
17. Butler DC, Heller MM, Murase JE. Safety of dermatologic medications in pregnancy and lactation. Part II. Lactation. J Am Acad Dermatol. 2014;70:e1-10.
18. Fernandes JD, Machado MCR, Oliveira ZNP. Children and newborn skin care and prevention. An Bras Dermatol. 2011; 86:102-10.

EXAMINATION QUESTIONS

1. Discuss the various stages of percutaneous absorption of drugs.
2. What are the advantages and disadvantages of topical therapy?
3. Discuss the drug and host factors determining the action of drugs.
4. Discuss the topical rapamycin in dermatology.

144 CHAPTER Topical Corticosteroids

Abhishek De, Sonal Singh, Aarti Sarda

INTRODUCTION

- The modern era of dermatotherapy began with the introduction of topical corticosteroids (TCS).
- They are effective for conditions involving hyperproliferation, immunological, and inflammatory properties.
- Safe and effective use of TCS requires extensive knowledge of their various formulations and potencies.
- TCS have a long list of potential side effects; physicians need to know the strategies to minimize them.

HISTORY AND EVOLUTION OF TOPICAL STEROIDS

- Kendall et al. in 1948 isolated extracts of bovine adrenal glands and marked the compounds from A to F. Of these six compounds, E (cortisone) and F (hydrocortisone) were found to be medically effective.
- Sulzberger and Witten created a milestone in 1952 by successfully treating eczematous eruptions with topical hydrocortisone.[1,2]

STRUCTURE

- Hydrocortisone is considered to be the prototype of all TCS molecules.
- Hydrocortisone is made up of 21 carbon atoms constituting the cyclo-pentano-perhydro-phenanthrene nucleus and a 17,21-dihydroxy (OH)-20-keto (O) side chain **(Fig. 1)**.
- Efficacy and adverse effects of TCS depend on multiple factors including molecular structure, the vehicle, area of application and condition of the skin.

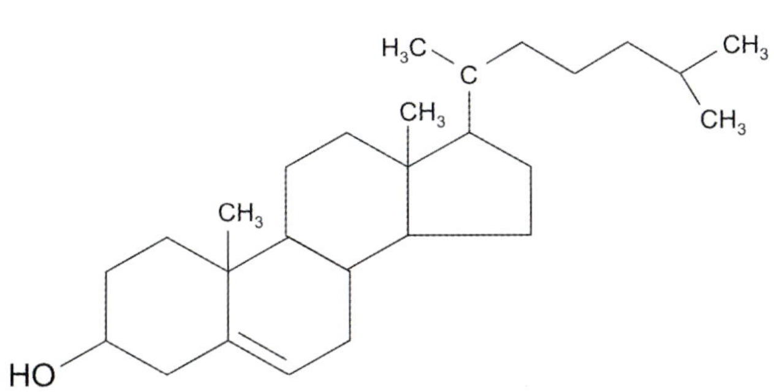

Fig. 1: Structure of hydrocortisone.

- Different types of TCS molecules are created by placing hydroxyl groups into the 11-β, 17-α, and 21 positions; ketone groups into the 3 and 20 positions; and a double-bond into the four position of the glucocorticoid nucleus.
- The intrinsic potency of TCS may be augmented by esterification and halogenation.
- Fluorination at C6 and C9 atoms of this molecule increases potency while addition of an acetonide group enhances penetrability and percutaneous absorption.[3,4]

MECHANISM OF ACTION

- TCS exert biological effects by binding to the glucocorticoid receptor.
- The receptor is cytoplasmic in the unbound state and is translocated to the nucleus after glucocorticoid binding **(Fig. 2)**.[4-6]
- The action of TCS can be divided into mainly two groups: I. Anti-inflammatory effects; II. Antiproliferative effect **(Flowchart 1)**.[4-6]

ANTI-INFLAMMATORY EFFECTS

Direct effects: These impart immediate effect:

- Stabilize cell membrane and lysosomal membranes preventing release of lysosomal contents and phospholipid precursors.
- Inhibits of IgE-induced mast cell sensitization and release of mast cell mediators including histamine.

GCR-mediated effects: These impart delayed effects:

- Induce anti-inflammatory proteins such as lipocortins, vasocardin, and vasoregulin.
- Inhibit phospholipase A_2 and blocks release of arachidonic acid metabolites, leading to depletion in inflammatory mediators such as prostaglandins, leukotrienes, etc.
- Decrease vascular permeability.

ANTIPROLIFERATIVE EFFECTS

- Both direct and GCR-mediated effects are important.
- *Epidermal actions:*
    - Decrease keratinocyte mitosis
    - Reduce stratum corneum thickness

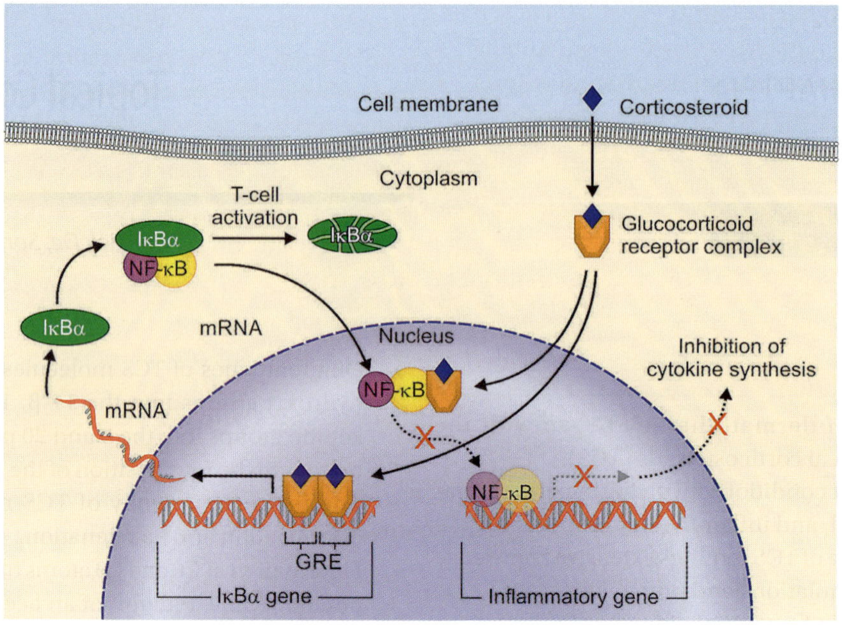

Fig. 2: The double-pronged inhibitory effect of corticosteroids on NF-kB.
(GRE: glucocorticoid responsive element; IkBa: inhibitory nuclear factor-kappa B alpha; NF-kB: nuclear factor-kappa B)

Flowchart 1: Mechanism of action of topical corticosteroids.

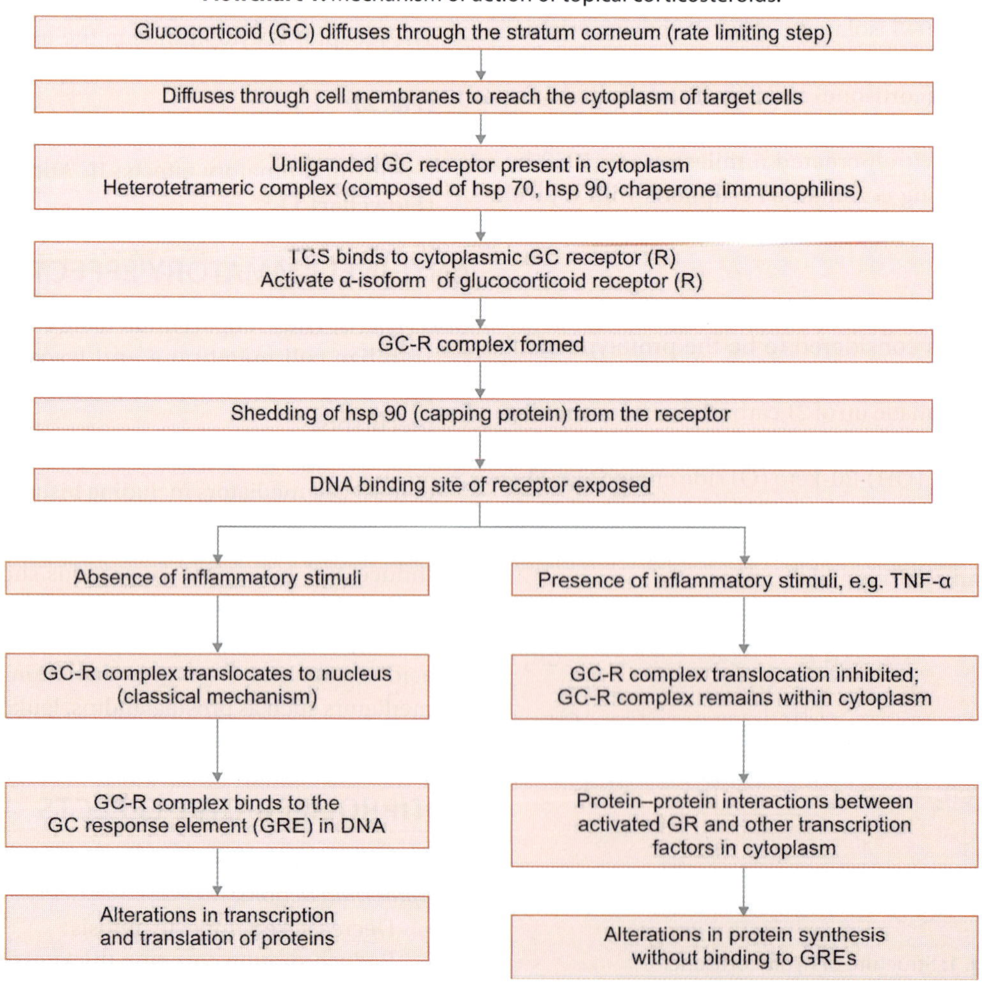

- Reduce granular layer
- Flatten basal layer of keratinocytes
- Inhibit pigment production from melanocytes

- *Dermal actions:*
  - Decrease dermal volume by reducing water content and loss of glycosaminoglycans
  - Decrease fibroblasts activity
  - Reduce collagen and elastic fibers (late)
  - Makes dermal vessels fragile and dilated through loss of fibrous and ground substance.

PHARMACOKINETICS

Percutaneous Absorption

- Thickness of the stratum corneum and the vascular supply regulates penetration of the TCS.
- Corticosteroids are better absorbed and more permeable in regions of thin epidermis, such as the eyelid, compared to thicker regions of epidermis, such as the sole. The penetration difference between the two varies by 300 fold.
- The condition of the skin also affects bioavailability. In inflamed or diseased skin the penetration of TCS increases.
- TCS may get stored in stratum corneum up to 5 days.[7-11]

Metabolism

- Intraepidermal de-esterification is one of the main mechanisms of metabolism of TCS.
- It may be one of the causes for tachyphylaxis.
- Biotransformation of TCS in the skin can be modulated advantageously to enhance potency.[9-11]

Potency Assessment

- Most commonly used method for assessing potency of TCS is human vasoconstrictor assay of McKenzie and Stoughton. It measures the degree of visible blanching caused by various dilutions of TCS applied to human skin.
- *Other methods include:*
  - *Measurement of anti-inflammatory property*: Dumas and Scholtz small plaque psoriasis bioassay, Rat thymus involution assay, and antigranuloma assay
  - *Measurement of atrophogenicity*: Fibroblast assay
  - *Other*: Histamine pin-prick bioassay.[12,13]

VEHICLES AND FORMULATIONS

- The vehicle is the carrier of the drug. Vehicles and formulations of TCS play an important role in graded efficacy and safety of the TCS preparation.
- Physicians must be careful in choosing a right vehicle or formulations for the drug delivery keeping in mind the conditions, area of affection, age of the patients, and comfort of application. Choice of proper vehicle also increases compliance **(Table 1)**.

TABLE 1: Examples of different vehicles.

Vehicle/Formulation	*Drug name*	*Strength (%)*
Cream	Hydrocortisone	0.5–2.5
	Fluocinolone acetonide	0.01, 0.025
	Triamcinolone acetonide	0.025, 0.1
	Desoximetasone	0.1, 0.25
Ointment	Hydrocortisone	0.5–2.5
	Triamcinolone acetonide	0.025
Lotion	Hydrocortisone	0.5–2.5
	Triamcinolone acetonide	0.025, 0.1
Gel	Hydrocortisone	0.1, 0.2

- Ointments—administered for thick hyperkeratotic lesions; the most potent vehicle since they are the most occlusive and should not be administered on hair-bearing regions because it may result in folliculitis.
- Creams—less potent than ointment but cosmetically more appealing since they leave no residue; the drying, nonocclusive nature leads to their administration for acute exudative inflammation and dermatitis within the intertriginous areas.
- Lotions—less occlusive and greasy; work well in hair-bearing regions.
- Gels-like lotions, less occlusive and greasy; work well in hair-bearing regions; more beneficial for the scalp as they do not cause matting of the last occlusive and greasy hair.
- Foams—highly effective for steroid delivery to the scalp but are costly.[14,15]

CLASSIFICATION OF TOPICAL CORTICOSTEROIDS

- There are two important systems of classification of TCS.
- The United States classification consists of seven classes, with class 1 super potent and class 7 least potent **(Box 1)**.[4]

The other classification by the British National Formulary is simpler and involves a four-point scale of mild, moderate, potent, and very potent **(Table 2)**.[4]

Different factors affect the choices of TCS, which have been described in **Box 2**.

INDICATIONS

Topical corticosteroids are one of the most commonly used dermatological drugs. The most indications are as follows:[4]

- *Dermatitis and eczema*: Atopic dermatitis, seborrheic dermatitis, contact dermatitis, dyshidrotic eczema, nummular dermatitis, lichen simplex chronicus, stasis dermatitis, prurigo nodularis.
- *Papulosquamous disorders*: Psoriasis, pityriasis rosea, lichen planus.

- *Bullous dermatoses*: Bullous pemphigoid, pemphigus, pemphigoid gestationis, familial benign pemphigus.
- *Connective tissue diseases*: Lupus, dermatomyositis, morphea.
- *Neutrophilic dermatoses*: Sweet syndrome, Behçet's disease, pyoderma gangrenosum.
- *Hair disorder*: Alopecia areata, lichen planopilaris.

BOX 1: United States classification of topical corticosteroids (TCS).

Class 1 (super potent):
- Clobetasol propionate
- Halobetasol propionate ointment and cream 0.05% (optimized vehicle)

Class 2 (high potency):
- Betamethasone dipropionate cream, lotion 0.05
- Mometasone furoate ointment 0.1%

Class 3 (high potency):
- Betamethasone valerate ointment 0.1%
- Fluticasone propionate ointment 0.005%

Class 4 (medium potency):
- Desoximetasone cream 0.05%
- Fluocinolone acetonide ointment 0.025%
- Hydrocortisone valerate ointment 0.2%

Class 5 (medium potency):
- Betamethasone dipropionate lotion 0.05%
- Fluticasone propionate cream and lotion 0.05%

Class 6 (low potency):
- Desonide 0.05% in any vehicle
- Fluocinolone acetonide cream 0.01%

Class 7 (low potency): Hydrocortisone 1% and 2.5% cream or lotion or ointment

TABLE 2: British National Formulary classification of topical corticosteroids (TCS).

Potency	*Drugs*	*Formulation/ Concentration*
Very potent	Clobetasol propionate	0.05%
	Fluocinolone acetonide	0.2%
Potent	Betamethasone valerate	0.1%, 0.025%
	Mometasone furoate	0.1%
Moderately potent	Beclomethasone dipropionate	0.025%
	Clobetasone butyrate	0.05%
Mild	Dexamethasone	0.1–0.2%
	Methylprednisolone acetate	0.25%

BOX 2: Factors affecting the choice of topical corticosteroids (TCS).

- Anatomic area of application
- Disease responsiveness
- Severity of disease
- Extent of body surface area involvement
- Age of patient
- Suitability of vehicle
- Potency of corticosteroid molecule

- *Inflammatory conditions*: Sarcoidosis, granuloma annulare, lichen sclerosus et atrophicus, pruritic urticarial papules and plaques of pregnancy, necrobiosis lipoidica diabeticorum, chondrodermatitis nodularis helicis.
- *Pigmentary diseases*: Vitiligo, lichen planus pigmentosus, melasma (as a part of triple combination with retinoids and hydroquinone).
- *Malignant and premalignant condition*: Cutaneous T-cell lymphoma, Jessner's lymphocytic infiltrate.
- *Others*: perianal or vulval pruritus, keloids, hypertrophic scars.

FINGERTIP UNIT TECHNIQUE

- To standardize the amount of TCS to be applied, Long and Finlay developed the fingertip unit technique (FTU) **(Table 3)**.
- One FTU is defined by the amount of TCS that comes after squeezing the cream or ointment from a tube having a nozzle diameter of 5 mm along an adult index finger starting from the tip down to the first joint crease.
- One FTU weighs 0.49 g and covers 312 cm^2 in adult males, and weighs 0.43 g and covers 257 cm^2 in adult females. Roughly one FTU covers two palm sizes.
- The relationship between "rule of hand" and "fingertip unit" can be expressed in a simple formula. "4 hand areas = 2 fingertip units = 1 g ointment."[16,17]

Duration of Use

- Super potent TCS such as clobetasol and halobetasol propionate should not be used for the duration greater than 14 days with the total dose not exceeding 50 g per week for halobetasol and 60 g per week for clobetasol.
- Usage of betamethasone dipropionate should not exceed 45 g per week.
- It is generally recommended to switch over to a corticosteroid of lower potency or nonsteroidal preparations for maintenance therapy after 2 weeks use of potent or super potent steroids.[4]

TABLE 3: Estimating the necessary amount of topical corticosteroid for adults.

Anatomical area	*Number of FTU required to cover*	*Amount for 1 week of bid application (g)*
Face and neck	2.5	17.5
Anterior or posterior trunk	7	49
Arm	3	21
Hand (both sides)	1	7
Leg	6	42
Foot	2	14

Wet-wrap Therapy

- Wet-wrap therapy is a technique where TCS are applied followed by wet gauze or cotton pads being rolled over affected body areas with the aim of enhancing penetration and efficacy.
- Use of wet-wrap with diluted TCS has been found to be more efficacious as a short-term intervention than only emollients in children with atopic dermatitis.[4]

ADVERSE EFFECTS OF TOPICAL STEROID

- The side effect of TCS is directly related to their potencies. When used in large amounts for longer duration TCS can cause systemic side-effects.
- Skin atrophy leads to epidermal thinning and increased resorption within the dermis ground substance. This is the most common side effect of TCS and it is related to the antimitotic effect of TCS.
- The loss of connective tissue leads to erythema, telangiectasias, and purpura.
- Atrophy is usually reversible with steroid withdrawal; but may take months for recovery.
- Tachyphylaxis is development of tolerance to the TCS, due to loss of vasoconstriction at the level of the capillaries. Capillaries usually regain the ability to vasoconstrict after 4 days of stoppage of TCS; therefore TCS should be discontinued for 4 days if it has lost its effectiveness.
- Formation of acne by the use of TCS occurs due to the degradation of the follicular epithelium and an increase in the concentration of free fatty acids on the skin surface. This fosters an environment for bacteria growth, ultimately leading to comedogenesis.
- Perioral dermatitis occurs due to prolonged use of potent corticosteroids on the face. It presents as follicular pustules and papules on an erythematous base surrounding the perioral region but sparing the vermillion border **(Table 4)**.[18]

CONTACT ALLERGY TO TOPICAL CORTICOSTEROIDS

- Contact allergy to TCS should be suspected in typical steroid responsive dermatoses when there is worsening of the existing skin lesion while on treatment with TCS; especially if the condition has improved and then worsened.
- To prove contact sensitivity to TCS, one needs to do a patch test with TCS, most commonly done with Tixocortol pivalate as reagent.
- Pathogenesis of contact allergy due to topical corticosteroid use has been depicted in **Flowchart 2**.
- Based on the patch test reactivity the TCS are grouped into four, within which cross reactivity is common.

TABLE 4: Side effects of topical corticosteroids (TCS).

Systemic	*Local*
Hypothalamic-pituitary-adrenal axis suppression	Immediate effects include stinging and irritation
Iatrogenic Cushing's syndrome	Epidermal atrophy
Growth retardation in children	Hypo/hyperpigmentation, photosensitivity, loss of skin barrier, and premature aging
Eye side effects: Glaucoma, posterior subcapsular cataract	Fixed erythema
New onset diabetes mellitus/ hyperglycemia	Rebound flares of psoriasis, pustular psoriasis, reactivation of Kaposi's sarcoma and rebound erythema of the face (after sudden withdrawal of steroids)
Mineralocorticoid effects (edema, hypocalcemia, hypokalemia, hypertension)	Tachyphylaxis
Osteoporosis and avascular necrosis of bones in elderly	Hypertrichosis
	Allergic and irritant contact dermatitis, contact urticaria and granuloma gluteale infantum
	Exacerbation of infections
	Perioral dermatitis
	Steroid-induced rosacea and acne
	Delayed wound healing, telangiectasias, ulcerations, Bateman's purpura, easy bruising, and stellate scars
	Striae distensae
	Topical steroid damaged facies

Flowchart 2: Pathogenesis of contact allergy to topical corticosteroids.

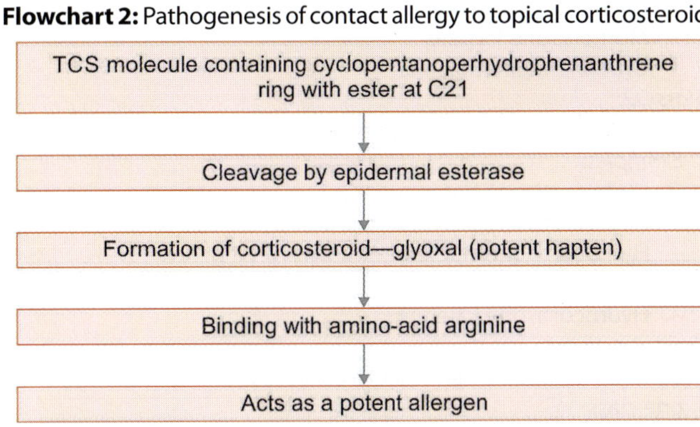

- When patch tests show allergy to a specific topical steroid, it is likely that the patient will also be allergic to others in the same class **(Box 3)**.
- Confirmation of corticosteroid allergy requires the prompt removal of the causative agent and then management as for any acute dermatitis/eczema; this may include treatment with TCS (one which you are not allergic to) emollients.[19,20]

BOX 3: Classes of corticosteroid according to their structure and sensitivity pattern.

Class A:
- *Test substance*: Tixocortol pivalate
- *Examples*:
  - Hydrocortisone (acetate)
  - Methylprednisolone
  - Prednisolone
  - Tixocortol pivalate
  - Oral cloprednol
  - Oral fludrocortisone acetate
  - Oral methylprednisolone
  - Oral prednisolone

Class B:
- *Test substance*: Budesonide and triamcinolone
- *Examples*:
  - Amcinonide
  - Desonide
  - Fluocinolone acetonide
  - Halcinonide
  - Triamcinolone (acetonide, diacetate)
  - Oral budesonide
  - Oral triamcinolone

Class C:
- *Examples*:
  - Clocortolone pivalate
  - Desoximetasone
  - Oral betamethasone
  - Oral dexamethasone

Class D1:
- *Test substance*: Clobetasol-17-propionate
- *Examples*:
  - Alclometasone dipropionate
  - Betamethasone dipropionate
  - Betamethasone valerate
  - Clobetasol propionate
  - Clobetasone butyrate
  - Diflorasone diacetate
  - Fluticasone propionate
  - Mometasone furoate
  - Oral/IM betamethasone

Class D2:
- *Test substance*: Hydrocortisone-17-butyrate
- *Examples*:
  - Hydrocortisone buteprate
  - Hydrocortisone butyrate
  - Hydrocortisone valerate
  - Prednicarbate
  - Hydrocortisone valerate

Cross-reactions:
- Sometimes, people can react to corticosteroids in more than one class
- Class A cross-reacts with Class D2
- Budesonide cross-reacts with Class D2

Contraindications

- Active bacterial infections including impetigo, furuncles and carbuncles, cellulitis, erysipelas, lymphangitis, and erythrasma.
- Relative contraindications include candida and dermatophytes.

MONITORING THE TCS THERAPY

- Like most prescription drugs, TCS therapy requires supervision to optimize benefits and minimize adverse effects.
- The most effective form of supervision is the follow-up visit.
- High-potency steroids should not be administered for a longer than 2 weeks, and after this period, should be tapered to avoid adverse effects.
- More emphasis must be placed on educating the patient at the first visit.
- Pertinent instructions must be given in each visit, regarding the frequency of application, duration of application, and amount to be applied.
- Strategies to prevent adverse effects include the use of lower-potency steroids, morning-only applications, alternate-day treatment, and decreasing the extent of occlusion.
- TCS should be used with utmost caution in children. TCS use should be restricted to as mild a steroid as possible, for as short a period as possible, over as small an area as possible.
- Infants are particularly at risk because of higher ratio of skin surface area to body weight, higher absorption due to thinner skin and due to lesser ability to metabolize the absorbed drug.[4]

USE IN PREGNANCY

- An estimated 6% of pregnant women receive prescription of TCS, which are pregnancy risk category C. Animal studies show teratogenic effects, but data are limited and conflicting regarding use in pregnant women.
- Pregnant women can be reassured that there is no apparent increased risk of adverse fetal effects when using TCS during pregnancy, although some data do suggest fetal growth restriction with more potent TCS. Overall, women should be prescribed the lowest potency required whenever possible.
- Mild-to-moderate potency TCS should be preferred to more potent corticosteroids during pregnancy.
- Potent to very potent TCS should be used as second-line therapy for as short a time as possible.
- The risk of adverse events is increased, theoretically, with use on high-absorption areas like the eyelids, genitals, and flexures.
- Currently, there is no data to determine the fetal safety of the newer potent lipophilic TCS (e.g., mometasone, fluticasone, and methylprednisolone) and whether they are associated with less risk of fetal growth restriction.[9,21]

KEY POINTS

- TCS exert biological effects by binding to the glucocorticoid receptor. The receptor is cytoplasmic in the unbound state and is translocated to the nucleus after glucocorticoid binding.

- Thickness of the stratum corneum and the vascular supply regulates penetration of the TCS.
- TCS may get stored in stratum corneum up to 5 days.
- Intraepidermal de-esterification is one of the main mechanisms of metabolism of TCS.
- Most commonly used method for assessing potency of TCS is human vasoconstrictor assay of McKenzie and Stoughton.
- The United States classification of TCS consists of seven classes, with class 1 super potent and class 7 least potent.
- British National Formulary is a simpler classification of TCS and involves a four-point scale of mild, moderate, potent, and very potent.
- One fingertip unit is approximately equivalent to 0.49 g and 0.43 g of ointment by weight for males and females, respectively.
- The side-effect of TCS is directly related to their potencies. When used in large amounts for longer duration TCS can cause systemic side effects.
- A classification system based on the structural features of topical corticosteroid compounds has been devised to predict cross-sensitivity on patch testing. This consists of four groups; namely, group A (hydrocortisone type), group B (triamcinolone acetonide type), group C (betamethasone type), and group D (hydrocortisone butyrate type).
- All TCS are included under pregnancy category C (benefit outweighs risk) and these should be prescribed with caution during lactation.

REFERENCES

1. Cooney WP 3rd. Compound F: the history of hydrocortisone and hand surgery. J Hand Surg Am. 2013;38:774-8.
2. Sulzberger MB, Witten VH. The effect of topically applied compound F in selected dermatoses. J Invest Dermatol. 1952;19:101-2.
3. Chaffman MO. Topical corticosteroids: a review of properties and principles in therapeutic use. Nurse Practitioner Forum. 1999;10:95-105.
4. Mehta AB, Nadkarni NJ, Patil SP, Godse KV, Gautam M, Agarwal S. Topical corticosteroids in dermatology. Indian J Dermatol Venereol Leprol. 2016;82(4):371-8.
5. Norris DA. Mechanisms of action of topical therapies and the rationale for combination therapy. J Am Acad Dermatol. 2005;53(1 Suppl 1):S17-25.
6. Ahluwalia A. Topical glucocorticoids and the skin—mechanisms of action: an update. Mediators Inflamm. 1998;7:183-93.
7. Stoughton RB. Vasoconstriction activity and percutaneous absorption of glucocorticosteroids. Arch Dermatol. 1969;99:753-6.
8. Feldmann RJ, Maibach HI. Regional variation in percutaneous penetration of 14C cortisol in man. J Invest Dermatol. 1967;48(2):181-3.
9. Tadicherla S, Ross K, Shenefelt PD, Fenske NA. Topical corticosteroids in dermatology. J Drugs Dermatol. 2009;8(12):1093-105.
10. Brattsaud R. Influence of 16, 17 acetyl substitution and steroid corticosteroids. J Steroid Biochem. 1982;16:779-86.
11. Vickers CFH. Existence of a reservoir, i.e., the stratum corneum. Arch Dermatol. 1963;88:20-3.
12. Ashworth J. Potency classification of topical corticosteroids: modern perspectives. Acta Derm Venereol Suppl (Stockh). 1989;151:20-5.
13. Dumas KJ, Scholtz JR. The psoriasis bio-assay for topical corticosteroid activity. Acta Derm Venereol. 1972;52:43-8.
14. Purdon CH, Haigh JM, Surber C, Smith EW. Foam drug delivery in dermatology: beyond the scalp. Am J Drug Deliv. 2003;1:71-5.
15. Goa KL. Clinical pharmacology and pharmacokinetic properties of topically applied corticosteroids. A review. Drugs. 1988;36(Suppl 5):51-61.
16. Long CC, Finlay AY. The fingertip unit: a new practical measure. Clinic Exp Dermatol. 1991;16:444-7.
17. Stoughton RB, Cornell RC. Topical steroids in dermatology. In: Christophers E, Schopf E, Kligman AM (Eds). Topical Corticosteroid Therapy: A Novel Approach to Safer Drugs. New York: Raven Press; 1988. pp. 1-12.
18. Coondoo A, Phiske M, Verma S, Lahiri K. Side-effects of topical steroids: a long overdue revisit. Indian Dermatol Online J. 2014;5(4):416-25.
19. Saraswat A. Contact allergy to topical corticosteroids and sunscreens. Indian J Dermatol Venereol Leprol. 2012;78:552-9.
20. Coopman S, Degreef H, Dooms-Goossens A. Identification of cross-reaction patterns in allergic contact dermatitis from topical corticosteroids. Br J Dermatol. 1989;121:27-34.
21. Chi CC, Wang SH, Mayon-White R, Wojnarowska F. Pregnancy outcomes after maternal exposure to topical corticosteroids: a UK population-based cohort study. JAMA Dermatol. 2013;149(11):1274-80.

EXAMINATION QUESTIONS

1. Classify topical corticosteroids.
2. Describe briefly the MOA and adverse effects of topical corticosteroids.
3. Write a brief note on contact allergy to topical corticosteroids.

145 CHAPTER

Topical Antibiotics

Sonal Singh, Aarti Sarda, Abhishek De

INTRODUCTION

Topical antibiotics are not only used to treat superficial bacterial infections of skin but also to prevent it. Advantages of topical antibiotics over systemic treatment are high level of local drug concentration and minimum systemic absorption, hence the chance of systemic adverse effects decreases.

They are divided into two broad categories as shown in **Flowchart 1**.

Overall microbiologic coverage of various antibiotics is shown in **Table 1**.

Pregnancy category of various topical antibiotics is shown in **Table 2**.

Flowchart 1: Types of topical antibiotics.

Topical antibiotics

Drugs used for minor bacterial infections and wound care
- Bacitracin
- Polymyxin B
- Neomycin
- Framycetin
- Mupirocin
- Retapamulin
- Fucidic acid
- Indolmycin
- Gentamicin
- Silver sulfadiazine
- Iodoquinol
- Mafenide
- Chloramphenicol
- Clioquinol

Drugs used for acne and rosacea
- Benzoyl peroxide
- Clindamycin
- Erythromycin
- Metronidazole
- Azelaic acid
- Dapsone
- Sodium sulfacetamide

TABLE 1: Microbiologic coverage of antibiotics.

Microorganism	*Effective antibiotic*
Gram-positive bacteria	Mupirocin, retapamulin, fusidic acid, and erythromycin
Gram-positive and gram-negative bacteria	Neomycin, gentamicin, iodoquinol, silver sulfadiazine, nadifloxacin, and metronidazole
Gram-negative bacteria	Polymyxin B
Corynebacterium	Macrolide
Anaerobes	Metronidazole and clindamycin
Propionibacterium acnes	Benzoyl peroxide, azelaic acid, sodium sulfacetamide, etc.

COMMON DRUGS USED FOR MINOR BACTERIAL INFECTIONS AND WOUND CARE

Mupirocin

- *Origin*: Isolated from *Pseudomonas* fluorescens as pseudomonic acid.
- *Mechanism of action*: Bactericidal by inhibition of bacterial isoleucyl transfer ribonucleic acid (tRNA) synthetase, and hence blocking bacterial RNA, protein, and cell wall synthesis.[1]
- *Microbiologic activity*:
  - Active against gram-positive bacteria including methicillin-resistant *Staphylococcus aureus* (MRSA).
  - Ineffective against anaerobes, *Pseudomonas aeruginosa*, fungi, and normal skin flora.
  - Recently resistance reported in MRSA and methicillin-resistant *Staphylococcus epidermidis* (MRSE) is due to mutations in *ileS* gene encoding isoleucyl tRNA synthetase.
- *Formulations*: 2% ointment in polyethylene glycol or cream or newer calcium salt of mupirocin for intranasal use.
- *Systemic absorption*: Minimal <3%
- *Efficacy*: Less effective on weeping wounds as it is 95% protein bound.
- *Clinical usage*:
  - For treatment of impetigo, impetiginized eczema, folliculitis, burns, lacerations, and leg ulcers
  - To prevent chronic carrier state of *Staphylococcus aureus* by intranasal twice daily application.
- *Adverse effects*:
  - Pain, itching, and burning (due to vehicle base, i.e., polyethylene glycol; as intranasal formulation does not contain this vehicle, so is less irritating).
  - It does not cross-react with other topical antibiotics.

TABLE 2: Pregnancy category of topical antibiotics.

Pregnancy category	*Topical antibiotics*
B	Polymyxin B, mupirocin, retapamulin, silver sulfadiazine, clindamycin, erythromycin, metronidazole, and azelaic acid
C	Bacitracin, gentamicin, iodoquinol, benzoyl peroxide, dapsone, sodium sulfacetamide
D	Neomycin

Retapamulin

- *Origin*: It belongs to pleuromutilins derived from *Pleurotus mutilus* (edible mushroom).
- *Mechanism of action*:
  - *Bacteriostatic*: Selectively inhibiting bacterial protein synthesis by:
    - Binding to protein L3 (on 50S ribosomal subunit)
    - Inhibiting ribosomal peptidyl transferase
    - Preventing translation by blocking interaction of fMet-tRNA to the P-site of the ribosome
- *Microbiologic activity*:
  - Gram-positive aerobic cocci including MRSA and mupirocin-resistant *Staphylococcus* (macrolide-resistant strains) as well as anaerobic bacteria such as clostridia and *Propionibacterium acnes*.[2]
  - Stepwise mutation in gene encoding protein L3 is needed for resistance (although rare, is still reported).
- *Formulation*: 1% ointment
- Systemic absorption is minimum (by hepatic microsomal CYP3A4).
- *Clinical usage*[3] *[Food and Drug Administration (FDA) approved]*: Impetigo (due to methicillin susceptible *S. aureus* or *S. pyogenes* only) in children >9 months of age and adults (twice daily application for 5 days).
- *Adverse effect*: Local irritation is the most common one.

Fusidic Acid

- *Origin*: It is derived from *Fusidium coccineum* (fungus).
- *Mechanism of action*: It inhibits bacterial protein synthesis by interfering with translocation elongation factor G.
- *Microbiologic activity*: Against coagulase negative *S. aureus*, beta-hemolytic *Streptococcus*, *Corynebacterium*, and *Clostridium*[4]
- *Clinical usage*: Infected eczema
- *Adverse effects*: Sensitization (uncommon)

Indolmycin

- *Origin*: It is tryptophan analog.
- *Mechanism of action*: Bacterial tryptophanyl-tRNA synthetase is selectively inhibited by it.
- *Microbiologic action*: Active against even fusidic acid and mupirocin-resistant *Staphylococcus*
- *Clinical usage*: Nasal carriage of MRSA is treated effectively.

Bacitracin

- *Origin*: This polypeptide is produced by *Bacillus subtilis* (Tracy I strain).
- *Mechanism of action*: It inhibits bacterial cell wall formation by complexing with carrier protein C55-isoprenyl pyrophosphate.
- *Formulation*: When complexed with zinc (decreased water solubility), the self-life of drug increases to 2–5 years.
- *Microbiologic activity*: Mostly against gram-positive bacteria.
- *Clinical usage*:
  - Bacitracin in combination with polymyxin B and neomycin (called as "double antibiotics" and "triple antibiotics", respectively) is used for superficial infection.
  - In triple combination bacitracin, polymyxin and neomycin is added respectively for gram-positive bacteria, *Pseudomonas* species, and gram-negative bacteria coverage.
  - It does not eliminate nasal carriage of *S. aureus*.
- *Adverse effects*: Contact dermatitis (common sensitizer), nephrotoxicity anaphylaxis, and also reported to cross-react with neomycin.

Polymyxin B

- *Origin*: It is isolated from aerobic gram-positive *Bacillus polymyxa*. It is combination of polymyxin B1 and B2.
- *Mechanism of action*: It increases permeability of bacterial cell wall.
- *Microbiologic action*: It is bactericidal against all gram-negative bacteria except *Proteus* group.
- *Formulation*: 0.1–1% cream
- *Clinical usage*: Treat minor skin wounds
- *Adverse effect*: Almost minimum risk of sensitization and resistance.

Neomycin and Framycetin

- *Origin*: This aminoglycoside is isolated from *Streptomyces fradiae*.
- *Mechanism of action*: It binds to 30S subunit of ribosome and hence inhibition of bacterial protein synthesis.
- *Microbiologic action*: It is broad-spectrum antibiotic which covers both gram-positive and gram-negative bacteria, but does not act against *P. aeruginosa* and anaerobes.[5]
- *Formulation*: 1%
- *Clinical usage*: To treat superficial skin infection used in triple combination (to minimize sensitization and resistance).
- *Adverse effects*:
  - Sensitization, ototoxicity, and nephrotoxicity
  - To minimize these adverse effects no >1 g/day of topical preparation be used for more than 7 days.

Framycetin is a broad-spectrum aminoglycoside antibiotic available as cream and gauze dressing.

Gentamicin Sulfate

- *Origin*: This aminoglycoside antibiotics is isolated from *Micromonospora purpurea* (gram-positive bacteria).
- *Mechanism of action*: Protein synthesis inhibition by binding to 30S ribosomal subunit.
- *Microbiologic action*: Bactericidal against both gram-positive (*S. aureus*) and gram-negative bacteria (*E. coli*, *Proteus* species, and *P. aeruginosa*) as well as on fungi and yeast. Although it does not act against streptococci.

- *Formulation*: 0.1–0.3% ointment
- *Clinical usage*: Hidradenitis suppurativa
- *Adverse effects*:
  - Vestibulotoxic, nephrotoxic, sensitization, and contact allergy when used in chronic otitis media.
  - Cross sensitivity has been reported in aminoglycosides.

Silver Sulfadiazine

- *Origin*: It is structurally similar to para-aminobenzoic acid (PABA) and hence competitively inhibits folic acid synthesis.
- *Mechanism of action*: Inhibits bacterial replication by binding to bacterial deoxyribonucleic acid (DNA) (silver has a role in bactericidal activity).
- *Microbiologic activity*: Acts against both gram-positive (MRSA) and gram-negative bacteria (*P. aeruginosa*).
- *Formulation*: 1% topical formulation
- *Clinical usage*: Burn wound (most common)
- *Adverse effects*:
  - Relatively low sensitization but its vehicle causes most of toxicity and allergic reactions.
  - Uncommonly sulfur moiety can lead to hemolysis (also methemoglobinemia and hyperosmolarity) in glucose-6-phosphate dehydrogenase (G6PD) deficient patients.
  - Argyria, local site discoloration, and deposition in kidney, liver, and retina.

Iodoquinol

- *Origin*: It is a halogenated quinolone derivative.
- *Mechanism of action*: Unknown
- *Microbiologic action*: Broad spectrum of coverage (*Propionibacterium acnes*, MRSA, *Pseudomonas aeruginosa*, *Corynebacterium aquaticum*; dermatophytes, and yeasts—*Candida albicans* too)
- *Formulation*: 1% cream or gel
- *Clinical usage*: It is used as three to four applications daily for superficial infections caused by bacterial or fungus.
- *Adverse effects*: No data is available on the topical application side effects of it. But systemic formulation can cause iodine hypersensitivity, neurotoxicity, and dysfunctional thyroid gland.

Mafenide

- *Origin*: Sulfonamide
- *Microbiologic action*: Bacteriostatic for gram-positive and gram-negative bacteria (including *P. aeruginosa*)
- *Clinical usage*: Burn
- *Adverse effects*:
  - Secondary candidal infection
  - Contraindicated in renal impairment

Chloramphenicol

- *Mechanism of action*: Inhibition of protein synthesis by blocking 50S subunit of ribosome
- *Adverse effects*: Fatal aplastic anemia and bone marrow toxicity on long-term topical use.

Clioquinol

- *Origin*: Iodochlorhydroxyquin[6]
- *Mechanism of action*: Inhibition of enzymes and DNA replication
- *Microbiologic action*: Broad-spectrum antibiotic, antifungal, and antiprotozoal
- *Clinical usage*: Superficial infection of leg
- *Adverse effects*:
  - Stain skin, hair, and nail
  - Dysfunctional thyroid gland

TOPICAL ANTIBIOTICS USED FOR ACNE AND ROSACEA[1,6]

Benzoyl Peroxide

- *Mechanism of action*: Broad-spectrum antibiotic
  - Powerful oxidizing agent
  - Reduces inflammation by inhibition of triglyceride hydrolysis and bactericidal for *P. acnes*
  - Keratolytic and comedolytic activity
- *Microbiologic action*: *P. acnes*, *S. capitis*, *S. epidermidis*, and *P. granulosum*.
- *Formulation*: 2.5–20% washes, lotions, creams, and gel. It may oxidize tretinoin if applied simultaneously.
- *Clinical usage*: Effective on both inflammatory and noninflammatory lesions in acne and rosacea.
- *Adverse effects*: Irritant dermatitis (erythema, burning, peeling, and dryness) (2.5% formulation is preferred to 5% or 10% as both are equally effective), contact allergy, and bleaching of fabric and hair.

Clindamycin

- *Origin*: It is indirectly isolated from *Streptomyces* species (synthetic derivative of lincomycin which is isolated from this bacteria).
- *Mechanism of action*: It interferes with bacterial protein synthesis by irreversibly binding to 50S subunit of ribosome.
- *Microbiologic action*: It is broad-spectrum antibiotic (covers both aerobic gram-positive cocci and anaerobic gram-positive and gram-negative bacteria).
- *Formulation*: 1% lotion or gel
- *Clinical usage*: It is used in treatment of acne, erythrasma, folliculitis, periorificial facial dermatitis, rosacea, Fox-Fordyce spots, and pitted keratolysis.
- *Adverse effects*:
  - Itching, erythema, burning, stinging, dryness, peeling, and oily skin (mostly due to vehicle, clindamycin itself rarely causes contact dermatitis)
  - Gram-negative folliculitis

  - *Pseudomembranous colitis* (extremely rare due to clindamycin as only 4–5% of drug is systemically absorbed; systemic absorption is also decreased by zinc acetate addition to topical clindamycin).

Erythromycin

- *Origin*: Isolated from *Streptomyces erythraeus* as macrolide antibiotic.
- *Mechanism of action*: It also inhibits bacterial protein synthesis by binding to 50S subunit of bacterial ribosome.
- *Microbiologic action*: Broad-spectrum coverage of gram-positive cocci, *Corynebacterium, Haemophilus influenzae, Legionella pneumophila, Mycoplasma pneumoniae, Ureaplasma urealyticum, Treponema pallidum*, and *Chlamydia* spp.
- *Formulation*: 1.5%, 2%, and 5% formulations. Liposomal forms are more permeative than emulsions and hydro-alcoholic solutions in decreasing order.
- *Clinical usage*: Acne and rosacea
- *Adverse effects*: It is a weak sensitizer so may present with contact dermatitis features (erythema, scaling, irritation, and dryness).

Metronidazole

- *Origin*: It belongs to nitroimidazole group.
- *Mechanism of action*: Kills bacteria by DNA disruption and inhibition of nucleic acid synthesis
- *Microbiologic action*: Active against anaerobic bacteria and protozoa (not acting against gram-positive bacteria and demodex)
- *Formulation*: 0.75%/1%/2% cream or gel
- *Clinical usage*: Acne and rosacea, cutaneous ulcers, seborrheic dermatitis
- *Adverse effects*:
  - Rarely dryness, itching, burning, and stinging (low sensitization possibility)
  - Cross-reactivity is noted with isothiazolinones and contact allergy to tioconazole.

Azelaic Acid

- *Origin*: It is saturated dicarboxylic acid.
- *Mechanism of action*:
  - By serendipity, it was noted that dicarboxylic acids produced by tinea versicolor are competitive inhibitors of tyrosinase.
  - Suppression of ultraviolet B-induced expression of interleukin-1β (IL-1β), IL-6, and tumor necrosis factor-alpha (TNF-α) and inhibitory interaction with peroxisome proliferators activated receptor-γ (mechanism in rosacea).
  - Inhibition of protein synthesis
  - Inhibition of multiplication and differentiation of keratinocytes
- *Microbiologic action*: Acts against *Staphylococcus, Propionibacterium, Pseudomonas*, and *Candida*
- *Formulation*: 3%/15%/20% gel or cream
- *Clinical usage*: Acne, rosacea, perioral dermatitis, plaque psoriasis, and hyperpigmentation disorders
- *Adverse effects*: Mild itching, burning, and scaling (which is decreased by once daily application for initial 1–2 weeks).

Dapsone

- *Mechanism of action*:
  - Interferes with neutrophilic function, IL-8 release and production of TNF-α
  - Inhibition of dihydropteroate synthetase (antimicrobial activity)
- *Microbiologic action*: Active against *Mycobacterium, Pneumocystis, Leishmania*, and *Toxoplasma*
- *Formulation*: 5% gel
- *Clinical usage*: Acne, cutaneous lupus, and rosacea
- *Adverse effects*:
  - Transient erythema, dryness, or sunburn
  - G6PD-deficient patients can have hemolytic anemia and methemoglobinemia.
  - In combination with benzoyl peroxide, it may lead to orange-brown discoloration of clothes but not skin.

Sodium Sulfacetamide

- *Mechanism of action*: It prevents conversion of PABA into folic acid by inhibition of dihydropteroate synthetase.
- *Microbiologic action*: Nonspecific antifungal and antibiotic
- *Clinical usage*: Acne, rosacea, and tinea versicolor
- *Adverse effects*:
  - Dryness and transient itching
  - It might stain clothes to orange brown but not skin when combined with benzoyl peroxide.

KEY POINTS

- While using topical antibiotics, both microbiologic spectrum and adverse effects should be kept in mind.
- Most of topical antibiotics are safe with least possibility of contact dermatitis except bacitracin (0.9%), neomycin (0.09–1.1%), and benzoyl peroxide (0.2–1%).
- Broad-spectrum antibiotics should be preferred for superficial wounds while *Propionibacterium*-specific antibiotics should be preferred in acne management.

REFERENCES

1. Motaparthi S, Hsu S. Topical antibacterial agents. Wolverton ES (Ed). Comprehensive Dermatologic Drug Therapy, 3rd edition. China: Elsevier Publishing House; 2013. pp. 445-59.
2. Dhingra D, Parkh A, Ramachandran S. Retapamulin: a newer topical antibiotic. 2013;59(20):127-30.
3. Mhlaba JM, Immaneni S, Vashi NA, Kundu RV. Commonly used drugs and medication guidelines. In: Vashi NA (Ed). The

Dermatology Handbook: A Clinician's Guide. Berlin, Germany: Springer; 2019. pp. 149-89.
4. Drucker CR. Update on topical antibiotics in dermatology. 2012;25(1):6-11.
5. Condoo A, Sengupta S. Topical therapy in dermatology. Sacchidanand S (Ed). IADVL Textbook of Dermatology, 4th edition. Mumbai: Bhalani Publishing House; 2013. pp. 2280-3.
6. Berth-Jones J. Topical therapy (antibiotics). In: Burns T, Breathnach S, Cox N, Griffiths C (Eds). Rook's Textbook of Dermatology, 8th edition. Oxford: Wiley-Blackwell; 2008.

EXAMINATION QUESTION

1. Write a short note on newer topical antibiotics.

146 CHAPTER Topical Immunomodulators

Abhishek De, Aarti Sarda, Sachi Gupta

INTRODUCTION

- Topical immunomodulators are drugs that are used topically to regulate the local immune response of the skin.
- Compared to systemic immunomodulatory agents, these agents have the advantages of ease of application, and greater safety for use of longer periods without requiring stringent monitoring.
- Based on their mechanism of action, they can be divided into two categories—immunostimulatory or immunosuppressive.
- They can also be classified into steroidal and nonsteroidal immunomodulatory agents, but in this chapter, we will only discuss nonsteroidal topical immunomodulators.

IMMUNOSTIMULATORS

Imiquimod

Introduction

- Imiquimod, a synthetic immunomodulator, stimulates innate and adaptive immune response pathways, resulting in antiviral, antitumor, and immunoregulatory properties.
- It was first approved in 1997 for the treatment of genital and perianal warts in 1997.[1]

Mechanism of Action

- Imiquimod is a Toll-like receptor-7 (TLR-7) agonist and binds with the receptors on antigen-presenting cells (e.g., Langerhans cells, other dendritic cells, macrophages).
- This leads to the interaction of the cytoplasmic portion of the receptor with MyD88.
- This facilitates association of MyD88 with interleukin (IL)-1 receptor-associated kinase (IRAK), which in turn activates TNF receptor-activated 6 (TRAF6) and ultimately results in stimulation of nuclear factor-κB-mediated signaling.
- This induces various proinflammatory cytokines, including interferon-alpha (IFN-α), tumor necrosis factor-alpha (TNF-α), interleukin (IL)-6, and IL-8.
- In addition, imiquimod can enhance acquired immunity by indirectly stimulating the production of T-helper type 1 (TH1) cytokine interferon IFN-γ.
- Imiquimod, at higher concentrations, also induces apoptosis of tumor cells through activation of Bcl-2 (Bcl-2 proteins) proteins and caspase family of proteases **(Fig. 1)**.[2]

Dosages and Formulation

- It is commercially available as 2.5, 3.75, and 5% creams, though it is the last strength that is more universally available.
- *Dosage for anogenital warts:* 5% cream three times weekly for up to 16 weeks, or 3.75% cream daily for up to 8 weeks.
- *Dosage for actinic keratoses:* 5% cream twice weekly for 16 weeks, or 2.5–3.75% cream daily for two 2-week cycles separated by 2 weeks without treatment.
- *Dosage for superficial BCC:* 5% cream five times weekly for 6 weeks.[1]

Indications

- The Food and Drug Administration (FDA)-approved indications for imiquimod use in cutaneous disorders are:
  - Anogenital warts
  - Basal cell carcinoma (superficial)
  - Actinic keratosis
- *Off-label uses of imiquimod in cutaneous disorders:* In addition to its FDA-approved indications, topical imiquimod has been used off-label in the treatment of several infectious, neoplastic, and other cutaneous disorders **(Table 1)**.[3]

Side Effects of Topical Imiquimod

- *Cutaneous side effects:*
  - *Common:* Erythema, itching, burning, irritation, tenderness, pain, scabbing/crusting, erosions/ulceration, and cellulitis
  - *Rare:* Eczema, vitiligo-like depigmentation, telogen effluvium, angioedema, mycosis fungoides-like histologic changes, eruptive epidermoid cysts, and erosive pustular dermatosis of the scalp
- *Systemic side effects:*
  - Constitutional symptoms (fever, fatigue, nausea, myalgias, and arthralgias)

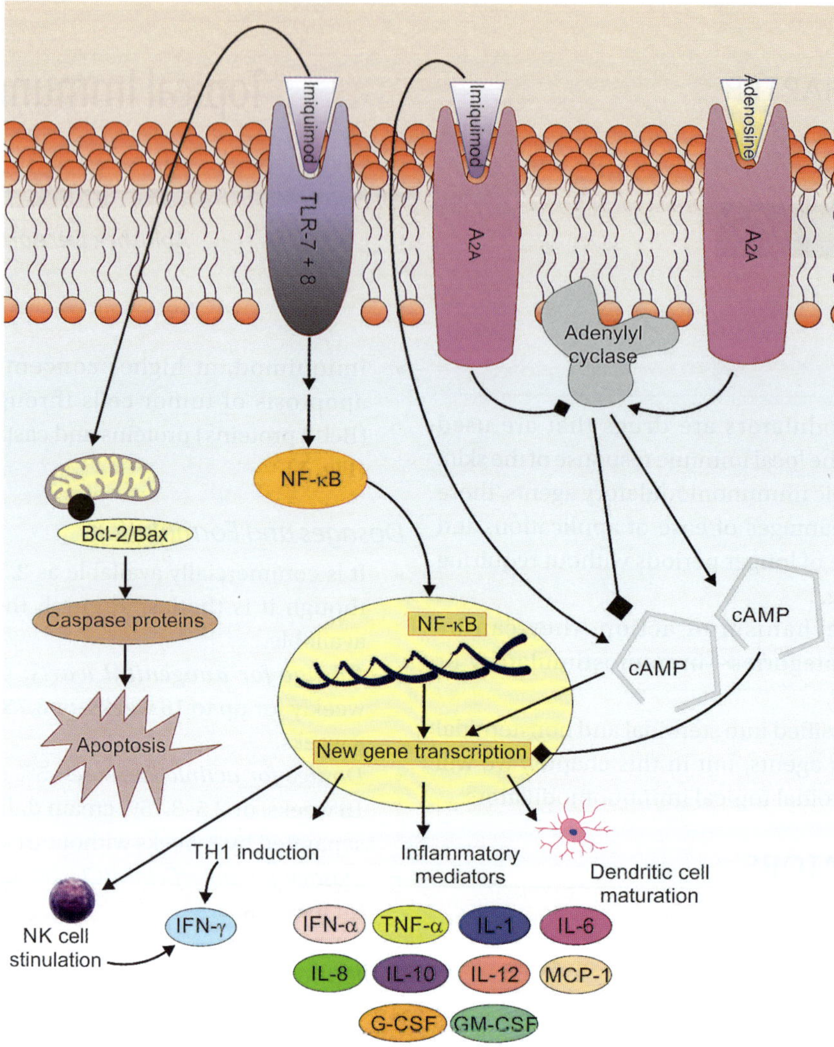

Fig. 1: Mechanism of action of topical imiquimod.

TABLE 1: Off-label uses of imiquimod in cutaneous disorders.

Infectious	*Neoplastic*	*Inflammatory*	*Others*
• Nongenital warts • Epidermodysplasia verruciformis • Molluscum contagiosum • Human orf • Herpes • Leishmania	• Bowen's disease • Melanoma *in situ* • Nodular basal cell carcinoma • Keratoacanthoma • Extramammary Paget's • Oral leukoplakia • Verrucous carcinoma • Kaposi's sarcoma • Pyogenic granuloma • Hemangioma of infancy • Angiolymphoid hyperplasia with eosinophilia • Mycosis fungoides • Lymphomatoid papulosis • B-cell lymphomas	• Granuloma annulare • Morphea	• Keloid • Porokeratosis of Mibelli • Follicular mucinosis • Tattoo removal

- Influenza-like symptoms
- Insignificant transient shifts in white blood cells and hemoglobin
- Conjunctivitis, ocular stinging (in periocular use)
- Chronic neuropathic pain
- Headache and postural hypotension[1]

Use in Pregnancy

Pregnancy (Category C)

Resiquimod (R-848)

- Imidazoquinoline amine 0.01% gel
- It is a potent, soluble analog of imiquimod.
- It showed effectiveness in the treatment of recurrent genital herpes by reducing the frequency of mucosal HSV-2 reactivation (genital shedding).[4]

MACROLACTAM IMMUNOMODULATORS

Tacrolimus (FK 506)

Introduction

- Tacrolimus is produced by a type of soil bacterium *Streptomyces tsukubaensis* in the Tsukuba region of Japan.
- The name tacrolimus was abbreviated from the words "*T*sukuba," "M*acrol*ide," and "Im*mu*nosuppressive."
- Topical tacrolimus was launched in 2000.[5]

Mechanism of Action

- Both tacrolimus and pimecrolimus bind to the FK506-binding protein (FKBP), forming complexes that inhibit calcineurin.
- Calcineurin normally dephosphorylates the cytoplasmic subunit of nuclear factor of activated T-cells (NFAT), which then translocates to the nucleus and forms a complex that promotes transcription of proinflammatory cytokines, including the T-cell mitogen IL-2 **(Fig. 2 and Table 2)**.[6,7]

Dosages and Formulation

- Topical tacrolimus is available in 0.1 and 0.03% ointments.
- Tacrolimus 0.1 and 0.03% ointments are approved in patients ≥16 and ≥2 years of age, respectively.

Properties of Tacrolimus

Absorption:

- Despite the relatively high molecular weight of 822 Da, tacrolimus is well absorbed topically by intact skin.
- Tacrolimus is absorbed at a significantly higher rate in damaged skin.
- The bioavailability of topical tacrolimus is lower than 0.5%.
- Tacrolimus does not accumulate, either in the skin or blood, following repeated applications.
- When applied topically, compared with cyclosporin A, tacrolimus has a significantly better penetration due to lower lipophilicity and the lower molecular weight of tacrolimus compared with cyclosporin A (1,202 Da).
- It has been shown that liposomal formulations of tacrolimus have a 9-fold increase in skin levels compared to the systemic agents.

Metabolism:

- There is no evidence of cutaneous metabolism of topical tacrolimus.
- Systemically, tacrolimus metabolism is mediated by the cytochrome P450 3A4 isoenzyme.

Elimination: Tacrolimus is eliminated in bile with a systemic half-life of 40 hours.[5,6]

Indications

- *FDA-approved indications for use of topical calcineurin inhibitors in cutaneous disorders*: Atopic dermatitis (AD)
- *Off-label dermatologic uses:*
    - Contact dermatitis
    - Psoriasis
    - Seborrheic dermatitis
    - Oral and cutaneous lichen planus
    - Psoriasis
    - Ichthyosis linearis circumflexa
    - Lichen sclerosus
    - Pigmentary abnormalities

TABLE 2: Mechanism of action of pimecrolimus, tacrolimus, and topical corticosteroids.

Parameters	*Pimecrolimus*	*Tacrolimus*	*Corticosteroids*
Cells affected	• T-lymphocytes • Mast cells	• T-lymphocytes • Mast cells • Eosinophils, basophils • Langerhans cells	• T-lymphocytes • Mast cells • Eosinophils, basophils • Langerhans cells • Keratinocytes • Endothelial cells • Fibroblasts
Cytokines	IL-2, IL-3, IL-4, IL-5, INF-γ, TNF-α	IL-2, IL-3, IL-4, IL-5, INF-γ, TNF-α	IL-2, IL-3, IL-4,IL-5, INF-γ, TNF-α, INF-α, GM-CSF
Apoptosis of Langerhans cells	–	+	+
Absorption through the skin	+	++	+++
Atrophogenic activity	–	–	+++

(INF-γ: interferon-gamma; IL: interleukin; GM-CSF: granulocyte macrophage-colony stimulating factor; TNF-α: tumor necrosis factor-alpha)

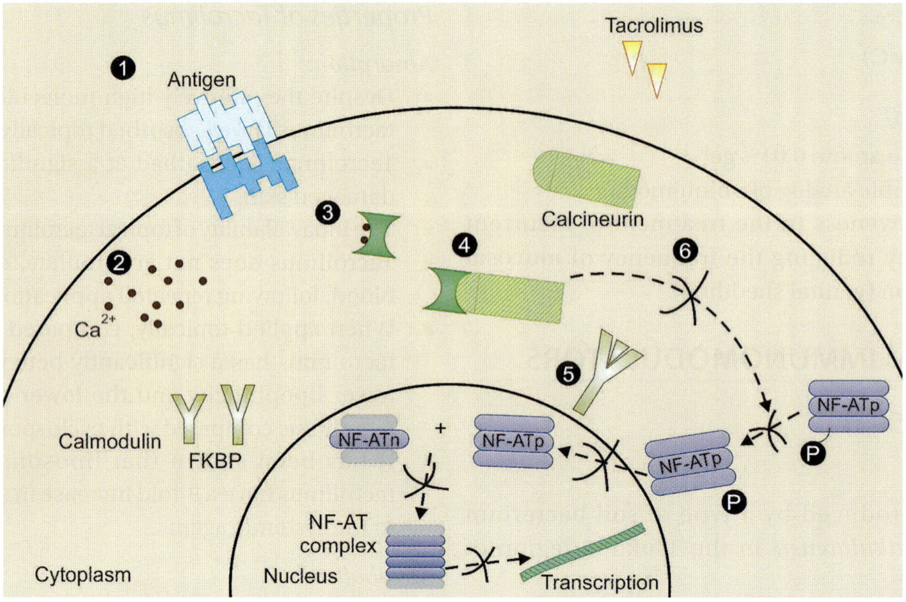

Fig. 2: *The mechanism of action of tacrolimus (FK506):* (1) Antigen binding; (2) Increase in cellular Ca^{2+}; (3) Ca^{2+} binds to calmodulin; (4) Calcineurin is activated; (5) Tacrolimus binds to FK-binding protein (FK-BP); (6) Prevention of dephosphorylation of nuclear factor of activated T-cells p (NF-ATp). NF-ATp cannot enter the nucleus, NFAT complex does not form, transcription is inhibited.

  - Steroid-induced rosacea
  - Vitiligo
  - Autoimmune dermatoses-like cutaneous lupus erythematosus
  - Morphea
  - Pyoderma gangrenosum
  - Chronic leg ulcers in a rheumatoid arthritis patient
  - Granuloma annulare
  - Cutaneous Crohn's disease
  - Granuloma faciale
  - Balanitis xerotica obliterans, zoon balanitis
  - Chronic actinic dermatitis[8,9]
- *The guidelines for use of topical tacrolimus in AD:*
  - The long-term efficacy of tacrolimus was studied in patients with AD and it was found that over time the symptoms of AD decreased significantly. The effectiveness of tacrolimus ointment 0.1% was maintained throughout
  - Treatment of moderate-to-severe AD in case, there is no satisfactory response or no tolerance to conventional treatment, such as topical corticosteroids
  - From 2 to 16 years, first, 0.03% ointment twice daily for 3 weeks, then once daily until disappearance of lesions
  - From 16 years, 0.1% ointment until the disappearance of lesions
  - Supportive treatment of moderate-to-severe AD to prevent recurrence and extend periods without recurrence in patients with frequent exacerbations (4 or more times a year) who initially responded to treatment with tacrolimus ointment twice daily for maximum 6 weeks
  - Use once daily 2 days a week (e.g. Monday and Thursday) on the affected surface
  - 0.1% ointment in adults, 0.03% in children[10]

Side Effects

- Tacrolimus ointment is generally well tolerated.
- When used in a topical formulation, tacrolimus has a low systemic absorption rate below 0.25 ng/mL. The bioavailability of topical tacrolimus was found to be lower than 0.5%. Topical tacrolimus, therefore, has no systemic toxic effects in animals or humans.
- The most common side effects are burning of the skin, stinging, pruritus, sensation of warmth at sites of application, flu-like symptoms, skin erythema, and headaches. A local flushing reaction in association with alcohol consumption can also occur.
- Burning of the skin and pruritus are frequent in patients with severe or extensive disease and are generally transient.
- Allergic contact dermatitis and a rosacea-like granulomatous reaction on the face are rarely reported due to topical tacrolimus.
- In 2006, the US FDA released a boxed warning regarding a theoretical concern for risk of malignancy. However, there has been no short-term or intermediate-term (>15 years) evidence of systemic immunosuppression or an increased risk for malignancy in clinical studies, systematic reviews, or post-marketing surveillance of topical tacrolimus.

- An international task force recommended the removal of the boxed warning.[5,6]

Contraindications

- *Absolute:* Hypersensitivity to pimecrolimus or any components of the cream
- *Relative:*
    - Children <2 years of age
    - Active skin infection (at the site to be treated)

Use in Pregnancy

Pregnancy (Category C)

Pimecrolimus

Introduction

- Pimecrolimus is an ascomycin macrolactam.
- It is produced by the fermentation of *S. hygroscopicus* var. *Ascomycetous.*
- Topical pimecrolimus was introduced in 2001.[11]

Mechanism of Action

- Similar to tacrolimus
- Compared to tacrolimus, pimecrolimus shows lower skin penetration, higher affinity to epithelial structures, lower affinity to lymphoid structures, lower immunosuppressive effects, and threefold lower affinity to macrophilin-12 (FKBP12).[12]

Dosages and Formulation

- Pimecrolimus is available as 1% cream; each gram cream contains 10 mg of pimecrolimus.
- Pimecrolimus cream is applied twice daily for no longer than 6 weeks continuously.
- Pimecrolimus 1% cream is approved for treatment of "mild-to-moderate" AD in individuals ≥2 years of age.
- However, pimecrolimus has also been studied extensively in infants 3–23 months of age, and the American Academy of Dermatology's current guidelines recommend off-label use of pimecrolimus 1% cream and tacrolimus 0.03% ointment for children <2 years of age with mild-to-severe AD.

Indications

- *FDA-approved indication:* Atopic dermatitis
- *Off-label dermatologic uses:*
    - Erosive oral and genital lichen planus
    - Vulvar lichen sclerosus
    - Fox–Fordyce disease
    - Intertriginous psoriasis
    - Seborrheic dermatitis
    - Erosive circinate balanitis
    - Cutaneous lupus erythematosus
    - Cutaneous dermatomyositis
    - Vulvar pruritus
    - Vitiligo
    - Cutaneous chronic graft-versus-host disease (GVHD)
    - Eczematous dermatitis of the eyelids, intertriginous (skin fold) areas, or hands[4]
    - Perioral dermatitis
    - Pyoderma gangrenosum
    - Rosacea[12,13]
- The guidelines for use of topical pimecrolimus in AD:
    - Mild-to-moderate AD when topical corticosteroids are not recommended or not possible
    - Adults and children older than 2 years, twice daily until lesions disappear, not longer than 6 weeks
    - Pimecrolimus has similar efficacy as low-to-moderately potent topical corticosteroid creams for mild-to-moderate AD during the first 5–6 years of life, with similar rates of adverse events.
    - In the treatment of pediatric AD in a short-term, continuous-use course, pimecrolimus 1% cream versus tacrolimus 0.03% ointment has a similar efficiency as assessed by the improvement in the Investigator's Global Assessment (IGA) scale and is equally well tolerated.[14]

Side Effects

- Pimecrolimus showed a good safety profile in children >3 months of age.
- Studies indicate that the use of pimecrolimus cream results in minimal systemic absorption.
- Long-term intermittent treatment of adults with extensive dermatitis using pimecrolimus cream is associated with minimal systemic exposure and no evidence of drug accumulation over time.
- The most common side effects are burning, stinging, or a sensation of heat at sites of application. This may happen, especially when the site of the application is acutely inflamed.
- There are reports of enhancement of alcohol-induced facial flushing, facial acne, and molluscum contagiosum after the use of topical pimecrolimus.
- Topical calcineurin inhibitors (TCIs) including pimecrolimus received a black-box warning for the theoretical risks of skin malignancies in animal studies. Although there has been no definite establishment of a causal relationship, skin malignancies and lymphomas have rarely been reported in patients using topical pimecrolimus.

Contraindications

- *Absolute:* Hypersensitivity to pimecrolimus or any components of the cream
- *Relative:*
    - Children <2 years of age

- Areas of skin with active premalignant or malignant lesions [such as cutaneous T-cell lymphoma (CTCL)] or skin infections (bacterial or viral)
- Patients who are immunocompromised or are taking systemic immunosuppressive medications
- Patients who have severely impaired skin barrier function that may be at higher risk for increased systemic absorption (i.e., Netherton syndrome)

Use in Pregnancy

- Pregnancy (Category C)
- There is an absence of adequate studies in pregnant women.

Sirolimus (Rapamycin)

- It is isolated from *S. hygroscopicus* in Rapa Nui Island.
- Sirolimus exerts immunosuppressive effects after building with macrophilin-12 (FKBP12).
- The target protein of this complex is serine-kinase, "mammalian target of rapamycin (mTOR)" that regulates cell growth.
- By inhibition of this protease, sirolimus inhibits the cytokine-dependent proliferation of T-cells.
- Beneficial therapeutic effects of sirolimus were reported in the treatment of tuberous sclerosis.
- When used in the treatment of children ≥36 weeks of age, applied once a day, three times per week for 9 months, it has shown efficacy in regression of facial angiofibroma.[15]

Cyclosporine

- Cyclosporine is a lipophilic cyclic polypeptide isolated from *Tolypocladium inflatum* gams.
- Cyclosporine is a prodrug that becomes active only after forming a complex with an intracytoplasmic immunophilin known as cyclophilin.
- Topical cyclosporine had been used successfully in:
  - Oral pemphigus (5 mL of solution, 100 mg/mL, 5-minute mouthwash three times daily)
  - Lichen planus (erosive, oral, and vulvar)
  - Pyoderma gangrenosum
  - Benign familial pemphigus
- It does not penetrate the skin probably due to its large molecular size (about 1,200 Da)[16]

PHOSPHODIESTERASE 4 INHIBITOR

Crisaborole

Introduction

- Crisaborole (Eucrisa) is a novel anti-inflammatory inhibitor of phosphodiesterase 4 (PDE4) that is now licensed for the topical treatment of mild-to-moderate AD in patients aged 2 years or more.[17]

Mechanism of Action

- Crisaborole is a boron-containing, small molecule (251.1 Da) inhibitor of PDE4.
- The low molecular weight of crisaborole permits effective skin penetration and target cell access.
- PDE4 is the most prevalent PDE in keratinocytes and the cells of the immune and nervous systems.
- The inhibition of PDE4 by crisaborole results in increased intracellular cyclic adenosine monophosphate (cAMP) levels and the subsequent inhibition of pro-inflammatory and T-cell cytokine production including Th2 [interleukin (IL)-4, IL-13, IL-31] and Th22 (IL-22) cytokines.
- Specifically, in human peripheral blood mononuclear cells, crisaborole inhibited the production of tumor necrosis factor-α, interferon-c, IL-2, IL-5, and IL-10.

Dosages and Formulation

Crisaborole is available as 2% ointment.

Pharmacokinetics

- Crisaborole is systemically absorbed, but systemic exposure following topical administration is minimal, albeit rapid, and increases as the area of application.
- Following systemic uptake, crisaborole is rapidly and substantially metabolized into inactive metabolites, either by hydrolysis or by oxidation. In vitro, crisaborole is highly bound (97%) to human plasma proteins. Systemically absorbed crisaborole is eliminated via renal excretion as metabolites.

Indications

It is now US FDA approved for the topical treatment of mild-to-moderate AD in patients aged 2 years or more.

Therapeutic Efficacy

- In two phase III studies, topical therapy with crisaborole ointment 2% reduced disease severity and pruritus severity of AD when compared with vehicle.
- Improvements in the other signs of AD (erythema, exudation, excoriation, induration/papulation, and lichenification) were also seen.
- Crisaborole ointment 2% was generally well tolerated in the short-term studies, with its favorable safety profile maintained over the longer-term (up to 52 weeks) in a multicenter, extension study.

Side Effects

- Crisaborole ointment 2% is generally well tolerated.
- Most treatment-emergent adverse events (TEAEs) were of mild-to-moderate severity and considered unrelated to the study medication.
- Moreover, the incidence of application-site pain following short- and long-term topical therapy with crisaborole ointment 2% was low.[18]

CONTACT SENSITIZERS

- Topical immunotherapy is defined as the induction and periodic elicitation of allergic contact dermatitis by applying a potent contact allergen.
- Contact immunotherapy was introduced in 1976, by Rosenberg and Drake.
- Later, potent contact allergens, namely dinitrochlorobenzene (DNCB), squaric acid dibutyl ester (SADBE), and diphencyprone (DPCP) superseded the earlier used allergens.
- The immunotherapeutic effectiveness of contact allergens in alopecia areata (AA), now understood to be a consequence of immunomodulation.
- DPCP affects T-cell activation and cytokine release.
- SADBE exerts extravasation and recruitment of activated autoreactive T-cells.

Diphenylcyclopropenone

- Diphencyprone was first synthesized in 1959.
- It is a potent contact allergen.
- *Uses:*
  - *Most commonly used in AA:* In AA, DPCP induces allergic response in 98–99% and a cosmetically acceptable hair regrowth in 28–80%.
  - Common warts
  - *In melanomas:*
    - Metastatic cutaneous melanoma with exclusively cutaneous metastases
    - Refractory melanomas unresponsive to conventional treatment methods
  - Basal and squamous cell carcinoma
  - Bowen's disease
  - Actinic keratoses
- *Castling phenomenon:* Denser and faster hair regrowth observed over the untreated site. This can rarely happen with AA treated with contact immunotherapy.
- *Mechanism of action:*
  - In the past, its effect was exclusively attributed to "competitive antigen inhibition."
  - However it is now understood, DPCP is not strictly "contact allergic," but also has "immunomodulatory" effects.
  - Mainly, a decrease in CD4 to CD8 lymphocyte count from 4:1 to 1:1 occurs.
  - A decrease in intrabulbar CD6 lymphocytes and Langerhans cells is also noted.
- *Method of application of diphencyprone in AA:*
  - The scalp is the usual sensitization site.
  - A cotton-tipped applicator saturated with 2% DPCP in acetone is applied to an area of at least 10 cm^2.
  - Patients are advised to avoid washing the area and protect it from sunlight for 48 hours.
  - Applications of the contact allergen are repeated weekly with increasing concentrations.
  - The usual initial concentration of DPCP is 0.001–0.1% and the concentration is adjusted according to the response.
  - An eczematous response (which may occur after 5 days or more) indicates that sensitization has taken place.
  - A second application may be made if necessary.
- *Side effects:*
  - Persistent dermatitis
  - Painful cervical lymphadenopathy
  - Generalized eczema
  - Blistering
  - Contact leukoderma
  - Urticarial reaction[19]

Dinitrochlorobenzene

- Dinitrochlorobenzene (DNCB) is a potent-contact allergen.
- It is used mainly in refractory AA and in viral warts.
- DNCB is also used less commonly in Bowen disease, actinic keratosis, and basal cell carcinoma.
- DNCB contains contaminants that are mutagenic and carcinogenic to animals.
- When topically applied, >40% of the drug is absorbed systemically. Systemic manifestations such as fever, arthralgia, and yellowish discoloration of gray hair are noted more often with DNCB than any other contact sensitizers.
- Although no evidence of carcinogenicity is reported in patients treated with DNCB, it has been largely replaced by DPCP and SADBE.[20]

Squaric Acid Dibutyl Ester

- Squaric acid dibutyl ester (SADBE) is a universal topical sensitizer.
- It is popular in Europe and south-east Asia.
- It is widely used in the treatment of AA and viral warts.
- SADBE is more expensive than other contact allergens.
- No identifiable contaminants of its preparations have been discovered.
- It is not mutagenic in the Ames assay. Nevertheless, additional testing in animals is required to ascertain the mutagenicity and safety of SADBE.
- Persistent contact dermatitis at the site of application and singular pigmentary metamorphosis observed in the newly grown scalp hair has been noted with the use of SADBE.[20]

TOPICAL VITAMIN D3

- There are three topical vitamin D3 analogs used in dermatology: Calcipotriene (originally named calcipotriol), calcitriol, and tacalcitol.

- Studies have demonstrated the superior efficacy of calcipotriene over calcitriol and tacalcitol.

Calcipotriene (Calcipotriol)

- Calcipotriene is a synthetic analog of calcitriol.
- It exhibits immunomodulatory effects by binding to vitamin D receptors with the same affinity as calcitriol, but it is less likely to cause hypercalcemia due to its rapid local metabolism.
- It inhibits cellular proliferation and induces cellular differentiation of the cells.
- It acts on monocytes, macrophages, and B- and T-lymphocytes to inhibit thymocyte proliferation induced by IL-1 and the release of IL-6 and IFN-γ from activated mononuclear cells.
- It does not induce skin atrophy or photosensitization; it is well tolerated in children, and it is not teratogenic.
- Calcipotriene is available in 0.005% ointment, cream, and solution
- It showed therapeutic efficacy in the treatment of:
  - Plaque psoriasis (US FDA-approved indication)
  - Other keratinization disorders, such as pityriasis rubra pilaris, congenital ichthyosis, hereditary palmoplantar keratoderma, disseminated superficial actinic porokeratosis
  - Vitiligo
  - Morphea
  - Cutaneous T-cell lymphoma
  - *Miscellaneous skin disorders:* Acanthosis nigricans, keratosis pilaris, and Darier's disease, Grover's disease, erythema annulare centrifugum, prurigo nodularis
- Its side effect is skin irritation, especially on the face.
- *Contraindications:*
  - *Absolute:* None
  - *Relative:* Conditions causing hypercalcemia
- Pregnancy (Category C)[21]

Calcitriol

- Hormonally active vitamin D3 (1a, 25-dihydroxyvitamin D3) is a metabolite, also called calcitriol, which is synthesized in keratinocytes.
- It is available as 3 μg/g ointment.
- Studies have shown calcitriol is safe and effective for the treatment of psoriasis.
- It is suitable for the treatment of psoriasis on the face, neck, and flexural areas, where it exhibits better efficacy than calcipotriol.
- In the treatment of psoriasis, it may be used as monotherapy or as an adjuvant therapy with a topical corticosteroid or UVB phototherapy.
- The maximum recommended dose of calcitriol ointment should not exceed >200 g per week in adults and 100 g in children.
- When used in combination with corticosteroids, it reduces their side effects by:
  - Restoring the epidermal permeability by increasing lipids
  - Increasing antimicrobial peptides
- It is not recommended for children younger than 15 years of age
- It is not recommended in pregnancy.[22]

Tacalcitol

- It has limited hypercalcemic activity, unlike calcitriol.
- It is available as a 0.0002% ointment, cream, and solution.
- The main indication is topical treatment of psoriasis.

MISCELLANEOUS TOPICAL AGENTS

Topical Zinc Sulfate

- Available as 2.5% cream
- It has anti-inflammatory effects as it inhibits the release of inflammatory cytokines such as IL-1 and IL-6 from keratinocytes.
- It has been used with reasonable efficacy alone or in combination with topical steroids in the treatment of chronic eczema, eczematous psoriasis, and lichen planus.
- It was also used in the treatment of acne in a formulation with erythromycin (1.2% zinc + 4% erythromycin) where besides inhibition of IL-6 release from keratinocytes, it also lowers 5-alpha reductase in the sebaceous glands.[23-25]

Anthralin

- Anthralin is an immunomodulator that was mainly used in plaque psoriasis and AA.
- It exerts an antimitotic effect by inhibiting DNA synthesis, repair, and replication within keratinocytes, lymphocytes, and fibroblasts.
- It is available as an ointment, cream, or gel (0.1–5%).
- Liposomal aqueous gel-based formulation causes minimal coloration and no irritation in comparison to regular formulation.

KEY POINTS

- Topical immunomodulators are agents that regulate the local immune response of the skin.
- Topical immunomodulators include the following agents: macrolactams, contact sensitizers, immunostimulants, and miscellaneous agents.
- Imiquimod is a toll-like receptor-7 (TLR-7) agonist and binds with the receptors on antigen-presenting cells.
- The Food and Drug Administration (FDA)-approved indications for imiquimod use in cutaneous disorders are: anogenital warts, basal cell carcinoma (superficial) and actinic keratosis.

- Both tacrolimus and pimecrolimus bind to the FK506-binding protein (FKBP), forming complexes that inhibit calcineurin.
- FDA-approved indications for use of topical calcineurin inhibitors in cutaneous disorders: atopic dermatitis.

REFERENCES

1. Hanna E, Abadi R, Abbas O. Imiquimod in dermatology: an overview. Int J Dermatol. 2016;55(8):831-44.
2. Ahmed I, Berth-Jones J. Imiquimod: a novel treatment for lentigo maligna. Br J Dermatol. 2000;143(4):843-5.
3. DiBiagio JR, Pyle T, Green JJ. Reviewing the use of imiquimod for molluscum contagiosum. Dermatol Online J. 2018;24(6):13030/qt3b4606qt.
4. Mark KE, Corey L, Meng T-C, Magaret AS, Huang M-L, Selke S, et al. Topical resiquimod 0.01% gel decreases herpes simplex virus type 2 genital shedding: a randomized, controlled trial. J Infect Dis. 2007;195(9):1324-31.
5. Nasr IS. Topical tacrolimus in dermatology. Clin Exp Dermatol. 2000;25(3):250-4.
6. Khandpur S, Sharma VK, Sumanth K. Topical immunomodulators in dermatology. J Postgrad Med. 2004;50(2): 131-9.
7. Mandelin JM, Remitz A, Virtanen HM, Malmberg LP, Haahtela T, Reitamo S. A 10-year open follow-up of eczema and respiratory symptoms in patients with atopic dermatitis treated with topical tacrolimus for the first 4 years. J Dermatolog Treat. 2010;21(3):167-70.
8. Woo DK, James WD. Topical tacrolimus: a review of its uses in dermatology. Dermatitis. 2005;16(1):6-21.
9. Guenther L, Lynde C, Poulin Y. Off-label use of topical calcineurin inhibitors in dermatologic disorders. J Cutan Med Surg. 2019;23(4_suppl):27S-34S.
10. Cury Martins J, Martins C, Aoki V, Gois AF, Ishii HA, da Silva EM. Topical tacrolimus for atopic dermatitis. Cochrane Database Syst Rev. 2015;2015(7):CD009864.
11. Fiorillo L, Marcoux D, Ramien M. Contemporary role of topical calcineurin inhibitors: a pediatric dermatology perspective. J Cutan Med Surg. 2019;23(4_suppl):11S-18S.
12. Sehgal VN, Pahwa M. Pimecrolimus, yet another intriguing topical immunomodulator. J Dermatolog Treat. 2007;18(3): 147-50.
13. Fabroni C, Lotti T. Pimecrolimus in dermatology. G Ital Dermatol Venereol. 2009;144(3):321-5.
14. Rajagopalan M, De A, Godse K, Shankar DSK, Zawar V, Sharma N, et al. Guidelines on management of atopic dermatitis in India: an evidence-based review and an expert consensus. Indian J Dermatol. 2019;64(3):166-81.
15. Sandbank S, Molho-Pessach V, Farkas A, Barzilai A, Greenberger S. Oral and topical sirolimus for vascular anomalies: a multicentre study and review. Acta Derm Venereol. 2019; 99(11):990-6.
16. Jitsukawa K, Ring J, Weyer U, Kimmig W, Radloff H. Topical cyclosporine in chronic benign familial pemphigus (Hailey-Hailey disease). J Am Acad Dermatol. 1992;27(4): 625-6.
17. Ramachandran V, Cline A, Feldman SR, Strowd LC. Evaluating crisaborole as a treatment option for atopic dermatitis. Expert Opin Pharmacother. 2019;20:1057-63.
18. Yosipovitch G, Gold LF, Lebwohl MG, Silverberg JI, Tallman AM, Zane LT. Early relief of pruritus in atopic dermatitis with crisaborole ointment, a non-steroidal, phosphodiesterase 4 inhibitor. Acta Derm Venereol. 2018;98:484-89.
19. Jang YH, Jung HJ, Moon SY, Lee WJ, Lee SJ, Lee WK, et al. Systematic review and quality analysis of studies on the efficacy of topical diphenylcyclopropenone treatment for alopecia areata. J Am Acad Dermatol. 2017;77(1): 170-2.e1.
20. Yoshimasu T, Furukawa F. Modified immunotherapy for alopecia areata. Autoimmun Rev. 2016;15(7):664-7.
21. Patel NU, Felix K, Reimer D, Feldman SR. Calcipotriene/betamethasone dipropionate for the treatment of psoriasis vulgaris: an evidence-based review. Clin Cosmet Investig Dermatol. 2017;10:385-91.
22. Sigmon JR, Yentzer BA, Feldman SR. Calcitriol ointment: a review of a topical vitamin D analog for psoriasis. J Dermatolog Treat. 2009;20(4):208-12.
23. Peters DC, Balfour JA. Tacalcitol. Drugs. 1997;54(2):265-71; discussion 272.
24. Cervantes J, Eber AE, Perper M, Nascimento VM, Nouri K, Keri JE. The role of zinc in the treatment of acne: a review of the literature. Dermatol Ther. 2018;31(1):e12576.
25. Torsekar R, Gautam MM. Topical therapies in psoriasis. Indian Dermatol Online J. 2017;8(4):235-45.

EXAMINATION QUESTIONS

1. Write a brief note on imiquimod.
2. Write a brief note on topical tacrolimus.

147 CHAPTER

Topical Antifungals

Vandana Mehta

INTRODUCTION

Topical antifungals are considered as first-line therapy for uncomplicated superficial dermatophytic infections owing to their superior efficacy and low potential for side effects. The choice of agent is determined by the site and extent of the infection and by the causative organism. Their other potential indications include pregnancy, pediatric dermatophytic infections, concomitant liver, renal, and cardiovascular disease and as an adjuvant to systemic antifungals.[1]

Topical antifungals are broadly classified into:[2]

- *Polyenes*: Nystatin, amphotericin B
- Imidazoles (e.g., miconazole, ketoconazole, clotrimazole, eberconazole, sertaconazole) and triazoles (fluconazole)
- *Allylamines/benzylamines*: Terbinafine, naftifine
- *Morpholines*: Amorolfine
- *Miscellaneous antifungals*: Selenium sulfide, ciclopirox olamine, Whitfield's ointment, Castellani paint, tolnaftate
- *New antifungals*: Tavaborole, efinaconazole, ME1111

CLASSIFICATION OF ANTIFUNGALS BASED ON MECHANISM OF ACTION

Classification of antifungals based on mechanism of action is given in **Table 1**.

MISCELLANEOUS ANTIFUNGALS

Ciclopirox Olamine

It is a hydroxypyridone derivative and acts by disrupting the cell membrane integrity by preventing the active transport of essential molecules. It is available as a 1% cream, shampoo and as 8% nail lacquer for twice daily application against yeasts and dermatophytes.[3,4]

Selenium Sulfide

It possesses a cytostatic effect on keratinocytes and follicular epithelium by causing increased corneocyte shedding. It is effective in seborrheic dermatitis, tinea versicolor, confluent, and reticulate papillomatosis of Gougerot and Carteaud. It is available as 1% and 2.5% lotion.

Castellani's Paint

It has antibacterial, antifungal, and local anesthetic properties. Hence, it is useful in the treatment of intertriginous dermatoses such as tinea cruris, candidiasis, and pustular dermatoses of hands and feet. It comprises basic carbol fuchsin (300 mg/100 mL) which stains the skin red, phenol (4.5 g/100 mL), and resorcinol (10 g/100 mL). Irritation of the skin with staining and stinging are its limitations.

Whitfield's Ointment

It is a combination of benzoic acid 6% and salicylic acid 3%. It is useful in the treatment of dermatophytic infections when applied twice daily in view of its keratolytic property, however, it has a strong propensity for causing irritant reactions.

Tolnaftate

It is effective when used topically as a lotion against dermatophytes, however, its mode of action is unknown. It must be used daily on the affected area for 2–6 weeks.

Amorolfine

It is a morpholine derivative and acts by inhibiting the ergosterol synthesis by acting on the delta 14-reductase enzyme. It is effective against dermatophytes, molds, yeasts, and other pathogenic fungi and is available as 5% nail lacquer to be applied on the affected nails once or twice weekly for 6 months.[3,4]

AVAILABLE ANTIFUNGAL FORMULATIONS

Available antifungal formulations are given in **Tables 2**.

ADVERSE EFFECTS

Almost all the topical antifungals are well tolerated with <1% of patients showing adverse effects such as stinging, burning, and itching at the site of application.[3]

NEWER ANTIFUNGALS

- *Efinaconazole*: It demonstrates broad-spectrum antifungal activity against molds, dermatophytes and non

TABLE 1: Classification of antifungals based on mechanism of action.

Class	*Drugs*	*Mechanism*	*Organisms*
Polyenes	Nystatin	Fungistatic and fungicidal in vitro. Acts by binding to cell membrane sterols causing change in membrane permeability and subsequent leakage of cellular components	Yeasts (*Candida*)
Azoles	Miconazole, clotrimazole, ketoconazole, econazole, oxiconazole, luliconazole	Fungistatic. Acts by blocking the biosynthesis of ergosterol by interfering with lanosterol 14α-demethylase which is CYP450 dependent	Dermatophytes *Candida* *Malassezia furfur*
Allylamines	Naftifine, terbinafine	Fungistatic and fungicidal. These are highly lipophilic and act by inhibiting ergosterol synthesis by squalene epoxidase inhibition which is CYP450 independent	Dermatophytes *Candida*
Benzylamines	Butenafine	Fungicidal. Acts by squalene epoxidase inhibition leading to ↓ ergosterol synthesis and increased accumulation of squalene	Dermatophytes *Candida*

TABLE 2: Antifungal formulations.

Polyenes	*Formulation*	*Pregnancy safety status*
Nystatin	Cream, ointment twice daily application	Category B
Amphotericin B	0.1% liposomal cream: 2 weeks	Category B
Azoles	*Formulation (once or twice daily application)*	*Pregnancy safety status*
Miconazole	2% cream, powder, spray	Category B
Clotrimazole	1% cream, solution	Category B
Ketoconazole	2% cream, shampoo	Category B
Oxiconazole	1% cream, lotion	Category B
Econazole	1% cream	Category B
Sulconazole	1% cream, solution	Category B
Sertaconazole	2% cream	Category C
Luliconazole	1% cream	Category B
Allylamines/benzylamines	*Formulation (once or twice daily application)*	*Pregnancy safety status*
Naftifine	1% cream, gel	Category B
Terbinafine	1% cream, spray	Category B
Butenafine	1% cream	Category B

dermatophytes and may be effective as a 10% solution in mild-to-moderate onychomycosis.[5]

- *Tavaborole*: It is a highly specific fungal protein synthesis inhibitor that is capable of penetrating the thick nail plate effectively in view of its relatively low molecular weight. It is active against both dermatophytes and nondermatophytic molds and could be an effective adjuvant to oral therapy.[6]
- *ME1111*: It is a relatively new fungicidal antifungal agent that selectively inhibits the mitochondrial respiratory enzymes leading to blockade of ATP production. It has a very small molecular size that enhances its penetration into the nail plate.[7]

SPECIAL CONSIDERATIONS

- Members of the Azole family (ketoconazole, bifonazole), allylamines (naftifine), and ciclopirox olamine possess an additional anti-inflammatory activity comparable to hydrocortisone via their ability to inhibit polymorphonuclear chemotaxis, and the release of inflammatory cytokines.
- Some molecules such as miconazole, clotrimazole, and ciclopirox olamine work against the gram-positive and gram-negative bacteria which makes them an excellent adjuvant in the treatment of mixed bacterial and fungal infections such as impetigo, folliculitis, and erythrasma.

Example: A BPO (benzoyl peroxide) and miconazole combination has been studied in acne vulgaris.

The Allylamine family of antifungals is highly lipophilic and more potent than azoles in the management of dermatophytes. Owing to their "reservoir effects", the patients continue to improve even after cessation of therapy with low relapse rates.[8]

KEY POINTS

- Majority of the topical antifungals available belong to azoles and allylamines.
- Efficacy-wise the allylamines are superior to azoles in activity against dematophytes. The reverse is true against yeasts such as candida and malassezia.
- Antifungal potency in dermatophyte infections butenafine > terbinafine > ciclopirox olamine = naftifine > azoles.
- Antifungal potency in candidiasis ciclopirox olamine = azoles > butenafine > naftifine > terbinafine.
- Nail lacquers are a valuable tool in management of onychomycosis when given in combination with oral antifungals.
- Amorolfine nail lacquer used every 2 weeks was found to be an effective prophylactic agent in onychomycosis treated earlier with oral antifungals.
- In case of nonresponsiveness to topical therapy or irritancy, physician must check for "propylene glycol" which is a vehicle and often added to the formulation to enhance its percutaneous penetration.

REFERENCES

1. Kyle AA, Dahl MV. Topical therapy for fungal infections. Am J Clin Dermatol. 2004;5:443-51.
2. Gupta AK, Cooper EA. Update in antifungal therapy of dermatophytosis. Mycopathologica. 2008;166:353-67.
3. Sahoo AK, Mahajan R. Management of tinea corporis, tinea cruris and tinea pedis: a comprehensive review. Indian Dermatol Online J. 2016;7:77-86.
4. Zane LT, Chanda S, Coronado D, Del Rosso J. Antifungal agents for onychomycosis: new treatment strategies to improve safety. Dermatol Online J. 2016;22(3). pii: 13030.
5. Tatsumi Y, Nagashima M, Shibanushi T, Iwata A, Kangawa Y, Inui F, et al. Mechanism of action of efinaconazole, a novel triazole antifungal agent. Antimicrob Agents Chmother. 2013;57:2405-9.
6. Elewski BE, Aly R, Baldwin SL. Efficacy and safety of tavaborole topical solution 5%, a novel boron based antifungal agent for the treatment of toe nail onychomycosis: results from 2 randomized phase III studies. J Am Acad Dermatol. 2015;73:62-9.
7. Ghannoum M, Isham N, Long L. In vitro antifungal activity of ME1111, a new topical agent for onychomycosis, against clinical isolates of dermatophytes. Antimicrob Agents Chemother. 2015;59:5154-8.
8. Schäfer-Korting M, Schoellmann C, Korting HC. Fungicidal activity plus reservoir effect allow short treatment courses with terbinafine in tinea pedis. Skin Pharmacol Physiol. 2008;21(4):203-10.

EXAMINATION QUESTION

1. Write a short note on newer topical antifungals.

148 CHAPTER

Topical Retinoids

Surajit Gorai

INTRODUCTION

Retinoids are vitamin A derivatives. It includes all natural and synthetic compounds that have activity like vitamin A. It is not a single molecule, rather few fat soluble naturally occurring biological compounds having similar action. Retinol (vitamin A alcohol form), retinal (vitamin A aldehyde from), and retinoic acid (vitamin A acid form) are collectively termed as vitamin A.[1] The first topically used retinoid was all-trans retinoic acid, called as tretinoin (naturally occurring form). It came to the market for commercial use in acne vulgaris, in 1970. Later on in 1986, its effect on photoaging was found and use in fine wrinkles started. Both the property was discovered by Dr Albert Kligman at the University of Pennsylvania.[2] Gradually, other forms of topical retinoids were discovered and used in various other skin conditions such as psoriasis, Kaposi's sarcoma, and cutaneous T-cell lymphoma (CTCL).[3]

TYPES[4,5]

	Topical	*Systemic*
First generation (Nonaromatic)	Tretinoin (all-trans retinoic acid)	Isotretinoin (13-cis retinoic acid) Alitretinoin (9-cis retinoic acid)
Second generation (Monoaromatic)	–	Etretinate, acitretin
Third generation (Polyaromatic)	Tazarotene, bexarotene, adapalene	Bexarotene

PHARMACOLOGY

All topically applied retinoids penetrate through upper layer of skin and hair follicle. Then it gets distributed within keratinocytes with minimal absorption to dermis or systemic circulation. Every topical form is active except topical tazarotene which is converted to tazarotenic acid. In all cases, excretion occurs through skin desquamation and hepatobiliary system. Tazarotene is excreted through skin desquamation, urine, and feces.[6]

MECHANISM OF ACTION (FLOWCHART 1)

This complex binds to RARE (retinoic acid responsive element) within DNA and influence gene transcription.[7] A number of responsive elements are identified now.

Flowchart 1: Mechanism of action.

Topically applied retinoic acid enters keratinocytes

↓

Excess retinoic acid is stored as retinyl ester (as it is stored in liver) within keratinocytes

↓

When in need, free retinol comes and gets oxidized to retinoic acid

↓

Retinoic acid binds to cytosolic retinoic acid-binding protein (CRABP)

↓

CRABP II is predominant in human skin

↓

Then it enters to the nucleus and binds with retinoic acid receptor (RAR) and retinoid X receptor (RXR) (two forms of retinoic acid receptor)

Through gene transcription it changes cell proliferation, normalizes keratinization, causes epidermal hyperplasia, and reduces inflammation. Thus, it shows beneficial action on acne, psoriasis, photoaging, and hyperpigmentation, and keratinization disorder.[8]

USES

All-trans retinoic acid: Acne vulgaris, chronic photoaging, hyperpigmentation, and actinic keratosis.

Adapalene: Acne vulgaris and hyperpigmentation

Tazarotene: Acne vulgaris, psoriasis, CTCL, and ichthyotic disorders

Alitretinoin: Kaposi's sarcoma, photoaging, and hand dermatitis

Bexarotene: CTCL, lymphomatoid papulosis, hand dermatitis, psoriasis, and alopecia areata.[9]

SIDE EFFECTS

- Erythema
- Burning
- Stinging, photosensitivity
- Desquamation, dryness, and irritation

These are termed as "retinoid dermatitis." It may lead to discontinuation of therapy. Prior counseling regarding minimal application, avoidance of rubbing, avoidance of irritant cosmetic products is important.[10]

KEY POINTS

- Retinoids are derivatives of vitamin A. Three compounds namely: (1) retinol (vitamin A alcohol form), (2) retinal (vitamin A aldehyde from), and (3) retinoic acid (vitamin A acid form) are collectively termed as vitamin A.
- First topical form was all-trans retinoic acid/tretinoin (naturally occurring form).
- Topically applied drug enters the nucleus of keratinocytes; binds with RAR (retinoic acid receptor) modify the gene transcription. Thus, they normalize keratinization, epidermal proliferation, and controls acne.
- They are mainly used in acne vulgaris, chronic photoaging, hyperpigmentation, and actinic keratosis.
- Topical retinoids may have some side effects such as erythema, burning, stinging, photosensitivity, desquamation, dryness, and irritation. These are termed as "retinoid dermatitis."

REFERENCES

1. Bollag W, Geiger JM. The development of retinoids in dermatology. In: Cunliffe WJ, Miller AJ (Eds). Retinoid therapy: a review of clinical and laboratory research, 1st edition. Dordrecht, Netherlands: Springer; 1984. pp. 1-7.
2. Kligman LH, Duo CH, Kligman AM. Topical retinoic acid enhances the repair of ultraviolet damaged dermal connective tissue. Connect Tissue Res. 1984;12(2):139-50.
3. Orfanos CE, Zouboulis CC, Almond-Roesler B, Geilen CC. Current use and future potential role of retinoids in dermatology. Drugs. 1997;53(3):358-88.
4. Kagechika H, Shudo K. Synthetic retinoids: recent developments concerning structure and clinical utility. J Med Chem. 2005;48(19):5875-83.
5. Mukherjee S, Date A, Patravale V, Korting HC, Roeder A, Weindl G. Retinoids in the treatment of skin aging: an overview of clinical efficacy and safety. Clin Interv Aging. 2006;1(4): 327-48.
6. Roos TC, Jugert FK, Merk HF, Bickers DR. Retinoid metabolism in the skin. Pharmacol Rev. 1998;50(2):315-33.
7. Sporn MB, Roberts AB, Roche NS, Kagechika H, Shudo K. Mechanism of action of retinoids. J Am Acad Dermatol. 1986;15(4):756-64.
8. Marill J, Idres N, Capron CC, Nguyen E, Chabot GG. Retinoic acid metabolism and mechanism of action: a review. Curr Drug Metab. 2003;4(1):1-10.
9. Verschoore M, Bouclier M, Czernielewski J, Hensby C. Topical retinoids: their uses in dermatology. Dermatologic Clinics. 1993;11(1):107-15.
10. Ellis CN, Krach KJ. Uses and complications of isotretinoin therapy. J Am Acad Dermatol. 2001;45(5):S150-7.

EXAMINATION QUESTION

1. Write a short note on topical retinoids.

149 CHAPTER Moisturizers

Dipayan Sengupta

INTRODUCTION

Moisturizers are not only one of the most commonly prescribed medications by dermatologists, but probably one of the best-selling OTC (over-the-counter) products as well.[1] Unfortunately many dermatologists view moisturizers as an adjuvant therapy for most of its indications and often lack the comprehensive knowledge regarding its proper use in different scenarios. In this chapter, we will present a practical overview of different classes of moisturizers and how to use them in practice, individually or in combination.

DIFFERENT TYPES OF MOISTURIZERS

Moisturizers are usually classified in four categories:[1]

1. Occlusives
2. Humectants
3. Emollients
4. Rejuvenators

They have been summarized in **Table 1**.

Additionally, some moisturizers have been described as therapeutic moisturizers which are often combined with different adjuvants to enhance their functions.[2]

Occlusives

Occlusive moisturizers physically form a layer over the skin and reduce transepidermal water loss (TEWL).[3] There are many occlusive agents available, but most important are *petrolatum* and *dimethicone*.

Petrolatum: The most powerful occlusive agent.[3] Other common moisturizers such as mineral oil and liquid paraffin are derived from petrolatum. *Cons*: Greasy feel, can cause occlusive folliculitis so cannot be given over face/acne prone skin, also should be avoided in rosacea and sensitive skin.

Dimethicone: Chemically silicone. *Pros*: It can be used in face, over sensitive skin or rosacea, often combined with sunscreen. *Cons*: It is an occlusive and much weaker compared to the petroleum group.

Others: There are many other groups of occlusives such as fatty acids, fatty alcohols, wax and wax esters, sterols, and some triglycerides. *Lanolin*, a fatty alcohol may cause allergic contact dermatitis (ACD)[4] and contact urticaria. Most occlusives are comedogenic, so caution is to be taken specially before applying over the face.

Best uses of occlusive are:

- When barrier defect is the key pathological event such as atopic dermatitis, xerotic dermatitis (However, in these cases, it should be combined with an emollient that also repairs the physiological defect).
- To protect skin from external allergen/irritants such as hand eczema (occlusive should be applied before work, when gloves cannot be used).

Humectants

Humectants are hygroscopic (attract water) substances and draw water from the environment (in a humid environment). However, they also draw water from epidermis and may actually increase TEWL. To prevent that, they are usually combined with occlusive agents.[5]

Some important humectants with their special properties are mentioned here.

Glycerine: It is by far the most effective humectant available.

Propylene glycol: An alcohol. It may cause irritation/ACD and poisoning in burn patients.

Alpha-hydroxy acids: They are also considered as therapeutic moisturizers. Most notable examples are sodium pyrrolidone carboxylic acid (PCA), hyaluronic acid, and lactic acid. Also the salts of lactic acids (sodium, potassium, and ammonium lactate) are very effective humectants.

Urea: Mostly effective for foot eczema.

Note: Urea (20% and above) and lactic acid may also cause keratolysis and is an ideal choice for hyperkeratotic eczema or other conditions with dryness along with excess keratin.

Best uses for humectants are:

- As a maintenance moisturizer in normal to dry skin (glycerine).
- In keratinizing disorders such as psoriasis and ichthyosis (urea, lactic acid)
- In facial dryness and as a rejuvenator (α-hydroxy acids such as glycolic acid)
- Moisturizer for acne prone skin as mostly they are noncomedogenic. However, some may cause irritation

(propylene glycol, urea, lactic acid, and PCA) and better be avoided in sensitive skin.

Emollients

Emollients are lipid molecules that infiltrate into stratum corneum to repair the defective skin barrier more physiologically (contrasting with mechanical protection of an occlusive). They make the skin soft and smooth so have more cosmetic appeal.[6]

Note: In practice, most occlusive has some function as emollients and vice versa. For example, cetyl alcohol has both properties.

Examples of emollients are essential fatty acids, fatty alcohols, and vegetable oils (palm oil, coconut oil, etc.).

Best uses for emollients are:

- To repair physiological defects (pseudoceramide mimics ceramide, the most important intracellular lipid in stratum corneum), in atopic dermatitis[7] and asteatotic dermatitis.
- Some of them are highly economical to use as long-term maintenance over a large area. *Example*: Pure coconut oil in asteatotic eczema due to old age (*Note*: try to avoid synthetic components in the commercial brands and lean more toward pure form).
- Some of them are noncomedogenic (e.g., cyclomethicone) and mostly devoid of their occlusive property. They can be used for acne and over the face as a cosmetic product (as they make the skin soft and smooth, it adds to the cosmetic appeal).

Rejuvenator

They are mostly small molecular weight proteins[8] (collagen, elastin, and keratin molecules) and used to replenish important proteins in skin. However, contrary to the claims of many commercial products, such added collagen cannot fully compensate for the loss of collagen due to the aging process.

Best use: Photoaged skin, senile dryness of skin, and asteatotic dermatitis. Usually to be combined with other classes of moisturizers.

SOME ADJUVANTS TO MOISTURIZERS

Apart from the major classes of moisturizers described earlier, earlier marketed products often combine various adjuvants, to increase efficacy or stability of the product.[9] Some important classes of adjuvants are mentioned here below:

- *Preservatives*: They are used to prevent bacterial contamination. Some of them like paraben may cause ACD. Phenoxyethanol has least irritant potential among preservatives.
- *Fragrance*: It is used to attract users. Unfortunately, they are the most common cause of ACD with moisturizers.
- *Sunscreen*: TiO_2 and ZnO_2
- *Botanical substances*: Example, aloe and oatmeal
- *Vitamins and antioxidants*: Vitamin A, E, C, and niacin
- Chelating agents such as EDTA
- Emulsifying agents

A PRACTICAL ALGORITHM TO SELECT MOISTURIZER

Primary Agents

- *Face/acne prone skin/sensitive skin*: Humectant or select dimethicone as occlusive. Added sunscreen may be beneficial. Avoid paraben-containing products.
- *Other areas*: An occlusive agent may or may not be combined with a humectant.

Additional Agents

- Where loss of physiological lipid is the primary pathology (atopic dermatitis, asteatotic dermatitis) → emollients specially ceramides.
- Keratinizing disorders → keratolytic moisturizers such as urea, lactic acid
- Senile and photoaged skin, where loss of protein causes skin defects → protein rejuvenators
- Physiological defects that require maintenance rather than active treatment are best targets for emollients (some are very economical especially vegetable oils).

TABLE 1: Summary of different groups of moisturizers (for details, see text).

Name	*Mechanism of action*	*Advantage*	*Disadvantage*	*Example*
Occlusive	Physically form a layer over the skin and reduces TEWL	Most effective in reducing TEWL	May cause occlusive folliculitis	Petrolatum and dimethicone
Humectants	Hygroscopic (attracts water) substances and draw water from environment (in humid environment)	Can be used for maintenance, nonocclusive. Specific functions in special conditions (see text)	Needs to be combined with an occlusive	Glycerine, urea, lactic acid
Emollient	Infiltrates into stratum corneum to repair the defective skin barrier	Makes skin soft and shiny (increases cosmetic appeal)	Not enough for highly compromised barrier defect	Vegetable oils, such as coconut oil
Rejuvenator	Replenish important proteins in skin	Helps to recover physiological functions of skin	Acts only as an adjuvant agent	Collagen, elastin

(TEWL: transepidermal water loss)

Practical tips: There are a huge number of moisturizers available in the market in various combinations. Practitioners should select one or two moisturizers available in his/her practice area for each purpose such as acne [retinoid dermatitis/topical steroid-dependent face (TSDF)], psoriasis, hand eczema, and atopic dermatitis. A good practice is to ask patients to apply a small amount of sample to see if there is any allergy before selecting a product.

KEY POINTS

- Moisturizers are one of the most commonly prescribed agents by dermatologists.
- Moisturizers are classified based on their mechanism of action into four classes.
- Occlusive moisturizers physically form a layer over the skin and reduce transepidermal water loss. Examples of occlusive agents are petrolatum and dimethicone.
- Humectants are hygroscopic agents that draw water from the environment as well as epidermis.
- Emollients are lipid molecules that infiltrate into stratum corneum to repair the defective skin barrier more physiologically.
- Protein rejuvenators are mostly small molecular weight proteins used to replenish important proteins in skin such as collagen.
- Additionally, many agents are combined with moisturizers for various purposes.
- In practice, different moisturizers and their combinations are used in different disorders that dermatologists need to be familiar with.

REFERENCES

1. Sethi A, Kaur T, Malhotra SK, Gambhir ML. Moisturizers: the slippery road. Indian J Dermatol. 2016;61(3):279-87.
2. Draelos ZD. Therapeutic moisturizers. Dermatol Clin. 2000;18(4):597-607.
3. Ghadially R, Halkier-Sorensen L, Elias PM. Effects of petrolatum on stratum corneum structure and function. J Am Acad Dermatol. 1992;26(3):387-96.
4. Miest RY, Yiannias JA, Chang YH, Singh N. Diagnosis and prevalence of lanolin allergy. Dermatitis. 2013;24(3):119-23.
5. Kraft N, Lynde CW. Moisturizers: What they are and a practical approach to product selection. Skin Therapy Lett. 2005;10:1-8.
6. Rawlings AV, Canestrari DA, Dobkowski B. Moisturizer technology versus clinical performance. Dermatol Ther. 2004;17(1):49-56.
7. Chamlin SL, Kao J, Frieden IJ, Sheu MY, Fowler AJ, Fluhr JW, et al. Ceramide-dominant barrier repair lipids alleviate childhood atopic dermatitis: changes in barrier function provide a sensitive indicator of disease activity. J Am Acad Dermatol. 2002;47(2):198-208.
8. Nolan K, Marmur E. Moisturizers: reality and the skin benefits. Dermatol Ther. 2012;25(3):229-33.
9. Sarkar R, Garg S. Moisturizers, 1st edition. New Delhi: Jaypee Brothers Medical Publishers; 2017.

EXAMINATION QUESTIONS

1. Write a short note on different types of moisturizers.
2. Discuss applications of moisturizers in dermatology.

150 CHAPTER Sunscreen

Varsha Vaidyanathan, Aarti Sarda, Abhishek De

INTRODUCTION

Chronic sun exposure can accelerate the aging process and can lead to the development of skin disorders, malignancies, and aggravation of pre-existing dermatoses. Sunscreens are topical agents which either absorb or reflect the sun's ultraviolet (UV) radiation and help protect against the harmful effects of sun exposure. Judicious application of sunscreens helps to mitigate the deleterious effects of sun exposure.

CLASSIFICATION OF SUNSCREENS

Topical Sunscreens

These contain UV filters which scatter and absorb the UV radiation. They may be organic or inorganic. The organic agents act by absorbing the UV rays and getting excited to a higher energy state. Upon return to the ground state, the energy is dissipated in the form of heat. The inorganic agents primarily absorb but also reflect and scatter the UV rays.

Organic Sunscreens[1,2]

Based on the absorption spectrum, they are further classified as UVB, UVA, and mixed filters.

Ultraviolet B filters:

- *Para-aminobenzoic (PABA) derivatives*: These are highly effective, especially padimate O. However, since it stains clothing and is a **(Flowchart 1)** contact allergen, it is no longer used in modern sunscreens.

Flowchart 1: Classification of sunscreens.

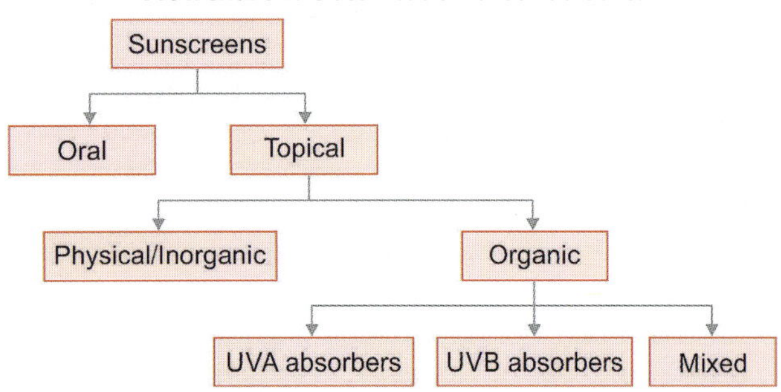

(UVA: ultraviolet A; UVB: ultraviolet B)

- *Benzophenones*: Dioxybenzone (benzophenone-8) is a good UVB filter. Other benzophenones like oxybenzone block both UVA2 and UVB.
- *Salicylates*: Octisalate, homosalate, and trolamine salicylate are weak UVB filters as compared to PABA derivatives and are used in conjunction with other agents. Alone, they are not very effective sunscreens.
- *Cinnamates*: Cinoxate and octinoxate (octyl methoxycinnamate) are powerful UVB filters and have replaced PABA derivatives. Octinoxate can destabilize in the presence of avobenzone (a UVA filter) when used together.
- *Others*:
    - *Octocrylene*: Unlike other UVB filters, octocrylene can stabilize avobenzone and hence is a part of broad-spectrum sunscreens.
    - *Ensulizole (phenylbenzimidazole sulfonic acid)*: Unlike other oil-based sunscreen ingredients, ensulizole is water-based and hence renders the sunscreen lighter, less greasy, and more cosmetically acceptable. It is also photostable.
    - Enzacamene, octyl triazone (Uvinal T), amiloxate, and are some other newer UVB filters which are awaiting Food and Drug Administration (FDA) approval.

Ultraviolet A filters:

- *Avobenzone*: It provides protection against both UVA1 and UVA2. It is photolabile and has a tendency to degrade other sunscreen ingredients, especially octinoxate, when used in combination. Hence, it is combined with octocrylene which can help to stabilize avobenzone, or with non-sunscreen agents like dimethyl 2,6-naphthalate. Sulisobenzone is another UVA filter similar to avobenzone.
- *Ecamsule (terephthalylidene dicamphor sulfonic acid/ Mexoryl SX)*: This is a good UVA absorber and is one of the new FDA approved sunscreen agents.
- Bisdisulizole and diethylamino hydroxybenzoyl hexyl benzoate (Uvinal A) are some other UVA filters awaiting FDA approval.

Mixed/combination filters:

- *Oxybenzone*: It can absorb UVA2 spectrum well along with UVB. As it provides protection against both UVB and short-range UVA, it is considered to be broad-spectrum sunscreen.

- *Meradimate*: Like oxybenzone, this too is effective against both UVA2 and UVB. However, it is weaker and less effective than oxybenzone.
- Other broad-spectrum agents include drometrizole trisiloxane (Mexoryl XL), bemotrizinol (Tinosorb S), and bisoctrizole (Tinosorb M).

Inorganic/Insoluble/Physical Sunscreens

They consist of opaque particles that both absorb and reflect and scatter the UV rays reaching the skin. Inorganic agents include titanium dioxide and zinc oxide. As the application of these agents gave a ghostly-white appearance which was found to be esthetically displeasing, the agents were micronized and nanosized to give a better look. This however resulted in less protection in the UVA range of titanium dioxide. The protection factor of zinc oxide was virtually unchanged.

Oral Sunscreens[3]

- *Fern extract (polypodium leucotomos)*: This has been studied for its utility as an adjunct to topical sunscreens. It contains polyphenolic compounds such as benzoate and cinnamates along with caffeic acid and ferulic acid. Along with photoprotective effects, it also has anti-inflammatory and antioxidant properties. More research is required to judge its effectiveness as an oral sunscreen. It is available in some countries under the trade names Fernblock and Heliocare.
- *Antioxidants*: Although antioxidants such as ascorbate, tocopherol, and beta carotenoids have been used for photoprotection, it is as yet unknown how effective they are.

RATING OF SUNSCREENS

- *UVB rating*:[4]
    - Sun protection factor (SPF) is determined by cutaneous phototesting with artificial sunlight.
    - SPF = minimum erythema dose (MED) of the sunscreen-protected skin (after application of 2 mg/cm^2 of the product)/MED of unprotected skin.
      Example, a sunscreen with SPF 15 would allow 15 times as much sun exposure with the same level of erythema as compared to without the sunscreen in the same individual.
    - SPF 15 provides 94% protection from UVB whereas SPF 30 provides more than 97% protection.
    - SPF categorization is as follows:
        - *Low protection:* 2–6
        - *Medium:* 8–12
        - *High:* 15–25
        - *Very high:* 30–50
        - *Ultra:* 50+
    - In general practice, SPF of 30+ is recommended.
- *UVA rating*:[5] There are no internationally accepted standards for UVA rating. Various in vivo and in vitro tests are used including immediate pigment darkening (IPD), persistent pigment darkening (PPD), and critical wavelength (CW). For CW, the sunscreen is dissolved in a solvent and a spectrophotometer is used to determine the absorption spectrum. CW is the wavelength at which the cumulative absorption of radiation above 290 nm is 90%. FDA mandates that in order for a sunscreen to be classified a broad-spectrum, the CW must be at least 370 nm.
- *PA rating*: Protection grade of UVA is a methodology initially established in Japan in 1996 and has now been accepted in some non-Asian countries as well. It is based on PPD. The rating is as follows:

PA+	some UVA protection	PPD 2–4
PA++	moderate	4–8
PA+++	high	8–16
PA++++	extremely high	>16

- *Boots star rating*: It measures the percentage of UVA absorbed as compared to UVB. It gives an indication of how broad spectrum a sunscreen is. The closer the ratio of UVA/UVB is to 1, the higher the Boots star rating and hence more broad spectrum the sunscreen is.

SUBSTANTIVITY

This determines how well the sunscreen adheres to the skin, especially after contact with water. Depending upon this adherence property, sunscreens can be:

- *Water-resistant*: Retain their SPF after 40 minutes of water exposure.
- *Water-proof*: Retain their SPF after 80 minutes of water exposure.

SUNSCREEN VEHICLES[6]

Sunscreens are available in the following forms:

- *Emulsions*: Most effective UV absorbers are oils so they are incorporated into the oil phase of the emulsion (creams and lotions). Higher the SPF, greater is the oil content leading to a greasy and heavy feel. In order to lighten the feel, silica is used to make "ultrasheer" sunscreens.
- *Gels*: Water-soluble sunscreen ingredients such as ensulizole and trolamine salicylate can be made into gel formulations. Although they are lighter, they are easily washed away by sweating or swimming. They are of utility in those with oily and acne-prone skin.
- *Sprays*: These are convenient however there is a potential for less protection if applied in a patchy and uneven manner. Overall, it is less effective as compared to other vehicles.

- *Sunscreen sticks*: These are used for special areas such as nose, lips, and eyes.
- *Cosmetics*: Most of the recent foundations contain some amount of sunscreen (SPF 15). These are esthetically pleasing and provide better compliance among women. However, as the SPF is still relatively low, cosmetics alone cannot be relied upon for complete photoprotection.

INSTRUCTIONS FOR SUNSCREEN USE

- Sunscreens should be used in all weather and not just in the summers.
- Sunscreen usage must be diligent between the hours of 10 AM and 4 PM.
- Sunscreen should be applied 30 minutes before any anticipated sun exposure and reapplied every 2–3 hours.
- Water-resistant or water-proof sunscreens should be used during swimming.
- For prolonged sun exposure, a broad-spectrum sunscreen of SPF 30 and above is recommended.
- 25–50 mL of sunscreen is required during one application for adequate protection for the body. In practical terms, two to three tablespoons of sunscreen for the entire body and one to two teaspoons for the face and neck is recommended.[6] If using a spray, it should be used liberally without any patchy areas.
- Umbrellas, hats, sunglasses, and tightly woven clothing should be used as additional shields along with sunscreens.

ADVERSE EFFECTS OF SUNSCREENS

- Irritant contact dermatitis
- Allergic contact dermatitis
- Stinging sensation in the eyes
- Folliculitis
- Can induce or worsen acne
- Some compounds may act as photoallergens.

SUNSCREEN USE IN SPECIAL POPULATIONS[7]

- *Children*: Sunscreens are not recommended in children less than 6 months of age. For toddlers and slightly older children, adequate application of physical sunscreen is used. In school-age children, the American Academy of Dermatology recommends application of a broad-spectrum sunscreen every 2 hours.[8]
- *Pregnant women*: Physical sunscreens are recommended.
- *Patients with photosensitive conditions*: Patients with lentigines, melasma, polymorphous light eruption, etc., need more UVA, especially UVA1 protection. They should be prescribed sunscreens containing avobenzone, ecamsule, or physical sunscreens.
- *Patients with sunscreen intolerance*: Patients with allergic reactions, urticaria, and stinging eyes should be offered physical sunscreens.
- *Patients with acne-prone oily skin*: Oil-free and gel-based sunscreens are ideal in such situations.

CHARACTERISTICS OF AN IDEAL SUNSCREEN

- Broad-spectrum coverage (ability to block both UVA and UVB)
- Nonirritant
- Inexpensive
- Water-resistant
- Cosmetically pleasing
- Safe for both humans and the environment.

CONCLUSION

Sunscreens are a key weapon in a dermatologist's arsenal. A thorough understanding of sunscreens with their uses and limitations is essential so that the appropriate sunscreen can be offered to the patients based on their requirements.

KEY POINTS

- Sunscreens are topical agents which either absorb or reflect the sun's UV radiation and help protect against the harmful effects of sun exposure.
- Organic agents absorb the UV rays and dissipate it in the form of heat. Inorganic agents scatter and reflect the rays along with absorption.
- UVB filters include PABA derivatives, benzophenones, salicylates, cinnamates, and others such as octocrylene and ensulizole.
- UVA filters include avobenzone and ecamsule.
- Broad-spectrum sunscreens are those which are effective against both UVA and UVB.
- Physical sunscreens are titanium dioxide and zinc oxide. They are of use in children, pregnant women, and those that are allergic to the organic sunscreens.
- UVB sunscreens are rated by SPF while UVA sunscreens are rated by CW, IPD, and PPD.
- Water-resistant sunscreens retain SPF after 40 minutes of water immersion while water-proof sunscreens retain their SPF after 80 minutes of water immersion.

REFERENCES

1. Mancuso JB, Maruthi R, Wang SQ, Lim HW. Sunscreens: an update. Am J Clin Dermatol. 2017;18(5):643-50.
2. DeLeo VA. Sunscreens and photoprotection. In: Bolognia JL, Schaffer JV, Cerroni L (Eds). Dermatology, 4th edition. Philadelphia: Elsevier; 2018. pp. 2310-17.
3. El-Haj N, Goldstein N. Sunprotection in a Pill: the photoprotective effects of *Polypodium lecotomos*. Int J Dermatol. 2015;54(3):362-6.

4. Khanna N, Sugandhan S. Photodermatology and photodermatoses. In: Valia RG, Valia AR (Eds). IADVL Textbook of Dermatology, 3rd edition. New Delhi: Bhalani Publishing House; 2008. pp. 614-41.
5. Diffey BL, Tanner PR, Matts PJ, Nash JF. In vitro assessment of the broad-spectrum ultraviolet protection of sunscreen products. J Am Acad Dermatol. 2000;43:1024-35.
6. Li H, Colantonio S, Dawson A, Lin X, Beecker J. Sunscreen application, safety, and Sun protection: the evidence. J Cutan Med Surg. 2019;23(4):357-69.
7. Mori S, Wang SQ. Sunscreens. In: Wolverton SE (Ed). Comprehensive Dermatologic Drug Therapy, 4th edition. Philadelphia: Elsevier; 2021. pp. 565-75.
8. Julian E, Palestro AM, Thomas JA. Pediatric sunscreen and Sun safety guidelines. Clin Pediatr (Phila). 2015;54(12):1133-40.

EXAMINATION QUESTION

1. Classify sunscreens with a short note on broad-spectrum sunscreens.

151 CHAPTER

Miscellaneous Topical Therapy

D Dinesh Kumar, Anoosha P

INTRODUCTION

Topical therapy has always been an integral part of a dermatologist's prescription due to the advantage of direct drug delivery to the affected area with minimal systemic effects.

This chapter entails to cover the following among topical therapies:

- Keratolytics agents
- Skin-lightening agents
- Antipruritic agents
- Topical anesthetics
- Topical antivirals
- Shampoos and conditioners

KERATOLYTIC AGENTS[1-4]

Keratolytic agents act by reducing the thickness of stratum corneum by means of eliminating the corneocytes, thereby being particularly beneficial in hyperkeratotic disorders characterized by either accelerated epidermal proliferation or reduced desquamation.

Salicylic Acid

Salicylic acid is derived from the bark of the willow tree *Salix alba*. It is a β-hydroxy acid with a wide variety of uses in dermatology. Topical salicylic acid is available as creams, lotions, ointments, gels, foams, solutions, shampoos, cleansers, pads, and plasters.

Salicylic acid acts on the desmosomal elements and reduces the cell-to-cell adhesion among the corneocytes, although it may also have antimicrobial and mild anti-inflammatory effects **(Table 1)**. They are commonly co-prescribed with other topical medications as it enhances their penetration.

Irritation, peeling, and sometimes even erosions can occur based on the concentration and site of application.

TABLE 1: Uses of topical salicylic acid based on its concentration.

Concentration of topical salicylic acid	*Uses*
0.5–2%	Acne (comedolytic)
1–6%	Hyperkeratotic dermatosis (psoriasis and ichthyosis)
10–40%	Warts, corns, and calluses

Allergic contact dermatitis is uncommon but has been described. Salicylism is a complication, which can occur due to systemic absorption, when salicylic acid is applied over extensive areas, particularly in neonates and infants and presents with gastrointestinal and neurologic toxicity. Salicylic acid is pregnancy category C and premature closure of the ductus arteriosus in the fetus has been reported with extensive use in late pregnancy.

Urea

At lower concentrations (10–25%), topical urea acts as a humectant and mild keratolytic agent, while it is a hygroscopic keratolyic at higher concentrations (40–50%). Topical urea is available as creams, lotions, gels, solutions, and foams.

Urea is a hygroscopic agent and hence increases the water-binding capacity of desmosomal proteins. It absorbs water from the atmosphere and enhances barrier function by decreasing transepidermal water loss. By increasing the skin hydration, it helps in reducing the effect of topical irritants on the skin. In the process of water absorption, urea causes mechanical alteration in the intercellular connections thereby leading to desquamation.

Generally, well tolerated, may rarely cause irritation or burning sensation at sites of application, especially on inflamed or eroded/fissured skin. Urea is pregnancy category B.

Alpha-hydroxy Acids

Alpha-hydroxy acids (AHAs) include glycolic, lactic, mandelic, tartaric, malic, and citric acids. Glycolic and lactic acids are most commonly used in dermatology. These are available as cleansers, shampoos, lotions, creams, gels, masks, and peeling agents in various concentrations. AHAs are used in the management of ichthyoses, xerosis, acne vulgaris, rosacea, and photoaging.

Alpha-hydroxy acids act by decreasing the strength of intercellular bonding, thereby weakening corneocyte cohesion and leading to exfoliation. They tend to have an effect on the lower newly forming keratinocytes in contrast to the other keratolytics, which tend to affect the layers of stratum corner predominantly. Higher concentrations of AHAs may have dermal addition to the epidermal effects.

They are generally well tolerated, but can cause irritation and/or burning when used over inflamed or fissured skin.

Propylene Glycol

Propylene glycol commonly used as a preservative and a penetration enhancer, acts as a keratolytic agent at a concentration of 10–20%. Irritation occurs at higher concentrations.

SKIN-LIGHTENING AGENTS[5-7]

Kojic Acid

Kojic acid is a tyrosinase inhibitor in melanin synthesis as it chelates the copper ions. It has only a moderate benefit when used alone and hence is usually combined with other agents in topical formulations. Used in 1–4% concentrations, it can cause contact dermatitis, stinging, and erythema.[5]

Arbutin

Although a natural derivative of hydroquinone, arbutin is less cytotoxic than it on melanocytes. Sources of arbutin include cranberries, blueberries, bearberry leaves, wheat, and pear skin. It acts by inhibiting tyrosinase and melanosome maturation. There is a risk of paradoxical hyperpigmentation when used in higher concentrations. It is generally used in combination with other agents.

Ascorbic Acid

Ascorbic acid acts by reducing dopaquinone to dihydroxyphenylalanine (DOPA) and also inhibits tyrosinase thus interfering with melanogenesis. Its unstable nature is one its major disadvantages. It may cause a stinging or burning sensation when applied on skin sometimes.[6]

Hydroquinone

Hydroquinone (1,4-dihydroxybenzene) is a skin-lightening agent commonly used along with other topical agents such as tretinoin and steroid for treating melasma and other pigmentary disorders. Available in concentrations of 2%, 3%, and 4% as creams, gels, and solutions.

Hydroquinone acts by interfering with the melanin synthesis by inhibiting the conversion of tyrosine to DOPA. Thereby it reduces the melanosome production and also reduces the transfer of melanin to keratinocytes by production of highly reactive oxygen radicals.

They can cause allergic contact dermatitis. Prolonged usage in high concentration can cause exogenous ochronosis. Hydroquinone is pregnancy category C.

Monobenzyl Ether of Hydroquinone

In cases of extensive vitiligo, in order to attain a uniform appearance, monobenzyl ether of hydroquinone (MBEH) is infrequently used to depigment remaining normal skin. MBEH acts by competitive inhibition of tyrosinase enzyme and free-radical-mediated damage of melanocytes. Irritant and allergic contact dermatitis represents possible side effects.

Mequinol

Mequinol (4-hydroxyanisole) is a competitive inhibitor of melanin biosynthesis. A combination of mequinol 2% and tretinoin 0.01% is Food and Drug Administration (FDA)-approved for the treatment of solar lentigines. The mequinol–tretinoin combination product is pregnancy category X.

Liquorice

Commonly used in Chinese medicine, liquorice extracts contain a component called glabridin, which mediates its effect on epidermal skin pigmentation by decreasing tyrosinase activity as well as by limiting the ultraviolet B (UVB)-induced skin damage. They may cause skin irritation, which usually subsides on discontinuation.

Retinoids

Retinoids function in several ways as skin lightening agents. They induce an accelerated epidermal turnover and cause desquamation of corneocytes by reducing the intercellular cohesions. They also cause dispersion of keratinocyte pigment granules and interference with pigment transfer to keratinocytes. Retinoic acid (0.05% and 0.1%), adapalene (0.1%), and tazarotene all have use in skin lightening and antiaging topical preparations.

Azelaic Acid

Azelaic acid was thought to act by competitive inhibition of tyrosinase, but however has been found to be a free radical scavenger. It has been found to be predominantly active on malignant or hyperactive melanocytes with very little or no action on normal melanocytes. Hence, it may arrest the progression or even cause disappearance of melanoma in lentigo maligna. It is moderately effective as a depigmenting agent in melasma and postinflammatory hyperpigmentation. It has been approved for use in rosacea more due to its antioxidant effect. Azelaic acid may cause burning, stinging and itching over application sites although it has an overall good safety profile.

Niacinamide

Topical niacinamide causes dose-dependent reversible decrease in hyperpigmentation by inhibiting the melanosome transfer from melanocytes to keratinocytes without affecting tyrosinase activity, melanin production, melanocyte number, or cell viability.

ANTIPRURITIC AGENTS[8]

The "itch" pathway includes both central as well as peripheral receptors and nerve fibers. The most effective way to reduce

TABLE 2: Topical antipruritic agents.

Agent	*Mechanism of action*	*Uses*	*Side effects*
Camphor (0.25–0.5%)	Local anesthetic effect	Mild pruritus	Irritation when used over inflamed skin
Capsaicin (0.025–0.075% cream, gel, lotion, and 8% patch)	Depresses the synthesis, storage, transfer, and release of substance P	Localized chronic pruritus, dialysis-related pruritus, and brachioradial pruritus	Transient burning sensation
Doxepin (5% cream)	Antihistamine (H1 and H2) Anticholinergic effect	Pruritus in atopic dermatitis	Drowsiness and allergic contact dermatitis
Diphenhydramine (2% cream, lotion, gel, and spray)	Antihistamine (H1) Local anesthetic effect	Not recommended due to poor antipruritic effect	Allergic contact dermatitis
Calamine lotion		Acute and subacute dermatitis	
Menthol (up to 16% cream and gel)	Activation TRPM8 on C fibers, producing a cooling sensation	Patients in whom itch is relieved by cold showers	Irritation
Pramoxine (1% gel and lotion)	Anesthetic effect	Histamine-induced itch and uremic pruritus	Allergic contact dermatitis
Phenol	Acts directly on cold receptors	Used in throat sprays	Irritation; contraindicated in pregnancy
Tacrolimus/pimecrolimus	Calcineurin inhibitors which block proinflammatory cytokines	Pruritus in atopic dermatitis	Transient burning sensation
Barrier repair creams	Decrease TEWL and form a physical barrier to the exposure to irritants	Pruritus in atopic dermatitis	None

(TEWL: transepidermal water loss; TRPM8: transient receptor potential cation channel subfamily M member 8)

pruritus involves treatment of the underlying dermatologic or systemic condition. Antipruritic agents act by several mechanisms such as substituting a different sensation for itching, anesthetizing cutaneous nerve endings, and blocking molecular mediators of pruritus **(Table 2)**.

TOPICAL ANESTHETICS[9]

Topical anesthetic agents play an important role in decreasing the pain associated with superficial dermatological, esthetic, and laser procedures. Topical anesthetics may also be administered for postherpetic neuralgia and painful ulcers. Ensuring the cleansing of treatment sites is important as skin contaminants and other topical medications can alter absorption and effectiveness. These agents act by reversibly blocking the free nerve endings near the site of application thereby temporarily producing loss of sensation over a limited area.

Eutectic Mixture of Lidocaine and Prilocaine

Eutectic mixture of local anesthetics (EMLA) is a eutectic mixture of lidocaine (2.5%) and prilocaine (2.5%), both sodium channel-blocking amide anesthetics. For maximal benefit, it is typically applied under occlusion 1 to 1.5 hours prior to a procedure. Transient blanching or erythema at the application site, burning, and irritation may be its side effects. The prilocaine component is most often responsible for contact urticaria or allergic contact dermatitis. Systemic exposure can occur when applied over a large surface area, especially in infants and children and methemoglobinemia represents a potential complication. Hence, should be used with caution in the younger age group and avoided in those with glucose-6-phosphate dehydrogenase (G6PD) deficiency.

Lidocaine

Lidocaine (4% or 5%) cream is often used for 30–60 minutes with or without occlusion to attain cutaneous anesthesia. Again, it should be used with caution when applying over large surface areas.

Benzocaine

Topical benzocaine is an ester anesthetic that is found in a variety of over-the-counter topical preparations used for temporary amelioration of pain on the skin and mucous membranes. It is a potent contact sensitizer.

TOPICAL ANTIVIRALS[10]

Antivirals available for topical usage include acyclovir, penciclovir, and docosanol available as creams in varying concentrations. Acyclovir is found to decrease the viral shedding in genital herpes when used for the first episode. It is sometimes used in combination with hydrocortisone in orolabial herpes in order to shorten the healing time **(Table 3)**.

Penciclovir has been found to be effective in treating infections caused by herpes simplex virus 1 (HSV-1), herpes simplex virus 2 (HSV-2), varicella-zoster virus (VZV), and Epstein–Barr virus (EBV). Penciclovir as well as docosanol are indicated in recurrent orolabial herpes infections.

SHAMPOOS AND CONDITIONERS[11,12]

Hair Shampoos

Shampoos are cleansing agents formulated to remove sweat, sebum, squames, dirt, and styling products from scalp and hair. They contain several additives, which include foaming agents, detergents, sequestering agents, conditioners, fragrances, and preservatives in varying combinations. Based on their chemical composition, shampoos can be classified as anionics, cationics, nonionics, amphoterics, and natural surfactants **(Table 4)**.

Shampoos contain higher concentration of sequestering agents, which are needed to chelate calcium and magnesium ions, in order to prevent the formation of insoluble salts known as soap scum, thus distinguishing them from bar soaps.

TABLE 3: Topical antiviral agents.

Antiviral	*Dose and uses*	*Side effects*
Acyclovir (5% cream and ointment)	Six times/day for 1 week	Burning, stinging, erythema, and itching
Penciclovir (1% cream)	Six times/day for 4 days	Burning, stinging, erythema, headache, and dysgeusia
Docosanol (10% cream)	Five times/day until the episode is resolved	Burning, pruritus, xerosis, erythema, edema, and acne

TABLE 4: Chemical classification of shampoos.

Surfactant type	*Characteristics*	*Result on hair*
Anionics	Deep cleansers	Hair may be rough
Cationics	Poor cleansers	Hair is soft and manageable
Nonionics	Very mild cleansers	Improves manageability
Amphoterics	Mild cleansers	Easy on eyes and improves manageability
Natural surfactants	Poor cleansers	Hair may be dry if product is overused

TABLE 5: Types of conditioners.

Type	*Method of usage*
Instant	Apply after shampoo and then rinse
Deep	Apply for 20–30 minutes before shampoo and then rinse
Leave on	Apply after towel drying the hair
Rinse off	Apply after shampoo, leave on for 2–3 minutes and then rinse off

Hair Conditioners

In the process of cleansing, when shampoos tend to remove too much of the sebum from scalp and hair, the hair tends to become dry, rough, and difficult to comb or manage. This is where conditioners have a role. Conditioners function to restore the sheen, increase the strength, and repair the degradation of hair protein, thereby reversing the overall damage to the hair. There are different types of conditioners based on their method of usage **(Table 5)**.

KEY POINTS

- Topical therapies deliver the drug to the desired site of action with minimal systemic absorption.
- This chapter covers topical agents, which not discussed much and are generally used in combination but nevertheless play an important role in dermatological topical therapy.
- These agents cover a wide variety of indications and it is essential to know their mechanism of action and also their adverse event profile.

REFERENCES

1. Lin AN, Nakatsui T. Salicylic acid revisited. Int J Dermatol. 1998;37:335-42.
2. Imayama S, Ueda S, Isoda M. Histologic changes in the skin of hairless mice following peeling with salicylic acid. Arch Dermatol. 2000;136:1390-5.
3. Van Scott EJ, Yu RJ. Control of keratinization with alpha-hydroxy acids and related compounds. I. Topical treatment of ichthyotic disorders. Arch Dermatol. 1974;110:586-90.
4. Smith WP. Epidermal and dermal effects of topical lactic acid. J Am Acad Dermatol. 1996;35(3 Pt 1):388-91.
5. Dogra S, Kanwar AJ, Parsad D. Adapalene in the treatment of melasma: a preliminary report. J Dermatol. 2002;29:539-40.
6. Solano F, Briganti S, Picardo M, Ghanem G. Hypopigmenting agents: an updated review on biological, chemical and clinical aspects. Pigment Cell Res. 2006;19:550-71.
7. Hakozaki T, Minwalla L, Zhuang J, Chhoa M, Matsubara A, Miyamoto K, et al. The effect of niacinamide on reducing cutaneous pigmentation and suppression of melanosome transfer. Br J Dermatol. 2002;147:20-31.
8. Hercogova J. Topical anti-itch therapy. Dermatol Ther. 2005; 18:341-3.
9. Railan D, Alster TS. Use of topical lidocaine for cosmetic dermatologic procedures. J Drugs Dermatol. 2007;6:1104-8.
10. Loveless M, Sacks SL, Harris JRW. Famciclovir in the management of first-episode genital herpes. Infect Dis Clin Pract. 1997;6:S12-16.
11. Garcia ML, Epps JA, Yare RS, Hunter LD. Normal cuticle-wear patterns in human hair. J Soc Cosmet Chem. 1978;29:155-75.
12. Corbett JF. Hair conditioning. Cutis. 1979;23:405-13.

EXAMINATION QUESTIONS

Write short notes on the following:

1. Tacrolimus.
2. Pimecrolimus.
3. Topical demelanizing agents.

152 CHAPTER Systemic Corticosteroids

Aayushi Mohan, Aarti Sarda, Abhishek De

INTRODUCTION

Since the discovery of steroid by Philip Hench and Edward Kendall in 1935, steroids have served a wide range of uses. Initially, these isolates from adrenal glands were thought to be useful only in patients suffering from Addison disease.[1] Corticosteroids (CSs) have numerous applications in treating inflammation and diseases of immune function based on their significant anti-inflammatory and immunosuppressive effects.[2]

PHARMACOLOGY

Structure

Corticosteroids being synthesized from cholesterol, their basic structure consist of three hexane rings and 1 pentane ring, also known as cyclopentanoperhydrophenanthrene nucleus. All steroidal CSs are variations of this basic structure and require an 11-hydroxyl group. The positions of this group differentiate the potency, half-life, metabolism, and effects of the drug.[3,4]

Figures 1 and 2 present structures of hydrocortisone, prednisone, prednisolone, and methylprednisolone. **Table 1** represents classification of different corticosteroids according to potency, half life and duration of action.

ABSORPTION AND DISTRIBUTION

- Exogenous CS absorbed in upper jejunum.
- The two carrier proteins of glucocorticoids in plasma are:
  - *Cortisol-binding globulin (CBG)/transcortin*:
    - Low capacity and high affinity
    - About 80–90% endogenous CS bound to CBG and the free fraction represent active form.[5,6]

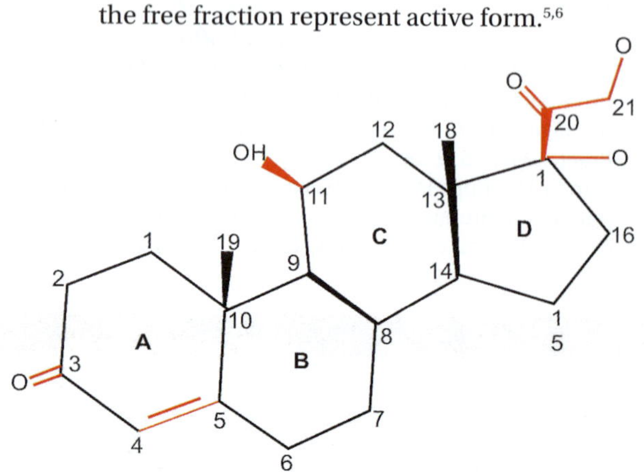

Fig. 1: Structure of hydrocortisone.

  - *Albumin*:
    - Low affinity and high capacity
    - Binds excess exogenous CS, but still most of them remain free (as affinity of exogenous CS < endogenous CS)
- ↓*CBG; increased CS fraction:*
  - Hypothyroidism
  - Liver disease
  - Renal disease
  - Obesity
- ↑*CBG; decreased CS fraction:*
  - Estrogen therapy
  - Pregnancy
  - Hyperthyroidism.

All CS are widely distributed to most body tissues even in fetal tissue except prednisolone.

METABOLISM AND EXCRETION

- All CS can be metabolized by liver to produce inactive substance.
- 3-ketone substituent → 3-hydroxyl substituent → conjugated with sulfate or glucuronic acid → water-soluble metabolite formed, which is excreted by kidney.[7]
- In case of CS, plasma half-life is a poor indicator of duration of action (biologic activity) of drug. So, the better indicator is the period of suppression of adrenocorticotropic hormone (ACTH) secretion from pituitary gland after single administration of glucocorticoid. This duration of activity correlates well with glucocorticoid and anti-inflammatory effects. There is an inverse correlation between duration of action and the relative mineralocorticoid (MC) effect of various CS.

MECHANISM OF ACTION OF EXOGENOUS CORTICOSTEROID AT MOLECULAR LEVEL

Normal Hypothalamic–Pituitary–Adrenal Axis Function

It is important to understand the normal hypothalamic-pituitary-adrenal (HPA) axis to better understand the effect of its suppression by synthetic CS **(Fig. 3)**.[7]

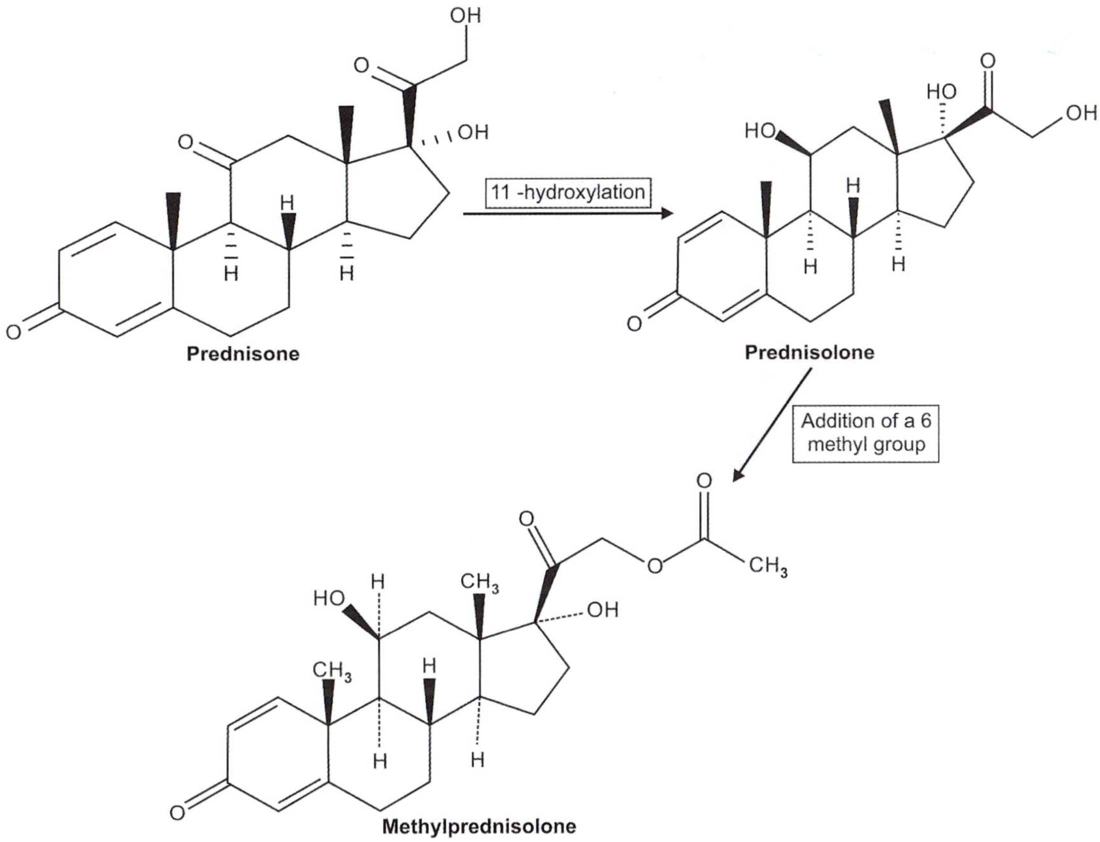

Fig. 2: Structures of prednisone, prednisolone, and methylprednisolone.

TABLE 1: Classification of corticosteroids.

	Equivalent GC dose (mg)	*GC potency (relative)*	*Mineralocorticoid potency (relative)*	*Duration of action (hours)**	*Plasma half-life (minutes)*
Short-acting					
Cortisone	25	0.8	1.0	8–12	60
Hydrocortisone	20	1	0.8	8–12	90
Intermediate-acting					
Prednisone	5	4	0.25	24–36	69
Prednisolone	5	4	0.25	24–36	200
Methylprednisolone	4	5	0	24–36	180
Triamcinolone	4	5	0	24–36	300
Long-acting					
Dexamethasone	0.75	25–30	0	36–54	200
Betamethasone	0.6	30–35	0	36–54	200

* Differs with intramuscular injection.
(GC: glucocorticoid)

Glucocorticoid and Mineralocorticoid Effects

Table 2 depicts glucocorticoid and mineralocorticoid effects.

Immunosuppressive and Anti-inflammatory Effects[8,9]

Figure 4 shows immunosuppressive and anti-inflammatory effects.

Vascular Effects

- Angiogenesis in wound healing
- Vasoconstriction
- Increased fragility of vascular smooth muscle.

CLINICAL INDICATIONS

- *Bullous dermatoses*:
  - Pemphigus vulgaris

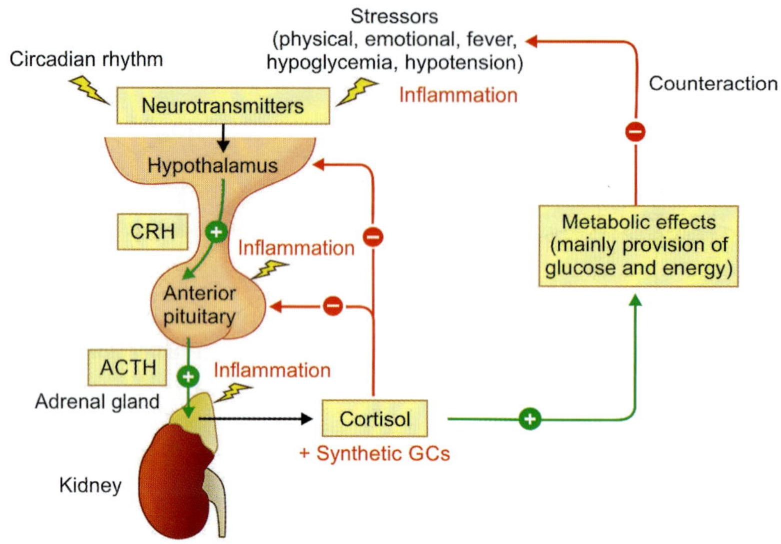

Fig. 3: Hypothalamic–pituitary–adrenal axis.
(ACTH: adrenocorticotropic hormone; CRH: corticotropin-releasing hormone; GCs: glucocorticoids)

TABLE 2: Glucocorticoid (GC) and mineralocorticoid (MC) effects.

GC effects	*MC effects*
Gluconeogenesis by protein catabolism	Sodium and water retention
Increases insulin resistance	Increase potassium excretion
Glycogen storage in liver	
Lipolysis and release of triglycerides	

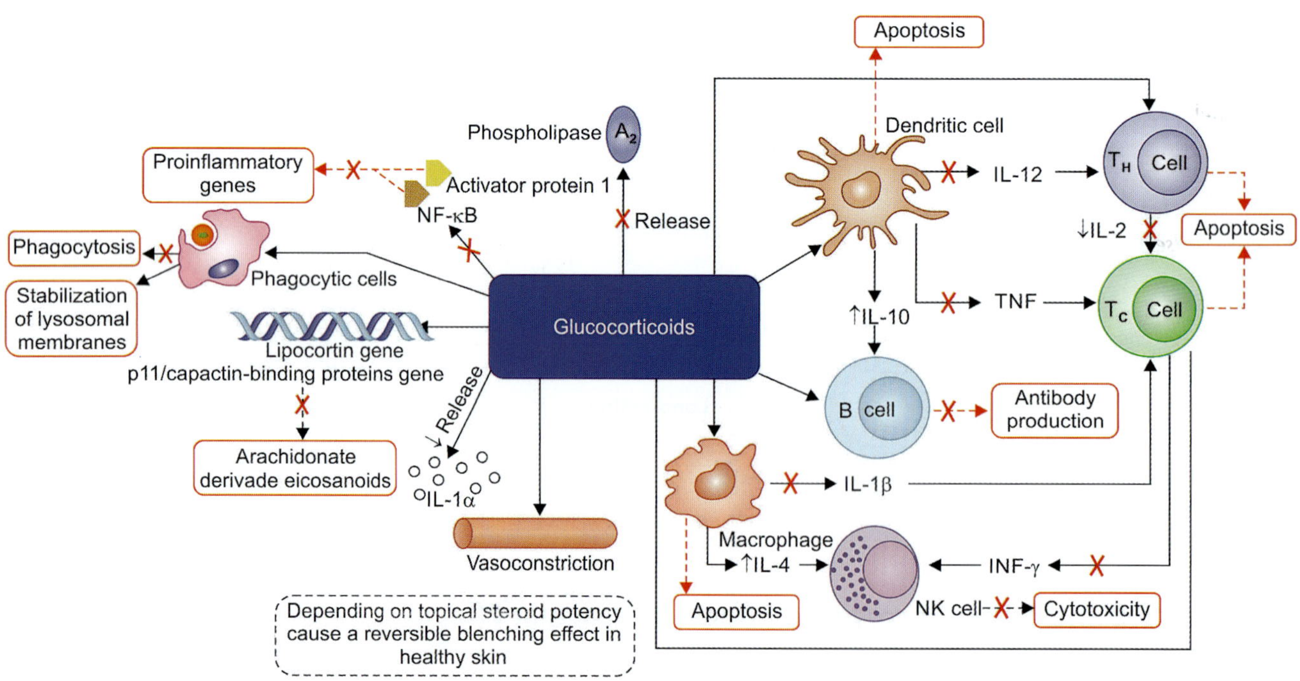

Fig. 4: Immunosuppressive and anti-inflammatory effects of corticosteroids.
(IL: interleukin; INF-γ: interferon-γ; NK: natural killer; TNF: tumor necrosis factor)

- Bullous pemphigoid
- Cicatricial pemphigoid
- Herpes gestationis
- Epidermolysis bullosa acquisita
- Linear immunoglobulin A (IgA) bullous dermatosis
- Erythema multiforme

- *Autoimmune connective tissue disease*:
    - Lupus erythematosus
    - Dermatomyositis
- *Vasculitis*:
    - Cutaneous
    - Systemic
- *Neutrophilic dermatosis*:
    - Pyoderma gangrenosum
    - Behçet's disease
    - Sweet syndrome
- *Severe dermatitis*:
    - Contact dermatitis
    - Atopic dermatitis
    - Photodermatitis
    - Exfoliative erythroderma
- *Others*:
    - Sarcoidosis
    - Severe urticaria
    - Postherpetic neuralgia prevention.

MODE OF ADMINISTRATION

- Short-term oral therapy
- Long-term oral therapy
- *Intramuscular (IM)*: Given as a supervised dose for acute dermatosis. In IM route, betamethasone and dexamethasone duration of action is first week; while triamcinolone is long acting (duration of action—3 weeks).
- Intravenous (IV)
- Intralesional (like triamcinolone in keloid and alopecia areata)
- *Pulse IV CS administration*: Used in life-threatening conditions and for rapid relief.
    - *IV pulse therapy*: Methylprednisolone given in dose of 0.5–1 g over in 5% dextrose over 2 hours for 5 days followed by oral maintenance therapy.

DEXAMETHASONE-CYCLOPHOSPHAMIDE PULSE THERAPY

The introduction of dexamethasone-cyclophosphamide pulse (DCP) therapy for the pemphigus group of disorders by Pasricha et al. in 1981 has revolutionized the therapy of pemphigus.[10]

The entire treatment was divided into four phases:

1. *Phase I*: DCP therapy was given in the presence of signs and symptoms. Patients received monthly doses of 100 mg of dexamethasone dissolved in 500 mL of 5% dextrose by slow IV infusion over 2 hours on 3 consecutive days along with 500 mg of cyclophosphamide in the infusion on day 2. In between, the patients received 50 mg of oral cyclophosphamide daily.
2. *Phase II*: Patients were in remission but monthly DCP therapy and daily oral cyclophosphamide were continued for 9 months.
3. *Phase III*: Only oral cyclophosphamide 50 mg was given to patients for an additional 9 months.
4. *Phase IV*: All treatments were withdrawn and patients were followed up for relapse.

Monitoring for pulse IV methylprednisolone therapy:

- Cardiac monitoring—blood pressure (BP) and pulse
- Daily electrolyte levels
- Daily glucose levels
- Baseline investigations.

CONTRAINDICATIONS

- *Absolute*:
    - Systemic fungal infection
    - Herpes simplex keratitis
    - Hypersensitivity
    - Active tuberculosis (TB)
- *Relative*:
    - *Cardiovascular system (CVS):* Hypertension and congestive heart failure (CHF)
    - *Central nervous system (CNS):* History of psychosis and severe depression
    - *Gastrointestinal (GI):* Active peptic ulcer disease (PUD) and recent anastomosis
    - *Metabolic:* Diabetes mellitus
    - *Musculoskeletal:* Osteoporosis
    - *Ocular:* Cataracts and glaucoma
    - Pregnancy.

ADVERSE EFFECTS[11]

- *Due to short-term therapy*:
    - Psychiatric—mood changes, anxiety, and insomnia
    - GI symptoms—GI intolerance
    - Metabolic—hyperglycemia, fluid/sodium retention, increased appetite, and weight gain
- Based on long-term therapy, the adverse effects are given in **Table 3**.
- Opportunistic infection—caused by multidrug immunosuppressives; alternate morning therapy should be used
- Opportunistic malignancy—CS in transplant patients; malignancy such as Kaposi's sarcoma and non-Hodgkin's lymphoma
- *Corticosteroids in pregnancy:*
    - Pregnancy category C
    - Cleft lip and palate in animal studies
    - Fetal HPA axis suppression
    - Benefit risk ratio to be assessed.

TABLE 3: Adverse effects due to long-term therapy.

Category	*Adverse effect*	*Risk factor*	*Mechanism of action*	*Prevention and management*
HPA axis	Adrenal crisis—hypoglycemia and HTN	Stress, surgery, and trauma	Abrupt cessation of CS after prolonged high dose	IV hydrocortisone (night before surgery and every 8 hours)
	Withdrawal syndrome—lethargy, myalgia, mood disorder, anorexia		Rapid tapering after prolonged high dose	Rise dose to initial level and slow tapering
GI effects	Bowel perforation, peptic ulcer, pancreatitis—mild pain to severe abdominal pain	• Recent bowel anastomosis • Use of NSAIDs/smoking alcohol • History of PUD	• ↓Mucus production • ↓Wound healing	• H_2 receptor antagonist and PPI • Prompt surgical referral
Musculo-skeletal	Myopathy—proximal muscle weakness	Lack of exercise	• Increase protein catabolism • Decrease glucose and amino acid uptake	• Exercise • Correct tapering • Alternate morning therapy
	• Osteoporosis • Osteonecrosis	• Age >50 years • Postmenopausal women • Trauma • Smoking • Hypercoagulability	• Decrease osteoblast and increase osteoclast activity • Decrease serum calcium and increase PTH	• DEXA scan every 1–3 years • Oral bisphosphonate • Teriparatide • HRT
	Growth retardation	Early puberty	Decrease GH, IGF-1, protein, and collagen	Alternate morning therapy
Metabolic	• Hyperglycemia hyperlipidemia • Cushingoid changes	• DM, HTN, and hypothyroidism • Elderly • Family history of hyperlipidemia	Increase gluconeogenesis, lipoprotein lipase, and insulin resistance	Monitor glucose, exercise, and low calorie intake
CVS	CHF and HTN	Elderly	Sodium retention, vasoconstriction, and fluid overload	• CS with least MC effect • Diuretics • Alternate morning therapy
CNS	Pseudotumor cerebri	Headache and nausea vomiting	Rapid tapering	Gradual tapering
Psychiatric	Depression and psychosis	History of psychiatric disorder	Electrolyte imbalance	Atypical antipsychotics
Ocular	Cataract and glaucoma	Extreme of age	Altered lens protein	Slit-lamp examination every 6–12 months
Cutaneous	Atrophy, striae, acne, and hirsutism		• Decrease collagen, ground substance • Increase androgen	

(CHF: congestive heart failure; CNS: central nervous system; CS: corticosteroid; CVS: cardiovascular system; DEXA: dual energy X-ray absorptiometry; DM: diabetes mellitus; GI: gastrointestinal; GH: growth hormone; HPA: hypothalamic–pituitary–adrenal; HRT: hormone replacement therapy; HTN: hypertension; IGF: insulin-like growth factor; IV: intravenous; MC: mineralocorticoid; NSAIDs: nonsteroidal anti-inflammatory drugs; PPI: proton-pump inhibitor; PTH: parathyroid hormone; PUD: peptic ulcer disease)

DRUG INTERACTIONS

- *Increased serum CS levels:*
  - Macrolides and azoles (CYP3A4 inhibitors)
  - Hormonal contraceptives
- *Decreased serum CS levels:*
  - Rifampicin, phenytoin, and phenobarbitone (CYP3A4 inducer)
- *Increase serum levels of other drugs:*
  - Immunosuppressive agent
- *Decrease serum levels of other drugs:*
  - Isoniazid and salicylates
- *Oppose therapeutic benefit of other drugs:*
  - Insulin
- *Specific side effect potentiated:*
  - Nonsteroidal anti-inflammatory drugs (NSAIDs)
  - Diuretics such as thiazide and furosemide.

MONITORING GUIDELINES

Baseline:

- Blood pressure and weight
- Height and weight on a growth curve in children
- Ophthalmoscopic examination for cataracts
- TB screening (tuberculin testing and chest X-ray)
- Fasting glucose, triglycerides, and potassium levels.

FOLLOW-UP

Follow-up on corticosteroid treatment is presented in **Table 4**.

TABLE 4: Follow-up on corticosteroid treatment.

At 1 month, then every 3 months	Every 6 months	At cessation of long-term therapy
Through history and BP	Ophthalmic examination	Morning cortisol level
Height weight on a growth curve in children	DEXA scan for elderly	
FBS, lipid profile, and electrolyte		

(BP: blood pressure; DEXA: dual energy X-ray absorptiometry; FBS: fasting blood sugar)

PRINCIPLES FOR TAPERING SYSTEMIC CORTICOSTEROIDS

- *Tapering in long-term therapy:*
  - *>60 mg:* 20 mg decrement
  - *30–60 mg:* 10 mg decrement
  - *10–30 mg:* 5 mg decrement
  - *<10 mg:* 2.5 mg decrement
- *Tapering in short-term therapy:*
  - Off therapy by 2–3 weeks
  - Attempt to reach physiological doses by 3–4 weeks
  - Alternate day therapy with steroid sparing.

IMPORTANT PRINCIPLES TO MAXIMIZE THE SAFETY OF SYSTEMIC CORTICOSTEROIDS

- Proper indication
- Patient compliance assured
- Risk factors and relative contraindications known
- Start with lowest possible dose
- Risk-benefit ratio
- Proper monitoring
- Proper dose tapering methods.

KEY POINTS

- *Equivalent dose of corticosteroid:* 1.2 mg betamethasone = 1.5 mg dexamethasone = 8 mg methylprednisolone = 10 mg predisolone = 40 mg hydrocortisone = 12 mg deflazacort.
- Oral steroids are absorbed in upper part of jejunum and are bound to CBG, metabolized by liver and excreted through kidney.
- *Absolute contraindications:* Systemic fungal infection, herpes simplex keratitis, hypersensitivity.
- *Relative contraindications:* Hypertenson, congestive cardiac failure, psychosis, depression, active TB, diabetes mellitus, osteoporosis, cataract, glaucoma, pregnancy.

REFERENCES

1. Kendall EC. (1950). The development of cortisone as a therapeutic agent. [online] Available from: https://www.nobelprize.org/prizes/medicine/1950/kendall/lecture/. [Last accessed February, 2021].
2. Alfred GS, Goodman LS. The Pharmacological Bases of Therapeutics, 10th edition. New York: McGraw Hill; 2003.
3. Schäcke H, Döcke WD, Asadullah K. Mechanisms involved in the side effects of glucocorticoids. Pharmacol Ther. 2002;96(1):23-43.
4. Pereira ALC, Bolzani FCB, Stefani M, Charlin R. Systemic use of corticosteroids: literature review. Rev Med Cutan Iber Lat Am. 2007;35:35-50.
5. Lin H-Y, Muller YA, Hammond GL. Molecular and structural basis of steroid hormone binding and release from corticosteroid-binding globulin. Mol Cell Endocrinol. 2010;316:3-12.
6. Siiteri PK, Murai JT, Hammond GL, Nisker JA, Raymoure WJ. The serum transport of steroid hormones. Recent Prog Horm Res. 1982;38:457-510.
7. Steimer T. Steroid Hormone Metabolism. Geneva, Switzerland: Geneva Foundation for Medical Education and Research; 2003.
8. Nicolaides NC, Charmandari E, Kino T, Chrousos GP. Stress-Related and Circadian Secretion and Target Tissue Actions of Glucocorticoids: Impact on Health. Front Endocrinol (Lausanne). 2017;8:70.
9. Zannas AS, Chrousos GP. Epigenetic programming by stress and glucocorticoids along the human lifespan. Mol Psychiatry. 2017;22:640-6.
10. Pasricha JS, Srivastava G. Cure in pemphigus a possibility. Indian J Dermatol Venereol Leprol. 1986;52:185-6.
11. McDonough AK, Curtis JR, Saag KG. The epidemiology of glucocorticoid-associated adverse events. Curr Opin Rheumatol. 2008;20(2):131-7.

EXAMINATION QUESTIONS

1. Write a short note on systemic steroids.
2. Classify systemic steroids and briefly describe their applications.

153 CHAPTER Antihistamines

Prerna Raj, Aarti Sarda, Abhishek De

HISTAMINE

Histamine is synthesized from histidine by mast cells through the process of decarboxylation, and stored inside them, covalently bound to its granules. Stimulation of cutaneous mast cells cause release of granule-linked histamine, along with other chemoreactants such as chymase, tryptase, eicosanoids, and cytokines. Cutaneous mast cells can get stimulated immunologically or nonimmunologically. For immunological stimulation, they express on its surface FcER1 receptors, which binds to IgE, anti-FcER1 IgG, or anti-IgE antibodies.[1] However, they may also get stimulated nonimmunologically by substance-P, complements C3a, C4a, C5s, radiocontrast media, stem cell factor, salicylates, and NSAIDs.

Histamine Receptors

Histamine expresses its effect through histamine receptors. Both H_1 and H_2 receptors are expressed in human skin.[2,3] Histamine-induced itching and axon reflex is evoked by H_1 receptors whereas both H_1 and H_2 receptors produce vaso-dilatation and increased vascular permeability in the skin.[4-9] H_2 receptors also regulate T-lymphocyte activity by decreasing its proliferation and cytotoxicity thereby showing effectiveness in treatment of verruca vulgaris with cimetidine,[10-12] an H_2 antihistamine. Gastric parietal cells also express H_2 receptors thereby establishing the role of H_2 selective antihistamines for treatment of peptic ulcer disease and gastroesophageal reflux. H3 receptors express negative feedback effect on biosynthesis and release of histamine at the axon terminal. H_4 receptors are expressed on skin mast cells and neurons.[4]

Pharmacological attempts to block histamine synthesis has been largely unsuccessful. Thus, antihistamines serve the mainstay in blocking the action of histamine in the body once released.

ANTIHISTAMINES

Chronic idiopathic urticaria patients have an elevated tissue histamine levels producing the triple response of Lewis, characterized by erythema, edema, and axon reflex flare.[5] Histamine also plays a role in urticarial vasculitis where increased vessel permeability causes extravasation of inflammatory cells, neutrophils, complements thereby causing vessel wall damage and extravasation of RBCs at the site. Substances which reverse the effects of histamine, are called antihistamines. Earlier believed to be competitive antagonist of histamine, they are now known to be inverse agonists of the same, at their respective receptor sites.[13]

First Generation Antihistamines

First generation antihistamines consist of ethers based on the imidazole ring structure of histamine. Mepyramine was the first ever clinically used H_1 antihistamine, followed by diphenhydramine which got FDA approval. Cimetidine was the first ever H_2 antihistamine.

The 1st generation H_1 antihistamine can be divided into five categories **(Table 1)**.

Being highly lipophilic, they readily cross the blood-brain barrier inducing sedation by blocking the histamine stimulatory effects on brain H_1 receptors. They reach peak plasma concentration in about 2 hours, therefore used as preventives, then rescue medication. Metabolism occurs by cytochrome P450, including CYP2D6. Thus, their plasma half-life can be prolonged in patients of liver disease or those taking CYP3A4 inhibitors such as erythromycin and ketoconazole. Because of their persistence in tissues, the therapeutic effect can last longer than their plasma half-life **(Table 2)**. They may interfere with hypothalamic function, thus causing increased appetite and weight gain. Cyproheptadine in addition has anti-serotonin property as well, thereby being more effective in cold-induced urticaria and other physical urticarias.[14]

Adverse Effects

- *Central nervous system*: Sedation, impaired cognition, increased appetite
- *Gastrointestinal*: Dry mouth, constipation
- *Genitourinary*: Urinary retention, dysuria, erectile dysfunction

TABLE 1: Categories of 1st generation H_1 antihistamine.

Ethanolamine	Diphenhydramine
Piperidine	Cyproheptadine
Phenothiazine	Promethazine
Alkylamine	Chlorpheniramine
Piperazine	Hydroxyzine

- *Cardiac*: Arrythmia, tachycardia
- *Others*: Blurred vision

Second Generation Antihistamines

Developed by alteration of the imidazole ring structure of histamine. They are poorly lipophilic, thus do not cross blood-brain barrier, making them less sedative as a class. Also, they are highly selective at H_1 receptor, having negligible anticholinergic effect **(Table 2)**.

Currently five molecules are in use:

Active drug	*Derived from*
1. Fexofenadine	Terfenadine
2. Cetirizine	
3. Levocetirizine	Hydroxyzine
4. Loratadine	
5. Desloratadine	Loratadine

Fexofenadine

- Active metabolite of terfenadine that got discontinued due to cardiotoxicity.
- Readily absorbed orally, peak plasma concentration achieved in 1–3 hours.[15]
- Elimination half-life is 11–15 hours.[16]
- Single therapeutic dose of 40 mg can suppress wheal flare reaction of CIU by 80%.
- Does not undergo liver metabolism, no adverse cardiac effects.

Cetirizine

- Carboxylic acid metabolite of hydroxyzine
- Excreted unchanged in urine
- Peak onset of action in 1 hour.[17,18]
- Plasma half-life is 8 hours
- Pharmacological action lasts for 24 hours
- Normal therapeutic dosage is 10 mg in patients of hepatic or renal failure, 5 mg is sufficient.[19-21]
- Despite having minimal anticholinergic activity, drowsiness has been reported.
- Additionally it also inhibits eosinophil accumulation in tissues.

TABLE 2: Different drug and their uses.

Drug	*Peak plasma levels in (hours)*	*Half-life*	*Metabolism*	*Excreted in*	*Sedation*	*Pregnancy class*
1st Generation Antihistamines						
Diphenhydramine	0.6–2.8	4	Hepatic	Minimal renal	Yes	B
Cyproheptadine	2–3	1–4	Hepatic	40% renal	Yes	B
Promethazine	2–3	10–14	Hepatic	Predominantly renal	Yes	C
Chlorpheniramine	2–3.6	15–25	Liver	Predominantly renal	Yes	B
Hydroxyzine	1.7–2.5	20–25	Cetirizine is active metabolite	70% renal	Yes	C
2nd Generation Antihistamines						
Fexofenadine	1–3	14.4	Terfenadine is prodrug	80% feces	Minimal	C
Cetirizine	0.5–1.5	8.3	Levocetirizine is active metabolite	70% renal	Minimal	B
Levocetirizine	0.75	11	Active metabolite of cetirizine	Largely renal	Minimal	B
Loratadine	0.7–1.3	2–14	Desloratadine is active metabolite	Negligible in urine	Minimal	B
Desloratadine	2–3	19–34	No interaction with CYPs	Minimal renal	Minimal	C
Bilastine	1	14.5	No interaction with CYPs	Unchanged in urine and stool	No	
TCAs						
Doxepin	2	11–23	Nordoxepin an active metabolite	Minimal in urine	Yes	C
Mirtazapine						
Mast cell stabilizer						
Cromolyn sodium	0.25	1–2		Significant renal	No	B
Olopatadine		2.9–3.4		Significant renal	No	
Bepotastine	1	2.4	Piperidine derivative	Unchanged in urine	No	

Levocetirizine

- New 2nd generation H_1 antihistamine[22-24]
- R-enantiomer of cetirizine, and its active metabolite
- It is more potent than others even at 5 mg
- It has minimal sedative and anticholinergic side-effects

Loratadine

- It is a tricyclic, piperidine derivative, long-acting selective H_1 antihistamine.
- Peak plasma concentration of 10 mg therapeutic dose achieved by 0.7–1.3 hours.
- Its plasma half-life 8–11 hours, action lasts up to 12 hours.[25]
- Safe in renal hepatic impairment or advanced age.
- Minimal sedative or anticholinergic effect.

Desloratadine

- Active metabolite of loratadine
- Therapeutic dose of 5 mg is sufficient.[26-28]
- 5 times more potent than loratadine.
- It has no sedative, anticholinergic or cardiac side-effect
- Not metabolized by CYP enzyme, thus no drug interaction.

Bilastine

- It is a novel 2nd generation H_1 antihistamine. Got approval for use in chronic urticaria and allergic rhinitis in 2015[29]
- Has highly selective H_2 receptor action. Thus, minimal or no adverse effects. Safe for long-term administration
- Therapeutic dose of 20 mg once daily for as long as 52 weeks showed no reduction in efficacy or tachyphylaxis
- Safe in patients aged >12 years, or in patients with hepatic or renal compromise, and in elderly.

Olopatadine

- Structural analog of doxepin
- Selective H_1 antagonist and mast cell stabilizer.[30]
- Efficient in attenuating inflammatory and allergic reactions of chronic spontaneous urticaria.

Bepotastine

- Topical and oral 2nd generation H_1 antihistamine with mast cell stabilizing properties[31]
- In addition also have other immunoactive properties, such as inhibition of eosinophil migration, interleukin-5 (IL-5), leukotrienes (e.g., LTB4), and platelet-activating factor (PAF)
- Approved as a safe and effective treatment option for use in allergic rhinitis and urticaria in Japan
- Non-sedative, minimal side-effect, does not cross blood–brain barrier.
- Quick onset of action with prolonged effect

Contraindications

- Hypersensitivity to drug or its component.
- Newborn or premature infants (1st generation only)
- Pregnancy or lactating (1st generation only)
- Angle closure glaucoma (1st generation only)

Warnings/Precautions

- Promethazine should be avoided in <2 years children for the fear of respiratory depression
- *Neurologic*: Neuroleptic malignant syndrome
- *Cardiac*: Ischemic heart disease
- *Metabolic*: Thyroid dysfunction
- *BPH*: May cause urine retention
- COPD/sleep apnea

Pregnancy/Lactation

- Among 1st generation antihistamines, diphenhydramine and chlorpheniramine has maximum evidence supporting safety (Classified as Pregnancy Category B).[32,33]
- Among 2nd generation antihistamines, cetirizine and loratadine are Category B classified
- Doxepin, hydroxyzine, fexofenadine and desloratadine are Category C classified, and should be avoided
- Cetirizine and loratadine are excreted least in breast milk, thus safer alternatives in lactating mothers.[34-36]

H_2 ANTIHISTAMINES

They are selective inverse agonist on H_2 receptor downregulating its activity on epithelial, endothelial and parietal cells of gastric mucosa. They have also been implicated in altering cellular recruitment, antigen presentation, inflammatory mediator release because of presence of H_2 receptor on lymphocyte, monocyte, neutrophils, mast cells and dendritic cells. H_2 antihistamines available are:

- Cimetidine
- Ranitidine
- Famotidine
- Nizatidine

Their peak plasma concentration is achieved within 2 hours of oral intake. They do not cross blood–brain barrier, thus have low risk of CNS side-effect. However, dosage reduction maybe required in patients of hepatic or renal compromise[37,38] Unique adverse effect of cimetidine at high doses include galactorrhea, decreased libido, and decreased sperm count. Famotidine carries risk of QT prolongation and Torsades de pointes.[39,40] Because of CYP metabolism, they have huge drug interactions, thus increases serum levels of warfarin, BB, SSRI, metformin.

Tachyphylaxis/Subsensitivity

It is the development of a reduced response to prolonged antihistamine therapy perceived by patients. However, clear evidence for tachyphylaxis or subsensitivity in patients taking daily antihistamines is unsubstantiated, and recent reviews have either omitted mention of this condition or denied its existence.[41-43]

Miscellaneous Drugs

Doxepin

- It is a tricyclic antidepressant with H_1 and H_2 antihistamine activity, seen to be 800 times more potent than diphenhydramine. Thus, used in refractory cases of chronic idiopathic urticaria (CIU), physical urticarias and systemic disease associated pruritus.[44-46]
- Topical doxepin is found to be effective in atopic dermatitis (AD) and lichen simplex chronicus (LSC).[46]
- Sedation is the most common adverse effect, although this improved with continued use.
- Oral doxepin is Category-C whereas topical doxepin is considered Category-B drug.[47]
- Avoided in pregnancy, lactating, elderly, and children <12 years of age.

Mirtazapine

- It is a tetracyclic antidepressant with H_1 antihistamine property[48]
- Beneficial in reducing nocturnal itch in patients with chronic pruritus[49]

Mast Cell Stabilizer: Cromolyn Sodium

- It blocks mast cell degranulation, thereby preventing wheal flare reactions
- It is and extremely rapidly acting drug. Reaches peak plasma levels in 0.25 hours, and has a half-life of 1–2 hours.
- Produces no sedation
- It is pregnancy category B drug.

Uses

In Urticaria

H_1 antihistamines remain the cornerstone of treatment in chronic idiopathic urticaria or even in other physical urticarias.[50-52] However, they are seen to be less effective in preventing angioedema episodes, that occur in about 40% patients of CIU. In refractory cases, higher doses of 2nd generation. H_1 antihistamines are prescribed, up to four-folds.[53] In cases suffering from insomnia or anxiety, 10–25 mg of doxepin can be prescribed. A preferred strategy is prescription of fexofenadine in the morning and cetirizine at night, to deal with sedative effects relating to cetirizine.[54] Another strategy is of using a combination of H_1 and H_2 receptor antagonist in resistant CIU. Beyond urticaria, concomitant H_1 and H_2 antihistamines have been found to be effective in relieving abdominal pain of cutaneous mastocytosis.[55-57]

In Atopic Dermatitis

The effectiveness of H_1 antihistamines as antipruritics in AD is at best ambiguous.[58,59] One study, however, did demonstrate decreased pruritus in AD patients treated with four times the recommended dose of cetirizine, but the reduction in pruritus was attributed to cetirizine's sedative effects.[60] Yet, H_1 antihistamines may be beneficial for AD patients with other manifestations of atopy, such as allergic rhinitis or allergy induced asthma.

KEY POINTS

- Histamine is synthesized from histidine by the process of decarboxylation, and stored inside the mast cells.
- Antihistamines act as inverse agonists rather than antagonist of histamine. They form the mainstay of treatment in urticaria.
- The older first generation H1 antihistamines penetrate readily into the brain causing sedation, drowsiness, fatigue and impaired concentration.
- The newer second generation H1 antihistamines are safer, more efficacious and cause less side effects.
- Though every drug in pregnancy carries the risk of teratogenicity, cetirizine, levocetirizine and loratidine are relatively safer in pregnancy.
- Cardiotoxicity is an observed adverse effect. Fexofenadine, cetirizine, loratidine are relatively safer in children.

REFERENCES

1. Bain WA, Hellier FF, Warin RP. Some aspects of histamine antagonists. Lancet. 1948;2(6538):964-9.
2. Ash AS, Schild HO. Receptors mediating some actions of histamine. 1966. Br J Pharmacol. 1997;120(Suppl 4):302-4.
3. Bleehen SS, Thomas SE, Greaves MW, Newton J, Kennedy CT, Hindley F, et al. Cimetidine and chlorpheniramine in the treatment of chronic idiopathic urticaria: a multicentre randomized double blind study. Br J Dermatol. 1987;117(1):81-8.
4. Dunford PJ, Williams KN, Desai PJ, Karlsson L, McQueen D, Thurmond RL. Histamine H4 receptor antagonists are superior to traditional antihistamines in the attenuation of experimental pruritus. J Allergy Clin Immunol. 2007;119(1):176-83.
5. Hide M, Francis DM, Grattan CE, Hakimi J, Kochan JP, Greaves MW. Autoantibodies against the high-affinity IgE receptor as a cause of histamine release in chronic urticaria. N Engl J Med. 1993;328(22):1599-604.
6. Fiebiger E, Maurer D, Holub H, Reininger B, Hartmann G, Woisetschläger M, et al. Serum IgG autoantibodies directed against the alpha chain of Fc epsilon RI: a selective marker and pathogenetic factor for a distinct subset of chronic urticaria patients? J Clin Invest. 1995;96(6):2606-12.
7. Dinh QT, Cryer A, Dinh S, Peiser C, Wu S, Springer J, et al. Transcriptional up-regulation of histamine receptor-1 in epithelial, mucus and inflammatory cells in perennial allergic rhinitis. Clin Exp Allergy. 2005;35(11):1443-8.
8. Greaves MW, Marks R, Robertson I. Receptors for histamine in human skin blood vessels: a review. Br J Dermatol. 1997;97(2):225-8.
9. Rocklin RE. Histamine induced cell response in normal and atopic subjects. In: Ganellin CR, Schwartz JC (Eds). Frontiers in Histamine Research. Oxford: Pergamon; 1985:357-64.
10. Yilmaz E, Alpsoy E, Basaran E. Cimetidine therapy for warts: a placebo-controlled, double-blind study. J Am Acad Dermatol. 1996;34(6):1005-7.

11. Rogers CJ, Gibney MD, Siegfried EC, Harrison BR, Glaser DA. Cimetidine therapy for recalcitrant warts in adults: is it any better than placebo? J Am Acad Dermatol. 1999;41(1):123-7.
12. Glass AT, Solomon BA. Cimetidine therapy for recalcitrant warts in adults. Arch Dermatol. 1996;132(6):680–682.
13. Simons FE. Advances in H_1-antihistamines. N Engl J Med. 2004;351(21):2203-17.
14. Wanderer AA, Ellis EF. Treatment of cold urticaria with cyproheptadine. J Allergy Clin Immunol. 1971;48(6):366-71.
15. Lippert C, Ling J, Brown P, Burmaster S, Eller M, Cheng L, et al. Mass balance and pharmacokinetics of fexofenadine HCl in healthy male volunteers. Pharm Res. 1995;12:S390.
16. Russell T, Stolz M, Eller M, Eller MG, Weir S. Acute and subchronic dose tolerance of fexofenadine HCl in healthy male subjects (abs p. 41). British Society of Allergy and Clinical Immunology Meeting; 1996.
17. Kassem N, Roman I, Gural R, Dyer JG, Robillard N. Effects of loratadine (SCH 29851) in suppression of histamine-induced skin wheals. Ann Allergy. 1988;60(6):505-7.
18. Delpón E, Valenzuela C, Tamargo J. Blockade of cardiac potassium and other channels by antihistamines. Drug Saf. 1999:11-8.
19. Wood SG, John BA, Chasseaud LF, Yeh J, Chung M. The metabolism and pharmacokinetics of 14C-cetirizine in humans. Ann Allergy. 1987;59(6Pt2):31-4.
20. Juhlin L, de Vos C, Rihoux JP. Inhibiting effect of cetirizine on histamine-induced and 48/80-induced wheals and flares, experimental dermagraphism, and cold-induced urticaria. J Allergy Clin Immunol. 1987;80(4):599-602.
21. Michel L, De Vos C, Rihoux JP, Burtin C, Benveniste J, Dubertret L. Inhibitory effect of oral cetirizine on in vivo antigen-induced histamine and PAF-acether release and eosinophil recruitment in human skin. J Allergy Clin Immunol. 1988;82(1):101-9.
22. Benedetti MS, Plisnier M, Kaise J, Maier L, Baltes E, Arendt C, et al. Absorption, distribution, metabolism and excretion of [14C]levocetirizine, the R enantiomer of cetirizine, in healthy volunteers. Eur J Clin Pharmacol. 2001;57(8):571-82.
23. Monroe EW, Fox RW, Green AW, Izuno GT, Bernstein DI, Pleskow WW, et al. Efficacy and safety of loratadine (10 mg once daily) in the management of idiopathic chronic urticaria. J Am Acad Dermatol. 1988;19(1Pt 1):138-9.
24. Powell RJ, Leech SC, Till S, Huber PAJ, Nasser SM, Clark AT, et al. BSACI guideline for the management of chronic urticaria and angioedema. Clin Exp Allergy. 2015;45(3):547-65.
25. Clissold SP, Sorkin EM, Goa KL, Loratadine: a preliminary review of its pharmacodynamic properties and therapeutic efficacy. Drugs. 1989;37(1):42-57.
26. McClellan K, Jarvis B. Desloratadine. Drugs. 2001;61(6):789-96.
27. Ring J, Hein R, Gauger A, Bronsky E, Miller B. Once-daily desloratadine improves the signs and symptoms of chronic idiopathic urticaria: a randomized, double-blind, placebo-controlled study. Int J Dermatol. 2001;40(1):72-6.
28. Monroe E, Finn A, Patel P, Guerrero R, Ratner P, Bernstein D, et al. Efficacy and safety of desloratadine 5 mg once daily in the treatment of chronic idiopathic urticaria: a double-blind, randomized, placebo-controlled trial. J Am Acad Dermatol. 2003;48(4):535-41.
29. Papadopoulos NG, Zuberbier T. The safety and tolerability profile of bilastine for chronic urticaria in children. Clin Transl Allergy. 2019;9:55.
30. Yamamoto H, Yamada T, Kubo S, Osawa Y, Kimura Y, Oh M, et al. Efficacy of oral olopatadine hydrochloride for the treatment of seasonal allergic rhinitis: a randomized, double-blind, placebo-controlled study. Allergy Asthma Proc. 2010;31(4):296-303.
31. Godse K, Kumari N. Bepotastine besilate: a novel antihistamine. Indian J Drugs Dermatol. 2017;3(2):64-8.
32. Murase JE, Heller MM, Butler DC. Safety of dermatologic medications in pregnancy and lactation: Part I. pregnancy. J Am Acad Dermatol. 2014;70(3):401.e1-e14.
33. Kar S, Krishnan A, Preetha K, Mohankar A. A review of antihistamines used during pregnancy. J Pharmacol Pharmacother. 2012;3(2):105-8.
34. American Academy of Pediatrics Committee on Drugs. The transfer of drugs and other chemicals into human milk. Pediatrics. 1994;93(1):137-50.
35. Hilbert J, Radwanski E, Affrime MB, Perentesis G, Symchowicz S, Zampaglione N. Excretion of loratadine in human breast milk. J Clin Pharmacol. 1988;28(3):234-9.
36. Briggs GG, Freeman RK, Towers CV, Forinash AB. Drugs in Pregnancy and Lactation: A Reference Guide to Fetal and Neonatal Risk, 11th edition. Philadelphia: Lippincott Williams & Wilkins; 2017.
37. Drayer DE, Romankiewicz J, Lorenzo B, Reidenberg MM. Age and renal clearance of cimetidine. Clin Pharmacol Ther. 1982;31(1):45-50.
38. Penston J, Wormsley KG. Adverse reactions and interactions with H_2-receptor antagonists. Med Toxicol. 1986;1(3):192-216.
39. Famotidine: Drug information. In: UpToDate. Waltham, MA: UpToDate Inc. [online] Available from: https://www.uptodate.com. [Last accessed March, 2021].
40. Poluzzi E, Raschi E, Moretti U, De Ponti F. Drug-induced torsades de pointes: data mining of the public version of the FDA Adverse Event Reporting System (AERS). Pharmacoepidemiol Drug Saf. 2009;18(6):512-8.
41. Bousquet J, Chanal I, Murrieta M, Stalla-Bourdillon A. Lack of subsensitivity mizolastine over an 8-week treatment. Allergy. 1996;51(4):251-6.
42. Bousquet J, Chanal I, Skassa-Brociek W, Lemonier C, Michel FB. Lack of subsensitivity to loratadine during long-term dosing during 12 weeks. J Allergy Clin Immunol. 1990;86(2):248-53.
43. Long WF, Taylor RJ, Wagner CJ, Leavengood DC, Nelson HS. Skin test suppression by antihistamines and the development of subsensitivity. J Allergy Clin Immunol. 1985;76(1):113-7.
44. Richelson E. Tricyclic antidepressants and histamine H_1 receptors. Mayo Clin Proc. 1979;54(10):669-74.
45. Greene SL, Reed CE, Schroeter AL. Double-blind crossover study comparing doxepin with diphenhydramine for the treatment of chronic urticaria. J Am Acad Dermatol. 1985;12(4):669-75.
46. Drake LA, Fallon JD, Sober A. Relief of pruritus in patients with atopic dermatitis after treatment with topical doxepin cream. The doxepin study group. J Am Acad Dermatol. 1994;31(4):613-6.
47. Doxepin: Drug information. In: UpToDate. Waltham, MA: UpToDate Inc. [online] Available from: https://www.uptodate.com. [Accessed March, 2021].
48. Anttila SA, Leinonen EV. A review of the pharmacological and clinical profile of mirtazapine. CNS Drug Rev. 2001;7(3):249-64.
49. Hundley JL, Yosipovitch G. Mirtazapine for reducing nocturnal itch in patients with chronic pruritus: a pilot study. J Am Acad Dermatol. 2004;50(6):889-91.
50. Grattan CE, Humphreys F. British Association of Dermatologists Therapy Guidelines and Audit Subcommittee. Guidelines for

evaluation and management of urticaria in adults and children. Br J Dermatol. 2007;157(6):1116-23.

51. Zuberbier T, Asero R, Bindslev-Jensen C, et al. EAACI/GA(2) LEN/EDF/WAO guideline: definition, classification and diagnosis of urticaria. Allergy. 2009;64(10):1417-26.
52. Nelson HS, Reynolds R, Mason J. Fexofenadine HCl is safe and effective for treatment of chronic idiopathic urticaria. Ann Allergy Asthma Immunol. 2000;84(5):517-22.
53. Staevska M, Popov TA, Kralimarkova T, Lazarova C, Kraeva S, Popova D, et al. The effectiveness of levocetirizine and desloratadine in up to 4 times conventional doses in difficult-to-treat urticaria. J Allergy Clin Immunol. 2010;125(3):676-82.
54. Church MK, Maurer M, Simons FE, Bindslev-Jensen C, van Cauwenberge P, Bousquet J, et al. Risk of first-generation H(1)-antihistamines: a GA(2)LEN position paper. Allergy. 2010; 65(4):459-66.
55. Friedman BS, Santiago ML, Berkebile C, Metcalfe DD. Comparison of azelastine and chlorpheniramine in the treatment of mastocytosis. J Allergy Clin Immunol. 1993;92(4):520-6.
56. Morgan M, Khan DA. Therapeutic alternatives for chronic urticaria: an evidence-based review, part 1. Ann Allergy Asthma Immunol. 2008;100(5):403-12.
57. Fedorowicz Z, van Zuuren EJ, Hu N. Histamine H_2-receptor antagonists for urticaria. Cochrane Database Syst Rev. 2012; 3:CD008596.
58. Klein PA, Clark RA. An evidence-based review of the efficacy of antihistamines in relieving pruritus in atopic dermatitis. Arch Dermatol. 1999;135(12):1522-5.
59. Hannuksela M, Kalimo K, Lammintausta K, Mattila T, Turjanmaa K, Varjonen E, et al. Dose ranging study: cetirizine in the treatment of atopic dermatitis in adults. Ann Allergy. 1993;70(2):127-33.
60. Sidbury R, Davis DM, Cohen DE, Cordoro KM, Berger TG, Bergman JN, et al. Guidelines of care for the management of atopic dermatitis: section 3. Management and treatment with phototherapy and systemic agents. J Am Acad Dermatol. 2014;71(2):327-49.

EXAMINATION QUESTIONS

1. Write a short note on second generation antihistamincs.
2. Discuss antihistamines.

154 CHAPTER

Dapsone

Deepika Halder, Aarti Sarda, Abhishek De

INTRODUCTION

Dapsone is 4,4′-diamino-diphenyl sulfone, or DDS, an aniline derivative belonging to the group of synthetic sulfones **(Fig. 1)**. It was synthesized a century ago and continues to be a powerful therapeutic agent in many skin diseases. Dapsone has got antimicrobial, antiprotozoal, and anti-inflammatory effects.

Dapsone has been the principal drug in various regimens recommended by the WHO for the treatment of leprosy. As an anti-infective agent, it is also used for treating malaria and, more recently, for *Pneumocystis carinii* pneumonia in HIV patients. Beyond these, dapsone is also used in various noninfectious conditions.

HISTORY

- Fromm and Whittman first formulated Dapsone in 1908.[1]
- The first effective drug for leprosy was an injectable sulfone named Promin (glucosulfone sodium), reported from Carville, USA in 1943.[2]
- Dapsone was used for leprosy later in the 1940s by Cochrane and Muir in India, Lowe and Davey in Nigeria and Souza Lima in Brazil.[3]

MECHANISM OF ACTION

Dapsone as Bacteriostatic Agent

Dapsone acts against bacteria and protozoa in the same way as sulfonamides that is by inhibiting the synthesis of dihydrofolic acid through competition with para-amino-benzoate for the active site of dihydropteroate synthetase. Dapsone similarly acts by inhibiting folate metabolism in *M. leprae*.[4]

Dapsone as an Anti-inflammatory Agent

The anti-inflammatory action of the drug is unrelated to its antibacterial action and is still not fully understood.

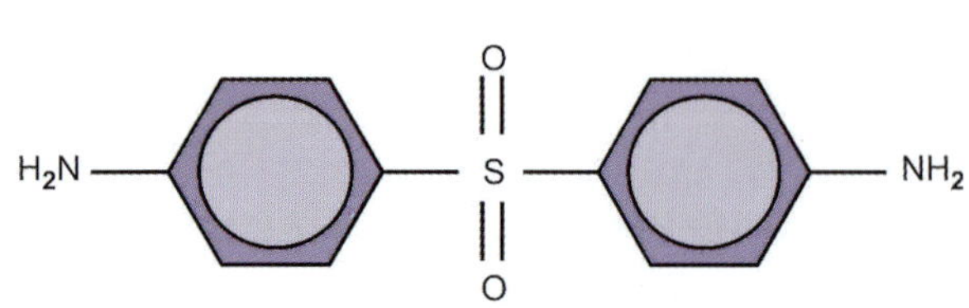

Fig. 1: Structure of Dapsone.

Dapsone is effective in dermatoses with abnormal neutrophil accumulation, through many potential mechanisms. Also, by multiple mechanisms, dapsone reduces the release of prostaglandins and leukotrienes and blocks their inflammatory effects.

- Dapsone interferes with neutrophil chemotactic migration and β_2 integrin (CD11b/CD18)-mediated adherence of neutrophils.
- It inhibits the production of reactive oxygen species directly and reversibly inhibits the myeloperoxidase enzyme thus decreasing hypochlorous acid formation
- Dapsone protects cells from neutrophil- and eosinophil-mediated injury by directly inhibiting myeloperoxidase (MPO) in neutrophils and eosinophil peroxidase.
- Dapsone has a potent activity in reducing the effect of eosinophil peroxidase on mast cells, which results in a decreased liberation of histamine.
- Dapsone inhibits the binding of LTB4 to receptors on neutrophils and inhibits neutrophil chemotactic response to LTB4.
- Dapsone inhibits the generation of 5-lipoxygenase products
- Dapsone also inhibits lysosomal enzymes
- Additionally, dapsone inhibits the release of inflammatory mediators, including interleukin (IL)-8,12 prostaglandin D2, and TNF-α.
- Dapsone also inhibits the myeloperoxidase H_2O_2-halide-mediated cytotoxic system
- Dapsone was shown to inhibit the alternative pathway of complement activation *in vitro*.[5]

Pharmacokinetics

Absorption and Bioavailability[5,6,7]

- Dapsone is readily absorbed from gut completely with a bioavailability of 86%.
- After intake of 100 mg of oral dapsone, peak serum dapsone concentrations between 1.10 and 2.33 mg/L is reached within 0.5–4 hours.
- The therapeutic range of serum concentration is 0.5–5 mg/L for leprosy.
- Dapsone has got long elimination half-life (average 24–36 hours) because of significant enterohepatic circulation and

strong protein binding of both dapsone and its metabolite monoacetyl diamino-diphenyl sulfone (MADDS).

Distribution[5-7]

- Dapsone is approximately 70% protein-bound, and its monoacetylated metabolite is almost entirely protein-bound.
- Dapsone is distributed to all body organs including skin, liver, kidneys, and erythrocytes.
- Dapsone can cross the placenta and it is excreted in breast milk.

Metabolism[5-7]

- There are two major metabolic pathways of orally ingested dapsone.
- In the liver, dapsone is metabolized by either N-hydroxylation to produce toxic hydroxylamines or by acetylation to produce nontoxic acetyl-dapsone.
- Acetyl-dapsone includes monoacetyl dapsone (MADDS) and biacetyl dapsone **(Fig. 2)**.
- Hydroxylamine metabolites are responsible for the hematological adverse effects of dapsone.

Excretion[5]

- Dapsone and its metabolites are conjugated in the liver as dapsone glucuronide (water soluble) and excreted via kidneys.
- No dose adjustment needed in liver failure as minor changes in dapsone metabolism have been noted.

Clinical Uses of Dapsone in Dermatology

In dermatology, the FDA-approved indications for dapsone are leprosy, dermatitis herpetiformis, and acne vulgaris **(Box 1)**.[8]

Use of Dapsone in Leprosy

Both regimens advised by the WHO for paucibacillary leprosy and multibacillary leprosy contain dapsone. Monotherapy with dapsone is avoidable leprosy because of higher risk of resistance.[8]

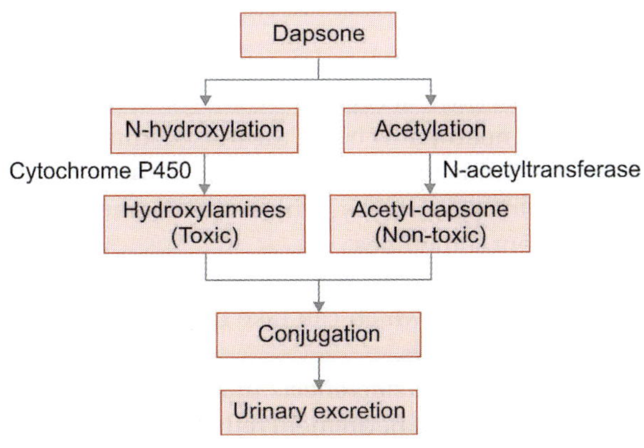

Fig. 2: Metabolic pathway of dapsone.

Use of Dapsone in Dermatitis Herpetiformis

Dapsone is the only FDA-approved drug for treating dermatitis herpetiformis. It is to be used along with a gluten-free diet. It is prescribed at a starting dose of 50 mg/day and gradually increased up to 200 mg/day until the disease is controlled.[8]

Use of Dapsone in Acne Vulgaris

Topical dapsone 5% gel has been approved for the use in many clinical indications, including acne vulgaris. In 2017, the FDA approved the use of topical dapsone 7.5% gel for acne vulgaris which has a better compliance than 5% gel because of its easier once daily application. Oral dapsone is an effective and safe alternative to isotretinoin when treating severe acne (nodulocystic or conglobata acne).[8]

Dosage

A therapeutic dose of dapsone varies from 25 to 200 mg/day, usually given as a single dose. The recommended starting dose is between 50 and 100 mg/day to minimize potential adverse effects. Dapsone has been used safely in infants and children at doses of 1–2 mg/kg/day.

Topical dapsone (5% gel, 7.5% gel) is FDA approved for acne vulgaris in adults and adolescents up to the age of

BOX 1: Dermatological used of dapsone.

US FDA approved indication:
- Acne vulgaris (Topical 5% and 7.5% formulation)
- Leprosy
- Dermatitis herpetiformis (DH)

Off-label uses of dapsone in cutaneous disorders
Infectious diseases:
- Toxoplasmosis
- *Plasmodium falciparum*

Inflammatory diseases:
- Acne inversa
- Rosacea
- Granuloma annulare
- Lupus miliaris disseminatus faciei
- Familial Mediterranean fever
- *Neutrophilic diseases*: Sweet syndrome, pyoderma gangrenosum, Behçet's syndrome/aphthous stomatitis
- *Eosinophilic diseases*: Eosinophilic cellulitis (Wells' syndrome) and eosinophilic annular erythema, eosinophilic folliculitis (Ofuji's disease), chronic idiopathic
- Urticaria or delayed pressure urticaria, eosinophilic fasciitis
- *Pustular diseases*: Acropustulosis of infancy and subcorneal pustular dermatosis (Sneddon-Wilkinson), localized (palmoplantar) pustular psoriasis, erosive pustular dermatosis
- *Vasculitis*: Cutaneous vasculitis (leukocytoclastic), urticarial vasculitis, erythema elevatum diutinum (EED)
- *Bullous diseases*: Pemphigus vulgaris, IgA pemphigus, linear IgA dermatosis, bullous pemphigoid, mucous membrane pemphigoid, lichen planus pemphigoides, and dermatitis herpetiformis (Duhring's disease).
- *Genetic diseases*: Hailey–Hailey disease
- *Miscellaneous*: Brown recluse spider bite (loxoscelism), idiopathic thrombocytopenic purpura.

12 years. It has not been reported to cause hemolysis even in the patients with G6PD deficiency. However, in a few cases of G6PD methemoglobinemia were found, and the FDA decided to change the label in July 2015 to "caution of use."[8,9]

Adverse Effect

Dapsone is associated with both pharmacologic and idiosyncratic side effects **(Box 2)**.

Hematological

Hemolytic Anemia

- Hemolysis of red blood cells is the most important side-effect of dapsone
- Mild hemolysis with a drop in hemoglobin of 1–2 g/dL occurs in most patients at a standard therapeutic dose.
- N-hydroxy metabolites of dapsone (N-hydroxy dapsone hydroxylamine and N-hydroxy monoacetyl dapsone hydroxylamine) are potent oxidants and cause persistent oxidative stress to RBC membranes and finally hemolysis.
- G6PD-deficient individuals are more susceptible to dapsone metabolite induced oxidative stresses. Other risk factors are dosage of dapsone, and advancing age.
- Patients present with fatigue, dyspnea, weakness and laboratory tests reveal anemia, increased reticulocytes, lactate dehydrogenase (LDH), and indirect bilirubin.[10]

BOX 2: Important adverse effects of dapsone.

- *Pharmacologic adverse effect*:
  - Hemolytic anemia
  - Methemoglobinemia
- *Idiosyncratic*:
  - *Hematologic*:
    - Leukopenia
    - Agranulocytosis
  - *Hepatic*:
    - Hepatitis (predominantly transaminase elevations)
    - Infectious mononucleosis-like syndrome (dapsone hypersensitivity syndrome)
    - Prehepatic jaundice
    - Cholestatic jaundice (rarely)
    - Hypoalbuminemia (rarely)
    - Hepatic coma (rarely)
  - *Cutaneous*:
    - Morbilliform eruption (exanthematous, maculopapular)
    - Exfoliative erythroderma
    - Erythema multiforme
    - Erythema nodosum
    - Urticaria
    - Scarlatiniform exanthem
    - Photosensitivity
    - Fixed drug eruption
    - Toxic epidermal necrolysis
  - *Gastrointestinal*:
    - Gastric irritation with nausea, vomiting
    - Anorexia
    - Abdominal pain
  - *Renal*:
    - Albuminuria
    - Electrolyte imbalance
  - *Cardiac*:
    - Atrioventricular block
  - *Neurologic and psychiatric*:
    - Psychosis
    - Peripheral neuropathy (predominantly motor effect)
    - Blindness
    - Insomnia

Methemoglobinemia

- Methemoglobinemia is the second most common dose related adverse effect of dapsone.
- Presents with headache, shortness of breath, lethargy, and a bluish discoloration of lips and fingertips
- The formation of methemoglobin is related to the N-hydroxy (hydroxylamine) metabolites of dapsone.
- Vitamin E (800 IU daily) has been demonstrated to provide a small amount of protection against the formation of methemoglobin and hemolysis.
- Cimetidine (400 mg three times daily) can reduce methemoglobin levels by inhibition of CYP450, which reduces synthesis of the toxic hydroxylated metabolites.
- Ascorbic acid, which can be administered both orally and intravenously, is effective in reducing methemoglobin nonenzymatically.
- More severe cases need treatment with oxygen and IV methylene blue 1% solution to restore the iron in hemoglobin to its reduced oxygen carrying state.[11]

Agranulocytosis

- Agranulocytosis is the most serious idiosyncratic adverse effect of dapsone.
- The median duration of therapy with dapsone before the development of agranulocytosis was 7 weeks (between 3 and 12 weeks), with an average of 100 mg daily dosage.
- Agranulocytosis has occurred as early as 3 weeks of therapy.
- Most patients recover after cessation of dapsone, typically within 7 to 14 days.
- Granulocyte-colony stimulating factor (G-CSF) has been used for speedy recovery of normal granulocyte number.[12]

Neurological

- Dapsone has also been associated with a variety of neurological side effects.
- Peripheral neuropathy being the most common one.
- Dapsone-induced peripheral neuropathy is primarily distal motor neuropathy, with some degree of sensory involvement sometimes.
- Most of the patients recover completely with discontinuation of the drug, which can take from a few weeks to a maximum of 2 years.
- Other neurological side effects include acute psychosis, mood changes, and permanent retinal damage with optic atrophy.[8]

Dapsone Hypersensitivity Syndrome

- *Synonym*: "DDS syndrome" or "sulfone syndrome" or "five week dermatitis"
- *History*: In 1950, Lowe first reported cases of hypersensitivity to dapsone. Allday and Barnes in 1951 gave it the name "dapsone syndrome."
- Dapsone hypersensitivity syndrome is an idiosyncratic reaction initially described as an infectious mononucleosis-like eruption in lepromatous leprosy patients.
- Classically, it consists of exfoliative dermatitis and/or other skin rashes, generalized lymphadenopathy, hepatosplenomegaly, fever, hepatitis, and mononucleosis (lymphocytes and monocytes 70%)
- Cutaneous involvement of dapsone syndrome is always present, though others may be absent.
- The cutaneous manifestations of this syndrome show wide variations including erythroderma, papular erythematous eruptions, erythema multiforme, toxic epidermal necrolysis and Stevens-Johnson syndrome. Erythematous maculopapular rash and exfoliative dermatitis are present in the majority of cases.
- Patch testing with dapsone tablet or injection form and the delayed type intradermal skin test with 0.05% dapsone in saline may be undertaken for confirmation; though these tests are, however, unreliable.
- The conditions of most patients improve after cessation of dapsone therapy. For more severe cases; prednisolone in the range of 30 to 60 mg/day may be given.[13]

Pregnancy and Lactation

- Dapsone is a pregnancy category C drug.
- Dapsone can be secreted in breast milk and rarely can cause hemolytic anemia in infants breastfeeding from mothers on dapsone.

Contraindications

- Absolute contraindication to dapsone is hypersensitivity to the dapsone including agranulocytosis and hypersensitivity syndrome.
- Relative contraindications are:
  - G6PD deficiency
  - Allergy to sulfonamide antibiotics
  - Severe cardiopulmonary disease
  - Severe hepatic or renal impairment
  - Peripheral neuropathy

DRUG INTERACTIONS WITH DAPSONE[8]

- *Drugs those may decrease dapsone serum levels (loss of efficacy) due to CYP3A4 enzyme induction*: Rifampin, anticonvulsants (carbamazepine, oxcarbazepine, phenobarbital, phenytoin), griseofulvin, antiretroviral (nevirapine, efavirenz).
- *Drugs those may decrease dapsone serum levels (loss of efficacy) by decreasing absorption*: Antacids, didanosine.
- *Drugs that may increase serum levels (and potential toxicity) of dapsone*: Probenecid.
- *Drugs those may inhibit enzymes in the folate metabolic pathway and may increase hematologic risk of dapsone*: Sulfonamide, methotrexate, pyrimethamine, trimethoprim.
- *Drugs (oxidants) those may increase oxidative stress to RBC—result in hemolysis or methemoglobinemia*: Sulfonamides, local anesthetics, antimalarials.
- *Others*: Zalcitabine increases the risk for peripheral neuropathy.

Drug Monitoring[8]

Baseline

- Extensive history and examination to rule cardiopulmonary, gastrointestinal, neurologic, and renal impairment
- Complete blood count
- Liver function tests
- Renal function tests
- Urine routine
- G6PD level

Follow-up

- History and examination to rule out peripheral neuropathy, methemoglobinemia, and other adverse effects
- Complete blood count every week for 4 weeks, then every 2 weeks until week 12, then every 3 to 4 months
- Reticulocyte count as needed to assess degree of response to dapsone-induced hemolysis
- Liver function tests every 3–4 months
- Renal function tests and urinalysis every 3–4 months
- Methemoglobin levels if indicated

REFERENCES

1. Fromm E, Wittmann J. Derivate des p-nitrophenols. Berichte Deutsch Chem Ges. 1908;41:2264-73.
2. Faget G, Pogge R, Johansen F, Dinan J. The promin treatment of leprosy. Pub Health Rep. 1943;58:1729-41.
3. Cochrane R, Ramanujam H, Paul H, Russell D. Two-and-a-half years' experimental work on the sulphone group of drugs. Lepr Rev. 1949;20:4-64.
4. Seydel JK, Richter M, Wempe E. Mechanisms of action of the folate blocker diamino-diphenylsulfone (dapsone, DDS) studied in comparison to sulfonamides. Int J Leprosy. 1980;48:18-29.
5. Zhu YI, Stiller MJ. Dapsone and sulfones in dermatology: overview and update. J Am Acad Dermatol. 2001;45(3):420-34.
6. Pieters FA, Zuidema J. The absolute oral bioavailability of dapsone in dogs and humans. Int J Clin Pharmacol Ther Toxicol. 1987;25:396-400.
7. Venkatesan K. Clinical pharmacokinetic considerations in the treatment of patients with leprosy. Clin Pharmacokinet. 1989;16:365-86.

8. Ghaoui N, Hanna E, Abbas O, Kibbi AG, Kurban M. Update on the use of dapsone in dermatology. Int J Dermatol. 2020;59(7): 787-95.
9. Draelos Z, Carter E, Maloney J, Elewski B, Poulin Y, Lynde C, et al. Two randomized studies demonstrate the efficacy and safety of dapsone gel 5% for the treatment of acne vulgaris. J Am Acad Dermatol. 2007;56:439.e1-e10.
10. Jollow DJ, Bradshaw TP, McMillan DC. Dapsone-induced hemolytic anemia. Drug Metab Rev. 1995;27(1-2):107-24.
11. Dawson AH, Whyte IM. Management of dapsone poisoning complicated by methemoglobinemia. Med Toxicol Adverse Drug Exp. 1989;4(5):387-92.
12. Coleman MD. Dapsone-mediated agranulocytosis: risks, possible mechanisms and prevention. Toxicology. 2001;162(1): 53-60.
13. Thappa DM, Sethuraman G. Dapsone (sulfone) syndrome (CME). Indian J Dermatol Venereol Leprol. 2000;66: 117-20.

EXAMINATION QUESTIONS

1. Write a note of dapsone.
2. Discuss dapsone hypersensitivity syndrome.

155 CHAPTER Antimalarial Drugs

Manjyot Gautam, Suyomi Shah

INTRODUCTION

The antimalarial drugs used for the treatment of dermatologic disorders include hydroxychloroquine (HCQ) and chloroquine (CQ). Earlier an antimalarial drug called quinacrine was also used, but because of its toxicity and ineffectiveness it was replaced by better drugs. HCQ and CQ are 4-aminoquinoline compounds and derivatives of quinine. Quinine is a naturally occurring white crystalline alkaloid derived from the bark of cinchona trees, originally found in South America. Infusions of cinchona bark have been used for the treatment of malaria since 1630s.[1] Quinine was isolated in 1820 and remained the drug of choice for malaria until 1940s when other drugs with fewer adverse effects replaced it. It was first used in dermatology by Payne in 1894 to treat discoid lesions in lupus erythematosus. CQ phosphate was synthesized in 1934.[1] It was introduced in 1947 for the prophylactic treatment of malaria. HCQ sulfate was synthesized in 1946. Quinacrine hydrochloride was introduced in 1930 and was first used by Francis Page for the treatment of lupus in 1951.[2]

STRUCTURE[3]

Hydroxychloroquine and CQ both are 4-aminoquinoline compounds. Quinacrine has an extra benzene ring and is an acridine compound **(Fig. 1)**.

BIOAVAILABILITY[4]

All antimalarials are:

- Bitter
- Water soluble and crystalline powder
- Absorbed from the gastrointestinal tract
- Bind to tissue proteins
- Highest concentrations present in the eye and skin followed by liver, kidneys, muscles, heart, and brain.

PHARMACOKINETICS[5]

Pharmacokinetics of antimalarial drugs has been given in **Table 1**.

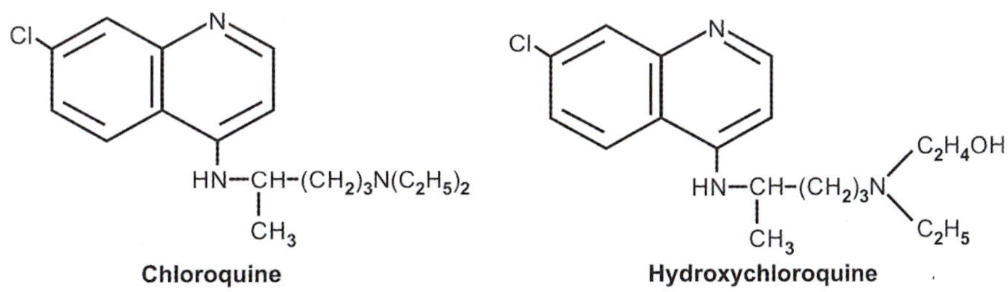

Fig. 1: Structure of hydroxychloroquine and chloroquine.

TABLE 1: Pharmacokinetics of antimalarial drugs.

Name	*HCQ*	*CQ*	*Quinacrine*
Peak effect (hour)	4	5	1–3
Bioavailability (%)	74	50	100
Protein binding (%)	45	50–65	80
Half-life (days)	40–50	40–50	5–14
Metabolism	Desethylchloroquine and desethylhydroxychloroquine metabolites	Desethylchloroquine metabolite	None
Excretion	20% excreted unchanged in urine; also biliary excretion	42–47% excreted unchanged in urine	Urine, bile, sweat, and saliva

MECHANISM OF ACTION

Anti-inflammatory and Immunomodulatory

- Stabilization of lysosomal membranes[6]
- Decrease proinflammatory cytokines—interleukin-1 (IL-1), IL-2, IL-6, and tumor necrosis factor (TNF-α).[6]
- Lysosomal pH is increased.
- Lysosomal protease activity is decreased.
- The binding of autoantigens to the class to major histocompatibility complex (MHC) is reduced.
- There is decreased stimulation of toll-like receptor (TLR) 9.
- TLRs 3, 7, and 8 activated
- There is increased loading of class 1 MHC antigens.

Antiproliferative

- Decreased lymphocyte proliferation
- Interference with natural killer cell activity
- Alteration of autoantibody production

Photoprotective Effect

- Antioxidant
- Bind to porphyrin → facilitate their clearance
- Solubilize and mobilize hepatic porphyrins and their clearance

INDICATIONS

FDA-approved Indications

- *Dermatologic*: Lupus erythematosus (in selected cases)[6]
- *Nondermatologic*:
  - Malaria (all three antimalarials)
  - Rheumatoid arthritis (HCQ)

Off-label Dermatological Uses

- *Photosensitive dermatoses*:
  - Porphyria cutanea tarda
  - Polymorphous light eruption (PMLE)
  - Discoid lupus erythematosus
  - Solar urticaria[6]
  - Dermatomyositis (cutaneous features)[6]
- *Granulomatous dermatoses*:
  - Sarcoidosis
  - Granuloma annulare (generalized)[6]
  - Rosacea
  - Lepra reactions type 1 and 2
  - Other granulomatous dermatoses
- *Panniculitis*:
  - Chronic erythema nodosum[6]
  - Lupus panniculitis[6]
- *Other dermatoses*:
  - Oral lichen planus
  - Chronic ulcerative stomatitis[4]
  - Reticular erythematous mucinosis
  - Atopic dermatitis
  - Urticarial vasculitis
  - Localized scleroderma
  - Follicular mucinosis
  - Primary Sjögren's syndrome[4]
  - Eosinophilic fasciitis[4]
  - Hereditary bullous epidermolysis[4]
  - Lichen sclerosus et atrophicus[4]
  - Morphea
  - Necrobiosis lipoidica[4]
  - Lymphocytic infiltrates

CONTRAINDICATIONS

- *Absolute*:
  - Hypersensitivity to the drug[6] (theoretical potential for cross-reactions between CQ and HCQ)
  - Retinal or visual field changes[6]
- *Relative*:
  - Severe blood dyscrasias
  - Significant hepatic dysfunction
  - Significant neurologic disorders
  - Psoriasis
- Pregnancy prescribing status—category C[7]

ADVERSE EFFECTS

- *Gastrointestinal*:
  - Nausea, vomiting, diarrhea, and flatulence
  - Liver function test—uncommon transaminase elevations
- *Ocular*:
  - *Reversible:*
    - Corneal deposition—halos, blurred vision, and photophobia
    - Loss of accommodation
    - Premaculopathy—retinal pigment deposition and paracentral and pericentral scotoma
  - *Irreversible:* True retinopathy—bull's eye pigment deposition, central scotoma, and visual acuity changes
- *Hematologic*:
  - Rarely agranulocytosis or pancytopenia
  - Hemolysis with glucose-6-phosphate dehydrogenase (G6PD) patients
  - Severe thrombocytopenia
- *Neuromuscular*:
  - Irritability, psychosis, and insomnia
  - Headache
  - Seizures, vertigo, tinnitus, and anxiety[4]
  - Skeletal muscle weakness[4]
- *Cardiac*: Drop in blood pressure, T-wave depression and inversion, and decreased cardiac muscle response[4]
- *Cutaneous*:
  - Bluish-gray pigmentation (sun-exposed areas)
  - Bleaching of hair roots[4]
  - Hypersensitivity reactions—morbilliform, lichenoid, eczema, urticarial, exfoliative erythroderma[4]
  - Psoriasis
  - Anhidrosis, alopecia, and nail changes[4]
  - Lemon yellow discoloration of the skin and sclera (quinacrine)

- *Others*:
    - Neuromyopathies and exacerbation of porphyria[4]
    - Teratogenic defects such as deafness, mental retardation, and convulsions[3]

DOSAGE

- CQ—3.5 mg/kg/day
- HCQ—6.5 mg/kg/day (risk of retinopathy seen when daily dosage exceeds 5 mg/kg/day for several years)
- HCQ—400 mg/day for dermatological diseases[8]
- HCQ—125 mg two to three times a week for 6–18 months is given for porphyria cutanea tarda.[3]

BASELINE MONITORING GUIDELINES

- *Ocular*:[3]
    - Baseline slit-lamp and fundoscopic examination and assessment of visual acuity
    - Visual field testing by both static and kinetic techniques with a 3-mm red test object
- *Laboratory*:[3]
    - Complete blood count (CBC)
    - G6PD screening (only needed in selected clinical settings)
    - Automated chemistry profile (emphasis on liver function tests)
    - Random or 24-hour urinary porphyrin screening (alternatively may order serum porphyrins)

FOLLOW-UP

- *Ocular*:
    - Reviewing subjective visual complaints, slit-lamp and fundoscopic test results, and visual acuity (in the first year of commencing therapy and in the absence of risk factors screening should be performed after 5 years).
    - Discontinuing CQ or HCQ treatment if bilateral field defects are confirmed.
- *Laboratory*:
    - CBC count (monthly for 3 months, then every 4–6 months).
    - Renal profile (baseline, after 1 month, after 3 months, and then every 4–6 months).

DRUG INTERACTIONS[6]

- CQ and HCQ should not be given together as it causes additive retinal toxicity.
- Antimalarials increase the levels of digoxin and D-penicillamine, metoprolol.
- CQ can reduce the bioavailability of ampicillin.
- Kaolin and antacids may decrease the absorption of CQ.

TABLE 2: Difference between chloroquine (CQ) and hydroxychloroquine (HCQ).

Characteristics	*CQ*	*HCQ*
Salt	Phosphate	Sulfate
Dose	250–500 mg/day	200–400 mg/day
Bioavailability	30%	75%
Ocular toxicity	More common	Less common
Gastrointestinal tolerance	Poor	Better
Excretion	Urine	Bile

DIFFERENCE BETWEEN CHLOROQUINE AND HYDROXYCHLOROQUINE

Table 2 presents difference between CQ and HCQ.

KEY POINTS

- The antimalarial drugs used for the treatment of dermatologic disorders include HCQ and CQ.
- HCQ and CQ both are 4-aminoquinoline compounds.
- Antimalarials have anti-inflammatory, immunomodulatory, antiproliferative, and photoprotective effect.
- The FDA-approved dermatological condition in which antimalarials can be used is lupus erythematosus.
- Bluish-gray pigmentation, bleaching of hair roots, hypersensitivity reactions, and psoriasis are some of the cutaneous adverse effects of antimalarials.
- HCQ dose is 400 mg/day for all dermatological diseases except porphyria cutanea tarda wherein the dose is 125 mg two to three times a week for 6–18 months.
- Overall, HCQ is better tolerated with less chances of ocular toxicity as compared to CQ.

REFERENCES

1. O'Neill P, Barton V, Ward S, Chadwick J. 4-Aminoquinolines: Chloroquine, Amodiaquine and Next-Generation Analogues. In: Staines H, Krishna S (Eds). Treatment and Prevention of Malaria. Germany: Springer; 2011. pp. 19-44.
2. Tanenbaum L. Antimalarial agents. Arch Dermatol. 1980; 116(5):587-91.
3. Koranda F. Antimalarials. J Am Acad Dermatol. 1981;4(6): 650-5.
4. Ochsendorf F. Use of antimalarials in dermatology. J Dtsch Dermatol Ges. 2010;8(10):829-45.
5. Callen J, Camisa C. Antimalarial agents. In: Wolverton S, Wu J (Eds). Comprehensive Dermatologic Drug Therapy, 4th edition. Amsterdam: Elsevier; 2020.
6. Kalia S, Dutz J. New concepts in antimalarial use and mode of action in dermatology. Dermatol Ther. 2007;20(4):160-74.
7. Phillips-Howard P, Wood D. The safety of antimalarial drugs in pregnancy. Drug Saf. 1996;14(3):131-45.
8. Fernandez A. Updated recommendations on the use of hydroxychloroquine in dermatologic practice. J Am Acad Dermatol. 2017;76(6):1176-82.

EXAMINATION QUESTIONS

1. Write a short note on hydroxychloroquine.
2. Discuss the applications and monitoring guidelines of hydroxychloroquine.

156 CHAPTER

Immunosuppressive Drugs in Dermatology

Sachi Gupta, Vrushali Lonikar

INTRODUCTION

Immunosuppressive and cytotoxic drugs are useful therapeutic tools in dermatology, which are being used with increasing frequency in various diseases.

Severe and life-threatening complications are associated with these agents and it is therefore imperative to have a complete understanding of their pharmacology and be able to recognize and treat the adverse reactions.

METHOTREXATE

Introduction

Methotrexate, an antimetabolite and antifolate drug, was first synthesized in 1940s for treatment of malignancies and subsequently found useful in psoriasis and many other dermatoses.

Pharmacokinetics and Pharmacodynamics

- *Absorption:* Enteric
- *Distribution:*
  - *Peak plasma concentration:* 1 hour
  - Throughout body, except brain
- *Metabolism:* Intracellular, hepatic
- *Elimination:* Kidneys.

Mode of Action

- Transported into cells as MTX-monoglutamate, which gets converted to MTX-polyglutamates (active form) that cannot get transported extracellularly leading to intracellular accumulation (basis for once weekly efficacy).
- These have three effects:
  1. *DNA synthesis*: Prevents conversion of folic acid into tetrahydrofolate by inhibiting *Dihydrofolate reductase* and the conversion of tetrahydrofolate into RNA/DNA, by inhibiting *Thymidylate synthase*
  2. *Immunosuppressive*: Inhibition of DNA synthesis in immune cells
  3. *Anti-inflammatory:* Block:
     - *AICART:* Causes increased adenosine (anti-inflammatory mediator)
     - *Methionine synthetase*: Decreases S-adenyl methionine (proinflammatory mediator)

Indications

FDA approved:

- *Psoriasis:* All subtypes, selection criteria vary
- Sézary syndrome

Off-label:

- Lupus erythematosus, dermatomyositis, systemic sclerosis, morphea
- Sarcoidosis
- Atopic dermatitis
- Bullous pemphigoid, pemphigus vulgaris
- Others

Contraindications

Absolute	*Relative*
Women attempting to conceive, pregnancy, breastfeeding	Male partners of women wishing to conceive
Bone marrow dysfunction or failure	Recent live vaccinations
Dialysis	Excessive alcohol intake
Severe renal dysfunction	Mild-to-moderate renal impairment
Severe hepatic dysfunction/ cirrhosis	Mild-to-moderate liver dysfunction
Immunodeficiency	History of hepatitis B, C
Active peptic ulceration	Gastritis
Concurrent trimethoprim	Patient unreliability
MTX hypersensitivity	
Active tuberculosis or hepatitis	
Pulmonary fibrosis or significantly reduced lung function	

Pregnancy: FDA Category X.

Side Effects and their Management

Side-effect	*Comment/Management*
Cutaneous	
T-Therapy PUVA-radiation recall	
-TEN	
X-Loss of hair (alopecia)	

Contd...

Contd...

Side-effect	*Comment/Management*
Systemic	
Pancytopenia	• Highest cause of mortality • Due to renal dysfunction, concomitant drugs such as NSAIDs, dehydration causing intercurrent infections
Hepatotoxicity	• Drug-induced hepatitis • Fibrosis (long-term use)
Nausea, anorexia (most common); vomiting, diarrhea	*Treatment:* Ondansetron, divided doses, parenteral
Reproductive	Teratogenic, reversible oligospermia
Pulmonary	• Acute pneumonitis—Rare, idiosyncratic at low doses, life-threatening • Pulmonary fibrosis on chest X-ray-Uncommon
Nephrotoxicity	High doses
Malignancy induction (lymphoma)	Unproven but vigilance advised
Overdose	• Mucositis, fever, diarrhea, erythema, ulceration 6–23 days Rx: Calcium folinate (folinic acid) within 24 hours-Initial dose up to 100 mg/m^2 IV infusion, if dose of MTX unknown. To be continued till MTX <0.05 µmol/L or side effects regressed

Drug Interactions

- *NSAID:* Increase MTX
- *Tetracyclines:* Increase MTX
- *Trimethoprim/Sulfamethoxazole:* Increase hematological toxicity
- *Dapsone:* Increase hematological toxicity
- *Retinoids:* Increase hepatotoxicity.

Formulations

- *Tablets:* 2.5 mg, 5.0 mg, 7.5 mg, 10 mg, 15 mg
- *Parenteral (subcutaneous, intramuscular, intravenous, intrathecal, intra-arterial):* 2 mL vials with 2.5 mg/mL to 25 mg/mL.

Dosage and Suggested Regimens

- *Test dose:*
  - A small test dose of 5–10 mg is given and full blood count (FBC) is checked after 1 week (to detect sensitivity)
  - If FBC remains stable, MTX can be administered once a week
- *Initiation dose*: 5 and 15 mg weekly
- *Increments:* 2.5 mg or 5 mg per week
- *Maintenance dose:* Once remission achieved, use lowest possible dose
- *Clinical considerations:*
  - *Folic acid supplementation:* Regimens vary from 5 mg daily to 5 mg weekly to be given on or excluding MTX days (no consensus).
  - Consider alternatives or subcutaneous, if minimal efficacy by 12–16 weeks
  - Maximum dose in psoriasis is 30 mg per week but usually controllable at 10–15 mg
  - Low risk of hepatotoxicity, if dose does not exceed 15 mg per week.

Investigations

- *Baseline:*
  - FBC
  - Liver function test (LFT)
  - Urea and electrolytes (U&Es)/estimated glomerular filtration rate (eGFR)
  - Hepatitis B, C serology
  - HIV serology, especially in high risk
  - Varicella zoster virus (VZV) serology (if no history of varicella)
  - Chest X-ray
  - Pregnancy test (where appropriate)
  - Procollagen III N-terminal peptide (PIIINP)
- *Monitoring:*
  - FBC, LFT, U&Es—every 1–2 weeks for the first month until steady dose reached, after which can be reduced to every 2–3 months
  - PIIINP-3 monthly
  - Recommended actions for abnormal test results

Total WBC count <3 × 10^9 cells L^{-1}	Withhold/decrease dose of MTX; consider discussing with hematologist
Neutrophils <1.0 × 10^9 cells L^{-1}	Withhold/decrease dose of MTX; consider discussing with hematologist
Platelets < 100 x cells L^{-1}	Withhold/decrease dose of MTX; consider discussing with hematologist
MCV >105 fL	Consider withholding/decreasing dose of MTX; check serum B$_{12}$, folate and thyroid function tests; consider discussing with hematologist
AST and ALT increased by less than two times the normal	Repeat LFTs in 2–4 weeks
AST and ALT greater than 2–3 times the normal	Withhold/decrease dose of MTX; consider other risk factors and consider discussing with gastroenterologist
New or increasing dyspnea or dry cough	Withhold/decrease dose of MTX; repeat chest X-ray and pulmonary and discuss with respiratory team function tests
Severe sore throat, abnormal bruising	Withhold MTX; check FBC immediately

Contd...

Contd...

If PIIINP: • >8 mg L^{-1} on two occasions • If three measurements are >4.2 mg L^{-1} in a 12-month period; or • If >10 mg L^{-1} on one occasion	Refer onward for further specialist assessment

*WBC: white blood cells; MTX: methotrexate; MCV: mean corpuscular volume; AST: aspartate aminotransferase; ALT: alanine transaminase; LFT: liver function test; FBC: full blood count.

Steps for Prescribing

1. Take a full history to establish indications and drug intake especially NSAIDs, cotrimoxazole
2. Rule out contraindications
3. Request and check baseline investigations
4. Additional considerations in special circumstances:
   a. *Children:*
      i. Indications—Same as adults; obesity-relative contraindication
      ii. Dose—0.2–0.4 mg per kg weekly; maximum 25 mg per week
      iii. Side effects similar to adults
      iv. PIIINP higher in growing children
   b. *Renal impairment:*
      i. Reduced dose; avoid in dialysis
   c. *Conception:*
      i. Women should not conceive whilst taking MTX and 3 months after stopping
      ii. Two forms of contraception throughout treatment
      iii. MTX to be avoided during breastfeeding
      iv. Men to delay planning family for at least 3 months following last dose
   d. Immunization—Live vaccines at least 4 weeks prior to starting
   e. Alcohol—Should be below national guidelines
   f. TB—Screen for latent or active TB and treat prior to commencing
5. *Counseling:*
   a. Weekly dose regime
   b. Contraception and pregnancy advise
   c. Clinical response takes 6–12 weeks
   d. Should seek urgent medical advice, if develop signs of toxicity:
      i. Fever/flu-like illness
      ii. Mouth ulceration
      iii. Tiredness
      iv. Unexplained bruising or bleeding gums
      v. Nausea, vomiting, abdominal pain or dark urine
      vi. Breathlessness or cough
6. Prescribe in appropriate dose and regimen
7. Monitoring and recommended actions

CYCLOSPORINE

Introduction

Cyclosporine is a neutral, hydrophobic, cyclic polypeptide containing 11 amino acids with a molecular weight of 1203 Da which was first isolated from the soil fungus *Tolypocladium inflatum* in 1970.

Pharmacokinetics and Pharmacodynamics

- *Metabolism:* Cytochrome P450 enzyme system
- *Elimination:* Bile and feces with a minor proportion (approximately 3–6%) being excreted in the urine.

Mode of Action

- Suppression of the T-helper (Th) cell response (Th1/Th2) by binding to cytoplasmic cyclophilin, thus inhibiting calcineurin phosphatase and reducing lymphocyte activation and production of lymphokines
- Inhibit the function of antigen-presenting cells
- Inhibition of the release of mast cell mediators including histamine and prostaglandins
- Inhibition of keratinocyte proliferation and keratinocyte cytokine secretion

Indications

Licensed	• Atopic dermatitis (in persons aged 16 years or older) • Psoriasis (in persons aged 16 years or older)
Good evidence outside its license	• Atopic dermatitis (in persons younger than 16 years) • Behçet disease • Chronic spontaneous (idiopathic) urticaria • Graft versus host disease • Palmoplantar pustulosis • Pyoderma gangrenosum
To be used as last resort and unlikely to be beneficial	• Alopecia areata • Discoid lupus erythematosus • Pemphigus foliaceous • Pemphigus vulgaris

Contraindications and Cautions

- Impaired renal function
- Uncontrolled hypertension
- Malignancy
- Active infection
- Concomitant UVB or PUVA therapy
- Severe hepatic dysfunction
- Immunodeficiency

Side Effects

Side effects	*Comment/Management*
Cutaneous	
Hypertrichosis	
Hirsutism	

Contd...

Contd...

Hyperplasia-gingival	
Hyperplasia-sebaceous	
Acneiform eruption	
Systemic	
Hypertension	
Nephrotoxicity, hyperuricemia	
Hypertriglyceridemia	
Metabolic	Hyperkalemia, hypercalciuria, hypomagnesemia
Malignancy	Increased risk of nonmelanoma skin cancers especially squamous cell carcinoma
Neurological	Paresthesia, tremors, lowered seizure threshold Hepatoxicity
Miscellaneous	Fatigue, headache, flu-like symptoms, GI disturbances

Drug Interactions

CYP450 inducers (reduce cyclosporine levels)	• Rifampicin • Phenobarbital • Carbamazepine • Phenytoin • St John's wort
CYP450 inhibitors (increase cyclosporine levels)	• Macrolide antibiotics (erythromycin, clarithromycin) • Ciprofloxacin • Fluoxetine • Ketoconazole/Itraconazole/ Fluconazole • Omeprazole • Cimetidine • Grapefruit juice
Acyclovir and other antiviral drugs	Increased risk of nephrotoxicity
Antimalarials	Increase plasma concentration of cyclosporine
Methotrexate	Reduce elimination of cyclosporine
Statins	Increased risk of myopathy
Nephrotoxic drugs	

Baseline Investigations and Monitoring

- Blood pressure should be monitored on at least two occasions, preferably 2 weeks apart for the first 2 months of treatment and then monthly thereafter.
- Physical examination to exclude infection and skin malignancy
- Serum creatinine eGFR and electrolytes should be measured every 2 weeks for the first 2 months then every 2 months.
- Complete blood count (CBC), electrolytes, uric acid, LFTs fasting lipids.

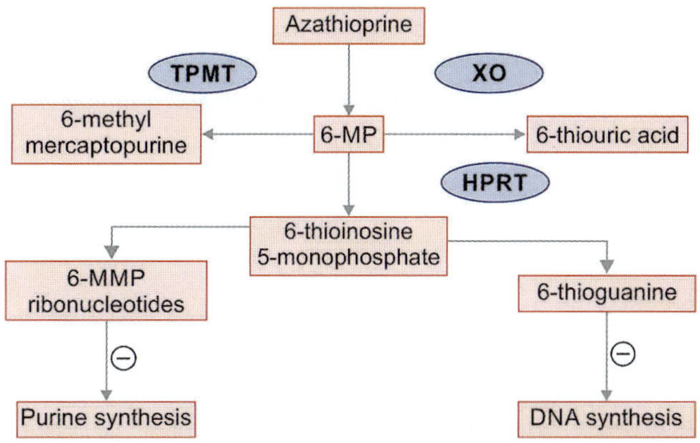

Fig. 1: Metabolism of azathioprine.
(6-MMP: 6-methyl mercaptopurine; HPRT: hypoxanthine guanine phosphoribosyl transferase; TPMT: thiopurine methyl transferase; XO: xanthine oxidase)

Dosing

2.5–5 mg/kg per day in two divided doses.

AZATHIOPRINE

Introduction

Azathioprine (AZA) is an antimetabolite thiopurine analog drug with immunomodulating action.

Pharmacokinetics and Pharmacodynamics and Mode of Action

- Following oral administration, azathioprine is rapidly, and almost completely absorbed from the gut.
- AZA undergoes rapid nonenzymatic conversion to 6-mercaptopurine (6-MP), the active compound, and imidazole derivatives which compete with their endogenous counterparts in many biochemical pathways thus resulting in immunosuppressive effect and cytotoxicity.
- 6-MP has a long half-life and is metabolized by three competing pathways **(Fig. 1)**.
- Impairment of these pathways, due to inherent low enzyme activity or drug interactions can lead to accumulation of potentially toxic levels of thioguanine nucleotides and the risk of life-threatening bone marrow suppression.

Indications

Licensed	• Systemic lupus erythematosus • Dermatomyositis/polymyositis • Pemphigus vulgaris
Unlicensed	• Bullous pemphigoid • Atopic dermatitis • Psoriasis • Lichen planus • Chronic actinic dermatitis • Pyoderma gangrenosum • Pityriasis rubra pilaris • Wegener's granulomatosis • Cutaneous vasculitis

TABLE 1: Recommended dose of azathioprine according to thiopurine methyl transferase (TPMT) activity.

TPMT activity	*Recommended dose of azathioprine*
<5.1 U/mL	Do not administer
5.1–13.7 U/mL	<0.5 mg/kg/day
13.8–18.0 U/mL	<1.5 mg/kg/day
18.1–26.0 U/mL	<2.5 mg/kg/day
26.1–40 U/mL	<3.0 mg/kg/day

Side Effects

Cutaneous	*Systemic*
Pellagroid dermatitis	• Gastrointestinal • Idiosyncratic hypersensitivity reactions • Hepatitis • Hematological—bone marrow suppression • Malignancy • Infection • Pancreatitis

Dosing

- Recommended dosage for dermatological indications is 1–3 mg/kg daily, adjusted within these limits according to response
- Recommended dose of azathioprine according to thiopurine methyl transferase (TPMT) activity is given in **Table 1**.

Baseline Investigations and Monitoring

- Weekly monitoring of CBC and LFTs for the first 4 weeks of therapy, or until the maintenance dose is achieved; reducing to a minimum of once every 3 months for the duration of therapy.
- Increase in dosage of AZA should be accompanied by return to weekly CBC and LFTs for 4 weeks, reducing to a minimum of once monthly or every 2 months for the duration of therapy.

Contraindications and Cautions

- Hypersensitivity to AZA or 6-MP
- Very low/absent or unknown TPMT levels
- Severe infection
- Pancreatitis
- Severely impaired hepatic function or bone marrow depression
- Pregnancy (unless benefits outweigh risks)
- Lactation
- Malignancy.

Drug Interactions

Angiotensin-converting enzyme (ACE) inhibitors	Increase risk of anemia/leukopenia in patients with renal impairment
Allopurinol	• Potentially life-threatening myelotoxicity due to inhibition of XO and accumulation of active metabolites • In case of co-administration, dose of azathioprine should be reduced to one-quarter or one-third of routine dose with careful hematological monitoring
Live-attenuated vaccines	
Ribavirin	Severe pancytopenia
Warfarin	• Resistance reported • Increased warfarin dosing with close monitoring of anticoagulation required
Drugs causing bone marrow suppression	Other immunosuppressants, trimethoprim, cotrimoxazole, clozapine

CYCLOPHOSPHAMIDE

Introduction

Cyclophosphamide is an antineoplastic drug from the nitrogen mustard group of alkylating agents.

Pharmacokinetics and Pharmacodynamics

- *Absorption:* Well absorbed after oral administration with bioavailability of more than 75%
- *Metabolism:* Liver to active metabolites by specific cytochrome P450 isoenzymes
- *Excretion:* Urine and have irritant effect on bladder mucosa.

Mode of Action

- Inhibition of DNA replication and cell division by DNA cross-linking
- Suppression of T cell mediated and humoral immunity.

Indications

Licensed	Advanced mycosis fungoides
Unlicensed	Immunobullous diseases—Pemphigus (vulgaris, foliaceus), pemphigoid (bullous, cicatricial)
	Vasculitis—refractory cutaneous vasculitis, polyarteritis nodosa, ANCA-associated vasculitis, cryoglobulinemic vasculitis, autoimmune connective tissue disease associated vasculitis
	Connective tissue diseases—systemic and cutaneous lupus erythematosus, dermatomyositis, Behçet disease Pyoderma gangrenosum

Side Effects

Cutaneous	
Alopecia (anagen effluvium)	
Diffuse hyperpigmentation (palmoplantar, nail)	
Stevens-Johnson syndrome/ toxic epidermal necrolysis (SJS/TEN)	

Contd...

Contd...

Systemic	
Hematological	Leukopenia, anemia, thrombocytopenia
Bladder toxicity and hemorrhagic cystitis	
Malignancy	Increased risk of bladder cancer, acute leukemia, nonmelanoma skin cancer, solid tumors
Infection	
Gastrointestinal	Nausea, vomiting, anorexia
Cardiac and pulmonary	Pulmonary fibrosis, interstitial pneumonitis, cardiomyopathy
Hypersensitivity	
Infertility	Amenorrhea, azoospermia, irreversible sterility

Dosing

- 50–200 mg/day rarely more than 2.5 mg/kg/day
- Pulse regimen with corticosteroids in pemphigus:
    - Days 1–3, 100 mg dexamethasone in 500 mL of 5% glucose as an IV infusion over 2 hours
    - Day 2, 500 mg of cyclophosphamide added to dexamethasone IV infusion
    - Days 4–28, oral cyclophosphamide 50 mg daily with conventional daily doses of oral corticosteroids
    - The cycle is repeated every 28 days until clinical remission is achieved and oral steroids are withdrawn.

Baseline Investigations and Monitoring

- CBC weekly for first month 2 weekly for next 2 months then monthly consider to decrease to every 3 months if stable after 3–6 months
- Renal function, LFTs monthly for 3–6 months, then every 3 months if stable
- Urine analysis monthly after 3–6 months every 3 months if stable
- Urine cytology if hematuria or after cumulative dose of 50 g.

Contraindications

- Previous urinary malignancy
- Hemorrhagic cystitis
- Bone marrow suppression/severe leukopenia
- Pregnancy and lactation
- Hypersensitivity to cyclophosphamide
- Serious underlying infection.

Cautions

- Previous or concurrent mediastinal irradiation—risk of cardiotoxicity
- Hepatic impairment—reduce dose
- Hepatitis B and C virus
- Previous tuberculosis (TB) or risk of TB
- Renal impairment—dose reduction
- Elderly—dose reduction.

Drug Interactions

Sulphonyl urea	Potentiation of hypoglycemic effects leading to altered glycemic control
Allopurinol	Increased bone marrow toxicity
Barbiturates and clozapine	Increased risk of agranulocytosis
Digoxin	Absorption reduced due to cyclophosphamide
Itraconazole and fluconazole	Increased risk of adverse effects
Live vaccinations	Contraindicated during and for 3 months after cyclophosphamide therapy

MYCOPHENOLATE MOFETIL

Introduction

Mycophenolate mofetil (MMF) an ester form of mycophenolic acid (MPA), was synthesized as a prodrug with greater bioavailability and lesser side effects than MPA. It is being increasingly recognized as an immunosuppressant with long-term safety profile and relative lack of toxicity.

Pharmacokinetics and Pharmacodynamics

- Absorption and bioavailability
    - *Peak levels:* 6–12 hours
    - *Bioavailable:* Nearly 100%
    - *Protein binding:* 97%
- *Elimination:*
    - *Half-life:* 16
    - *Metabolism:* MPA (active metabolite), MPAG (nonactive)
    - *Excretion:* Urine

Mode of Action

- There are two mechanisms for purine synthesis in nucleated cells-Salvage pathway and the De novo pathway. T- and B-lymphocytes are unique in being solely dependent on the latter.
- MMF (pro-drug) gets converted into MPA (active form) which blocks inosine monophosphate dehydrogenase, in activated lymphocytes, which is a key enzyme of the de novo pathway.
- Thus, production of purine metabolites necessary for proliferation of lymphocytes, is disrupted leading to selective immunosuppression whilst having minimal effects on other cells.

Indications

FDA approved

Renal, cardiac and liver allograft rejection prevention

Non-FDA approved:

- Psoriasis
- Dermatitis

- Bullous dermatoses
- Lupus erythematosus, dermatomyositis, systemic sclerosis
- Vasculitis, pyoderma gangrenosum
- GVHD
- Others—Lichen planus

Contraindications

Absolute	*Relative*
Pregnancy (teratogenic)	Lactation
Drug allergy	Peptic ulcer disease
	Hepatic/Renal disease
	Azathioprine
	Lesch-Nyhan and Kelley-Seegmiller syndromes

Pregnancy: FDA Category D

Side Effects and their Management

Lesser nephrotoxic, hepatotoxic, and neurotoxic than other immunosuppressants.

Cutaneous	*Comment*
Not reported	
Systemic	
Nausea, vomiting and diarrhea (Most common)	Mild *Treatment:* Divided dosing; with food; MPA delayed release tablets
Systemic	*Comment*
Myelosuppression	• Mild, dose-dependent • Rx: Reversible with dose reduction or discontinuation
Urinary (urgency, frequency, dysuria)	• Decrease in frequency after one year • Does not cause nephrotoxicity
Infections	In transplant patients
Carcinogenicity (Lymphoma, nonmelanoma)	Controversial
Neurological (Weakness, fatigue, tinnitus)	

Drug Interactions

- *Antacids:* Decrease MMF
- *Amoxicillin:* Decrease MMF
- *Anti-inflammatory (Salicylates):* Increase MMF
- *Acyclovir and valaciclovir:* Levels increased by MMF
- *Azathioprine:* Increased toxicity
- *Cyclosporine:* Levels increased of MMF
- *Contraceptives (Hormonal)*: Efficacy reduced by MMF.

Formulations

- *Capsules:* 250 mg, Tablets: 500 mg
- *Oral suspension:* 1 g/5 mL
- *IV injections:* 500 mg vials
- *MPA delayed release tablets:* 180 mg, 360 mg.

Dosage and Suggested Regimens

- *Initiation dose*: 500 mg BD
- *Increments:* 500 mg
- *Maintenance dose:* 1 g BD, max 1.5 g BD.

Investigations

- *Baseline:*
  - FBC and differential WBC and platelets
  - LFT
  - Urea and electrolytes and creatinine
  - Hepatitis B, C serology
  - HIV serology, especially in high risk
  - VZV serology (if no history of varicella)
  - Chest X-ray
  - Pregnancy test (where appropriate)
  - Cutaneous examination to rule out malignancy; lymphadenopathy, breast lumps and organomegaly; up-to-date cervical screening
- *Monitoring:* FBC, LFT, U&Es- weekly for 4 weeks and then twice a month for 2 months and then monthly for the first year and then 3 monthly
- *Recommended actions:*
  - Total WBC <4 × 10^9/L—Stop or withhold
  - Neutrophil count <2 × 10^9/L—Stop or withhold
  - Platelet count <150 × 10^9/L—Stop or withhold
  - ALT/AST> 2 x the normal limit—Stop or withhold
  - Hypogammaglobulinemia—Stop or withhold.

FUMARIC ACID ESTERS

Introduction

In 1959, German chemist, Schweckendieck first reported effective use of fumaric acid esters (FAE) in psoriasis and in 1994 it was approved in Germany for it, where it continues to be widely used as a first line drug.

Mode of Action

- Immunomodulatory without immunosuppressive actions
- *In psoriasis:* Shift toward IL-10 instead of IL-12, 23 and stimulation of IL-4 producing Th-2 cells.

Indication

Psoriasis (only licensed in Germany).

Contraindications

- Chronic gastritis, peptic ulcer disease
- Pregnancy and lactation
- Severe liver disease
- Severe kidney disease.

Pregnancy: FDA Category C

Side Effects and their Management

	Comments
Diarrhea, abdominal pain, nausea	Very common (Up to two-third of patients) Worst in first 3 months, improves with time Rx: Give with milk/dairy products
Flushing	Mild to severe Rx-Aspirin

Drug Interactions

Not known; avoid nephrotoxic drugs

Formulations

Tablet: 30 mg, 120 mg.

KEY POINTS

	Methotrexate	*Cyclosporine*	*Azathioprine*	*Cyclophosphamide*	*MMF*
MOA	1. *DNA synthesis:* Inhibits a. Dihydrofolate reductase b. Thymidylate synthase 2. *Anti-inflammatory:* Inhibits a. AICART b. Methionine synthetase	It inhibits *calcineurin* which is present within T-cells and responsible for its activation and production of *IL-2*	Is a prodrug of 6MP, which undergoes metabolism by 3 competing enzymatic pathways: 1. *TPMT*→Inactive metabolite 2. *XO*→ Inactive metabolite 3. *HGPRT*→Active metabolite inhibits purine synthesis (antiproliferative)	Inhibits DNA synthesis by causing *DNA cross-linking*	Blocks purine synthesis by inhibiting *IMPDH* (Inosine monophosphate dehydrogenase)
Dose	5–15 mg/week	2.5–5 mg/kg/day in two divided dose	1–3 mg/kg/day	1–2 mg/kg/day	30–40 mg/kg/day
Pregnancy category	Category X	Category C	Category D	Category D	Category C
Side effects					
Skin	*M*-Mouth ulcers; Ulcers in psoriatic plaques *T*-Therapy PUVA-Radiation recall; TEN *X*-Loss of hair (alopecia)	*Hy*pertrichosis *Hi*rsutism *Hy*perplasia—gingival Acneiform eruption	Pellagroid dermatitis	Nail—Pigmentation Hair—Anagen effluvium Teeth—Pigmented bands	Not reported
Systemic (Most common)	Nausea, anorexia		Nausea, vomiting	Nausea, vomiting	Nausea, vomiting, Diarrhea
		*Hy*pertension		Cardiac arrhythmias	
		*Hy*pertriglyceridemia			
	Hepatotoxicity		Hepatotoxicity		
	Pancytopenia		Pancytopenia	Pancytopenia	
				Hemorrhagic cystitis	Urinary
		Nephrotoxic	Nephrotoxicity		
Gonadal dysfunction	Yes		No	Yes	

BIBLIOGRAPHY

1. Archer CB, Maibach HI, Wakelin SH (Eds). Handbook of Systemic Drug Treatment in Dermatology, 2nd edition. CRC Press, 2015.
2. Berth-Jones J, Exton LS, Ladoyanni E, Mohd Mustapa MF, Tebbs VM, Yesudian PD, Levell NJ. British Association of Dermatologists guidelines for the safe and effective prescribing of oral ciclosporin in dermatology 2018. Br J Dermatol. 2019;180(6):1312-38.

3. Meggitt SJ, Anstey AV, Mohd Mustapa MF, Reynolds NJ, Wakelin S. British Association of Dermatologists' guidelines for the safe and effective prescribing of azathioprine 2011. Br J Dermatol. 2011;165(4):711-34.
4. Warren RB, Weatherhead SC, Smith CH, Exton LS, Mohd Mustapa MF, Kirby B, Yesudian PD. British Association of Dermatologists' Guidelines for the safe and effective prescribing of methotrexate for skin disease 2016. Br J Dermatol. 2016;175(1):23-44.
5. Wolverton, Stephen E. Comprehensive Dermatologic Drug Therapy. Philadelphia: Saunders, 2001.

EXAMINATION QUESTIONS

1. Write a short note on systemic steroids.
2. Classify systemic steroids and briefly describe their applications.

157 CHAPTER Antibiotics in Relation to Dermatology

Sonal Singh, Aarti Sarda, Abhishek De

PENICILLIN

Penicillin G (benzylpenicillin) was discovered in 1928 and is obtained from *Penicillium chrysogenum*. There are many semisynthetic penicillins and classified as in **Table 1**.

CLASSIFICATION

Pharmacokinetics

As penicillin undergoes gastric acid degradation, therefore it is taken 1 hour before or after a meal and its elimination half life is <1.5 hours.[1] Except for nafcillin, oxacillin, and piperacillin, which are eliminated through the biliary system, rest are excreted renally **(Table 2)**.

CEPHALOSPORINS

It is mainly derived from mold *Cephalosporium acremonium*.

Antimicrobial Activity

Generations of cephalosporin based on their antimicrobial activity spectrum is given in **Table 3**.[5]

TABLE 1: Classification of penicillins.

Source	*Route of administration*	*Based on spectrum of activity*	*Resistant to hydrolyzing enzyme*	*Resistant to acids*
Natural	*Oral*	*Narrow spectrum*	*Resistant to beta-lactamase*	*Acid stable*
Penicillin G	*Amoxycillin*	Methicillin	Methicillin	Penicillin G
Penicillin V	Oxacillin	Oxacillin	Oxacillin	Oxacillin
Biosynthetic	*Cloxacillin*	Dicloxacillin	Cloxacillin	Cloxacillin
Penicillin G	Dicloxacillin	Nafcillin	Dicloxacillin	Ampicillin
Penicillin V	*Ampicillin*	*Broad spectrum*	*Nonresistant to beta lactamase*	*Acid unstable*
Penicillin X	*Parenteral*	Ampicillin	Penicillin G	Ticarcillin
Penicillin F	*Penicillin G*	*Amoxycillin*	Penicillin V	Methicillin
Penicillin K	Methicillin	*Intermediate spectrum*	Ampicillin	Piperacillin
Semisynthetic	*Nafcillin*	Penicillin G and V	Amoxycillin	
Oxacillin, cloxacillin, dicloxacillin, ampicillin, methicillin	Carbenicillin, *ticarcillin*	*Extended spectrum*	Carbenicillin	
		Carbenicillin, ticarcillin		

TABLE 2: Uses and adverse effects of penicillin.

Dermatologic uses	*Adverse effects*	*Drug interactions*
• Antibacterial indications such as erysipelas, cellulitis, impetigo, folliculitis, furunculosis, bacterial paronychia, ecthyma, anthrax, lymes, and actinomycosis • Staphylococcal scalded skin syndrome	• GI disturbances including nausea and antibiotic-associated diarrhea • Cholestasis	Probenecid retards its renal excretion
STD—syphilis and chlamydial infections	Seizures, electrolyte disturbances	Alters the anticoagulant effects of warfarin
To treat dermal fibrosis in patients with circumscribed and systemic sclerosis	Hemolytic anemia, neutropenia, and platelet dysfunction	
• Pityriasis rubra pilaris • Oral and genital aphthae and erythema nodosum-like lesions in patients with Behçet's disease • Guttate psoriasis[2,3]	• Hypersensitivity reactions, local skin reactions, phlebitis, myositis, and vasospasm[4] • Shore nails	

(GI: gastrointestinal; STD: sexually transmitted diseases)

TABLE 3: Generations of cephalosporin based on their antimicrobial activity spectrum.

First generation (active against gram-positive cocci)		*Second generation (increase activity against gram-negative, lesser against gram positive)*	
Oral	*Parenteral*	*Oral*	*Parenteral*
Cephalexin	Cephalothin	Cefaclor	Cefuroxime
Cephradine	Cefazolin	Cefuroxime axetil	Cefoxitin
Cefadroxil		Cefprozil	
Third generation (good against both)		*Fourth generation (broad spectrum)*	
Oral	*Parenteral*	*Parenteral*	
Cefixime	Cefotaxime	Cefepime	
Cefdinir	Ceftizoxime	Cefpirome	
Ceftibuten	Ceftriaxone		
Cefpodoxime proxetil	Ceftazidime		
Ceftamet pivoxil	Cefoperazone		

TABLE 4: Uses and adverse effects of cephalosporins.

Dermatological uses	*Adverse effects*	*Drug interactions*
Impetigo, folliculitis, furuncles, carbuncles, cellulitis, ecthyma, erysipelas	• GI toxicities, nausea, vomiting, or diarrhea, antibiotic-associated colitis • Mild elevation of liver transaminases[8]	• Disulfiram-like reactions • Prolong prothrombin time
Postoperative wound infections, necrotizing fasciitis	• Hypersensitivity reactions, skin eruption • Vaginal infections from overgrowth of *Candida* spp.	Aminoglycosides or potent diuretics increase the risk of nephrotoxicity
Diabetic foot infections and Lyme disease[6,7]	• Headache and insomnia • Hemolytic anemia[9]	
STD	Nephrotoxicity	

(GI: gastrointestinal; STD: sexually transmitted diseases)

TABLE 5: Uses and adverse effects of β-lactam and β-lactamases inhibitor combinations.

Dermatologic indications	*Adverse effects*	*Drug interactions*
Polymicrobial infections	GI complaints—diarrhea, transient elevation of transaminases. Cholestatic injury	Oral probenecid slows the rate of renal tubular secretion
Animal or human bites	Positive Coombs' test, thrombocytopenia, neutropenia, and eosinophilia[12]	
Diabetic foot ulcers, infected decubiti, and burn wounds[11]	Hypersensitivity reactions	

Pharmacokinetics

The absorption of cephalosporins vary greatly and is dependent on food intake. First- and second-generation cephalosporins are excreted mainly by the kidneys and therefore dose needs to be adjusted in renal insufficiency **(Table 4)**.

β-LACTAM AND β-LACTAMASES INHIBITOR COMBINATIONS

Amoxicillin/Clavulanate and Others

β-lactamase enzymes irreversibly hydrolyze the amide bond of the β-lactam ring. The production of a β-lactamase is transferable and is done by either chromosomal or plasmid genes. β-lactamase inhibitors inhibit β-lactamase produced by *Enterobacteriaceae*, *Staphylococcus aureus*, and gram-negative anaerobes. These include β-lactam antibiotic and β-lactamase inhibitor include amoxicillin-clavulanate, ampicillin-sulbactam, ticarcillin-clavulanate, and piperacillin-tazobactam.

Antibacterial Activity

- Active against—methicillin-susceptible *Staphylococcus aureus* (MSSA), *Haemophilus* spp., *Klebsiella* spp., *Escherichia coli*, *Proteus* spp., *Bacteroides fragilis*.
- Not active against—*Pseudomonas aeruginosa*, *Enterobacter*, and *Citrobacter* spp.[10]

Pharmacokinetics (Table 5)

Rapidly absorbed orally, with peak concentrations achieved 40–60 minutes after ingestion. Dosage adjustment is required in patients with renal disease.

CARBAPENEMS AND MONOBACTAMS

Both of these drug groups have limited applicability in dermatology as they are available only in parenteral forms.

Carbapenems

Imipenem is combined with cilastatin, a natural inhibitor of renal dehydropeptidase enzyme. Other carbapenems include meropenem and ertapenem. They are active against most aerobic and anaerobic gram-negative bacteria.[13]

Monobactams

Aztreonam, the only monobactam, which exhibits an antimicrobial activity limited to aerobic gram-negative organisms. Aztreonam can be safely given to patient allergic to penicillin.[14]

OTHER SYSTEMIC AGENTS AFFECTING THE BACTERIAL CELL WALL

Vancomycin

Vancomycin, a glycopeptide antibiotic derived from the actinomycetes, *Streptomyces orientalis*, inhibits synthesis of the bacterial cell wall.[15]

Pharmacology and Antibacterial Activity

Antibacterial spectrum includes gram-positive organisms, methicillin-resistant *Staphylococcus aureus* (MRSA) and methicillin-resistant coagulase-negative *Staphylococci*.

Pharmacokinetics

It is given parenterally and is used orally only for the treatment of *Clostridium difficile* diarrhea. The half-life is 4–8 hours. Dose modification is required in patients with marked renal insufficiency **(Table 6)**.

MACROLIDES

- Macrolides include erythromycin, azithromycin, and clarithromycin.
- Macrolides are bacteriostatic antibiotics which inhibit RNA-dependent protein synthesis.[16]
- They also have anti-inflammatory properties which help in inflammatory facial dermatoses.[17]

Pharmacology and Antimicrobial Activity

They are effective against most gram-positive organisms. Clarithromycin and azithromycin also act against gram-negative pathogens.

Pharmacokinetics

They are given orally and undergo renal elimination whereas azithromycin is primarily metabolized by the liver **(Table 7)**.

FLUOROQUINOLONES

They inhibit DNA gyrase and topoisomerase IV thus inhibiting DNA replication.[18,19]

Pharmacology and Antimicrobial Activity

They act against gram-negative organisms and some gram-positive bacteria. They are active against *Mycobacterium* species.

TABLE 6: Uses and adverse effects of vancomycin.

Dermatologic indications	*Adverse effects*	*Drug interactions*
SSTI	Red man syndrome and shock secondary to histamine release	With aminoglycosides increases the risk of nephrotoxicity
HA-MRSA	• Toxic epidermal necrolysis • Linear IgA bullous dermatosis • Renal failure • Fever, neutropenia, thrombocytopenia	Increase the activity of nondepolarizing muscle relaxants

(HA-MSRA: hospital-associated methicillin-resistant *Staphylococcus aureus*; SSTI: skin and soft-tissue infections)

TABLE 7: Uses and adverse effects of macrolides.

Dermatologic indications	*Adverse effects*	*Drug interactions*
Pyodermas, abscesses ulcers	Nausea, abdominal pain, and diarrhea	Inhibits the hepatic and intestinal CYP3A4
Lyme disease, erythrasma, anthrax	Hepatic or renal dysfunction	
Nongonococcal urethritis, syphilis, chancroid, and lymphogranuloma venereum	Risk of hearing loss	
Leprosy, atypical mycobacterial skin infection	Allergic reactions	
• Acne vulgaris, rosacea, perioral dermatitis • Guttate psoriasis • Confluent and reticulated papillomatosis • Pityriasis rosea	Cardiac conduction defect	

TABLE 8: Uses and adverse effects of fluoroquinolones.

Dermatologic indications	*Adverse effects*	*Drug interactions*
USSTI	• GI tract—such as nausea, vomiting, and diarrhea • Liver toxicity	Decreased bioavailability with calcium, aluminum and magnesium-containing antacid
Gonorrhea	Hypersensitivity and photosensitivity reactions	Metabolism is reduced of theophylline, warfarin, cyclosporine
Donovanosis and chancroid, cutaneous anthrax	Headaches, dizziness, agitation, and sleep disturbances	Increase the risk of torsades de pointes

(GI: gastrointestinal; USSTI: uncomplicated skin and soft-tissue infections)

TABLE 9: Uses and adverse effects of tetracyclines.

Dermatologic indications	*Adverse effects*	*Drug interactions*
Acne vulgaris, rosacea	• Acute vestibular side effects • Benign intracranial hypertension	Increase pharmacologic effects of warfarin, lithium, theophylline, digoxin
Rickettsial diseases, spirochete atypical mycobacterial infections	• *GI tract:* Nausea, vomiting, and abdominal discomfort • Hepatitis and pancreatitis	Pseudotumor cerebri with retinoids
Immunobullous dermatoses	• Photosensitivity • Dyspigmentation	
Granulomatous dermatoses, oral lichen planus	Hypersensitivity reaction	

(GI: gastrointestinal)

Pharmacokinetics

With the exception of norfloxacin, the oral bioavailability of the FQ is good. Half-lives vary from 3 to 13 hours. FQ are mainly excreted renally, and thus require dosage adjustment in renal disease patients **(Table 8)**.

TETRACYCLINES

Tetracyclines (TCNs)—doxycycline and minocycline.

Bacteriostatic and inhibit bacterial protein synthesis. They have a variety of direct and indirect anti-inflammatory properties as they inhibit production of neutrophil chemoattractants, neutrophil migration, granuloma formation, and multiple matrix metalloproteinases (MMP).[20,21]

Pharmacology and Antibacterial Activity

They show activity against many gram-positive and gram-negative bacteria.

Pharmacokinetics (Table 9)

Tetracyclines are lipophilic and are well absorbed regardless of food intake.

Renal failure prolongs the half-life of most TCNs, except doxycycline.

RIFAMYCINS

Rifampin inhibits bacterial DNA-dependent RNA polymerase. Rifampin exhibits a broad-spectrum of antibiotic activity against *Mycobacterium* spp., staphylococci, *Neisseria*, *Haemophilus influenzae*.

TABLE 10: Uses and adverse effects of rifamycins.

Dermatologic indications	*Adverse effects*	*Drug interactions*
Mycobacterial infections	• Orange-red discoloration of liquid body excretions • CNS side effects such as headache • GI discomfort	Potent inducer of multiple CYP isoforms, including CYP1A2, 2C9, 2C19, 2D6, and 3A4
Cutaneous leishmaniasis rhinoscleroma	*Immunologic side effects:* Cutaneous, gastrointestinal and flu-like thrombocytopenia, hemolytic anemia, etc.	
Bartonella	Liver toxicity	

(CNS: central nervous system; GI: gastrointestinal)

PHARMACOKINETICS (TABLE 10)

Gastrointestinal (GI) absorption is reduced by when taken with food. It has extensive hepatic metabolism.

FOLATE SYNTHESIS INHIBITORS

Trimethoprim-sulfamethoxazole

Trimethoprim-sulfamethoxazole (TMP-SMX) consists of dihydrofolate reductase inhibitor (TMP) and a dihydropteroate synthetase inhibitor (SMX).

Clinical Use and Dermatologic Indications

- Acne vulgaris
- Hidradenitis suppurativa
- Granuloma inguinale

Adverse effects:
- GI and CNS side effects
- Hypersensitivity reactions
- Hematologic toxicity

LINCOSAMIDES

Clindamycin

Clindamycin (lincosamide) is obtained from *Streptomyces lincolnensis*. It inhibits ribosomal translocation.

Pharmacology and Antimicrobial Activity

Active against aerobic gram-positive cocci and variety of anaerobes.

Pharmacokinetics

Clindamycin can be administered orally or parenterally, metabolized in the liver, with a plasma half-life of 2.4–3.0 hours in adults.

Clinical use and dermatology indications:
- Uncomplicated skin and soft-tissue infections (USSTI)
- Deep soft-tissue infections

Adverse effects:
- Nausea, vomiting
- Metallic taste
- Arthritis
- Thick mucosal discharge

OXAZOLIDINONES

Linezolid

It binds to the 23S portion of the 50S ribosomal subunit active against MRSA, vancomycin intermediate, and resistant strains of staphylococci, and vancomycin-resistant enterococci.

Adverse effects: Elevations in serum transaminases and creatinine, and myelosuppression.

REFERENCES

1. Kadurina M, Bocheva G, Tonev S. Penicillin and semisynthetic penicillins in dermatology. Clin Dermatol. 2003;21(1):12-23.
2. Naldi L, Chalmers RJ. Psoriasis. In: Williams H, Bigby M, Diepgen T, Herxheimer A, Naldi L, Rzany B (Eds). Evidenced-Based Dermatology, 2nd edition. Malden, Massachusetts: Blackwell Publishers; 2008. p. 183.
3. Vincent F, Ross JB, Dalton M, Wort AJ. A therapeutic trial of the use of penicillin V or erythromycin with or without rifampin in the treatment of psoriasis. J Am Acad Dermatol. 1992; 26(3 Pt 2):458-61.
4. Torres MJ, Blanca M. The complex clinical picture of β-lactam hypersensitivity: Penicillins, cephalosporins, monobactams, carbapenems, and clavams. Medical Clinics of North America. 2010;94(4):805-20.
5. Del Rosso JQ. Cephalosporins in dermatology. Clin Dermatol. 2003;21(1):24-32.
6. Gustaferro CA, Steckelberg JM. Cephalosporin anti-microbial agents and related compounds. Mayo Clin Proc. 1991;66: 1064-73.
7. Nadelman RB, Luger SW, Frank E, Wisniewski M, Collins JJ, Wormser GP. Comparison of cefuroxime axetil and doxycycline in the treatment of early Lyme disease. Ann Intern Med. 1992;117(4):273-80.
8. Steed ME, Rybak MJ. Ceftaroline: A new cephalosporin with activity against resistant Gram-positive pathogens. Pharmacotherapy. 2010;30(4):375-89.
9. Lopez AJ, O'Keefe P, Morrissey M, Pickleman J. Ceftriaxone-induced cholelithiasis. Ann Intern Med. 1991;115(9):712-4.
10. Maddux MS. Effects of beta-lactamase-mediated antimicrobial resistance: The role of beta-lactamase inhibitors. Pharmacotherapy. 1991;11(2 (Pt 2)):40S-50S.
11. Lee N, Yuen KY, Kumana CR. Clinical role of beta-lactam/beta-lactamase inhibitor combinations. Drugs. 2003;63(14):1511-24.
12. Sensakovic JW, Smith LG. Beta-lactamase inhibitor combinations. Med Clin North Am. 1995;79(4):695-704.
13. Hellinger WC, Brewer NS. Imipenem. Mayo Clin Proc. 1991; 66:1074-81.
14. Zhanel GG, Johanson C, Embil JM, Noreddin A, Gin A, Vercaigne L, et al. Ertapenem: Review of a new carbapenem. Expert Rev Anti-infect Ther. 2005;3(1):23-39.
15. Finch RG, Eliopoulos GM. Safety and efficacy of glycopeptide antibiotics. J Antimicro Chemother. 2005;55(Suppl 2):5-13.
16. Fernandez-Martin J, Leport C, Moriat P, Meyohas MC, Chauvin JP, Vilde JL. Pyrimethamine-clarithromycin combination for therapy of acute toxoplasma encephalitis in patients with AIDS. Antimicrob Agents Chemother. 1991;35:2049-52.
17. Franck N, Cabie A, Villette B, Amor B, Lessana-Leibowitch M, Escande JP. Treatment of Mycobacterium chelonae induced skin infection with clarithromycin. J Am Acad Dermatol. 1993;28(6):1019-20.
18. Sable D, Murakawa GJ. Quinolones in dermatology. Clin Dermatol. 2003;21(1):56-63.
19. MacDougall C, Harpe SE, Powell JP, Johnson CK, Edmond MB, Polk RE. *Pseudomonas aeruginosa, Staphylococcus aureus*, and fluoroquinolone use. Emerg Infect Dis. 2005;11(8):1197-204.
20. Sapadin AN, Fleischmajer R. Tetracyclines: Nonantibiotic properties and their clinical implications. JAAD. 2006;54(2): 258-65.
21. Del Rosso JQ. Update on rosacea pathogenesis and correlation with medical therapeutic agents. Cutis. 2006;78(2):97-100.

EXAMINATION QUESTION

1. Write a short note on tetracycline in dermatology.

158 CHAPTER

Systemic Antifungals

Ishad Agarwal

INTRODUCTION

Dermatophytosis, the most common superficial fungal infection, is caused by keratinophilic fungi. There has been an increase in the occurrence of difficult to treat recalcitrant, recurrent, and chronic dermatophytosis in India over the last few years. The current face of dermatophytosis in India has possibly been an outcome of a complex and intrigued interplay between the host, fungus, drug, and environment, contributed by multiple factors, including more humid and warmer climate, the absurd use of topical corticosteroid-based combinations, the increased use of broad-spectrum antibiotics, the increasing burden of immunocompromised population, the widespread use of antifungals in the agricultural industry, and the questionable role of antifungal drug resistance.[1] Systemic antifungal agents, such as griseofulvin, terbinafine, ketoconazole, fluconazole, and itraconazole have been known to be active against dermatophytes, terbinafine being the only fungicidal drug.

Before understanding the indications of systemic antifungals in treatment of dermatophytoses, it is pertinent to understand the key pharmacological aspects of these drugs.

PHARMACOLOGY OF SYSTEMIC ANTIFUNGALS

Classification

Systemic antifungals are classified upon the basis of their mechanism of action. **Table 1** presents a brief summary of systemic antifungals used in dermatology along with their salient pharmacological characteristics.

Let us now review some systemic antifungals in a greater detail.

Griseofulvin

This is an oral fungistatic[2] agent derived from a number of *Penicillium* species. It inhibits cell division and nucleic acid synthesis in fungi. Griseofulvin is active against dermatophytes, but has no effect against yeasts or other fungi.

The drug is poorly absorbed orally, varying between 25 and 70% of an oral dose. Peak plasma levels are attained approximately after 4 hours of ingestion. Absorption is significantly enhanced by fatty meal. The smaller microcrystalline and ultramicronized forms are better absorbed.

Griseofulvin is usually well tolerated. Adverse effects include headache, gastrointestinal disturbance and, less commonly, urticaria, diarrhea, and photosensitivity. The drug should be avoided during pregnancy and in patients with liver disease. Griseofulvin can diminish the anticoagulant effect of warfarin and concurrent administration of phenobarbitone may decrease griseo-fulvin bioavailability. Griseofulvin may also interact with alcohol, causing a disulfiram-type reaction. Therefore, alcohol will be a contraindication to its use in many patients.

Dosage and indications: Dosage of griseofulvin is discussed in greater detail in **Table 2**.

Ketoconazole

Ketoconazole is an oral or topical synthetic dioxolane imidazole compound that interferes with the biosynthesis of ergosterol, leading to alterations in certain membrane-associated cell functions. It has a high affinity for keratin and a broad spectrum of activity which includes both dermatophytes and yeasts.

Peak plasma concentration is attained within 1–2 hours of a single oral dose. The absorption depends upon the gastric pH and shows variable absorption with food. The drug is highly protein bound. It cannot penetrate the cerebrospinal fluid (CSF).

Ketoconazole is not absorbed systemically following topical application, but is well absorbed orally under acid conditions. It is poorly absorbed in patients with achlorhydria and in those taking antacids or H2-receptor antagonists. Liver function must be monitored in patients receiving treatment for more than 30 days. The most common adverse effects are nausea, anorexia, and vomiting occurring in about 20% of patients. Adrenal or testicular steroid metabolism may be affected. Coadministration of ketoconazole with either terfenadine or astemizole has been associated with potentially fatal cardiac arrhythmias. Ketoconazole also enhances the effects of warfarin, oral hypoglycemics, and phenytoin. Ketoconazole blocks androgen synthesis by interfering with cytochrome P450 at high doses and causes gynecomastia, impotence, and irregular menstrual cycles.

TABLE 1: Systemic antifungals used in dermatology along with their salient pharmacological characteristics.

S. No.	*Drug name*	*Mechanism of action*	*Salient features*	*Side effects*
			Triazoles	
1.	Itraconazole	Blocks ergosterol synthesis by inhibiting 14α-demethylase	Fungistatic, lipophilic, and needs acidic milieu for absorption	Cardiotoxicity, worsening of congestive heart failure, hepatic dysfunction, reduction of WBC, nephrotoxicity, and increased triglycerides
2.	Voriconazole		Has a broad spectrum of activity. It can be taken both orally and intravenously	Liver damage, ocular symptoms, and dermatologic reactions Inhibits cytochrome P450 (↑ levels of digoxin, cyclosporine, etc.) Causes visual disturbances
3.	Fluconazole		Fungistatic, crosses blood–brain barrier	Nausea, headache, pain abdomen, and diarrhea. QT prolongation with or without torsade de pointes have been reported
			Imidazoles	
4.	Ketoconazole	Inhibits 14α-demethylase	Fungistatic, lipophilic, and needs acidic milieu for absorption. It cannot penetrate the CSF	Inhibits CYP3A, increases concentration of drugs such as cyclosporin and atorvastatin. CYP3A inducers such as phenytoin and rifampicin decrease the concentration of ketoconazole. Gynecomastia and fulminant hepatitis
			Allylamines	
5.	Terbinafine	Inhibits squalene epoxidase	Fungicidal, biotransformed in liver, does not inhibit cytochrome P450	Nausea, metallic taste, liver damage, and drug-induced LE
			Polyenes	
6.	Amphotericin B	Binds ergosterol and forms membrane pores		Acute reaction after infusion (fever, chills, nausea, and tachypnea), nephrotoxicity, agranulocytosis, seizures, and arrhythmias
			Others	
7.	Griseofulvin	Disrupts microtubule function (metaphase arrest)	Fungistatic, increased absorption with fatty meal, and induces cytochrome P450	Headache, paresthesia, photosensitivity, drug-induced LE, and worsens acute intermittent porphyria
8.	Caspofungin	Inhibits synthesis of glucan (fungal cell wall)		

(CSF: cerebrospinal fluid; LE: lupus erythematosus; WBC: white blood cell)

TABLE 2: Dosage of oral griseofulvin.

Oral dosing of griseofulvin			
	Adult		*Pediatric (over 2 years of age)*
	Tinea corporis and cruris	*Tinea pedis, manuum, unguium, and capitis*	
Griseofulvin microsize (125 mg/5 mL suspension; 250 and 500 mg tablets)	500–1,000 mg daily	750–1,500 mg daily	15–20 mg/kg daily (usual maximum 1 g); use higher range (20–25 mg/kg daily) for tinea capitis
Griseofulvin ultramicrosize (125 and 250 mg tablets)	375–500 mg daily	500–750 mg daily	10–15 mg/kg/day (maximum usually 750 mg/day)
Duration of treatment			
2–4 weeks for tinea corporis, 6–12 weeks for tinea capitis, 4–8 weeks for tinea pedis, 4 months for fingernail onychomycosis, and 6 months for toenail onychomycosis			

The risk of hepatitis,[3,4] albeit rare (1 in 10,000 to 1 in 15,000 of patients treated with a medium time of onset of 1 month), makes ketoconazole a secondary choice for dermatophyte infections. However, ketoconazole has become the drug of choice for treating *Malassezia* infections and is an important adjunct in the treatment of acquired immunodeficiency syndrome (AIDS) patients with fluconazole-resistant *Candida* infections.

Dosage and indications: Ketoconazole is available in 200 mg tablets. Adults take one or two tablets daily. Children over 2 years of age take 6.6 mg/kg orally once daily (typically for 5 days) for pityriasis versicolor. For other tinea infections and cutaneous candidiasis, children over 2 years of age take 3.3–6.6 mg/kg/day orally for 2–4 weeks. For mucocutaneous candidiasis in children, the dose is 5–10 mg/kg/day divided into two doses; the maximum dose is 400 mg a day. Absorption is improved with an acidic stomach pH.

Fluconazole

Fluconazole is an oral synthetic bistriazole compound that inhibits the cytochrome P450-dependent 14α-demethylation

TABLE 3: Dosing of oral fluconazole.

Indication	*Pediatric dosage*	*Adult dosage*
Pityriasis versicolor		400 mg once *or* 300 mg once, with possible second dose in 1 week, depending on clinical response
Tinea corporis and tinea cruris		5,150 mg per week for 2–4 weeks
Tinea pedis		Pulse doses of 150 mg per week for 2–6 weeks
Tinea capitis		6 mg/kg/day for 2–3 weeks
Oropharyngeal candidiasis	6 mg/kg on day 1 then 3 mg/kg 24–72 hours for 14 days	200 mg on day 1 then 100 mg per day for at least 2 weeks
Vaginal candidiasis		150 mg once
Esophageal candidiasis	6 mg/kg on day 1 then 3–12 mg/kg per day 24–72 hours for 21 days	200 mg on day 1 then 100 mg per day for at least 3 weeks Treat for at least 2 weeks after symptoms resolve
Systemic candidiasis	6–12 mg/kg per day for 28 days	Up to 400 mg per day

step in the formation of ergosterol. This leads to alterations in a number of membrane-associated cell functions. Fluconazole has a broad spectrum of activity that includes both dermatophytes and yeasts.

Its absorption is not pH-dependent like ketoconazole. The drug has a longer half-life thus permitting its single dose regimen. Fluconazole is predominantly excreted through the renal route and the dose should be adjusted according to the creatinine clearance.

The common side effects are nausea, headache, pain abdomen, and diarrhea.[5,6] Unlike ketoconazole and itraconazole, fluconazole has few significant drug interactions. However, the effects of warfarin, oral hypoglycemics, phenytoin, and theophylline may be increased by fluconazole when given in doses of 200 mg/day or higher.

Dosage and indications: Fluconazole is available as 50 mg, 100 mg, and 200 mg tablets and as an orange-flavored suspension in 10 mg/mL and 40 mg/mL strengths. The usual adult doses range from 100 to 400 mg/day, depending on the immune status of the patient, the infecting organism, and the patient's response to therapy. With most mucocutaneous diseases in immunocompetent patients, the recommended adult dose is 150 mg/week for 4 weeks. Vaginal candidiasis usually responds to a single dose of 150 mg **(Table 3)**.

Itraconazole

This is an oral synthetic dioxolane triazole compound that functions in much the same way as fluconazole. It has a broad spectrum of activity that includes both dermatophytes and yeasts. Itraconazole can be used to treat various cutaneous infections, including dermatophytosis, pityriasis versicolor, and oral and vaginal forms of candidiasis. It is more specific for fungal cytochrome P450 than ketoconazole resulting in less toxicity and greater efficacy than the latter.

TABLE 4: Adult dosage of itraconazole.

Tinea corporis and tinea cruris	100 mg po qd for 2 weeks *or* 200 mg po qd for 1 week
Tinea pedis	100 mg po qd for 2 weeks *or* 200 mg po qd for 1 week
Onychomycosis of toenails	200 mg po qd for 12 weeks *or* 200 mg po bid for 1 week, then 3 weeks without treatment, repeated twice more for a total of three pulses of therapy
Onychomycosis of fingernails	200 mg po qd for 6 weeks *or* 200 mg po bid for 1 week, then 3 weeks without treatment, then 200 mg po bid for 1 week

Itraconazole has been described as causing a unique triad of hypertension, hypokalemia, and edema, mostly in older adults. A negative inotropic effect resulting in congestive heart failure has also been described and has prompted changes to the package labeling to avoid administration of itraconazole to patients with a history of heart failure. Itraconazole enhances the anticoagulant effect of coumarin-like drugs. It may increase the concentration of cyclosporin if given together, thus enhancing renal toxicity. The most frequently observed side effects are nausea, headache, abdominal pain, and constipation.[7]

Dosage and indications: Itraconazole is available as 100 mg capsules and a 10 mg/mL solution. The solution should be taken on an empty stomach and the capsules should be taken with a full meal to enhance absorption. Pediatric dosing is 3–5 mg/kg daily. Doses over 200 mg should be divided into two doses per day. For tinea capitis in children, itraconazole may be given continuously for 2–4 weeks or as 1- to 3-week-long pulses (with 3 weeks without drug in between each pulse) **(Table 4)**.

Terbinafine

This is an oral or topical synthetic allylamine compound that inhibits the action of squalene epoxidase, a crucial enzyme in the formation of ergosterol, leading to membrane disruption and cell death. It is a fungicidal agent with a limited clinical spectrum of activity primarily against dermatophytes.

The drug is well-absorbed and is strongly lipophilic, being concentrated in the dermis, epidermis and adipose tissue.[8] Terbinafine is metabolized by the liver and the inactive metabolites are excreted in the urine. The drug should be given cautiously in patients with deranged hepatic or renal function tests. It can precipitate or exacerbate subacute cutaneous lupus erythematosus. Acute exanthematous pustulosis has been reported with terbinafine therapy. Cimetidine decreases its elimination, whereas rifampicin increases its elimination of drug; hence the dose should be regulated when given along with these drugs.

Terbinafine is generally well tolerated with the most common adverse effects being nausea and abdominal pain, and allergic skin reactions, but these are often mild and transient. Taste disturbance and hepatic toxicity have also been reported.

Dosage and indications: The usual adult dose is 250 mg/day with the duration of treatment dependent on the site and extent of the infection, ranging from 2 weeks for inter digital tinea pedis, 4–6 weeks for widespread or chronic nonresponsive dermatophytosis of skin and/or scalp, to 12 weeks for nails.

Amphotericin B

Amphotericin B (AmB) pregnancy category B is a polyene macrolide antibiotic first obtained from *Streptomyces nodosus*. The drug is available mainly for intravenous use. The drug is fungicidal. It acts by interfering with the permeability of the fungal cell membrane by forming pores after binding to sterols.

The antifungal spectrum of AmB includes *Candida* spp., *Cryptococcus neoformans*, dimorphic fungi (*Histoplasma capsulatum*, *Coccidioides immitis*, and *Blastomyces dermatitidis*), and *Aspergillus* spp. It is used to treat severe fungal infections including disseminated systemic candidiasis, cryptococcal meningitis, blastomycosis, disseminated histoplasmosis, extra-cutaneous sporotrichosis, coccidioidomycosis, paracoccidioidomycosis, mucormycosis, and aspergillosis. Dosing of intravenous AmB varies depending upon the formulation of the medication (e.g., 0.75–1 mg/kg/day of conventional AmB versus 3–5 mg/kg/day of lipid formulations).[9]

An acute hypersensitivity reaction may occur 1–3 hours after infusion that may partially contribute to an increased synthesis of prostaglandin and histamine liberation. Other side effects include phlebitis, ventricular fibrillations, hypokalemia, pulmonary dysfunction, thrombocytopenia, renal dysfunction, and anaphylaxis. The most serious adverse effect is nephrotoxicity. A dosage of more than 5 mg may produce irreversible renal damage.

NEWER ANTIFUNGALS

The increase in the number and types of fungal pathogens and especially the emergence of azole resistant fungi

TABLE 5: Newer antifungals.

Agents	*Mechanism of action*	*Indications*	
Echinocandins[10]			
Caspofungin	Interfere with cell wall synthesis/ permeability via inhibition of β-(1,3)-D-glucan synthesis	Invasive aspergillosis in patients refractory to or intolerant of other antifungals, candidemia, and esophageal candidiasis	Caspofungin acetate is given as a slow intravenous infusion over 1 hour. For treatment of *Aspergillus* infections, the loading dose on the first day is 70 mg. The dose is 50 mg intravenously per day thereafter. Patients who do not respond to this dose may respond to 70 mg intravenously per day. Caspofungin must not be mixed with solutions containing dextrose, and patients with moderate hepatic insufficiency should receive 35 mg per day after the 70 mg loading dose. This drug has not been adequately studied in children
Micafungin		Prophylaxis for *Candida* infections in hematopoietic stem cell transplant patients, esophageal candidiasis	Micafungin is only available in an intravenous form. For esophageal candidiasis, it is administered as 150 mg intravenously daily. In hematopoietic stem cell transplant patients, as prophylaxis for *Candida* infections, it may be given at a dose of 50 mg intravenously daily
Anidulafungin		Candidemia, esophageal candidiasis, intra-abdominal *Candida* infections, and peritonitis	Anidulafungin is also available in an intravenous form for *Candida* infections. In candidemia, the dose is 100 mg intravenously daily after a loading dose of 200 mg; treatment should continue until 2 weeks after the most recent positive blood culture. For esophageal candidiasis, the dose is 50 mg daily
Pradimicins	Unique antifungals that act through calcium binding to mannans in the fungal wall	Pradimicin in the form of BMS-181184 has broad spectrum in vitro antifungal activity against *Candida* spp., *Cryptococcus neoformans*, *Aspergillus* spp., dematiaceous molds, and the zygomycetes	Early studies indicate an excellent therapeutic index with no major end-organ toxicity. Pradimicins warrant further investigation for treatment of opportunistic mycoses in immunocompromised hosts

TABLE 6: The newer azoles.[11]

Agents	*Indications and dosage*
Posaconazole	Prevention of invasive aspergillosis and *Candida* infections in immunosuppressed hosts. Posaconazole is a 40 mg/mL suspension, given with food. It is indicated for prophylaxis of invasive fungal infections in immunocompromised patients. The dosage is 200 mg orally three times daily in patients over 13 years of age. For oropharyngeal candidiasis, it may be given as 100 mg orally twice daily (on the first day) and then 100 mg daily for 12 days In cases refractory to fluconazole or itraconazole, the dose is increased to 400 mg orally twice daily
Voriconazole	Voriconazole is used for invasive aspergillosis at 4 mg/kg intravenously every 12 hours or 100–200 mg orally every 12 hours. A loading dose of 6 mg/kg intravenously, given twice, 12 hours apart, is administered prior to the intravenous or oral regimen. Dose adjustments must be made in patients with renal or hepatic dysfunction
Pramiconazole	In preclinical studies, pramiconazole exhibited similar or superior antifungal activity to ketoconazole and itraconazole, and selectively inhibited ergosterol synthesis with a broad-spectrum activity. Pramiconazole was absorbed rapidly and had a long half-life, allowing for once-daily dosing. In phase I and II clinical trials, pramiconazole reduced the growth of *Candida albicans, Malassezia globosa, Microsporum canis, Trichophyton mentagrophytes*, and *Trichophyton rubrum*, and was generally well-tolerated

has prompted a continuing search for new therapeutic options. These drugs with their mechanism of actions and salient features are discussed in greater details in **Tables 5 and 6**.

CONCLUSION

Although the chapter provides insight into the pharmacotherapy and pharmacology of dermatophytoses with systemic antifungals, the discussion of principles of management of these infections has seen a vast change over last few years and is beyond the scope of this chapter. Superficial dermatophytosis are a public health problem of vast importance due to ever increasing prevalence and resistance, therefore the students reading the text are advised to read consensus guidelines for treatment of fungal infections in a greater detail.

KEY POINTS

- Dermatophyte infections are no longer simple and may need long treatments with systemic antifungals, like Itraconazole.
- Side effects of oral itraconazole must be borne in mind, especially in patients with co-morbidities, hence pretreatment testing is important.
- Triazoles and imidazoles are fungustatic while terbinafine is fungicidal.
- Echinocandins and pradimicins are newer antifungals.

REFERENCES

1. Rajagopalan M, Inamadar A, Mittal A, Miskeen AK, Srinivas CR, Sardana K, et al. Expert Consensus on The Management of Dermatophytosis in India (ECTODERM India). BMC Dermatol. 2018;18:6.
2. Hay RJ, Roberts SOB, Mackenzie DWR. Mycology. In: Champion RH, Burton JL, Ebling FJG (Eds). Textbook of Dermatology. Oxford: Blackwell Scientific Publications; 1992. p. 1128.
3. Kauffman CA, Carver PL. Antifungal agents in 1990's: current status and future development. Drugs. 1997;53:539-49.
4. Lewis JH, Zimmerman HJ, Benson GD, Ishak KG. Hepatic injury associated with ketoconazole therapy: analysis of 33 cases. Gastroenterology. 1984;80:503-13.
5. Kotogyan A, Harmanyeri Y, Gunes AT, Erboz S, Palali Z, Sabuncu I, et al. Efficacy and safety of oral fluconazole in the treatment of patients with tinea corporis, cruris and pedis or cutaneous candidiasis. Clin Drug Invest. 1996;12:59-66.
6. Faergemann J. Use of fluconazole in the treatment of human fungal infections of the skin. Int J Dermatol. 1992;12:59.
7. Gupta AK, Doncker PD, Heremans A, Stoffels P, Piérard GE, Decroix J, et al. Itraconazole for the treatment of tinea pedis: a dosage of 400 mg/day given for 1 week is similar in efficacy to 100 or 200 mg/day given for 2 to 4 weeks. J Am Acad Dermatol. 1997;36(5 Pt 1):789-92.
8. Ryder NS. Terbinafine: mode of action and properties of the squalene epoxidase inhibition. Br J Dermatol. 1992; 126(suppl 39):2-7.
9. Hiemenz JW, Walsh TJ. Lipid formulations of amphotericin B. Recent progress and future directions. Clin Infect Dis. 1996;22 (suppl):133-44.
10. Vazquez JA, Sobel JD. Anidulafungin: a novel Echinocandin. Clin Infect Dis. 2006;43:215-22.
11. Cornely OA, Maertens J, Winston DJ, Perfect J, Ullmann AJ, Walsh TJ, et al. Posaconazole vs. fluconazole or itraconazole prophylaxis in patients with neutropenia. N Engl J Med. 2007;356(4):348-59.

EXAMINATION QUESTIONS

1. Write a short note on newer antifungals.
2. Classify systemic antifungals used in dermatology and write about itraconazole in detail.
3. Uses of Amphotericin B in dermatology.
4. Treatment of onychomycosis.
5. Write short notes of fluconazole, terbinafine, and ketoconazole.
6. Explain antifungal resistance in dermatology and newer drug therapies.

159 CHAPTER

Antiviral Drugs

Abhijit Saha, Maitreyee Sengupta

INTRODUCTION

Viral diseases, while fairly common, can be one of the most challenging for a dermatologist to treat. Dermatological manifestations are commonly caused by viruses belonging to the poxvirus, herpesvirus, and papillomavirus families. Human immunodeficiency virus (HIV) infection is also associated with varied cutaneous presentations. Even though patient education and prevention are essential to control the spread of these infections, once acquired, antiviral drugs remain the mainstay of treatment. However, most viral exanthems (measles, rubella, and hand-foot-mouth disease) are treated symptomatically where antiviral drugs have little to no role. Antiviral agents currently used may be systemic or topical.

SYSTEMIC ANTIVIRAL DRUGS

Drugs for Human Herpesvirus Infections

Human herpesviruses (HHVs) are large linear double-stranded deoxyribonucleic acid (DNA) viruses with an icosahedral capsid, tegument, and envelope glycoprotein. HHV-1 and HHV-2 (herpes simplex virus-1 and 2) and HHV-3 [varicella-zoster virus (VZV)] primarily cause cutaneous disease. The systemic antivirals available are acyclovir, valacyclovir, and famciclovir.

Acyclovir

Acyclovir most widely used antiviral drug. Chemical structure of acyclovir is shown in **Figure 1**.

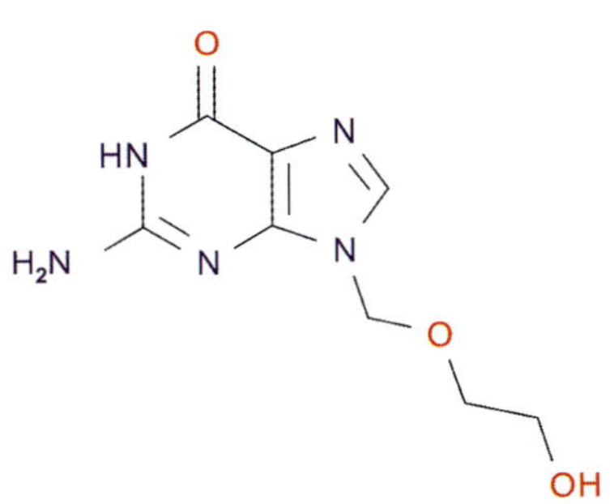

Fig. 1: Chemical structure of acyclovir.

Pharmacology (**Flowchart 1**):

- Guanosine analog [(9-(2-hydroxyethoxymethyl)guanine or acycloguanosine].[1]
- Once inside the host cell, it is phosphorylated by herpes-specific thymidine kinase to acyclovir monophosphate.
- Bi- and tri-phosphorylation is then carried out by host cellular enzymes.
- Acyclovir triphosphate is then incorporated into viral DNA by viral DNA polymerase resulting in chain termination.
- Acyclovir is postulated to have much higher affinity for viral DNA polymerase than cellular DNA polymerase.

Valacyclovir

- Valacyclovir is a prodrug of acyclovir, available only in oral form.
- Its bioavailability is nearly three to five times that of oral acyclovir.

Famciclovir

- Famciclovir, another oral prodrug, is converted to penciclovir in vivo.
- Like acyclovir, penciclovir is phosphorylated to penciclovir triphosphate and incorporated into viral DNA by viral DNA polymerase, resulting in chain termination.
- Its bioavailability is higher than that of both acyclovir and valacyclovir.[2]

Flowchart 1: Pharmacology of acyclovir.

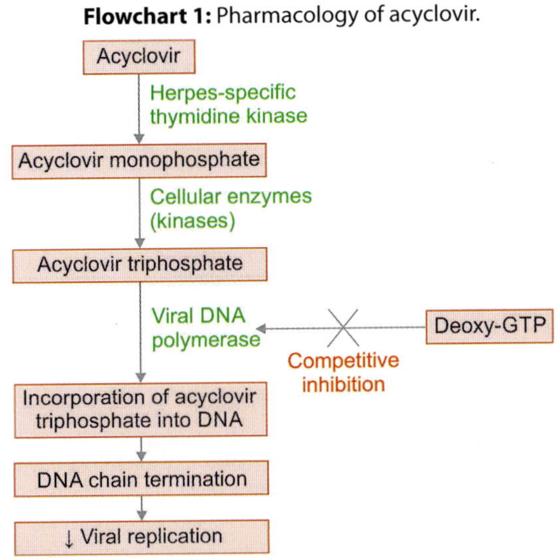

(DNA: deoxyribonucleic acid; GTP: guanosine-5'-triphosphate)

Indications

- Systemic acyclovir can be administered orally or intravenously, valacyclovir and famciclovir are available only in oral forms.
- The systemic anti-herpetic drugs are indicated for:[2,3]
  - Primary and recurrent episodes of genital herpes simplex infection
  - Chronic suppression of genital herpes
  - Orolabial herpes
  - Varicella caused by Varicella-zoster virus infection
  - Herpes zoster
  - HSV encephalitis
  - Recurrent mucocutaneous herpes simplex in the immunocompromised
- *Off-label indications:* Herpes associated erythema multiforme, eczema herpeticum, primary herpes gingivostomatitis, herpetic whitlow and neonatal herpes.
- In pregnancy, acyclovir should be started before 36 weeks of gestation to reduce the chances of perinatal transmission and the need for cesarean delivery. It is a pregnancy category B drug.

Flowchart 2: Indications and dosages of systemic anti-herpetic drugs.

Primary genital herpes/orolabial herpes
- Acyclovir 400 mg thrice daily for 7–10 days
- Valacyclovir 1 g twice daily for 7–10 days
- Famciclovir 250 mg thrice daily for 7–10 days

↓

Recurrent genital herpes/orolabial herpes
- Acyclovir 200 mg five times a day for 5–10 days
- Valacyclovir 500 mg twice daily for 3 days or 1 g daily for 5 days
- Famciclovir 125 mg twice daily for 5 days

↓

Chronic suppression of genital herpes
- Acyclovir 400 mg twice daily or 200 mg 3–5 times a day, reassess after 12 months
- Valacyclovir 500 mg daily for 10 or fewer recurrences per year
- Valacyclovir 1 g daily for over 10 recurrences per year
- Famciclovir 250 mg twice daily

↓

Varicella
- Patients over 2 years of age, over 40 kg: Acyclovir 800 mg five times daily for 5 days
- Patients over 2 years of age, under 40 kg: Acyclovir 20 mg/kg five times daily for 5 days (maximum 800 mg per dose)

↓

Herpes zoster
- Acyclovir 800 mg five times a day for 7–10 days
- Valacyclovir 1 g thrice daily for 7 days
- Famciclovir 500 thrice daily for 7 days
- Disseminated herpes zoster: Acyclovir 5–10 mg/kg IV q 8 hours for 7–10 days

↓

Recurrent mucocutaneous herpes simplex in the immunocompromised
- Acyclovir 5 mg/kg IV q 8 hours for 7 days
- Acyclovir 400 mg orally five times a day for 14–21 days
- Valacyclovir 1 g thrice daily for 7 days

↓

HSV encephalitis: Acyclovir 10 mg/kg iv q 8 hours for 10 days

Contraindications

There are no major contraindications to any of the three drugs except for hypersensitivity to the drug itself or any component of the formulation.

Adverse Effects

All three drugs have excellent patient tolerance. They may rarely cause headaches and nausea.

Drug Interactions

- Since none of the drugs are metabolized by hepatic microsomal enzymes, drug interactions are few. However, famciclovir increases the levels of digoxin by ≈19%.
- Probenecid increases the bioavailability of acyclovir and famciclovir by reducing renal clearance.
- Zidovudine can also increase acyclovir levels leading to severe drowsiness and lethargy.

Drug Resistance

- Drug resistance is extremely rare in immunocompetent individuals.
- But, in immunocompromised individuals, like those with HIV infections or organ transplant recipients, may develop acyclovir-resistant strains. These usually show cross-resistance with valacyclovir and famciclovir.
- Resistance occurs as a result of mutation in viral thymidine kinase. Intravenous foscarnet and cidofovir may be used in these patients. They act by direct inhibition of viral DNA polymerase. Foscarnet is the oral drug of choice for acyclovir-resistant herpes simplex virus infections.

Vaccines for Human Herpesvirus Infections

Varicella-zoster Vaccines

- The varicella vaccine is a live-attenuated vaccine consisting of a lyophilized preparation of Oka/Merck strain of VZV.
- It can be administered at 9 months of age along with the measles, mumps, and rubella (MMR) vaccine with a booster 3–4 years later. It is also indicated in the elderly to reduce the occurrence and duration of herpes zoster.[4]

Herpes Simplex Vaccines

No clinically successful vaccines have yet been developed.

ANTIRETROVIRAL DRUGS

- The diagnosis of HIV infection is often first suspected from its cutaneous manifestations. These can range from viral exanthems to concomitant sexually transmitted infections (STIs) to papulosquamous disorders.

- Antiretroviral drugs can be classified into seven categories. They include:
  1. Nucleoside reverse transcriptase inhibitors—zidovudine, lamivudine, didanosine, zalcitabine, stavudine, abacavir, and emtricitabine;
  2. Nucleotide reverse transcriptase inhibitor—tenofovir;
  3. Non-nucleoside reverse transcriptase inhibitors—nevirapine, delavirdine, efavirenz, and etravirine;
  4. Protease inhibitors—saquinavir, indinavir, ritonavir, nelfinavir, amprenavir, fosamprenavir, atazanavir, lopinavir, tipranavir, and darunavir;
  5. Fusion inhibitor—enfuvirtide;
  6. Entry inhibitor/CCR5 coreceptor antagonist—maraviroc; and
  7. Integrase inhibitor—raltegravir.

TOPICAL AND INTRALESIONAL ANTIVIRAL DRUGS

The topical and intralesional antiviral drugs can be divided into three categories: (1) Viricidal drugs, (2) immune-enhancing drugs, and (3) cytodestructive drugs.

Viricidal Drugs

Acyclovir

- Topical acyclovir is available as 5% cream and 5% ointment formulations.
- Acyclovir 5% ointment applied six times daily for 7 days in genital herpes and herpes labialis reduces viral shedding but does not affect time to healing or recurrence.
- Acyclovir 5% cream applied within 24 hours of onset of symptoms reduces time to healing by 1.5 days. It is useful in ocular herpes.
- Oral acyclovir is preferred to topical acyclovir in recurrent herpes due to greater efficacy.

Penciclovir

- Penciclovir is available only in topical form due to poor oral bioavailability. The mechanism of action is similar to acyclovir.
- 1% cream has to be applied every 2 hours on herpes simplex lesions. It is not preferred due to inconvenience of frequent application.

Cidofovir

- Cidofovir is available in injectable form and can be compounded into a topical preparation.
- Off-label uses of topical cidofovir include molluscum contagiosum, condyloma acuminata, verruca vulgaris, and herpes simplex.

Idoxuridine

Topical idoxuridine is only indicated as an ophthalmic solution in herpes keratitis.

Immune-enhancing Drugs

Imiquimod

Imiquimod, a non-nucleoside heterocyclic amine, is an immune modulator that was Food and Drug Administration (FDA) approved in 1997. It has potent antitumor and antiviral effects.

Mechanism of action:

- Imiquimod activates toll-like receptor (TLR) 7 and 8 leading to activation of nuclear factor-κβ resulting in influx of dendritic cells and other mononuclear inflammatory and cytotoxic cells.
- Imiquimod induces secretion of tumor necrosis factor-α (TNF-α), interferon-γ (IFN-γ), IFN-α, interleukin-6 (IL-6), IL-1α, IL-1β, IL-8, IL-12, granulocyte-macrophage colony-stimulating factor (GM-CSF), and granulocyte colony-stimulating factor (G-CSF) which mounts a T helper type 1 (Th1) immune response. It also reduces adenylyl cyclase activity, thus suppressing the regulatory negative feedback.[5]
- It inhibits angiogenesis, interfering with viral neovascularization and at higher concentrations, causes apoptosis of tumor cells.

Indications:

- *External genital and perianal warts:* Imiquimod 5% cream is applied thrice weekly (at bedtime on alternate days) for up to 16 weeks. It is also safe and effective in immunocompromised patients on highly active antiretroviral therapy (HAART). The advantages include ease of self-application and lack of systemic absorption.
- Imiquimod has also been used with somewhat less success in cutaneous warts and molluscum conta-giosum.
- Other nonviral indications include actinic keratoses and small superficial nonfacial basal cell carcinoma (BCC) (<2 cm). It has also been tried in melanoma in situ (lentigo maligna type).

Contraindications: Hypersensitivity to the drug or any of its components. It is a pregnancy category C drug.

Adverse effects: Imiquimod is a safe drug but may cause local reactions such as erythema, pruritus, ulceration, and pain.

Interferon-α

Intralesional IFN-α is indicated in genital warts and acquired immunodeficiency syndrome (AIDS)-associated Kaposi's sarcoma. It binds to cell surface receptors leading to macrophage activation.

Intralesional Bacillus Calmette–Guérin Vaccine

- Intralesional immunotherapy with Bacillus Calmette-Guérin (BCG) vaccine utilizes the ability of the immune system to mount a delayed-type hypersensitivity

response to certain viral antigens leading to infiltration of CD4 T-lymphocytes and macrophages in wart lesions and activation of cytotoxic and natural killer cells. Immunotherapy not only clears the treated wart but also the distant warts.[6]
- Various studies have shown its safety and efficacy in multiple and recurrent warts.

Cytodestructive Drugs

Bleomycin

Bleomycin is a complex of sulfurated glycopeptides antibiotics derived from *Streptomyces verticillus*. It is an anticancer drug with antibacterial and antiviral activity.

Mechanism of action: It binds to DNA during M and G2 phases of cell cycle leading to a single-strand break, thus hindering protein synthesis.

Indications: Intralesional bleomycin has been used in human papillomavirus (HPV) warts with variable success (14–99%). It is administered as a 0.1% solution with normal saline of 1 U/mL injectable bleomycin. Each individual lesion receives 0.1 mL of the diluted solution up to a maximum of 2 mL per treatment session. Since the injections are painful, it may be diluted with local anaesthetic instead.[7]

Contraindications: Pregnancy, children, immunocompromised patients, and patients with vascular compromise.

Adverse effects:
- The most common adverse effect is injection site pain. There may be erythema, swelling, and pain with eschar formation. Scarring and Raynaud's phenomenon are uncommon.
- A disadvantage is rapid deterioration of the reconstituted solution at room temperature.

Podophyllin and Podofilox

Podophyllin is a compounded extract of podophyllotoxin from the Mayapple plant (*Podophyllum* spp.). Podofilox is a commercially available 0.5% podophyllotoxin preparation that is safe for self-application.

Mechanism of action: Podophyllotoxin is an antimitotic agent that binds reversibly to tubulin and halts cells in metaphase stage.

Indications: Condyloma acuminata—Both office-applied podophyllin and self-applied podofilox are effective in clearing genital warts. Multiple sessions are required. But in large or pedunculated perianal warts, office-applied podophyllin is far more effective, both as monotherapy and in combination with other cytodestructive procedures such as cryotherapy and CO_2 laser.[8]

Contraindications: It is contraindicated in pregnancy due to its teratogenic potential.

Adverse effects: Local irritant reactions, i.e., burning, erythema, pain, and erosions.

Trichloroacetic Acid

- Trichloroacetic acid (TCA) acts by causing proteolysis leading to necrosis of cells. This effect is not specific to virus-infected cells so the surrounding area has to be protected.
- TCA is used in external genital warts and for smaller nongenital warts (verruca plana). It can be safely used in pregnancy.
- TCA has also been tried in molluscum contagiosum (along with extraction) and in cervical HPV infection.

Cantharidin

Cantharidin, derived from Spanish fly, was a colloidal solution causing a blistering reaction. It is no longer commonly used.

Salicylic Acid

- Salicylic acid is a keratolytic agent available as an ointment. It is also available as a collodion in combination with lactic acid.
- It is indicated for the treatment of palmar and plantar warts, with or without occlusion. It is also beneficial in treating corns and calluses.

5-Fluorouracil

- 5-fluorouracil (5-FU) is an antimetabolite (pyrimidine analog) that disrupts ribonucleic acid (RNA) synthesis.
- Topical 5-FU has been used for treating resistant genital warts, plane warts, and common warts.

Sinecatechin

Sinecatechin is a green tea polyphenol extract which has been used in the treatment of external genital and perianal warts.

KEY POINTS

- Systemic antiviral drugs in dermatology are primarily used to treat HHV infections. Antiretroviral drugs are prescribed by health professionals other than dermatologists.
- Oral acyclovir, valacyclovir, and famciclovir are more effective and potent against HSV infections than topical preparations. VZV infections always require oral antivirals. They are all pregnancy category B.
- Topical acyclovir is indicated in ocular herpes. Intravenous acyclovir is reserved for severe illness and the immunocompromised.
- Imiquimod acts by enhancing immunity by activating TLR 7 and 8 and is used in condyloma acuminata, actinic keratosis, and small superficial BCC.
- Intralesional BCG and bleomycin are now being used in verruca vulgaris.

- Podophyllin (office-applied) is one of the most effective in genital warts.
- TCA application is used in viral warts and molluscum contagiosum. It is safe in pregnancy.
- Salicylic acid is used in hyperkeratotic warts and topical 5-FU in recurrent warts.

REFERENCES

1. Wagstaff AJ, Faulds D, Goak L. Acyclovir, a reappraisal of its antiviral activity, pharmacokinetic properties and therapeutic efficacy. Drugs. 1994;47:153-205.
2. Tyring SK. Advances in the treatment of herpes virus infections: the role of famciclovir. Clin Ther. 1998;20:661-70.
3. Sampathkumar P, Drage LA, Martin DP. Herpes zoster (shingles) and postherpetic neuralgia. Mayo Clin Proc. 2009;84(3):274-80.
4. Oxman MN, Levin MJ, Johnson GR, Schmader KE, Straus SE, Gelb LD, et al. A vaccine to prevent herpes zoster and postherpetic neuralgia in older adults. N Engl J Med. 2005; 352:2271-84.
5. Kwok CS, Gibbs S, Bennett C, Holland R, Abbott A. Topical treatments for cutaneous warts. Cochrane Database Syst Rev. 2012;9:CD001781.
6. Jaisinghani AK, Dey VK, Suresh MS, Saxena A. Bacillus Calmette-Guerin immunotherapy for recurrent multiple warts: an open-label uncontrolled study. Indian J Dermatol. 2019;64:164.
7. Dhar SB, Rashid MM, Islam A, Bhuiyan M. Intralesional bleomycin in the treatment of cutaneous warts: a randomized clinical trial comparing it with cryotherapy. Indian J Dermatol Venereol Leprol. 2009;75(3):262-7.
8. Lacey CJ, Goodall RL, Tennvall GR, Maw R, Kinghorn GR, Fisk PG, et al. Randomised controlled trial and economic evaluation of podophyllotoxin solution, podophyllotoxin cream, and podophyllin in the treatment of genital warts. Sex Transm Infect. 2003;79:270-5.

EXAMINATION QUESTIONS

1. Name and classify the antiretroviral drugs.
2. Classify the drugs that are used in treatment of HSV infection.
3. Write a short note on cidofovir.

160 CHAPTER Oral Retinoids

Binod Kumar Thakur

INTRODUCTION

The term retinoids include all synthetic and natural compounds that have biological activity like that of vitamin A and structural similarity of vitamin A; that comprises retinol, retinal, and its isoform retinyl ester, and retinoic acid.

HISTORY

Early observations documented that deficiency of vitamin A causes hyperkeratosis of the skin and squamous metaplasia of mucous membranes and vitamin A replacement reverses these epithelial changes. The first dermatologic use of vitamin A was in 1943 by Straumfjord for acne vulgaris.[1]

High doses of vitamin A were initially used to treat skin conditions such as acne, psoriasis, ichthyoses, Darier's disease, and pityriasis rubra pilaris (PRP). However, therapeutic doses were accompanied by unacceptable side effects (skin and mucous membrane changes; and bone, liver, and neurologic complications). All-trans-retinoic acid, tretinoin was the first retinoid to be synthesized. However, it did not have significant advantage over vitamin A.

There are now three generations of synthetic retinoids. Isotretinoin (13-cis-retinoic acid) was first synthesized in 1955 and has been used in Europe since the early 1970s for the treatment of acne. Isotretinoin was approved by United States Food and Drug Administration (FDA) in 1982 to treat severe nodulocystic acne. Alitretinoin is a first-generation retinoid recently approved for chronic hand eczema.

The second-generation retinoids, etretinate and acitretin, also known as aromatic retinoids, are most effective in treating psoriasis and keratinizing disorders. In 1998, etretinate was phased out and largely replaced by its metabolite acitretin.

The third-generation retinoids include bexarotene.

PHARMACOKINETICS

Absorption and Distribution

The oral bioavailability of retinoids is enhanced when administered with food particularly fatty meal. Etretinate is approximately 50 times more lipophilic than acitretin resulting in increased storage in adipose tissue from which it is slowly released.

The metabolism of retinoids is mainly via oxidation and chain shortening to biologically inactive, water soluble products in the liver which is eliminated through bile and urine. Isotretinoin is completely cleared from the body within 1 month the drug is stopped. Though the elimination t1/2 for acitretin is 2 days, there is possibility of reverse metabolism to etretinate. Alcohol indirectly enhances the re-esterification of acitretin to etretinate, which is detectable only after a few days of an acitretin regimen **(Table 1)**.[2]

MECHANISM OF ACTION

Retinoids elicit its biological effects by activating nuclear receptors and regulating gene transcription. The retinoid receptors belong to a superfamily of nuclear receptors that

TABLE 1: Key pharmacology concepts—systemic retinoids.

Drug name	*Bioavailability (%)*	*Protein binding (%)*	*Elimination half-life*	*Receptors*	*Standard dosage range*
Tretinoin	--	Albumin 99	40–60 minutes	RAR	45 mg/m²/day
Isotretinoin	25	Albumin 99	10–20 hours	No clearly identified affinity for any retinoid nuclear receptor	0.5–2 mg/kg/day
Alitretinoin	Unknown	Plasma protein	2–10 hours	RXR and RAR	30 mg/day
Etretinate	44	Lipoprotein 99	80–160 days	No clearly identified affinity for any retinoid nuclear receptor	0.25–1 mg/kg/day
Acitretin	60	Albumin 95	50 hours	RAR (weak interaction)	25–50 mg/day
Bexarotene	No data	Plasma proteins 99	7–9 hours	RXR	300 mg/m²/day

(RAR: retinoic acid receptor; RXR: retinoid X receptor)

Note: Acitretin and etretinate activate the RARs in spite of binding poorly to them.

act as ligand-activated transcription factors and include the steroid, vitamin D3, and thyroid hormone receptors as well as peroxisome proliferator-activated receptors.

Transport of Retinoids

Cytosolic retinoic acid-binding protein (CRABP) is the intracellular carrier which transports retinoic acid to nucleus. CRABP-I modulates the levels of retinoic acid in various tissue while CRABP-II is predominant form in human epidermis and markedly elevated in lesional skin of psoriasis and other keratinizing disorders. CRABP-II stimulates the retinoic acid-induced transcriptional activity.

Mechanism at Nuclear Level

Mechanism at nuclear level is shown in **Flowchart 1**.

The antiproliferative and anti-inflammatory actions of retinoids are result of antagonizing the action of other transcription factor specifically activator protein-1 (AP1).[3]

The clinical effects of systemic retinoids in dermatology are related to their ability to affect pathways involved in inflammation, cellular differentiation, apoptosis, and sebaceous gland activity.[4]

FDA-approved Indications

FDA-approved indications are given in **Table 2**.

Psoriasis

The retinoid treatment is effective in localized and generalized pustular psoriasis. The initial dose of acitretin is 25 mg daily and increasing the dose based on effectiveness or patient tolerance, maximum 0.5–1 mg/kg/day. In chronic plaque psoriasis, the complete clearance is achieved in around 30% of patients; however, it often leads to decreased thickness, scaling and itching of the plaques.

Flowchart 1: Mechanism at nuclear level.

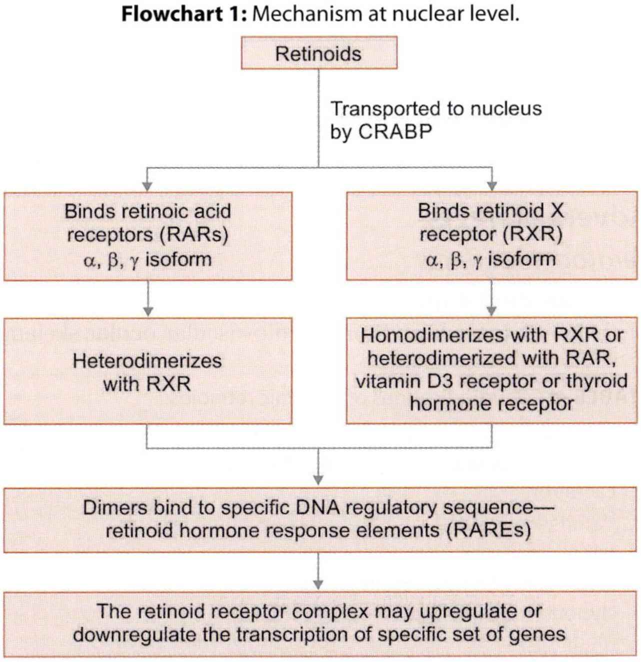

(CRABP: cytosolic retinoic acid-binding)

TABLE 2: FDA-approved indications.

Psoriasis (acitretin): • Severe plaque-type psoriasis • Pustular psoriasis—localized and generalized
Combination therapy: • With UVB or PUVA • With cyclosporine • With biologic therapies
Acne vulgaris (isotretinoin): • Nodulocystic acne • Recalcitrant, especially if any scarring tendency
Mycosis fungoides (bexarotene): Resistant to at least one systemic therapy

(PUVA: psoralen and ultraviolet A; UVB: ultraviolet B)

Psoriasis: Retinoids in Combination Therapy

Retinoid and phototherapy

Combination therapy with systemic retinoids and phototherapy is more effective than either modality alone. Current recommendations for combination acitretin-UV therapy include initiating low dose (25 mg) acitretin 2 weeks prior to the initiation of phototherapy. The initial dose of UV light and subsequent increments should be adjusted downward to accommodate the acitretin effect.

Acitretin with Methotrexate or Cyclosporine

This combination can be used in specific situations. The duration of this combination should be as minimum as possible to reduce the potential side effects such as hepatotoxicity with methotrexate and increased triglycerides with cyclosporine. Combination therapy can be planned as sequential regimen.

Acitretin in Combination with Biologic Agents

As retinoids are not considered as immunosuppressive, it may be considered ideal agent for combination therapy with biologic agents. In a randomized trial, the combination of acitretin with etanercept 25 mg once weekly was superior to acitretin alone and was equivalent to etanercept 25 mg twice weekly, with similar safety profiles.[5]

Acne Vulgaris

Isotretinoin is the only retinoid approved for treatment of severe recalcitrant nodular acne. With increasing experience, isotretinoin is also used in less severe disease who responds unsatisfactorily to conventional therapies such as long-term antibiotics.

A reasonable therapeutic plan is to start isotretinoin at a dose of 0.5–1 mg/kg daily until a total cumulative dose of 120–150 mg/kg is attained. The relapse rate tends to reduce with higher cumulative dose.

Cutaneous T-cell Lymphoma-Mycosis Fungoides and Sezary Syndrome

FDA approved bexarotene in 1999 for the treatment of CTCL that is refractory to at least one systemic therapy. The dose is 300 mg/m^2. The mechanism of action may be induction of apoptosis of malignant cells.[6]

Off-label Dermatologic Use

Off-label dermatologic use is given in **Table 3**.

Rosacea

Isotretinoin at 10 mg/day is usually effective in severe form or in treatment resistant rosacea. Continuous "microdoses" as low as 20–30 mg per week after low daily doses of isotretinoin for 4–6 months also prevented relapses in rosacea patients.[7]

Ichthyosiform Dermatoses

Lamellar ichthyosis responds well to acitretin. Other conditions where moderate response seen are bullous congenital ichthyosiform erythroderma, congenital ichthyosiform erythroderma, and X-linked ichthyosis.

Hidradenitis Suppurativa and Dissecting Cellulitis of Scalp

Isotretinoin has limited effect on HS and dissecting cellulitis of scalp. However, higher doses 0.7–1.2 mg/kg is required for therapeutic response.

TABLE 3: Off-label dermatologic use.

Follicular disorders: • Rosacea and acne-related conditions: – Gram-negative folliculitis – AIDS-associated eosinophilic folliculitis – Acne with solid facial edema – Granulomatous rosacea – Hidradenitis suppurativa (HS) – Dissecting cellulitis of scalp
Disorders of keratinization and related disorder: • Darier's disease • Pityriasis rubra pilaris • Ichthyosis, different forms • Keratodermas
Chemoprophylaxis of malignancies: • Organ transplantation patients • Bazex syndrome • Nevoid basal cell carcinoma syndrome • Muir–Torre syndrome • Xeroderma pigmentosa
Recurrent BCC or SCC (nonimmunosuppressed) Kaposi's sarcoma
Other dermatoses: • Lupus erythematosus (cutaneous features) • Lichen planus • Lichen sclerosus et atrophicus • Graft-versus-host disease • Human papillomavirus infections

(BCC: basal cell carcinoma; AIDS: acquired immunodeficiency syndrome; SCC: squamous cell carcinoma)

Darier's Disease

Improvement is usually noted in Darier's disease with acitretin and isotretinoin. Acitretin should be initiated at low dose 10 mg/day in moderate to severe form and may increase up to 20 mg/day. Combination of retinoids and antibiotic may enhance the clinical effects.

Pityriasis Rubra Pilaris

Significant improvement is seen in 70% of patients with isotretinoin at a dose 1–1.5 mg/kg/day. Acitretin in combination with narrow band UVB is reported as beneficial in PRP.

Chemoprevention of Malignancies

Systemic retinoids may prevent nonmelanoma skin cancer. However, the preventive action of retinoids does not persist upon discontinuation of retinoids.

Lupus Erythematosus

Both isotretinoin and acitretin gives good response in various forms of cutaneous lupus erythematosus. However, the lesions recur after completion of treatment.

Lichen Planus

There may be a role of systemic retinoids such as acitretin in widespread, hypertrophic, or oral erosive lichen planus. In these situations, retinoids alone or in combination with low-dose corticosteroids may be beneficial.

Chronic Hand Eczema

Alitretinoin is the first systemic treatment to be approved in the EU (European Union) for the treatment of severe chronic hand eczema unresponsive to potent topical corticosteroids. The recommended dosage of alitretinoin is 10 or 30 mg once daily, with a recommended starting dosage of 30 mg once daily; dosage adjustments may be required based on efficacy and tolerability.

Contraindications of Systemic Retinoids

Contraindications of systemic retinoids are given in **Table 4**.

Adverse Effects

Teratogenic Effects

This is the most important adverse effect. Retinoids induced birth defects include auditory, cardiovascular, ocular, skeletal,

TABLE 4: Contraindications of systemic retinoids.

Absolute: • Pregnancy or woman who is likely to become pregnant • Lactation • Hypersensitivity to parabens (in isotretinoin capsules)
Relative: • Leukopenia (in bexarotene) • Hypothyroidism (in bexarotene patients) • Moderate-to-severe cholesterol or triglyceride elevation • Significant hepatic and renal dysfunction

thymic abnormalities and central nervous system (CNS) (hydrocephalus, microcephaly).[8] Women in childbearing age must be counseled properly about birth control and they must not become pregnant during the therapy and up to 1 month and 2 years of stoppage in isotretinoin and acitretin respectively. It must be ensured that the women are not pregnant at the initiation of therapy. There is little, if any, risk of retinoid embryopathy in fetus fathered by men taking systemic retinoids.

iPLEDGE Registry Requirement

All patients must be registered in the iPLEDGE system (followed in United States of America) by the prescriber and must sign the informed consent. It dictates that the women in childbearing age must use two forms of contraception while on isotretinoin.

Mucocutaneous Adverse Effect

Cheilitis is most frequent and others include blepharo-conjunctivitis, dry eyes, dry nose, dry mouth, xerosis of the skin, and photosensitivity. Bexarotene appears to induce fewer mucocutaneous and ocular side effects than other retinoids.

Hair and Nail Effect

Telogen effluvium is dose dependent and is reversible. Nail fragility with onychorrhexis and onychoschizia is common.

Ocular Side Effects

The most common side effect is blepharoconjunctivitis, most likely due to decreased meibomian gland secretion. Patients should be counseled for possibility of developing dry eyes. Artificial tears can be used in symptomatic patients.

Other effects include decreased night vision, corneal opacities, and bacterial conjunctivitis.

Musculoskeletal Adverse Effects

Diffuse idiopathic skeletal hyperostosis may develop rarely in patients taking high dose of systemic retinoids for long periods of time. Premature epiphyseal closure is rare and occurs only in higher doses. In the setting of short course of oral retinoids, there are virtually no adverse effects on bone or ligaments.

Myalgias are seen roughly in 15% of isotretinoin treated patients. It is rare in patients with etretinate and acitretin.

Hyperlipidemia

Isotretinoin, etretinate, and acitretin elevate triglycerides in 50% of patients and cholesterol in 30%.[9] Disturbance of blood lipid levels is generally higher with isotretinoin and bexarotene than with acitretin. The current recommendation is to put all the patients taking bexarotene on lipid-lowering agents prior to initiation of therapy and to monitor serum lipid regularly.

Depression

There appears to be no direct link between isotretinoin and depression or anxiety, with the Swedish study suggesting that severe acne itself is a risk for depression and suicide.[10]

Central Nervous System

Pseudotumor cerebri though infrequent is important CNS side effect. Combined therapy with isotretinoin and tetracycline, doxycycline, or minocycline should be avoided.

Inflammatory Bowel Disease

There are several reports with conflicting results regarding isotretinoin use as a cause of inflammatory bowel disease (IBD). The patients need to be informed about sign and symptom of IBD and stop medication if it occurs.

Liver Effects

Elevated transaminases have been reported with both acitretin and isotretinoin use. Monitoring of liver transaminases is advisable and if the value increases more than threefold, discontinuation is recommended.

Thyroid Effect

Abnormalities in thyroid function have only been reported for bexarotene. Current recommendations include obtaining baseline thyroid-stimulating hormone (TSH) and free thyroxine studies, starting low-dose levothyroxine in all patients, and monitoring the free thyroxine level during therapy.

Hematologic Toxicity

A high incidence (up to 43%) of dose related neutropenia has been reported with bexarotene therapy. Leukopenia and neutropenia resolve within 30 days after dose reduction or discontinuation.

Drug Interactions

Drug interactions are given in **Table 5**.

MONITORING GUIDELINES FOR SYSTEMIC RETINOIDS

Baseline Examination

- Careful history and physical examination.
- Identify patients at increased risk for toxicity or adverse effects: For example, liver disease or cirrhosis, biliary tract disease, excessive alcohol consumption, prior pancreatitis, thyroid disease, uncontrolled hyperlipidemia, uncontrolled diabetes mellitus, human immunodeficiency virus (HIV), leukopenia, chronic infection, and cataracts.
- Document concomitant medications that may interact with retinoids.

TABLE 5: Examples of interacting drugs.

Interacting drug or group	*Examples and comments*
The following drugs may increase the serum levels (and potential toxicity) of retinoids:	
Vitamin A	Induces hypervitaminosis A-like toxicities
Tetracycline, doxycycline, and minocycline	May increase intracranial pressure pseudotumor cerebri risk
Gemfibrozil	Increased bexarotene levels due to CYP3A4 inhibition
Macrolides, azoles, etc.	Other CYP3A4 inhibitors
The following drugs may reduce the serum levels of retinoids via CYP3A4 induction:	
Antituberculosis drugs	Rifampin, rifabutin
Anticonvulsants	Phenytoin, phenobarbital, carbamazepine
Retinoids may increase the drug levels (and potential toxicity) of the following drugs:	
Cyclosporine	Increased cyclosporine levels via competition with retinoids for CYP3A4 metabolism
Retinoids may reduce the drug levels of the following drugs:	
Progestin only contraceptives	Reduced efficacy of these contraceptives when prescribed along with acitretin
Other potentially important drug interactions:	
Alcohol	Acitretin "reverse metabolism" to etretinate increased when acitretin used in combination with alcohol or other products such as mouth washes, cough syrup which may contain ethanol

Follow-up Examination

- Clinical evaluation every 2 weeks for first 4–8 weeks.
- Then monthly for the next 3 months; long-term clinical evaluation every 2–3 months.

Baseline Laboratory

- Serum or urine pregnancy test (in women of childbearing potential)
- Complete blood count (CBC)
- Liver function tests
- Fasting lipid profile
- Renal function tests
- *Thyroid function tests*: TSH, T4 in case of bexarotene therapy
- Optional urinalysis (if patients have renal diseases, proteinuria, diabetes, or hypertension).

Follow-up Laboratory

- Above tests monthly for the first 3–6 months, then every 3 months.
- But in bexarotene therapy fasting lipid profile every 1–2 weeks until the lipid response is established (usually 2–4 weeks).

Baseline Special Tests

- Baseline ophthalmologic examination if patients have a history of cataracts.
- Baseline X-ray of wrist, ankles or thoracic spine if long-term plan for retinoids.

Follow-up Special Tests

Repeat ophthalmologic examination periodically during treatment if patients have a history of abnormal ocular findings prior to retinoid therapy.

In case of isotretinoin and acitretin: Consider yearly X-rays of wrists, ankles or thoracic spine with long-term retinoids and radiographic studies of significantly symptomatic joints.

KEY POINTS

- The term retinoids include all compounds, synthetic and natural, that possesses vitamin A activity.
- Retinoids elicit its biological effects by activating nuclear receptors, a retinoic acid receptor (RAR), and retinoid X receptor (RXR) and regulating gene transcription.
- Oral retinoids (isotretinoin) are most effective drugs available for severe nodular acne and in many disorder such as pustular psoriasis, psoriatic erythroderma, and PRP (acitretin > isotretinoin) is effective.
- Bexarotene is approved for cutaneous T-cell lymphoma and alitretinoin is recently approved for chronic hand eczema.
- Teratogenicity is the most important adverse effect.
- Proper counseling to women of childbearing age about contraception is necessary. Hypertriglyceridemia, elevated transaminases, ocular, musculoskeletal, and hematologic adverse effect may occur.
- Oral retinoids have many drug interactions. Tetracycline group of drugs should not be combined as it may increase intracranial pressure.
- Systemic retinoids needs proper patient selection and monitoring regularly.

REFERENCES

1. Wolverton SE. Systemic drug for skin diseases. Philadelphia: WB Saunders; 1991. pp. 187-218.
2. Koo J, Nguyen Q, Gambla C. Advances in psoriasis therapy. Adv Dermatol. 1997;12:47-72.
3. Nagpal S, Chandraratna RA. Vitamin A and regulation of gene expression. Curr Opin Clin Nutr Metab Care. 1998;1: 341-6.
4. Patton TJ, Ferris LK. Systemic retinoids. In: Wolverton SE (Ed). Comprehensive Dermatologic Drug Therapy, 3rd edition. Philadelphia: Elsevier; 2013. p. 255.
5. Gisondi P, Del Giglio M, Cotena C, Girolomoni G. Combining etanercept and acitretin in the therapy of chronic plaque psoriasis: a 24-week, randomized, controlled,

investigator-blinded pilot trial. Br J Dermatol. 2008;158: 1345-9.
6. Budgin JB, Richardson SK, Newton SB, Wysocka M, Zaki MH, Benoit B, et al. Biological effects of bexarotene in cutaneous T-cell lymphoma. Arch Dermatol. 2005;141: 315-21.
7. Hofer T. Continuous 'microdose' isotretinoin in adult recalcitrant rosacea. Clin Exp Dermatol. 2004;29:204-5.
8. Lammer EJ, Chen DT, Hoar RM, Agnish ND, Benke PJ, Braun JT, et al. Retinoic acid embryopathy. N Engl J Med. 1985;313:837-41.
9. David M, Hodak E, Lowe NJ. Adverse effects of retinoids. Med Toxicol Adverse Drug Exp. 1988;3:273-88.
10. Sundström A, Alfredsson L, Sjölin-Forsberg G, Gerdén B, Bergman U, Jokinen J. Association of suicide attempts with acne and treatment with isotretinoin: retrospective Swedish cohort study. BMJ. 2010;341:c5812.

EXAMINATION QUESTIONS

1. Write a short note on systemic retinoids.
2. Classify systemic retinoids and briefly describe their MOA and applications in dermatology.

161 CHAPTER Biologics in Dermatology

Manas Chatterjee, Surbhi Rajput

INTRODUCTION

The term "biologics" refers to those protein molecules derived from natural sources which are therapeutically used to target various events in the inflammatory cascade. It can be a serum, vaccine, virus, antitoxin, antibodies, blood or blood products being used to cure various diseases.[1] They are large molecules, 100–1000 times greater than the size of a small molecule drug and have a complex structure. As the knowledge in the etiopathogenesis of various disorders become robust, biologics are being used extensively as immune modulating agents in the field of dermatology.

CLASSIFICATION OF BIOLOGICS USED IN DERMATOLOGY[2]

- Monoclonal antibody
- Recombinant antibody fusion proteins
- Human cytokines and growth factors

MONOCLONAL ANTIBODIES

Monoclonal antibodies target cell-specific receptors. They are made of human and animal products. Therapeutically, they are predominantly of IgG1 class. Previously, only murine antibodies were used which led to the formation of anti-murine antibodies and blocked the action of monoclonal antibodies. Presently, the antibodies being used have minimal quantity of murine antibody in the variable region.[3]

They are categorized as:

- Murine antibodies
- Humanized antibodies
- Fully human antibodies

Monoclonal Antibodies of Dermatological Importance

Monoclonal Antibodies against TNF-α

Infliximab: Infliximab is a human mouse chimeric IgG1 antibody which specifically binds to and blocks the action of TNF-α. It has 75% human constant region and 25% murine variable region. It neutralizes the soluble TNF-α and block the action of membrane bound TNF-α. Infliximab also causes complement mediated lysis of cells producing TNF-α. It has a molecular weight of 150 kDa. It has a terminal half-life of 10 days and is metabolized by proteolysis. There is a risk of immunogenicity due to its chimeric component and long-term usage of infliximab leads to antidrug antibody production thereby reducing its effectiveness.

US FDA approved dermatologic indications:
Psoriasis and psoriatic arthritis: 5 mg/kg IV at 0, 2, and 6 weeks, and 8 weekly thereafter.[4]

Off-label dermatological uses:

- *Hidradenitis suppurativa*: Given at a dose of 10 mg/kg every 6 weeks
- *Neutrophilic dermatosis*: Sweet's syndrome, pyoderma gangrenosum
- Vasculitis
- Granulomatous dermatosis
- Atopic dermatitis
- Sarcoidosis

Adalimumab: It is a fully human IgG1 antibody directed against TNF-α. It can lyse cells expressing TNF-α like infliximab. It targets both soluble and membrane-bound TNF-α. It has a half like of around 12 days and metabolized by proteolysis. It is given in a dose of 40 mg SC every other week. As it is a fully human monoclonal antibody, risk of immunogenicity and anti-drug antibody production is minimal.[5]

US FDA approved indications:

- *Psoriasis*: 80 mg SC once and after 1 week, then 40 mg SC at every 2 weeks.
- *Hidradenitis suppurativa*: *Induction*: 160 mg SC on day 1 then 80 mg 2 weeks later

Maintenance: 40 mg SC every week (as HS lesions have five times higher levels of TNF-α than any other condition).

Off-label uses:

- Vasculitis
- Neutrophilic dermatoses
- Granulomatous dermatoses

Golimumab: It is a fully human antibody against TNF-α being approved for psoriatic arthritis at a dose of 50 mg SC monthly.

Certolizumab pegol: It is a recombinant humanized monoclonal antibody where in the Fab portion is attached to polyethylene glycol (PEG) thereby increasing its terminal half-life.[6] Unlike other antibodies, this does not have a Fc portion. Due to the absence of Fc portion, it does not fix complement, does not cause complement-mediated cytotoxicity or antibody dependent cellular cytotoxicity. It is safe in pregnancy as it is not being transported through the placenta due to lack of Fc portion. It is approved by US FDA for plaque psoriasis at a dosage of 400 mg every other week.

Monoclonal Antibodies against B-cells

Rituximab: It is a monoclonal chimeric antibody directed against B-cell specific antigen CD20 and triggers B-cell depletion. It was first approved for treatment of CD20+ B-cell non-Hodgkin's lymphoma. Rituximab causes depletion of B-cells through antibody-dependent cellular cytotoxicity, complement-mediated cytolysis and signaling-induced apoptosis of B-cells.[7] It has a molecular weight of 145 kDa. The terminal half-life is 18 days and is metabolized by proteolysis.

Other anti-CD-20 antibodies that are under clinical trial: Ofatumumab, veltuzumab, ocrelizumab (type 1), tostimumab, and obintuzumab (type 2).

US FDA approved dermatological indications
Pemphigus vulgaris: *Induction*: 1,000 mg IV on day 1 and then after 2 weeks

Maintenance: 500 mg IV on 12th month and then every 6 months based on clinical evaluation.

Off-label uses:

- *Autoimmune bullous dermatosis*: Pemphigus foliaceus, paraneoplastic pemphigus, epidermolysis bullosa acquisita, bullous pemphigoid, and mucus membrane pemphigoid.
- Dermatomyositis
- Cutaneous lupus erythematosus
- Graft versus host disease
- Eosinophilic granulomatosis with polyangiitis

Belimumab: Belimumab is a fully human recombinant IgG1 monoclonal antibody directed against B-cell activating factor which in turn prevents the interaction of BAFF with its receptor and indirectly decreases B-cell survival and production of autoantibodies. It is approved by US FDA for the treatment of systemic lupus erythematosus. The recommended dose of belimumab is 10 mg/kg at 2-week intervals for the first three doses and at 4-week intervals thereafter.[8]

Other Monoclonal Antibodies of Dermatological Significance

Omalizumab: It is a recombinant humanized IgG1k monoclonal antibody directed against free human IgE. It prevents interaction of IgE molecule with the high affinity FceRI receptors on mast cells and basophils thereby preventing the release of histamine and other mediators leading to allergy and urticaria. It forms immune complexes, i.e., cyclic hexamers with free IgE which are cleared by the reticuloendothelial system.[9]

US FDA approved dermatological indications: Patients >12 years of age with chronic idiopathic urticarial refractory to H_1 antihistamine treatment.

Off-label uses:

- Bullous pemphigoid
- Hyper-IgE syndrome
- Peanut or latex allergy
- Severe delayed pressure angioedema
- Recurrent idiopathic angioedema
- Physical urticaria
- Urticarial vasculitis
- Mastocytosis

Ustekinumab: It is a human IgG1 antibody targeting the shared p40 subunit of IL-12 and IL-23, and hence stops its interaction with the IL-12 receptor thereby preventing T-cell activation and inflammatory pathway. It was approved by US FDA for psoriasis in 2009 and for psoriatic arthritis in 2013. However, it is yet to be available in India.

Monoclonal Antibodies against IL-17

Secukinumab: It is a fully human antibody against IL-17 indicated for treatand for psoriatic arthritis in 2013. Howeverent of psoriasis and psoriatic arthritis. The recommended dose of secukinumab is 300 mg SC at weeks 0, 1, 2, 3, 4 followed by every 4 weeks. The placebo-controlled study (FIXTURE) demonstrated that induction and maintenance therapy with secukinumab had great results in moderate-to-severe psoriasis.[10]

Ixekizumab: It is a humanized IgG4 antibody against IL-17 A which prevents its interaction with IL-17 receptor. It is being used for moderate-to-severe psoriasis and psoriatic arthritis, not available in India.

Brodalumab: It is a fully human IgG2 human IL-17A receptor antagonist indicated for moderate-to-severe plaque psoriasis.

Monoclonal Antibodies against IL-23

Guselkumab: It is a recombinant monoclonal antibody against IL-23 and was approved in 2017 for treatment of moderate-to-severe plaque psoriasis. Two phase III studies (VOYAGE) were conducted to assess the pharmacokinetics and safety of guselkumab and its administration in psoriasis.[11] It is currently approved by USFDA for the treatment of patients with moderate-to-severe plaque psoriasis who are candidates for systemic therapy or phototherapy.

Tildrakizumab and Risankizumab are two other novel IL-23 inhibitors approved for use in moderate-to-severe plaque psoriasis in patients who are candidates for systemic therapy.

Efalizumab: It is a recombinant humanized monoclonal antibody against CD11 a, subunit of LFA-1 thus blocking the immunological synapse. It was FDA approved for psoriasis in 2003 and also being used for eruptive lichen planus. It was withdrawn from the market in 2009.

Daclizumab: Daclizumab is a humanized monoclonal antibody against CD25 subunit of the IL-2 receptor. It blocks the T-cell proliferation and activation. Its efficacy was in psoriasis. It has been withdrawn from the market in 2018.

Siplizumab: It is a monoclonal humanized antibody against CD2 which blocks the immunological synapse by preventing the interaction of CD2 with LFA-3 thereby stopping the inflammatory cascade. It has potential use in psoriasis.

Basiliximab: It is monoclonal chimeric antibody which is directed IL-2 (CD25), being studied for severe psoriasis and generalized pustular psoriasis.

Duplimumab: Duplimumab is a fully human monoclonal antibody which is directed against α-subunit of IL-4 receptor. By inhibiting the IL-4 receptor which is shared by both IL-4 and IL-13, type 2 (Th 2) cytokines are inhibited which have a major role in the pathogenesis of atopic dermatitis. It is FDA approved for moderate-to-severe atopic dermatitis in adults and adolescents more than 12 years of age refractory to topical therapy. It is also being used for alopecia areata and chronic idiopathic eczematous eruption of aging.

Nemolizumab: It is a monoclonal antibody that antagonizes the IL-31 receptor which in turn blocks the IL-31 signaling on T-cells, macrophages and neurons. It is being experimented for use in cases of recalcitrant atopic dermatitis. US FDA has granted breakthrough therapy designation to the drug for the treatment of pruritus associated with prurigo nodularis in December 2019.

Anakinra: Anakinra is the non-glycosylated form of IL-1R antagonist and works by blocking the action of IL-1. It is being used for psoriatic arthropathy, familial cold autoinflammatory syndromes and Schnitzler's syndrome, Still's disease, generalized pustular psoriasis, and palmoplantar pustulosis. It is given as 100 mg subcutaneous injection once daily in psoriasis and along with thalidomide in Schnitzler's syndrome.

Gevokizumab and Canakinumab: These are two IL-1β antagonists which have shown efficacy in generalized pustular psoriasis and urticarial, respectively.

Fusion Proteins

Fusion proteins are the combination product of constant region of human IgG with receptor domain of human protein. The resultant fusion protein binds to a receptor or a ligand thereby blocking its action.[12]

The commonly used fusion proteins in dermatology are:

Alefacept: It is a bivalent human recombinant fusion protein containing hinge portion of LFA-3 with human IgG. The LFA-3 portion of alefacept binds to the CD2 receptor thereby breaking the immunological synapse. The US FDA approved alefacept for the treatment of psoriasis in 2002, given intramuscularly or intravenously at a dose of 10 mg/kg IM or 7.5 mg/kg IV. Other off-label indications are neutrophilic dermatoses, lichen planus, alopecia areata and chronic graft versus host disease.[13] It is currently not being marketed.

Etanercept: It is a recombinant dimeric fully human fusion protein of p75 TNF-α with Fc portion of human IgG. It is a TNF-α inhibitor and binds to both soluble and membrane bound TNF-α thus preventing its actions on its receptors. It also binds to TNF-β and hence has a very high affinity for TNF. Its molecular weight is 150 kDa. The terminal half-life of etanercept is 4.8 days. It is metabolized by proteolysis with the by-products being eliminated in bile or urine.[14]

US FDA approved indications:
Plaque psoriasis.

Off-label uses:

- Neutrophilic dermatosis
- Granulomatous dermatoses
- Vasculitis
- Severe drug reaction psoriasis
- Psoriatic arthritis

Abatacept: It is a fusion protein combination of extracellular portion of CTLA4 with Fc portion of human IgG4. It binds on the surface of antigen presenting cells hence stopping T-cell activation. It is being used for psoriasis vulgaris and rheumatoid arthritis. Belatacept is a second generation CTLA4 protein being studied for allograft rejections.

Denileukin diftitox: It is a recombinant fusion protein consisting of fragments of diphtheria toxin combined with human IL-2 which works by blocking the IL-2 receptors. It was being tried for recalcitrant psoriasis. It is approved for cutaneous T-cell lymphoma.

Onercept: It is a novel soluble p55 tumor necrosis factor binding protein used for psoriasis and psoriatic arthritis. However, trials have been stopped due to unfavorable safety profile.

Recombinant Human Cytokines and Growth Factors

Cytokines are nonimmunoglobin proteins or glycoproteins being used as immunomodulators in response to immune stimulus.[15]

Interferons: Interferons are a group of proteins being produced by virus-infected leukocytes. They have immunomodulatory, antiproliferative, antineoplastic, and antiviral activity.

Interferon-α: Recombinant interferon-α is being used in verruca vulgaris, condyloma acuminate, AIDS-related Kaposi's sarcoma, basal cell carcinoma, melanoma, hemangioma, and keloids.

Interferon-γ: It is FDA approved for the treatment of chronic granulomatous disease. It is also being used for atopic dermatitis and cutaneous T-cell lymphoma.

Interleukin-2: Recombinant IL-2 has antitumor activity and being used in cutaneous T-cell lymphoma and metastatic melanoma.

Interleukin-11: It is being used in the treatment of psoriatic arthritis.

Granulocyte-Monocyte Colony Stimulating Factor (GM-CSF): It works by stimulating the granulocytes, monocytes, and macrophages. It is used in melanoma, Sezary syndrome, and to accelerate wound healing.

ADVERSE EFFECTS OF BIOLOGICS[16,17]

- *Allergic reaction and antibody formation*: Seen with TNF-α inhibitors
- Hypersensitivity
- *Injection site reactions*: Mild erythema, edema, bruising and burning can be noticed especially with TNF-α inhibitors.
- *Acute flu-like illness*: Mild fever, chills and myalgia is seen in 20% of the patients, more commonly with infliximab.
- *Reactivation of tuberculosis*: Seen with TNF-α inhibitors.
- *Infections*: Hepatitis B, hepatitis C, sepsis to *Listeria*, *Histoplasma capsulatum* have been also been reported.
- *Demyelinating disorders*: Worsening of multiple sclerosis is noticed with anti TNF-α therapy.
- *Malignancy*: Hematogenous malignancies and non-melanoma skin cancers are known to occur with prolonged use of biologics
- *Activation of lupus*: ANA and lupus-like syndrome may develop during treatment with anti-TNF-α therapy but generally does not show signs and symptoms.
- *Thrombocytopenia*: May occur 6–8 months after initiation of efalizumab and may require discontinuation of therapy.
- *Autoimmune hemolytic anemia*: Seen with efalizumab therapy.
- Hepatitis has been reported with infliximab therapy and the treatment should be withheld in case of jaundice or elevation of enzymes to more than five times the upper limit.
- *Congestive cardiac failure*: Worsening of congestive cardiac failure is known to occur with anti-TNF α therapy.

PATIENT SCREENING FOR BIOLOGICS[18,19]

Patients before being put on biologics therapy should undergo a thorough evaluation including history, clinical examination, and investigations. The investigations routinely advised are:

Baseline Investigations

- Full blood count
- Renal and liver function tests
- Screening for hepatitis B, C, and HIV infection
- Antinuclear antibodies
- Urine analysis
- Chest X-ray
- Tuberculin skin testing and/or Interferon Gamma Release Assay (IGRA)

Follow-up Investigations

- Liver and renal function tests should be done every month for first 3 months and then at 6 months.
- Chest X-ray and tuberculin skin testing/IGRA should be done every year.

Contraindications

- Active tuberculosis
- Pre-existing hepatitis or liver failure
- Premalignant conditions or active malignancy
- Previous treatment with >200 PUVA therapies
- Hepatitis B, C or HIV positivity
- Pre-existing congestive cardiac failure
- Active infections
- Pregnancy and breastfeeding

Assessment of Response to Biologics

Various scoring systems and indices can be used for assessment of response of biologic therapy. For example, psoriasis area and severity index (PASI) is used to assess the clinical response in psoriasis. Reduction in the baseline score of >75% (PASI75) is the standard used by FDA to assess the response of biologic therapy.[20] PASI and DLQI is recommended to be recorded initially for 3 months and then every 6 months.

KEY POINTS

- Biologics represent the modern day therapy not only in dermatology but in various other fields.
- Among the various conditions of dermatology, the most common condition where biologics are being exercised is psoriasis.
- However, the various adverse effects and high cost of the drugs limit their routine use in the present state in our country.
- Use should be judicious in situations where there are adverse effect of conventional therapy or the conventional drugs have failed to produce desired results.

REFERENCES

1. Feldman M, Steinman L. Design of effective immunotherapy for autoimmunity. Nature. 2005;435:612-9.
2. Stern DK, Tripp JM, Ho VC, Lebwohi M. The use of systemic immune moderators in dermatology. In: Mclean DI, Maddin WS (Eds). Dermatologic Clinics, Vol 23. Amsterdam, Netherlands: Elsevier; 2005. p. 275.

3. Waldmann TA. Immunotherapy: past, present and future. Nat Med. 2003;9:269-77.
4. Winterfield L, Menter A. Psoriasis and its treatment with infliximab-mediated tumour necrosis factor α blockade. Dermatol Clin. 2004;22:437-44.
5. Scheinfeld N. Adalimumab (HUMIRA): a review. J Drugs Dermatol. 2003;2:375-7.
6. Pasut G. Pegylation of biological molecules and potential benefits: pharmacological properties of certolizumab pegol. Biodrugs. 2014;28:S15-S23.
7. Reff ME, Carner K, Chambers KS, Chinn PC, Leonard JE, Raab R, et al. Depletion of B cells on vivo by a chimeric mouse human monoclonal antibody to CD20. Blood. 1994;83(2):435-45.
8. Srivastava A. Belimumab in Systemic Lupus Erythematosus. Indian J Dermatol. 2016;61(5):550-3.
9. Kaplan AP, Gimenez-Arnau AM, Saini SS. Mechanism of action that contribute to efficacy of omalizumab in chronic spontaneous urticarial. Allergy. 2017;72(4):519-33.
10. Langley RG, Elewski BE, Lebwohl M, Reich K, Griffiths CEM, Papp K, et al. Secukinumab in plaque psoriasis: results of two phase 3 trials. N Engl J Med. 2014;371(4):326-38.
11. Blauvelt A, Papp KA, Griffiths CE, Randazzo B, Wasfi Y, Shen YK, et al. Efficacy and safety of guselkumab, an anti-interleukin 23 monoclonal antibody, compared with adalimumab for continuous treatment of patients with moderate-to-severe psoriasis: results from phase III, double blinded, placebo- and active-comparator controlled VOYAGE I clinical trial. J Am Acad Dermatol. 2017;76(3):405-17.
12. Krueger JG. The immunological basis of treatment of psoriasis with new biological agents. J Am Acad Dermatol. 2002;46: 1-23.
13. Krueger GG. Current concepts and review of alefacept in the treatment of psoriasis. Dermatol Clin. 2004;22:407-22.
14. Goldsmith DR, Wagstaff AJ. Etanercept: a review of its use in the management of plaque psoriasis and psoriatic arthritis. AM J Clin Dermatol. 2005;6:121-36.
15. Holman DM, Kallaji AN. Cytokines in dermatology. J Drug Dermatol. 2006;5:520-4.
16. Kormieli T, Lowe Nj, Yaamuchi PS. Psoriasis immunopathogenesis and evolving immunomodulators and systemic therapies; US experiences. Br J Dermatol. 2004;151: 3-15.
17. Koo J, Khera P. Update on the mechanisms and efficacy of biological therapies for psoriasis. J Dermatol Sci. 2005;38:75-87.
18. Asadullah K, Sterry W, Ebeling M, Friedrich M, Leopold M, Jasulaitis D, et al. Clinical and immunological effects of IL-10 therapy in psoriasis. Br J Dermatol. 1999;141:989.
19. Sukal SA, Nadiminti L, Granstein RD. Etanercept and demyelinating disease in a patient with psoriasis. J Am Acad Dermatol. 2006;54:160-4.
20. Scheinfeld N. Adalimumab: a review of side effects. Exp Opin Drug Saf. 2005;4:637-41.

EXAMINATION QUESTIONS

1. Describe the mechanism of action, indications and adverse effects of TNF-alpha inhibitors.
2. Describe the role of newer biologics used in psoriasis.
3. Discuss biologicals in AD.

Write short notes on the following:

4. Rituximab.
5. Omalizumab.
6. Infliximab.

162 CHAPTER

Miscellaneous Systemic Drugs in Dermatology

Priyankar Misra

INTRODUCTION

This chapter will cover drugs which are used less frequently and in unique conditions for dermatologic care. Most of them are second or third line drugs of choice for that particular disease. The list is as follows:

- Thalidomide
- Colchicine
- Potassium iodide
- Gold
- Biotin
- Attenuated androgens (stanozolol and danazol)
- Anticholinergics (glycopyrrolate and oxybutynin)
- Fumaric acid esters
- Penicillamine
- Pregabalin and gabapentin
- Zinc sulphate

THALIDOMIDE

This was initially introduced in Europe in late 1950s as a sedative but was subsequently withdrawn because of its dreaded teratogenic side effects that were reported after a few years. Later encouraging results were seen in the management of erythema nodosum leprosum. Finally in 1998, it received approval from FDA for ENL but with caution and strict monitoring.

Pharmacokinetics

- Thalidomide is a synthetic derivative of glutamic acid with one chiral center and consists of a glutarimide ring (responsible for sedative effects) and a pthalidimide ring (responsible for teratogenic effects).[1]
- *In vivo*, it is present in interchangeable racemic mixtures of R and S isomers where R is responsible for the sedative effects and S is responsible for the teratogenic effects.[2]
- Its oral bioavailability is low and reaches a peak blood concentration after 6 hours and has highest distribution in skin and kidneys.

Mechanism of Action

The exact mechanism is still unknown but the possible hypotheses are as follows:

- *Hypnosedative actions*: It can penetrate the blood–brain barrier and causes sedation by affecting the deeper centers of forebrain and this perhaps explains its efficacy in conditions such as prurigo nodularis.
- *Immunomodulatory actions*: It leads to specific inhibition of TNF-α and suppression of IL12 and INF-γ and enhances the humoral immunity by increased production of IL4 and IL5.
- *Anticancer effects*: *In vitro* research has revealed that thalidomide has a cytostatic activity, anti-angiogenic properties via inhibition of VEGF and anti-emetic activity in patients receiving chemotherapy for cancer.[1]

Indications

- *Erythema nodosum leprosum*: This the only FDA approved indication of thalidomide. An average daily dose of 100 mg has been found to be effective, although higher initial dose of 400 mg daily and maintenance with 50–100 mg daily have also been tried. Combining with steroids permits reduction of dose of thalidomide.
- Other conditions where it has reported to be useful are as follows:
  - Severe and recalcitrant aphthous stomatitis
  - Behçet's disease
  - Prurigo nodularis
  - Actinic prurigo
  - Discoid lupus erythematosus
  - Systemic lupus erythematosus
  - Pyoderma gangrenosum
  - Jessner's lymphocytic infiltrate
  - Histiocytosis X
  - Toxic epidermal necrolysis
  - Lichen planus
  - Kaposi sarcoma
  - Post-herpetic neuralgia
  - HIV infection
  - Graft versus host disease
  - Malignant melanoma
  - Sarcoidosis
  - Uremic pruritus
  - Rheumatoid arthritis
  - Waldenstrom macroglobulinemia

Adverse Effects

The common adverse effects are as follows:

- Teratogenicity
- Somnolence and fatigue

- Dizziness
- Peripheral neuropathy
- Skin rash
- Constipation
- Thromboembolism

Contraindications[3]

Absolute	Relative
• Hypersensitivity to the drug • Pregnancy • Peripheral neuropathy	• Existing renal dysfunction • Existing hepatic dysfunction • Hypertension • Hypothyroid • Existing gastrointestinal dysfunction

Monitoring and Precautions

- A written, informed consent must be obtained and patient must be explained in detail about adverse effects.
- Females must follow two methods of contraception, a barrier method along with another highly effective method, starting 1 month before the start of thalidomide and up to 1 month after the end of treatment.
- Males should follow one method of contraception for the same duration.
- Blood donation during the period of treatment is discouraged.
- Before starting treatment, complete clinical examination especially neurological examination should be performed.
- Routine investigations and some specific ones such as baseline pregnancy test, complete blood count with an absolute neutrophil count, HIV RNA, electromyography (EMG) or nerve conduction velocity (NCV) study should be conducted.
- While on treatment, pregnancy is ruled out by repeating pregnancy tests initially at weekly intervals for 1 month and then monthly thereafter. Detailed neurological testing is repeated monthly for 3 months and then every 6 months. It is also recommended that EMG and NCV be repeated biannually or with every 10 g increase in the cumulative dose. In HIV positive patients, HIV RNA must be repeated at 1 month, 3 months, and every 3 months thereafter.
- *Treatment should be discontinued under following circumstances*:
  - Positive pregnancy test
  - Absolute neutrophil count going below 750/cubic mm
  - Development of paresthesia
  - Noncompliant patient
  - Decrease in sensory nerve action potential by 40%

Colchicine

- Colchicine is an alkaloid extracted from the seeds and tubers of *Colchicum autumnale* and has to be protected from sunlight as UV radiation since it degrades into inactive products.
- It gets concentrated in leukocytes and bind to microtubules leading to metaphase arrest and also prevents chemotaxis and cell motility. It also prevents PMN adhesiveness to endothelial cells and interferes with lysosomal degranulation. Thus it has both antimitotic and anti-inflammatory actions.
- *Indications*:
  - Acute gout and familial Mediterranean fever are the only FDA approved indication.
  - Off-label indication for dermatological conditions are as follows:
    - Neutrophilic dermatosis such as Behçet disease, erythema nodosum, aphthous stomatitis, dermatitis herpetiformis, Sweet's syndrome, linear IgA bullous, etc.
    - Papulosquamous disorders such as psoriasis
    - Connective tissue disorders such as dermatomyositis and progressive systemic sclerosis
    - Vasculitis
- *Adverse effects*:
  - Gastrointestinal effects are most common like abdominal cramps and diarrhea which generally gets tolerated by slowly increasing the dose.
  - Colchicine overdose can be serious. Acute overdose leads to cholera-like syndrome with dehydration, hypokalemia, hyponatremia, metabolic acidosis, renal failure, and ultimately shock. Respiratory distress syndrome, disseminated intravascular coagulation, and bone marrow failure may ensue. Other toxic manifestations include hepatic failure and late central nervous system disorders. Myopathy, hypocalcemia, alopecia, stomatitis, and porphyria cutanea tarda have been reported in acutely intoxicated patients who ultimately survived.[4,5] Chronic intoxication may occur after prolonged therapy with at least 1 mg daily. Complications include leukopenia, aplastic anemia, myopathy, and alopecia.[4]
- *Dose*: For dermatological indications, dose is generally 0.6 mg twice or thrice daily.
- *Contraindications*:
  - *Absolute*: Blood dyscrasias and hypersensitivity to the drug. Regular monitoring of routine blood parameters is important to avoid hematological complications.
  - *Relative*: Any concurrent severe gastrointestinal, hepatic, or cardiac disorders.

Potassium Iodide

- *Mechanism of action*:
  - In vitro studies have found that the drug has no effect on effect on *Sporothrix schenckii*. Its efficacy is probably due to alteration in the host's immunologic or nonimmunologic response to the organism. Iodides concentrate in infected granulomas and necrotic tissue and have been shown to inhibit further granuloma formation.[6]

- The other mechanism is by release of large quantities of heparin from the mast cell by iodide that leads to suppression of delayed hypersensitivity.
- Potassium iodide can also suppress the generation of inflammatory oxygen intermediate from activated PMNs.[7]

- *Indications*: There are no FDA approved indications in dermatology but the off-label ones are as follows:
  - *Deep fungal infections like sporotrichosis*: The initial dose for sporotrichosis is 5 drops of the saturated solution (each drop contains 67 mg of potassium iodide) three times daily in milk or juice. This dose is gradually increased by 3–5 drops (with roughly weekly increments) until a dose of at least 15 drops three times daily is reached. Doses up to 50 drops three times daily may be required in occasional patients. Lesions usually heal within 2–4 weeks, and therapy is continued for an additional 2–4 weeks.[8] Efficacy is also seen in other deep fungal infections such as mucormycosis and zygomycosis.
  - Erythema nodosum
  - Nodular vasculitis
  - Pyoderma gangrenosum
  - Erythema multiforme
  - Sweet's syndrome
  - Wegener's granulomatosis
  - Granuloma annulare
- *Contraindications*:[3]

Absolute	*Relative*
Hypersensitivity to the drug	• Hypothyroidism • Cardiac disease • Renal insufficiency • Addison's disease • Hyperkalemia

- *Adverse effects*:
  - *Hypothyroidism*: Generally seen with high doses and prolonged therapy and most patients have underlying hypothyroidism.[9]
  - *Cutaneous side-effects*: Skin lesions of various morphologies are remarkably common and include acneiform, dermatitic, and vascular eruptions.[10] A distinctive, vegetating eruption known as iododerma may occur with chronic low-dose ingestion.
  - *Other systemic side effects*: Chronic intoxication begins with an unpleasant brassy taste, a burning sensation in the mouth, and increased salivation. Coryza, sneezing, and eye irritation are common. Mild iodism simulates a head cold. Parotid and submaxillary glands may become enlarged and tender. Gastric irritation is common. Diarrhea, fever, anorexia, and depression may occur.[11]
- *Monitoring*: Before initiating potassium iodide therapy, patients should be closely questioned regarding previous history of thyroid disease and size of thyroid gland to be assessed. Note should be taken of concurrent medications, such as lithium and amiodarone, that can also affect thyroid function. Baseline thyroid-stimulating hormone (TSH), T4 level, antithyroglobulin, and antimicrosomal antibodies should be checked in patients suspected of having an underlying thyroid disease.[9]

Gold

- Gold was parenterally administered until 1985, when oral auranofin became available. The two parenteral agents, aurothioglucose and aurothiomalate. It is accumulated in reticuloendothelial cells, kidneys, and adrenal gland. Oral gold is excreted by hepatobiliary route whereas parenteral gold is excreted mainly in urine.
- *Mechanism of action*:
  - Its anti-inflammatory action is due to inhibition of chemotaxis and phagocytosis of macrophages and PMNs. It also inhibits compliment cascade and synthesis of prostaglandings.[12,13]
  - The beneficial effect of gold in treating pemphigus may relate to interference with blister formation by inhibition of degradative epidermal lysosomal enzymes and normalizes the defective Langerhans' cell antigen presentation.[14]
- *Indications*:
  - Connective tissue diseases such as DLE, SLE
  - Psoriatic arthritis
  - Bullous disease such as pemphigus foliaceus and vulgaris, epidermolysis bullosa acquisita and cicatricial pemphigoid.
- *Adverse effects*:
  - Mucocutaneous reactions such as stomatitis, cheilitis, lichen planus such as or PR like eruptions are seen in 40% cases.[12,15]
  - Gastrointestinal effects such as diarrhea is seen in 35–40% cases whereas severe enterocolitis and intrahepatic cholestasis have been rarely reported.[12]
  - Hematologic adverse effects, most common with parenteral administration, occur in approximately 1–2% of patients and include leukopenia, thrombocytopenia, eosinophilia, and in rare instances, aplastic anemia.
  - Renal adverse effects include proteinuria and nephritis seen in 2–10% cases.
  - The nitritoid reaction is a vasomotor response characterized by flushing, dizziness, metallic taste, hypotension, and syncope occurring within 10 minutes of gold injection. The nitritoid reaction occurs almost exclusively with the aqueous gold sodium thiomalate formulation.
  - Sudden dyspnea with diffuse bilateral pulmonary infiltrates is rare reaction that can progress to chronic pulmonary fibrosis. Infrequent neurologic complications include acute progressive polyneuropathy and diffuse fasciculations.[12]

- *Contraindications*:
  - Prior anaphylactic reaction to gold
  - Exfoliative dermatitis
  - Aplastic anemia or other severe hematologic disorder
  - Necrotizing enterocolitis
  - Pulmonary fibrosis
- *Therapeutic guidelines*:
  - Parenteral therapy in adults begins with a 10-mg intramuscular injection. This is followed 1 week later by a 25-mg injection and subsequent biweekly 50-mg injections. Once a clinical response is obtained, the interval between doses may be lengthened or the weekly dose reduced. Children initially receive 1 mg/kg weekly, and the interval between injections is subsequently lengthened to 2–4 weeks.[12]
  - In adults, oral gold therapy is initiated at 3 mg twice daily.[12] A total daily dose of 9 mg may be required for selected patients. When disease control is attained, a single daily auranofin dose of 3 mg may maintain adequate control.

Biotin

- Biotin (also known as vitamin H, vitamin B_7, and co-enzyme R) is a water-soluble, B-complex vitamin essential for the function of a number of carboxylase enzymes. Food sources of biotin include organ meats, egg yolk, milk, fish, and nuts; biotin may also be synthesized by intestinal flora.
- Cutaneous signs of biotin deficiency are similar to those of multiple carboxylase deficiency, namely thinning of the hair and poliosis. A seborrheic dermatitis-like eruption may occur around the eyes, nose, and mouth, mimicking the rash seen in zinc deficiency.
- The daily requirement of biotin for an adult is between 100 and 200 mg.[35] The most frequently used dose for hair and nail problems is 2.5–3.0 mg daily. Higher doses have been used to treat dermatitic eruptions (5 mg daily) and keratodermas (50 mg daily). Duration of therapy ranges from several weeks to months. Time to response is variable, and supplementation must be continued indefinitely to maintain improvement.

Attenuated Androgens (Danazol and Stanozolol)

- These are synthetic derivatives of testosterone alkylated at 17-alpha position which reduces hepatic metabolism that increases oral bioavailability and the attached pyrazole ring increases the anabolic activity and reduces the androgenic properties.[16]
- *Mechanism of action*:
  - Potent fibrinolytic activity by alteration of synthesis of hepatic proteins.
  - Stanozolol has also been shown to increase collagen synthesis of cultured dermal fibroblasts, which may have a beneficial effect on wound healing.[17]
- *Indications*:[3]
  - *Hereditary angioedema*: Stanozolol therapy is initiated at a dose of 2 mg three times daily; danazol at a dose of 200 mg two or three times daily. After edematous episodes are successfully prevented, the doses are slowly titrated downward. Long-term prophylaxis is typically obtained with doses not exceeding 2 mg daily of stanozolol or 200 mg daily of danazol.
  - Cryofibrinogenemia
  - Lipodermatosclerosis
  - Livedoid vasculopathy
  - Lichen sclerosus et atrophicus of the penis
  - There has been reports showing improvement of chronic urticaria, Raynaud's phenomenon, autoimmune progesterone dermatitis, and refractory pruritus associated with myeloproliferative disorders with attenuated androgens.
- *Adverse effects*:
  - Mild hirsutism, deepening of the voice, alopecia, acne, menstrual irregularities, weight gain, and dyspareunia have all been reported to occur in female patients.[16,18]
  - Neuromuscular dysfunction in the form of muscles cramps and myalgia
  - Microscopic hematuria and even hemorrhagic cystitis is a rare and worrisome side effect.
  - Insulin resistance and mild deterioration of glucose tolerance may occur.[19]
  - Episodes of anxiety, tremulousness, and exacerbations of underlying migraine headaches have been described.[20]
  - Because of the sodium-retaining effects of these drugs, worsening of hypertension, and congestive heart failure may occur.
- Therapeutic monitoring

Because androgen derivatives can cause cholestatic jaundice, peliosis hepatis, and liver tumors, monitoring of liver function is advised. If hepatotoxic effects arise, then it is judicious to shift to oxandrolone which is an anabolic steroid with less hepatotoxic effects.

Anticholinergics (Glycopyrrolate and Oxybutynin)

- Systemic anticholinergic drugs for the symptomatic treatment of hyperhidrosis have been used for decades. Atropine is avoided because of its numerous ophthalmic side effects. Glycopyrrolate and propantheline bromide appear to be the most frequently used anticholinergic agents in the sparse literature available on this topic.[21]
- Glycopyrrolate is usually prescribed in doses of 1–2 mg, two to three times daily. Propantheline's initial dose is

usually 15 mg, two to three times daily. These medications can be gradually titrated to higher doses if anticholinergic symptoms are tolerated.

- Mild side effects such as dryness of mouth and blurring of vision is common at therapeutic doses but fortunately serious side effects such as glaucoma is rare.

Fumaric Acid Esters

- Esters of fumaric acid (FAEs) such as monoethylfumarate (MEF), monomethylfumarate (MMF), diethylfumarate (DEF) and dimethylfumarate (DMF) are potent chemicals and have been used in the treatment of psoriasis in European countries for over 30 years.
- In 1994, Fumaderm, an enteric-coated tablet containing DMF and calcium, magnesium and zinc salts of MEF was approved for the treatment of psoriasis in Germany.[2] DMF is rapidly metabolized to monomethyl fumarate (MMF) which, together with DMF, is regarded as the main bioactive metabolite.
- The mechanism of action is still unclear but the hypotheses are as follows:[22]
  - It inhibits the cytokine-induced expression of adhesion molecules such as VCAM-1, ICAM-1, and E-selectin on dermal fibroblasts and endothelial cells.
  - Enhancement in formation of anti-inflammatory cytokines such as IL-10 and reduction in formation of T-helper cells and proinflammatory cytokines such as TNF-α and IFN-γ.
  - Promoting apoptosis in dendritic and the antigen presenting cells.
  - Induction of apoptosis in various other immune cells including activated T-cells which is accompanied by a strong induction of the anti-inflammatory stress protein heme oxygenase 1 (HO-1).
  - Through the above mechanisms they exert anti-inflammatory, immune-modulatory, and antiproliferative effects.
- *Indications*:
  - *Psoriasis*: Each tablet of Fumaderm has 30 mg of DMF. Initially, patient is started on one tablet daily and dose escalation is done till peak response is reached. Then the dose is reduced and a steady maintenance dose is continued.
  - Disseminated granuloma annulare.[23-26]
  - Sarcoidosis[27,28]
  - Necrobiosis lipoidica[29]
- *Contraindications*:[22]
  - Significant gastrointestinal diseases such as chronic gastritis or active or recent gastric or duodenal ulcers.
  - Severe liver or kidney diseases
  - Less than 18 years age
  - Women during pregnancy or lactation
- *Adverse effects*:[22]
  - *Most common side-effects*: Gastrointestinal complaints and flushes
  - *Frequent*: Lymphopenia
  - *Infrequent*: Eosinophilia and proteinuria
  - *Rare*: Raised liver enzymes and bilirubin levels

Penicillamine

- Penicillamine is a breakdown product of penicillin. It is a potent chelator of heavy metals (i.e., copper, gold, lead, mercury, and zinc), promoting their excretion in urine.
- The oral absorption of penicillamine ranges between 40 and 70% and is diminished by food and antacids containing magnesium–aluminum salts. Hepatic metabolism occurs, transforming most penicillamine to disulfides and inorganic sulfate. The disulfides play major roles in both therapeutic and toxic effects. The disulfide products readily bind to plasma proteins and are not excreted renally. These metabolic products accumulate during the first few weeks of therapy and are slowly eliminated once therapy is stopped.
- Dermatological use includes dermatologists treatment of various forms of PSS, primarily for localized versions of the condition. In most cases of PSS adult dosing is initiated at 125–250 mg daily, with increases of 125–250 mg daily occurring incrementally every 1–3 months until satisfactory remission or toxicity occurs (usually at levels between 750 and 1,500 mg daily). Therapy is commonly required for several months, with time to response and remission varying widely.
- Nondermatologic indications for the drug's use include the treatment of heavy metal poisoning, cystinuria, Wilson's disease, primary biliary cirrhosis, and rheumatoid arthritis.
- *Contraindications*: Dose adjustments and extra caution should be used in those allergic to penicillin or with renal dysfunction, during pregnancy, and in the pediatric population.
- *Adverse effects*: Common adverse effects of therapy include nausea, vomiting, abdominal pain, and diarrhea. Mucocutaneous side effects include bullous dermatoses (including several forms of pemphigus, cicatricial and bullous pemphigoid, and epidermolysis bullosa acquisita), a lupus-like syndrome, lichen planus, elastosis perforans serpiginosa, and pseudoxanthoma elasticum.

Pregabalin and Gabapentin

- These are anticonvulsant agents which are used in various dermatological conditions. The other indications of pregabalin and gabapentin are presented in the **Box 1**.[30]
- The initial dosage of gabapentin is 300 mg/day and can be increased up to 1200 mg three times a day.[31,32] It can be started at its effective dose rather than gradually titrated

upwards in dosage.[33] It should not be discontinued abruptly, but rather tapered gradually, because it can lead to withdrawal-related side-effects.[8] It has a high toxicity ratio, minimizing the chance of adverse effects with even very high overdoses, hence, routine monitoring of clinical laboratory parameters is not required. Pregabalin is started at an initial dose of 150 mg/day and can be increased up to 600 mg/day.

- The most common side effect is sedation and drowsiness which improves with continuous use. The other side effects are dizziness, malaise/lassitude and ataxia.

Rarely, they can cause pancytopenia, causing fever, sore throat and ulcers in the mouth, or unusual bleeding and easy bruising, fluid retention in the legs and weight gain.[31,32] A few cases of allergic eruptions[34] and Stevens–Johnson syndrome[35] have also been reported.

Zinc Sulfate

- Zinc being a trace element has a role in various cellular processes and its deficiency is seen in those on total parenteral nutrition and breastfed infants especially during weaning.

BOX 1: Indications of gabapentin and pregabalin.

- *Neuropathic pain*:
  - Postherpetic neuralgia
  - HIV neuropathy
  - Diabetic neuropathic pain
- *Neuralgia*:
  - Glossopharyngeal neuralgia
  - Trigeminal neuralgia
  - Facial neuritis
- *Skin hypersensitivity*:
  - *Allodynia*:
    - Buccofacial allodynia
    - Mechanical allodynia
  - Reflex sympathetic dystrophy
- *Dynia*:
  - Glossodynia
  - Carotidynia
  - Vulvodynia
  - Orchidynia
  - Prostatodynia
  - Coccygodynia
  - Proctodynia
  - Scalp dysesthesia
- Hot flashes
- Temperature-sensitive dermatosis
- Dysesthetic pain after reconstruction surgery
- *Pruritus*:
  - Brachoradial pruritus
  - Uremic pruritus
  - Pruritus of unknown origin
- Seizure due to AIP
- Self-injurious behavior in Lesh-Nyhan syndrome
- Steroid-induced mania
- Piloleiomyoma-related pain
- *Pain of vasolabile conditions*: Erythromelalgia

(HIV: human immunodeficiency virus; AIP: acute intermittent porphyria)

- True dietary deficiencies and acrodermatitis enteropathica can be readily detected by obtaining serum zinc levels. Both usually respond rapidly to zinc supplementation. Common doses of zinc replacement are in the range of 1–2 mg/kg daily of elemental zinc in three divided doses.
- Zinc has been used with inconsistent success in the treatment of various acneiform conditions, alopecia, and verrucae. Recent publications suggest that zinc sulfate may be useful in treating acute cutaneous leishmaniasis and perhaps leg ulcers in persons with low zinc levels.[36,37]

KEY POINTS

- Thalidomide has numerous role in dermatology especially in the management of leprosy reactions.
- The interesting mechanism of action of colchicine enables it to be used in neutrophillic dermatoses.
- Biotin has an important role to play in skin and hair disorders.
- Potassium iodide stands as a time-tested therapy in management of deep fungal infections.
- Zinc has multiple role in various cellular processes that can help in management of many diseases.

REFERENCES

1. Hassan I, Dorjay K, Anwar P. Thalidomide in dermatology: revisited. Indian J Dermatol. 2015;60:213.
2. Man HW, Corral LG, Stirling DI, Muller GW. Alpha-Fluoro-substituted thalidomide analogues. Bioorg Med Chem Lett. 2003;13:3415-7.
3. Wolverton SE (Ed). Comprehensive Dermatologic Drug Therapy; 3rd edition. Philadelphia, Pa: WB Saunders; 2013. p. 429.
4. Famaey JP. Colchicine in therapy: state-of-the-art and new perspectives for an old drug. Clin Exp Rheumatol. 1988;6: 305-17.
5. Simons RJ, Kingma DW. Fatal colchicine toxicity. Am J Med. 1989;86:356-7.
6. Sandhu K, Gupta S. Potassium iodide remains the most effective therapy for cutaneous sporotrichosis. J Dermatolog Treat. 2003;14:200-2.
7. Schulz EJ, Whiting DA. Treatment of erythema nodosum and nodular vasculitis with potassium iodide. Br J Dermatol. 1976;94:75-8.
8. Cabezas C, Bustamante B, Holgado W, Begue RE. Treatment of cutaneous sporotrichosis with one daily dose of potassium iodide. Pediatr Infect Dis J. 1996;15:352-4.
9. Heymann WR. Potassium iodide and the Wolff-Chaikoff effect: relevance for the dermatologist. J Am Acad Dermatol. 2000;42:490-2.
10. Farwell AP, Braverman LE. Iodide. In: Hardman JG, Limbird LE, Molinoff PB, et al. (Eds). Goodman and Gilman's: The Pharmacological Basis of Therapeutics, 9th edition. New York: McGraw-Hill; 1996. pp. 1402-4.
11. Eeckhout E, Willemsen M, Deconinck A, Somers G. Granulomatous vasculitis as a complication of potassium iodide treatment for Sweet's syndrome. Acta Derm Venereol (Stockh). 1987;67:362-4.
12. Thomas I. Gold therapy and its indications in dermatology. J Am Acad Dermatol. 1987;16:845-54.

13. Penneys NS. Gold therapy: dermatologic uses and toxicities. J Am Acad Dermatol. 1979;1:315-20.
14. Penneys NS, Ziboh V, Gottlieb NL, Katz S. Inhibition of prostaglandin synthesis and human epidermal enzymes by aurothiomalate in vitro: possible actions of gold in pemphigus. J Invest Dermatol. 1974;63:356-61.
15. Wilkinson SM, Smith AG, David MJ, Mattey D, Dawes PT. Pityriasis rosea and discoid eczema: dose related reactions to treatment with gold. Ann Rheum Dis. 1992;51:881-4.
16. Helfman T, Falanga V. Stanozolol as a novel therapeutic agent in dermatology. J Am Acad Dermatol. 1995;33:254-8.
17. Falanga V, Greenberg AS, Zhou L, Ochoa SM, Roberts AB, Falabella A, et al. Stimulation of collagen synthesis by the anabolic steroid stanozolol. J Invest Dermatol. 1998;111: 1193-7.
18. Purvis RS, Tyring SK. Cutaneous and subcutaneous endometriosis: surgical and hormonal therapy. J Dermatol Surg Oncol. 1994;20(10):693-5.
19. Wynn V. Metabolic effects of danazol. J Int Med Res. 1977; 5(Suppl):25-35.
20. Hosea SW, Santaella ML, Brown EJ, Berger M, Katusha K, Frank MM. Long-term therapy of hereditary angioedema with danazol. Ann Intern Med. 1980;93:809-12.
21. Knable AL Jr. Miscellaneous systemic drugs. In: Wolverton SE, (Ed). Comprehensive Dermatologic Drug Therapy, 1st edition. Philadelphia: Saunders; 2001. p. 461.
22. Roll A, Reich K, Boer A. Use of fumaric acid esters in psoriasis. Indian J Dermatol Venereol Leprol. 2007;73:133-7.
23. Breuer K, Gutzmer R, Volker B, Kapp A, Werfel T. Therapy of noninfectious granulomatous skin diseases with fumaric acid esters. Br J Dermatol. 2005;152:1290-5.
24. Eberlein-Konig B, Mempel M, Stahlecker J, Forer I, Ring J, Abeck D. Disseminated granuloma annulare: treatment with fumaric acid esters. Dermatology. 2005;210:223-6.
25. Kreuter A, Gambichler T, Altmeyer P, Brockmeyer NH. Treatment of disseminated granuloma annulare with fumaric acid esters. BMC Dermatol. 2002;2:5.
26. Schulze-Dirks A, Petzoldt D. Granuloma annulare disseminatum: successful therapy with fumaric acid ester. Hautarzt. 2001;52:228-30.
27. Gutzmer R, Kapp A, Werfel T. Successful treatment of skin and lung sarcoidosis with fumaric acid ester. Hautarzt. 2004;55: 553-7.
28. Nowack U, Gambichler T, Hanefeld C, Kastner U, Altmeyer P. Successful treatment of recalcitrant cutaneous sarcoidosis with fumaric acid esters. BMC Dermatol. 2002;2:15.
29. Kreuter A, Knierim C, Stucker M, Pawlak F, Rotterdam S, Altmeyer P, et al. Fumaric acid esters in necrobiosis lipoidica: results of a prospective non-controlled study. Br J Dermatol. 2005;153:802-7.
30. Mittal A, Agarwal C, Balai M, Taneja A. Gabapentin and pregabalin in dermatology. Indian J Dermatol Venereol Leprol. 2018;84:634-40.
31. Scheinfeld N. The role of gabapentin in treating diseases with cutaneous manifestations and pain. Int J Dermatol. 2003; 42:491-5.
32. Yesudian PD, Wilson NJ. Efficacy of gabapentin in the management of pruritus of unknown origin. Arch Dermatol. 2005;141:1507-9.
33. Ferrendelli JA. Concerns with antiepileptic drug initiation: safety, tolerability, and efficacy. Epilepsia. 2001;42(Suppl 4): 28-30.
34. University of Michigan Health System. [online] Available from: http://www.med.umich.edu/1libr/prescrpt/epil12.htm#side. [Last accessed on March, 2021].
35. DeToledo JC, Minagar A, Lowe MR, Ramsay RE. Skin eruption with gabapentin in a patient with repeated AED-induced Stevens-Johnson syndrome. Ther Drug Monit. 1999;21: 137-8.
36. Sharquie KE, Najim RA, Farjou IB, Al-Timimi DJ. Oral zinc sulfate in the treatment of acute cutaneous leishmaniasis. Clin Exp Derm. 2001;26(1):21-6.
37. Wilkinson EAJ, Hawke C. Oral zinc for arterial and venous leg ulcers. The Cochrane Library. 2004;(4)CD001273.

EXAMINATION QUESTIONS

Write short notes on the following:

1. Thalidomide.
2. Role of zinc in dermatology.
3. Role of potassium iodide in dermatology.
4. Colchicine.

15 SECTION | Procedural Dermatology

163 CHAPTER Phototherapy and Photochemotherapy

CR Srinivas, Sathish Pai B

INTRODUCTION

Phototherapy is a very useful treatment modality for a large number of dermatological conditions. Ultraviolet radiation (UV) consists of UVC (200–290 nm), UVB (290–320 nm), and UVA (320–400 nm) rays. When ultraviolet radiation is used for treating dermatological conditions, it is termed as phototherapy. It may be used with or without an external photosensitizer. The various forms are narrow band UVB phototherapy, psoralen photochemotherapy, targeted phototherapy, UVA1 phototherapy, and photodynamic therapy.[1]

HISTORY

Sunlight had been used for therapeutic purposes by Egyptians, Romans, and Greeks.

1925: William Goeckerman used ultraviolet rays with crude coal tar in treating psoriasis.

1950: John Ingram developed treatment modality using UVB radiation along with coal tar and anthralin paste.

1970: Broadband UVB and psoralen photochemotherapy (PUVA) (oral and topical) were introduced.

1980: Narrow band UVB was discovered.

TYPES OF PHOTOTHERAPY

- Psoralen photochemotherapy
- Narrow band UVB phototherapy
- Targeted phototherapy
- Excimer laser
- Photodynamic therapy
- Turbo-PUVA[2]
- Band pass filter cream[3]
- Digital UV photochemotherapy[4]

PHOTOCHEMOTHERAPY

The use of psoralens (P) along with ultraviolet A radiation (UVA) is termed as PUVA and both are required for it to be effective in treating skin conditions. When used in conjunction it induces a phototoxic reaction which brings about improvement in various skin diseases. Psoralens are furocoumarin compounds that are present in fruits and vegetables.

Types of Psoralens

- 8-methoxypsoralen (methoxsalen) (8-MOP)
- Trimethylpsoralen (trioxsalen)
- 5-methoxypsoralen (5-MOP)

Methods of PUVA Administration

- Oral PUVA
- Oral PUVASOL
- Topical PUVA
- Bath PUVA
- Turban PUVA

Sources of UVA

- Sunlight
- UVA chambers **(Fig. 1)**

Indications for PUVA[1]

- Psoriasis
- Atopic dermatitis
- Vitiligo
- Generalized lichen planus
- Generalized granuloma annulare
- Pityriasis rubra pilaris
- Prurigo nodularis

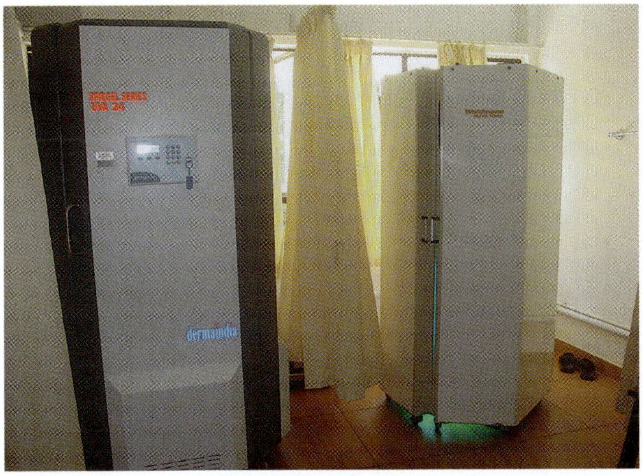

Fig. 1: UVA chambers.

- Polymorphic light eruptions
- Solar urticaria
- Chronic actinic dermatitis

Oral PUVA

8-methoxypsoralen is given orally in the dose of 0.6–0.8 mg per kg body weight. One and half to two hours later the skin is exposed to UVA in a whole body phototherapy chamber. The starting dose of UVA is based on the skin type or minimal phototoxic dose (MPD). As it is difficult to determine the MPD on Indian skin, the starting dose[5] is 2–3 J/cm^2 with increments of 0.5 J /cm^2. Psoralens are better absorbed on empty stomach but to avoid nausea, in practice patients are advised to take it after food. Oral PUVA therapy is given two to three times a week till clearance is achieved and then maintenance therapy is given once or twice weekly for 2–3 months. In psoriasis the clearance is usually seen with 20–25 treatment sessions whereas vitiligo patients need 150–200 treatment sessions for complete or near total repigmentation.

Oral PUVASOL

UVA rays present in sunlight can be used along with oral psoralen. This method of treatment is termed as PUVASOL therapy. It is an inexpensive treatment modality, can be used in places where artificial chambers are not available and patients need not travel to hospitals for receiving treatment. There are some disadvantages like it is difficult to monitor the amount of UVA rays present in sunlight and adverse effects may occur with UVB, visible, and infra-red rays present in the sunlight.

The best time for PUVASOL therapy[6] is between 9.15 AM to 11.15 AM and 2.30 PM to 3.30 PM. The exposure time to sunlight varies with place, season, and atmospheric conditions. The starting exposure time is 4 minutes[6] in the month of summer at 11 AM with increments of 1 minute every week till a maximum of 30 minutes is reached. Treatment is given 2–3 times a week.

Instructions for patients receiving PUVA and PUVASOL therapy:

- UVA protective goggles to be worn [B2 Torid **(Fig. 2)** or Green 60] during therapy and for atleast 12 hours on the day when psoralen tablets are taken, if the patient is going out in the sun.
- Patients should minimize going out on the days of therapy to protect the skin from psoralen induced phototoxic reaction.

Topical PUVA

It is indicated in vitiligo when it involves less than 5% of the body surface area. The vitiligo patch is painted with 0.01–0.1% 8-MOP solution. After 30 minutes the patch is exposed to UVA radiation. The normal surrounding skin can be protected with a sunscreen or zinc oxide cream to prevent tanning. Sunlight can also be used as a source of UVA, but care has to be taken to avoid phototoxic reaction. The patch needs to be exposed to sunlight for 1 minute and increments of 1 minute are given every week till mild erythema is seen after which the exposure time to sunlight is kept constant. Therapy is given 2–3 times a week.

Bath PUVA[7]

Bath PUVA was developed in the treatment of psoriasis and has been found to be as effective as oral PUVA in various studies. It involves soaking the body in psoralen (8-MOP) solution, which can be of various concentrations ranging from 0.5–4.6 mg per liter followed by exposure to UVA in a whole body phototherapy chamber.[7]

Procedure

To 100 liters of water in a bath tub 37.5 mL of 8-methoxy-psoralen solution is added so as to obtain a concentration of 3.75 mg per liter. The patient then soaks himself for 10 minutes in supine position **(Fig. 3)** and 10 minutes in prone position **(Fig. 4)** in the solution, then comes out of the tub pat dries his skin and is immediately exposed to UVA radiation in a phototherapy unit. Bath PUVA therapy is administered three times in a week. Psoriasis usually clears with 12–15 treatments **(Figs. 5 and 6)**, after which maintenance therapy is given twice weekly for a month and then once weekly. UVA irradiation is started with 0.5–1 J/cm^2 and for subsequent treatments the dose is increased

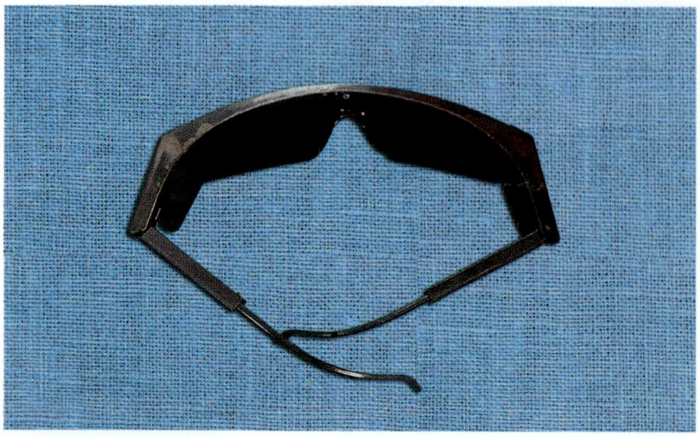

Fig. 2: UVA protective B2 Torid glasses.

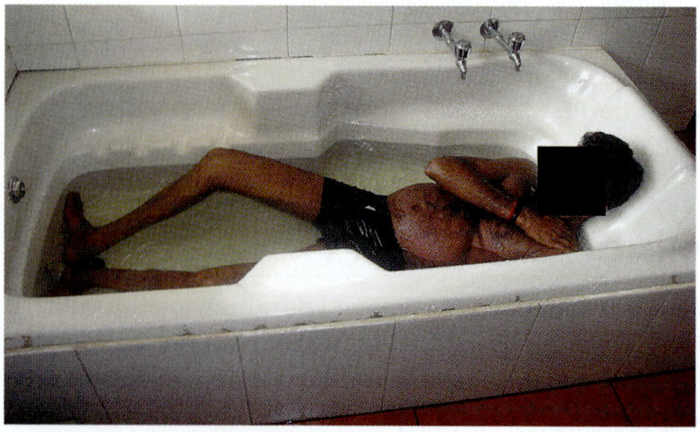

Fig. 3: Patient receiving psoralen bath in supine position.

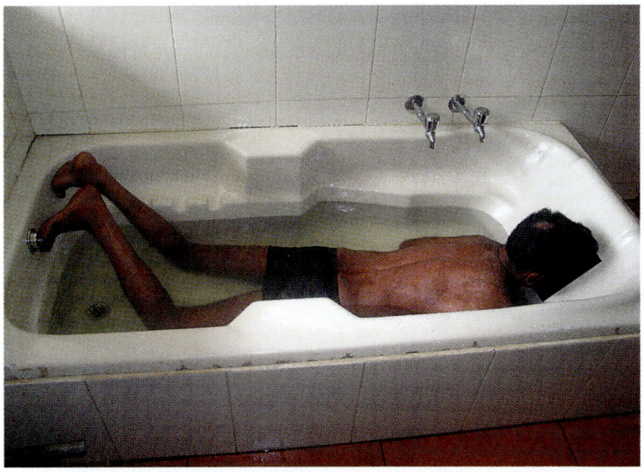

Fig. 4: Patient receiving psoralen bath in prone position.

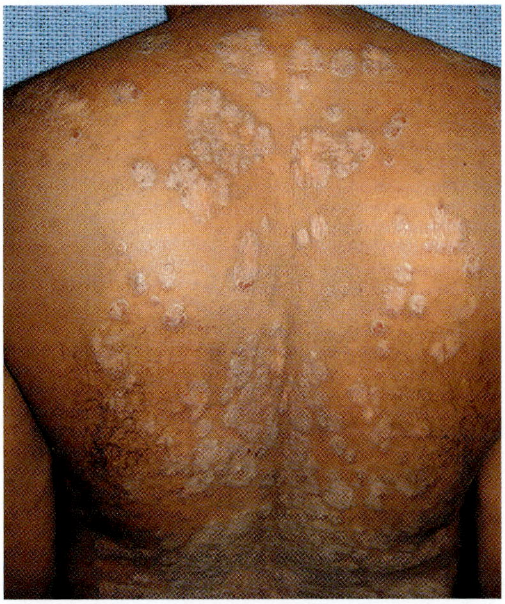

Fig. 5: Plaque type of psoriasis before bath PUVA.

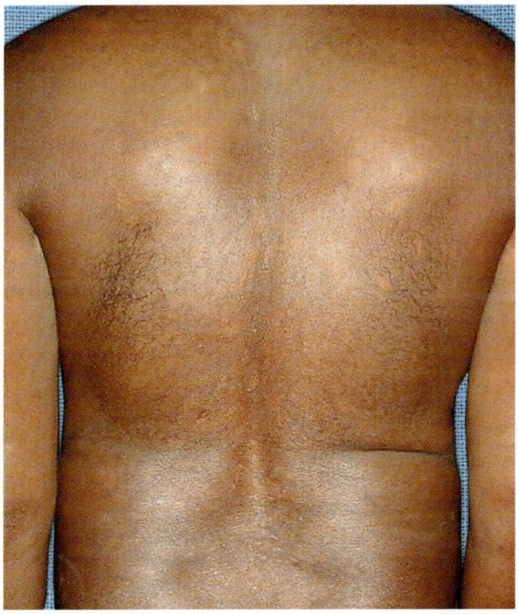

Fig. 6: Complete clearance of psoriasis after 15 bath PUVA treatments.

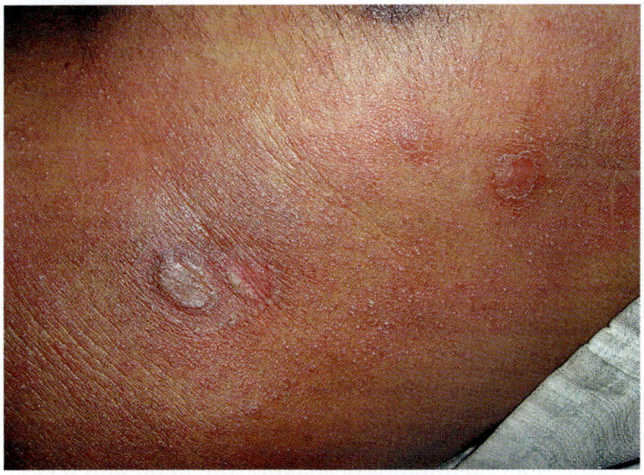

Fig. 7: Phototoxic reaction following bath PUVA.

by 0.5 J/cm^2 provided there are no adverse reactions such as erythema and burning.

When compared to oral PUVA there are no systemic side effects with bath PUVA and also the cumulative dose of UVA is lower than oral PUVA. But it can be associated with minor adverse events such as phototoxicity **(Fig. 7)**, pruritus, folliculitis, and pigmentation.

Indications

- Psoriasis (strength of recommendation A)
- Scleroderma (strength of recommendation D)
- Mycosis fungoides (strength of recommendation D)
- Urticaria pigmentosa (strength of recommendation D)
- Lichen planus (strength of recommendation D)
- Subacute prurigo (strength of recommendation B).

Turban PUVA[1]

It is used in the treatment of alopecia areata. To 2 liters of water 1 mL of 8-MOP solution is added to obtain a concentration of 3.75 mg per liter. A water absorbing cotton cloth is dipped in the solution for 30 seconds and then gently squeezed to remove excess water and later wrapped around the head like a turban for 5 minutes. This is repeated four times and then the area is exposed to UVA rays or sunlight. Treatment is given 3–4 times a week for 10–12 weeks. There is good regrowth of hair after 12 weeks of treatment.

Soak PUVA[7]

Psoralen soak PUVA is indicated in the treatment of palmoplantar psoriasis, chronic hand and feet eczema, 20 nail dystrophy, palmoplantar pustulosis, and vitiligo of hands and

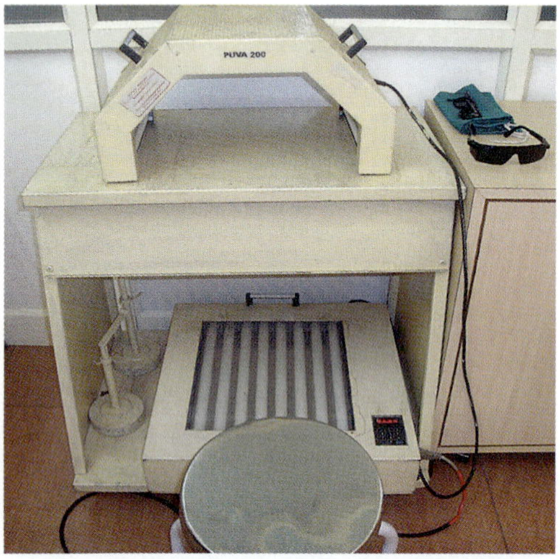

Fig. 8: UVA hand and foot unit.

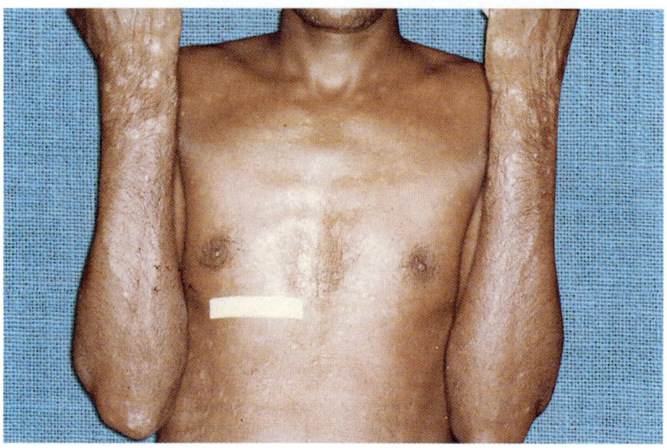

Fig. 10: Complete clearance after 15 bath suit PUVA treatments.

feet. The hands and feet are soaked for 20 minutes in psoralen solution, which is prepared by adding 1 mL of 8-MOP to 2 liters of water. After 20 minutes of soaking, the hand and feet are removed pat dried and then exposed to UVA in a hand and foot unit **(Fig. 8)** after a lag time of 30 minutes. The initial UVA dose is 1–2 J/cm^2 with increments of 0.5 J/cm^2. Sunlight can also be used as a source of UVA. Therapy is given 3–4 times a week.

Bathing Suit PUVA

Bathing suit PUVA has been found to be effective in the treatment of stable plaque type of psoriasis **(Figs. 9 and 10)**.[8] A suit made up of water absorbing material is stitched to suit the patient. Two liters of water is taken in a bucket to which 1 mL of 8-MOP solution is added to obtain a concentration of 3.75 mg per liter. The suit is dipped for 5 minutes, removed, gently squeezed so that water is not running. The patient then wears the suit for 15 minutes. After 20 minutes, suit is removed and the skin is immediately exposed to UVA rays in a whole body phototherapy chamber. The starting dose and increments of UVA are the same as for bath PUVA.

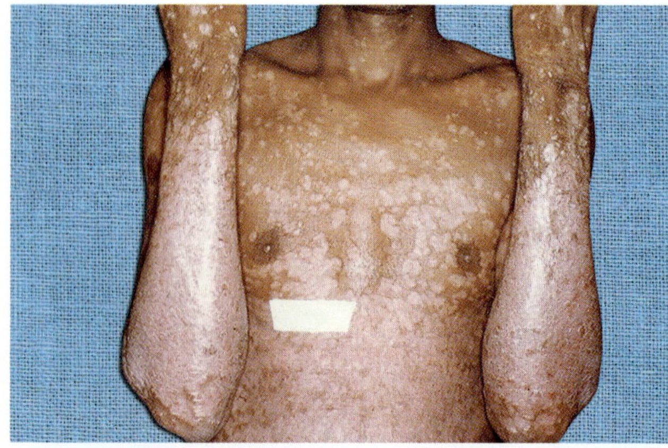

Fig. 9: Psoriasis before bath suit PUVA.

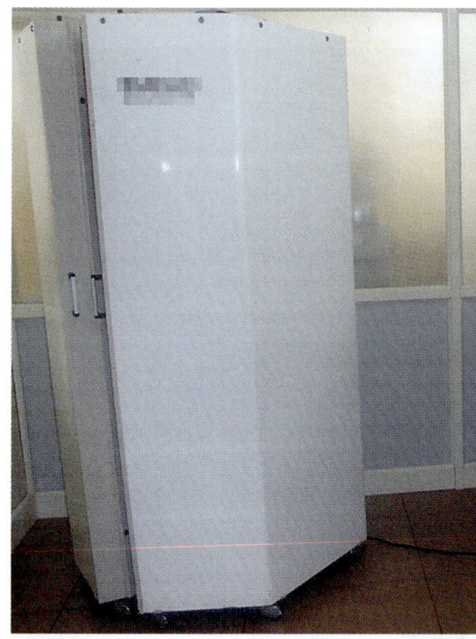

Fig. 11: NBUVB chamber.

Soap PUVA[9]

Soap PUVA is a method where psoralen solution is mixed with cleansing lotion. In this study by Srinivas et al., MED was determined to concentration of 1:60 and they observed MED at 2.5 J/cm^2. They proposed to use this psoralen and cleansing solution mixture in the treatment of psoriasis either using UVA from phototherapy chambers (soap PUVA) or sunlight as the source of UVA (soap PUVASOL).

NARROW BAND UVB PHOTOTHERAPY (FIG. 11)

The narrow band UVB (NBUVB) fluorescent bulbs were developed in the mid-1980s and it emitted a narrow spectrum of UVB rays in the range of 311–313 nm. Ever since its introduction, it has become one of the most commonly used treatment modalities in dermatology.

Indications

- Psoriasis vulgaris
- Palmoplantar psoriasis
- Vitiligo
- Atopic dermatitis
- Polymorphic light eruptions
- Pityriasis rosea
- Pityriasis rubra pilaris
- Pityriasis lichenoides chronica
- Generalized pruritus
- Generalized granuloma annulare
- Lichen planus
- Mycosis fungoides patch stage

Methods of Administration

- MED based
- Skin type based

MED-based Protocol

MED determination is recommended in all patients receiving NBUVB phototherapy. In our country, preirradiation MED is not done in most of the centers. There are few studies on MED on Indian skin and the MED ranged from 150 to 1,100 mJ/cm^2 in these studies. Robert Dawe et al. stated that in populations with a broad range of erythemal sensitivity the MED-based protocol could have an important impact on treatment effectiveness.[10]

MED determination: A template with 8 windows of 2 × 2 cm each is applied on the upper back. The rest of the body is adequately protected from irradiation by using protective gown and glasses. The windows are irradiated with geometric series of NBUVB starting with 300–1,080 mJ/cm^2. First all the windows are irradiated with 300 mJ/cm^2. Then the first window is closed and other windows are irradiated with an additional 60 mJ so that the second window will receive 360 mJ. Windows are closed one by one and the required doses are delivered. The reading is done after 24 hours. The window which shows just perceptible erythema is the MED **(Fig. 12)**.

In MED-based protocol, the starting dose is 70% of MED. Increments ranges from 105 to 20% based on the erythema response.

Frequency: Three times a week is optimal.

Duration: 25–30 sessions for clearance in psoriasis. Maintenance once weekly for 4 weeks. 150–200 sessions for vitiligo.

Skin Type Based Protocol

Here the starting dose and increments vary with the skin types. For example, in skin type IV the starting dose is 330 mJ/cm^2 with increments of 45 mJ/cm^2.

NBUVB combination

NBUVB plus topical preparations	*NBUVB plus systemic drugs*
• Topical steroids • Dithranol • Calcipotriol • Tazarotene	• Methotrexate • Acitretin • Etanercept

TARGETED PHOTOTHERAPY

It is otherwise called as microphototherapy. Here the light is undiffused, concentrated and of high energy. There are many advantages of targeted phototherapy. The treatment can be given only to affected area without causing any damage to unaffected normal skin. As the energy is high treatment duration is short, frequency is less, and outcome is better.

Types:

- Excimer laser
- Excimer light
- UV light **(Fig. 13)**

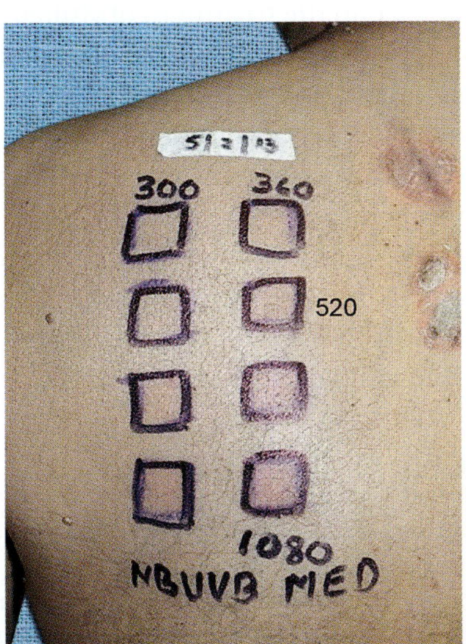

Fig. 12: MED to NBUVB seen at 520 mJ as just perceptible erythema.

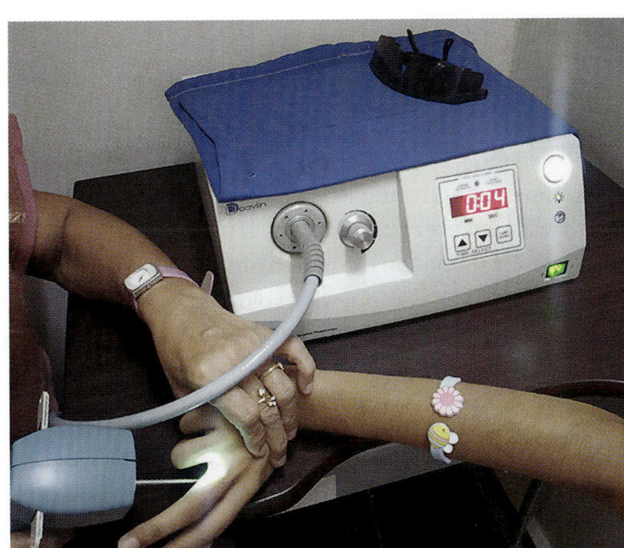

Fig. 13: Lumera targeted phototherapy unit.

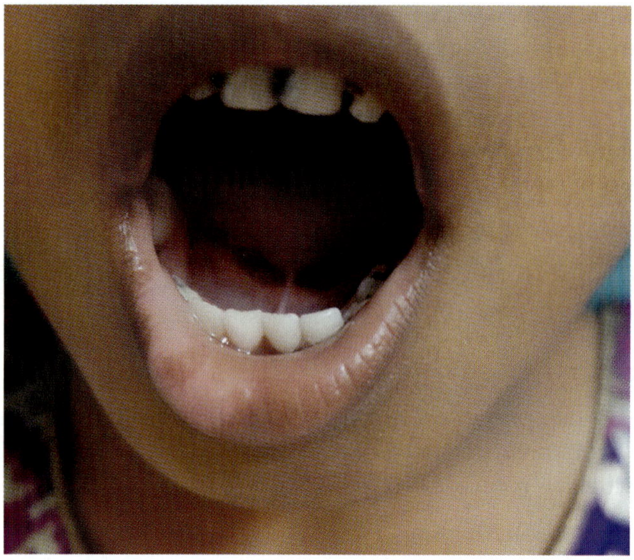

Fig. 14: Lip vitiligo before targeted phototherapy.

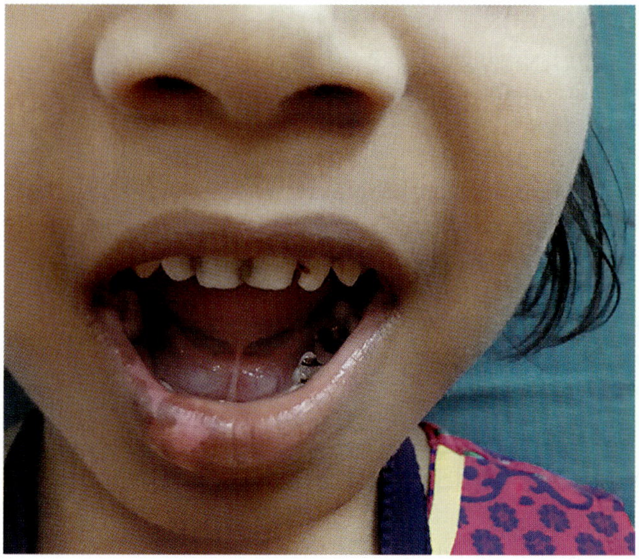

Fig. 15: Repigmentation of lip vitiligo after 12 weeks of targeted phototherapy.

Indications:
- Vitiligo **(Figs. 14 and 15)**
- Psoriasis localized
- Alopecia areata
- Lichen simplex chronicus

Treatment schedule:
- MED determination
- Start with one MED
- Increments are given by 50 mJ/cm^2
- Treatment is continued till mild erythema is seen
- This mildly erythematous dose is then given till the lesions improve. Frequency of treatment is twice weekly. Improvement usually occurs with 12 weeks of treatment.

Side effects:
- Burning
- Severe erythema
- Blistering.

Dos and Don'ts for Phototherapy Chambers

- Machines without inbuilt dosimetry the irradiation should be measured every 25–50 hours of use
- The meter should be calibrated once in a year
- Always check the output when old tubes are replaced
- Do not put two new tubes together. Swap with the old ones and rearrange the tubes.

CONCLUSION

- Phototherapy is one of the most effective treatment modalities in skin conditions especially psoriasis and vitiligo
- MPD determination is difficult on Indian skin so for PUVA therapy the dose of UVA is based on skin type
- MED determination is advisable for NBUVB phototherapy
- Phototherapy can be combined with topical or systemic medications to optimize the outcome
- Sunlight can be used as a source of UVA for psoralen photochemotherapy.

KEY POINTS

- Phototherapy is the use of ultraviolet radiation in the treatment of dermatological conditions.
- PUVA involves the use of the drug psoralen orally, topically or as bath followed by exposure to UVA radiation or sunlight (PUVASOL).
- PUVA is effective only when the drug psoralen and UVA are combined.
- PUVASOL therapy can be carried out at home and is commonly used in the treatment of vitiligo.
- The most commonly used phototherapy in practice is Narrow band UVB (NBUVB).
- MED-based protocol is recommended while using NBUVB.
- PUVA and NBUVB can be combined with various topical or systemic agents.
- Phototherapy chambers need to be maintained with regard to measuring the output, change of tubes, etc.
- Targeted phototherapy is recommended in localized psoriasis and vitiligo.

REFERENCES

1. Rai R, Srinivas CR. Phototherapy: An Indian perceptive. Indian J Dermatol. 2007;52:169-75.
2. Taylor CR, Kwangsukstith C, Wimberly J, Kollias N, Anderson RR. Turbo-PUVA: dihydroxyacetone-enhanced photochemotherapy for psoriasis: a pilot study. Arch Dermatol. 1999; 135:540-4.

3. Wang X, McCoy J, Lotti T, Goren A. Topical cream delivers NB-UVB from sunlight for the treatment of vitiligo. Expert Opin Pharmacother. 2014;15:2623-7.
4. Reidel U, Bechstein S, Asschenfeldt BL. Treatment of localized MF with digital photochemotherapy. Photodermatol Photoimmunol Photomed. 2015;31:333-40.
5. Shenoi SD, Prabhu S. Photochemotherapy (PUVA) in psoriasis and vitiligo. Indian J Dermatol Venereol Leprol. 2014;80: 497-504.
6. Srinivas CR, Devadiga R, Parashar TR, Chandras. Exposure time to sunlight for ultraviolet light therapy. Indian J Dermatol Venereol Leprol. 1991;57:17-18.
7. Pai SB, Shetty S. Guidelines for bath PUVA, bathing suit PUVA and soak PUVA. Indian J Dermatol Venereol Leprol. 2015;81:559-67.
8. Pai S, Srinivas CR. Bathing suit delivery of 8-methoxypsoralen for psoriasis: A double blind placebo controlled study. Int J Dermatol. 1994:33;576-8.
9. Srinivas CR, Sekar CS. SOAP PUVA. Indian Dermatol Online J. 2018;9:175-6.
10. Dawe RS, Cameron HM, Yule S, Ibbotson SH, Moseley HH, Ferguson J. A randomized comparison of methods of selecting narrowband UV-B starting dose to treat chronic psoriasis. Arch Dermatol. 2011;147:168-74.

EXAMINATION QUESTIONS

1. Describe the indications, mechanism of action, types, and side effects of psoralen photochemotherapy.
2. Discuss the indications, mechanism of action, treatment protocol and side effects of narrow band UVB (NBUVB) phototherapy.
3. Write short note on targeted phototherapy.
4. Describe the role and indications of phototherapy in dermatology.
5. Write short note on excimer laser.
6. Describe uses and side effects of psoralens.

164 CHAPTER

Basics of Dermatosurgery

Thurakkal Salim, Laila Achampat

INTRODUCTION

Dermatologic surgery or dermatosurgery is a subspecialty of dermatology devoted to the treatment of disease and disorders of the skin, soft tissues, mucosal tissues, and skin appendages that medical treatment cannot resolve, thus requiring the use of surgical techniques. Dermatology is a procedure-based practice that requires the understanding of techniques in dermatologic surgery, postoperative patient care and managing complications.

Every dermatologist should be familiar with the principles of dermatologic surgery and should be capable of carrying out the basic set of procedures. These range from diagnostic biopsies to excisions, scar revision, vitiligo surgeries, hair transplantation, and many more. This chapter will cover some of the common dermatosurgical procedures of practical importance including different techniques of excision and skin grafts.

SUTURE MATERIAL

One of the cornerstones of dermatologic surgery is suturing. Mastering good suturing techniques is paramount to achieve both good aesthetic and functional outcome.[1] Nonabsorbable sutures are primarily used for superficial skin closures as these causes least tissue reaction and thereby a cosmetically acceptable scar. Polypropylene and Nylon are the most commonly used for this purpose. Absorbable sutures are commonly used in buried dermal suturing technique and to close the dead spaces. **Tables 1 and 2** outline the features and properties of different suture materials.[2,3]

TABLE 1: Suture material: Non-absorbable.

Generic or Trade name	*Material*	*Configuration*	*Tensile strength*	*Tissue reactivity*	*Handling*	*Knot security*	*Memory*
Silk	Silk	Braided or twisted	Good	High	Good	Good	Poor
Ethilon	Polyamide (nylon)	Monofilament	High	Low	Poor	Poor	High
Prolene	Polyolefin (polypropylene)	Monofilament	Fair	Low	Poor	Poor	High
Novafil	Poly-butester	Monofilament	High	Low	Fair	Poor	Low
Ethibond	Polyester	Braided	High	Moderate	Good	Good	Fair
Stainless steel	Stainless steel	Monofilament, twisted or braided	High	Low	Poor	Good	Poor

TABLE 2: Suture material: Absorbable.

Property	*Gut*	*Polyglycolic acid (Dexon)*	*Polyglactin (vicryl)*	*Polydioxanone (PDS)*	*Polytrimethylene carbonate (Maxon)*	*Poliglecaprone (Monocryl)*
Handling	Fair	Fair-good	Good	Poor	Good	Excellent
Knot security	Poor	Fair-good	Fair	Poor	Good	Good
Tensile strength	Low	High	High	Moderate	High	High
Coefficient of friction	High	High	Medium	Low	Low	Low
Memory	Low	Low	Low	High	Low	Low
Tissue reactivity	High	Low	Low	Low	Low	Low
Rate of absorption	Unpredictable (60–90 days, 2–4 weeks for fast-absorbing gut)	Predictable (90–120 days)	Predictable (60–90 days)	Predictable (180–210 days)	Predictable (180–210 days)	Predictable (90–210 days)

EXCISION AND REPAIR

Fusiform (Elliptical) Excision

Elliptical excision is the mainstay of cutaneous excisional and reconstructive surgery. This is one of the simplest and oldest techniques used in removal of various cutaneous lesions, growths, and scar revision. It can be used in removing small-to-medium sized benign or premalignant lesions or scars.

Basic understanding of anatomy of skin, wound healing, tumor biology, relaxed skin tension lines, and functional considerations of head and neck will help the dermatosurgeon to execute the procedure meticulously, giving excellent cosmetic outcome.[4,5]

Indications of elliptical excision are given in **Box 1**.

Technique

The scar is excised in a fusiform pattern parallel to the RSTLs and the wound edges are undermined and closed in 2 layers. The ratio of length and breadth of the incision should be 1:3 to 1:4 as shown in **Figures 1 and 2**. The tip of ellipse should meet at 30° angle. Enough of free margins should be left while treating malignant lesions to prevent further spread and recurrence.

A well-planned incision line running parallelly to the RSTL will not only make the scar inconspicuous but also gives high tensile strength to the wound and, heals faster. **Figures 3A and B** show the RSTL over the face. Variations of ellipse may occur as we follow the RSTLs on curved surfaces. Lazy S and crescentic pattern of excision is required in these areas **(Figs. 4 and 5)**.

BOX 1: Indications for simple excisions.

Simple excisions without suturing (small benign lesions)
- Small hamartomas
- Mucoceles
- Small epidermal inclusion cysts

Elliptical excision (moderate-to-large lesions)
- *Benign lesions*: Sebaceous cyst, lipoma, fibroma, epidermoid cyst, nevi
- *Malignant and premalignant lesions*: Basal cell carcinoma, squamous cell carcinoma, Bowen's disease, keratoacanthoma, large hamartomas

Modification in simple excision
- *Punch incision and closure*: Sebaceous cyst, lipoma
- *Excision with full thickness graft or rotation flap*: Large malignant lesions

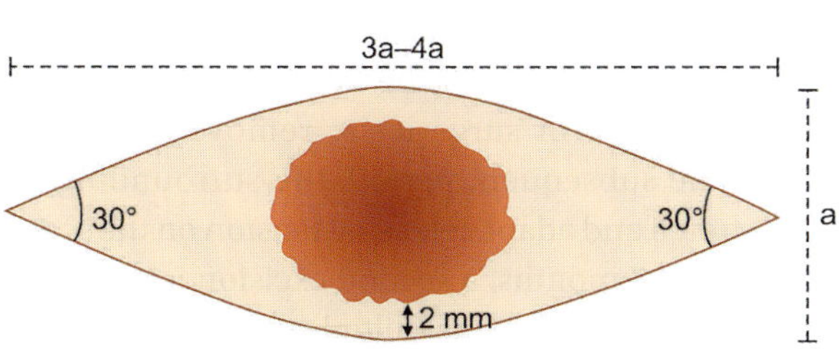

Fig. 1: Ratio of length and breadth in elliptical incision.

Remove the specimen with uniform thickness and avoid beveling the wound edges when making your incision, to minimize "scooping" or "boating" of the specimen and wound

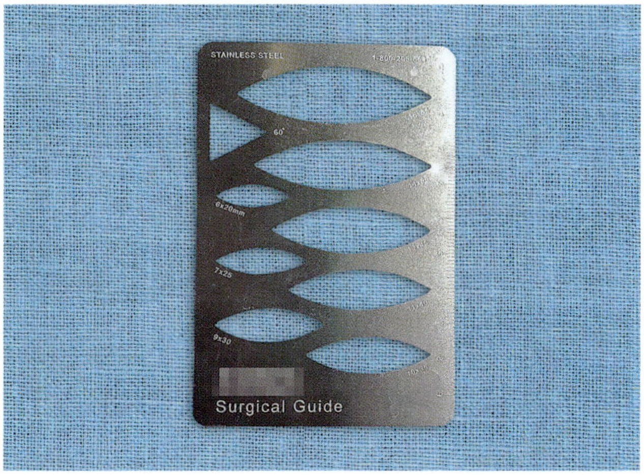

Fig. 2: Surgical incision guide for elliptical incision.

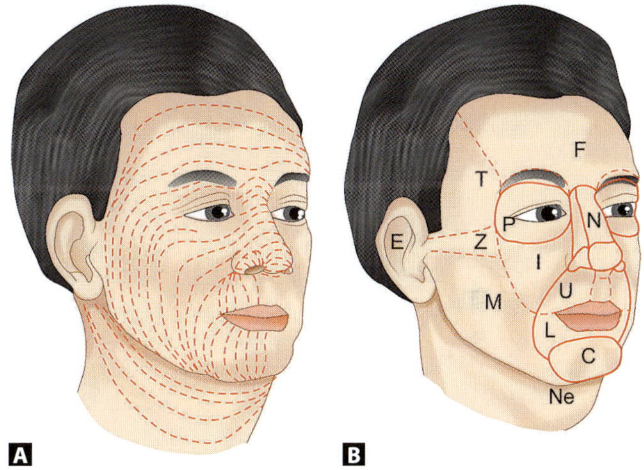

Figs. 3A and B: (A) RSTLs of face; (B) Facial cosmetic units.
(F: forehead; T: temple; Z: zygomatic; I: infraorbital; M: mandibular; N: nose; U: upper lip; L: lower lip; C: chin; E: ear; Ne: neck)

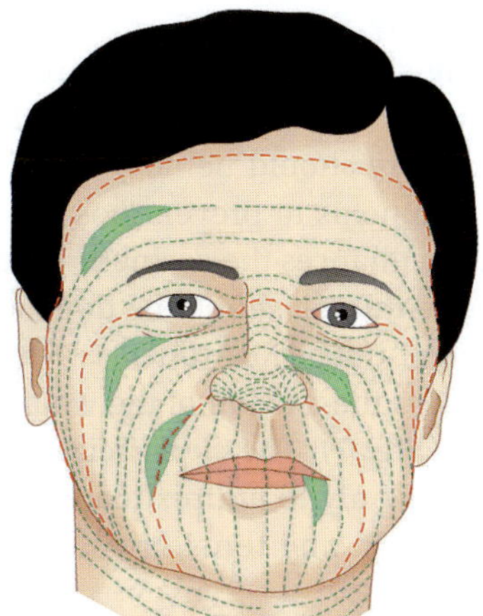

Fig. 4: Variations of ellipse over on curved surfaces.

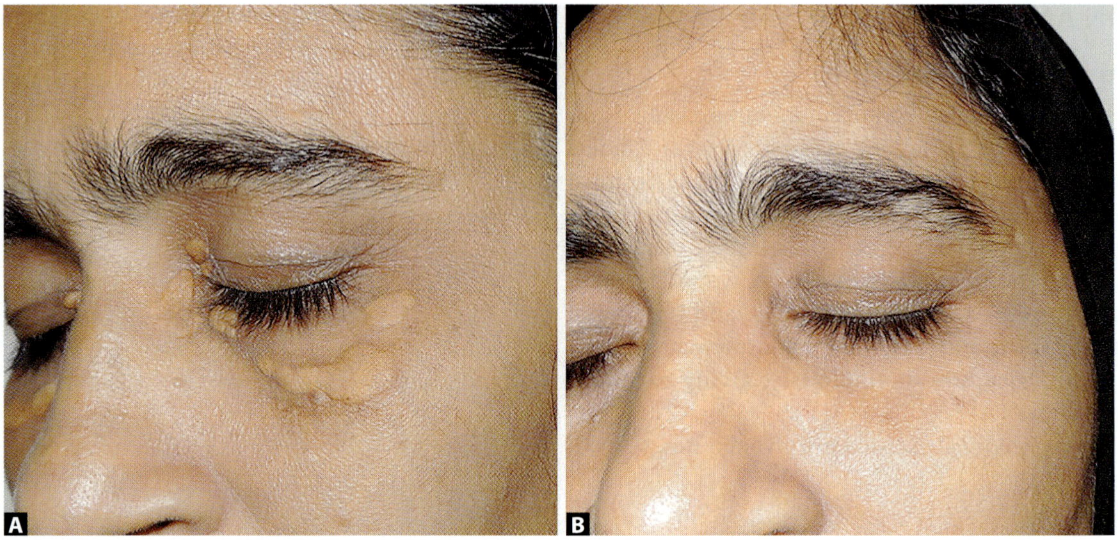

Figs. 5A and B: (A) Multiple xanthelasma over the face before excision; (B) Complete clearance of lesions with least scarring after modified fusiform excision.

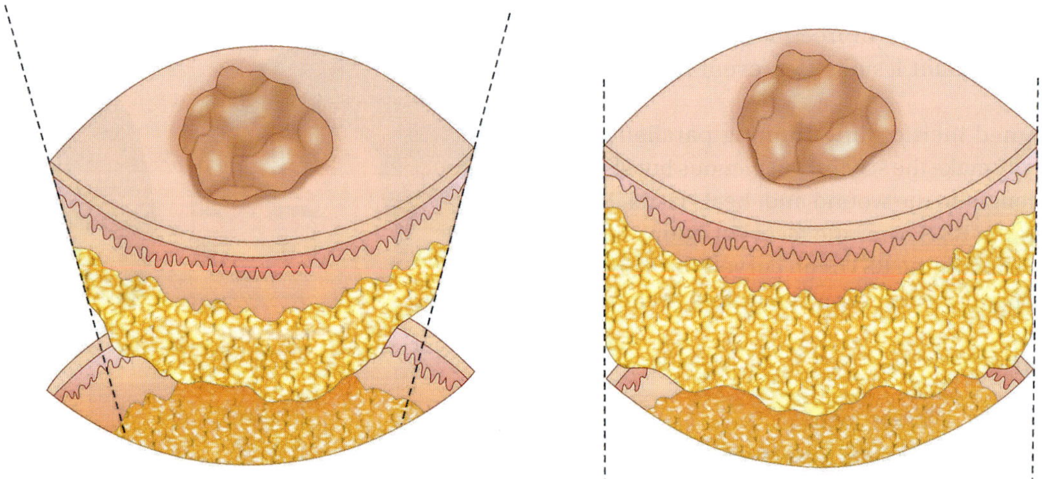

Fig. 6: Correct method of excision avoiding beveling the wound edges.

edges, as this will ultimately affect the proper apposition of the wound edges **(Fig. 6)**.

Undermining should be done all around the wound including the two ends. After undermining, the edges should be everted and there should be no tension on the wound margins. This also helps to prevent postoperative vascular compromise and enhances the cosmetic outcome after scar contraction. Undermining should be done as superficial as possible using blunt-tipped instruments. Deep buried dermal sutures should bear the tension of the wound while closing larger excisions **(Fig. 7)**. The superficial skin closure with everted margins is only to approximate the wound edges and should not hold any tension so as to prevent scar widening.[6]

Instruments required for excision and closure are given in **Figures 8 and 9**. **Box 2** explains various tips to improve the outcome in elliptical excision. Stages of various elliptical excision are illustrated in **Figures 10 to 12**.

Serial Excision

This technique is employed while treating large lesions or scars in which the surrounding tissue laxity is insufficient for a single excision.[7,8]

Serial excision involves the removal of one portion of the lesion with primary closure of the wound followed by a similar additional surgery or surgeries to remove the remaining lesion. In the subsequent period, the surrounding skin is going to stretch and adapt, releasing tension on the scar. After a minimum of 3 months, a second excision is performed to remove the rest of the lesion. Multiple serial excisions may be required in case very large lesions **(Figs. 13A to F)**.

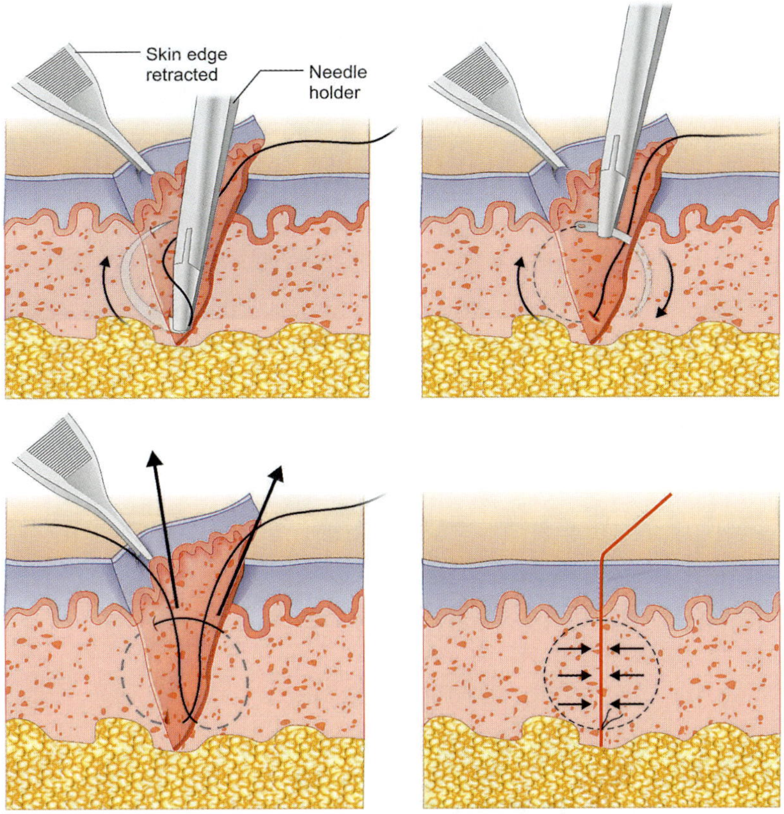

Fig. 7: Subcutaneous buried sutures.

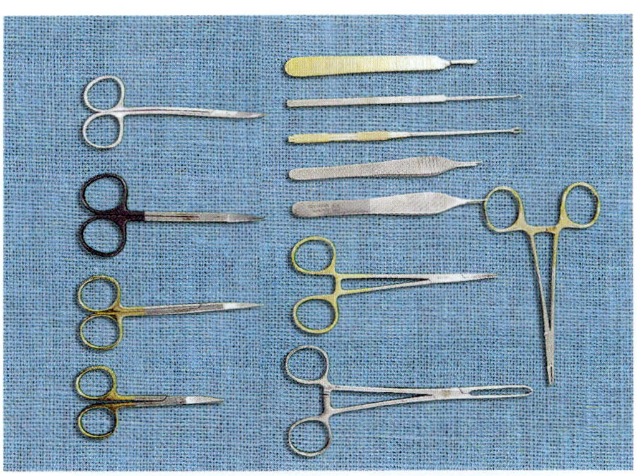

Fig. 8: Instruments required for excision. Brad Parker knife, kin hooks, artery forceps, tissue-holding forceps, needle holder, scissors, etc.

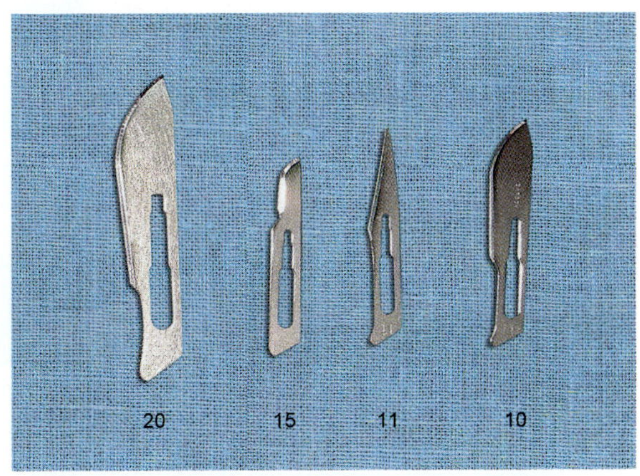

Fig. 9: Surgical blades of different sizes. 15 number blade is commonly used for small to medium sized excisions.

BOX 2: Preoperative evaluation.

Bleeding disorders:
- History of current administration of anticoagulant or antiplatelet drugs
- Bleeding tendencies

Abnormal wound healing:
- Keloidal tendency
- Causes of delayed wound healing

Hypersensitivity reactions:
- Drug hypersensitivity including anesthetic agents
- Contact dermatitis to topical medicaments and dressings and adhesives

Chances for postoperative infection:
- Diabetes, debilitation, anemia, malnutrition, emotional stress
- Damaged or infected skin, poor hygiene
- Immunocompromised states, corticosteroid therapy

Transmission of infections:
- Human immunodeficiency virus infection
- Hepatitis B and C infections

Investigations:
- Complete blood count
- Bleeding time, clotting time, prothrombin time
- Blood sugar level
- Serological screening of HIV, Hepatitis B and C

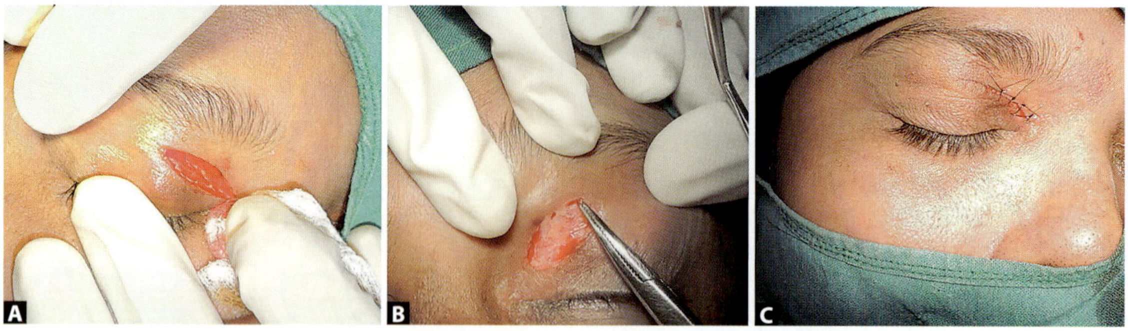

Figs. 10A to C: (A) Elliptical incision made; (B) Undermining; (C) Immediately after closing the wound.

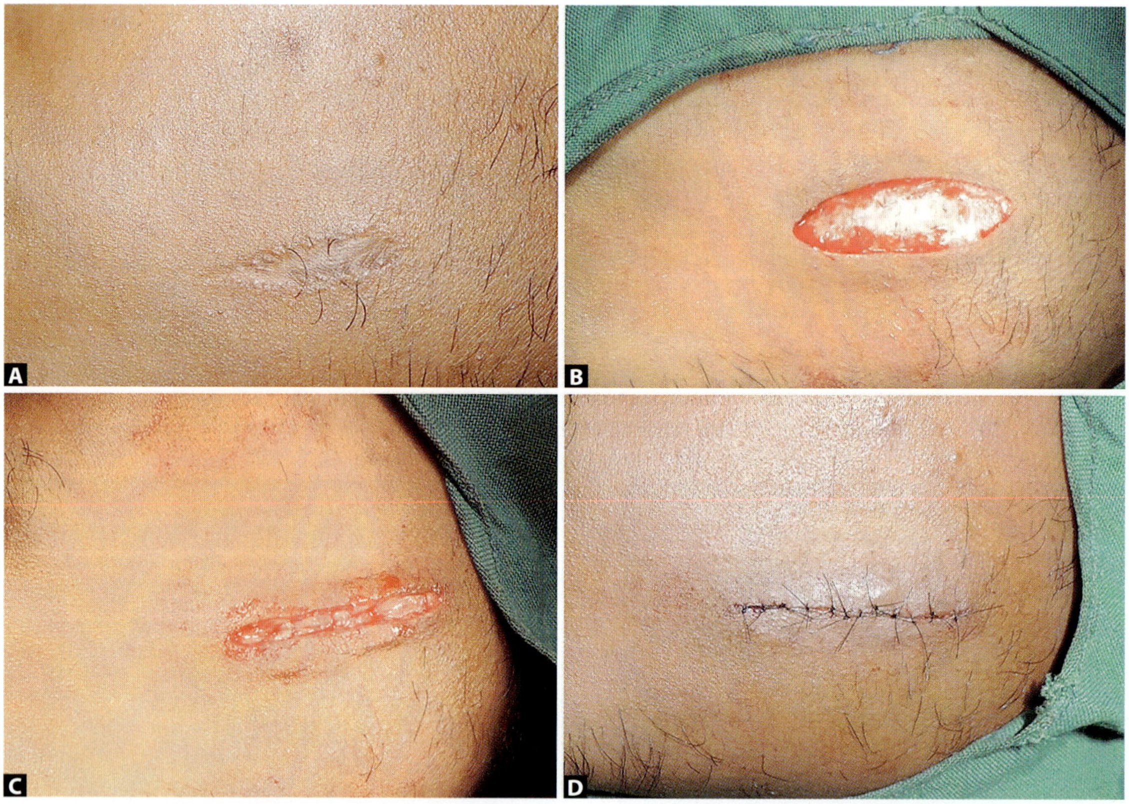

Figs. 11A to D: (A) A depressed scar before treatment; (B) After making incision; (C) After applying the deep buried sutures. Note the approximation of tissue; (D) Skin closure made with nylon sutures without any tension.

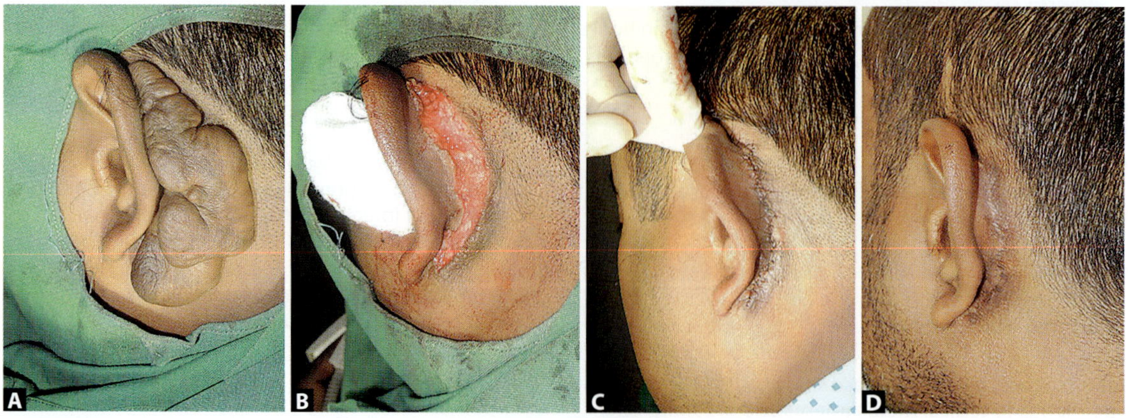

Figs. 12A to D: (A) Posterior auricular keloid before treatment; (B) After excision and application of deep buried sutures; (C) Immediately after skin closure; (D) After 3 months.

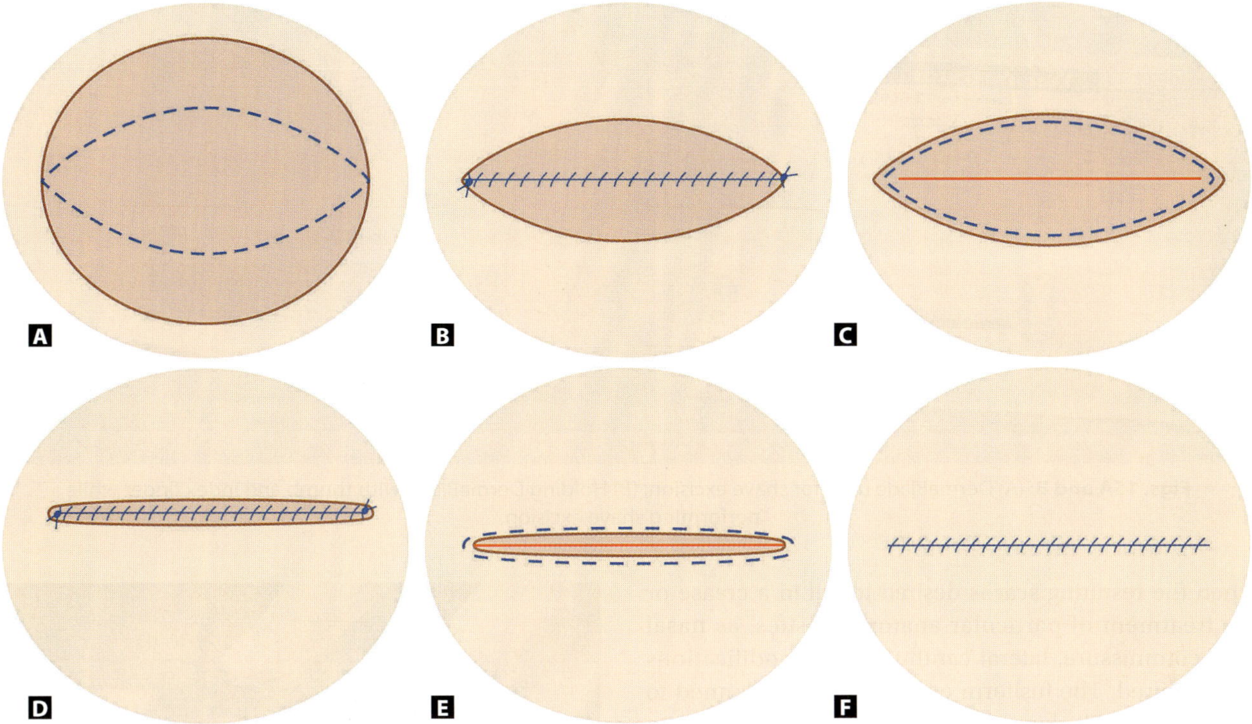

Figs. 13A to F: Serial excision steps: (A) Elliptical incision made on the lesion; (B) First-stage excision done and the lesion has reduced in size; (C) Second-stage excision; (D) Further reduction in size; (E) Third-stage excision; (F) Complete removal of the initial lesion.

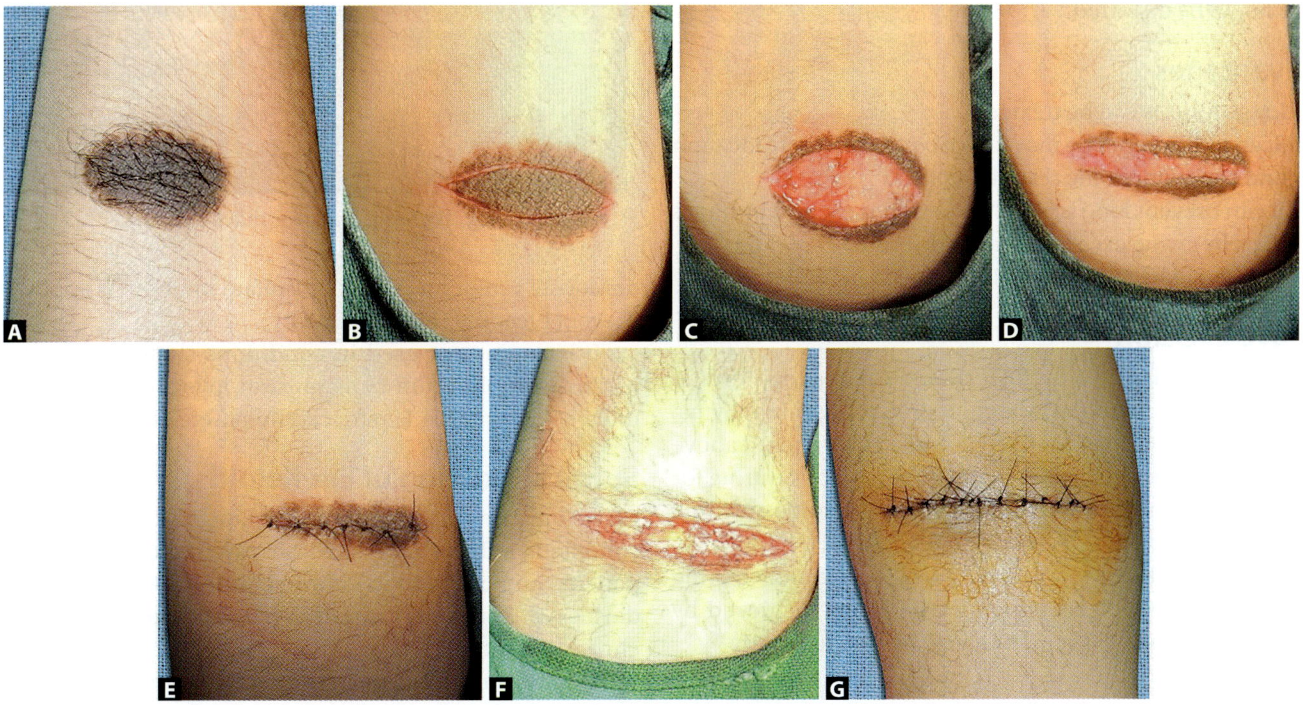

Figs. 14A to G: Serial excision of hairy melanocytic nevi: (A) Before serial excision; (B) Elliptical incision made on the lesion; (C) First-stage excision done; (D) After application of deep buried sutures; (E) Skin closure done; (F) Second-stage excision; (G) Complete removal of the initial lesion.

Technique

A symmetric, fusiform ellipse is drawn within the lesion, parallel to the RSTLs and the margins are undermined enough to obtain a tension-free suture and the lesion is partially excised. Remaining part of the lesion is excised in the next sitting with complete removal **(Figs. 14A to G)**.

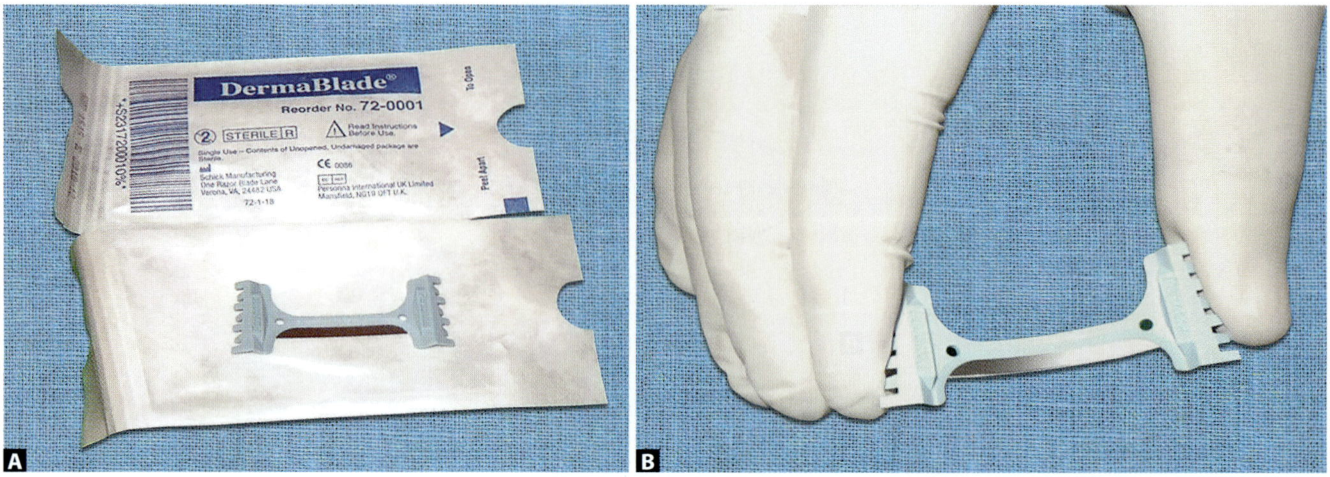

Figs. 15A and B: (A) DermaBlade used for shave excision; (B) Holding DermaBlade with thumb and index finger while performing shave excision.

When the resulting scar is desired to fall in a crease or for the treatment of particular anatomical sites, as nasal ala, oral commissure, lateral canthus, some modifications may be required. The fusiform excision may be planned to be eccentric and the skin undermined more on one side, to move the tissue in one direction rather than the opposite one. The direction of the prevalent movement can be towards a natural crease, the border of an aesthetic unit or an anatomical area not to be distorted.

Advantages

- Large lesions can be treated.
- Scar or lesion can be moved to a better anatomic location and can reorient the scar along RSTL.
- It can prevent long scars as the lesion is excised in stages thereby giving excellent cosmetic results.
- Scar could be moved to hairline and kept hidden.

Shave Excision

Shave excision is a very useful technique in treating elevated lesions from simple moles to large lesions such as rhinophyma. It is suitable for lesions confined to epidermis or raised above skin. It is less time consuming, does not require suturing for closure, faster healing and results in good cosmetic outcome **(Figs. 15 to 19)**.

Lesions heals with secondary intension without scarring in expert hands. Effective hemostasis can be achieved by chemical hemostatic agents or a bipolar electrocautery.[9]

Curettage

It is a procedure where the skin lesion is removed *in toto* or partly by the act of physical scraping and scooping with dermal curette. Superficial growths, soft tumors or tissues are removed by scraping or scooping technique using spoon curet and ring curet which are available in different sizes.[10] After removal of the lesion, hemostatic agents such as silver nitrate or Monsel's solution (Ferric subsulfate solution) is applied to prevent bleeding **(Figs. 20 and 21)**.

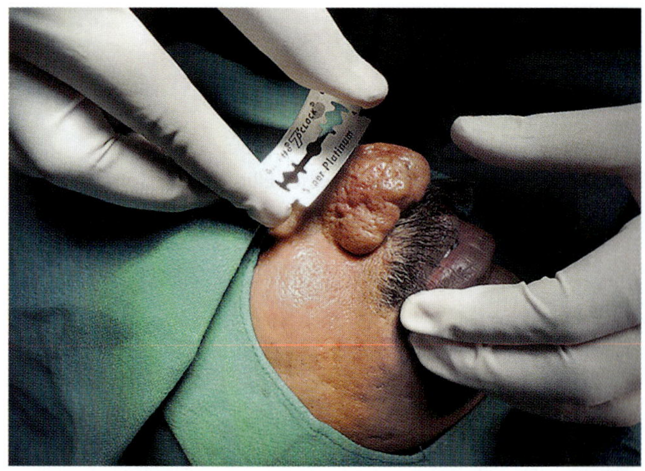

Fig. 16: Razor blade for shave excision.

It is commonly used in conditions such as seborrheic keratosis, molluscum contagiosum, pyogenic granuloma, milia, solar keratosis, keratoacanthoma, etc. **(Figs. 22 and 23)**.

Surgical Excision of Ear Keloids

Ear keloids are among the most challenging dermatosurgical conditions and may have significant psychosocial impact to the patient. Surgical excision followed by postoperative pressure devices with or without intralesional pharmacotherapy is the choice of treatment **(Box 3)**.

Surgical removal of excessive scar tissue returns the wound to the initial state. Further postoperative scaring can be reduced by adjunctive therapies. Multimodal therapy (excision followed by combination of intralesional steroid, silicone gel therapy and compression) entailing less recurrence.[11,12]

Simple excision and closure with least tension, core extirpation, flap closure and intramarginal excision and fillet flap closure are choices of surgery for such keloids.[13]

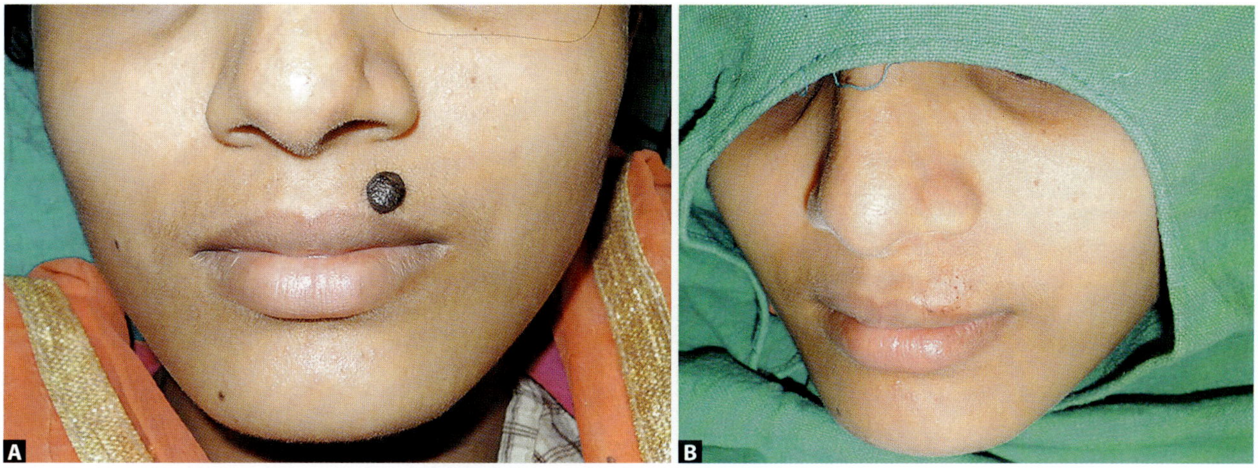

Figs. 17A and B: Shave excision of mole—before (A) and after (B).

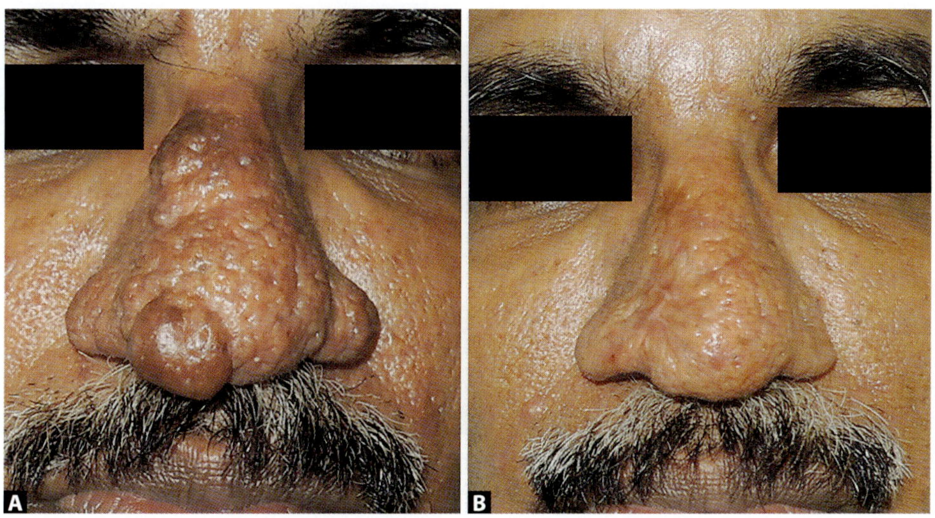

Figs. 18A and B: Shave excision of rhinophyma—before (A) and after (B).

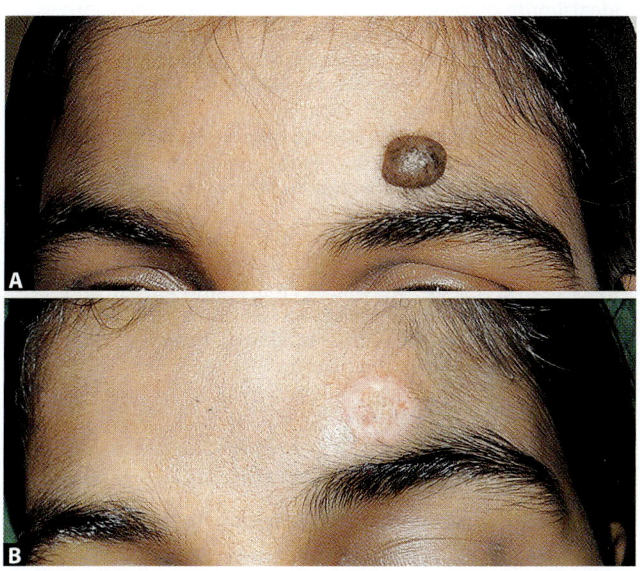

Figs. 19A and B: Shave excision of compound nevus—before (A) and after (B).

Each case should be dealt in a personalized approach. The deformity may vary in size, cosmetic disfigurement, and area of occurrence. Hence, the surgical technique may vary from cases to cases. Some cases may require a simple excision and closure others may require an intramarginal excision followed by simple, advancement flaps. **Figures 24 to 28** show the steps of different types of ear keloid managed using different techniques. Compilations of keloid surgeries are enumerated in **Box 4**.

Skin Grafts

Skin grafting involves removal of intact piece of skin that has been completely separated from one part of the body and transferred to another part where it continues to survive by re-establishing new blood supply.[14]

Indications

Skin grafts are used to close skin defects regardless of the cause.

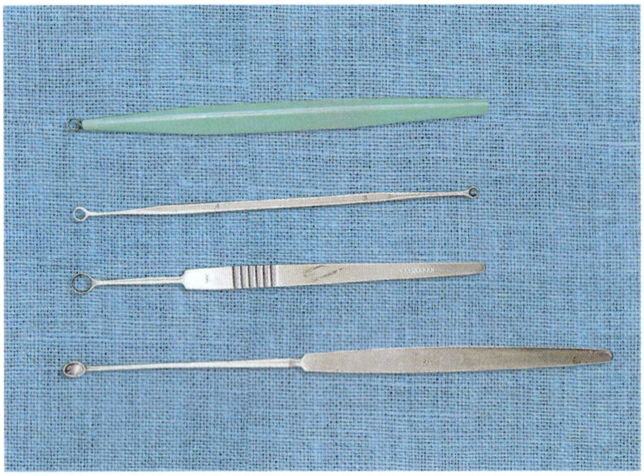

Fig. 20: Dermal curettes. Ring curettes and spoon curettes of different sizes.

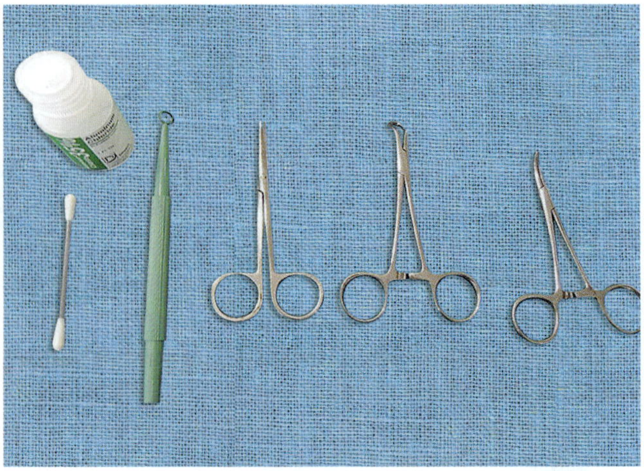

Fig. 21: Topical hemostatic solution and instruments required for curettage.

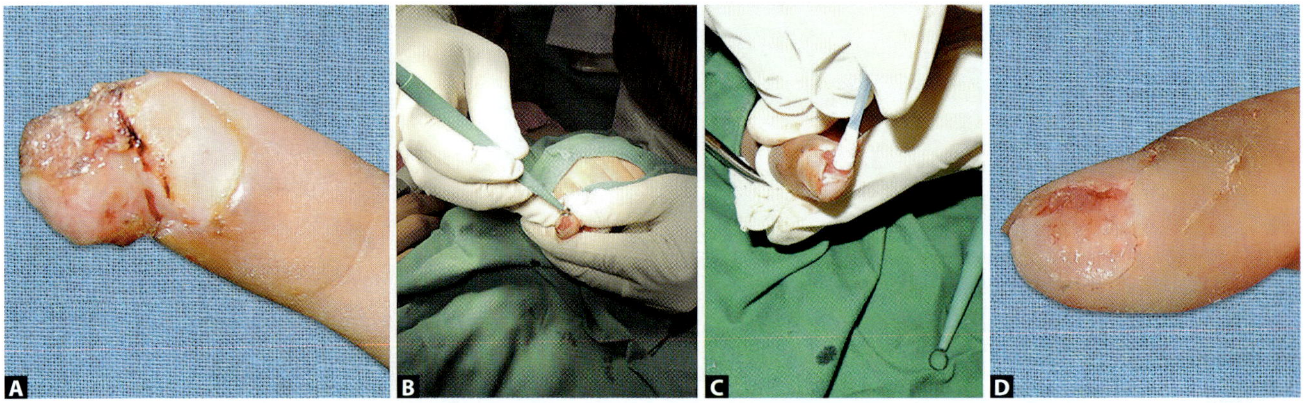

Figs. 22A to D: Removal of granuloma pyogenicum over finger by curettage. (A) Before; (B) Curettage being performed; (C) Application of hemostatic agent to prevent bleeding; (D) After treatment.

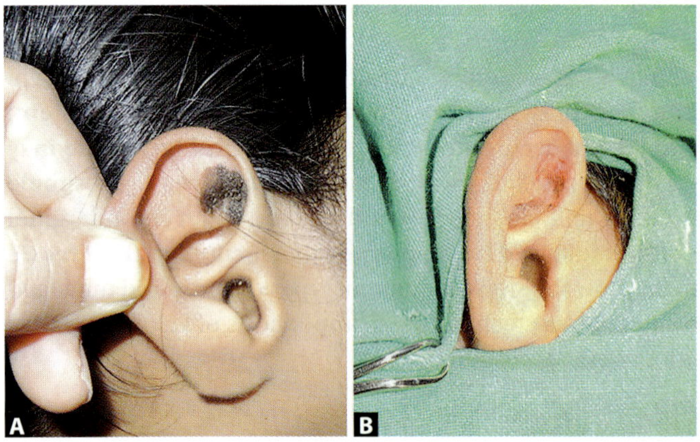

Figs. 23A and B: Removal of seborrheic keratosis by curettage.

BOX 3: Elliptical excision: Tips.

- Ideal length of the ellipse should be three times the width
- The angle of the ellipse should be 30° or less in order to prevent the possible exuberant tissue, called "dog-ear" formation. This dog-ear can be corrected by extending the ellipse or removing the excess skin with a L or Y incision
- The scalpel handle should be held perpendicular to the skin at the initiation of the incision. Right angle incision through the dermis up to the subcutaneous fat is must to get a good alignment of suture line **(Fig. 5)**
- Undermining the wound edges is essential to reduce the tension at wound margins
- Deep buried dermal sutures takes the wound tension and thereby prevent scar widening. Skin closure done with nonabsorbable sutures such as proline or nylon, without any tension along with everted margins gives excellent cosmetic outcome

It is commonly used in nonhealing ulcer management, postsurgical wound closure, cicatricial alopecia and surgical correction of depigmenting disorders with the use of suction blister grafts and split-thickness grafts. **Box 5** shows different indications of skin grafting.

Types of Grafts

Skin grafts are divided into three major categories depending on their histologic depth.

1. *Split-thickness skin grafts (STSGs):* These are the most commonly used grafts in dermatosurgical practice. STSGs

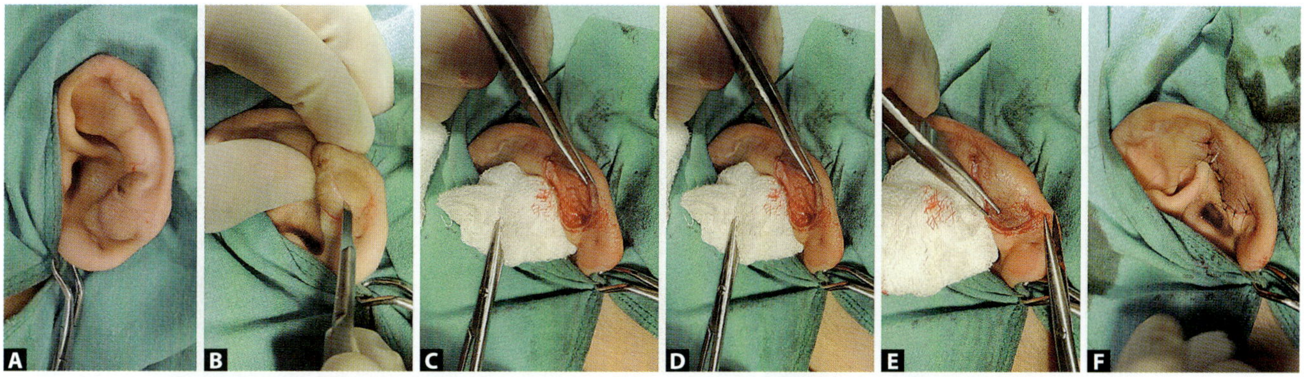

Figs. 24A to F: Ear keloid treated by Intramarginal excision followed by flap closure.

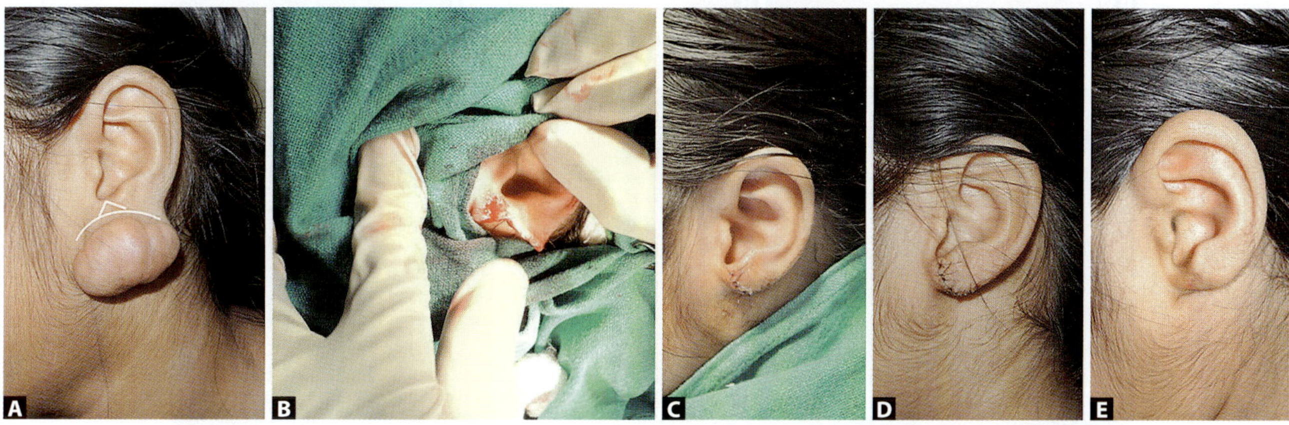

Figs. 25A to E: Earlobe keloid treated by total excision and closed with tension-free sutures. Before treatment and after 6 months.

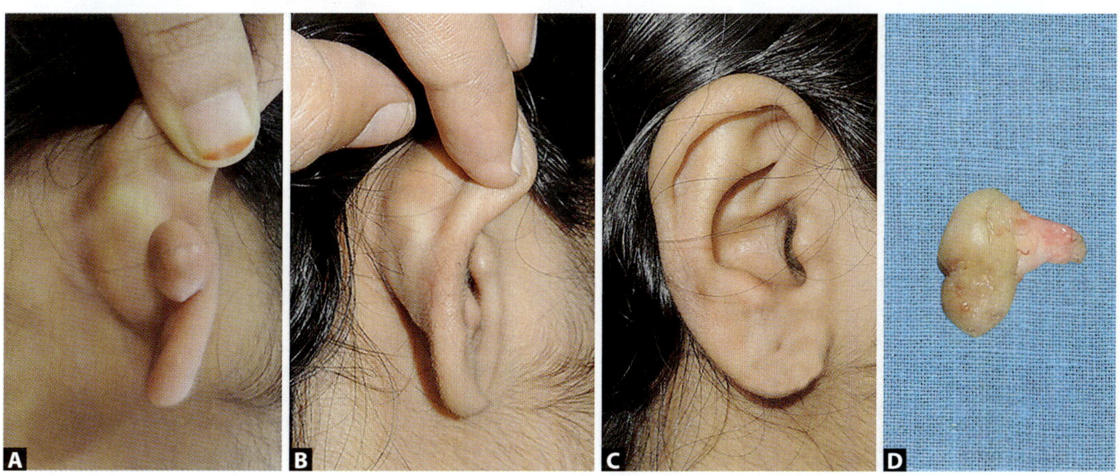

Figs. 26A to D: Ear keloid over pierced site, "dumbbell keloid" excised. Before and after 1 year. The excised keloid lesion has interconnecting bridge following the pierced area.

may be subdivided into thin (0.008–0.012 mm), medium (0.012–0.018 mm), and thick (0.018–0.030 mm) grafts.

2. *Full-thickness skin grafts (FTSGs):* These consist of epidermis and full thickness dermis. It is also called whole skin grafts or Wolffe's grafts.
3. *Composite grafts:* These consists of both epidermis and full thickness dermis along with additional components such as subcutaneous fat, cartilage, etc.

Apart from this the grafts can be classified depending on the techniques by which they are obtained. These include pinch grafts and postage stamp grafts used in ulcer management, and punch grafts and suction blister epidermal grafts used in vitiligo treatment.

Procedure

- Instruments required for skin grafting are given in **Box 6**.

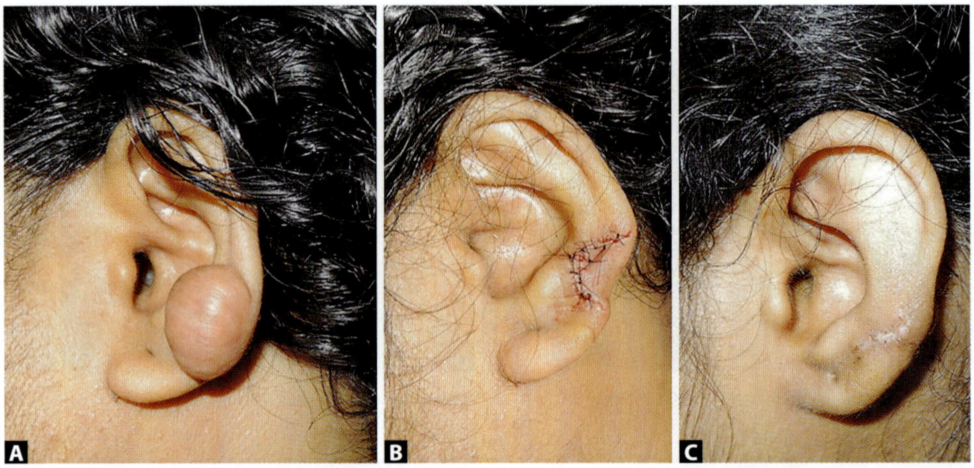

Figs. 27A to C: Ear keloid treated by intramarginal excision followed by flap closure.

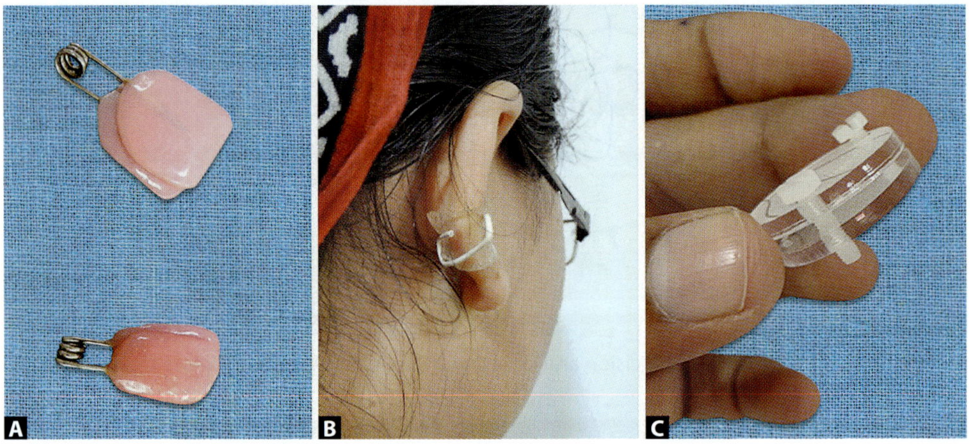

Figs. 28A to C: Compression devices for ear keloids. (A) Costume-made acrylic device; (B) Silicone gel applied and kept in position with the help of paper clips; (C) Commercially available pressure device.

BOX 4: Advantages of elliptical excision.

- Good cosmetic results
- Minimal or no tissue destruction
- Not a blind procedure
- Costly instruments are not required
- Quality specimen is available for histopathologic examination

BOX 5: Complications of keloid surgery.[7,8]

- Hemorrhage, hematoma formation
- Pain
- Infection
- Reactivation of keloid
- Cosmetic disfigurement

- Procedure is done under local anesthesia or general anesthesia depending on the extend of the area to be grafted. Grafts are harvested from anterolateral aspect of thigh, the arms or abdomen.
- Donor area is cleaned with povidone-iodine and surgical spirit.

BOX 6: Skin grafting: Indications.

- *Acute skin loss*: Traumatic injury, surgical wound after excision of tumors
- *Chronic conditions*: Nonhealing ulcers of various etiology, burn injuries, postoperative wound dehiscence
- As a biological cover to prevent heat and fluid loss in large areas of burns
- Stable vitiligo, piebaldism
- Tattoo removal closed with skin grafts
- After excision of large epidermal malformations such as verrucous epidermal nevus, nevus sebaceous, cicatricial alopecia, etc.

- Tumescent anesthesia is administered over the donor area so as to reduce the bleeding and to keep the area stretched during harvesting. The size of the graft required is measured before harvesting.
- The skin over the donor area is stretched and cutting edge of the dermatome is held at 15–30° angle to the skin surface and sunk to desired depth and the device is moved with uniform pressure and speed. The blade is moved back and forth gently by sawing movement to obtain translucent thin graft as required **(Figs. 29A to C)**.

- The harvested graft is transferred into a petri dish containing normal saline.
- If the grafts are large, small incisions are made on the graft so as to drain the wound fluid drainage.

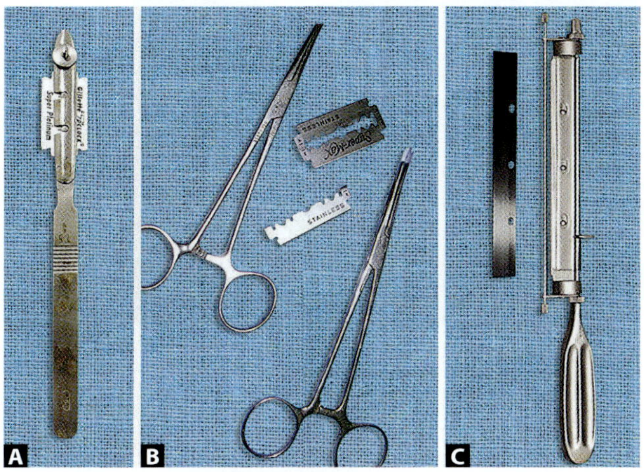

Figs. 29A to C: Instruments required for skin grafting. (A) Modified silver's knife; (B) Straight artery forceps and Razor blade; (C) Humby's knife.

- The graft is placed and spread uniformly on the prepared healthy ulcer bed with dermal side facing downward. The grafts are secured using proline stay sutures or surgical glue.
- A pressure dressing is given. The site is dressed with a paraffin tulle dressing and further with surgical pads and dressings to keep the area secured and immobilized.
- The dressings on both donor and recipient areas are removed after a week. Stay sutures are also removed **(Figs. 30 to 32)**.

Complications

Donor site: Bleeding, pain, secondary infection, and delayed wound healing.

Recipient site: Hematoma, seroma, infection, graft rejection, cosmetic mismatch, and scarring.

Pinch Grafts

Pinch grafting involves harvesting small disks of skin and applying them evenly over the prepared ulcer bed. As multiple skin pieces are placed over the surface of the ulcer,

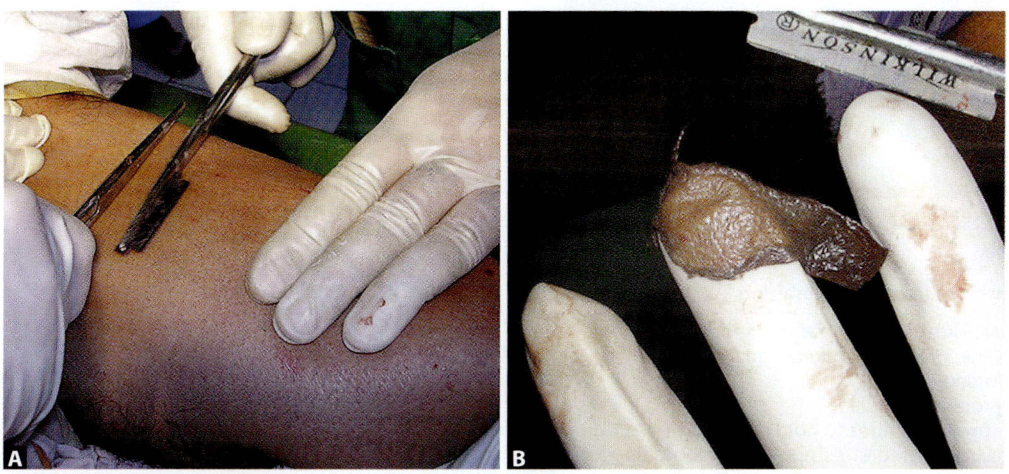

Figs. 30A and B: (A) Harvesting donor skin for STSG; (B) Thin harvested skin.

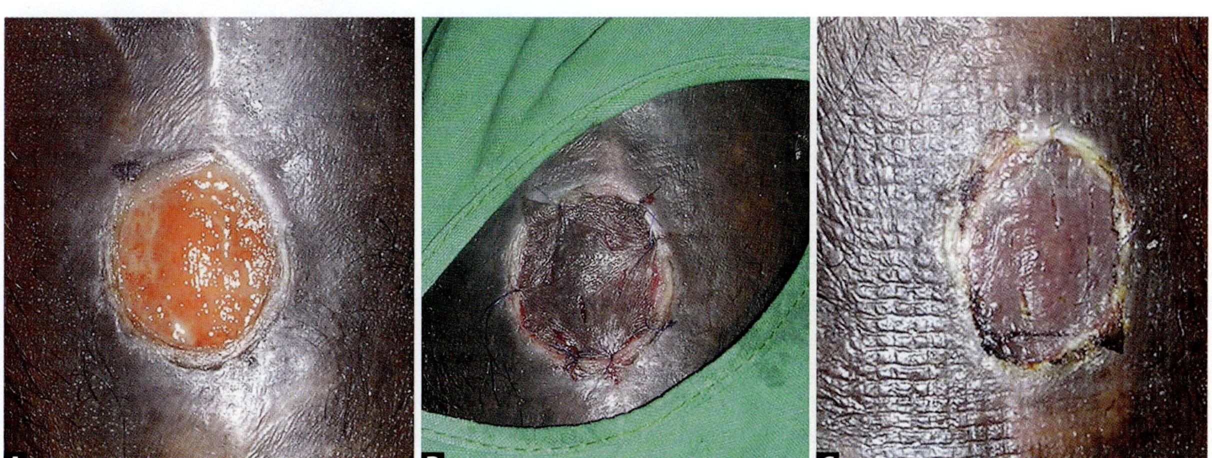

Figs. 31A to C: STSG on nonhealing ulcer: (A) Before; (B) Graft secured with sutures; (C) After.

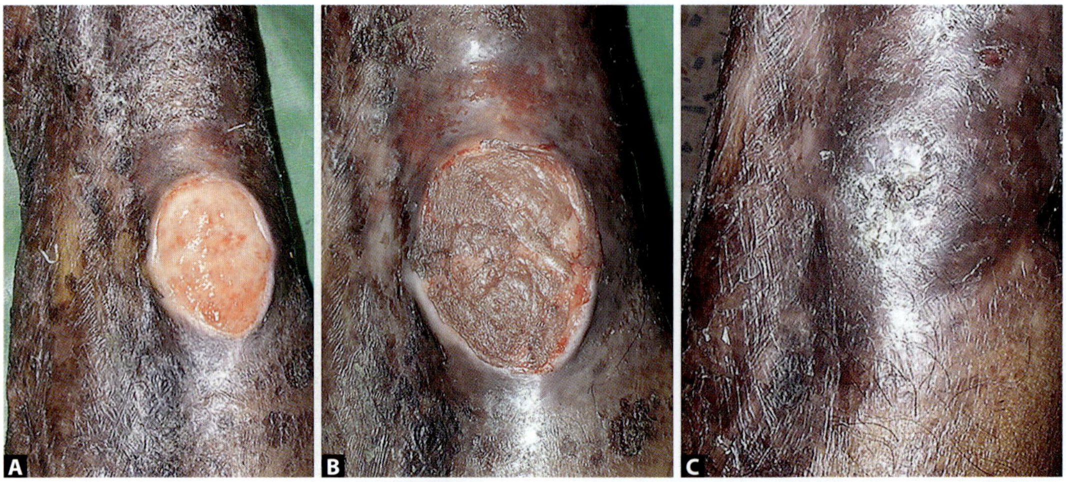

Figs. 32A to C: STSG: (A) Before; (B) Immediately after; (C) After 2 months.

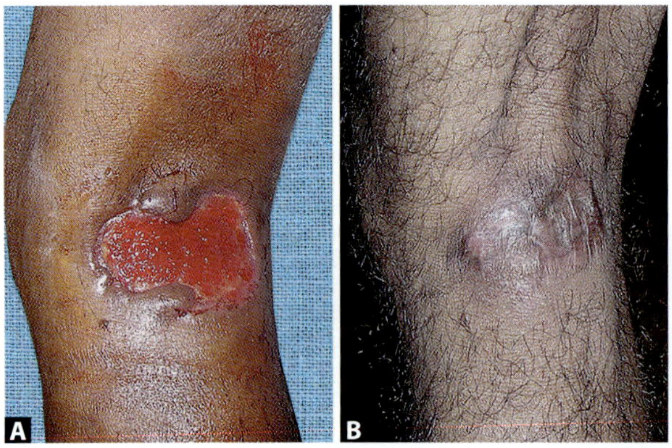

Figs. 33A and B: STSG on ulcer before (A) and after 6 months (B).

BOX 7: Instruments required for skin grafting.

- *Skin grafting knife*: Humby's skin grafting knife, Padget's or Davol's dermatome, or Silver's knife or a razor blade on a straight artery forceps
- Graft spreading rods or spatula
- Surgical glue or proline sutures to hold the graft in position
- Sterile Petri dishes, dermal curettes, non-traumatizing ring forceps, iris scissors

re-epithelization happens around the grafts as well so as to cover the ulcer in a short period **(Figs. 33A and B)**.[15]

This is an easy and inexpensive method to treat nonhealing ulcers. As there are multiple small grafts placed, even if few grafts are lost due to necrosis or secondary infection, the others survive and re-epithelize. **Figures 34 and 35** show the technique and outcome of pinch grafts.

Patch Grafts/Postage Stamp Grafts

Split-thickness skin grafts are cut into postage stamp size and placed over the prepared wound bed at uniform distance. A large ulcer can be treated by using smaller donor skin. As in case of pinch graft, there are multiple grafts placed individually; hence, the chance of complete graft rejection is rare **(Figs. 36 and 37)**, explains the technique of patch grafting and outcome **(Box 7)**.[16,17]

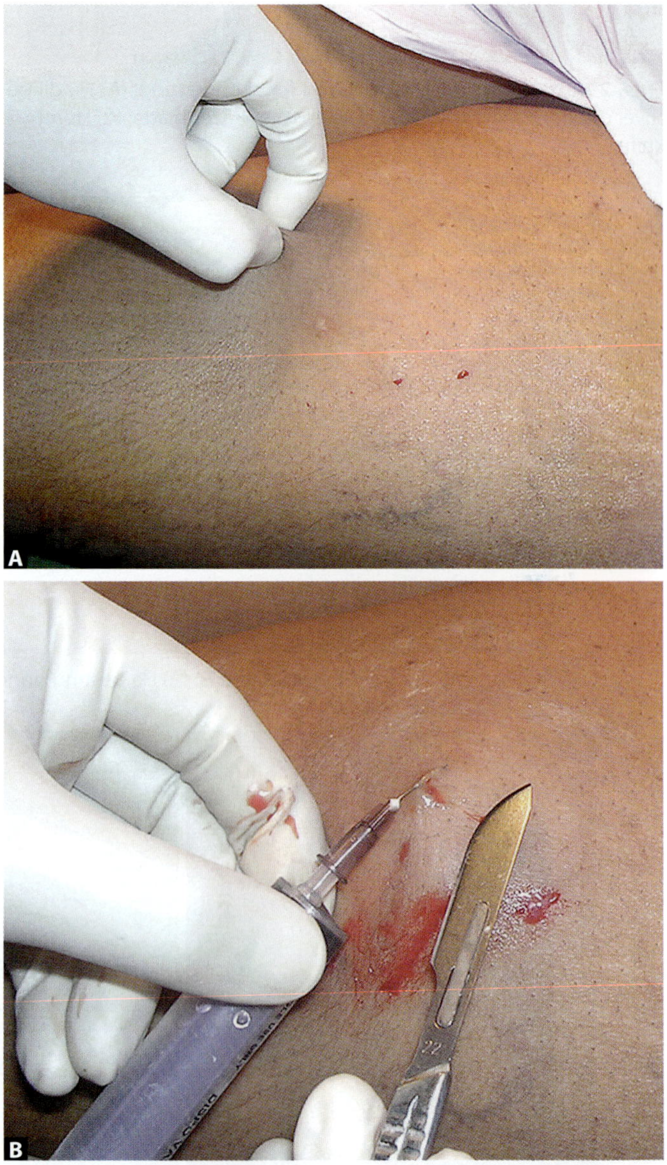

Figs. 34A and B: (A) Skin is pinched to elevate the skin; (B) With the help of a needle, skin is elevated and cut with scalpel blade.

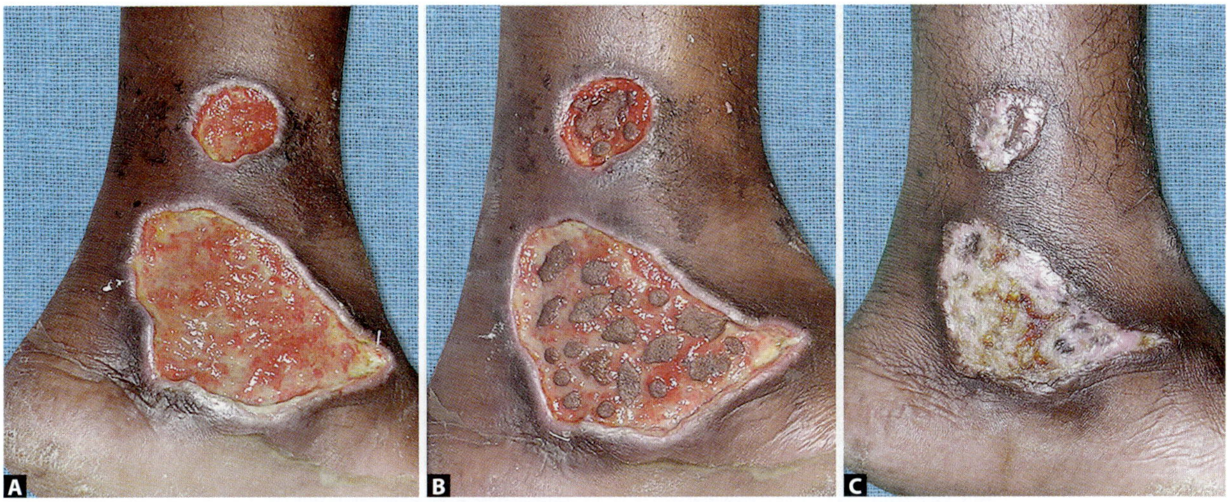

Figs. 35A to C: (A) Ulcer before pinch grafting; (B) Pinch grafts placed over the ulcer; (C) After 4 weeks.

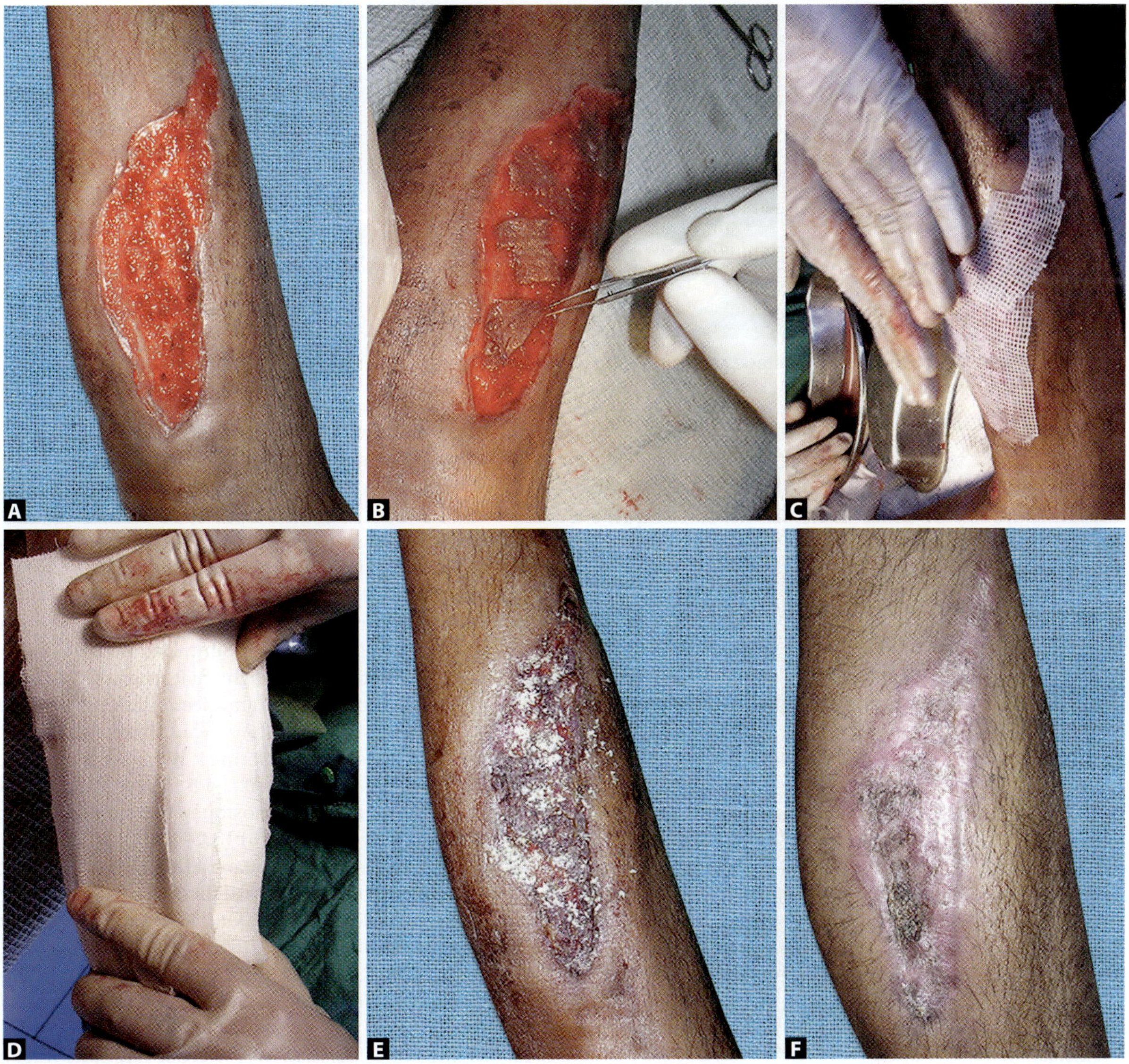

Figs. 36A to F: Patch or postage stamp grafting in ulcer treatment. (A) Ulcer before treatment; (B) Placing patch grafts; (C and D) Dressings given; (E) After 7 days. Collagen powder being applied over the uncovered areas; (F) After 3 months.

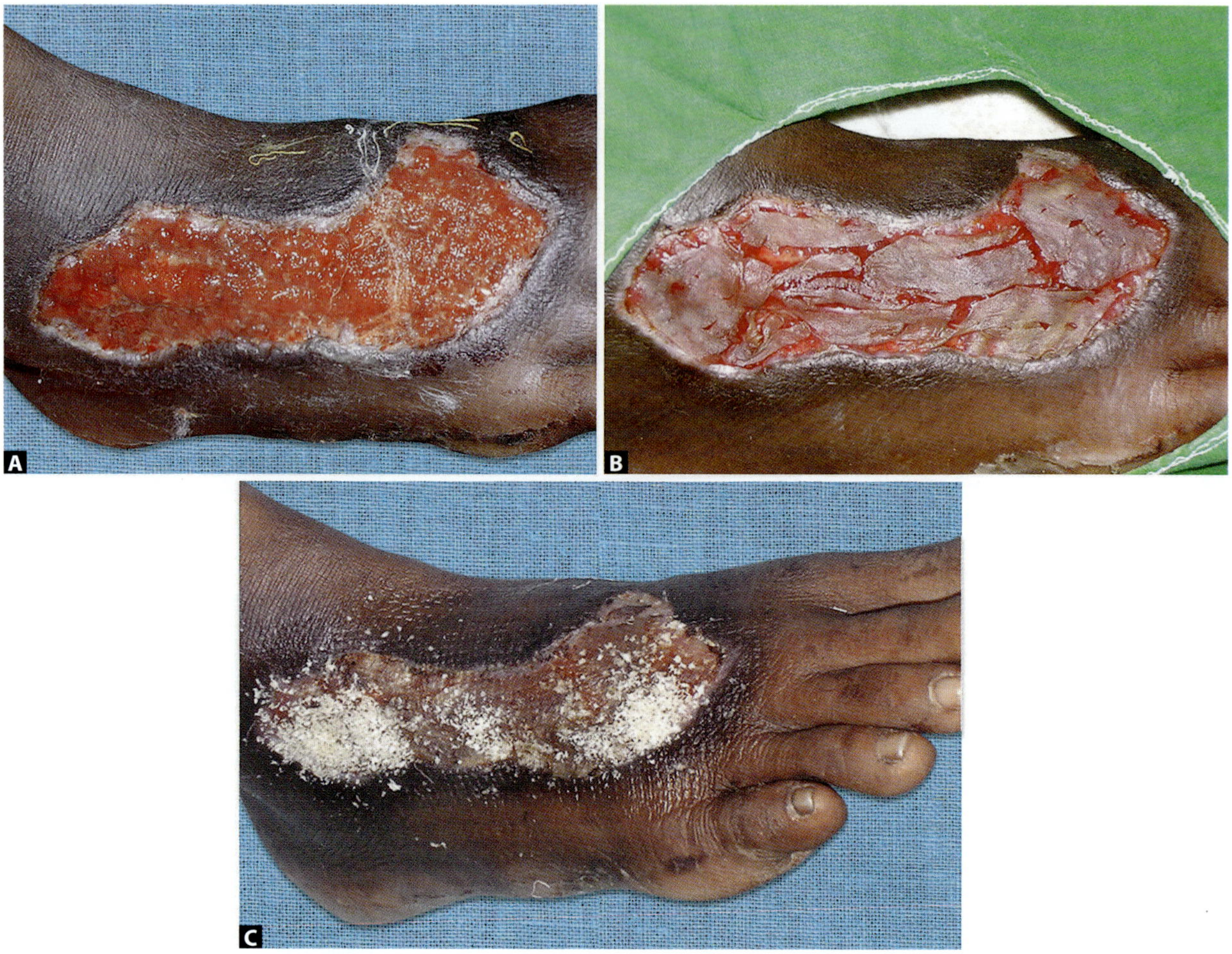

Figs. 37A to C: Patch or postage stamp grafting: (A) Before; (B) After placing the grafts; (C) After 10 days.

KEY POINTS

- Basic dermatosurgical procedures help the dermatologists to tackle majority of the conditions which require a surgical referral.
- As dermatology is a procedure-based practice, it requires the understanding of techniques in dermatologic surgery, postoperative patient care and managing complications.
- Good excision and grafting skills should be developed and adequate training is mandatory to tackle various conditions.

REFERENCES

1. Tajirian AL, Goldberg DJ. A review of sutures and other skin closure materials. J Cosmet Laser Ther. 2010;12(6):296-302.
2. Ammirati CT. Advances in wound closure materials. Adv Dermatol. 2002;18:313-38.
3. Moy RL, Waldman B, Hein DW. A review of sutures and suturing techniques. J Dermatol Surg Oncol. 1992;18(9):785-95.
4. Pardasani AG, Leshin B, Hallman JR, White WL. Fusiform incisional biopsy for pigmented skin lesions. Dermatol Surg. 2000;26:622-4.
5. Sonthalia S, Sharma P, Agrawal M. How to perform an elliptical excision of the skin. N Engl J Med. 2019;381(5):490-2.
6. Boyer JD, Zitelli JA, Brodland DG. Undermining in cutaneous surgery. Dermatologic Surgery. 2001;27:75-8.
7. Altchek ED. A technical consideration in the serial excision of a nevus. Plast Reconstr Surg. 1980;66:849-50.
8. Arneja JS, Gosain AK. Giant congenital melanocytic nevi of the trunk and an algorithm for treatment. J Craniofac Surg. 2005;16:886-93.
9. Emmett AJ, Broadbent GD. Shave excision of superficial solar skin lesions. Plast Reconstr Surg. 1987;80(1):47-54.
10. Edens BL, Bartlow GA, Haghighi P, Astarita RW, Davidson TM. Effectiveness of curettage and electrodesiccation in the removal of basal cell carcinoma. J Am Acad Dermatol. 1983;9:383-8.
11. Rosen DJ, Patel MK, Katherine F, Weiss PR. A primary protocol for the management of ear keloids: results of excision combined with intraoperative and postoperative steroid injections. Plast Reconstr Surg. 2007;120(5):1395-400.
12. Tanaydin V, Beugels J, Piatkowski A. , Colla C, Kerckhove E van den, Hugenholtz GCG, et al. Efficacy of custom-made pressure clips for ear keloid treatment after surgical excision. J Plast Reconstr Aesthet Surg. 2016;69(1):115-21.
13. Lee Y, Minn KW, Baek RM, Hong JJ. A new surgical treatment of keloid: keloid core excision. Ann Plast Surg. 2001;46(2):135-40.
14. Kirsner RS, Eaglstein WH, Kerdel FA. Split-thickness skin grafting for lower extremity ulcerations. Dermatol Sur. 1997;23(2):85-91.

15. Oien RF, Hansen BU, Håkansson A. Pinch graft skin transplantation for leg ulcers in primary care. J Wound Care. 2000; 9(5):217-20.
16. Biswas A, Bharara M, Hurst C, Armstrong DG, Rilo H. The micrograft concept for wound healing: strategies and applications. J Diabetes Sci Technol. 2010;4(4):808-19.
17. Miyanaga T, Kishibe M, Yamashita M, Kaneko T, Kinoshita F, Shimada K. Minced skin grafting for promoting wound healing and improving donor-site appearance after split-thickness skin grafting: a prospective half-side comparative trial. Plast Reconstr Surg. 2019;144(2): 475-83.

EXAMINATION QUESTION

1. Write short note on local anesthetics used in dematosurgery.

165 CHAPTER

Wound Repair

Varsha M Shetty

INTRODUCTION

Skin, being the outer barrier is subjected to a variety of stress factors resulting in frequent cell and barrier damage.[1] Wound healing is very crucial for survival as it is responsible for restoring the integrity of skin, at the same time preventing infection and dehydration.[2] Tissue regeneration and repair occurs in response to a stimulus which disrupts the physical continuity in functional tissues. The stimuli can be external or internal, physical, chemical, or thermal.[3]

Ideally the repair process should result in regeneration of the injured tissues with structural, functional, and esthetic properties resembling uninjured skin. However, the skin integrity is restored at the cost of replacing the damaged tissues by fibrotic material ultimately resulting in scarring. Wound healing in oral mucosa and fetal skin is different in that it does not result in scarring owing to the limited inflammatory response during the repair.[4]

STAGES OF WOUND HEALING

Tissue injury triggers a series of overlapping and highly orchestrated phases of hemostasis, inflammation, proliferation, and remodeling **(Figs. 1A and B)**. Alteration in any one or more of these phases can give rise to impaired wound healing. Moreover, wound repair is also influenced by several external factors and diseases such as diabetes, renal failure, malnutrition, and infection. Sometimes the repair process may be exaggerated causing formation of fibroproliferative scars such as hypertrophic scars and keloids.

Hemostasis

The immediate response following injury is to contain the blood loss by vasoconstriction and formation of a hemostatic plug to seal the vessel. This phase begins with the adherence and aggregation of platelets following which there is activation of coagulation and complement pathway ultimately resulting in the formation of a fibrin clot.

The fibrin network thus formed not only helps in arresting the blood loss but also acts as a barrier against microbes and serves as a matrix for cellular migration. There is release of various chemoattractants and growth factors such as thrombin, CCL5, transforming growth factor β (TGF-β), platelet-derived growth factor (PDGF), and vascular endothelial growth factor (VEGF) which promote migration of inflammatory cells and fibroblast proliferation.

The degradation of fibrin and the subsequent complement activation plays a crucial role in influx of inflammatory cells, angiogenesis, and stromal proliferation.[2,3]

Inflammation

This stage involves the influx of neutrophils, macrophages, and lymphocytes which coincides with the appearance of signs of inflammation namely erythema and edema at the site of the lesion. This neutrophilic cellular response is

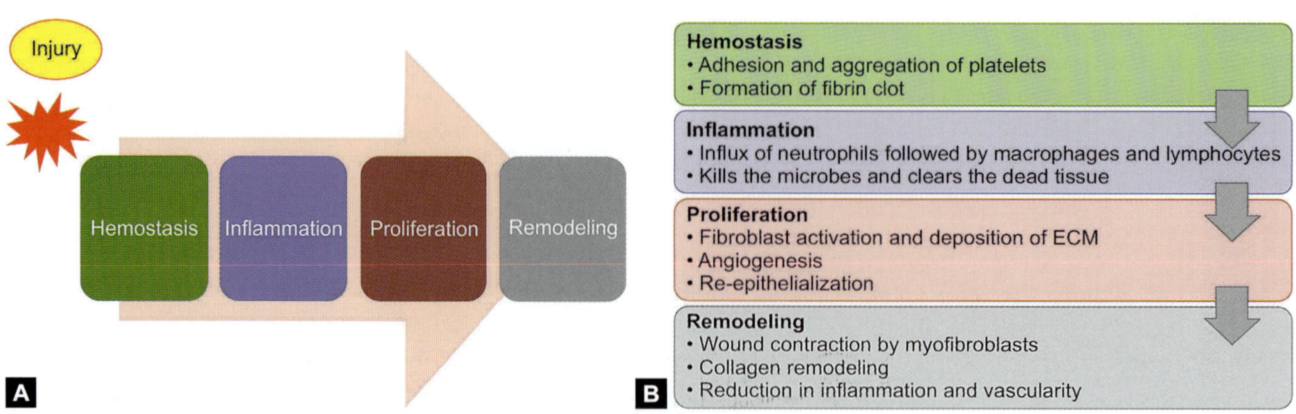

Figs. 1A and B: (A) Stages of wound repair and; (B) Schematic representation of all the changes occurring during different stages of wound repair. (ECM: extracellular matrix)

established within first 24 hours of the wound but may last up to 2 days.

Bradykinin, C3a and C5a (anaphylatoxins) generated by the complement cascade, platelet degranulation and bacterial degradation products recruit neutrophils which are the first cells to appear at the site of the wound.

The main purpose of neutrophils is to eliminate the bacteria and clean up the injured tissue. This they achieve by secretion of proteases, antimicrobial peptides, and generation of reactive oxygen species. The neutrophils also promote fibrin degradation, angiogenesis, and re-epithelialization.

Monocytes infiltrate the area within 2–3 days thus becoming the predominant cell population. The chemokines such as CCL2 released by the neutrophils, keratinocytes attract the circulating monocytes into the tissue where they differentiate into macrophages. Macrophages help in clearing the dead cells and apoptotic neutrophils thereby removing the cytokines and hence preventing further leukocyte influx into the area. Macrophages play a key role in wound repair as they are known to secrete cytokines and growth factors such as TGF-α, TGF-β, PDGF, and fibroblast growth factor (FGF) which trigger and propagate tissue proliferation by activating endothelial cells, keratinocytes, and fibroblasts. Hence, macrophages by causing cell proliferation, extracellular matrix (ECM) synthesis, and angiogenesis trigger the transition from an exudative phase to proliferation phase in tissue repair. Thus, macrophage depletion can result in impaired wound healing.[2,3]

Lymphocytes being the last cells to arrive exert specific response against microbes either by producing antibodies (B-cell mediated) or by secretion of cytokines and causing cytolysis (T-cell mediated). Mast cells are also known to appear later in the course of wound healing, however, their specific role in wound healing requires further research. But mast cells are known to be associated with hyperproliferative states such as keloid and hypertrophic scars.[2]

Proliferation

This phase begins around 2 days after injury and can last up to 3 weeks. The principal events in this phase are recruitment of fibroblasts, ECM deposition, angiogenesis, and re-epithelialization.

Platelet-derived growth factor and TGF-β synthesized by macrophages and mast cells activate fibroblasts which in turn proliferate and lay down matrix proteins such as hyaluronic acid, collagen, fibronectin, and proteoglycans. This acts as a provisional ECM for keratinocyte migration and gets ultimately replaced by granulation tissue.

Granulation tissue comprises blood vessels, macrophages and fibroblasts distributed in a loose matrix of collagen, fibronectin, and hyaluronic acid.[2] Angiogenesis is crucial for the formation of granulation tissue which starts with endothelial proliferation, rearrangement of basement membrane, and recruitment of pericytes ultimately resulting in the formation of a microvascular network. This network supplies the essential nutrients and oxygen to the repairing tissues.[3,5] The key angiogenic factors are produced by macrophages, fibroblasts, keratinocytes, and endothelial cells which include VEGF, CXCL8, basic FGF, and angiopoietin 1. Type III collagen replaces the provisional fibrin matrix which in turn will be replaced by type I collagen during remodeling.[2]

Fibroblasts enable connective tissue contraction which is greatly reinforced when fibroblasts are driven to differentiate into α-smooth muscle actin expressing myofibroblasts in the presence of TGF-β and CXCL8. The myofibroblasts tend to draw the wound close and aligns the collagen bundles, which is a primary constituent of scar tissue.[5]

Re-epithelialization occurs by the proliferation and migration of keratinocytes to cover the wound. Various cytokines and growth factors such as TGF-β, epidermal growth factor (EGF), FGF, PDGF, and keratinocyte growth factor (KGF) synthesized by platelets, neutrophils, macrophages, endothelial cells, and fibroblasts initiate and maintain keratinocyte proliferation and migration. Proteases of cysteine, serine, and matrix metalloproteinase (MMP) family ensure keratinocyte migration through the fibrin matrix and over underlying dermal tissue inducing re-epithelialization.[2]

Remodeling

The remodeling phase begins within 2–3 weeks of the onset of the wound and can last till a year **(Fig. 2)**. It is characterized by the following events:

- Significant reduction in inflammatory cells and vascularity
- Wound contraction mediated by myofibroblasts
- *Collagen remodeling*: During which type III collagen is replaced by type I collagen, collagen fibers get thicker and come to lie parallel to one another, undergo cross-linking with the help of lysyl oxidase. These remodeling changes help in restoring the tensile strength of skin to 80% of the unwounded skin.

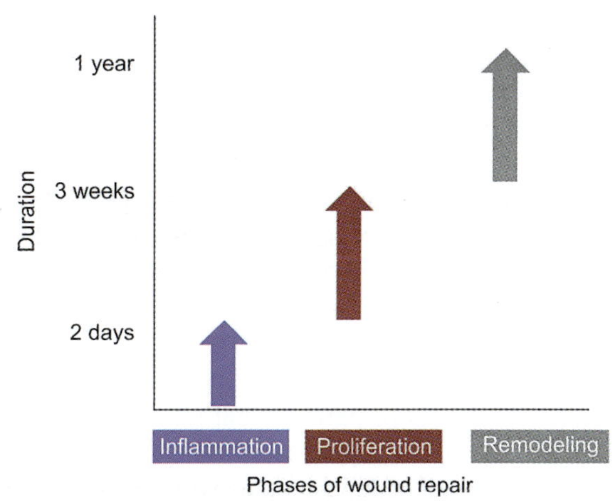

Fig. 2: Duration of different phases of wound repair.

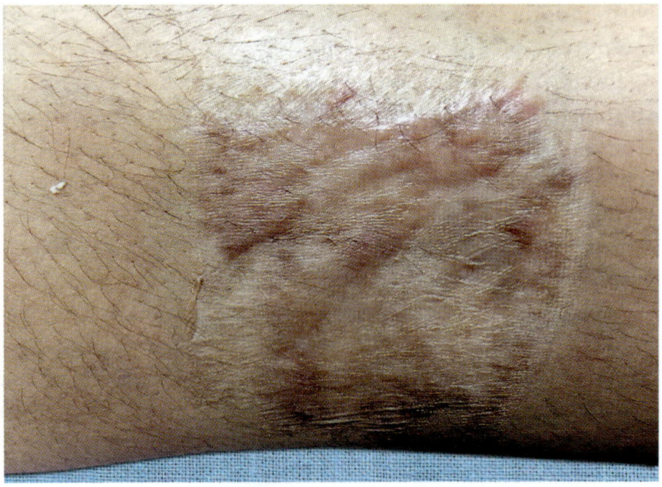

Fig. 3: Post-traumatic scar showing atrophic and hypertrophic areas.

The collagen synthesis is regulated by growth factors such as TGF-β and FGF ultimately resulting in the formation of scar[2] **(Fig. 3)**.

IMPAIRED WOUND HEALING

There could be two possible outcomes of impaired wound healing—an ulcerative defect (chronic wound) or excessive formation of scar (keloid or hypertrophic scar).

Chronic Wounds

These are nothing but defects in the continuity of skin resulting when the process of wound repair does not occur in an orderly and timely manner. Very often the disruption in tissue repair occurs as a result of a faulty inflammatory phase with some of the reasons being illustrated in **Box 1**. The persistent inflammation, high bacterial load, and high amount of protease secretion favor tissue degradation over repair.[1,4]

BOX 1: Common causes of chronic wounds.[1,4]

- Vascular insufficiency
- Diabetes mellitus
- Local pressure effects
- Malnutrition
- Immunocompromised status
- Old age
- Chronic mechanical stress
- Infection

Venous leg ulcers are one of the common examples of chronic nonhealing wounds which arise as a result of persistent inflammation, defective keratinocyte migration and improper signaling or expression of microRNA.

Atherosclerosis is the second most common cause of nonhealing leg ulcer due to vascular insufficiency. Diabetes is the most common metabolic disease associated with impaired wound healing resulting in diabetic foot ulcer (DFU). Chronic nonhealing ulcers are responsible for significant mortality and morbidity **(Fig. 4)**. It is observed that the 5-year mortality associated with DFU and ischemic ulcers is higher than that due to prostate or breast cancer.[1]

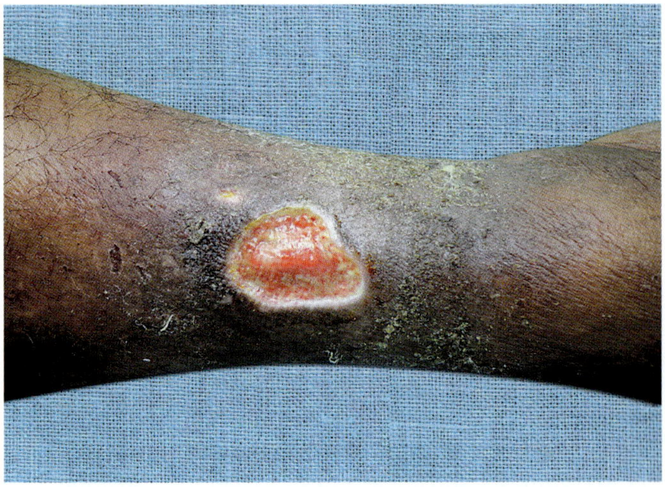

Fig. 4: Chronic leg ulcer secondary to venous insufficiency.

Scarring

There are two forms of pathological scarring reported in human skin: (1) hypertrophic scars and (2) keloid **(Fig. 5)**. Both arise as a result of deposition of excessive ECM causing tissue fibrosis. These can cause significant discomfort to the patient as for example if found over a joint can result in restriction of movement **(Table 1)**.

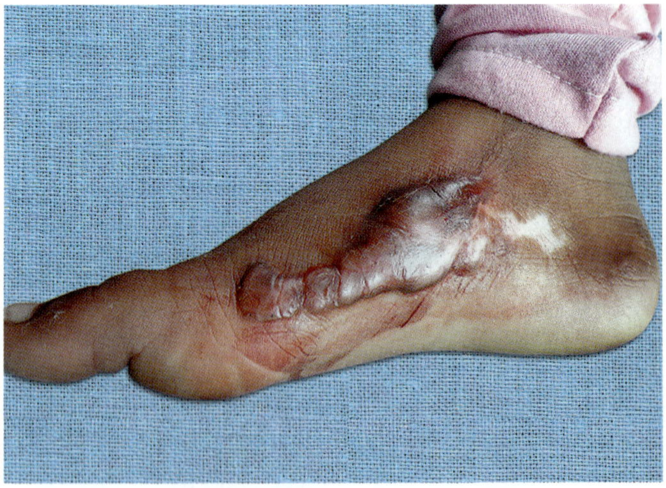

Fig. 5: Keloid on the medial border of the right foot.

Moreover, pathological scars are known to occur with greater incidence in dark-skinned individuals and are not common before puberty. TGF-β is one of the key growth factors implicated in scarring. It is observed that persistent inflammation induces fibroblasts to increase the production of osteopontin which causes bundling up of collagen fibers and pathological scarring.[1]

TABLE 1: Differences between hypertrophic scar and keloid.[1]

Hypertrophic scar	*Keloid*
Follows a surgery, trauma or burns	Arises spontaneously in most of the cases
Restricted to the site of injury	Extend beyond the margins of the original tissue damage
Has a tendency for spontaneous regression (usually within 6 months)	No tendency for spontaneous regression
No genetic predisposition	Genetic predisposition present
Less chance of recurrence after treatment	Greater chances of recurrence following treatment

RECENT ADVANCES IN WOUND HEALING

There has been a steady progress in the management of chronic wounds in the last decade with most approaches focusing on the local wound environment. Dressings promote healing of the wound by protecting it from further trauma, absorbing excess exudate at the same time providing adequate moisture. There are complex dressings available in the market nowadays which apart from serving the basic functions exert an antibacterial action, cause synthesis of ECM, and promote proliferation and migration of the local cells.

Role of Growth Factors in Wound Healing

Various recombinant growth factors have been used locally to stimulate wound healing with limited success.

Becaplermin, a recombinant human PDGF was approved in 1997 by United States Food and Drug Administration (USFDA) for the treatment of DFU. They act by promoting epithelial migration, angiogenesis, and ECM deposition. However, large randomized controlled trials are necessary to establish its safety and efficacy in other types of ulcers.

Keratinocyte growth factor-1 (KGF-1) received FDA approval in 2004 to prevent oral mucositis in patients receiving chemotherapy. It acts by targeting the epidermal cells and is being marketed under the names palifermin or kepivance.

Clinical trials are being conducted to study the role of other growth factors such as FGF and VEGF (telbermin—VEGF-A165) in wound healing.

Cell-based Therapies

It is been observed that mesenchymal stem cells (MSCs) derived from bone marrow and adipose tissue help in promoting the repair process when applied topically onto the chronic wounds. This has been particularly useful in augmenting the healing in chronic wounds of recessive dystrophic epidermolysis bullosa (RDEB).

Recent developments include production of induced pluripotent stem cells (iPSCs) from keratinocytes and other differentiated cells. These cells are capable of synthesizing human skin equivalent; hence, they have been tried in regenerating genetically reprogrammed healthy cells in RDEB children. However, all these stem cell-based therapies are still in the stage of clinical trial and none have been approved by FDA as of now.[1]

KEY POINTS

- Wound repair is an essential physiological process which involves a multicellular and well-orchestrated phase of hemostasis, inflammation, proliferation, and remodeling.
- Wound repair in adult human skin results in the formation of a scar with the extent of scarring depending upon the degree of inflammation.
- Impaired wound healing occurs when there is fault in any one or more phases of wound repair.
- The outcome of impaired wound healing can either be a chronic wound or hypertrophic scars and keloids.

REFERENCES

1. Eming SA, Martin P, Tomic-Canic M. Wound repair and regeneration: mechanisms, signaling, and translation. Sci Transl Med. 2014;6(265):265sr6.
2. Thiruvoth FM, Mohapatra DP, Sivakumar DK, Chittoria RK, Nandhagopal V. Current concepts in the physiology of adult wound healing. Plast Aesthet Res. 2015;2:250-6.
3. Gonzalez AC, Costa TG, Andrade ZA, Medrado ARAP. Wound healing—A literature review. An Bras Dermatol. 2016;91(5): 614-20.
4. Rajan V, Murray RZ. The duplicitous nature of inflammation in wound repair. Wound Pract Res. 2008;16(3):122-9.
5. Shaw TJ, Martin P. Wound repair at a glance. J Cell Sci. 2009; 122:3209-13.

EXAMINATION QUESTIONS

1. Discuss the stages of wound healing and add a note on impaired wound healing.
2. Enumerate the causes of impaired wound healing and add a note on role of growth factors in wound repair.
3. Explain novel therapies in wound healing.

166 CHAPTER Nail Surgery

Sushil Tahiliani, Harsh Tahiliani

INTRODUCTION

Nail unit surgery is in a stage of infancy in India. Having a sound knowledge of the surgical anatomy of the nail unit is a pre-requisite before one can start the practice of nail surgery.

SURGICAL ANATOMY

The nail unit (nail complex) consists of nail matrix, nailbed, nail plate, proximal nail fold (PNF), lateral nail fold (LNF), and hyponychium. It can be subdivided in to three structures:

1. Matrix with nail plate being its product
2. Nailbed that firmly attaches the plate to the underlying connective tissue and bone
3. Paronychium (PNF and LNF) that acts as a frame for the nail plate.

In addition, distal interphalangeal joint and distal phalanx are a part of "nail organ".

Blood supply: Arterial supply is derived from lateral digital arteries which supply the nail unit through formation of superficial, proximal, and distal arcades.

Venous drainage follows arterial vasculature, the only difference being that it combines proximally forming two digital veins on either side.

Nerve supply: Innervation of the nail unit is through two laterally positioned sensory nerves, i.e., dorsal and ventral. The nail unit is richly innervated.

Indications for surgery of the nail unit:

- To help in diagnosis
- To treat infection
- To alleviate pain
- To correct/prevent deformities
- To treat localized neoplasms

Relative contraindications for surgery of the nail unit: They are few due to availability of better medical care and refinement of the technique.

- Peripheral vascular disease
- Collagen vascular disease
- Disorders of hemostasis
- Uncontrolled diabetes mellitus
- Acute infection/inflammation of the nail unit.

Preoperative considerations:

- Rule out contraindications
- Concurrent medication that may cause blood thinning
- Drug allergies
- Discuss duration of functional impairment
- Discuss risk of short-term/long-term nail dystrophy
- Good clinical image
- Informed and written consent.

Instruments

General instruments:

- Binocular magnifying loupe that magnifies 2.5–3.5 times at a distance of 35–45 cm
- Delicate Adson's forceps with one by two teeth/Castroviejo forceps
- Double prong Guthrie retractors
- Delicate needle holder
- Stevens/Gradle scissors
- Straight mosquito forceps
- Curette
- *Digital tourniquet*: Penrose drain wrapped around the base of digit with the 2 ends clamped together with a hemostat. It is not ideal and the pressure created can be excessive. Should be released every 10 minutes if the surgery goes on longer. Digital pressure applied by the assistant on the lateral aspect of proximal phalanx of the digit may suffice for shorter procedures. In case of hand digit surgery, it is best to use a sterile glove 1 size smaller than the appropriate size which is put on the patient's hand that is cleansed and injected with local anesthetic. The appropriate fingertip of the glove is cut and rolled back till it reaches the base of the digit.

Specific instruments:

- *Nail elevator*: Lempert (2–3 mm wide)/Freer septum elevator/dental spatula
- English anvil-action nail splitter
- Nail nipper

Sutures:

- Biopsies and excisions with a diameter 3 mm do not require suturing
- For nail matrix/nailbed,4-0 to 6-0 absorbable suture
- For PNF/LNF 4-0 to 5-0 absorbable or non-absorbable suture.

Surgical Setting

Nail avulsions, biopsies and simple excisions can safely be performed in dermatologist's office under same conditions as basic skin surgery procedures. Advanced nail surgical procedures should be performed in operation theater.

Anesthesia

- A good knowledge of the techniques of anesthesia of the nail apparatus is mandatory to have surgery at that site comfortable, both for the patient and surgeon.
- *Agents*: Plane lidocaine is a reference anesthetic agent (2% preferred over 1%).
- Ropivacaine and bupivacaine may be used for longer lasting postoperative effect (4–8 hours) though these molecules are used more commonly for regional blocks.
- Lidocaine with adrenaline is safe but not preferred as bleeding control measures are still necessary.
- *Syringe*: Luer lock or dental syringe
- Needle 27–30 gauge
- *Techniques*: Distal digital block (wing-block)/proximal digital block are the most preferred methods. They offer total nail unit anesthesia.

Ring block is not a desirable method of injecting local anesthetic agent.

	Distal digital block ***(Fig. 1)***	*Proximal digital block* ***(Fig. 2)***
Point of insertion	2–3 mm proximal to junction of PNF and LNF both sides of digit	Base of digit both sides of digit
Onset of effect	<1 minute	8–10 minutes
	More painful, may cause swelling of operative field, may be inadequately effective for the whole operative field in more extensive surgeries	Less painful
	Induces compression hemostasis	
Amount of agent needed	1–1.5 mL	5–10 mL
C.I.	Local infection, vasculopathies	
	Low risk of neurovascular compromise	

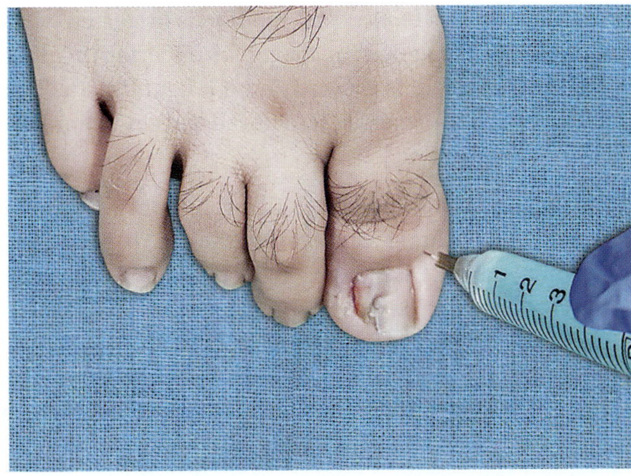

Fig. 1: Point of insertion for distal digital block.

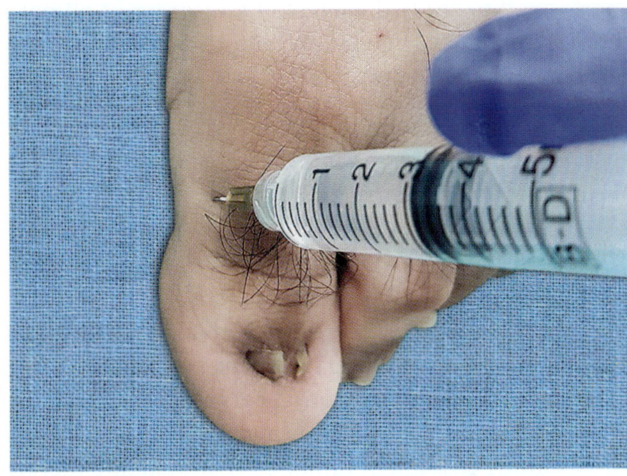

Fig. 2: Point of insertion for proximal digital block.

Operative Techniques

Nail Biopsy

Nail unit biopsy is a useful and simple procedure that helps in the treatment and diagnosis of various nail diseases. A biopsy becomes necessary when routine medical history, clinical examination and diagnostic tests fail to establish a diagnosis. It is the most primitive type of nail unit surgery that should be a part of every dermatologist's armamentarium.

Nail biopsies may be classified based on:

- *Site of biopsy*: Nail plate, nailbed, matrix, nail-fold, combination of these.
- *Sampling method*: Punch, incisional, shave biopsy
- *Axis of incision*: Longitudinal, transverse
- *Preparation of biopsy site*: With avulsion of nail-plate, without avulsion of nail plate.

Punch biopsy: A punch biopsy is useful to obtain sample from the nail plate, nailbed or both. Soaking the nail in tepid water for 10–15 minutes prior to punching is useful. For specimen from the nailbed, a 4-mm punch should be used and pushed till it reaches the periosteum of the distal phalanx. Firm pressure on the nail plate or a 30-gauge needle helps in upward popping of the tissue cylinder.

Siegle and Swanson have developed a two-punch technique for biopsy of the nailbed. A larger 5- or 6-mm punch is used to make a circular defect in the nail plate. A smaller 3- or 4-mm punch is used to acquire tissue sample from the nailbed. Extraction of the nailbed tissue is easier with this double punch method. The punched-out nail plate is placed in its original position after the specimen has been obtained.

Longitudinal nailbed biopsy: This method is preferred when a larger sample is needed for diagnosis of certain nailbed tumors. The nail plate is avulsed and a longitudinal ellipse parallel to the ridges of nailbed is removed and closure is done with absorbable sutures.

Nail matrix biopsy: A transverse nail matrix biopsy should be performed when a larger sample from the matrix is needed. The proximal nail fold has to be reflected and proximal third of the nail plate has to be removed while performing a matrix biopsy. The distal curved configuration of the lunula should not be disturbed while performing a nail matrix biopsy. Even a 3-mm punch biopsy of the matrix heals without a significant deformity when performed correctly.

A lateral longitudinal wedge-shaped nail matrix and nailbed biopsy from the hyponychium to the matrix may be performed to study the effect of a disorder of all parts of the nail apparatus. This method is more beneficial to study the extent of malignancies.

Nail-fold biopsy: A 2-mm punch biopsy, shave excisional biopsy or crescent excision 4 mm at its greatest width may be done to study tumors of the PNF.

Nail Plate Surgery (Nail Avulsion)

Removing the nail plate is indicated in:

- Accessing underlying nailbed/nail matrix for visualizing pathology/biopsy/surgical treatment
- Treatment of retronychia, onychogryphosis, etc.

It is combined with some other surgical procedures (matrixectomy, excision of tumor etc.) or systemic therapy (onychomycosis). Certain nail disorders like retronychia are an exception to this rule.

Nail avulsion may be classified as:

- Total nail plate avulsion
- Partial nail plate avulsion
- Curled nail plate avulsion
- Trapdoor nail plate avulsion

Total Nail Plate Avulsion

Total nail plate avulsion is indicated in a very few nail disorders such as removal of a dermatophytoma in total dystrophic onychomycosis. Total nail plate avulsion may also be carried out to expose the nailbed or matrix for removal of underlying growths, however it is not a popular method as the opposing force exerted on the nailbed is lost leading to distal embedding. Total nail avulsion may be carried under the cover of a distal digital block using just a nail elevator and a hemostat.

Techniques:

- *Proximal approach*: Done when the distal part of nail plate is too thick or is so firmly attached to nailbed that the level of cleavage cannot be established.
- *Distal approach*: Usual approach. Used for exposure and surgical removal of large nailbed lesions and removal of onychomatricoma/dermatophytoma.

Nail Plate Avulsion Followed by Replacement (Fig. 3)

Advantages:

- The ventral aspect of nail plate has some nailbed and nail matrix keratinocytes and replacement acts as a partial thickness graft
- Postoperative pain is lesser
- New nail alignment is better
- In cases where the matrix has been operated and sutured, it prevents formation of pterygium.

Techniques:

- *Trap-door avulsion*: Distal to proximal separation
- *Curled avulsion*: From one of the lateral sides of nail-plate

Partial Nail Plate Avulsion

Partial nail plate avulsion (PNA) results in a large portion of the nail plate remaining in place, thereby reducing the risk of distal embedding. Partial nail avulsion is a part of many nail procedures such as surgery of ingrown toe-nails, surgery for nail spicules, and partial matrixectomy. A partial nail avulsion may be performed under a distal digital block or a proximal digital block. Postoperative pain is lesser and healing is usually faster.

Indications:

- Biopsy
- Matrixectomy
- Linear melanonychia
- Acute infections of nailbed/nailfolds
- Some cases of onychomycosis
- For removal of nail unit "space-occupying lesions."

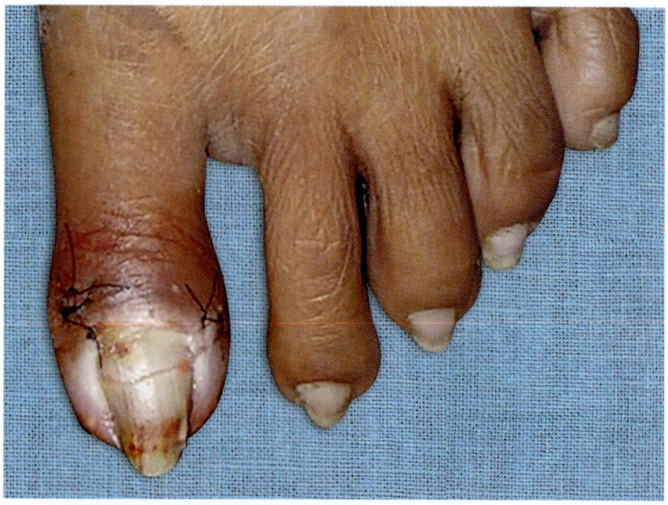

Fig. 3: Repositioning the avulsed nail plate after surgery.

Matrixectomy (Surgery of the Nail Matrix)

Matrix rests on the distal phalanx and is covered by ventral part of PNF. The part of matrix not covered by the PNF is visualized as lunula.

Distal part of matrix forms ventral part of nail plate, and hence removal of distal matrix does not lead to a significant nail plate dystrophy as the dorsal part of nail plate produced by proximal matrix will cover the defect.

Partial Matrixectomy

Indication: Ingrown nail (onychocryptosis)

Tourniquet application: Techniques—

- Chemical
- Surgical
- Radiofrequency
- CO_2 laser vaporization.

Of above-mentioned methods, chemical matrixectomy is the most preferred, widely used and by far carries least chances of complications/recurrence.

The lateral most part of the nail plate is separated from the PNF, LNF and corresponding part of nailbed, using a nail elevator/dental spatula (2–3 mm width). Separation is extended under PNF till the proximal end of nail matrix. Complete hemostasis is a must as blood will get coagulated by the chemical and matrix will not get effectively destroyed. Chemical (88% phenol, 10% NaOH, 100% TCA) is taken on cotton-tipped applicator and applied in the lateral sulcus and pushed under the PNF **(Figs. 4 to 9)**.

Time of contact of chemical: 88% Phenol-3 minutes, 10% NaOH and 100% TCA-1 minute.

The tourniquet is removed and nonadherent gauze applied. This is covered by a bulky dressing kept for 2 days. Limb should be elevated for 1 day.

Complications: Uncommon

- Secondary infection
- Recurrence
- Nail spicule
- Periostitis (only in surgical approach, if accompanied by vigorous "deep" curettage).

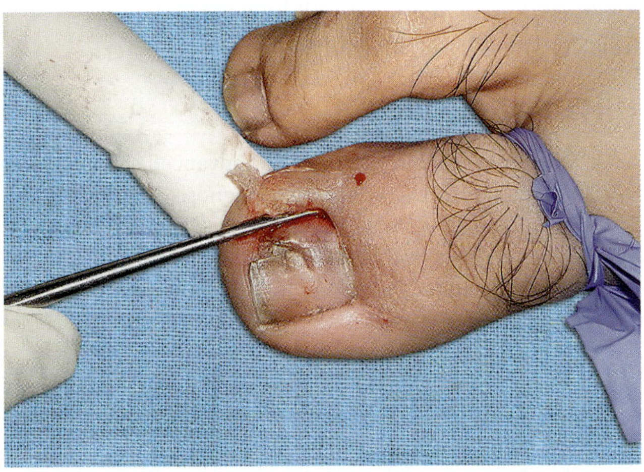

Fig. 4: Separation of LNF and nail plate using a nail elevator.

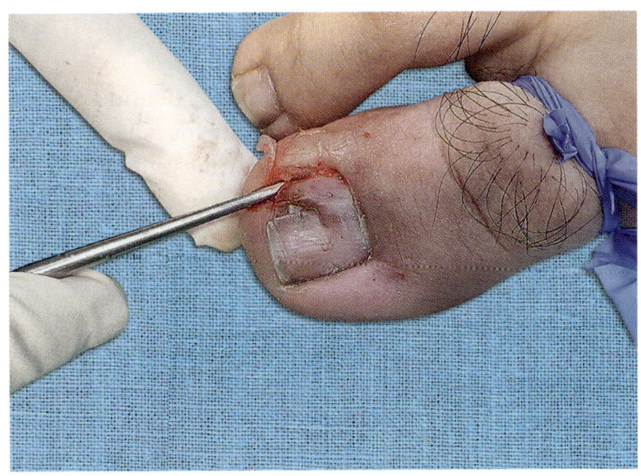

Fig. 5: Nailbed and nail plate separation using a nail elevator.

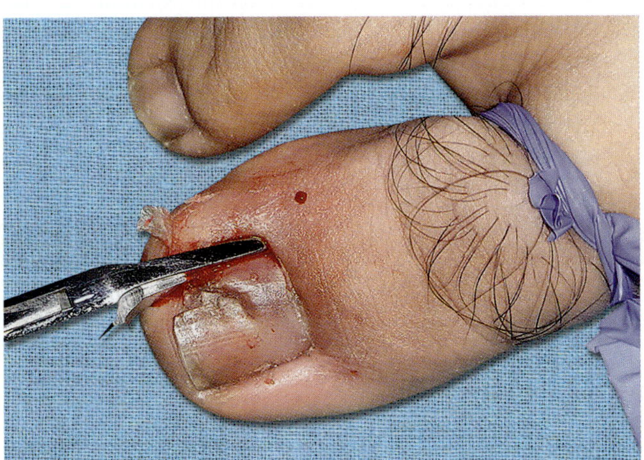

Fig. 6: Splitting the lateral part of nail plate using a nail splitter.

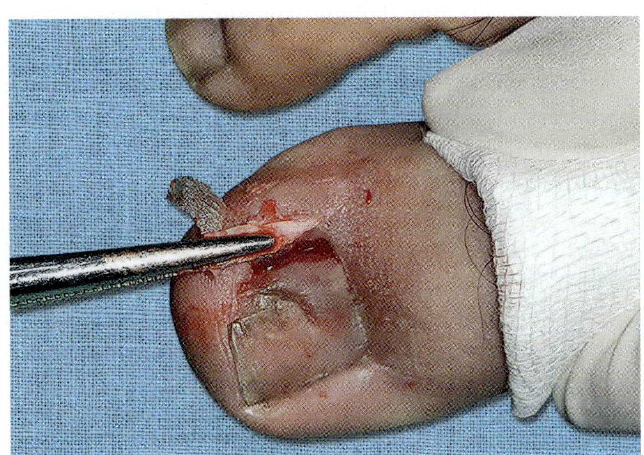

Fig. 7: Removal of the partially avulsed nail plate with an artery forceps.

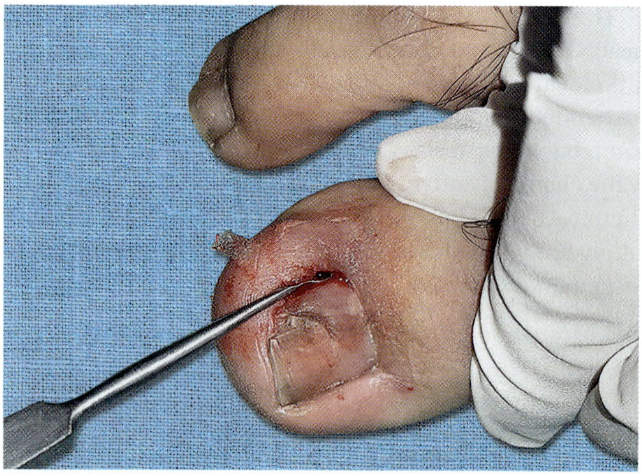

Fig. 8: Check curettage to look for remnants of nail plate.

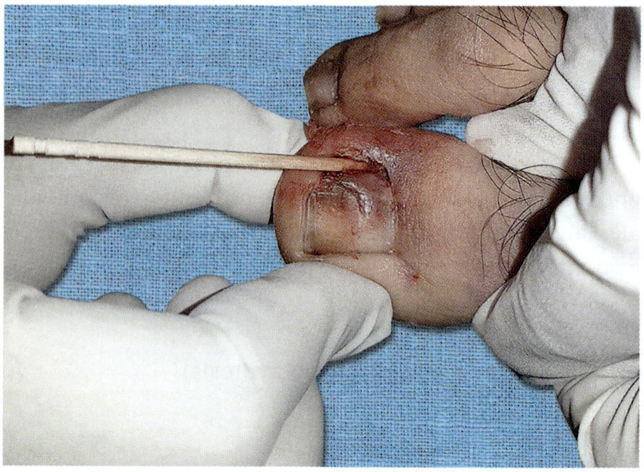

Fig. 9: Chemical matrixectomy with 88% phenol.

Total Matrixectomy

It will lead to permanent loss of nail plate.

Indications: Onychauxis, onychogryphosis, severe hereditary/acquired onychodystrophies, severe cases of pincer nails.

Techniques: Same as partial matrixectomy.

Incision and Reflection of PNF

An incision starting at the junction of PNF and LNF and extended proximally at an angle of 45° helps reflect the PNF and visualize underlying matrix as well as the ventral surface of PNF. Nail elevator must be inserted under the area to be incised to ensure prevention of accidental injury to underlying matrix.

KEY POINTS

- Nail surgeries are an integral part of dermatosurgery, though a lot needs to be done to integrate it in dermatology training.
- A thorough knowledge of anatomy, pathology and local anesthesia techniques is mandatory for practicing nail surgery.
- Proper sterilization, lighting, magnifying loupes, hemostasis as well as proper instruments are a prerequisite.
- Basic surgical procedures can be done as office procedures whereas a proper OT set-up is mandatory for advanced nail surgeries.
- Nail plate avulsion, biopsy of various components of nail unit, matrixectomy, and nail-fold surgery are the mainstay of nail unit surgery.
- Emphasis should be given to proper dressing of the operated nail unit, elevation of the limb, analgesia and counseling the patient about long lay over period before desired results can be achieved.

FURTHER READING

1. Abimelec P, Dumontier C. Basic and advanced nail surgery. In: Scher RK, Daniel CR (Eds). Nails: Diagnosis Therapy, Surgery, 3rd edition. Philadelphia: Saunders; 2005. pp. 265-306.
2. Dawber RP, Baran R, Berker D. Science of the nail: gross anatomy. In: Baran R, Dawber RP (Eds). Diseases of the Nails and their Management. Oxford, England: Blackwell Science; 1994. pp. 1-34.
3. Richert B, Chiacchio ND, Caucanas M (Eds). Management of Ingrowing Nails: Treatment Scenarios and Practical Tips. Switzerland: Springer; 2016.
4. Richert B. Surgery of the nail plate. In: Richert B, Chiacchio ND, Haneke E (Eds). Nail Surgery. London: Informa Healthcare. 2011.
5. Salasche SJ. Nail unit surgery. In: Robinson JK, Arndt KA, LeBoit PE, Wintroub BU (Eds). Atlas of Cutaneous Surgery, 1st edition. Philadelphia: Saunders; 1996. pp. 189-200.
6. Scher RK. The Nail. In: Roenigk RK, Roenigk HH, Ratz JL (Eds). Dermatologic surgery: principles and practice. New York: Marcel Dekker; 2006. pp. 281-8.

EXAMINATION QUESTIONS

1. Describe surgical management of ingrown nails.
2. Describe indications and different techniques of nail unit biopsy.
3. Write short note on nail biopsy.
4. Write short note on nail block.

167 CHAPTER

Acne Scar Surgery

R Raghunatha Reddy, Savitha AS, Shashi Kumar BM

INTRODUCTION

Acne is a common chronic inflammatory disorder affecting the pilosebaceous glands in about 80% adolescents and few adults. Acne scars are a common unfortunate sequence of acne which is preventable to some degree. Scarring occurs due to the severe inflammatory response and the degree of scarring depends on the depth and severity of inflammation, however, its incidence and severity varies from person to person due to various reasons. The severity of acne scars proportionally causes psychological distress to the patient. Acne scars can either be keloidal/hypertrophic with excess tissue or atrophic with loss of tissue. Atrophic scars are more common in acne.

CLASSIFICATION

Acne scars are classified to help in assessment of severity and to plan the treatment **(Flowchart 1)**.

Macular or pigmented scars: These are macules and actually not scars, early scars are erythematous, more common in sensitive skin, and rosacea prone skin. Hyperpigmented scars are common in darker skin patients and acne excoriee. Erythematous scars may evolve into hyperpigmented scars with time.

Atrophic Scars[1]

Ice pick scars: Severe inflammation causes complete destruction of the follicle. These scars are deep, narrow, and sharply defined epithelial tracts that extend vertically to the deep dermis or subcutaneous tissue. These types of scars occur more with comedonal acne. The surface opening is wider than the deeper portion as it tapers into a "V" shape. They are difficult to treat because of the depth and fibrosis **(Fig. 1)**.

Rolling scars: As the inflammation spreads to surrounding periadnexal areas, wide deep scars, tethering the dermis to underlying tissue occur. The overlying skin is relatively normal. The scar depth tends to change on stretching the scar. The therapeutic results are better compared to ice pick scars and boxcar scars due to their superficial nature and less fibrosis **(Fig. 2)**.

Boxcar scars: These are deep and punched out depressions with sharp vertical edges. They may be shallow (0.1–0.5 mm) or deep (>0.5 mm) and are most often 1.5–4.0 mm in diameter. Usually, their depth does not change on stretching the skin and they are resistant to treatment **(Fig. 3)**.

Elevated Scars

Papular scars: Skin colored, hypo- or hyperpigmented elevated scars occur due to destruction of elastic and collagen fibers in dermis around hair follicles, they commonly occur on back, chin, and nose **(Fig. 4)**.

Hypertrophic scars: These appear as firm, elevated nodular/plaque-type lesions more over the mandibular area, shoulders chest, and back **(Fig. 5)**.

Flowchart 1: Classification of acne scars.

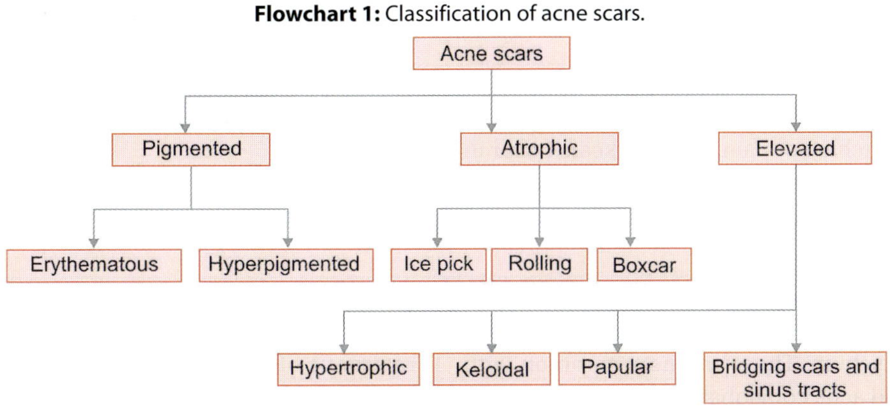

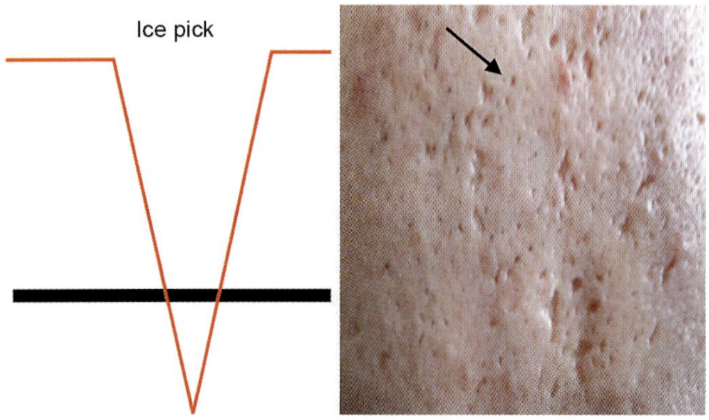

Fig. 1: Ice pick scars.

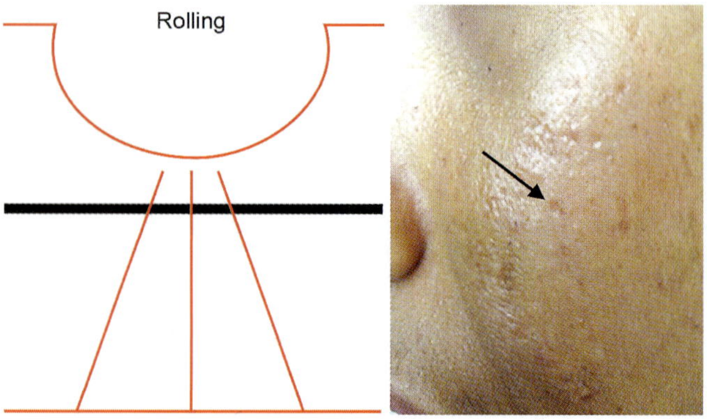

Fig. 2: Rolling scars.

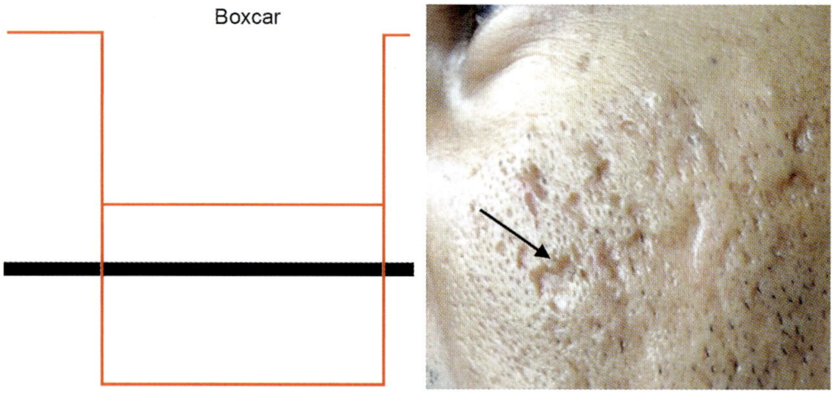

Fig. 3: Boxcar scars.

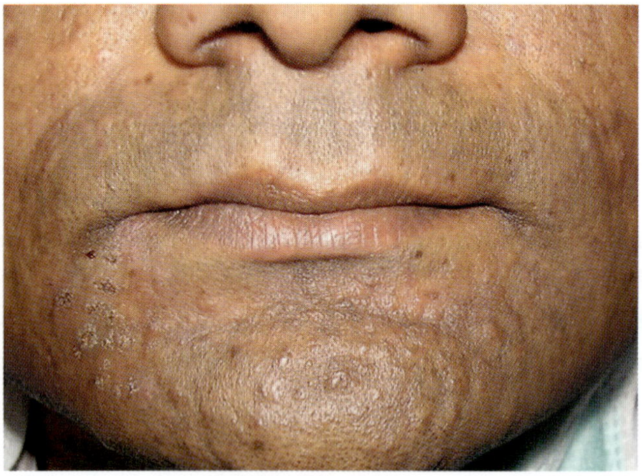

Fig. 4: Papular scars.

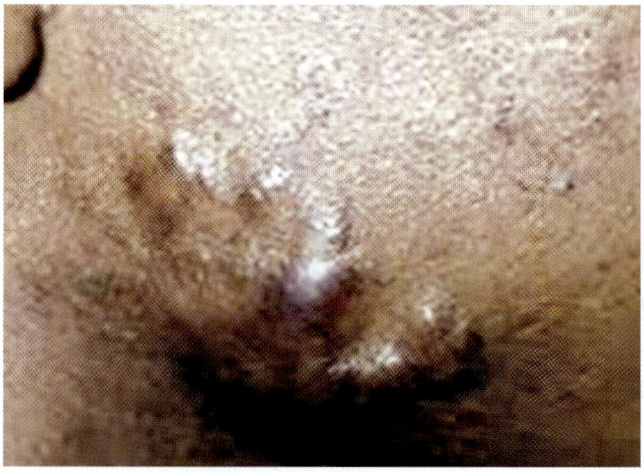

Fig. 5: Hypertrophic scars.

Keloidal scars: Keloids develop over acne lesions and may be symptomatic causing itching or pain. Keloidal scars occur in persons with genetic predisposition to keloids and with severe inflammatory type of acne, acne keloidalis is more common over the upper back.

Bridging scars and sinus tracts: These are multiple linear scars joined together by epithelial tracts containing foul-smelling products of sebum. These are more common with nodulocystic acne and acne conglobata **(Fig. 6)**.

QUALITATIVE GRADING

Goodman and Baron grading of acne scars is discussed in **Table 1**.[2]

Figure 7 summarizes the types of acne scars.

TREATMENT

Treatment of scars has to be individualized taking into consideration, type of scars, skin type, presence of active

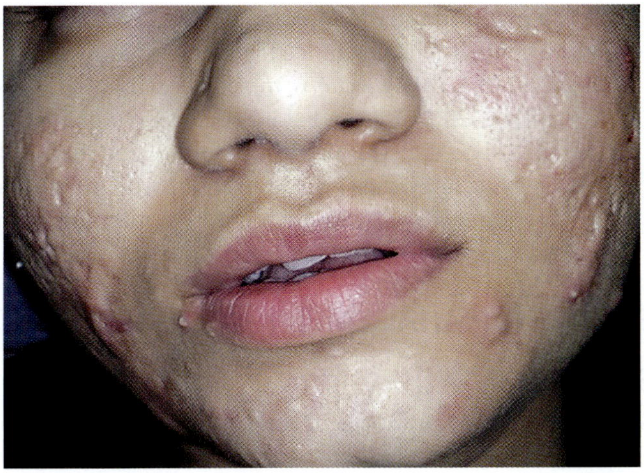

Fig. 6: Bridging scars.

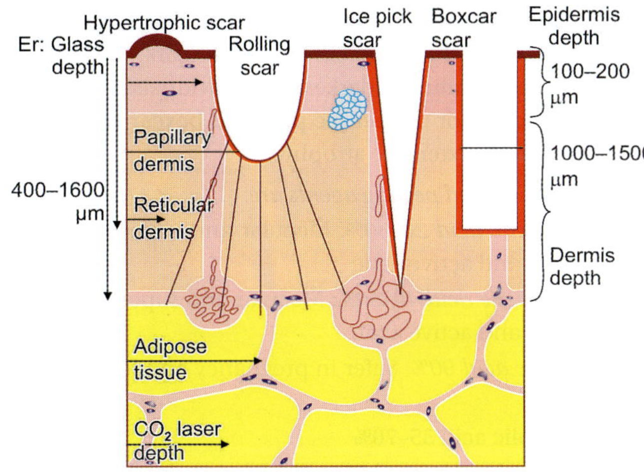

Fig. 7: *Acne scars:* Schematic representation of acne scars.[3]

TABLE 1: Goodman and Baron grading of acne scars.

Grade	*Level of disease*	*Characteristics*
1	Macular disease	Erythematous, hyper- or hypopigmented flat marks visible to patient or observer irrespective of distance
2	Mild disease	Mild atrophy or hypertrophy that may not be obvious at social distances of 50 cm or greater and may be covered adequately by makeup or the normal shadow of shaved beard hair in males or normal body hair if extrafacial
3	Moderate disease	Moderate atrophic or hypertrophic scarring that is obvious at social distances of 50 cm or greater and is not covered easily by make-up or the normal shadow of shaved beard hair but is still able to be flattened by manual stretching of the skin
4	Severe disease	Severe atrophic or hypertrophic scarring that is obvious at social distances of 50 cm or greater and is not covered easily by make-up or the normal shadow of shaved beard hair in males or body hair (if extrafacial) and is not able to be flattened by manual stretching of the skin

inflammation, and psychological morbidity. As multiple types of scars are commonly present in a patient, there is no single ideal procedure. A combination of different modalities and multiple treatments is necessary in any given patient. The golden rule of "A scar cannot be removed but can be modified and improved"—should be properly explained while counseling the patients before undertaking any treatment.

Patient assessment before the procedure should take into consideration the following points:

- Type, size, severity, and location of acne scars
- Skin type of patient
- General health assessment
- Psychological assessment to know the patient's expectations
- Presence of herpes simplex infections
- Tendency of the patients skin to heal with postinflammatory hyperpigmentation
- Presence of active acne
- Keloidal tendencies
- Counsel the patient regarding the types of procedures, downtime, risk of postinflammatory hyperpigmentation, sun protection, requirement for multiple sittings and what percentage of improvement can be expected.
- Detailed informed consent and photographic recording at each visit is essential.

Topical and Minimally Invasive Procedures

Though management of acne scar is mainly surgical, topical therapy has a role in mild scarring and as an adjuvant therapy.

- *Sunscreens:* Broad-spectrum noncomedogenic gel-based sunscreen helps to prevent postinflammatory hyperpigmentation after a procedure; they are also used during priming.
- *Skin priming and depigmenting agents: Topical agents like retinoic acid* 0.025–0.05% and glycolic acid 12% help to reduce fine scars with antiaging properties when applied for long term. It can also be used as a priming agent. Depigmenting agents such as topical hydroquinone, kojic acid, and azelaic acid in various concentrations help to reduce pigmentation and thus help in reducing the impact of appearance of scar.
- *Cryotherapy (cryopeeling)*: Cryoroller dipped in liquid nitrogen is rapidly rolled over the face for 2–4 seconds after cleaning the face with acetone. Erythema and light edema of the skin is seen which may last for 24 hours. The process has to be repeated every 2–3 weeks till a satisfactory response is seen.
- *Chemical peels*: Chemical peels are advised in erythematous hyperpigmented scars, acne excoriee, and

atrophic mild scars. Though medium depth and deep peels were used traditionally for acne scars, they have a risk of pigmentation in darker skin individuals. Superficial peels are not for deeper ice pick and boxcar scars or in patients with extensive atrophy.

Commonly used peeling agents are:

- *Salicylic acid 20–30%*: Macular and superficial acne scars and active acne
- *Mandelic acid 40–50%*: Macular and superficial acne scars and active acne
- *Lactic acid 90%:* Safer in pregnancy and for sensitive skin
- Glycolic acid 35–70%
- *Jessner's solution*: 14% salicylic, 14% lactic, and 14% citric acid
- Trichloroacetic acid (TCA) 15–35%

Priming the patient 2 weeks before the procedure and use of sunscreens and noncomedogenic moisturizers after the procedures are important. Chemical peels can be combined with other treatment such as subcision, microneedling, and lasers for additive effect.

- *CROSS technique:* Chemical reconstruction of skin scars (CROSS) is a technique where high concentrations (50–100%) of TCA are applied focally on the depth of the scars. This causes full thickness skin necrosis followed by re-epithelialization from adnexae as well as collagen remodeling. This method is best suited for ice pick scars **(Fig. 8)**.

Procedure: After cleansing the skin with acetone, the skin is stretched to reach the bottom of the scar and TCA is applied with sharpened tooth pick, applying pressure on the depressed area until frosting is seen. Avoid spillage of TCA to surrounding skin as it can cause hyperpigmentation. A crust forms after 2–3 days which may last up to 10 days. Patients are advised not to peel the scab. Strict sun protection is advised after the procedure. Procedure is repeated every 2–4 weeks, until four sittings **(Fig. 9)**.

Commonly encountered side effects are postinflammatory hypo- and hyperpigmentation, and 3–4 weeks of healing time, which is a major limitation in working class, otherwise the results are good, especially for ice pick scars.

- *Intralesional steroid injections:* Injections of triamcinolone acetonide 5–20% into the keloids or hypertrophic scars help to reduce the size of the scars and make them soft and flat and later they can be treated with fractional CO_2, microneedle radiofrequency (RF) or microneedling techniques.

SURGICAL MANAGEMENT

Subcision

Subcision is the workhorse of any surgical procedure for acne scars. Subcision (subcutaneous incision less surgery) is a process of elevation of depressed scars by breaking the vertically-oriented subcutaneous fibrous adhesions tethering the scars. This is the best procedure for rolling scars to release the scar and make them elevated.

Procedure: After surgically preparing the area, marking is done with the patient in sitting position. Lying down position alters the morphology of scars. Topical anesthesia is not an ideal choice since the procedure involves subcutaneous cutting of collagen fibers. Local anesthesia is infiltrated locally or as field block depending the number of scars to be treated in the area. For large areas, the procedure can be done under nerve blocks. Nokor needle or hypodermic needle size 18 or 22 is used. Nokor needle is the ideal choice to break the fibrous bands due to its shape and sturdy nature; however, the entry hole size will be slightly larger. After stretching and fixing the skin, the needle is inserted 1 or 2 mm away from the edge of the scar with the bevel pointing upward. Then, it is moved back and forth and also in fanning motion to break all adhesions (grating sound is heard due to breakage of adhesions) beneath the scar keeping the needle parallel to the skin surface. Multiple entry points can be used to cover entire area. Firm pressure is applied for 10–15 minutes immediately after subcision to prevent large hematoma **(Figs. 10 to 12)**.

The danger areas are the temporal and preauricular areas as the branches of the facial nerve are superficial and can be injured and one should be cautious in those areas.

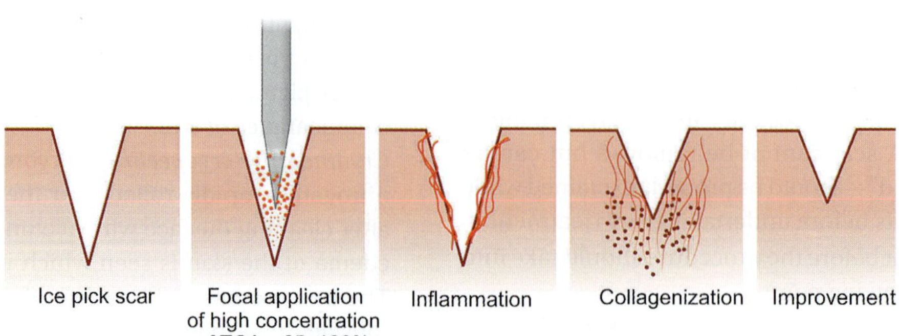

Fig. 8: TCA CROSS mechanism of action.
(CROSS: chemical reconstruction of skin scars; TCA: trichloroacetic acid)

Postprocedure

Topical antibiotics and sun protection to be advised. Patients notice immediate improvement due to edema. Procedure may be repeated every 4–6 weeks until optimum response is seen.

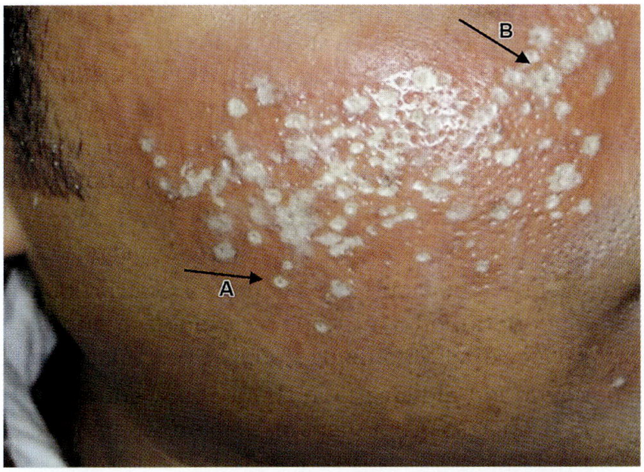

Fig. 9: A: Frosting after application of trichloroacetic acid (TCA); B: Avoid spillage to surrounding areas.

Complications

Bruising and swelling, which resolves in 1–2 weeks. Hematoma formation, if large will have to be evacuated, hematoma will resolve in 4–6 weeks' time.

Subcision can be combined with other procedures such as CROSS, punch excision, lasers, fat fillers, and dermal grafts in the same sitting or different sitting.

Punch Excision Techniques

Punch excision is indicated for large depressed scars with abnormal surface texture. They are best suited for punched out scars with sharp adherent walls that cannot be treated by resurfacing procedures.

Procedure: Each scar has to be assessed individually. Subcision can be done on preceding days or on same sitting. Procedure is done under local infiltration anesthesia. Scars have to be marked before the procedure, and with appropriate size of the

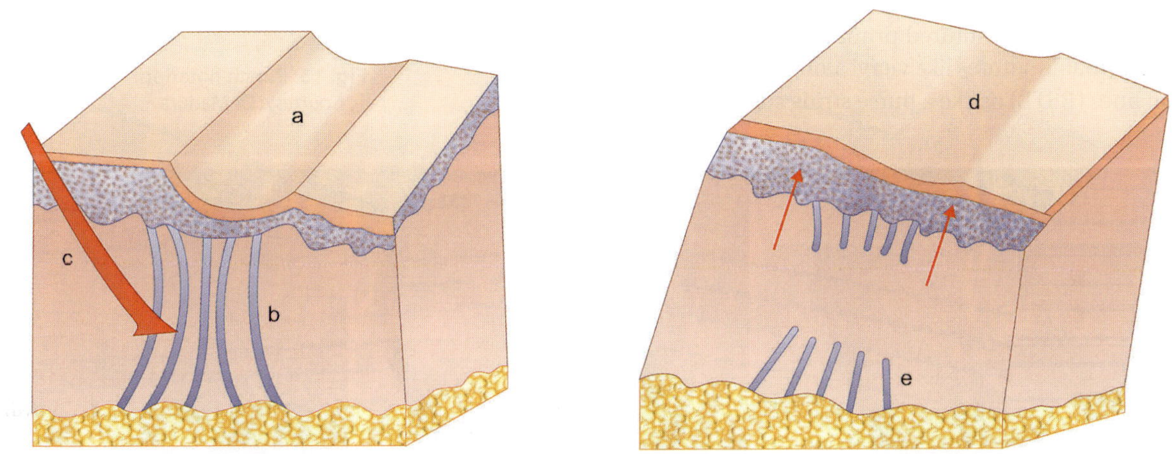

Fig. 10: Schematic representation of subcision: a—Depressed scar, b—Strands of scar, c—Needle used for subcision, d—Elevated scar following release of fibrotic strands, e—Fibrotic strands after release.

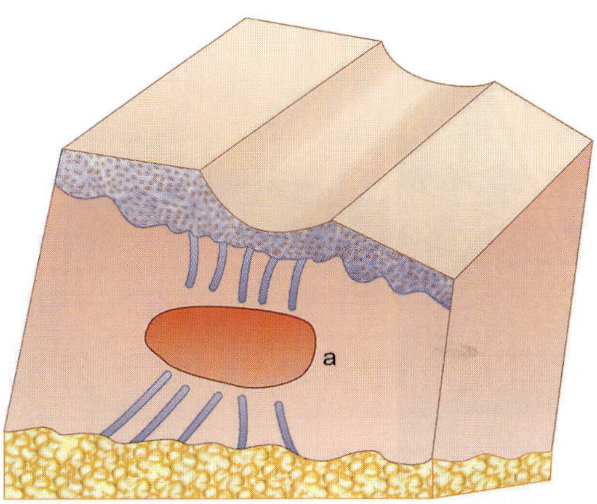

Fig. 11: Schematic representation of hematoma formation (a—Depressed scar).

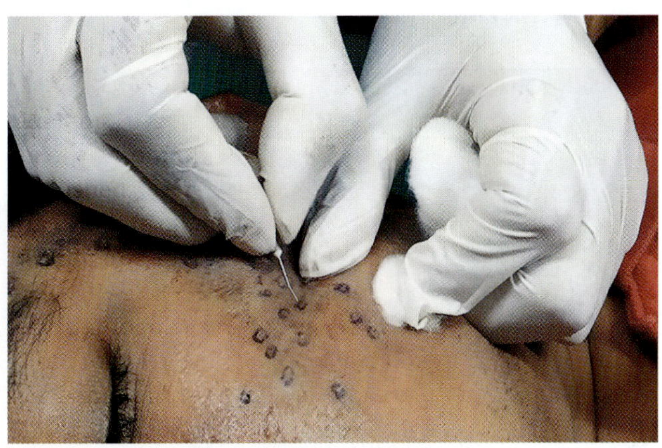

Fig. 12: Marking the scars prior to anesthesia, using a bent needle for adequate depth.

punches, the scar should be punched out up to the depth of subcutis and excised. The defect may be closed with suturing or may be replaced with full thickness skin graft harvested from postauricular nonhair-bearing area.

Punch Incision and Elevation or Flotation

- This is best suited for depressed scars 2–4 mm in diameter, with normal surface texture.
- After choosing the appropriate size punch which fits the scar, the punch is advanced till the subcutaneous tissue. The punch is then raised to the surface without cutting the base with fine forceps or needle. Skin plug is held for 1–2 minutes for fixation **(Fig. 13)**.
- Subcision done 4–4 weeks before this procedure will be a great advantage for better results.
- About 70–80% improvement is expected since mild depression can result from ensuing fibrosis.
- Advantages are that it is a quick procedure with excellent color matching.
- Complications are ring scar, partial improvement.

Punch Excision

- If there are very few scars or scars which are >4 mm, they can be excised and defect sutured primarily with 6-0 prolene or 6-0 absorbable sutures like vicryl along the relaxed skin tension lines (RSTL) or like a purse string suture.
- This procedure cannot be performed if scars are very close to each other **(Figs. 14A to C)**.

Punch Excision and Graft Placement

- If the surface of the scars is atrophic and >4–5 mm, then such scars can be excised and replaced with punch grafts taken from postauricular area.
- The graft should be flush with the epidermis and fit snugly **(Figs. 15A to C)**.

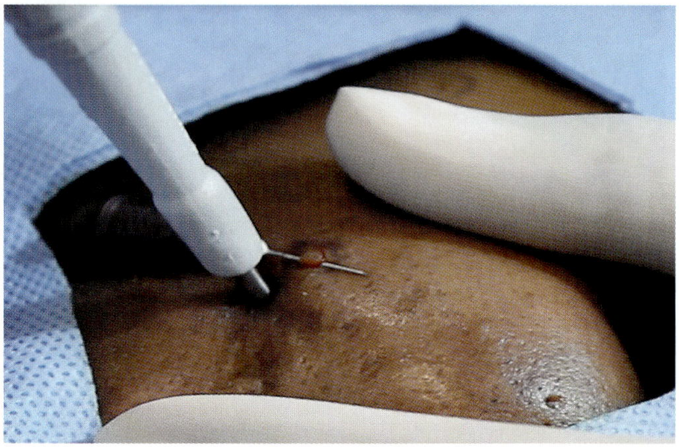

Fig. 13: Punch flotation.
Courtesy: Dr Madura

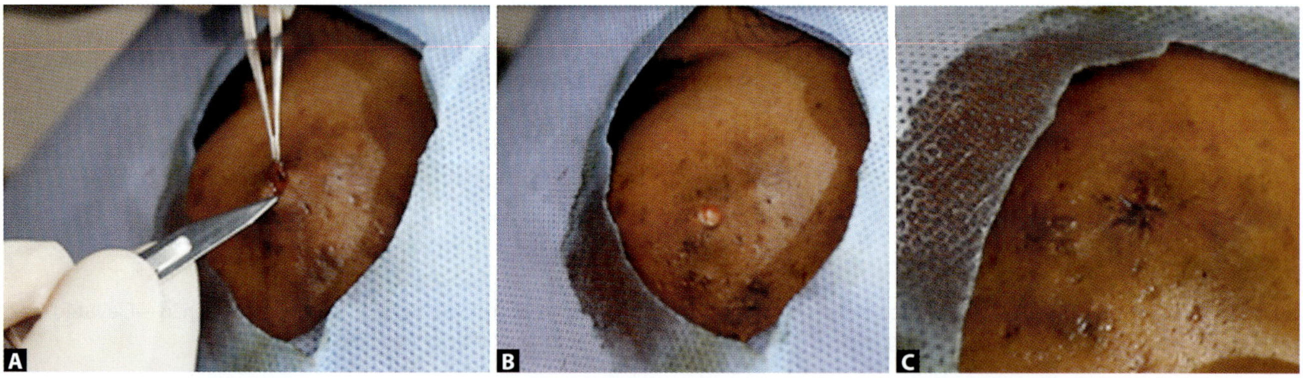

Figs. 14A to C: Punch excision and closure.

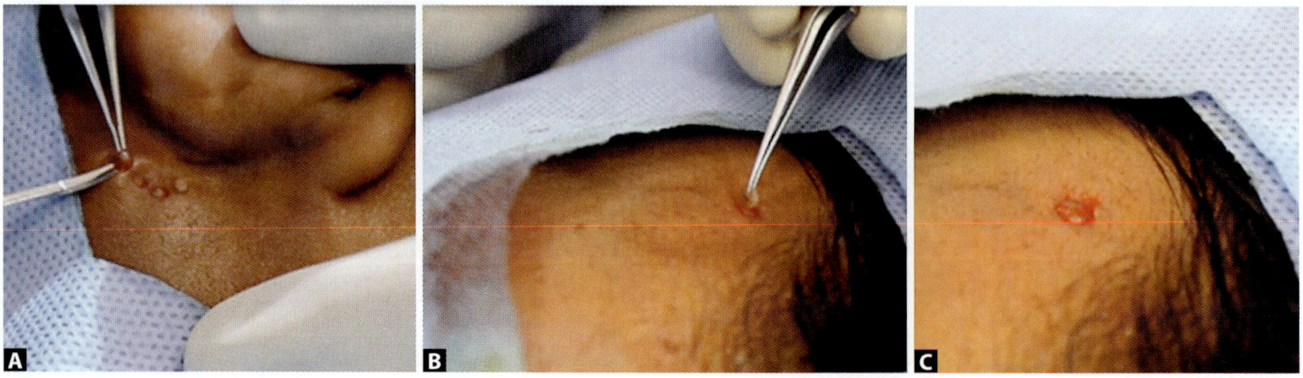

Figs. 15A to C: Graft taken from postauricular area and placed in the excised scar area.
Courtesy: Dr Madura

- Complications are color mismatch, cobblestoning, and scarring in the donor area.

Microneedling

Microneedling is simple office-based procedure suited for rolling scars and shallow box scars. The dermaroller contains a plastic handle with a drum-shaped cylindrical instrument at its end, tiny stainless steel needles are placed over the cylinder. The length of the needles varies from 0.5 to 2 mm. 1.5 mm is the commonly used needle size. Rolling the instrument with tiny needles creates multiple superficial puncture wounds in the skin. This stimulates production of collagen and elastin, improving the texture of the skin. The procedure is performed under topical anesthesia. After preparing the area, the skin is stretched with nondominant hand and the instrument is rolled back and forth 6–8 times in four directions till fine pinpoint bleeding spots are seen. The depth of penetration depends on the pressure applied. Rolling is repeated every 4–6 weeks. It may be combined with procedures such as subcision, topical vitamin C application, and fractional laser ablation.

Dermabrasion[4]

Dermabrasion is a skin resurfacing technique that involves mechanically removing the epidermis and papillary dermis to create new wound which heals by secondary intention. Re-epithelialization of dermabraded skin occurs by upward migration of cells from the adnexal structures including hair follicles, sebaceous glands, and sweat ducts. Dermabrasion can be done either manually or motorized, using a rapidly rotating wire brush or diamond fraise. With the advent of fractional lasers, the utility of dermabrasion has reduced considerably. Though the lasers cause lesser erythema and faster re-epithelialization, their efficacies in treating scars hardly match dermabrasion. The disadvantage of dermabrasion is that it is operator dependent and has a long learning curve. While resurfacing, if there is accidental injury to the reticular dermis, it results in additional scarring. Full-face dermabrasion requires oral or intramuscular sedation in conjunction with the use of cryoanesthesia, local, or tumescent anesthesia, and nerve blocks. Dermabrasion is done till fine red papillary bleeding dots are seen. After dermabrasion, the application of gauze soaked in 1% lidocaine with epinephrine (1:100,000) under prechilled ice packs helps to achieve hemostasis and soothes postoperative stinging. The abraded area is covered with semipermeable dressing to enhance re-epithelialization. Infections, acne flares and milia are potential complications after the procedure. Postprocedure hyperpigmentation is common in Fitzpatrick skin types 5 and 6. Patients are advised strict sun protection for 6 weeks postprocedure.

Lasers and Lights

Fractional CO_2, fractional Er:YAG lasers and microneedling radiofrequency techniques are most effective for atrophic acne scars. They can be combined with procedures such as subcision and CROSS for better results. The fractional device delivers light in microscopic columns sparing normal skin in between, producing an array of microthermal treatment zones (MTZs). This creates small microscopic columns of thermal damage in the epidermis and dermis up to a depth of 300–400 µg in regularly space arrays over a fraction of the skin surface. This is in contrast to ablative resurfacing where the entire epidermis and part of the dermis is removed. Since a major portion of intervening skin is left unaffected, healing occurs quickly, thereby reducing the downtime. At each subsequent session, such fractions are treated and over 3–6 sittings with an interval of 4 weeks between sessions, treatment is completed. For deeper scars, subcision done prior to use of LASERS is always an advantage for better results **(Table 2)**.

TABLE 2: Lasers for acne scars.[5]

Laser, light device and wavelength	*Chromophore and mode of action*	*Clinical application*
CO_2 laser 10600 nm ablative and fractional CO_2	Water, nonselective tissue ablation, thermal damage and collagen shrinkage	Grade 4 atrophic and hypertrophic scars
Er:YAG 2940 nm ablative and fractional Er:YAG	Water, nonselective ablation, minimal thermal damage	Grade 2–3 atrophic and hypertrophic scars
Er: Glass 1540/1550 nm nonablative fractional	Water, nonablative, columns of thermal damage in dermis	Grade 1–2 atrophic and hypertrophic acne scars
1320/1440 nm nonablative fractional	Water, nonablative, columns of thermal damage in dermis	Grade 1–2 atrophic and hypertrophic acne scars
Pulse dye laser 585 nm	Selective photothermolysis; oxyhemoglobin	Hypertrophic scars and keloids
IPL	Selective photothermolysis; hemoglobin, melanin	Hypertrophic scars, erythematous and hyperpigmented macular scars
Nd:YAG 1064 nm	Hemoglobin, water	Grade 1 atrophic scars
Diode 1450 nm	Water	Grade 1 atrophic scars

(IPL: intense pulsed light; Nd:YAG: neodymium-doped yttrium aluminum garnet)

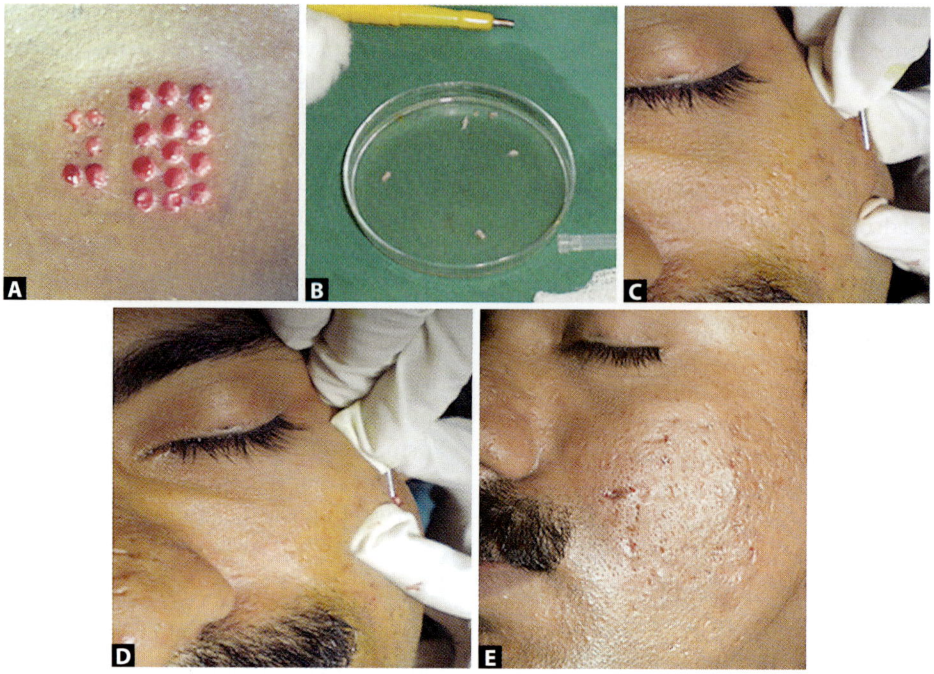

Figs. 16A to E: (A) Dermis is punched out; (B) Graft in petri dish; (C) Subcision to create a pocket; (D) Placing the dermal graft; and (E) After surgery.

Fillers

The principle of scar correction using fillers is to elevate the depressed scar to level of surrounding skin. Space is created underneath the scar by subcision and the filler is placed in the pocket. Hyaluronic acid (HA), dermis and fat, has been used as fillers to raise the acne scars.

Hyaluronic acid: It is a highly hydrophilic, natural, linear polysaccharide component of connective tissue in all mammals and is not tissue or species specific. It displays isovolemic degradation in which molecules of HA degrades allowing those remaining to absorb more water. The duration of effect for acne scars is roughly a year or more. Fillers are ideal for larger and deeper scars, but are more expensive and need to be done repeatedly.

Autologous fat: Autologous fat is obtained by liposuction from the patient's abdomen, thigh, or gluteal area. It is advisable to do overcorrection, as a percentage of matter is nonviable. The reabsorption rate varies by location, amount injected, technique, and other factors. Variable reports of 6–18 months' duration may be seen.

Dermal grafts: Dermal grafts act as natural fillers. It is best suited for larger, depressed scars >3 mm, linear scars (soft and distensible), and scars with normal skin without sharp walls.

The epidermis behind the ear is dermabraded and dermis is punched out, or the skin is punched and the epidermis is cut to harvest the dermis. The dermis can be treated with trypsin and antitrypsin to make the dermis soft and malleable to enable easy insertion and deposition in the subcutaneous plane underneath the scar. Subcision is done beneath the scars creating a pocket to receive the dermal graft and the grafts are inserted into subcutaneous pocket with a blunt needle or with cannulas. All aseptic precautions to be followed and postsurgical care to be given importance to avoid infection. Dermal grafts have a longer longevity and most ideal graft since it is the most natural replacement of the damaged tissue compared to other material used **(Figs. 16A to E)**.

KEY POINTS

- Treating the acne optimally and continually to prevent scar formation is very important, procedures such as comedone extraction, intralesional triamcinolone acetonide in low concentrations 5-10 mg/mL, concentration will help prevent or minimize scar formation.
- All patients must be counseled properly with clear explanation of procedure, number of sittings required, and the possible outcome.
- It should be emphasized clearly to all patients the golden rule, "once a scar—it cannot be completely removed or brought to complete normalcy." However, it can be improved with different procedures selected suitable to the type of scars and the procedure repeated multiple sittings.
- Any given patient will usually have different types of scars—so a combination of different procedures is a rule in any given patient. A single procedure is not an ideal option.
- Combination of different techniques such as topical applications, chemical peels, spot peels, surgical

procedures, and fractioned lasers if combined judiciously as per the patient's needs is the ideal method.

REFERENCES

1. Jacob CI, Dover JS, Kaminer MS. Acne scarring: a classification system and review of treatment options. J Am Acad Dermatol. 2001;45(1):109-17.
2. Goodman GJ, Baron JA. Postacne scarring: a qualitative global scarring grading system. Dermatol Surg. 2006;32(12):1458-66.
3. Khunger M, Khunger N. Pathophysiology of acne scars. In: Khunger N (Ed). Step by Step® Treatment of Acne Scars. New Delhi: Jaypee Brothers Medical Publishers; 2014. pp. 1-16.
4. Harmon CB, Thiel JJ. Dermabrasion for acne scars. In: Tosti A, De Padova MP, Beer KR (Eds). Acne Scars. Classification and Treatment. UK: Informa HEALTH CARE; 2010. pp. 42-9.
5. Aurangabadkar S. Lasers and light devices. In: Khunger N (Ed). Step by Step® Treatment of Acne Scars. New Delhi: Jaypee Brothers Medical Publishers; 2014. p. 130.

EXAMINATION QUESTIONS

1. Explain classification and management of acne scars.
2. Write briefly on dermal graft technique for acne scars.

168 CHAPTER Mohs Micrographic Surgery

Marisa Pongprutthipan

INTRODUCTION

Nonmelanoma skin cancers especially basal cell carcinoma (BCC) and squamous cell carcinoma (SCC) are the most common skin cancers worldwide. The treatments include topical imiquimod, topical and intralesional 5-fluorouracil, photodynamic therapy, surgical removal, and nonsurgical procedural treatments, i.e., electrosurgery with curettage, cryotherapy, and radiation. Treatment guidelines differ among countries. The common approach is the classification of low- versus high-risk tumor and the staging of the tumor invasion. The commonly used treatment guidelines include National Comprehensive Cancer Network (NCCN) guideline, British Association of Dermatologists (BAD) guideline[1] and American Academy of Dermatology guidelines.[2] The selection of treatment depends on the risk classification and availability of each practice-based country.

Treatment decision making is important since patient expectation of total removal of the skin cancer is high and the final wound appearance after the surgery is also high concern especially when tumor is located in the visible area, especially on the face.

Mohs micrographic surgery (MMS) is a staged excision with total margin visualization under microscopic frozen section in each stage, until complete control of tumor extension. It could be used for many skin cancers and some benign neoplasms that well demonstrate by frozen section technique. It is performed in outpatient setting by a physician specially trained in cutaneous surgery and pathology. The residual extensions of the tumor margins are mapped and selectively removal. This allows preservation of surrounding healthy tissue and thus smaller defects. MMS has highest cure rates when compared with conventional procedure, especially the high risk and recurrent skin cancers. For recurrent BCC, the 5-year recurrent rate is 2.4% for MMS, compared with 12.1% for standard excision and 10-year recurrent rate is 3.9% for MMS, compared with 13.5% for standard excision.[3]

HISTORY

In 1930s, Frederic E. Mohs developed a technique of mapping and excisional surgery in which chemical fixation in situ before excision, so called "chemosurgery", to maintain cytological detail for microscopic margin evaluation of the excised specimen. The precision of tumor margin removal is achieved and significant higher cure rates.[2] Later, the chemical fixation is replaced by frozen section processing which provide more rapid tissue fixation and ready for the next stage of excision within a few hours.[4]

INDICATIONS

The common indications of MMS are shown in **Box 1**.

BOX 1: Indications for Mohs micrographic surgery.

Types of skin cancers:
- *Nonmelanoma skin cancers (NMSCs):* Basal cell carcinoma (BCC) and squamous cell carcinoma (SCC)
  - Recurrent skin cancers
  - Positive margin after primary excision
  - Poorly defined clinical margin
  - At high risk for local recurrence and/or metastasis, sclerosing (morpheaform), infiltrative, micronodular, metatypical subtypes of BCC
  - Perineural BCC or SCC
- Malignant melanoma (MM)
- Merkel cell carcinoma
- Dermatofibrosarcoma protuberans
- Atypical fibroxanthoma
- Malignant fibrous histiocytoma
- Microcystic adnexal carcinoma
- Sebaceous carcinoma
- Extramammary Paget's disease (EMPD)

*In an area where tissue conservation is important demonstrate in red (Area H)(**Fig. 1**)*

Area H (high-risk area, demonstrate in red): "Mask areas" of face [central face, eyelids (including inner/outer canthi), eyebrows, nose, lips (cutaneous/mucosal/vermillion), chin, ear, and periauricular skin/sulci, temple]; genitalia (including perineal and perianal), hands, feet, nail units, ankles, and nipples/areola.

Less indications on the following area:
- *Area M (intermediate-risk area, demonstrate in yellow):* Cheeks, forehead, scalp, neck, jawline, and pretibial surface
- *Area L (low-risk area):* Trunk and extremities (excluding pretibial surface, hands, feet, nail units, and ankles)

The other conditions that consider risk factors for recurrence include:
- *Immunocompromised:* Patient with human immunodeficiency virus (HIV), organ transplant, hematologic malignancy, or pharmacologic immunosuppression
- *Genetic syndromes:* Basal cell nevus syndrome, xeroderma pigmentosum, or other syndromes at high risk for skin cancer
- *Prior radiated skin:* Patient has previously received therapeutic radiation in this area of the body

PREOPERATIVE EVALUATION

A thorough history of medical conditions, previous skin condition, allergies, and physical examination should be performed at the time of consultation. The pathology should be reviewed and confirmed. Indications of prophylactic antibiotics should be evaluated. Prophylactic antibiotics may be considered when the surgical area involves lip, nose, and nasal cavity. Patient with implanted cardiac pacemaker or defibrillator should be evaluated by cardiologist. For the patient, who take "blood thinners", aspirin, novel anticoagulants, clopidogrel, and warfarin, the risk of surgery should be discussed but usually there is no need to stop the medication. Plan for closure should be well prepared and discussed with the patient.

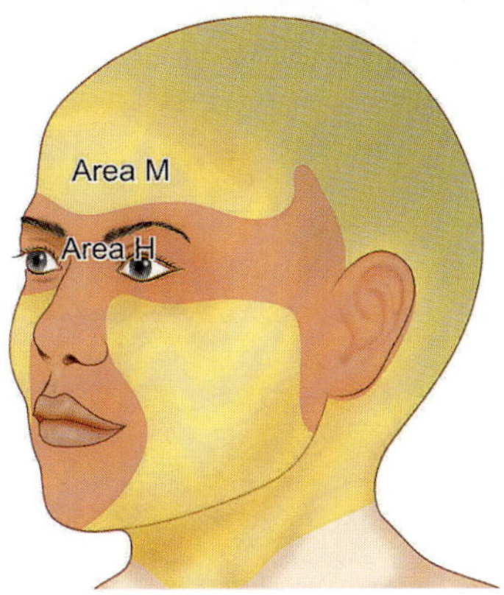

Fig. 1: Anatomic risk areas of the head and neck.

OPERATIVE TECHNIQUE

The consultation between doctor and patient should be done before the procedure since this procedure is a repeated surgical procedure and take hours in the outpatient office. The contraindication is the patient who cannot receive local anesthesia and who cannot tolerate surgery.

The fundamental of MMS is the microscopic mapping of tumor margin. The visible tumor is usually removed by shave excision or curettage to provide better demonstration of true margin. Then peripheral tumor margins are mapped by score marks on the surrounding tissue and across the specimen to serve as markers for subsequent stages. The required tissue margin for each skin cancer is different. For BCC, 1–3 mm tissue margin and for SCC, 2–4 mm tissue margin,[4] tissue is removed in the first stage. For MM, at least 5–10 mm tissue margin for thin lesion (≤1 mm in depth) and 10–20 mm tissue margin in thicker lesion (1–2 mm in depth) is removed for the first stage.[5] The excision with a beveled 45° angle technique is advised for processing horizontal section **(Figs. 2A to E)**. Colored staining with indelible ink of each tissue margin is recommended to assure mapping information under microscopic examination. The tissue is frozen, mounted, and serial sectioned by the technician. The *en face* section is

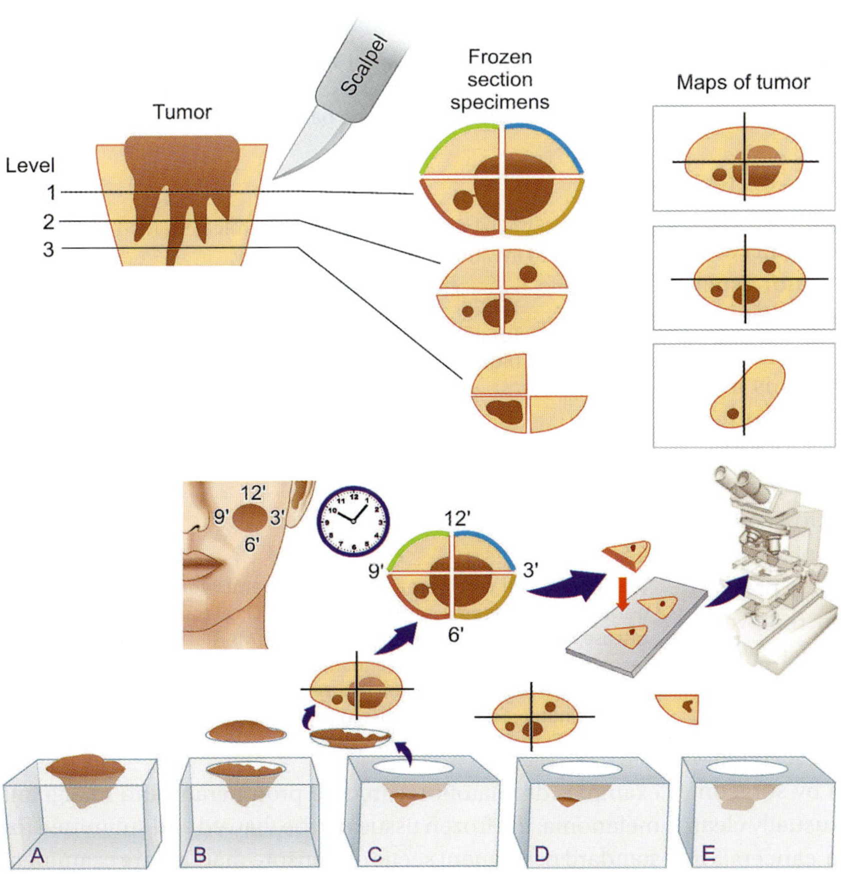

Figs. 2A to E: Mohs micrographic surgery procedure. (A and B) Tumor is identified and removal by shave excision, blade excision, or curettage; (C) Mapping anatomical location and 1–2 mm tissue margin specimen is removed for microscopic examination; (D) Residual tumor is identified under microscopic examination and mapping with the anatomical location; and (E) Further removal of residual tumor in the next stage is done and repeated the microscopic examination until margin is clear.

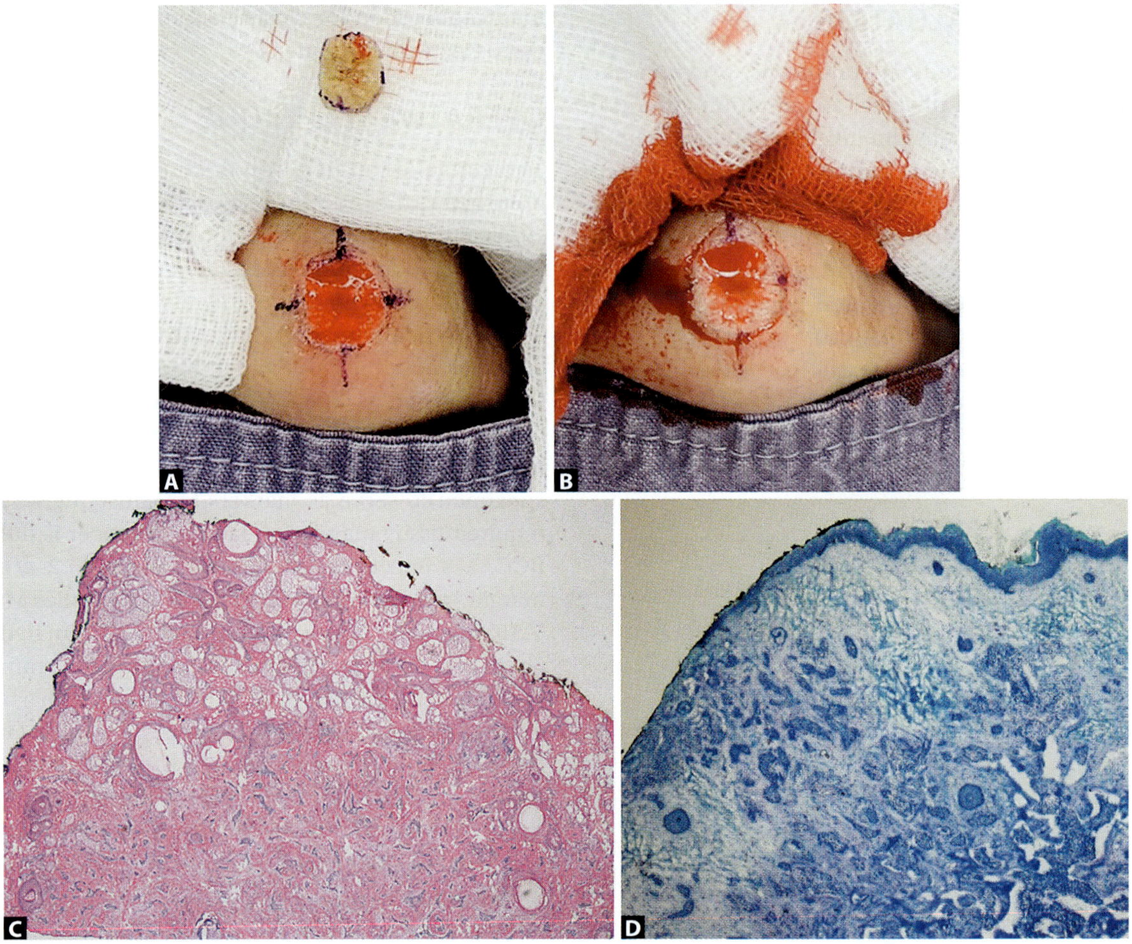

Figs. 3A to D: (A) Basal cell carcinoma is clinically identified and removed by shave excision; (B) Peripheral and deep is taken for frozen section; (C) Hematoxylin and eosin (H&E) stain in horizontal section demonstrate islands of basal cell carcinoma and its lateral tumor margin. The deeper section will demonstrate the deep margin; and (D) Special quick stain using methylene blue demonstrate basal cell carcinoma, micronodular type, at the margin of resected tissue.

prepared to represent deep and peripheral margin tissues. The slides are stained by hematoxylin and eosin, unless otherwise other special stain recommended for each tumor types **(Figs. 3A to D)**. Currently, MMS using immunohistochemical stains for MM is more commonly use, melanoma antigen recognized by T cells (MART-1) on frozen section is used for melanoma in situ and superficially invasive MM (<1 mm Breslow depth). Other special and immunohistochemical stains in frozen section are shown in **Table 1**. Microscopic examination with anatomical mapping is done to carefully identify residual tumor, failure of mapping is one of the main causes of recurrence after MMS. If residual tumor is present, the positive tissue margin is marked and further removal is performed in the next stage. The process is repeated until tumor is clear from surrounding tissue. The awareness of inflammatory cells infiltration that possible obscures the tumor is mentioned in the studies.[7] The surgical repair or secondary intention is managed with appropriate decision by surgeon. Most of the BCC and SCC that treated with MMS usually clear after two stages. In selected cases of some skin cancers for examples dermatofibrosarcoma protuberans and malignant melanoma, the frozen tissue can be thawed and submitted for standard permanent section to ensure margins are examined.

TABLE 1: Special and immunohistochemical stains for specific tumors used in Mohs micrographic surgery.

Tumors	*Special stains*	*Immunohistochemical stains*
BCC	Toluidine blue	AE1/AE3, Ber-EP4
SCC	–	AE1/AE3
MM	–	MiTF, MART-1, Mel-5, S-100, SOX10, HMB45[8]
DFSP	–	CD34
EMPD	PAS	CK7, CEA

(BCC: basal cell carcinoma; CEA: carcinoembryonic antigen; DFSP: dermatofibrosarcoma protuberans; EMPD: extramammary Paget's disease; HMB45: human melanoma black-45; MART-1: melanoma antigen recognized by T-cells; MM: malignant melanoma; MiTF: microphthalmia-associated transcription factor; PAS: periodic acid–Schiff; SCC: squamous cell carcinoma; SOX10: Sry-related HMG-Box gene 10)

POSTOPERATIVE MANAGEMENT

Standard wound care is applied. Postoperative antibiotics may be required in cases that have large defect and in the anatomical area that have higher risk of infection such as nose, lip, ear, inguinal area, and axilla. The suture removal date is assigned by anatomical location of surgical wound. In the facial area, suture removal could be done on day 5th–10th after surgery, depends on the tension of the wound edge and to prevent wound dehiscence. While the lesion on the lower extremities and back could be delayed up to 14 days after surgery. Since the patient has a history of skin cancer, skin cancer screening should be performed regularly at least once a year.

COMPLICATIONS

Mohs micrographic surgery is known as a safe surgical procedure with low complication. The risk of infection is similar to clean wound surgery; prophylactic antibiotic is usually does not required.[8] Over 95% of patients were deemed to have good or excellent functional and esthetic outcomes in the British study.[9] The most common reported complication of MMS is surgical wound infection,[8] less common is hematoma, wound dehiscence, scarring, decrease in function, and recurrence.[10]

In the future, the increasing of noninvasive imaging, immunostaining, and digital technology accompanying with MMS technique will provide more precision excision and best outcome for the patients.

KEY POINTS

- Mohs micrographic surgery provides the highest cure rate and tissue sparing.
- To complete microscopic margin control, the frozen histologic sections of the excised tumor are examined to determine the clearance of the skin cancers at the margin.
- Mohs surgery is commonly indicated for nonmelanoma skin cancers, especially BCC and SCC.
- The advantages of MMS are the highest cure rate for high risk of recurrent or rapidly progressive tumors and for tumors in anatomical areas where tissue sparing is critical.
- Mohs surgery requires a training in the surgery and pathology field to accurately excise, map tumor extensions for pathology, and reconstruction.

REFERENCES

1. Telfer NR, Colver GB, Morton CA. Guidelines for the management of basal cell carcinoma. Br J Dermatol. 2008; 159(1):35-48.
2. American Academy of Dermatology; American College of Mohs Surgery; American Society for Dermatologic Surgery Association; American Society for Mohs Surgery; Ad Hoc Task Force, Connolly SM, et al. AAD/ACMS/ASDSA/ASMS 2012 appropriate use criteria for Mohs micrographic surgery: a report of the American Academy of Dermatology, American College of Mohs Surgery, American Society for Dermatologic Surgery Association, and the American Society for Mohs Surgery. Dermatol Surg. 2012;38(10):1582-603.
3. Murray C, Sivajohanathan D, Hanna TP, Bradshaw S, Solish N, Moran B, et al. Patient indications for Mohs micrographic surgery: a systematic review. J Cutan Med Surg. 2019;23(1): 75-90.
4. Schell AE, Russell MA, Park SS. Suggested excisional margins for cutaneous malignant lesions based on Mohs micrographic surgery. JAMA Facial Plast Surg. 2013;15(5):337-43.
5. Hui AM, Jacobson M, Markowitz O, Brooks NA, Siegel DM. Mohs micrographic surgery for the treatment of melanoma. Dermatol Clin. 2012;30(3):503-15.
6. Alam M, Khan M, Veledar E, Pongprutthipan M, Flores A, Dubina M, et al. Correlation of inflammation in frozen sections with site of nonmelanoma skin cancer. JAMA Dermatol. 2016;152(2):173-6.
7. Beaulieu D, Fathi R, Srivastava D, Nijhawan RI. Current perspectives on Mohs micrographic surgery for melanoma. Clin Cosmet Investig Dermatol. 2018;11:309-20.
8. Levin EC, Chow C, Makhzoumi Z, Jin C, Shiboski SC, Arron ST. Association of postoperative antibiotics with surgical site infection in mohs micrographic surgery. Dermatol Surg. 2019;45(1):52-7.
9. Hussain W, Affleck A, Al-Niaimi F, Cooper A, Craythorne E, Fleming C, et al. Safety, complications and patients' acceptance of Mohs micrographic surgery under local anaesthesia: results from the U.K. MAPS (Mohs Acceptance and Patient Safety) Collaboration Group. Br J Dermatol. 2017;176(3): 806-8.
10. Etzkorn JR, Gharavi NM, Carr DR, Tope WD, Bordeaux JS, Maher IA. Examining the relevance to patients of complications in the American College of Mohs Surgery Registry: results of a Delphi Consensus Process. Dermatol Surg. 2018;44(6):763-7.

EXAMINATION QUESTION

1. Write a brief note on Mohs micrographic surgery.

169 CHAPTER Hair Transplant

Kavish Chouhan, Gillian Roga

INTRODUCTION

Hair plays a vital role, especially in today's society which is obsessed with esthetics and appearance. This has resulted in hair transplantation becoming one of the most sought after procedure with tremendous technological advancement in this field. Patterned hair loss (PHL) represents the most common cause for baldness in men and the past decade has seen significant developments in its management. While medical therapy with both minoxidil and finasteride has a definite place in the treatment of PHL, its effect is temporary and the results are not satisfactory in advanced hair loss. Surgical management remains the only permanent method of restoring hair in PHL. The ability to provide natural looking results has encouraged larger number of balding men and women to opt for this surgical solution.

ETIOPATHOGENESIS OF PATTERNED HAIR LOSS

Patterned hair loss also known as androgenetic alopecia, is probably multifactorial and may be inherited as an autosomal dominant trait with variable penetrance.[1] In androgenetic alopecia, follicles undergo miniaturization, shrinking from terminal to vellus hair about 1 cm in length.[1,2] In miniaturization, the duration of anagen may shrink from the normal of 3–5 years to as less as 1 month, but the duration of telogen (3 months) remains the same. For reasons unknown, occipital scalp is not androgen-dependent. One hypothesis is that the dermis in the occipital area is derived from cephalic mesoderm, whereas the dermis over the rest of the scalp comes from neural crest derivatives. Whatever the reason, the fact that occipital hair is permanent serves as the basis of hair transplantation. A difference in the distribution of androgen receptors has been noted on the female scalp. It has also been hypothesized that the presence of enzyme aromatase in the female scalp may result in peripheral conversion of testosterone to estrogen, thus decreasing the severity of hair loss.[3,4] Thus, hair transplantation is based on this "theory of donor dominance in androgenic alopecia." If a graft is taken from an area destined to be permanently hair bearing and transplanted to an area suffering from male patterned baldness, it will, after an initial period of effluvium, grow hair in its new site as long as it would have at its original site.

HISTORY

In late 19th century, a German surgeon performed the first transplant and is said to have remarked that very soon, baldness would be a thing of the past. In the early 1950s, Dr Norman Orentreich, a dermatologist from New York introduced punch graft transplants for hair restoration.[4] To overcome the doll look appearance, from the early 1980s, smaller grafts called mini- and micrografts were introduced. In 1984, Headington[5] demonstrated that hair does not occur singly but as naturally occurring groups which were referred to as the follicular unit (FU). The concept of FU paved the way for follicular unit transplantation (FUT) in the 1990s and the recent follicular unit extraction (FUE) technique which proposed the dream of "no visible scarring."[6] In FUE, the grafts are extracted as individual FUs in a two-step or three-step technique whereas the method of implantation remains the same as in the traditional FUT. The addition of latest automated FUE technique seeks to overcome some of the limitations in this relatively new technique and it is now possible to achieve more than a thousand grafts in 1 day in trained hands.

METHODS OF HAIR TRANSPLANTATION

Follicular Unit Transplantation (Strip Technique)

In this method, donor harvesting was done by single-strip method with elliptical excision of donor, followed by suturing. The significant disadvantage of single-strip harvesting was the resultant linear donor scar. Though it is possible to provide a very fine linear scar with the newly described trichophytic closure, it does pose cosmetic problems for many patients particularly those who wish to wear short hair.

Follicular Unit Extraction

Bernstein and Rassman[7] started developing the FOX procedure, heralding a new surgical hair restoration procedure without strip harvesting. The FOX procedure, also known as FUE (follicular unit extraction), FUSE (follicular unit separation extraction) method,[8] Wood's technique,[9] and FU isolation method, is fast becoming an alternative method of extraction of grafts as FUs in selected cases.

The differences between follicular unit transplantation and follicular unit extraction methods of hair transplantation are given in **Table 1**.

TABLE 1: Differences between FUT and FUE.

	FUT strip method	*FUE procedure*
Harvesting technique	Single strip	Individual follicular units
Microscopic dissection	Required	Not required
Stitches	Required	Not required
Postoperative bleeding/pain	May occur	Uncommon
Nerve damage	Possible	Uncommon
Reaction to suture material	May occur	Uncommon
Duration of procedure	Short	Long
Fatigue	Not tiring due to shorter procedure	Tiring due to longer procedure
Shaving of head prior to surgery	Not required	Required
Hairstyle in donor area	Short hair not possible	Short hair possible
Healing time: *Donor area* *Recipient area*	 2–3 weeks 10–14 days	 1 week 10–14 days
Recovery time	2–3 weeks	1 week
Patient is fit to return to work	5–7 days	The day after
Visible scarring	Present	Absent
Large areas	Possible faster	Tedious
Cost	Cheaper	Expensive
Staff requirement	More	Less
Natural result in recipient area	Yes	Yes

Note: Transection rates in both FUT and FUE method depends on the expertise of the surgeon but preferably should be <5%.
(FUT: follicular unit transplantation; FUE: follicular unit extraction)

HAIR TRANSPLANT CONSULTATION

Candidate Selection

Proper patient selection is extremely important. Patients in their early 20s with early thinning of hair are not good candidates as the pattern of hair loss is yet to be established. Further, though highly motivated, these patients are often obsessed about their disability and have unrealistic expectations. Hence, they need to be properly counseled and given medical therapy. Likewise, patients with advanced baldness may not have sufficient donor hair and hence may not represent good candidates. The ideal candidates are patients with established baldness in their late 20s, 30s, or 40s, without significant systemic health problems and with realistic expectations.[10]

Ideal Candidates

- Realistic goals
- Stable and high-quality donor hair
- Recipient area that will support growth of the transplanted hair.

Poor Candidates

- Unrealistic expectations
- Mental illness
- Donor area—miniaturization, low donor density, retrograde alopecia, scarring
- Recipient area—unusual hair loss pattern, rapid progression, low residual hairline
- Many broken hairs, excessive shedding, fine hair, low density grafts.

Counseling and Informed Consent

Informed consent should be obtained after detailed counseling session which includes:

- Discussion on the different management options available
- Detailed explanation about the surgical procedure and possible postoperative complications
- Specific instructions that result would be seen only after 8–9 months
- In young patients, the specific instruction that continued drug therapy is necessary to preserve the existing hair
- Patients should not expect to get the same amount of hair that they had before balding
- Patients should understand that hair transplantation is a cosmetic procedure and will not affect the underlying process of baldness, which may continue in future
- Any allergies or medical condition that the patient may have should be recorded.

PREOPERATIVE EVALUATION AND WORK-UP

The surgeon must take into account the patient's age, medical history, family history of alopecia, facial features, and hair characteristics (caliber, texture, color) that may have an effect on the final outcome. Examination such as hair pull test can be used to check for effluvium. Typically, a cluster of 30–40 hairs is grasped at the base then pulled slowly. If five or more telogen hairs are pulled out, it is considered a positive test, and surgery should be postponed until the cause of the hair loss is discovered. Routine blood investigations—complete blood count, liver function tests, renal function tests, urine routine, blood sugar, bleeding and clotting times, prothrombin time, hepatitis B, ECG.[10] Advice of physician may be sought if there is any underlying systemic illness **(Fig. 1)**.

These are routine and include:

- Advice to stop smoking as smoking increases intraoperative bleeding
- Avoidance of vigorous exercise
- Use of ketoconazole shampoo if the patient has dandruff
- To avoid oral nonsteroidal anti-inflammatory drugs (NSAIDs) as they may increase intraoperative bleeding

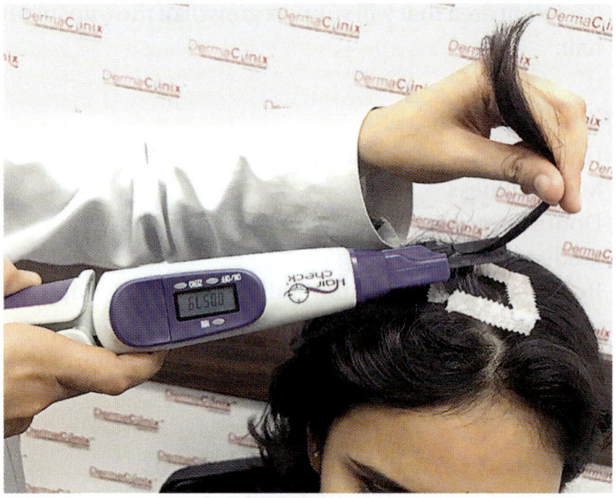

Fig. 1: Hair mass index measurement using hair check device.

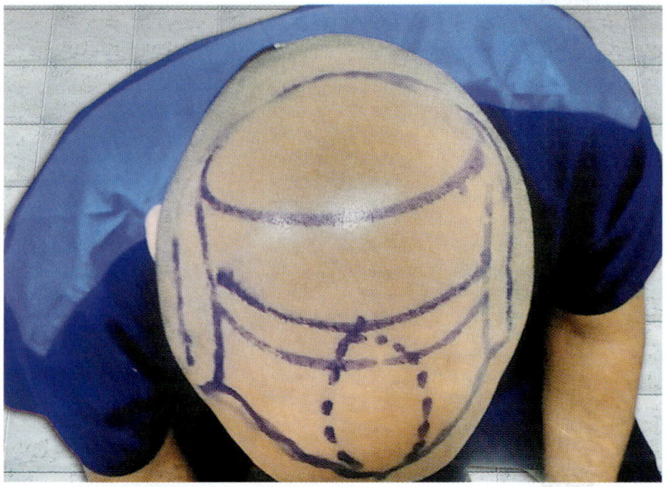

Fig. 2: Hairline designing preoperatively.

- The use of minoxidil should be suspended 2 weeks before surgery.

Preparation of the Patient

The patients hair is trimmed short prior to the surgery. Anxiolytics, painkiller, and antibiotics are administered prior to starting the surgery. Strict surgical asepsis is taken care of.

- Preoperative antibiotic such as amoxicillin and a preoperative tranquilizer such as diazepam or lorazepam can be used.
- The donor site hairs are trimmed to a length of about 2–4 mm. The location of the strip is just above the occipital protuberance, extending from one ear to the other. Too low a strip will lead to poor healing while too high a strip will lead to the possibility of donor hair being in the androgen-dependent balding area. Likewise, temporal hairs are not included as the scar may be visible. The length of the strip depends on the number of grafts required. Generally, for a 1,500 FU session, a strip 15 cm long and 1.2 cm wide would be sufficient in a patient with an FU density of 100 units.

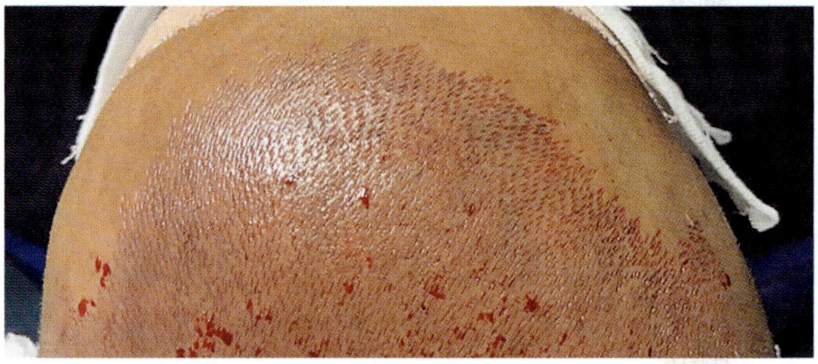

Fig. 3: Frontal hairline designing showing micro- and macroirregularities.

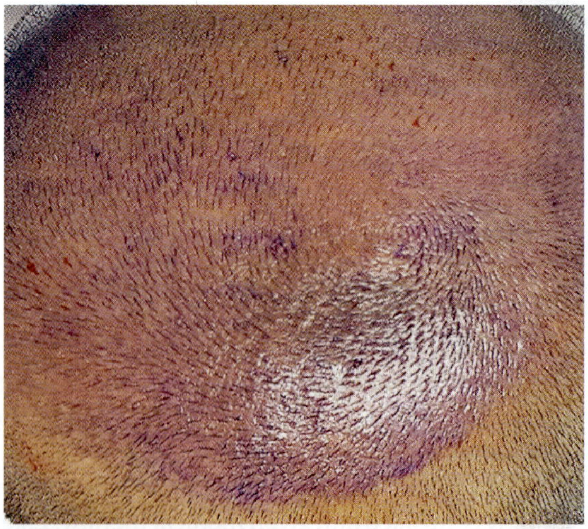

Fig. 4: Vertex designing.

Hairline Designing

The planning of the hairline is one of the most important steps in hair transplantation. The hairline is the most visible landmark and the quality of work of a surgeon is often judged by the quality of the hairline. As proposed by Michelangelo, to locate the ideal hairline in a bald patient, it is necessary to divide the face into three equal segments. In the midline, the hairline starts at least 8 cm from the glabella. A curve sweeps around to the lateral side of the forehead from the center. At this point, the sides of the hairline should be oriented parallel to the curve when the subject is looking straight ahead. The lateral hairlines are usually 9.5–11.5 cm above the lateral canthus of the eyes. The temporal angles should form moderately sharp right angles or acute angles in most men, but these angles should be more rounded in women **(Fig. 2)**. The micrografts in the hairline should be placed in an irregular saw-toothed pattern of macro- and microirregularity to give a natural appearance **(Fig. 3)**. The designing of the vertex requires much more expertise along with reconstruction in a whorled pattern. The whorl may be clockwise/counter clockwise in direction **(Fig. 4)**.

Anesthesia

Supraorbital and supratrochlear nerve blocks are given to anesthetize the recipient area. Ring block anesthesia was administered to the recipient area using a combination of xylocaine and bupivacaine **(Fig. 5)**. This is followed by the tumescent injection which is a mixture of bupivacaine with adrenaline, saline/ringer lactate, and triamcinolone acetate **(Fig. 6)**. Similarly, a ring block anesthesia followed by tumescent solution was administered to the donor area **(Fig. 7)**

Donor Harvesting

- *FUT strip*: In the strip method, a strip of scalp is harvested just below the hair follicles. Care must be given to prevent transection of the follicles. The length of the strip is determined by the hair density and the required number of FUs. After hemostasis of the bed, trichophytic closure can be done where a 1 mm edge is removed from the lower edge of the wound. It is important to take the bites only up to the dermis so that the deeper hair roots are not damaged, and thus can be utilized in subsequent surgery. Wounds are closed with continuous sutures. This allows hairs to grow through the residual scar and scars are therefore more acceptable.

Graft preparation in FUT: The harvested donor strips are immediately immersed in chilled normal saline. This is achieved by keeping the tray containing the grafts, immersed in saline on ice. Proper hydration of the donor grafts with cold saline is very important throughout the surgery as it influences the survival rate of the grafts. If a single large strip has been harvested, it can be divided into smaller pieces or slivers before the cutting of individual grafts. The subcutaneous fatty tissue below the hair roots or bulbs is stripped leaving up to 2 mm of fat below the hair bulb. Follicular unit grafts (**FUGs**) are made having 1–4 hairs. Grafts are immersed in saline in a petridish **(Fig. 8)** or are kept on a moist wet gauze over chilled ringer lactate **(Fig. 9)**. Good illumination is essential during the cutting of the grafts. The grafts may be cut on

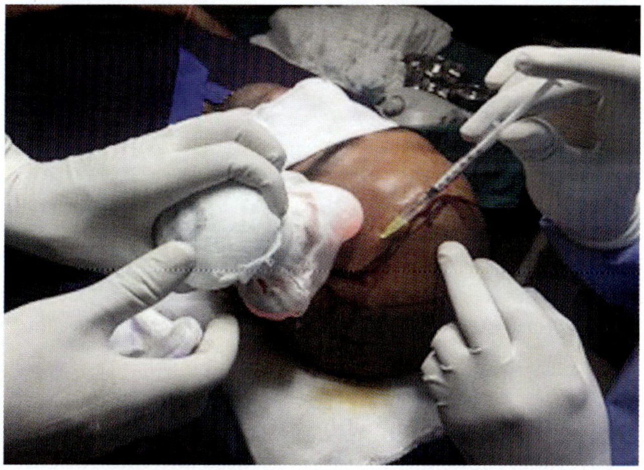

Fig. 5: Ring block anesthesia in recipient area.

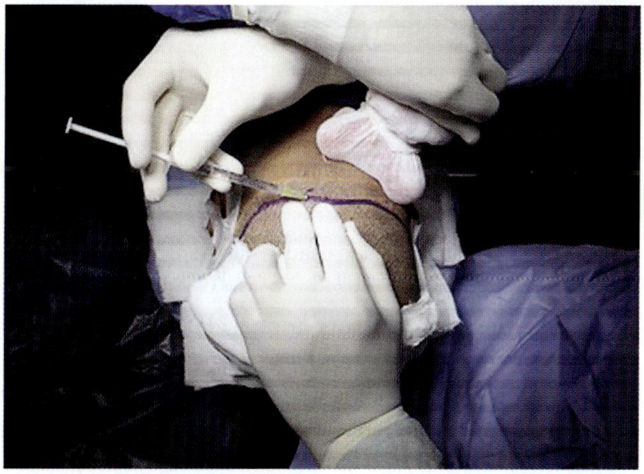

Fig. 7: Ring block anesthesia in the donor area.

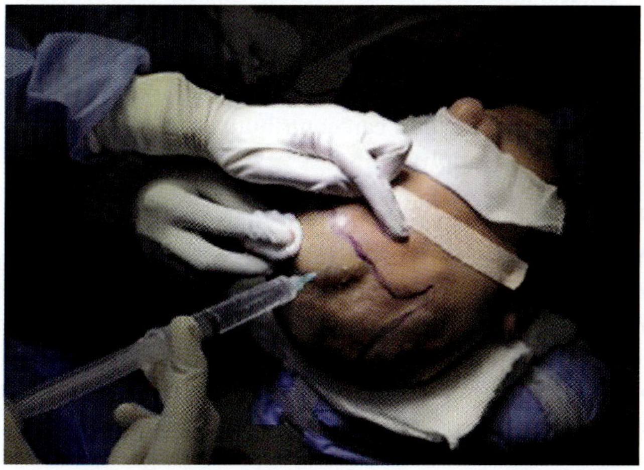

Fig. 6: Tumescent anesthesia in the recipient area.

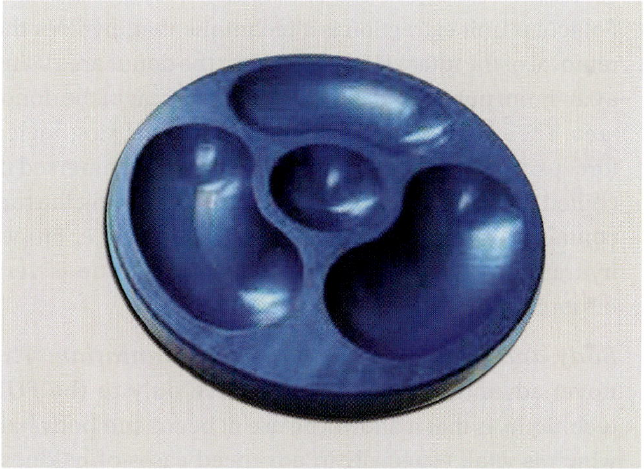

Fig. 8: Petridish used for graft holding.

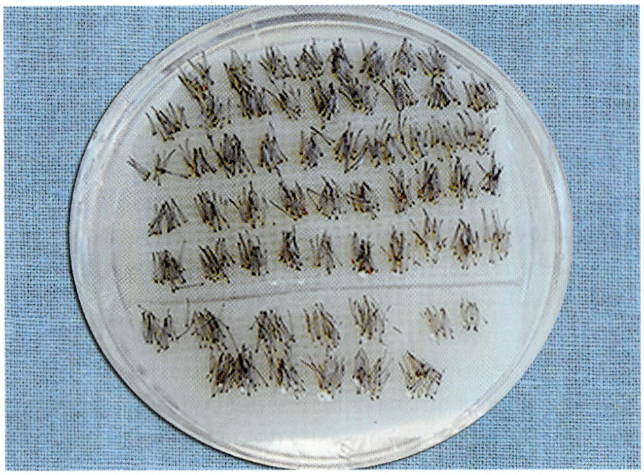

Fig. 9: Grafts placed on moist cotton gauze.

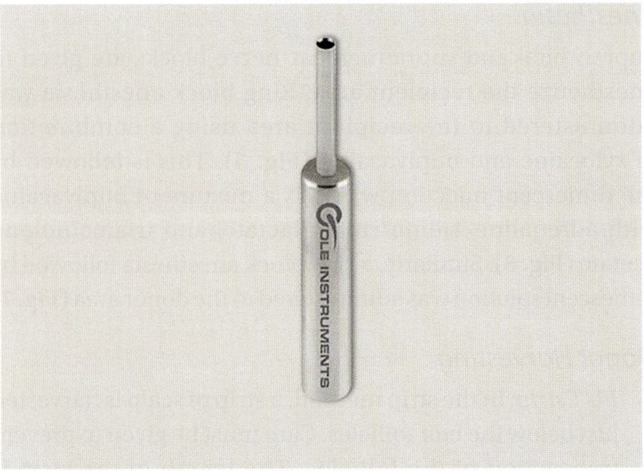

Fig. 11: Surrounded Coles punch used for extraction.

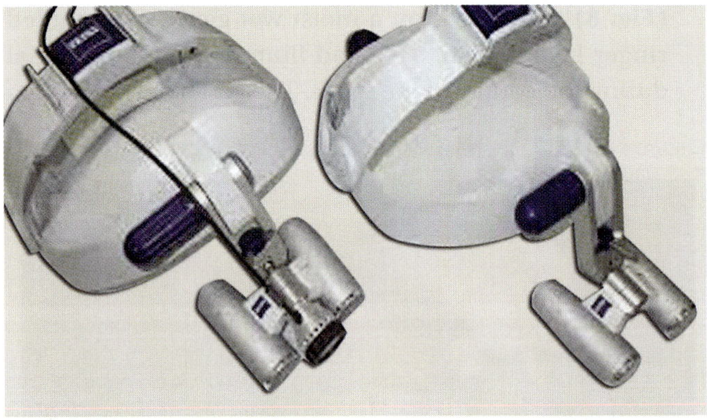

Fig. 10: Loupe magnification used in hair transplant surgery.

wooden tongue depressors or on a clear vinyl dissecting surface with a backlighting system. It is important that no piece of wood sticks to the grafts after they have been cut, because these foreign bodies can later form troublesome epidermal cysts. Loupe magnification of 2X or 3X power is useful in creating FUGs **(Fig. 10)**. Graft preparation with a dissecting stereomicroscope makes the dissection a little slower, but it is much more accurate.

- Follicular unit extraction is a technique that involves the removal of the intact FU directly from the donor area using a 0.8–1 mm punch **(Fig. 11)** that leaves no scar in the donor area. The scored grafts can then be extracted using angled forceps. The harvested FUs are immediately immersed in chilled normal saline. This is achieved by keeping the tray containing the grafts, immersed in saline on ice. Proper hydration of the donor grafts with cold saline is very important **(Fig. 12)**.

  Body and beard hair in hair transplantation: The novel advantage, which is exclusive only to the FUE technique, is that it allows the use of beard and body hair which is vital, especially in advanced cases of baldness with limited scalp donor area. Beard hair which is coarse can be mixed along with scalp hair to provide better coverage, especially in the vertex area and midfront area. Body hair (chest, leg, back, etc.) can be used along with scalp hair, especially in the frontal hairlines due to their shorter and finer characteristics, which in turn provides a more natural hairline. In this aspect, FUE definitely scores over FUT since majority of the advanced grade baldness cases have a limited scalp donor supply and it is in these cases that body hair can contribute tremendously to the donor hair supply.[10]

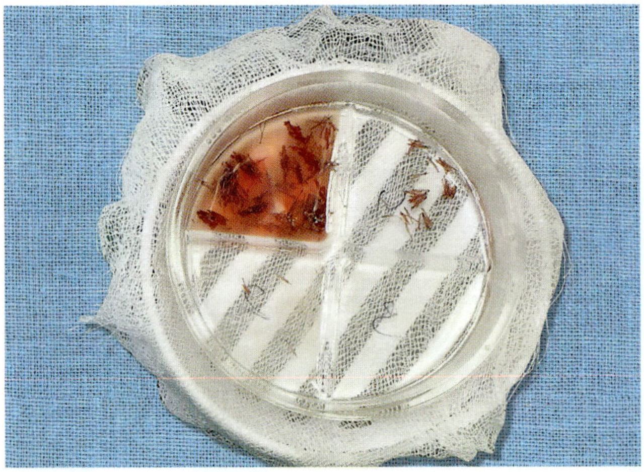

Fig. 12: Harvested follicular units stored in chilled normal saline directly after extraction.

Preparation of the Recipient Area

While making slits or holes in the recipient area, it is very important to follow the direction of the existing hair in that particular region. While making the holes, it is important to keep in mind the angle at which the native hair is coming out of the scalp, as well as the direction of the hairs. In order to adjust the length of the blade before designing the recipient area a few follicles can be extracted and the length of the blade can be adjusted accordingly **(Fig. 13)**. The hairline should

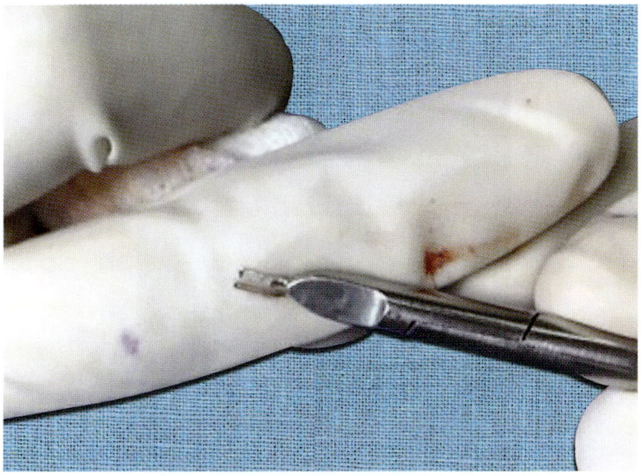

Fig. 13: Length of blade being adjusted according to the length of the hair follicles.

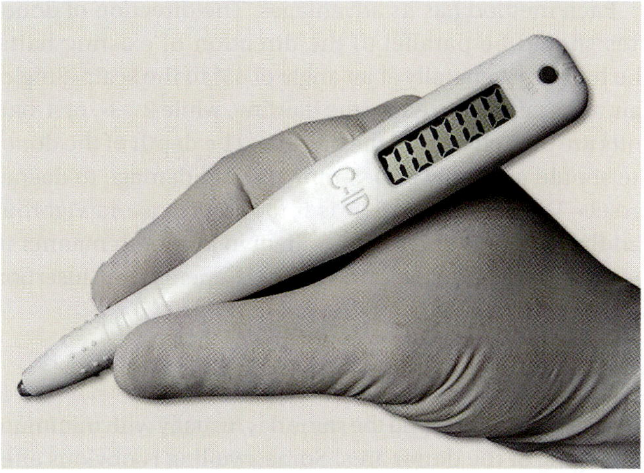

Fig. 15: Incision counting device used for counting the number of slits.

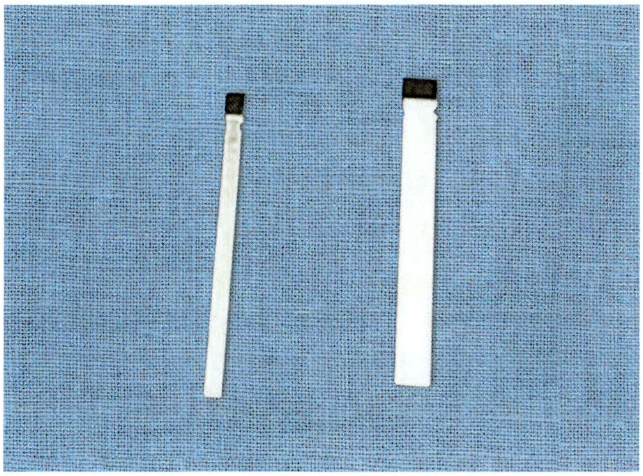

Fig. 14: Cut-to-size blade used for designing the recipient area.

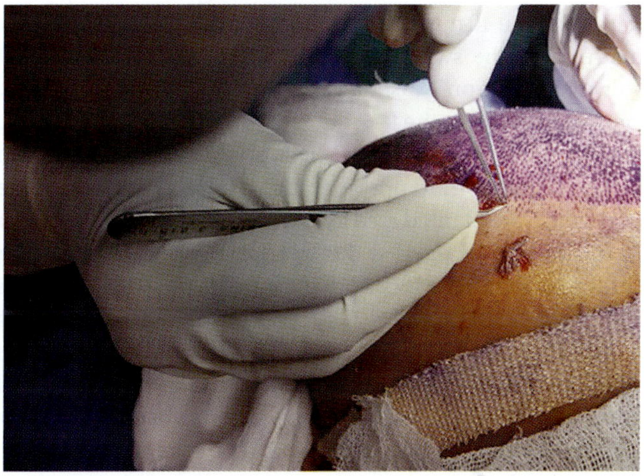

Fig. 16: Implantation using two fine-angled forceps.

have a ragged, saw-toothed natural look. Slits are made with a No. 18/20/23-gauge needle or cut-to-size blades as preferred by the author **(Fig. 14)**. Alternatively, a counting incision device can also be used for automatically counting the number of incisions made **(Fig. 15)**.

Graft Insertion

The grafts are placed into the recipient slits using fine-angled forceps **(Fig. 16)**. It is important to employ an atraumatic technique for graft placement. To avoid damage, the FUs are grasped by the 2 mm of subcutaneous tissue left below the hair bulbs to position them into the recipient sites and not by the follicle end in the case of FUT. In FUE, the author advocates a "no root touch" technique where the FU are held by the upper one-third region without damaging the bulb. A steady pressure is applied to ensure that the grafts are flush with the surrounding skin. Burying the grafts beneath the level of the skin must be avoided because it can give a pitted appearance and also lead to the formation of epidermal cysts. A cobblestone appearance is seen if the grafts are too elevated from the surface. There are several methods for insertion:

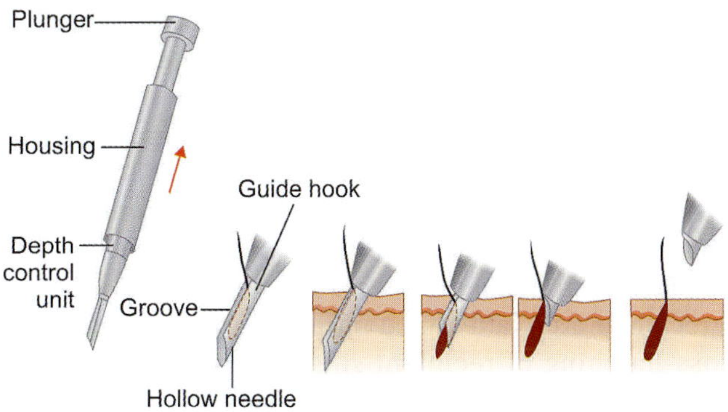

Fig. 17: Implanters being used for designing the hairline.

- The "stick and place method" involves making a recipient site, followed immediately by insertion of hairs into the site by an assistant.
- Creating all the required recipient sites at one time and then placing the grafts one by one.
- The use of implanters which involves the use of preloaded pen-like instruments with an extracted graft in its hollow end, directly into the scalp **(Fig. 17)**.

Each method has its advantages. The direction of donor sites should be parallel to the direction of existing hairs. The hairs are generally at an angle of 45° to the scalp. Single-hair units are preferred for the hairline, while 2-, 3-, or 4-hair units are packed behind the hairline. The depth of the donor site should generally be 4–5 mm to avoid damage to deeper vessels. During insertion, it is important to avoid vigorous handling of grafts and to insert them in a smooth manner in the direction of the creation of the site. Generally, the insertion is done from back to front to avoid popping.

POSTOPERATIVE CARE

The patient is discharged the same day, usually with minimum bandaging of the donor area. Some swelling is obvious after a hair transplantation surgery and the patient should be informed of this prior to the procedure. Oral steroids for 3–5 days can minimize the edema. Some surgeons use injection triamcinolone 40 mg in the tumescent solution and claim that this reduces the swelling. A head-band worn immediately after the operation is useful in preventing the swelling from coming down on to the face and creating a puffy appearance. The patient is instructed to wash his hair with a mild shampoo on the second or third postoperative day. While combing the hair in the transplanted area for 3 weeks, the tooth of the comb should not strike against the transplanted grafts. Wearing clothes such as T-shirts or pullovers which have to be taken off over the head should also be avoided for 3 weeks. Hair oils or other stronger shampoos as well as helmets are also to be avoided for the same period. After the transplant, 5% minoxidil lotion is applied once the shampooing has begun. This has been shown to promote earlier growth of the transplanted hair.

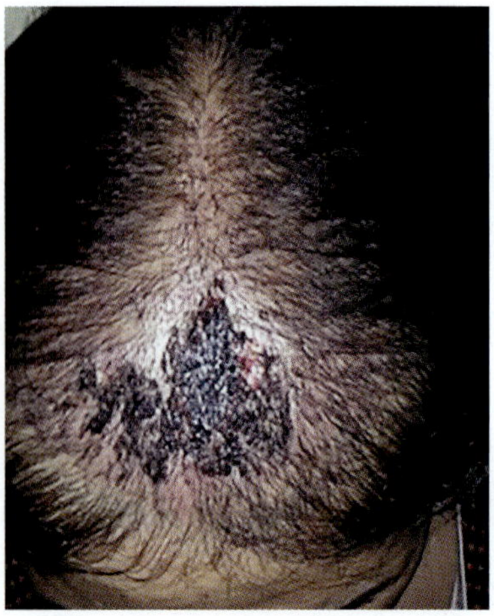

Fig. 18: Necrosis seen in recipient area.

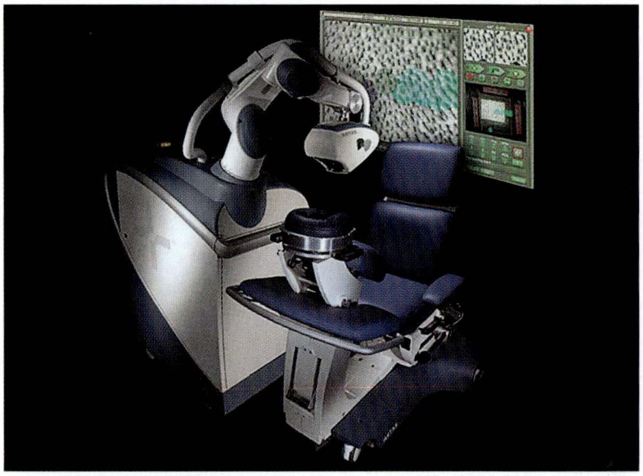

Fig. 19: ARTAS machine used for robotic hair transplantation surgery.

POSTOPERATIVE COMPLICATIONS

The most common complication is postoperative pain, which needs to be managed by proper use of analgesics. Swelling over the forehead occurs in about 25% of patients on day 3 of surgery due to postoperative edema and the presence of large amount of saline injected during anesthesia. This is temporary and can be managed with ice compresses and administration of a short course of oral steroids. Infection is rare. Some case may develop frontal central necrosis due to excessive damage to recipient area (attempted ultra-high density transplant, cross-hatching of recipient sites) or excessive usage of adrenaline **(Fig. 18)**. Drug-induced gastritis, persistence of crust at the recipient sites, persistent pain at the donor site, and sterile pustules during the second month (caused by an irritant reaction during hair growth) are some of the other common but minor complications. Keloid formation is rare. Delayed hair growth is another complication.

CONCLUSION

In view of the psychological aspects of hair loss, hair transplantation requires a thorough preoperative assessment to understand the patient's expectations, a careful examination to determine if surgery is appropriate and, most importantly, the establishment of realistic goals. If the surgical route is chosen, meticulous attention to detail is required in every aspect of the procedure, so that these goals may be realized. Nowadays with the progress in technology robotic hair transplant in the form of ARTAS is available and Food and Drug Administration (FDA) approved for male pattern hair loss (MPHL) but the punch size used is 1 mm or more with reported transection rate varies from 8 to 23%. It is not approved for usage in females and in parietal/temporal areas transection rates are very high **(Fig. 19)**. It is a daunting task for the hair restoration surgeon and team to develop the necessary expertise for perfecting surgical hair restoration; but when they do the procedure can be extremely satisfying to patients **(Figs. 20A and B)**.

KEY POINTS

- Advancement in hair restoration technology today has led to advanced grade of androgenetic alopecia, being successfully treated with an exceptionally natural looking and esthetic result.

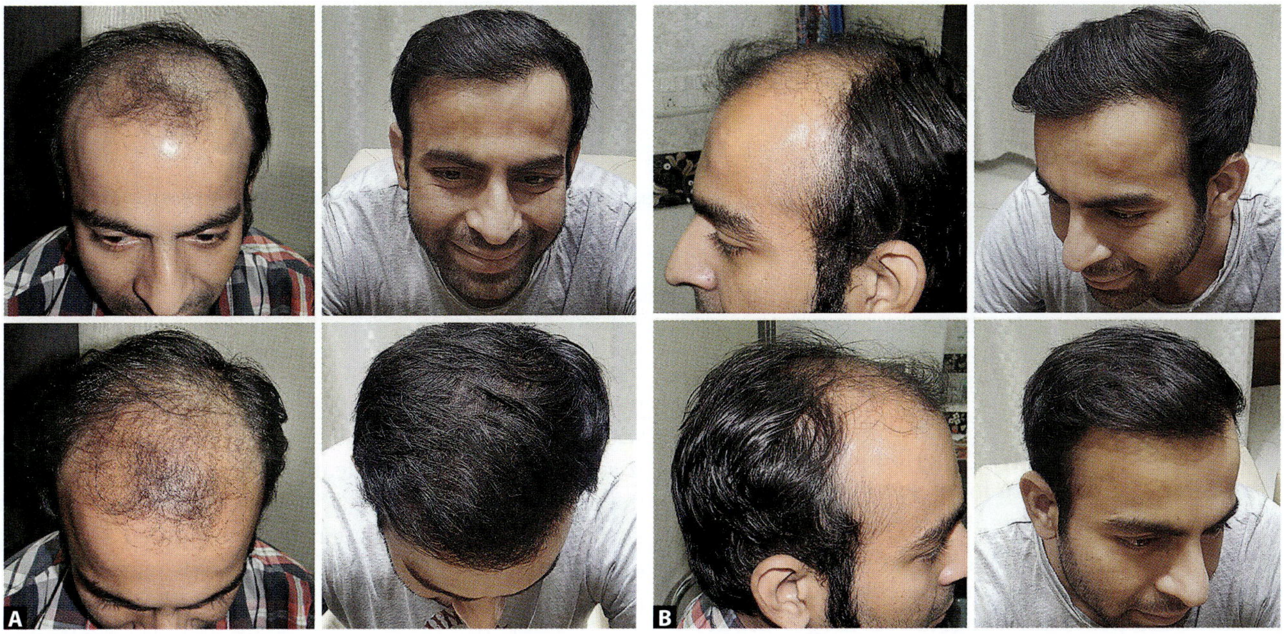

Figs. 20A and B: Result of frontal and mid-frontal coverage post-FUE in Grade 5 baldness (lateral view) after 9 months.

- Time management, graft management and staff management play an important role in a successful surgical outcome.

REFERENCES

1. Whiting DA. Possible mechanisms of miniaturization during androgenetic alopecia or pattern hair loss. J Am Acad Dermatol. 2001;45:81-6.
2. Rebora A. Pathogenesis of androgenetic alopecia. J Am Acad Dermatol. 2004:50;777-9.
3. Chartier MB, Hoss DM, Grant-Kels JM. Approach to the adult female patient with diffuse nonscarring alopecia. J Am Acad Dermatol. 2002;47:809-18.
4. Orentreich N. Autografts in alopecias and other elected dermatological conditions. Ann NY Acad Sci. 1959;83:463-79.
5. Headington JT. Transverse microscopic anatomy of the human scalp. Arch Dermatol. 1984;120:449-56.
6. Bernstein RM, Rassman WR. Follicular transplantation. Patient evaluation and surgical planning. Dermatol Surg. 1997;23: 771-84.
7. Rassman WR, Bernstein RM, McClellan R, Jones R, Worton E, Uyttendaele H. Follicular unit extraction: minimally invasive surgery for hair transplantation. Dermatol Surg. 2002;28:720-7.
8. Poswal A. Donor sealing: a novel method in hair transplant surgery. Indian J Dermatol. 2006;51:55-6.
9. Woods A. Chest hair micrografts display extended growth in scalp tissue: a case report. Br J Plast Surg. 2004;57:789-91.
10. Chouhan K, Roga G, Kumar A, Gupta J. Approach to hair transplantation in advanced grade baldness by follicular unit extraction: a retrospective analysis of 820 cases. J Cutan Aesthet Surg. 2019;12(4):215-22.

EXAMINATION QUESTIONS

1. Write a brief note on FUT.
2. Write a brief note on FUE.

170 CHAPTER

Radiosurgery in Dermatology

Karalikkattil T Ashique, Feroze Kaliyadan

INTRODUCTION

Radiofrequency (RF) device is one of the first things that a dermatologist in the residency period places his hands in the procedure room with a lot of awe and expectations. Radiosurgery has generally replaced older electrocautery units; radiosurgery uses a frequency of 3.8 MHz and is generally considered superior to electrosurgery, with an added, more powerful coagulation mode. Modern radiosurgery machines are compact, easy to handle, and fresh dermatologists can master the art quickly and start doing with ease the myriad of procedures with the small machine in the office. RF surgery can aptly be called a poor man's magic wand in view of the large number of indications and the ease of acquiring and using even in a poor resource setting.

Why RF in the First Place? (Advantages)

- The capital investment is low (around 20K INR for a decent machine commercially available at present in India, although there are more costly devices available). Maintenance costs are also very low. The electrodes are the only part which needs replacements and these are usually not very costly.
- The machines are quite versatile and the learning curve is small. Needless to say, the results are reasonably good even in the hands of a beginner. The precision of the good machines is really very useful in doing procedures on cosmetically important areas. The cut and coagulate mode is of immense use to do the excision without much of a bleeding.
- The machines are compact and portable. They can be carried along for those people who have freelance practice in more than one place and again reduces the investment burden.
- Low lateral heat is an advantage of a good RF machine and the resultant tissue necrosis is very minimal. Which means even biopsy specimen can be collected with an RF machine (although this requires practice).[1]

HISTORICAL PERSPECTIVE

Dr GE Ward who was a tumor surgeon was one of the pioneers in electrosurgery. He defined electrosurgery as "the use of heat generated in body tissue through tissue resistance to high-frequency alternating current for the destruction and removal of diseased tissue or for cutting through normal tissue with minimal bleeding."[2] He used electrosurgery for cutting tissues. In 1907, Walter de Keating-Hart and Pozzi introduced the term fulguration. In 1970, CO_2 laser came into existence. Dr Irving Ellman (DDS, Engineer) was granted a US patent on his 3.8 MHz high-frequency four-waveform dental radiosurgical device in 1976.[3]

PHYSICS AND ELECTROPHYSIOLOGY

All electrosurgical units basically produce oscillating electromagnetic radiation. The frequency of the waves used is in the same bandwidth as those used of radiotransmission and hence these machines are also called RF units and the procedure is also called radiosurgery.[4,5] The older machines (like the hyfrecator) emit waves in the 500 kHz range while the newer RF units generate waves in the 2.5–4 MHz range. The most effective RF is considered to be 3.8 MHz. When the RF waves encounter resistance (impedance) while passing through tissues, it generates heat, boiling the water, leading to steam producing which in turn ultimately causes the cutting or coagulation of the tissue.[4,5]

Basic Terms Related to Current

Ampere: Measures rate of current flow. Higher amperage means faster current flow

Voltage: Force which drives current against resistance. Higher the voltage more the amount of current flow in a circuit.

Damping: A damped wave is one in which the amplitude decreases with time. The more rapidly the oscillations decrease to reach zero, the more damped a wave. The word rectified waves are sometimes used as a synonym for damped waves.[4,5]

Terminology: Monopolar, Monoterminal, and Bipolar

In *monopolar electrosurgery*, the patient is part of the circuit. Monopolar electrosurgery uses two electrodes—one placed at the surgical site (the active electrode) and the other (dispersive/patient return electrode) elsewhere on the patient's body. The dispersive electrode is often referred to as the grounding plate, which is a misnomer as the purpose of the dispersive electrode is to complete the circuit and return the current to the machine, rather than to ground it.

In *monoterminal* units such as hyfrecators (where a dispersive plate is not used), patient self-capacitance is used so that the current flows through the patient, to the ground, and back to the electrosurgery unit.

In *bipolar units*, the patient is not a part of a circuit. The current is delivered using a forceps-like device with the current flowing between the two ends only through the target tissue (because of this bipolar units are generally safer in the context of implantable electronic devices such as pacemakers).[4,5]

Terminology: Electrodessication, Electrofulguration, Electrocoagulation, and Electrosection

Electrodessication: High-frequency, high-voltage, low-amperage current is used in a monoterminal application with the electrode in contact with the skin leading to tissue destruction.

Electrofulguration: Monoterminal, high-voltage current is used. Here the electrode is kept some distance away from the skin. The electrode produces a spark which reaches the skin. Damage is generally less compared to electrodessication.

Electrocoagulation: This is a biterminal method using lower voltage (but higher amperage) as compared to electrodessication. The main purpose is hemostasis.

Electrosection: Low-voltage, high-amperage, biterminal method. The waves are either completely undamped or very slightly damped. If completely undamped, it produces a pure cutting effect (with very less lateral damage) and if slightly undamped, it produces a combination of cutting and coagulation which is best for most dermatological indications. It is this method which is mainly used in most radiosurgery procedures.

Components and Care of the Machine and Loops

The machine predominantly comprises a base unit powered by 220-V electric current, a patient plate, and the operator hand piece to which the electrodes and loops are attached when operational **(Figs. 1A to C)**. The RF device delivers optimal performance when the machine runs without any fluctuations. Frequent power failures may also adversely affect the life of the machine. Hence, it is always desirable to operate the device under live UPS (uninterrupted power supply) support.

An ideal RF procedure room should be well lit and the machine is placed on the facing wall at overhead level of the operator. This makes the machine safe and also helps the operator to adjust the setting during the procedure **(Fig. 2)**. The electrodes may get charred very easily with the necrotic debris. They can be cleaned by rubbing them in a wet gauze with the machine in operation intermittently. All the electrodes can be sterilized by ethylene oxide (ETO) (gas sterilization) for reuse. Some suppliers have made the disposable loops available for those who can afford them. Electrodes are available in various sizes and shapes. There are disposable and reusable and are freely available in the market **(Fig. 3)**.[4,5]

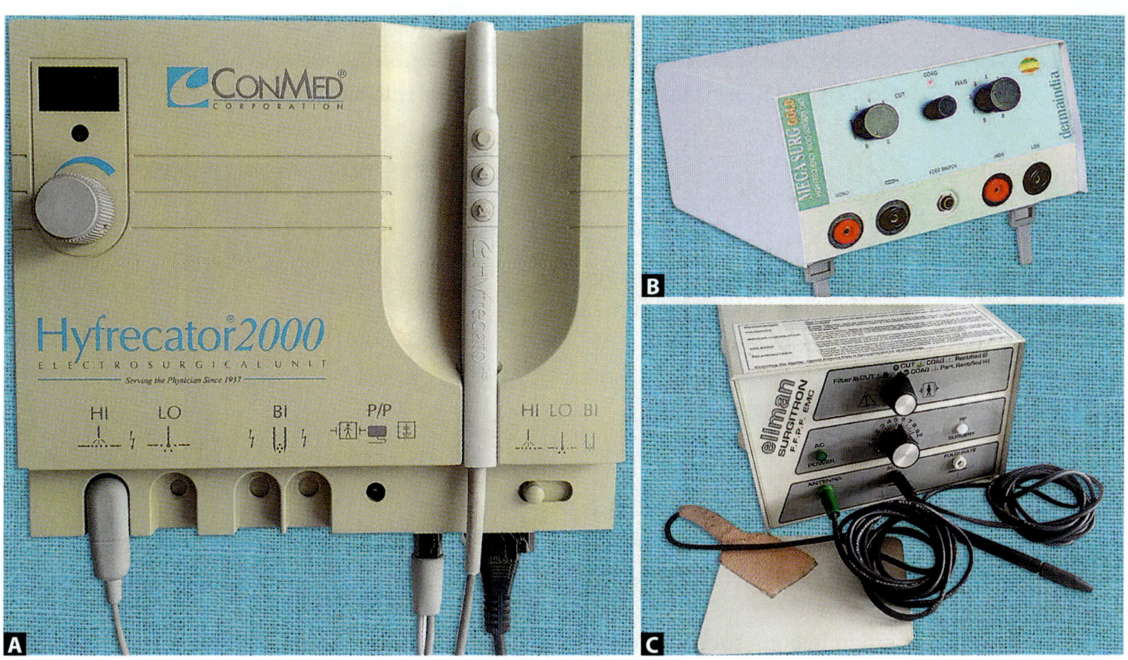

Figs. 1A to C: Three of the popular radiofrequency machines commercially available in India; (A) Hyfrecator™ (CONMED); (B) Megasurg Gold™ (DERMAINDIA); and (C) Surgicon™ (ELLMAN).

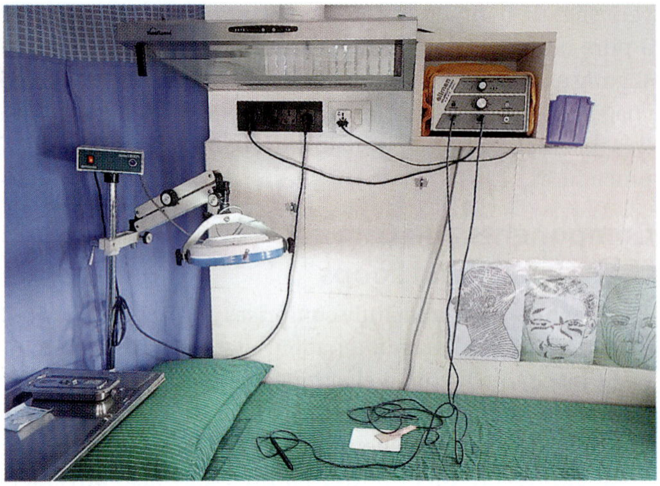

Fig. 2: An ideal setting for the radiofrequency unit in the operator room. Note the placement of the base unit at overhead level.

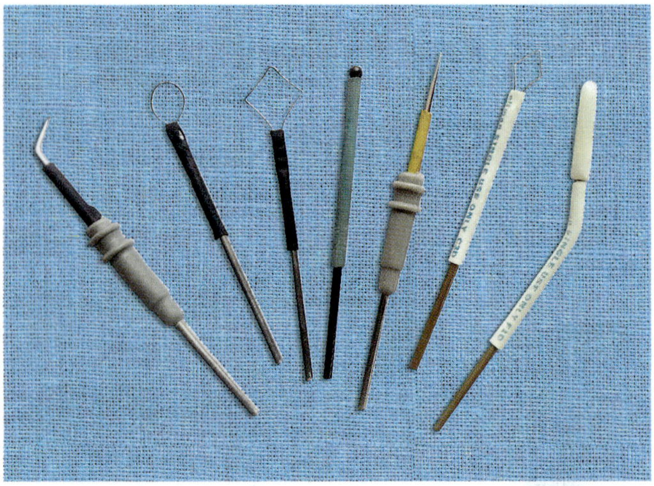

Fig. 3: Electrodes of various sizes and shapes available in the market. The white and blue sleeved ones are disposable electrodes from Ellman™.

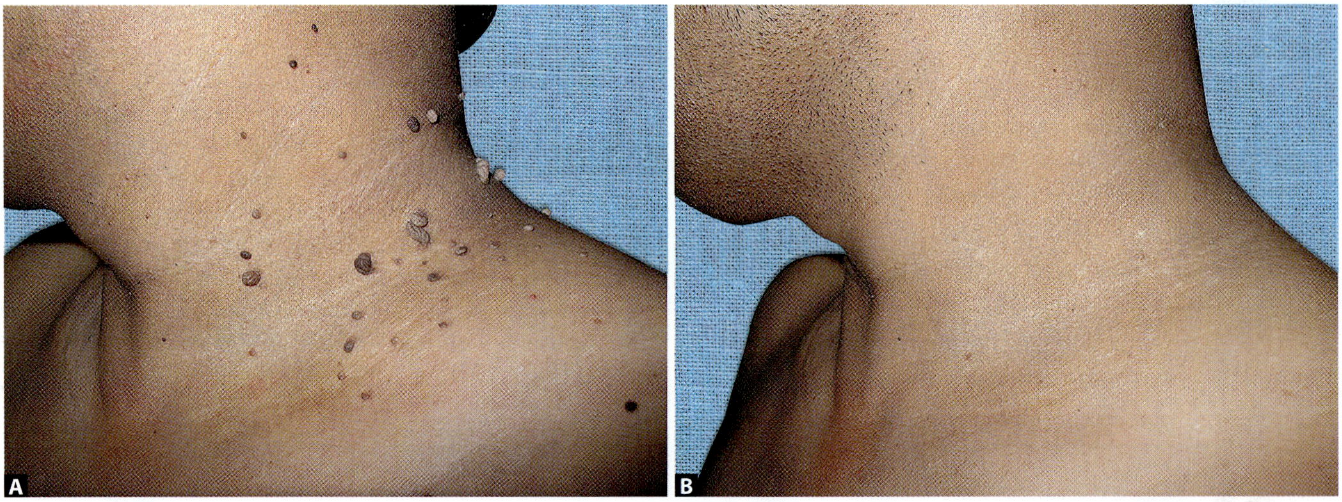

Figs. 4A and B: Skin tags before and after removal with radiofrequency.

INDICATIONS[1,6-10]

Cosmetic

- Removal of benign lesions such as moles, skin tags, dermatoses papulosa nigra (DPNs), spider angiomas, cherry angiomas, seborrheic keratoses, etc.
- Mole excision
- Freckles can be removed at very low energy mode.

Therapeutic

- Removal of warts, skin tags, DPN, seborrheic keratosis, calluses, and molluscum contagiosum **(Figs. 4 to 6)**
- Removal of vascular lesions such as pyogenic granuloma and cherry angioma
- Ablating and/or excising benign lesions such as xanthelasma palpebrarum, steatocystoma multiplex, mucocele on the lips, and syringomas

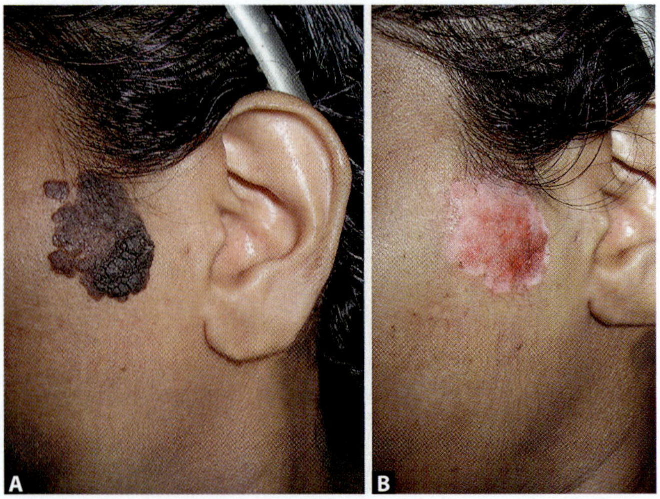

Figs. 5A and B: Seborrheic keratosis immediately after removal with radiofrequency.

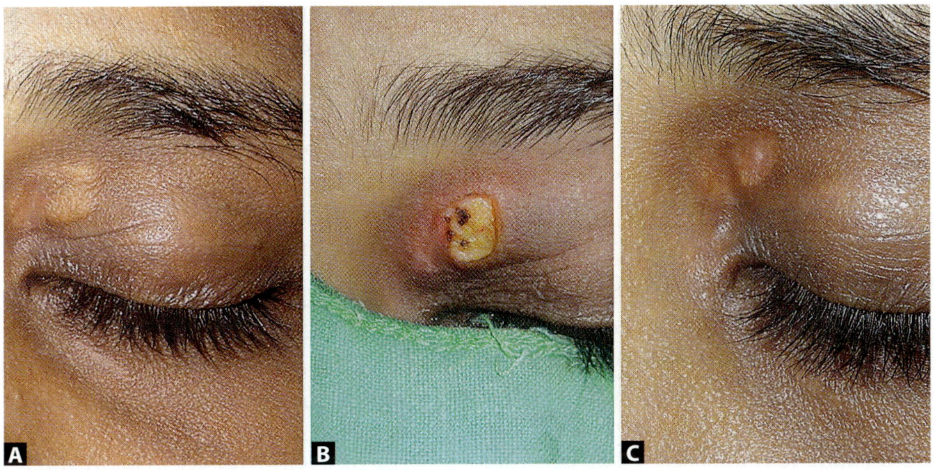

Figs. 6A to C: Preoperative, intraoperative, and postoperative images of xanthelasma palpebrarum treated with radiofrequency.

- Rhinophyma correction
- Matrixectomy in nail surgery
- Tattoo removal
- Removal of ticks from the skin
- *Other miscellaneous indications include* Hailey-Hailey disease, preparation of graft sites in vitiligo surgery, mole removal, diagnostic, and therapeutic excision of malignant skin tumors such as basal cell carcinoma.

Miscellaneous

- Vitiligo surgery recipient bed preparation
- Removal of cobblestones formation after punch grafting in vitiligo surgery
- Debulking keloids during the surgery such as ear lobe keloids

HEALTH HAZARDS FOR THE OPERATING PHYSICIAN

One of the most common problems faced in the operating room is the obnoxious smell of the burnt skin during and immediately after the procedure. A review by Lewin et al. opined that surgical smoke poses potential health risks to the operating dermatologists who perform procedures using electrocautery and lasers. They recommended use of high-filtration masks in addition to smoke evacuation systems to dermatologists performing laser surgery and using electrocautery.[11] We had deviced a simple modification by using a domestic chimney as a tool to reduce the smoke and smell in the operating room. This is in no way an alternative to a full-fledged smoke evacuator.[12]

INTRAOPERATIVE AND OTHER PRECAUTIONS

- This is one very important aspect that acetone or surgical spirit should never be used to clean the area being operated irrespective of the procedure. This may trigger burns and injure the skin very bad.
- Although the procedure may seem very simple in the operating room, the patient should always be reclined and relaxed in the operating table and never seated in a chair, etc. Taking a written consent and following all standard aseptic precautions are mandatory before RF also as in any other procedure.
- Never attempt a procedure when the lighting is poor or the electricity is fluctuating.
- The electrode, even if it is not in direct contact, is likely to disperse some electric signals and heat and hence should be cautiously used when working near vital organs such as the eye.
- Patient who reports allergic reaction to topical anesthetics should be warned about an increased erythema after the procedure to avoid a confusion and displeasure.
- It is desirable to avoid any procedure if the patient has active herpes labialis to avoid a prospective dissemination of virus.
- Radiofrequency has been reported to affect function of implanted electronic devices such as pacemakers. Pacemakers can be affected in various ways including inhibition, reprogramming, depleted battery, and destruction. The effect on pacemakers may lead to various rhythm abnormalities such as skipped beats, asystole, bradycardia, ventricular fibrillation, and unspecified tachyarrhythmia. The effect on pacemakers is more with monopolar mode as compared to bipolar mode as mentioned earlier.
- The British Cochlear Implant Group (BCIG) who come out with guidelines about the use of cochlear implants have put forth this guideline which states that: it is advised that monoterminal electrosurgery "should not be used in the head and neck region in patients with cochlear implants." Biterminal electrosurgery can be used safely but "should not be used within 2 cm of the implant." In regards to

"therapeutic diathermy," there is "potentially a very serious risk to health for implant users from short-wave diathermy and microwave diathermy" and these should *never* be used. Ultrasound diathermy is acceptable below the head and neck.[4,5,13,14]

COMPLICATIONS AND SOLUTIONS

Postinflammatory Hyperpigmentation

This is one of the worst and unpredictable complications after any radiosurgery. To some extent, we can prevent them by taking adequate care during and immediately after the procedure. Using very less or optimal voltage is by far the first and foremost thing to be done to reduce the tissue charring and the resultant unwelcome PIH. Using the ball tip of the can helps in a blunt injury unlike a sharp cut, especially while undertaking RF removal of freckles, etc. Generous use of ice packs immediately after the procedure and plenty of sunscreens in addition to sun protection measures is the "must do" instruction which the clinician should advise the patient before he leaves the operating room.

Innovations

Poor light for the operating field is a big drawback for any RF device. The need for an external light source again demands additional space for the operating room. This becomes very difficult in small clinics and poor resource settings. We had deviced the use of an LED (light-emitting diode) light source with a gooseneck mechanism to overcome this limitation. The said modifications can even work on a 5-V battery power from a portable energy bank used to charge mobile phones.[15] Gingival pigmentation has been treated with RF devise successfully by Mahesh et al. They have stated that if RF is used judiciously, it can be valuable clinically as a safe and effective method for depigmentation, in conjunction with aesthetic dentistry.[16]

TIPS AND PRECAUTIONS

- Keep the lesions wet (normal saline or water can be used and completely avoid inflammable antiseptics)
- Always ask for a history of pacemaker insertion
- Use smoke evacuators
- Avoid keeping the foot switch pressed continuously as it leads to damage to the machine
- Select the appropriate electrode (e.g., loops for excising skin tags and needle electrodes for making incisions)
- Use appropriate power settings (charring indicates that the power is too much, stickiness of the electrode may indicate a lower power)
- With smaller electrodes use lower power
- In general, start with lower power settings initially till you are familiar with the machine.
- Use good lighting. The basic surgical principle of "cut only what you see and see what you cut" applies to radiosurgery too.
- Select the appropriate waveform. It is good to be oriented with the basic physics of RF surgery.
- Make sure that the electrode is fully inserted.
- Avoid pressure when applying the electrode and use light circular motion for coagulation

KEY POINTS

- Radiofrequency surgery is a simple and effective treatment options for many indications, which were earlier treated with electrosurgery.
- The procedure is easy to learn and is associated with low complications if basic principles of care are applied.
- Radiosurgery uses a frequency of 3.8 MHz and has a strong coagulation mode and low lateral heat damage, thereby giving bloodless fields and aesthetically better results.
- Radiosurgery is contraindicated in patients who are on pacemakers.

REFERENCES

1. Turner RJ, Cohen RA, Voet RL, Stephens SR, Weinstein SA. Analysis of tissue margins of cone biopsy specimens obtained with "cold knife," CO_2 and Nd:YAG lasers and a radiofrequency surgical unit. J Reprod Med. 1992;37(7):607-10.
2. Ward GE. Electricity in medicine: electrosurgery. Am J Surg. 1932;17:86-93.
3. Pollack SV, Carruthers A, Grekin RC. The history of electrosurgery. Dermatol Surg. 2000;26:904-8.
4. Tawade YV. Radiofrequency in dermatology. In: Mysore V (Ed). ACSI Textbook on Cutaneous and Aesthetic Surgery Aesthetics, Lasers and Dermatosurgery. New Delhi, India: Jaypee Brothers Medical Publishers; 2012. pp. 255-60.
5. Sarkar R, Nair V. Electrosurgery. In: Mysore V (Ed). ACSI Textbook of Cutaneous and Aesthetic Surgery Aesthetics, Lasers and Dermatosurgery. New Delhi, India: Jaypee Brothers Medical Publishers; 2012. pp. 245-54.
6. Aferzon M, Millman B. Excision of rhinophyma with high-frequency electrosurgery. Dermatol Surg. 2002;28(8): 735-8.
7. Kaliyadan F. Using the ball-shaped attachment of a radiofrequency ablation device for preparation of recipient site in vitiligo surgery. Indian J Dermatol. 2011;56:459-60.
8. Lahiri K, Sengupta SR. Steatocystoma Multiplex, Treatment With Electrosurgery—A Novel Approach. Indian J Dermatol. 1998;(43)4:148-51.
9. Ashique KT, Kaliyadan F. Radiofrequency device for tick removal. J Am Acad Dermatol. 2015;72(6):e155-6.
10. Küçüktaş M, Kutlubay Z, Yardimci G, Khatib R, Tüzün Y. Comparison of effectiveness of electrocautery and cryotherapy in partial matrixectomy after partial nail extraction in the treatment of ingrown nails. Dermatol Surg. 2013;39(2): 274-80.
11. Lewin JM, Brauer JA, Ostad A. Surgical smoke and the dermatologist. J Am Acad Dermatol. 2011;65(3):636-41.
12. Ashique KT, Kaliyadan F. "Something better than nothing" using the house hold electric chimney in the procedure room as an

attempt to reduce the smell and biohazard. J Cutan Aesthet Surg. 2014;7:46-8.
13. Frampton SJ, Ismail-Koch H, Mitchell TE. How safe is diathermy in patients with cochlear implants? Ann R Coll Surg Engl. 2012;94:585-7.
14. British Cochlear Implant Group (2014). Recommended Guidelines on Safety for Cochlear Implant Users. [online] Available from: https://www.bcig.org.uk/wp-content/uploads/2014/12/BCIG-safety-document-2014.pdf [Last accessed January, 2021].
15. Ashique KT, Kolakkadan K, Kaliyadan F. Assembling a make-shift light source for a Radiofrequency device for skin ablation. Indian J Dermatol Venereol Leprol. 2017;83:268-9.
16. Mahesh HV, Harish MR, Shashikumar BM, Ramya KS. Gingival pigmentation reduction: A novel therapeutic modality. J Cutan Aesthet Surg. 2012;5:137-40.

EXAMINATION QUESTION

1. Write a short note on radiofrequency in dermatology.

171 CHAPTER

Cryotherapy

Niteen Dhepe, Shrenik Balger

INTRODUCTION

Cryotherapy is defined as application of cryogens (cooling agents) locally for controlled destruction of living tissues thereby helping in treatment of variety of conditions. In cryotherapy, the target tissue is rapidly cooled to extreme low temperature followed by rewarming or thawing. This causes destruction or cryonecrosis of the tissue. It is an easy, safe and effective office procedure for removal of various benign and malignant growths.

HISTORY

Egyptians used cold application to reduce pain and inflammation. Hippocrates doctored the use of cold to reduce signs of inflammation. James Arnott considered the Father of Modern Cryotherapy first used refrigeration as local analgesia for treatment of variety of skin diseases.

White in 1899 used cold refrigerants for treating benign, premalignant, and malignant lesions. William Pusey promoted the use of CO_2 snow. Allington was the first to use liquid nitrogen in the treatment of skin diseases. Since 1960s liquid nitrogen (LN_2) has become the popular tool in cryotherapy.

CRYOGENS

Cryogens are substances which freeze the tissue by withdrawal of heat and cause cryonecrosis **(Table 1)**.

TABLE 1: Different cryogens.

Cryogen	*Cooling temperature*
Ice	0°C
Salt-ice	–20°C
Fluorocarbons	–30°C
Nitrous oxide	–75°C
Carbon dioxide	–20°C (Slush) –79°C (Snow)
Liquid nitrogen	–20°C (Swab) –196°C (Spray/probe)
Dimethyl ether	–24°C

Factors Affecting Freezing

- Proximity and temperature of cryogen
- Tissue conductivity
- Volume
- Water content
- Vascularity of tissue.

  Liquid nitrogen is the most commonly used cryogen.

Advantages of liquid nitrogen:

- Nontoxic
- Easily available
- Cost effective
- Easily stored
- Can be used in malignant skin lesions.

Mechanism of Action of Cryotherapy

Tissue injury is caused by extraction of heat and subsequent freezing of the target tissue.

- Cellular injury is caused by the following:
  - *Ice crystal formation*: Rapid freezing causes micro-crystal formation both within and outside the cell. This causes rupture of cell membrane and damage to cellular organelles respectively.
  - *Osmolarity changes*: It causes cell shrinkage during cooling and rupture of cell membrane during thawing.
  - Thermal shock
  - Denaturation of proteins.
- *Vascular injury*: Local vasoconstriction endothelial damage, vascular stasis, platelet aggregation, microthrombi formation all occur during freezing. Vasodilation occurs during thawing which leads to increased flow of emboli and blockage of small vessels which causes ischemia and necrosis.
- *Immunomodulation*: Cold injury is known to induce apoptosis of tumor cells and also stimulates immune response (cryoimmune response).

Cell type	*Lethal temperature*
Keratinocytes	–20°C to –30°C
Melanocytes	–4°C to –8°C
Dermal connective tissue and fibroblasts	–30°C to –40°C

Lethal Temperature of Different Cells

From above table, we can notice that melanocytes are the first cells to die during cryotherapy, and hence depigmentation is a common side effect following cryotherapy.

INDICATIONS

- *Infections*: Viral warts, molluscum contagiosum
- *Vascular lesions*: Cherry angiomas, hemangiomas, pyogenic granuloma
- *Benign lesions*: Acrochordons or skin tags, keloids, milia, syringomas, myxoid cysts, mucoid cysts, seborrheic keratoses, epidermal nevus, dermatosis papulosa nigra (DPN)
- *Premalignant lesions*: Actinic keratoses, Bowen's disease, actinic cheilitis, leukoplakia, keratoacanthoma
- *Malignant lesions*: Basal cell carcinoma, squamous cell carcinoma in situ, lentigo maligna, lentigo maligna melanoma
- *Miscellaneous*: Cutaneous leishmaniasis, hypertrophic lichen planus, prurigo nodularis

CONTRAINDICATIONS

Absolute Contraindications

- Cold urticaria
- Cryoglobulinemia
- Blood dyscrasias
- Lesions for which histopathology is required
- Lesions with vascular compromise
- Sclerosing BCC

Relative Contraindications

- Collagen vascular disease
- Raynaud's disease
- Multiple myeloma
- Sensory loss at lesional site
- Sensitive areas such as eyelid margins, pretibial area and ala nasi.

CRYOSURGICAL EQUIPMENT

- *Cryopen* ***(Fig. 1)***: This device uses cartridges of nitrous oxide under high pressure and has got different probes through which tissue can be freezed with pinpoint precision.

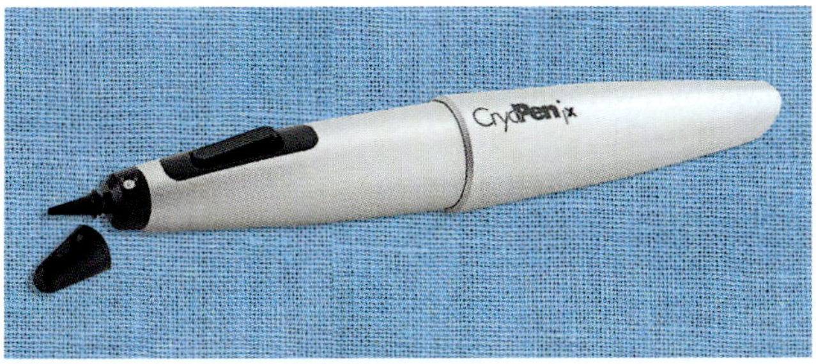

Fig. 1: Cryopen.

- *Cryogun*: CO_2 cylinders are attached to gun, probes, and tubings and can be delivered as slush.
- *Hand-held cryosurgical unit* ***(Fig. 2)***: They are vacuum-assisted LN2 devices and are used in various premalignant and malignant lesions.
- *Table-top cryosurgical unit*: These are compact liquid nitrogen devices which allow fine regulation of volume of spray with gun trigger.
- *Cryoprobes* ***(Fig. 3)***: These are of two types—open-end and closed-end cryoprobes.

Sterilization of all cryosurgical equipment can be done by autoclaving or chemical (2% glutaraldehyde) sterilization.

STEPS IN CRYOTHERAPY

Preprocedure

Photography, written informed consent stating the details of the procedure, complications, post-treatment pain, blistering, and chance of recurrence. Biopsy if needed should be done prior to the procedure.

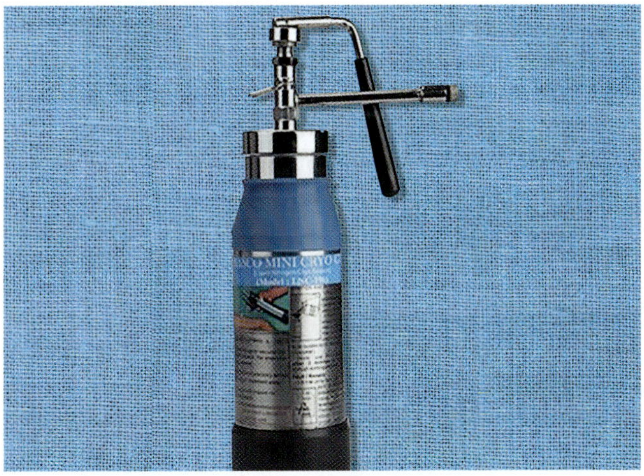

Fig. 2: Hand-held cryosurgical unit.

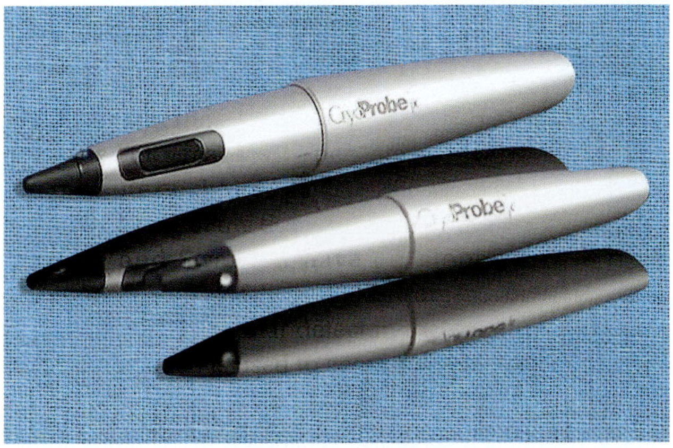

Fig. 3: Cryoprobes.

Procedure

Cryogen	Techniques available
LN2	Dipstick, roller, cryospray, cryoprobe, intralesional
CO_2	Cryoslush, pencil stick, probe
Nitrous oxide	Probe

Methods of Cryotherapy

Cryospray Method

It is also called timed spot-freeze technique and is the most popular method used. In this, cryogen (LN2) is sprayed from a hand-held gun. The nozzle is held at a distance of 1 cm from the surface of the lesion and triggered till uniform layer of ice is formed over the surface of lesion and also a rim of normal tissue around it. This ensures adequate destruction. Spray is continued for optimum period depending on the type of lesion and then allowed to thaw completely. Adequate thawing is confirmed by palpation of the tissue. The spray method can again be divided into four different ways:

1. *Direct freeze/spot freeze method* **(Fig. 4)**: Spray is aimed at the center of the lesion in case of small, discrete, rounded lesions of size <2 cm.
2. *Open spray method*: Used when the larger areas are treated. It is done by paint-brush method, spiral or rotation method.
3. *Confined spray method*: Cryogen is sprayed through cones to restrict the ice field to minimal.
4. *Cryopeel spray technique*: Special acne tips are used to spray LN2 over whole face in the treatment of nodulocystic acne, acne scarring, photo-damaged skin, actinic keratoses, lentigines, and rhytids.

Cryoprobes

In this, LN2 is circulated so as to cool the tip of the probe which is then applied over the lesion. Different types of probes such as flat, pointed, and rounded are available. Precooling of the probe is necessary and conducting gel is used during the procedure. Probe touches the skin through the gel and gently lifted along with the skin to prevent collateral damage to normal tissue. Depth of destruction can be controlled by maintaining the pressure.

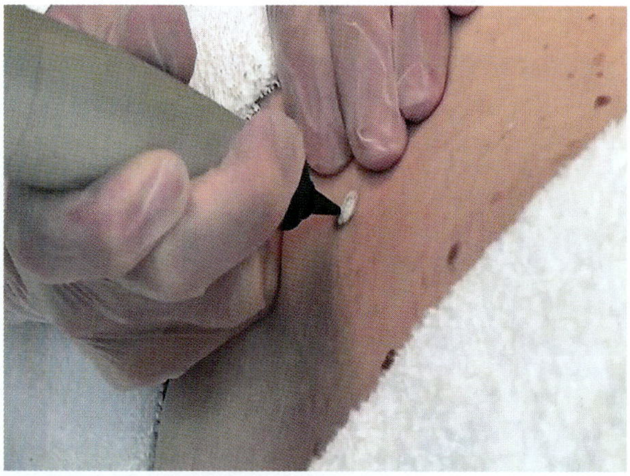

Fig. 4: Treatment of seborrheic keratoses with cryoprobe using spot freeze technique.

Intralesional Technique (Washahy's Technique)

In this injection, needles are passed through the lesion and LN2 is passed through the lumen of needles which cause cryonecrosis. There is no epidermal damage and chances of hyperpigmentation is less. This method is suitable for keloid and hypertrophic scars.

Dipstick Technique

A cotton-tipped applicator is dipped in cryogen and applied with pressure on the target tissue. This technique is inexpensive but less efficacious. Multiple freeze thaw cycles are required.

Cryoroller Technique

A cylindrical roller is dipped in cryogen and applied over the tissue. It is useful in larger lesions.

Forceps/Clamp Technique

A needle holder or hemostat forceps is dipped in liquid nitrogen and the lesion is held at the base for 10–15 seconds. The lesion dies and falls off in a week. It is useful in pedunculated lesions.

Gross Changes Postcryotherapy

After thawing, there is erythema of the lesion within few minutes. In few hours, there is brown or violaceous discoloration at the margins which moves centripetally. There is hemorrhagic blister formation on the surface in and finally eschar is formed and lasts for a few days to weeks.

Postprocedure

Non-steroidal anti-inflammatory drugs (NSAIDs), antibiotics should be given; sterile antibiotic dressing for 48–72 hours. Large blisters if formed should be drained. There is formation of crust which falls off in 1–2 weeks. In case of malignant lesions, they become dry, hard and adherent crust is formed after 10–14 days. In benign lesions, patient is followed up after 10–15 days. In malignant cases, patient is followed weekly till crust falls off, then every 3–6 months for 4–6 years to detect recurrence.

Freeze-thaw cycle (FTC): Time taken for actual freeing of tissue followed by rewarming of the tissue back to room temperature **(Table 2)**.

BENIGN SKIN LESIONS

Warts

Spray technique depending on type, site and size of the wart is recommended. Paring is done in plantar warts before

TABLE 2: Recommended freeze thaw cycle for common conditions.

Type of lesion	*Freeze time in seconds*	*No. of freeze thaw cycles*	*No. of sessions and interval between treatments*
Common warts	15–20	1	1–3 weeks
Plane warts	5–10	1	1–3 weeks
Filiform warts	5–10	1	Usually single session required
Plantar	30–60	2	2–4 weeks
Condyloma acuminata	10	1	1–3 weeks
Molluscum	5–10	1	Single session
Seborrheic keratoses	10–15	1	1 session
Acne cysts and scars	2–7	1	4 weeks
Skin tags	5–10	1	Single treatment
Keloids	20–30	2–31	2–4 weeks
Prurigo nodularis	20–30	1	1–2 weeks
Actinic keratoses		1–2	3
Bowen's disease		1–2	3
SCC, BCC, Lentigo maligna	30–90	2–3	2–4 weeks

cryotherapy and 2–3 freeze cycles are needed. Whereas lower freeze time with single freeze thaw cycle is sufficient in nonplantar warts.

Keloids

They respond well to cryotherapy. Usually single cycle of 20–30 seconds is necessary for effective treatment of keloids. The extent of resolution depends on number of treatment rather than that of duration of freeze-thaw cycles. Can be combined with intralesional steroids for better results.

MALIGNANT SKIN LESIONS

SCC, BCC, and lentigo maligna melanoma can all be treated with cryotherapy. Thermocouple needles are used to monitor the temperature. Border is marked along with 5–10 mm of normal skin around the tumor tissue. Infiltrative anesthesia is given. Cryogen is evenly sprayed on the lesion till the marked border. Freeing is continued till -50°C temperature is reached. Usually freeze time of 30–90 seconds is applied followed by thaw time of 3 minutes. Second cycle of same time is carried out after 3–5 minutes.

COMPLICATIONS OF CRYOTHERAPY

Immediate

- Edema and blistering
- Pain during and after the procedure.
- Hemorrhage
- Syncope
- Headache when lesions are present on head.

Delayed

- Infection
- Delayed wound healing
- Hypertrophic scar or keloid formation
- Pseudoepitheliomatous hyperplasia.

Protracted Complications

- Hypopigmentation
- Atrophy
- Scarring alopecia
- Nerve damage leading to paresthesias
- Ectropion of eyelids.

ADVANTAGES

- Simple outpatient procedure
- High cure rate
- Good cosmesis
- Cost-effective and safe equipment
- Lesions on sites of poor skin mobility can be treated
- Multiple tumors can be treated at same time

DISADVANTAGES

- Pain and burning sensation during the procedure
- Long recovery period
- Complications such as hypopigmentation and scarring
- Need for multiple sessions

RECENT ADVANCES IN CRYOTHERAPY

Cryolipolysis: This is noninvasive method of cold application. It was observed that children who suck a large number of ice candy or "popsicles" developed loss of cheek fat, that was defined as popsicle panniculitis. This principle is used to destroy fat cells in localized areas of fat deposition that do not respond to diet and exercise. The device involves a suction cup that sicks a fold of skin, a coupling medium that is antifreeze membrane that transfers cooling without epidermal damage and inbuilt temperature sensors. It cools the fat in skin fold to -4 to 10°C. This induces natural death of certain fraction of adipocytes by apoptosis. The dead adipocytes are cleared by body's scavenging system. Many studies have shown visible change in body contour and also by ultrasound assessment. Various protocols with different contact time, different target temperature are trying and most of them yield satisfactory results. Addition of manual massage immediately after removal of cryoprobe adds to the efficacy, probably by intracellular ice crystals disrupting adipocyte cell wall. Cryolipolysis is indicated for excess localized fat depositions in waist (love handles), thighs, abdomen, side of the chest (bra-bulges). Maintenance of the shape with strict diet and exercise is indicated along with the treatment without which results are very difficult to achieve.

Cryopen: It is an innovative method of cryosurgery which has been FDA approved in April, 2002. The base unit cools the pens and the pens have disposable and inexpensive nitrous oxide cartridges. When removed from the wells the temperature of the pen reaches approximately -90°C, and it stays at these extreme temperatures and high pressures for approximately 10 minutes. It has different sized applicators and thus can treat lesions ranging from 1 to 10 mm accurately without damaging the surrounding tissue. It can reach to a depth of 2-3 mm. It comes with a temperature indicator. It lights green when ready for use and is at desired temperature and lights red when not ready for use. It can be used in treating keloids, warts, molluscum contagiosum, condyloma acuminata, porokeratoses and lentigines.

KEY POINTS

- Cryotherapy is utilization of cryogens to destruct tissue by cryonecrosis.
- It is useful in treating many benign, premalignant and malignant conditions.
- Melanocytes are the first cells to die during cryotherapy, and hence depigmentation is a common side effect following cryotherapy.
- Cold urticaria, cryoglobulinemia, blood dyscrasias, sclerosing BCC are absolute contraindications for cryotherapy.
- Various methods of cryotherapy are cryospray, cryoprobe, cryopen and cryoroller, dipstick, intralesional and clamp technique.
- Recurrence of keloids can be prevented with combination of intralesional steroids and cryotherapy.
- Edema, pain and hemorrhagic blistering are the immediate complications whereas, scarring, depigmentation, atrophy, paresthesia are delayed and protracted complications.

FURTHER READING

1. Andrews MD. Cryosurgery for common skin conditions. Am Fam Physician. 2004;69(10):2365-72.
2. Bernstein EF. Longitudinal evaluation of cryolipolysis efficacy: two case studies. J Cosmet Dermatol. 2013;12(2):149-52.
3. Blume-Peytavi U, Zouboulis CC, Jacobi H, Scholz A, Bisson S, Orfanos CE. Successful outcome of cryosurgery in patients with granuloma annulare. Br J Dermatol. 1994;130:494-7.
4. Cooper SM, Dawber RPR. The history of cryosurgery. JR Soc Med. 2001;94(4):196-201.
5. Damstra RJ, Van Vloten WA. Cryotherapy in the treatment of condylomata acuminata: a controlled study of 64 patients. J Dermatol Surg Oncol. 1991;17:272-6.
6. Dover J, Burns J, Coleman S, Fitzpatrick R, Garden J, Goldberg D, et al. A prospective clinical study of noninvasive cryolipolysis for subcutaneous fat layer reduction: interim report of available subject data. Lasers Surg Med. 2009;41(S21):43.
7. Ghodsi SZ, Reziei M, Taheri A, Karami M, Mansoor P, Farnaghi F. Comparison of cryotherapy and curettage for the treatment of pyogenic granuloma: a randomized trial. Br J Dermatol. 2006;154(4):671-5.
8. Graham GF. Cryosurgery for benign, premalignant and malignancy lesions. In: Wheeland RG (Ed). Cutaneous Surgery, 1st edition. Philadelphia: WB Saunders; 1994. pp. 835-69.
9. Guan H, Zhao Z, He F, Zhou Q, Meng Q, Zhu X, et al. Cryobiology. 2007;55:52-9.
10. Har-Shai Y, Amar M, Sabo E. Intralesional cryotherapy for enhancing the involution of hypertrophic scars and keloids. Plast Reconstr Surg. 2003;111(6):1841-52.
11. Ranawaka RR, Weerakoon HS, Opathella N. Liquid nitrogen cryotherapy on *Leishmanial donovani* cutaneous leishmaniasis. J Dermatolo Treat. 2011;22(4):241-5.
12. Rusciani L, Rossi G, Bono R. Use of cryotherapy in the treatment of keloids. J Dermatol Surg Oncol. 1993;19(6):529-34.
13. Savant SS. Cryosurgery. In: Textbook of Dermatosurgery and Cosmetology, 3rd edition. Mumbai: Bhalani Publishing House; 2018. pp. 182-202.
14. Sharma VK, Khandpur S. Guidelines for cryotherapy. Indian J Dermatology Venereol Leprol. 2009;75(Suppl 2):90-100.
15. Sheperd JP, Dawber R. Cryosurgery: history and scientific basis. Clin Exp Dermatol. 1982;7:321-8.
16. Sinclair RD, Dawber RP. Cryosurgery of malignant and premalignant diseases of skin: a simple approach. Australas J Dermatol. 1995;36(3):133-42.
17. Torre D. Alternative cryogens for cryosurgery. J Dermatol Surg. 1975;1:156-8.

EXAMINATION QUESTION

1. Write a short note on cryotherapy.

172 CHAPTER

Lasers in Dermatology

Rajat Kandhari, Himanshu Gupta

INTRODUCTION

The term **LASER** is an acronym for **L**ight **A**mplification by **S**timulated **E**mission of **R**adiation. The first laser was invented by TH Maiman in 1959, which was a ruby laser emitting red light with a wavelength of 694 nm,[1] subsequently in 1963, Dr Leon Goldman first used a ruby laser for various dermatological conditions.[2] The next two decades witnessed the emergence of the CO_2 laser and the argon laser, but these were plagued by high rates of scarring. It was not until 1983 that the theory of "selective photothermolysis" was unveiled by R Anderson and JA Parrish, which revolutionized the use of lasers in dermatology. In 2003, the theory of "Fractional photothermolysis" led to further advancement in the field of laser resurfacing.[3]

LASER BASICS

Laser light represents a part of electromagnetic spectrum and has three unique characteristics **(Fig. 1)**:

1. *Monochromaticity*: Lasers emit light of a single wavelength or very narrow band of wavelengths. The wavelength is defined by the lasing medium (e.g., solid, liquid or gas) **(Table 1)**
2. *Coherence*: Laser light waves are in phase with respect to time and space, i.e., the emitted photons are "in step" and have a definite phase relation to each other.
3. *Collimation*: Light waves are parallel, thus laser beam has narrow diameter without any divergence. Even with increasing distance, diameter does not increase. Thus energy of laser light is not lost even after travelling long distances.

TABLE 1: Varying lasing mediums.

Solid	Alexandrite	755 nm
	Er:YAG	2490 nm
	Nd:YAG	1064 nm
	Ruby	694 nm
	Diode	800–810 nm
Liquid	Pulse dye laser	585–595 nm
Gas	Argon	418 nm
	Excimer	308 nm
	CO_2	10,600 nm

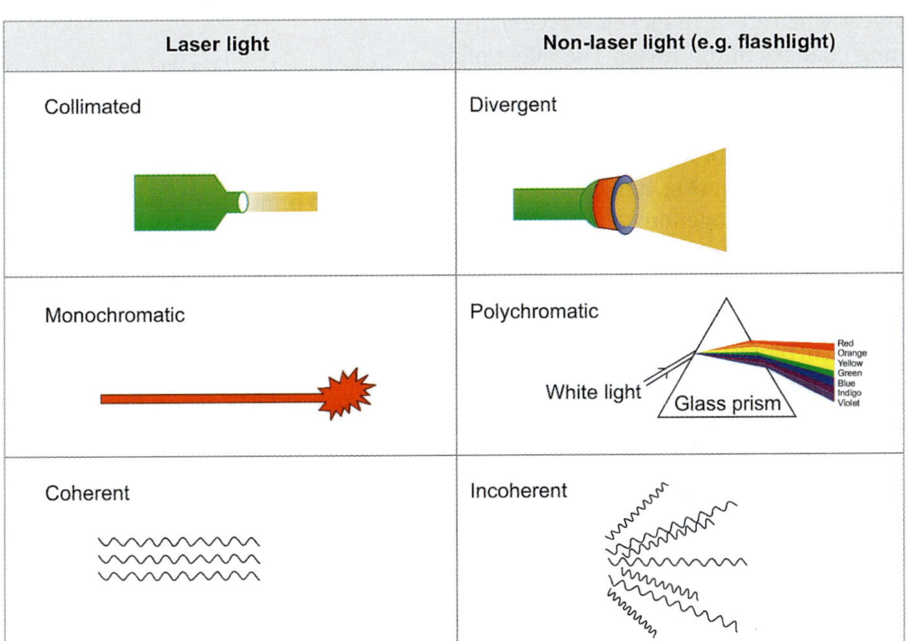

Fig. 1: Unique characteristics of a laser light.

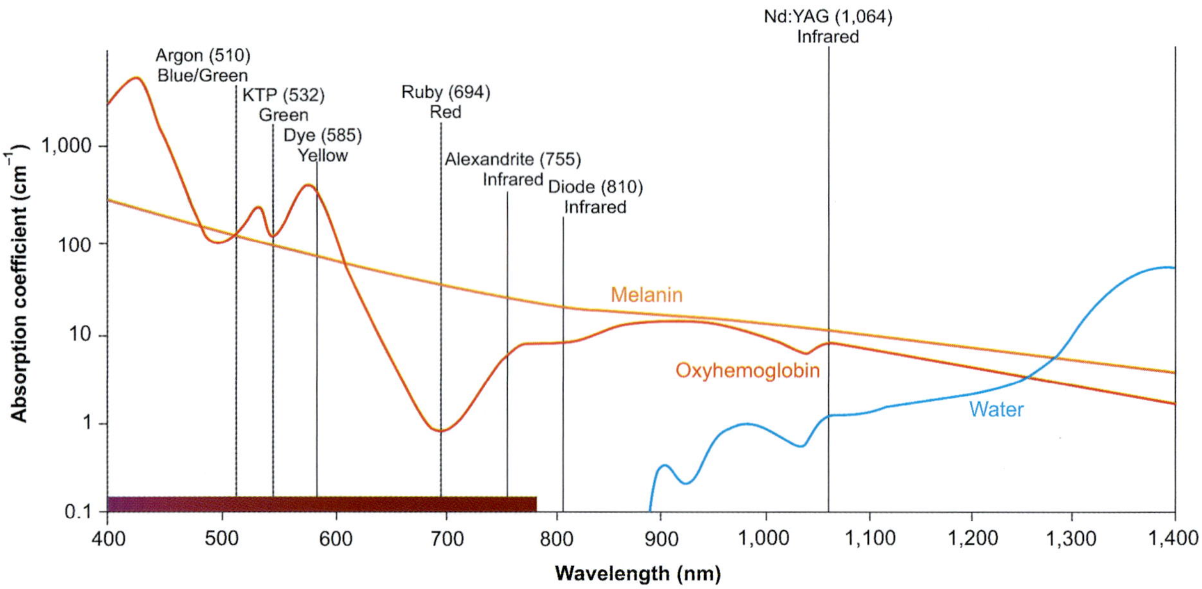

Fig. 2: Absorption spectrum of endogenous chromophores in the skin.*

*The peak absorption of melanin (400–750 nm), hemoglobin (400–600 nm) and water (mid infrared—3000–8000 nm and far infrared—15,000–1000,000 nm).

Nonlaser light sources, e.g., intense pulsed light (IPL) devices generate pulsed polychromatic high intensity light by using flash lamps. An IPL emits light of a wide range of wavelengths usually ranging from 500 to 1300 nm, with in built cut-off filters, which are used to tailor the wavelength as per the indication to be treated or the target structure. IPL devices have pulse durations in the millisecond range and the spot sizes are usually large.

A laser beam incident on skin tissue may be absorbed, reflected, transmitted, or scattered. Further, for a laser to be effective, the light must be absorbed by the tissue, and the amount of light absorbed is chromophore dependent. Chromophores are targets which absorb a specific wavelength of light thereby exerting changes in the tissue. The effect of a laser directly correlates to the wavelength used and the absorptive characteristics of a particular chromophore. The skin has three main endogenous chromophores, in the form of melanin*, oxyhemoglobin and water*, **(Fig. 2)** whereas *tattoo ink* represents an example of an exogenous chromophore. The peak absorption of these chromophores of a particular wavelength dictate their use in a particular indication, e.g., the peak absorption of oxyhemoglobin lies between 400 and 700 nm, which makes treatment of blood vessels with a pulsed dye laser, an appropriate choice. There are three basic effects which may occur subsequent to the absorption of the laser light[3]:

1. *Photothermal*: Absorption of the incident light by a chromophore leading to destruction of the target via conversion of the absorbed energy into heat. This forms the basis of selective photothermolysis, e.g., laser hair reduction.
2. *Photochemical*: Photosensitizer mediated reactions—the light is absorbed by a molecule mediating a reaction for effect, e.g., photodynamic therapy.

TABLE 2: Varying sizes of absorbing chromophores and their thermal relaxation time (TRT).

	Size (in μm)	*TRT (Approx)*
Tattoo ink particle	0.5–4	10 ns
Melanosome	0.5–1	1 μs
Erythrocyte	7	2 μs
Blood vessel	50	1 ms
	100	5 ms
	200	20 ms
Hair follicle	200	10–100 ms

3. *Photomechanical*: Rapid thermal expansion leading to acoustic waves and subsequent photomechanical destruction of the absorbing tissue, e.g., laser tattoo removal, which demonstrates not only photomechanical but also photothermal and photochemical effects.

Chromophores absorb energy and lead to damage of the collateral structures, and this is dependent on the thermal relaxation time (TRT) of a particular chromophore **(Table 2)**. The time taken by the chromophore to lose 50% of its heat after being heated up is known as the TRT. Different chromophores have different TRTs depending upon their size. Moreover, the TRT predicts the pulse width to be used for destruction of a particular target.

LASER PROPERTIES AND PARAMETERS

The different types of lasers include:[3]

- *Continuous wave (CW)*: A constant light beam with long durations of exposure resulting in nonselective tissue injury, e.g., CW CO_2 laser.

- *Quasi-CW*: Segment the continuous wave into interrupted emissions of constant laser energy, e.g. potassium-titanyl-phosphate (KTP).
- *Pulsed lasers*: Emit high energy in ultrashort pulse durations with long intervening time periods (0.1–1 second) between each pulse.
    - *Long-pulsed:* Pulsed dye laser (PDL), 450 s to 40 ms.
    - *Very short-pulsed:* Quality-switched (QS) neodymium (Nd): yttrium-aluminum-garnet (YAG) lasers (5–100 ns)
    - *Superpulsed:* Very short pulses in a repeat pattern to decrease the amount of collateral damage adjacent to the vaporized tissue, e.g., CO_2 lasers.

Laser Terminology and Important Parameters

- *Energy*: Number of photons delivered in a single pulse, measured in Joules (joules = watts × seconds)
- *Fluence* (energy density) = joules/cm^2 = watts × seconds/cm^2
- *Power*: Amount of energy released by laser per unit time watts = joules/second
- *Irradiance* (power density) = watts/cm^2
- *Pulse duration/pulse width*: Time over which energy is actually delivered:
    - Long pulsed laser—Milliseconds
    - Short pulsed laser—Nanoseconds
    - Picosecond laser—Picoseconds
- *Frequency*: Pulse repetition rate (Hertz = pulses per second)
- *Spot size*: Determines the diameter of the laser beam. Fluence (energy density) and irradiance (power density) of the laser is inversely proportional to square of spot size radius. Larger spot size decreases the scattering and thus increases the penetration depth. However, this is not true for microscopic spot sizes, e.g., in fractional resurfacing, spot size of 100 to several hundred micrometers penetrates very deep.
- *Beam profiles*: How the intensity of laser light is distributed across the beam diameter is represented by the beam profile **(Figs. 3A to C)**?
    - *Gaussian profile*: Intensity peaks at center of the diameter. From the center, intensity falls off toward sides with a bell-shaped curve (Gaussian distribution).
    - *Doughnut-shaped*: Intensity is greatest at the edge of the beam diameter. The intensity fluctuates across the beam diameter in a target-shaped manner.
    - *Top hat*: A near-uniform fluence (energy density) within a circular disk. They deliver a more constant intensity across the beam diameter.

PRACTICAL TIPS BEFORE COMMENCING LASER PROCEDURES

Preprocedure:

- Informed consent for the procedure must be taken.
- Preprocedure photographs of the treatment area must be recorded.
- Advise the patient to use a broad-spectrum sunscreen and counsel regarding the importance of preprocedure priming.

Precautions during procedure:

- Use of protective eyewear for the patient and physician.
- Area to be treated must be marked with white skin marker.

CONTRAINDICATIONS FOR LASER TREATMENT

Although the contraindication may vary for certain lasers for simplicity a table comprising common contraindications for all laser treatment with appropriate comments has been illustrated in **Box 1**.

LASER HAIR REMOVAL

Laser hair reduction (LHR) is probably the one of the most vastly carried out cosmetic procedures worldwide. LHR achieved US-FDA approval in 1995, and the definition of *"permanent hair removal"* coined by the US-FDA is "A significant reduction in the number of terminal hairs after a given treatment, which is stable for a period of time longer

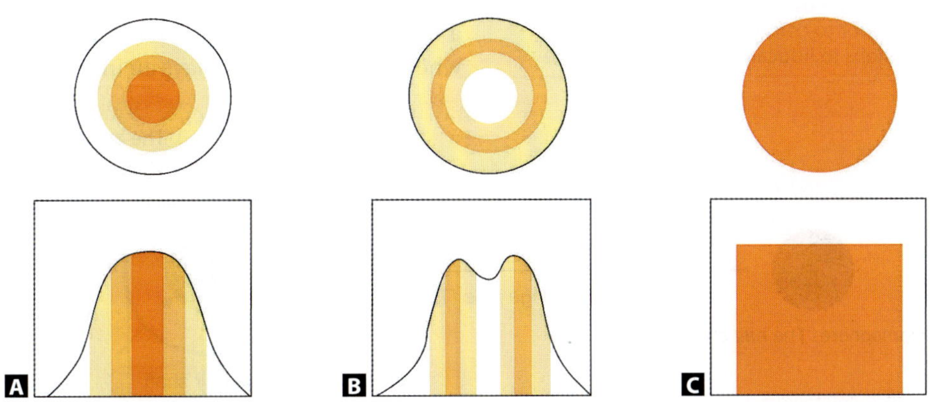

Figs. 3A to C: Differing beam profiles of laser lights. (A) Gaussian; (B) Doughnut-shaped; (C) Top hat.

than the complete growth cycle of hair follicles at the given body site."[4]

Mechanism

Laser hair reduction works on the principle of selective photothermolysis with melanin as the primary chromophore. Increased understanding in the domain of LHR in recent years suggests the importance of the follicular stem cells in the bulge area of the outer root sheath (ORS), which appears to be the target for LHR. This observation led to the concept of "extended selective photothermolysis" wherein there is diffusion of heat from the primary chromophore (melanin in the hair shaft) to the actual target (follicular stem cells in the ORS) by heat diffusion from melanin in the hair shaft **(Fig. 4)**. This also unveiled the term "thermal damage time," which appears to be the time required for the heat to propagate from the primary chromophore to the actual target.[4]

BOX 1: Contraindications for laser procedures.

Contraindications (appropriate comments)

Absolute contraindications:
- Unrealistic expectations
- Active HSV infection/bacterial or fungal infections at treatment site
- Pregnancy and lactation
- Appendageal abnormality (particularly for ablative fractional resurfacing for large areas)
- Open wounds

Relative contraindications:
- History of keloids or scarring ("test area" is recommended)
- Skin grafts, deep chemical peels or deep dermabrasion (particularly for ablative fractional resurfacing or traditional ablative resurfacing)
- Active collagen vascular disease
- Pigmented lesions such as moles/freckles/lentigines/tattoo's must be avoided (crucial during laser hair reduction)
- Excessively dry, irritated or sensitive skin (*moisturize the skin, reassess the skin and be cautious in your approach*)
- History of epilepsy
- Use of photosensitizing drugs
- History of herpes simplex (consider oral antiviral prophylaxis)
- Using high fluences on patients with low pain threshold (consider topical or local anesthesia and/or oral analgesics prior to treatment)
- Patients with higher phototypes (use low densities in fractional lasers and low fluences in laser hair reduction/pigment lasers and consider "test area" prior to commencing treatment)
- Patients with drug reactions to lidocaine/tetracaine mixture

The theory of extended selective photothermolysis has resulted in treatments with low fluences and repetitive millisecond pulses which achieve heat stacking in the hair bulb and bulge (ORS, with stem cells). This model works on not using melanin as a chromophore but helps heat the subdermal layer of the skin. Low fluences and repetitive pulse treatments are considered equally efficacious to traditional stamping modalities with lesser pain.[5] The various lasers and lights used for LHR have been enumerated **(Table 3)**.

Indications

Laser hair reduction is no longer considered restricted to hair removal on the face or body. The various indications for LHR have been enumerated in **Table 4**.

Practical Tips for LHR

- Advise the patient to avoid waxing, bleaching or plucking prior to treatment.
- Adhesive tape/saline-soaked gauze may be used to remove loose hairs after shaving.
- One may consider the addition of topical eflornithine, (hirsutism and pseudofolliculitis barbae) spironolactone and/or combined OCPS (confirmed cases of hirsutism) for enhancing outcomes.[6]
- There is no specific data regarding the precise age for LHR. After taking all factors into consideration, the Indian Task Force recommends that laser hair removal may be performed above 15 years of age. In the authors, experience if the benefits outweigh the risk or the procedure is undertaken to improve the quality of life of an individual it may be performed earlier with due consent of the parents or legal guardians and the opinion of an endocrinologist.[7]

Complications of LHR

With the advent of new technology complications with LHR are usually mild provided the procedure is carried out by a skilled professional. The side effects with LHR have been enumerated **(Table 5)**.

LHR is here to stay and although the patients' desire for a persistent solution for their unwanted hair is understandable, a cautious approach to persistent hair removal is prudent, wherein "counseling" plays an important role.

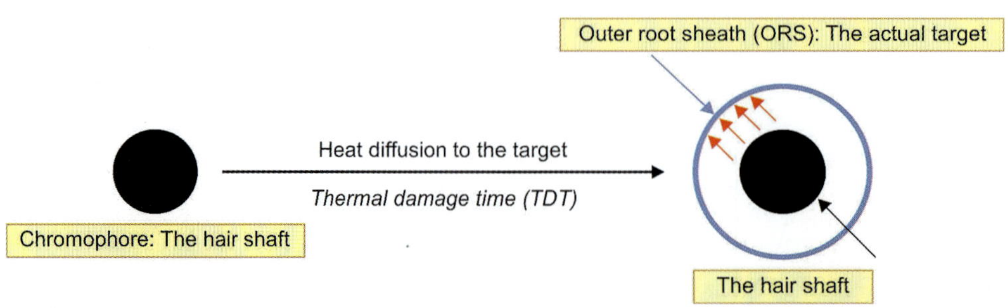

Fig. 4: Theory of extended selective photothermolysis and thermal damage time (TDT).

TABLE 3: Lasers and lights for laser hair reduction.

Lasers/Light source	*Comment*
Long pulsed Ruby (694 nm)	Not widely used in India due to short wavelength and heightened melanin absorption
Long pulsed Nd:YAG (1064 nm)	Good for darker skin types, deep penetration and lower melanin absorption, good for thick hair
Long pulsed Alexandrite (755 nm)	Powerful melanin absorption, good for thin and superficial hair. Practice caution in darker phototypes
Long pulsed diode (810 nm)	Considered the gold standard for LHR in India. Moderate melanin absorption and deep penetration (bulge and bulb) makes it an ideal choice **(Fig. 5)**
Dual wavelengths (1064 nm/755 nm)	*Limited data:* The synergy of two wavelengths claims to offer improved safety and less pain
Triple wavelengths (1064 nm/755 nm/ 810 nm)	Limited data
Q-switched Nd: YAG	Used rarely, helps in LHR for very fine hair
IPL	Nonselective, tough to cover larger body areas

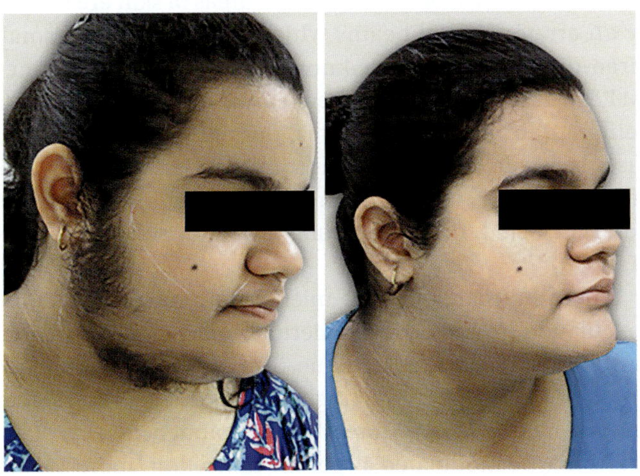

Fig. 5: Laser hair reduction via diode laser (810 nm).

TABLE 4: Indications of LHR.

Common/Cosmetic	*Uncommon/Therapeutic*
Females (hirsutism/ hypertrichosis) • Face (neck, upper lip, chin, cheeks, side locks, uni-brow) • Underarms • Lower limbs • Abdomen • Upper body—back, arms, chest • Full body hair reduction	• Pseudofolliculitis (beard area/neck) • Pilonidal sinus • Acne keloidalis nuchae • Hidradenitis suppurativa • Becker's nevus • Keloids on the sternum • Sex change operations Hypertrichosis post-topical corticosteroid abuse/ cyclosporine usage • Reconstructive myocutaneous flaps
Males • Beard shaping • Upper body • Ear • Uni-brow • Back	

TABLE 5: Side effects of LHR.

Common
Mild • Pain, transient erythema and perifollicular edema. These are not side effects in the true sense as some pain is essential as a temperature of up to 60–70 °C is required to heat the bulge region of the hair follicle. Moreover, erythema and perifollicular edema are desirable end points of LHR • Induction or aggravation of acne **Severe** Thermal burns **(Fig. 6)**, blisters, hyperpigmentation, persistent hypopigmentation, and permanent scarring can also occur—common in cases with use of high fluences and higher phototypes
Uncommon
• Paradoxical hypertrichosis—use of suboptimal fluences leading to subtherapeutic injury to the follicle may result in the release of factors that alter follicular angiogenesis and influence hair cycling—common in jawline in women and back/shoulders in males (personal observation) • Inflammatory and pigmentary changes of pre-existing nevi • Prolonged diffuse redness and edema of the face
Very uncommon
Rosacea-like rash, premature graying of hair, tunneling of hair[8]

PIGMENT-SPECIFIC LASERS

Treatment of a variety of pigmentary lesions **(Table 6)** is carried out with melanin specific, high energy, and Q-switched lasers.

Mechanism of Pigment-specific Lasers

Q-switched laser systems work on the principle of selective photothermolysis, which induces damage in the form of necrosis confined to the melanosomes, thereby preventing damage to the surrounding structures. Selective photothermolysis is largely dependent upon two main parameters:

1. *Wavelength*: This should match the absorption spectrum of the pigment with minimal absorption by hemoglobin and melanin. This is particularly crucial while treating tattoos as different colors of the tattoo will require different wavelengths for optimal outcomes **(Table 7)**.
2. *Pulse duration*: This should be shorter than TRT of the pigment. Pulse width of Q-switched lasers is in the nanoseconds range.

The mechanism of tattoo removal has been elaborated in **Flowchart 1**. In recent years, our understanding of mechanism

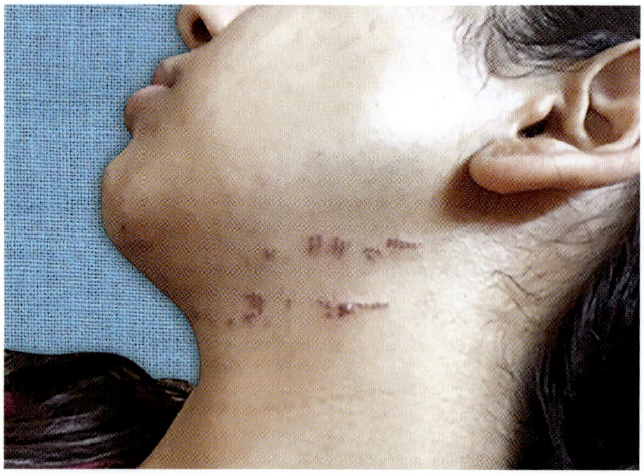

Fig. 6: Thermal burns around the jawline secondary to laser hair reduction.

TABLE 6: Indications where pigment specific lasers are used.

Epidermal lesions	Solar lentigines, ephelides, café-au-lait macules, and seborrheic keratoses
Dermal and mixed epidermal/dermal lesions	• Melanocytic nevi, blue nevi, nevi of Ota/Ito, infraorbital hyper-pigmentation, drug-induced hyperpigmentation, Becker's nevi, and nevus spilus • Melasma (Laser toning, use with caution, recurrence is common) • Rejuvenation (laser toning with laser genesis, carbon peeling)
Tattoo	• Amateur and professional tattoos
Laser hair removal	• Photomechanical effect on the hair shaft—good for fine hair and causing a delay in the hair growth cycle
Vascular lesions	• Rarely used for indications such as telangiectasias, cherry angiomas and small spider nevi
Dark lips[9]	• Q-switched Nd:YAG 532 nm has shown promise.

TABLE 7: Wavelength used according to tattoo pigment.

Q-switched lasers	*Wavelength (nm)*	*Pulse duration (ns)*	*Tattoo pigment*
Frequency doubled Nd:YAG	532	5–10	Red
Ruby	694	25–40	Blue, black, green
Alexandrite	755	50–100	Blue, black, green
Nd:YAG	1064	5–10	Blue, black

of Q-switched lasers working in melasma has grown by leaps and bounds. Data reveal that low fluence (1.6–3.5 J/cm^2), large spot size (6–8 mm), and treatment with multiple passes, performed in 5–10 sessions at weekly to monthly intervals are safe and effective in treating refractory melasma. The "low-dose" QS Nd:YAG laser theoretically causes melanin granule fragmentation with minimal thermal damage, and has been popularly referred to as *laser toning*. This treatment should be regarded as an effective method for treating melasma through subcellular-selective photothermolysis, i.e., a decrease in melanocytic dendrites occurred because of the thermolytic effect of the laser on melasma. [10,11]

Complications of Pigment-specific Lasers

Although, the commonly encountered complications are transient and do not require termination of treatment, few complications would warrant modification of treatment parameters or termination of treatment. These have been elaborated in **Table 8**.

FRACTIONAL LASERS

It was in 2003, that the concept of "Fractional Photothermolysis (FP)" was unveiled, subsequent to which Manstein et al. introduced their prototype FP device.[12]

Mechanism of Fractional Photothermolysis

Fractional photothermolysis capitalizes on the concept of tissue sparing, i.e., only microscopic areas of skin are treated by an array of small beams which creates multiple small three-dimensional zones known as microthermal zones (MTZs). The chromophore here is tissue water with targets being epidermal keratinocytes, dermal collagen, dermal vascular structures and sebaceous glands. About 25–50% of the surface is treated at one time leaving the rest of the skin unaffected, unlike the bulk heating of ablative devices **(Table 9)**.[13]

Microthermal zones are microscopic zones of thermal coagulation characterized by dermal collagen denaturation, surrounded by unharmed tissue. Size of each MTZ depends on pulse energy per MTZ (higher the pulse energy, deeper and wider is the MTZ). Moreover, the treatment density of the MTZs maybe modulated as per the indication (more MTZs/cm^2 in one pass result in lesser intervening normal tissue, and hence more social and clinical downtime).

The formation of these MTZs further leads to[14]:

- *MENDs (Micro-Epidermal Necrotic Debris)*: Accumulation of button-shaped necrotic debris below the intact stratum corneum over each MTZ which forms after treatment. MENDs are removed by transepidermal elimination process, removing coagulated tissue of epidermal and dermal origin.
- *TGF-beta release by inflammatory cells around the MTZs*: Increases the synthesis of fibronectin, collagen, myofibroblast transformation, angiogenesis, the heat shock response.

Flowchart 1: Mechanism of tattoo pigment via Q-switched lasers.

Due to *photothermal effect*, pigment particle undergoes thermal expansion

↓

Acoustic shock waves are generated, audible as popping sound with each pulse *(photoacoustic effect)*

↓

Tensile strength of shock waves is greater than the fracture threshold of the tattoo pigment, leading to fragmentation of the particles

↓

Gas bubbles formed at fast rate under unstable pressure conditions can undergo cavitation further fracturing the tattoo pigment *(photochemical effect)*

↓

High temperatures cause rapid vaporization of water leading to formation of gas bubbles, this leads to epidermis turning white after the laser pulse

↓

In days to weeks, acute inflammatory infiltrate (sequestering phagocytes) surrounds the pigment and debris from fragmented cells resulting in clearing of fragmented pigment

↓

Free pigment is intracellular again within approximately 4 weeks, thus sitting can be repeated at an interval

TABLE 8: Complications associated with the use of pigment-specific lasers.

Transient complications	• Immediate erythema • Physical urticaria • Acneiform eruption • Minute petechiae • Whitening of fine hair • Rebound hyperpigmentation
Complications warranting termination of treatment	• Mottled hypo- and hyperpigmentation • Leukoderma • Severe urticaria • Severe acneiform eruption • Herpes simplex activation • Scarring and keloids **(Fig. 7)**

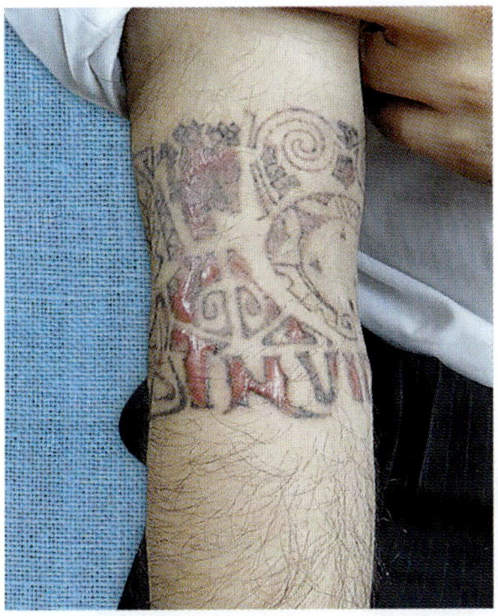

Fig. 7: Keloidal scarring post Q-switched Nd:YAG treatment for tattoo.

- *Increased heat shock protein expression*: Increased procollagen and collagen I and III deposition.

TABLE 9: Traditional ablative resurfacing vs fractional resurfacing.

	Ablative resurfacing	*Fractional resurfacing*
Epidermal repair/ thermal damage	Re-epithelialization is delayed—long migratory path lengths for keratinocytes.	Epidermal repair is fast due to microscopically small volumes of thermal damage (MTZs)
S. Corneum intact	No (epidermal vaporization and coagulation of underlying dermis)	Yes (NAFR)/No (AFR)
Clinical downtime	Upto 1 week	None, 48 hours
Social downtime	Upto 1 month	1–5 days

(AFR: ablative fractional resurfacing; NAFR: nonablative fractional resurfacing)

TABLE 10: Chronological events after FP treatment: Histopathology.

Number of days	*Chronological event*
1 day	MEND is formed
3 days	Complete re-epithelialization
5 days	MEND entirely within stratum corneum
1 month	Complete MEND exfoliation
3 months	Complete replacement of MTZs by new collagen formation

- *Increased matrix metalloproteinase inhibitor expression and photothermolysis of the scar microvasculature.*

All the afore-mentioned factors lead to a continued dermal remodeling. The chronological histological event after a single FP session have been elaborated in **Table 10**.

Types

- *Ablative fractional lasers:*
  - Fractional CO_2 (10,600 nm)
  - Fractional erbium: YAG (2940 nm)
- *Nonablative fractional lasers:*
  - Fractional erbium glass 1540 nm, 1550 nm
  - Fractional erbium fiber 1565 nm
  - Fractional thulium fiber 1927 nm

Indications

The indications of fractional lasers have been delineated in **Table 11**.

Complications

Complications with the use of fractional lasers have been enumerated **(Table 12)**. It was earlier believed that the rate of complications, particularly scarring maybe increased while using fractional technology in patients on isotretinoin. Although recent data demonstrates that performing dermatosurgical and laser procedures in patients receiving or recently received isotretinoin is safe.

VASCULAR LASERS

The use of vascular-specific lasers has been limited in the Indian subcontinent due to fear of complications owing to the superficial penetration of these lasers and the absorption by melanin, which acts a competing chromophore particularly in higher phototypes.

These systems work on the principle of selective photothermolysis and target intravascular oxyhemoglobin to effect destruction of various congenital and acquired vascular lesions. The absorption peaks for oxyhemoglobin are within 418, 542, and 577 nm. The flashlamp-pumped PDL (585 nm) revolutionized the treatment of vascular lesions and is now available in differing wavelengths (590, 595, and 600 nm) and longer pulse durations to allow deep penetration and safe and effective use in darker skin tones. The indications which can be addressed by the PDL have been briefly enumerated **(Box 2)**.

TABLE 11: Indications of fractional lasers.

Category	*Indications*	*Level of evidence*	*Comments*
Aesthetic	Photoaging, periorbital wrinkles	B	Efficacy and safety well established
	Acne scarring **(Fig. 8)**	B	
	Post burn and surgical scars	C	Moderate benefit—fractional ablative lasers—better results
	Stretch marks	C	Moderate benefit, counseling required, photography challenging, requires learning. NAFR is currently considered first line treatment for stretch marks.[15]
	Melasma, PIH, nevus of Ota, poikiloderma of civatte, other dyschromias	C	Routine use not recommended, few studies show benefit, relapse is a rule
	Residual hemangiomas	C	Few reports, more data required
Nonaesthetic	Granuloma annulare, colloid milium, DSAP, etc.	C	Isolated case reports, use at your own discretion.

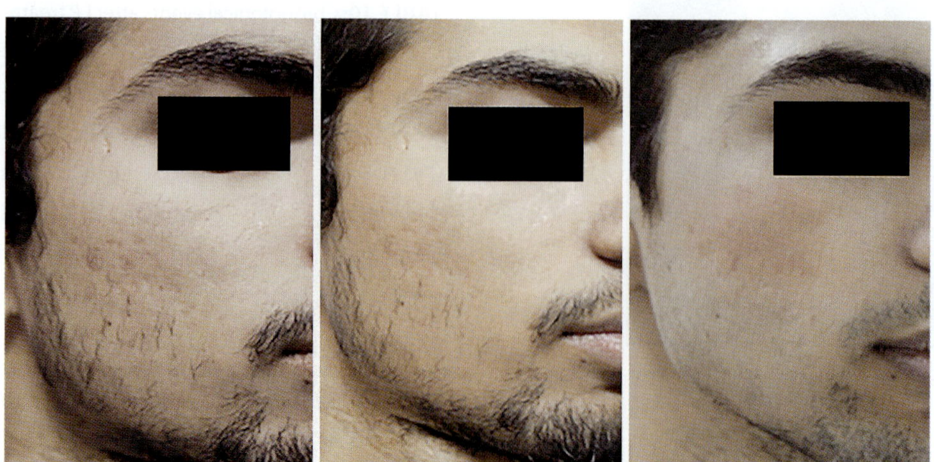

Fig. 8: Treatment with nonablative fractional erbium glass 1540 nm laser (2 sessions) combined with erbium fiber 1565 nm laser (2 sessions).

TABLE 12: Complications associated with fractional laser use.

Common	*Uncommon*	*Rare*
Erythema	Prolonged erythema (more than 4 days for NAFR)	Dermatitis
Edema and crusting	Prolonged edema (longer than 2 days for NAFR)	Impetigo
Acneiform eruptions	Postinflammatory hyperpigmentation (PIH)—transient/rarely persistent	Purpura
	HSV outbreaks	Scarring
	Superficial erosions	Ectropion

BOX 2: Indications addressed by vascular specific lasers.

Commonly treated conditions:
- *Benign congenital and acquired vascular lesions:* Port-wine stains, facial telangiectases, hemangiomas, pyogenic granulomas, Kaposi's sarcoma
- *Hypertrophic and keloid scars*
- *Striae distensae (striae rubra)*

Less commonly treated conditions:
Poikiloderma of Civatte, warts, angiofibromas, lymphangiomas, Goltz's syndrome, inflammatory linear verrucous epidermal nevus, eccrine hidrocystoma, lupus pernio, lupus erythematosis, morphea, granuloma faciale, necrobiosis lipoidica diabeticorum, elastosis perforans serpiginosa, sebaceous gland hyperplasia, and molluscum contagiosum

KEY POINTS

- In selective photothermolysis, the therapeutic response is primarily adjusted by wavelength, fluence, and pulse duration, whereas in fractional photothermolysis the therapeutic response is adjusted by MTZ shape, density, depth, and pattern.
- The depth is the variable factor that plays a predominant role in fractional laser efficacy—the type/depth of the scar will dictate your settings, e.g., rolling and superficial boxcar scars responded the best while ice-pick scars are less amenable to fractional technology, hence combining treatments is prudent.
- Appropriate selection of wavelength, pulse duration, and fluence are important in optimizing the hair removal—higher fluences are associated with greater permanent hair removal in practice.

REFERENCES

1. Maiman T. Stimulated optical radiation in ruby. Nature. 1960;187(4736):493-4.
2. Goldman L, Blaney DJ, Kindel DJ, Franke EK. Effect of the laser beam on the skin. J Invest Dermatol. 1963;40(121):2.
3. Tanzi EL, Lupton JR, Alster TS. Lasers in dermatology: four decades of progress. J Am Acad Dermatol. 2003;49(1):1-34.
4. Dierickx C. Laser-assisted hair removal: state-of-the-art. Dermatol Ther. 2000;13(1):80-9.
5. Pai GS, Bhat PS, Mallya H, Gold M. Safety and efficacy of low-fluence, high-repetition rate versus high-fluence, low-repetition rate 810-nm diode laser for permanent hair removal: a split-face comparison study. J Cosmet Laser Ther. 2011;13(4):134-7.
6. Weaver III SM, Sagaral EC. Treatment of pseudofolliculitis barbae using the long-pulse Nd: YAG laser on skin types V and VI. Dermatol Surg. 2003;29(12):1187-91.
7. Buddhadev RM. Standard guidelines of care: laser and IPL hair reduction. Indian J Dermatol Venereol Leprol. 2008;74(Suppl S1):68-74.
8. Nisar MS, Lloyd JR, Khan T. Laser hair removal put in the wrong hands. Dermatol Surg. 2013;39(3 pt1):480-2.
9. Kunachak S, Kunachakr S, Kunachakr S, Leelaudomlipi P, Wongwaisayawan S. An effective treatment of dark lip by frequency-doubled Q-switched Nd: YAG laser. Dermatol Surg. 2001;27(1):37-40.
10. Mun JY, Jeong SY, Kim JH, Han SS, Kim IH. A low fluence Q-switched Nd: YAG laser modifies the 3D structure of melanocyte and ultrastructure of melanosome by subcellular-selective photothermolysis. J Electron Microsc. 2010;60(1):11-8.
11. Hofbauer CP, Careta MF, Valente NY, Torezan LA. Clinical and histopathologic assessment of facial melasma after low-fluence Q-switched neodymium-doped: yttrium aluminium garnet laser. Dermatol Surg. 2016;42(4):507-12.
12. Manstein D, Herron GS, Sink RK, Tanner H, Anderson RR. Fractional photothermolysis: a new concept for cutaneous remodeling using microscopic patterns of thermal injury. Lasers Surg Med. 2004;34(5):426-38.
13. Laubach HJ, Tannous Z, Anderson RR, Manstein D. Skin responses to fractional photothermolysis. Lasers Surg Med. 2006;38(2):142-9.
14. Ross NA, Ho D, Fisher J, Mamalis A, Heilman E, Saedi N, et al. Striae distensae: preventative and therapeutic modalities to improve aesthetic appearance. Dermatol Surg. 2017;43(5):635-48.
15. Mahadevappa OH, Mysore V, Viswanath V, Thurakkal S, Majid I, Talwar S, et al. Surgical outcome in patients taking concomitant or recent intake of oral isotretinoin: a multicentric study—ISO-AIMS study. J Cutaneous Aesthetic Surg. 2016;9(2):106.

EXAMINATION QUESTIONS

1. Write a short note on laser in dermatology.
2. Write the principle of laser hair reduction (LHR) and types of lasers used in LHR.
3. Write a short note on selective photothermolysis.
4. Discuss lasers used in pigmentary disorders.
5. Discuss lasers used in removal of tattoos.
6. Discuss lasers used in various vascular disorders.
7. What are the recent advances in laser management of acne and rosacea.

173 CHAPTER Sclerotherapy

S Sacchidanand, Sujala Sacchidanand Aradhya

INTRODUCTION

Sclerotherapy is the targeted elimination of small vessels, varicose veins, and vascular anomalies by the injection of a sclerosant.[1] Aim of sclerotherapy is to damage the vessel wall and transform it into a fibrous cord that cannot be recanalized.[1] This is a simple, quick, efficacious, cost-effective, and esthetically acceptable modality for both therapeutic and esthetic conditions associated with a varicose vein.

MECHANISM OF ACTION

A sclerosant causes damage to the endothelium of vessels and possibly of entire vascular wall. Subsequently, a secondary, local thrombus attached to vessel wall is generated and the vessel is transformed into a fibrous cord.[1] Rather than merely thrombosing a vessel that may be amenable to recanalization, sclerosing a vessel transforms it into a fibrous cord, which cannot be recanalized.[2]

INDICATIONS[1]

The indications of sclerotherapy are given in **Table 1**.

CONTRAINDICATIONS[1]

The contraindications of sclerotherapy are described in **Table 2**.

TABLE 1: Indications and level of evidence of sclerotherapy.

Indications	*Level of evidence*
Varicose veins: Truncal veins, major tributaries of greater and lesser saphenous veins, lateral venous system varicosities, collateral veins' varicose veins associated with incompetent perforating veins, reticular veins, residual and recurrent varicose veins, complications such as stasis dermatitis and venous ulcers	Level A
Vascular malformations: Low-flow lesions (venous or lymphatic malformations), rapidly growing or noninvoluting hemangiomas	Level A
Benign vascular tumors: Angiolymphoid hyperplasia with eosinophilia	Level C
Others: Pyogenic granuloma, mucous cysts, sebaceous cysts, venous lakes	Level C
Esthetic indications: Telangiectasias, spider veins, reticular veins	Level A

Sclerotherapy is contraindicated in an immobile patient because ambulation postprocedure is important to minimize risks of thrombosis. While in diabetes and edema, there is compromised circulation and prolonged healing.[3]

SCLEROSANTS[2]

The characteristics of sclerosants are explained in **Table 3**.

Comparison of Sclerosants[2,4]

The comparison of sclerosants is shown in **Table 4**.

PREPROCEDURE WORKUP[5]

History

- General condition, physical activity, pregnancy, use of hormone replacement therapy or oral contraceptive pills (OCPs), smoking, intake of alcohol, and comorbidities should be recorded.
- Nonsteroidal anti-inflammatory drugs (NSAIDs) or anticoagulants must be stopped 1 week prior.

TABLE 2: Absolute and relative contraindications of sclerotherapy.

Absolute contraindications	*Relative contraindications*
• Acute superficial or DVT • Local infection in treatment area or generalized infection • Immobility • Advanced peripheral arterial occlusive disease (stage 3 or 4) • High flow lesions such as AV fistula and large varicose vein with incompetent saphenofemoral junction • Hyperthyroidism (sclerosant containing iodine) • Pregnancy in first trimester and after 36th week of gestation • Known allergy to sclerosant • Severe systemic disease	• Flat port-wine stains • Saphenofemoral junction incompetence • Thrombophilia; history of DVT • Leg edema • Diabetes • Peripheral arterial occlusive disease stage 2 • Poor general health • Myocardial decompensation • Migraine • Bronchial asthma • Marked allergic diathesis • Known hypercoagulability

(AV: arteriovenous; DVT: deep vein thrombosis)

TABLE 3: Characteristics of detergents, osmotic agents, and chemical irritants (sclerosants).

Detergents	*Osmotic agents*	*Chemical irritants*
Act by *protein theft mechanism,* they cause vascular injury by altering the surface tension (by loss of cell surface lipids) and disrupting endothelial cells • Sodium tetradecyl sulfate (STS) • Polidocanol (POL) • Sodium morrhuate • Ethanolamine oleate	Cause endothelial cell damage through an osmotic gradient created by *dehydration* • Hypertonic sodium chloride solution 23.4% • 10% sodium chloride with 5% dextrose solution	Cause endothelial cell damage by their *direct corrosive action* • Chromated glycerin • Polyiodinated iodine • Alcoholic solution of zein • OK-432 (Picibanil) • Bleomycin

- Results of any previous treatments and whether the primary or recurrent lesion is being treated must be noted.

Examination

- Physical examination to assess evidence of stasis dermatitis, stasis ulcer, examination of venous system to determine types of varicosity and status of perforators.
- Check for previous deep vein thrombosis (DVT) and arterial pulses.
- *Vascular malformation:* Check extent of malformation, pulsations and bruit.

Investigations

- CBC, BT, CT, RBS, and ECG
- Venous color Doppler scans of venous system for location and patency of perforators.

TABLE 4: Comparison of sclerosants.

Sclerosing solution	*Brand names*	*FDA approval*	*Vessel treated*	*Concentrations*	*Maximum volume/dose of sclerosant*	*Advantages*	*Disadvantages*
Sodium tetradecyl sulfate	Setrol, Sotradecol, Fibro-vein	1946	All sizes	*0.1–0.2%:* Telangiectasias *0.2–0.5%:* Reticular *0.5–1.0%:* Varicose *1.0–3.0%:* Axial varicose	10 mL of 3%	Minimal pain, unless injected extravascularly	Necrosis occasionally (at >1%), anaphylaxis (0.1–0.3% cases), moderate risk of pigmentation
Polidocanol	Asklerol, Asclera®, Eth-oxysclerol	2010	Small to medium	*0.25–0.5%:* Telangiectasias *0.5–1.0%:* Reticular *1.0–3.0%:* Varicose	20 mL of 3% Not to exceed 2 mg/kg	Minimal pain, necrosis rarely, low risk of pigmentation even at high concentrations	Anaphylaxis (0.2% cases)
Sodium morrhuate	Scleromate	1930	Small	*Undiluted:* Telangiectasias *Undiluted:* Reticular	10 mL of 5%	Moderate pain, moderate risk of pigmentation	Necrosis frequently, allergic reactions and anaphylaxis (10% cases, highest reported)
Hypertonic saline 23.4% (NaCl)	Hypertonic saline	Off-label, used for esophageal varices only	Small	*23.4–11.7%:* Telangiectasias *23.4%:* Reticular	20 mL Restrict volume in salt restricted diets	No allergic reactions, low risk of pigmentation	Painful, muscle cramps, significantly ulcerogenic if extravasated
10% saline + 5% dextrose	Sclerodex	No	Small	*Undiluted:* Telangiectasias *Undiluted:* Reticular	20 mL	Low risk of pigmentation and allergic reaction	Painful, significantly ulcerogenic if extravasated
Chromated glycerin	Chromex, Scleremo	No	Smallest	*Undiluted:* Telangiectasias	10 mL	Moderate risk of pain, necrosis rarely, low risk of pigmentation, allergic reaction rarely	Very weak sclerosant
Polyiodinated iodine	Varigloban, Variglobin, Sclerodine	No	Largest	1–2%, for up to 5 mm veins 2–6%, for the largest veins	3 mL of 6%	Necrosis occasionally, low risk of pigmentation	Painful, avoid use in iodine allergy and renal insufficiency

- Arterial Doppler studies, if necessary
- Doppler study in vascular malformations to indicate flow of lesion; CT scan, or preferably MRI to assess extent and depth of malformation.

Counseling

Counseling includes number of sessions needed, duration of procedure, limitations of activity after sessions, need for compression therapy, potential adverse events, and expected results.

Documentation of Case

- Specific informed consent, always
- Pre- and postoperative photographs
- Operative record should include the type, concentration, and volume of sclerosant used and anatomical site treated.
- Complications during procedure must be noted **(Fig. 1)**.

PROCEDURE

Techniques[5,6]

The method used to inject a sclerosant basically depends on the size of vein to be treated.

- *Fegan's technique:*
  - Patient sits at end of bed with leg in dependent position and varicosities are marked.
  - Varicosity is cannulized with a needle attached to syringe filled with sclerosant.
  - Leg is elevated above cardiac level for 2 minutes.
  - Blood is drawn into syringe to ensure needle remained in vein's lumen **(Fig. 2)**.
  - Inject 0.5–1.0 mL sclerosant per site
  - Immediately apply firm pressure above and below site of injection for 1 minute, to confine sclerosant to affected site.
  - Next apply compression with a foam pad secured by elastic tape.
  - Particularly effective for incompetent perforators (mark their sites during venous Doppler study).
- *Sigg's technique*: Preferred for sclerosing saphenous junctions. An open needle (not attached to syringe) is inserted into the skin and manipulated until blood drips from hub, then sclerosant is injected.
- *Reticular veins*:
  - Fegan's technique with reduced concentration, strength, and volume of sclerosant.
  - Subdermal reticular veins are treated only after all sources of reflux have been treated prior. Less than 0.5 mL of 0.2–0.5% sodium tetradecyl sulfate (STS) is used per injection site.

POSTPROCEDURE CARE[1,7]

- After procedure continuous compression must be maintained.

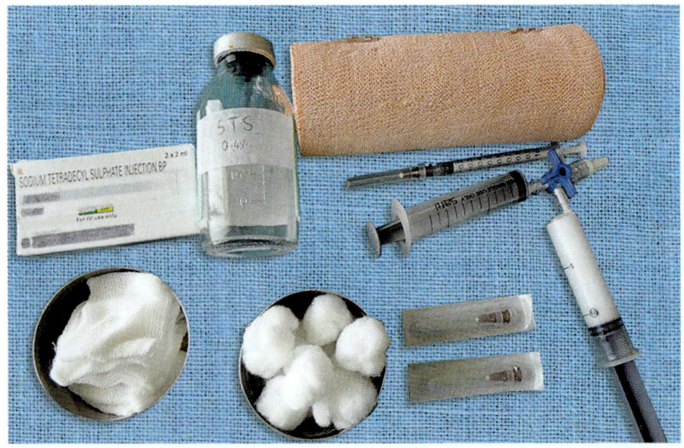

Fig. 1: Sclerotherapy tray.

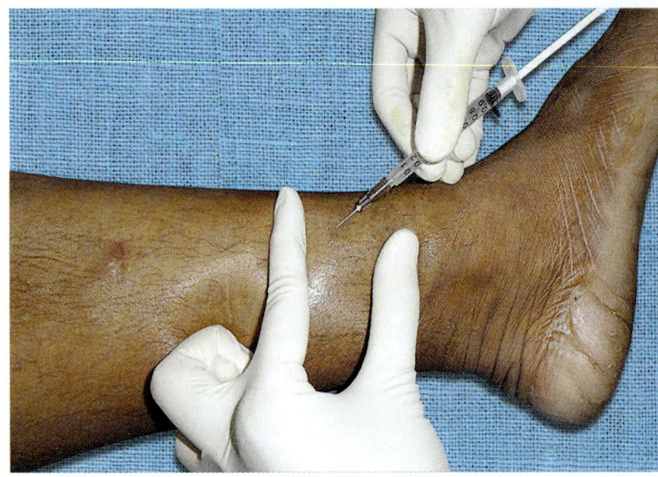

Fig. 2: Position of noninjecting hand, to stabilize the vein to be injected.

- *Compression*: Cotton ball taped at injection site and elastocrepe compression bandage over it, 16 mm Hg compressions for smaller veins, or graduated 20–30 mm Hg support hose for larger veins.
- Duration of compression depends on size of vessel injected and varies from 1 day for spider veins to 3 weeks for larger veins.
- Patient must walk for 30 minutes immediately after procedure and daily for 2 weeks.
- Avoid blood thinners, intensive workouts, hot baths, saunas, strong UV radiation for 2 weeks.

TIPS FOR A GOOD PROCEDURE AND RESULTS

- Mark all varicosities with patient standing but insert needle only with patient recumbent or in slight reverse Trendelenburg position.
- Empty blood in vein prior to injecting[1]
- Use motorized table with height and position adjustments[5]

TABLE 5: Complications of sclerotherapy.

Possible complications	*Tips to avoid them*
Allergic reaction	• Anaphylaxis and systemic allergic reactions occur rarely • More common with marked allergic diathesis • Consider using only hypertonic saline • Observe patient for 30 minutes after procedure
DVT, pulmonary embolism	• Avoid large volume of liquid or foam sclerosant at single site • Patient must ambulate immediately and daily after procedure
Arterial injection	• Extremely rare, but can lead to large areas of skin necrosis with damage to subcutaneous tissue and muscle; takes months to heal • *Emergency treatment:* Immediate application of ice, flushing injected artery with normal saline and heparin, injection of procaine 3% to inactivate STS, vascular surgeon consultation for intravenous anticoagulation
Thrombophlebitis	• Avoid treatment of larger diameter veins • Compressions after treatment • *Superficial thrombophlebitis:* Very tender, indurated, and linear erythematous swelling. Transdermal glyceryl trinitrate speeds resolution
Cutaneous ulceration, necrosis	• Occurs if sclerosant spills outside vessel into skin • Though rare, occurrence is serious and treatment may be difficult • Common with STS but very rarely with polidocanol • Use lowest concentration and volume of sclerosant • Normal saline 10:1 should be injected at site • Application of 2% nitroglycerine paste at extravasation site greatly reduces risks of necrosis
Neurologic symptoms: Transient migraine-like symptoms, scintillating scotomas, TIA, stroke	• Avoid foam in patients with patent foramen ovale • Use lowest concentration and volume of sclerosant
Hyperpigmentation	• Pigmentation along the course of a treated vein • Initially due to perivascular hemosiderin deposition, later, hemosiderin is replaced by melanin • Compression helps. Use lowest concentration and volume of sclerosant • Removal of postsclerotherapy coagulant by a 21G needle after small incision decreases incidence of pigmentation • Pigmentation clears within 6 months and rarely persists >1 year • Weekly subcutaneous administration of desferrioxamine mesylate 500 mg reduces pigmentation
Matting	• Appearance of new fine bluish telangiectasia groups surrounding or replacing a previously treated area • Spontaneous resolution in 3–12 months with 70–80% resolution in 6 months • Use lowest concentration and volume of sclerosant • Consider laser therapy instead
Bruising	Use compression bandage postsclerotherapy
Blister	Usually from ill-fitting compression stockings and bandages
Others	Nerve damage, scarring, vision disturbances, orthostatic collapse

(DVT: deep vein thrombosis; STS: sodium tetradecyl sulfate; TIA: transient ischemic attack)

- Always inject proximal to distal; larger vein before smaller veins.[1]
- Reflux points should be determined initially and treated specifically.[1]
- Exert direct finger pressure to spread and compress over injected vein.
- Ensure adequate ambulation immediately after treatment.[1]
- Using a bent needle to inject can help in keeping the injecting hand more stable.
- Always withdraw to look for blood in needle hub before injecting sclerosant.
- Start with lower concentrations and lower volumes of sclerosants in initial sessions.
- Not >1 mL of sclerosing agent should be injected at each site and only a total of 10 mL may be injected in a single session.
- Patient can mark vessels which they feel are more troublesome.
- Resulting vessel size is the best prognostic indicator of treatment response and complications.
- Allow 4–8 weeks between treatments.

COMPLICATIONS[2,8]

The complications of sclerotherapy are described in **Table 5**.

SPECIAL TECHNIQUES OF SCLEROTHERAPY

Sclerotherapy Guided by Duplex Ultrasonography[9]

- Recommended for saphenous junctions, truncal veins next to saphenous junctions, perforating veins, and low-flow vascular malformations.
- Vein is visualized by duplex ultrasonography with patient lying down and is punctured during visualization.
- Needle is visible in ultrasound image and intravascular injection can be controlled.
- Aim is to achieve a controlled procedure that results in fewer complications and increased effect.

Foam Sclerotherapy[10]

- Sclerosing foam is a mixture of gas bubbles in a liquid solution that contains surface-active molecules.
- Gas bubbles should be <100 μ. According to bubble diameter, foams can be *froth, macrofoam, minifoam,* and *microfoam.*
- If relative volume fraction of liquid is <5%, the foam is *dry,* whereas >5% is *wet.*
- Wet foam (Tessari's foam) has maximum stability. Uniform bubble diameter provides more stability.

Techniques of Foam Sclerotherapy

- *Monfreux method*: Foam is produced in glass syringe filled with 0.3–0.5 mL of sclerosant. Negative pressure is created by closing tip of syringe with sterile plug and holding tension on piston until 2–3 mL of foam is generated. The consistency is low due to large size of bubbles and also this technique has a higher rate of side effects.
- *Cabrera method*: Juan Cabrera used CO_2 for producing foam.
- *Benigni–Sadoun method*: Plastic syringes are used with repeated fast pulling and release of piston. But foam is very short lasting.
- *Lorenzo Tessari's Tourbillon method*: Two plastic syringes are connected by a three-way stop-cock. Foam is formed by mixing liquid sclerosant with four or five parts of air, through 20 passes between syringes with the hub at a 30° rotation. This rotation narrows the stopcock passage generating high turbulence, producing high quality microfoam. Most frequently used techniques **(Fig. 3)**.
- *Frullini method*: It is similar to Tessari method, but connecter is inserted into vial of STS and other end is connected to syringe. Vial is positioned upside down and quick injections and aspirations of solution are performed.

Advantages and Disadvantages of Foam Sclerotherapy[10]

Advantages and disadvantages of foam sclerotherapy are given in **Table 6**.

Figures 4 to 6 are before procedure and after procedure photographs to depict the results with sclerotherapy.

KEY POINTS

- Sclerotherapy is a simple, safe, and effective procedure for treatment of varicose veins and low-flow vascular malformations.
- It may be superior to other treatments to relieve symptoms and reach optimal cosmetic results for small, localized, primary varices of lower extremity.
- Advantages are low morbidity, almost no mortality and no necessity for hospitalization, therefore avoiding loss of work time.
- Proper training in technique, dilution and amount of sclerosant injected is vital for optimal, risk-free outcomes.
- When procedure is done with adequate precautions, there are relatively very few complications.
- *Greatest advantage* is even if it fails it can be safely repeated any number of times.

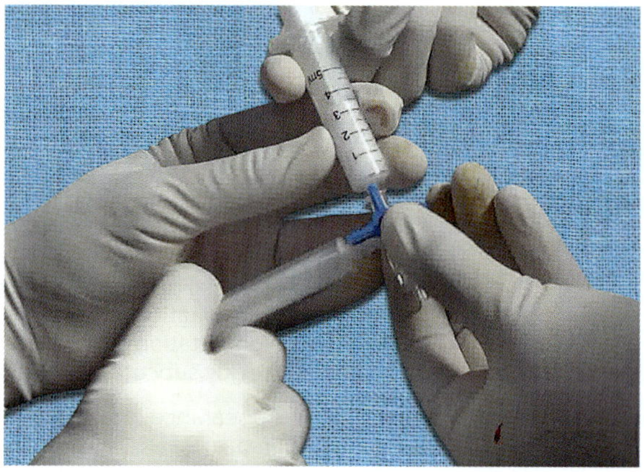

Fig. 3: Preparation of foam for sclerotherapy.

TABLE 6: Advantages and disadvantages of foam sclerotherapy.

Advantages	*Disadvantages*
Foam is 3–4 times more potent than equivalent concentrations and volumes of liquid sclerosants	Difficulty in standardization (main disadvantage)
There is an increase in the effective surface area of sclerosant	Foam can lodge in lungs and produce pulmonary fibrosis in patients of ductus arteriosus
Displacement of blood at treatment site, allowing undiluted intimal contact for a longer time	Deep vein thrombosis (DVT) and superficial thrombophlebitis
Increased vasospasm and sclerosis occurs even at a distance farther away from site of injection	Pain and pigmentation are relatively more common
Smaller volumes and concentrations are used	
Enhanced visibility on duplex imaging due to increased echogenicity of foam	

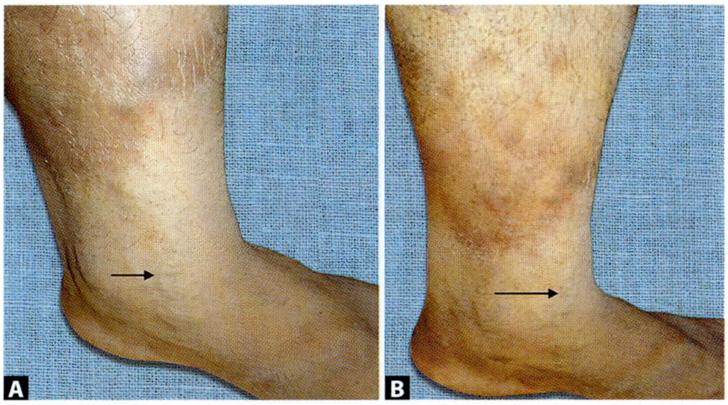

Figs. 4A and B: Before and 3 weeks after one session of sclerotherapy with 1.5% sodium tetradecyl sulfate (STS).

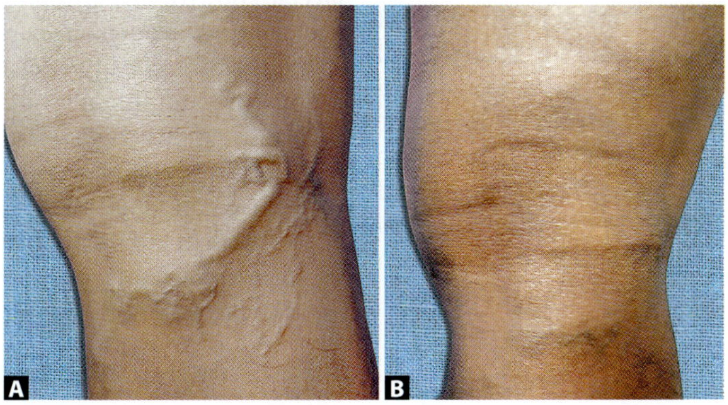

Figs. 5A and B: Before and 6 weeks after two sessions of sclerotherapy with 1.5% sodium tetradecyl sulfate (STS) given 3 weeks apart.

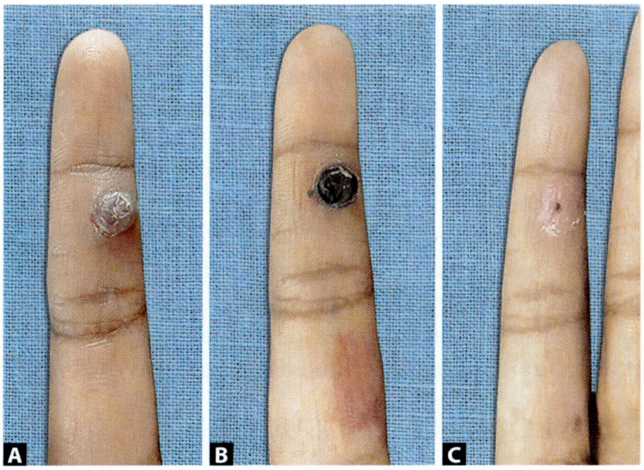

Figs. 6A to C: Before, 1 week and 2 weeks after two sessions of sclerotherapy with 1.0% sodium tetradecyl sulfate (STS) given 1 week apart.

REFERENCES

1. Khunger N, Sacchidanand S. Standard guidelines for care: Sclerotherapy in dermatology. Indian J Dermatol Venereol Leprol. 2011;77:222-31.
2. Mann MW. Sclerotherapy: it is back and better. Clin Plast Surg. 2011;38:475-87.
3. Rabe E, Pannier-Fischer F, Gerlach H, Breu FX, Guggenbichler S, Zabel M, et al. Guidelines for sclerotherapy of varicose veins (ICD 10: I83.0, I83.1, I83.2, and I83.9). Dermatol Surg. 2004;30:687-93; discussion 693.
4. Subbarao NT, Sacchidanand S, Veerabhadrappa NH. Sclerotherapy in the management of varicose veins and its dermatological complications. Indian J Dermatol Venereol Leprol. 2013;79:383-8.
5. Sacchidanand S, Nagesh TS. Sclerotherapy. In: Venkataram M, (Ed). ASC(I) Textbook on Cutaneous and Aesthetic Surgery. New Delhi: Jaypee Brothers Medical Publishers; 2012. pp. 452-62.
6. Goldman MP, Weiss RA, Bergan JJ. Diagnosis and treatment of varicose veins: a review. J Am Acad Dermatol. 1994;31:393-413; quiz 414-6.
7. Goldman MP. How to utilize compression after sclerotherapy. Dermatol Surg. 2002;28:860-2.
8. Goldman MP. Complications and adverse sequelae of sclerotherapy. In: Bergan JJ (Ed). The Vein Book. USA: Elsevier Academic Press; 2007. pp. 149-53.
9. Yamaki T, Nozaki M, Iwasaka S. Comparative study of duplex-guided foam sclerotherapy and duplex-guided liquid sclerotherapy for the treatment of superficial venous insufficiency. Dermatol Surg. 2004;30:718-22.
10. Sacchidanand S, Nagesh TS, Sujala SA. Sclerotherapy. In: Venkataram M (Ed). ASC(I) Textbook on Cutaneous and Aesthetic Surgery. New Delhi: Jaypee Brothers Medical Publishers; 2017. pp. 559-68.

EXAMINATION QUESTION

1. Describe sclerotherapy and foam sclerotherapy. List the indications, side effects, complications, advantages and disadvantages of conventional sclerotherapy.

174 CHAPTER Liposuction

BC Sharath Kumar, Namratha C Manjunath,
Kusuma MR, Harsha Siddappa, Dinesh Jayaram

INTRODUCTION

Since ancient times, surgeons have sought after different ways to alter the body contour. Body contouring by fat removal began in the late 1970s. Liposuction is the surgical removal of subcutaneous fat by means of a suction-assisted aspiration cannula, which is introduced through small skin incisions. Body contouring by liposuction was initially done by plastic surgeons, but recently dermatologists have also started performing this technique. Advances in this technique has made it safe and it can be performed as a day-care procedure under local anesthesia.

NOMENCLATURE

Liposuction, also known as liposuction surgery, suction-assisted lipectomy, fat suction, liposculpting, suction lipoplasty, and blunt suction lipectomy.

HISTORY

Charles Dujarrier in 1921, was the first to attempt localized removal of excess fat from calves and knees using a uterine curette.[1] Injury to the femoral artery during this lead to amputation. In 1964, Schrudder revised this procedure and extracted fat from the leg, using a curette, but it lead to a hematoma and seroma. Subsequently, Pitanguy performed en bloc removal of both fat and skin to remove excess thigh fat, but wide incisions did not allow this technique to become popular. Modern liposuction began with Giorgio Fischer and his father Arpad Fischer from Rome, Italy in 1974.[2] Pierre Fournier of Paris, France introduced a "dry technique" in which no fluids were infiltrated prior to liposuction. Illouz introduced the "wet technique" by introducing hypotonic saline into adipose tissue before liposuction. Jeffery Klein, described the tumescent technique for lipo-aspirations in 1987.[3] In 1996, Michael Zocchi developed Ultrasonic liposuction.[4]

BASIC PRINCIPLE

Liposuction requires knowledge of the anatomic, biochemical, and physiological basis of fat layer. The female silhouette is recognized by concavity below the rib cage that changes to a convexity over the hips and thighs, forming a gynoid pattern of obesity. In contrast, men have a linear silhouette, with only relative concavities in the pelvic region and convexity in the buttocks area forming an android type of obesity. When a person puts on weight, there will be an increase in the size of fat cell, known as hypertrophic obesity. With continued weight gain, there will be an increase in the number of fat cells, known as hyperplastic obesity. Diet and exercise help in reducing fat cell size but not the number, which are known as "resistant fat." Liposuction acts on resistant fat. Liposuction removes the resistant fat by following mechanisms:

- It breaks the fat cells by the to-and-fro motion of the cannula.
- Suctioning out the fat and the fluid to shape up the area.
- Remaining damaged fat cells get absorbed slowly through the lymphatics.

Anatomical Considerations

Subcutaneous fat is arbitrarily divided into three layers: (1) Superficial, (2) intermediate, and (3) deep compartment.[5,6] The deeper layer contains a larger proportion of the subcutaneous fat in the abdominal, gluteal, and thigh regions and is responsible for the bulges associated with weight gain. Liposuction is focused more on the middle or deeper fat layers. The superficial fat layer should be avoided due to increased risk of contour irregularities, skin dimpling, risk of hyperpigmentation, and necrosis. The anatomic "zones of adherence," have to be identified preoperatively which are areas of dense fibrous attachment to the underlying deep fascia, as they are more prone to contour deformities. They are gluteal crease, lateral gluteal depression, mid medial thigh, inferolateral-iliotibial tract, and distal posterior thigh.

TECHNIQUES OF LIPOSUCTION

- Dry liposuction
- *Wet liposuction*:
  - Microcannular tumescent liposuction
  - Suction-assisted liposuction
  - Syringe-assisted liposuction
- Ultrasound-assisted liposuction (UAL)
- VASER-assisted liposuction (VAL)
- Power-assisted liposuction
- Laser-assisted liposuction

Dry Liposuction

Dry liposuction is done under general anesthesia using a large cannula. It requires hospitalization and is associated with high mortality. The recovery time is prolonged and is associated with significant scarring.

This is a quick method and can remove large amounts of fat (up to 8–10 liters) in a single session. In this technique, large incisions (about 1.5 cm) are made and large cannulas (6–10 mm in diameter) are used to aspirate the fat. It is not commonly practiced nowadays due to the complications. It is mainly performed by plastic surgeons.

Wet Liposuction

Microcannular Tumescent Liposuction

It was developed by Dr Jeffrey A Klein . It involves infiltrating the subcutaneous tissue with large amounts of tumescent solution, followed by aspiration of fat with small cannula (1–3 mm) through small adits. In a single session 4–5 liters of fat can be extracted.

Suction-assisted Liposuction

It is the standard method of liposuction. In this approach, a small cannula is inserted through an incision (0.5 cm), which is attached to a vacuum device to create the negative pressure for liposuction. Here the surgeon prefers the radial tunneling method of fanning out the cannula, creating tunnels in multiple layers, from which the fat is removed sequentially at different levels.

Syringe-assisted Liposuction

Toledo popularized this technique.[7] In this technique, the tip of the syringe is connected to the liposuction cannula and a locking ring holds the plunger back, creating the vacuum for suctioning. There is no tubing attached, which enables the operator freedom, improved control, and enhanced precision.

Advantages are low cost, ideal for small local areas (face, neck), and also to harvest fat. The disadvantage is the suction can be lost at the access sites, particularly when using the short cannula or in small areas.

Ultrasound-assisted Liposuction

It was first promoted by Zocchi in the early 1990s.[4] This technique uses ultrasound waves to damage fat cells. Clinical end point of UAL is the loss of tissue resistance with cannula movement and the presence of blood in the aspirate.[5]

It is effective in fibrous body areas such as male breasts and back and in reduction of cellulite and skin tightening. Disadvantages are seromas, thermal injury, bruising, and prolonged postoperative bleeding.

VASER-assisted Liposuction

VASER-assisted liposuction employs a newer generation ultrasound-assisted liposuction device that uses less energy with more efficient, solid probes. Advantage is less blood loss and is recommended in large-volume liposuction procedures and areas of fibrous fatty tissue where excess blood loss is expected (VASER: vibration amplification of sound energy at resonance).

Power-assisted Liposuction (PAL)

The device operates with either compressed air or electric driven cannulas which produces rapid to-and-fro movements of the cannula facilitating easy breakdown of fat cells. It is effective when large volumes of fat are to be removed in a tight area. The advantages are less surgeon fatigue, greater emulsification of fat, decrease in operative time, less pain, and hematomas.

Disadvantages are rapid fat extraction resulting in irregularities in the thighs, buttocks, arm and the vibration of the machine may lead to discomfort for the surgeon and patient.

Laser-assisted Liposuction

The major lasers used are the 1064-nm Nd:YAG, 980-nm diode, and the 1064-/1320-nm Nd: YAG.[8] It destroys the fat and induces skin tightening due to its thermal effect. Even though it is expensive and it is a good option for fibrous tight areas such as upper chest, male breast, flanks in abdomen and in small areas such as double chin, neck, arms, and periumbilical area.

PATIENT SELECTION AND COUNSELING

Indications, contraindications, and counseling of liposuction have been shown in **Boxes 1 to 3**.

BOX 1: Indications for liposuction.

Cosmetic:
- Localized fat deposits which cannot be lost by dieting or exercise (face, chins, cheeks, arms)
- Adjunct to rhytidectomy, abdominoplasty, medial thigh lift, breast reduction

Noncosmetic: Lipomas, gynecomastia, pseudogynecomastia, lipodystrophy, axillary hyperhidrosis, and bromhidrosis

Reconstruction of the skin: Flap elevations, subcutaneous debulking, correction of trap door deformity, and mobilization of flaps

Autologous fat transplantation: Depressed and atrophic scar, furrows, wrinkles and tissue augmentation

BOX 2: Contraindications for liposuction.

- Patient with unrealistic expectation
- Body dysmorphic disorder
- BMI >35
- Bleeding disorders
- Coagulation disorders including thrombophilia
- Chronic smokers
- Overlying skin infections
- Pregnancy
- Keloidal tendency
- Hepatic and renal impairment
- Uncontrolled diabetes and hypertension
- Cardiovascular diseases

(BMI: body mass index)

BOX 3: Patient counseling.

- Patient should be explained about all the available options
- Patient should be explained in detail regarding the steps of the procedure and possible postprocedural complications and consent must be obtained
- Role of diet and exercise postprocedure and chances of recurrence, if not adhered to it should be explained
- To expect results after 6–12 weeks
- Not to have unrealistic expectations
- Weight lost will be equal to the amount of fat aspirated
- The procedure will improve the shape of body, but not necessarily any cellulite or striae.

PROCEDURE

Preoperative Work-up of the Patient

- *Physical evaluation*: Assessment of the general physical health to determine whether the patient is a suitable candidate for surgery and examination of specific sites under consideration for liposuction to check for any potential problems.
- *Psychosocial evaluation*: Enquire about diet and exercise habits, history of weight gain and loss, familial body shape. Evaluate the patient's emotional ability to endure the procedure, his or her understanding of the limitations of liposuction, and whether the patient has realistic expectations.
- *Medical history*: The use of all medications, vitamins and herbs that affect blood clotting (e.g., aspirin, nonsteroidal anti-inflammatory agents, vitamin E, anticoagulants) should be stopped 3 weeks prior.
- History of bleeding diathesis, emboli, thrombophlebitis, infectious disease, and prior abdominal surgery should be evaluated.
- *Laboratory investigations*: Routine blood investigations such as a complete blood count, coagulation profile, blood sugar, serology, and liver function test should be performed.
- Patient should be advised to stop smoking.
- Vitamin-K injection to be given to reduce bleeding.
- Preoperative anxiolytics to be given the night before the surgery.

Preoperative Marking

The markings are made in standing position **(Fig. 1)** in front of a mirror, if possible. Areas to be suctioned are marked with a circle and "Zones of adherence" and areas to avoid are marked with hash marks.

Instruments Required for Liposuction

- Cannulas for infiltration and suction
- Vacuum pump or syringes to produce the suction pressure
- Connecting tubings
- Tumescent anesthesia **(Box 4)**

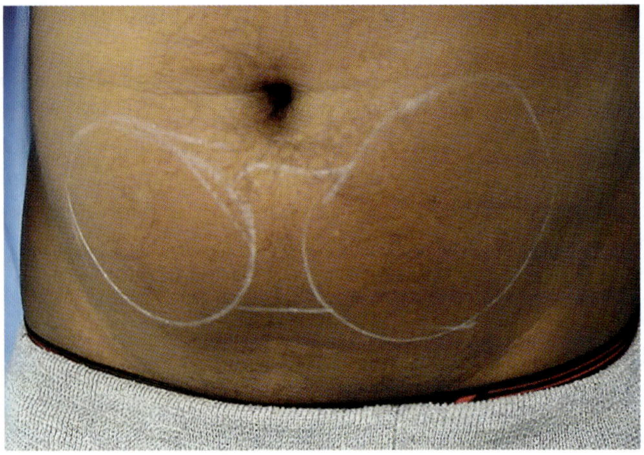

Fig. 1: Area to be suctioned is marked in a topographic pattern. *Courtesy:* Cutis Academy.

BOX 4: Tumescent anesthesia/Klein solution.[5]

Composition
- 50 mL of 1% or 2% lidocaine (0.05–0.1% lidocaine)
- 1 mL of 1:1,000 epinephrine
- 12.5 mL of 8.4 mEq of sodium bicarbonate
- 1 L of normal saline

Principle

Lignocaine in the form of tumescent anesthesia is given in large doses (up to 45–55 mg/kg) over a large area to provide anesthesia and analgesia. Klein demonstrated that tumescent anesthesia containing higher doses of lignocaine is safe as the rate of absorption of lignocaine is slow leading to smaller peak values and less toxicity.

Causes for Slow Absorption of Lignocaine
- Lignocaine is lipophilic and is easily sequestrated in fat
- Subcutaneous fat has less blood flow volume
- Epinephrine causes vasoconstriction and reduces systemic absorption of lignocaine
- Vasoconstriction occurs due to increased hydrostatic pressure by large volume of solution injected
- While aspirating fat, most of the tumescent solution is removed along with it thereby reducing the duration for systemic absorption

Advantages of Tumescent Anesthesia
- It creates a blood less field
- Tumescence magnifies defects, making the need for a secondary procedure less likely
- Very large areas can be treated under local anesthesia

Steps of Tumescent Liposuction

- Infiltration of tumescent anesthesia
- Aspiration of fat
- Postoperative dressing

Infiltration of Tumescent Anesthesia

- First, the adits should be created. These are small holes created for the insertion of infiltration cannula (0.5–1 mm) and aspiration cannula (1–3 mm). The size of the adit should be slightly larger than the size of the largest cannula. The site is infiltrated with 1 mL of 2% lignocaine just before making the adit. Dermal punches

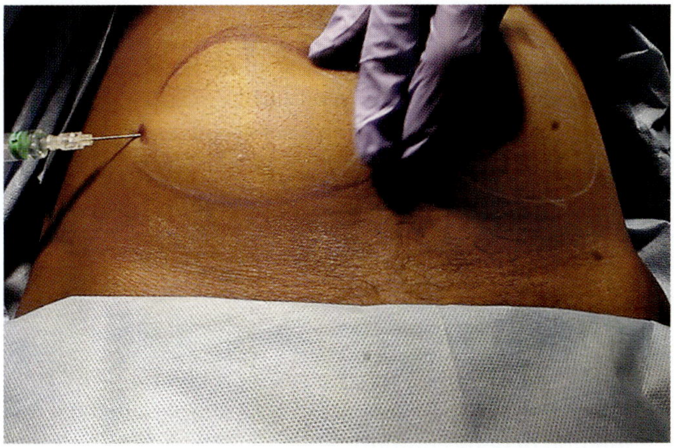

Fig. 2: Infiltration of tumescent anesthesia.
Courtesy: Cutis Academy.

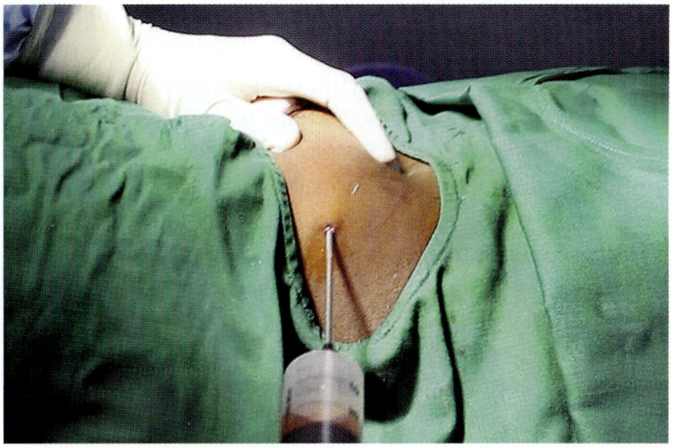

Fig. 4: Aspiration of fat with syringe.
Courtesy: Cutis Academy.

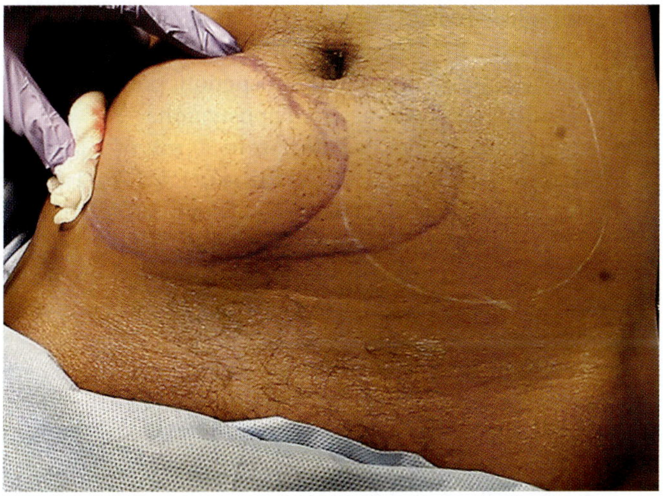

Fig. 3: End point of tumescence is indicated when skin becomes swollen and firm.
Courtesy: Cutis Academy.

of appropriate size or a number 11 blade can be used to create the adit. The number of adits to be made depends on the area involved.

- Tumescent solution is infiltrated with the help of infiltration cannula or using a lumbar puncture needle (23G) **(Fig. 2)**. The delivery can be accelerated, by using infiltration pumps or pressure cuffs. It is important to deliver the solution slowly, uniformly in all directions, across the involved area. Faster, sudden movements can cause pain. First the deeper layers should be infiltrated and then the superficial layers. It takes about 1 hour for proper anesthesia to be delivered. The end point is indicated when the skin becomes swollen, difficult to grasp and has a firm feel **(Fig. 3)**.
- *Detumescence:* It is important to wait for 30–60 minutes after infiltration of tumescence anesthesia, for its full effect to take place. It is indicated by a slight decrease in firmness of the skin and ability to grasp it.

Aspiration of Fat

After proper tumescence and detumescence, aspiration cannula is inserted into the adits to aspirate the fat.

- Aspiration cannulas range from 1 to 3 mm in diameter. Smaller cannulas are inserted first to create tunnels. Then large cannulas can be used to aspirate fat faster. The various shapes of cannulas available are blunt (least aggressive), bullet (moderately aggressive), and spatula (most aggressive).
- The aspiration cannula should always be at an angle to the skin and never tangential to it. It should be moved in a to-and-fro motion, slowly in a rhythmic and in a fan-like pattern in all directions. Deeper layers are aspirated first and then superficial layers.
- The nonoperating hand should be used to guide to lead the fat in the direction of aspiration and prevent the cannula from going beyond the affected area or injure the superficial layers.
- Aspiration can be done connecting the cannulas to a suction pump (for large areas) or to Luer-lock syringes (for smaller areas) **(Fig. 4)**. About 2–4 mL of suction pressure is sufficient for aspiration. Higher pressure can damage the fat cells. This method is called syringe liposuction.
- It is also important not to aspirate too much fat as it can lead to dimpling and asymmetry. After aspirating, the areas should be compared for symmetry and then proceed further. The patient can be asked to stand for comparing symmetry as the procedure is done under tumescent anesthesia and patient is conscious.
- It takes up to 90–120 minutes to aspirate 2–4 liters of fat. If the tumescence is proper, there is minimal blood loss (30–50 mL).

Postoperative Dressing

- Postprocedure a small amount of tumescent solution is always left behind to provide anesthesia in the post-operative period.

- The adits are covered with antiseptic ointment and gauze swab.
- Tight pressure dressing (Bimodal compression) should be put to ensure proper drainage of remaining fluid that continues for 3–5 days postoperatively. Patient should be advised to wear compression garments over the dressing. The pressure dressings can be removed after 3 days, but patient must continue to use compression garments for 2–3 weeks.

POSTOPERATIVE COURSE AND FOLLOW-UP

- Mild fatigue and discomfort is noted during the first few days postoperatively.
- Patient should be advised complete rest for 1–2 days.
- Postoperative antibiotics and analgesics are given for 1 week.
- Compression garments in the form of binders, girdles, or elastic tape must be used postoperatively to ensure proper drainage of the tumescent fluid and to minimize bruising, discomfort, hematoma or seroma formation.
- Compression also helps to improve the aesthetic outcome.
- Patient is followed up on Day 2 and Day 7 to look for any swelling and healing of adits.
- Patient is advised to resume his normal activities and exercise after 2 weeks.

COMPLICATIONS

Tumescent liposuction

Intraoperative
- Damage to muscles or blood vessels
- Lidocaine toxicity
- Abdomen wall perforation
- Blood loss

Postoperative
- *Immediate:*
  - Pain
  - Bleeding/bruising
  - Hematoma/seroma
  - Edema
  - Vasovagal syncope
  - Infection
  - Menstrual irregularities
- *Late:*
  - Prolonged numbness of skin
  - Contour irregularity
  - Excessive skin laxity and sagging
  - Postinflammatory hyper- or hypopigmentation
  - Liponots and lipotrops
  - Skin necrosis
  - Scar
  - Erythema ab lipoaspiration
  - Postliposuction panniculitis
  - Necrotizing fasciitis
  - Increased risk of thromboembolic events

CONCLUSION

Liposuction has many clinical applications both in the field of aesthetic surgery and in functional and reconstructive surgery. Proper case selection, counseling, selection of proper technique and following principles of surgery are the key to success. In the last few decades, numerous studies have demonstrated the wide differentiation and regenerative capacity of adipose-derived stem cells making liposuction an interesting field.

KEY POINTS

- Liposuction has evolved tremendously over the past three decades. Liposuction is a safe, simple, and effective method of body contouring.
- Five zones of adherence should be avoided to prevent contour deformities.
- Liposuction performed with wetting solution-like Klein's solution has more advantages than dry liposuction
- Other liposuction techniques include ultrasound-assisted liposuction, VASER-assisted liposuction, power-assisted liposuction, and laser-assisted liposuction.
- Composition of Klein's solution is 50 mL of 1% or 2% lidocaine (0.05%–0.1% lidocaine), 1 mL of 1:1,000 epinephrine, 12.5 mL of 8.4 mEq of sodium bicarbonate in 1 L of normal saline.
- Advantages of tumescent anesthesia are: (1) creates a blood less field, and (2) very large areas can be treated under local anesthesia.
- Steps of tumescent anesthesia are infiltration of tumescent anesthesia, aspiration of fat, and postoperative dressing.
- Postoperatively rest is advised for 1–2 days and compression garments to ensure proper drainage of the tumescent fluid and to minimize bruising, discomfort, hematoma, or seroma formation.

REFERENCES

1. Dolsky RL, Newman J, Fetzek JR, Anderson RW. Liposuction: history, techniques, and complications. Dermatol Clin. 1987;5:313-33.
2. Fischer G. Liposculpture: the correct history of liposuction—part I. J Dermatol Surg Oncol. 1990;16:1087-9.
3. Klein JA. The tumescent technique for liposuction surgery. Am J Cosmet Surg. 1987;4:263-7.
4. Zocchi M. Ultrasonic liposculpting. Aesthetic Plast Surg. 1992;16:287-98.
5. Rohrich RJ, Beran SJ, Kenkel JM. Ultrasound-assisted liposuction. St Louis, MO: Quality Medical Publishing; 1998.
6. Kenkel JM, Janis JE, Rohrich RJ, Beran SJ. Aesthetic body contouring: ultrasound-assisted liposuction. Operat Tech Plast Reconstr Surg. 2003;8:180-91.
7. Toledo L, Lewis CM. Why I use the syringe in superficial liposculpture? New York: Springer-Verlag; 1993.
8. Fakhouri TM, El Tal AK, Abrou AE, Mehrega DA, Barone F. Laser-assisted lipolysis: a review. Dermatol Surg. 2012;38:155-69.

EXAMINATION QUESTION

1. Describe the steps of tumescent liposuction and its indications.

175 CHAPTER

Chemical Peels

Niti Khunger, Kumar Abhishek

INTRODUCTION

Chemical peeling is one of the most commonly performed aesthetic procedures by dermatologists. This is a preferred technique by young dermatologists early in their practice as it does not incur any heavy financial burden to the doctor and the patient, it is easy to learn, and can be performed as an office procedure.

Chemical peeling is defined as the controlled destruction of the layers of the skin followed by skin regeneration and remodeling, accomplished by application of a chemical agent.[1] It is also referred to as chemoexfoliation, as it removes the outer layers of the skin leading to improvement in overall skin appearance. This concept of using various chemicals for enhancing skin beauty has been used since ancient times. Chemical peeling is a time-tested procedure, and various peeling agents have been introduced over time[2] **(Table 1)**.

CLASSIFICATION OF PEELS

Chemical peels are classified according to their depth of penetration which defines their use in various concentrations and indications **(Table 2)**. Peels which act at the stratum corneum or till the upper layers of stratum spinosum are classified as very superficial peels. Those peels which penetrate the entire depth of the epidermis and possibly the upper papillary dermis are classified as superficial peels. Most of the peels that are used in darker skin, types 4 and 5, belong to the above two categories. The peels which penetrate to the level of the upper reticular dermis and mid reticular dermis are classified as medium-depth and deep peels, respectively. These two categories of peels should be used with utmost care and expertise as the risk of complications in darker skin types 4, 5, and 6 is higher with these peels.

TABLE 1: History of chemical peels.[2]

Physician (year)	*Work*
Fox (1871)	Phenol for freckles
Unna (1882)	Salicylic acid, resorcinol, phenol, TCA Description
Monash (1945)	TCA peels
MacKee (1952)	Phenol for face scars
Van Scott and Yu (1984)	Alpha-hydroxy acids

(TCA: trichloroacetic acid)

Peels can also be classified according to their chemical structure **(Table 3)**. Most of the chemical peels are classified as alpha-hydroxyl acids (AHAs) which are basically derived from fruits. These peels do not have the self-neutralizing properties; hence, they have to be neutralized. Salicylic acid is a beta-hydroxy acid (BHA) derived from willow tree bark, wintergreen oil, and sweet birch. Apart from these two peels, there is trichloroacetic acid (TCA), phenol, Jessner's peel, and various combination peels. Unlike the AHAs, TCA or salicylic acid peels are self-neutralizing.

MECHANISM OF ACTION[3-6]

Chemical peels act by exfoliating the superficial layers of skin which eventually leads to stimulation of skin regeneration and rejuvenation. All the peels act by causing one of the following actions: metabolic, caustic, or toxic. Some peels act in multiple ways and hence give multitude of effects while some act in a specific manner and hence are used for particular indications.

- Interfere with enzyme function—AHAs
- Reduce intercellular adhesions—AHAs, salicylic acid

TABLE 2: Classification of chemical peels according to depth.

Depth	*Examples*
Very superficial	Glycolic acid 30–50%, TCA 10%, Jessner's solution (1–3 coats), salicylic acid 20–30%, lactic acid 50%, tretinoin 1–5%
Superficial	Glycolic acid 50–70%, TCA 10–30%, Jessner's solution (4–7 coats)
Medium	Glycolic acid 70%, TCA 35–50%, phenol 88%
Deep	Baker–Gordon phenol formula

TABLE 3: Classification of peels according to structure.

Chemical structure	*Examples (source)*
Alpha-hydroxy acids	Glycolic acid (sugarcane), malic acid (apples), tartaric acid (grapes), mandelic acid (almonds), lactic acid (milk)
Beta-hydroxy acids	Salicylic acid, beta-lipohydroxy acid
Alpha-keto acids	Pyruvic acid 40–70%
Others	TCA, phenol, Jessner's peel, tretinoin or retinol peels

- Stimulate epidermal growth—AHAs, retinoic acid
- Induce inflammation and deposition of glycosaminoglycans (GAGs) and neocollagenosis—AHAs
- Antimicrobial action—azelaic acid, phenol
- Coagulation of proteins—TCA

Factors affecting the activity and penetration of the peel: The depth of peeling can be controlled by modifying the concentration of the peeling agent, which is the single most important factor in controlling peel depth. The other factors that can modify the action of the peel include pH of solution, application time, application technique, quantity applied, skin preparation, skin type, and location of the peel.

INDICATIONS

There are various indications of chemical peels **(Box 1)**.

CONTRAINDICATIONS

Contraindication to peels includes the presence of active bacterial, viral, fungal, or herpetic infection at the site of peeling. These should be treated before undertaking the peels. In patients with a history of recurrent herpes simplex, prophylactic acyclovir should be given. A history of drug ingestion with photosensitizing potential is a contraindication as it can lead to increased risk of postinflammatory hyperpigmentation (PIH). Any pre-existing inflammatory dermatoses, such as psoriasis, atopic dermatitis, and seborrheic dermatitis, can aggravate due to Koebner's phenomenon. An uncooperative patient who is careless about sun exposure or application of medicine or patients with unrealistic expectations are relative contraindications to any aesthetic procedure. They should be adequately counseled and informed regarding outcomes of peelings, associated risks, and importance of adherence to postprocedure instructions so that complications are minimized. A history of abnormal scarring, keloids, and atrophic skin are relative contraindications. Medium-depth and deep peels should be performed cautiously or avoided in patients using isotretinoin in the last 6 months.

CHOICE OF PEELS

Choosing the right peel to treat the disorder is often a source of stress to the beginner as there is a wide variety available. The choice should be guided by the pathology and depth of the disorder and the patient's skin type.

BOX 1: Indications of chemical peels.

- Acne
- Acne scars
- *Pigmentary conditions:* Melasma, postinflammatory hyperpigmentation
- *Aging:* Fine wrinkles
- Dilated pores
- Keratosis pilaris
- Photodamage

Melasma is one of the most common pigmentary conditions for which chemical peels have been tried with reasonable success. While glycolic acid peels are widely used for melasma, the risk of complications can limit their utility in dark-skinned individuals. For melasma peeling, glycolic acid is used in a concentration of 30–70%. Beyond this, TCA 15%, phenol 8%, and Jessner's solution have also been used as peeling agents in melasma with variable success.[7-9]

Periorbital melanosis is a very common aesthetic condition, yet there is no definite treatment modality. Glycolic acid, lactic acid, arginine peels, and retinoid peels give favorable results.

Postinflammatory hyperpigmentation usually responds well to glycolic acid or TCA peels. Even salicylic acid, either alone or in combination with glycolic acid, yields good results in acne-induced PIH.[10]

Acne is another very common indication for chemical peels. Not only to treat active acne, but also for management of superficial acne scars or postinflammatory pigmentation due to acne, chemical peels have proven efficacious. Glycolic acid, salicylic acid, mandelic acid, retinol peels, and Jessner's peels are the ones which show improvement in active acne, reduce inflammation, minimize PIH risk, and eventually improve acne scarring.[11-14] For superficial acne scars, chemical peeling is a good modality of treatment. Since it causes controlled destruction of a part of or the entire epidermis, with or without the dermis, followed by regeneration of new epidermal and dermal tissues and collagen, it improves acne scars. Deep phenol peels are required for deep scars, which are risky in darker skins; hence, other methods are preferred. The most frequently used peeling agents are salicylic acid, glycolic acid, pyruvic acid, lactic acid, mandelic acid, Jessner's solution, TCA, and phenol.[15-18] The appropriate peel is chosen based on the patient's skin type, acne activity, and type of acne scars.

Antiaging and skin rejuvenation: Chemical peels for wrinkles and photodamaged skin have been widely used and studied. Glycolic acid and TCA when used as superficial peels have given good improvement in photodamaged skin, and noticeable improvement has been recorded in the wrinkles.

Prepeel Asssessment

The patient should also be counseled adequately regarding the indication for which the peel is performed, necessary precautions, natural course of results, and the possible complications. Prior written consent and photographs should be taken before performing the procedure.

Priming: It is the most essential and vital step which has a significant bearing on the results and the incidence of complications. It is essential to prime the patients for better outcomes. The common priming agents are glycolic acid creams 6–12%, kojic acid 2%, hydroquinone 2–4%, tretinoin 0.025%, and adapalene 0.1% as topical preparations for home use. The patient should be asked to use these agents for at least

4–6 weeks before starting the peels. They should be stopped a day before the intended session.

Apart from priming, the choice of peels according to the indication and the skin type is important. In India, most of the population is Fitzpatrick skin type 4–5. The risk of complications such as PIH are higher when medium-depth or deep peels are used. Hence, they should be used carefully and judiciously. The choice of peels also depends on the vehicle of the peel, like solution or gel based.

TECHNIQUE

Preparation of skin: The skin should be cleaned with a mild cleanser or degreasing should be done using acetone which helps remove unwanted sebum and dirt from the skin surface.

Applying the peel: Before applying the peel, the sensitive areas of the skin should be covered by applying petrolatum jelly **(Fig. 1)**. The application of the peel should be done using a paint brush or a cotton bud in a unidirectional manner **(Fig. 2)**. The brush or cotton bud should carry just an adequate amount of the peeling agent. Excess chemical agent application can lead to undesirable side effects such as burns. Feathering should be done at the margins of the peeled areas so as to avoid appearance of demarcation lines.

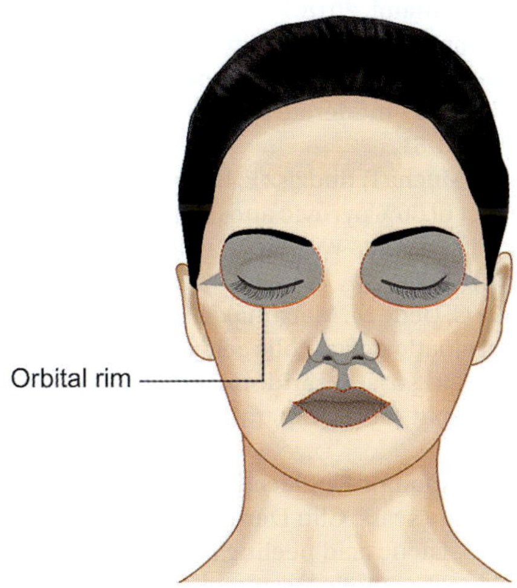

Fig. 1: Sensitive areas of the skin (gray areas).

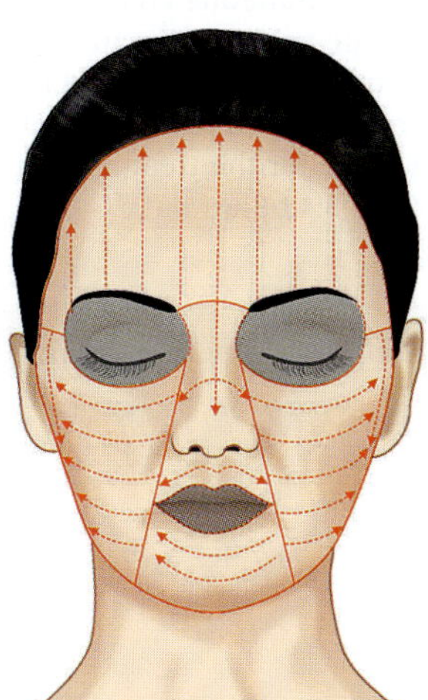

Fig. 2: Direction of strokes of the peeling agent.

Termination: To terminate the peeling, identification of the end point of the peeling session is important. With most of the AHAs, mild perceptible erythema with stinging sensation is the end point. These peels should be terminated using a neutralizer (sodium bicarbonate solution) rather than using water. There may be mild stinging sensation while neutralizing which is because neutralization is an exothermic reaction which releases heat. Salicylic acid and TCA peels are self-neutralizing peels. In salicylic acid peels, the end point is indicated by the appearance of pseudofrost, which is not a true frost but crystallization of the salicylic acid. In TCA peels, the appearance of tiny speckles of white-gray areas indicates frosting that is due to the coagulation of tissue proteins, which indicates the end point of the session.

Postpeel care: The patient should be counseled regarding the course of action as the peel takes the effect. He/she should be advised to use moisturizers and sun protection in the peeling phase. Once the peeling phase ends, the daily care home maintenance regimen should be restarted till the nest session.

COMPLICATIONS

Persistent erythema and burning sensation can occur, particularly if peels are done frequently and can be a sign of overpeeling. Chemical burns with strong peels, PIH, and appearance of demarcation lines can occur in dark-skinned patients. Rarely ulcerations may occur due to deeper penetration. The risk of systemic absorption with salicylic acid causing salicylism may occur with salicylic acid peels applied over large body surface areas.

Newer Peels

Ferulic acid, mandelic acid, kojic acid, lactic acid, pyruvic acid, citric acid, polyhydroxy acids (PHAs), lactobionic acid, phytic acid, lipohydroxy acid (LHA), tartaric acid, malic acid, and jasmonic acid are some of the newer peels that have been introduced, mostly as combination peels. Combination peels that contain multiple peeling agents in a compatible vehicle are safer as they permit lower concentrations of individual peels with increased efficacy. Lowering the concentration reduces the risk of side effects. Newer peels also contain additives that lower the risk of side effects and improve healing. Peels can also be sequential, that is, applying one peel, neutralizing it, and applying the second peel, thus giving added benefit in the same session.

CONCLUSION

Chemical peeling is a relatively easy, minimally invasive, and cost-effective procedure for the patient. Also, it requires minimal investment from the physician to perform a chemical peel for a patient and gives manifold benefits. The traditional peeling agents such as glycolic acid, salicylic acid and TCA are still being used, but combination peels with multiple agents are preferred as they offer multiple benefits with reduced risk and concentration. Adequate training and knowledge about chemical peels is essential to give the best results to the patients. However, multiple sessions are required to give optimum results and maintenance peels are required to sustain them.

KEY POINTS

- Chemical peels cause controlled exfoliation followed by regeneration leading to smoother skin, improved skin texture, and uniform skin tone and color.
- Peels are classified according to the depth of penetration into very superficial, superficial, medium-depth, and deep peels.
- Chief indications include acne, superficial acne scars, pigmentary conditions such as melasma, PIH, fine wrinkles, and photoaging.
- Glycolic acid, trichloroacetic acid, salicylic acid, and retinoic acid are traditional peels while newer combination peels are increasingly becoming popular due to an increased safety margin.
- Prepeel priming increases efficacy and reduces the risk of side effects. Postpeel skin care regimens are important to maintain results.
- Complications include burning sensation, persistent erythema, PIH, and rarely scarring with deeper peels.
- Chemical peeling is a cost-effective, easy-to-perform procedure with little downtime.

REFERENCES

1. Khunger N. Importance of chemical peels. Step by Step Chemical Peels, 2nd edition. New Delhi: Jaypee Brothers Medical Publishers; 2014. pp. 7-15.
2. Brody HJ, Monheit GD, Resnik SS, Alt TH. A history of chemical peeling. Dermatol Surg. 2000;26:405-9.
3. Dewandre L. The chemistry of peels and a hypothesis of action mechanisms. In: Rubin MG (Ed). Chemical Peels, 1st edition. Philadelphia: Elsevier Inc; 2006. pp. 1-12.
4. Brody HJ. Skin response to chemical peeling. In: Coleman WP, Lawrence N (Eds). Skin Resurfacing, 1st edition. Baltimore: Williams and Wilkins; 1998. pp. 37-44.
5. Savant SS. Superficial and medium depth chemical peeling. In: Savant SS (Ed). Textbook of Dermatosurgery and Cosmetology, 2nd edition. Mumbai: ASCAD; 2005. pp. 177-95.
6. Baumann L. Chemical peeling. In: Baumann L (Ed). Cosmetic Dermatology. Principles and Practice, 1st edition. New York: McGraw-Hill; 2002. pp. 173-86.
7. Safoury OS, Zaki NM, El Nabarawy EA, Farag EA. A study comparing chemical peeling using modified Jessner's solution and 15% trichloroacetic acid versus 15% trichloroacetic acid in the treatment of melasma. Indian J Dermatol. 2009;54(1):41-5.
8. Grover C, Reddu BS. The therapeutic value of glycolic acid peels in dermatology. Indian J Dermatol Venereol Leprol. 2003;69:148-50.
9. Faghihi G, Shahingohar A, Siadat AH. Comparison between 1% tretinoin peeling versus 70% glycolic acid peeling in the treatment of female patients with melasma. J Drugs Dermatol. 2011;10:1439-42.
10. Ahn HH, Kim IH. Whitening effect of salicyclic acid peels in Asian patients. Dermatol Surg. 2006;32:372-5.
11. In Jae J, Dong Ju H, Dong Hyun K, Yoon MS, Lee HJ. Comparative study of buffered 50% glycolic acid (pH 3.0) + 0.5% salicylic acid solution vs Jessner's solution in patients with acne vulgaris, J Cosmet Dermatol. 2018;17(5):797-801.
12. Dayal S, Amrani A, Sahu P, Jain VK. Jessner's solution vs. 30% salicylic acid peels: a comparative study of the efficacy and safety in mild-to-moderate acne vulgaris. J Cosmet Dermatol. 2017;16(1):43-51.
13. Marczyk B, Mucha P, Budzisz E, Rotsztejn H. Comparative study of the effect of 50% pyruvic and 30% salicylic peels on the skin lipid film in patients with acne vulgaris. J Cosmet Dermatol. 2014;13(1):15-21.
14. Kaminaka C, Uede M, Matsunaka H, Furukawa F, Yamomoto Y. Clinical evaluation of glycolic acid chemical peeling in patients with acne vulgaris: a randomized, double-blind, placebo-controlled, split-face comparative study. Dermatol Surg. 2014; 40(3):314-22.
15. Kontochristopoulos G, Platsidaki E. Chemical peels in active acne and acne scars. Clin Dermatol. 2017;35(2):179-82.
16. Sachdeva S, Lactic acid peeling in superficial acne scarring in Indian skin. J Cosmetic Dermatol. 2010;9(3):246-8.
17. Leheta TM, Abdel Hay RM, El Garem YF. Deep peeling using phenol versus percutaneous collagen induction combined with trichloroacetic acid 20% in atrophic post-acne scars: a randomized controlled trial. J Dermatol Treat. 2014;25(2):130-6.
18. Puri N. Efficacy of modified Jessner's peel and 20% TCA versus 20% TCA peel alone for the treatment of acne scars. J Cutan Aesthet Surg. 2015;8:42-5.

EXAMINATION QUESTIONS

1. Discuss the procedure of chemical peels in aesthetic practice.
2. Write short note on chemical peeling.

176 CHAPTER

Botulinum Toxin

Aarti Sarda, Abhishek De

INTRODUCTION

Botulinum toxin (BT) is responsible for causing botulism, a paralyzing and potentially fatal foodborne illness.

The name botulinum is derived from the latin word botulus meaning sausage because the illness was once believed to originate from consumption of sausages.

Botulinum toxin is produced by the bacteria *Clostridium botulinum*.[1] The bacteria elaborate eight exotoxins (A, B, C1, C2, D, E, F, and G).

Among the several types of BT, subtype A is the most potent toxin produced by the bacterium. Exotoxin A is available as Botox, Dysport, and Xeomin, Exotoxin B as Myobloc.[2,3]

Box 1 shows the Food and Drug Administration (FDA)-approved preparations.

MECHANISM OF ACTION[1,3]

Botulinum toxin blocks the release of acetylcholine, which is the principal neurotransmitter at the neuromuscular junction, thus causing muscle paralysis.

More specifically, botulinum toxin type A (BT-A) and BT-B target a group of proteins called SNARE (soluble NSF attachment protein receptor). The function of this SNARE protein is to release neurotransmitters from the storage vesicles by helping the membranes of the vesicles fuse with the cell membrane. Because SNARE is also involved in the release of other neurotransmitters, BTs have additional effects. By preventing the release of glutamate and substance P, BT also decreases the sensation of pain. **Figure 1** depicts the mechanism of action of BT by binding to SNARE proteins.

In addition to its effects on muscles, BT-A also denervates sweat glands. This makes it an effective alternative treatment for hyperhidrosis.

FORMULATION

Three preparations of BT-A exist—Dysport, Botox, and Xeomin. Myobloc is a BT-B preparation.[7,8]

BOX 1: The FDA-approved preparations.[4-6]

- OnabotulinumtoxinA (Botox)
- AbobotulinumtoxinA (Dysport)
- IncobotulinumtoxinA (Xeomin)
- RimabotulinumtoxinB (Myobloc)

RECONSTITUTION AND STORAGE[9]

Botulinum toxin should be stored in a freezer at or below –5°C. It is reconstituted with sterile saline without preservative.

As the toxin may be denatured by shaking the bottle, the diluent should be gently injected onto the inside wall of the toxin vial. 100 units is generally reconstituted with 1–10 mL of the diluent. More dilute solutions can lead to diffusion of the toxin, may cause undesired side effects.

After reconstitution, the toxin should be kept in the refrigerator at 2–8°C. The reconstituted Botox should be used within 6 weeks.

In mesotherapy with BT, the toxin is diluted with 5–10 mL of 0.9% preservative-free normal saline. This is used to treat fine wrinkles.

INDICATIONS

Dynamic lines result from the repeated contraction of muscles perpendicular to the rhytides. The approved indications of BT include the esthetic use to reduce the activity of hyperfunctional facial muscles which cause facial lines **(Table 1)** and the treatment of focal hyperhidrosis (axillary, palmar, and plantar hyperhidrosis). It is currently FDA-approved for the treatment of rhytides occurring in the upper face.[8-10]

Indications currently being studied:

- Hypertrophic scar and keloid
- Postherpetic neuralgia
- Facial erythema and blushing
- Hidradenitis suppurativa

MODE OF ADMINISTRATION[16,17]

A proper knowledge of the functional anatomy of muscles is necessary to correctly use BT in clinical practice. Facial assessment should be made during rest, and muscle contraction and asymmetry should be kept in mind during injections

Botulinum toxin is injected into affected muscles or glands using an insulin syringe. Injections for esthetic indications may be given intramuscularly, subcutaneously, or intradermally. Doses should be individualized and the dose depends on the bulk of the muscle being injected. Higher doses are required for larger muscles.

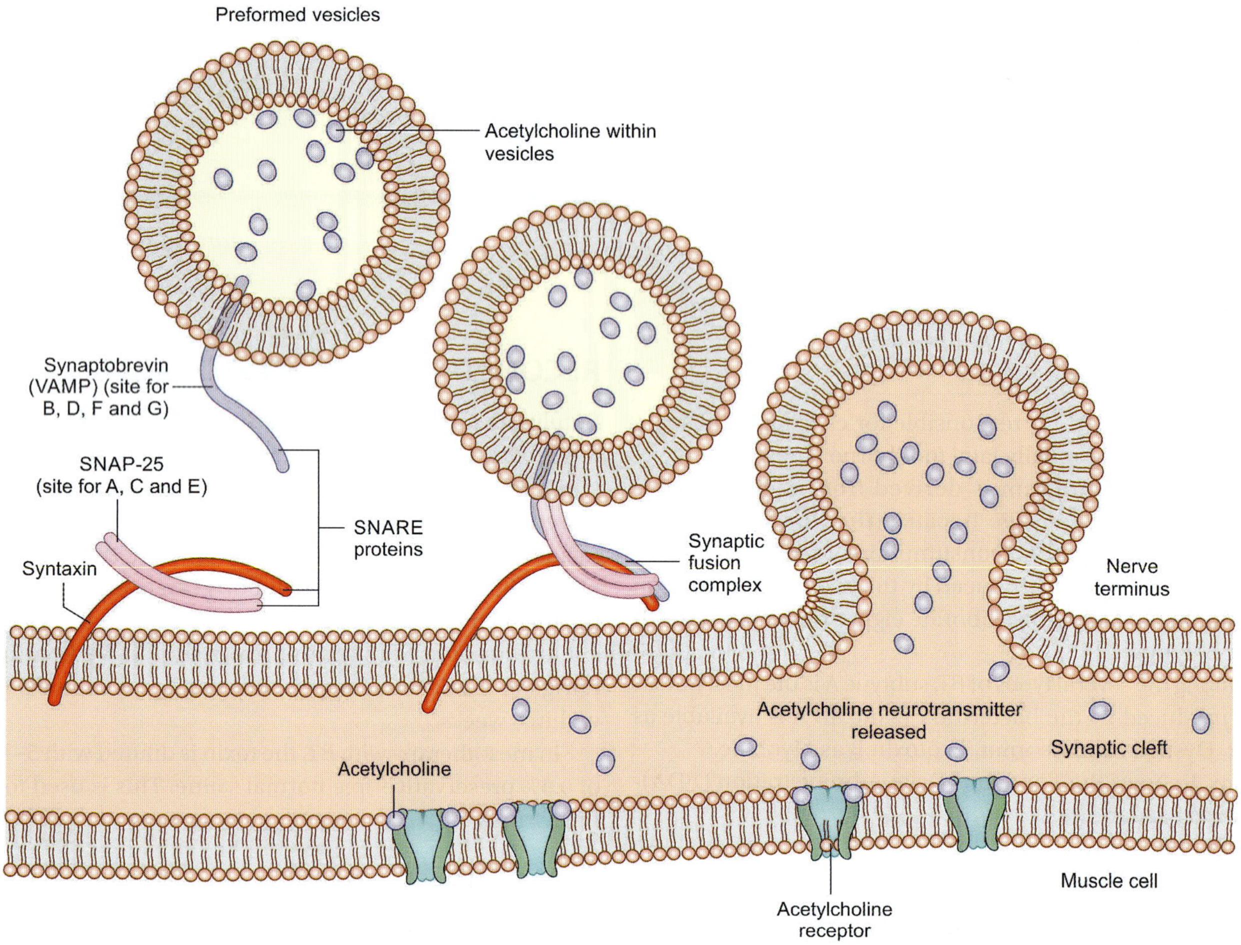

Fig. 1: The mechanism of action of botulinum toxin by binding to SNARE proteins.

TABLE 1: Clinical indications of botulinum toxin in esthetic dermatology.[10-15]

Esthetic indication	*Muscle targeted*
Forehead lines (worry lines)	Frontalis
Glabellar frown lines (vertical)	Corrugator, orbicularis oculi
Horizontal creases across the bridge of the nose	Procerus
Crow's feet (lateral canthal rhytides)	Lateral orbicularis oculi
Bunny lines/Nasal flare	Nasalis
Nasal tip droop	Depressor septi nasi
Nasolabial fold	Nasolabial groove
Gummy smile	Levator labii superioris alaeque nasi
Mouth frown	Depressor anguli oris (DAO) muscle and mentalis
Marionette lines	Depressor anguli oris
Mental crease	Mentalis
Smokers lip lines	Orbicularis oris
Puckering of the chin	Mentalis
Neck bands	Platysma
Masseter hypertrophy	Masseter
To increase eye aperture	Lower pretarsal orbicularis

It takes approximately 2 weeks to see the results of the injections and the effects last for 3–5 months.

Since an element of atrophy (muscle wasting) occurs with each injection, the interval needed for a second treatment can gradually lengthen following repeated injections.

An uncommon side-effect of BT-A is the unintended weakness of the surrounding muscles (occurring in fewer than 10% of treatments). This weakness results from the spread of the toxin from the injection site into adjacent muscle groups.

Use of careful injection technique to target the toxin to the appropriate muscles and the use of concentrated low doses to limit its diffusion to nontargeted muscles or glands are recommended to try to prevent the occurrence of these adverse effects. In general, a higher concentration allows for more accurate placement, greater duration of effect, and fewer side effects, since lower concentrations may encourage the spread of toxin. Injections with BT are generally well-tolerated and side effects are few.

CONTRAINDICATIONS[1]

- Infection at the injection site
- Pre-existing motor neuron disease

- Myasthenia gravis
- Lambert-Eaton syndrome
- Neuropathies
- History of hypersensitivity to BT or albumin
- Pregnancy/lactation
- Unrealistic expectations

DRUG INTERACTIONS

- Aminoglycosides and tetracyclines may potentiate the effect of BT.
- Penicillamine, quinine, chloroquine, and hydroxychloroquine may reduce the effect of BT.

PREREQUISITES

- Realistic expectation
- Awareness about transient nature of therapy
- Photographic documentation of pre- and post-treatment appearance
- Patients should not be on aminoglycosides or other neuromuscular blockers which may potentiate the effect of BT.

TECHNIQUE OF INJECTION[1,18]

Local anesthesia can be achieved with the help of EMLA cream or application of ice cubes. Regional nerve blocks and field blocks are required for palmoplantar and axillary hyperhidrosis, respectively.

Botulinum toxin is given under aseptic condition. Patient should be in sitting position. The toxin is administered with the help of an insulin syringe with a 30 G needle.

Figure 2 shows the muscles targeted by botulinum toxin.

Figure 3 shows the points of injection in palmar hyperhidrosis.

POSTPROCEDURE CARE[19,20]

- Area injected should not be massaged.
- Patient should not recline for 3–6 hours to avoid undesired diffusion of toxin.
- Patient should refrain from rubbing or manipulating the area for 24 hours.
- There is evidence suggesting that BT binds preferentially at actively stimulated muscles and hence patients are also asked to contract and relax the treated muscles as much as possible for 2–3 hours following the injections.
- Touchups may be required after 1–2 weeks if results are suboptimal.

ADVERSE EFFECTS/COMPLICATIONS[1-3]

The main causes for adverse effects from BT injections are poor injection technique, inappropriate dose selection, and incorrect injection site. Poor results may be improved by further injection, e.g., into compensatory muscles.

- Pain, headache
- Infection
- Bruising occurs most frequently in periorbital region. It can be avoided by mitigating injection in patients taking medications or supplements which increase bruising tendency such as aspirin, nonsteroidal anti-inflammatory agents, anticoagulant drugs, omega-3 and omega-6 fish oil supplements, and alcohol.
- Eyelid ptosis occurs when Botox is accidentally injected or diffuses into levator palpebrae superioris while treating the glabellar frown. It can be counteracted to some extent by administering apraclonidine 0.5% or phenylephrine 2.5% eye drops at regular intervals.
- Brow ptosis occurs when treating horizontal forehead lines. Excess Botox paralyzes the frontalis leading to brow drop.

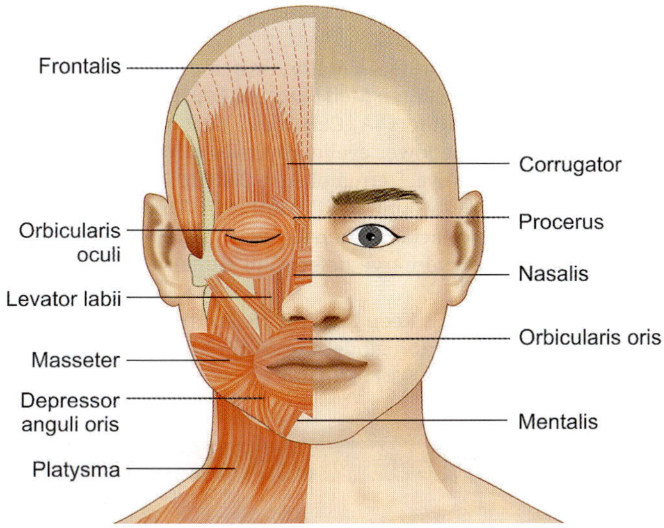

Fig. 2: Muscles targeted by botulinum toxin.

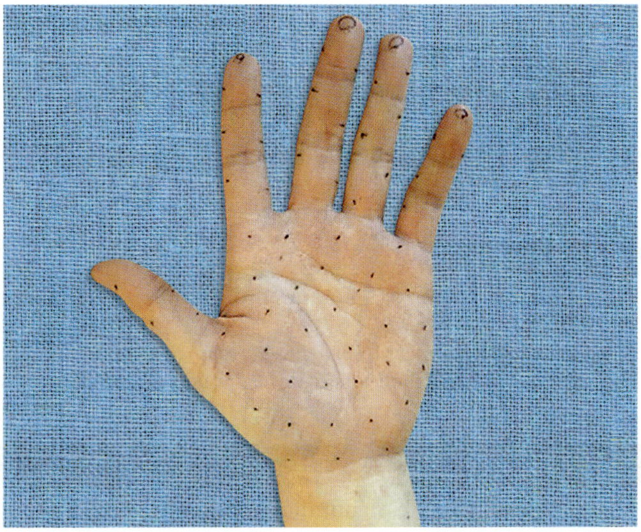

Fig. 3: Points of injection in palmar hyperhidrosis.

- Ectropion occurs while treating crow's feet in a patient with weak tarsal tone.
- A quizzical or "cockeyed" appearance can occur in the brow when the lateral fibers of the frontalis muscle have not been injected adequately and these untreated lateral fibers pull upward on the brow.
- Other side effects are lower eyelid laxity, epiphora, diplopia, decreased strength of eye closure, and dry eye.
- Lower face asymmetry and lateral lip ptosis occur if injections in the lower periocular area are too lateral and too low to the infraorbital areas, encroaching on the zygomatic areas.
- Dysphagia can occur when treating platysmal folds.
- Mouth incompetence, difficulties in speech, and the inability to whistle can rarely occur.
- Weakness of hands may occur when treating for palmar hyperhidrosis.
- Suboptimal response or resistance can occur due to development of neutralizing antibodies.

KEY POINTS

- A proper knowledge of the functional anatomy of muscles is necessary to correctly use BT in clinical practice.
- The use of aminoglycoside antibiotics or drugs interfering with neuromuscular transmission (e.g., tubocurarine-type muscle relaxants) can usually potentiate the effect of BT. Therefore, a detailed drug history should be elicited before injection of the toxin.
- Precautions should be taken when BT-A is utilized for the treatment of disorders such as myasthenia gravis, Lambert–Eaton syndrome, and others which produce a depletion of acetylcholine.
- There is the possibility of anaphylactic reaction as occurs with all biologic products. Necessary precautions should be taken and epinephrine should be available.
- No data is available on the use of BT-A in pregnant women or of its excretion in human milk. Therefore, one should be cautious about the use of BT in pregnant and lactating women.
- It is not established to be safe for use in children under 12 years of age.
- Patients with BT administration should resume activity gradually.

REFERENCES

1. Nigam PK, Nigam A. Botulinum toxin. Indian J Dermatol. 2010;55(1):8-14.
2. Patel KB, Cai S, Adler M, Singh BK, Parmar VS, Singh BR. Natural compounds and their analogues as potent antidotes against the most poisonous bacterial toxin. Appl Environ Microbiol. 2018;84(24):e01280-8.
3. Bentivoglio AR, Del Grande A, Petracca M, Ialongo T, Ricciardi L. Clinical differences between botulinum neurotoxin type A and B. Toxicon. 2015;107(Pt A):77-84.
4. Zakin E, Simpson D. Evidence on botulinum toxin in selected disorders. Toxicon. 2018;147:134-40.
5. Patil S, Willett O, Thompkins T, Hermann R, Ramanathan S, Cornett EM, et al. Botulinum toxin: pharmacology and therapeutic roles in pain states. Curr Pain Headache Rep. 2016; 20(3):15.
6. Park J, Park HJ. Botulinum toxin for the treatment of neuropathic pain. Toxins (Basel). 2017;9(9):260.
7. Coté TR, Mohan AK, Polder JA, Walton MK, Braun MM. Botulinum toxin type A injections: adverse events reported to the US Food and Drug Administration in therapeutic and cosmetic cases. J Am Acad Dermatol. 2005;53(3):407-15.
8. Cliff SH, Judodihardjo H, Eltringham E. Different formulations of botulinum toxin type A have different migration characteristics: a double-blind, randomized study. J Cosmet Dermatol. 2008;7(1):50-4.
9. Trindade de Almeida AR, Marques E, de Almeida J, Cunha T, Boraso R. Pilot study comparing the diffusion of two formulations of botulinum toxin type A in patients with forehead hyperhidrosis. Dermatol Surg. 2007;33(1 Spec No.): S37-43.
10. Walker TJ, Dayan SH. Comparison and overview of currently available neurotoxins. J Clin Aesthet Dermatol. 2014;7(2):31-9.
11. Ranoux D, Gury C, Fondarai J, Mas JL, Zuber M. Respective potencies of Botox and Dysport: a double blind, randomized, crossover study in cervical dystonia. J Neurol Neurosurg Psychiatry. 2002;72:459-62.
12. Simonetta Moreau M, Cauhepe C, Magues JP, Senard JM. A double-blind, randomized, comparative study of Dysport vs. Botox in primary palmar hyperhidrosis. Br J Dermatol. 2003;149:1041-5.
13. Ahn MS, Catten M, Maas CS. Temporal brow lift using botulinum toxin A. Plast Reconstr Surg. 2000;105:1129-35.
14. Huang W, Rogachefsky AS, Foster JA. Browlift with botulinum toxin. Dermatol Surg. 2000;26:55-60.
15. Huilgol SC, Carruthers A, Carruthers JD. Raising eyebrows with botulinum toxin. Dermatol Surg. 1999;25:373-6.
16. Carruthers A, Carruthers J. Eyebrow height after botulinum toxin type A to the glabella. Dermatol Surg. 2007;33(1 Spec No.): S26-31.
17. Carruthers J, Carruthers A. Botox use in the mid and lower face and neck. Semin Cutan Med Surg. 2001;20:85-92.
18. Flynn TC, Carruthers JA, Carruthers JA. Botulinum-A toxin treatment of the lower eyelid improves infraorbital rhytides and widens the eye. Dermatol Surg. 2001;27:703-8.
19. Armstrong MW, Mountain RE, Murray JA. Treatment of facial synkinesis and facial asymmetry with botulinum toxin type A following facial nerve palsy. Clin Otolaryngol Allied Sci. 1996;21:15-20.
20. Blitzer A, Brin MF, Keen MS, Aviv JE. Botulinum toxin for the treatment of hyperfunctional lines of the face. Arch Otolaryngol Head Neck Surg. 1993;119:1018-22.

EXAMINATION QUESTION

1. Write a short note on botulinum toxin in dermatology.

177 CHAPTER

Soft Tissue Augmentation

Madhuri Agarwal

INTRODUCTION

Dermal fillers or soft tissue fillers are a noninvasive treatment approved by the US-Food and Drug Administration (USFDA) to restore youth and volume to the face and for increasing the volume of the back of the hand.

As the facial skin ages, there is a significant volume loss due to fat atrophy and bony resorption which leads to contour irregularities and folds that define the signs of aging. There is flattening of midface, nasolabial folds deepen, the tear trough hollows under the eyes appear and corner of the mouth droop. Use of soft tissue fillers improves or corrects all the effects of aging due to volume loss.

Filler injections are quick and simple, and provide instant results with a minimal amount of discomfort and downtime. They are administered via tiny injections and the results are visible instantly. The natural soft tissue gel is completely safe, and actually encourages the skin to produce more collagen (biostimulation) to restore a youthful appearance.

Dermal fillers can last anywhere between 6 and 18 months, depending on the type of the filler material used and the area where it is injected.

HISTORY[1,2]

The search for an ideal soft tissue filler to correct various facial folds and wrinkles has been going for years and in the recent times we have seen a number of new products for soft tissue augmentation. The practice of soft tissue augmentation was started by Neuber in 1893, who took fat from the arms and transplanted it into facial defects. In 1899, Paraffin was used and was later given up due to side effects. In the 1940s and 1950s, silicone was used extensively until the commissioner of USFDA declared the use of injectable silicone to be illegal. The field underwent a revolutionary change in early 1970s when researchers at Stanford University worked on the use of animal and human collagen as implant materials. In 1996, hyaluronic acid derivatives (Restylane™) was introduced. In 2004, first hyaluronic acid HYLAFORM® was approved by USFDA. In 2006, first uniform consistency hyaluronic acid was approved by USFDA (JUVÉDERM® injectable gel). Since then a series of revolutionary changes took place in the field of Fillers.

CLASSIFICATION[3,4]

Fillers can be classified based on different criteria:

- *Based on longevity* **(Table 1)**:
  - *Temporary fillers* stay in the tissue for less than a year. These fillers stay for less than 12 months, hence spontaneously disappearing, if the patient is not satisfied with the results. Adverse event with such fillers is also temporary. However, rare permanent side effects have been reported even with temporary fillers.
  - *Semi-permanent fillers* stay for up to 1–2 years
  - *Permanent fillers* are substances that remain in the tissue more than 2 years
- *Based on the origin:* Knowing the source of the filler is important, to know about the need for pre-skin testing and the patient's preference. Many patients may not wish to use animal products for religious or personal reasons.
  - *Collagen-based:* Can be animal or human origin
    - *Bovine collagen-based products:* Zyderm/Zyplast
    - *Human tissue-derived collagen:* Cosmoderm/Cosmoplast
    - *Tissue-bank collagen material:* Cymetra/Fascian

TABLE 1: Dermal fillers classification by longevity.

Temporary biodegradable (<1 year)	*Semipermanent biodegradable (1–2 years)*	*Permanent nonbiodegradable (>2 years)*
• Autologous fat transfer (AFT) • Acellular dermis—cadaver	• Calcium hydroxylapatite (CaHA) • Dextran particles (DEAE)	• Collagen implant— porcine • Silicone oil (polydimethylsiloxane oil) (LIS)
• Collagen—human, bovine, porcine • Cultured fibroblasts—human • Fascia autograft—human	• Hydroxyethylmethacrylate (HEMA) • Polylactic acid (PLA) • Polyvinyl alcohol (PVA)	• Polyacrylamide gel (PAAG) • Polymethylmethacrylate (PMMA) • Expanded polytetrafluoroethylene (ePTFE)
Hyaluronic acid (HA)—avian, bacterial		Polytetrafluoroethylene (PTFE)

TABLE 2: Various hyaluronic acid fillers currently available in India and their characteristics.

Product	*Description*	*Site of placement*
Juvederm Ultra Plus XC	24 mg/mL with 0.3% lidocaine	Mid dermis
Juvederm Ultra XC	24 mg/mL with 0.3% lidocaine	Superficial dermis
Juvederm Voluma	20 mg/mL with 0.3% lidocaine	Deep dermis/ Supraperiosteal
Volift	17.5 mg/mL with 0.3% lidocaine	Mid dermis
Volbella	17.5 mg/mL with 0.3% lidocaine	Superficial dermis
Restylane	20 mg/mL	Mid dermis
Perlane	20 mg/mL	Deep dermis
Emervel	20 mg/mL with 0.3% lidocaine	Superficial dermis
Belotero Hydro	18 mg/mL	Superficial dermis
Belotero Soft	20 mg/mL	Mid dermis
Belotero Balance	22.5 mg/mL	Mid dermis
Belotero Volume	26 mg/mL	Deep dermis/ Supraperiosteal

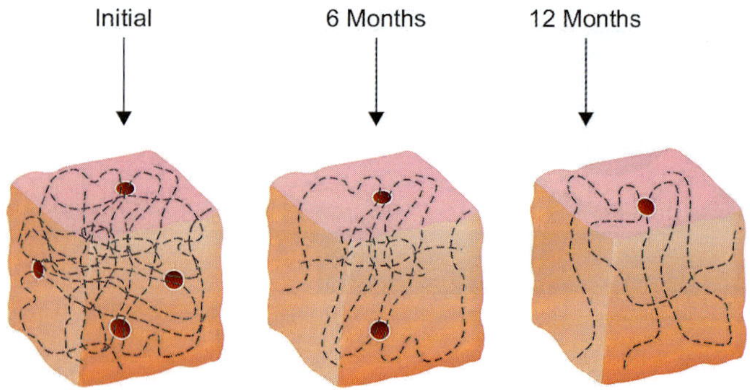

Fig. 1: Hyaluronic acid (HA) fillers are isovolemically degraded, the volume is maintained until the product is completely degraded.

TABLE 3: Comparison of allopathic implants.

Products	*Description*	*Indication*	*Site of placement*
Sculptra	Poly-L-lactic acid	Volume filler	Deep dermis, subcutis
Radiesse	Calcium hydroxylapatite	Volume enhancement	Deep dermis
Bioin blue	Polyvinyl alcohol	Volume enhancement	• Hypodermis Deep dermis • Intramuscular • Subfascial

- *Synthetic fillers:* Nonimmunogenic and are not associated with the risk of allergic reactions.
  - Hyaluronic acid-based fillers
  - *Allopathic implants:* Calcium hydroxyl apatite or poly-L-lactic acid.

Hyaluronic Acid-based Fillers

A wide range of hyaluronic acid products are available with varying concentrations and cross-linking structure and hence, also differ in their indications. All of the hyaluronic acid fillers are supplied as clear colorless transparent gels packaged in a disposable syringe.

Table 2 shows the various hyaluronic acid fillers currently available in India and their characteristics.

Hyaluronic acid fillers are available in two forms non-animal or animal source derivatives.

1. *Nonanimal source hyaluronic acid (NASHA):* Juvéderm™ (Allergan) and Restylane/Perlane™ (Medicis; Scottsdale, Arizona)
2. *Animal-based:* Hylaform™ (Biomatrix, Inc; Ridgefield).

Principle of Hyaluronic Acid Filler (Fig. 1)

- After injection, the hyaluronic acid gel binds the water and thus adds volume to the tissue, thereby restoring the skin contours to the desired level of correction.
- The implant is naturally integrated into the tissue and will in time undergo isovolemic degradation.
- The implant will last for 6–12 months, after which a repeat procedure will be essential to maintain the desired cosmetic results.
- Concern areas show improvement within few seconds of the injection, with the complete effect to be observed after 6 hours.

Allopathic Implants

Comparison of allopathic implants is shown in **Table 3**.

Sculptra: US-FDA approved for AIDS lipodystrophy.

- It is composed of powder of poly-L-lactic acid microspheres, sodium carboxymethylcellulose, nonpyrogenic mannitol, and sterile water for injection. Sculptra is available as a sterile freeze-dried preparation for injection in a clear glass vial. A pack of Sculptra consists two vials (367.5 mg of powder each).
- The filler triggers an ingrowth of type I collagen in the region of accumulated particles while the polylactic acid microspheres go through dissolution. This effect occurs for weeks to months after injection and a long-term filling effect is achieved.

Radiesse™: Made of calcium hydroxyl apatite (CaHA) microspheres, US-FDA approved:

- The microspheres (particles) form a scaffold through which body's own collagen grows.
- Correction for up to 12–24 months. Used for deeper lines, volume enhancement

TABLE 4: Optimal filler characteristics.

Dermal Filler Characteristic Checklist *Optimal characteristics—temporary fillers*	
• Long duration/persistence • Performance promise • Painless • Reasonable cost • Nontoxic • Noninflammatory • Noncarcinogenic	• No migration • Non-animal origin • Easy to inject • Easy to store • Ease of learning how to inject • Minimal side effects • Biodegradable (in case of temporary and semipermanent fillers)

- For the first three months after injection, Radiesse performs as a filler substance by plumping up the skin, later due to its collagen-generating properties. Radiesse stimulates new tissue development for extended correction.

As a physician, there are certain ideal characteristics that are sought out in soft tissue fillers. The properties of an ideal soft tissue filler are enumerated in **Table 4**.

INDICATIONS

Dermal filler can be used for the following indications:[3]

Facial Areas

- Wrinkles and folds
- Lip augmentation
- *Depressed scars:* Postsurgical, traumatic, post-acne, chickenpox, and other diseases
- Enhancement of facial contour
- Periocular melanosis and sunken eyes
- *Dermatological diseases:* Angular cheilitis, dermal atrophy, AIDS lipodystrophy
- Earring ptosis, atrophic earlobes
- Nasal depressions

Nonfacial Areas

- Neck
- Décolleté rejuvenation
- Hands
- *Corns and calluses:* To reduce contact points, pain, and risk of ulcer formation

CONTRAINDICATIONS

Contraindications of fillers are generally rare; they include:
Absolute:

- Hypersensitivity to products
- Unrealistic expectations

Relative:

- Keloidal tendency
- Patients with autoimmune diseases
- Pregnancy and lactation
- Patients with localized infection or herpes
- Patients on blood thinners.

Preprocedure

- Medical and aesthetic assessment of the patient is a must.
- It is very important that the patient is educated about the filler, technique of administration, outcome, side effects, postprocedure care, need for maintenance and any other additional procedures required to achieve optimum results. A handout on these aspects can be given to patients for reference.
- Written informed consent has to be signed after counseling and adequate briefing of the patient. However, consent has to be taken specifically for facial photographs where identity could be revealed.
- Document any asymmetry present between two sides.
- Well-focused, pretreatment photographs should be taken not only for a better assessment of defects, but also for legal purposes.
- Longevity of results is a crucial issue in the use of fillers. Patients should always know fully the duration of results expected for proper planning. Both this and the fact that individual results may vary should be explained to the patient.
- Need for touch up after few days must be informed to the client.

Procedure

Strict asepsis has to be maintained during filler administration. The area to be treated has to be disinfected with the spirit-povidone iodine-spirit method. Sterile cotton and gauze has to be used.

Any medical intervention has to be as painless as possible, more so when an enhancement procedure likes filler procedure is being done. To alleviate the pain, infraorbital nerve block or use of topical anesthetic creams has to be deployed. Fillers premixed with lidocaine are available which can be chosen. Always check for hypersensitivity to anesthetic agent for every patient.

Injection Depth

- The depth of hyaluronic acid injection is an essential factor for achieving the optimal aesthetic outcome **(Fig. 2)**.
- Hyaluronic acid may be placed in the mid-dermal plane—between the papillary and the reticular dermis.
- In some cases, in the reticular dermis or upper subcutaneous tissue.
- Often the subdermal plane is a critical plane for contouring the skin.

Techniques[5]

The choice of the injection technique depends on the indication, its location, the filler substance, size of the needle, and the experience of the injector. The techniques include:

- Linear threading technique
- Serial puncture
- Fanning
- Cross-hatching
- Depot
- Fern
- Cone

The first four techniques are used commonly, whereas the last three are only used in special situations. It is important to place the filler in the right place and the bevel orientation is not a significant issue at any site.

Serial puncture technique: Multiple injections are placed serially along the length of the wrinkle. The serial placements of the product within the skin should join together into a smooth, continuous line **(Fig. 3)**. There should be no spaces between the injected materials. Serial puncture technique is suitable for the nasolabial folds, fine lines, marionette lines, and glabella.

Linear threading technique: The full length of the needle is inserted into the middle of the line or fold. The product can

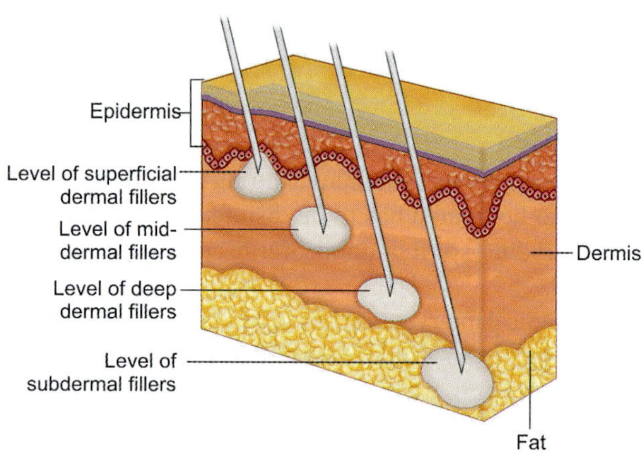

Fig. 2: The illustration shows the various levels/depths of filler placement.

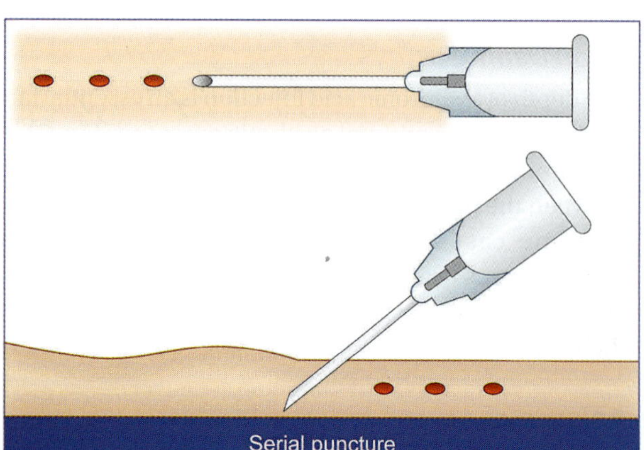

Fig. 3: Serial puncture technique for soft tissue filler.

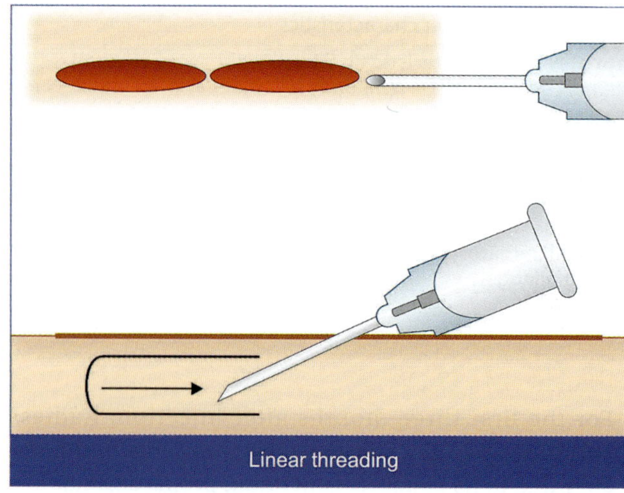

Fig. 4: Linear threading technique for soft tissue filler.

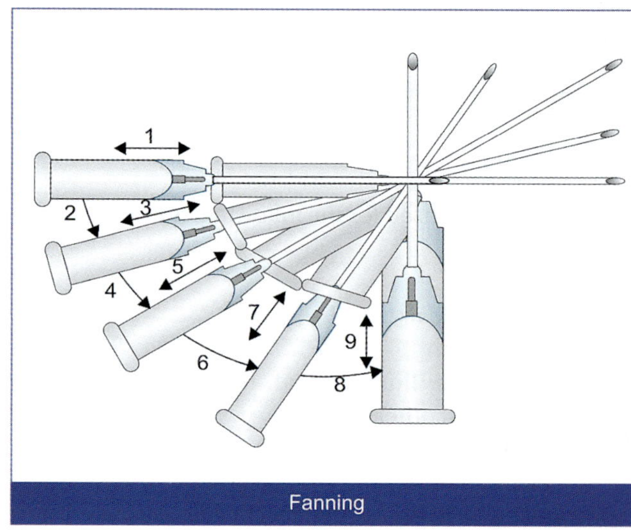

Fig. 5: Fanning technique for soft tissue filler.

be injected in anterograde or retrograde manner **(Fig. 4)**. Anterograde linear threading is filler injected while the needle is slowly introduced forward and the filler product is deposited along the length of the wrinkle or fold. In retrograde technique, the full length of the needle is inserted as far as needed. The filler product is injected while pulling the needle slowly backward. The physician can use the approach dependent on comfort and preference.

Fanning: This technique is good for filling deep volume loss areas with a single entry point to maximize the use of filler product. The needle is inserted in the same manner as the linear threading technique but before withdrawing the needle out from the fold, its direction is altered to the adjacent area and the filler product is injected in this new area **(Fig. 5)**. The entire area is treated in a fan-like manner to give a smooth even contour.

Cross hatching: Cross-hatching is a technique in which the product is injected in the volume loss area in a grid pattern.

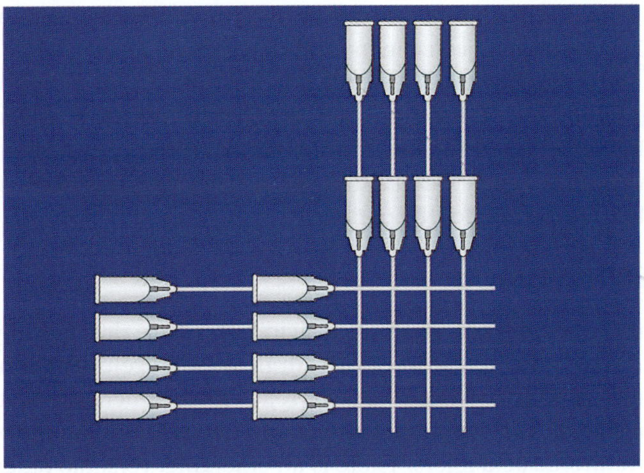

Fig. 6: Cross-hatching technique for soft tissue filler.

TABLE 5: Optimum amount of filler used, but this may vary according to the need of the client and amount of correction required.[4]

Facial region	*Volume*
Glabellar wrinkles	0.5 mL
Nasolabial folds	0.5–1.0 mL (each side)
Lips	0.5–1.0 mL (each lip)
Nose	0.5–1.0 mL
Infraorbital area	1.0–2.0 mL (each side)

It is useful in areas with low bone and ligament support, e.g., perioral area. The needle is inserted in the same manner as the linear threading technique. Then the product is placed serially in a grid manner to achieve a lift and reduce the volume deficit **(Fig. 6)**.

Injecting the Proper Amount of Filler

- The amount of filler injected should be based on age-appropriate contours **(Table 5)**.
- Over correction is most noticeable in the tear troughs, upper cutaneous lip region, and body of the lips.
- For patients who require filling of deep wrinkles, folds, or scars, better results are likely if the clinician is conservative in the amount of filler injected **(Fig. 7)**. If necessary, additional filler can be injected at a follow-up visit in 2 weeks to 2 months.

Documentation of the Procedure Done

The name of the filler and quantity injected in different areas should be mentioned in a chart which contains a sketch of the body part treated. This is not only of relevance for follow-up but also very important if the patient is being considered for any other antiaging procedures such as laser, radiofrequency, etc.

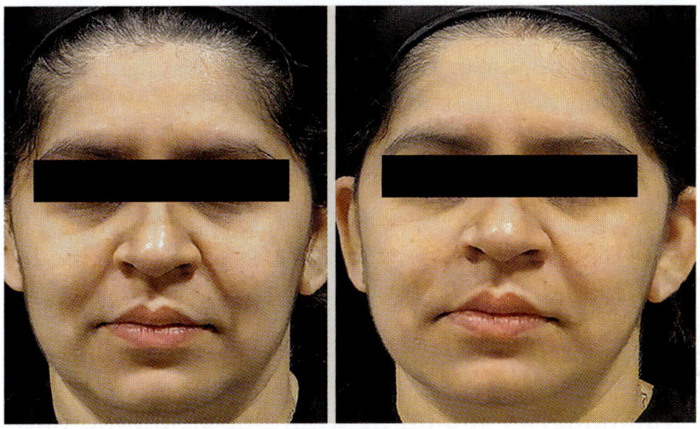

Fig. 7: Nasolabial fold correction with conservative use of Juvederm Ultra Plus XC to soften the lines.

Postprocedure Care

Postprocedure care plays a vital role in the achievement of optimal results, and hence it is essential to educate patients on this aspect.

- Avoid massaging in the area of the filler injection for 2 weeks
- Avoid exposure to direct sunlight, excessive cold weather, outdoor activities until redness, swelling subsides
- Avoid exposing to extremes of temperatures such as sauna or skiing
- Peels, microdermabrasion can be done after a gap of one week, photofacial, laser hair reduction should be done after 2 weeks
- To avoid fillers when the client is on fractional laser services
- No dental work for 2 weeks is also recommended
- Client can be called for a follow-up for touch up after 4–5 days. In case of lips touch up is advisable after 10–14 days as swelling and bruising can last longer.

SIDE EFFECTS

Dermal fillers do come with some side effects which tend to occur immediately after injection, but these are usually temporary and disappear within a few days. According to the FDA, normal side effects include redness, swelling, bruising, itching and tenderness, but on extremely rare occasions more serious side effects requiring early management can occur.

Common Transient Side Effects[7-10]

- Bruising
- Redness
- Swelling
- Pain
- Tenderness
- Itching, rash
- Difficulty in performing activities (only observed when injected into the back of the hand)

Less Common Side Effects

- Raised bumps in or under the skin (nodules or granulomas) that may need to be surgically removed
- Infection
- Open or draining wounds
- A sore at the injection site
- Allergic reaction
- Necrosis (tissue death)

COMPLICATIONS[6–9]

Dermatologists should be aware of all the potential complications that could arise either by the injection itself or the implanted material. Special precautions need to be carried out especially on the glabella, periorbital area, and tip of the nose. Strict asepsis throughout the procedure is advised to avoid infections. One should be able to manage complications without any adverse sequel, or be able to refer the patient to an appropriate center for further management. Proper patient selection, proper technique and right choice of fillers would minimize the incidence of complications.

Following can be the possible complications arising:

- Inflammatory nodule
- Tyndall effect (blue bump)
- Allergic reactions
- Vascular occlusion
- Granulomas

AUTOLOGOUS FAT TRANSPLANT[10]

Autologous fat transfer is a century-old method popularized by Coleman decade ago, which is now considered by many plastic surgeons a valuable tool for soft tissue augmentation in both aesthetic surgery and reconstructive surgery. The procedure is used worldwide as it is simple, less expensive, permanent, and effective. It is considered by many plastic surgeons the ideal body filler to treat volume and contour defects. Furthermore, atrophic scars, lipodystrophy, and scleroderma en coup de sabre can be treated.

Indications

- *Fill defects:*
  - Congenital
  - Traumatic
  - Disease (acne)
  - Iatrogenic
- *Cosmetic:*
  - Furrows (rhytids, wrinkles)
  - Refill of lost supportive tissue (aging)
  - Enhancement

Successful fat transfer involves appropriate fat harvesting, cleansing, and injecting. Harvesting is performed by liposuction in areas of fat which respond poorly to diet. The fat is then cleansed with a physiologic solution of normal saline or Ringer lactate. Fat can be concentrated with the use of centrifugation. The fat is then injected in multiple layers to fill the defect.

Autologous fat transfer has been very successful with good patient satisfaction. However, major disadvantage of this technique remains unpredictable fat resorption rates. A second or even third fat transfer may be necessary to reach the volume best for the patient.

CONCLUSION

In the last decade, hyaluronic acid fillers have dramatically changed the scenario of nonsurgical facial rejuvenation. In the arena of nonsurgical facial rejuvenation, there is a rapid onslaught of newer innovations and newer formulations of hyaluronic acid fillers. There is an emerging, versatile range of soft tissue fillers that can be utilized to treat the customized needs of individuals. A thorough knowledge of the different soft tissue fillers, their various characteristics and optimal utility in the facial rejuvenation is essential to obtain a desirable aesthetic outcome.

KEY POINTS

- Dermal fillers or soft tissue fillers are a noninvasive treatment approved by Food and Drug Administration to restore youth and volume to the face and for increasing the volume of the back of the hand.
- Filler injections are quick and simple, and provide instant results with a minimal amount of discomfort and downtime.
- Hyaluronic acid fillers are the most commonly used fillers in India.
- The choice of the injection technique depends on the indication, its location, the filler substance, size of the needle, and the experience of the injector.
- It is very important that the patient is educated about the filler, technique of administration, outcome, side effects, postprocedure care, need for maintenance and any other additional procedures required to achieve optimum results.
- Dermal fillers do come with some side effects which tend to occur immediately after injection, but these are usually temporary and disappear within a few days.

REFERENCES

1. Naoum C, Dasiou-Plakida D. Dermal filler materials and botulin toxin: review. Int J Dermatol. 2001;40:609-21.
2. Roenigk HH Jr. Treatment of the aging faces. In: Roenigk and Roenigk's Dermatologic Surgery: Principles and Practice, 2nd edition. New York: Marcel Dekker; 1996. pp. 1057-76.
3. Baumann L. Soft tissue augmentation in cosmetic dermatology: principles and practice. New York: Tata McGraw Hill; 2003. pp. 155-72.
4. Hanke WC. Filler materials. In: Theirs BH, Lang PG Jr (Eds). Yearbook of Dermatology and Dermatologic Surgery. St Louis, Missouri: Mosby; 2004. pp. 1-15.

5. Rohrich RJ, Ghavami A, Crosby MA. The role of hyaluronic acid fillers (Restylane) in facial cosmetic surgery: review and technical considerations. Plast Reconstr Surg. 2007:120;6S.
6. Lupton JR, Alsters TS. Cutaneous hypersensitivity reaction to injectable hyaluronic acid gel. Dermatol Surg. 2000;26:135-7.
7. Schanz S, Schippert W, Ulmer A, Rassner G, Fierlbeck G. Arterial embolisation caused by injection of hyaluronic acid (Restylane). Br J Dermatol. 2002;146:928.
8. Piacquadio D, Jarcho M, Goltz R. Clinical and laboratory studies: evaluation of hylan B gel as a soft tissue augmentation implant material. J Am Acad Dermatol. 1997;36:544-9.
9. Michaels P. Human anti-hyaluronic acid antibiotics: is it possible? Dermatol Surg. 2001;27:185-91.
10. Pendergrast PM, Shiffman MA. Facial augmentation with autologous fat. Aesthetic Medicine: Art and Techniques. Amsterdam, The Netherlands: Elsevier; 2012. pp. 347-54.

EXAMINATION QUESTIONS

1. Write a brief note on hyaluronic acid fillers.
2. Write a brief note on dermal fillers.

178 CHAPTER Platelet Rich Plasma Therapy

Gagan Jot Kaur, Aarti Sarda, Abhishek De

INTRODUCTION

Platelet-rich plasma (PRP) is defined as "abundant platelets concentrated into a small volume of plasma."[1]

HISTORY

The concept and of PRP was introduced in the field of hematology in 1970s when hematologists described it as the plasma with a platelet count above that of peripheral blood. Initially, PRP was used as a transfusion product to treat patients with thrombocytopenia.

Later, PRP was used in maxillofacial surgery as platelet-rich fibrin (PRF). Fibrin with its homeostatic properties and the potential for adherence along with complemented PRP thus stimulating cell proliferation. Later PRP was found to have good role in the musculoskeletal field in sports injuries as it stimulates osteoblasts and hence rejuvenation.

More recently, PRP has got many applications in dermatology and aesthetics and has been explored in various indications.

DEFINITION

Platelet-rich plasma is defined as a highly concentrated solution of plasma prepared from patient's own blood which contains platelets above the baseline.

It is a concentration of several growth factors (GFs) by virtue of platelets alone (stored as α-granules in platelets) and plasma proteins, namely fibrin, fibronectin, etc.

This cocktail of GFs **(Fig. 1)** plays a pivotal role in tissue repair and regeneration **(Table 1)**,[2] whereas the plasma proteins act as a scaffold for the connective tissue, bone, and epithelial migration.

PRINCIPLE OF PRP TREATMENT

In a typical blood sample, cells are present in the following percentages: 93% red blood cells (RBCs), 6% platelets, and 1% white blood cells. The principle behind PRP treatment is to reverse the RBC-to-platelet ratio by increasing the platelets in plasma through centrifugation so that a concentration of 94% platelets and 5% RBCs is obtained as depicted in **Figure 2**.

The high level of growth factors and cytokines in PRP help in tissue repair and rejuvenation. The platelet concentration of approximately 1 million platelets/μL, which is approximately 5 times the normal concentration of platelets, has demonstrated tissue repair efficacy.

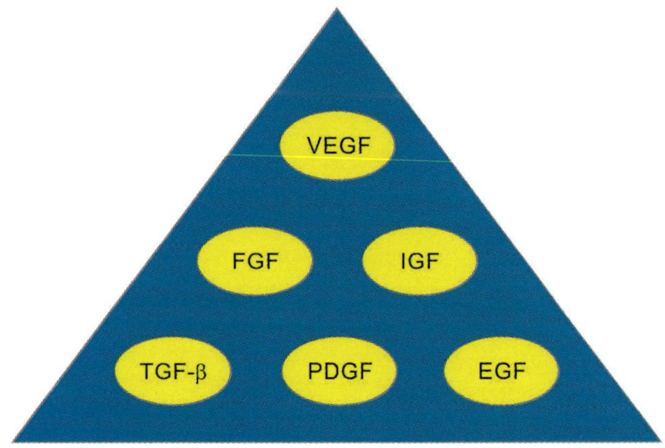

Fig. 1: Principal growth factors released after degranulation from platelets (EGF: epidermal growth factor; FGF: fibroblast growth factor; IGF: insulin growth factor; PDGF: platelet derived growth factor; TGF-β: transforming growth factor-β; VEGF: vascular endothelial growth factor).

TABLE 1: Platelet growth factors and their functions.[2]

Growth factors	*Functions*
Transforming growth factor (TGF-α/β)	• Extracellular matrix synthesis • Keratinocyte regulation in re-epithelization • Stimulation of angiogenesis • Stimulation of type I and type III collagen production • Stimulation of fibroblasts and mesenchymal stem cells proliferation
PDGF	• Mitogenetic for fibroblasts, smooth muscle cells, mesenchymal stem cells, and osteoblasts • Stimulation of macrophage and neutrophil chemotaxis; activation of macrophages
VEGF	Stimulation of angiogenesis
EGF	• Stimulation of epithelial/mesenchymal mitogenesis • Stimulation of chemotaxis of keratinocytes • Stimulation of endothelial chemotaxis, mitogenesis and angiogenesis • Regulation of the secretion of collagenase
FGF	Promotion of angiogenesis, endothelial and fibroblast proliferation and migration, fibronectin synthesis and secretion

(EGF: epidermal growth factor; FGF: fibroblast growth factor; IGF: insulin growth factor; PDGF: platelet-derived growth factor; VEGF: vascular endothelial growth factor)

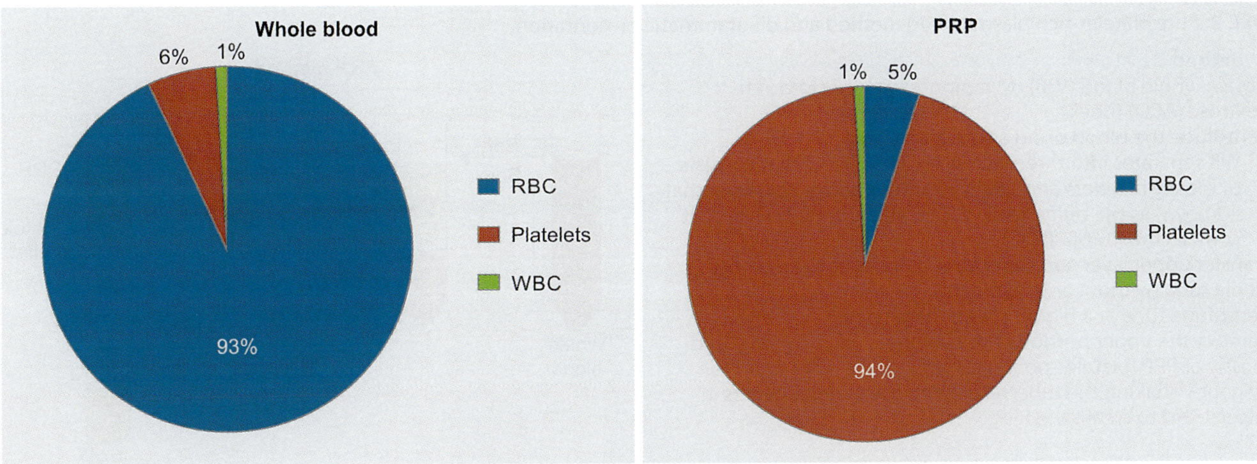

Fig. 2: Pie chart comparing whole blood and PRP.

PREPARATION OF PRP

Aim

To obtain the platelets in high concentrations and in a viable state so that they can actively secrete growth factors and achieve desired therapeutic effect.

Principle of PRP Preparation

Preparation of PRP is based on the concept of differential centrifugation. In this process, acceleration force during centrifugation is adjusted to sediment certain cellular constituents according to their different specific gravities.[3]

Concentration of PRP

The mean blood platelet count is 200,000 ± 75,000/μL.[4] The optimum PRP platelet count has not yet been defined but still a platelet concentration of >1 million/μL (approximately 4–7 times the mean levels) is accepted as the therapeutically effective concentration of PRP.[1,5]

Precautions

- Strict aseptic conditions to be maintained
- Optimum temperature, i.e., 20–22°C to be regularized
- *Use of anticoagulant:* Most commonly acid citrate dextrose solution formula A (ACD-A) is used as it prevents aggregation of platelets and their premature activation (binds free calcium in blood thus preventing clotting cascade).

Method

Around 30 mL blood sample is withdrawn in a conical tube containing anticoagulant. The yield can vary depending upon the baseline platelet count of the patient, the device and the technique used.

Blood is then centrifuged to separate blood components according to their different specific gravities. RBCs being the heaviest will settle down, followed by WBCs, and platelets being the lightest will be collected in upper layer. The first centrifugation is kept slow to avoid spinning down platelets and also to isolate plasma. Platelets get mostly concentrated right on top of the buffy coat layer. Second centrifugation is faster and platelets are spun down. They separate as a pellet at the bottom of the tube and gets separated from platelet-poor plasma (PPP) above. Approximately three-fourths of the supernatant is discarded. Then the platelet-rich pellet is resuspended in the remaining amount of plasma. Thus PRP is obtained. Approximately, 3–5 cc of PRP is obtained from 30 cc of blood.

Next step is to "activate PRP." Calcium chloride ($CaCl_2$) or thrombin is used as an "activator." The purpose is to trigger coagulation, and hence degranulation of GFs which brings in therapeutic effect. The procedure has been illustrated in a simplified manner in **Flowchart 1**.

Flowchart 1: Basic steps for preparation and mechanism of action of "activated" PRP.

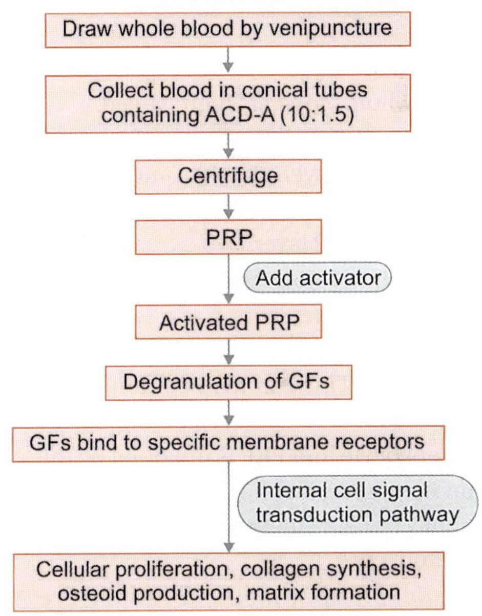

TABLE 2: Pure platelet-rich plasma (PRP) method and diagrammatic presentation.

PRP method

1. Obtain whole blood (WB) by venipuncture in acid citrate dextrose (ACD) tubes.
2. Centrifuge the blood using a soft spin.
   - WB separates into three layers: An upper layer that consists of mostly platelets and WBCs, an intermediate thin layer that is known as the buffy rich in WBCs, and a bottom layer that consists mostly of RBCs.
3. Transfer upper layer and superficial buffy layer to an empty sterile tube (without anticoagulant).
4. Centrifuge tube at a higher speed (hard spin).
5. Remove the upper portion of the volume which is composed mostly of PPP (platelet-poor plasma).
6. By gently shaking the tube, resuspend the platelet pellets in lower 1/3rd to create the PRP.

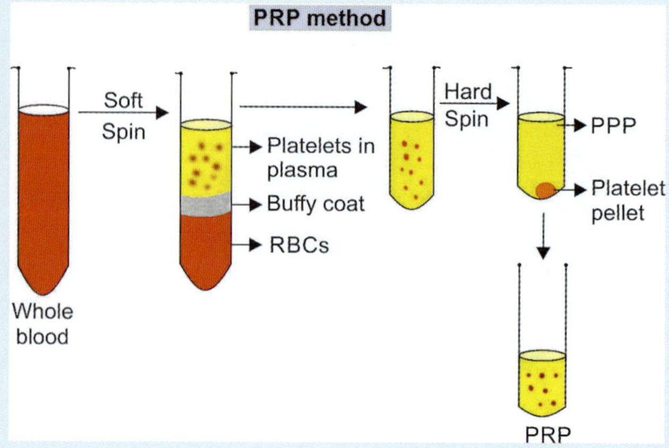

There are many ways of preparing PRP. It can be prepared by the PRP method or by the buffy-coat method **(Table 2)**.

Buffy Coat Method

- Centrifuge whole blood at "high" speed.
- *Three layers are formed:* The bottom layer contains mostly RBCs, the middle layer platelets and WBCs, and the top PPP layer.
- Remove the top PPP layer.
- Transfer the buffy-coat along with superficial RBCs to another sterile tube.
- Further centrifugation can be done at low speed to separate WBCs. This can also be done using leukocyte filtration filter. Reduce suspension to ¼ and resuspend.
- *L-PRP:* Leukocyte and PRP is obtained by this method.
- PRP can be prepared either by using automated devices or manually by using methods such as PRP method, buffy coat method, etc.
- *Manual double spin method:* As per the American Association of Blood Banks (AABB) technical manual,[4] "platelet-rich plasma can be separated from the whole blood using 'light-spin' centrifugation and can be further concentrated using 'heavy-spin' centrifugation and subsequent removal of the supernatant plasma."
- Soft spin ~ 1,200 rotations/min for 10 min
- Hard Spin ~ 2,400 rotations/min for 10 min
- A handmade PRP can be prepared in a cost effective manner without using a commercial kit.
- Automated devices

Various commercial devices of varying standards are available for the preparation of PRP though their application is a bit confusing because machines employ different techniques thus leading to a different product which may have dissimilar biology and variable relative efficacy.

Though these commercial kits are time saving but these can be quite expensive as compared to the manual process.

Factors Influencing PRP Yield

- *Technique of drawing blood:* The clotting process is influenced from the time the blood is withdrawn. Most protocols advocate use of large bore needles (>22) to withdraw the blood so as to avoid activation of platelets.
- *Anticoagulants:* For preserving the platelet's functionality, morphology and integrity, choice of anticoagulant is important.

  Most authors agree that EDTA should not be used as it can damage the platelet membrane. The use of anticoagulants such as ACD-A is recommended as it prevents premature activation of platelets.
- *Centrifugation:* Yield of PRP depends on speed and time of centrifugation. When an ordinary centrifuge (mainly used for diagnostic purposes) is used to obtain PRP, sufficient platelet yield may not be obtained. The double spin method is preferred over the single spin method because in some studies therapeutic concentration of platelets was not obtained.
- *Temperature:* Temperature maintenance is important to prevent platelet activation. As per AABB, temperature of 21–24°C is acceptable during centrifugation for obtaining PRP.[5,6]
- *Activation of PRP:* PRP can be activated exogenously by thrombin, calcium chloride, or mechanical trauma. Collagen is a natural activator of PRP, thus when PRP is used in soft tissue, it does not need to be exogenously activated.

The active secretion of prepackaged GFs begins within 10 minutes of clot initiation and 95% of the secretion is completed within 1 hour. Hence, PRP must be used on the treated site within 10 minutes of activation.

In addition to above factors, the hematocrit value and total platelet count influence the final platelet concentration of the PRP.

TABLE 3: Types of PRP.

	Pure PRP	*L-PRP (Leukocyte and PRP)*	*P-PRF/PRFM*	*L-PRF (Leukocyte and platelet-rich fibrin)*
Cell content	Rich in platelets	Rich in platelets and leukocytes	Rich in platelets	Rich in platelets and leukocytes
Fibrin architecture	Low-density fibrin network	Low-density fibrin network	High-density fibrin network	High-density fibrin network

(PRF: platelet-rich fibrin; PRFM: platelet-rich fibrin matrix)

CLASSIFICATION OF PRP CONCENTRATES

Dohan Ehrenfest et al.[7] classified PRP in 2009 in four types **(Table 3)** following two principle parameters:

1. Cell content
2. Fibrin architecture

INDICATIONS IN DERMATOLOGY

Alopecia (Androgenic Alopecia, Alopecia Areata, in Hair Transplantation)[8-10]

Mechanism of Action

↑*Bcl-2 levels*: Antiapoptotic
↑*B-catenin:* Differentiation of stem cells into hair follicles
↑*Expression of FGF-7 in dermal papilla cells:* Prolongs anagen
↑*PDGF and VEGF:* Proangiogenic

Procedure

- *Interfollicular injection of PRP:* The amount injected is around 0.05–0.1 mL/cm^2
- *PRP mesotherapy:* Scalp is punctured with dermaroller and then PRP is sprayed.
- *In hair transplantation:* (1) Follicular grafts are dipped into PRP for 15 minutes before implantation as it might increase their survival rate; (2) PRP may be applied over the recipient area before implanting the grafts.

Skin Rejuvenation

Mechanism of Action

Dermal elasticity: Stimulates the removal of photodamaged extracellular matrix (ECM) components.

Expression of MMPs (matrix metalloproteinases): Induces the synthesis of new collagen by dermal fibroblasts.

- Traumatic, postsurgical, and acne scars
- Wound healing
- Striae distensae
- Dermal volume augmentation
- Lipodermatosclerosis and lichen sclerosus.

SAFETY OF PRP

- PRP is autologous preparation, hence it is devoid of any serious side effects. However, pain during injection or secondary infection can occur.
- There is no risk of transmission of infections such as HIV or Hepatitis B, C.
- The mitogenic effects of PRP are theoretically not mutagenic and are only limited to augmentation of the normal healing process.

CONCLUSION

Owing to the plethora of growth factors, cytokines and chemokines it contains, PRP is being widely used as a new therapeutic option in the field of dermatology, wound healing, trichology, and aesthetic dermatology. Being autologous, the therapy is general well tolerated. Despite numerous studies in various peer-reviewed journals, still no standard guidelines regarding the exact concentration, dosing parameters, frequency of application, and duration of therapy are available. PRP is a promising and evolving therapy and to use it to its full potential, standard guidelines about its preparation and administration are the need of the hour.

KEY POINTS

- Platelet rich plasma (PRP) is defined as a highly concentrated solution of plasma prepared from patient's own blood which contains platelets above the baseline.
- PRP is being used as a new therapeutic option for different pathologies in the field of dermatology, such as trichology, wound healing, and aesthetic dermatology.
- It is an effective concentration of multiple fundamental growth factors (GFs) which play a pivotal role in modulation of tissue repair and regeneration.
- Preparation of PRP is based on the concept of differential centrifugation. In this process, acceleration force during centrifugation is adjusted to sediment certain cellular constituents according to their different specific gravities.
- *"All PRPs are not the same":* PRP concentrates have been classified into P-PRP, L-PRP, P-PRF and L-PRF types depending on the cell types present and fibrin architecture.
- Standardization of PRP preparation and administration will help to use it to its full potential.

REFERENCES

1. Marx RE, Garg AK. Dental and craniofacial applications of platelet-rich plasma. Chicago: Quintessence Publishing; 2005.
2. Steed DL. The role of growth factors in wound healing. Surg Clin North Am. 1997;77:575-86.

3. Dhurat R, Sukesh MS. Principles and methods of preparation of platelet-rich plasma: a review and author's perspective. J Cutaneous Aesthet Surg. 2014;(4):189-97.
4. American Association of Blood Banks Technical Manual Committee. Method 6.11: Preparation of platelets from whole blood. In: Vengelen-Tyler V (Ed). AABB Technical Manual, 13th edition. Bethesda, MD: American Association of Blood Banks; 1999. p. 725.
5. Arshdeep, M Sendhil Kumaran. Platelet-rich plasma in dermatology: boon or a bane? Ind J Dermatol Venereol Leprol. 2014;80(1):5-14.
6. Sweeny J, Grossman BJ. Blood collection, storage and component preparation methods. In: Brecher M (Ed). Technical Manual, 14th edition. Bethesda, MD: American Association of Blood Banks (AABB); 2002. pp. 955-8.
7. Dohan Ehrenfest DM, Rasmusson L, Albrektsson T. Classification of platelet concentrates: from pure platelet-rich plasma (P-PRP) to leucocyte- and platelet-rich fibrin (L-PRF). Trends Biotechnol. 2009;27:158-67.
8. Alves R, Grimalt R. A review of platelet rich plasma: history, biology, mechanism of action and classification. Skin Appendage Disord. 2018;4:18-24.
9. Takakura N, Yoshida H, Kunisada T, Nishikawa S, Nishikawa SI. Involvement of platelet-derived growth factor receptor-alpha in hair canal formation. J Invest Dermatol. 1996;107:770-7.
10. Uebel CO, da Silva JB, Cantarelli D, Martins P. The role of platelet plasma growth factors in male pattern baldness surgery. Plast Reconstr Surg. 2006;118:1458-66.

EXAMINATION QUESTION

1. Write a brief note on platelet rich plasma in dermatology.

179 CHAPTER Camouflage

Rasya K Dixit, Vandini Kabra

INTRODUCTION

Skin is an embodiment of beauty and often skin diseases evoke social stigma and cause patients significant psychological distress and a decreased quality of life. Most of these skin conditions are often chronic or recurrent, and need a long time for remission or to achieve good results. Camouflaging skin lesions can be a useful option in such patients, offering better quality of life with proper use of products or techniques. This following chapter will discuss different camouflage options for patients with different dermatological conditions **(Box 1)**.

The noun form of the word "camouflage" can mean either "concealment by some means that alters or obscures the appearance" or "a device/stratagem used for concealment." Medical camouflage is now commonly used to cover scars, imperfections and pigmentary abnormalities and hair disorders.[1] Camouflage techniques can be especially useful in patients who do not achieve complete or immediate attractive results from dermatologic therapy for their conditions.

VITILIGO

Vitiligo is a condition associated with significant social stigma. Patients often suffer from decreased self-esteem and low quality of life due to the psychosocial effects of the disease. Studies show that cosmetic camouflage shows a significant improvement in the quality of life in patients with vitiligo and must be part of the counseling offered to the patients **(Box 2)**.[2-4]

As it is difficult to get a good color match with liquid dyes and indigenous preparations, and as they are easily washed away, these methods of temporary camouflage have been more or less replaced by foundation-based camouflage products.[5,6]

Foundation-based camouflage products fulfill most of the criteria for being an ideal camouflage agent **(Box 3)**.[7] They are available in a range of colors and are highly pigmented when compared to traditional makeup foundation. Most camouflage foundations are manufactured as creams, as it is possible to incorporate increased concentrations of iron oxide to provide better coverage. They are usually available in a matt finish, and last up to 24 hours after a single application.[8,9]

The application of these camouflage products is different from traditional cosmetic use and patient has to be educated about how to choose the product and apply it. The patient may need to purchase more than one shade of color as there may be differing shades of skin color on face and body parts, and also one shade might not correctly match the skin. The product is ideally applied by patting over the affected areas and blended over the edges to conceal the vitiligo. The product has to be removed with a water soluble makeup remover and the skin cleansed at bedtime to prevent any irritation of the skin due to alcohol or acetone-based makeup removers.[8]

Though these products offer good cover, they cannot be used over large areas or over irritated and infected or ulcerated skin areas. Also they tend to wear off quickly over hands and feet due to friction.[9]

Self-tanning products containing dihydroxyacetone (DHA) have also been used in vitiligo camouflage.[10] These work in temporarily staining the skin by forming brown chromophores called melanoidins in the stratum corneum. However, proper color match is not possible with this product.[11]

BOX 1: Dermatological conditions which can be camouflaged by procedures.

- Vitiligo
- Pigmentary conditions—melasma, postinflammatory hyperpigmentation, tattoos
- Vascular conditions—vascular malformations, telangiectasia
- Hair conditions—alopecia of various causes
- Scars

BOX 2: Camouflage products in vitiligo.

- *Temporary camouflage:*
  - Liquid dyes—potassium permanganate, henna, indigo carmine, Bismarck brown
  - Indigenous preparations
  - Foundation-based cosmetic camouflage
  - Self-tanning products
- *Permanent camouflage:*
  - Micropigmentation

BOX 3: Characteristics of an ideal camouflage agent.

- Color matching ability or multiple colors available
- Must look natural while also able to conceal deformity
- Waterproof and sweat proof
- Long wear
- Easily applicable
- Nonallergic/noncomedogenic
- Cost-effective

Micropigmentation or medical tattooing can be used as a permanent camouflage technique in recalcitrant vitiligo lesions, especially over distal digits, lips, hands, wrists, axillae, elbows, perianal areas, lower legs, mucosae, and mucocutaneous junctions.[12] Pigments such as iron oxide, (light and dark brown), white (titanium dioxide), yellow (cadmium sulfide), and red (mercuric sulfide/cinnabar) with cadmium sulfide are used alone or in combination, and deposited in between the superficial and middle dermis. Over the years, a small amount of this pigment may migrate to the regional lymph nodes with resultant fading. It has been observed on histopathology that the initial pigment, which is largely intracellular, gradually becomes extracellular and lies among collagen bundles, blood vessels, and hair follicles without causing foreign body inflammation in the majority of cases.[13,14] Though micropigmentation offers quick results, the complications such as poor color match, color fading, granuloma formation, and oxidation of pigment to cause blackish deposits make dermatologist usually adopt this treatment only for treatment of smaller areas recalcitrant to treatment.[15] However, with the use of noncultured melanocyte cell suspensions which yield superior results, these techniques are now used only sparingly.

DISORDERS OF HYPERPIGMENTATION AND VASCULAR ETIOLOGY (MELASMA, POSTINFLAMMATORY HYPERPIGMENTATION, NEVI, SPIDER NEVI, TELANGIECTASIA)

Visible skin conditions are a cause of emotional distress to the patients, especially if they are over socially visible areas such as face and extremities. Even children are socially handicapped when they have skin lesions which they are unable to explain to their peers. There are many papers which talk about the psychological effects of medical treatment on such conditions. Similarly, using an appropriate camouflage offers significant emotional benefits to such patients.[16,17]

Cosmetic camouflage agents can be used appropriately in patient with acne, rosacea, melasma, hemangiomas, and telangiectasia as in these conditions systemic and topical therapies may take several weeks to months of consistent use to achieve noticeable improvement. Although patients are often dissatisfied knowing that there are no "quick fixes" available, it is important that there is a clear discussion regarding the planned therapeutic regimen and the importance of close clinical follow-up, and that meticulous commitment to treatment be emphasized by the practitioner. Perhaps the most notable benefit of cosmetic camouflage is the immediate results and instant gratification that can be achieved after application of the product which allows the patient to return to social activities immediately.[18] Studies have shown significant improvement in dermatology life quality index (DLQI) post-camouflage in skin conditions, such as discoid lupus erythematosus (DLE), acne, and melasma, confirming that the use of decorative cosmetics in subjects with disfiguring skin disease is an effective, well-tolerated treatment to help increase quality of life and that decorative cosmetics should complement medical treatment protocols.[4,19]

SCARS

Camouflaging pigmentary conditions tend to be easier than camouflaging uneven scars as rough scars are more difficult to conceal because unevenness may be exaggerated after camouflaging. For contouring, several products have to be applied. Hypertrophic scars appear lighter than the surrounding skin and have to be camouflaged applying a darker product than the surrounding skin. Atrophic scars, however, appear darker than the surrounding skin and have to be corrected using a lighter product.[20,21]

Patients have also discovered novel techniques to camouflage their surgical and accidental scars with tattoos. Tattoos no longer carry social taboos and this can be offered to patients, especially if they already have another tattoo.[22]

HAIR CAMOUFLAGE

Hair loss can cause psychological distress to both women and men. In studies, both patients with alopecia areata and androgenetic alopecia scored similarly on emotional assessment. Patients in both groups were less motivated to pursue personal interests and experienced difficulty in coping with stress compared to the controls.[23] Often patients with hair loss also believe that their hair loss was a barrier to gainful employment.[24] Even patients on chemotherapy felt that the most burdensome part of their chemotherapy was alopecia.[25] Chemotherapy-induced alopecia can lead to anxiety, depression, reduced quality of life, and decreased self-esteem.[26]

Treatment of hair loss in many patients takes time and some camouflage techniques can be offered in the interim **(Box 4)**.

Hair complement devices such as wigs may be wefted, which is the most common and least expensive; or net, the more expensive but more natural-looking option. They use synthetic or human hair which are weaved into

BOX 4: Hair camouflage devices and treatments.

- *Hair complement devices:*
  - Wigs
  - Hair extensions
- Pigmented powders, sprays, and lotions
- *Surgical methods:*
  - Hair transplantation
  - Micropigmentation

the foundation. The cost of these devices depends on how natural they look.[27,28]

Hair extensions can be used for patients with patchy hair loss or to increase volume in patients with long hair. However, hair extensions may make alopecia worse because of traction. Traction alopecia can result from constant tension of hair extension on natural hairs and cause the hair shaft to separate from the ostium, resulting in hair loss. Traction alopecia in these cases was initially nonscarring but may lead to scarring or permanent alopecia.[29]

Pigmented Powders, Lotions, and Sprays

Patients often innovate and do use pigmented substances such as kajal and mascara to not only enhance but also fill gaps in eyebrow hair. They also use these over the thinning scalp for hiding the early patterned hair loss. Powders, lotion, and sprays are available in different colors and help to camouflage the onset of hair loss. However, they need to be reapplied daily and are often distorted by getting hair wet as it may happen accidentally during a rain shower.[27]

Hair fibers, which are positively charged particles of wool keratin that adhere to the negatively charged terminal and vellus hair fibers on the scalp, can be used over the hairy areas of the scalp. They are ineffective over the bald areas. These are derived from wool or rice keratin, rayon, or human hair, and have to be reused daily for results.[27]

SURGICAL METHODS

Hair transplant and scalp micropigmentation are permanent methods of hair camouflage. Van der Velden et al. described the medical use of tattooing, specifically in alopecia areata of the eyebrows.[30] Traquina first reported the use of micropigmentation of the scalp specifically for scalp scars.[31]

The process involves the insertion of a pigment through the skin in the upper dermis, using conventional tattoo instruments and artistic and objective judgment on dot placement. The patient will need approximately two to four sessions for completion, with each session lasting up to 8 hours. Risks include infection and allergies to pigment. Needle use carries a risk of infectious disease transmission, such as HIV, hepatitis, and skin infections. In addition to the risk of infection, disadvantages to micropigmentation include the fact that natural hair may gray over time and hair may need to be dyed to match the changing pigment. Also, the final product may need touch-ups over time due to fading and progression of hair loss.[32]

CONCLUSION

Cosmetic camouflage has a definitive role in the management of chronic skin conditions which often need long-term treatments. Dermatologists and their staff must be aware of these options and offer them to patients to help them cope with their psychosocial issues and to improve their quality of life.

KEY POINTS

- Camouflage is an important tool for helping cover scars, imperfections, and hair disorders till such time they can be treated.
- Camouflage should be part of medical and surgical treatment options.
- Skin and hair conditions can be effectively camouflaged by various techniques.

REFERENCES

1. Kaliyadan F, Kumar A. Camouflage for patients with vitiligo. Indian J Dermatol Venereol Leprol. 2012;78(1):8-15.
2. Talsania N, Lamb B, Bewley A. Vitiligo is more than skin deep: a survey of members of the Vitiligo Society. Clin Exp Dermatol. 2010;35:736-9.
3. Kent G, Al'Abadie M. Psychologic effects of vitiligo: a critical incident analysis. J Am Acad Dermatol. 1996;35:895-8.
4. Holme SA, Beattie PE, Fleming CJ. Cosmetic camouflage advice improves quality of life. Br J Dermatol. 2002;147:946-9.
5. Sarveswari KN. Cosmetic camouflage in vitiligo. Indian J Dermatol. 2010;55:211-4.
6. Sugathan P, Nejeeba R. A new camouflage for vitiligo. Indian J Dermatol Venerol Leprol. 1991;57:45-6.
7. Draelos ZD. The multifunctional value of sunscreen-containing cosmetics. Skin Therapy Lett. 2011;16:1-3.
8. Antoniou C, Stefanaki C. Cosmetic camouflage. J Cosmet Dermatol. 2006;5:297-301.
9. Tanioka M, Miyachi Y. Waterproof camouflage for vitiligo of the face using Cavilon 3M as a spray. Eur J Dermatol. 2008;18:93-4.
10. Hsu S. Camouflaging vitiligo with dihydroxyacetone. Dermatol Online J. 2008;14:23.
11. Rajatanavin N, Suwanachote S, Kulkollakarn S. Dihydroxy-acetone: a safe camouflaging option in vitiligo. Int J Dermatol. 2008;47:402-6.
12. Vassileva S, Hristakieva E. Medical applications of tattooing. Clin Dermatol. 2007;25:367-74.
13. Mazza JF Jr, Rager C. Advances in cosmetic micropigmentation. Plast Reconstr Surg. 1993;92:750-1.
14. Savant SS. Tattooing versus punch grafting for nipple-areola vitiligo. Indian J Dermatol Surg. 2000;2:9-25.
15. Patrizi A, Raone B, Savoia F, Bacci F, Pileri A, Gurioli C, et al. Tattoo-associated pseudolymphomatous reaction and its successful treatment with hydroxychloroquine. Acta Derm Venereol. 2009;89:327-8.
16. Cotterill JA, Cunliffe WJ. Suicide in dermatological patients. Br J Dermatol. 1997;137(2):246-50.
17. Pawaskar MD, Parikh P, Markowski T, McMichael AJ, Feldman SR, Balkrishnan R. Melasma and its impact on health-related quality of life in Hispanic women. J Dermatolog Treat. 2007;18(1):5-9.
18. Cunliffe WJ. Strategy of treating acne vulgaris. J Eur Acad Dermatol Venereol. 1992;1:43-52.
19. Hayashi N, Imori M, Yanagisawa M, Seto Y, Nagata O, Kawashima M. Make-up improves the quality of life of acne patients without aggravating acne eruptions during treatments. Eur J Dermatol. 2005;15(4):284-7.

20. Bouloc A. Camouflage techniques. In: Draelos ZD (Ed). Cosmetic dermatology: products and procedures, 1st edition. Oxford: Wiley-Blackwell; 2010. pp. 176-83.
21. Rayner VL. Camouflage therapy. Dermatol Clin. 1995;13: 467-72.
22. Spyropoulou GA, Fatah F. Decorative tattooing for scar camouflage: patient innovation. J Plast Reconstr Aesthet Surg. 2009;62(10):e353-5.
23. Monselise A, Bar-On R, Chan L, Leibushor N, McElwee K, Shapiro J. Examining the relationship between alopecia areata, androgenetic alopecia, and emotional intelligence. J Cutan Med Surg. 2013;17(1):46-51.
24. Tischer B. Influence of hair loss on employment decisions. Abstract presented at: American Academy of Dermatology Meeting. March 2000; San Francisco, CA. 2000.
25. Baxley KO, Erdman LK, Henry EB, Roof BJ. Alopecia: effect on cancer patients' body image. Cancer Nurs. 1984;7(6):499-503.
26. Hesketh PJ, Batchelor D, Golant M, Lyman GH, Rhodes N, Yardley D. Chemotherapy-induced alopecia: psychosocial impact and therapeutic approaches. Support Care Cancer. 2004;12(8):543-9.
27. Donovan JC, Shapiro RL, Shapiro P, Zupan M, Pierre-Louis M, Hordinsky M. A review of scalp camouflaging agents and prostheses for individuals with hair loss. Dermatol Online J. 2012;18(8):1.
28. Banka N, Bunagan MJ, Dubrule Y, Shapiro J. Wigs and hairpieces: evaluating dermatologic issues. Dermatol Ther. 2012;25(3):260-6.
29. Yang A, Iorizzo M, Vincenzi C, Tosti A. Hair extensions: a concerning cause of hair disorders. Br J Dermatol. 2009; 160(1):207-9.
30. van der Velden EM, Drost BH, Ijsselmuiden OE, Baruchin AM, Hulsebosch HJ. Dermatography as a new treatment for alopecia areata of the eyebrows. Int J Dermatol. 1998;37(8):617-21.
31. Traquina AC. Micropigmentation as an adjuvant in cosmetic surgery of the scalp. Dermatol Surg. 2001;27(2):123-8.
32. Rassman WR, Pak JP, Kim J, Estrin NF. Scalp micropigmentation: a concealer for hair and scalp deformities. J Clin Aesthet Dermatol. 2015;8(3):35-42.

EXAMINATION QUESTION

1. Name some methods of camouflaging hair loss. Describe their advantages and disadvantages.

180 CHAPTER

Recent Advances in Drug Therapy in Dermatology

Shashank Bhargava, Anupam Das

INTRODUCTION

Dermatology is an ever-expanding medical branch owing to discovery of new entities almost every day. Also due to continuous research activities, the pathogenesis of diseases is better understood and hence new molecules are discovered. Several old known drugs are being used for new indications and are used as repurposed drugs in dermatology. There are many more areas in which repurposed drugs can potentially fulfill unmet needs in future. The summary of new molecules along with new dermatological indications of known drugs (drug repositioning or repurposing) has been provided for the readers.

APREMILAST FOR NEWER INDICATIONS

Apremilast is a known inhibitor of phosphodiesterase 4 (PDE4) and binds to Toll-like receptor 4 in peripheral blood cells. It results in elevation in the levels of cyclic adenosine monophosphate (cAMP) which ultimately decreases the proinflammatory cytokines [tumor necrosis factor-alpha, interleukin-23 (IL-23), IL-12, leukotriene B4)] and increases IL-10 which is anti-inflammatory.

Apart from the known indications, it is now employed for Behçet's disease,[1] hidradenitis suppurativa (HS),[2] atopic dermatitis,[3] and recalcitrant pyoderma gangrenosum.[4,5] It can be used for 16 weeks and 12 weeks (30 mg twice daily) in HS and Behçet's disease, respectively. In a case of pyoderma gangrenosum, apremilast 30 mg twice daily was added to a conventional regimen of oral prednisone 7.5 mg daily and subcutaneous methotrexate 18 mg weekly, for 4 months with remarkable improvement.[5]

BETA-BLOCKERS IN AUTOIMMUNE BLISTERING DERMATOSIS

Beta-blockers also act by blocking vascular endothelial growth factor (which is endothelial cell mitogen) and arrest the progression of keloids. This growth factor is located in the dermis, keratinocytes, and fibroblasts of keloids when compared to normal skin, hence beta-blockers should be used for keloids.[6]

BIOLOGICS (NEWER MOLECULES)

There have been various biologic agents which are introduced into practice for numerous dermatological conditions such as psoriasis, atopic dermatitis, etc. These have been arranged in order of their approval by the Food and Drug Administration (FDA) in chronological order.

Newer Biological Agents for Chronic Plaque Psoriasis/Psoriatic Arthritis

- *Ixekizumab*: It was approved by the FDA in March 2016 and December 2017 for chronic plaque psoriasis and psoriatic arthritis, respectively. It is a humanized monoclonal antibody with neutralizing activity against IL-17RA. It is to be given by subcutaneous route at a dose of 160 mg at week 0 and 80 mg on weeks 2, 4, 6, 8, 10, and 12 followed by 80 mg every 4 weeks for the maintenance.[7]
- *Brodalumab*: This monoclonal antibody got approval in July 2016 for plaque psoriasis. It is human monoclonal IgG2K antibody against IL-17RA. It is to be given at a dose of 210 mg subcutaneously at weeks 0, 1, and 2 and 210 mg every 2 weeks safely.[8]
- *Guselkumab*: This biologic is a human monoclonal antibody against IL-23 receptor and was approved for use in plaque psoriasis in July 2017. It is given at a dose of 100 mg subcutaneously at weeks 0, 4, and every 8 weeks later.[9]
- *Tildrakizumab*: It was also approved for plaque psoriasis in March 2018. It is IgG1/K antibody against IL-23. The dosage of this agent is 100 mg at weeks 0, 4, and later 100 mg every 12 weeks subcutaneously.[10]
- *Risankizumab*: It got approval by the FDA in April 2019 for use in plaque psoriasis. It is again a human monoclonal IgG antibody against IL-23. It is given via subcutaneously route at 150 mg weeks 0, 4, and every 12 weeks later.[11]
- *Bimekizumab*: This agent is in phase 3 trial for chronic plaque psoriasis and psoriatic arthritis. It is directed against IL-17A and IL-17F, and tried at a loading dose of 320 mg and later 160 mg every 4 weeks subcutaneously.[12]
- *Mirikizumab*: It is directed against IL-23 and in phase 3 trial for plaque psoriasis and psoriatic arthritis. It is given at a dose of 300 mg every 4 weeks.[13]

Newer Biological Agents for Atopic Dermatitis

- *Dupilumab*: It was approved by the FDA for atopic dermatitis in March 2017. Other conditions where it has been prescribed successfully are prurigo nodularis and bullous pemphigoid. It is a fully humanized antibody which inhibits IL-4 and IL-3 and binds to the alpha subunit of IL-4 receptor. It also reduces immunoglobulin E (IgE) secretion by downregulating eosinophil chemotaxis and TH2-associated chemokine activity. It also inhibits preactivated B-cells, directing B-cells toward IgG4 production. It is also hypothesized that it may improve pruritus by reducing peripheral itch sensory neuron signaling through its direct effect on IL-4 and IL-13 which ultimately hampers IL-31 production.[14-16]
- *Lebrikizumab*: It is a monoclonal antibody (humanized) which inhibits IL-13. It is given subcutaneously at a dose of 125 mg once weekly for 12 weeks. It is in phase 3 trial presently.[17]
- *Nemolizumab*: It is also one of the newer biologic agents in phase 3 trial for atopic dermatitis. It is a humanized monoclonal antibody that inhibits IL-31. It is given at a dose of 0.5–1 mg/kg subcutaneously for 6–12 months safely.[18]

Other Newer Biologic Agents

- *Spartalizumab*: It is a biologic agent used in melanoma and is still in phase 3 trial. It binds to programmed cell death receptor 1 (PD-1) and interferes with interaction with programmed death ligand 1 (PD-L1) and PD-L2. It works as an immune checkpoint inhibitor.[19]
- *Cemiplimab-rwlc*: It was approved by the FDA in September 2018 for locally advanced and metastatic squamous cell carcinoma (SCC). It inhibits PD-1 and is prescribed at a dose of 350 mg as intravenous infusion every 3 weeks.[20]
- *Selumetinib*: It was approved recently in April 2020 for patients with neurofibromatosis 1 having symptomatic and inoperable plexiform neurofibromas. It can be used for everyone above the age of 2 years. It inhibits mitogen-activated protein kinases and hence reduces extracellular signal-regulated kinase (ERK) phosphorylation.[21]
- *Ligelizumab*: It is in phase 2b trials for chronic spontaneous urticaria. It binds to IgE and has immunomodulatory action. It is to be used at doses of 24, 72, and 240 mg monthly subcutaneously.[22]
- *Avelumab*: This biologic agent got its approval in March 2017 for metastatic Merkel cell carcinoma for patients aged above 12 years. It is a fully human IgG1 anti-PD-L1 antibody which blocks PD-1 and PD-L1 interaction. It is given by intravenous route every 2 weeks safely.[23]
- *Lanadelumab*: It is indicated in hereditary angioedema (to prevent attacks) and was approved in August 2018. It inhibits active plasma kallikrein and hence reduced bradykinin. It is administered at a dose of 150–300 mg once in 2 weeks subcutaneously.[24]

INTRALESIONAL BLEOMYCIN FOR LYMPHANGIOMA CIRCUMSCRIPTUM

Bleomycin is an antineoplastic, antibacterial, and antiviral drug. It breaks the basic skeleton of DNA by generating free radicals and also has a sclerosant action on endothelial cells. It also inhibits the incorporation of thymidine into the DNA. It is used by reconstituting with 5 mL of distilled water and then mixing 1 mL of the solution with 2 mL of 2% lignocaine and finally injecting with a 26 G needle, the endpoint being blanching of the site.[25] A recent study combined it with triamcinolone and bevacizumab to treat lymphangioma circumscriptum of the tongue.[26]

TOPICAL CETIRIZINE IN ANDROGENETIC ALOPECIA

Topical cetirizine might be one of the adjuvant therapeutic options for androgenetic alopecia by suppressing the prostaglandin D2 and inflammatory infiltrate in the affected area.[27]

CHLORINE DIOXIDE IN KERATOSIS PILARIS

Chlorine dioxide complex (simply clear acne gel with Dioxicare) is a broad-spectrum antimicrobial and a keratolytic compound. It neutralizes the reactive oxygen molecules and degrades the intramolecular and intermolecular disulfide bonds that stabilize the keratin, thereby acting as a keratolytic and hence can be used in treating keratosis pilaris.[28]

CLASCOTERONE CREAM IN ACNE VULGARIS

Androgens bind to their receptors on the keratinocytes, sebaceous glands, and dermal papilla cells. Clascoterone inhibits the binding of dihydrotestosterone to the receptors. It penetrates the skin and metabolizes to cortexolone, thus limiting the potential side-effects. Clascoterone cream, 1%, is a novel investigative topical androgen receptor blocker.[29]

CRISABOROLE IN ATOPIC DERMATITIS

It was approved in December 2016 by the US FDA, for the treatment of atopic dermatitis. Crisaborole is also a PDE4 similar to apremilast and suppresses the release of cytokines by downregulating nuclear factor kappa B. It comes a topical preparation, unlike topical corticosteroids and calcineurin inhibitors, which have potential adverse side-effects with continued use; it can be used safely for long duration without any adverse effects.[30]

DICLOFENAC GEL FOR ACTINIC KERATOSIS AND SEBORRHEIC KERATOSIS

Diclofenac gel is a nonsteroid anti-inflammatory drug that blocks cyclo-oxygenase pathway in turn reduces prostaglandin E2 production.[31] In actinic keratosis, the proliferative tissue is not able to increase due to blockage of this pathway.[32] The exact mechanism of action in seborrheic keratosis is unknown.

GENTAMICIN (TOPICAL) IN HEREDITARY HYPOTRICHOSIS OF SCALP

Gentamycin reduces the synthesis of corneodesmosin by the read-through activity of nonsense mutation which accumulates and damages hair follicles in hypotrichosis of scalp. It can be applied topically for 6 months twice daily safely.[33]

GENTIAN VIOLET FOR NEWER INDICATIONS

Gentian violet activates the extrinsic apoptotic pathway by increasing caspase 8, death receptors 4 and 5, tumor necrosis factor (TNF) receptor, and Fas ligand. This has been published as an in vitro study and these preclinical findings open up the avenues for research on antineoplastic features of gentian violet, thus providing a rationale for clinical studies of the use of this molecule as a novel, inexpensive, topical therapy for cutaneous T-cell lymphoma.[34] Gentian violet acts as a nicotinamide adenine dinucleotide phosphate oxidase inhibitor thereby downregulating the production of angiopoietin 2 and in turn helps in the management of erythema multiforme.[35]

GLYCOPYRRONIUM AND SOFPIRONIUM BROMIDE GEL IN AXILLARY HYPERHIDROSIS

Glycopyrronium tosylate is a topical anticholinergic approved by the FDA for primary axillary hyperhidrosis for age > 9 years. It is to be applied once daily in the axilla with a premoistened towelette for 4 weeks for visible results.[36]

Sofpironium bromide is an ester analog of glycopyrrolate that inhibits muscarinic receptors including sweat glands. This novel formulation is available as 5%, 10%, or 15% active drug, can help in reduction of axillary hyperhidrosis.[37]

HEPATITIS B VIRUS VACCINE IN WARTS

Hepatitis B virus vaccine can also be given intralesionally to get rid of warts. The exact mechanism of action is not clearly understood but the most likely mechanism is the stimulation of Th1 cytokine profile such as IL-2, IL-12, and interferon-gamma (IFN-γ). It can be given in the dose of 0.2 mL in the largest wart and repeated every fortnight, for a maximum of five sessions.[38]

HYDROGEN PEROXIDE FOR SEBORRHEIC KERATOSIS

Hydrogen peroxide 40% lotion can be used topically to reduce seborrheic keratosis. It oxidizes the tissue and generates reactive oxygen species, further it leads to lipid peroxidation and generates high oxygen concentrations to kill the pathological cells.[39]

LIDOCAINE FOR PERISTOMAL DERMATITIS

Lidocaine gel is to be applied on the affected area and cleansed followed by a warm water rinse. Owing to its anti-inflammatory effect, erythema and weepiness is reduced along with sting sensation caused due to usage of adhesives.[40]

LOSARTAN FOR EPIDERMOLYSIS BULLOSA

Losartan, an angiotensin 1 receptor antagonist, reduces transforming growth factor-beta (TGFβ) signaling in dystrophic epidermolysis bullosa and dermal fibroblasts and help reduce progressive fibrosis and contractures. It is beneficial in dystrophic epidermolysis bullosa and other such conditions where TGFβ and inflammation are the major drivers for fibrosis.[41]

MELATONIN IN ATOPIC DERMATITIS

Melatonin has sleep-inducing properties and is anti-inflammatory as well, that helps in atopic dermatitis. Melatonin regulates circadian rhythm and improves sleep latency. Melatonin also has an anti-inflammatory effect by inducing synthesis of IL-2, IL-6, and IL-12. It upregulates the antioxidant enzymes, thereby neutralizing free radicals and protecting cell membranes, possibly leading to improvement of the condition of the patient. It is a safe drug and can be given at a dose of 3 mg/day for 4 weeks in the night as an adjunct.[42]

METFORMIN (TOPICAL) IN MELASMA

Topical metformin can be readily prepared by mixing 30 g of metformin powder with 70% alcohol and propylene glycol in 30% weight:volume ratio. The resultant 30% lotion is dispensed in an amber-colored bottle. It has to be applied once at night. It decreases the cAMP accumulation and phosphorylation of cAMP responsive element binding protein, leading to decreased expression of microphthalmia-associated transcription factor (MITF) and other melanogenic proteins such as tyrosinase-related protein-1, tyrosinase-related protein-2, and tyrosinase. It also inhibits diacylglycerol and prevents the anchorage of protein kinase to melanosomes, thereby acts as a topical melanopenic agent.[43]

MINOCYCLINE FOR NEWER INDICATIONS

Topical Minocycline

To overcome the known side effect of pigmentation with oral minocycline, a novel topical 4% minocycline foam preparation has been formulated to correct inflammatory lesions of non-nodular moderate-to-severe acne in adults and children aged 9 years or older. It has been approved by the US FDA in 2019, also it is nonphotoallergic in nature unlike the oral preparation.[44]

ORAL MINOXIDIL

Minoxidil is a potassium channel opener that causes hyperpolarization of the membranes, ultimately leading to vasodilation. It decreases the entry of calcium into the cells, thereby inhibiting epidermal growth factor (EGF)-induced inhibition of hair growth. It also activates prostaglandin-1 synthetase enzymes that stimulate hair growth. It can be safely prescribed in low dose (0.5–1 mg/day) to manage chemotherapy-induced alopecia, monilethrix, female and male pattern alopecia.[45-48] In women with alopecia, it is given at a dose of 0.25–1.25 mg/day and in men with alopecia, it is given at a dose of 2.5–5 mg/day.

MOLECULES (NEWER) FOR HEREDITARY ANGIOEDEMA

Numerous nonbiologic agents have been introduced to treat hereditary angioedema over last decade.

- *Berinert*: It was approved in 2009 for hereditary angioedema (on demand treatment). It is C1 esterase inhibitor which is plasma derived. It is given at the dose of 20 IU/kg per dose intravenously.[49]
- *Ruconest*: It has been used for management of acute attacks of hereditary angioedema after its approval in July 2014. It is a recombinant C1 esterase inhibitor. It is to be given as slow infusion over 5 minutes in the dosage of 50 IU/kg. It is a recombinant and inhibitor of C1 esterase enzyme.[50]
- *Haegarda*: It is used to prevent attacks of hereditary angioedema. It is plasma-derived concentrate of C1 esterase inhibitor. It is to be used at a dose of 60 IU/kg twice weekly and given subcutaneously.[51]
- *Berotralstat (BCX7353)*: It is indicated for both prevention and treatment of attacks of hereditary angioedema. It is presently in phase 3 trial. It is to be taken at 35 mg QID for 28 days orally.[52]

TOPICAL MUPIROCIN FOR BALANITIS CIRCUMSCRIPTA PLASMA CELLULARIS-ZOON'S BALANITIS

Zoon's balanitis results from a complex interplay of various factors such as chronic irritant dermatitis, heat, hypospadias, and *Mycobacterium smegmatis* infection. Mupirocin acts by irreversible inhibition of isoleucyl-transfer RNA synthetase, thereby inhibiting bacterial protein and RNA synthesis. The effectiveness of mupirocin in Zoon's balanitis raises the possibility that this condition could be triggered by a bacterial infection or a superantigen.[53] Successful treatment of Zoon's balanitis has been observed with topical 2% mupirocin when applied for 3 months.

NARROW-BAND ULTRAVIOLET B FOR VERRUCA PLANA

Narrow-band ultraviolet B is effective in extensive verruca plana as shown in one of the studies. It most likely works by inhibiting replication of viral DNA, leading to cell cycle arrest.[54] A dose of 0.3 J/cm^2 was given in an 11-year-old boy without any significant adverse effects apart from the darkening of the skin in verruca plana. Complete resolution was noted after 12 exposures.

NORMAL SALINE INJECTION FOR STEROID-INDUCED ATROPHY

Saline injection has been used for steroid-induced atrophy. Normal saline injection converts the precipitated steroid into a solution. Eventually, macrophages treat the solution as foreign bodies, leading to the removal of steroids from the affected area.[55]

OLEOGEL-S10 FOR EPIDERMOLYSIS BULLOSA

Dry extract from birch bark and its active marker substances have also been shown to increase the migration of primary human keratinocytes, accelerate wound closure, and promote differentiation of keratinocytes in vitro and in vivo processes that are essential for re-epithelialization and maintenance of the skin barrier. Phase 2 trials have been conducted in cases of dystrophic epidermolysis bullosa for faster re-epithelialization of superficial wounds.[56]

OLUMACOSTAT GLASARETIL: SEBUM-SUPPRESSING AGENT

Olumacostat glasaretil alters the composition of sebum which is involved in the growth of *Propionibacterium acnes*, biofilm formation, comedogenesis, and pilosebaceous inflammation. It is in phase 2a clinical trial conducted on patients with moderate-to-severe facial acne vulgaris.[57] Topical preparation as 5% gel is in phase 3 trial.[58]

OZENOXACIN CREAM FOR IMPETIGO

Ozenoxacin is a nonfluorinated quinolone that is bacteriostatic and bactericidal against most of the gram-positive pathogenic organisms. It inhibits bacterial enzymes such as DNA gyrase A and topoisomerase IV.[59] Ozenoxacin 1% cream applied twice daily for 5 days helps in the treatment of impetigo.

RANITIDINE IN MOLLUSCUM CONTAGIOSUM

Ranitidine at a dose of 5 mg/kg/day in two divided doses is an effective alternative for widespread molluscum in immunocompetent children. One of the old proton-pump inhibitors (cimetidine) has been shown to provide benefit by immunomodulatory effects (enhancement of T-cell immunity by inhibition of suppressor lymphocyte function). This has been extrapolated to ranitidine, and the molecule has been utilized in the treatment of molluscum contagiosum. It is supposed to increase the activity of natural killer, lymphokine-activated killer cells, and interferon-activated killer cells. Ranitidine may exert its antiviral effects, by increasing the activity of these cells.[60] Since the evidence of the role of ranitidine in molluscum contagiosum remains dicey, studies with a larger sample size must be done, in order to have a better idea regarding its efficacy.

TOPICAL RAPAMYCIN AND CALCITRIOL FOR ANGIOFIBROMAS IN TUBEROUS SCLEROSIS

Rapamycin is mixed with vitamin D for topical use in angiofibromas in tuberous sclerosis. Rapamycin calcitriol combination is made by combining 1 g of rapamycin powder, 1 g of 0.3% calcitriol ointment with 998 g of petroleum. It is stored at 4°C and it is to be used within 3 months. The ointment can be applied safely twice daily for 24 weeks. It helps in faster resolution of erythema. The reduction in the size of papules is significant and the durability is longer (after discontinuation of treatment).[61] It can be applied even after ablating the lesions for quicker results. Vitamin D analogs reduce TGFβ-induced fibroblast proliferation and acts synergistically with rapamycin.

SARECYCLINE IN ACNE

Sarecycline is a narrow-spectrum tetracycline and has notable fewer gastrointestinal side-effects compared to broad-spectrum tetracyclines. It is indicated in moderate-to-severe acne vulgaris at a single daily dose of 1.5 mg/kg/day.[62]

SERLOPITANT FOR PSORIATIC PRURITUS

Serlopitant is a potent neurokinin 1 receptor antagonist that helps in the reduction of pruritus. It is to be prescribed at a dose of 5 mg once daily and does not have somnolence which is a side effect of conventional antihistamines. It is in phase 2 trials at multiple centers.[63]

SILYMARIN PREVENTS THE RISE OF ALANINE AMINOTRANSFERASE AND ASPARTATE TRANSAMINASE LIVER ENZYMES IN PATIENTS TAKING ISOTRETINOIN

Silymarin is extracted from the plant. It is also known as milk thistle and belongs to the Asteraceae family. It inhibits free radicals, promotes DNA polymerase and increases glutathione levels, thereby preventing further liver damage. It also binds to hepatocytes, thereby altering the cellular uptake of toxins by altering the phospholipid bilayer. It is given at a dose of 140 mg/day.[64] Hence, patients on hepatotoxic drugs like isotretinoin should be coadministered with silymarin.

TOPICAL TIMOLOL IN CHRONIC, RECALCITRANT FISSURES, AND EROSIONS OF HAND ECZEMA

Timolol increases the migration of keratinocytes, phosphorylation of ERKs, and increases the re-epithelialization. It restores the damaged skin barrier. Application of 1–2 drops of timolol 0.5% ophthalmic solution at bedtime can effectively correct hand eczema.[65]

TOFACITINIB IN ALOPECIA AREATA AND ATOPIC DERMATITIS

It is well known that topical and oral tofacitinib is used in the treatment of atopic dermatitis. Oral tofacitinib 5–10 mg twice daily can be given in alopecia universalis which otherwise is a difficult to treat condition. Tofacitinib is an inhibitor of the enzyme Janus kinase 1 and 3, thus interfering with the Janus kinase-signal transduction and activation of a transcription signaling pathway. Therefore, it blocks a cluster of differentiation 8 (CD8) cell-mediated destruction of hair follicles in alopecia areata.[66,67]

TRANEXAMIC ACID (5%) FOR POSTACNE ERYTHEMA

In acne, postinflammatory erythema occurs due to the release of inflammatory mediators and cytokines, it is a common problem faced once the active acne is cleared. Tranexamic acid suppresses TNFα and IL-6, and angiogenesis. The injectable tranexamic acid is diluted with 0.9% sodium chloride and the obtained solution (tranexamic acid 5%) can be applied topically once at night.[68]

TRANEXAMIC ACID FOR STEVENS–JOHNSON SYNDROME/TOXIC EPIDERMAL NECROLYSIS

Stevens–Johnson syndrome and toxic epidermal necrolysis are the conditions which often have mucosal involvement. It can lead to oral hemorrhages which are very difficult to manage at times. A solution of 5% tranexamic acid applied to gauze and placed in the buccal cavity, can be used as a technique to manage oral hemorrhagic lesions. It inhibits the conversion of plasminogen to plasmin, by preventing the attachment of plasminogen to fibrin molecules. The 5% solution of tranexamic acid is prepared by diluting the intravenous preparation (500 mg in 5 mL) with 5 mL of sterile water.[69]

TRIFAROTENE CREAM FOR ACNE

Trifarotene is a novel topical retinoid that can be applied once daily at night for truncal and facial acne vulgaris.[70] It was approved by the US FDA in October 2019. Trifarotene acts on the retinoic acid receptor-gamma (RAR-γ) receptor; and the side effects such as irritation, pruritus, and burning which are noted with tretinoin and adapalene, are not seen with trifarotene.

VALACYCLOVIR AS A MODALITY FOR ZOSTERIFORM MYCOSIS FUNGOIDES

Zosteriform mycosis fungoides is a rare variant characterized by lesions in a zosteriform distribution. It is hypothesized to be triggered by the varicella zoster virus. Valacyclovir, when given at a dosage of 500 mg daily, helps in quicker resolution of the disease.[71]

ZOLIFLODACIN IN GONORRHEA

Zoliflodacin is a newer drug in trials to treat uncomplicated gonorrhea. It acts by inhibiting microbial biosynthesis by halting cleavage of covalent gyrase complex and formation of fused circular DNA required for synthesis. It is given as a single dose of 2–3 g orally.[72]

CONCLUSION

In this chapter, we have summarized the newer therapeutic options in dermatological conditions. We have also tried to include newer uses of older molecules; apart from enlisting the names and indications of the recently approved molecules. However, we would like to mention that the aforementioned options should be considered, only after giving due importance to the availability, side effect profile, and the cost factor and these options shall be very useful in the future.[73]

KEY POINTS

- Dermatology is an evolving branch of medicine with discovery of new entities daily.
- New molecules are used for various known diseases for better and quicker management.
- Numerous known drugs are used for newer indications and are termed as repurpose drugs.

REFERENCES

1. De Luca G, Cariddi A, Campochiaro C, Vanni D, Boffini N, Tomelleri A, et al. Efficacy and safety of apremilast for Behçet's syndrome: a real-life single-centre Italian experience. Rheumatology (Oxford). 2020;59:171-5.
2. Vossen AR, van Doorn MB, van der Zee HH, Prens EP. Apremilast for moderate hidradenitis suppurativa: results of a randomized controlled trial. J Am Acad Dermatol. 2019;80:80-8.
3. Simpson EL, Imafuku S, Poulin Y, Ungar B, Zhou L, Malik K, et al. A phase 2 randomized trial of apremilast in patients with atopic dermatitis. J Invest Dermatol. 2019;139:1063-72.
4. Vernero M, Ribaldone DG, Cariti C, Ribero S, Susca S, Astegiano M, et al. Dual-targeted therapy with apremilast and vedolizumab in pyoderma gangrenosum associated with Crohn's disease. J Dermatol. 2020;47:e216-7.
5. Laird ME, Tong LX, Lo Sicco KI, Kim RH, Meehan SA, Franks AG Jr. Novel use of apremilast for adjunctive treatment of recalcitrant pyoderma gangrenosum. JAAD Case Rep. 2017; 3:228-9.
6. Abdelmaksoud A, Vestita M. Beta-blockers for treatment of autoimmune blistering dermatosis. J Eur Acad Dermatol Venereol. 2018;32:e458-9.
7. Kemény L, Berggren L, Dossenbach M, Dutronc Y, Paul C. Efficacy and safety of ixekizumab in patients with plaque psoriasis across different degrees of disease severity: results from UNCOVER-2 and UNCOVER-3. J Dermatolog Treat. 2019; 30:19-26.
8. Lebwohl M, Strober B, Menter A, Gordon K, Weglowska J, Puig L, et al. Phase 3 studies comparing brodalumab with ustekinumab in psoriasis. N Engl J Med. 2015;373:1318-28.
9. Reich K, Armstrong AW, Langley RG, Flavin S, Randazzo B, Li S, et al. Guselkumab versus secukinumab for the treatment of moderate-to-severe psoriasis (ECLIPSE): results from a phase 3, randomised controlled trial. Lancet. 2019;394:831-9.
10. Reich K, Papp KA, Blauvelt A, Tyring SK, Sinclair R, Thaçi D, et al. Tildrakizumab versus placebo or etanercept for chronic plaque psoriasis (reSURFACE 1 and reSURFACE 2): results from two randomised controlled, phase 3 trials. Lancet. 2017;390:276-88.
11. Gordon KB, Strober B, Lebwohl M, Augustin M, Blauvelt A, Poulin Y, et al. Efficacy and safety of risankizumab in moderate-to-severe plaque psoriasis (UltIMMa-1 and UltIMMa-2): results from two double-blind, randomised, placebo-controlled and ustekinumab-controlled phase 3 trials. Lancet. 2018;392: 650-61.
12. Ritchlin CT, Kavanaugh A, Merola JF, Schett G, Scher JU, Warren RB, et al. Bimekizumab in patients with active psoriatic arthritis: results from a 48-week, randomised, double-blind, placebo-controlled, dose-ranging phase 2b trial. Lancet. 2020; 395:427-40.
13. Reich K, Rich P, Maari C, Bissonnette R, Leonardi C, Menter A, et al. Efficacy and safety of mirikizumab (LY3074828) in the treatment of moderate-to-severe plaque psoriasis: results from a randomized phase II study. Br J Dermatol. 2019;181:88-95.
14. Simpson EL, Paller AS, Siegfried EC, Boguniewicz M, Sher L, Gooderham MJ, et al. Efficacy and safety of dupilumab in adolescents with uncontrolled moderate to severe atopic dermatitis: a phase 3 randomized clinical trial. JAMA Dermatol. 2019;156:44-56.
15. Napolitano M, Fabbrocini G, Scalvenzi M, Nisticò SP, Dastoli S, Patruno C. Effectiveness of dupilumab for the treatment of generalized prurigo nodularis phenotype of adult atopic dermatitis. Dermatitis. 2020;31(1):81-4.

16. Abdat R, Waldman RA, de Bedout V, Czernik A, Mcleod M, King B, et al. Dupilumab as a novel therapy for bullous pemphigoid: a multicenter case series. J Am Acad Dermatol. 2020;83(1):46-52.
17. Guttman-Yassky E, Blauvelt A, Eichenfield LF, Paller AS, Armstrong AW, Drew J, et al. Efficacy and safety of lebrikizumab, a high-affinity interleukin-13 inhibitor, in adults with moderate to severe atopic dermatitis: a phase 2b randomized clinical trial. JAMA Dermatol. 2020;156:411-20.
18. Silverberg JI, Pinter A, Pulka G, Poulin Y, Bouaziz JD, Wollenberg A, et al. Phase 2B randomized study of nemolizumab in adults with moderate-to-severe atopic dermatitis and severe pruritus. J Allergy Clin Immunol. 2020;145:173-82.
19. Naing A, Gainor JF, Gelderblom H, Forde PM, Butler MO, Lin CC, et al. A first-in-human phase 1 dose escalation study of spartalizumab (PDR001), an anti-PD-1 antibody, in patients with advanced solid tumors. J Immunother Cancer. 2020;8:e000530.
20. Migden MR, Khushalani NI, Chang AL, Lewis KD, Schmults CD, Hernandez-Aya L, et al. Cemiplimab in locally advanced cutaneous squamous cell carcinoma: results from an open-label, phase 2, single-arm trial. Lancet Oncol. 2020;21:294-305.
21. Espírito Santo V, Passos J, Nzwalo H, Carvalho I, Santos F, Martins C, et al. Selumetinib for plexiform neurofibromas in neurofibromatosis type 1: a single-institution experience. J Neurooncol. 2020;147:459-63.
22. Maurer M, Giménez-Arnau AM, Sussman G, Metz M, Baker DR, Bauer A, et al. Ligelizumab for chronic spontaneous urticaria. N Engl J Med. 2019;381:1321-32.
23. D'Angelo SP, Russell J, Lebbé C, Chmielowski B, Gambichler T, Grob JJ, et al. Efficacy and safety of first-line avelumab treatment in patients with stage IV metastatic Merkel cell carcinoma: a preplanned interim analysis of a clinical trial. JAMA Oncol. 2018;4:e180077.
24. Banerji A, Riedl MA, Bernstein JA, Cicardi M, Longhurst HJ, Zuraw BL, et al. Effect of lanadelumab compared with placebo on prevention of hereditary angioedema attacks: a randomized clinical trial. JAMA. 2018;320:2108-21.
25. Sharma RK, Gupta M. Intralesional bleomycin in lymphangioma circumscriptum of tongue. Indian J Drugs Dermatol. 2018;4:82-4.
26. Hwang J, Lee YK, Burm JS. Treatment of tongue lymphangioma with intralesional combination injection of steroid, bleomycin and bevacizumab. Arch Craniofac Surg. 2017;18:54-8.
27. Sharma RK, Gupta M, Sood S, Gupta A. Dyskeratosis congenita: presentation of cutaneous triad in a sporadic case. BMJ Case Rep. 2018;11:149-51.
28. Zirwas MJ, Fichtel J. Chlorine dioxide complex cleanser: a new agent with rapid efficacy for keratosis pilaris. J Drugs Dermatol. 2018;17:554-6.
29. Hebert A, Thiboutot D, Stein Gold L, Cartwright M, Gerloni M, Fragasso E, et al. Efficacy and safety of topical clascoterone cream, 1%, for treatment in patients with facial acne: two phase 3 randomized clinical trials. JAMA Dermatol. 2020;156:1-10.
30. Callender VD, Alexis AF, Stein Gold LF, Lebwohl MG, Paller AS, Desai SR, et al. Efficacy and safety of crisaborole ointment, 2%, for the treatment of mild-to-moderate atopic dermatitis across racial and ethnic groups. Am J Clin Dermatol. 2019;20:711-23.
31. Aktaş H, Ergin C, Keseroğlu HÖ. Diclofenac gel may be a new treatment option for seborrheic keratosis. Indian Dermatol Online J. 2016;7:211-2.
32. Thomas GJ, Herranz P, Cruz SB, Parodi A. Treatment of actinic keratosis through inhibition of cyclooxygenase-2: potential mechanism of action of diclofenac sodium 3% in hyaluronic acid 2.5. Dermatol Ther. 2019;32:e12800.
33. Peled A, Samuelov L, Sarig O, Bochner R, Malki L, Pavlovsky M, et al. Treatment of hereditary hypotrichosis simplex of the scalp with topical gentamicin. Br J Dermatol. 2019;183:114-20.
34. Wu J, Wood GS. Analysis of the effect of gentian violet on apoptosis and proliferation in cutaneous T-cell lymphoma in an in vitro study. JAMA Dermatol. 2018;154:1191-8.
35. Murthy RK, Van L, Arbiser JL. Treatment of extensive erythema multiforme with topical gentian violet. Exp Dermatol. 2017;26:431-2.
36. Baker DM. Topical glycopyrrolate reduces axillary hyperhidrosis. J Eur Acad Dermatol Venereol. 2016;30:2131-6.
37. Kirsch B, Smith S, Cohen J, DuBois J, Green L, Baumann L, et al. Efficacy and safety of topical sofpironium bromide gel for the treatment of axillary hyperhidrosis: a phase II, randomized, controlled, double-blinded trial. J Am Acad Dermatol. 2020;82(6):1321-7.
38. Nofal A, Elsayed E, Abdelshafy AS. Hepatitis B virus vaccine: a potential therapeutic alternative for the treatment of warts. J Am Acad Dermatol. 2021;84(1):212-3.
39. Baumann LS, Blauvelt A, Draelos ZD, Kempers SE, Lupo MP, Schlessinger J, et al. Safety and efficacy of hydrogen peroxide topical solution, 40% (w/w), in patients with seborrheic keratosis: results from 2 identical, randomized, double-blind, placebo-controlled, phase 3 studies (A-101-SEBK-301/302). J Am Acad Dermatol. 2018;79:869-77.
40. Neill BC, Favata ME, Neill JA, Rajpara MD, Aires DJ. A novel technique using lidocaine 2% topical gel for peristomal dermatitis. J Am Acad Dermatol. 2018; S0190-9622(18)30431-6.
41. Nyström A, Thriene K, Mittapalli V, Kern JS, Kiritsi D, Dengjel J, et al. Losartan ameliorates dystrophic epidermolysis bullosa and uncovers new disease mechanisms. EMBO Mol Med. 2015;7:1211-28.
42. Chang YS, Lin MH, Lee JH, Lee PL, Dai YS, Chu KH, et al. Melatonin supplementation for children with atopic dermatitis and sleep disturbance: a randomized clinical trial. JAMA Pediatr. 2016;170:35-42.
43. Banavase Channakeshavaiah R, Andanooru Chandrappa NK. Topical metformin in the treatment of melasma: a preliminary clinical trial. J Cosmet Dermatol. 2020;19:1161-4.
44. Raoof TJ, Hooper D, Moore A, Zaiac M, Sullivan T, Kircik L, et al. Efficacy and safety of a novel topical minocycline foam for the treatment of moderate-to-severe acne vulgaris: a phase 3 study. J Am Acad Dermatol. 2020;82:832-7.
45. Jimenez-Cauhe J, Saceda-Corralo D, Rodrigues-Barata R, Hermosa-Gelbard A, Moreno-Arrones OM, Fernandez-Nieto D, et al. Effectiveness and safety of low-dose oral minoxidil in male androgenetic alopecia. J Am Acad Dermatol. 2019;81:648-9.
46. Yang X, Thai KE. Treatment of permanent chemotherapy-induced alopecia with low dose oral minoxidil. Australas J Dermatol. 2016;57:e130-2.
47. Sinclair R. Treatment of monilethrix with oral minoxidil. JAAD Case Rep. 2016;2:212-5.
48. Sinclair RD. Female pattern hair loss: a pilot study investigating combination therapy with low-dose oral minoxidil and spironolactone. Int J Dermatol. 2018;57:104-9.
49. Arora NK, Swaminathan S, Mohapatra A, Gopalan HS, Katoch VM, Bhan MK, et al. Research priorities in maternal, newborn, and child health and nutrition for India: an Indian Council of Medical Research-INCLEN initiative. Indian J Med Res. 2017;145:611-22.

50. Cruz MP. Conestat alfa (ruconest): first recombinant C1 esterase inhibitor for the treatment of acute attacks in patients with hereditary angioedema. P T. 2015;40:109-14.
51. Bernstein JA, Li HH, Craig TJ, Manning ME, Lawo JP, Machnig T, et al. Indirect comparison of intravenous vs. subcutaneous C1-inhibitor placebo-controlled trials for routine prevention of hereditary angioedema attacks. Allergy Asthma Clin Immunol. 2019;15:13.
52. Longhurst H, Farkas H. Biological therapy in hereditary angioedema: transformation of a rare disease. Expert Opin Biol Ther. 2020;20:493-501.
53. Bari O, Cohen PR. Successful management of zoon's balanitis with topical mupirocin ointment: a case report and literature review of mupirocin-responsive balanitis circumscripta plasmacellularis. Dermatol Ther. 2017;7:203-10.
54. Zhang K, Ren J, Ren J, Xiang LC, Sun L. Successful treatment of verruca plana with NB-UVB: a case report. Dermatol Ther. 2020;33:e13207.
55. Sadat Sadati M, Hemmatian Boroujen N, Sepaskhah M. Normal saline injection; a promising method to treat steroid-induced atrophy. Iran J Dermatol. 2018;21:20-2.
56. Schwieger-Briel A, Ott H, Kiritsi D, Laszczyk-Lauer M, Bodemer C. Mechanism of oleogel-S10: a triterpene preparation for the treatment of epidermolysis bullosa. Dermatol Ther. 2019;32: e12983.
57. Bissonnette R, Poulin Y, Drew J, Hofland H, Tan J. Olumacostat glasaretil, a novel topical sebum inhibitor, in the treatment of acne vulgaris: a phase IIa, multicenter, randomized, vehicle-controlled study. J Am Acad Dermatol. 2017;76:33-9.
58. US National Library of Medicine. A study of olumacostat glasaretil gel in subjects with acne vulgaris. [online] Available from: https://clinicaltrials.gov/ct2/show/NCT03028363 [Last accessed August, 2021].
59. Rosen T, Albareda N, Rosenberg N, Alonso FG, Roth S, Zsolt I, et al. Efficacy and safety of ozenoxacin cream for treatment of adult and pediatric patients with impetigo: a randomized clinical trial. JAMA Dermatol. 2018;154:806-13.
60. Chitalia AJ, Agarwal SA, Pilani A, Madke B. Oral ranitidine in molluscum contagiosum: a novel common treatment modality for a common disease. Clin Dermatol J. 2018;3:166.
61. Chen PL, Hong JB, Shen LJ, Chen YT, Wang SJ, Liao YH. The efficacy and safety of topical rapamycin-calcitriol for facial angiofibromas in patients with tuberous sclerosis complex: a prospective, double-blind, randomized clinical trial. Br J Dermatol. 2020;183(4):655-63.
62. Moore A, Green LJ, Bruce S, Sadick N, Tschen E, Werschler P, et al. Once-daily oral sarecycline 1.5 mg/kg/day is effective for moderate to severe acne vulgaris: results from two identically designed, phase 3, randomized, double-blind clinical trials. J Drugs Dermatol. 2018;17:987-96.
63. Pariser DM, Bagel J, Lebwohl M, Yosipovitch G, Chien E, Spellman MC. Serlopitant for psoriatic pruritus: a phase 2 randomized, double-blind, placebo-controlled clinical trial. J Am Acad Dermatol. 2020;82:1314-20.
64. Mirnezami M, Jafarimanesh H, Rezagholizamenjany M, Alimoradian A, Ranjbaran M. The effect of silymarin on liver enzymes in patients taking isotretinoin: a randomized clinical trial. Dermatol Ther. 2020;33:e13236.
65. Pawar M. Topical timolol in chronic, recalcitrant fissures and erosions of hand eczema. J Am Acad Dermatol. 2021;84(3): e125-6.
66. Ibrahim O, Bayart CB, Hogan S, Piliang M, Bergfeld WF. Treatment of alopecia areata with tofacitinib. JAMA Dermatol. 2017;153:600-2.
67. Bissonnette R, Papp KA, Poulin Y, Gooderham M, Raman M, Mallbris L, et al. Topical tofacitinib for atopic dermatitis: a phase IIa randomized trial. Br J Dermatol. 2016;175:902-11.
68. Jakhar D, Kaur I. Topical 5% tranexamic acid for acne-related post inflammatory erythema. J Am Acad Dermatol. 2020; 82(6):e187-8.
69. Adams L, Creamer D. Controlling oral hemorrhages in Stevens-Johnson syndrome/toxic epidermal necrolysis. J Am Acad Dermatol. 2020;82:e3-4.
70. Tan J, Thiboutot D, Popp G, Gooderham M, Lynde C, Del Rosso J, et al. Randomized phase 3 evaluation of trifarotene 50 μg/g cream treatment of moderate facial and truncal acne. J Am Acad Dermatol. 2019;80:1691-9.
71. Lewis DJ, Hinojosa T, Chan WH, Wu JH, Duvic M. Successful suppression of recurrent zosteriform mycosis fungoides with maintenance valacyclovir. Actas Dermosifiliogr (Engl Ed). 2018;109:757-60.
72. Taylor SN, Marrazzo J, Batteiger BE, Hook EW 3rd, Seña AC, Long J, et al. Single-dose zoliflodacin (ETX0914) for treatment of urogenital gonorrhea. N Engl J Med. 2018;379:1835-45.
73. Das A, Toshniwal A, Madke B. What is new in dermatotherapy? Indian J Dermatol Venereol Leprol. 2021;87(1):135-43.

EXAMINATION QUESTIONS

1. Write a short note on recent advances in drug therapy in dermatology.
2. Explain the role of HLA in predicting drug reactions.
3. Write a short note on DRESS.

Question Papers
(From Various Universities)

Disclaimer: *Questions were collected from faculty of various universities as suggested practice paper, so pattern of these questions may vary from actual university examination. Students are requested to be familiar with the recent trends of their respective board examination.*

[Time: 3 Hours] [Max. Marks: 100]

DERMATOLOGY, VENEREOLOGY AND LEPROSY BASIC SCIENCES AS APPLIED TO DERMATOLOGY, VENEREOLOGY AND LEPROSY PAPER – I

Your answers should be specific to the questions asked
Draw neat, labeled diagrams wherever necessary

Answer all the Questions **10 × 10 = 100 Marks**

1. Antigen presenting cells.
2. Skin microbiome.
3. Embryological milestones in development of various components of skin.
4. Describe immunohistochemistry technique. Enumerate dermatological diseases where it is used in diagnosis with the corresponding markers.
5. Draw a neat labeled diagram depicting the ultrastructure of the cell envelope of *Mycobacterium leprae*.
6. Normal genital flora in females.
7. Chlamydia trachomatis.
8. Describe collagen biosynthesis. Enumerate types of collagen present in the skin.
9. Anatomy and physiology of Sebaceous glands.
10. Psoriasiform changes in histopathology.

[Time: 3 Hours] [Max. Marks: 100]

DERMATOLOGY, VENEREOLOGY AND LEPROSY DERMATOLOGY PAPER – II

Your answers should be specific to the questions asked
Draw neat, labeled diagrams wherever necessary

Answer all the Questions **10 × 10 = 100 Marks**

1. Describe in detail the porphyrin metabolism. Discuss clinical features, diagnosis and management of Gunther's disease.
2. Classify cutaneous vasculitis. Describe the clinical features, diagnosis and management of Henoch-Schönlein purpura.
3. Sweet's syndrome.
4. Mixed connective tissue disease.
5. Idiopathic photodermatoses.
6. Cholinergic urticaria.
7. Noneczematous contact dermatitis.
8. Describe painful skin tumors.
9. Hydroa vacciniforme.
10. Lipoid proteinosis.

[Time: 3 Hours] [Max. Marks: 100]

DERMATOLOGY, VENEREOLOGY AND LEPROSY
S.T.D. AND LEPROSY PAPER – III

Your answers should be specific to the questions asked
Draw neat labeled diagrams wherever necessary

Answer all the Questions **10 × 10 = 100 Marks**

1. Explain in detail pathogenesis of trophic ulcer and its management.
2. Discuss in detail the structure and immunopathogenesis of human immunodeficiency virus (HIV) infection.
3. Vaccines in leprosy.
4. Kaposi's sarcoma.
5. Clofazimine.
6. Multiplex polymerase chain reaction.
7. Microcellular rubber footwear.
8. Buschke-Löwenstein tumor.
9. Pregnancy and syphilis.
10. Management of nerve abscess in leprosy.

[Time: 3 Hours] [Max. Marks: 100]

DERMATOLOGY, VENEREOLOGY AND LEPROSY
BASIC SCIENCES OF DERMATOLOGY, S.T.D. AND LEPROSY PAPER – I

Your answers should be specific to the questions asked
Draw neat labeled diagrams wherever necessary

Answer all the Questions **10 × 10 = 100 Marks**

1. Role of skin in thermoregulation.
2. Describe in detail about epidermal attachment complexes.
3. Norwegian scabies.
4. Cleavage lines in skin.
5. Chromhidrosis.
6. Cytodiagnosis.
7. Wood's lamp and skin.
8. Langerhans cell.
9. Odland bodies.
10. Keratinization in nail unit.

[Time: 3 Hours] [Max. Marks: 100]

DERMATOLOGY, VENEREOLOGY AND LEPROSY BASIC SCIENCES AS APPLIED TO DERMATOLOGY, VENEREOLOGY AND LEPROSY PAPER – I

Your answers should be specific to the questions asked
Draw neat, labeled diagrams wherever necessary

Answer all the Questions **10 × 10 = 100 Marks**

1. Draw neat labeled diagrams of the eccrine sweat glands showing their position in a section of skin and the ultrastructure of the glandular element. Mention the components of human sweat.
2. Littre's glands.
3. Specialized nerve endings in skin and their role.
4. Use of various experimental animals in leprosy.
5. Antimicrobial peptides.
6. Discuss keratins.
7. Heat shock proteins.
8. Genitourinary defenses against STIs.
9. Use of immunofluorescence in dermatology.
10. Emulsifiers used in topical therapy.

[Time: 3 Hours] [Max. Marks: 100]

DERMATOLOGY, VENEREOLOGY AND LEPROSY PAPER – IV

Your answers should be specific to the questions asked
Draw neat, labeled diagrams wherever necessary

Answer all the Questions **10 × 10 = 100 Marks**

1. Cutaneous manifestation of diabetes mellitus.
2. Management of acne scars.
3. Skin lesions in SLE.
4. Lasers in pigmented lesions.
5. Paraneoplastic pemphigus.
6. Porphyria cutanea tarda.
7. Mycophenolate mofetil (MMF).
8. Topical calcineurin inhibitors.
9. Cryotherapy.
10. Kyrle's disease.

[Time: 3 Hours] [Max. Marks: 100]

DERMATOLOGY, VENEREOLOGY AND LEPROSY
DERMATOLOGY INCLUDING DISEASES
PAPER – II

Your answers should be specific to the questions asked
Draw neat labeled diagrams wherever necessary

Answer all the Questions **10 × 10 = 100 Marks**

1. Discuss approach to a patient with fever and rash.
2. Classify and discuss cutaneous markers of internal malignancy.
3. List water soluble vitamins. Discuss the etiology, clinical features and treatment of Pellagra.
4. Discuss the various manifestations of cutaneous sarcoidosis. Add a note on treatment.
5. Enumerate the psychiatric disorders associated with dermatologic symptoms. Discuss the clinical features and management of trichotillomania.
6. Classify dermatoses of pregnancy. Discuss clinical features and treatment of polymorphic eruptions of pregnancy.
7. Classify systemic sclerosis. Discuss pseudoscleroderma.
8. Write notes on (a) Piedra; (b) Trumpet nails.
9. Write notes on (a) Colchicine in dermatology; (b) Acropustulosis of infancy.
10. Acantholytic disorders.

[Time: 3 Hours] [Max. Marks: 100]

DERMATOLOGY, VENEREOLOGY AND LEPROSY
DERMATOLOGY PAPER – II

Your answers should be specific to the questions asked
Draw neat, labeled diagrams wherever necessary

Answer all the Questions **10 × 10 = 100 Marks**

1. Management of hidradenitis suppurativa.
2. Investigative techniques in hair disorders.
3. Lichen planus pemphigoides.
4. Pigmentary demarcation lines.
5. Discuss etiology, clinical features and management of erythema nodosum.
6. Familial benign chronic pemphigus.
7. Androgenic alopecia in women.
8. Cheilitis granulomatosa.
9. Griscelli syndrome.
10. Management of oral lichen planus.

[Time: 3 Hours] [Max. Marks: 100]

DERMATOLOGY, VENEREOLOGY AND LEPROSY S.T.D. AND LEPROSY PAPER – III

Your answers should be specific to the questions asked
Draw neat, labeled diagrams wherever necessary

Answer all the Questions **10 × 10 = 100 Marks**

1. Discuss the natural course of syphilis briefly.
2. Diagnosis of donovanosis. Describe Pund-Greenblatt cell.
3. Discuss the causes of resistance in gonorrhea. How will you manage such a case?
4. What is phagedenic chancroid? Discuss the management.
5. Management of a case of current genital herpes in pregnancy.
6. Discuss Indian classification of leprosy and its importance.
7. What is Lazarine leprosy and how will you manage?
8. WHO classification of deformities in leprosy. How to prevent them?
9. Discuss relapse in leprosy. How will you distinguish reinfection?
10. Discuss the complication in dapsone therapy. Describe dapsone syndrome.

[Time: 3 Hours] [Max. Marks: 100]

DERMATOLOGY, VENEREOLOGY AND LEPROSY S.T.D. AND LEPROSY PAPER – III

Your answers should be specific to the questions asked
Draw neat labeled diagrams wherever necessary

Answer all the Questions **10 × 10 = 100 Marks**

1. Discuss multidrug therapy and its effects in controlling leprosy in India.
2. Prenatal syphilis.
3. Lucio phenomenon.
4. Trichomoniasis.
5. Dapsone syndrome.
6. Write a note on biology of *Neisseria gonorrhoeae.*
7. Immune reconstitution inflammatory syndrome.
8. Discuss systemic involvement leprosy.
9. Clutton's joints.
10. Childhood leprosy.

[Time: 3 Hours] [Max. Marks: 100]

DERMATOLOGY, VENEREOLOGY AND LEPROSY
PAPER – IV

Your answers should be specific to the questions asked
Draw neat labeled diagrams wherever necessary

Answer all the Questions **10 × 10 = 100 Marks**

1. Cutaneous manifestation of hepatitis C virus infection.
2. Classify dyslipidemias, mentioning the corresponding lipid abnormality and relevant cutaneous manifestations.
3. Recent advances in the management of rosacea.
4. Discuss cutaneous adverse reactions to anti-malignancy drugs.
5. Cutaneous manifestations of diabetes mellitus.
6. Bowel-associated dermatitis-arthritis syndrome.
7. Skin changes due to liver disease.
8. Janus kinase inhibitors.
9. Topical anti-aging agents.
10. Myxedema in thyroid diseases.

[Time: 3 Hours] [Max. Marks: 100]

DERMATOLOGY, VENEREOLOGY AND LEPROSY BASIC SCIENCES OF DERMATOLOGY, S.T.D. AND LEPROSY PAPER – I

Your answers should be specific to the questions asked
Draw neat labeled diagrams wherever necessary

Answer all the Questions **10 × 10 = 100 Marks**

1. Write in detail about keratinization and regulation of epidermopoesis.
2. Write in detail structure of HIV and it's immunology.
3. Write short notes on Kveim's test.
4. Write briefly about NBUVB in dermatology.
5. Write briefly about elastic fibers in health and disease.
6. Write briefly on use of azathioprine in dermatology.
7. Brief note on microbiology of *Mycobacterium Leprae*.
8. Write short note on histopathology of cutaneous tuberculosis.
9. Glomus bodies.
10. Ultra structure of gonococci.

[Time: 3 Hours] [Max. Marks: 100]

DERMATOLOGY, VENEREOLOGY AND LEPROSY DERMATOLOGY INCLUDING DISEASES PAPER – II

Your answers should be specific to the questions asked
Draw neat labeled diagrams wherever necessary

Answer all the Questions **10 × 10 = 100 Marks**

1. Classify pustular psoriasis. Describe the clinical features and management of generalized pustular psoriasis.
2. Classify vasculitis. Describe the etiology, clinical features and management of Kawasaki disease.
3. Pyoderma faciale.
4. Macular amyloidosis.
5. Onycholysis.
6. Scleredema adultorum.
7. Circinate balanitis.
8. Pompholyx.
9. *Corynebacterium* species in dermatology.
10. Atypical mycobacterial infections.

[Time: 3 Hours] [Max. Marks: 100]

DERMATOLOGY, VENEREOLOGY AND LEPROSY S.T.D. AND LEPROSY PAPER – III

Your answers should be specific to the questions asked
Draw neat, labeled diagrams wherever necessary

Answer all the Questions **10 × 10 = 100 Marks**

1. Describe clinical features, diagnosis and treatment of granuloma inguinale.
2. Describe the immunology and pathogenesis of leprosy.
3. Bacillary angiomatosis.
4. Syndromic approach to vaginal discharge.
5. Lucio leprosy.
6. Management of neurosyphilis.
7. Lepromin test.
8. AIDS-related malignancies.
9. Post-exposure prophylaxis.
10. Foot care in leprosy.

[Time: 3 Hours] [Max. Marks: 100]

DERMATOLOGY, VENEREOLOGY AND LEPROSY PAPER – IV

Your answers should be specific to the questions asked
Draw neat labeled diagrams wherever necessary

Answer all the Questions **10 × 10 = 100 Marks**

1. Describe the skin manifestations of subacute LE. Write a note on ANA.
2. Discuss the clinical features and pathology of trans-epidermal elimination disorders.
3. Acanthosis nigricans.
4. Granuloma faciale.
5. Calcineurin inhibitors.
6. Moisturisers.
7. Skin and smoking.
8. Botox for non-cosmetic indications in dermatology.
9. Genetic counseling in genodermatoses.
10. Acute skin failure.

[Time: 3 Hours] [Max. Marks: 100]

DERMATOLOGY, VENEREOLOGY AND LEPROSY BASIC SCIENCES AS APPLIED TO DERMATOLOGY, VENEREOLOGY AND LEPROSY PAPER – I

Your answers should be specific to the questions asked
Draw neat labeled diagrams wherever necessary

Answer all the Questions **10 × 10 = 100 Marks**

1. Discuss the cutaneous vasculature. Discuss its importance in clinical dermatology.
2. Discuss cutaneous inflammation and its mediators.
3. Bartholin's gland.
4. Trichelemmal keratinization.
5. Synthesis of melanin.
6. Valaciclovir.
7. Immunology of leprosy.
8. *Treponema pallidum* heme agglutination assay.
9. Bedside test to assess motor nerve functions in leprosy.
10. Super antigens.

[Time: 3 Hours] [Max. Marks: 100]

DERMATOLOGY, VENEREOLOGY AND LEPROSY DERMATOLOGY PAPER – II

Your answers should be specific to the questions asked
Draw neat, labeled diagrams wherever necessary

Answer all the Questions **10 × 10 = 100 Marks**

1. Discuss differential diagnosis of vesicular lesions in a neonate. Discuss staphylococcal scalded skin syndrome.
2. Discuss the clinical features, investigations and management of Langerhans cell histiocytosis.
3. Perioral dermatitis.
4. Discuss psoriatic arthritis and its management.
5. Discuss various causes of generalized hypermelanosis.
6. Sclerema adultorum of Buschke.
7. Pathogenesis of allergic contact dermatosis.
8. Premalignant skin diseases.
9. Bacillary angiomatosis.
10. Jogren Larsen syndrome.

[Time: 3 Hours] [Max. Marks: 100]

DERMATOLOGY, VENEREOLOGY AND LEPROSY
S.T.D. AND LEPROSY PAPER – III

Your answers should be specific to the questions asked
Draw neat, labeled diagrams wherever necessary

Answer all the Questions **10 × 10 = 100 Marks**

1. Classify neurosyphilis. Discuss the clinical features and management of tabes dorsalis.
2. Classify deformities in leprosy. Discuss the management and prevention.
3. Acute complications of gonorrhea.
4. Erythema necroticans.
5. Ocular manifestation in leprosy.
6. Subclinical leprosy.
7. Balanoposthitis.
8. Dimorphous leprosy.
9. Adverse drug reactions to HAART.
10. Differential diagnosis of skin lesions in leprosy.

[Time: 3 Hours] [Max. Marks: 100]

DERMATOLOGY, VENEREOLOGY AND LEPROSY
BASIC SCIENCES OF DERMATOLOGY, S.T.D. AND LEPROSY
PAPER – I

Your answers should be specific to the questions asked
Draw neat labeled diagrams wherever necessary

Answer all the Questions **10 × 10 = 100 Marks**

1. Write in detail about development and structure of sebaceous gland. What is the etiopathogenesis of acne vulgaris?
2. Describe the solar spectrum. Classify photodermatoses. Discuss management of polymorphic light eruptions.
3. Describe the anatomy of male urethra. What is the pathogenesis of gonococcal urethritis?
4. Describe the structure of eccrine gland with the help of a diagram. Discuss management of palmar hyperhidrosis.
5. Classify normal flora of the skin. What are the factors which affect the normal flora?
6. Discuss the physiological function of adipose tissue. Add a note on obesity and skin.
7. Describe the sense organs of the skin with suitable diagram.
8. Write notes on (a) Epidermotropism (b) Functions of sebum.
9. Whiff test.
10. Mosaicism and chimerism.

[Time: 3 Hours] [Max. Marks: 100]

DERMATOLOGY, VENEREOLOGY AND LEPROSY
DERMATOLOGY INCLUDING DISEASES
PAPER – II

Your answers should be specific to the questions asked
Draw neat labeled diagrams wherever necessary

Answer all the Questions **10 × 10 = 100 Marks**

1. Classify cutaneous amyloidosis. Discuss etiology, clinical features, histopathology, diagnosis and management of primary localized cutaneous amyloidosis.
2. Discuss in detail cutaneous aspects of renal disease.
3. Discuss cutaneous manifestations of immunosuppressive therapy.
4. List the causes of cheilitis. Describe the clinical feature of actinic cheilitis.
5. Enumerate premalignant skin conditions. Discuss the clinical features and management of Bowen's disease.
6. Describe the clinical features of cutaneous T cell lymphoma.
7. Dapsone in dermatology—Indications, mechanism of action, dosage and side effects.
8. Write short notes on (a) Pemphigoid nodularis (b) Syringoma.
9. Perforating disorders.
10. Pseudoxanthoma elasticum.

[Time: 3 Hours] [Max. Marks: 100]

DERMATOLOGY, VENEREOLOGY AND LEPROSY S.T.D. AND LEPROSY PAPER – III

Your answers should be specific to the questions asked
Draw neat labeled diagrams wherever necessary

Answer all the Questions **10 × 10 = 100 Marks**

1. Enumerate the causes of abnormal vaginal discharge. Discuss approach to a patient with abnormal vaginal discharge.
2. Discuss pregnancy and leprosy.
3. Describe the histopathology and treatment of condyloma acuminate.
4. Describe the atypical presentations of herpes genitalis in patients with AIDS. Add a note on laboratory diagnosis of herpes virus infection.
5. Discuss Jarisch-Herxheimer reaction.
6. Discuss the pathogenesis, clinical features, diagnosis and management of type 1 lepra reaction.
7. Discuss role of physiotherapy in leprosy.
8. Write notes on (a) Acetic acid test (b) SFG index.
9. IRIS.
10. Newer drugs in leprosy.

[Time: 3 Hours] [Max. Marks: 100]

DERMATOLOGY, VENEREOLOGY AND LEPROSY BASIC SCIENCES AS APPLIED TO DERMATOLOGY, VENEREOLOGY AND LEPROSY PAPER – I

Your answers should be specific to the questions asked
Draw neat, labeled diagrams wherever necessary

Answer all the Questions **10 × 10 = 100 Marks**

1. Enumerate the physiological skin changes in pregnancy.
2. Discuss in detail about interface dermatitis.
3. Keratinocytes.
4. Cryotherapy.
5. Merkel's cells.
6. Wood's lamp.
7. Delayed type hypersensitivity tests in dermatology.
8. Cutaneous vasculature.
9. Dermoscopy in hair disorders.
10. Structure and function of sebaceous glands.

[Time: 3 Hours] [Max. Marks: 100]

DERMATOLOGY, VENEREOLOGY AND LEPROSY DERMATOLOGY PAPER – II

Your answers should be specific to the questions asked
Draw neat, labeled diagrams wherever necessary

Answer all the Questions **10 × 10 = 100 Marks**

1. Mycetoma.
2. Herpes zoster.
3. Xeroderma pigmentosum.
4. Hemangiomas of infancy.
5. Pityriasis rubra pilaris.
6. Stasis dermatitis.
7. Principles of topical therapy in psoriasis.
8. Chemical peeling agents in dermatology.
9. Granuloma annulare.
10. DEGO's disease.

[Time: 3 Hours] [Max. Marks: 100]

DERMATOLOGY, VENEREOLOGY AND LEPROSY S.T.D. AND LEPROSY PAPER – III

Your answers should be specific to the questions asked
Draw neat, labeled diagrams wherever necessary

Answer all the Questions **10 × 10 = 100 Marks**

1. Evaluation and management of a male patient with genital ulcer disease.
2. Discuss the problem of drug resistance in leprosy and its management.
3. Serological diagnosis of leprosy.
4. Discuss the differences between reversal reactions and relapse in leprosy.
5. Indeterminate leprosy.
6. Management of anogenital warts.
7. Syphilis in HIV.
8. Clinical variants of chancroid.
9. Syndromic approach for urethral discharge in male.
10. Conjugal leprosy.

[Time: 3 Hours] [Max. Marks: 100]

DERMATOLOGY, VENEREOLOGY AND LEPROSY
PAPER – IV

Your answers should be specific to the questions asked
Draw neat, labeled diagrams wherever necessary

Answer all the Questions **10 × 10 = 100 Marks**

1. Cutaneous manifestations of renal disorders.
2. Surgical management of vitiligo.
3. Dermatoses of pregnancy.
4. Role of diet in dermatological disorders.
5. Rituximab.
6. Hair removal lasers.
7. Photodynamic therapy.
8. Newer topical antifungal agents.
9. Surgery for acne scar.
10. Ataxia telangiectasia.

[Time: 3 Hours] [Max. Marks: 100]

DERMATOLOGY, VENEREOLOGY AND LEPROSY
BASIC SCIENCES OF DERMATOLOGY, S.T.D. AND LEPROSY
PAPER – I

Your answers should be specific to the questions asked
Draw neat labeled diagrams wherever necessary

LONG ESSAYS **2 × 20 = 40 Marks**

1. Describe the steps of collagen synthesis. Classify Ehler's Danlos syndrome and describe the clinical features of classical Ehler's Danlos syndrome.
2. Describe briefly the complement cascade and give an account of hereditary familial angioedema.

SHORT ESSAYS **6 × 10 = 60 Marks**

3. Draw the coronal section of male genital organs. Add a note on the lymphatic drainage.
4. Describe the ultrastructure of *M. leprae*. Add a note on transmission of leprosy.
5. Discuss barrier function of the skin.
6. Describe ultrastructure of hair with a diagram. Discuss trichogram.
7. Discuss the principles of immunofluorescence.
8. Write notes on (a) Acanthosis (b) Civatte bodies.

[Time: 3 Hours] [Max. Marks: 100]

DERMATOLOGY, VENEREOLOGY AND LEPROSY
DERMATOLOGY INCLUDING DISEASES
PAPER – II

Your answers should be specific to the questions asked
Draw neat labeled diagrams wherever necessary. Answer all questions

LONG ESSAY **2 × 20 = 40 Marks**

1. Discuss in detail about keratinization and briefly classify ichthyosis.
2. Discuss in detail about hypermelanosis in India; mention about lichen planus pigmentosus.

SHORT ESSAY **6 × 10 = 60 Marks**

3. Write short note on fixed drug eruption.
4. Write briefly on IVIg (intravenous immunoglobulin) in dermatology.
5. Write short note on microdermabrasion.
6. Write short note on Melkersson-Rosenthal syndrome.
7. Write briefly about calcineurin inhibitors.
8. Write short note about pyoderma gangrenosum.

[Time: 3 Hours] [Max. Marks: 100]

DERMATOLOGY, VENEREOLOGY AND LEPROSY S.T.D. AND LEPROSY PAPER – III

Your answers should be specific to the questions asked
Draw neat labeled diagrams wherever necessary. Answer all questions

LONG ESSAY **2 × 20 = 40 Marks**

1. Define complicated gonorrhoea and describe the manifestations and the management of it in males.
2. Discuss the clinical features and the management of reversal reactions in leprosy.

SHORT ESSAY **6 × 10 = 60 Marks**

3. Hairy penis.
4. Rifampicin in venereology and leprosy.
5. Early diagnostic signs of lepromatous leprosy.
6. Chancre - Mou valant.
7. Heinz bodies.
8. Write notes on following:
   (a) Amsel's criteria.
   (b) Lichen sclerosis et atrophicus.

[Time: 3 Hours] [Max. Marks: 100]

DERMATOLOGY, VENEREOLOGY AND LEPROSY BASIC SCIENCES OF DERMATOLOGY, S.T.D. AND LEPROSY PAPER – I

Your answers should be specific to the questions asked
Draw neat, labeled diagrams wherever necessary

Answer all the Questions **10 × 10 = 100 Marks**

1. Describe in detail the syndromic approach to genital ulcer disease (GUD).
2. Describe in detail about eye involvement in leprosy.
3. Granulomas.
4. Anatomy of male urethra.
5. Treponema pallidum.
6. Tzanck test.
7. Barrier function of skin.
8. Role of polymerase chain reaction (PCR) in dermatology.
9. Lymphatic drainage of female external genitalia.
10. TRUE test.

[Time: 3 Hours] [Max. Marks: 100]

DERMATOLOGY, VENEREOLOGY AND LEPROSY
DERMATOLOGY INCLUDING DISEASES
PAPER – II

Your answers should be specific to the questions asked
Draw neat, labeled diagrams wherever necessary

Answer all the Questions **10 × 10 = 100 Marks**

1. Discuss clinical manifestations, diagnosis and management of sarcoidosis.
2. Discuss the differential diagnosis of bullous eruption in children.
3. a. Apoptosis b. Sporotrichosis
4. a. LE cell b. Plasma cell
5. a. Napkin dermatitis b. Perioral dermatitis
6. a. Tuberculosis b. Lyme disease
7. a. Pediculosis capitis b. Favus
8. a. Erythema annulare centrifugum b. Lichen sclerosus et atrophicus
9. a. Kerion b. Botryomycosis
10. a. Follicular occlusion tetrad b. Epidermotropism

[Time: 3 Hours] [Max. Marks: 100]

DERMATOLOGY, VENEREOLOGY AND LEPROSY
S.T.D. AND LEPROSY
PAPER – III

Your answers should be specific to the questions asked
Draw neat, labeled diagrams wherever necessary

Answer all the Questions **10 × 10 = 100 Marks**

1. Discuss clinical features and treatment of urethral discharge in male.
2. Discuss the differential diagnosis of annular lesions on the trunk and clinical features and management of borderline lepromatous leprosy.
3. a. Leprosy vaccine b. Nine banded armadillo
4. a. False positive VDRL b. Romberg's sign
5. a. Plasma cell b. Ape thumb
6. a. Retro virus b. Acetoacetic acid whitening
7. a. Clofazimine b. Bartholin's gland
8. a. Congenital syphilis b. Split skin smear
9. a. Mitsuda reactions b. Stigmata of leprosy
10. a. Contact tracing in STI b. Conjugal leprosy

[Time: 3 Hours] [Max. Marks: 100]

DERMATOLOGY, VENEREOLOGY AND LEPROSY BASIC SCIENCES AS APPLIED TO DERMATOLOGY, VENEREOLOGY AND LEPROSY PAPER – I

Your answers should be specific to the questions asked
Draw neat, labeled diagrams wherever necessary. Answer all questions

LONG ESSAYS **2 × 20 = 40 Marks**

1. Discuss the structure of hair. Briefly mention the various stages of hair.
2. Discuss the control of sebum. Briefly mention its contents.

SHORT ESSAYS **6 × 10 = 60 Marks**

3. Elastic fibers.
4. Phenyl alanine.
5. Effects of solar radiation on skin.
6. Serum proteins.
7. Armadillo.
8. Toll like receptors.

[Time: 3 Hours] [Max. Marks: 100]

DERMATOLOGY, VENEREOLOGY AND LEPROSY DERMATOLOGY PAPER – II

Your answers should be specific to the questions asked
Draw neat labeled diagrams wherever necessary. Answer all questions

LONG ESSAY **2 × 20 = 40 Marks**

1. A 40-year-old patient present with painful nodules over the leg, how do you approach for the diagnosis? What investigations do you perform? Describe the general lines of management.
2. Classify palmoplantar keratoderma. Name the syndromes associated with PPK. Write in brief about palmoplantar psoriasis.

SHORT ESSAY **6 × 10 = 60 Marks**

3. Albinism.
4. Gunther's disease.
5. Tinea unguium.
6. Lichen planopilaris.
7. Hidradenitis suppurativa.
8. Medical management of hirsutism.

[Time: 3 Hours] [Max. Marks: 100]

DERMATOLOGY, VENEREOLOGY AND LEPROSY S.T.D. AND LEPROSY PAPER – III

Your answers should be specific to the questions asked
Draw neat labeled diagrams wherever necessary

LONG ESSAYS **2 × 20 = 40 Marks**

1. Describe the clinical stages of HIV infection.
2. Describe the epidemiology of leprosy.

SHORT ESSAYS **6 × 10 = 60 Marks**

3. Pelvic inflammatory disease.
4. Plasma cell balanitis.
5. Bowenoid papulosis.
6. Virchow cells.
7. PCR in leprosy diagnosis.
8. Bone involvement in leprosy.

[Time: 3 Hours] [Max. Marks: 100]

DERMATOLOGY, VENEREOLOGY AND LEPROSY PAPER – IV

Your answers should be specific to the questions asked
Draw neat labeled diagrams wherever necessary

LONG ESSAYS **2 × 20 = 40 Marks**

1. Discuss androgen pathophysiology in hirsutism.
2. Discuss nail manifestations of systemic diseases.

SHORT ESSAYS **6 × 10 = 60 Marks**

3. Oral care in bed ridden patients.
4. Pseudo xanthoma elasticum.
5. Langerhans cell histiocytosis.
6. Classification of antihistamines.
7. Mode of action of azathioprine.
8. Psychologic interventions in dermatology.

[Time: 3 Hours] [Max. Marks: 100]

DERMATOLOGY, VENEREOLOGY AND LEPROSY BASIC SCIENCES AS APPLIED TO DERMATOLOGY, VENEREOLOGY AND LEPROSY PAPER – I

Your answers should be specific to the questions asked
Draw neat, labeled diagrams wherever necessary

Answer all the Questions **10 × 10 = 100 Marks**

1. Discuss the embryology of skin. Write a note on dermatoglyphics.
2. Write in detail the lymphatic drainage of the female genitalia.
3. Cytoid bodies.
4. Structure of *M. leprae.*
5. Kveim test.
6. Innate immunity and skin.
7. Lipid mantle in skin.
8. Cutaneous microflora.
9. Hair cycle.
10. Anatomy of nail.

[Time: 3 Hours] [Max. Marks: 100]

DERMATOLOGY, VENEREOLOGY AND LEPROSY DERMATOLOGY PAPER – II

Your answers should be specific to the questions asked
Draw neat labeled diagrams wherever necessary

Answer all the Questions **10 × 10 = 100 Marks**

1. Describe the pathogenesis of atopic dermatitis.
2. Discuss the dermatoses related to mechanical injury to skin.
3. Pseudolymphomas.
4. Azathioprine in skin disease.
5. Tungiasis.
6. Pyoderma gangrenosum.
7. Histopathology of granuloma annulare.
8. Sarcoidosis.
9. Approach to patient with palpable purpura.
10. Thalidomide in dermatology.

[Time: 3 Hours] [Max. Marks: 100]

DERMATOLOGY, VENEREOLOGY AND LEPROSY PAPER – IV

Your answers should be specific to the questions asked
Draw neat, labeled diagrams wherever necessary

Answer all the Questions **10 × 10 = 100 Marks**

1. Fever with rash in children. Discuss the causes and management.
2. Cutaneous changes in thyroid disorders.
3. IVIg (Intravenous immunoglobulin).
4. Excimer lasers.
5. Hepatitis C virus and skin.
6. CREST syndrome.
7. Paraneoplastic pemphigus.
8. Neonatal lupus.
9. Photo dynamic therapy.
10. Skin resurfacing techniques.

[Time: 3 Hours] [Max. Marks: 100]

DERMATOLOGY, VENEREOLOGY AND LEPROSY
BASIC SCIENCES OF DERMATOLOGY, S.T.D. AND LEPROSY
PAPER – I

Your answers should be specific to the questions asked
Draw neat labeled diagrams wherever necessary

LONG ESSAYS **2 × 20 = 40 Marks**

1. Describe the structure of an eosinophil. Enumerate the eosinophilic dermatoses and describe the clinical features of Well's syndrome.
2. Discuss role of the skin in thermoregulation. Mention the factors which control temperature regulation by the skin.

SHORT ESSAYS **6 × 10 = 60 Marks**

3. Describe the stages of hair cycle with suitable diagram.
4. Describe the structure of human immunodeficiency virus.
5. Discuss type IV hypersensitivity reaction.
6. Describe the lymphatic drainage of female genital tract.
7. Classify antihistamines. List the side effects.
8. Write notes on (a) Marginal band (b) Desmosomes.

DERMATOLOGY, VENEREOLOGY AND LEPROSY
DERMATOLOGY INCLUDING DISEASES
PAPER – II

Your answers should be specific to the questions asked
Draw neat, labeled diagrams wherever necessary. Answer all questions

LONG ESSAYS **2 × 20 = 40 Marks**

1. Describe in detail the pathogenesis, clinical features and management of mycosis fungoides.
2. Describe in detail the mode of action and uses of synthetic retinoids in dermatology.

SHORT ESSAYS **6 × 10 = 60 Marks**

3. Parthenium dermatitis.
4. Myiasis.
5. Uses of cyclosporine.
6. Write short notes on (a) Pediculosis capitis (b) Phthirus pubis.
7. Write short notes on (a) Antinuclear antibody (b) CREST syndrome.
8. Henoch-Schonlein purpura.

DERMATOLOGY, VENEREOLOGY AND LEPROSY
S.T.D. AND LEPROSY
PAPER – III

Your answers should be specific to the questions asked
Draw neat, labeled diagrams wherever necessary. Answer all questions

LONG ESSAYS **2 × 20 = 40 Marks**

1. Describe clinical features, diagnosis and treatment of lymphogranuloma venerum.
2. Describe the clinical features and management of lepromatous leprosy.

SHORT ESSAYS **6 × 10 = 60 Marks**

3. Kaposi's sarcoma.
4. Protease inhibitors.
5. Newer antileprosy drugs.
6. VDRL.
7. Clofazimine.
8. Jarisch-Herxheimer reaction.

[Time: 3 Hours] [Max. Marks: 100]

DERMATOLOGY, VENEREOLOGY AND LEPROSY
BASIC SCIENCES OF DERMATOLOGY, S.T.D. AND LEPROSY
PAPER – I

Your answers should be specific to the questions asked
Draw neat, labeled diagrams wherever necessary. Answer all questions

LONG ESSAYS **2 × 20 = 40 Marks**

1. Discuss the effect of ageing on the skin.
2. Define granuloma. Give a histopathological account of the various types of granulomatous infiltrates of the skin.

SHORT ESSAYS **6 × 10 = 60 Marks**

3. a. Woods Lamp b. Pediculosis capitis
4. a. Langerhan cell b. Dark field examination
5. a. Actinic elastosis b. Seminal fluid
6. a. Chloroquine b. Acne fulminans
7. a. Dapsone syndrome b. Tzanck cell
8. a. Nonveneral genital ulcers b. Intertrigo

[Time: 3 Hours] [Max. Marks: 100]

DERMATOLOGY, VENEREOLOGY AND LEPROSY DERMATOLOGY INCLUDING DISEASES PAPER – II

Your answers should be specific to the questions asked
Draw neat labeled diagrams wherever necessary

LONG ESSAYS **2 × 20 = 40 Marks**

1. Discuss approach to a 25-year-old lady presenting with red face.
2. Discuss the transient neonatal skin disorders.

SHORT ESSAYS **6 × 10 = 60 Marks**

3. Enumerate the premature aging syndromes. Describe the clinical features of pseudoxanthoma elasticum.
4. What are the drugs causing alopecia? Discuss trichorrhexis invaginata.
5. Discuss the pathogenesis of psoriasis.
6. What are the causes of erythroderma? Discuss the complications and management of erythroderma.
7. Bath water PUVA therapy—Indications, procedure and side effects.
8. Write notes on (a) Pseudofolliculitis barbae (b) Bromhidrosis.

[Time: 3 Hours] [Max. Marks: 100]

DERMATOLOGY, VENEREOLOGY AND LEPROSY S.T.D. AND LEPROSY PAPER – III

Your answers should be specific to the questions asked
Draw neat, labeled diagrams wherever necessary. Answer all questions

LONG ESSAYS **2 × 20 = 40 Marks**

1. Discuss clinical features and management of AIDS.
2. Clinical features, differential diagnosis, management of trophic ulcer.

SHORT ESSAYS **6 × 10 = 60 Marks**

3. a. Animal models in leprosy b. Indices in leprosy
4. a. ROM b. Clue cell
5. a. Mitsuda reaction b. Jarisch-Herxheimer reaction
6. a. BUBO b. Peyronie's disease
7. a. Genital warts b. Neonatal herpes simplex infection
8. a. Congenital syphilis b. Fitz-Hugh-Curtis syndrome

[Time: 3 Hours] [Max. Marks: 100]

DERMATOLOGY, VENEREOLOGY AND LEPROSY BASIC SCIENCES AS APPLIED TO DERMATOLOGY, VENEREOLOGY AND LEPROSY PAPER – I

Your answers should be specific to the questions asked
Draw neat labeled diagrams wherever necessary

LONG ESSAYS **2 × 20 = 40 Marks**

1. Discuss epicutaneous skin tests.
2. Describe percutaneous absorption.

SHORT ESSAYS **6 × 10 = 60 Marks**

3. Matrix metallo proteinases.
4. Anatomy of female genitalia.
5. Immunity against leprosy infection.
6. Chromosome.
7. UV induced immunosuppression.
8. Antimicrobial peptides and skin.

[Time: 3 Hours] [Max. Marks: 100]

DERMATOLOGY, VENEREOLOGY AND LEPROSY DERMATOLOGY PAPER – II

Your answers should be specific to the questions asked
Draw neat labeled diagrams wherever necessary

LONG ESSAYS **2 × 20 = 40 Marks**

1. Describe the cutaneous manifestations of collagen vascular diseases.
2. Describe the venous system of legs and mention the consequences of venous hypertension.

SHORT ESSAYS **6 × 10 = 60 Marks**

3. Histopathology of cutaneous B-cell lymphoma.
4. Hurler's syndrome.
5. Kaposi's varicelliform eruption.
6. Pigmented contact dermatitis.
7. Milroy's disease.
8. Salt-split technique.

[Time: 3 Hours] [Max. Marks: 100]

DERMATOLOGY, VENEREOLOGY AND LEPROSY
S.T.D. AND LEPROSY PAPER – III

Your answers should be specific to the questions asked
Draw neat labeled diagrams wherever necessary. Answer all questions

LONG ESSAY **2 × 20 = 40 Marks**

1. Describe the immunology of leprosy. Write about serological tests for leprosy.
2. Management of pregnant lady with anemia and HIV.

SHORT ESSAY **6 × 10 = 60 Marks**

3. Claw hand.
4. Histoid Hansen's.
5. Leprous osteitis.
6. VDRL.
7. Epididymitis.
8. Esthiomene.

[Time: 3 Hours] [Max. Marks: 100]

DERMATOLOGY, VENEREOLOGY AND LEPROSY
PAPER – IV

Your answers should be specific to the questions asked
Draw neat labeled diagrams wherever necessary

LONG ESSAYS **2 × 20 = 40 Marks**

1. Classify hypertriglyceridemias and outline management.
2. Discuss the differential diagnosis of peripheral neuropathy.

SHORT ESSAYS **6 × 10 = 60 Marks**

3. Sneddon's syndrome.
4. Management of post-herpetic neuralgia.
5. Moh's microscopic surgery.
6. Eflornithine.
7. Cutaneous manifestations of Crohn's disease.
8. Extramammary Paget's disease.

[Time: 3 Hours] [Max. Marks: 100]

DERMATOLOGY, VENEREOLOGY AND LEPROSY
BASIC SCIENCES AS APPLIED TO DERMATOLOGY

Your answers should be specific to the questions asked
Draw neat labeled diagrams wherever necessary

LONG ESSAYS **2 × 20 = 40 Marks**

1. Discuss about nerve damage in leprosy.
2. What measures can you take to control sexually transmitted diseases?

SHORT ESSAYS **6 × 10 = 60 Marks**

3. Ultrastructure of epidermis.
4. Transmission of itch sensation.
5. Stuart's medium.
6. Skin as an immunological organ.
7. Macrophage.
8. Glycosaminoglycans.

[Time: 3 Hours] [Max. Marks: 100]

DERMATOLOGY, VENEREOLOGY AND LEPROSY
DERMATOLOGY PAPER – II

Your answers should be specific to the questions asked
Draw neat labeled diagrams wherever necessary. Answer all questions

LONG ESSAY **2 × 20 = 40 Marks**

1. Classify fungal infections of skin. Discuss in detail the clinical features, diagnosis and management of cryptococosis.
2. Describe the various premature ageing syndromes.

SHORT ESSAY **6 × 10 = 60 Marks**

3. Dercum's disease.
4. Para neoplastic pemphigus.
5. Kaposi's varicelliform eruptions.
6. Graft versus host disease.
7. SHARP syndrome.
8. Eosinophilic granuloma.

[Time: 3 Hours] [Max. Marks: 100]

DERMATOLOGY, VENEREOLOGY AND LEPROSY
S.T.D. AND LEPROSY PAPER – III

Your answers should be specific to the questions asked
Draw neat labeled diagrams wherever necessary

LONG ESSAYS **2 × 20 = 40 Marks**

1. Discuss the differential diagnosis of genital bubo.
2. Describe the structure of Myco leprae.

SHORT ESSAYS **6 × 10 = 60 Marks**

3. Counseling in HIV/AIDs.
4. Dhat syndrome.
5. Bacterial vaginosis.
6. Ofloxacin in leprosy.
7. Unstable leprosy.
8. Armadillo.

[Time: 3 Hours] [Max. Marks: 100]

DERMATOLOGY, VENEREOLOGY AND LEPROSY
PAPER – IV

Your answers should be specific to the questions asked
Draw neat labeled diagrams wherever necessary

LONG ESSAYS **2 × 20 = 40 Marks**

1. Discuss management of toxic epidermal necrolysis.
2. What are the cutaneous manifestations of cardiac diseases?

SHORT ESSAYS **6 × 10 = 60 Marks**

3. Laser hair removal.
4. Indications for radiotherapy in skin diseases.
5. Klinefelter's syndrome.
6. Botulinum toxin.
7. Sclerotherapy.
8. Excisional skin biopsy.

Paper I – Basic Sciences in Dermatology, Venereology and Leprosy

SECTION I

Long answer questions **[16 × 2 = 32]**

1. Describe the structure and functions of neutrophils. Enumerate the dermatological diseases with tissue neutrophilia.
2. Evaluate the role of cytokines as inflammatory mediators in dermatological diseases.

Short answer questions **[6 × 3 = 18]**

3. Analyze ichthyosis in relation to BRICK and MORTOR theory.
4. Correlate the basement membrane zone antigens with vesiculobullous disorders in dermatology.
5. Role of Odland bodies in the keratinization process.

SECTION II

Long answer questions **[16 × 2 = 32]**

1. How will you interpret slit skin smear for AFB in leprosy.
2. Describe the lymphatic drainage of the female external genitalia.

Short answer questions **[6 × 3 = 18]**

3. Principles of Q switched lasers.
4. Antigens of *Neisseria gonorrhoeae*.
5. Sertoli's rosette and streptocytes.

Paper I – Basic Sciences in Dermatology, Venereology and Leprosy

SECTION I

Long answer questions **[16 × 2 = 32]**

1. Evaluate the role of direct immunofluorescence in autoimmune vesiculobullous diseases.
2. Describe the structure and functions of Langerhan cells. Analyze the immunological role of these cells in contact dermatitis.

Short answer questions **[6 × 3 = 18]**

3. Interleukins in psoriasis.
4. Interface dermatitis.
5. Mechanism of apocrine sweat formation.

SECTION II

Long answer questions **[16 × 2 = 32]**

1. Describe the ultrastructure of *M. leprae*.
2. Analyze antibiotic resistance in gonococcal infections.

Short answer questions **[6 × 3 = 18]**

3. Immunology of Type II lepra reaction.
4. Interpretation of VDRL in pregnancy.
5. Etymology of tacrolimus.

Paper II – Dermatology

SECTION I

Long answer questions **[16 × 2 = 32]**

1. How will you manage a woman with adult acne?
2. Debate the role of corticosteroids in the management of toxic epidermal necrolysis.

Short answer questions **[6 × 3 = 18]**

3. Pautrier's microabscess should be called as Darier's epidermal nests – substantiate the statement.
4. Role of moisturizers in atopic dermatitis.
5. Managing cutaneous infections due to methicillin-resistant *Staphylococcus aureus* [MRSA].

SECTION II

Long answer questions **[16 × 2 = 32]**

1. Enumerate and describe the various cutaneous manifestation of systemic lupus erythematosus.
2. Describe the various types of acanthosis nigricans.

Short answer questions **[6 × 3 = 18]**

3. Morphology of oral lichen planus.
4. Management of alopecia universalis.
5. Pathogenesis of bulla formation in bullous pemphigoid.

Paper II – Dermatology

SECTION I

Long answer questions **[16 × 2 = 32]**

1. Analyze the various theories of bulla formation in pemphigus group of vesiculobullous diseases.
2. Critically evaluate the role of dermatologist in preventing topical steroid abuse.

Short answer questions **[6 × 3 = 18]**

3. Histopathology of lichen sclerosus et atrophicus.
4. Analyze the concept of Ruocco's immunocompromised cutaneous district.
5. Precautions while prescribing isotretinoin in acne.

SECTION II

Long answer questions **[16 × 2 = 32]**

1. How will you evaluate a patient for methotrexate in the management of psoriasis?
2. Enumerate various painful tumors of the skin and evaluate the pathogenesis of pain in these diseases.

Short answer questions **[6 × 3 = 18]**

3. Norwegian scabies.
4. Leser-Trelat sign.
5. Ophiasis.

Paper III – Leprosy, Sexually Transmitted Diseases

SECTION I

Long answer questions **[16 × 2 = 32]**

1. How will you manage leprosy in a pregnant woman?
2. Evaluate the immunopathogenesis of type I lepra reaction.

Short answer questions **[6 × 3 = 18]**

3. Lazarine leprosy.
4. Armadillos.
5. Eye in leprosy.

SECTION II

Long answer questions **[16 × 2 = 32]**

1. Debate the use of syndromic approach in the management of sexually transmitted infections.
2. Immune reconstitution inflammatory syndrome – Analyze the pathogenesis.

Short answer questions **[6 × 3 = 18]**

3. Clue cells and false clue cells.
4. How will you differentiate bubos of LGV from chancroid?
5. Extra genital cutaneous manifestations of lymphogranuloma venereum.

Paper III – Leprosy, Sexually Transmitted Diseases

SECTION I

Long answer questions **[16 × 2 = 32]**

1. Describe the pathomechanism of plantar ulcer in leprosy and discuss the management.
2. Evaluate the role of dermatologist in the management of severe and recurrent type II lepra reaction.

Short answer questions **[6 × 3 = 18]**

3. Morphology of cutaneous lesions in mid borderline leprosy.
4. Hematological side effects of dapsone.
5. Fluoroquinolones in leprosy.

SECTION II

Long answer questions **[16 × 2 = 32]**

1. How will you manage herpes progenitalis infection during pregnancy?
2. How will you evaluate a patient with balanoposthitis?

Short answer questions **[6 × 3 = 18]**

3. Desquamative vulvovaginitis.
4. Penicillinase resistant *Neisseria gonorrhoeae* management.
5. Atypical manifestation of syphilis in HIV infection.

Paper IV – Recent Advances in Dermatology, Venereology and Leprosy

Long answer questions (4 out of 5) **[25 × 4 = 100]**

1. Analyze the use of omalizumab in chronic urticaria.
2. Discuss parainflammatory pyoderma gangrenosum.
3. Evaluate the role of various lasers used in hair removal.
4. How will you interpret ANA profile results in various collagen vascular diseases?
5. The use of chemical peels in acne.

Paper IV – Recent Advances in Dermatology, Venereology and Leprosy

Long answer questions (4 out of 5) **[25 × 4 = 100]**

1. Evaluate the role of biologics in the management of psoriasis.
2. How will you investigate a women aged 25 years with hirsutism?
3. Recent concepts of paraneoplastic pemphigus.
4. How will you evaluate a patient as treatment with ISOTRETINOIN for nodulocystic acne?
5. Analyze the surgical modalities of management of stable segmental vitiligo.

Paper I – Basic Sciences in Dermatology

SECTION I

Long answer question **[20 × 1 = 20]**

1. Itch pathway and causes of pruritus.

Short answer questions **[10 × 3 = 30]**

2. Ultrastructure of *M. leprae*.
3. Venous drainage of lower limb.
4. Wood's lamp in dermatology.

SECTION II

Long answer question **[20 × 1 = 20]**

1. Describe the ZN staining method and interpretation of slit skin smear for AFB in Hansen's disease.

Short answer questions **[10 × 3 = 30]**

2. Palisading granuloma.
3. Principles of dermatoscopy.
4. Microbiology of nongonococcal urethritis.

Paper I – Basic Sciences in Dermatology

SECTION I

Long answer question **[20 × 1 = 20]**

1. Analyze the epidermal keratinization process.

Short answer questions **[10 × 3 = 30]**

2. Describe VDRL test and its interpretation.
3. Anatomy of ulnar nerve and its involvement in Hansen's disease.
4. Structure of mast cell.

SECTION II

Long answer question **[20 × 1 = 20]**

1. Structure of human immunodeficiency virus.

Short answer questions **[10 × 3 = 30]**

2. Giant cells in dermatology.
3. Sensory nerve end organs in skin.
4. Immunology of type II lepra reaction.

Paper 4 – Advances in Dermatology

SECTION I

Long answer question **[20 × 1 = 20]**

1. Discuss the various surgical modalities of therapy for acne scarred face.

Short answer questions **[10 × 3 = 30]**

2. Secukinumab in psoriasis.
3. Drug hypersensitivity syndrome.
4. Platelet rich plasma in dermatology.

SECTION II

Long answer question **[20 × 1 = 20]**

1. How will you manage a case of pemphigus vulgaris resistant to conventional methods of treatment?

Short answer questions **[10 × 3 = 30]**

2. Acitretin in psoriasis.
3. Uniform MDT in Hansen's disease.
4. Atypical presentation of primary chancre.

Paper 4 – Advances in Dermatology

SECTION I

Long answer question **[20 × 1 = 20]**

1. Enumerate antiretroviral drugs. Discuss the various combination of these drugs in the management of HIV infection.

Short answer questions **[10 × 3 = 30]**

2. Nonsedative antihistamines.
3. EMLA cream.
4. Minocycline in Hansen's disease.

SECTION II

Long answer question **[20 × 1 = 20]**

1. Analyze the advantages and disadvantages of various hair removal lasers.

Short answer questions **[10 × 3 = 30]**

2. Side effects of isotretinoin.
3. Immunohistochemistry of malignant melanoma.
4. Acute generalized exanthematous pustulosis.

Paper 2 – Clinical Dermatology

SECTION I

Long answer question **[20 × 1 = 20]**

1. Describe the various cutaneous manifestation of tuberous sclerosis.

Short answer questions **[10 × 3 = 30]**

2. Condyloma lata.
3. Immune reconstitution syndrome.
4. How will you perform a nerve biopsy in a case of suspected neural Hansen's disease.

SECTION II

Long answer question **[20 × 1 = 20]**

1. Analyze the spectral concept in cutaneous tuberculosis.

Short answer questions **[10 × 3 = 30]**

2. Histopathology of histoid leprosy.
3. Role of hydroxychloroquine in dermatology.
4. Cutaneous side effects of systemic cyclosporine.

Paper 2 – Clinical Dermatology

SECTION I

Long answer question **[20 × 1 = 20]**

1. Justify the statement that psoriasis is a metabolic syndrome.

Short answer questions **[10 × 3 = 30]**

2. Etanercept in psoriatic arthritis.
3. Histopathology of pityriasis rubra pilaris (PRP).
4. Morphology of cutaneous lesions in borderline tuberculoid Hansen's disease.

SECTION II

Long answer question **[20 × 1 = 20]**

1. Management of eumycotic mycetoma.

Short answer questions **[10 × 3 = 30]**

2. Role of doxycycline in sexually transmitted infection.
3. a. Castling phenomenon b. Nanogen hair
4. Paraneoplastic pyoderma gangrenosum.

MD/MS DEGREE EXAMINATION

DERMATOLOGY, VENEREOLOGY AND LEPROSY

Basic Sciences Related to Dermatology Venereology and Leprosy

November/May 2019 Maximum: 100 Marks (Time: 3 Hours)

Instructions to Candidates

1. Answer all the questions
2. Draw diagrams wherever necessary

....

1. Analyze the itch pathway
2. Describe soaking, bathing and wet dressings in dermatology
3. Role of special stains in dermatology
4. Describe stratum conjunctum and disjunctum
5. Direct immunofluorescence
6. BRICK and MORTAR theory in ichthyosis
7. Ultrastructure of *M. leprae*
8. Inguinal lymph nodes
9. Screening tests for HIV infection
10. Streptocytes and sertoli rosette

MD/MS DEGREE EXAMINATION

DERMATOLOGY, VENEREOLOGY AND LEPROSY

Basic Sciences Related to Dermatology, Venereology and Leprosy

November/May 2019 Maximum: 100 Marks (Time: 3 Hours)

Instructions to Candidates

1. Answer all the questions
2. Draw diagrams wherever necessary

....

1. Sensory end organs in the skin
2. Palisading granulomas
3. Role of streptococci in various dermatological disorders
4. Hemidesmosomes
5. Structure and function of Langerhans cell
6. Interpretation of slit skin smear in leprosy
7. Epidermal melanin unit
8. Immunology of disseminated gonococcal infection
9. Holocrine secretion
10. Transepidermal water loss

MD/MS DEGREE EXAMINATION

DERMATOLOGY, VENEREOLOGY AND LEPROSY
Dermatology

November/May 2019 | Maximum: 100 Marks | (Time: 3 Hours)

Instructions to Candidates

1. Answer all the questions
2. Draw diagrams wherever necessary

Essay **[2 × 20 = 40]**

1. Debate the role of corticosteroids in the management of toxic epidermal necrolysis. Write a note on setting up an intensive care unit for dermatology
2. How will you correlate results of ANA profile in collagen vascular diseases?
3. **Write short note on following:** **[6 × 10 = 60]**
   a. Etymology of tacrolimus
   b. Diabetic dermopathy
   c. Topical anesthesia in dermatology
   d. Parainflammatory pyoderma gangrenosum
   e. Epidermotropism
   f. Igneous rock sign

MD/MS DEGREE EXAMINATION

DERMATOLOGY, VENEREOLOGY AND LEPROSY
Dermatology

November/May 2019 | Maximum: 100 Marks | (Time: 3 Hours)

Instructions to Candidates

1. Answer all the questions
2. Draw diagrams wherever necessary

Essay **[2 × 20 = 40]**

1. Enumerate the various factors to be considered for vitiligo surgery. How will you analyze the stability of vitiligo?
2. Enumerate the causes of tissue neutrophilia. How will you manage a patient with generalized sterile pustular eruption?
3. **Write short note on following:** **[6 × 10 = 60]**
   a. Welsch regimen
   b. Histopathology of seborrheic keratosis
   c. Invisible lichen planus
   d. Pseudo-pseudoxanthoma elasticum
   e. Ruocco's immunocompromised cutaneous district
   f. Analyze the "Multiple hit hypothesis" in the pathogenesis of pemphigus

MD/MS DEGREE EXAMINATION

DERMATOLOGY, VENEREOLOGY AND LEPROSY

Venereology and Leprosy

November/May 2019 Maximum: 100 Marks (Time: 3 Hours)

Instructions to Candidates

1. Answer all the questions
2. Draw diagrams wherever necessary

Essay **[2 × 20 = 40]**

1. How will you differentiate between late reversal reaction and relapse in leprosy?
2. Analyze the relationship between syphilis and HIV infection. Describe the atypical manifestation of syphilis in HIV.
3. **Write short note on following:** **[6 × 10 = 60]**
   a. Immune reconstitution inflammatory syndrome
   b. Extra-genital cutaneous manifestation of LGV
   c. Hematological side effects of dapsone
   d. (1) Immune area of wade (2) Lazarine leprosy
   e. Management of genital herpes during pregnancy
   f. Uniform MDT

MD/MS DEGREE EXAMINATION

DERMATOLOGY, VENEREOLOGY AND LEPROSY

Venereology and Leprosy

November/May 2019 Maximum: 100 Marks (Time: 3 Hours)

Instructions to Candidates

1. Answer all the questions
2. Draw diagrams wherever necessary

Essay **[2 × 20 = 40]**

1. Critically analyze the present scenario of leprosy in India.
2. Discuss HPV infection during pregnancy.
3. **Write short note on following:** **[6 × 10 = 60]**
   a. Penicillinase-producing *Neisseria gonorrhoeae* (PPNG)
   b. Histopathology of lepromatous leprosy
   c. Clinical features of mid-borderline leprosy
   d. Newer anti-leprosy drugs
   e. Post-exposure prophylaxis in HIV
   f. Candidal balanoposthitis

MD/MS DEGREE EXAMINATION

DERMATOLOGY, VENEREOLOGY AND LEPROSY

Dermatology in Internal Medicine and Recent Advances

November/May 2019 Maximum: 100 Marks (Time: 3 Hours)

Instructions to Candidates

1. Answer all the questions
2. Draw diagrams wherever necessary

Essay **[2 × 20 = 40]**

1. Analyze the role of RITUXIMAB in the management of pemphigus group of diseases.
2. Define the role of skin in diagnosing internal malignancies.
3. **Write short note on following:** **[6 × 10 = 60]**
   a. Diode laser
   b. Glycolic acid peels
   c. Dermoscopy in alopecia areata
   d. Porphyria cutanea tarda
   e. Topical steroid abuse
   f. Systemic mastocytosis

MD/MS DEGREE EXAMINATION

DERMATOLOGY, VENEREOLOGY AND LEPROSY

Dermatology in Internal Medicine and Recent Advances

November/May 2019 Maximum: 100 Marks (Time: 3 Hours)

Instructions to Candidates

1. Answer all the questions
2. Draw diagrams wherever necessary

Essay **[2 × 20 = 40]**

1. How will you manage recurrent/resistant dermatophytoses? Analyze the current scenario of dermatophytoses in India.
2. Enumerate the painful tumors of the skin with reference to the mnemonic BLEND TAN EGG. Describe any one among these tumors.
3. **Write short note on following:** **[6 × 10 = 60]**
   a. Secukinumab
   b. Acute generalized exanthematous pustulosis
   c. CO_2 fractional lasers in acne scars
   d. Rhinoentomophthoromycosis
   e. Polymorphic eruption of pregnancy
   f. SIROLIMUS in dermatology

DERMATOLOGY, VENEREOLOGY AND LEPROSY PAPER-II
CLINICAL DERMATOLOGY

Total Marks: 100

Instructions:

- Answer all questions
- Draw neat labeled diagrams wherever necessary
- Answers to each section to be written on separate answer books

SECTION I

1. Discuss skin changes in diabetes mellitus (20)
2. Write short note on following: (30)
   a. Cyclophosphamide
   b. Antinuclear antibodies
   c. Kasabach Merritt syndrome

SECTION II

3. Discuss the clinical features and management of reactions in leprosy. (20)
4. Write short note on following: (30)
   a. Nail patella syndrome
   b. Trichoepithelioma
   c. Senear Usher syndrome

DERMATOLOGY, VENEREOLOGY AND LEPROSY PAPER-I
BASIC SCIENCES IN DERMATOLOGY

Total Marks: 100

Instructions:

- Write legibly and to the point
- Draw diagrams to support your answer
- Marks are indicated on right

SECTION I

1. Discuss the ultrastructure of dermoepidermal junction. Write clinical features and management of chronic bullous disease of childhood. (20)
2. Write short note on following: (30)
   a. Diascopy
   b. Bacteriological index
   c. Structure of HIV

SECTION II

3. Discuss histopathological differential diagnoses of psoriasiform dermatoses (20)
4. Write short note on following: (30)
   a. Elastic fibers
   b. Langerhans cell
   c. Hair cycle

DERMATOLOGY VENEREOLOGY AND LEPROSY PAPER-III
ADVANCES IN DERMATOLOGY

Total Marks: 100

Notes:
- All questions are compulsory
- Draw neat labeled diagrams wherever necessary
- Your answer should be specific to the questions asked

SECTION I

1. Discuss the recent advances in the pathogenesis and management of vitiligo (20)
2. Write short note on following: (30)
   a. Beta blockers in hemangioma
   b. Apremilast
   c. Bleach bath

SECTION II

3. Discuss the surgical management of acne (20)
4. Write short note on following: (30)
   a. LASERS for Tattoo removal
   b. Dolutegravir
   c. Newer drug delivery systems

SUBJECT: PAPER-III
LAPROSY, SEXUALLY TRANSMITTED DISEASE, HIV

Total Marks: 100

Notes:
- All questions are compulsory
- Draw neat labeled diagrams wherever necessary
- Your answer should be specific to the questions asked

SECTION I

1. Describe in detail the structure of vulva and vagina. Discuss vaginal microflora (20)
2. Write short note on following: (30)
   a. Cutaneous infections in HIV disease
   b. Differential diagnosis of urethral discharge in male
   c. IRIS in HIV infections

SECTION II

3. Discuss investigations to be done in a case of lepromatous leprosy (20)
4. Write short note on following: (30)
   a. Management of type 1 lepra reaction
   b. Animal models in leprosy
   c. Persisters in leprosy and their importance

SUBJECT: PAPER-IV
RECENT ADVANCES IN DERMATOLOGY, VENEREOLOGY AND LEPROSY

Total Marks: 100

Instructions:

- All questions are compulsory
- Draw net labeled diagrams whenever necessary
- Each question has 10 marks

1. Discuss dermatological manifestations of autoimmune thyroid disease
2. Targeted phototherapy
3. Janus kinase (JAK) inhibitors in dermatology
4. Fillers in dermatology
5. Nanotechnology
6. Immunotherapy of melanoma
7. Recent advances in pathogenesis and management of chronic spontaneous urticarial
8. Gluten free diet and its place in dermatology
9. Pathogenesis of pemphigus
10. Discuss utility of cohort studies in dermatology

DERMATOLOGY, VENEREOLOGY AND LEPROSY
SUBJECT: PAPER-I BASIC SCIENCES IN DERMATOLOGY

Total Marks: 100

Notes:

- All questions are compulsory
- Draw net labeled diagrams whenever necessary
- Your answer should be specific to the question asked

SECTION I

1. Enumerate the disorders hair follicle. Describe clinical features and diagnosis of them. (20)
2. Write a short note of epidermopoiesis. (30)

SECTION II

3. Describe the structure of HIV and laboratory diagnoses of HIV (20)
4. Write short note on following: (30)
   a. Dark proud microscopy
   b. Bacterial index on legacy
   c. Three glass urine test

DERMATOLOGY, VENEREOLOGY AND LEPROSY PAPER-II DERMATOLOGY

Total Marks: 100

Notes:
- All questions are compulsory
- Draw neat labeled diagrams whenever necessary
- Your answer should be specific to the question asked

SECTION I

1. Describe the emergencies in dermatology (20)
2. Write short note on following: (30)
    a. Management of palmoplantar hyperhidrosis
    b. Angiolymphoid hyperplasia
    c. Epidermolysis bullosa acquisita

SECTION II

3. Discuss cutaneous manifestations of diabetes mellitus (20)
4. Write short note on following: (30)
    a. Hirsutism
    b. Kawasaki disease
    c. Milkers nodule

DERMATOLOGY, VENEREOLOGY AND LEPROSY PAPER-III ADVANCES IN DERMATOLOGY

Total Marks: 100

Notes:
- All questions are compulsory
- Draw neat labeled diagrams whenever necessary

SECTION I

1. Describe the management of hidradenitis suppurativa (20)
2. Write short note on following: (30)
    a. Secukinumab
    b. Tranexamic acid
    c. Carbon peel

SECTION II

3. Describe the role of dermatoscopy in dermatology (20)
4. Write short note on following: (30)
    a. HIV vaccine
    b. Complications of laser therapy in tattoo removal
    c. Microneedling

DERMATOLOGY, VENEREOLOGY AND LEPROSY
SUBJECT: PAPER-I BASIC SCIENCES IN RELATION TO DERMATOLOGY, VENEREOLOGY AND LEPROSY

Total Marks: 100

Instructions:
- All questions are compulsory
- Draw net labeled diagrams whenever necessary

SECTION I

1. Describe in detail the microanatomy of keratinocyte. Write a short note on epidermal cell kinetics (20)
2. Write short note on following: (30)
   a. Special stains in dermatology
   b. Tissue smears in dermatology
   c. Palisading granulomas

SECTION II

3. Discuss in detail formation of eccrine sweat. Classify hyperhidrosis (20)
4. Write short note on following: (30)
   a. Mast cell
   b. Superantigens
   c. Cryoglobulins and cold agglutinins in dermatology

PAPER-I BASIC SCIENCES IN DERMATOLOGY

Total Marks: 100

Notes:
- All questions are compulsory
- Draw neat labeled diagrams whenever necessary
- Your answer should be specific to the question asked

SECTION I

1. Describe the anatomy of nail. Describe nail changes in systemic diseases (20)
2. Write short note on following: (30)
   a. Koebner's phenomenon
   b. Ozone layer and skin
   c. Structure of *Treponema pallidum*

SECTION II

3. Describe epidermal melanin unit and etiopathogenesis of vitiligo (20)
4. Write short note on following: (30)
   a. Serodiagnosis of leprosy
   b. Boosted protease inhibitors
   c. Dendritic cells

PAPER-II DERMATOLOGY

Total Marks: 100

Notes:

- All questions are compulsory
- Draw neat labeled diagrams whenever necessary
- Your answer should be specific to the question asked

SECTION I

1. Enumerate systemic causes of generalized pruritus. Write the clinical features, diagnosis and treatment of cutaneous T-cell lymphoma. (20)
2. Write short note on following: (30)
   a. Onychomycosis
   b. Role of patch test in dermatology
   c. Monilethrix

SECTION II

3. Discuss pregnancy induced dermatoses. (20)
4. Write short note on following: (30)
   a. Latrogenic hyperhidrosis
   b. Epidermodysplasia verruciformis
   c. Toxic epidermal necrolysis

PAPER-III LEPROSY, SEXUALLY TRANSMITTED DISEASES, HIV

Total Marks: 100

Notes:

- All questions are compulsory
- Draw neat labeled diagrams whenever necessary
- Your answer should be specific to the question asked

SECTION I

1. Describe the differential diagnosis of Inguinal bubo in a sexually active male and add a note on LGV bubo and its management. (20)
2. Write short note on following: (30)
   a. Post exposure prophylaxis in HIV
   b. Pruritus vulvae
   c. Role of Gram stain in STI clinic

SECTION II

3. Discuss in detail Claw hand in leprosy. (20)
4. Write short note on following: (30)
   a. Thalidomide in leprosy
   b. Lepra vaccine
   c. MCR footwear

PAPER-IV RECENT ADVANCES IN DERMATOLOGY, VENEREOLOGY AND LEPROSY

Total Marks: 100

Notes:
- All questions are compulsory
- Draw neat labeled diagrams whenever necessary
- Your answer should be specific to the question asked

Write short note on following: 10 marks each

1. Bilastine
2. Oral skin lightening agents
3. Fillers in dermatology
4. Follicular unit extraction
5. The 5 alpha reductase inhibitors
6. Immunotherapy of warts
7. Teledermatology
8. Role of confocal microscopy in dermatology
9. Lasers for hair removal
10. Superantigens in dermatology

PAPER-I BASIC SCIENCES IN RELATION TO DERMATOLOGY, VENEREOLOGY AND LEPROSY

Total Marks: 100

Notes:
- All questions are compulsory
- Draw neat labeled diagrams whenever necessary
- Your answer should be specific to the question asked

SECTION I

1. Describe the structure and function of Langerhans cell. Add a note on Langerhans cell histiocytosis. (20)
2. Write short note on following: (30)
   a. Nail capillaroscopy
   b. Interface dermatitis
   c. Atypical mycobacteria

SECTION II

3. Describe the anatomy of male genital tract. Add a note on pathogenesis of gonococcal urethritis (20)
4. Write short note on following: (30)
   a. Animal models in leprosy
   b. Integrase inhibitors
   c. Fenticonazole

DERMATOLOGY, VENEREOLOGY AND LEPROSY
PAPER-I

Time: 3 Hours | Full Marks: 100

The figures in the margin indicate full marks for the questions

Answer all questions

1. Describe the development of hair with the hair cycle. (10)
2. Melanocyte and melanogenesis. (10)
3. Write in brief about tight junction and gap junction of skin. (10)
4. Write short notes on mast cell. (10)
5. Antimicrobial peptide. (10)
6. Thermoregulatory function of skin. (10)
7. Write about cutaneous lymphatics. (10)
8. Type IV hypersensitivity reaction. (10)
9. Write about dyskeratosis and dyskeratotic cells. (10)
10. KOH examination of the skin. (10)

DERMATOLOGY, VENEREOLOGY AND LEPROSY
PAPER-II

Time: 3 Hours | Full Marks: 100

The figures in the margin indicate full marks for the questions

Answer all questions

1. Enumerate and discuss Epidermolytic Hyperkeratosis as a histopathological findings. (10)
2. Discuss immunopathogenesis of psoriasis. (10)
3. Classify neutrophilic dermatoses. Discuss about pyoderma gangrenosum. (10)
4. Histopathology of basal cell carcinoma.
5. Discuss about the evaluation and treatment of a patient of paraneoplastic pemphigus. (10)
6. Discuss about the pre malignant skin condition. (10)
7. Approach to a case of severe cutaneous drug reaction. (10)
8. Write brief notes on following: (10)
   a. Mycetoma
   b. Atopic March
9. Write brief notes on following: (10)
   a. Acrodermatitis enteropathica
   b. Tuberculosis
10. Write brief notes on following: (5 + 5 = 10)
   a. Porokeratosis
   b. Iontophoresis

DERMATOLOGY, VENEREOLOGY AND LEPROSY
PAPER-IV

Time: 3 Hours | Full Marks: 100

The figures in the margin indicate full marks for the questions

Answer all questions

1. Give a brief account on scoring system in dermatology. (10)
2. Recent advance in management of urticaria. (10)
3. Management of acute skin failure. (10)
4. Management of rifampicin-resistant *Mycobacterium leprae*. (10)
5. Role of CO_2 laser in dermatology. (10)
6. Discuss about dermal fillers. (10)
7. Recent advance in pathogenesis and management of vitiligo. (10)
8. Write brief notes on following: (5 + 5 = 10)
   a. Omalizumab
   b. Antihistamines in pregnancy
9. Write brief notes on following: (5 + 5 = 10)
   a. Newer topical antifungals
   b. Contact sensitizers
10. Write brief notes on following: (5 + 5 = 10)
   a. Platelet rich plasma
   b. Dermoscopy

DERMATOLOGY, VENEREOLOGY AND LEPROSY
PAPER-I

Time: 3 Hours | Full Marks: 100

The figures in the margin indicate full marks for the questions

Answer all questions

1. Describe with neat labeled diagram the anatomy of eccrine gland. Discuss functions of these glands. (6 + 4 = 10)
2. Write about hemidesmosomes. (10)
3. Discuss direct immunofluorescence (DIF). (10)
4. Describe and discuss epidermolytic hyperkeratosis as a histopathological findings. (10)
5. Discuss teledermatology. (10)
6. Write briefly on types of epidemiological study. (10)
7. Explain—Mosaicism. (10)
8. Write in brief about—Cytokines. (10)
9. Compare and write about—“physical and chemical sunscreens”. (10)
10. Discuss—“Dermatology Life Quality Index”. (10)

DERMATOLOGY, VENEREOLOGY AND LEPROSY
PAPER-III

Time: 3 Hours Full Marks: 100

The figures in the margin indicate full marks for the questions

Answer all questions

1. Discuss immune reconstitution inflammatory syndrome (IRIS) in context of HIV-AIDS. (10)
2. Strategy for laboratory diagnosis of HIV infection. (10)
3. Dark field microscopy (10)
4. Write briefly on "stigmata" of congenital syphilis. (10)
5. Discuss differential diagnosis of unilateral inguinal swelling in a 30-year-old female sex worker. (10)
6. Elaborate on advantages and disadvantages of "syndromic management". (10)
7. Comment on management of leprosy in persons with type II reaction, but unable to tolerate rifampicin. (10)
8. Describe histopathology of lapromatous leprosy. (10)
9. Differentiate BT Hansen from BL Hansen by their clinical features. (10)
10. Discuss "hematological profile" in leprosy. (10)

DERMATOLOGY, VENEREOLOGY AND LEPROSY
PAPER-II

Time: 3 Hours Full Marks: 100

The figures in the margin indicate full marks for the questions

Answer all questions

1. Classify T-cell lymphoma. Describe clinical features of mycosis fungoides and its management. (3 + 4 + 3 = 10)
2. Describe cutaneous features, systemic complications and investigations in Pseudoxanthoma elasticum. (4 + 3 + 3 = 10)
3. Cutaneous manifestations of rheumatoid arthritis. (10)
4. Describe clinical features, investigations and treatment of actinomycosis. (4 + 3 + 3 = 10)
5. Pathogenesis of psoriasis and atopic dermatitis. (5 + 5 = 10)
6. Spiradenoma. (10)
7. Describe briefly parvovirus B19 associated disorder. (10)
8. Scleroderma. (10)
9. Disorders associated with sporotrichoid lesions. (10)
10. Describe the clinical features, variants and management of dermatofibrosarcoma protuberans. (10)

DERMATOLOGY, VENEREOLOGY AND LEPROSY PAPER-IV

Time: 3 Hours | Full Marks: 100

The figures in the margin indicate full marks for the questions

Answer 10 out of the 12 questions:

1. Describe the role of zinc in dermatology. (10)
2. Role of β-blockers in dermatology. (10)
3. Newer treatment of leprosy. (10)
4. Outline the probable causes and remedies of sudden volcanic appearance of Tinea. (10)
5. Immunotherapy in recurrent wart. (10)
6. Elaborate the newer treatment of acne vulgaris. (10)
7. Describe the role of autophagy in dermatology. (10)
8. Complications and treatment of hyperlipidemia (10)
9. Describe the role of rituximab in dermatology. (10)
10. Role of laser for vascular disorder. (10)
11. Write brief notes on following: (5 + 5 = 10)
    a. Cutaneous larva migrans
    b. Pseudoepitheliomatous hyperplasia
12. Write brief notes on following: (5 + 5 = 10)
    a. Pathogenesis of bullous pemphigoid
    b. Acanthosis nigricans.

DERMATOLOGY, VENEREOLOGY AND LEPROSY PAPER-I

Time: 3 Hours | Full Marks: 100

The figures in the margin indicate full marks for the questions

Answer all questions

1. Briefly describe the anatomy of the nail unit. (10)
2. Elaborate barrier function of the skin. (10)
3. Write about innate immunity of the skin. (10)
4. Indirect immunofluorescence test. (10)
5. Cutaneous photobiology. (10)
6. Nerve supply of the skin. (10)
7. Describe the anatomy and function of the sebaceous glands. (10)
8. Write about cornoid lamella. (10)
9. Tonofilaments desmosome complex. (10)
10. Telomere.

DERMATOLOGY, VENEREOLOGY AND LEPROSY
PAPER-IV

Time: 3 Hours | Full Marks: 100

The figures in the margin indicate full marks for the questions

Answer all questions

1. Discuss evidence-based dermatology. (10)
2. Recent advance in management of psoriasis. (10)
3. Discuss about skin manifestation in chronic kidney disease. (10)
4. Discuss about facial rejuvenation. (10)
5. Discuss about biologics in immune-bullous disorders. (10)
6. Discuss FAS and FAS ligand. (10)
7. Write brief notes on following: (10)
   a. Lichen planus
8. Write brief notes on vaccines in Human Papilloma virus. (10)
9. Describe the immunology and treatment of type 1 lepra reaction. (10)
10. Write about disability prevention in leprosy. (10)

DERMATOLOGY, VENEREOLOGY AND LEPROSY
PAPER-III

Time: 3 Hours | Full Marks: 100

The figures in the margin indicate full marks for the questions

Answer all questions

1. Describe the method of specimen collection for the diagnosis of STIs. (10)
2. Write clinical manifestation and management of neonatal HSV infection. (10)
3. Describe oral manifestation of syphilis. (10)
4. Syndromic management of genital discharge. (10)
5. HAART. (10)
6. Describe etiopathogenesis and management of trophic ulcer of leprosy. (10)
7. Histoid Leprosy and management. (10)
8. Manifestation of relapse in lepromatous leprosy. (10)
9. Write brief notes on following: (5 + 5 = 10)
   a. Cutaneous larva migrans
   b. Pseudoepitheliomatous hyperplasia
10. Write brief notes on following: (5 + 5 = 10)
    a. Pathogenesis of bullous pemphigoid
    b. Acanthosis nigricans.

Paper I

Duration: 3 Hours
Marks: 100

Instruction:

- All questions are compulsory except wherever option is given.
- Answers must be specific to the questions.
- Give neat, labeled and schematic diagram wherever applicable.
- Mobile phones, pagers, blue tooth or any other such communication devices are not allowed in the examination premises and in all adjacent area.

Long Questions (Compulsory): **25 Marks each**

1. Correlate the various antigens present in the basement membrane zone with various vesiculobullous and autoimmune diseases.
2. Describe the structure and functions of eosinophils. Enumerate dermatological disorders with tissue eosinophils.

Write Short Notes on ANY FIVE of the following: **10 Marks each**

1. Propionobacteria in acne.
2. Inflammatory mediators in mast cell.
3. Histopathological importance of colloid bodies.
4. Wood's lamp examination in dermatology.
5. Describe the apocrine gland secretion.
6. Role of interleukins in psoriasis.

Paper II

Duration: 3 Hours
Marks: 100

Instruction:

- All questions are compulsory except wherever option is given.
- Answers must be specific to the questions.
- Give neat, labeled and schematic diagram wherever applicable.
- Mobile phones, pagers, blue tooth or any other such communication devices are not allowed in the examination premises and in all adjacent area.

Long Questions (Compulsory): **25 Marks each**

1. How will you manage a middle aged man presenting with purpuric lesions, foot drop and peripheral eosinophilia?
2. Analyze the role of dermatologist in the management of cutaneous T-cell lymphoma.

Write Short Notes on ANY FIVE of the following: **10 Marks each**

1. Psoriatic arthritis mutilans.
2. Mucous membrane lichen planus.
3. Histopathology of benign familial pemphigus.
4. Drug induced pyogenic granuloma.
5. Dermarollers in acne scars.
6. Welsch's regimen in actinomycotic mycetoma.

Paper III

Duration: 3 Hours
Marks: 100

Instruction:

- All questions are compulsory except wherever option is given.
- Answers must be specific to the questions.
- Give neat, labeled and schematic diagram wherever applicable.
- Mobile phones, pagers, blue tooth or any other such communication devices are not allowed in the examination premises and in all adjacent area.

Long Questions (Compulsory): **25 Marks each**

1. Critically analyze post eradication scenario of leprosy in India.
2. Critically evaluate the atypical manifestations of syphilis in HIV patients.

Write Short Notes on ANY FIVE of the following: **10 Marks each**

1. Management of balanitis xerotica obliterans.
2. Protease inhibitors in HIV infection.
3. Penicillin resistant *Neisseria gonorrhoeae*.
4. Lazarine leprosy.
5. Interpretation of slit skin smear for AFB in leprosy.
6. Fluoroquinolones in leprosy.

Dermatology – Paper – I

[Time: 3 Hours] **[Max. Marks: 100]**

Notes:

- Answer all questions
- Draw neat labeled diagram wherever necessary

LONG ESSAYS **[2 × 20 = 40 Marks]**

1. Analyze the role of various cytokines in dermatological disorders.
2. What is brick and mortar therapy in relation to Ichthyosis? Substantiate the various genetically inherited ichthyosis in relation to this theory.

SHORT ESSAYS **[6 × 10 = 60 Marks]**

3. Role of dermoscopy in analyzing seborrheic keratoses.
4. Utility of Odland bodies in epidermal keratinization process.
5. Analyze the importance of transepidermal water loss in exfoliative dermatitis.
6. Autosomal recessive genodermatoses with DNA repair abnormalities.
7. Role of mast cells in dermatological disorders.
8. Mechanism of laser hair removal.

Dermatology – Paper – II

[Time: 3 Hours] **[Max. Marks: 100]**

Notes:

- Answer all questions
- Draw neat labeled diagram wherever necessary

LONG ESSAYS **[2 × 20 = 40 Marks]**

1. Debate the role of corticosteroids in the management of toxic epidermal necrolysis.
2. Analyze the various theories of bullae formation in pemphigus group of disorders.

SHORT ESSAYS **[6 × 10 = 60 Marks]**

3. Role of secukinumab in the management of psoriasis.
4. Write a note on etymology of tacrolimus.
5. Your suggestions to prevent abuse of topical steroid creams.
6. Pathogenesis of Darier's disease and chronic benign familial pemphigus.
7. a. Igneous rock sign.
   b. Brocq's phenomenon.
8. Chemical peels with glycolic acid.

Dermatology – Paper – III

[Time: 3 Hours] **[Max. Marks: 100]**

Notes:
- Answer all questions
- Draw neat labeled diagram wherever necessary

LONG ESSAYS **[2 × 20 = 40 Marks]**

1. Analyze the effect of pregnancy on various sexually transmitted infections. Describe the role of dermatologist in the management of delivery of a patient with genital warts.
2. Describe the pathomechanism of nerve damage in leprosy.

SHORT ESSAYS **[6 × 10 = 60 Marks]**

3. Enumerate the differences between reversal reaction and relapse in leprosy.
4. Interpretation of AFB smear in leprosy.
5. Role of thalidomide in type II lepra reactions.
6. Immune reconstitution inflammatory syndrome.
7. Protease inhibitors in HIV infection.
8. Management of drug resistance in gonorrhea.

Dermatology – Paper – IV

[Time: 3 Hours] **[Max. Marks: 100]**

Notes:
- Answer all questions
- Draw neat labeled diagram wherever necessary

LONG ESSAYS **[2 × 20 = 40 Marks]**

1. Enumerate the various factors to be considered for vitiligo surgery. How will you analyze the stability of vitiligo?
2. Analyze the pathomechanism of pain in various benign painful tumors of the skin.

SHORT ESSAYS **[6 × 10 = 60 Marks]**

3. Omalizumab.
4. Ruocco's immunocompromised cutaneous district.
5. Dariers epidermal ness.
6. Diode laser.
7. MAGIC syndrome.
8. Cutaneous manifestations of chronic renal failure.

Index

Page numbers followed by *b* refer to box, *f* refer to figure, *fc* refer to flowchart, and *t* refer to table.

B

C

E

F

G

H

I

J

K

N

O

P

S

T

U

W

X

Y

Z